Gynaecology

To our wives, Mae, Winnie and Julia
for their patience, understanding and support.

For Churchill Livingstone

Commissioning Editor: Sheila Khullar
Project Editor: Antonia Seymour
Copy Editors: Jennifer Bew, Teresa Brady
Indexer: Liza Weinkove

Gynaecology

Edited by

Robert W. Shaw MD FRCOG FRCS(Ed) MFFP

Professor and Head, Department of Obstetrics and Gynaecology, University of Wales College of Medicine, Cardiff, UK

W. Patrick Soutter MD MSc FRCOG

Reader in Gynaecological Oncology, Institute of Obstetrics and Gynaecology, Royal Postgraduate Medical School, Hammersmith Hospital, London, UK

Stuart L. Stanton FRCS FRCOG

Professor and Chair in Reconstructive Pelvic Surgery and Urogynaecology, Department of Obstetrics and Gynaecology, St George's Hospital, London, UK

SECOND EDITION

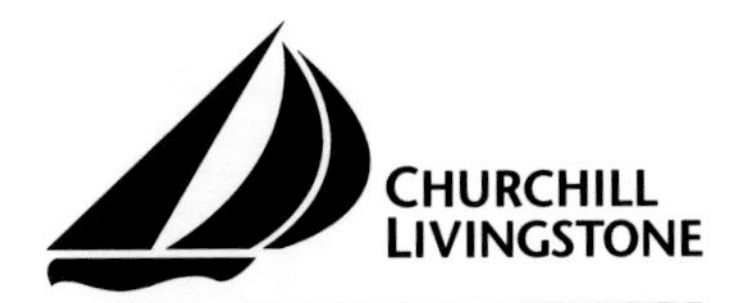

EDINBURGH LONDON NEW YORK PHILADELPHIA ST LOUIS SYDNEY TORONTO 1997

CHURCHILL LIVINGSTONE
An imprint of Harcourt Publishers Limited

First edition 1992
Second edition 1997
Reprinted 1998
Reprinted 1999
Reprinted 2000

ISBN 0 443 05231X

British Library Cataloguing in Publication Data
A catalogue record for this book is available from the British Library.

Library of Congress Cataloging in Publication Data
A catalog record for this book is available from the Library of Congress.

Note
Medical knowledge is constantly changing. As new information becomes available, changes in treatment, procedures, equipment and the use of drugs become necessary. The editors and contributors and the publishers have, as far as it is possible, taken care to ensure that the information given in this text is accurate and up to date. However, readers are strongly advised to confirm that the information, especially with regard to drug usage, complies with latest legislation and standards of practice.

The publishers have made every effort to trace holders of copyright in original material and to seek permission for its use. Should this have proved impossible, them copyright holders are asked to contact the publishers so that suitable acknowledgment can be made at the first opportunity.

Printed in China

The publisher's policy is to use paper manufactured from sustainable forest

Contents

Section Three: Benign and malignant tumours

Section Four: Urogynaecology

Section Five: Genitourinary infections

Section Six: Legal and general

Contributors

Mostafa I. Abuzeid MD MRCOG FACOG
Director of Reproductive Endocrinology and Infertility, Hurley Medical Center; Associate Professor in Obstetrics and Gynecology, Michigan State College of Human Medicine, Flint, USA

Masoud Afnan MRCOG
Senior Lecturer in Obstetrics and Gynaecology, University of Birmingham; Consultant, Birmingham Women's Hospital, Edgbaston, Birmingham, UK

Nazar N. Amso MBChB MRCOG MFFP PhD
Consultant Obstetrician and Gynaecologist; Director, Centre for Assisted Reproduction, Queen Elizabeth Hospital, Gateshead, UK

Malcolm C. Anderson FRCOG FRCPath
Senior Lecturer, Department of Histopathology, University Hospital, Queen's Medical Centre, Nottingham, UK

Yves Muscat Baron MD MRCOG MRCPI
Senior Registrar, Department of Obstetrics and Gynaecology, St Luke's Hospital Medical School, Gwardamangia, Malta

Michael Baum ChM FRCS
Professor of Surgery, University College, London; Consultant Surgeon, UCCH Trust, London, UK

Colin D. Bevan MRCOG
Senior Registrar in Obstetrics and Gynaecology, Southampton University NHS Trust, Southampton, UK

Mark Brincat PhD(Lond) MRCOG
Director, Department of Obstetrics and Gynaecology, St Luke's Hospital Medical School, Msida, Malta

Graeme M. Bydder BSc MBChB FRACP FRCP FRACR
Professor and Director, Magnetic Resonance Imaging Robert Steiner Unit, Hammersmith Hospital, London, UK

Linda Cardozo MD FRCOG
Professor of Urogynaecology, King's College, London; Consultant Gynaecologist, King's Healthcare Trust, London, UK

Rashna Chenoy MBBS MRCOG
Consultant Obstetrician and Gynaecologist, Newham General Hospital, London

Roger V. Clements FRCS(Ed) FRCOG FAE
Consultant Obstetrician and Gynaecologist; Risk Management Consultant; Editor-in-Chief, 'Clinical Risk', London, UK

David O. Cosgrove MA MSc FRCP FRCR
Senior Lecturer, Royal Postgraduate Medical School and Honorary Consultant, Hammersmith Hospital, London, UK

Carmel A. E. Coulter FRCP FRCR
Consultant in Clinical Oncology, St Mary's Hospital, London, UK

Sarah M. Creighton MD MRCOG
Consultant, Department of Obstetrics and Gynaecology, University College Hospital, London, UK

Nicholas E. Day PhD MRCPath
Professor of Public Health Medicine, Department of Community Medicine, Institute of Public Health, University Forvie Site, Cambridge

Nandita M. DeSouza MD FRCR
Senior Lecturer in Radiology, Royal Postgraduate Medical School, Hammersmith Hospital, London, UK

Sheila L. B. Duncan MD FRCOG
Reader and Honorary Consultant in Obstetrics and Gynaecology, Jessop Hospital for Women, Sheffield, UK

D. Keith Edmonds FRCOG FRACOG
Consultant Obstetrician and Gynaecologist, Queen Charlotte's and Chelsea Hospital, London, UK

Anthony J. France MA MB BChir FRCP(Ed)
Consultant Physician, Infection, Immunodeficiency and Respiratory Medicine, King's Cross Hospital, Dundee, UK

Stephen Franks MD FRCP HonMD(Uppsala)
Professor of Reproductive Endocrinology, Imperial College of Medicine at St Mary's, London, UK

John R. Friend MA DM FRCOG
Senior Consultant Obstetrician and Gynaecologist, Derriford Hospital, Plymouth, UK

Ray Galea MD MRCOG
Senior Registrar, Department of Obstetrics and Gynaecology, St Luke's Hospital Medical School, Gwardamangia, Malta

Raymond Garry MD FRCOG
Consultant Gynaecologist, South Cleveland Hospital, Middlesbrough, UK

Carole Gilling-Smith MA MRCOG
Lecturer/Honorary Senior Registrar in Obstetrics and Gynaecology, St Mary's Hospital, London

Joanna C. Girling MA MRCP MRCOG
Senior Registrar in Obstetrics and Gynaecology, Hammersmith Hospital, London, UK

Anna Glasier BSc MD FRCOG
Director of Family Planning and Well Woman Services, Edinburgh Healthcare NHS Trust; Senior Lecturer, Department of Obstetrics and Gynaecology, University of Edinburgh, Edinburgh, UK

Lawrence Goldie MD DPM FRCPsych MAE Grad Member Brit. Psychol Soc
Honorary Consultant Psychiatrist, The Tavistock Clinic, London; formerly Consultant Medical Psychotherapist, The Royal Marsden Hospital, The Royal National Throat Nose and Ear Hospital, the Institute of Obstetrics and Gynaecology, Hammersmith Hospital, London, UK

J. Geddes Grudzinskas MD FRCOG FRACOG
Professor of Obstetrics and Gynaecology, St Bartholomew's Hospital and Royal London Hospital School of Medicine and Dentistry, University of London, London, UK

Michael M. Henry MB FRCS
Consultant Surgeon, Chelsea, Westminster and Royal Marsden Hospitals, London

Paul Hilton MD BS FRCOG
Consultant Gynaecologist (Sub-specialist in Urogynaecology), Royal Victoria Infirmary, Newcastle upon Tyne; Senior Lecturer in Urogynaecology, University of Newcastle upon Tyne, Newcastle upon Tyne, UK

Michael G. R. Hull MD FRCOG
Professor of Reproductive Medicine and Surgery, Department of Obstetrics and Gynaecology, University of Bristol, Bristol, UK

James E. Jackson MRCP FRCR
Senior Lecturer (Honorary Consultant), Department of Imaging, Royal Postgraduate Medical School, Hammersmith Hospital, London, UK

Ian J. Jacobs MD MRCOG
Consultant Gynaecological Oncologist and Senior Lecturer, Director, Gynaecological Cancer Research Unit, Department of Gynaecological Oncology, St Bartholomew's/Royal London Hospital and Medical School, London, UK

Gerald J. Jarvis MA FRCS(Ed) FRCOG
Consultant Obstetrician and Gynaecologist, St James's University Hospital, Leeds, UK

Frank D. Johnstone MD FRCOG
Consultant Gynaecologist, Royal Infirmary of Edinburgh; Senior Lecturer in Obstetrics and Gynaecology, University of Edinburgh, Edinburgh, UK

George R. Kinghorn MD FRCP
Clinical Director for Communicable Diseases, Royal Hallamshire Hospital, Sheffield, UK

Stephen Kirkham MA MB BChir FRCP
Consultant in Palliative Medicine, Poole Hospital NHS Trust, Poole, UK

Eswar Krishnan MBBS MPhil
Research Fellow, Division of Cancer Epidemiology, Regional Cancer Centre, Tivandrum Medical College Hospitals, Tivandrum, India

Joanna Lambert FRCOG FRCR
Senior Lecturer (Consultant), Hammersmith Hospital, London, UK

Frances Lewington OBE BSc PhD
Medical Training Organiser, Metropolitan Police Forensic Medical Services Branch, Wellington House, London, UK

B. Victor Lewis MD FRCS FRCOG
Senior Consultant Gynaecologist, Department of Obstetrics and Gynaecology, Watford and Mount Vernon NHS Trust, Watford, UK

Mary Anne Lumsden MD MRCOG
Senior Lecturer/ Honorary Consultant, University of Glasgow, Western Infirmary, Glasgow, UK

John Lynn MS FRCS
Consultant Endocrine Breast and General Surgeon, Department of Surgery, Hammersmith Hospital Trust; Honorary Senior Lecturer in Surgery, Royal Postgraduate Medical School, London, UK

Raul A. Margara MD
Consultant and Senior Lecturer in Fertility Studies, Royal Postgraduate Medical School, Hammersmith Hospital, London, UK

Joanne Marsden BSc FRCS(Lond)
Clinical Research Fellow, Department of Surgery, The Royal Marsden and St George's Hospitals Trusts, London, UK

Peter Mason FRCS FRCOG
Consultant Gynaecologist, St Mary's Hospital and Samaritan Hospital for Women, London, UK

Neil McClure MD MRCOG
Consultant Obstetrician and Gynaecologist, Royal Maternity Hospital, Belfast; Senior Lecturer, Obstetrics and Gynaecology, The Queen's University of Belfast, Belfast, UK

J. McCue FRCS
Senior Registrar in Surgery, Hammersmith Hospital, London, UK

G. Angus J. McIndoe PhD FRCS MRCOG
Consultant in Gynaecological Oncology, Hammersmith Hospital; Honorary Senior Lecturer, Royal Postgraduate Medical School, London, UK

Ash K. Monga MRCOG
Consultant Gynaecologist, Princess Anne Hospital, Southampton, UK

Adam Moors MRCOG
Senior Registrar, Royal Hampshire County Hospital, Winchester; Formerly MRC Research Fellow, Princess Anne Hospital, Southampton, UK

Jane Norman MD MRCOG
Senior Lecturer/ Honorary Consultant, University of Glasgow, Glasgow Royal Infirmary, Glasgow, UK

P. M. Shaughan O'Brien MD FRCOG
Consultant Obstetrician and Gynaecologist, North Staffordshire Hospital (NHS) Trust; Professor and Head of Obstetrics and Gynaecology, Keele University, Keele, UK

Anthony D. Parsons MBBS FRCOG MFFP
Consultant Gynaecologist, Hospital of St Cross, Rugby; Senior Lecturer in Gynaecology, University of Warwick, Coventry, UK

R. John Parsons BSc Tech PhD FIPEMB
Head of Department of Medical Physics and Biomedical Engineering, Plymouth General Hospital, Plymouth, UK

Alison B. Peattie MRCOG
Consultant in Obstetrics and Gynaecology, Countess of Chester Hospital, Chester, UK

Jennifer Peebles MBBS MIPSM
Hospice Physician, The Pilgrim Hospice, Canterbury, UK

Bruce A. J. Ponder PhD FRCP
Professor of Clinical Oncology, University of Cambridge; Director, Cancer Research Campaign, Human Cancer Genetics Research Group; Honorary Consultant Physician, Addenbrooke's Hospital, Cambridge, UK

Cecilia J. F. Priestley MB MRCP
Director of Genitourinary Medicine, West Dorset Hospitals NHS Trust, Weymouth, UK

John P. Pryor MS FRCS
Consultant Uroandrologist, Senior Urologist, St Peter's Hospital, London; Reader in Urology, Institute of Urology, London University, London, UK

Margaret Puxon Queen's Counsel MD FRCOG
Medical/Legal Consultant, London

Michael A. Quinn MBChB MGO MRCP MRCOG FRACOG CGO
Director of Oncology, Royal Women's Hospital; Associate Professor, University of Melbourne, Melbourne, Australia

Raine E. I. Roberts MBChB DCH DMJ(Clin.) FRCGP
Clinical Director of the Sexual Assault Referral Centre, St Mary's Hospital, Manchester, UK

Gordon J. S. Rustin MD MSc FRCP
Director of Medical Oncology, Mount Vernon Centre for Cancer Treatment, Mount Vernon Hospital, Northwood, UK

Khaldoun Sharif MRCOG MFFP FICS
Lecturer in Obstetrics and Gynaecology, University of Birmingham; Senior Registrar, Birmingham Women's Hospital, Edgbaston, Birmingham, UK

Robert W. Shaw MD FRCOG FRCS(Ed) MFFP
Professor and Head, Department of Obstetrics and Gynaecology, University of Wales College of Medicine, Cardiff, UK

W. Patrick Soutter MD MSc FRCOG
Reader in Gynaecological Oncology, Institute of Obstetrics and Gynaecology, Royal Postgraduate Medical School, Hammersmith Hospital, London, UK

Stuart L. Stanton FRCS FRCOG
Consultant Urogynaecologist, Pelvic Floor Reconstruction Centre, St George's Hospital, London, UK

William E. Svensson LRCPSI FRCSI FRCR
Consultant Radiologist and Honorary Senior Consultant, Ealing Hospital and Hammersmith Hospital, London, UK

E. Malcolm Symonds MD FRCOG
Foundation Professor, Department of Obstetrics and Gynaecology, University of Nottingham; Dean, Faculty of Medicine and Health Sciences, University of Nottingham, Nottingham, UK

Eric J. Thomas MD MRCOG
Professor of Obstetrics and Gynaecology, University of Southampton, Princess Anne Hospital, Southampton, UK

William Thompson BSc MD FRCOG
Professor of Obstetrics and Gynaecology, The Queen's University, Belfast, UK

John A. Tidy BSc MD MRCOG
Senior Lecturer in Gynaecological Oncology, Northern General Hospital, University of Sheffield, Sheffield, UK

Geoffrey H. Trew MBBS MRCOG
Consultant in Reproductive Medicine, Institute of Obstetrics and Gynaecology, Hammersmith Hospital, London, UK

Jean-Pierre van Besouw BSc (Hons) MBBS FRCA
Consultant Anaesthetist, Honorary Senior Lecturer, Department of Anaesthesia, St George's Hospital, London

Ian D. Vellacott MB BCh FRCOG
Consultant Obstetrician and Gynaecologist, Lincoln and Louth NHS Trust, Lincoln, UK

Clare C. Vernon MA FRCR
Consultant in Clinical Oncology, Hammersmith Hospital, London, UK

Kathleen G. Waller BM BCh MRCOG
Senior Registrar, Department of Obstetrics and Gynaecology, Hammersmith and Ealing Hospitals, London, UK

Christine P. West MD FRCOG
Consultant Obstetrician and Gynaecologist, Royal Infirmary, Edinburgh; Part-time Senior Lecturer in Obstetrics and Gynaecology, University of Edinburgh, Edinburgh, UK

Fred C. W. Wu BSc MD FRCP(Ed.) FRCP
Senior Lecturer, Department of Medicine, University of Manchester; Honorary Consultant Endocrinologist, Manchester Royal Infirmary and St Mary's Hospital, Manchester, UK

Preface

It may be only five years since the first edition of *Gynaecology* was published but many important advances have occurred in our speciality and we hope that this second edition encompasses them comprehensively.

The philosophy of our textbook remains as before – we have a general introductory section with chapters on anatomy, investigative techniques, and pre- and post-operative care. Subsequent sections are subspeciality based – Physiology and Reproductive Medicine; Benign and Malignant diseases of the reproductive organs and Urogynaecology disorders, their investigation and treatment. The final sections contain subjects less easily ascribed to any of the above, but reflect the interdependence of gynaecology with other specialities such as general surgery, psychiatry, anaesthesia and infective diseases, not forgetting to mention the ethical and medicolegal dilemmas we face.

Since our first edition we have seen major advances in our speciality, particularly in the field of minimal access surgery. These innovative procedures have been introduced into practice and the relevance and role of each are being compared against our long-established surgical procedures. For these reasons, we have expanded the chapters on endoscopy into separate sections for hysteroscopy and laparoscopy and have tried to emphasise the complications inherent to minimal access surgery and how to avoid them!

All the other chapters have been extensively revamped and rewritten; often from new internationally recognised experts who have joined our established team of contributors.

Our first edition proved an instant hit with trainees and specialists alike. We believe this second edition goes even further, providing a comprehensive, informative, up-to-date, and readable textbook. The keynotes at the end of each chapter encompass the salient points and, together with the extended reference lists, should provide a useful source for further in depth review of each of the subject chapter headings.

Gynaecology Second Edition, will take you knowledgably into the next millenium. It will provide trainees with a substantive text in preparation for their speciality exams and qualified specialists with a definitive tome to refer to when preparing for teaching, lecturing or as a source of reference. We have enjoyed rewriting this edition and we sincerely hope you enjoy reading it!

Robert Shaw
Pat Soutter
Stuart Stanton

April 1997

SECTION 1

Basic principles and investigations

1

Embryology of the female genital tract: its genetic defects and congenital anomalies

S. L. B. Duncan

INTRODUCTION

An understanding of the development of the female genital tract is important in the practice of gynaecology. The mechanisms by which sexual differentiation is established long before birth are complex and remarkable. They are also easily perturbed. Advances in genetics and in our understanding of steroidogenesis, together with painstaking experimental work on mammalian embryos, have combined to improve our understanding of some of the derangements of the female genital tract seen in clinical practice. Errors of development which result in intersex states, though rare, are distressing but careful study of sporadic cases has provided knowledge out of proportion to their frequency.

In this chapter some of the key events in the development of the female genital tract are discussed, especially where these relate to clinical abnormalities. Genetic conditions and congenital abnormalities of the genital tract affecting gynaecological practice are outlined. A basic understanding of the development of the gut and urogenital system is assumed, as is an understanding of the formation of gametes, cell division and of female and male chromosome complements. This chapter does not include discussion of disorders where development is so disorganized that it is incompatible with life, nor does it deal with conditions diagnosed in infancy and primarily dealt with by the paediatric surgeon. Reference is made to male development only in so far as it is of relevance in understanding congenital anomalies in the female or where the phenotype is female. Thus, disorders of virilization or of spermatogenesis in phenotypic males are not discussed.

EMBRYOLOGY

Development of the mesonephros and kidneys

Both the urinary and genital systems develop from a common mesodermal ridge running along the posterior abdominal wall. Although the systems are less intimately connected in the female compared with the male, the external openings of the two systems eventually reach the same urogenital sinus.

During the 5th week of embryonic life (i.e. from fertilization) the nephrogenic cord develops from the mesoderm and forms the urogenital ridge and mesonephric duct (later to form the wolffian duct). The mesonephros consists of a comparatively large ovoid organ on each side of the midline with the developing gonad on the medial side of its lower portion. The paramesonephric duct, later to form the müllerian system, develops as an ingrowth of coelomic epithelium anterolateral to the mesonephric duct. The primordial germ cells migrate from the yolk sac along the dorsal mesentery of the hindgut and reach the primitive gonad by the end of the 6th week (42 days; Fig. 1.1). The fate of the mesonephric and paramesonephric ducts is critically dependent on gonadal secretion. Assuming female development, the two para-

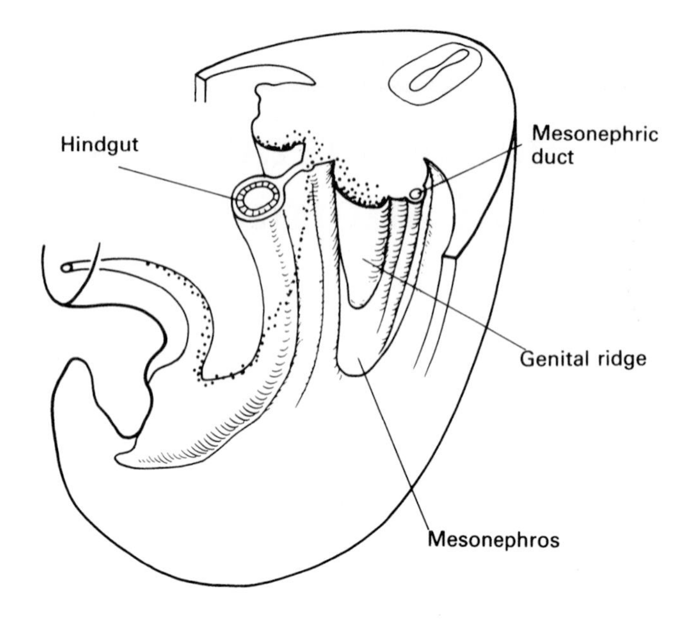

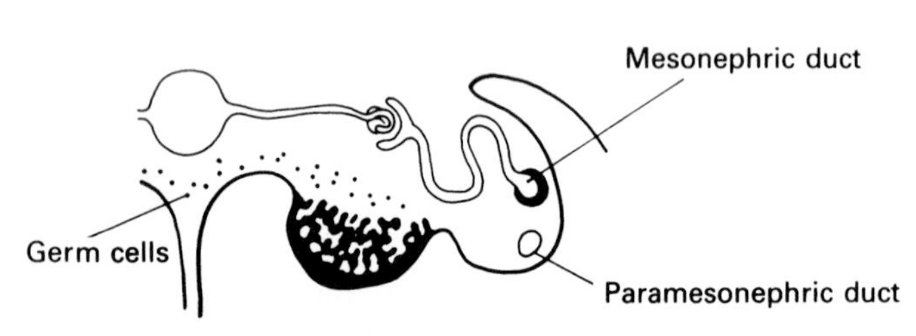

Fig. 1.1 Cross-sectional diagram of posterior abdominal wall in embryo. **Top** Migration of germ cells into genital ridge, overlying the mesonephros, with mesonephric duct on lateral aspect. **Bottom** Paramesonephric (müllerian) duct lying anterolaterally to the mesonephric duct.

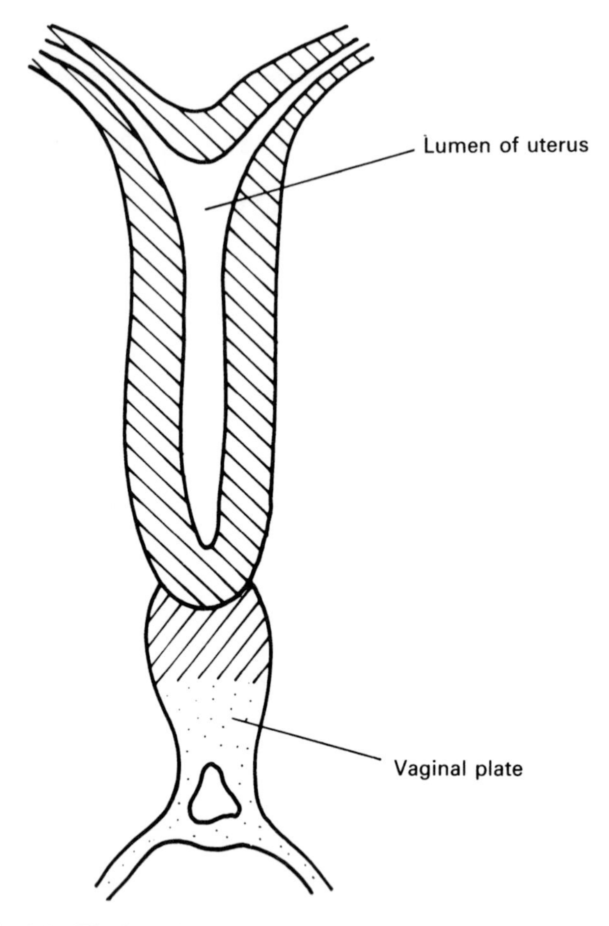

Fig. 1.2 The fused lower paramesonephric ducts later form the uterus, cervix and upper vagina. The müllerian tubercle has invaginated but not opened into the urogenital sinus.

mesonephric ducts extend caudally to project into the posterior wall of the urogenital sinus as the müllerian tubercle. There is degeneration of the wolffian system. The lower ends of the müllerian system fuse, later to form the uterus, cervix and upper vagina, while the cephalic ends remain separate, forming the fallopian tubes (Fig. 1.2).

The ureter develops as an outgrowth of the mesonephric duct close to its lower end, and grows outward and upward to penetrate the metanephric mesoderm which ultimately forms the definitive kidney. Unilateral renal aplasia is usually due to degeneration of the ureteric bud and this failure is frequently associated with failure of müllerian development on the same side, since both are dependent on adequate development of the mesonephric system. Splitting of the ureteric bud results in partial or complete duplication of the ureter. If a developing ureter fails to connect with the bladder it may retain its connection with the wolffian duct and thus open into the vagina or vestibule. This is more likely to occur if there has been splitting of the bud and abnormal ureteric development. The kidney starts off much more caudally than the gonads, and failure to ascend accounts for its occasional pelvic location and for supernumerary renal vessels which result from the persistence of embryonic vessels.

The cloaca

Meanwhile, and usually before the 7th week, the urorectal septum divides the cloaca into the urogenital sinus and the anorectal canal. When the urogenital septum reaches the cloacal membrane, the perineum is formed (Figs 1.3 and 1.4). An ectodermal anal pit forms to meet the anorectal canal and an opening forms here during the 9th embryonic week. Thus, the lower third of the anal canal forms from ectoderm and consists of stratified squamous epithelium and is supplied by the internal pudendal artery. Where the anal pit fails to form or there is atresia of the lower end of the rectum, the thickness of the intervening layer is very variable. Sometimes the rectal opening is in the perineum or even in the vagina (Fig. 1.5).

The urogenital sinus may be divided into:

1. An upper part which forms the urinary bladder. The early connection superiorly with the allantois obliterates

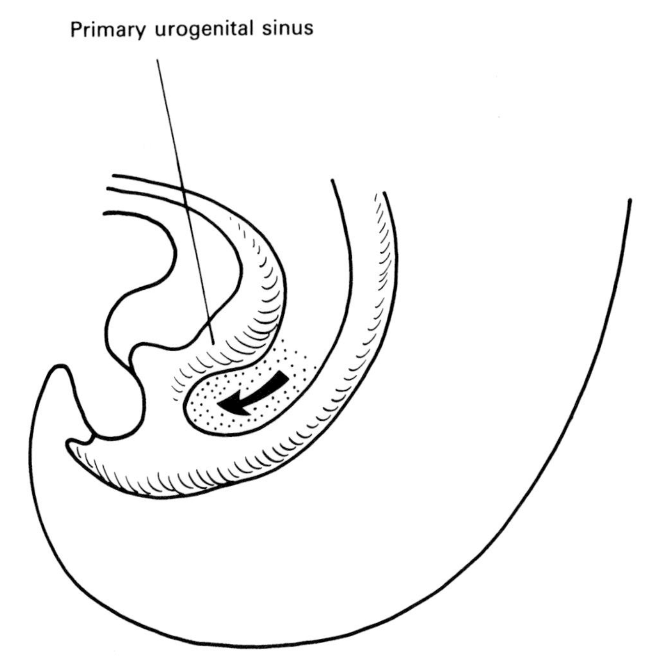

Fig. 1.3 Development of the urorectal septum (arrowed), eventually separating the bladder and vagina from the rectum.

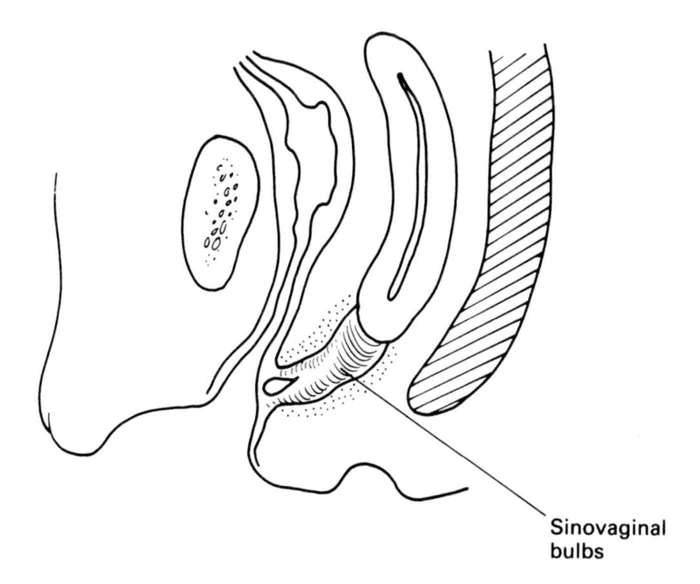

Fig. 1.4 A later stage in development where the müllerian tubercle and the sinovaginal bulbs (not yet canalized) are elongating and lying within the urorectal septum. In this diagram, the anorectal canal has failed to connect with the anal pit; this would later present as an imperforate anus.

and forms the urachus which connects the apex of the bladder to the umbilicus. If mesoderm fails to invade the cloacal membrane anteriorly, extrophy of the bladder results.

2. A pelvic part which forms the urethra and lower vagina. This is intimately connected with the development of the lower part of the müllerian system.

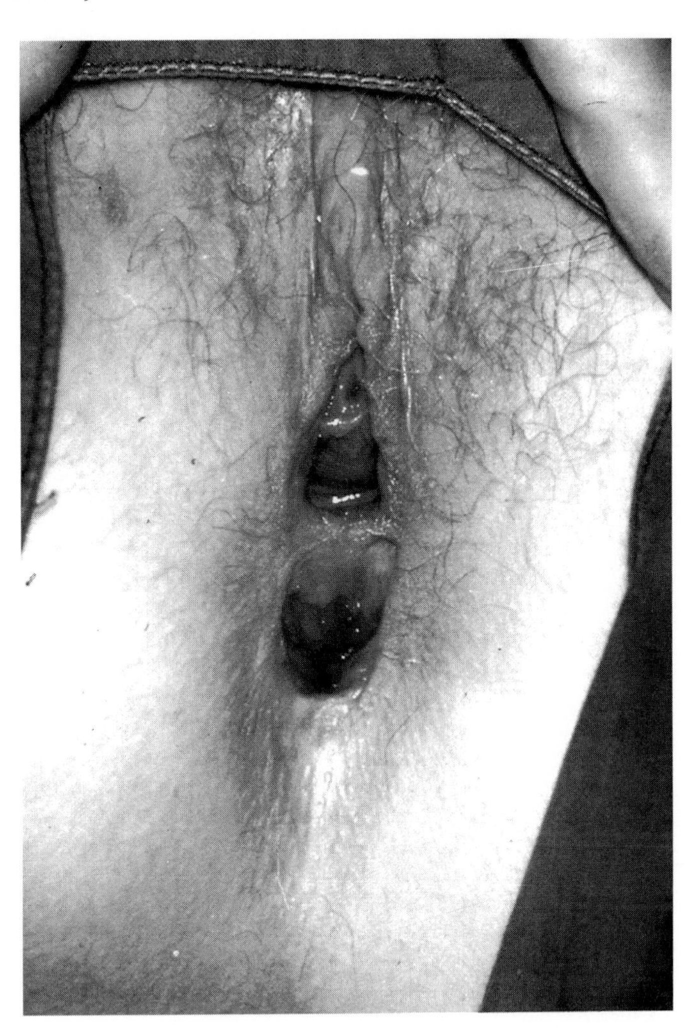

Fig. 1.5 Incomplete development of urorectal septum resulting in perineal anus with deficient perineum.

Development of the müllerian system

The müllerian ducts, which have fused in their lower part, reach and invaginate the urogenital sinus in the 9th week (30-mm stage). The end is solid and single and forms the müllerian tubercle which does not open into the sinus but makes contact with sinovaginal bulbs which are solid outgrowths from the sinus. As the hind part of the fetus unfolds and the pelvic region elongates, the sinus and the müllerian tubercle become increasingly distanced from the tubular portion of the ducts and a solid epithelial cord forms which provides length for the future vagina (Fig. 1.4). Thereafter lacunae appear which eventually join up to canalize the future vagina. How much of the original solid plate and epithelium of the vagina comes from the original urogenital sinus has long been a matter of dispute among embryologists. The current view is that most of the upper vagina is of müllerian origin and that there is metaplasia of müllerian epithelium to form its stratified squamous epithelium (Gray & Skandalakis

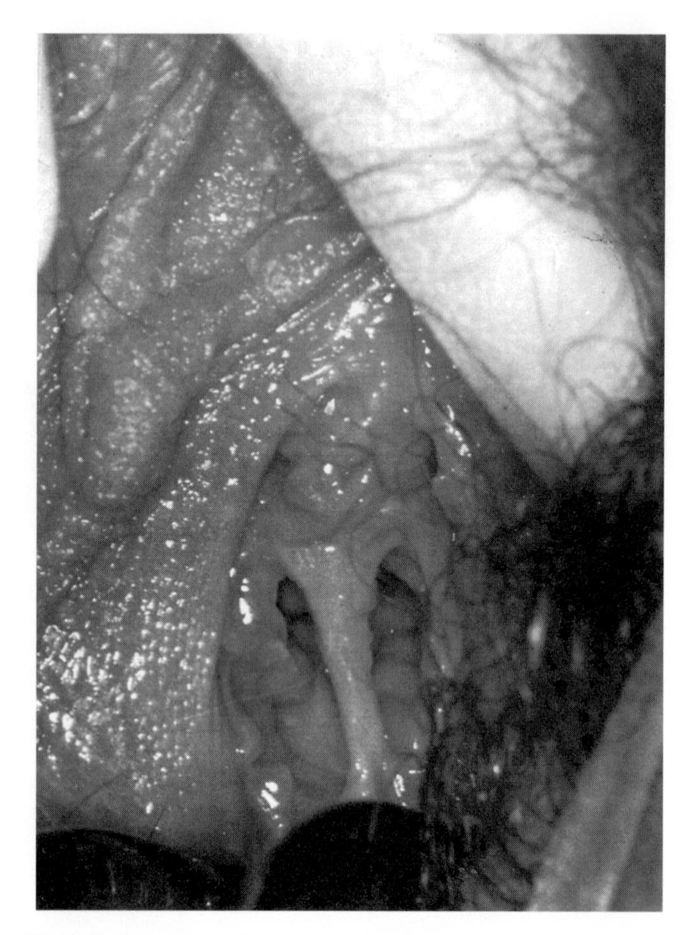

Fig. 1.6 Anteroposterior septum at introitus.

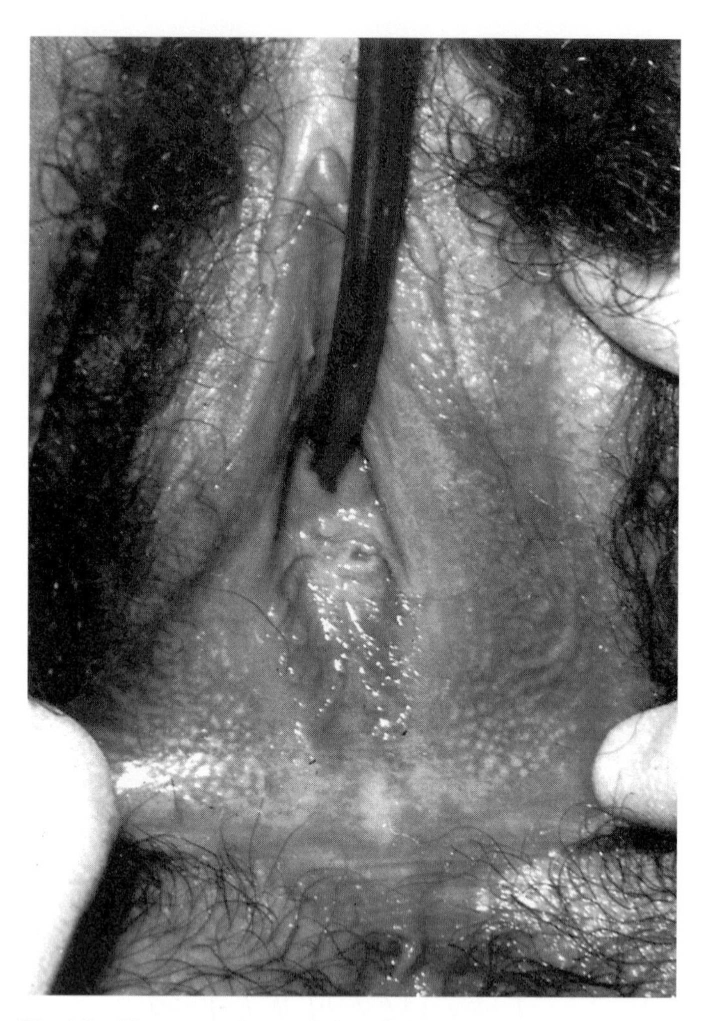

Fig. 1.7 Almost complete occlusion of introitus with small opening about 2 cm posterior to the urethra and slightly to the left. There had been no obstruction to menstrual flow but there was apareunia and inability to insert a tampon.

1972). The solid sinovaginal bulbs also have to canalize to form the lower vagina and this occurs above the level of the eventual hymen so that the epithelia of both surfaces of the hymen are of urogenital sinus origin.

Complete canalization of the vagina is a comparatively late event (occurring in the 6th and 7th month), and failure may occur at a variety of levels and for variable depth. If the tubular portions of the müllerian ducts develop to form a uterus and cervix, there is usually a patent upper vagina. If there is no development of the urogenital sinus, the subsequent vaginal atresia involves most of the vagina. Where there is müllerian agenesis, the urogenital sinus still forms but does not lengthen as much as normally and the vagina is short though of variable length. Correct early formation with failure of complete canalization (essentially failure of the lacunae to join up fully) can leave a variety of septae: transverse, sagittal, coronal or oblique, of varying thicknesses (Fig. 1.6). The mildest abnormality of this sort to cause complete obstruction is a lower vaginal transverse membrane (imperforate hymen) which is generally just above the anatomical hymen. Partial obstruction may result in apareunia or inability to insert a tampon but no obstruction to menstrual flow (Fig. 1.7).

Duplication or failure of fusion at uterine level

Fusion of the ducts occurs at an early stage of müllerian development before organ differentiation into cervix or uterine body. Thus, there is no point at which a formed uterus and cervix fuse. A true duplication of the uterus, cervix and tubes can occur but this involves splitting of the müllerian duct at an early stage. This can occur on one or both sides but is rare. More common is incomplete development of the fused ducts indicating their bilateral origin, i.e. incomplete fusion of two halves. These variations form a series of well recognized uterine anomalies of varying clinical significance (Rock & Schlaff 1985).

Remnants of the mesonephric duct

The distal portion of the regressing wolffian duct may leave remnants in the mesovarium (epoopheron) or in the cervical or vaginal walls (Gartner's duct). These may form cysts. The incidence of some remnant is estimated to be about 20%, but they are less often of clinical significance.

Mechanism and timescale of gonadal development

To understand the development of the external genitalia and some of the derangements of internal structures, it is necessary to consider some of the factors which control gonadal development. This complex area has been much clarified by the studies of many workers in the last decades, notably Jost & Wachtel (for references see Wilson et al 1981a). This topic is dealt with in Chapter 11 but reference is necessary here to understand the importance of timing in deviations of embryological development. The basic sequence is chromosomal sex, gonadal differentiation and phenotype. Essentially, whatever chromosome complement is present, it is the endocrine effects of the gonads which determine phenotype.

The germ cells arise outside the gonad and if they do not arrive at the genital ridge during the 6th week of embryonic development, the gonad forms only a fibrous streak. By this stage the gonad is bipotential and consists essentially of primordial germ cells, connective tissue of the genital ridge and covering epithelium. It is a structure with cortical and medullary potential.

What happens then depends on whether there is sufficient testicular component to induce somatic cells to form all or part of a male system. Normally this occurs when there is a Y chromosome and the relevant genes are carried in the pericentric region of the short arm. Exceptions to this situation are recognized, e.g. 46XX males where there is no recognizable Y chromosome.

The precise connection between the Y chromosome and the somatic cells is not clear. It is certain that formation of the testis precedes any other sexual development. A serologically determined male antigen, on the plasma membrane of the cells of the male embryo, has been recognized as a Y-induced histocompatibility antigen (H-Y; Wachtel 1983). This substance is essential for the organization of seminiferous tubules and subsequent male development. Without it, no male gonadal development proceeds. Recent monoclonal antibody techniques have shown that this Y-inducer substance is not necessarily contained in the Y chromosome, as it is present in XX males, but the concept of its presence to induce male development is still valid. The testis-determining DNA sequence is now known to be located on the short arm of the Y chromosome and is called the sex-determining region on the Y (SRY). It is possible that interchange of material or copy of this sequence may occur on an X chromosome (Ferguson-Smith 1988). The subsequent testicular development is one of cortical regression and medullary growth leading to the development of spermatic cords, seminiferous tubules and Leydig cells. Human chorionic gonadotrophin stimulates the Leydig cells and testosterone synthesis is well under way by 9 weeks from fertilization.

The differentiation of the gonad determines the hormonal environment and, in turn, the differentiation of the internal duct system, the external genitalia and perhaps the embryonic brain (Wilson et al 1981b). The timing of these steps is shown in Figure 1.8.

Mechanism and timescale of ovarian development

Morphological development of the ovary starts about 2 weeks later than the testis and proceeds more slowly. Development of the female internal duct system is not dependent on ovarian formation and proceeds ahead of development of the germ cells. Nevertheless, oestrogen is produced from the ovary prior to germ cell growth and it is presumed that the primitive Leydig cells produce oestrogen by conversion from testosterone – a process that has been shown to occur before differentiation.

If no H-Y antigen is formed, the cortical zone of the gonad develops and contains the germ cells, whereas the medullary zone regresses to form a compressed aggregation of tubules and Leydig cells in the hilus of the ovary. The germ cells divide and by 20 weeks of gestation there are primordial follicles with oocytes. The peak formation of primordial follicles occurs at about this time, reaching about 5–7 million by 20 weeks. Atresia starts around that time, and by birth there are about 1–2 million germ cells surrounded by a layer of follicular cells. The germ cells enter the first meiotic division and are arrested in prophase.

Development of the duct systems

Provided that the genital ridge develops, all embryos have wolffian and müllerian systems. Normally one system develops and the other regresses. Development of the müllerian system is passive and will usually occur unless positively inhibited. In contrast, the wolffian system is controlled by the presence of sufficient androgens.

The process of determining duct development is controlled by the fetal gonad. The first interactive event between gonad and duct system is the production of müllerian inhibition. The hormone involved was formerly called müllerian-inhibiting factor (MIF), but is now characterized as a glycoprotein formed by the Sertoli cells of the spermatogenic tubules very early in the development of the fetal testis, and is called anti-müllerian hormone (AMH). If this function fails, a female genital tract will form internally regardless of chromosomal sex. The production of AMH precedes and is separate from, androgen production. It acts locally and deficiency can be unilateral. A hereditary disorder of persistent müllerian duct syndrome exists where a fallopian tube and hemiuterus may occur on one or both sides and coexist with normal

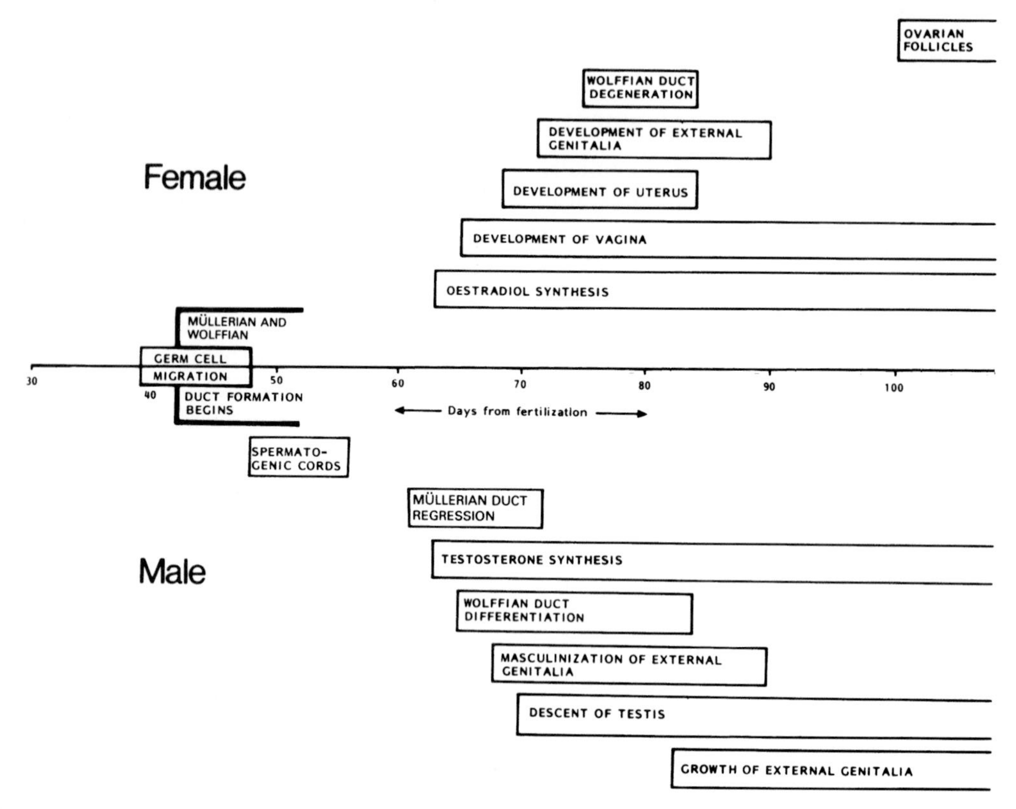

Fig. 1.8 Timing of anatomical, gonadal and endocrine events. Data from Coulam (1979) and Wilson et al (1981b).

wolffian development in otherwise normal genetic and phenotypic males. It is not clear whether this results from failure to produce AMH or from tissue unresponsiveness. Suboptimal testicular function is probable since there is often failure of testicular descent.

Another feature indicative of the independence of these processes is that there is usually regression of the müllerian ducts even when defective testosterone synthesis results in an under-masculinized male. If there is no functional testis, no AMH is produced, the müllerian system develops and there is no stimulation of the wolffian system. This is the normal event in the female and proceeds whether there is a normal ovary or not. The two genital duct systems and the urinary tract have a common opening between the genital folds. Their fate depends on the formation of the external genitalia.

Development of the external genitalia

There is an overlap in the timing of the formation of the external genitalia and the internal duct system (Fig. 1.9). There is a common indifferent stage, consisting of two genital folds, two genital swellings and a midline, anterior genital tubercle. The female development is a simple progression from these structures:

genital tubercle → clitoris
genital folds → labia minora
genital swellings → labia majora.

In the male, the genital folds elongate and fuse, with the following formation:

genital tubercle → glans
genital folds → penis and urethra
genital swelling → scrotum.

This process is normally dependent on fetal testosterone production. Agents or inborn errors that prevent the synthesis or action of androgens inhibit formation of the external genitalia.

By the end of the first trimester of pregnancy, fusion of the genital folds has occurred in the male but with little differential growth. Hence at this stage of gestation inspection of the genitalia may be misleading. It is during the second trimester that most of the differential male growth occurs.

The external genitalia are very sensitive to androgen effects during development, the end-result depending on both androgen availability and local tissue sensitivity. This can account for a variable degree of ambiguity of the basic female phenotype. If sufficient local androgen activity is not achieved by the 10th week from fertilization, incom-

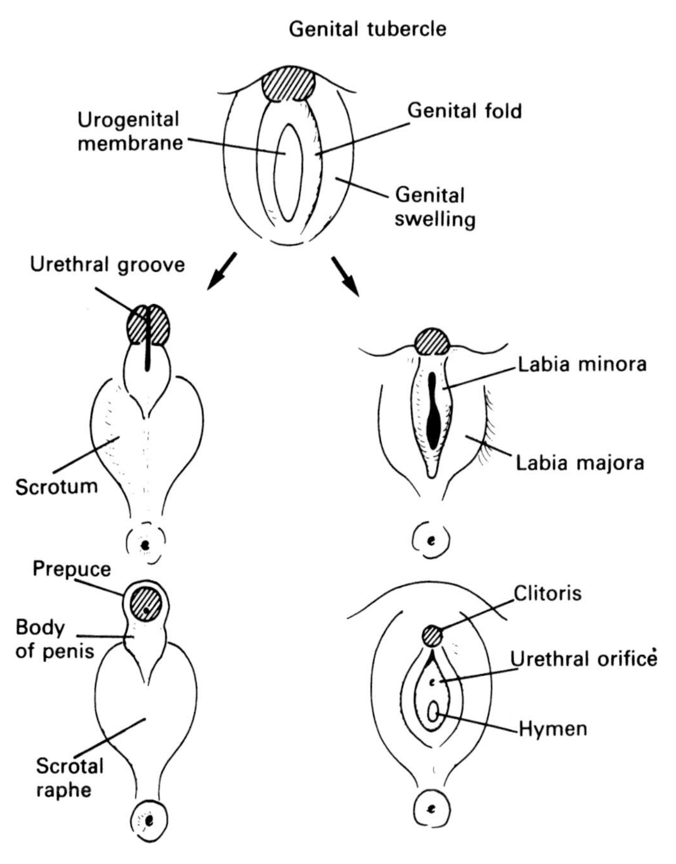

Fig. 1.9 Development of female and male external genitalia from the different stages.

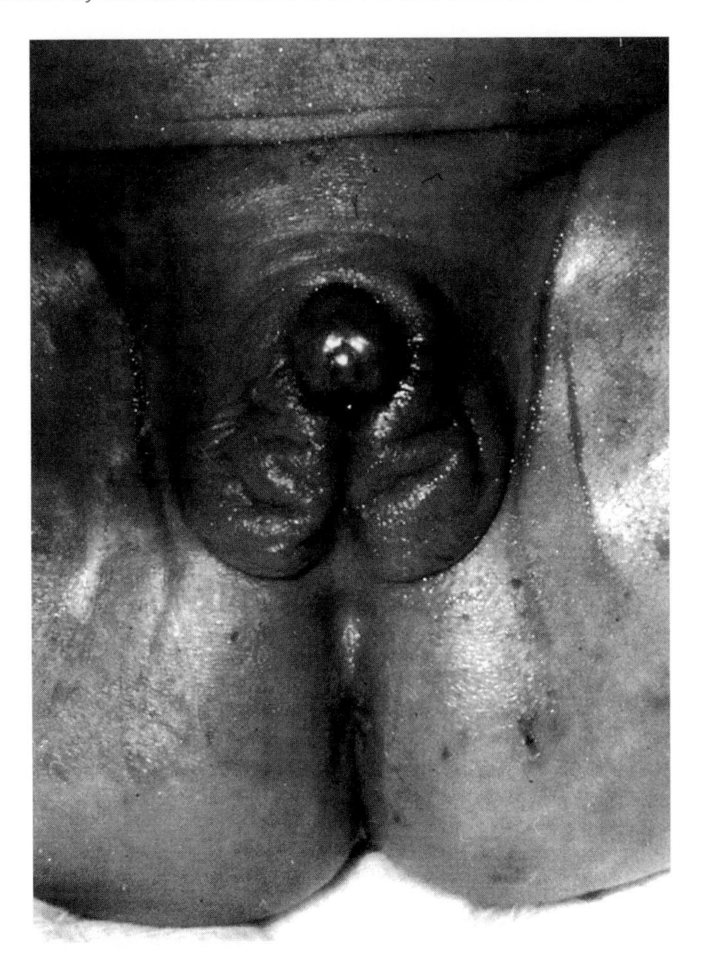

Fig. 1.10 Masculinized female genitalia in congenital adrenal hyperplasia.

pletely masculinized genitalia will result in the male. Equally, exposure to sufficient androgens can result in a very similar appearance in the female. In congenital adrenal hyperplasia in the female, the degree of masculinization is variable (Fig. 1.10) but full scrotal and penile development may take place. However, the timing of adrenal development means that the androgenic stimulus arrives too late to affect the internal duct system. Once the external genitalia are fully developed, future androgen stimulus in the female will cause clitoral hypertrophy but not fusion of the labia.

Defective virilization resulting in female phenotype

There are several mechanisms by which defective virilization in a genetic male may occur. Although this range of conditions is quite uncommon, their existence has helped elucidation of the mechanism of differentiation. They are of importance to the gynaecologist where the end-result is one of female or ambiguous external genitalia. Because awareness of these conditions arose by sporadic reports in different countries, an assortment of terminology developed, including 'XY gonadal dysgenesis', 'agonadism', 'vanishing testes', 'anatomical testicular failure', 'male pseudohermaphrodism', and 'testicular feminization'. There are several subgroups.

1. Chromosomal anomaly, e.g. some cases of 45X/46XY.
2. Gonadal failure: testicular regression due to, for example, viral infection or vascular accident.
3. Defect of testosterone biosynthesis; enzyme defects.
4. End-organ resistance: complete androgen insensitivity, incomplete androgen insensitivity, 5a-reductase deficiency, androgen receptor failure.

Better sense can be made of the component of gonadal failure in this spectrum of conditions, by recognition of critical stages in testicular development, with the final effect depending on the embryonic stage at the time of testicular failure (Coulam 1979). It is important to distinguish testicular failure from androgen insensitivity (see Ch. 11) and this section refers only to individuals who are agonadal by the time of birth.

The spectrum of clinical effects depends on whether the fetal testis produced enough AMH to suppress the müllerian system, and whether there was enough androgen pro-

Table 1.1 Classification of XY agonadal individuals

	Embryonic testicular regression		Fetal testicular regression				
Timing	Early	Late	Early			Mid	Late
Days from fertilization		43	60	69	75	84	120
Embryological consequence of testicular failure	No genital ridge development	Müllerian regression not yet started; no testosterone production	Müllerian regression not complete; testosterone synthesis *just* started	Müllerian regression still not complete; testosterone enough for duct development	Müllerian regression complete; testosterone production too little to develop duct system but some for external genitalia	Müllerian regression complete; wolffian development complete; incomplete external genitalia; rudimentary testes	Complete wolffian duct system; complete external genitalia; no testes or epididymis
Müllerian system	–	+	+	+	–	–	–
Wolffian system	–	–	–	+	–	+	+
External genitalia	Female	Female	Ambiguous	Ambiguous	Ambiguous	Ambiguous Male	Male

Adapted from Coulam (1979).

duction to develop both the wolffian system and male external genitalia. There are seven different clinical entities (Table 1.1). In this group of conditions, to have a female phenotype there has to be failure of testicular development before androgen is secreted, but not necessarily before AMH is produced. Therefore such a girl would not be expected to have wolffian duct development. Whether or not there is a female genital tract depends on whether there was AMH (or enough AMH) before gonadal failure occurred. To have ambiguous or male genitalia, there must have been some secretion of androgen before gonadal failure occurred. The amount and duration of androgen production determines the anatomical result. Müllerian and wolffian ducts can coexist if gonadal failure occurred before müllerian regression was complete yet after androgen secretion had started. The clinical effects can be seen as a consequence of loss of testicular function at different stages of intrauterine development. The possible range extends from complete failure of development of the genital ridge (and therefore no internal duct system of either kind) to a male phenotype with anorchia.

The cause of these testicular insults is not usually known. They can be experimentally induced by drugs such as cyproterone acetate. In the human situation some may be viral or a consequence of torsion or vascular occlusion. This group of conditions is best described as the testicular regression syndrome, classified further according to the timing of the failure in development (Table 1.1).

Testosterone failure

The group of individuals with a Y chromosome, gonadal formation but some abnormality of testosterone production or effect are not discussed further here. However some of the latter abnormalities (e.g. androgen insensitivity syndrome) result in an entirely female phenotype and are relevant to disorders of puberty (see Ch. 13).

GENETICS – SEX CHROMOSOME ANOMALIES

Although sexual development is essentially gonadal, this is influenced by the sex chromosome complement. There are many derangements of the X and Y chromosomes and some of these have important anatomical and functional effects. The problem may reside in the number or in the structure of the chromosomes and variations may occur in mosaic or non-mosaic form. The main non-mosaic forms are summarized in Table 1.2 in order of the number of X chromosomes and of extra Y chromosomes.

Aneuploidy

Aneuploidy may result from non-disjunction of either meiotic division in either parent or in an early cleavage of the zygote. Some are more common in older women (e.g. 47XXX and 47XXY) and the non-disjunction is presumed to arise mainly in maternal meiosis. The occurrence of 45X does not seem to be related to maternal age (Therman 1986).

Table 1.2 Identified non-mosaic patterns of sex chromosomes; normal male and female karyotypes highlighted

Female phenotype	Male phenotype	Barr bodies
45X	**46XY** 47XYY 48XYYY	0
46XX	46XX 47XXY 48XXYY 49XXYYY	1
47XXX	48XXXY 49XXXYY	2
48XXXX	49XXXXY	3
49XXXXX		4

Although there is a wide range of clinical effects, some generalizations can be made:

1. If there is a Y chromosome, the phenotype is usually male.
2. If the number of sex chromosomes increases beyond three (i.e. more than one extra), there is a strong tendency to some degree of mental retardation.
3. Additional Y chromosome material tends to increase height.
4. Provided there is at least one Y chromosome, one or more extra chromosomes result in hypogonadism.
5. In each somatic cell, all but one X chromosomes are inactivated (lyonized).

Both Klinefelter's syndrome (XXY) and XYY occur in about 1 in 700 newborn males. The clinical features are well recognized but are outside the scope of this chapter. The higher-order anomalies with a male phenotype are very rare.

X chromosome aneuploidy with a female phenotype

Many of the abnormal X chromosomal complements are associated with gonadal dysgenesis and abnormalities of stature.

One X less

The 45X chromosome constitution accounts for more than half of the number of girls with Turner's syndrome. The overall incidence of this condition is about 1 in 2500 live female births but nearly half have a mosaic pattern or some other X chromosome aberration (de la Chapelle 1983). Short stature is invariable in 45X; sexual infantilism is usual, and other somatic features such as webbed neck, low hairline, cubitus valgus, pigmented naevi and cardiovascular anomalies are variably expressed but useful diagnostically. There is no systematic impairment of IQ, at least by verbal testing, but scoring on spatial ability tends to be lower. Classically, by the time of birth (or puberty) the gonads are non-functioning streaks but ovarian function has been described in about 3% and even fertility (especially in those with mosaicism or structural anomalies of a second X). Pregnancy loss and karyotype anomalies of the fetus are common when pregnancy does occur.

One extra X

Triple X arises in about 1 in 1200 live female births and often passes unnoticed. There is no consistent clinical syndrome, thus accounting for the lack of ascertainment, but an increased incidence of psychosis has been noted. Phenotype, puberty and fertility are normal though there is a higher incidence of secondary amenorrhoea and early menopause. There is a tendency to increased height. Conception may result in XXX or XXY (or mosaic) progeny, but this occurs much less often than the predicted 50% and it is clear that in the meiotic division of the oocyte, the extra X chromosome ends up in the polar body more often than would be predicted by chance.

More than one extra X

This is rare. Dysmorphism and mental retardation are usual but psychosis and aggression are not features. There may be some resemblance to Down's syndrome (de Grouchy & Turleau 1984). Phenotype, external genitalia and puberty are usually normal. Menstrual disorders are common. Fertility is possible and the incidence of chromosomal abnormalities in the progeny, though not well assessed, is likely to be high.

Mosaicism

This is more common for sex chromosomes than for autosomes. Two cell lines can arise from a single zygote due to non-disjunction in an early mitosis. The commonest are 46XX or 46XY accompanied by a 45X cell line, but an enormous variety is possible and there can be more than two cell lines. The mechanisms which control their origin are extremely complicated and not well understood (Simpson et al 1982).

The clinical effects are wide-ranging and especially complex when there is both an XX and an XY cell line. The relative proportion of the different cell lines tends to determine the phenotype, but this can vary in different organs and some result in hermaphrodite or intersex states.

Structural abnormalities of X chromosomes

Apart from the number of X chromosomes and mosaic

cell lines, there are many possible variations in the X chromosome pattern in the female. Developments in banding techniques and in other methods of studying DNA sequences have enabled the identification of locations, on the X chromosome, of genes determining gonadal and somatic features (Fig. 1.11). Technical progress has necessitated frequent revision of concepts of karyotype–phenotype correlation, and this process is developing rapidly (Migeon 1994). Undetected mosaicism is always a possibility and any generalizations are subject to early revision. The basic conventions of banding and nomenclature of chromosomes with respect to deletion and isochromy should be understood (Fig. 1.12).

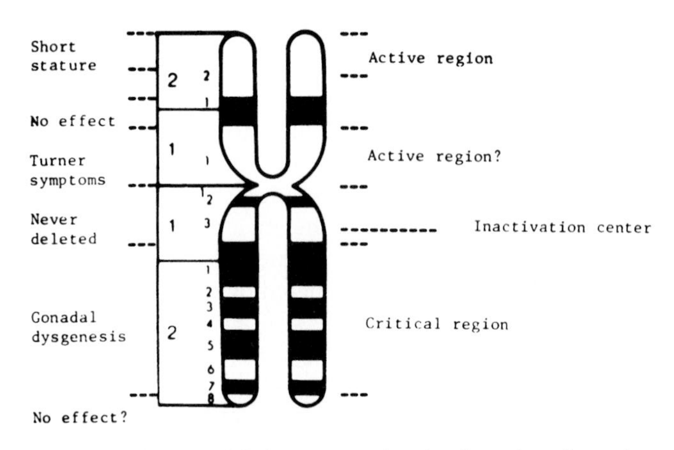

Fig. 1.11 Diagram of X chromosome showing the main active regions. On the left, the main phenotypic effects of various deletions are shown. (From Therman 1986, with permission.)

The generalizations in Table 1.3 are relevant to an understanding of the clinical effects.

If there is one normal X and the other is abnormal, inactivation of the abnormal X occurs in the somatic cells and this tends to diminish the effect of the abnormality.

Gonadal function, stature and the stigmata of Turner's syndrome depend on the nature of the second X chromosome and this clinical effect is further varied by the existence of a mosaic cell line (usually 45X). Despite the fact that the second X is usually inactivated, both X chromosomes are required for female fertility. Whether deletion of portions of either arm of one X chromosome results in gonadal dysgenesis depends critically on exactly what genetic material is missing. Deletion of all or part of the short or long arm can occur. If most or all of the short arm

Table 1.3 General effects of structural abnormalities of X chromosomes

	Aspects of phenotype affected	Effect of loss of material	Effect of extra material
Short arm	Ovarian function	Gonadal dysgenesis	
	Somatic features of Turner's	Turner's phenotype	
	Growth	Short stature	
Long arm	Ovarian function	Gonadal dysgenesis	
	Growth	Reduced growth	Increased growth

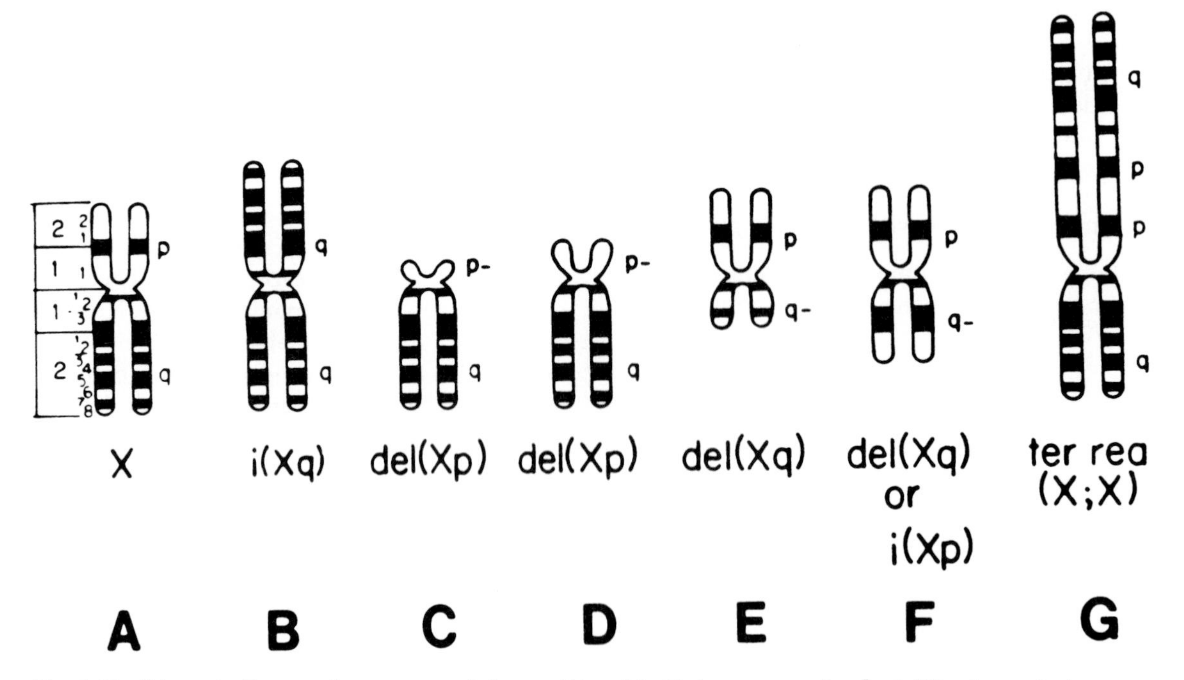

Fig. 1.12 Schematic diagram of some structural abnormalities of the X chromosome. **A** normal; **B** isochrome for long arm; **C** deletion of most of the short arm; **D** probable interstitial deletion of the middle portion of the short arm; **E** interstitial deletion of the long arm; **F** deletion of a portion of the long arm; **G** short-arm end-to-end terminal rearrangement. (From de la Chapelle 1983, with permission.)

Table 1.4 Correlation of X karyotype, phenotype and gonadal development

Sex chromosomes				
Problem	Example of karyotype	Stature	Primary amenorrhoea	Breast development
Monosomy for X	45X	Short	Almost certain	Absent or minimal
Short arm material missing				
Isochromy of long arm	46X, i(Xq) or 45X/46X, I(Xq)	Short	Almost certain	Absent or minimal
Most of short arm	46X, del(X)(p11)	Short	Variable	May be some
Terminal part of short arm	46X, del(X)(p22)	Short	Not likely	Usually some
Long arm material missing				
Isochromy of short arm (rare or doubtful mosaic)	46X, i(Xp)	Reduced	Certain	None
Most of long arm	46X, del(X) (q13)	Reduced	Likely	Minimal
Terminal part of long arm	46X, del(X)(q22)	Reduced	Likely	Minimal
Mosaic	45X/46XX	Variable	Variable	Variable*
	46XX/range of deletions/isochromy	Variable	Variable	Variable*

* The effect of these depends very much on the proportion and distribution of the normal cell line.
Compiled from data in Simpson et al (1982).

is deleted, then short stature and Turner's features are usual. Deletion of most or all of the long arm is nearly always associated with gonadal dysgenesis.

A ring chromosome can form if part of both ends is missing. The clinical effect will depend on the amount of genetic material lost but the effect tends to be less than if a whole arm is absent. Isochromy, due to misdivision at the centromere, can result in two long arms i(Xq) instead of a short (p) and a long (q) arm. In effect this results in three long arms and one short one and the effect on gonadal function and stature is the same as 45X.

Gonadal determinants appear to be located on both arms but it is not a question of total amount, since duplication of one fails to compensate for loss of the other and each arm must carry different functions. There appear to be components determining stature on both arms, but loss of short arm material seems to result more consistently in short stature.

Although this area remains complex and only partially understood, a reasonable prediction of stature and potential for gonadal function can be made from consideration of the karyotype (Table 1.4).

XX gonadal dysgenesis

There need not be a demonstrable abnormality of sex chromosome pattern for gonadal dysgenesis to occur. The gonads and genitalia look exactly the same in this condition as in 45X, though most such girls are of normal stature without Turner features. This condition is usually autosomal recessive and developments in genetics may clarify the mechanism in the future.

Translocations

Translocation can occur between an X chromosome and an autosome. The effect on ovarian function and phenotype varies (position effect). The normal X is inactivated and the parts of the other X attached to the autosomal segments remain active (Zakharov & Baranovskaya 1983). If the translocation is unbalanced there is mental retardation and ovarian failure. If balanced, mental retardation is still likely.

X-X translocations

One X chromosome may be replaced by a very long X consisting of two X chromosomes attached by either their long or short arms. This results in a variable amount of X genetic material being deleted or being present in a double dose. Where long arm material is lost there is usually gonadal dysgenesis, despite the extra X material. The translocation X is late replicating and it is the structurally normal X which is genetically active (Fig. 1.13; Dewald & Spurbeck 1983).

True hermaphrodites

This condition is characterized by the demonstration of both ovarian and testicular tissue. From the genetic point of view it is heterogeneous. The commonest single chromosome pattern is 46XX but there is often more than one cell line and this may be due to chimaerism (two cell lines at fertilization) or mitotic non-disjunction. Recognized cell lines include 46XX/46XY and 46XX/47XXY. Essentially, the more testicular tissue there is, the more likely is gonadal descent. Usually there is at least a hemi-uterus, and if ovarian tissue is present it is more likely to be on the left side.

The management depends on the phenotype (see Ch. 11). Ovulation and, where the anatomy is appropriate, conception and delivery can occur.

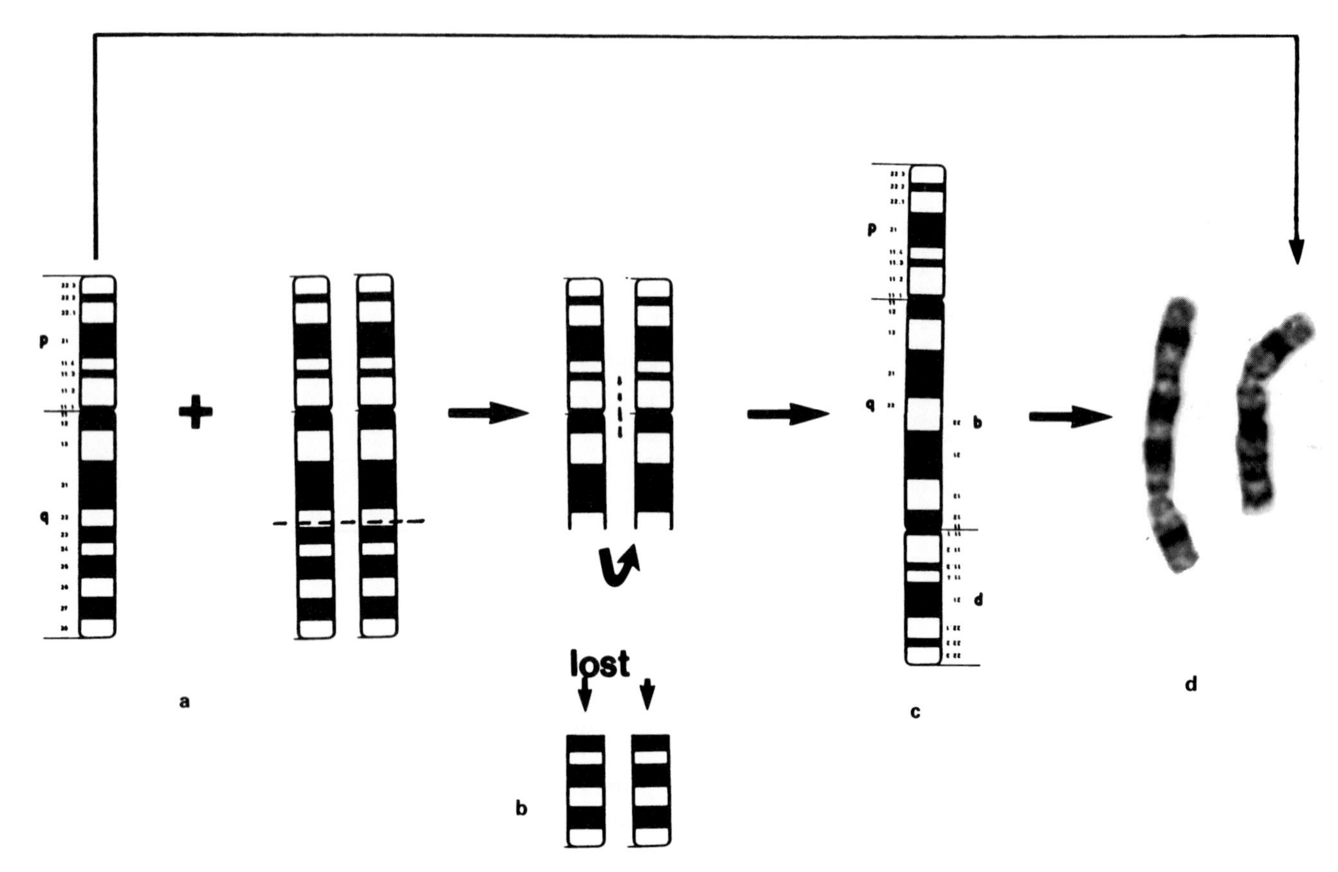

Fig. 1.13 Formation of an isodicentric X chromosome idic(X)q(22). **a** Chromatid breakage at band q22. **b** Reunion of sister chromatids with loss of acentric segment. **c** Division of centromere to form end-to-end fusion chromosome. One centromere becomes inactive. **d** Chromosomes form a 46X idic(X)(q22) cell.

CONGENITAL ABNORMALITIES OF FEMALE DEVELOPMENT

Anomalies of female development may present to the gynaecologist in many ways and at different stages of life. The preceding sections have aimed to set out a basis for understanding variations in terms of chromosomal sex, gonadal development (including inappropriate hormone production), sex duct development and external genitalia. Some of the resulting conditions are mainly the concern of the paediatric surgeon (e.g. cloacal anomalies), the urologist (e.g. bladder extrophy, abnormal ureters) or the paediatrician (e.g. disorders of growth). There is necessarily overlap between specialties in conditions such as ambiguous genitalia (see Ch. 11) and disorders of puberty (see Ch. 13).

This section deals with anatomical disorders of the genital tract in the phenotypic female. Fetal diagnosis, although possible for some conditions, is not considered further here. Conditions with a genetic but no anatomical genital abnormality, e.g. 45X, and other conditions presenting with primary amenorrhoea, e.g. complete androgen insensitivity, are discussed later (see Ch. 13).

Some of the anatomical abnormalities seen are an arrest of a stage of normal development, e.g. vaginal atresia, while others, e.g. bladder extrophy, do not represent a stage through which the normal fetus ever passes.

The most common times of presentation of abnormalities of the genital tract are:

1. newborn, if there are external abnormalities or obstruction of bladder or bowel;
2. childhood, if there is no external abnormality but there is disturbance of function;
3. puberty, particularly if menstrual function is affected;
4. because of attempted coitus, where there is relative obstruction during intercourse;
5. adulthood, because of infertility or during pregnancy or parturition.

It is not possible to estimate the incidence of genital tract anomalies accurately, since the age of ascertainment, the thoroughness of surveillance and the inclusion of minor anomalies will influence this. In pregnancy, an incidence of müllerian anomalies of 1 in 600 women has been estimated but this excludes the very important groups who cannot conceive. Perhaps a reasonable estimate would be some abnormality of the genital tract in 1% of phenotypic females.

The neonate or child

Neonates and children with congenital abnormalities of female development may present in one of several ways:

1. ambiguous genitalia;
2. imperforate vagina, with a large abdominal mass due to mucocolpos;
3. duplication of the vulva;
4. cloaca (often involving spinal defects);
5. ectopia vesicae;
6. imperforate anus;
7. disorders of renal system affecting micturition or drainage.

Need for gynaecological assessment

Although recognition, diagnosis and management are the province of the paediatrician and paediatric surgeon, there are several reasons why a gynaecologist should be involved.

1. Study of the original anatomy aids comprehension of the problem.
2. Familiarity with the surgery on the infant helps with reconstructive surgery at puberty or later.
3. Where there are anomalies of the urinary or bowel systems, liaison improves the investigation of the anatomy of the genital tract.
4. Diagnosis of the abnormal vulva is not easy and improves with practice.

Where there are abnormalities of the urinary or bowel systems in the female, concomitant anomalies of the genital tract are quite common. However, the need to consider the function of the genital tract is less pressing and its investigation in these conditions presenting early in life is often incomplete (Fleming et al 1986).

Multiple abnormalities

These include persistent cloaca (Fig. 1.14), bladder exstro-

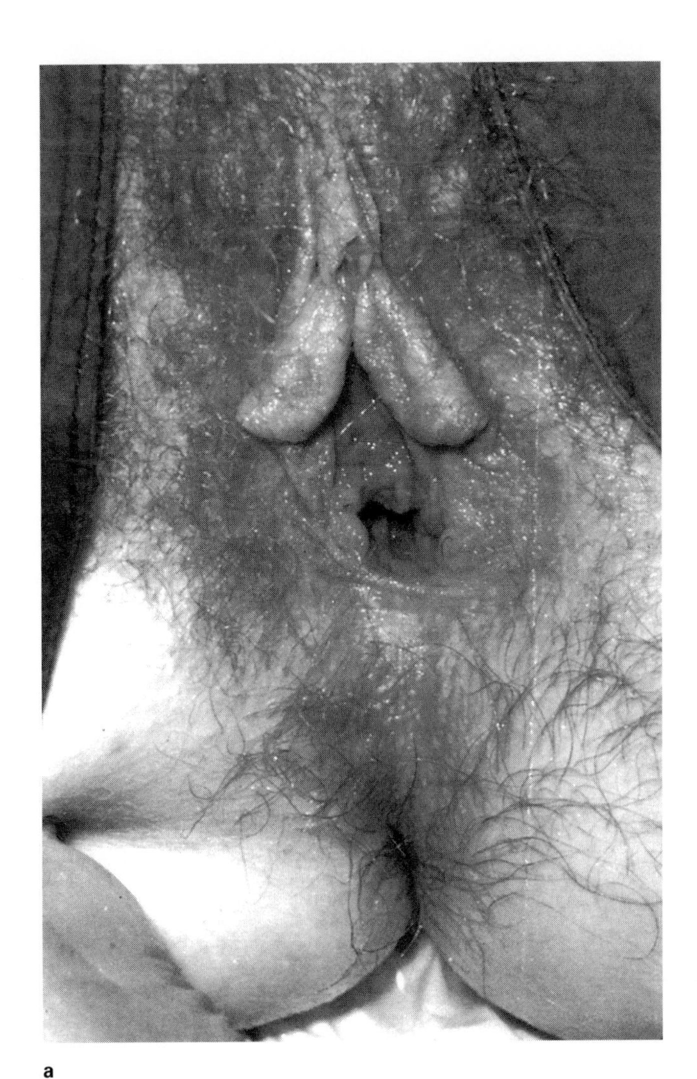

a

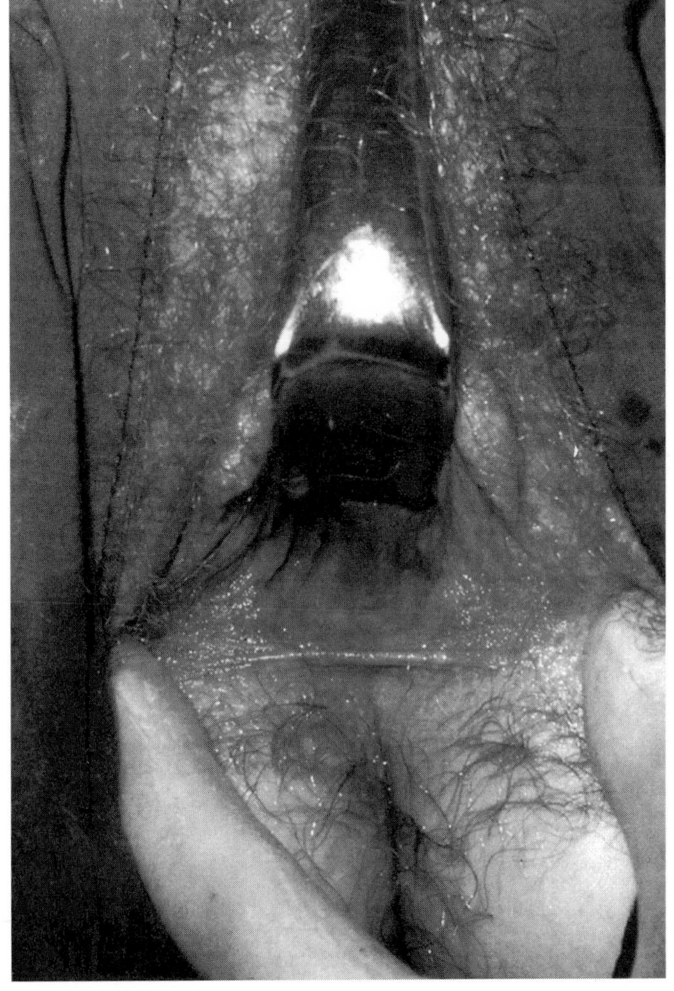

b

Fig. 1.14 Cloaca: **a** single opening with absence of anus; **b** rectal columns posteriorly in cloaca.

phy and ectopic ureter. The anatomy of the genital tract can be clarified in the course of investigation using endoscopy, ultrasound, contrast vaginogram (or sinogram) and, where necessary, laparotomy. More recently magnetic resonance imaging (MRI) has proved useful. The primary concern is function of the bladder and bowel but free drainage of the genital tract is also important as obstruction is often a feature. Careful recording of the genital anatomy is valuable for prognosis and later reference.

Imperforate vagina

Mucocolpos due to an imperforate vagina may cause a large abdominal mass in the newborn. It is not clear why this occurs only occasionally when there is obstruction, or whether a minor degree occurs in all girls with an imperforate vagina but passes unnoticed. Although the clinical problem is rare in the newborn, it is important in the differential diagnosis of an abdominal mass in a newborn girl.

Duplication of vulva

This is rare, and full paediatric surgical investigation is required to establish other abnormalities and effective drainage. A didelphic uterus is likely. If there is no functional problem then an acceptable cosmetic effect would be the aim.

Ambiguous genitalia

This conditions arises in:

1. virilized females, e.g. on account of congenital adrenal hyperplasia, high maternal androgen levels, maternal drug ingestion;
2. under-masculinized males;
3. true hermaphrodites.

The diagnosis and management are essentially paediatric and clinical aspects of abnormal sexual development are discussed in Chapter 11. At birth, ambiguity is a management problem requiring high priority (Gearhart 1992).

Puberty or later

Of the conditions with gynaecological relevance considered here some result from embryological failure, some are a consequence of mutant genes and in others a genetic factor is suspected but not certain. Reporting of these conditions has not been systematic and has been more likely where there have been family aggregates. The close relation between urinary tract and genital anomalies should be remembered.

In müllerian agenesis, there is no corpus or cervix and no upper vagina (Fig. 1.15). There may or may not be fallopian tubes representing the upper separate ends of the müllerian duct system. There may also be remnants of müllerian tissue. The condition has been reported in siblings but not with enough consistency to suggest that it is due to single gene defect. Müllerian agenesis accounts for over 80% of occurrences of no vagina.

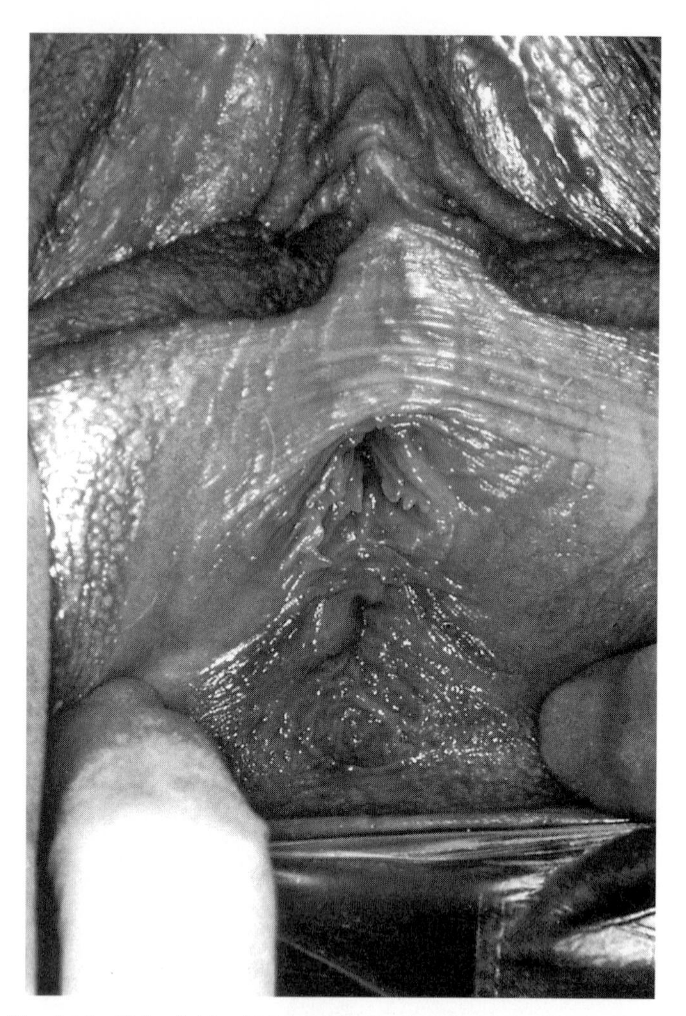

Fig. 1.15 Vulva (labia widely retracted) of a girl with müllerian agenesis. The urethra is abnormally patulous and there is very little formation of the urogenital sinus portion of the vagina.

Vaginal atresia with development of the müllerian system is a distinct condition, with no reporting of family aggregates except where the atresia is part of multiple anomalies (Simpson et al 1982). The failure of the urogenital sinus to form the lower vagina may be complete or there may be a lower vagina with an obstruction of variable thickness in the mid-portion. True duplication, due to splitting of the müllerian duct or even of the genital ridge early in embryogenesis, does not have any family aggregates whereas incomplete fusion may be one component of a congenitally determined malformation. Even if it occurs as the only abnormality, incomplete fusion seems to have a polygenic or multifactorial basis resulting in some family aggregation.

Presentation

Abnormalities not diagnosed in infancy may become of clinical relevance around the time of puberty or later and are more likely to affect the vagina or upper genital tract. Vulvar abnormalities, however, may become evident because of hormonal stimulation. Failure of pubertal development is discussed in Chapter 13. Where there is primary amenorrhoea with secondary sexual development, absence of the uterus or obstruction to menstrual flow should be considered. Other presenting complaints include apareunia or inability to insert a tampon.

Vaginal atresia or obstruction

Where this condition has not been diagnosed in infancy, failure to menstruate is the likeliest presenting symptom. The crucial clinical question is whether or not there is haematocolpos. Higher levels of obstruction, at the cervix or upper vagina, will tend to cause symptoms early and also cause more serious backflow and endometriosis. Any recurrent abdominal pain (not necessarily regular or monthly) in a pubertal girl with secondary sexual development should be investigated adequately. Ultrasound of the pelvis and kidneys is very useful. Inspection of the introitus, although important, may be misleading where there is a high obstruction (Figs 1.16–1.19).

Where the obstruction is low and thin, usually just above the hymen, a simple cruciate incision to allow free drainage of retained menses is all that is required initially.

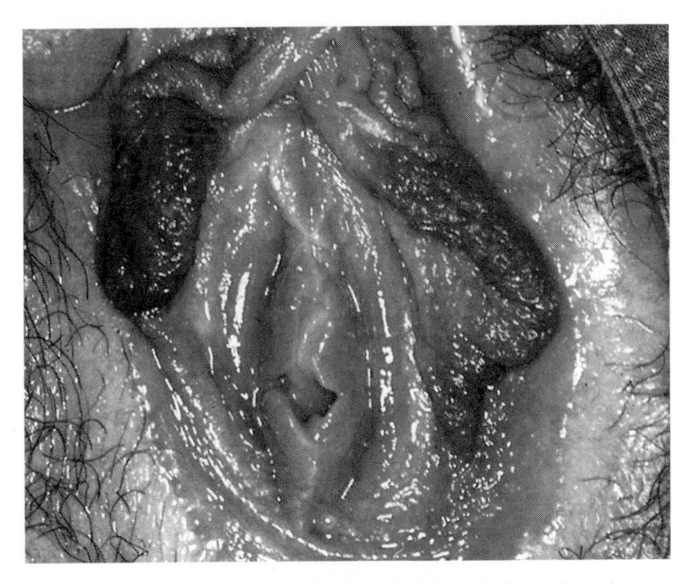

Fig. 1.16 Normal-looking vulva of a girl with vaginal atresia and haematocolpos and haematometra. There was a short lower vagina.

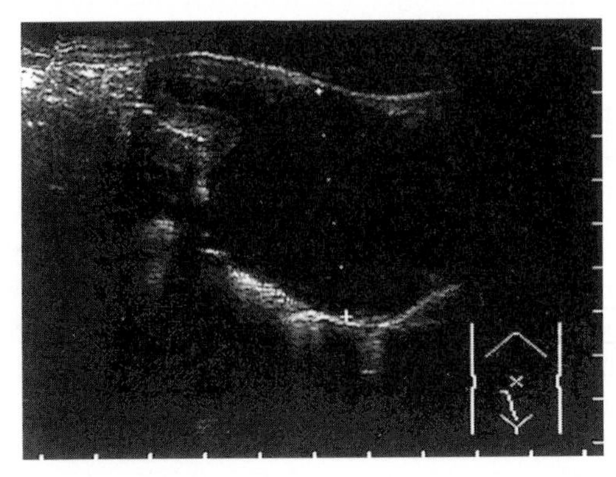

Fig. 1.17 Ultrasound scan of the same girl, showing distended upper vagina and distended uterus.

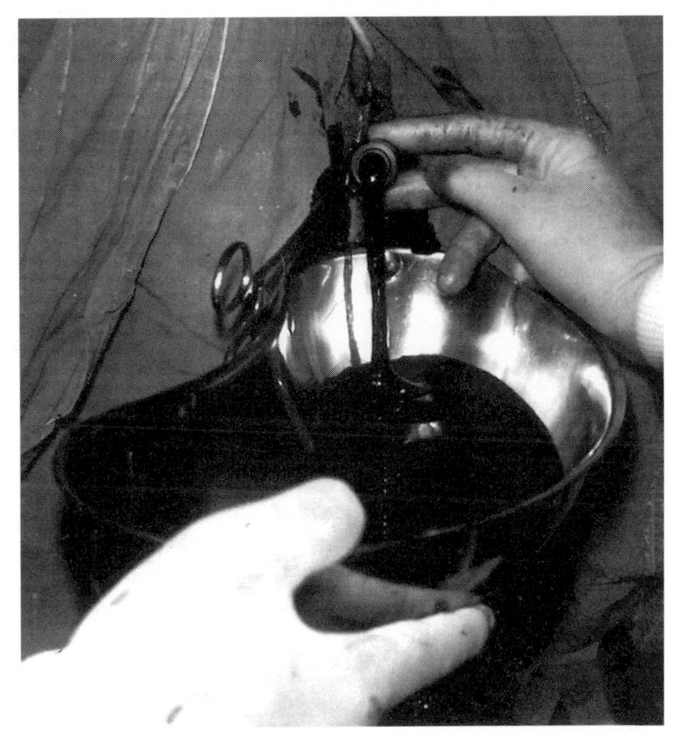

Fig. 1.18 Drainage of haematocolpos required dissection and insertion of a trocar.

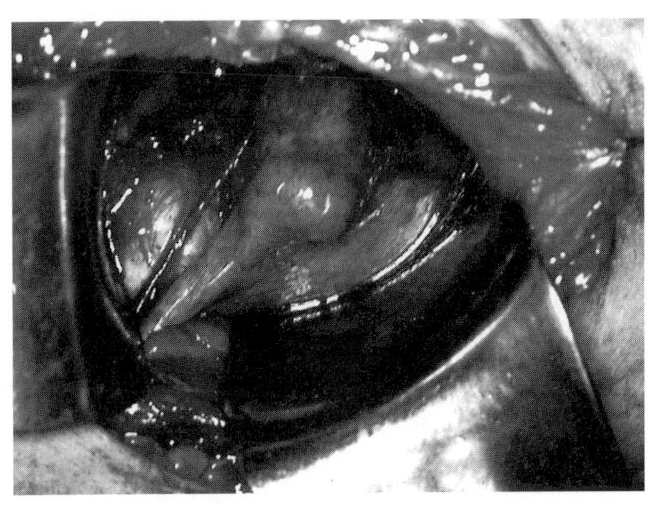

Fig. 1.19 Associated haematosalpinx.

After two or three further periods, by which time the anatomy will probably be restored to normal, laparoscopy is indicated to diagnose and treat any endometriosis. The anatomy of the renal tract should be established.

Where there is vaginal atresia, management can be difficult. If it is not possible to reach the upper vagina from the perineum, an abdominoperineal approach may be required. Achieving drainage is not usually difficult and should be effected from the vagina if possible. The difficulty is to maintain subsequent patency. Much patience and ingenuity may be required. Continuous oestrogen/ progestogen treatment may provide a respite.

Atresia of the cervix

This condition is due to failure of development of the cervical portion of the fused müllerian ducts. It is rare and serious. The uterus may be normal or didelphic. If initial attempts to create a cervical opening are not effective it may be better to resort to hysterectomy before serious intraperitoneal infection occurs since the resulting tubo-ovarian masses and peritonitis may become life-threatening (Geary & Weed 1973). Unless this condition is diagnosed and treated very early, the tubes are unlikely to function. Indeed, access to the uterus and ovaries may be quite impossible after episodes of peritonitis. In one of the present author's own cases, a patient who had large, bilateral hydrosalpinges, after years of conservative efforts, removal of the diseased tubes because of severe peritonitis led to quiescence with continuing ovarian and uterine function and at least a prospect of in vitro or donor egg fertility.

Vaginal agenesis as part of müllerian agenesis

Where vaginal agenesis is part of müllerian duct failure, the clinical picture is different. The introitus may look normal or there may be hypoplasia of the entire urogenital component. Usually there is a short (1–2 cm) vagina. The incidence is about 1 in 10 000 female births. Ureterorenal anomalies occur in about 50%. A rudimentary uterus is quite common but it may be just a thin band of tissue on one or both sides and is not usually canalized. The appearances on ultrasound have sometimes been deceptive but with better resolution a false impression of canalization is less likely. However, it should be noted that ultrasound of the uterus is more difficult where there is no vagina.

The presentation is generally with amenorrhoea and well developed secondary sex characteristics. Care is required if the girl is seen soon after the time of expected menarche to establish for certain whether or not there is a functioning uterus. If not, the question of a neovagina is best deferred until there is an interest in sexual activity. A range of techniques is available (Edmonds 1993, Lesavony 1985) but the extent to which a small vagina can be enlarged by non-surgical means should not be underestimated where motivation is high.

Where there is a short blind vagina and müllerian agenesis, androgen insensitivity must be included in the differential diagnosis. Small breasts and poorly developed axillary and pubic hair are important accompanying features. There may be a family history. Virilization at puberty is a feature of partial androgen insensitivity. Chromosome analysis is helpful in these circumstances and should be done when there is müllerian agenesis without well developed secondary sexual characteristics.

Persistent urogenital sinus

A common genitourinary channel is the normal arrangement in a male infant and occurs to some degree during development in all female infants. Failure of development and caudal movement of the lower vagina results in a higher common channel than usual. The confluence of the vagina and urethra may be at a very variable level. The condition is present in most girls with infantile congenital adrenal hyperplasia; all individuals with an intersex condition brought up as girls, and spontaneous incomplete development (see Ch. 13).

The presentation depends on whether there is, or has been, masculinization (which is not necessarily a feature), and on prior surgery, possibly in infancy. The typical feature is a small, single opening with no visible separate urethra and fusion of the labia majora. A minor degree of the condition may interfere with coitus or use of tampons. When the degree is severe, surgery is necessary to enable coitus.

Virilization occurring at puberty

There are a number of causes.

1. An intersex problem rectified in infancy but leaving a slightly enlarged clitoris. This tends to enlarge at puberty during spontaneous or replacement hormone stimulation, even only by oestrogens (Fig. 1.20).
2. Incomplete androgen insensitivity; there may have been only slight clitoral enlargement which responds further to the greater androgen boost at puberty.
3. 5a-reductase deficiency; this is always relative and again the puberty levels of testosterone cause growth.
4. Gonadoblastoma in a dysgenetic gonad.

The hormonal, gonadal and anatomical status must be completely evaluated. Inappropriate androgen secretion must be removed, except in some cases of 5a-reductase deficiency, where reinforcement of the male gender has been successful. If clitoral hypertrophy remains a problem, and it will tend not to regress much if oestrogen replacement is effected, some form of clitoral reduction should be offered (Kogan 1993).

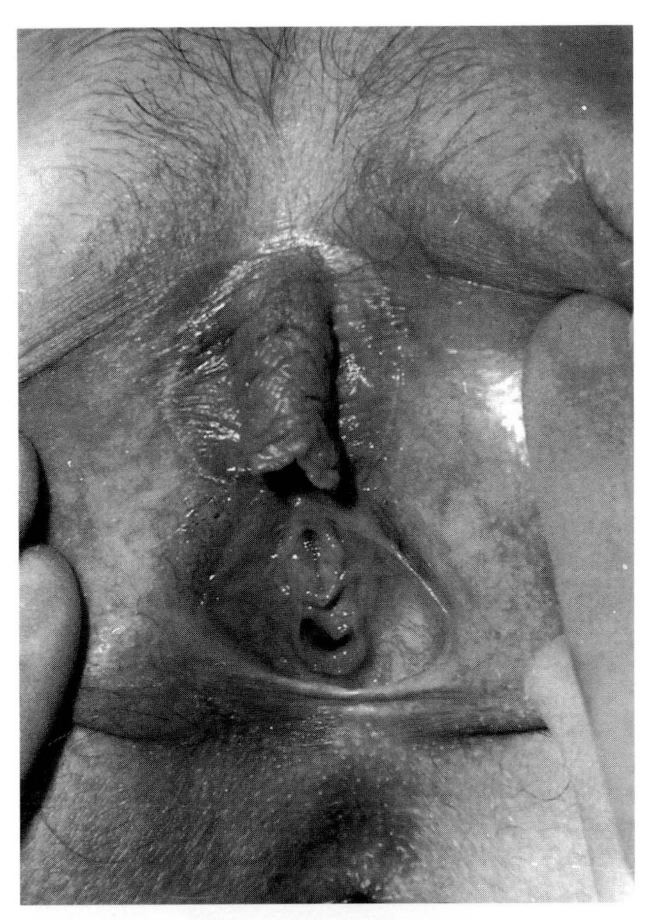

Fig. 1.20 Hypertrophy of clitoris occurring at puberty due to oestrogen administration, in an otherwise phenotypic female (XY). There had been minimal hypertrophy in infancy associated with intersex (mainly scrotal development with testes) and the gonads had been removed in the neonatal period. Note that the androgenic stimulus in utero had not been sufficient to fuse the genital folds.

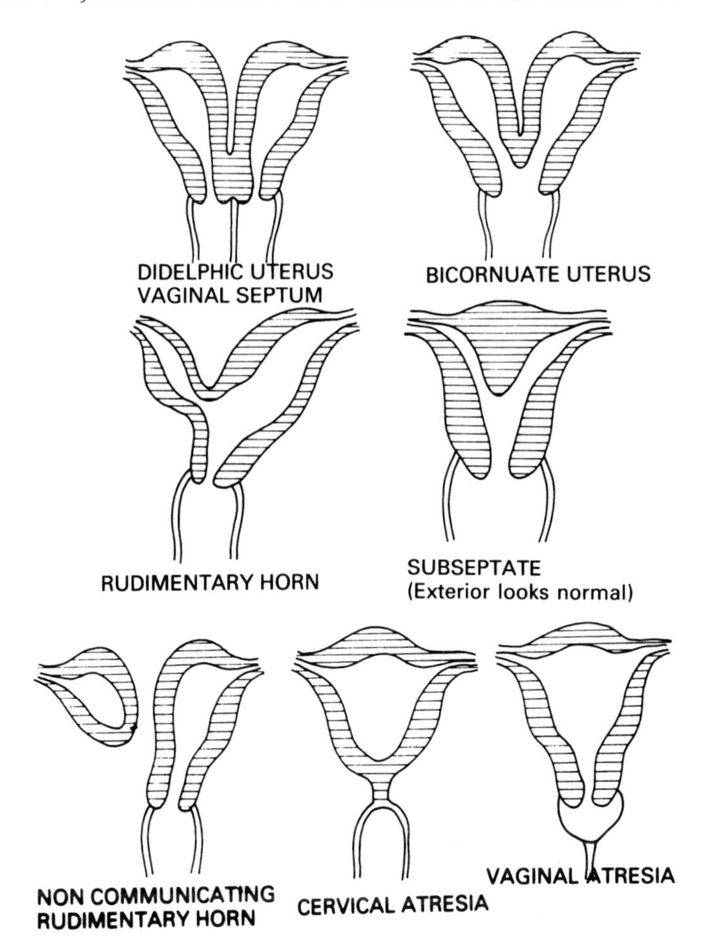

Fig. 1.21 Varieties of uterine anomaly.

Uterine anomalies

Absence of the uterus is an important cause of primary amenorrhoea and is discussed more fully in Chapter 13. Since it is essentially due to failure of development of the lower part of the paramesonephric (müllerian) ducts, the cervix and upper vagina are also absent. There may be a vestigial uterus and cervix without canalization and without function.

True duplication of the müllerian ducts with doubling of reproductive structures on one or both sides is rare.

Fusion anomalies are more common and result in a variety of well recognized uterine shapes (Fig. 1.21) (American Fertility Society 1988). Where there is atresia of one of the paramesonephric ducts there is a unicornuate uterus with a single tube. The kidney on the side of the defective duct is often absent. If the unilateral atresia is partial, the rudimentary part may be an appendage to the well developed side and, if it fails to communicate, the rudimentary horn causes complications. Where there is a didelphic uterus, the uterine cavities are completely separate (Fig. 1.22) but the two cervices are often united externally. The vagina may or may not be septate. In this condition, asymmetry of the vagina may result in complete closure of only one-half, with subsequent cryptomenorrhoea and haematometra but with apparently normal

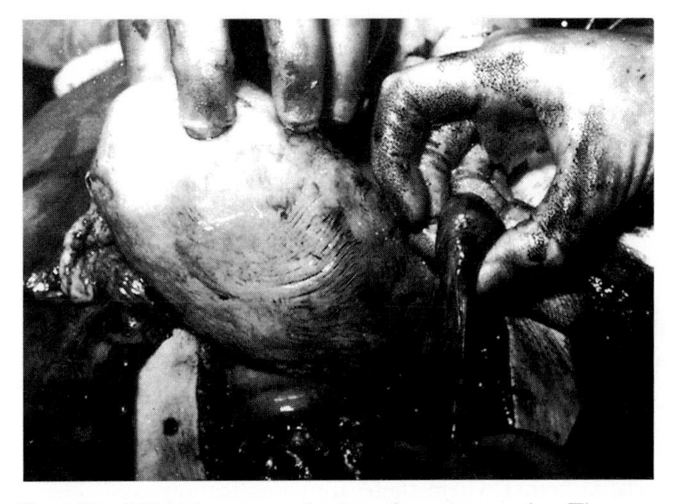

Fig. 1.22 Didelphic uterus at the time of caesarean section. The non-pregnant right uterus is attached externally at the cervix

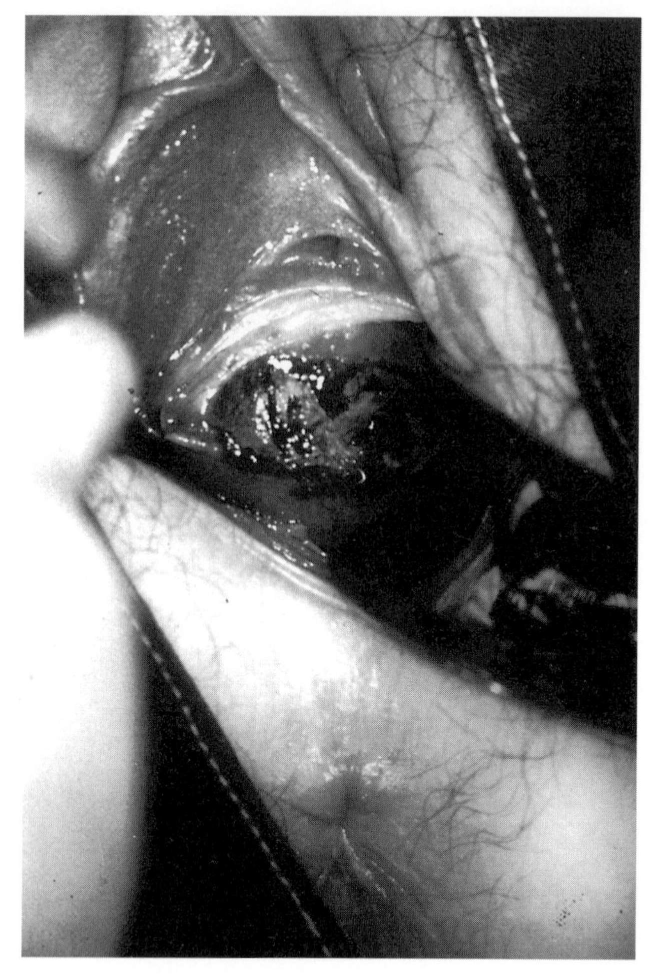

Fig. 1.23 Partially exposed haematocolpos of right hemivagina. The speculum is in the normal left hemivagina.

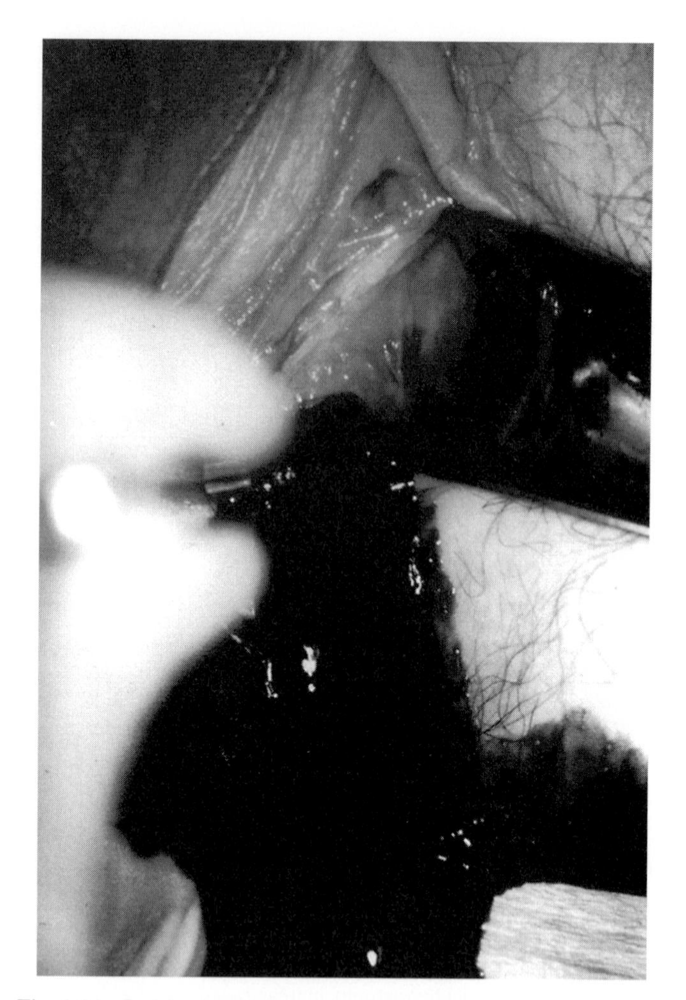

Fig. 1.24 Incision and drainage.

menstrual function (Figs 1.23–1.25). Curiously, when this condition occurs, the occluded side is nearly always on the right. There is ipsilateral absence of the kidney (Rock & Jones 1980). Failure of complete müllerian duct fusion and failure to form a ureter are both a consequence of a defective mesonephric duct.

Provided there is no obstruction to menstrual flow, these uterine anomalies present few problems in the absence of pregnancy. An increased incidence of miscarriage, poor fetal growth, malpresentation and placental adherence is recognized. The incidence of abnormalities and the complication rate are ill defined since ascertainment is higher where there are complications and operative delivery (Rock & Schlaff 1985). Pregnancy may occur

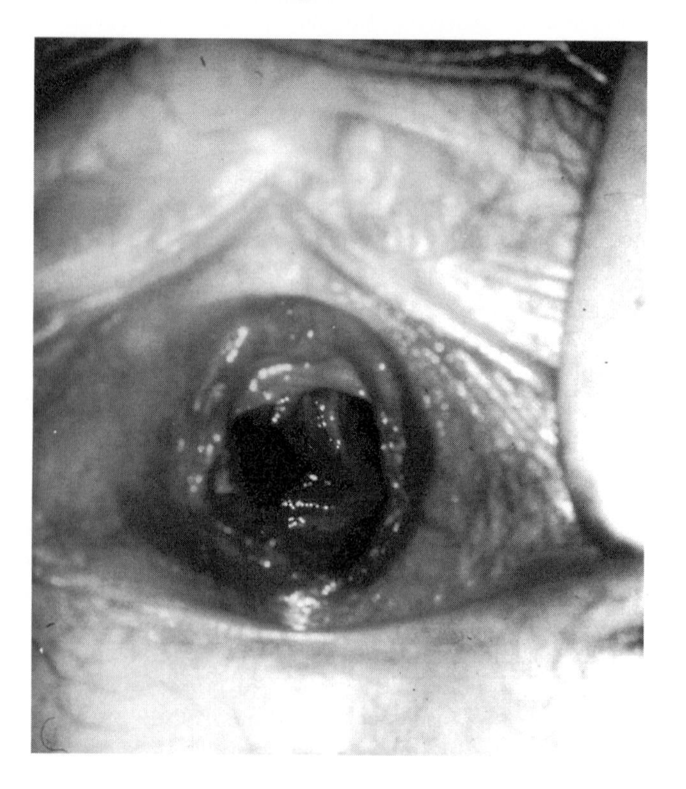

Fig. 1.25 Septum in the same girl after drainage.

in a non-communicating rudimentary horn by transperitoneal sperm passage and can result in a difficult diagnostic and management problem.

For many of the anatomical congenital anomalies, the event which caused developmental failure is not clear even if the stage of arrest can be recognized. Much has been discovered about the controlling mechanisms in recent decades and further elucidation is likely.

KEY POINTS

1. The nephrogenic cord develops from the mesoderm and forms the urogenital ridge and mesonephric duct (later to form the wolffian duct).
2. The paramesonephric duct, later to form the müllerian system, develops as an ingrowth of coelomic epithelium anterolateral to the mesonephric duct.
3. In the normal female, the wolffian system degenerates, and the lower ends of the müllerian system fuse to form the uterus, cervix and upper vagina while the cephalic ends remain separate, forming the fallopian tubes.
4. Unilateral renal aplasia is frequently associated with failure of müllerian development on the same side, since both are dependent on adequate development of the mesonephric system.
5. If the tubular portions of the müllerian ducts develop to form a uterus and cervix, there is usually a patent upper vagina.
6. If there is no development of the urogenital sinus, the subsequent vaginal atresia involves most of the vagina.
7. Where there is müllerian agenesis, the urogenital sinus still forms but does not lengthen and the vagina is short though of variable length.
8. Chromosomal sex determines the development of the gonad and this, in turn, ordains the sexual phenotype.
9. The wolffian system is dependent upon androgens for its development.
10. The müllerian system will develop in the absence of a glycoprotein, secreted by the fetal testis, called anti-müllerian hormone (AMH) and does not require a normal ovary.
11. The development of external genitalia depends upon both the presence of androgens and local tissue sensitivity to androgens.
12. If a Y chromosome is present, the phenotype is usually male.
13. Although the second X chromosome is usually inactivated, both X chromosomes are required for fertility.
14. Gonadal dysgenesis can occur in an XX individual.
15. The primary concern in the management of pelvic abnormalities recognized in childhood is function of the bladder and bowel, but free drainage of the genital tract is also important as obstruction is often a feature, and permanent damage may result if this is not corrected before puberty.
16. Müllerian agenesis is the commonest cause for an absent vagina in girls.
17. Recurrent abdominal pain in a pubertal girl with definite secondary sexual development should be investigated to exclude haematocolpos. Ultrasound of the pelvis and kidneys is very useful.
18. If correction of cervical atresia is unsuccessful, hysterectomy should be employed to avoid the potentially lethal peritonitis that may result.

REFERENCES

American Fertility Society 1988 The American Fertility Society classifications of adnexal adhesions, distal tubal occlusion, tubal occlusion secondary to tubal ligation, tubal pregnancies, Müllerian anomalies and intrauterine adhesions. Fertility and Sterility 49: 944–954

Coulam C B 1979 Testicular regression syndrome. Obstetrics and Gynecology 53: 44–49

de Grouchy J, Turleau C 1984 Sex chromosomes. In: Clinical atlas of human chromosomes, 2nd edn. John Wiley, New York, pp 375–409

de la Chapelle A 1983 Sex chromosome anomalies. In: Emery A E H, Rimoin D L (eds) Principles and practice of medical genetics. Churchill Livingstone, Edinburgh, p 197

Dewald G W, Spurbeck J L 1983 Sex chromosome anomalies associated with premature gonadal failure. Seminars in Reproductive Endocrinology 1: 79–90

Edmonds D K 1993 Surgical management of congenital abnormalities. In: Studd J, Jardine Brown C (eds) Yearbook of the Royal College of Obstetricians and Gynaecologists. RCOG Press, London, pp 43–54

Ferguson-Smith M 1988 Genes on the X and Y chromosomes controlling sex. British Medical Journal 297: 635–636

Fleming S E, Hall R, Gysier M, McLorie G A 1986 Imperforate anus in females. Frequency of genital tract involvement. Incidence of associated anomalies and functional outcome. Journal of Paediatric Surgery 21: 146–150

Gearhart J P 1992 Surgical management of genital ambiguity. In: Carpenter S E K, Rock J A (eds) Pediatric and adolescent gynaecology. Raven Press, New York, ch 6, pp 95–102

Geary W L, Weed J C 1973 Congenital atresia of the uterine cervix. Obstetrics and Gynecology 42: 213–217

Gray S W, Skandalakis J E 1972 The female reproductive tract. In: Gray S W, Skandalakis J E Embryology for surgeons. W B Saunders, Philadelphia, pp 633–664

Kogan S J 1993 Feminizing genital reconstruction for male pseudohermaphroditism. European Journal of Paediatrics 152 (suppl 2): S 85–87

Lesavony M A 1985 Vaginal reconstruction. Urological Clinics of North America 12: 369–379

Migeon B R 1994 X-chromosome inactivation: molecular mechanisms and genetic consequences. Trends in Genetics 10: 230–235

Rock J A, Jones H W 1980 The double uterus associated with an obstructed hemivagina and ipsilateral renal agenesis. American Journal of Obstetrics and Gynecology 138: 339–342

Rock J A, Schlaff W D 1985 The obstetric consequences of uterovaginal anomalies. Fertility and Sterility 43: 681–692

Simpson J L, Golbus M S, Martin A 1992 Disorders of sex chromosomes and sexual differentiation. In: Genetics in obstetrics and gynecology, 2nd edn. Grune & Stratton, New York, pp 133–163

Therman E 1996 Abnormal human sex chromosome constitutions. In:

Human chromosomes; structure, behavior, effects, 3rd edn. Springer-Verlag, New York, pp 220–227
Wachtel S S 1983 H-Y antigen and the biology of sex determination. Grune & Stratton, New York
Wilson J D, Griffin J E, George F W, Leshin M 1981a The role of gonadal steroids in sexual differentiation. Recent Progress in Hormone Research 37: 1–39
Wilson J D, George F W, Griffin J E 1981b The hormonal control of sexual development. Science 211: 1278–1284
Zakharov A F, Baranovskaya L I 1983 X-X chromosome translocations and their karyotype-phenotype correlations. In: Sandbert A A (ed) Cytogenetics of the mammalian X chromosome. Part B. Alan R Liss, New York, pp 261–279

FURTHER READING

Gray S W, Skandalakis J E 1972 Embryology for surgeons – the embryological basis for the treatment of congenital defects. W B Saunders, Philadelphia
Sadler T W 1985 Langman's medical embryology, 5th edn. Williams & Wilkins, Baltimore
Simpson J L 1994 Disorders of abnormal sexual differentiation. In: Sanfilipo J S, Muran D, Lee P A, Dewhurst I (eds) Pediatric and adolescent gynaecology. W B Saunders, Philadelphia, pp 77–103
Wachtel S S 1994 Molecular genetics of sex determination. Academic Press, London
Westenfelder M, Whitaker R H 1981 Malformations of the external genitalia. Monographs in paediatrics 12. Karger, Basel

2

Pelvic anatomy

I. D. Vellacott

INTRODUCTION

A clear understanding of the anatomy of the female pelvis is essential to successful gynaecological surgery and the avoidance of surgical morbidity. The close relationships between the reproductive, urinary and gastrointestinal tracts must be appreciated together with the pelvic musculofascial support, vascular and lymphatic circulations and neurological innervation. An in-depth understanding becomes even more critical in this new era of changing surgical techniques and the introduction of minimally invasive surgery.

THE OVARY

The size and appearance of the ovaries depends on both age and the stage of the menstrual cycle. In the young adult, they are almond-shaped, solid and grayish-pink in colour; 3 cm long, 1.5 cm wide and about 1 cm thick. The long axis is normally vertical before childbirth; after this there is a wide range of variation, presumably due to considerable displacement in the first pregnancy.

The ovary is the only intra-abdominal structure not to be covered by peritoneum. Each ovary is attached to the cornu of the uterus by the ovarian ligament, and at the hilum to the broad ligament by the mesovarium, which contains its supply of vessels and nerves. Laterally, each is attached to the suspensory ligament of the ovary with folds of peritoneum which become continuous with that over the psoas major.

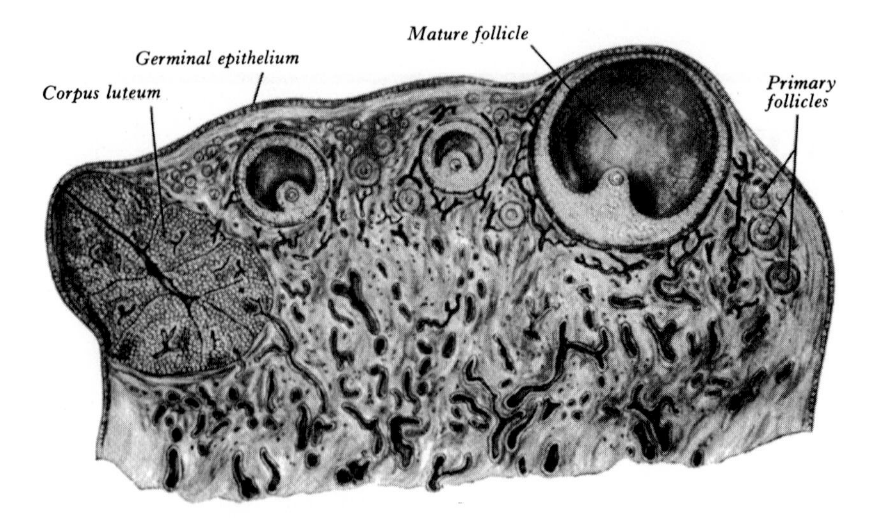

Fig. 2.1 Semi-diagrammatic section of an ovary.

Structure (Fig. 2.1)

The ovary has a central vascular medulla consisting of loose connective tissue containing many elastin fibres and non-striated muscle cells, and an outer thicker cortex, denser than the medulla and consisting of networks of reticular fibres and fusiform cells, although there is no clear-cut demarcation between the two. The surface of the ovary is covered by a single layer of cuboidal cells, the germinal epithelium. Beneath this is an ill defined layer of condensed connective tissue, the tunica albuginea, which increases in density with age. At birth, numerous primordial follicles are found, mostly in the cortex but some in the medulla. With puberty, some form each month into graafian follicles which at later stages of their development form corpora lutea and ultimately atretic follicles, the corpora albicantes.

Relations

Anteriorly lie the fallopian tubes, the superior portion of bladder and uterovesical pouch; posteriorly is the pouch of Douglas. The broad ligament and its content are related inferiorly whilst superior to the ovaries are bowel and omentum. The lateral surface of the ovary is in contact with the parietal peritoneum and the pelvic side walls.

Vestigial structures

The vestigial remains of the mesonephric duct and tubules are always present in young children, but are variable structures in adults. The epoophoron, a series of parallel blind tubules, lies in that part of the broad ligament between the mesovarium and the fallopian tube, the mesosalpinx. The tubules run to the rudimentary duct of the epoophoron, which runs parallel to the lateral fallopian tube. Situated in the broad ligament, between the epoophoron and the uterus, are occasionally seen a few rudimentary tubules, the paroophoron.

In a few individuals, the caudal part of the mesonephric duct is well developed, running alongside the uterus to the internal os. This is the duct of Gartner.

Age-related changes

During early fetal life, the ovaries are situated in the lumbar region near the kidneys. They gradually descend into the lesser pelvis and during childhood they are small and situated near the pelvic brim. They are packed with primordial follicles. The ovary grows in size until puberty by an increase in the stroma. Ova are first shed around the time of onset of menstruation and ovulation is usually established within a couple of years.

After the menopause, the ovary atrophies and assumes a smaller shrivelled appearance. The fully involuted ovary of old age contains practically no germinal elements.

THE FALLOPIAN TUBE

The uterine or fallopian tubes are two oviducts originating at the cornu of the uterus which travel a rather tortuous course along the upper margins of the broad ligament. They are around 10 cm in length and end in the peritoneal cavity close to the ovary. This abdominal opening is situated at the end of a trumpet-shaped lateral portion of tube, the infundibulum. This opening is fringed by a number of petal-like processes, the fimbriae, one of which closely embraces the tubal end of the ovary, the ovarian fimbria. This fimbriated end has an important role in fertility.

Medial to the infundibulum is the ampulla which is thin-walled and tortuous and comprises at least half the length of the tube. The medial third of the tube, the isthmus, is relatively straight. The tube has narrowed at

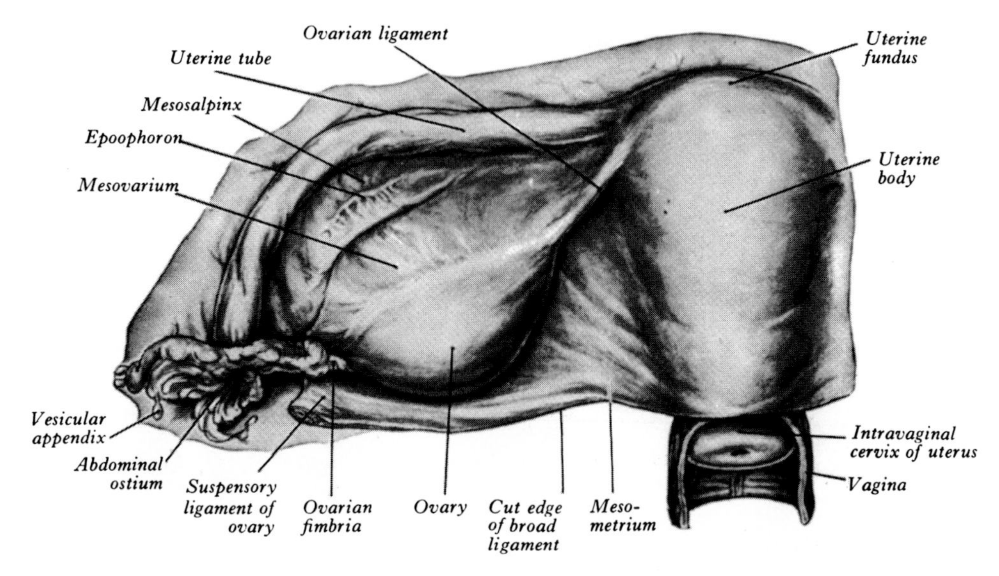

Fig. 2.2 Posterosuperior aspect of the uterus and the left broad ligament. The 'ligament' has been spread out and the ovary is displaced downwards.

this point, from around 3 mm at the abdominal opening to 1–2 mm. The final centimetre, the interstitial portion, is within the uterine wall.

Structure

The tubes are typical of many hollow viscera in that they contain three layers. The outer serosal layer consists of peritoneum and underlying areolar tissue. This covers the whole tube apart from the fimbriae at one end, and the interstitial portion at the other. The middle muscular layer consists of outer longitudinal fibres and inner circular ones. This is fairly thick at the isthmus and thins at the ampulla.

The mucous membrane is thrown into a series of plicae or folds, especially at the infundibular end. It is lined with columnar epithelium, much of which contains cilia, which, together with the peristaltic action of the tube, help in sperm and ovum transport. Secretory cells are also present as well as a third group of intercalary cells of uncertain function.

Relations (Fig. 2.2)

These are similar to those of the ovary (see above). Medially, the fallopian tube, after arching over the ovary, curves around its tubal extremity and passes down its free border.

THE UTERUS

The uterus is shaped like an inverted pear tapering inferiorly to the cervix and, in the non-pregnant state, is situated entirely within the lesser pelvis. It is hollow and has thick muscular walls. Its maximal external dimensions are about 9 cm long, 6 cm wide and 4 cm thick. The upper expanded part of the uterus is termed the body or corpus. The area of insertion of each fallopian tube is termed the cornu and that part of the body above the cornu, the fundus. The uterus tapers to a small central constricted area, the isthmus, and below this is the cervix, which projects obliquely into the vagina and can be divided into vaginal and supravaginal portions (Fig. 2.3).

The cavity of the uterus has the shape of an inverted triangle when sectioned coronally; the fallopian tubes open at the upper lateral angles (Fig. 2.4). The lumen is apposed anteroposteriorly. The constriction at the isthmus where the corpus joins the cervix is the anatomical internal os. Seen microscopically, the area where the mucous membrane of the isthmus becomes that of the cervix is the histological internal os.

Structure

The uterus consists of three layers — the outer serous layer (peritoneum); the middle muscular layer (myometrium) and the inner mucous layer (endometrium).

The peritoneum covers the body of the uterus and posteriorly, the supravaginal portion of cervix. This serous coat is intimately attached to a subserous fibrous layer, except laterally where it spreads out to form the leaves of the broad ligament.

The muscular myometrium forms the main bulk of the uterus and comprises interlacing smooth muscle fibres intermingling with areolar tissue, blood vessels, nerves and lymphatics. Externally these are mostly longitudinal but the larger intermediate layer has interlacing longitudinal, oblique and transverse fibres. Internally, they are mainly longitudinal and circular.

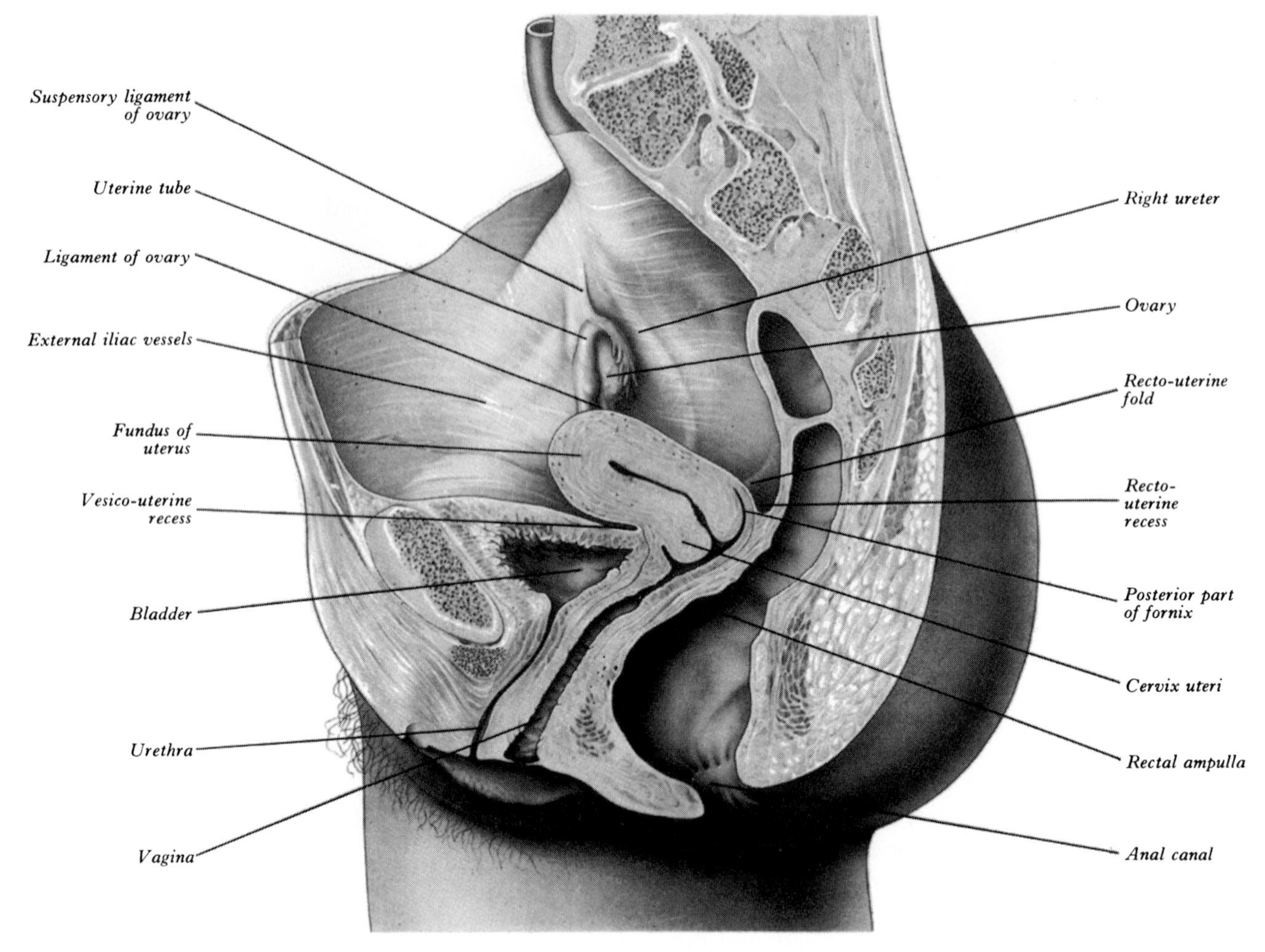

Fig. 2.3 Median sagittal section through a female pelvis.

The inner endometrial layer is not sharply separated from the myometrium: the tubular glands dip into the innermost muscle fibres. This is covered by a single layer of columnar epithelium. Ciliated prior to puberty, this columnar epithelium is mostly lost due to the effects of pregnancy and menstruation. The endometrium undergoes cyclical histological changes during menstruation and varies in thickness between 1 and 5 mm.

The cervix

The cervix is cylindrical in shape, narrower than the body of the uterus and around 2.5 cm in length. It can be divided into the upper, supravaginal and lower vaginal portions. Due to anteflexion or retroflexion, the long axis of the cervix is rarely the same as the long axis of the body. Anterior and lateral to the supravaginal portion is cellular connective tissue, the parametrium. The posterior aspect is covered by peritoneum of the pouch of Douglas. The ureter runs about 1 cm laterally to the supravaginal cervix. The vaginal portion projects into the vagina to form the fornices.

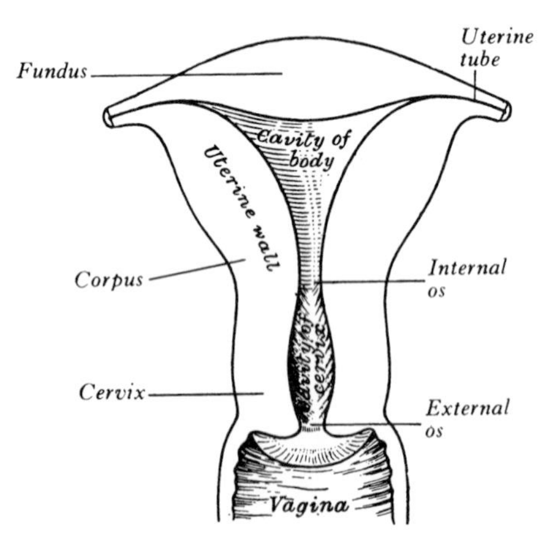

Fig. 2.4 Sectional diagram showing the interior divisions of the uterus and its continuity with the vagina.

The upper part of the cervix mostly consists of involuntary muscle, whereas the lower part is mainly fibrous connective tissue.

The mucous membrane of the endocervix has anterior

and posterior columns from which folds radiate out, the arbor vitae. It has numerous deep glandular follicles which secrete a clear alkaline mucus, the main component of physiological vaginal discharge. The epithelium of the endocervix is cylindrical and also ciliated in its upper two-thirds, and changes to stratified squamous epithelium around the region of the external os. This change may be abrupt or there may be a transitional zone up to 1 cm in width.

Position

The longitudinal axis of the uterus is approximately at right-angles to the vagina and normally tilts forwards: this is termed anteversion. The uterus is usually also flexed forwards on itself at the isthmus — anteflexion. In around 20% of women, this tilt is not forwards but backward — retroversion and retroflexion, respectively. In most cases, this does not have a pathological significance and the uterus is mobile.

Relations

Anteriorly, the uterus is related to the bladder, and is separated from it by the uterovesical pouch of peritoneum. Posteriorly is the pouch of Douglas plus coils of small intestine, pelvic colon and upper rectum. Laterally, the relations are the broad ligaments and that contained within it. Of special importance are the uterine artery and also the ureter, running close to the supravaginal cervix.

Age-related changes

The disappearance of maternal oestrogenic stimulation after birth causes the uterus to decrease in length by around one-third and in weight by about one-half. The cervix is then around twice the length of the body of the uterus. At puberty, however, the corpus grows much faster and the size ratio reverses; the body becomes twice the length of the cervix. After the menopause, the uterus undergoes atrophy, the mucosa becomes very thin, the glands almost disappear and the walls become relatively less muscular. These changes affect the cervix more than the corpus so that the cervical lips disappear and the external os becomes more or less flush with the vault.

THE VAGINA

The vagina is a fibromuscular tube which extends posterosuperiorly from the vestibule to the uterine cervix. It is longer in its posterior wall (around 9 cm) than anteriorly (around 7.5 cm). The vaginal walls are normally in contact except superiorly, at the vault, where they are separated by the cervix. The vault of the vagina is divided into four fornices — posterior, anterior and two lateral. These increase in depth posteriorly. The mid-vagina is a transverse slit, and the lower portion has an H-shape in transverse section.

Structure

The mucous membrane of the vagina is firmly attached to the underlying muscle and consists of stratified squamous epithelium. There are no glands present and the vagina is lubricated by mucus secretion from the cervix. The epithelium is thick and rich in glycogen, which increases in the postovulatory phase of the cycle. Doderlein's bacillus is a normal commensal of the vagina, breaking down the glycogen to form lactic acid and producing a pH of around 4.5. This pH has a protective role for the vagina in decreasing the incidence of pyogenic infection.

The muscle layers consist of an outer longitudinal and inner circular layer, but these are not distinctly separate and are mostly spirally arranged and interspersed with elastic fibres.

The hymen

The hymen is a thin fold of mucous membrane across the entrance to the vagina. It has no known function. There are usually one or more openings in it to allow menses to escape. If these are not present a haematocolpos will form with the commencement of menstruation. The hymen is usually, but not always, torn with first intercourse but can also be torn digitally or with tampons. It is certainly destroyed in childbirth and only small tags remain — carunculae myrtiformes.

Relations

The upper posterior vaginal wall forms the anterior peritoneal reflection of the pouch of Douglas. The middle third is separated from the rectum by pelvic fascia and the lower third abuts the perineal body.

Anteriorly, the upper vagina is in direct contact with the base of the bladder whilst the urethra runs down the lower half in the midline to open into the vestibule; its muscles fuse with the anterior vaginal wall.

Laterally, at the fornices, the vagina is related to the attachment of the cardinal ligaments. Below this are levator ani muscles and the ischiorectal fossa. Near the vaginal orifice, the lateral relations include the vestibular bulb, bulbospongiosus muscles and Bartholin's gland.

Age-related changes

Immediately after birth, the vagina is under the influence of maternal oestrogen so the epithelium is well developed. Acidity is similar to that of an adult and Doderlein's bacilli are present. After a couple of weeks, the effects of mater-

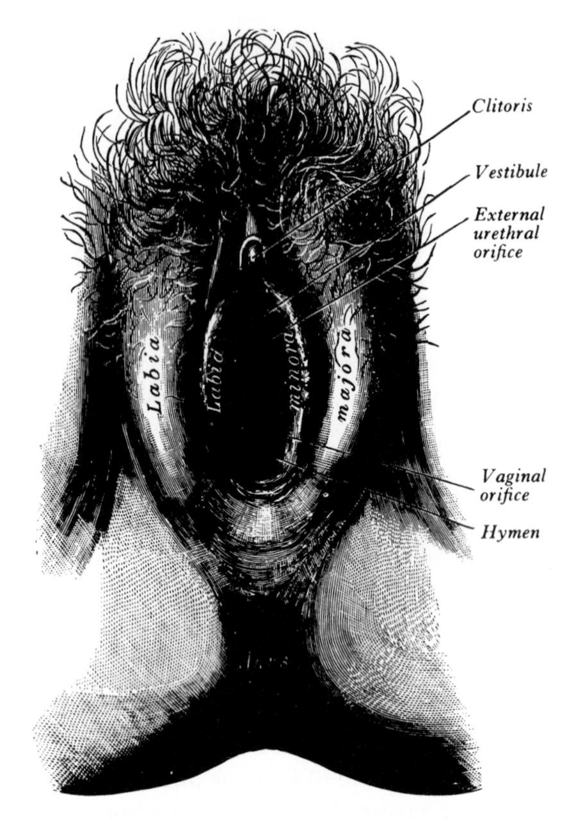

Fig. 2.5 Female external genitalia, with the labia majora et minora separated.

nal oestrogen disappear, the pH rises to 7 and the epithelium atrophies.

At puberty, the reverse occurs. The pH becomes acid again, the epithelium undergoes oestrogenization and the numbers of Doderlein's bacilli markedly increase. The vagina undergoes stretching during coitus, and especially childbirth, and the rugae tend to disappear.

At the menopause, the vagina tends to shrink and the epithelium atrophies.

THE VULVA

The female external genitalia, commonly referred to as the vulva, include the mons pubis, the labia majora and minora, the vestibule, the clitoris, and the greater vestibular glands (Fig. 2.5).

Labia majora

The labia majora are two prominent folds of skin with underlying adipose tissue bounding either side of the vaginal opening. They contain numerous sweat and sebaceous glands and correspond to the scrotum of the male. Anteriorly, they fuse together over the symphysis pubis to form a deposition of fat known as the mons pubis. Posteriorly, they merge with the perineum. From puberty onwards, the lateral aspects of the labia majora and the mons pubis are covered with coarse hair. The inner aspects are smooth but have numerous sebaceous follicles.

Labia minora

The labia minora are two small vascular folds of skin, containing sebaceous glands but devoid of adipose tissue, which lie within the labia majora. Anteriorly they divide into two to form the prepuce and frenulum of the clitoris. Posteriorly they fuse to form a fold of skin called the fourchette. They are not well developed before puberty and atrophy after the menopause. Their vascularity allows them to become turgid during sexual excitement.

Clitoris

This is a small erectile structure, about 2.5 cm long, homologous with the penis but not containing the urethra. The body of the clitoris contains two crura, the corpora cavernosa, which are attached to the inferior border of the pubic rami. The clitoris is covered by ischiocavernosus muscle, whilst bulbospongiosus muscle inserts into its root. The clitoris has a highly developed cutaneous nerve supply and is the most sensitive organ during sexual arousal.

Vestibule (Fig. 2.6)

The vestibule is the cleft between the labia minora. Into it open the vagina, urethra, the paraurethral (Skene's) duct and the ducts of the greater vestibular (Bartholin's) glands. The vestibular bulbs are two masses of erectile tissue on either side of the vaginal opening and contain a rich plexus of veins within bulbospongiosus muscle. Bartholin's glands, each about the size of a small pea, lie at the base of each bulb and open via a 2 cm duct into the vestibule between the hymen and the labia minora. These are mucus-secreting, producing copious amounts during intercourse to act as a lubricant. They are compressed by contraction of bulbospongiosus muscle.

Perineal body

This is a fibromuscular mass occupying the area between the vagina and the anal canal. It supports the lower part of the vagina and is of variable length. It is frequently torn during childbirth.

Age-related changes

In infancy, the vulva is devoid of hair and there is considerable adipose tissue in the labia majora and mons pubis which is lost during childhood but reappears during puberty, at which time hair grows. The vaginal opening tends to widen and sometimes shorten after childbirth. After the menopause, the skin atrophies and becomes

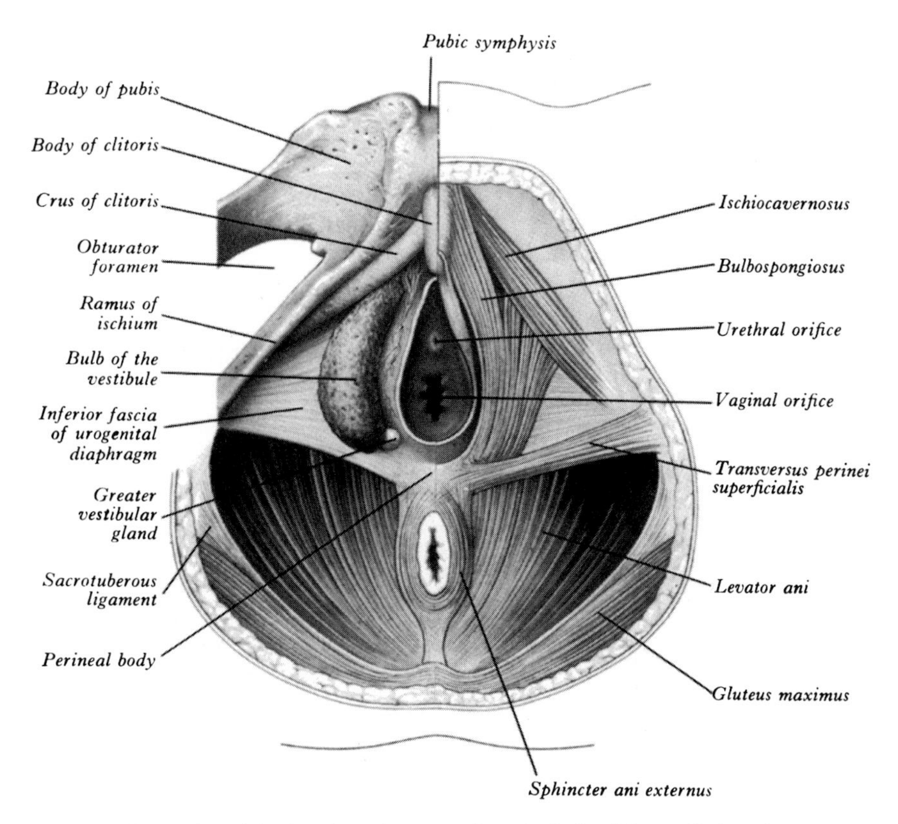

Fig. 2.6 Dissection of the female perineum to show the bulb of the vestibule and greater vestibular gland on the right; on the left side of the body the muscles superficial to these structures have been left in situ.

thinner and drier. The labia minora shrink, subcutaneous fat is lost and the vaginal orifice becomes smaller.

THE URETER

The ureters are a pair of muscular tubes which convey urine to the bladder by peristaltic action. They are between 25 and 30 cm in length, about half abdominally and half within the pelvis. Each has a diameter of around 3 mm but there are slight constrictions as they cross both the brim of the lesser pelvis and when they enter the bladder.

Structure

The ureter has three layers. The outer fibrous coat merges inferiorly with the bladder wall. The middle muscular one has outer circular and inner longitudinal non-striated fibres plus a further outer longitudinal layer along the lower third of the ureter. The inner mucous coat is lined with transitional epithelium and is continuous with the mucous membrane of the bladder below.

Relations and course

Throughout its abdominal course, the ureter travels retroperitoneally along the anteromedial aspect of psoas major and is crossed by the ovarian vessels. The right ureter passes down just laterally to the inferior vena cava and must be carefully retracted away if dissection of the nodes of the inferior vena cava is necessary.

The ureter enters the pelvis anterior to the sacroiliac joints and crosses the bifurcation of the common iliac artery. It then passes along the posterolateral aspect of the pelvis, running in front of and below the internal iliac artery and its anterior division, medial to the obturator vessels and nerves.

On reaching the true pelvis, the ureter turns forwards and medially, passing lateral to the uterosacral ligaments. It then travels through the base of the broad ligament and, lateral to the cervix, is crossed superiorly from the lateral to the medial side by the uterine artery. It continues, running about 1.5 cm lateral to the cervix, anterolateral to the upper part of the vagina and, passing slightly medially, enters the bladder at the trigone.

Surgical injury

The ureter can be damaged during gynaecological surgery at a number of points in its course. It can be injured near the pelvic brim where it is adjacent to the ovarian vessels or lower, near the cervix, where it crosses the uterine vessels. The dangers are greater when the pelvis is distorted by fibroids or ovarian cysts or the ureter's course is displaced by a broad ligament cyst. Damage can occur through the ureter being cut, crushed, or ligated and occasionally it may be devitalized by extensive dissection, especially at Wertheim's hysterectomy. Occasionally, it is injured by high sutures near the cervix in a pelvic floor repair.

THE BLADDER

The bladder is a muscular reservoir capable of altering its size and shape depending on the amount of fluid within it. It is a retroperitoneal viscus and lies behind the symphysis pubis. When empty it is the shape of a tetrahedron, with a triangular base or fundus, and a superior and two inferolateral surfaces. The two inferolateral surfaces meet to form the rounded border which joins the superior surface at the apex. The base and the inferolateral surface meet at the urethral orifice to form the bladder neck. As the bladder fills, it expands upwards and outwards and becomes more rounded. Normal bladder capacity is between 300 and 600 ml but it can, in cases of urinary retention, contain several litres and extend as far as the umbilicus.

Vesical interior

The mucous membrane of the bladder is only loosely attached to the underlying muscular coat, so that it becomes irregularly folded when the bladder is empty. A triangular area, the trigone, is immediately above and behind the urethral openings; the posterolateral angles are formed by the ureteric orifices (Fig. 2.7). The mucous membrane here is redder in colour, smooth and attached firmly to the underlying muscle. The superior boundary is slightly curved — the interureteric ridge.

The ureteric orifices are slit-like and about 2.5 cm apart in the contracted bladder. They enter the bladder at an oblique angle which helps to prevent reflux of urine during filling.

Structure

The wall of the bladder is in three layers. The outer serous coat, the peritoneal covering, is only present over the fundus. The muscular layer, the detrusor muscle, consists of three layers of non-striated muscle, inner and outer longitudinal layers and a middle circular layer.

The mucous membrane is entirely covered by transitional epithelium which is responsive to ovarian hormonal stimulation. There are no true glands in this layer.

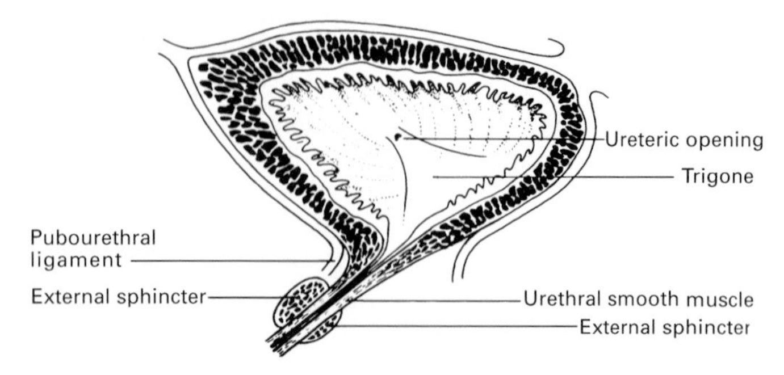

Fig. 2.7 Except where it is fixed at its base, the bladder is a highly distensible structure, and urinary continence probably depends on the physical relations of the fixed/mobile junction.

Relations

Superiorly, the bladder is covered by peritoneum. This extends forwards on to the anterior abdominal wall and sideways on to the pelvic side walls where there is a peritoneal depression, the paravesical fossa. As the bladder fills the peritoneum is displaced upwards anteriorly, so that suprapubic catheterization of the full bladder can take place without the peritoneal cavity being entered. Anteriorly, below the peritoneal reflection is the loose cellular tissue of the cave of Retzius.

Posteriorly the base of the bladder is separated from the upper vagina by pubocervical fascia. Above this is the supravaginal portion of cervix. The peritoneal reflection is at the isthmus of the uterus to form a slight recess, the uterovesical pouch, which often contains coils of intestine.

Surgical injury

The bladder may occasionally be opened during abdominal hysterectomy. The trigone, being in close relation with the upper vagina and anterior fornix, is fortunately rarely damaged and perforation is usually 3–4 cm above it and can be easily repaired without damage to the ureter. If the injury is not noted, however, a vesicovaginal fistula may result. Damage may also occur during anterior colporrhaphy or vaginal hysterectomy, especially if a previous repair has been performed.

THE URETHRA

The urethra begins at the internal meatus of the bladder and runs anteroinferiorly behind the symphysis pubis, immediately related to the anterior vaginal wall. It is around 4 cm long and about 6 mm in diameter. It crosses the perineal membrane and ends at the external urethral orifice in the vestibule, about 2.5 cm behind the clitoris. Skene's tubules, draining the paraurethral glands, open into the lower urethra. These glands are homologous to the male prostate.

There are no true anatomical sphincters to the urethra. The decussation of vesical muscle fibres at the urethrovesical junction acts as a form of internal sphincter and continence is normally maintained at this level. Urethral resistance is mostly due to the tone and elasticity of the involuntary muscles of the urethral wall, and this keeps it closed except during micturition. About 1 cm from its lower end, before it crosses the perineal membrane, the urethra is encircled by voluntary muscle fibres, arising from the inferior pubic ramus, to form the so-called external sphincter. This sphincter allows the voluntary arrest of urine flow.

Structure

The urethra has mucous and muscular coats. Near the bladder the mucous membrane is lined by transitional epithelium which gradually converts into non-keratinizing stratified squamous epithelium as it approaches the external urethral meatus. The muscular layer, consisting of inner longitudinal and outer circular fibres, is continuous with those of the bladder.

Relations

Anteriorly, the urethra is separated from the symphysis pubis by loose cellular tissue. Posteriorly is the anterior vaginal wall plus Skene's tubules. Laterally is the urogenital diaphragm, bulbospongiosus muscle and the vestibular bulb.

THE SIGMOID COLON

The pelvic or sigmoid colon is continuous with the descending colon and commences at the brim of the pelvis. It forms a loop around 40 cm in length and lies in the lesser pelvis behind the broad ligament. It is entirely covered by peritoneum, which forms a mesentery, the sigmoid mesocolon, which diminishes in length at either end and is largest at mid-segment. The lower end of the colon is continuous with the rectum at the level of the third sacral vertebra.

Structure

The mucous membrane of the colon is thrown into irregular folds and is covered by non-ciliated columnar epithelium. Separated from this layer by areolar tissue is the muscle layer. This is arranged as an inner circular layer and outer longitudinal layer which has three narrow bands, the taeniae coli. These bands are shorter than the general surface of the colon and therefore give it its typical sacculated appearance. The serous coat has attached a series of small pieces of fat, the appendices epiploicae.

Relations

The position and shape of the pelvic colon vary considerably and hence so do its relations. Inferiorly it rests on the uterus and bladder. Above and on the right are the coils of ileum; below and on the left is the rectum. Posterior relations also include the ureter, the internal iliac vessels, piriformis muscle and the sacral plexus, all on the left side. Lateral relations include the ovary, external iliac vessels and the obturator nerve.

THE RECTUM

The rectum, which begins at the level of the third sacral vertebra, moulds to the concavity of the sacrum and coccyx: its anteroposterior curve forms the sacral flexure of the rectum. It is around 12 cm in length. The lower end dilates to form the ampulla which bulges into the posterior vaginal wall and then continues as the anal canal. When distended, the rectum has three lateral curves, the upper and lower are usually convex to the right and the middle convex to the left. Peritoneum covers the front and sides of the upper third of rectum, and the front of the middle third. The lower third is devoid of peritoneum.

Structure

Unlike the sigmoid colon, there are no sacculations, appendices epiploicae or mesentery. The taeniae coli blend about 5 cm above the junction of the rectum and colon and form two bands, anterior and posterior, which descend the rectal wall. When the rectum is empty the mucous membrane is thrown into longitudinal folds which disappear with distension. Permanent horizontal folds are also present and are more pronounced during distension. The lining is of mucus-secreting columnar epithelium.

Anal canal

The anal canal is around 3 cm long and passes downwards and backwards from the rectum. It is slit-like when empty but distends greatly during defecation. This is aided by the presence of fat laterally in the ischiorectal fossa. Anteriorly the anal canal is related to the perineal body and lower vagina; posteriorly to the anococcygeal body.

For most of its length it is surrounded by sphincteric muscles which are involved in the control of defecation. The action of the levator ani muscles which surround it are also important in the control mechanism. The internal sphincter is involuntary and is a thickening of the circular muscle of the gut wall enclosing the anal canal just above the anorectal junction. The external sphincter is voluntary and composed of three layers of striated muscle.

Relations

The relations of the rectum are particularly important because they can be felt on digital examination. Posteriorly are related the lower three sacral vertebrae, the coccyx, median sacral and superior rectal vessels. Posterolateral relations are piriformis, coccygeus and levator ani muscles, plus third, fourth and fifth sacral and

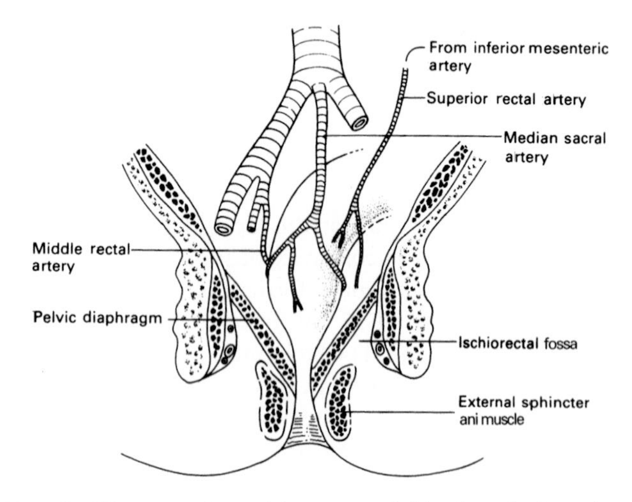

Fig. 2.8 The rectum has a rich anastomotic blood supply, from the median sacral, the internal iliac and the inferior mesenteric arteries and this arrangement is reflected in its venous drainage.

coccygeal nerves. Below and lateral to the levator ani muscle is the ischiorectal fossa (see Fig. 2.8).

Anteriorly, above the peritoneal reflection lie the uterus and adnexa, upper vagina and pouch of Douglas with its contents. Below the reflection it is related to the lower vagina.

PELVIC MUSCULOFASCIAL SUPPORT

Pelvic peritoneum

Posteriorly, the peritoneum is reflected from the rectum on to the posterior wall of the vagina, at which point it is in close contact with the outside world, a fact that can be used both diagnostically and therapeutically. It then passes upwards over the cervix and uterus to form the rectouterine pouch, the pouch of Douglas.

The peritoneum then passes over the fundus of the uterus and down its anterior wall to reach the junction of the body and cervix, where it reflects over the anterior wall of the bladder, forming a shallow recess, the uterovesical pouch. The peritoneum in front of the bladder is loosely applied to the anterior abdominal wall so that it strips away as the bladder fills. Suprapubic catheterization of the distended bladder can therefore be performed without entering the peritoneal cavity.

On either side of the uterus a double fold of peritoneum passes to the lateral pelvic side walls, the broad ligament. These two layers, anteroinferior and posterosuperior, enclose loose connective tissue, the parametrium. At the upper border, between the two layers, is the fallopian tube. The mesentery between the broad ligament and the fallopian tube is the mesosalpinx, and to the ovary, the mesovarium (Fig. 2.2). Beyond the fallopian tube, the upper edge of the broad ligament, as it passes to the pelvic side wall, forms the infundibulopelvic ligament, or suspensory ligament of ovary, and contains the ovarian blood vessels and nerves. Between the fallopian tube and the ovary, the mesosalpinx contains the vestigial epoophoron and paroophoron. After crossing the ureter, the uterine vessels pass between the layers of the broad ligament at its inferior border. They then ascend the ligament medially and anastomose with the ovarian vessels.

Pelvic ligaments

The round ligaments, a mixture of smooth muscle and fibrous tissue, are two narrow flat bands which arise from the lateral angles of the uterus and then pass laterally, deep to the anterior layer of the broad ligament, towards the lateral pelvic side wall. They then turn forwards towards the deep inguinal ring, crossing medial to the vesical vessels, obturator vessels and nerve, obliterated umbilical artery and the external iliac vessels. They finally pass through the inguinal canal to end in the subcutaneous tissue of the labia majora. Together with the uterosacral ligaments, the round ligaments help to keep the uterus in a position of anteversion and anteflexion.

The ovarian ligaments, which are fibromuscular cords of similar structure to the round ligament, lie within the broad ligament and each runs from the cornu of the uterus to the medial border of the ovary. The round and ovarian ligaments together form the homologue of the gubernaculum testis of the male.

In addition, there are also condensations of pelvic fascia on the upper surface of the levator ani muscles, the so-called 'fascial ligaments', comprised of elastic tissue and smooth muscle. They are attached to the uterus at the level of the supravaginal cervix and, being extensive and strong, have an important supporting role. The transverse cervical or cardinal ligaments pass laterally to the pelvic side walls, and their posterior reflection continues around the lateral margins of the rectum as the uterosacral ligaments. They insert into the periostium of the fourth sacral vertebra. These ligaments provide the major support to the uterus above the pelvic diaphragm, helping to prevent uterine descent. The uterosacrals also help to pull the supravaginal cervix backwards in the pelvis, to assist in anteflexion. Anteriorly, the pubocervical fascia is more of a fascial plane than a distinct ligament. It extends beneath the base of the bladder, passing around the urethra and inserting into the body of the pubis. It supports the bladder base and the anterior vaginal wall.

Pelvic musculature (Figs 2.9, 2.10)

The levator ani and coccygeus muscles on either side, together with their fascial coverings, form the pelvic diaphragm which separates the structures in the pelvis from the perineum and ischiorectal fossa. This diaphragm together with all the tissue between the pelvic cavity and the perineum makes up the pelvic floor. In lower mam-

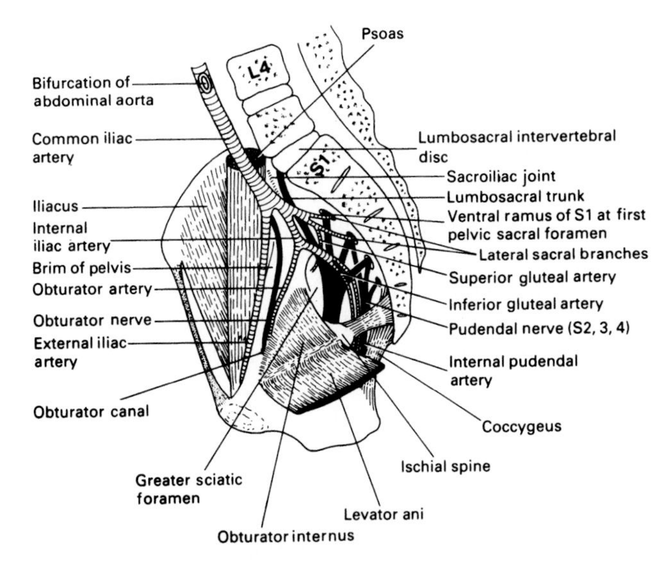

Fig. 2.9 Pelvic musculature. Muscles leave the pelvis either above the superior ramus of the pubis or through the greater or lesser sciatic foramina. Nerves and vessels also leave via the obturator foramen.

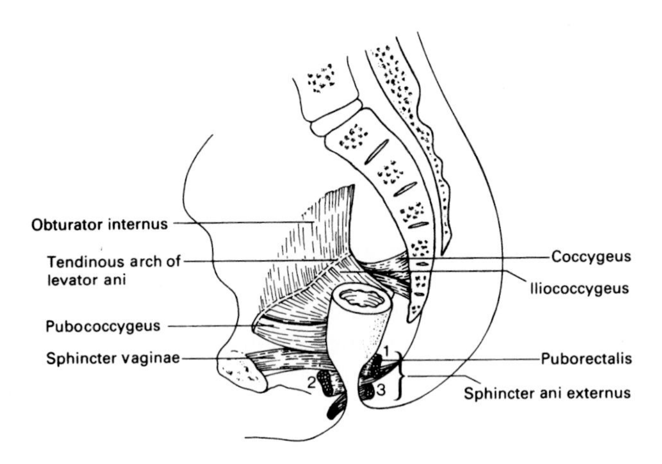

Fig. 2.10 Muscles of the pelvic floor. The slings of muscle that surround and separate the major body effluents have an important role as sphincters.

mals, the diaphragm represents the abductor and flexor muscles of the tail; in humans, who have an erect attitude, these muscles help provide support to the pelvic viscera.

Levator ani muscle is a wide, thin curved sheet of muscle which arises anteriorly from the pelvic surface of the body of the pubic bone, the ischial spine and the tendinous arch of the obturator fascia between the two. The muscle fibres converge across the midline. Levator ani can be divided into three parts: *puborectalis*, which is most medial, encircling the rectum and vagina and acting as support and additional sphincter for both; *pubococcygeus*, the strongest part of the muscular component, which is slung from the pubis to the coccyx; and *iliococcygeus*, the most posterior, also attached to the coccyx.

The posterior part of the pelvic floor is made up of coccygeus muscle, a thin flat triangular muscle, lying on the same plane as the iliococcygeal portion of levator ani. It

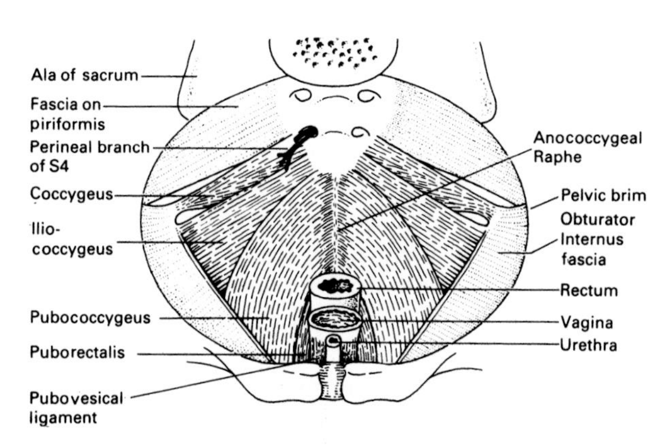

Fig. 2.11 The urogenital diaphragm. The floor of the pelvis slopes steeply forwards and plays an important role in continence and childbirth.

arises from the ischial spine and inserts into lower sacrum and upper coccyx. Like levator ani, it acts by supporting the pelvic viscera.

Most of the side wall of the lesser pelvis is covered by the fan-shaped obturator internus muscle which is attached to the obturator membrane and the neighbouring bone. The fibres run backwards and turn laterally at a right angle to emerge through the lesser sciatic foramen. The side wall is covered medially by obturator fascia (Fig. 2.11).

The ischiorectal fossa, the wedge-shaped space lateral to the anus, is bounded laterally by obturator internus and superomedially by the external surface of levator ani. The base is the perineal skin. The fossa extends forwards, almost to the pubis and backwards almost to the sacrum, where it is widest and deepest. The posterior boundary is made up by sacrotuberous ligament and gluteus maximus muscle, and the anterior boundary by the upper surface of the deep fascia of the sphincter urethrae muscle. It crosses the midline in front of the anal canal.

The musculature of the urogenital region can be divided into two groups, the superficial and deep muscles. Superficially, there are three: *bulbospongiosus*, the sphincter vaginae, which surrounds the vaginal orifice, posteriorly being continuous with the perineal body and anteriorly attaching to the corpora cavernosa of the clitoris; *ischiocavernosus*, covering the unattached surface of the crus of the clitoris; and *superficial transverse* perineal muscle. More deeply are the deep transverse perineal muscle, starting from the inner surface of the ischial ramus and passing to the perineal body, and sphincter urethrae, surrounding the membranous urethra. These layers, and their fascial component, constitute the urogenital diaphragm.

The perineal body or central perineal tendon is a fibromuscular mass lying between the anal canal and the vagina. Superficially it contains insertions of transverse perineal muscles and fibres of the external anal sphincter, and on a deeper plane levator ani muscle. It supports the lower part of the vagina, and is frequently torn during childbirth.

BLOOD SUPPLY TO THE PELVIS

Abdominal aorta

The abdominal portion of the aorta commences as it passes between the crura of the diaphragm at the level of the body of the 12th thoracic vertebra. It runs downwards to the left of the midline along the front of the vertebral column and bifurcates at the level of the body of the fourth lumbar vertebra to form the right and left common iliac arteries. The inferior vena cava runs immediately on its right. In the lower part of its course, ovarian and inferior mesenteric branches arise from the front of the aorta, and median sacral and lumbar branches arise from the back.

Ovarian artery

The ovarian arteries are long slender vessels which arise from the anterolateral aspect of the aorta just below the origin of the renal arteries. The right artery crosses the anterior surface of the vena cava, the lower part of the abdominal ureter and then, lateral to the ureter, enters the pelvis via the infundibulopelvic ligament. The left artery crosses the ureter almost immediately after its origin and then travels lateral to it, crossing the bifurcation of the common iliac artery at the pelvic brim to enter the infundibulopelvic ligament. Both arteries then divide to send branches to the ovaries through the mesovarium. Small branches pass to the ureter and fallopian tube and one branch passes to the cornu of the uterus where it freely anastomoses with branches of the uterine artery to produce a continuous arterial arch (Fig. 2.12).

The ovarian and uterine trunks drain into a pampiniform plexus of veins in the broad ligament near the mesovarium, which can occasionally become varicose. The right ovarian vein drains into the inferior vena cava, the left usually into the left renal vein.

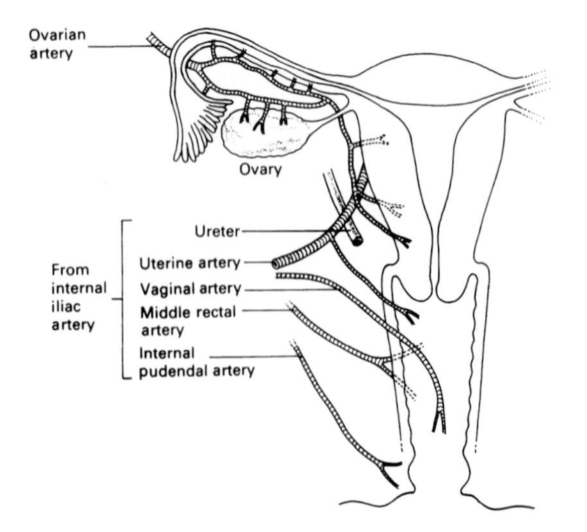

Fig. 2.12 Blood supply of the genitalia. The uterus has an anastomotic supply from both the ovarian and uterine arteries, both vessels running in the broad ligament.

Inferior mesenteric artery

The inferior mesenteric artery arises 3–4 cm above the bifurcation of the aorta. It descends at first in front of the aorta, then to the left of it, to cross the left common iliac artery medial to the left ureter and continues in the mesentery of the sigmoid colon into the lesser pelvis. During its course, it gives off a left colic branch which supplies the left half of the transverse colon and descending colon and a sigmoid branch supplying the sigmoid colon. In the lesser pelvis, it continues as the superior rectal artery, supplying upper rectum and anastomosing with the middle and inferior rectal branches. The inferior mesenteric artery can occasionally be traumatized during para-aortic lymph node dissection and will bleed freely. Transection however is not of serious consequence to the blood supply to the lower bowel due to considerable anastomotic connections.

Common iliac artery

After the aortic bifurcation, the two common iliac arteries run a distance of 4–5 cm before again bifurcating to form internal and external iliac branches on either side. The left artery runs partly lateral and partly in front of the corresponding iliac vein. On the right side, the slightly longer artery runs in front of the lowermost portion of inferior vena cava and the terminations of the two common iliac veins, and then lateral to the left common iliac vein. The bifurcation of the common iliac artery is in front of the sacroiliac joint. The ureter lies in front of the bifurcation at this point.

External iliac artery and its branches

These are larger than the internal iliac vessels and run obliquely and laterally down the medial border of psoas major. At a point midway between the anterior superior iliac spine and the symphysis pubis the artery enters the thigh behind the inguinal ligament and becomes the femoral artery. At this point it is lateral to the femoral vein but medial to the nerve. The ovarian vessels cross in front of the artery just below the bifurcation, as does the round ligament. The external iliac vein is partly behind the upper part of the artery, but medial in its lower part.

The external iliac artery gives off two main branches. The inferior epigastric artery ascends obliquely along the medial margin of the deep inguinal ring, pierces transversalis fascia and runs up between rectus abdominis muscle and its posterior sheath, supplying the muscle and sending branches to the skin. It anastomoses with the superior epigastric artery above the level of the umbilicus. The deep circumflex artery runs posteroinferior to the inguinal ligament to the anterior superior iliac spine and then pierces and supplies transversus abdominis and internal oblique muscles.

Once the external iliac artery has pierced the thigh and become the femoral artery it almost immediately gives off an external pudendal branch which supplies much of the skin of the vulva, anastomosing with the labial branches of the internal pudendal artery.

Internal iliac artery and its branches

The internal iliac arteries are both 4 cm long and descend to the upper margin of the greater sciatic foramen where they divide into anterior and posterior divisions (Fig. 2.13). In the fetus they are twice as large as the external iliac vessels and ascend the anterior wall to the umbilicus to form the umbilical artery. After birth, with the cessation of the placental circulation, only the pelvic portion remains patent; the remainder becomes a fibrous cord, the lateral umbilical ligament. The ureter runs anteriorly down the artery and the internal iliac vein runs behind.

The posterior division has three branches which mainly supply the musculature of the buttocks. The iliolumbar artery ascends deep to psoas muscle and divides to supply iliacus and quadratus lumborum. The lateral sacral arteries descend in front of the sacral rami and supply the structures of the sacral canal. The superior gluteal artery is the direct continuation and leaves the lesser pelvis through the greater sciatic foramen to supply much of the gluteal musculature.

The anterior division has seven main branches. The superior vesical artery runs anteroinferiorly between the side of the bladder and the pelvic side wall to supply the upper part of the bladder. The obturator artery passes to the obturator canal and thence to the adductor compartment of the thigh. Inside the pelvis it sends off iliac, vesical and pubic branches (Table 2.1).

The vaginal artery corresponds to the inferior vesical

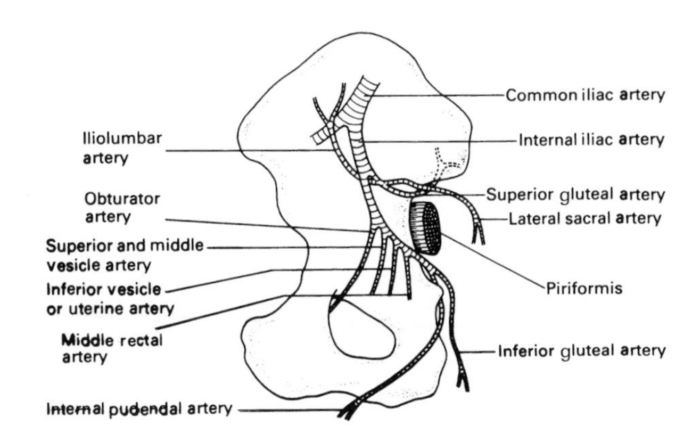

Fig. 2.13 The blood supply to the pelvic viscera is derived in the main from the internal iliac artery.

Table 2.1 Arterial supply of the pelvic organs

Organ	Artery	Origin
Ovary	Ovarian Uterine	Aorta Internal iliac
Fallopian tube	Ovarian Uterine	Aorta Internal iliac
Uterus	Uterine Ovarian	Internal iliac Aorta
Vagina	Vaginal Uterine Internal pudendal Middle rectal	Internal iliac Internal iliac Internal iliac Internal iliac
Vulva	Internal pudendal External pudendal	Internal iliac Femoral
Ureter	Renal Ovarian Uterine Superior vesical Inferior vesical	Aorta Aorta Internal iliac Internal iliac Internal iliac
Bladder	Superior vesical Inferior vesical	Internal iliac Internal iliac
Urethra	Inferior vesical Internal pudendal	Internal iliac Internal iliac
Sigmoid colon	Left colic	Inferior mesenteric
Rectum	Superior rectal Middle rectal Inferior rectal	Inferior mesenteric Internal iliac Internal pudendal (internal iliac)

artery of the male. It descends inwards, low in the broad ligament to supply the upper vagina, base of the bladder and adjacent rectum. It anastomoses with branches of the uterine artery to form two median longitudinal vessels, the azygos arteries of the vagina, one descending in front and the other behind.

The uterine artery passes along the root of the broad ligament and about 2 cm from the cervix crosses above and in front of the ureter. It then runs tortuously along the lateral margin of the uterus between the layers of the broad ligament. It supplies the cervix and body of the uterus, part of the bladder, and one branch anastomoses with the vaginal artery to produce the azygos arteries. It ends by anastomosing with the ovarian artery. The branches of the uterine artery pass circumferentially around the myometrium, giving off coiled radial branches which end as basal arteries supplying the endometrium.

The middle rectal artery is a small branch passing medially to the rectum to vascularize the muscular tissue of the lower rectum and anastomose with the superior and inferior rectal arteries.

The internal pudendal artery, the smaller of the two terminal trunks of the internal iliac artery, descends anterior to piriformis and, piercing the pelvic fascia, leaves the pelvis through the inferior part of the greater sciatic fora-

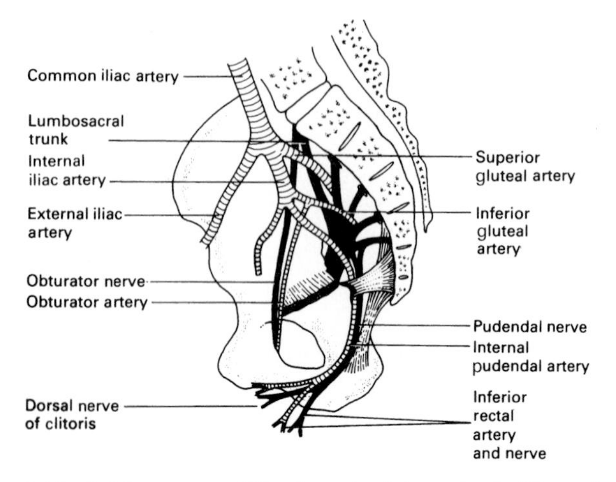

Fig. 2.14 Pelvic nerves and blood supply of the pudenda. The major nerve is the pudendal, but it is supplemented by the posterior cutaneous nerve of the thigh and the ilioinguinal and genitofemoral nerves.

men, crosses the gluteal aspect of the ischial spine and enters the perineum through the lesser sciatic foramen (Fig. 2.14). It then traverses the pudendal canal, with the pudendal nerve, about 4 cm above the ischial tuberosity. It then proceeds forwards above the inferior fascia of the urogenital diaphragm and divides into a number of branches. The inferior rectal branch supplies skin and musculature of the anus and anastomoses with the superior and middle rectal arteries: the perineal artery supplies much of the perineum, and small branches supply the labia, vestibular bulbs and vagina. The artery terminates as the dorsal artery of the clitoris.

The inferior gluteal artery, the larger terminal trunk, descends behind the internal pudendal artery, traverses the lower part of the greater sciatic foramen and with the superior gluteal artery supplies much of the buttock and back of the thigh.

NERVE SUPPLY TO THE PELVIS

Autonomic nerves (see Fig. 2.14)

The internal pelvic organs are supplied by both the sympathetic and the parasympathetic autonomic nervous system, and this is their sole innervation. As they descend into the pelvis, branches from the lower part of the lumbar sympathetic trunk join the aortic plexus of sympathetic nerves and ganglia as it continues downwards over the bifurcation of the aorta to form the superior hypogastric plexus. This then divides to form the right and left inferior hypogastric or pelvic plexuses, which lie lateral to the rectum and further subdivide into two — anteriorly innervating the base of the bladder and urethra and posteriorly innervating the uterus, cervix, vagina, sigmoid colon and rectum.

The parasympathetic nerves enter the pelvis through the second, third and fourth sacral nerves. The preganglionic fibres are distributed through the pelvic plexus and the parasympathetic ganglia are situated close to, or in the walls of, the viscera concerned. With the exception of the ovaries and fallopian tube which are supplied directly by nerves from the pre-aortic plexus travelling along the ovarian vessels, all internal pelvic organs are supplied via the pelvic plexuses.

Somatic nerves

The lumbar plexus is formed by the anterior primary rami of the first three lumbar nerves, part of the fourth and a contribution from the 12th thoracic (subcostal) nerve. It lies on the surface of psoas major and gives off a number of major branches.

The iliohypogastric and ilioinguinal nerves both arise from the first lumbar nerve. The former gives branches to the buttock, while the latter supplies the skin of the mons pubis and surrounding vulva. The genitofemoral nerve arises from the first and second lumbar nerves, its femoral branch supplying the upper thigh, whilst its genital branch supplies the skin of the labium majus. The lateral femoral cutaneous nerve arises from the second and third lumbar nerves and also supplies the thigh.

The femoral nerve is the largest branch, coming from second, third and fourth lumbar nerves. It descends in the groove between psoas and iliacus muscles and enters the thigh deep to the inguinal ligament, lateral to the femoral sheath, to supply the flexors of the hip, the extensors of the knee and numerous cutaneous branches including the saphenous nerve. The obturator nerve also comes from the second, third and fourth lumbar nerves and passes downwards medial to psoas into the pelvis, to supply the adductor muscles of the hip.

The lumbosacral trunk comes from the fourth and fifth lumbar nerves and passes medial to psoas into the pelvis to join the anterior primary rami of the first three sacral nerves to form the sacral plexus in front of piriformis muscle. From this plexus, a number of branches emerge. The most important of these are the sciatic nerve — a large nerve formed from the fourth and fifth lumbar and the first, second and third sacral nerves — which leaves the pelvis through the lower part of the greater sciatic foramen to supply the muscles of the back of the thigh and the lower limb, and the pudendal nerve, which forms from the second, third and fourth sacral nerves.

The pudendal nerve leaves the pelvis between piriformis and coccygeus muscles and curls around the ischial spine to re-enter the pelvis through the lesser sciatic foramen, where medial to the internal pudendal artery, it lies in the pudendal canal on the lateral wall of the ischiorectal fossa. The point where the nerve circles the ischial spine is the region in which a pudendal block of local anaesthetic is injected.

The pudendal nerve gives a number of terminal branches. The inferior rectal nerve gives motor and sensory fibres to the external anal sphincter, anal canal and skin around the anus. The perineal nerve passes forwards below the internal pudendal artery to give labial branches, supplying the skin of the labia majora, the deep perineal nerve supplying the perineal muscles and the bulb of the vestibule. The dorsal vein of the clitoris passes through the pudendal canal, giving a branch to the crus and piercing the perineal membrane 1–2 cm from the symphysis pubis. It supplies the clitoris and surrounding skin.

LYMPHATIC DRAINAGE TO THE PELVIS

In the pelvis, as elsewhere in the body, the lymph nodes are arranged along the blood vessels. The lateral aortic lymph nodes lie on either side of the aorta; their efferents form a lumbar trunk on either side which terminates at the cisterna chyli. Those structures which receive their blood supply directly from branches of the aorta, i.e. ovary, fallopian tube, upper ureter and, in view of arterial anastomoses, uterine fundus, drain directly into the lateral aortic group of nodes.

The lymph drainage of most other structures within the pelvis is via more outlying groups of lymph nodes associated with the iliac vessels. The common iliac lymph nodes are grouped around the common iliac artery and usually arranged in medial, lateral and intermediate chains. They receive efferents from the external and internal iliac nodes and send efferents to the lateral aortics (Fig. 2.15). The external iliac nodes lie on the external iliac vessels and are in three groups, lateral, medial and anterior. They collect from the cervix, upper vagina, bladder, deeper lower abdominal wall and from the inguinal lymph nodes. Inferior epigastric and circumflex iliac nodes are associated

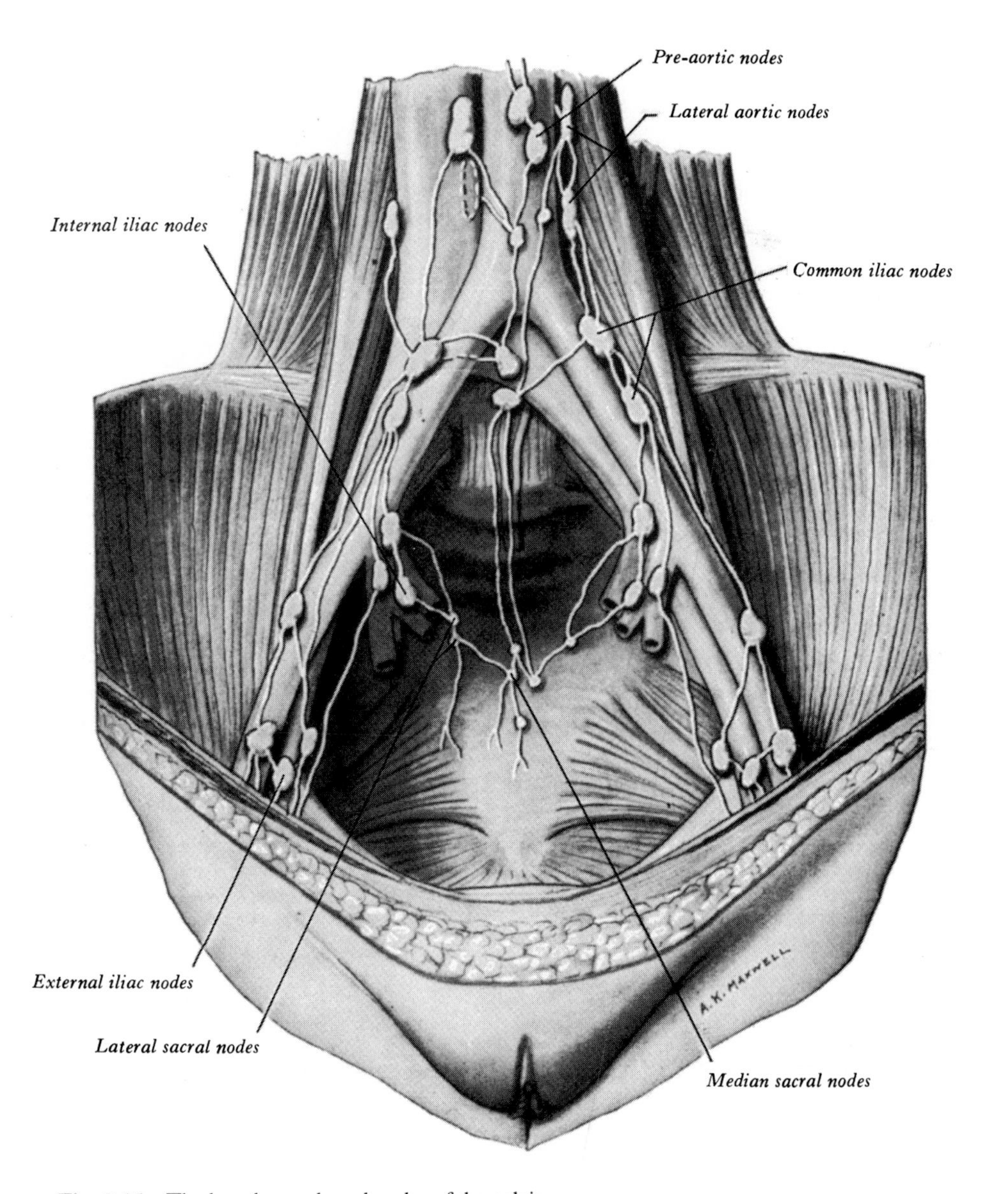

Fig. 2.15 The lymph vessels and nodes of the pelvis.

Table 2.2 Lymphatic drainage of the pelvis

Organ	Lymph nodes	Organ	Lymph nodes
Ovary	Lateral aortic nodes	Lower vagina	Superficial inguinal nodes
Fallopian tube	Lateral aortic nodes Superficial inguinal nodes External and internal iliac nodes	Vulva	Superficial inguinal nodes Internal iliac nodes (deep tissues)
Corpus uteri	External and internal iliac nodes Superficial inguinal nodes Lateral aortic nodes	Ureter	Lateral aortic nodes Internal iliac nodes
Cervix	External and internal iliac nodes Obturator node Sacral nodes	Bladder	External and internal iliac nodes
Upper vagina	External and internal iliac nodes Obturator node Sacral nodes	Urethra	Internal iiac nodes
		Sigmoid colon	Pre-aortic nodes
		Upper rectum	Pre-aortic nodes
		Lower rectum and canal	Internal iliac nodes
		Anal orifice	Superficial inguinal nodes

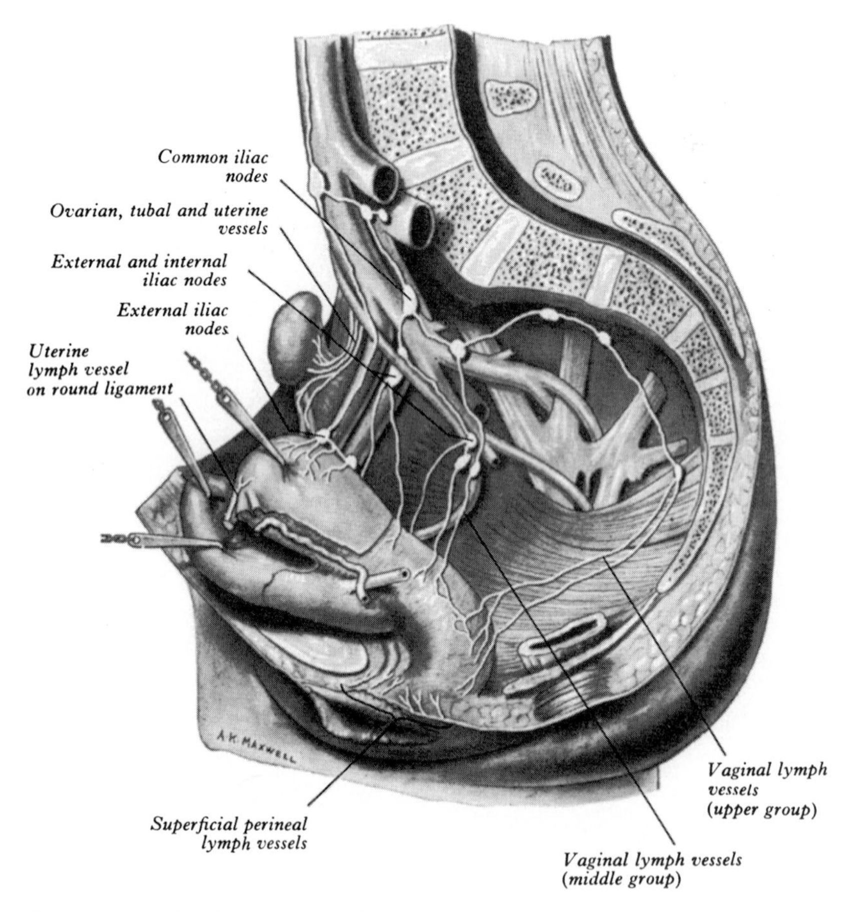

Fig. 2.16 The lymphatic drainage of the female reproductive organs (semi-diagrammatic after Cunéo & Marcille).

with these vessels and can be considered to be outlying members of the external iliac group (Table 2.2).

The internal iliac nodes, which surround the internal iliac artery, receive afferents from all the pelvic viscera, deeper perineum and muscles of the thigh and buttock. The obturator lymph node, sometimes present in the obturator canal, and the sacral lymph nodes on the median and lateral sacral vessels can be considered to be outlying members of this group (Fig. 2.16).

The upper group of superficial inguinal lymph nodes forms a chain immediately below the inguinal ligament. The lateral members receive afferents from the gluteal region and adjoining lower anterior abdominal wall. The medial members drain the vulva and perineum, lower vagina, lower anal canal, adjoining anterior abdominal wall and also from the uterus owing to lymph vessels that accompany the round ligament to the anterior abdominal wall. The lymphatics on either side of the vulva communicate freely, emphasizing the importance of removing the whole vulva in cases of malignant disease. The superficial lymph nodes send their efferents to the external iliac lymph nodes, passing around the femoral vessels or traversing the femoral canal.

The deep inguinal (femoral) lymph nodes, varying from one to three, are on the medial side of the femoral vein. They receive efferents from the deep femoral vessels, some from the superficial inguinal nodes; one, the node of Cloquet, is thought to drain the clitoris. Efferents from the deep nodes pass through the femoral canal to the external iliac group.

ACKNOWLEDGEMENTS

Figures 2.1–2.6, 2.15 and 2.16 are reproduced from Gray's Anatomy, 37th edn (eds: Williams P L et al 1989), and Figures 2.7–2.14 are reproduced from Obstetrics (eds: Turnbull A, Chamberlain G 1989), with permission of the authors and the publishers, Churchill Livingstone, Edinburgh

KEY POINTS

1. Knowing the course of pelvic migration of the ovaries is important in understanding the consequences of maldescent.
2. The round and ovarian ligaments together form the homologue of the gubernaculum testis in the male.
3. The sizes of the uterus and cervix, and their ratio, change with age and parity.
4. The uterine artery is a branch of the internal iliac artery that crosses above the ureter and passes medially in the base of the broad ligament to reach the supravaginal portion of the cervix. It divides to pass superiorly alongside the body of the uterus and inferiorly to supply the vagina and cervix.
5. The ovarian artery arises from the aorta at the level of the second lumbar vertebra. The right ovarian vein drains into the inferior vena cava while the left ovarian vein drains into the left renal vein.
6. The inferior epigastric artery is a branch of the external iliac artery and ascends between the rectus muscle and the posterior rectus sheath, where it should be avoided during insertion of laparoscopic cannulae.
7. The ureter crosses the pelvic brim at the bifurcation of the common iliac artery and descends on the lateral pelvic side wall, where it is at risk during oophorectomy.
8. The ureter runs beneath the uterine vessels in the base of the broad ligament and emerges close to the supravaginal portion of the cervix (1.0–1.5 cm), where it is at risk during the ligation of pedicles at hysterectomy.
9. The internal urethral sphincter comprises two loops of smooth muscle fibres that pass around the vesical neck.
10. The term external urethral sphincter refers to paraurethral striated muscle that is under voluntary control and includes the external, circular layer of urethral muscle together with the compressor urethrae and urethrovaginal sphincter.
11. The pudendal nerve leaves the pelvis between the piriformis and coccygeus muscles, passes around the ischial spine and re-enters the pelvis via the lesser sciatic foramen, where it lies medial to the internal pudendal artery in the lateral wall of the ischiorectal fossa.

3

Hysteroscopy

K. G. Waller   B. V. Lewis

INTRODUCTION

The first hysteroscopy was probably performed by Pantaleoni in 1869, using a narrow cylinder and a kerosene lamp for illumination (Lindemann 1973). The patient was a 60-year-old woman with severe postmenopausal bleeding who was found to have polyp-like growths. The widespread use of hysteroscopy only became practical with the development of high-powered fibreoptic light sources together with a method of distension for separating the walls of the uterine cavity (Lewis 1988).

Instruments

The standard 4-mm hysteroscope gives a panoramic view of the cervical canal and uterine cavity and is usually sufficient for diagnostic purposes. Most telescopes for hysteroscopy are rigid optical instruments with a distal lens, either at an angle of 0° to permit direct visualization, or at an angle of 30° in order to view the more inaccessible areas of the uterus such as the uterotubal ostia. Flexible hysteroscopes can also be used, but may suffer from inferior resolution because of the fibreoptics when compared to rigid telescopes with rod lens systems.

More complex instruments include the colpomicrohysteroscope, which possesses the properties of both a telescope and a compound microscope. The Hamou colpomicrohysteroscope has a direct ocular piece with two magnifications and an offset ocular piece with a further two magnifications. At high magnification, and with the lens in contact with the endometrium, magnification of 20–150× can be achieved to allow examination of the glandular and cellular structures of the endometrium and endocervix. This is the technique of contact hysteroscopy. It has only limited application in routine gynaecological practice, and will not be further described.

The uterine cavity must be distended to allow a clear view, and therefore the diagnostic hysteroscope incorporates a small diameter (5 mm) sheath through which gas or fluid is delivered to the tip. The sheath normally blocks the cervix and prevents escape of gas or fluid, but if leaks do occur, a portio adaptor can be placed over the cervix and held in place by suction. For intrauterine surgery, continuous flow hysteroscopes are used. These have a wider outer sheath of 7 mm in diameter, with a separate channel for introducing instruments such as biopsy forceps, scissors, suction tubes and laser fibres. There are also separate inflow and outflow channels, allowing clear fluid to continuously flush the tip of the telescope and maintain a clear field of view.

Distension media

Carbon dioxide gas is the medium of choice for diagnostic hysteroscopy, particularly when the latter is performed in the outpatient or office setting. It gives excellent visibility and is readily available and convenient. The gas must be delivered by an insufflator specially designed for hysteroscopy such as a Hysteroflator (Storz) or Metromat (Wolf). This controls the pressure, which should remain below 100 mmHg and the flow, which should be below 100 ml/min. In patients with patent fallopian tubes, the

CO_2 flow rate is usually between 40 and 60 ml/min, with an average intrauterine pressure of 60 to 80 mmHg. Carbon dioxide is, however, unsuitable for all but minor operative procedures because if there is bleeding, the resultant gas bubbles obliterate the view. Carbon dioxide is also unsuitable for use with laser surgery and electrocautery because of smoke.

High viscosity fluids such as dextran can be used for diagnostic hysteroscopy and simple operative procedures. Hyskon is a solution of Dextran 70 (32% dextran) in 10% dextrose which is electrolyte free and non-miscible with blood. It is, however a difficult medium to work with because it is so viscous, and it is rarely used. It can cause anaphylactic reactions and exerts a high osmotic pressure, with the risk of hypervolaemia if it is absorbed into the circulation. It has been withdrawn from the UK market.

Low viscosity fluids such as normal saline, 5% dextrose, sorbitol and 1.5% glycine are all used as distension media, particularly for operative hysteroscopy. They are miscible with blood, and a continuous flow of fluid under pressure is needed to keep the operating field clear. Delivery of fluid can be via an automatic rotary pump such as a Hysteromat (Storz), which automatically controls pressure and flow. However a gravity feed can be used, or a blood pressure cuff inflated to 80–120 mmHg placed around the bag, with care to avoid the risk of air embolus.

Because of its electrolyte content, normal saline cannot be used with electrosurgical equipment, as current can be transmitted through the fluid and cause burns. However, it has the advantage of being cheap and readily available, and fluid overload with normal saline does not cause electrolyte disturbance and can be easily reversed with diuretics. Dextrose 5% has no clinical advantage over 0.9% saline and, in addition, can cause dilutional electrolyte disturbance and fluid overload if absorbed in large quantities. The same is true for sorbitol, which is a 3% sugar solution. Excessive absorption of both fluids can cause hyperglycaemia. Glycine is an amino acid in a 1.5% solution, which is non-conducting and therefore an excellent medium for use with electrosurgical equipment. It can also cause dilutional electrolyte disturbance if fluid absorption is not carefully monitored and large volumes in excess of 1500 ml enter the circulation.

Technique

Hysteroscopy is best performed in the postmenstrual phase of the cycle, as a clear view is usually obtained without bleeding and there is no risk of pregnancy. Moreover, in the premenstrual phase the endometrium is often thrown into folds which produces a polypoid appearance.

Diagnostic and minor operative procedures can be performed in the outpatient setting. Most diagnostic hysteroscopy procedures will not require any anaesthetic, but administration of a prostaglandin synthetase inhibitor 1 to 2 h preoperatively may be useful in reducing uterine cramps. If cervical dilatation is required, or undue discomfort is experienced, a paracervical block can be administered. More major procedures, such as endometrial resection, are performed under local or general anaesthetic.

The cervix should first be cleaned with saline, because a foaming antiseptic can cause bubbles which obscure the view. When performing diagnostic hysteroscopy, the telescope, with carbon dioxide flowing, is gently inserted under direct vision into the endocervix. The flow of CO_2 creates a microcavity which allows the hysteroscope to enter the uterine cavity without trauma. In postmenopausal women and nulliparae, gentle cervical dilatation will usually be needed, but to avoid bleeding the dilators should not be inserted deeply.

The uterine fundus appears as saddle-shaped with a cornual orifice on each side. The colour of the endometrium varies with the menstrual cycle. The postmenstrual endometrium is pale (Fig. 3.1), and the vascular premenstrual endometrium is red. Postmenopausal endometrium is thin and avascular. A systematic survey should then be performed. The right tubal ostia is first identified and the proximal 1–2 mm of the intramural portion of tube is scrutinized. The instrument can then be withdrawn for a few centimetres and the fundus observed from right to left until the left tubal ostia is located and similarly evaluated. When normal tubal ostia are observed over a period of time, they are seen to open and close as gas enters the peritoneal cavity. The anterior, lateral and posterior walls are then inspected and finally, withdrawing the telescope to the level of the internal os allows a complete panoramic view of the uterine cavity. The uterus can be sounded after the procedure, as evaluating the length of the cavity by hysteroscopic means alone is difficult. This will be useful if endometrial ablation is contemplated.

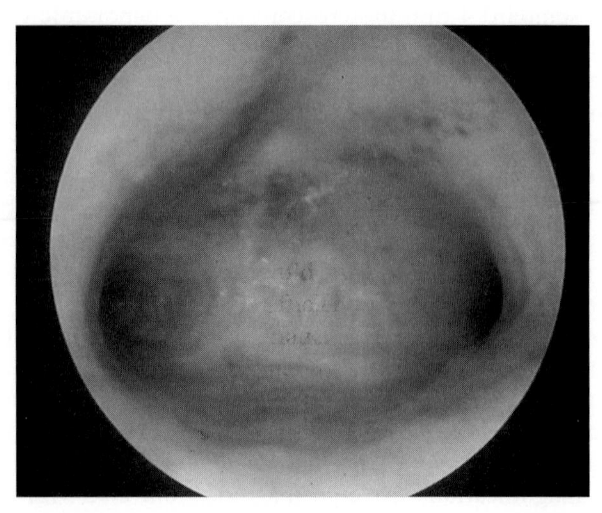

Fig. 3.1 Panoramic view of uterine cavity in postmenstrual patient.

INDICATIONS FOR DIAGNOSTIC HYSTEROSCOPY

Abnormal uterine bleeding

This is the commonest reason for hysteroscopy, and includes the investigation of menorrhagia, intermenstrual bleeding and postmenopausal bleeding. Hysteroscopy should now be replacing diagnostic curettage, which is particularly poor for the detection of focal endometrial lesions such as polyps or submucous fibroids (Fig. 3.2), and with the use of which small endometrial carcinomas may be missed (Gimpelson & Rappold 1988). Moreover it is now widely recognized that curettage alone has little therapeutic affect in women.

Infertility

Hysteroscopy should be considered as a procedure complementary to hysterosalpingography (HSG) in patients with infertility or recurrent pregnancy loss. It is questionable whether hysteroscopy is justified early in the work up of every infertility patient, as intrauterine disorders are rarely the primary cause of infertility. Hysteroscopy is indicated in infertile patients with a history of abnormal uterine bleeding, abnormalities of the uterine cavity or filling defects at HSG, unexplained infertility, or a history of uterine surgery or pregnancy related curettage (Siegler 1990).

Fallopian tube catheterization can also be performed hysteroscopically to investigate the patency of the intramural part of the tube.

Foreign bodies

Hysteroscopy is useful for visualizing misplaced intrauterine contraceptive devices (IUCD), when ultrasound has shown that the device is in the uterine cavity. Removal under direct visual control with grasping forceps can then be performed. This is particularly useful when the IUCD is embedded or fragmented.

Bony fragments may also occasionally be left in the uterus following incomplete abortion. These can be white or yellow in colour, and occasionally specific bones can be identified.

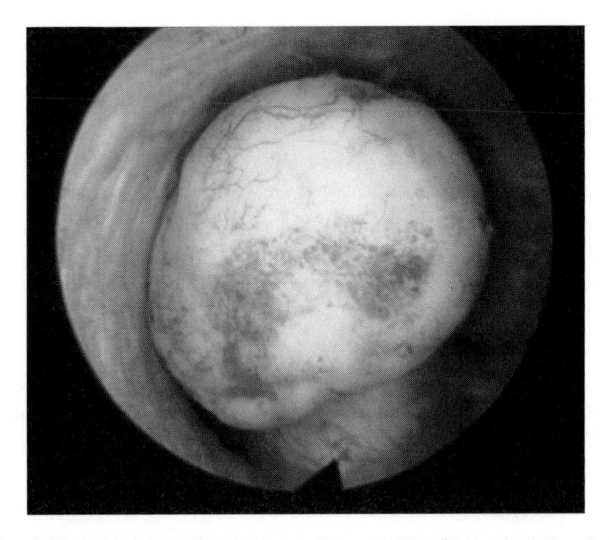

Fig. 3.2 Submucous fibroid polyp (from D. Van Herendael (Lewis & Magos 1993), with permission).

UTERINE ABNORMALITIES AT HYSTEROSCOPY

Benign endometrial polyps are smooth, soft and movable, and appear pink in colour, similar to endometrium. A benign polyp may be large enough to distort the uterine cavity but will not show signs of necrosis or ulceration. Multiple polyps cause irregularity of the uterine cavity. Submucous fibroids only are visible at hysteroscopy, appearing smooth in outline and paler in colour than the rest of the endometrium, because they are less vascular. They may also occupy most of the uterine cavity and their size and number should be recorded.

A polypoid endometrial carcinoma appears irregular in outline and is vascular. It may also show ulceration and bleeding. The extent of spread within the cavity can be assessed together with extension into the cervical canal. Visually directed biopsy is essential to confirm the diagnosis.

OPERATIVE HYSTEROSCOPY

Endometrial ablation

In recent years, minimally invasive hysteroscopic surgery to destroy the endometrium has become an alternative to hysterectomy for the treatment of functional menorrhagia. Hysteroscopy allows the endometrium to be treated selectively under direct vision. The endometrium has a remarkable capacity to regenerate, and any ablation technique must ensure adequate destruction of the basal layers of the endometrium. Many methods of causing endometrial destruction and scarring have been tried, including cryotherapy, superheated steam, intracavity radium, rigorous curettage, quinacrine methylcyanoacrylate, oxalic acid, paraformaldehyde and silicone rubber. These techniques have all been aimed at producing a therapeutic Asherman's syndrome (Asherman 1950), but none produced very satisfactory results. Newer methods of producing endometrial destruction are, however, more successful.

It is essential that the results of an endometrial biopsy are known prior to endometrial ablation, and in many clinical trials evaluation of the uterine cavity by hysteroscopy has also been performed.

Patient selection criteria for endometrial ablation are shown in Table 3.1. Patients are not suitable for endometrial ablation if they have atypical hyperplasia or malignancy, or very large submucous fibroids. Women with large endometrial cavities may not have such a good result from the procedure as resection is less likely to be com-

Table 3.1 Patient selection for endometrial ablation (Lewis 1994)

An alternative to hysterectomy for dysfunctional uterine bleeding
Uterine cavity <10 cm in length
Uterus not palpable per abdomen
Submucous fibroids <2 cm in diameter
Benign endometrial histology
Completed family
No other gynaecological problems indicating alternative surgery (e.g. prolapse, endometriosis, cervical intraepithelial neoplasia, pelvic inflammatory disease)
Preoperative counselling

plete. Postmenopausal women taking hormone replacement therapy who have heavy cyclical bleeding may also be treated by endometrial ablation.

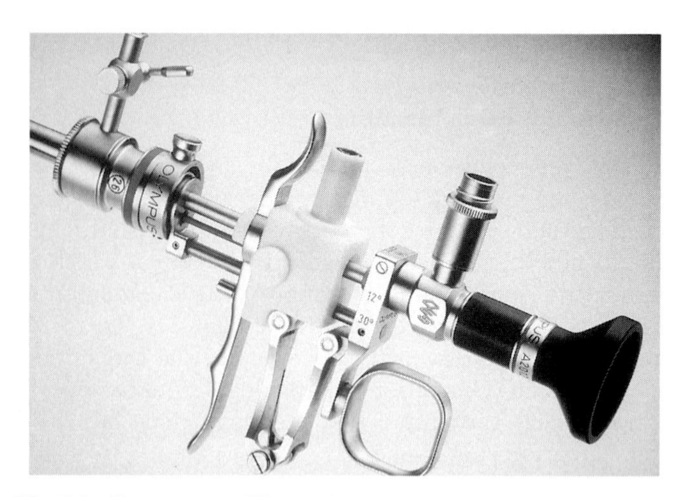

Fig. 3.3 Resectoscope (Olympus).

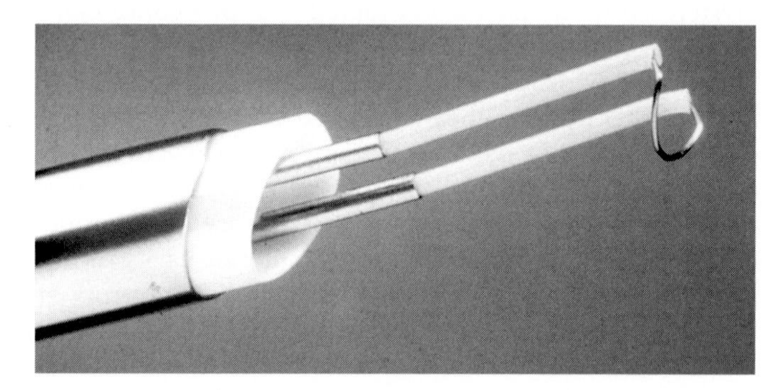

Fig. 3.4 Cutting loop of resectoscope.

Laser ablation

Goldrath et al in 1981 first described the technique of endometrial ablation using the neodymium:yttrium–aluminium–garnet (Nd-YAG) laser in women with intractable menorrhagia. Laser energy is widely scattered within deep tissue and produces destruction of the endometrium for a depth of 4 to 5 mm, while being contained within the 20-mm thickness of the myometrium. The contact or dragging technique can be used, where the laser fibre tip actually touches the surface of the endometrium, or the no-contact or blanching technique may be employed, where the fibre is kept 1 to 3 mm away from the surface of the endometrium (Lomano 1988). One advantage of the dragging technique is that the furrows made by the fibre clearly demarcate treated from non-treated areas.

Goldrath in 1989 described his 10-year experience with laser ablation, and reported that 93% of treatments were successful. A multicentre collaborative study, involving 859 women undergoing laser ablation, was reported by Garry et al in 1991. Of the women in this series, over half were followed up for more than 6 months. A satisfactory result was reported for 97%, although a few women (8%) required a second treatment. The rate of amenorrhoea was 60%, the mean operating time 24 min and 99% went home within 24 h. Erian (1994) reported similar results in 2342 women of whom 1866 had been followed up for over a year. Treatment was successful in 93%, and 56% of women remained amenorrhoeic. A few women underwent hysterectomy for treatment failure, and most of these were found to have adenomyosis on histological investigation. This is not easy to diagnose preoperatively, but a history of excessive pain with menstruation may indicate its presence.

Endometrial resection

Endometrial resection is the systematic excision of endometrium using the cutting loop of a resecting hysteroscope (Fig. 3.3). This technique was first described by DeCherney & Polan (1983), who used it in patients with intractable uterine bleeding in whom hysterectomy was contraindicated. The use of the continuous flow resectoscope was further developed by Hallez et al (1987) in France. Partial endometrial resection was performed at first, as it was thought that complete resection to the endocervix would cause cervical stenosis. However, total endometrial resection, where all the endometrium is removed is now the usual procedure in the United Kingdom (Fig. 3.4).

Studies on several large series of patients undergoing endometrial resection have been published (Fig. 3.5). Amenorrhoea rates ranging from 6 to 59% are reported, although the results in some series are difficult to interpret as postoperative hormonal suppression has been given. However, 80–97% of patients are reported as being satisfied with the procedure. Broadbent & Magos (1994) report that 80% of patients in their series were satisfied, at 2.5 years after the procedure, and that almost all had menstrual blood loss within the normal range. Less satisfactory results were reported for partial resections and for women younger than 35 years, which is likely to be because remnants of endometrium regenerate. In unsatisfactory cases, a repeat procedure can often be performed without resorting to hysterectomy.

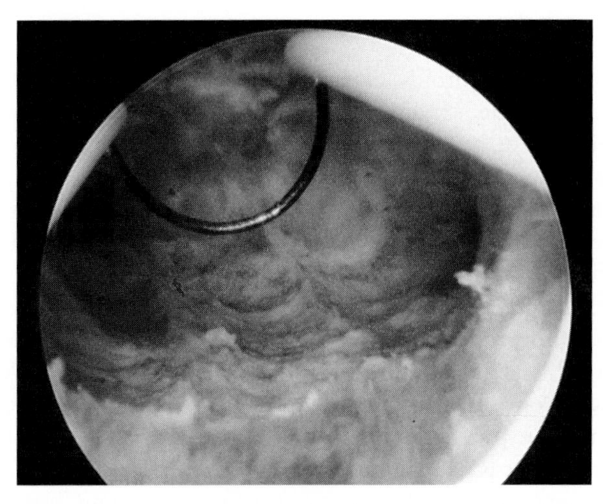

Fig. 3.5 Endometrial electroresection (from J. Hamou (Lewis & Magos 1993), with permission; see p. 44).

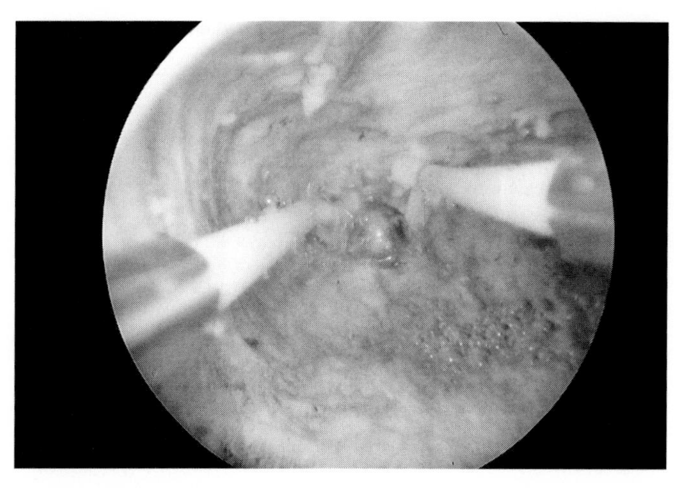

Fig. 3.6 Rollerball ablation (from J. Hamou (Lewis & Magos 1993), with permission; see p. 44).

Hysteroscopy performed several months after endometrial resection has shown a narrow fibrotic uterine cavity (Istre et al 1993). Histological examinations of biopsies of the uterine wall have revealed the presence of variable amounts of endometrium in many patients, even those who remain amenorrhoeic after the procedure.

Other methods of endometrial ablation

Endometrial ablation can also be performed electrosurgically using the technique of rollerball ablation (Vancaille 1989) (Fig. 3.6). The roller is either a 2–4-mm sphere or a cylinder on an electrosurgical resectoscope which can roll freely around its axis. A unipolar coagulating current is applied to the endometrium and this produces a zone of coagulation necrosis similar to that of the Nd-YAG laser. Daniell and colleagues, in 1992, reviewed 64 women 6 months after endometrial ablation using rollerball. Of these women, 30% had amenorrhoea and 80% were satisfied with the procedure.

Another method of endometrial destruction is radiofrequency-induced thermal endometrial ablation (RaFEA) (Phipps et al 1990). The cervix is dilated and a specially designed probe is inserted into the uterine cavity. Microwave energy at a power of 200 W is applied, which raises the temperature at the probe surface to about 60°C (Menostat, Rocket of London). Electromagnetic radiation relies on the interaction between the endometrium and an electric field generated around the treatment applicator, and is thus not direct heating. This technique is only suitable for women with dysfunctional bleeding and a normal uterus, therefore preoperative assessment by hysteroscopy and curettage is essential.

Preparation of the endometrium

The in vivo studies of Duffy and colleagues (1992) demonstrate that rollerball coagulation results in thermal necrosis to a depth of 3.3–3.7 mm. The depth of cut with a resection loop is 3–4 mm, and tissue is destroyed to a depth of 4–5 mm using the Nd-YAG laser. Endometrial thickness, however, varies from 3–12 mm during the menstrual cycle. Therefore satisfactory ablation can only be achieved if surgery is performed in the immediate postmenstrual phase. This would make scheduling of operations problematical, so the endometrium needs to be thinned prior to the procedure. Danazol and gonadotrophin-releasing hormone analogues (GnRH-a), such as goserelin, leuprorelin acetate or buserelin are effective at thinning the endometrium, and have now been compared in a randomized trial (Sutton & Ewen 1994).

Endometrial preparation is also important in that it reduces operating time, and therefore the risk of complications such as fluid overload.

Endometrial ablation versus hysterectomy

The results of randomized controlled trials comparing hysterectomy with endometrial resection have now been published (Dwyer et al 1993, Pinion et al 1994). These clearly show that postoperative morbidity (Table 3.2), length of hospital stay and the time taken to return to work, resume normal activities and sexual intercourse were significantly less after endometrial ablation when compared to hysterectomy. However, patient satisfaction may be slightly higher following hysterectomy, after only a few months of follow-up. Dysmenorrhoea and premenstrual symptoms were also improved in both groups (Pinion et al 1994). Previous studies have also shown that premenstrual symptoms are improved after laser ablation (Lefler 1989).

Publications of long-term results are awaited.

Table 3.2 Postoperative complications after abdominal hysterectomy and endometrial resection

Complications	Hysterectomy (n = 97)	Resection (n = 99)
No. with complications	46	4*
Type of complications		
Transfusion	6	2
Pyrexia	29	2*
Pelvic infection	5	2
Pelvic haematoma	8	1*
Wound infection	11	0*
Urinary infection	6	0*
Urinary retention	6	0*
Hb <10 g/dl	10	0*

*p = <0.001
Reproduced with permission from Dwyer et al 1993

Comparison of endometrial ablation techniques

Pinion et al (1994) compared the effectiveness and safety of endometrial laser ablation and endometrial resection with hysterectomy. No differences were observed between the two conservative technique groups, although the study was not large enough to exclude a difference.

All the techniques of endometrial ablation have their advantages and disadvantages, and they have not been compared in randomized controlled studies. The choice of technique depends on the availability of equipment, and more importantly, on the expertise of the surgeon. Endometrial resection is the only technique which provides an operative specimen for histology. Rankin & Steinberg in 1992 reported that four patients of 400 were found to have endometrial carcinoma after endometrial resection, although preoperative endometrial sampling was not performed routinely.

Analysis of data from the Royal College of Obstetricians and Gynaecologists (RCOG) MISTLETOE (minimally invasive surgical techniques, laser, endothermal or endoresection) study has shown that over 70% of women undergoing combined resection and rollerball procedures, or resection alone, were very satisfied with the results of surgery. Over 60% were very satisfied following rollerball alone or laser ablation. Cumulative failure rates at 1 year, including perioperative hysterectomy, subsequent repeat ablation, hysterectomy or listing for such procedures was lowest for combined resection and rollerball (15%) and highest for RaFEA (54%). The failure rate for women undergoing resection alone or rollerball alone was 20%, and for laser ablation the failure rate was 32%.

Recently there has been renewed interest in ablation performed by infusing hot fluid through a specially designed balloon which adapts to the shape of the uterine cavity. Initial studies suggest the technique is simple, safe and efficient.

Hysteroscopic myomectomy

Submucous fibroids cause menorrhagia and may impair fertility. The traditional management has been myomectomy or hysterectomy if childbearing is complete, but hysteroscopy now enables more precise diagnosis and treatment. Pretreatment with a GnRH-a for 2 months after the initial diagnostic hysteroscopy is often useful for shrinking fibroids greater than 2 cm in diameter.

Electroresection or the Nd-YAG laser can be used to resect fibroids. Large fibroids, or those where over half the fibroid is inside the uterine wall can be resected in a two-stage procedure (Donnez et al 1994). At the first hysteroscopy the protruding portion of the fibroid is resected. Further GnRH-a therapy can be given between the first and second procedure, and during the second hysteroscopy the myoma may again be seen to protrude thus allowing further resection. Complete resection of submucous fibroids seems to improve the long-term results (Wamsteker et al 1993).

Lysis of intrauterine adhesions

Asherman's syndrome is the total or partial occlusion of the endometrial cavity by adhesions, and 90% of cases occur following a pregnancy-related curettage. Endometrial adhesions can also occur following metroplasty and submucous myomectomy, or be caused by infection such as tuberculosis (Netter's syndrome). The symptoms of Asherman's syndrome vary according to the amount of cavity occluded and the type of adhesions, and include hypo- or amenorrhoea, infertility and dysmenorrhoea. Several classifications for intrauterine adhesions have been suggested, which are based on the extent of cavity involvement, whether the adhesions are filmy or dense and the pattern of menstruation.

Intrauterine adhesions can be divided mechanically with scissors, or using the Nd-YAG laser or electrosurgery. The division of synechiae begins at the cervical os if adhesions extend to that area, and a cavity is formed first before the hysteroscope is advanced. The uterine cavity is sculpted until symmetry is achieved. The adhesions are divided in the middle and then retract; removal is not necessary. The tubal ostia should be carefully inspected. Laparoscopy and dye procedures should also be performed if tubal blockage is suspected, or if the adhesions are extensive.

In order to prevent postoperative reformation of adhesions, an IUCD may be left in situ for 1–2 months. Prophylactic antibiotics are often administered, with cyclical oestrogens and progestogens, for 2–3 months. Restoration of normal menses occurs in 50–80% of patients and term pregnancy rates of up to 70% are reported (Siegler et al 1990). Those who become pregnant generally do well, but should be considered at risk from placenta accreta.

Hysteroscopic metroplasty

The most common uterine malformations are variants of the double uterus, i.e. bicornuate, didelphic and septate uteri (Fig. 3.7). These müllerian fusion defects, which are associated with pregnancy wastage, must be precisely defined before contemplating hysteroscopic resection. Only septate uteri (complete or incomplete) can be resected hysteroscopically as there is a much greater risk of perforating the myometrium and entering the abdominal cavity with a bicornuate or didelphic uterus. Therefore laparoscopy or ultrasound to examine the serosal surface of the uterus, in combination with either HSG or hysteroscopy is required to diagnose the abnormality. The septum is usually avascular and pretreatment with danazol or GnRH-a is not required. The septum can be transected using scissors, the electrosurgical resectoscope or the potassium-titanyl phosphate (KTP) or Nd-YAG laser (Fig. 3.8). Concomitant laparoscopy or ultrasound is advised. If a complete septum is resected, the other cervical os can be kept occluded with the balloon of a Foley catheter. The cervical septum can either be left in situ, or if transected, prophylactic cerclage may need to be considered in pregnancy. Insertion of an IUCD and postoperative hormone therapy is often advised (Gordon et al 1995).

Hysteroscopic transection is the treatment of choice for the septate uterus. Postoperative morbidity and discomfort are less than with transabdominal metroplasty. The peritoneum is not opened, and pelvic adhesions are less likely. Vaginal delivery is recommended. Pregnancy rates of about 70% occur after hysteroscopic metroplasty, of which about 80% go to term. This compares favourably with abdominal metroplasty (Fayez 1986).

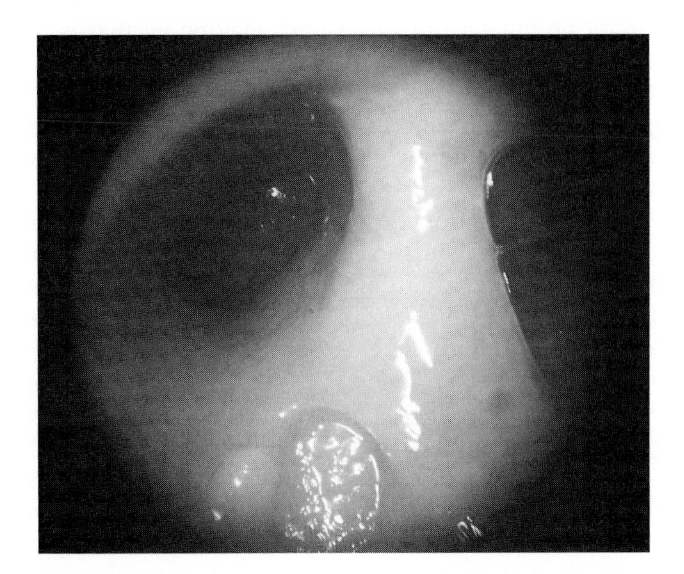

Fig. 3.7 Hysteroscopic view – septate uterus.

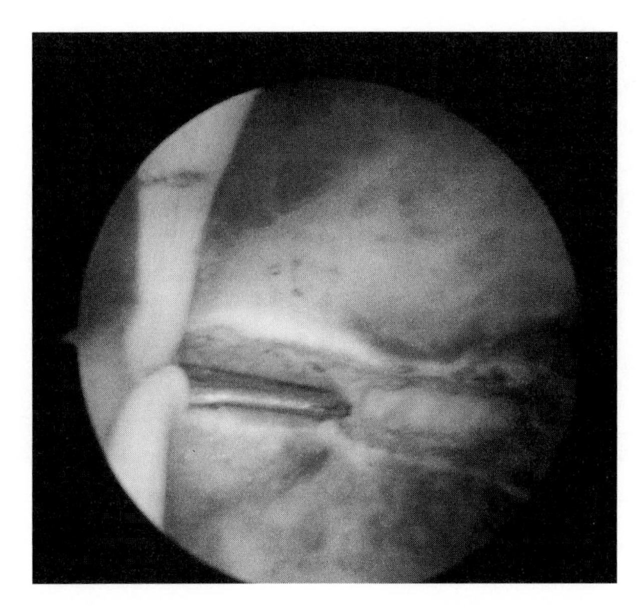

Fig. 3.8 Excision of septum with electrocautery knife.

Hysteroscopic sterilization

Hysteroscopically controlled methods of occluding the fallopian tubes have been investigated over many years. Methods have included the injection of sclerosing agents such as methlycyanoacrylate and quinacrine into the tubes, the destruction of the interstitial portion of the tubes and occlusion of the tube using plugs. The interstitial portion of the tubes can be destroyed using a blind thermal technique, the Nd-YAG laser or electrocoagulation. However, tubal patency rates were unacceptably high when these techniques were used, and complications such as peritonitis and ectopic pregnancies were not infrequent (Darabi & Richart 1977).

Various types of tubal plugs have been investigated, but most have a high rate of spontaneous expulsion. The Ovabloc system is the only one currently commercially available. The system involves the injection of liquid silicone into the tubes. Loffer & Loffer in 1992 reported a 5-year follow-up on a series of 265 patients who were sterilized using this procedure. A total of 88% were successfully sterilized, and 15% needed a repeat procedure. Only one pregnancy occurred, which was ectopic, giving a pregnancy rate of 0.0067 per 100 women-years. Removal of these plugs does not result in pregnancies as the tubes appear to scar closed in virtually all patients. The technique is not widely practised because it has an unacceptably high pregnancy rate, but more efficient methods are being investigated.

CONTRAINDICATIONS TO HYSTEROSCOPY

Hysteroscopy should not be performed in the presence of active pelvic infection. The only exception to this is when an IUCD is 'lost' and hysteroscopy is essential to

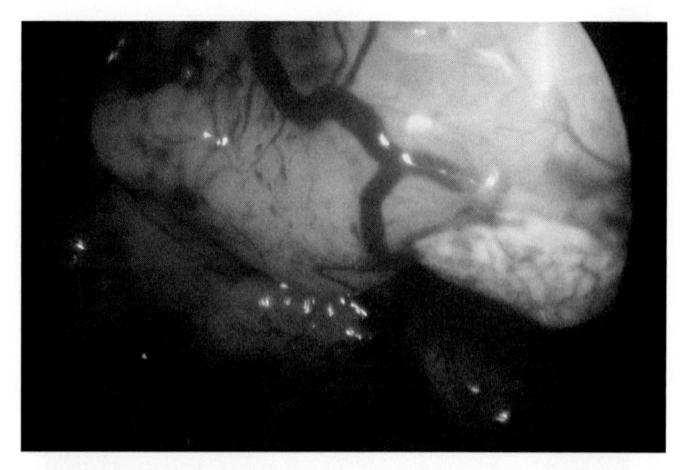

Fig. 3.9 Endometrial hyperplasia as viewed hysteroscopically – note prominent vessels and uneven surface (from R. Labastida (Lewis & Magos 1993), with permission).

locate and remove it. Antibiotic cover should be used for such a procedure.

Although pregnancy is generally a contraindication to hysteroscopy, experienced hysteroscopists can remove IUCDs in early pregnancy. The myometrium is more distensible and therefore the gas flow should be limited to 50 ml/min with a maximum pressure of 100 mmHg. The nervus opticus does not function before the 10th week, therefore hysteroscopy must be performed before then so there is no risk of damage.

Hysteroscopy in the presence of uterine bleeding requires more experience, but with a continuous flow hysteroscope good visibility can be obtained. Hysteroscopy should never be performed in the presence of cervical malignancy, and if endometrial carcinoma or atypical hyperplasia is suspected, biopsies should be taken and the extent of spread evaluated, and any planned operative procedure abandoned (Fig. 3.9).

The most important contraindication to hysteroscopy, however, is the inexperienced hysteroscopist.

COMPLICATIONS OF HYSTEROSCOPY

Hysteroscopy as a technique is associated with complications, particularly with more complicated operative procedures (Table 3.3). Operative hysteroscopy requires an intensive training period, and most complications occur in the hands of inexperienced surgeons. It is recommended that operative work is not carried out until the surgeon has become an experienced diagnostic hysteroscopist. Operative hysteroscopy should be taught using a video system under the supervision of an experienced surgeon. The RCOG (1994) has issued a classification of operative procedures, which indicates the different levels of training required (Table 3.4). The MISTLETOE initial analysis reported on overall complication rates of different endometrial ablation techniques, and included both perioperative and postoperative complications in the first 6 weeks. The complication rate was 11% for endometrial resection and 5% for laser and rollerball ablation.

Table 3.3 Complications of endometrial ablation techniques

Intraoperative	Early postoperative	Late postoperative
Uterine perforation	Infection	Recurrence of symptoms
Injury to intra-abdominal viscera and vessels	Secondary haemorrhage	Pregnancy
Primary haemorrhage	Haematometra	(Uterine malignancy)
Gas embolism	Cyclical pain	
	Treatment failure	

Reproduced with permission RCOG Working Party (1994)

Table 3.4 Stratification of hysteroscopic procedures by level of training

Level 1 Diagnostic procedures
Diagnostic hysteroscopy, plus target biopsy
Removal of simple polyps
Removal of intrauterine contraceptive devices (IUCDs)

Level 2 Minor operative procedures
Proximal fallopian tube cannulation
Minor Asherman's syndrome
Removal of pedunculated fibroid or large polyp

Level 3 More complex operative procedures requiring additional training
Division/resection of uterine septum
Endoscopic surgery for major Asherman's syndrome
Endometrial resection or ablation
Resection of submucous leiomyoma
Repeat endometrial resection or ablation

Reproduced with permission RCOG Working Party (1994)

Uterine perforation

This is the most common complication (Lewis 1994) and can occur when dilating the cervix, on insertion of the hysteroscope or during an operative procedure itself. Careful observation of the patient may be all that is required if perforation occurs during cervical dilation or insertion of the hysteroscope, but if there are clinical signs of ongoing haemorrhage then laparoscopy should be performed. Laparotomy or even hysterectomy may be required.

Uterine perforation occurs in around 1% of patients undergoing endometrial ablation (Lewis 1994). If perforation is suspected during the procedure, the operation must be stopped. Visualization of peritoneum or bowel through the hysteroscope is pathognomonic of a perforated uterus, but sudden loss of vision and rapid inflow of fluid distension media or abdominal distension are also suspicious.

Perforation occurs most easily at the cornual regions, which are also the most difficult to resect. Deaths have occurred after endometrial ablation, resulting from trauma to intra-abdominal organs, infection and haemorrhage. Such cases may have been under-reported in the literature. Laparotomy may be necessary to adequately assess and repair injury to major blood vessels, bowel or urinary tract.

Patients who have sustained uterine perforation during hysteroscopic fertility procedures may be at risk if they become pregnant. Spontaneous uterine rupture during pregnancy has been reported following hysteroscopic metroplasty (Lobaugh et al 1994), even when perforation has not occurred during the procedure.

Other forms of uterine trauma such as cervical laceration can occur during hysteroscopy. Prior cervical preparation is sometimes used using agents such as laminaria tents and prostaglandin E_2.

Hazards of liquid distension media

Significant fluid overload occurs in approximately 0.6% of endometrial ablation procedures (Lewis 1994). Liquid distension media are absorbed or intravasated from the uterine cavity into the uterine vasculature, as blood vessels are transected during operative procedures. Transtubal intra-abdominal absorption is probably of less significance as aspiration of fluid at concomitant laparoscopy does not seem to prevent complications. Fluid input should be carefully monitored when low viscosity liquids such as 1.5% glycine are used, as circulatory overload can occur, with complications such as pulmonary oedema and electrolyte disturbance.

Symptoms associated with the absorption of large volumes of distension media and consequent dilutional hyponatraemia have long been recognized by urologists as the 'post-TURP syndrome'. Symptoms include hypertension and bradycardia followed by nausea, vomiting, visual disturbances, headache, hypotension, agitation, lethargy and confusion. Seizures, coma and death may follow if the syndrome is not recognized and treated appropriately.

Acute hyponatraemia is tolerated by the body much less well than chronic hyponatraemia, and death can occur in the acute situation when the serum sodium is at a level of 120 mmol/l (Witz et al 1993). Central pontine myelinolysis is a danger if hyponatraemia is corrected too rapidly. Fluid input and output must be measured meticulously during operative hysteroscopy and surgery stopped at once if absorption exceeds target levels. Fit young women may easily absorb 1.5 l of glycine or normal saline but women with cardiovascular disease may become compromised. Elevated blood ammonia levels can occur with the use of glycine for hysteroscopy. Glycine should be used with caution in patients with impaired liver or renal function.

Adverse effects associated with the use of dextran-70 include anaphylactic shock which can occur when even small volumes of dextran are intravasated. Pulmonary oedema secondary to dextran use is most likely to be due to increased plasma volume due to dextran's effect as a plasma expander. The plasma volume can expand by 10 times the amount of dextran entering the circulation. Dextran is widely used as a thromboprophylactic agent as it reduces the level of a number of clotting factors and decreases platelet adhesiveness. Coagulation disorders such as disseminated intravascular coagulation have been reported after hysteroscopy with dextran.

Gas embolism

The rate of flow must always be carefully controlled as deaths have been reported from carbon dioxide embolism. Insufflating machines for laparoscopy, which have flow rates of 9 l/min are dangerous and must never be used. Air and other gases must never be used for hysteroscopy as fatal air embolism can occur (Baggish & Daniell 1989).

Haemorrhage

Haemorrhage can occur during procedures such as endometrial ablation and hysteroscopic myomectomy. It can be controlled by placing a 30-ml Foley catheter balloon in the uterus for 6–8 h. If haemorrhage continues when the balloon is deflated a hysterectomy might be needed; alternatively embolization of the uterine artery can be considered. In the MISTLETOE study, 1% of women undergoing endometrial resection required an emergency hysterectomy.

Infection

Postoperative infection after operative hysteroscopy is uncommon, but cases of tubo-ovarian abscesses have been reported (McCausland et al 1993). Patients with a history of pelvic inflammatory disease are likely to be more at risk from this complication. Necrotizing granulomatous endometritis has also been reported in specimens obtained at hysterectomy performed for continuing pain and bleeding after endometrial resection (Ferryman et al 1992).

Haematometra and cyclical pain

Haematometra is a rare late complication of endometrial resection in premenopausal women, and has also been reported in amenorrhoeic women who commence hormone replacement therapy (Dwyer et al 1991). Cyclical lower abdominal pain, worse than the preoperative dysmenorrhoea, can also occur following endometrial ablation in the absence of haematometra. Asherman (1950) described this phenomenon in his description of intrauterine synechiae. Pinion et al (1994), however, reported that dysmenorrhoea was relieved in most patients undergoing endometrial ablation. Erian (1994) reported that most women who had hysterectomies for pelvic pain following endometrial ablation had adenomyosis.

Pregnancy

Intrauterine and extrauterine pregnancies can occur following endometrial ablation, even after many months of amenorrhoea (Lam et al 1992). An intrauterine pregnancy may be advanced when first recognized and the risk of spontaneous abortion, premature delivery, placenta accreta, intrauterine growth retardation, fetal death and uterine dehiscence appear higher than average, although normal pregnancies do occur. It is not known whether cornual scarring increases the risk of ectopic pregnancy.

Women should be advised to be sterilized at the time of the procedure, or to continue using hormonal or barrier methods of contraception. An intrauterine contraceptive device is not recommended. Although the chances of conception are very small, the procedure may become less effective with time, and the chances of pregnancy higher.

Uterine malignancy

It is been shown that islands of endometrium remain after endometrial ablation procedures, even if total amenorrhoea is achieved (Broadbent & Magos 1994, Istre et al 1993). It is possible that endometrial carcinoma could develop in residual endometrium perhaps many years after endometrial ablation. In such a case, presentation and diagnosis might be delayed because of overlying scar tissue. Copperman et al (1993) reported a case of endometrial carcinoma after 5 years of amenorrhoea following rollerball ablation, in a postmenopausal woman not on hormone replacement therapy. At present, therefore, combined hormone replacement therapy is recommended for women who have undergone endometrial ablation, and any episode of bleeding that occurs after a long period of amenorrhoea should be treated as suspicious.

ACKNOWLEDGEMENT

Figures 3.1, 3.2, 3.3, 3.4, 3.5, 3.6 and 3.7 are reproduced with the permission of Professors van Herendael, Hamou and Labastida.

KEY POINTS

1. The indications for diagnostic hysteroscopy include abnormal uterine bleeding, infertility and the location of foreign bodies.
2. Uterine abnormalities detectable at hysteroscopy include: endometrial polyps, submucous fibroids, uterine septae, intrauterine adhesions, endometrial carcinoma and retained products of conception.
3. Hysteroscopic endometrial destruction can be partial or total, and techniques include the Nd-YAG laser, electroresection, rollerball or radiofrequency-induced endometrial ablation (RaFEA).
4. It is advantageous to thin the endometrium prior to endometrial ablation, using either danazol or GnRH analogues.
5. Endometrial ablation is associated with less postoperative morbidity, a shorter hospital stay and more rapid resumption of normal activities when compared with hysterectomy, but longer term results are awaited.
6. Hysteroscopic myomectomy using electroresection or the Nd-YAG laser is useful in the treatment of menorrhagia and infertility.
7. Lysis of intrauterine adhesions, metroplasty and sterilization can be performed hysteroscopically, although at present failure rates with hysteroscopic sterilization are unacceptably high.
8. Contraindications to hysteroscopy generally include pelvic infection, cervical malignancy and pregnancy.
9. Complications of hysteroscopy are more common with advanced operative procedures and operative work should only be carried out by an experienced diagnostic hysteroscopist.
10. Uterine perforation is the most common complication of hysteroscopy; others include gas embolism, haemorrhage, infection, haematometra and pregnancy.
11. Hazards of uterine distension media include hyponatraemia, pulmonary oedema and anaphylaxis.
12. Islands of endometrium remain after endometrial ablation procedures, and the long-term risk of uterine malignancy is unknown.

REFERENCES

Asherman J G 1950 Traumatic intrauterine adhesions. Journal of Obstetrics and Gynecology of the British Empire 57: 892–896

Baggish M S, Daniell J F 1989 Death caused by air embolism associated with neodymium-yttrium-aluminium-garnet laser surgery and artificial sapphire tips. American Journal of Obstetrics and Gynecology 161: 877–878

Broadbent J A M, Magos A L 1994 Transcervical resection of the endometrium. In: Sutton C, Diamond M (eds) Endoscopic surgery for gynaecologists. W B Saunders, London

Copperman A B, DeCherney A H, Olive D L 1993 A case of endometrial cancer following endometrial ablation for dysfunctional uterine bleeding. Obstetrics and Gynecology 4(2): 640–642

Daniell J F, Kurtz B R, Raymond W 1992 Hysteroscopic endometrial ablation using the rollerball electrode. Obstetrics and Gynecology 80(3): 329–332

Darabi K F, Richart R M 1977 Collaborative study on hysteroscopic sterilization procedures. A preliminary report. Obstetrics and Gynecology 49: 48–54

DeCherney A H, Polan M L 1983 Hysteroscopic management of

intrauterine lesions and intractable uterine bleeding. Obstetrics and Gynecology 61: 392–397
Donnez J, Nisolle M, Clerckx F, Casanas-Roux F, Saussoy P, Gillerot S 1994 Advanced endoscopic techniques used in dysfunctional bleeding, fibroids and endometriosis, and the role of gonadotrophin-releasing hormone agonist treatment. British Journal of Obstetrics and Gynaecology 101(suppl 10): 2–9
Duffy S, Reid P C, Sharp F 1992 In vivo studies of uterine electrosurgery. British Journal of Obstetrics and Gynaecology 99: 579–582
Dwyer N, Fox R, Mills M, Hutton J 1991 Haematometra caused by hormone replacement therapy after endometrial resection. Lancet 338: 1205
Dwyer N, Hutton J, Stirrat G M 1993 Randomized controlled trial comparing endometrial resection with abdominal hysterectomy for the surgical treatment of menorrhagia. British Journal of Obstetrics and Gynaecology 100: 237–243
Erian J 1994 Endometrial ablation in the treatment of menorrhagia. British Journal of Obstetrics and Gynaecology 101(suppl 11): 19–22
Fayez J A 1986 Comparison between abdominal and hysteroscopic metroplasty. Obstetrics and Gynecology 68: 399
Ferryman S R, Stephens M, Gough D 1992 Necrotising granulomatous endometritis following endometrial ablation therapy. British Journal of Obstetrics and Gynaecology 99: 928–930
Garry R, Erian J, Grochmal S A 1991 A multi-centre collaborative study into the treatment of menorrhagia by Nd-YAG laser ablation of the endometrium. British Journal of Obstetrics and Gynaecology 98: 357–362
Gimpelson R J, Rappold H O 1988 A comparative study between panoramic hysteroscopy with directed biopsies and dilatation and curettage. Journal of Obstetrics and Gynaecology 158: 489–492
Goldrath M H 1989 Intrauterine laser surgery. In: Keye W R Laser (ed) Surgery in Gynecology and Obstetrics. Year Book Medical Publishers, Chicago
Goldrath M H, Fuller T A, Segal S 1981 Laser photovaporization of endometrium for the treatment of menorrhagia. American Journal of Obstetrics and Gynecology 1981 140: 14–19
Gordon A G, Lewis B V, De Cherney A H 1995 Gynecologic endoscopy, 2nd edn. Mosby Wolfe, London
Hallez J, Netter A, Cartier R 1987 Methodical intrauterine resection. American Journal of Obstetrics and Gynecology 156: 1080–1084
Istre O, Skajaa K, Holm-Nielson P, Forman A 1993 The second-look appearance of the cavity after resection of the endometrium. Gynaecological Endoscopy 2: 159–163
Lam A M, Al-Jumaily R Y, Holt E M 1992 Ruptured ectopic pregnancy in an amenorrhoeic woman after transcervical resection of the endometrium. Australia and New Zealand Journal of Obstetrics and Gynaecology 32: 81–82
Lefler H T 1989 Premenstrual syndrome improvement after laser ablation of the endometrium for menorrhagia. Journal of Reproductive Medicine 34: 905–906
Lewis B V 1988 Hysteroscopy in clinical practice. Journal of Obstetrics and Gynaecology 9: 47–55
Lewis B V 1994 Guidelines for endometrial ablation. British Journal of Obstetrics and Gynaecology 101: 470-473
Lewis B V, Magos A L 1993 Endometrial ablation. Churchill Livingstone, Edinburgh
Lindemann H J 1973 Historical aspects of hysteroscopy. Fertility and Sterility 24: 230-242
Lobaugh M L, Bammel B M, Duke D, Webster B W 1994 Uterine rupture during pregnancy in a patient with a history of hysteroscopic metroplasty. Obstetrics and Gynecology 83: 838–840
Loffer F D, Loffer P S 1992 Hysteroscopic tubal occlusion with the use of formed-in-place silicone devices: a long-term follow-up. Gynaecological Endoscopy 1: 203–205
Lomano J M 1988 Dragging technique versus blanching technique for endometrial ablation with the Nd:YAG laser in the treatment of chronic menorrhagia. American Journal of Obstetrics and Gynecology 159: 152–155
McCausland V M, Fields G A, McCausland A M, Townsend D E 1993 Tubo-ovarian abscesses after operative hysteroscopy. Journal of Reproductive Medicine 38: 198–200
Phipps J, Lewis B V, Roberts T, Prior M V, Hand J W, Elder M, Field S B 1990 Treatment of functional menorrhagia by radiofrequency induced thermal endometrial ablation. Lancet 335: 374–376
Pinion S B, Parkin D E, Amramovich D R et al 1994 Randomised trial of hysterectomy, endometrial laser ablation and transcervical endometrial resection for dysfunctional uterine bleeding. British Medical Journal 309: 979–983
Rankin L, Steinberg L H 1992 Transcervical resection of the endometrium: a review of 400 consecutive patients. British Journal of Obstetrics and Gynaecology 99: 911–914
Royal College of Obstetricians and Gynaecologists (RCOG) Working Party 1994 Report of the RCOG working party on training in gynaecological endoscopic surgery. RCOG Press, London
Siegler A M 1990 Uterine causes of infertility. Current Opinion in Obstetrics and Gynecology 2: 173–181
Siegler A M, Valle R F, Lindemann H J, Mencaglia L 1990 In: Siegler A M et al Therapeutic hysteroscopy. Indications and Techniques. C V Mosby, St Louis
Sutton C J, Ewen S P 1994 Thinning the endometrium prior to ablation: is it worthwhile? British Journal of Obstetrics and Gynaecology 101(suppl 10): 10–12
Vancaillie T G 1989 Electrocoagulation of the endometrium with the ball end resectoscope. Obstetrics and Gynecology 74: 425–427
Wamsteker K, Emanuel M H, de Kruif J H 1993 Transcervical hysteroscopic resection of submucous fibroids for abnormal uterine bleeding: results regarding the degree of intramural extension. Obstetrics and Gynecology 82: 736–740
Witz C A, Silverberg K M, Burns W N, Schenken R S, Olive D L 1993 Complications associated with the absorption of hysteroscopic fluid media. Fertility and Sterility 60: 745–756

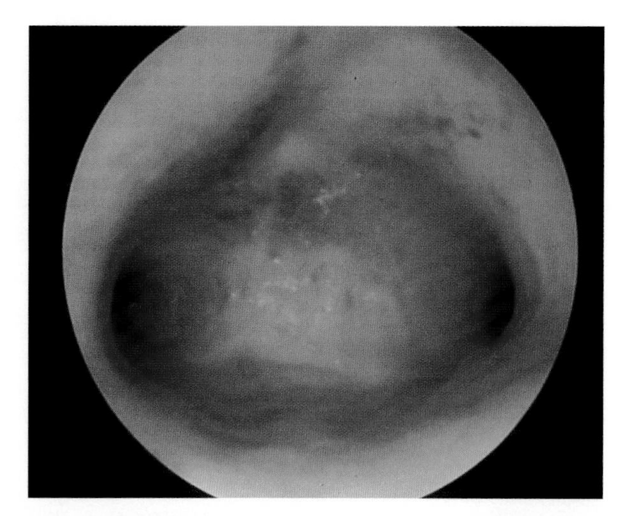

Fig. 3.1 Panoramic view of uterine cavity in postmenstrual patient.

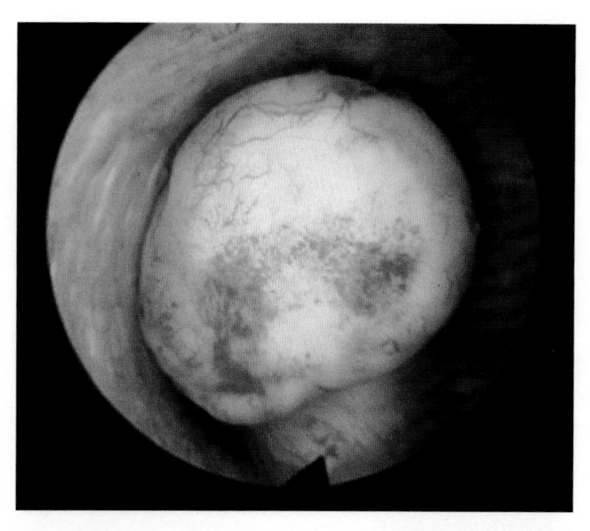

Fig. 3.2 Submucous fibroid polyp (from D. Van Herendael (Lewis & Magos 1993)).

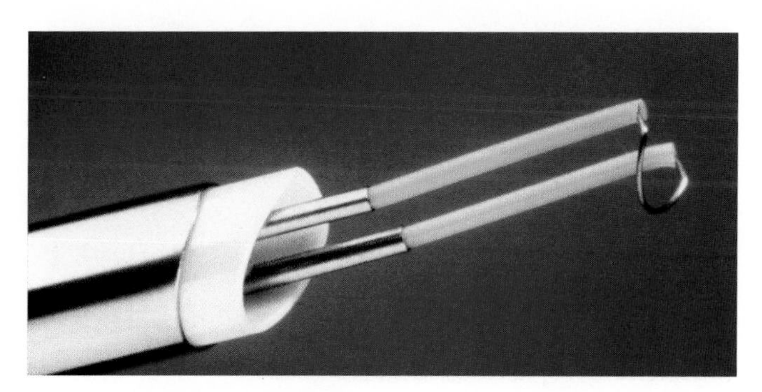

Fig. 3.4 Cutting loop of resectoscope.

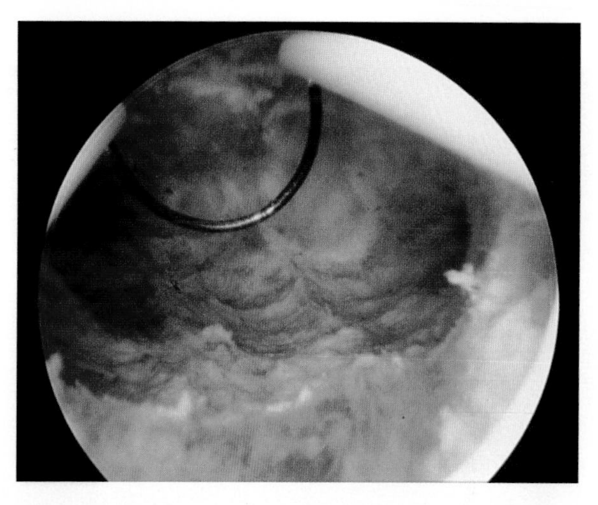

Fig. 3.5 Endometrial electroresection (from J. Hamou (Lewis & Magos 1993)).

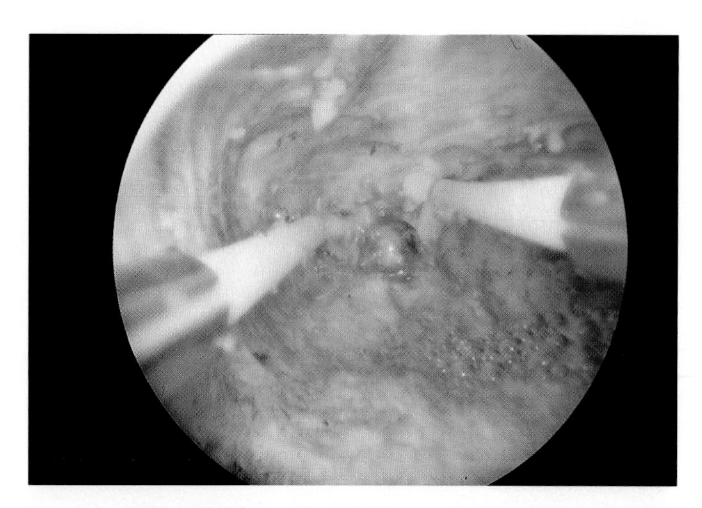

Fig. 3.6 Rollerball ablation (from J. Hamou (Lewis & Magos 1993)).

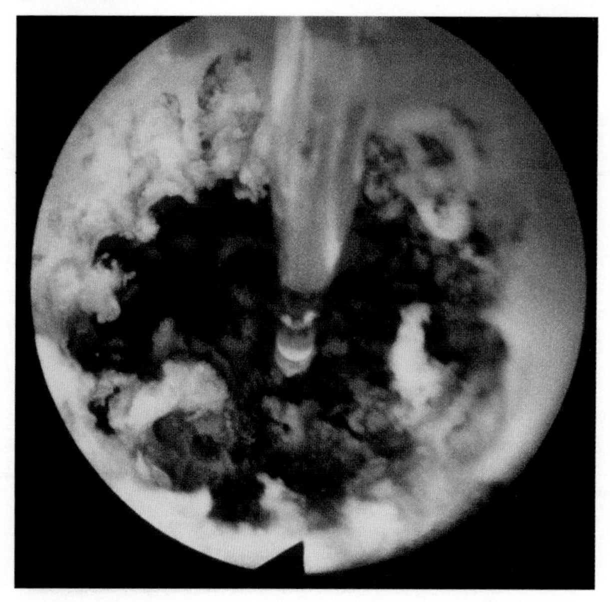

Fig. 28.12 A view of the uterine cavity during laser ablation. (By kind permission of Dr J. Davis)

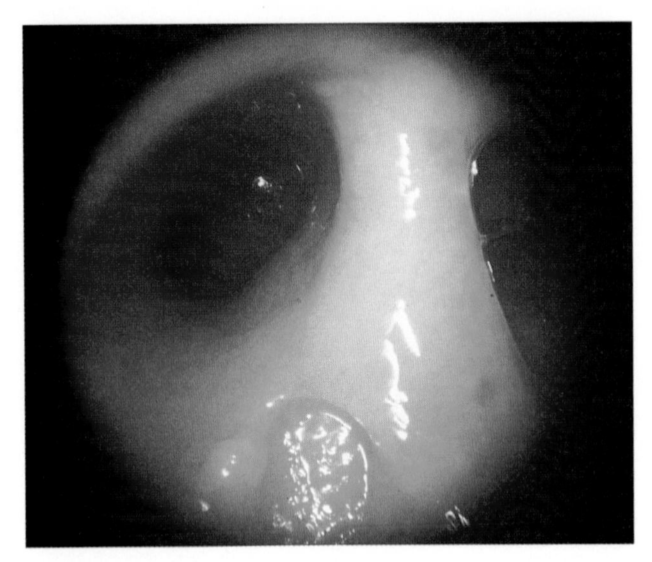

Fig. 3.7 Hysteroscopic view – septate uterus.

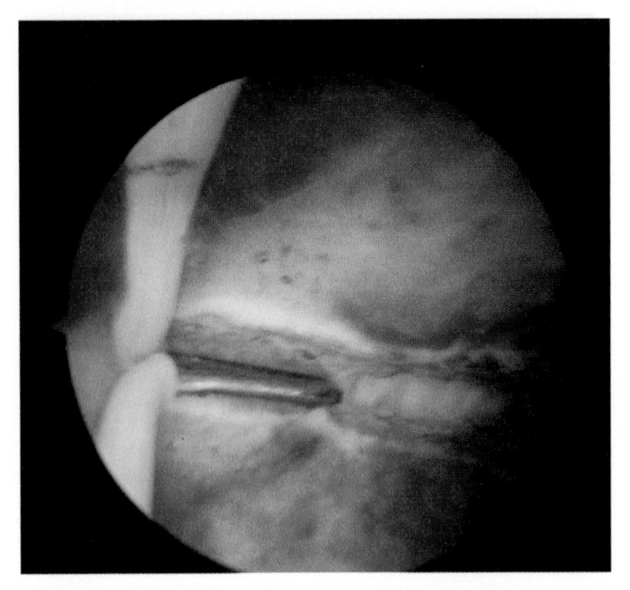

Fig. 3.8 Excision of septum with electrocautery knife.

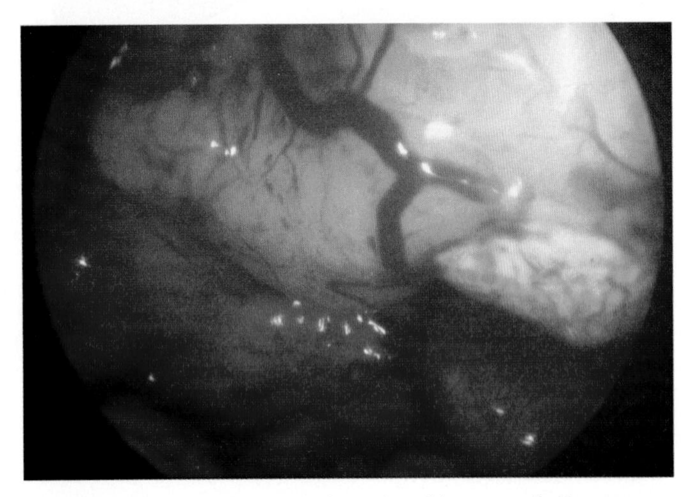

Fig. 3.9 Endometrial hyperplasia as viewed hysterocopically – note prominent vessels and uneven surface (from R. Labastida (Lewis & Magos 1993)).

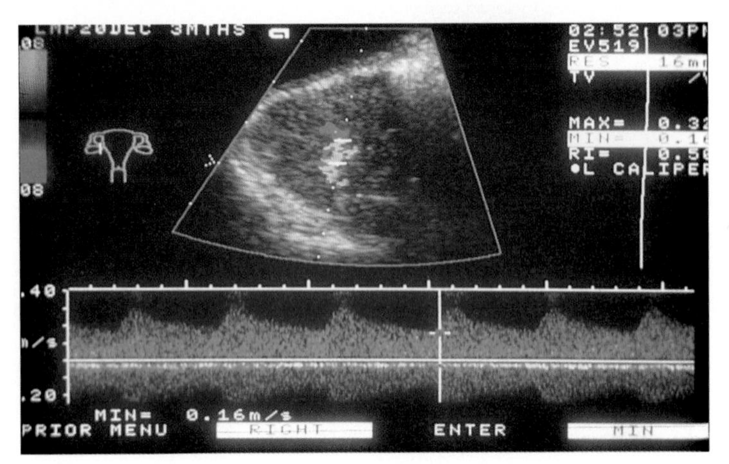

Fig. 6.2 Colour Doppler of a corpus luteum. On colour Doppler, flow signals are colour coded for direction and velocity. The neovascularization in this corpus luteum is shown as a knot of colour. Apart from providing a graphic display of vascularity, a useful feature of colour Doppler is to guide placement of the gate for spectral Doppler tracings. Shown in the lower portion of the figure is a low impedance trace with flow throughout diastole. This is typical of growing tissue.

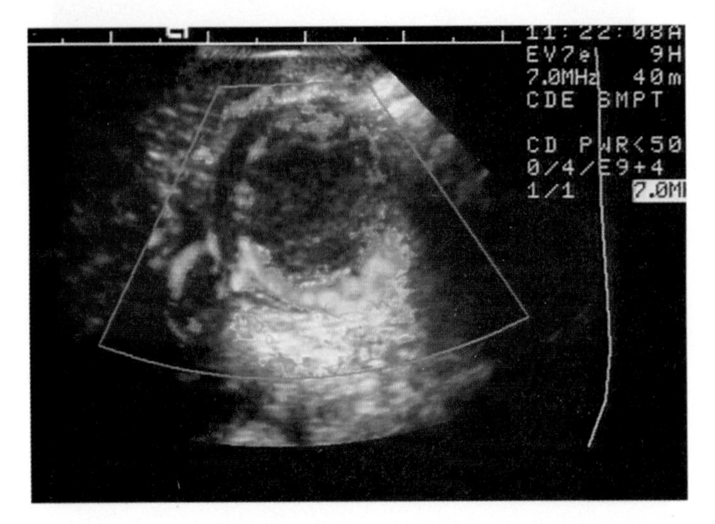

Fig. 6.13 Ectopic gestation. In this transvaginal scan, colour signals are seen around the ectopic sac. This scan was taken with the energy mode of colour Doppler a more sensitive type of signal processing.

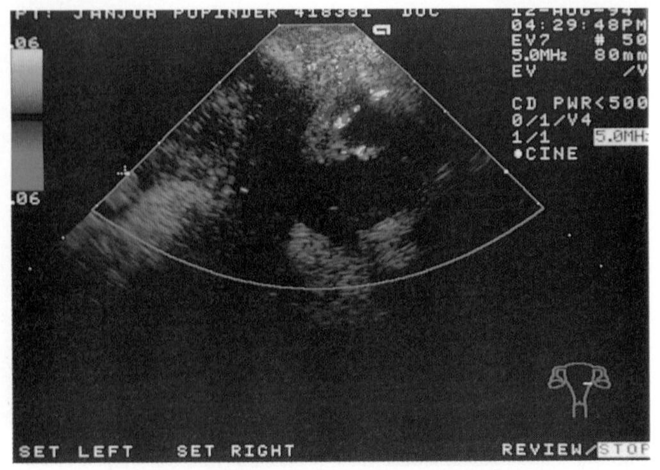

Fig. 6.15 Tubo-ovarian abcess. The marked colour signals within and around this abcess cavity are indicators of its inflammatory nature.

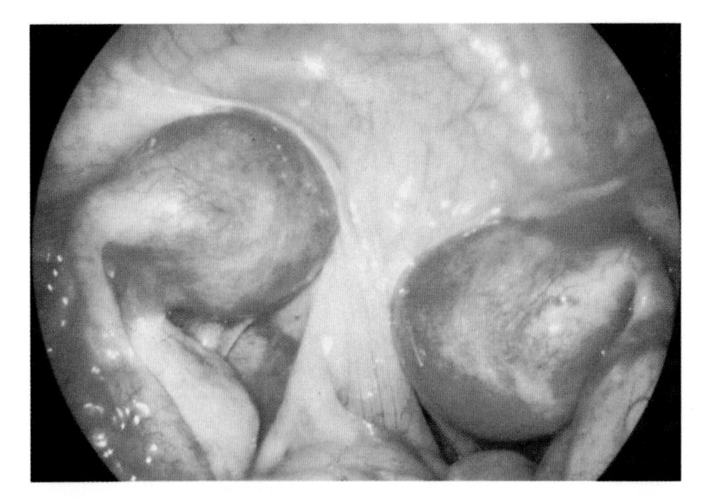

Uterus bicornis bicollis with double vagina (A. Auderbert).

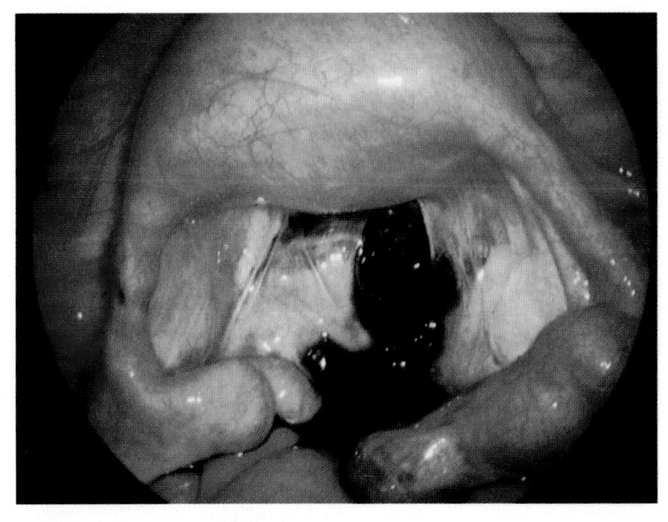

Extensive peritubal and periovarian adhesions. Spill and location of methylene blue dye (H. Frangenheim).

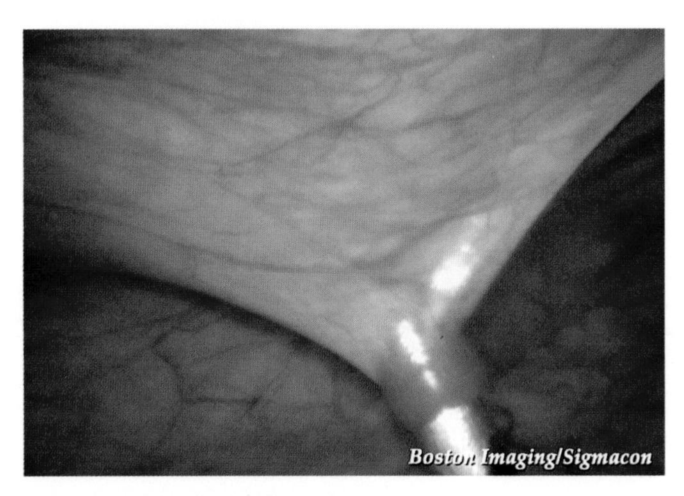

Fig. 4.8 Inferior epigastric vessels medial to the lower lateral port.

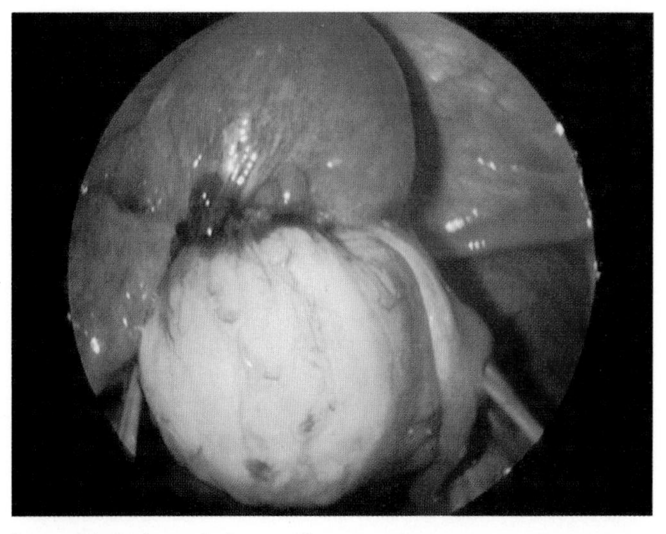

Large right endometriotic cyst adherent to the uterus (H. Frangenheim).

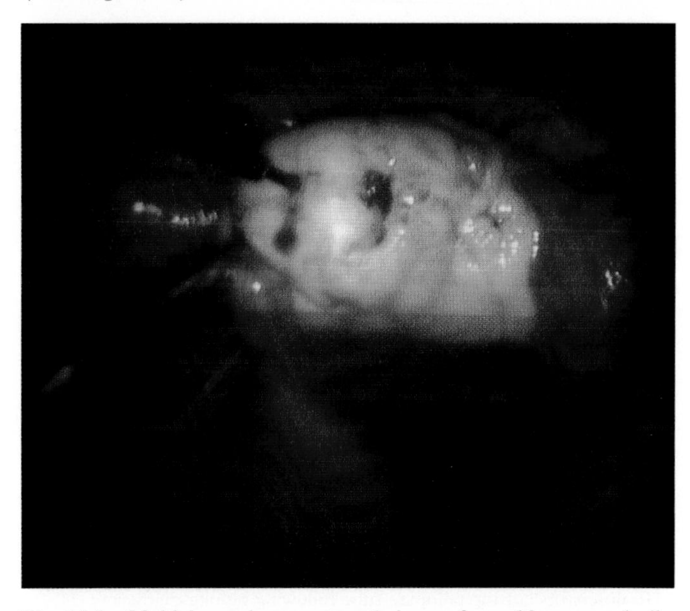

Fig. 15.9 Multiple ovarian punctures being performed laparoscopically on a polycystic ovary. (Photograph courtesy of Professor R W Shaw, Cardiff, UK.)

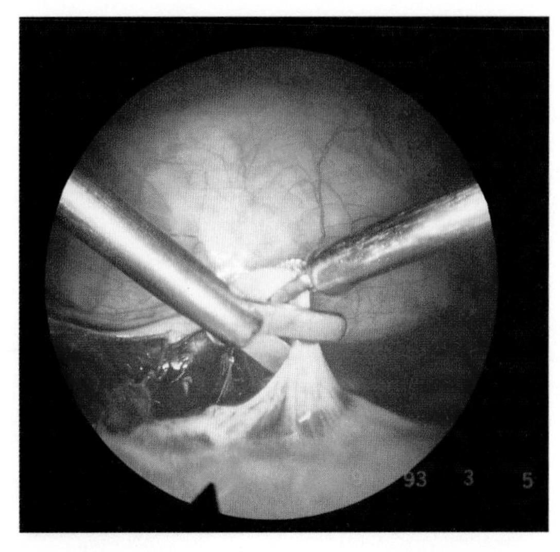

Fig. 4.13 Cutting the tissues of the infundibulopelvic ligaments, desiccated by bipolar diathermy using laparoscopic scissors.

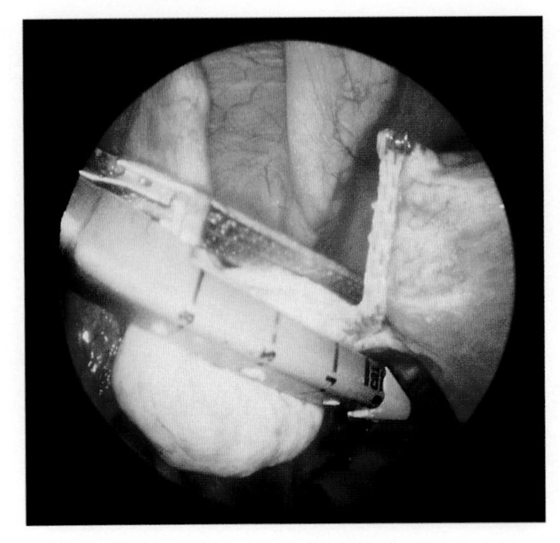

Fig. 4.16 Applying an automatic stapling device.

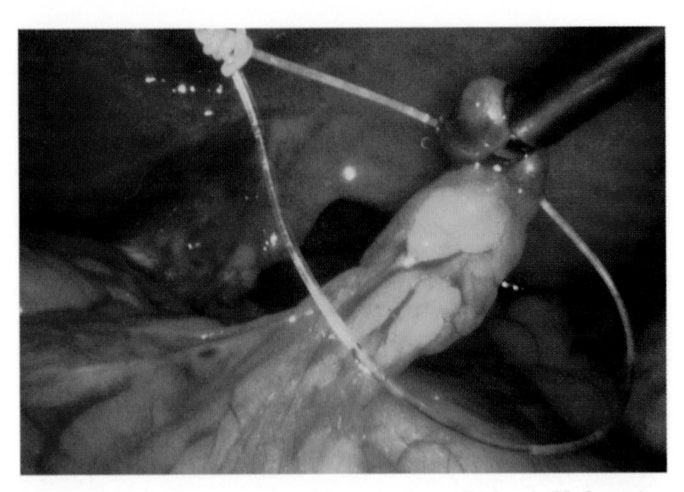

Ligation of vascular omentum with roeder loop (Ethicon) (K. Semm).

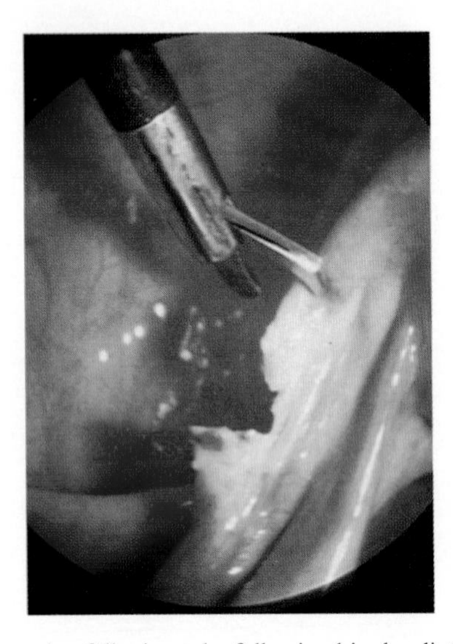

Hook scissors cutting fallopian tube following bipolar diathermy (H. Frangenheim).

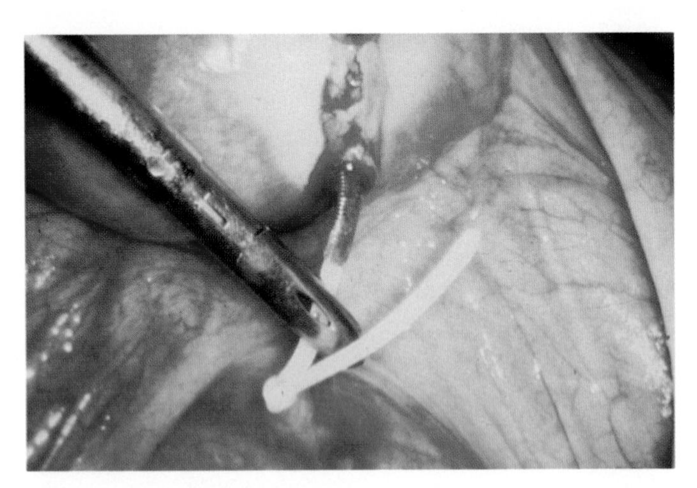

Perforation of fundus of the uterus by a Copper-7 contraceptive device. Laparoscopic recovery (K. Semm).

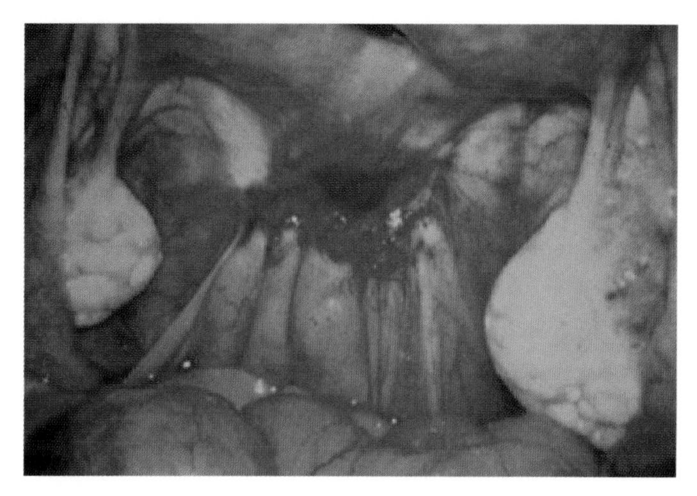

Haemorrhagic endometriosis in pouch of Douglas involving serosal surface of rectum.

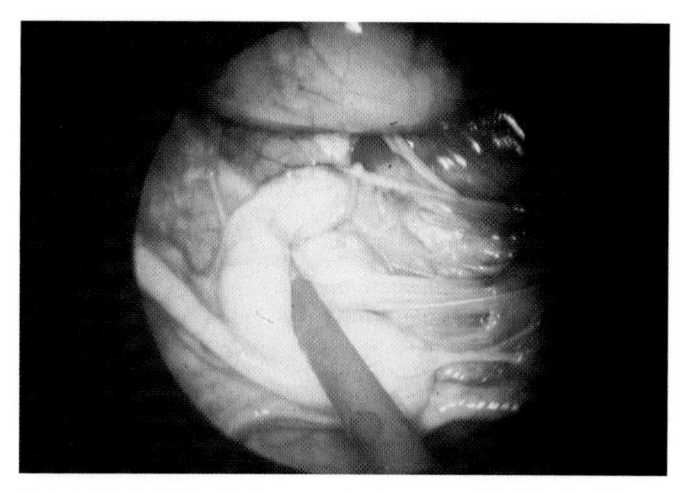

Peritubal and pelvic adhesions — endpoint in long-standing endometriosis producing infertility.

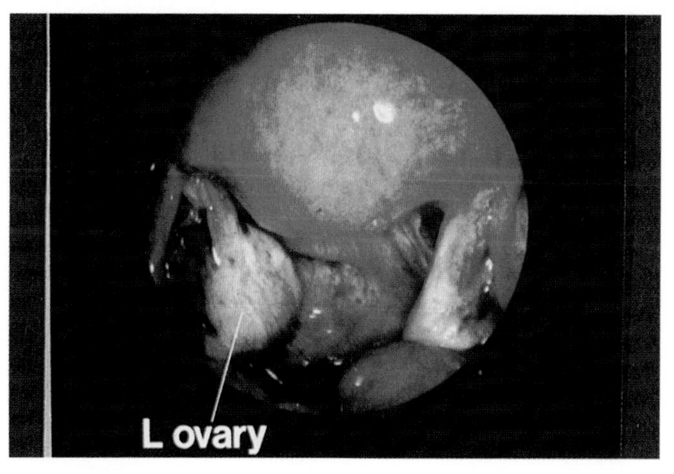

Fig. 30.7 Endometrioma in left ovary, superficial deposits on both ovaries and on uterosacral ligaments.

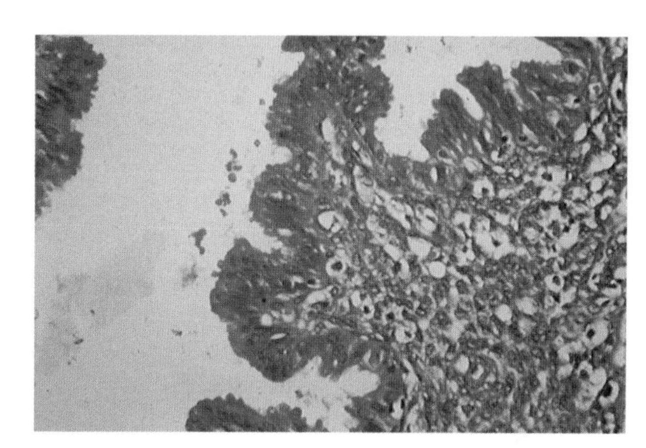

Fig. 30.2 High-power picture of biopsy from endometrial deposit demonstrating glandular structure and macrophages with lipid and haemosiderin accumulation (× 100). From Shaw & Marshall (1989) with permission.

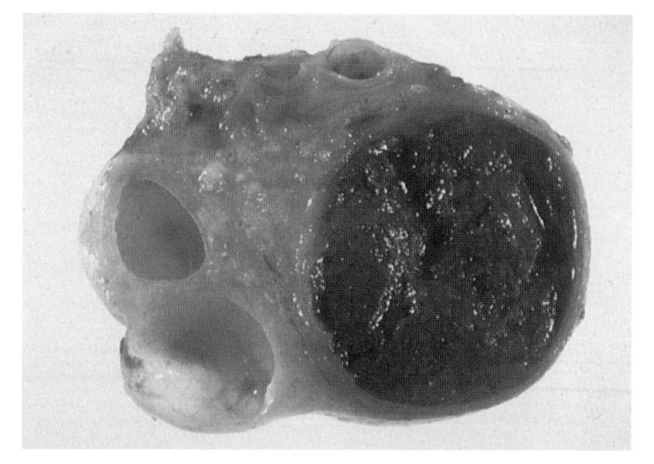

Fig. 30.8 Classical chocolate cyst of ovary (endometrioma) in an ovary containing two other fibrotic walled smaller cysts previously filled with 'chocolate' material prior to section

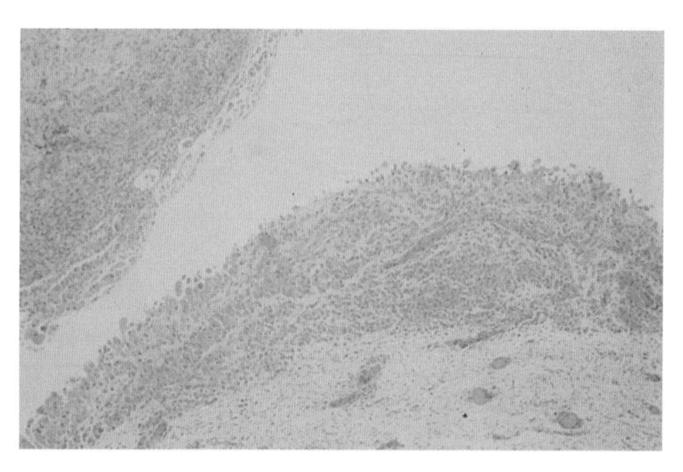

Fig. 30.4 Wall of an endometrial chocolate cyst with extensive fibrosis and haemorrhage but no recognisable endometrial glands or stroma.

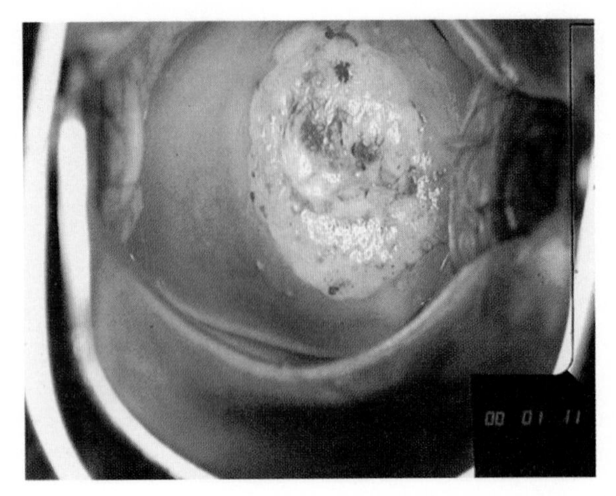

Fig. 34.6 CIN III showing strong acetowhite with clear, regular edges.

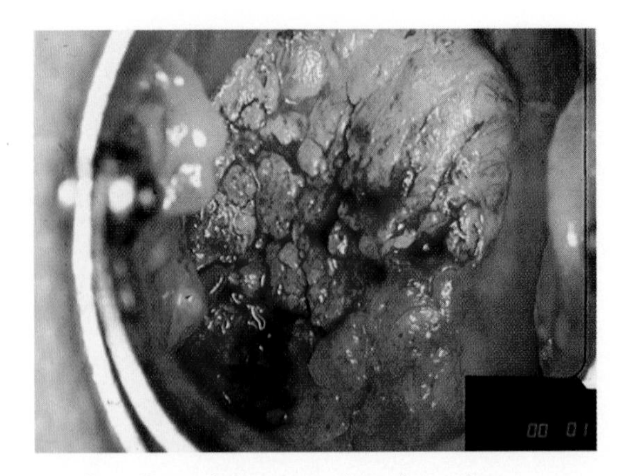

Fig. 34.8 Stage Ib cervical cancer —irregular surface.

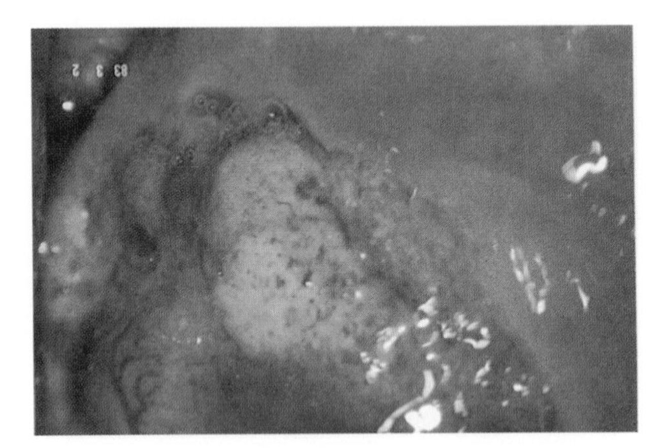

Fig. 34.9 Atypical vessels and irregular surface of invasion.

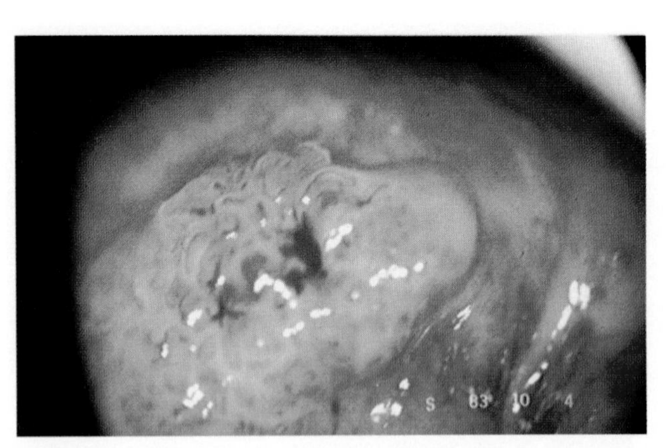

Fig. 34.10 Large cervical condyloma showing microvilli and looped capillaries.

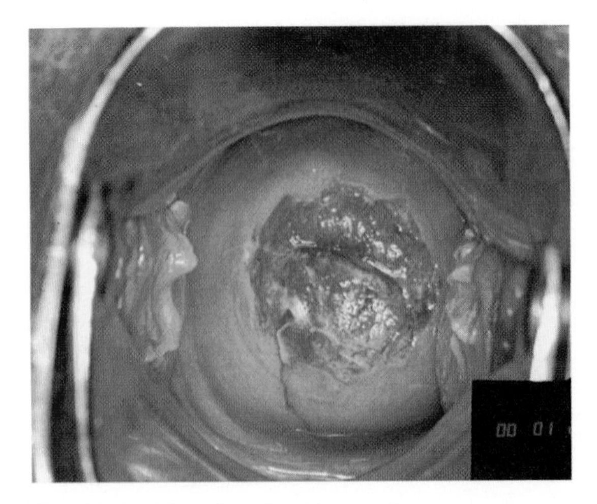

Fig. 34.11 Normal cervix with ectropion.

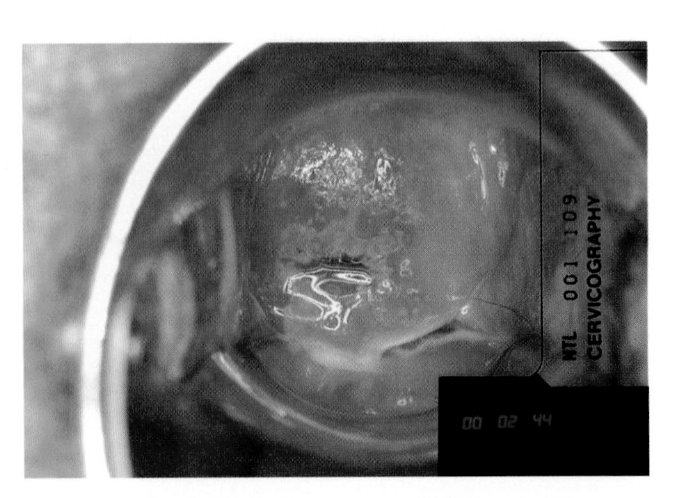

Fig. 34.12 This cervigram shows an area of faintly acetowhite epithelium around the cervical os; however, it is seen most clearly on the anterior lip in this photograph.

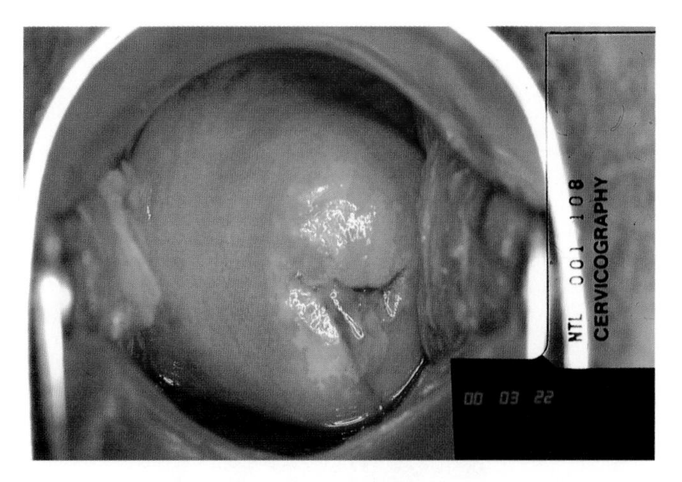

Fig. 34.13 A large, faintly acetowhite lesion with an irregular edge is visible on both lips of the cervix. Two satellite lesions are visible on the posterior lip at 6 o'clock below the main lesion.

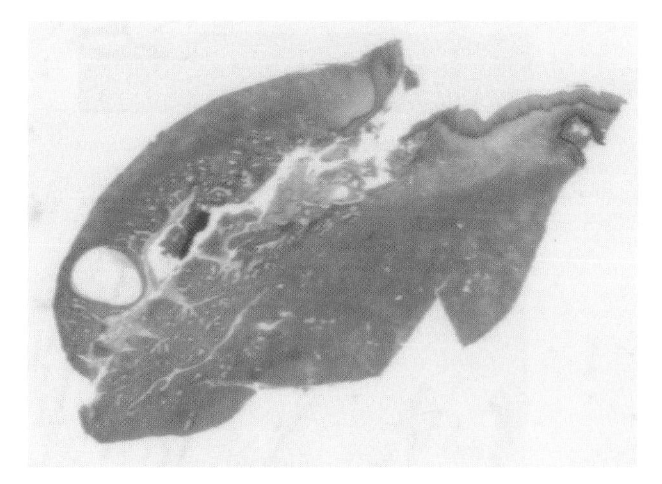

Fig. 34.15 An iatrogenic skip lesion can be seen in this cone biopsy performed in spite of a normal, satisfactory colposcopy because of severe dyskaryosis in a woman who had previously been treated with cervical electrodiathermy. The ectocervical end of this cone biopsy, to the bottom and left, is covered with normal squamous epithelium. The SCJ is near the external os and the lower canal is lined by columnar epithelium, but halfway up the canal, near the nabothian cyst on the right, is an isolated area of CIN III. In deeper sections this was shown to be an invasive tumour.

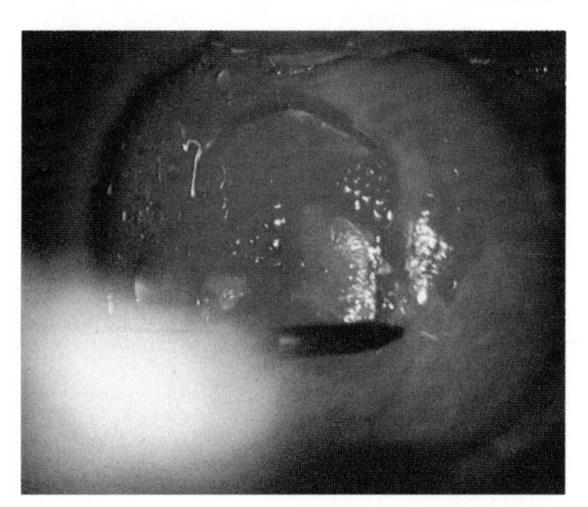

Fig. 34.17 Cone biopsy being performed with LLETZ. (Figure supplied by Valleylab UK)

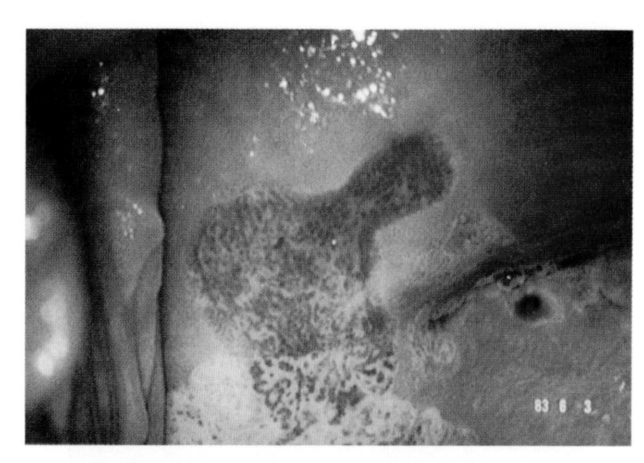

Fig. 34.14 Microinvasion with coarse punctation.

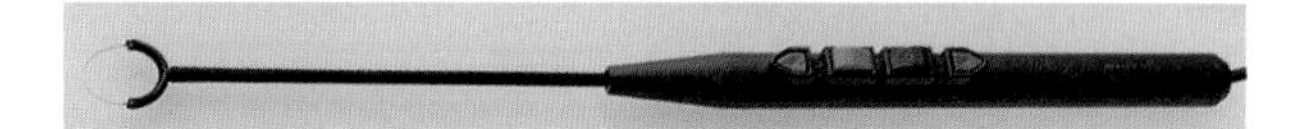

Fig. 34.16 One of the varieties of large wire loops used for LLETZ. (Figure supplied by Valleylab UK.)

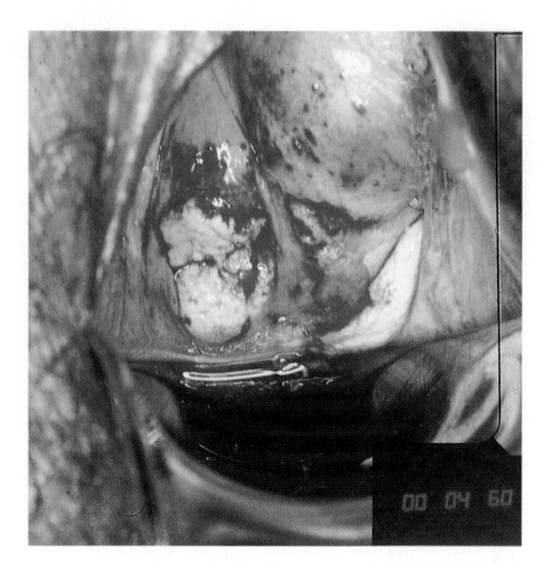

Fig. 34.19 VAIN after a hysterectomy. A patch of dense acetowhite epithelium is easily visible in the centre of the figure in the left vaginal angle. A second area of VAIN can be seen just above the speculum, spreading out of the right-angle.

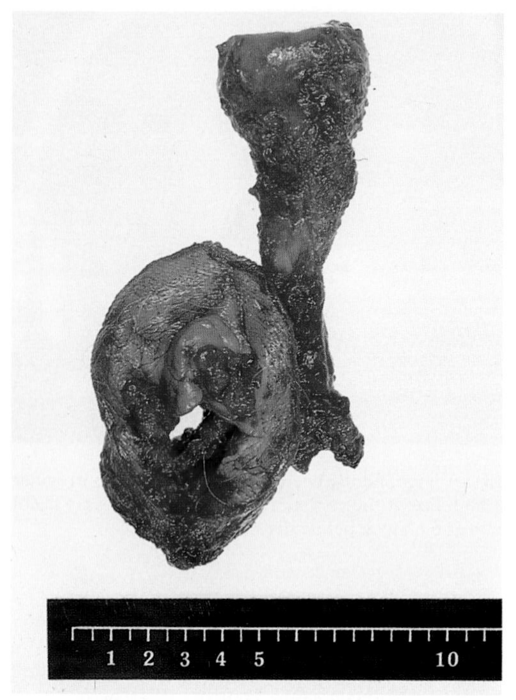

Fig. 34.20 A total vaginectomy, hysterectomy and vulvectomy performed by the vaginal route in an elderly woman with severe irritation from extensive VAIN and VIN 20 years after radiotherapy for cervical cancer (units in cm).

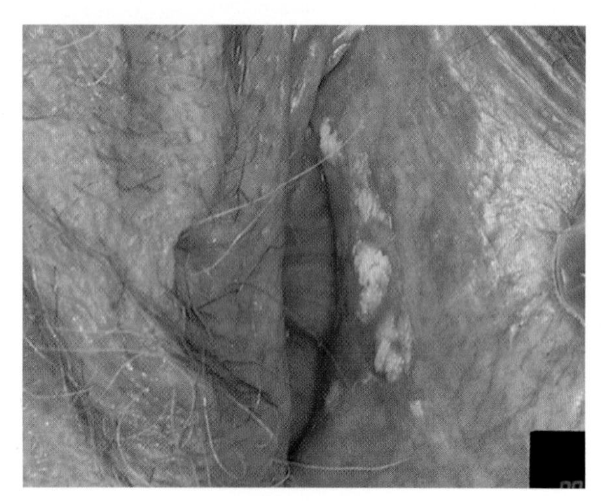

Fig. 34.21 Small patches of VIN III appearing as leukoplakia.

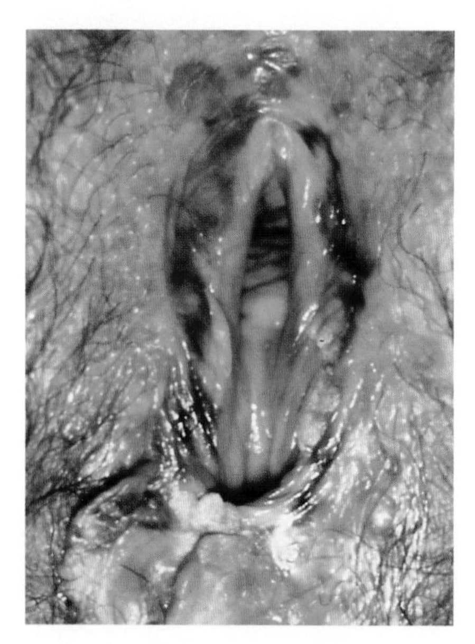

Fig. 34.22 A wide area of VIN III on the labia minora and the perineum seen as slightly raised, red lesion anteriorly, whitish lesions posteriorly and extensive dark brown lesions.

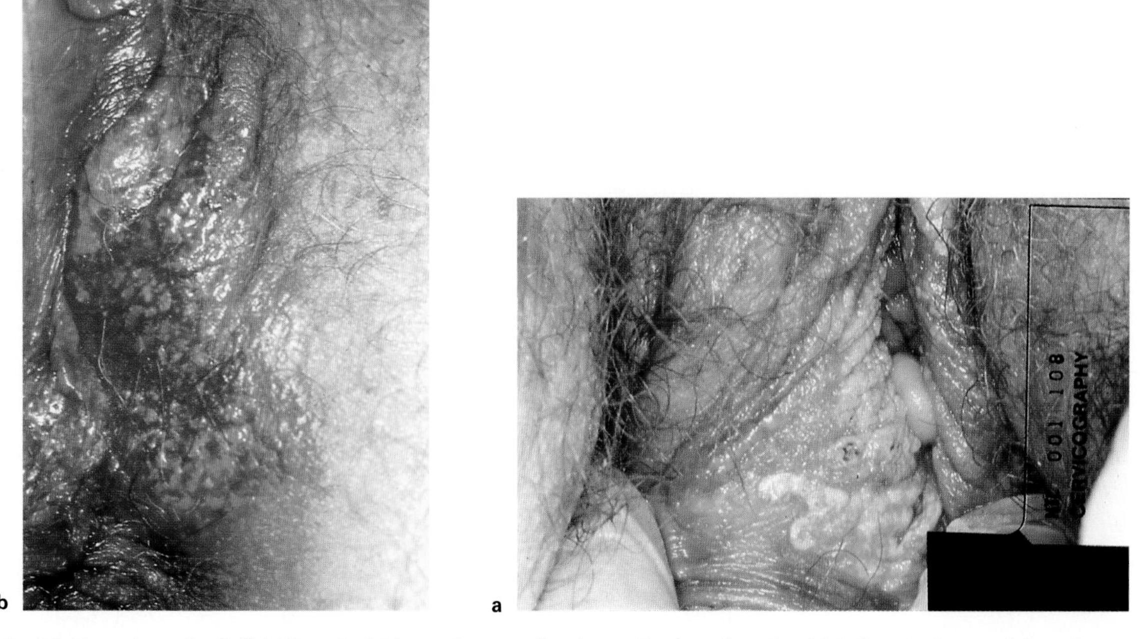

Fig. 34.23 **a** A patch of VIN III on the labium minorum after the application of acetic acid. **b** Paget's disease of the vulva. Note the red, crusted surface and clear margin.

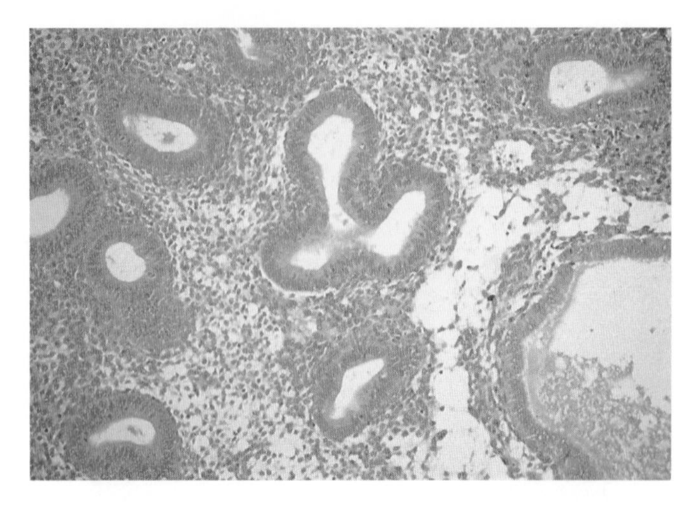

Fig. 34.24 Simple cystic hyperplasia. Haematoxylin and eosin × 100 (with kind permission of Dr Thomas Krausz).

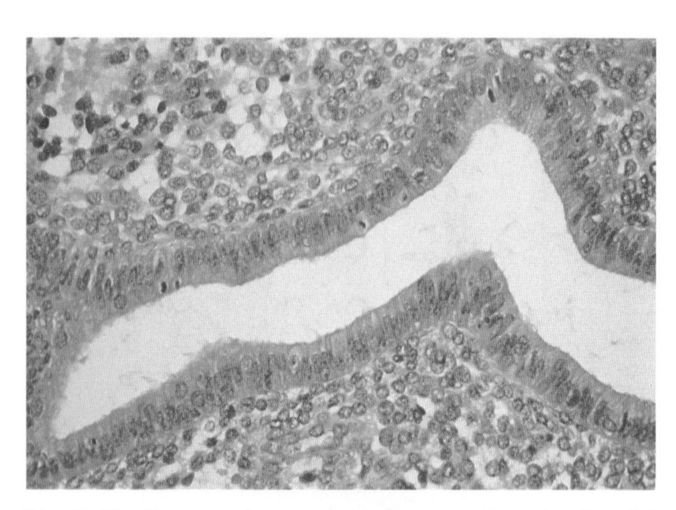

Fig. 34.25 Simple cystic hyperplasia. Haematoxylin and eosin × 250 (with kind permission of Dr Thomas Krausz).

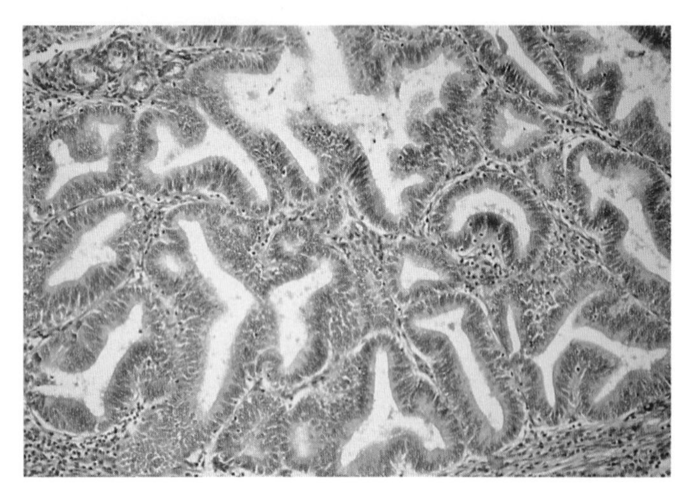

Fig. 34.26 Adenomatous hyperplasia without significant cytological atypia. Haematoxylin and eosin × 100 (with kind permission of Dr Thomas Krausz).

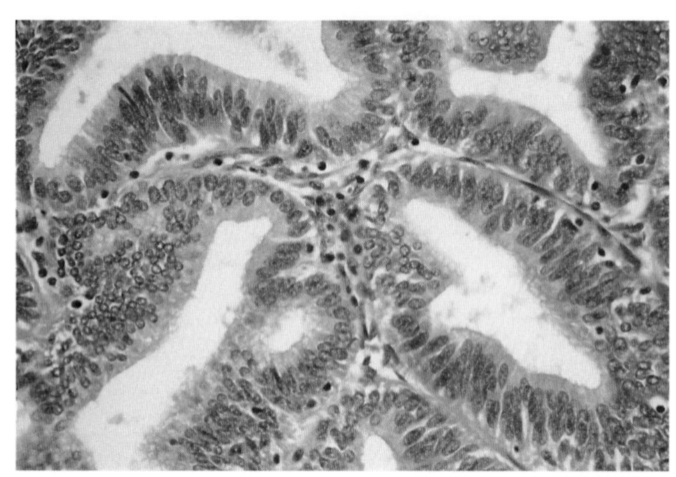

Fig. 34.27 Adenomatous hyperplasia without significant cytological atypia. Haematoxylin and eosin × 250 (with kind permission of Dr Thomas Krausz).

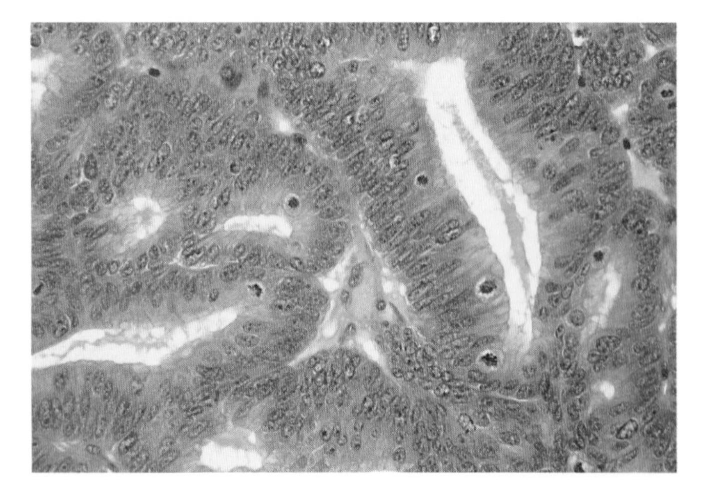

Fig. 34.28 Moderate atypical hyperplasia. Haematoxylin and eosin × 250 (with kind permission of Dr Thomas Krausz).

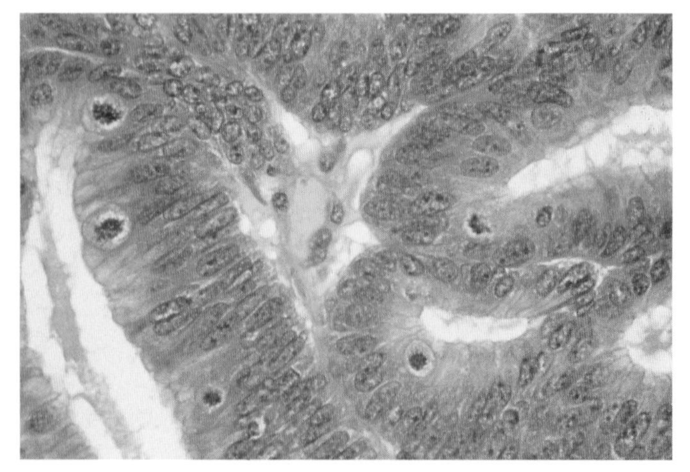

Fig. 34.29 Moderate atypical hyperplasia. Note the pseudostratification of the cells and the mitotic figures. The nuclei are plump, with some irregularity of the nuclear membrane and prominent nucleoli. Haematoxylin and eosin × 400 (with kind permission of Dr Thomas Krausz).

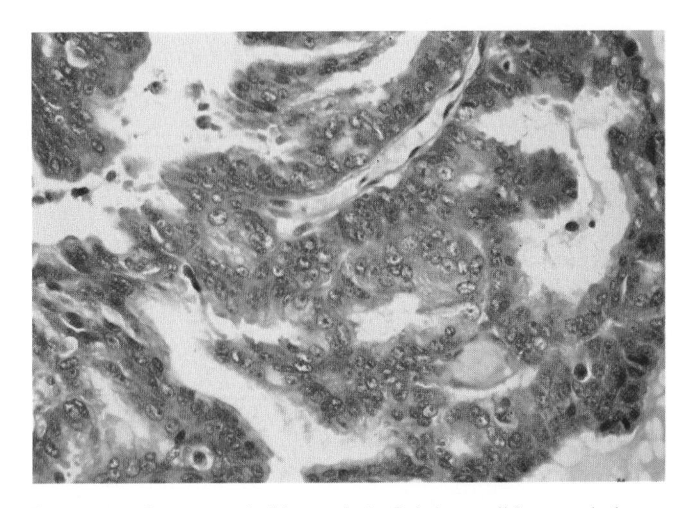

Fig. 34.30 Severe atypical hyperplasia. It is impossible to exclude invasive carcinoma from this material. Haematoxylin and eosin × 250 (with kind permission of Dr Thomas Krausz).

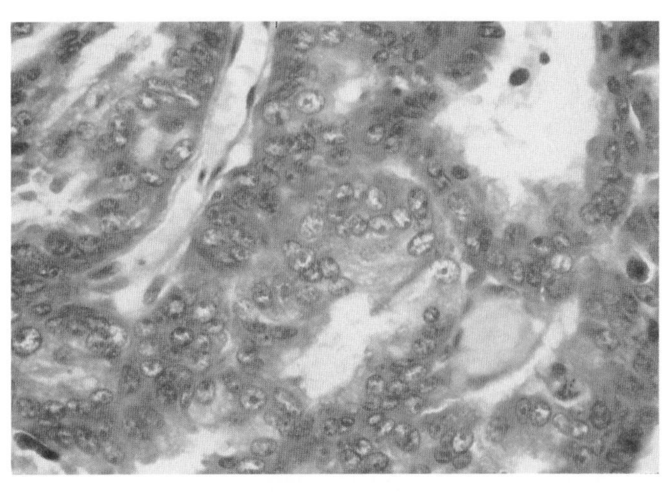

Fig. 34.31 Severe atypical hyperplasia. The nuclei are rounded and vesicular, with prominent nucleoli. Haematoxylin and eosin × 400 (with kind permission of Dr Thomas Krausz).

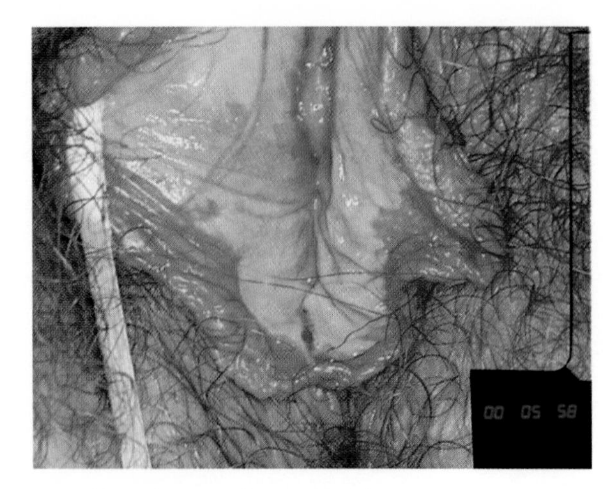

Fig. 36.2 Extensive area of acetowhite change.

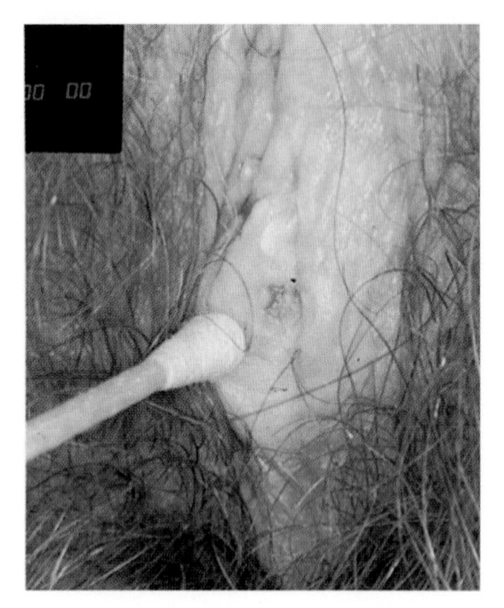

Fig. 36.4 Squamous hyperplasia with a small ulcer caused by scratching.

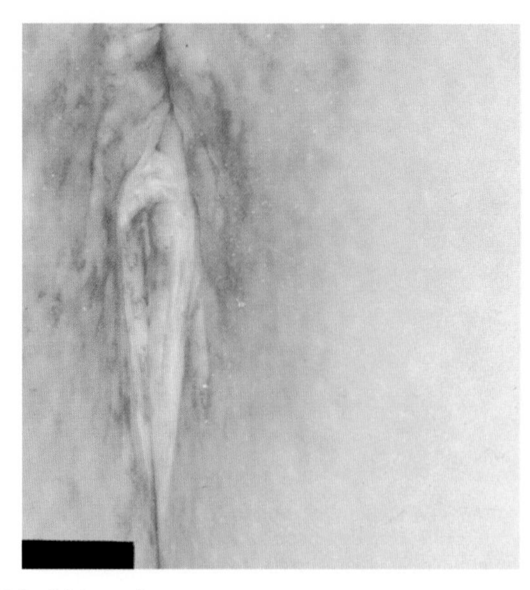

Fig. 36.3 Lichen sclerosus.

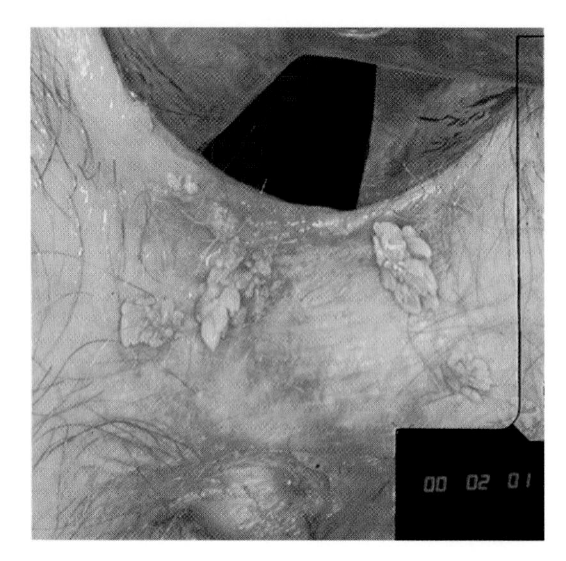

Fig. 36.6 Small genital warts at the fourchette.

Infections in Lower Genital Tract

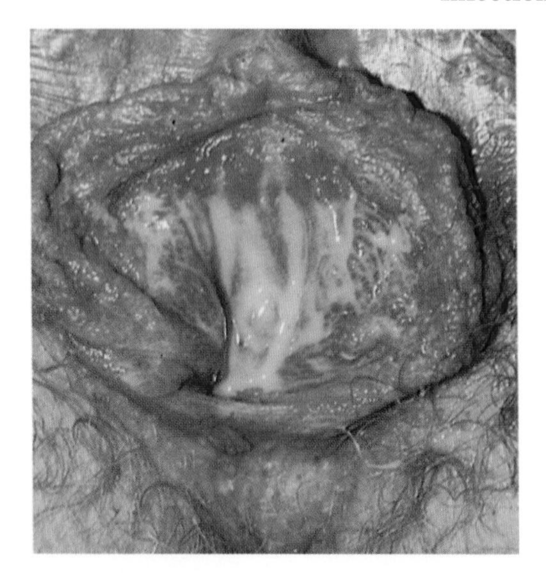

Fig. 56.17 Bacterial vaginosis.

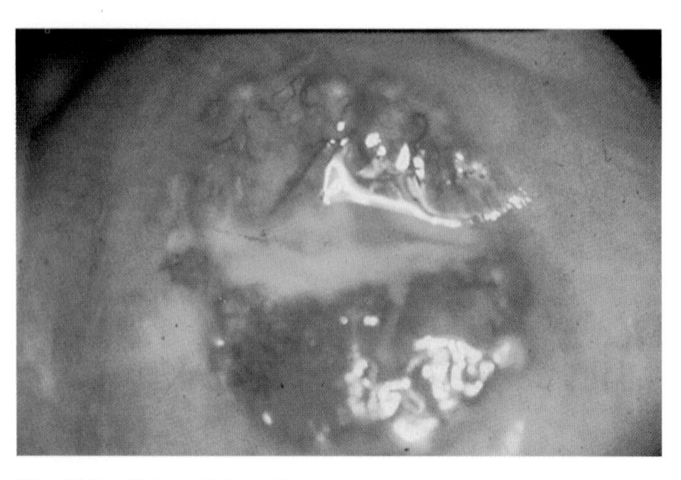

Fig. 56.8 Chlamydial cervitis.

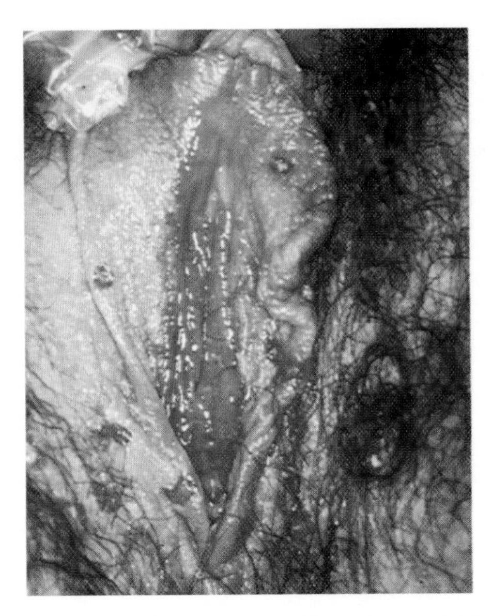

Fig. 56.13 Primary genital herpes—multiple ulcers on labia minora.

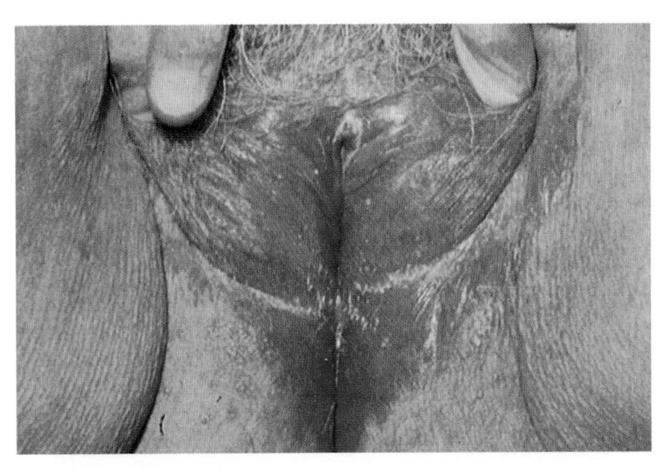

Fig. 56.19 Candida vulvitis.

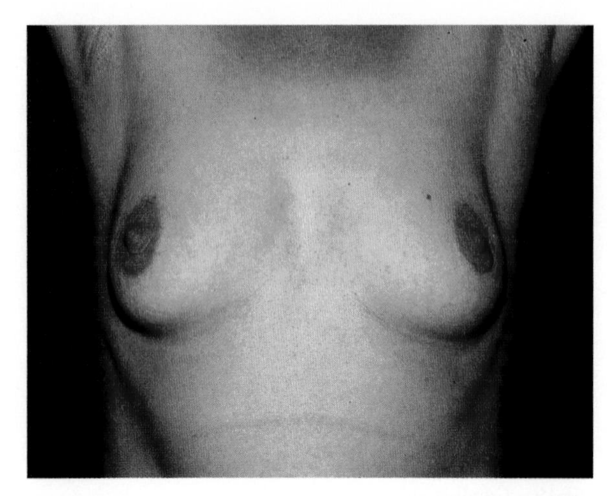

Fig. 43.4 A 34-year-old woman with a central tumour in her left breast. A biopsy was taken prior to referral.

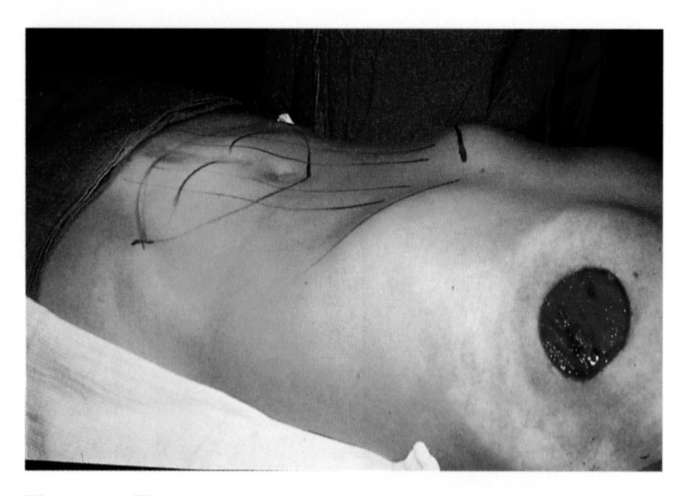

Fig. 43.5 The same patient after a periareolar mastectomy and axillary lymphadenectomy to level III. The preoperative marking of the TRAM flap is shown. A previous longitudinal incision did not interfere with the flap.

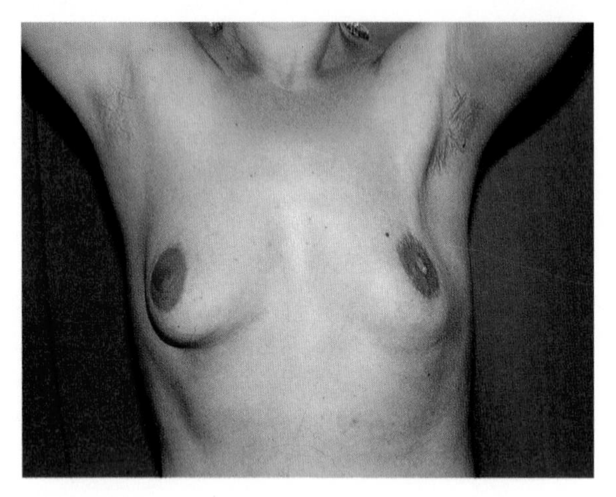

Fig. 43.6 The patient 4 months after the operation, with a reconstructed nipple and areola. The mastectomy scar is on the periareolar line.

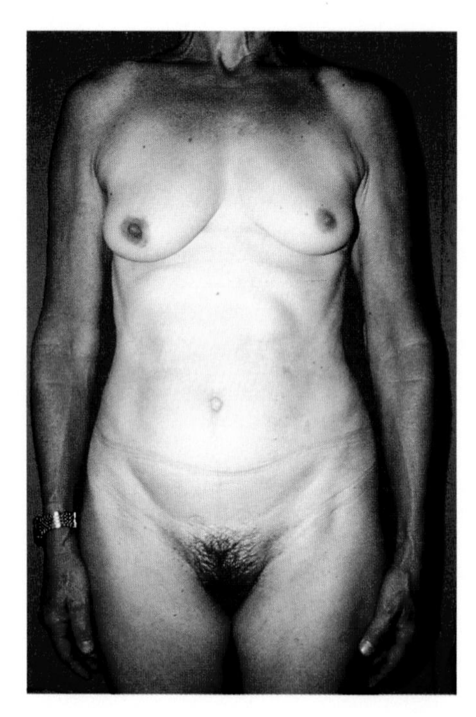

Fig. 43.7 A 42-year-old woman with a large central tumour in her right breast.

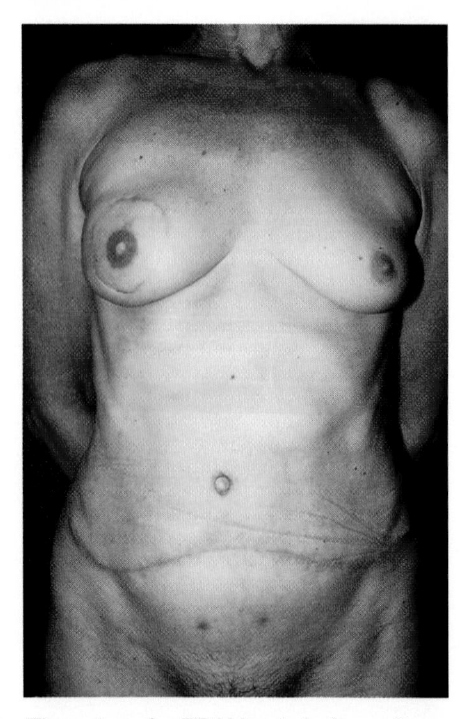

Fig. 43.8 The patient after TRAM and nipple–areola reconstruction. Note the scar on the donor area of the abdomen.

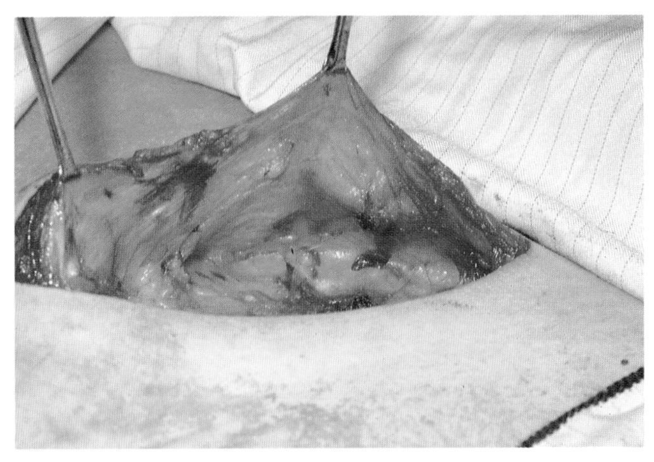

Fig. 37.3 The superficial plane deep to Camper's fascia is defined carefully, thus preserving sufficient subcutaneous fat to provide an adequate blood supply to the skin flap.

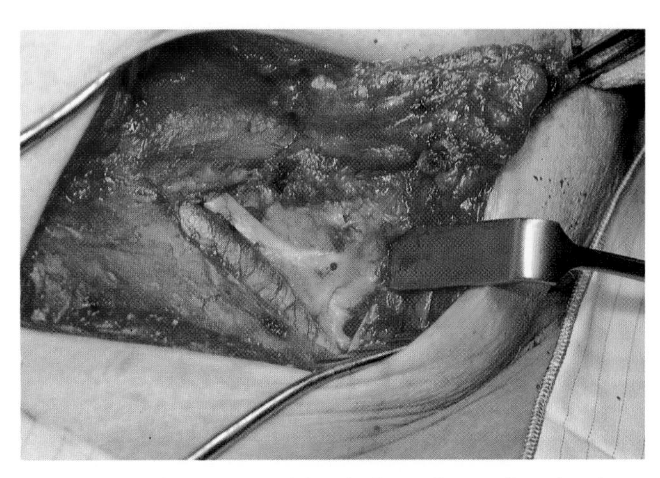

Fig. 37.4 The fascia lata overlying the femoral nerve, lateral to the femoral artery, has been preserved, but the femoral artery and the triangle medial to it have been meticulously dissected down to the surface of the adductor longus muscle posteriorly.

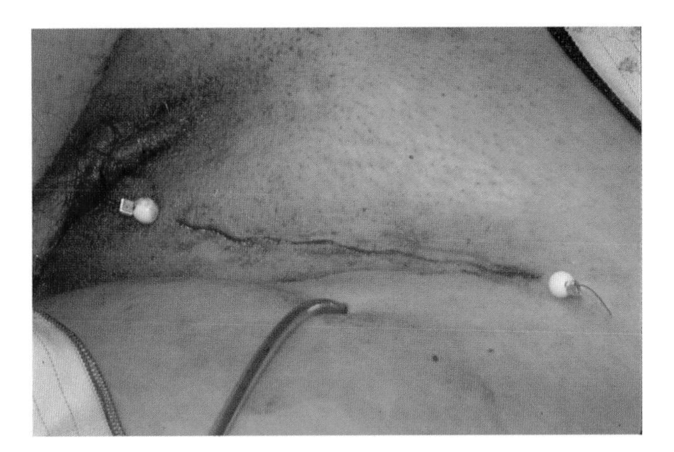

Fig. 37.5 The linear incision heals by first intention in the majority of cases, with greatly reduced morbidity.

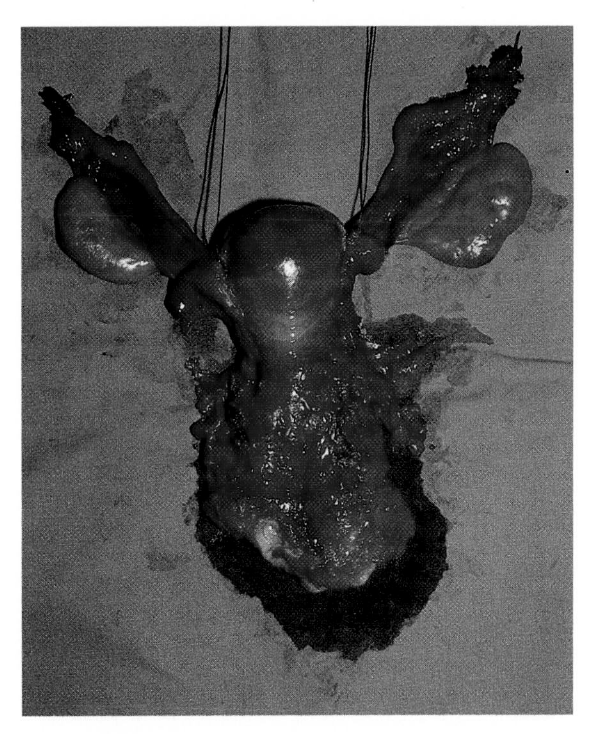

Fig. 37.6 Radical hysterectomy and total vaginectomy for Stage I carcinoma extending into the middle third of the vagina.

4

Laparoscopy

R. Garry

INTRODUCTION

The gynaecologist has long used the laparoscope for diagnostic and simple operative procedures such as tubal occlusion. Recent advances in optics, electronics and physics have allowed the development of excellent visualization systems which provide brilliant views of every part of the abdominal cavity. These new systems often provide close-up and magnified views far superior to those obtained at conventional open surgery. Such superb visualization techniques now make it possible to perform almost every type of intra-abdominal surgery through one or more small laparoscopic incisions.

The option of replacing long laparotomy incisions with small laparoscopic ones has several clear advantages. The laparoscopic incisions are much shorter and are associated with significantly less postoperative pain and less subsequent abdominal wall scarring. The laparoscopic approach also allows surgery to be performed without the need for retractors or packs. Tissue handling is avoided (thus non-touch) and tissue movements are minimized. The abdominal contents are not exposed to the air, and intra-abdominal moisture is retained preventing tissue dehydration. These benefits are all principles of good surgical technique, and the laparoscopic or minimal access approach to surgery facilitates good surgical practices (Garry 1992).

Reduced wound and intra-abdominal trauma is reflected in the need for less postoperative analgesia and consequently less postoperative drowsiness and nausea. The decrease in postoperative pain and upset is associated with rapid mobilization and reduced stay in hospital. Most patients can leave hospital within 2–4 days of surgery, no matter how extensive a laparoscopic procedure has been performed. Of even greater economic and social importance is the fact that the time required to recover and return to full activity is much reduced following laparoscopic surgery, when compared to surgery via laparotomy (Table 4.1).

These advantages are now being demonstrated daily in clinical practice. To obtain such optimal results, however, it is necessary to develop good laparoscopic techniques and to be adequately trained in this new approach to surgery. The author believes that the advantages of the minimal access approach to gynaecological surgery are so great that most operations will soon be performed in this manner.

Table 4.1 Advantages of the laparoscopic approach

More precise surgery because of superior view
Superior haemostasis
Less tissue handling and drying out
Avoids use of retractors and packs
Less pain and analgesic requirement
Less scarring
Quicker mobilization
Shorter convalescence
More rapid return to full activities
Reduced costs

ABDOMINAL DISTENSION TECHNIQUES

The abdominal cavity is only a potential space, and must be distended or elevated to permit diagnosis and surgery. It is usual to distend the cavity by infusing carbon dioxide under pressure and the most common way to introduce this gas is via a Veress needle (Veress 1938). This device consists of a sharp needle, containing within its lumen a spring-loaded gas-carrying channel. When the needle is inserted through the skin the blunt-ended gas channel is forced against its spring and into the central channel of the needle exposing the cutting edge of the needle. This sharp edge easily penetrates the various layers of the abdominal wall. When the tip enters the abdominal cavity, the gas channel, with its perforations, is released and protrudes beyond the needle tip to permit the free flow of gas.

The Veress needle minimizes, but does not totally avoid, the risk of damage to the vital structures inside the abdominal cavity. A variety of techniques have been described to ensure that the needle is correctly located in the cavity, and not placed either in the bowel or omentum or left within the layers of the abdominal wall. If a modern electronic gas insufflator is used, monitoring a combination of the gas flow rate and pressure recorded will give a good idea of accurate placement (Fig. 4.1). If the flow is rapid and the pressure does not rise substantially above preinfusion levels the needle is usually correctly located. If however the recorded pressure rises and the flow rate rapidly falls the needle must be incorrectly located and its position adjusted, and if satisfactory flow rates cannot be established in this site a different site, usually Palmer's point just below the 9th rib in the mid-clavicular line, should be chosen.

It is traditionally taught that about 2–3 l of CO_2 should be instilled prior to insertion of the primary cannula. The author, following the teaching of Harry Reich, does not agree with this advice. The single most catastrophic complication of laparoscopic surgery is the inadvertent insertion of the primary trocar into the major vessels which lie immediately below the umbilicus. Avoiding this calamity is the most essential aspect of laparoscopic technique. We believe that the larger the cushion of gas which is placed between the umbilicus and the aorta, the safer will be the insertion. We therefore recommend that the maximum infusion pressure on the insufflator be set *for the period of the first trocar insertion only* at a level of 25 mmHg pressure. Gas flow continues until this pressure is reached which may take from 4–12 l of CO_2. Such a volume ensures that the abdominal wall is stretched drum-tight, and is correspondingly much easier to penetrate in a controlled way than less tense abdominal walls. Such a volume also increases to a maximum the size of the 'gas bubble', and therefore ensures that the safety zone for insertion is as large as possible (Table 4.2).

Table 4.2 A technique for primary trocar insertion

Vertical intraumbilical skin incision
Initial intra-abdominal pressure at 25 mmHg
Large CO_2 gas bubble
Short length trocar
Shaft of trocar protected with extended index finger
Vertical insertion of trocar through thinnest part of abdominal wall

Theoretical objections to using this high infusion pressure include the risks of causing respiratory embarrassment and producing a CO_2 venous embolism. The former does not occur because all our patients undergoing laparoscopic surgery are mechanically ventilated, and careful monitoring of respiratory gases demonstrate no changes in the short time it takes to insert the first trocar. We have had no misadventures in many thousands of laparoscopies using this technique. It is important, however, to ensure that the intra-abdominal pressure is reduced to the conventional 15 mmHg pressure once the first trocar is satisfactorily in position.

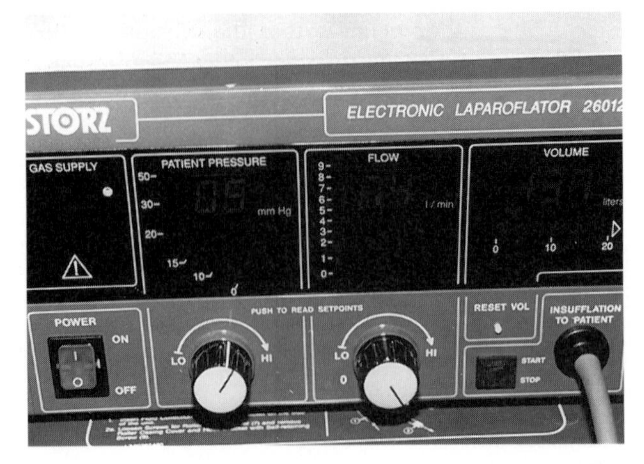

Fig. 4.1 A modern electronic insufflator with a maximum flow of 9 l/min, a large capacity gas store and facilities for measuring intra-abdominal pressure and rate of gas flow.

Gasless laparoscopy

An alternative technique for creating a workable abdominal cavity has recently been described (Chin et al 1993, Wood et al 1994). Instead of distending the cavity with gas under pressure, the anterior abdominal wall may be supported by a mechanical elevator. A variety of abdominal wall elevators are now available. Each works on the principle of inserting a rigid mechanical support through one or more holes in the abdomen. The elevator is then pulled vertically upwards and secured in such a position as to keep the anterior abdominal wall raised and under tension. Such elevators may use sophisticated electronic jacks or simpler suspensory chains attached under tension to a drip stand (e.g. the Maher elevator and the Phipps C arm).

The advantages of the gasless system include avoidance

of the need for CO_2 gas and the associated insufflators and their possible complications. This system also permits simpler and more economical trocars, without gas traps, to be used. It is also possible to open the vaginal vault and the abdomen without losing vision, raising the possibility of performing joint laparovaginal procedures in a way not possible with gas distension systems.

Disadvantages of this type of system include the risk of trauma and pressure ischaemia to the abdominal wall, and a triangular rather than cylindrical shape of cavity distension with possible adverse effects on lateral pelvic wall visualization. Gas under pressure also forces loops of small bowel into the upper abdomen. Lack of this pressure allows the bowel to 'creep' repeatedly into the operating field with impairment of access and operating conditions in the pelvis.

CHOICE OF TROCARS

Piston valve trocars

All gynaecologists will be familiar with the classical stainless steel reusable piston valve trocars (Fig. 4.2). These have been widely used and are well made and economical. They have, however, several design faults which make them, in the author's opinion, unsuitable for advanced operative laparoscopy. The piston valve must be depressed every time an instrument is inserted or withdrawn. As both the surgeon and the assistant are frequently already holding operative instruments, such an extra requirement is always inconvenient and often impractical. Improved and simplified valve mechanisms are preferred.

The traditional trocar and sheath is too long for most patients, so that it lies either too far inside the cavity, in a position which prevents the proper opening of the surgical instruments, or so far above the abdominal wall that its proximal end flaps about in a way which prevents easy insertion of instruments. In addition the shaft of the trocar sheath is polished steel and is inherently slippery. It therefore has a tendency to both slip into the wound up to the valve level and to be inadvertently pulled out of the incision with the removal of an instrument or specimen from the cavity. This can lead to frustration, loss of the pneumoperitoneum and delay.

In an attempt to overcome these positional problems and to prevent unintended removal of the sheath, some manufacturers have produced plastic fixation collars which can hold the trocar firmly in the desired position in the abdominal wall. This mixture of steel sheath and plastic collar is mechanically stable but electrically very dangerous, and should never be used. Such hybrid systems insulate the metal sheath from the earthed abdominal wall. In the event of a build-up of electrical charge, because of faulty insulation or capacitative coupling, the electrical energy cannot be harmlessly dissipated and may instead arc to intra-abdominal structures, such as bowel, with possibly catastrophic consequences.

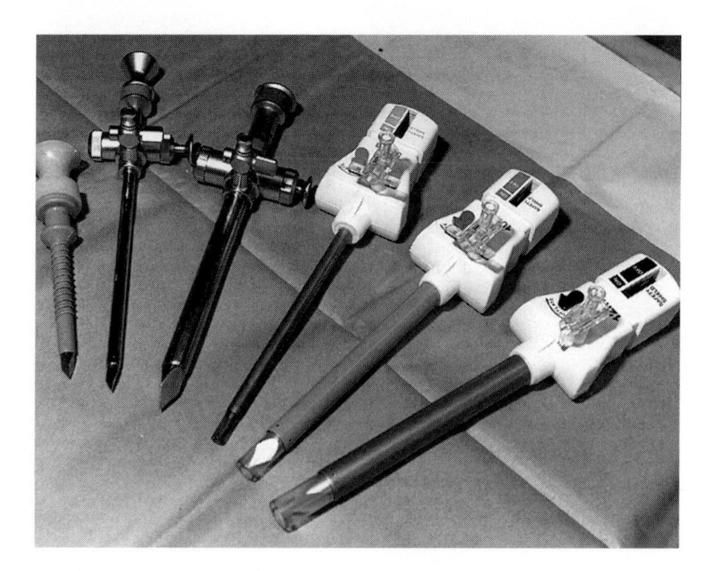

Fig. 4.2 A selection of trocars: left, a short 5-mm Apple trocar; centre, 5- and 10-mm piston valve trocars; right, 5-, 10- and 12-mm AutoSuture shielded trocars.

Shielded trocars

Some larger manufacturers have produced a new design of trocar, with flap valves to facilitate easy insertion and removal of instruments. Another major feature of this type of trocar is that the sharp tip of the trocar is covered or protected by a so-called 'safety shield'. The shield is a spring-loaded protective device which is pushed back to expose the sharp point of the trocar when it is forced through the firm tissues of the abdominal wall. The shield is then supposed to spring back instantly to cover the point of the trocar when it enters the low resistance abdominal cavity. The protection offered by this safety device is at best only partial, and there are many cases where damage to intra-abdominal structures has followed the use of 'safety shields'.

I believe that many designs for this type of shield in fact make the smooth and progressive insertion of the trocar more difficult, and hence potentially more dangerous. The greatest disadvantage of this type of trocar is, however, its cost. The protective shields are mechanically complex and expensive to make and this very complexity means that these well-made instruments cannot be adequately cleaned and so must be discarded after a single use. Recently, smaller manufacturers, spotting a niche market, have produced shielded but reusable devices which might make this approach more economical for those who believe it may be of value.

Miscellaneous trocar designs

An increasingly wide variety of novel designs for laparoscopic access are now becoming available. The features that these designs have in common include shorter trocar length, some form of atraumatic fixing device and a valve mechanism which facilitates easy instrument exchange (Reich & McGlynn 1990). Most abdominal walls are only a few centimetres thick and any trocar length greater than that required to pass through the wall is both unnecessary and a hindrance to good laparoscopic surgery. The standard trocar length is 10 cm, but in routine use lengths longer than 6–7 cm are seldom required.

Trocars can be fixed at the optimal level with a variety of different techniques including an inflatable balloon (e.g. Marlow), adjustable collar (Dexide), and screw threads (e.g. Apple). The author favours the simplest design which can be easily cleaned and reused, as he believes that it is good technique and not sophisticated design which will ensure the lowest risk of trocar-induced injury.

TECHNIQUES FOR PRIMARY TROCAR INSERTION

The initial skin incision for the first trocar is often made in a transverse manner just below the umbilicus. Hasson (1978) has clearly shown that the anatomy of the periumbilical area is such that a vertical incision actually in the umbilicus is to be preferred. At the umbilicus there is little fat no matter how obese the patient is. The abdominal wall is therefore at its thinnest at this point and easiest to enter. Moreover the parietal layer of peritoneum is firmly adherent at the umbilicus, but not elsewhere, on the anterior wall (Fig. 4.3). An insertion within the umbilicus is less likely to remain in an extraperitoneal position and in my opinion is the site of choice for insertion of the primary trocar.

It is most often advised that the first trocar should be inserted at an angle of 45° in the direction of the pelvis. Reference to Figure 4.3 will confirm that this route means the trocar passes a considerable, variable and inconsistent distance through the abdominal wall. Some authorities

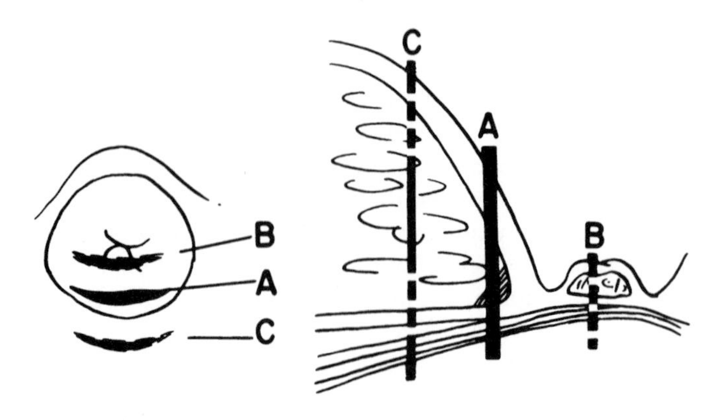

Fig. 4.3 The anterior abdominal wall at the level of the umbilicus (after Hasson 1978).

recommend a Z- or <-shaped type of insertion, with an even longer and less consistent distance through the abdominal wall. We recommend a vertical insertion through the umbilicus but *only when using a short trocar* down which an outstretched index finger can be laid to limit the maximum possible depth of insertion of the trocar to no more than 1 cm (Figs 4.4, 4.5).

We believe that the safest possible primary trocar entry is obtained with a combination of:

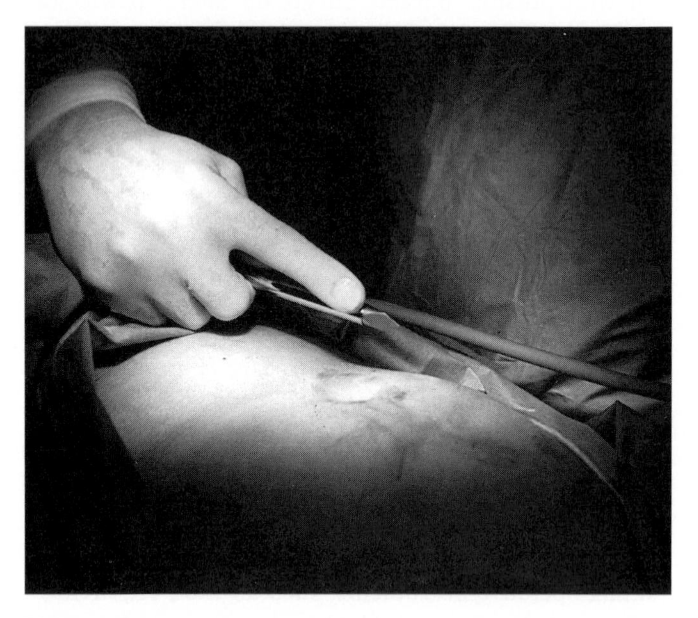

Fig. 4.4 Primary trocar, guarded by the extended index finger to leave only the sharp point of the trocar exposed.

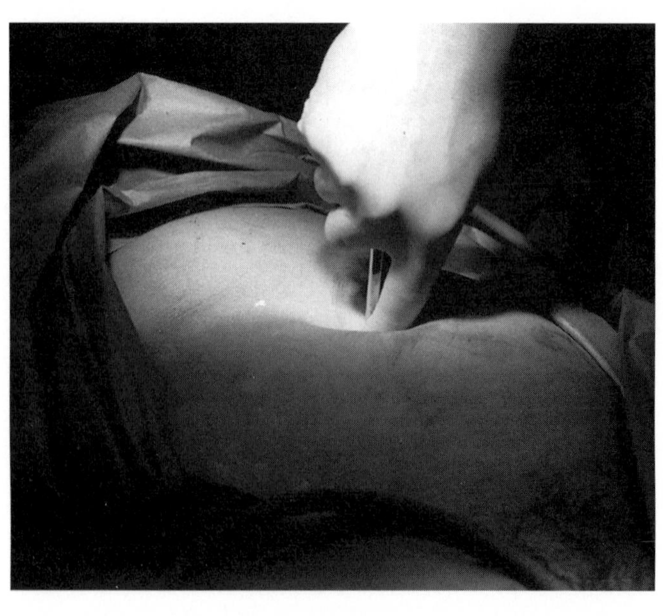

Fig. 4.5 Vertical insertion of the trocar through the intraumbilical incision. Note this must only be attempted with a high intra-abdominal pressure and a short trocar with the point guarded as shown.

1. the shortest possible route through the abdomen;
2. the largest possible distance between the umbilicus and the major vessels;
3. the shortest length of trocar;
4. the least unguarded length of trocar.

Open laparoscopy

Hasson described and developed an alternative system of laparoscopic entry which avoided the need to insert the first trocar blindly. He suggested a system of 'open laparoscopy' (Hasson 1978) in which the rectus sheath is incised and the peritoneum open under direct vision. A blunt-ended trocar sheath is then inserted down the tract and secured by a pair of sutures through the rectus sheath. Once the sheath is secured in an airtight position CO_2 is rapidly infused through the large diameter sheath and the contents of the abdomen visualized in the standard manner (Fig. 4.6).

This direct dissection technique was introduced to reduce the risk of trauma and damage to any loops of bowel morbidly adherent to the anterior abdominal wall. On occasions direct visualization may facilitate this, but as any surgeon who has inadvertently damaged the bowel during a standard laparotomy incision knows, direct vision in this manner does not necessarily guarantee that bowel damage will be avoided.

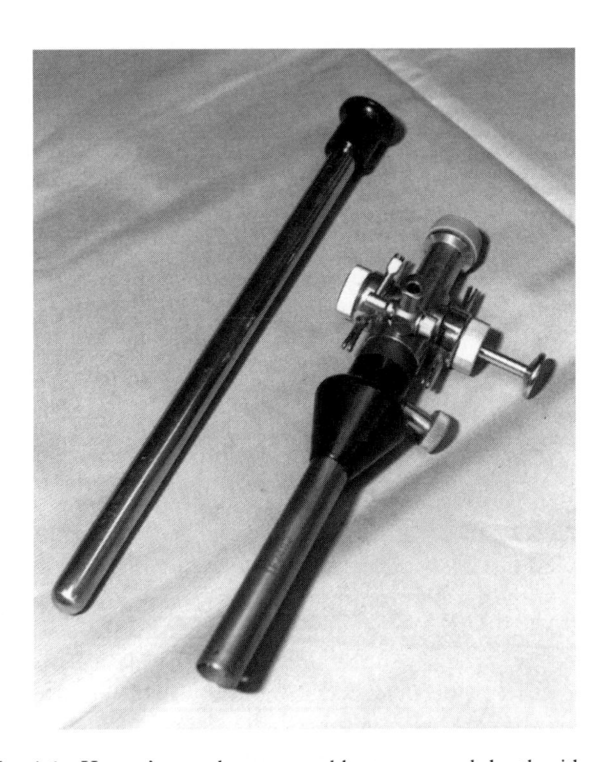

Fig. 4.6 Hasson's open laparoscopy blunt trocar and sheath with movable cone and fixing pegs on collar.

SECONDARY TROCAR INSERTION

It is often suggested that the right and left lower entry ports should be inserted medial to the inferior epigastric arteries in the so called 'safety triangle'. This position, however, greatly reduces the space for manoeuvre of the instruments and means that the trocars must go through the thickness of the rectus muscle. The author believes that lower quadrant trocars should be inserted laterally outside of the rectus muscle and through the thinner oblique muscles of the abdominal wall (Fig. 4.7).

The major danger when inserting lower lateral trocars is damage to the inferior epigastric vessels. It has traditionally been taught that these vessels can be visualized by 'transillumination'. With this technique the light source of the laparoscope is brought into contact with the abdominal wall in an attempt to outline the major vessels of the anterior abdominal wall. Unless the patient is extraordinarily thin the important deep epigastric vessels are not seen with this technique. Transillumination does often demonstrate the superficial epigastric vessels and should be used to identify and enable the operator to avoid these blood vessels. The deep epigastric vessels can usually be seen by direct laparoscopic inspection of the interior surface of the anterior wall where the artery will be seen to be arising from the region of the round ligament and ascending on the posterior surface of the rectus muscle. The artery will be accompanied on either side by a diagnostic pair of vennae commitantes (Fig. 4.8). If this vessel complex is identified laparoscopically, and the superficial vessels are visualized by simultaneous transillumination, an avascular area can be reliably identified, lateral to the line of the

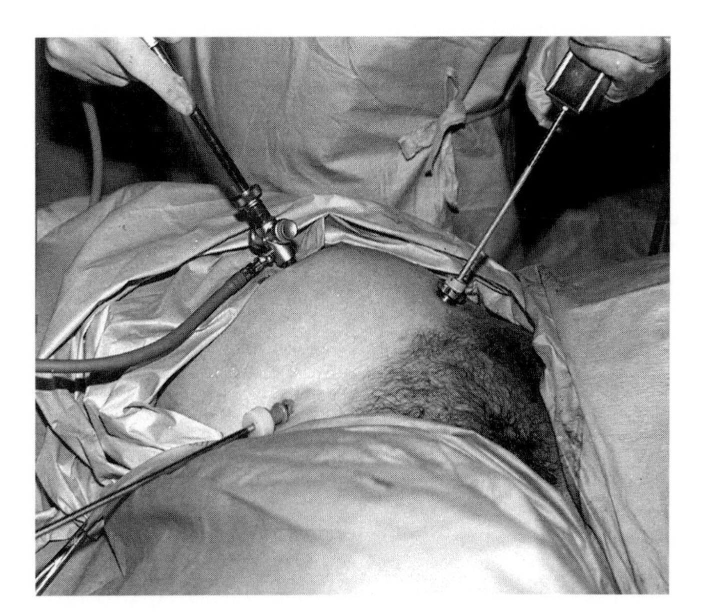

Fig. 4.7 Position of two 5-mm lower lateral ports inserted outside the line of the rectus muscle and the inferior epigastric vessels.

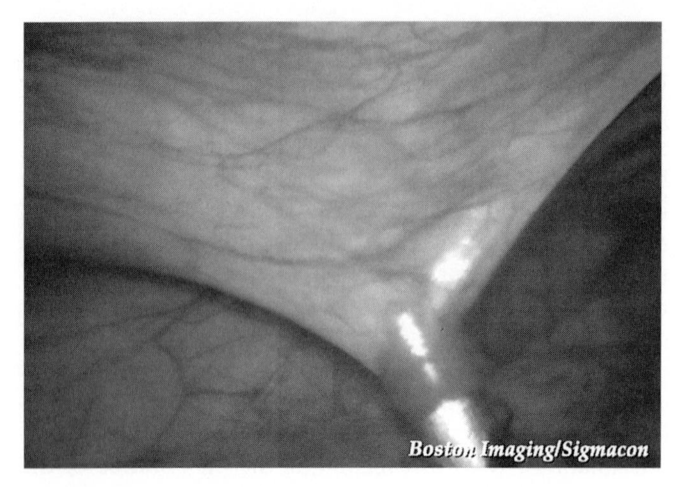

Fig. 4.8 Inferior epigastric vessels medial to the lower lateral port. (Reproduced in colour on Plate 3.)

outer border of the rectus muscle, for insertion of the lower right and left trocars.

MISCELLANEOUS EQUIPMENT

Insufflation equipment

The need for a modern electronically controlled CO_2 insufflator has already been implied. The most important feature of such a device is that the machine must communicate directly to a large volume cylinder of CO_2 gas. Early machines took gas from a cylinder and stored it in a second low-volume tank inside the insufflator. Such an internal tank usually had a capacity of 10–12 l. A difficult laparoscopic procedure may use many hundreds of litres of CO_2 during the surgery. It is clearly unacceptable that the tank should need to be refilled every minute or so during a prolonged procedure.

Gas is often lost at a rapid rate particularly during aspiration procedures. As suction aspiration is often performed to remove blood and provide a view of an actively bleeding damaged vessel, it is clearly inappropriate to lose vision because of aspiration of gas at such moments. Modern insufflators should be able to replace all the gas lost during aspiration, and must have the ability to pump in large volumes of gas rapidly. A maximum insufflation rate of 9 l/min is usually adequate although pumps with a capacity of 16 or even 32 l/min have been described (Fig. 4.1).

Laparoscopes

Excellent exposure and vision throughout the procedure is an essential prerequisite of any type of surgery. First-rate optics contribute to excellent vision during laparoscopy. Usually a 10-mm diameter optic is used with a sequence of Hopkins rod lenses relayed in the barrel of the laparoscope (Fig. 4.9). Replacing a series of thin glass lenses in a tube, separated by large distances of air, with long rod lenses separated by very little air improves the quality of the image significantly. Such 'Hopkin rod lenses' are now routinely used in solid endoscopes.

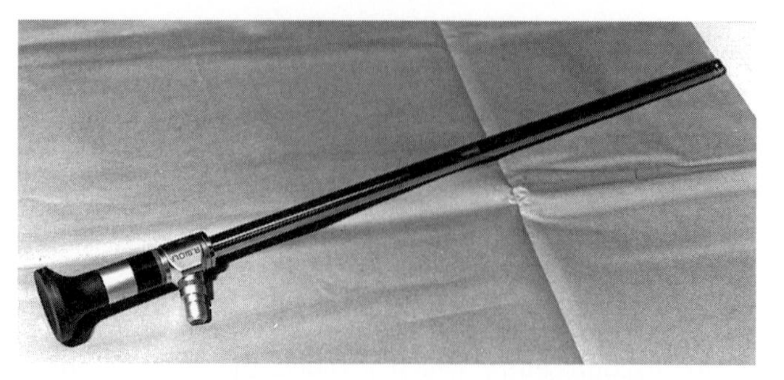

Fig. 4.9 A 10-mm laparoscope.

If lasers are to be used, and in some other circumstances, an 'operative laparoscope' is preferred. In this configuration a 10-mm outside diameter contains a 5-mm optic path combined with a 5-mm operating channel. This results in a somewhat smaller or poorer image which must be offset against the increased versatility of the operating laparoscope (Fig. 4.10). For diagnostic purposes, a 5-mm diameter laparoscope may be adequate, and such a smaller diameter scope should be on every major laparoscopic surgical tray.

Light sources

Light sources are important and a high intensity 'cold light' source is essential for videolaparoscopy. A 150 W xenon or halogen light is most commonly preferred. Such light sources are not at all 'cold' and indeed they generate considerable quantities of heat. They are so termed because the light box and its associated heat can be located a considerable distance from the patient, and the light is transmitted to the required place via a flexible quartz fibre light cable. These flexible cables consist of many individual quartz fibres each wrapped in light-reflecting cladding. These fibres may fracture and every fibre which breaks no longer transmits light. Care of, and periodic replacement of flexible light cables is essential to maintain optimal vision.

High quality CCD compact video systems are no longer expensive luxuries for the privileged laparoscopic surgeon. Complex laparoscopic surgical procedures, like conventional surgery, require informed medical and nursing assistance. The latter can only be provided if the assistant can see the operative view and the only practical way in which this can be provided is by the use of high quality small video camera systems. Such systems also allow the surgeon to adopt a reasonably comfortable upright position which is essential for performing prolonged surgery. It is

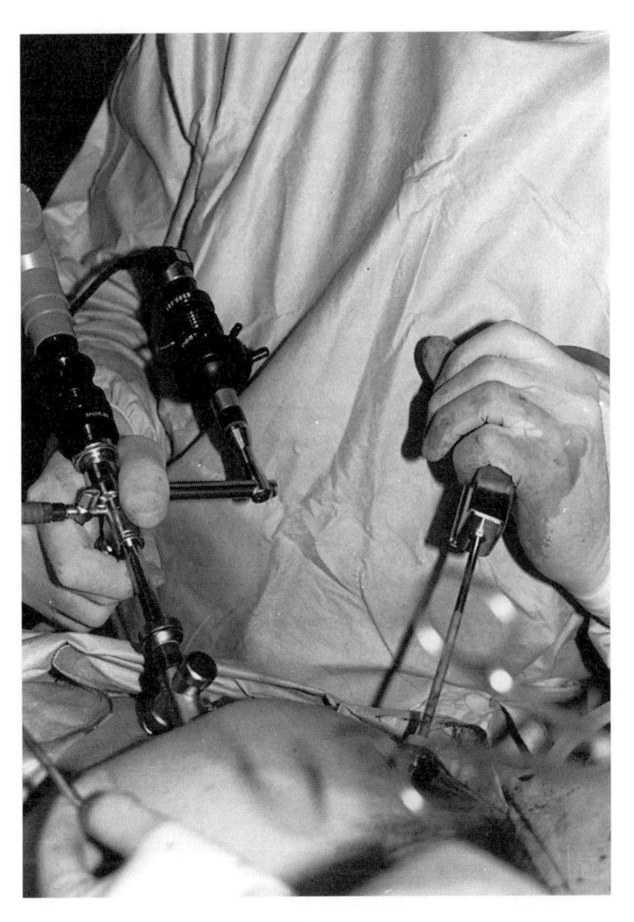

Fig. 4.10 An operating laparoscope with crank-handle type optic and a 5-mm operative channel connected to a carbon dioxide laser.

impossible to crouch over the patient for the many hours which some of these laparoscopic procedures require (Fig. 4.11).

Most systems used a very compact single-chip video camera. At the heart of such a system is a single chip made up of 500 × 600 individual pixels. Each pixel is covered by a coloured filter so that each is only sensitive to red, green or blue. Each three different coloured pixels are linked to form a single bit. Such 'single chip' cameras have become smaller and yet capable of giving better colour and resolution than was thought possible even a few years ago. These single-chip systems are the mostly widely used system at present.

Better colour resolution and picture quality can be obtained with 'three-chip' camera systems. With such a system, a prism splits the image into three separate components focused on different chips, each sensitive to a single colour. These systems are more bulky and more expensive, and these disadvantages must be offset against the more accurate image produced. Further advances in image quality will probably include the development of high definition television. At the time of writing, such excellent visualization systems are only a research tool and cost in excess of £500 000 each.

Three-dimensional laparoscopy is a theoretical advance in imaging. Depth perception is clearly improved with such systems, and several are now commercially available. They are, however, significantly more expensive and require viewers to wear active or passive Polaroid spectacles. The image brightness and quality is not yet as good as that

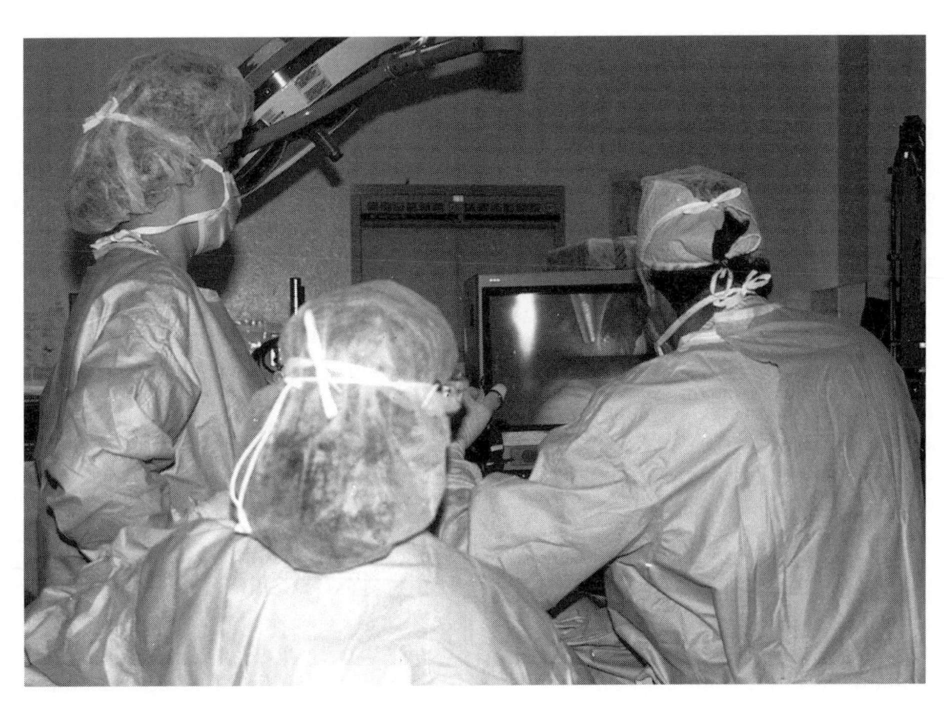

Fig. 4.11 The surgical field seen on the video screen.

achieved with two-dimensional systems; a three-dimensional system with an image quality equivalent to that available from more conventional, but highly developed, two-dimensional systems remains to be developed.

SURGICAL EQUIPMENT

The requirements for good surgery are similar whatever the mode of access. Tissues must be divided, haemostasis secured, the specimen removed and then the divided tissues repaired and wounds closed. A baffling array of high-tech devices and equipment have been suggested as desirable, or even essential, for performing these functions when the surgery is performed by the laparoscopic route. Some advanced technical equipment is helpful in laparoscopic surgery, but it is now clear that in the hands of skilled and appropriate trained surgeons even the most advanced procedures can be performed with the use of only laparoscopic scissors, grasping forceps, sutures, diathermy and a suction irrigator.

Tissue division and haemostasis

Tissue may be divided using scissors, electrodiathermy, a variety of lasers or a number of other mechanical and electronic devices. Division of living tissues is inevitably associated with division of blood vessels and the consequent problems of bleeding and haemostasis. The surgical ideal is to produce a fine and precise incision with simultaneous secure haemostasis. Unfortunately these two aims appear incompatible. A precise incision involves minimal lateral damage and thus no haemostasis. An incision with considerable lateral thermal or mechanical damage will occlude blood vessels and produce haemostasis but at the inevitable cost of a wider and less precise incision line. Any modality which produces precise cutting has poor haemostatic properties, and conversely any device which cuts with good haemostasis has relatively poor cutting properties. When choosing an instrument for laparoscopic tissue division the surgeon must select the modality or modalities which give the best compromise between cutting and haemostasis.

Laparoscopic scissors

The simplest, and in many surgeons' hands still the best tool for accurate tissue division, is a pair of scissors. Just as in open surgery, a variety of different types should be available for different purposes. Three or four main types should be available (Fig. 4.12):

1. a pair of sturdy hooked or 'Mayo' type scissors for cutting sutures and tough tissues;
2. a pair of curved scissors with round tips and smooth blades, or 'Metzenbam' type, for general tissue-cutting work;
3. a pair of flat scissors with rounded ends, which are often called 'peritoneal scissors', and are of particular value in cutting thinner structures such as peritoneum;
4. a pair of micro scissors that have small sharp blades and needle-sharp points.

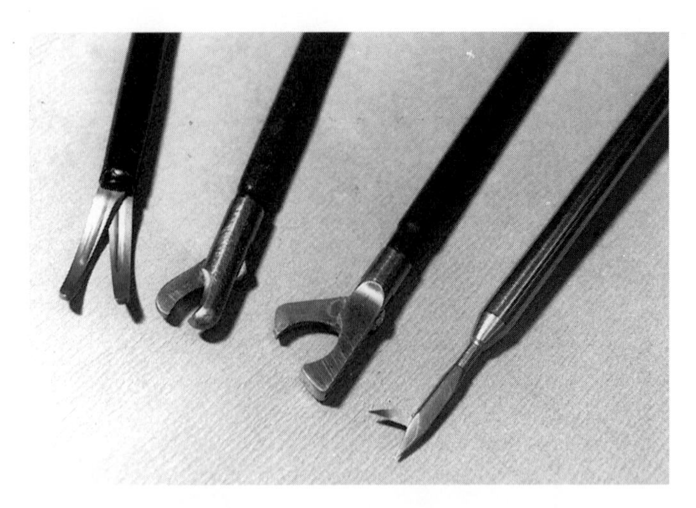

Fig. 4.12 Various types of laparoscopic scissors.

With good quality appropriately designed scissors, all types of surgical dissection can be accomplished. The incisions produced however will bleed. Smaller vessel bleeding can often be controlled by using scissors with a monopolar electrical facility. Application of electrical energy will produce some lateral tissue heating and consequent haemostasis. The blades of the scissors are first held slightly apart with the tissue containing the small vessels between. In this position passage of the current will produce a significant coagulation effect. Following this the blades can be closed and the tissues divided in a simple mechanical manner. Such a tool can be useful but produces a less precise incision. The other disadvantage of using such combined cutting and electrosurgical modalities is that the blades of the scissors become blunt very quickly, and so many enthusiasts for this combined technique often prefer the use of disposable single-use products.

An alternative way to utilize scissors is to use them in conjunction with separate bipolar diathermy forceps (Odell 1993). This technique, which is favoured by the author, requires the bipolar forceps to be used in a manner analogous to a haemostatic clamp in conventional surgery. The bipolar forceps are first applied to the tissue to be divided. A 'Kleppinger'-shaped forceps ensures that the tissues between the blades, including any vessels, are compressed. When the anterior and posterior walls of the vessels are coapted and then heated by the passage of electrical current between the forceps blades until desiccated, the tissue collagen fuses and occludes the vessels. There is significant spread of the thermal effect, as shown by

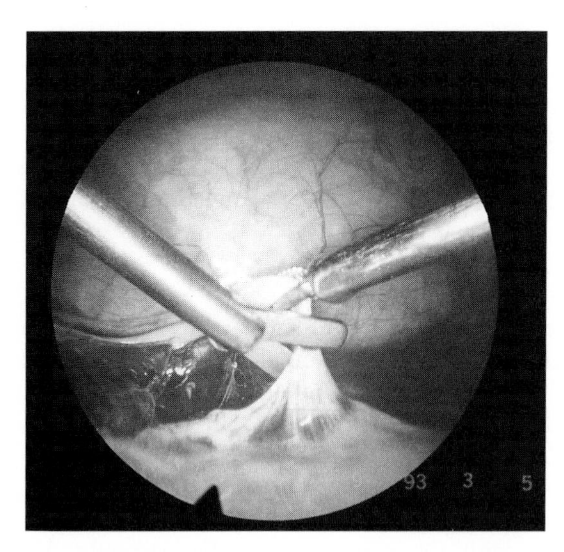

Fig. 4.13 Cutting the tissues of the infundibulopelvic ligaments, desiccated by bipolar diathermy using laparoscopic scissors. (Reproduced in colour on Plate 3.)

the lateral blanching which can be observed when this technique is employed. After producing tissue desiccation in this way, the tissues can be divided with curved scissors. Whole structures and organs can be removed by repeatedly 'clamping' (bipolar desiccation) and then cutting with scissors (Reich & McGlynn 1986) (Fig. 4.13).

When using a bipolar diathermy technique to produce large vessel haemostasis, it is essential to ensure that the current is applied for the optimal time. If the current used is inadequate, the centre of the vessels will not be heated and the procedure will fail to prevent bleeding. If too high a current is used, the outside of the pedicle will coagulate rapidly and char. This will raise the impedance and stop the passage of further current into the depth of the pedicle and the technique will fail. If an adequate current is chosen but applied for too long a time the coagulum will become stuck to the blades of the forceps and will be pulled away from the vessels when the blades are opened. To determine the optimal time of application, it is helpful to measure the flow of current with an ammeter built into the electrosurgical generator circuit. As soon as tissue desiccation is complete the tissue impedance rises and the flow of current falls. This change can either be visualized on an ammeter or computed automatically as in the Erbe Automatic electrosurgical generator system.

Lasers in laparoscopic surgery

The principles of lasers and their modes of action are discussed in detail in Chapter 5. Lasers can be effectively used in laparoscopic surgery to divide tissues and to achieve haemostasis.

Carbon dioxide laser

The carbon dioxide laser was the first and remains the most widely used laser in gynaecology (Bruhat et al 1979). It cannot easily be transmitted down a fibre and must be directed from the laser generator to the patient via a series of mirrors encased in an articulated tube. It can be guided into the abdominal cavity either down a second puncture as described by Sutton 1985 or more commonly down the 5-mm working channel of a 10-mm diameter operating laparoscope. An advantage of the latter approach is that the umbilical port can double as both an optic and operative port, reducing the need for other accessory ports. A further advantage of this approach is that the CO_2 beam will always be directed at the target as this will also coincide with the line of sight of the surgeon.

The beam must be directed down the centre of the operative channel and must not strike the wall of the tube. This is best achieved by connecting the articulated arm of the laser to the laparoscope using a Nezhat type of coupler (Fig. 4.10). The carbon dioxide wavelength is almost completely absorbed by water, and the cutting effect of the carbon dioxide laser is achieved by directing a very fine spot at tissue which is then heated so that the intracellular water is vaporized. The volume of tissue penetrated in this way is no more than 0.1 mm and so there is very little lateral thermal damage. Carbon dioxide lasers produce a very precise 'what you see is what you get' type of tissue damage and an accurate incision. They generally provide poor quality haemostasis, although by defocusing the beam some tissue heating and small vessel haemostasis can be achieved.

A practical disadvantage of the carbon dioxide laser is that tissue vaporization produces a great deal of 'plume' which can rapidly obscure vision in the confined space of the abdominal cavity. To overcome this problem, an efficient smoke evacuator must be used in conjunction with an effective fast-flow carbon dioxide insufflator to replace the aspirated contaminated gas. The precision of the incision and the lack of tissue charring can be further improved by pulsing the laser energy. With this approach, short bursts of very high carbon dioxide laser energy are alternated with considerable 'off' periods, to allow tissue cooling and to minimize further the already slight lateral spread.

Nd-YAG lasers

In contrast to the carbon dioxide wavelength laser, a Nd-YAG wavelength laser can penetrate deeply into tissues. It is not absorbed by water and produces its clinical effect by coagulation of tissue proteins. In its unmodified form, the Nd-YAG laser cuts very poorly, and conversely it produces a wide area of tissue heating and so good haemostasis. The poor cutting properties make the unmodified Nd-YAG laser unsuitable for laparoscopic use. This laser, however, possesses the clinically useful property of being transmittable down a flexible quartz fibre (Keckstein et al 1988). Another clinically useful property is that the Nd-YAG wavelength laser produces less smoke and 'plume' and so better vision is maintained during important stages of the surgery. As it is a contact laser system, there is no risk of past-pointing and unintended tissue damage beyond the target, which can be a problem with the carbon dioxide laser.

To exploit these useful features and to overcome the disadvantages of 'bare fibre' Nd-YAG laser energy special patented artificial ceramic 'sapphire tips' attached to specific laparoscopic handpieces have been developed (Fig. 4.14a,b). These specially shaped probes concentrate the Nd-YAG laser energy and convert it into heat so that a useful, fairly precise cutting effect combined with a reasonable haemostatic effect is obtained. These handpieces also give the laparoscopic surgeon some tactile feedback which is not available from the carbon dioxide beam laser.

The 'sapphire tips' become very hot and must be cooled, either with coaxial carbon dioxide gas or fluid. With these tips the maximum power required is 15 W. Higher powers will melt the tips. The cutting effect is achieved with the very tip of the probe which should be brushed if possible at right angles over the tissue to be divided.

This modality can be used to divide vascular and avascular adhesions and uterovesical peritoneum, for forming the bladder flap and for dividing most pedicles.

KTP, argon and holmium lasers

These, and lasers using other wavelengths, have physical and clinical properties falling between the carbon dioxide and Nd-YAG lasers. They are all transmissible down quartz fibres and can be used in ways similar to the Nd-YAG, but without the need for special tips. Each has its own combination of cutting and coagulation properties and the laparoscopic surgeon must be very familiar with the properties of the particular laser he chooses. Each system has advantages and disadvantages, but with clinical experience each seems to provide similar results and it is probable that the preference and experience of the individual surgeon is more important than the merits of a laser using a particular wavelength in influencing results.

a

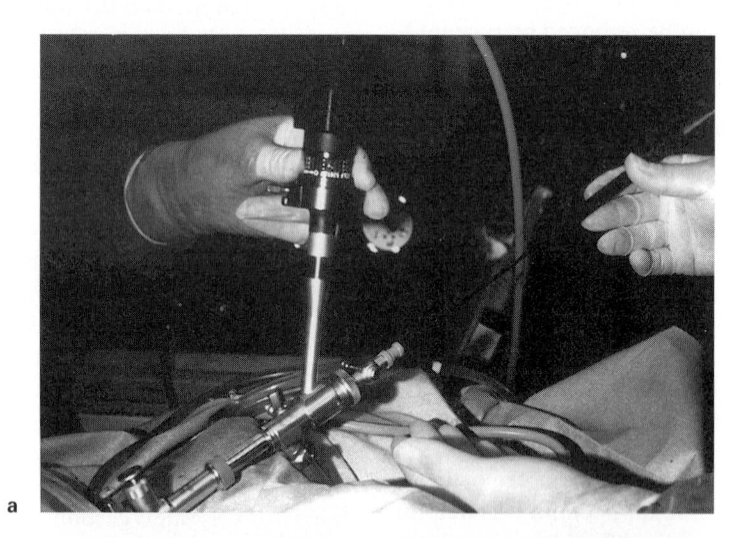

b

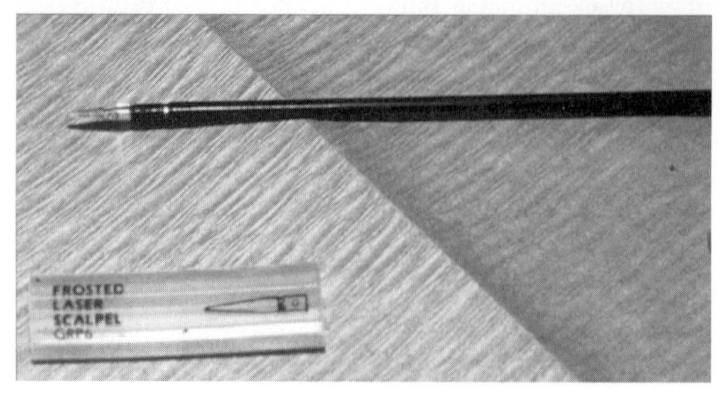

Fig. 4.14 a, b An operating laparoscope with a Nd-YAG laser handpiece down the operating channel.

Mechanical stapling devices

Another method of dividing tissue and simultaneously achieving haemostasis is that of using mechanical stapling devices. The Endo GIA 30 (Autosuture/USSC) and the Linear Cutter (Ethicon) each consist of a 12-mm diameter device which must be inserted down a similar diameter sheath. The device consists of a handle, a shaft and an anvil which can be used for several applications. To fire against the anvil there is a single-use stapling cartridge containing six layers of titanium staples and a self-contained knife blade. The staples are arranged in three rows on either side of the knife tract. The outer and inner row on each side are parallel and the middle row overlaps the spaces. This arrangement is intended to ensure that any vessel is occluded by at least one staple (Figs 4.15, 4.16).

These devices can provide a neat, quick and instantly haemostatic incision line, which has been found to be of particular benefit in securing the pedicles during a laparoscopic hysterectomy. There are disadvantages associated with this system, the main one being the considerable cost of these single-use items of equipment. The other major concern is related to their size, as they are 12 mm wide and this can bring them uncomfortably close to the ureters, particularly when used to secure the uterine arteries at the level of the cervix. Great care and appropriate additional techniques must be used if stapling devices are to be used in these situations.

Electrosurgical cutting

Tissues may also be divided using electrical energy. This is most easily achieved using unmodulated sinusoidal waveform electrical energy ('cutting current') in association with a needle-shaped electrode. Such a narrow electrode provides a high local current density which can then produce very high temperatures in a small area immediately adjacent to the tip of the electrode. The tissue in the treated area boils and is vaporized, thus dividing the structure. With this system there is very little lateral tissue heating and hence little haemostasis (Vancaillie 1994).

Small vessel haemostasis can be achieved with this type of electrode by changing the nature of the electrical input. The voltage should be increased and the current modu-

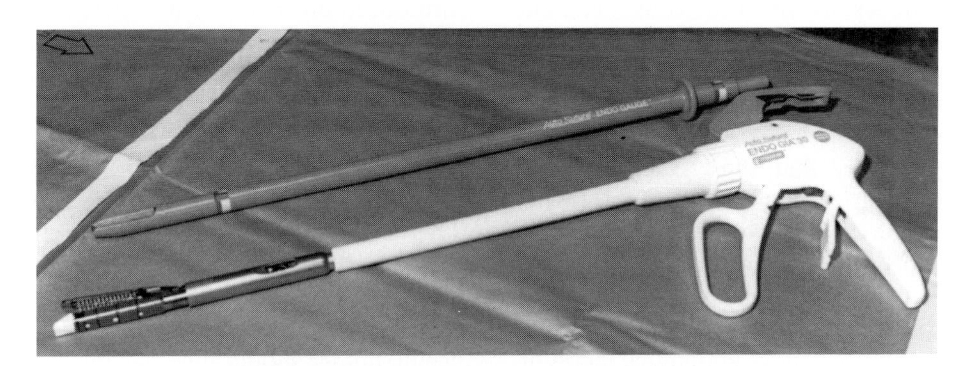

Fig. 4.15 An AutoSuture Endo-GIA automatic stapling device.

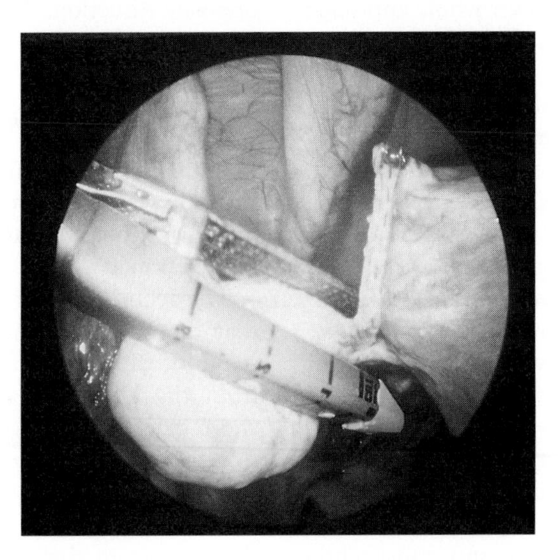

Fig. 4.16 Applying an automatic stapling device. (Reproduced in colour on Plate 4.)

lated (to provide, in the old terminology, 'coagulation current'). If the needle point is then placed a short distance from the tissue surface, an arc of this spray current will be produced which produces a diffuse but superficial tissue heating and coagulation effect. This method of producing haemostasis is known as 'fulguration'.

Laparoscopic suturing

In classical open surgery, haemostasis has traditionally almost always been obtained with appropriate suture ligation techniques. These techniques have stood the test of time and remain in most circumstances the method of choice. Why do we use such a wide variety of other methods to effect haemostasis when the laparoscopic mode of access is used?

The most probable explanation for this is that the techniques of laparoscopic suturing using a two-dimensional video screen are undoubtedly difficult and require considerable practice. Many established surgeons who are accomplished at open procedures are reluctant to submit themselves to the indignity of learning a new range of skills which they may find difficult. Initially at least laparoscopic suturing techniques are also time-consuming and add significantly to the time of the surgery. Thus other approaches, using electrosurgery, stapling devices etc., have been developed to avoid confrontation with these fundamental difficulties.

It is probable, however, that these alternative approaches considerably restrict the potential of the laparoscopic approach to surgery. Once every pedicle, structure, lesion and vessel can be as quickly and accurately sutured laparoscopically as at open surgery, then *every* intra-abdominal gynaecological surgical procedure will be able to benefit from the avoidance of large abdominal incisions. A few gynaecological endoscopists can already do this and this set of skills fundamentally alters their whole approach to gynaecological surgery. This change is as much a psychological as a technical one.

The author believes that the most important step a budding endoscopist can take is to continually practise laparoscopic suturing until they are proficient at this technique. There are a variety of intracorporeal and extracorporeal techniques available, and a number of different approaches should be mastered. New modifications to these basic approaches are being developed and more efficient needle-holders and graspers are being developed to facilitate these. The subsequent paragraphs will describe a few of these techniques, but they must essentially be learned at simulators and in practical courses.

The aim of all laparoscopic suturing techniques is to ligate major blood vessels and tissue pedicles with the same degree of security as would be acceptable at open surgery. When this can be confidently and consistently performed, the surgeon can carry out by laparoscopy virtually every procedure that can be accomplished by laparotomy.

Endoloop system

Perhaps the simplest technique to learn is the use of preformed Roeder loops attached to a plastic shaft (Ethicon). One end of the suture passes up the centre of the shaft and is fixed to the proximal end. This end can be snapped and thereby the suture can be pulled to tighten the loop and secure the pedicle. The pedicle to be secured is pulled through the loop with a grasping forceps and the loop pulled tight in the manner described above (Semm 1978).

A shaft, with suture and atraumatic needle attached, can be used to secure a pedicle and the needle can be withdrawn through the accessory trocar and a Roeder loop can be tied and then tightened in the manner described above.

Intracorporeal knot tying

A straight needle can be introduced down a standard 5-mm lateral port. Smaller diameter curved needles can be introduced down 10–12 mm ports. Once in the abdomen the needle is grasped by a second needle-holder and oriented at right angles to its shaft. This step, when performed with a curved needle from a two-dimensional screen, is difficult to learn.

When appropriately set up, the needle is placed through the tissues to be ligated and the suture pulled through. The needle is cut off and removed from the cavity. The suture is wrapped twice around the needle-holder which is held steady. With the free grasper, the end of the suture is removed from the jaws of the needle-holder. The looped needle-holder should then pick up the remaining free end of the suture and each end should then be pulled in the opposite direction. The procedure should then be repeated and the knot tightened.

Reich's extracorporeal knotting technique

A simple technique, using a knot-pusher, for laparoscopic suturing was first described by Clarke in 1972. This technique was then forgotten until rediscovered and published by Reich in 1992.

The technique, for any size of curved needle, requires that the suture material be grasped 1–2 cm behind the swath of the needle, after previously removing the sheath from the abdomen and backloading the suture into a short trocar sheath (Fig. 4.17). The needle-holder plus trocar sheath is inserted through the abdominal wall down the preformed track. The needle is repositioned in the holder and inserted through the pedicle. The needle is then cut from the suture and retained in the abdomen. The free end is pulled back up the primary trocar so that

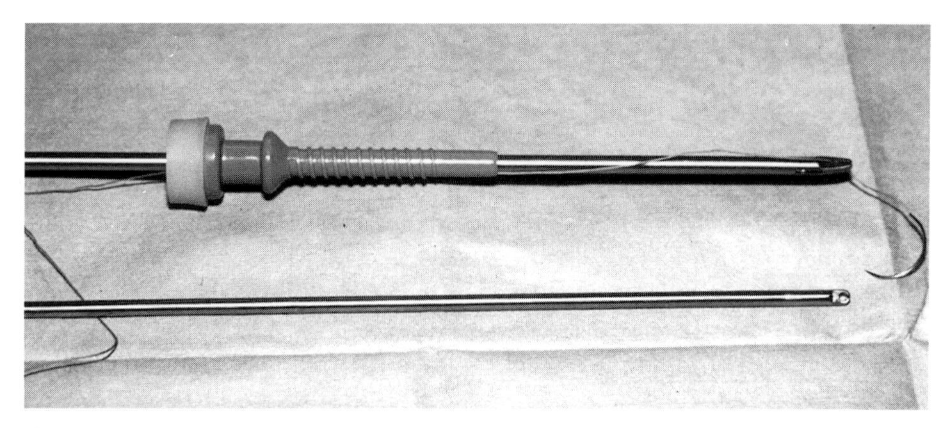

Fig. 4.17 A 5-mm port removed from the abdomen with needle-holder and suture assembled for reinsertion.

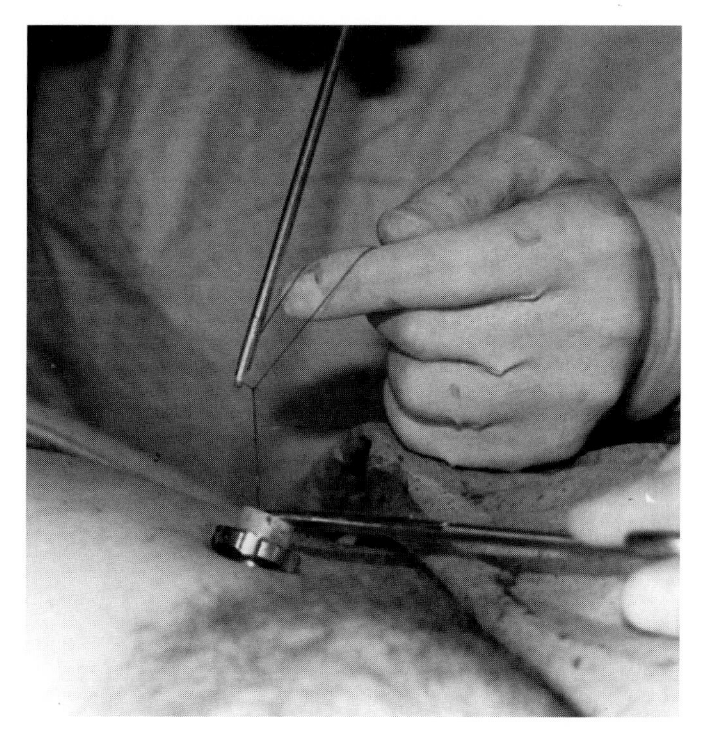

Fig. 4.18 Pushing a half-loop suture down the trocar with a Clarke–Reich knot-pusher.

the suture forms a loop down the trocar and through the tissue. A simple loop is cast and pushed firmly down the sheath with the knot pusher (Fig. 4.18).

Several additional throws are performed, the suture tails cut and then the needle is removed by dislodging the sheath and pulling the needle and holder upwards.

Additional equipment

Suction/irrigation system

A good suction/irrigation system is absolutely essential for effective laparoscopic surgery. Blood, cyst contents and debris must be removed and the operative field cleaned with warmed normal saline or Hartman's solution. The hydraulic energy from the pressurized fluid source can also be used as a most effective tissue dissector. This process of aquadissection is particularly useful as the force employed is a multidirectional one, which is more effective than undirectional forces such as a blunt probe in opening up tissue planes (Reich 1990).

Tissue forceps

As in open surgery, a variety of sizes and shapes of tissue forceps are required for endoscopic surgery. One or more designs of 5-mm atraumatic grasping forceps will be the standard tool to ensure optimum visualization of the operative field and to maintain optimum tissue tension. Single- and multiple-toothed forceps will be required in some circumstances, as will a more substantial 10-mm claw-tooth forceps for tissue removal.

Uterine mobilizer

Two rules of surgery are that excellent exposure is essential for excellent surgery and that tissues are best divided when held under an appropriate amount of tension. The uterus is a highly mobile organ and when suitably manoeuvred can be placed in acute anteversion to permit good views of the deep pelvis and pouch of Douglas and moved sharply laterally to place the contralateral side under tension to facilitate dissection and haemostasis. Many gynaecologists use a Spackman curette or a simple dilator to move the uterus.

I believe the Valtchev, or similar uterine manipulators, provide much superior operating conditions and a device of this type should be regarded as an essential tool for advanced laparoscopic surgery (Reich 1993) (Fig. 4.19).

Similarly the anterior and posterior vaginal fornices may be identified by placing opened sponge-holding forceps into the respective cul de sac. A rectal probe is also of

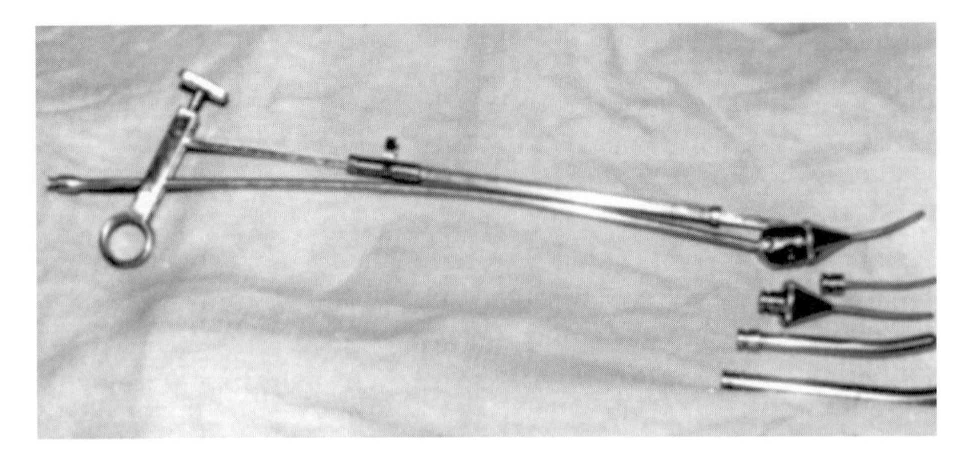

Fig. 4.19 A Valtchev uterine mobilizer with a number of tips of assorted sizes.

considerable help in moving and identifying the rectum in certain circumstances, particularly in the presence of advanced endometriosis.

CLINICAL USES OF THE LAPAROSCOPIC APPROACH

Diagnostic laparoscopy

Almost all gynaecologists are familiar with the use of laparoscopy in the diagnosis and management of infertility and pelvic pain. The improved resolution and quality of modern systems provide superior images and thus facilitate more precise and accurate diagnosis (Table 4.3).

Table 4.3 Indications for diagnostic laparoscopy

Infertility
Pelvic pain
Endometriosis
Pelvic inflammatory disease
Ectopic pregnancy
Unexplained pain
Assessment of pelvic masses
Ovarian cysts
Fibroids
Pelvic adhesions
Fertility problems
Location of lost intrauterine contraceptive device
Prior to in vitro fertilization
Prior to reversal of sterilization
Primary amenorrhoea
Congenital genital tract abnormalities
Polycystic ovarian syndrome
Second-look procedures
After malignancy therapy
After infertility surgery

Operative laparoscopy (Table 4.4)

Tubal surgery

The first and still the most widely performed operative laparoscopic procedure is tubal occlusion, either electrosurgically or mechanically. The advantages of the laparoscopic approach are such that throughout the world laparoscopic sterilization has almost completely replaced open procedures.

The best evaluated, more advanced laparoscopic procedures are laparoscopic salpingostomy and salpingectomy for the management of ectopic pregnancy (Bruhat et al 1980, Reich et al 1988). These approaches have been clearly shown, in many studies, to be associated with less pain and discomfort, to lead to a faster recovery and to be significantly cheaper than the open alternatives. Moreover the laparoscopic approach appears to encourage the less radical salpingostomy rather than salpingectomy.

Laparoscopic peritubal adhesiolysis and salpingostomy for distal tubal disease causing infertility, is a laparoscopic procedure which has been shown to be as effective as microsurgery but without the disadvantages of major abdominal surgery (Bruhat et al 1983, Dubuisson et al 1990, Gomel 1983).

Table 4.4 Operative laparoscopy

Tubal occlusion for sterilization
Peritubal adhesiolysis/salpingostomy
Salpingectomy/salpingotomy for ectopic pregnancy
Ovarian cystectomy/oophorectomy
Ovarian drilling for polycystic ovarian disease
Laparoscopic uterosacral nerve ablation/excision
Ablation or excision of endometriosis
Myomectomy/myolysis for fibroids
Total/subtotal hysterectomy
Colposuspension/pelvic support procedures
Infertility procedures
Pelvic and aortic lymphadenectomy

Ovarian cysts

Laparoscopic management of ovarian cysts is another common and well evaluated minimal access procedure (Audebert 1993, Johns 1991). Laparoscopic ovarian cystectomy and oophorectomy are technically straightforward procedures which can save patients considerable discomfort and convalescent time if performed instead of open procedures.

The main disadvantage of this approach is the small risk of inadvertently operating upon an undiagnosed ovarian cancer. Inadvertent contamination of the abdominal contents with malignant material alters the staging, and may alter the prognosis of the disease. With careful preoperative clinical and ultrasonic evaluation, the risk of this, and the clinical consequences, should be no worse for laparoscopic surgery than for open laparotomy removal. Care must be taken, however, to avoid contamination of the exit skin tract with possibly malignant tissue, as cases of malignant deposits developing in portal sites have been described. This can best be done by placing the intact cyst or ovary in a specially designed bag. These bags can be closed while in the cavity, and then pulled out through an abdominal port or a colpotomy incision. If the cyst is too large to remove easily in this way, the neck of the bag can be exteriorized and the contents morcellated inside the bag before extraction.

Gamete intrafallopian transfer and in vitro fertilization

Laparoscopic oocyte recovery is used in some circumstances as an alternative to ultrasound-directed oocyte recovery. The laparoscopic approach remains essential in intrafallopian gamete or zygote replacement.

Endometriosis

Perhaps the most common and important condition which can, with benefit, be managed laparoscopically is endometriosis. Superficial deposits can be excised or ablated (Martin & Diamond 1986). Ovarian endometriomata can be excised or opened and drained, and then the capsule removed with a carbon dioxide or KTP laser (Sutton 1993). Extensive cul-de-sac, deeply infiltrative endometriosis is a difficult and demanding condition, requiring the highest possible levels of surgical skill for effective management. The laparoscopic mode of access, with its excellent visualization and high magnification, represents the optimal way to deal with this problematic condition (Martin 1988).

Polycystic ovary syndrome

In patients with anovulation and infertility associated with resistant polycystic ovarian disease, ovulation can frequently be induced with a technique of ovarian drilling (Greenblatt & Casper 1987), using either electrosurgical or laser techniques.

Laparoscopic uterosacral nerve ablation (LUNA)

Patients with severe central pelvic pain, dysmenorrhoea and secondary dyspareunia may be helped by division of the uterosacral ligaments which contain some of the sensory nerve supply to the uterus. Doyle (1955) first described this procedure using laparotomy and others, including Sutton & Whitelaw (1993), have developed a laparoscopic version of this procedure using laser energy.

Uterine fibroids

Uterine fibroids of significant size can also be managed with a minimal access approach. The fibroids may be excised with a laparoscopic myomectomy technique (Dubuisson et al 1993), or may be reduced in size using a thermocoagulative necrosis technique called myolysis (Gallinat 1995).

Hysterectomy

Of most interest to general gynaecologists are the various techniques now being developed to perform laparoscopic hysterectomy. The whole uterus, with or without appendages, can be removed using laparoscopic techniques (Liu 1993a,b, Reich 1993). This surgically satisfying procedure is termed a total laparoscopic hysterectomy. Such an approach, however, requires considerable laparoscopic skills and takes a long time to perform. Most surgeons prefer to perform a proportion of the hysterectomy by the vaginal route (Wood et al 1994). Such a combined laparovaginal approach allows the upper pedicles to be secured by very simple laparoscopic techniques, after first mobilizing the adnexae and treating any associated disease, and then equally simple vaginal techniques may be used to complete the hysterectomy. This approach is called a laparoscopic-assisted vaginal hysterectomy (LAVH).

The extent of the laparoscopic component of the hysterectomy may be classified according to a system proposed by Garry, Reich & Liu (1993). The most difficult problem with laparoscopic hysterectomy is to secure the uterine vessels and those of the vaginal cuff without damage to the closely related ureter and bladder. If the upper uterine pedicles are secured by the laparoscopic route but the uterine artery is secured by the vaginal route, the method of hysterectomy will be termed a laparoscopic-assisted vaginal hysterectomy (LAVH). If the uterine artery is secured with laparoscopic techniques, the procedure is a laparoscopic hysterectomy (LH) and if, in addition, the attachments to the vagina and pelvis are divided laparoscopically the procedure is called a total laparoscopic hysterectomy (TLH) (Table 4.5). The exact proportion of the hysterectomy performed using the laparoscopic approach will depend on the patient and her pathology and on the surgeon and his relative skills and preference for laparoscopic and vaginal surgery. Some gynaecologists now prefer to retain the cervix and perform

Table 4.5 A classification system for laparoscopic hysterectomy

Vaginal hysterectomy with associated laparoscopy
Laparoscopic-assisted vaginal hysterectomy (LAVH)
Laparoscopic hysterectomy (LH)
Total laparoscopic hysterectomy (TLH)
Subtotal laparoscopic hysterectomy (SLH)
Subtotal laparoscopic assisted hysterectomy (SLAH)
Classical intrafascial subtotal hysterectomy (CISH)
Radical laparoscopic hysterectomy (RLH)

a laparoscopic subtotal hysterectomy (LSH) (Donnez & Nisolle 1993, Lyons 1993, Semm 1993).

Whatever minimal access technique is chosen for hysterectomy the major advantage of the approach is that it allows very accurate operative diagnosis and treatment of pathology such as endometriosis and pelvic adhesions. It allows very precise surgery, and also provides an excellent opportunity to ensure complete haemostasis at the end of the procedure. This facility may be of particular advantage after the use of a partial or complete vaginal approach to the hysterectomy. Small intra-abdominal bleeding points, not otherwise obvious externally, can readily be secured and complete haemostasis ensured.

Laparoscopic colposuspension and pelvic floor support procedures

Some urogynaecological (Liu 1993) and pelvic floor support procedures (Vancaillie & Butler 1993) are now being developed. Currently, particular interest is focused on the laparoscopic approach to Burch colposuspension, and some groups are reporting encouraging early results with this approach.

Laparoscopic gynaecological oncology procedures

Gynaecological oncologists are also becoming interested in the use of minimal access approaches to help in the management of various forms of gynaecological cancer. A few radical laparoscopic Wertheim-types of hysterectomy have been performed, but these really are a surgical tour de force. Of greater interest is the performance of bilateral pelvic laparoscopic lymphadenectomies as a staging technique for cervical and endometrial carcinoma (Querleu et al 1991). With this technique has come a reawakening of interest in the Schauta type of radical vaginal hysterectomy, for this procedure can, with great benefit, be performed in selected cases after a preliminary pelvic lymphadenectomy (Kadar & Reich 1993). With the excellent magnified view provided by modern laparoscopes, such lymphadenectomies can be as extensive as those performed at open surgery but again with much less associated morbidity. Para-aortic laparoscopic lymphadenectomy is technically rather more demanding, but is being increasingly used in the management of certain pelvic malignancies.

Relative merits of conventional and laparoscopic approaches

In summary almost every abdominal and vaginal gynaecological operation can now also be performed laparoscopically. Not every procedure may be better than its more conventional equivalent. Each must be evaluated and compared individually. Some minimal access procedures such as those for tubal occlusion, ectopic pregnancy and distal tubal infertility have already been convincingly shown to be superior to the open alternative. Others such as laparoscopic hysterectomy undoubtedly have advantages, but conventional approaches also retain a major role and the need here is to assess the indications for each of these procedures. Some of the newer procedures, such as laparoscopic myomectomy and colposuspension, have yet to be shown to be better than the standard approaches and the results of ongoing prospective studies in this area are keenly awaited.

CONTRAINDICATIONS TO LAPAROSCOPIC SURGERY

The major absolute contraindications are those which prohibit safe entry into the abdominal cavity. Severe shock, massive intra-abdominal bleeding, acute intestinal obstruction and/or cardiorespiratory compromise fall into this category (Table 4.6).

The known presence of very extensive intra-abdominal adhesions, particularly around the umbilicus, is a relative contraindication, as are bleeding diathesis and the presence of a very large pelvic mass. The ability to deal with these problems varies with the skill and determination of the surgeon and some may confidently and competently tackle such conditions, but most would be advised to avoid the laparoscopic approach in such circumstances.

Table 4.6 Contraindications to laparoscopy

Severe cardiorespiratory disease
Severe intra-abdominal bleeding
Acute intestinal obstruction
Severe intra-abdominal adhesions
Large intra-abdominal masses
Untreated advanced malignancy

COMPLICATIONS OF LAPAROSCOPIC SURGERY

Most of the complications encountered during laparoscopic surgery are similar to those expected from the conventional alternative procedure. The main complications specific to laparoscopic surgery are those related to the mode of access and the use of gas under pressure to distend the cavity (Table 4.7). These include damage to the major vessels or bowel by the Veress needle or primary trocar during the blind insertion of these sharp instru-

Table 4.7 Complications of laparoscopy

Complication
Primary trocar trauma
Major vessel trauma
Ileum/colon perforation
Bladder perforation
Lateral trocar trauma
Inferior epigastric vessel damage
Incisional hernia
Haematoma
Insufflation difficulties
Surgical emphysema
Venous gas embolism
Infection
Postoperative fever
Wound infection
Pelvic infection
Ureteric damage
Pulmonary embolism
Anaesthetic problems

ments. Damage to the vessels of the anterior abdominal wall, particularly the inferior epigastric vessels, can produce profuse haemorrhage and/or haematoma formation.

Incisional hernias, particularly if 10–12-mm lateral ports are used, are being seen with increasing frequency. To avoid this serious, and possibly fatal complication, it is now believed that all larger laparoscopic ports should be closed in layers to approximate the fascia.

Carbon dioxide may be forced into the tissues of the abdominal wall and produce extensive subcutaneous emphysema. The carbon dioxide gas under pressure may also be forced into opened blood vessels and, if this is unrecognized, may produce venous gas embolism with cardiac failure.

The use of electrosurgical energy may cause structural burns if care is not taken when using this powerful energy source. A problem peculiar to the laparoscopic use of electrical energy is the unintended discharge of capacitative coupled energy when monopolar electrical techniques are used down a sheath which is insulated from the patient.

All these specific risks may be avoided with careful use of good techniques and suitable equipment. Appropriate training will also minimize the risk of these problems, but in the end the laparoscopic approach like all other forms of surgery, will be associated with specific and non-specific complications. With these new approaches it is particularly important to counsel the patient about these risks, and to ensure that the consent she gives is truly informed.

ACKNOWLEDGEMENT

We are grateful to Blackwell Science Ltd for permission to use illustrations from Garry R, Reich H 1993 Laparoscopic hysterectomy. Blackwell Scientific, Oxford throughout this chapter.

KEY POINTS

1. The benefits of the laparoscopic approach to surgery include less pain, less scarring, less disability and quicker recovery.
2. To achieve these aims new equipment, new skills and new methods are required. These must be acquired by additional training, in the form of instructional courses, skills laboratories, video and multimedia demonstrations, but above all by a proctorship with a suitably experienced endoscopic surgeon.
3. Introduction of the primary trocar is a blind and potentially dangerous procedure. Attention to the technical detail of abdominal distension and trocar insertion is most important in reducing the risk of trocar injuries.
4. Good surgery requires good exposure and optimal vision at all times. Careful choice of modern laparoscopes, light sources and video systems can ensure good quality of vision.
5. The main function of the surgical approach is to divide tissues without haemorrhage. The laparoscopic mode of access requires new approaches in achieving these essential goals.
6. Electrosurgical energy and, to a lesser extent, lasers using various wavelengths are of help in performing laparoscopic surgery. It is essential to appreciate the physics and the clinical effects of these different energy sources, before using them in the potentially vulnerable environment of the closed abdominal cavity.
7. Attention to the details of this new mode of access should permit gynaecologists to bring the advantages of the minimal access approach to many of their patients.
8. A large number of gynaecological procedures may now be performed laparoscopically. The advantages and disadvantages of each minimal access approach must be individually assessed.

REFERENCES

Audebert A 1993 Laparoscopic ovarian surgery. Endoscopic surgery for gynaecologists. W B Saunders, London

Bruhat M A, Mage G, Manhes H 1979 Use of the CO_2 laser for laparoscopy. Proceedings of the Third International Congress in Laser Surgery: 275–281. Jerusalem Press, Tel Aviv

Bruhat M A, Manhes H, Mage G, Pouly J L 1980 Treatment of ectopic pregnancy by means of laparoscopy. Fertility and Sterility 33: 411–414

Bruhat M A, Mage G, Manhes H et al 1983 Laparoscopy procedures to promote fertility. Ovariolysis and salpingolysis results of 93 selected cases. Acta Europae Fertilitatis 14: 476–479

Chin A K, Moll F H, McColl M B, Reiv H 1993 Mechanical peritoneal retraction as a replacement for carbon dioxide pneumoperitoneum. Journal of the American Association of Gynecologic Laparoscopists 1: 62–66

Clarke H C 1972 Laparoscopy – new instruments for suturing and ligation. Fertility and Sterility 23: 274–277
Donnez J, Nisolle M 1993 Laparoscopic subtotal hysterectomy. Gynaecological Endoscopy 2: 77–78
Doyle J B 1955 Paracervical uterine denervation by transection of the cervical plexus for the relief of dysmenorrhoea. American Journal of Obstetrics and Gynecology 70: 1–5
Dubuisson J B, Bouquet de Jolinière et al 1990 Terminal tuboplasty by laparoscopy – 65 consecutive cases. Fertility and Sterility 54: 401–403
Dubuisson J B, Chapron C, Mouly M, Foulot H, Aubriot H 1993 Laparoscopic myomectomy. Gynaecological Endoscopy 2: 171–174
Gallinat A 1995 Myolysis. Gynaecological Endoscopy (in press)
Garry R 1992 Laparoscopic alternatives to laparotomy. Editorial. British Journal of Obstetrics and Gynaecology 99(8): 629–632
Garry R, Reich H 1993 Laparoscopic hysterectomy. Blackwell Scientific, Oxford
Gomel V 1983 Salpingo-ovariolysis by laparoscopy in infertility. Fertility and Sterility 340: 607–610
Greenblatt E, Cooper R F 1987 Endocrine changes after laparoscopic ovarian cautery in polycystic ovarian syndrome. American Journal of Obstetrics and Gynecology 156: 279–283
Hasson H M 1978 Open laparoscopy vs closed laparoscopy – a comparison of complication rates. Advances in Planned Parenthood 13: 41–50
Johns A 1991 Laparoscopic oophorectomy/oophorocystectomy. Clinical Obstetrics and Gynaecology 34: 460–466
Kadar N, Reich H 1993 Laparoscopically assisted radical Schauta hysterectomy for the treatment of bulky stage 1B carcinoma of the cervix. Gynaecological Endoscopy 2: 135–142
Keckstein J, Finger A, Steiner R 1988 Laser application in contact and non-contact procedures – sapphire types in comparison to 'bare fibre' argon laser in comparison to Nd-YAG laser. Lasers in Surgery and Medicine 4: 158–162
Liu CY 1993a Laparoscopic hysterectomy. Gynaecological Endoscopy 2: 73–75
Liu CY 1993b Laparoscopic retropubic colposuspension (Burch procedure): a review of 58 cases. Journal of Reproductive Medicine 38: 526–530
Lyons T 1993 Laparoscopic supravaginal hysterectomy using the Nd-YAG laser. Gynaecological Endoscopy 2: 79–83
Maher P, Hill D, Wood C 1994 Laparovaginal hysterectomy – a new approach. Gynaecological Endoscopy 3: 129–132
Martin D C 1988 Laparoscopic and vaginal colpotomy for the excision of infiltratory cul de sac endometriosis. Journal of Reproductive Medicine 33: 806–808
Martin D C, Diamond M P 1986 Operative laparoscopy: comparison of lasers with other techniques. Current Problems in Obstetrics, Gynaecology and Fertility 9: 563–601
O'Dell R 1993 Electrosurgery. Endoscopic surgery for gynaecologists. W B Saunders, London
Querleu D, LeBlanc E, Castelain B 1991 Laparoscopic pelvic lymphadenectomy in the staging of early carcinoma of the cervix. American Journal of Obstetrics and Gynecology 164: 579–581
Reich H 1990 Aquadissection. Laser endoscopy. Clinical practice of gynecology series. Elsevier, New York
Reich H 1993 New laparoscopic techniques. Endoscopic surgery for gynaecologists. W B Saunders, London
Reich H, McGlynn F 1986 Laparoscopic oophorectomy and salpingo-oophorectomy in the treatment of benign tubo-ovarian disease. Journal of Reproductive Medicine 31: 609–613
Reich H, McGlynn F 1990 Short self-retaining trocar sleeves for laparoscopic surgery. American Journal of Obstetrics and Gynecology 162(2): 453–456
Reich H, Johns D A, De Caprio J, McGlynn F, Reid E 1988 Laparoscopic treatment of 109 consecutive ectopic pregnancies. Journal of Reproductive Medicine 33: 885–890
Reich H, Clarke H C, Sekel L 1992 A simple method for ligating in operative laparoscopy. Obstetrics and Gynaecology 79: 143–147
Reich H, McGlynn F, Sekel L 1993 Total laparoscopic hysterectomy. Gynaecological Endoscopy 2: 59–64
Semm K 1978 Tissue puncher and loop ligations: new aids for surgical therapeutic pelviscopy (laparoscopy) – endoscopic intra-abdominal surgery. Endoscopy 10: 119–124
Semm K 1993 Classical abdominal Semm hysterectomy. Laparoscopic hysterectomy. Blackwell Scientific, Oxford
Sutton C J G 1985 Initial experience with carbon dioxide laser laparoscopy. Laser Medical Science 1: 25–31
Sutton C J G 1993 The role of laparoscopic surgery in the treatment of minimal to moderate endometriosis. Gynaecological Endoscopy 3: 131–134
Sutton C J G, Whitelaw N 1993 Laparoscopic uterine nerve ablation for intractable dysmenorrhoea. Endoscopic surgery for gynaecologists. W B Saunders, London
Vancaillie T G 1994 Electrosurgery at laparoscopy. Guidelines to avoid complications. Gynaecological Endoscopy 3: 143–150
Vancaillie T G, Butler D J 1993 Laparoscopic enterocele repair – description of a new technique. Gynaecological Endoscopy 3: 211–217
Veress J 1938 Neues instrument fur ausfuhrung von brust – oder brachpunktionen und pneumothoraxbehandlung. Deutsche Medizinische Wochenschrift 104: 1480–1481
Wood C, Maher P, Hill D 1994 Current states of laparoscopic associated hysterectomy. Gynaecological Endoscopy 3: 75–84

5

Diathermy and lasers

R. J. Parsons

INTRODUCTION

For many years diathermy was the technique of choice for tissue resection and destruction, both in gynaecology and general surgery. The advent of the laser in the 1960s threatened this supremacy; however during the last decade, advances in diathermy have led to a more balanced position between the two modalities. The aim of this chapter is to explain briefly the operation of the instruments, the tissue effects, the common system types, some of the safety aspects involved and the practical clinical use of both techniques in gynaecology.

DIATHERMY

The effects of high frequency electrical currents on tissue have been exploited in surgery for about 100 years (d'Arsonval 1893). They have been used for two main purposes: in surgical diathermy, for cutting and coagulation, and in shortwave diathermy, mostly in physiotherapy, for direct tissue heating.

Surgical diathermy

Early diathermy machines used a spark-gap generator where the breakdown of a spark gap in the machine caused resonance in the output circuit to which the patient was connected. The power output was controlled by varying the voltage between the two electrodes. Later diathermy sets, using a valve oscillator, were thought to give a superior waveform for cutting purposes. However, it was still electronically difficult to produce the subtle waveform changes which were known to influence tissue effects. The advent of the semiconductor generator made this task much easier and there is now a plethora of output parameters available to the surgeon.

When an alternating current is applied to the body, the effects depend on the frequency. From mains frequency (50 or 60 Hz) to about 50 kHz, muscle will contract and interfere with surgical procedures. It is necessary to exceed 100 kHz to prevent this happening, and in practice frequencies in the range of 400 kHz–10 MHz are used.

Electrode design is also very important, and the development of the loop electrode has enabled diathermy to challenge the laser, particularly in the excision of lesions of the cervix. A loop of wire acts as the active electrode and a blended output is employed to ensure both cutting and coagulation. Other types of electrode include a rollerball or barrel. The addition of a small jet of argon between the active electrode and the operating site will simultaneously direct the discharge to a precise area and keep the field clean.

Monopolar diathermy

In monopolar diathermy, one electrode is applied to the patient, who becomes part of the circuit. The surface area of the electrode plate is much greater than the contact area of the diathermy instrument to ensure that heating effects are confined to the end of the active electrode (Fig. 5.1).

The advantage of monopolar diathermy is that it can be used to cut as well as to coagulate tissues. Coagulation or cutting can be achieved by changing the area of contact or the waveform of the current. The area of contact is the main factor and a cutting effect is achieved when the cutting electrode is not quite in contact with the tissue, so that an electrical arc is formed. The cutting waveform is a low voltage but higher frequency current. The power and current levels will rise when cutting takes place inside a liquid-filled cavity such as the bladder or uterus.

When the electrode is brought into direct contact with tissue and the waveform is modulated, coagulation rather than destruction occurs. Power levels and voltages fall

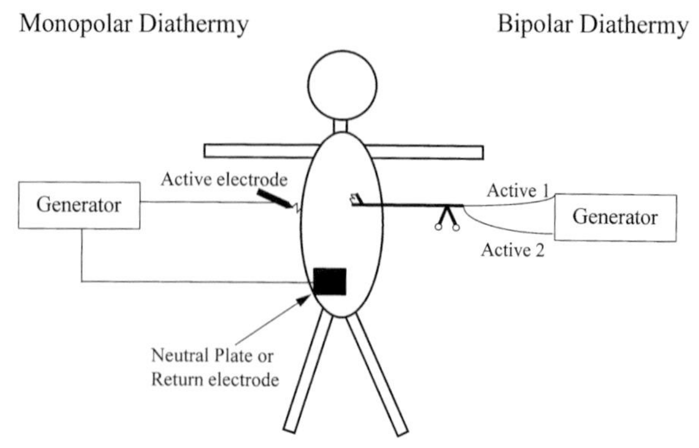

Fig. 5.1 Monopolar and bipolar diathermy systems.

but the current may well rise as the resistance is much lower. If a mixture of the two types of waveform is employed then the advantages of both techniques are exploited. This is normally termed 'blended' output and many combinations are possible.

The effect is usually confined to the tissue in contact with the instrument; however, this is not invariably the case. The current will follow the path of least resistance, and if a non-target tissue such as bowel lies in contact with target tissue, the current will flow through the tissue with least impedance. In addition, the impedance will rise as the target vessels desiccate and current may then flow to an alternate earth, usually but not necessarily in contact with the pedicle. If the current flows through bowel, damage will result which may not be recognized at the time.

Bipolar diathermy

In bipolar diathermy both contacts are on the surgical instrument (Fig. 5.1). This means that current flow is limited to a small area. This is safer, but a cutting effect cannot be achieved. Indeed, there is still a risk of aberrant current flow because the patient, table and diathermy machine are all earthed. In addition, the tissue temperatures are much higher (340°C), and this itself can cause unexpected effects.

Shortwave diathermy

Specific electrode design has led to an interest in the use of shortwave diathermy for tissue-destructive effects (Phipps et al 1990). Here the two electrodes form a capacitor in the output circuit, with the patient providing the dielectric medium between the two plates. Frequencies of around 27 MHz are employed, with power levels of about 500 W. By altering the shape and size of the electrodes, heating effects may be localized or diffused as required. However, care must be exercised as the effects are not always predictable.

Diathermy safety

The main requirement for diathermy safety, in addition to the obvious one of guaranteeing performance as set, is to prevent accidental discharge paths causing tissue effects remote from the operating site. It is not possible automatically to prevent inadvertent contact with the wrong organ, and the surgeon must activate the generator only when the electrode is in contact with, or in close proximity to, the target site.

The 'earth' plate must always be in broad contact with the patient and there must be a low-resistance path back to the generator. In most modern diathermy sets this is continuously monitored and operation of the machine is inhibited if the return path is broken. However, stray paths to earth can occur via metal objects, such as leg supports, and 'alternate site burns' result. This can be prevented by electrically isolating the diathermy output at the relevant frequencies, but the patient may still be at risk if the active electrode becomes 'earthed'. Steps must be taken to ensure that generator action is inhibited if this occurs. The risk of burns at a poorly applied return electrode can be reduced by dividing the electrode in two and monitoring the current returning to each half.

LASERS

A laser is a device capable of producing near-parallel beams of monochromatic light, either visible or invisible, at controlled intensities. This light can be focused, thus concentrating its energy, so that it can then be utilized to treat various conditions. The term 'laser' is an acronym for 'Light Amplification by the Stimulated Emission of Radiation'. The process of stimulated emission was foreseen by Einstein at the turn of the century, but it was not until 1960 that the first optical device was constructed (Maiman 1960). Since that time many lasers have been made but comparatively few have found their way into gynaecological practice.

Basic laser physics

A laser consists of three main elements: a power supply, an excitable medium and an optical resonator (Fig. 5.2). Atoms or molecules within the medium are raised to high energy states (Fig. 5.3a) by the power supply, and under normal circumstances these would decay to the ground state by the emission of the energy as photons (5.3b). By confining the process to an optical cavity and restricting the decay paths, stimulated emission (5.3c) can take place. This process produces a build-up of photons (light) at a particular wavelength inside the cavity. The laser output is a small fraction of this which is allowed to escape from one end of the cavity. Many substances have been found to be suitable laser media, including solids, liquids, gases or

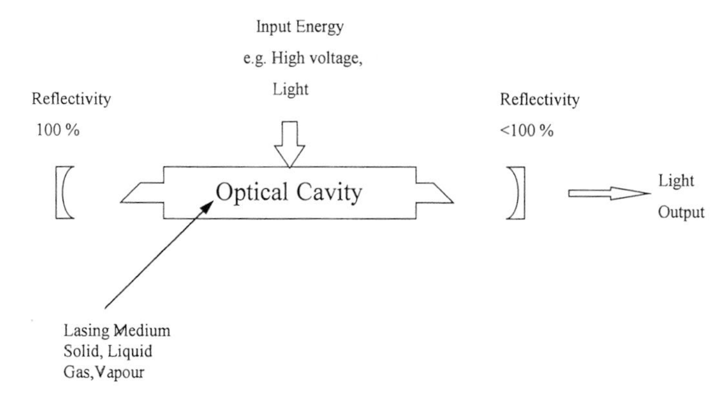

Fig. 5.2 Typical laser systems.

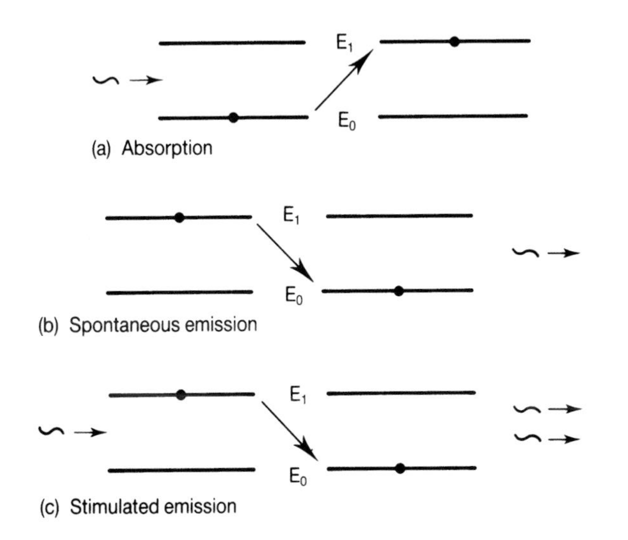

Fig. 5.3 Basic atomic processes. **a** absorption of a photon of energy; **b** spontaneous emission of a photon; **c** stimulated emission of an additional photon of energy. ~, photon; E_0, lower energy state; E_1, higher energy state; •, particle.

metallic vapours, but the basic principles remain the same. A more detailed explanation of laser physics is provided elsewhere (Carruth & McKenzie 1986).

The radiation emitted is monochromatic (if only one decay path is involved), coherent and collimated. Collimation, or the near-parallel nature of laser light, can be exploited in many ways and it is the main feature which makes such devices useful in the medical world. A single convex lens placed in the beam will bring it to a sharp focus, the size of which is dependent upon the width of the collimated beam. The use of different lenses or varying the lens-to-tissue distance alters the diameter of the beam at the point of contact with the tissue (Fig. 5.4). This is referred to as changing the spot size.

The most important determinant of the effects of a laser upon tissue is the power density (PD). This can be calculated roughly as:

$$PD = 100 \times W/D^2 \text{ watts/cm}^2$$

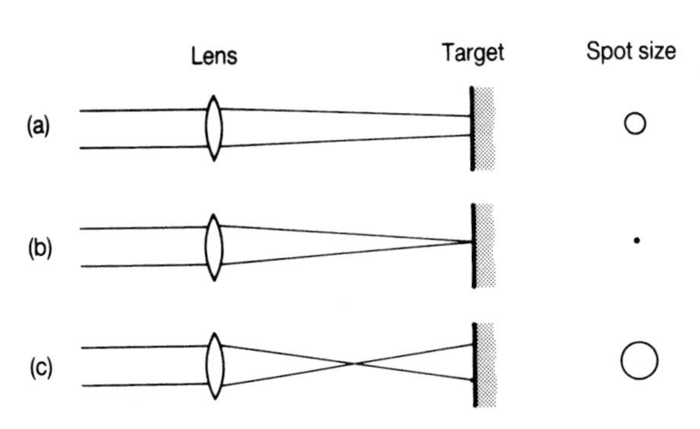

Fig. 5.4 Changing the focal length of the focusing lens while keeping the lens-to-tissue distance constant alters the spot size, i.e. the diameter of the beam at the point of contact with the tissue. **a** The focal length of the lens is greater than the lens-to-tissue distance; **b** the focal length of the lens is the same as the lens-to-tissue distance, i.e. the laser is focused on the tissue; **c** the focal length of the lens is less than the lens-to-tissue distance.

where PD is power density, W is power output in watts and D is the effective diameter of the spot in millimetres. D can be measured by firing a short low-power pulse at a suitable target. The power density can be altered by changing either the power or the spot size but the latter has the greater effect.

Light–tissue interaction

Light impinging on tissue is subject to the normal laws of physics. Some of the light is reflected and some is transmitted through the air–tissue barrier and passes into the tissue where it is scattered or absorbed. Obviously the extent to which each process dominates is dependent upon the physical properties of the light and the tissue. The theory of light–tissue interaction is not as well developed as that of ionizing radiation (Wall et al 1988) but enough is known to explain the macroeffects upon which most laser treatments depend.

At very low energy density levels (power density × time, joules/cm^2), say below 4 J/cm^2, a stimulating effect on cells has been observed, but above this level the effect is reversed and suppression occurs (Mester et al 1968). As the energy density rises to 40 J/cm^2, indirect cell damage can take place if any sensitizing agents present become activated (e.g. haematoporphorin derivative). Direct tissue damage does not take place until about 400 J/cm^2 when the first thermal effects appear and photocoagulation occurs. Another 10-fold increase in energy density results in complete tissue destruction as it is sufficient to raise the cell temperature rapidly to 100°C, causing tissue vaporization. Obviously these are general observations and other properties of the incident beam will have an influence, but the general 10-fold relationship alluded to above holds, even though other parameters may be varied. Amongst the most important of these are the wavelength and the pulsatile nature of the radiation involved.

The wavelength absorption characteristics of various body tissues are reasonably well understood, qualitatively if not quantitatively. Figure 5.5 shows the absorption curves for water, melanin and haemoglobin which, to a large extent, will determine the curves for tissue as a whole. In the ultraviolet and the middle-to-far infrared spectrum, absorption by water predominates whereas melanin and haemoglobin effects take over in the visible range. From this graph it is easy to see that a particular laser, operating at a fixed wavelength, will be preferentially absorbed by one tissue constituent and its effects will be different from those of another laser with a different wavelength.

So far in this description it has been implied that the laser is operated continuously for long enough for thermal effects to appear (continuous wave or CW mode). However, it is relatively simple, by means of a shutter or a controllable power supply, to switch the energy on and off rapidly: the pulse mode. In general, the medical definition of a pulse is a burst of energy lasting 0.25 s or less. This does not correspond to the definition of a pulse in physics and care must be taken to avoid confusion. Methods of generating these pulses differ according to the type of laser used, and the tissue effects can also vary. The reason for this phenomenon is shown in Figure 5.6.

Figure 5.6a shows the output from a CW laser which is modulated by a perfect shutter. The average power delivered to the tissue can be calculated from a knowledge of the CW power, the pulse repetition rate and pulse width. In the case of an electronically controlled high-pulse power system where the time–power curve is not so closely defined (Fig. 5.6b), it is much more difficult to determine the average power delivered. It is necessary to measure the energy of the pulse and the pulse repetition rate. The peak power, although impressive, is almost irrelevant.

The effects on tissue of this pulsatile radiation are to reduce the pure thermal effects (lower average power input) whilst maintaining and sometimes enhancing the vaporization potential. Provided the pulse repetition rate is sufficiently low to allow heat dissipation to take place between pulses, the tissue temperature will stabilize at a lower value. These effects are analogous to those induced by modulation in diathermy outputs, which lead to the differences between cutting and coagulation diathermy referred to earlier.

Very short pulses, such as those produced by Q-switched lasers, can cause electromechanical breakdown in tissues because of the extremely high energy densities obtainable. In the early days these lasers were tested in gynaecological situations but untoward side-effects were noted (Minton et al 1965).

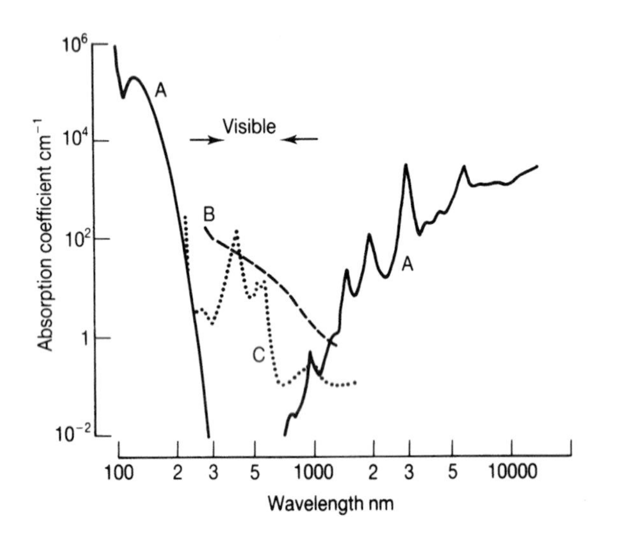

Fig. 5.5 Absorption characteristics, at different wavelengths of: **A** water; **B** melanin; **C** haemoglobin. After Boulnois (1986).

Common laser systems

Two lasers established themselves in gynaecological practice during the 1980s:

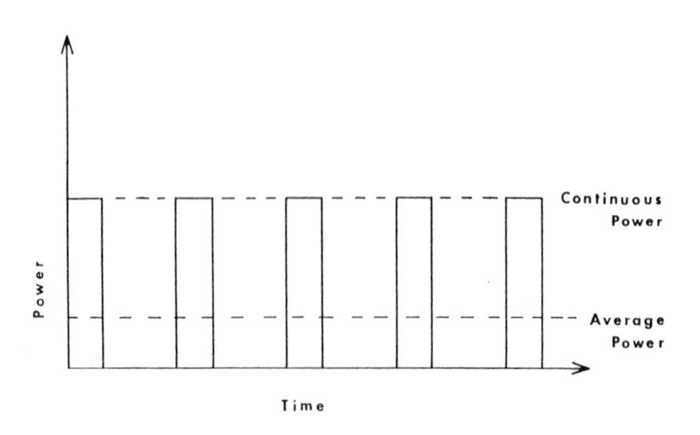

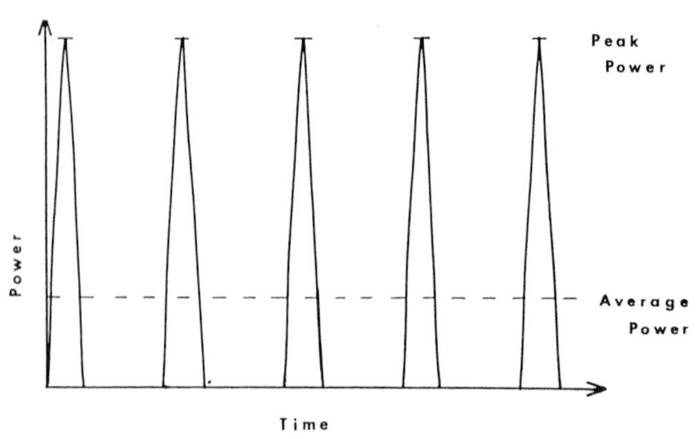

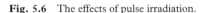

Fig. 5.6 The effects of pulse irradiation.

- the carbon dioxide laser,
- the neodymium:yttrium-aluminium-garnet (Nd:YAG) laser.

These will be described in detail with a further section devoted to other types which are now entering general usage after extensive research.

The carbon dioxide laser

This is the system which has been most used in gynaecology, since its introduction in the early 1970s. This has been because of its clinical suitability, ease of use, reliability and easy serviceability. Although it has the major drawback that its output cannot be transmitted by fibres, it has so far not been displaced by other lasers, but is now rivalled by some diathermy equipment.

As the name implies, the active lasing medium is carbon dioxide gas (CO_2). Efficiencies of 15% energy conversion to light output have been achieved. In fact, this ability has been used in an analyser to detect CO_2 in the breath! The first generation of CO_2 lasers used a flowing gas system with high-voltage direct-current excitation. A gas mixture of CO_2, nitrogen and helium was used to help achieve and maintain lasing conditions. Sealed tube lasers are now available, with radiofrequency low-voltage discharges being used for excitation. This has made the machines smaller and removed the need for gas bottles.

The output radiation, of wavelength 10.6 µm, is well into the infrared region of the spectrum. This radiation is absorbed rapidly by tissue water, and therefore cuts and vaporizes more easily than it coagulates. Most of the incident radiation is absorbed within about 0.03 mm of the surface and intense heating occurs. Coagulation will only take place in small blood vessels less than 0.5 mm in diameter, but haemostasis can be facilitated by reducing the power density so that the zone of thermal damage around the central crater is wider.

Because the 10.6 µm laser beam is invisible, an aiming beam must be used so that the operator can see where the therapeutic beam is going to have its effect. A helium–neon (HeNe) laser, emitting at 628 nm (red), is incorporated into the system and optically aligned so that it coincides with the therapeutic beam. This alignment can degenerate and should be checked regularly.

As yet there is no commercially available fibre which can transmit 10.6 µm light efficiently, so most commercial systems use some form of articulated arm. At each joint there is a mirror which is adjusted so that the beam stays central despite movement between the two adjacent limbs of the arm. The choice of the mirror material is limited because of the need to reflect both the infrared CO_2 beam and the red HeNe aiming beam. It is possible to use waveguide delivery systems to avoid the use of mirrors but this limits the manoeuvrability of the complete system.

The final delivery to the operation site can be carried out in two ways, both incorporating a focusing lens. For hand-held surgery, the lens at the end of a straight delivery tube focuses the beam on the operative field about 1 cm from the end of the tube. The lens-to-tissue distance can thus be varied at will so that the spot size will be changed within a narrow range (Fig. 5.7a). Colposcopic delivery involves a mirror positioned after the focusing lens which brings the beam into line with the viewing axis of the colposcope. This mirror is at the end of a joystick so that the beam may be moved around within the field of view (Fig 5.7b). Originally the spot size was changed by using lenses of different focal lengths and so was limited to three or four predetermined sizes. Now the use of zoom optics allows infinite adjustment over a limited range (0.5–4 mm).

The power outputs of these lasers can be from a few watts up to a continuous 100 W. Most commercial systems in gynaecology produce up to 25–35 W as this, coupled with a variable spot size, provides power densities of up to 6000 W/cm^2 sufficient for tissue-cutting and vaporization at a controllable rate. The extra power provided by instruments producing 40–60 W is useful for dealing with patients who bleed during the procedure. Higher peak powers are available with modulation being employed to keep tissue temperatures within acceptable limits but with 'cleaner' cuts.

The neodymium:YAG laser

This device is a solid-state laser with the active neodymium ions being incorporated in an artificial crystal of YAG. Pumping is achieved by energy input from a parallel gas discharge lamp, usually a water-cooled krypton tube, with the output radiation being refocused into the laser crystal. Output power levels up to a continuous 100 W can be achieved but with a conversion efficiency of 1% or so, nearly 10 kW of input power is needed.

The energy produced is at a wavelength of 1.06 µm and is thus in the near infrared. As such, it can be transmitted easily down a flexible fibreoptic delivery system and delivered to many more anatomical sites than can the CO_2 laser. The emergent radiation has lost its collimation and will diverge quite rapidly. However, sapphire tips can be added to the fibres, thus controlling the emerging beam to a certain extent and adding another dimension to laser surgery. Most fibres also have a coaxial flow of gas, usually CO_2, to keep debris away from the end of the fibre. This is particularly necessary where contamination with blood or blood products may make continuous operation difficult.

As with the CO_2 laser, 1.06 µm Nd:YAG radiation is invisible. A HeNe laser (or other light source) needs to be incorporated into the device as an aiming beam. This is also a very useful safety feature as near-infrared radiation

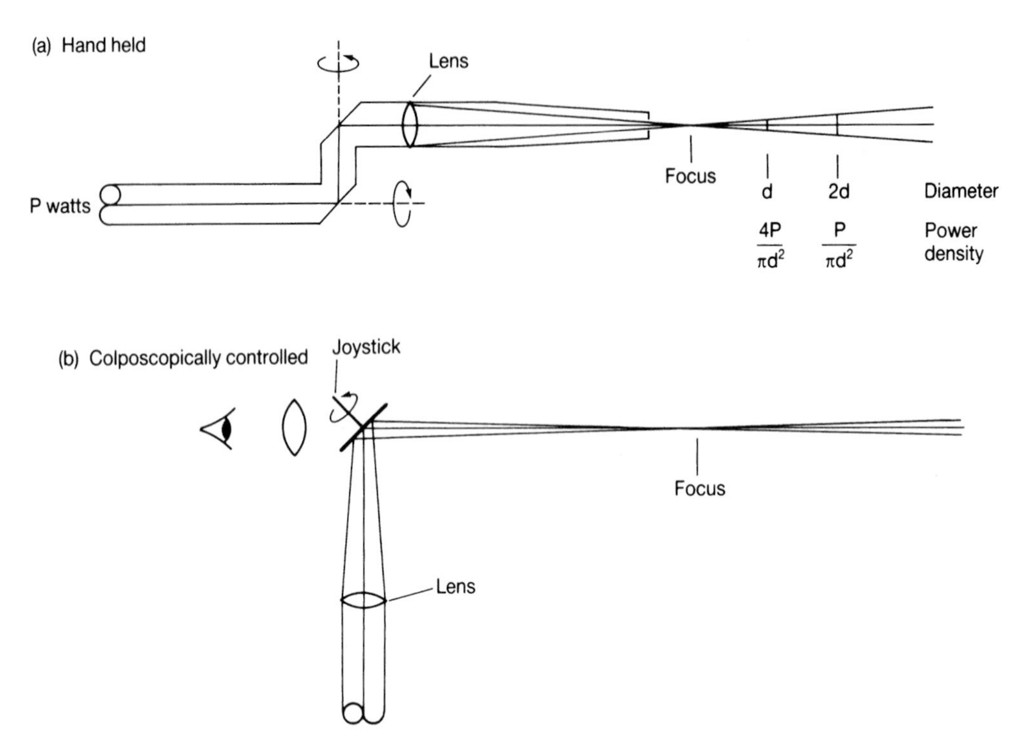

Fig. 5.7 Laser delivery systems: **a** hand-held; **b** colposcopically controlled.

can cause irreparable damage to the retina. The Nd:YAG laser is easy to operate as a Q-switched laser. An optoelectronic switch is incorporated inside the laser cavity and the lasing action prevented for a large percentage of the time. The photon energy therefore builds up to an even higher level than normal and when the switch is eventually opened a massive pulse of energy is delivered. The switch can then be closed and the process repeated. This type of action has found a use in ophthalmology where, by focusing the pulse to a very small spot, electromechanical breakdown of tissue can be induced with minimal surrounding damage.

Other laser systems

There are many other laser systems now being used in medicine and the length of time from research to common usage seems to be getting shorter. It is neither possible nor desirable to give a complete list but some of the following few examples may find an accepted place in gynaecological surgery.

Metal vapour lasers, as their name implies, consist of a container filled with a heated and vaporized metal in an inert gas atmosphere at low pressure. The electrical discharge used must be pulsed because the necessary conditions cannot be sustained long enough for true CW operation to take place. Two types of metal vapour laser have found a use in medicine: copper and gold. The copper vapour laser produces two beams at 510 and 578 nm at up to 25 W power output. These by themselves are not particularly useful, although the green output (510 nm) can be used as a substitute for the argon laser in dermatology. The output is ideally suited to act as an optical pumping source for a dye laser, which can be tuned to provide radiation for photodynamic therapy.

Photodynamic therapy is an experimental treatment for certain tumours (Spikes & Jori 1987). It relies upon selective retention in tumour tissues of a drug, such as haematoporphyrin derivative, which only becomes active on exposure to light of a particular wavelength. This can vary from drug to drug and the most suitable drug–wavelength combination is still being sought. The dye laser is useful in this research effort because the wavelength of its beam can be altered. Various dyes can be excited to form a population inversion between groups of energy states – not individual states as in a true laser – which allow a laser output to be generated. As there are many decay pathways available, the output is multi-wavelength but with suitable optical devices a narrow wavelength range can be selected. The copper vapour and dye laser combination can produce over 5 W of red light at 630 nm which is an absorption peak of haematoporphyrin derivative.

The other metal vapour device being investigated is the gold laser. The output of this is, at 627.8 nm, a close match to the dye laser, without the added complication of two devices in series.

The argon laser, producing light at 488 nm (blue) and 514.5 nm (blue-green), while favoured by ophthalmologists has not found a significant place in gynaecology, but the green output of the KTP laser (potassium titanyl-phosphate, 532 nm) has become more accepted. The output is derived by taking the neodymium:YAG beam and frequency-doubling it in a KTP crystal thus providing the surgeon with a choice of wavelengths (or even a mixture of the two).

Research into ultraviolet lasers has produced systems which seem to rely on non-thermal mechanisms for tissue destruction. These are the 'excimer' lasers, a term derived from 'excited dimer', where the active medium is made from a combination of two substances which do not normally combine, such as a rare gas and a halide. These lasers have found a place in ophthalmology and their potential for precise tissue removal could offer the microsurgeon a very powerful tool.

The early use of lasers in gynaecology was for the treatment of cervical intraepithelial neoplasia but they are now used in most other areas of the lower reproductive tract. The use of the laser in treatment of intraepithelial neoplasia of the genital tract is described in Chapter 34. Similar diathermy techniques are described in the same chapter.

Laser safety

All laser systems currently in use have no way of distinguishing between patient and operator. The desired effect on a patient can be a serious accident to the surgeon. The subject of safe construction and operation of lasers in medicine and surgery is thus very important, and must be understood by all involved. This section is biased in favour of UK regulations, but the situation is similar in most European countries and the USA although, of course, regulatory bodies and documents will have different guises.

As from January 1995 all lasers sold in the UK must conform to three basic standards. Electrical safety requirements are detailed in BS EN 60601-1 (British Standards Institution 1990), and non-ionizing radiation hazards are covered by BS EN 60825-1 and BS EN 60601-2-22 (British Standards Institution 1994, 1993). A further publication by the Medical Devices Agency (1995) outlines good laser practice together with some additional equipment safety features. All of these publications should be considered by a laser protection adviser (a health authority or trust appointee) who will assist each user in specifying and installing lasers in clinical surroundings. Although the requirements will vary from laser to laser and from site to site, the following sections outline the major considerations involved.

Nature of the hazard

The body is divided into two regions for hazard analysis: the eye and skin. In the visible region, which extends into the near infrared, the eye is the organ most at risk. Outside this range the eye is no different from skin except that corneal damage can lead to visual loss although the retina itself may be undamaged.

Radiation entering the eye is focused on to the retina and the power density can increase by up to 5×10^5 times so that a 50 W/m^2 corneal incident beam can become 25 MW/m^2 on the retina, with disastrous and irreparable results. Maximum permitted exposure (MPE) levels are laid down by the regulations and are set well below known damage thresholds. Manufacturing and administrative controls are written to prevent operators, assistants and patients from accidentally receiving radiation in excess of these limits. There are separate values for the skin and eye, with the latter being the more stringent.

Control of hazards

Lasers are currently classified into four groups from class 1 to 4, with class 1 being the least and class 4 the most hazardous. Class 3 is also subdivided into two classes, 3A and 3B. It is the manufacturers' responsibility to classify a laser but once this is done, the classification will rarely be changed. Stringent safety precautions must be introduced when class 3 and 4 lasers are in use. Most medical lasers are class 3B or 4 and do need such safeguards. Aiming beams are usually class 1 or 2 and present a minimal hazard.

In addition to classifying the laser, manufacturers must ensure that the equipment complies with the specification for its particular class. Generally all systems will have a key control and some way of monitoring the power being delivered to the patient. It should also indicate either visually or audibly when the laser shutter is opened and levels in excess of the MPE are being emitted.

Administrative controls are framed to ensure that the equipment is then used safely. A set of local rules must be drawn up which specify who is allowed to use a laser and where it can be used. A laser controlled area (LCA) must be defined and the activities within that area regulated. There must be no possibility of radiation in excess of the MPE passing out of the area, even if this means blocking windows and doors. Warning signs must be exhibited at the entrance to the LCA and door interlocks can be used but are not obligatory. Examples of such local rules can be found in other texts (Medical Devices Agency 1995, Stamp 1983).

All personnel within the LCA must either be protected from the radiation by the inherent optical properties of operating equipment or must wear appropriate spectacles. For example, any common translucent glass is impervious to CO_2 laser radiation. Precautions for the Nd:YAG laser are more complicated, and special eyewear for observers and filters to protect the operator from back-reflection through a delivery system are required. Obviously such devices cannot be used when the aiming beam is derived from the therapeutic beam. In this case an additional safety shutter is required to protect the surgeon during treatment. Precautions against eye damage must be rigorously implemented for all present, including the patient.

Fire is an ever-present hazard with the use of class 4 lasers and simple precautions must be observed. Aqueous instead of spirit-based solutions should be used and paper drapes should be avoided. CO_2 radiation is readily absorbed by water and by keeping swabs soaked in water or saline, tissues adjacent to the operation site can be protected. A suitable fire extinguisher should always be available. Great care must be exercised in the presence of inflammable anaesthetic gases. Endotracheal tubes have been ignited by a laser, with serious results (Bandle & Holyoak 1987). While the latter situation is not likely to be encountered in gynaecology, inflammable gases may be passed rectally by the patient during laser treatment of the lower genital tract, posing a theoretical risk of explosion.

A by-product of laser treatment (and diathermy to a certain extent) is a plume of smoke and debris, with a characteristic odour. This must be evacuated and collected from as near as possible to the impact zone for two important reasons. First, the emission of smoke is likely to obscure the operating site. This is particularly true in cervical or vaginal surgery. Second, doubts have been raised over the viability of particles contained within the plume (Garden et al 1988). Although the evidence is not overwhelming, it is essential that the smoke should be adequately extracted and filtered.

Unintentional reflections when the laser beam strikes an instrument can be dangerous. Although it is very unlikely that radiation reflected in this way will be sufficiently focused to cause damage, it is sensible to ensure that the instruments are not highly polished and thus scatter any incident radiation. It should not be assumed that the reflecting qualities of a surface are the same at visible and far-infrared wavelengths, so care should be exercised in the choice of specula and other operating instruments.

CONCLUSIONS

Diathermy techniques have improved markedly over the last few years and have replaced, on economic grounds, the laser techniques developed in the 1970s and 1980s. However, there is still a place for the use of lasers in gynaecology, particularly as new devices are made available and as yet unknown light–tissue interactions are discovered and exploited. Interactions between light, tissue and drugs hold much promise.

KEY POINTS

1. Monopolar diathermy uses electric currents to cut or coagulate. Dipolar diathermy can only be used for coagulation.
2. Great care must be taken to prevent accidental burns during diathermy usage. Current can flow to organs not in direct contact with the active electrode.
3. Lasers produce nearly parallel beams of monochromatic light.
4. The beam can be focused by a lens to alter the diameter of the beam at the point of contact with the tissue (the spot size) .
5. The power density (PD) is the most important determinant of the effects of the laser upon tissue.
6. The greater the power density the less the thermal effect and the less the haemostatic property of the beam.
7. The beam of a CO_2 or a Nd:YAG laser is invisible, so a guiding HeNe laser is required.
8. The eye must be protected from accidental exposure to laser energy. This is especially important with Nd:YAG endoscopic systems.

REFERENCES

Bandle A M, Holyoak B 1987 Laser incidents. In: Moseley H, Haywood J K (eds) Medical laser safety. Institute of Physical Sciences in Medicine, London, pp 47–57

Boulnois J 1986 Photophysical processes in recent medical laser developments: a review. Lasers in Medical Science 1: 47–66

British Standards Institution 1990 Medical electrical equipment part 1: specification for general safety requirements. BS EN 60601-1. British Standards Institution, London

British Standards Institution 1993 Medical electrical equipment part 2: particular requirements for the safety of diagnostic and therapeutic laser equipment. BS EN 60601-2-22. British Standards Institution, London

British Standards Institution 1994 Safety of laser products part 1: equipment classification, requirements and user's guide. BS EN 60825-1. British Standards Institution, London

Carruth J A S, McKenzie A L 1986 Medical lasers, science and clinical practice. Adam Hilger, Bristol

d'Arsonval M A 1893 Production de courants de haute fréquence et de grande intensité: leurs effets physiologiques. Comptes rendus Société de Biologie 9: 122–124

Garden J M, O'Banion M K, Shelnitz L S et al 1988 Papillomavirus in the vapour of carbon dioxide laser treated verrucae. Journal of the American Medical Association 259: 1199–1202

Maiman T H 1960 Stimulated optical radiation in the ruby. Nature 187: 493–494

Medical Devices Agency 1995 Guidance on the safe use of lasers in medical and dental practice. The Medical Devices Agency, London

Mester E, Ludany G, Vajda J et al 1968 Uber die Wirkung von Laser-Strahlen auf die Bakteriemphagozytose der Leukozyten. Acta Biologica et Medica Germanica 21: 317–321

Minton J P, Carlton D M, Dearman J R et al 1965 An evaluation of the physical response of malignant tumour implants to pulsed laser radiation. Surgery, Gynecology and Obstetrics 121: 538–544

Phipps J H, Lewis B V, Roberts T et al 1990 Treatment of functional menorrhagia by radiofrequency-induced thermal endometrial ablation. Lancet 335: 374–376

Spikes J D, Jori G 1987 Photodynamic therapy of tumours and other diseases using porphyrins. Lasers in Medical Science 2: 3–15

Stamp J M 1983 An introduction to medical lasers. Clinical Physics and Physiological Measurement 4: 267–290

Wall B F, Harrison R M, Spiers F N 1988 Patient dosimetry techniques in diagnostic radiology. Institute of Physical Sciences in Medicine, York

6

Imaging techniques in gynaecology

N. M. deSouza D. O. Cosgrove J. Jackson G. M. Bydder

INTRODUCTION

Since the discovery of X-rays by Roentgen in 1895, there has been an explosion in technology for imaging the human body; not only ionizing radiation but also high frequency sound, radiolabelled pharmaceuticals and non-ionizing radiation in strong magnetic fields are used. The parallel expansion in computer technology has enabled the development of cross-sectional imaging using computerized tomographic (CT) techniques, and 3-D imaging using magnetic resonance imaging (MRI) data.

METHODOLOGY

X-ray techniques

Standard radiographs are obtained by placing the patient between an X-ray source and a photographic film. Images are produced by the attenuation of X-ray photons by the patient. As a result, structures of interest are often obscured by the attenuation of photons by other overlying structures. A basic limitation of the standard X-ray technique is the effect of scattered photons adding to the image noise and degrading the quality of the final image. Various manoeuvres have been adopted to reduce this effect, for example scatter grids. The linear tomograph is obtained by the synchronous movement of the X-ray tube and the film, causing a blurring of the overlying and underlying structures while leaving the plane of interest in focus. This procedure increases the detection of lesions such as chest metastases.

Contrast studies

To increase contrast in the soft tissues, an iodine-containing agent may be injected into the lumen of a cavity such as the uterus and fallopian tubes (hysterosalpingogram) or blood vessels (angiogram). Such contrast agents are widely available both in ionic and more expensive non-ionic forms. The less toxic non-ionic preparations are preferred.

Ultrasound

Ian Donald in Glasgow in 1950 used an industrial flaw detector, designed for testing the integrity of steel boilers, to demonstrate that the massive abdominal swelling of one of his patients was fluid and not solid. A large ovarian cyst that proved to be benign was subsequently removed. Since then, the rapid and continuing evolution of ultrasound technology has lead to a proliferation of applications in almost all aspects of medicine and surgery.

Ultrasound waves are generated by a piezoelectric crystal mounted in a transducer housing, the whole construction being referred to as a probe. Piezo materials respond to an applied voltage by changing thickness and they produce electrical signals of a few millivolts when compressed. While the resolution along the beam is determined by the wavelength, resolution across it depends on the width of the beam, which is improved by focusing, using either lenses or electronic mechanisms, often in combination. Despite these devices, the lateral resolution is always poorer than the range resolution.

The time from the transmission of the ultrasound pulse

to the receipt of an echo is translated into depth using the speed of sound in tissue. Echoes arise whenever the pulse of ultrasound encounters an interface between tissues of different acoustic impedance. Thus, homogeneous materials such as clear fluids are echo-free, while low-level echoes are given by the interfaces between the various components of soft tissue structures. Stronger echoes result from the interface between fibrous tissue (high impedance) and fatty tissues (low impedance) and maximal echoes are given by interfaces between soft tissues and bone or gas, both of which are effectively opaque to ultrasound. To form a real-time image, the beam is electronically swept through a region of tissue and the images are pie-shaped (sector probes) or rectangular (linear probes).

The choice of frequency is usually a compromise between the image resolution and the depth of penetration required. The higher the frequency, the better the resolution but the greater the attenuation of the beam within the tissues. Hence, for abdominal scanning, frequencies of between 2.5 and 3.5 MHz are commonly employed. Probes designed for intracavitary and intraoperative use employ higher frequencies (5–8 MHz) because the organs of interest are closer to the transducer. This enables higher resolution images to be obtained.

The drawbacks of intravaginal probes are mainly an initial lack of observer familiarity with the anatomy in the transvaginal coronal and sagittal planes, and a depth of view limited to about 70 mm. Also the large-calibre probe may prove difficult for some postmenopausal women and for those in whom extensive surgery or radiotherapy to the pelvis has led to vaginal stenosis. However, the transabdominal approach may also be limited in such patients because of poor bladder filling. In these cases, transrectal scanning can be used and is often preferred in patients with suspected recurrent pelvic cancer.

The interactivity of ultrasound is another important feature: it is almost an extension of clinical examination and techniques such as probe palpation may be used to assess movement and compressibility. Ultrasound also provides numerous views during the real-time examination and facilitates guided-needle biopsies. However, it has many limitations, notably the variable image quality, that frustrate its application. The main problem is the complete barrier posed by gas in bowel which is why a full bladder is required for transabdominal scanning.

Doppler imaging operates by detecting the change in frequency of ultrasound echoes caused by movement of the target. In the simplest system, this is done continuously with only minimal control of the beam direction. Continuous wave Doppler is well suited to fetal heart monitoring, especially as movements of the fetus do not interrupt the signal. In gynaecology, the vessels of interest are small so that precise placement of the Doppler sample is a prerequisite. This is achieved with pulsed Doppler. The Doppler gate is superimposed on a real-time scan that allows the target to be pinpointed (Fig. 6.1). The Doppler signal depicts a range of blood velocities occurring in the selected vessel over time. Output can be audio or as a strip chart with intensity to indicate the strength of the signal at each velocity in the spectrum. A variety of measurements can be made from these tracings, the most useful of which are systolic/diastolic ratios. These are measures of the arteriolar resistance to flow, with a low value indicating low vasomotor tone, typical of the placenta and the corpus

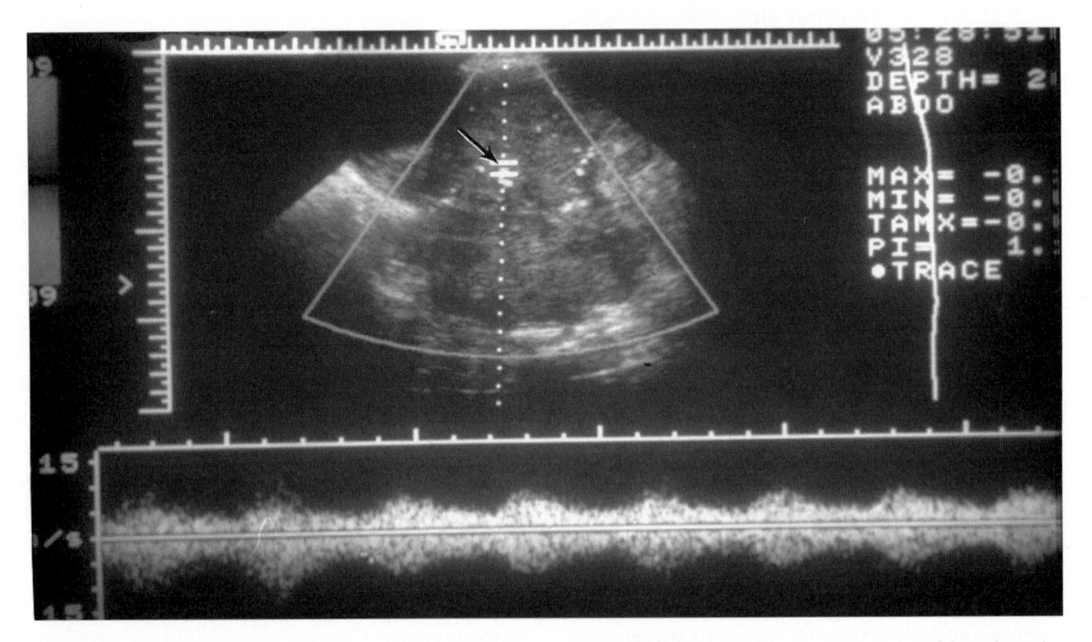

Fig. 6.1 Spectral Doppler. In this scan of an ovarian cancer, the Doppler gate (arrow) has been positioned on the tumour. The spectral tracing is in the lower portion of the figure and shows the typical low resistance pattern of malignant neovascularization with marked diastolic flow.

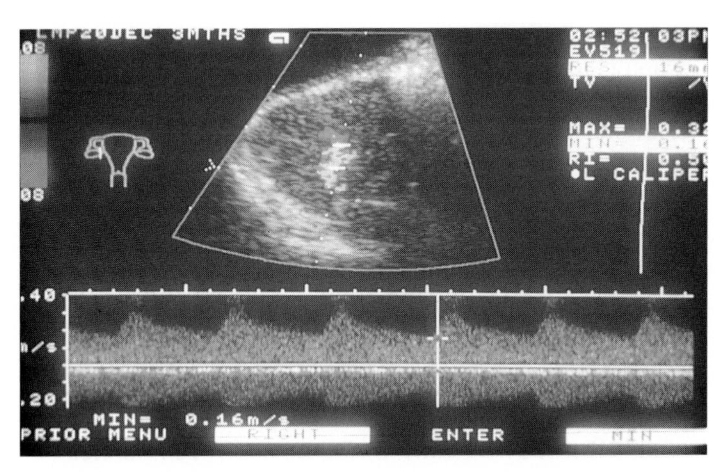

Fig. 6.2 Colour Doppler of a corpus luteum. On colour Doppler, flow signals are colour coded for direction and velocity. The neovascularization in this corpus luteum is shown as a knot of colour. Apart from providing a graphic display of vascularity, a useful feature of colour Doppler is to guide placement of the gate for spectral Doppler tracings. Shown in the lower portion of the figure is a low impedance trace with flow throughout diastole. This is typical of growing tissue.

luteum. This pattern also occurs in inflammation and malignancy. High indices are typical of inactive tissue, such as the resting uterus.

In colour Doppler scanning the same process is applied across an area of interest. The velocity signals are presented as a colour-coded overlay, superimposed on the real-time scan (Fig. 6.2). Though the Doppler information is less rich than with spectral Doppler (only the mean velocity is generally depicted), the angiogram-like map provides information on the morphological arrangement of the vascular tree and its sensitivity allows vessels as small as a millimetre or so in diameter to be detected. Often the colour Doppler map is used to locate a vessel to guide placement of the spectral Doppler gate for haemodynamic analysis. The addition of pulsed Doppler ultrasound has also made possible the measurement of fetal and uteroplacental blood flow, thereby producing physiological information from what was previously an anatomical imaging technique.

Computerized tomography

The sensitivity of conventional radiography may be improved by using a radiation detector such as a scintillation crystal and a photomultiplier tube. By measuring the attenuation of a finely collimated beam of radiation, passing through the patient at multiple angles, it has been possible to produce images of very high quality. A computer uses the attenuation of each beam passing through the patient to calculate the attenuation coefficient for each area of tissue in the cross-section of interest. The final images are reconstructed using a filtered back-projection technique and displayed in a grey scale as a series of attenuation units (with values between +500 and –500) in a matrix of 512 × 512 or 1024 × 1024 elements. The reconstruction of data is limited to the transverse (transaxial) plane. This technique of imaging revolutionized modern medicine in the 1970s but its impact on gynaecology has been less marked.

Magnetic resonance imaging (MRI)

MRI depends upon the magnetic properties of certain atomic nuclei which, when placed within a magnetic field and stimulated by radio waves of a specific frequency, will absorb and then re-emit some of this energy as a radio signal. This phenomenon of nuclear magnetic resonance (NMR) was first described by Felix Bloch and Edward Purcell in 1946. NMR as a basis for an imaging technique was proposed some 30 years later by Lauterbur.

Nuclei possessing magnetic properties have an odd number of protons or neutrons. The charged particles are spinning, which causes them to behave as tiny bar magnets. If placed within a magnetic field, a majority of protons will line up in the direction of the magnetic field. In addition their axes are tilted and caused to rotate like small gyroscopes. The frequency of this precessional movement is directly proportional to the strength of the applied field and is called the Larmor frequency. The hydrogen proton gives a relatively high signal due to its abundance in biological tissues. Other potential NMR isotopes include ^{13}C, ^{23}Na, ^{19}F, and ^{31}P.

If a pulse of radio waves is imposed on the nuclei, a strong interaction or 'resonance' will occur when the frequency coincides with the precessional frequency of the nuclei. The energy absorbed by the nuclei is then re-emitted as a signal that can be detected in a receiver coil situated around the sample. The initial strength of this signal is proportional to the proton density of the sample. It will then decay in an exponential fashion as the disturbed protons relax back to their original state. The T_1 relaxation time is described as the time taken for the stimulated protons to return to their initial state. The T_2 relaxation time is that taken for the precessing nuclei to get out of step with one another. A variety of sequences of radio wave pulses have been devised so that the resulting signal is weighted to different degrees by the proton density and the T_1 and T_2 relaxation times.

With MRI the contrast between different tissues can be manipulated by altering the pattern of radio waves applied. This is done by changing the time constants associated with the different sequences of radio waves: the inversion time (TI), echo time (TE), or repetition time (TR). A further advantage of MRI is the ability to obtain additional perspectives, such as sagittal or coronal views, without moving the patient.

The female pelvis is suitable for MRI examination because of the minimal effect of respiratory motion on the pelvic organs. By placing the receiver coil adjacent to the tissue of interest (e.g. endovaginally to maximize signal from the cervix), very high resolution images of an area of interest may be obtained. However, as the data to produce a set of images are accumulated over 5–10 min patients are required to remain still during this time. If multiple sequences and multiple planes are employed the total imaging time may exceed 60 min which reduces patient tolerance. However newer faster pulse sequences and improved computer software are greatly reducing scan times.

Radionuclide imaging

Unlike the other imaging modalities, radionuclide imaging provides physiological rather than anatomical detail. Modern gamma cameras are capable of accurately imaging the distribution of administered radiopharmaceuticals, and the use of tomographic systems for single photon emission tomography (SPECT) has improved image resolution. In gynaecological oncology, radiolabelled monoclonal antibodies may be employed in the localization of malignancies (radioimmunoscintigraphy) and in their treatment (radioimmunotherapy).

The purity and specificity of monoclonal antibodies gives them an important role in tumour detection and possibly in the targeting of antitumour agents. A murine monoclonal antibody (791T/36), initially developed for colorectal cancer, has subsequently been shown to localize in gynaecological cancers (Powell et al 1986a). Another monoclonal antibody produced against a cell surface antigen, CA125 is also proving invaluable for imaging ovarian cancer. Other monoclonal antibodies undergoing evaluation for imaging purposes include those against placental alkaline phosphatase (PLAP) and human milk fat globule (HMFG) antigen. Different malignancies may express the same antigens which may also be found in normal epithelial tissues, as is the case with HMFG. A monoclonal antibody OVLT3 is claimed to be specific for ovarian cancer.

The antibodies or antibody fragments are radiolabelled with a gamma-emitting radionuclide such as ^{99m}Tc, ^{131}I, ^{123}I or ^{111}In. A subcutaneous test dose is no longer given because of the immune response it may generate in the patient. If ^{131}I or ^{123}I is employed, oral potassium iodide is given to block thyroid uptake of free radioactive iodide. In addition, blood pool subtraction techniques are required for ^{131}I studies to simulate the non-tumour distribution of labelled antibody. This is not necessary for ^{123}I- or ^{111}In - labelled preparations.

Following injection of the antibody, a gamma camera provides serial images of the distribution and uptake of radiolabelled antibody between 18 and 72 h after the antibody has been administered. The radionuclide ^{111}In is ideally suited for tomographic studies using images produced by a gamma camera mounted on a gantry which rotates through 360°. The images are reconstructed by computer in the same manner as X-ray CT. ^{111}In tomography localizes the antibody uptake site more accurately, and may reduce the false-positive results. Figure 6.3 is an example of an ^{131}I-labelled antibody study of a patient with a palpable mass in the left iliac fossa, suspected to be recurrent ovarian tumour. This was subsequently confirmed by laparoscopy.

False-positive ^{131}I-imaging can arise as a result of incomplete subtraction of radio-iodide in the urinary bladder. ^{111}In-labelled antibody has a different biodistribution with uptake of radiolabel into the liver, spleen, bone marrow and occasionally the adrenal glands. Excretion of ^{111}In into the bladder has not been a problem. An example of an ^{111}In study is shown in Figure 6.4. A central area of increased uptake is apparent at the site of a primary ovarian cancer. ^{111}In is a more suitable radiolabel than ^{131}I and, together with ^{123}I and ^{99m}Tc, has largely replaced ^{131}I. However, ^{111}In is taken up by the reticuloendothelial system into the liver and spleen, preventing its use for the detection of liver metastases. Non-specific bowel uptake sometimes seen with ^{111}In may account for some false-positive results.

Angiography

Diagnostic and therapeutic angiography has made great strides in recent years, with the development of catheters whose tips can be manipulated. This allows considerable control over the guidance of these catheters into selected vessels. In parallel with this, ingenious devices have been devised which can be introduced via these catheters used for purposes as diverse as angioplasty and embolization.

In gynaecological practice, the main use of angiography is the control of pelvic bleeding but both the diagnosis of pelvic venous thrombosis and the prevention of subsequent pulmonary embolism are important roles for this exciting new technique. Pelvic arteriovenous malformations are most readily diagnosed and treated with angiography and pelvic varices causing chronic pain may be managed in the same way. Selective sampling of gonadal venous blood and steroid hormone assay can be most valuable in the preoperative assessment of phenotypic women with chromosomal abnormalities and intra-abdominal gonads of uncertain nature.

CLINICAL APPLICATIONS

Normal anatomy and variations

Uterus

The normal uterine cavity is delineated as a triangular structure on hysterosalpingography, with the cornua and the internal cervical os as the corners. Intracavitary abnormalities, both congenital and acquired, such as inter-

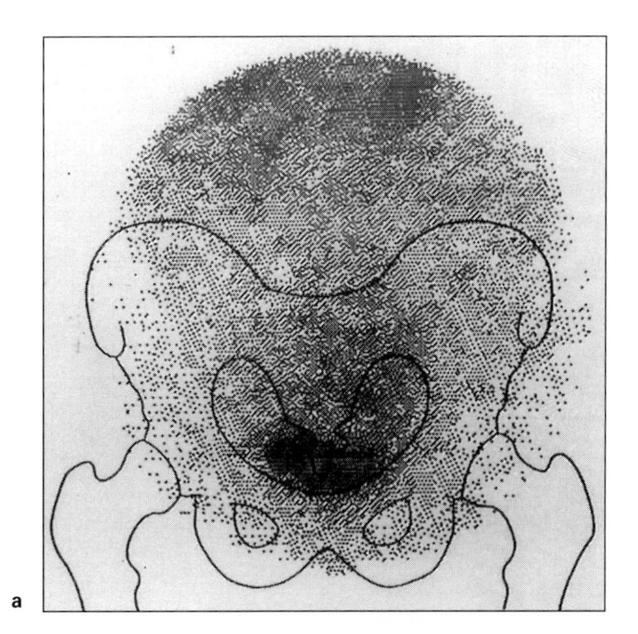

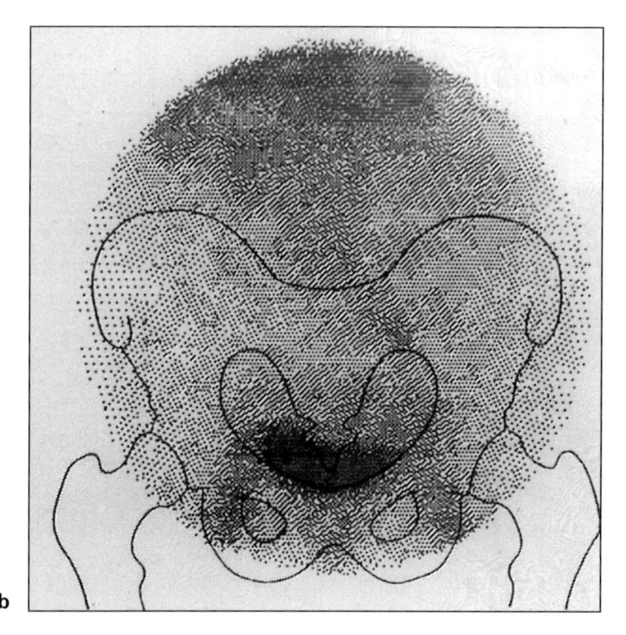

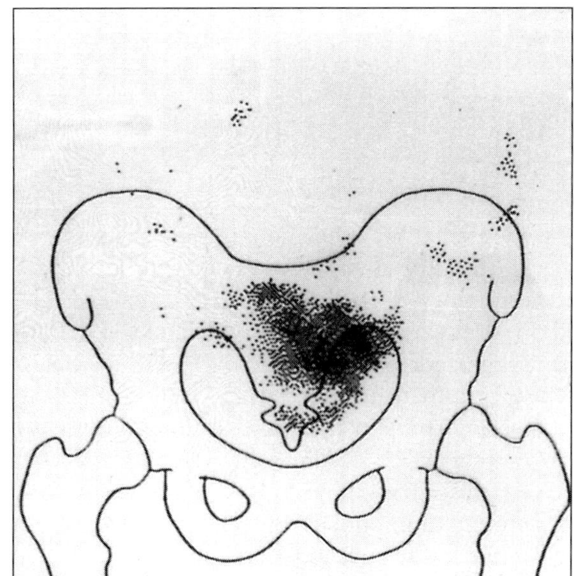
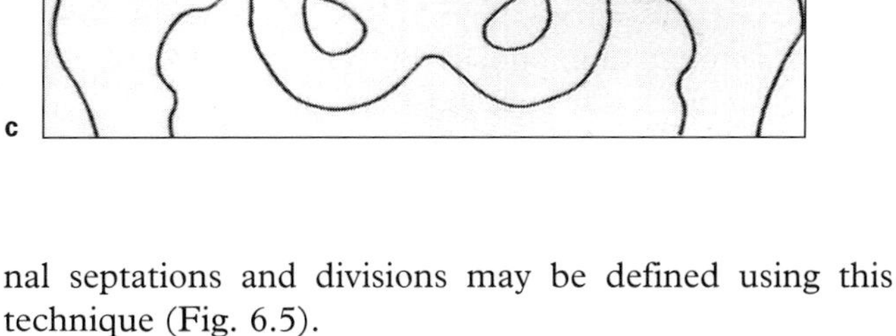

Fig. 6.3 Radionuclide scan of recurrent ovarian cancer. Anterior views of the pelvis with 80 Mbq ^{131}I-labelled antibody 791T/36. **a** The image before **b** subtraction of the ^{99m}Tc-labelled blood pool image; **c** after subtraction with an area of increased antibody uptake on the patient's left.

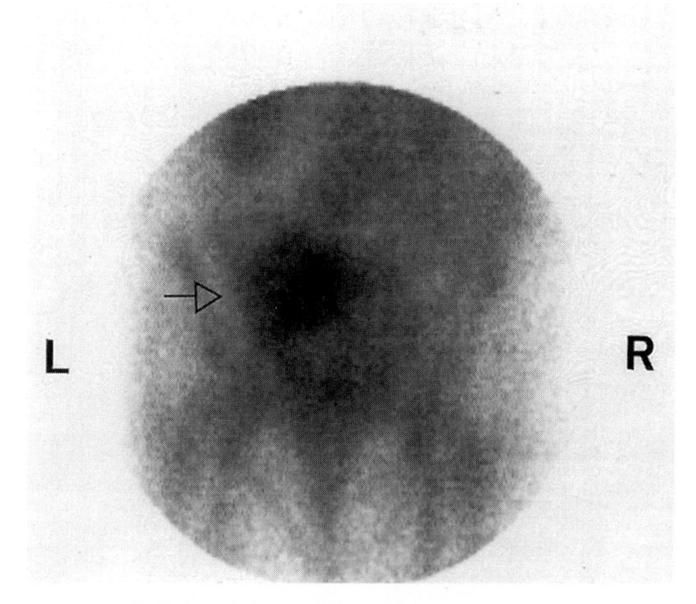

Fig. 6.4 Radionuclide scan: primary ovarian carcinoma. Anterior view of the pelvis with 80 Mbq ^{111}In-labelled OC-125.

nal septations and divisions may be defined using this technique (Fig. 6.5).

On ultrasound, the uterine cavity is normally represented by a bright line of apposition of the endometrial layers, though occasionally a trace of fluid can be seen at menstruation. Persistent fluid or fluid in a non-menstruating woman is abnormal. In adolescence, it may be caused by vaginal atresia, where the upper vagina dilates more than the uterus so that haematocolpos dominates the picture, while in postmenopausal women cervical stenosis, either fibrotic or malignant must be considered. Ultrasound is also useful in detecting the position of an IUCD; provided the coil lies in the uterus it is easily located, but a coil that has penetrated through the myometrium is obscured by echoes from bowel gas (Fig. 6.6).

The entire uterus can be imaged using ultrasound (Fig. 6.7) and the size measured accurately. This is useful in precocious or delayed puberty and in planning brachytherapy. The endometrium is seen as an echogenic layer of uniform texture, often with a fine echo-poor margin. Its thickness varies through the menstrual cycle from 12 mm premenstrually (double layer thickness) to a thin

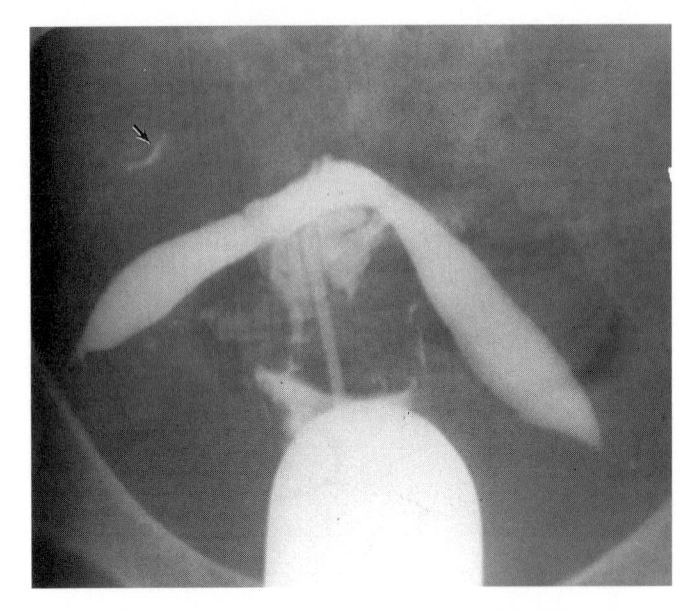

Fig. 6.5 Hysterosalpingogram: contrast outlining the cavities of a bicornuate uterus. Free spill into the peritoneal cavity can be seen on the right (arrow).

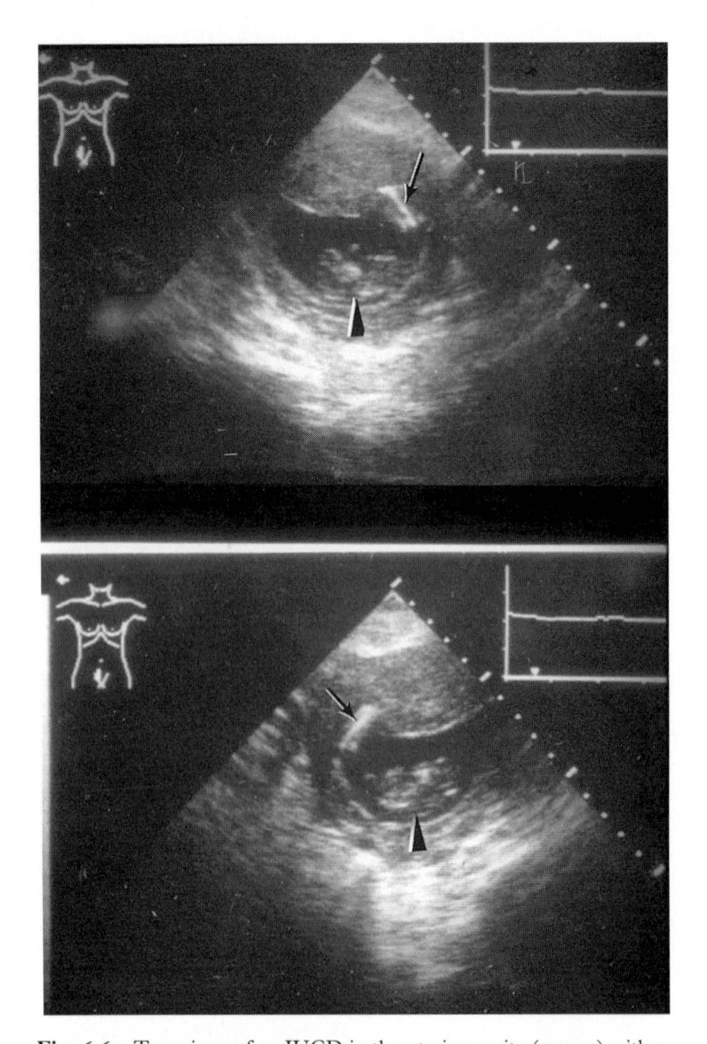

Fig. 6.6 Two views of an IUCD in the uterine cavity (arrows) with a coexisting pregnancy (arrowheads).

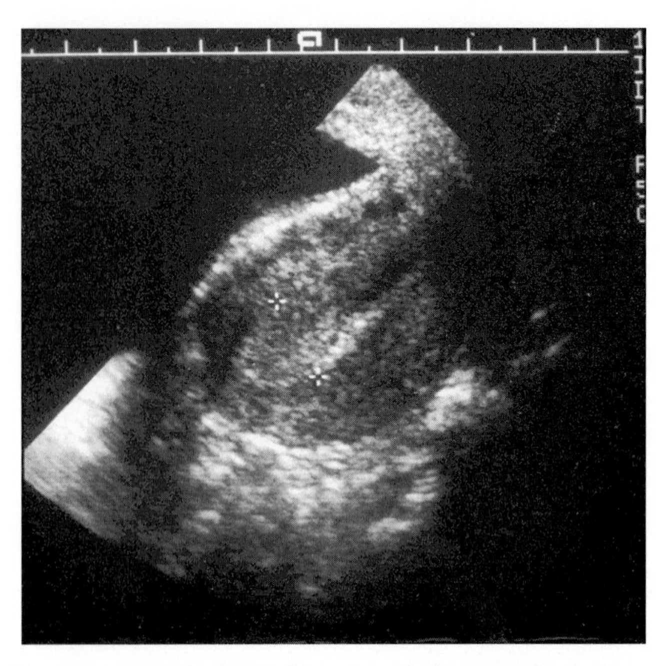

Fig. 6.7 Transvaginal scan of the uterus. In this scan, taken in the luteal phase of the cycle, the secretory endometrium is seen as an echogenic band by comparison with the relatively echo-poor myometrium.

line after menstruation. The endometrium gradually thins after menopause unless supported by hormones.

The morphology of the normal uterus, however is best defined on MRI where the zonal architecture of the uterus may be recognized (Hricak et al 1983). On T_2-weighted images the endometrium is seen as a central high-signal stripe which increases in thickness in the secretory phase of the menstrual cycle. The inner myometrium (junctional zone) is of lower signal intensity than the outer myometrium on T_2 weighting, and histologically correlates with a layer of more densely packed smooth muscle.

Fallopian tubes

The patency of the fallopian tubes may be demonstrated on hysterosalpingography where filling and free spill into the peritoneal cavity may be seen (Fig. 6.5). To reduce the radiation dose to the ovaries in patients trying to conceive, ultrasound salpingography is currently being evaluated. Normal uterine tubes cannot usually be demonstrated on ultrasound, but instillation of the newly developed echo-enhancing agents into the uterus and tubes permits their visualization and can be used as an initial screening test for tubal patency. The most effective echo-enhancing agents consist of microbubbles in the 2–5 micron range. They give intense echoes which can be seen both within the uterine cavity and flowing out along the tubes, eventually appearing in the adnexal region, following intrauterine injection. Though the anatomical detail is less than that offered by conventional X-ray salpingography, and false-positive results occur, this technique of ultrasound salpingography seems likely to find an important role as an initial screen; if the tubes are demonstrated to be patent, no further investigation is necessary and this should result in a reduction of radiation exposure.

The normal fallopian tubes are too small in calibre and of too variable a course to be reliably imaged using a cross-sectional technique such as CT or MRI.

Ovaries

The ovaries are best imaged with ultrasound (either trans-abdominal or preferably transvaginal). Changes in their appearances can be correlated with their functional status. Infantile ovaries are small (except in the neonate when hypertrophy and follicles stimulated by maternal hormones may be a surprising finding) and they enlarge before puberty. Follicular development begins before menstruation but these cycles and those at the menopause are often imperfect, so that follicles may persist and continue enlarging for several months. Normally ovulation occurs at a follicle size of 20–25 mm diameter and the echo-free follicle is replaced by a corpus luteum which can be cystic or solid. Corpora lutea produce a confusing variety of appearances, whose only consistent feature is their transience (Fig. 6.8a–c). In doubtful cases, a re-scan at 6 weeks to image them at a different phase of the cycle may be needed to resolve their identity.

On CT and MRI, the normal ovaries are often difficult

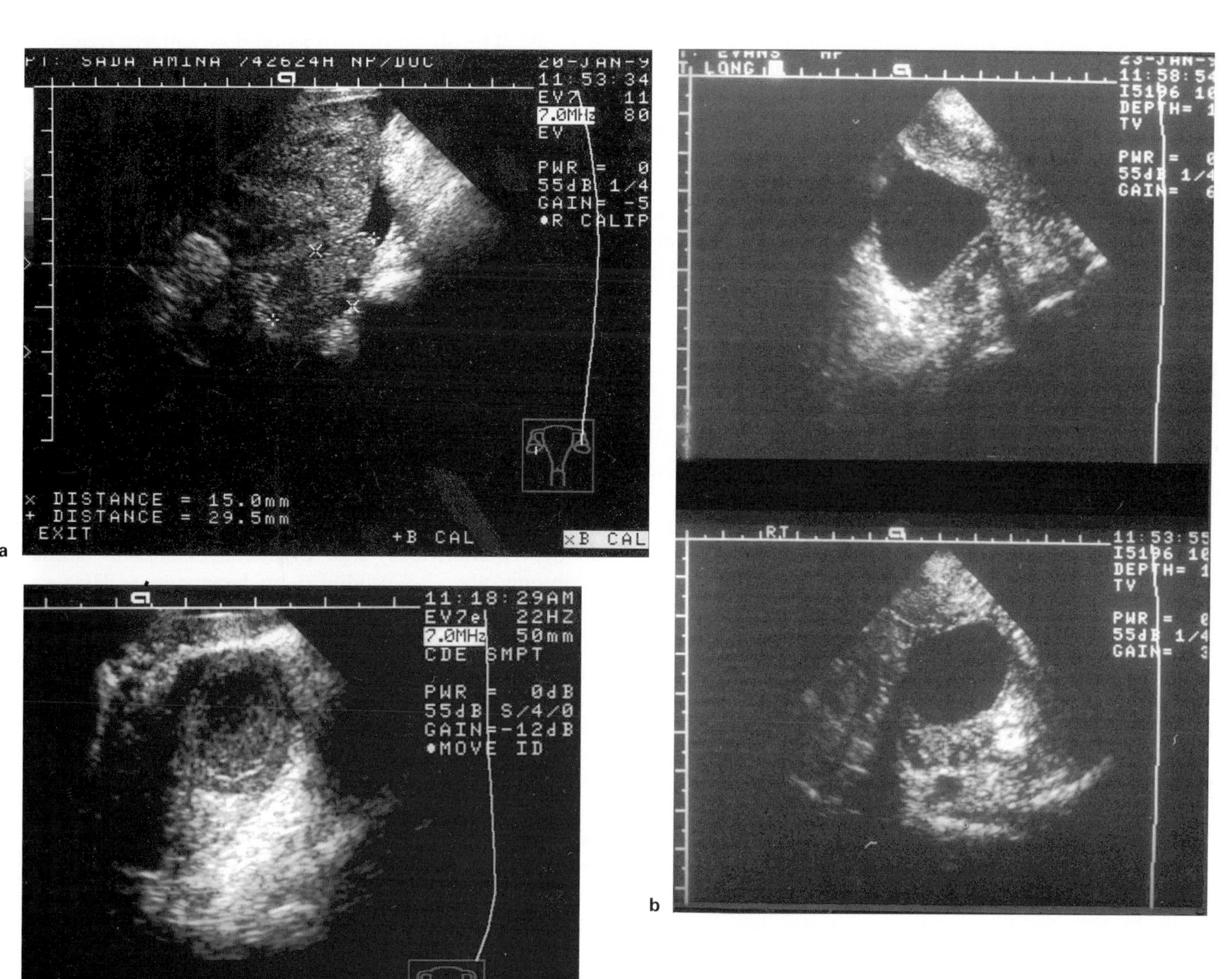

Fig. 6.8 Transvaginal scans of the ovary. **a** An inactive ovary is indicated by the calliper marks. It is surrounded by a small amount of free fluid and contains minute developing follicles. **b** Two views of an ovary containing a 3-cm simple cystic structure which presumably represents an unruptured follicle. **c** An ovary in the luteal phase containing a solid corpus luteum.

to define, but may be recognized on short inversion recovery (STIR) MRI sequences as very high signal foci in the adenexae.

Ovarian varices

The pelvic congestion syndrome is one of many causes of chronic pelvic pain and is associated with the presence of large varices within the broad ligaments (Hobbs 1990). When severe pelvic symptoms are present there may be gross dilatation of the ovarian veins, with reflux down into the pelvis and often into the legs. These vessels are best demonstrated by selective ovarian venography although they may also be imaged with duplex Doppler ultrasound. Venography is performed via a femoral or internal jugular venous approach and the ovarian veins are selectively catheterized with an appropriately shaped angiographic catheter. Satisfactory retrograde opacification of pelvic varices is achieved by injecting contrast medium through the selectively placed catheter with the patient almost upright on a tilting table, while Valsalva manoeuvre is performed.

Treatment of this condition is primarily surgical and consists of venous ligation. More recently symptomatic relief has been reported following transcatheter ovarian vein embolization (Sichlau et al 1994).

Investigation of female infertility

The success of in vitro fertilization (IVF) has been due in part to the correct timing of ovulation and subsequent oocyte recovery which ultrasound can provide. Using transabdominal scanning, ovarian follicles of 3–5 mm diameter can be visualized. They appear as echo-free structures amidst the more echogenic ovarian tissue. Their rate of growth is linear and the mean diameter prior to ovulation is 20.2 mm (range 18–24 mm, Bryce et al 1982). Structures within the follicle such as the cumulus oophorous can also be visualized. Following ovulation, internal echoes appear because of bleeding. Free fluid may also be observed in the pouch of Douglas.

Transvaginal sonography has largely replaced the transabdominal approach in infertility practice. Follicular aspiration is possible with a needle-guide attachment to the vaginal probe, as is fine-needle aspiration of fluid in the pouch of Douglas. A more precise measurement of follicular size is possible and the corpus luteum is easily recognized. In the mid-luteal phase it appears as an oval structure of 30–35 mm in length and 20–25 mm wide with a wide variety of sonographic appearances (Timor-Tritsch et al 1988). Endometrial reflectivity patterns have been proposed as another variable for the assessment of ovulation (Randall et al 1989). Ultrasound can only provide presumptive evidence of ovulation/pregnancy. The collection of secondary oocytes constitutes definitive evidence. The appearance of internal echoes before the follicle reaches 18 mm or continuous enlargement to 30–40 mm indicates follicular failure.

Ultrasound is also useful for accurate timing of artificial insemination, while a postcoital test can help differentiate between inadequate sperm penetration and poor mucus production in the presence of immature follicles. Ultrasound scanning is also employed to monitor patients on clomiphene therapy, and there is good correlation between follicular diameters and plasma estradiol concentrations. The hyperstimulation syndrome is uncommon if gonadotrophin therapy is monitored by ultrasound in conjunction with measurements of plasma estradiol levels.

The waveforms of blood flow in vessels supplying the ovaries of women undergoing IVF have been studied using transvaginal pulsed Doppler ultrasound (Barber et al 1988). The observation of blood flow patterns may help in the prediction of implantation failure.

MR imaging is valuable in the investigation of infertility where uterine pathology is suspected and it provides a particularly high diagnostic yield in patients with dysmenorrhoea and menorrhagia (deSouza et al 1995). It should be part of the investigation of patients with persistent unexplained infertility awaiting costly procedures such as gamete intrafallopian transfer (GIFT) and IVF. MR imaging should also be used before myomectomy in order to differentiate between leiomyoma and adenomyoma as attempts to perform a myomectomy on a localized adenomyoma often result in extensive uterine damage.

Adenomyosis and endometriosis

In infertility, where uterine conservation is paramount, the diagnosis of adenomyosis is often suggested by symptoms of hypermenorrhoea and dysmenorrhoea but similar symptoms are also produced by leiomyomas. Hysterosalpingography may show multiple small tracks of contrast extending into the myometrium but the results are often equivocal (Marshall & Eliasoph 1955) and the dose of pelvic radiation must be taken into consideration in patients trying to conceive. Laparoscopy may reveal a nodular, sometimes injected-looking uterine serosa. Myometrial biopsies taken at laparoscopy may be negative in focal disease and the diagnosis of adenomyosis may be missed. Ultrasound in skilled hands may be useful (Fedele et al 1992).

Adenomyosis is best demonstrated on T_2-weighted MR images, with which two patterns, a focal and a diffuse one, can be recognized (Hricak et al 1992, Togashi et al 1988). In focal adenomyosis there is a localized ill-defined mixed signal intensity mass (adenomyoma) within the myometrium (Fig. 6.9). Diffuse adenomyosis presents with diffuse or irregular thickening of the junctional zone, often with underlying high-signal foci (Fig. 6.10). Pathologically this represents smooth muscle hypertrophy and hyperpla-

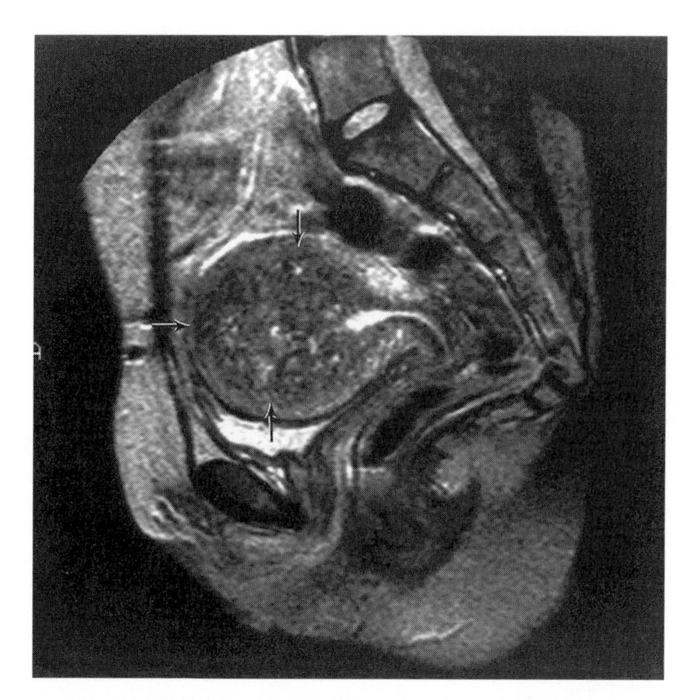

Fig. 6.9 Focal adenomyoma. T_2-weighted spin echo (SE2500/80) midline sagittal section through the uterus, demonstrating a large ill-defined mixed-signal intensity mass characteristic of an adenomyoma (arrows).

sia surrounding a focus of basal endometrium (Noval & deLima 1948). It is the smooth muscle changes that are easily recognized by MR rather than the foci of heterotopic glandular epithelium. In our experience, however, the thickening of the junctional zone that is described in adenomyosis (Togashi et al 1988) is not diagnostic of adenomyosis on its own; it may be seen in hypermenorrhoea where no pathological evidence for adenomyosis has subsequently been shown. In these instances, absolute values for junctional zone widths are unhelpful and ratios to the width of the outer myometrium or the cervical stroma may be more meaningful (Hricak et al 1983).

Like adenomyosis, the lesions of endometriosis are difficult to detect on ultrasound, mainly because of their small size. Larger endometriomas are seen as well defined spaces, most commonly in the adnexal region (Fig. 6.11). The role of MR imaging in the diagnosis of endometriosis also depends on the site of the endometriotic implants: deposits on the ovarian cortex are much more readily identified than small peritoneal deposits. The latter are recognized at laparoscopy but may be missed on MR imaging (Brosens 1993). MR imaging may, however, be valuable in detecting deep enclosed endometriosis typically found in the uterosacral ligaments and rectovaginal septum (Fig. 6.12). This type is associated with pelvic pain. It consists mainly of fibromuscular rather than endometrial tissue (Hamlin et al 1985) and because of its position often goes undetected on visual inspection of the pelvic cavity.

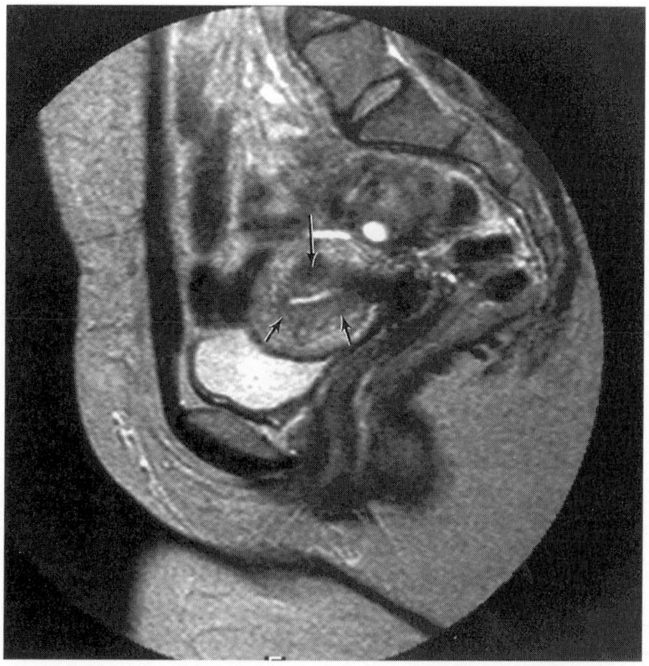

Fig. 6.10 Diffuse adenomyosis. T_2-weighted spin echo (SE2500/80) midline sagittal section through the uterus, showing thickening and irregularity of the low signal band of junctional zone (short arrows). Diffuse infiltration of a mixed-signal lesion (long arrow) is seen in the posterior wall.

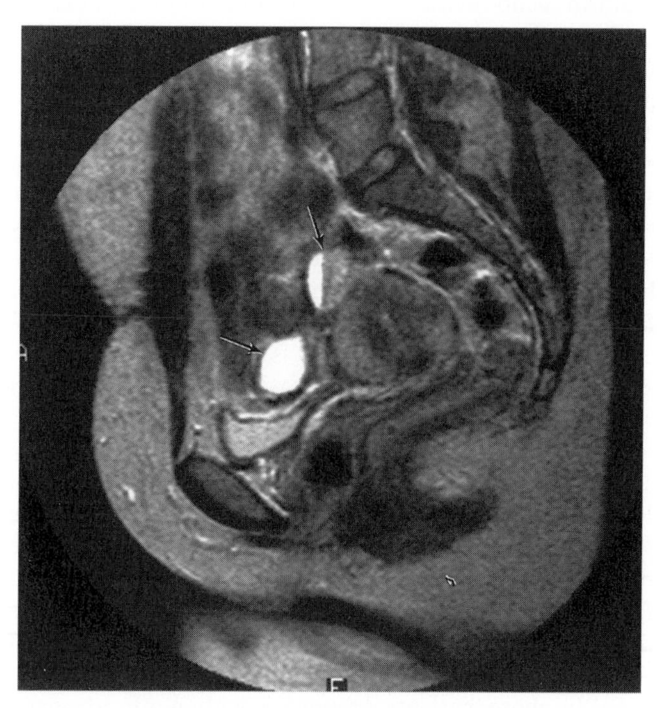

Fig. 6.11 Endometriotic deposits. T_2-weighted spin echo (SE2500/80) midline sagittal image; fluid levels are seen in cystic lesions with mixed signal intensity suggestive of haemorrhage (arrows).

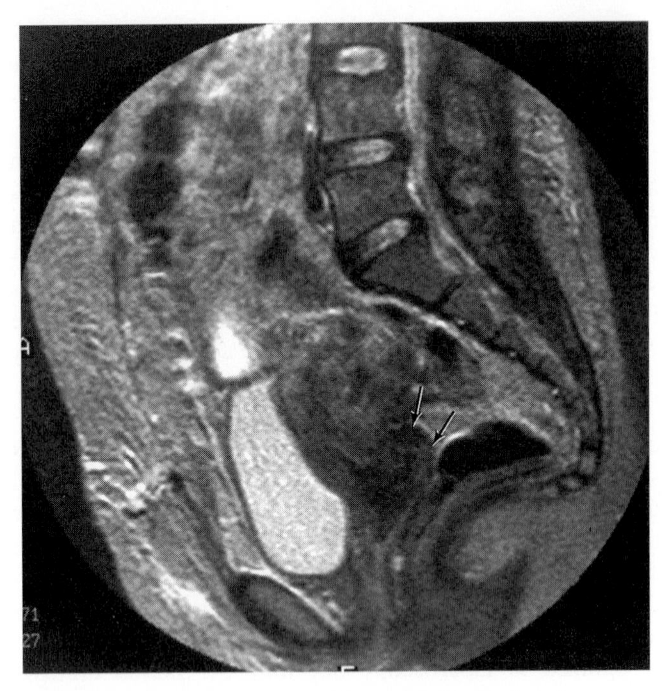

Fig. 6.12 Rectovaginal endometriosis. T_2-weighted spin echo (SE2500/80) sagittal section demonstrating a rectovaginal mass (arrows) in a patient with laparoscopically proven endometriosis. This was not detected at laparoscopy because it is retroperitoneal

Leiomyomas

The commonest cause of disturbance of the normal uniform echo texture of the myometrium is fibroids. Generally, a focal thickening occurs and their position in the uterus can be determined. Submucosal fibroids, or the polyps they may produce, can be mistaken for endometrial thickening, though occasionally the way they move with normal uterine contractions is diagnostic. Instillation of saline into the uterine cavity, a form of ultrasound contrast, provides much more information about intracavitary lesions. Pedunculated or broad ligament fibroids frequently masquerade as extrauterine masses. The echo texture of fibroids is very variable in accordance with their histological spectrum. A characteristic is calcification which is easily recognized on ultrasound, as intensely reflective foci with accompanying acoustic shadowing.

MR imaging has been reported to be superior to ultrasound for the diagnosis of leiomyomas (Ascher et al 1994, Hamlin et al 1985, Hricak et al 1992). Characteristic well defined low intensity masses are seen within the myometrium on T_2-weighted scans, often with high signal foci within them. There are no completely reliable features that distinguish fibroids from leiomyosarcomas on ultrasound or MRI and even Doppler has proved disappointing here. In those patients presenting with more advanced disease, alterations in the uterine configuration may suggest malignant change.

Ectopic pregnancy

Traditionally, ultrasound has been used to exclude an ectopic pregnancy by demonstrating an intrauterine pregnancy. The positive diagnosis of ectopic pregnancy requires the demonstration of an extrauterine fetal heart. Secondary features that may be recognized are an adnexal mass with peritrophoblastic Doppler signals, free fluid in the pelvis and increased endometrial thickness. With a combination of these features the negative predictive value of an ultrasound examination may be 96%. This figure is improved further with the addition of the measurement of β-hCG (Emerson 1992). However, significant problems can arise in distinguishing an ectopic pregnancy without a pseudogestational sac from an early normal or failed intrauterine pregnancy.

The role of ultrasound in the diagnosis of ectopic gestations has been strengthened by the use of transvaginal probes and the introduction of Doppler. A weakness of transabdominal scanning was the difficulty in demonstrating the sac itself, because of gas in overlying or adherent bowel. With transvaginal scanning, the adnexal sac can be demonstrated and women at high risk can be monitored through the first few weeks of pregnancy (Fig. 6.13). Early ectopic sacs can be treated by injection of potassium chloride or methotrexate under ultrasound guidance. This approach is especially useful in IVF programmes where sparing the uterine tubes is so important.

Infections

Ultrasound is useful in the diagnosis and management of ovarian abscesses, where shaggy walled cavities can be demonstrated in the adnexal region (Fig. 6.14). They

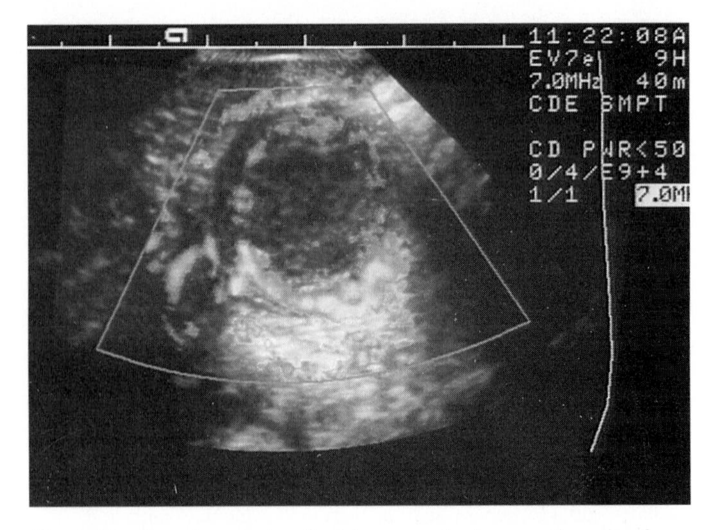

Fig. 6.13 Ectopic gestation. In this transvaginal scan, colour signals are seen around the ectopic sac. This scan was taken with the energy mode of colour Doppler, a more sensitive type of signal processing.

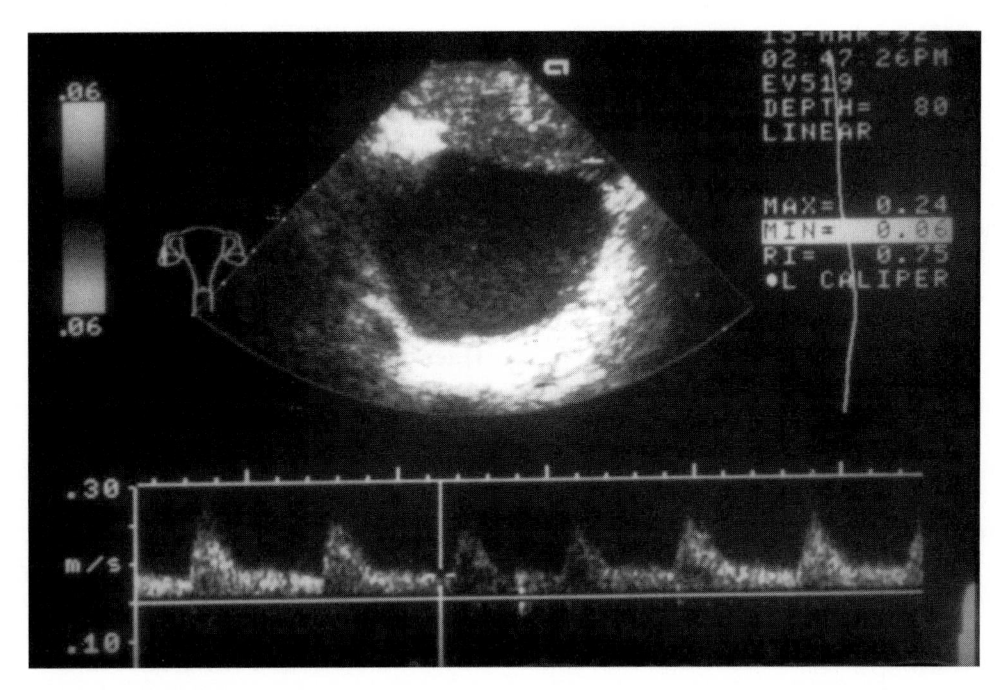

Fig. 6.14 Tubo-ovarian abscess. The irregular walls of this cavity are vascularized as part of the inflammatory response.

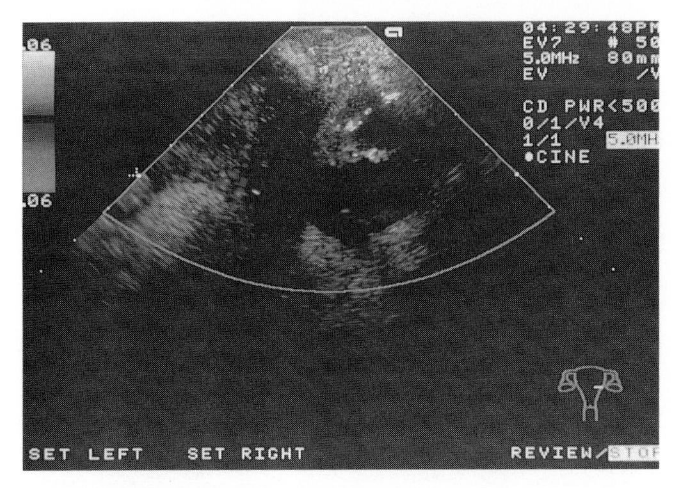

Fig. 6.15 Tubo-ovarian abscess. The marked colour signals within and around this abscess cavity are indicators of its inflammatory nature.

usually have a vascular pseudocapsule that can be demonstrated on colour Doppler (Fig. 6.15). However, in pelvic inflammatory disease without abscess formation, the ultrasonic changes are too subtle to make this a useful technique. Monitoring the effects of antibiotic treatment on tubo-ovarian abscesses may be useful, although in some cases sterile cavities persist for many weeks after signs of infection have been controlled. The hydrosalpinx that complicates pelvic inflammatory disease (PID) is seen as a funnel-shaped cavity in the adnexal region with thin walls and no internal echoes.

Venous thrombosis

Diagnosis

A relatively common complication of pregnancy and gynaecological malignancies, deep venous thrombosis is most easily diagnosed using colour Doppler ultrasound and this should be the investigation of first choice. Visualization of the iliac veins may be difficult and some patients will have to proceed to contrast venography. If colour Doppler ultrasound has shown the femoral veins to be clear of thrombus, venography is most easily performed by puncturing these vessels directly. This will allow excellent opacification of the iliac veins and thus a confident diagnosis or exclusion of thrombosis, which might be difficult on conventional venograms performed with injection of contrast medium through foot veins.

Inferior vena cava filter insertion

The indications for insertion of an inferior vena cava filter are listed in Table 6.1. The procedure is easily performed via femoral or jugular venous punctures, and some devices

Table 6.1 Indications for inferior vena cava filter placement

Recurrent pulmonary emboli despite anticoagulation
Pulmonary embolic disease in a patient in whom anticoagulation is contraindicated
Free-floating pelvic or inferior vena caval thrombus
Prophylaxis during surgery (see text)
Previous life-threatening pulmonary embolism

may even be inserted through a sheath introduced into an antecubital fossa vein. The majority of these filters are inserted permanently; short-term placement is possible, however, and is most commonly indicated in the late stages of pregnancy (when free-floating thrombus is demonstrated or when a recent pulmonary embolus has occurred), or prior to surgical removal of a large pelvic tumour which has caused compression and thrombosis of one or both iliac veins. Two types of short-term filter may be used:

1. *Temporary filters* are mounted on a long catheter and are placed via an internal jugular or antecubital fossa venous approach into the infrarenal inferior vena cava above the thrombus (Fig. 6.16). The device is then sutured in place. These devices can only remain in situ for a period of approximately 10 days and should then be removed because of the risk of infection.

2. *Retrievable filters* are designed for permanent placement but may be removed up to 10 days after their insertion via an internal jugular venous approach. One such device is the Günther Tulip filter (William Cook Europe, Bjaeverskov, Denmark) which has a hook on its superior aspect. This may be grasped with a loop snare and withdrawn into a sheath prior to its removal. Removal of these devices is possible after 10 days, but this is associated with more potential complications, as some endothelialization of the filter is likely to have occurred at this time and the filter limbs may be partially fixed to the caval wall.

Haemorrhage

Haemorrhage from the genital tract may complicate parturition or may be associated with benign (e.g. uterine arteriovenous malformation) or malignant (e.g. cervical carcinoma) disease. Traditional surgical therapy of severe pelvic haemorrhage consists most commonly of unilateral or bilateral internal iliac artery ligation, although in the case of primary postpartum haemorrhage (PPH) hysterectomy is performed more often than ligation (Shingawa 1964). In the largest series devoted to internal iliac artery

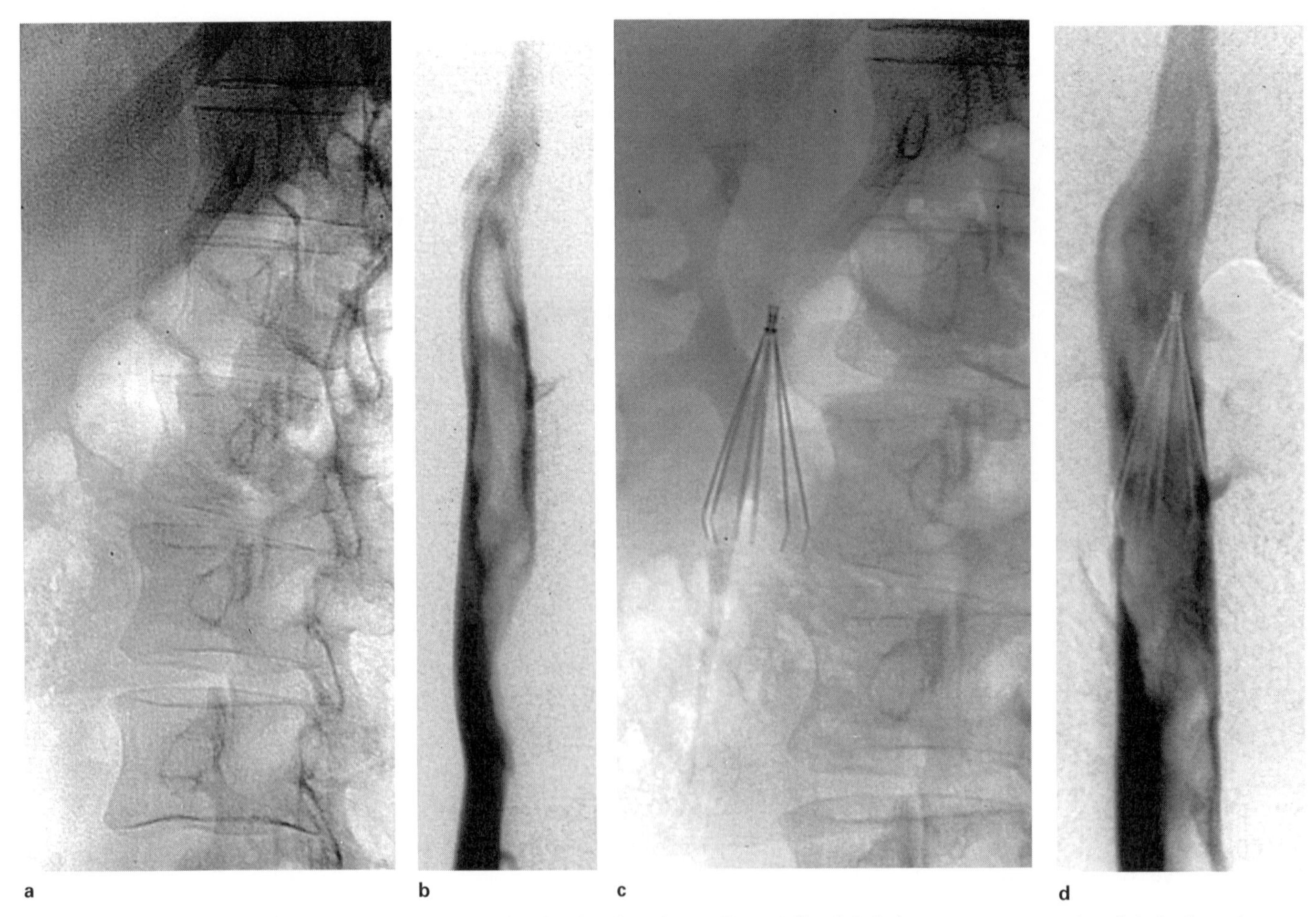

Fig. 6.16 Temporary vena caval filter insertion above free-floating thrombus. **a** Control film. **b** Inferior vena cavogram using digital subtraction demonstrates a large free-floating thrombus **c, d** A temporary filter has been placed on top of the thrombus using a right internal jugular approach. The plastic catheter on which the filter is mounted is barely visible.

ligation, however, the technique was successful in only eight out of 19 cases (Clark et al 1985).

There is a strong argument in favour of angiography and embolization being performed prior to arterial ligation or hysterectomy in hospitals where the expertise is available for this form of therapy. Bleeding sites are often impossible to localize at surgery (hence the necessity for non-specific ligation of the internal iliac artery) but are often easily identified at angiography; occlusion of the haemorrhaging vessel can then be performed very selectively, with a much higher likelihood of controlling bleeding (Fig. 6.17). Previous internal iliac artery ligation does not necessarily prevent successful arterial embolization but may make the procedure technically more difficult (Collins & Jackson 1995, Duggan et al 1991).

Embolization is very successful in a variety of gynaecological disorders complicated by bleeding (Collins & Jackson 1995). For certain conditions (e.g. uterine arteriovenous malformations, bleeding from recurrent cervical carcinoma) this therapy should probably be considered as the procedure of first choice (Fig. 6.18). In others it may be life-saving when more conventional treatment has failed.

a

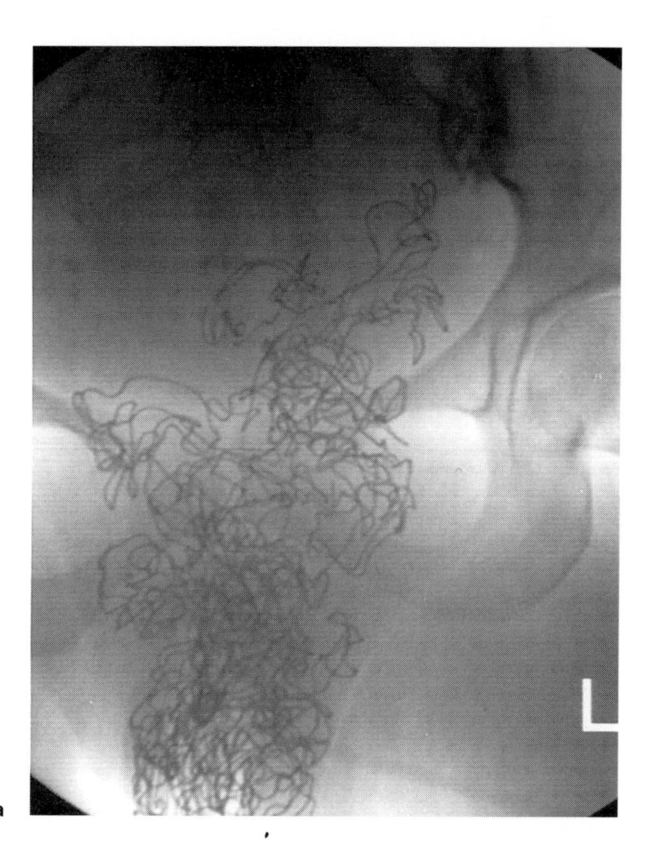

b

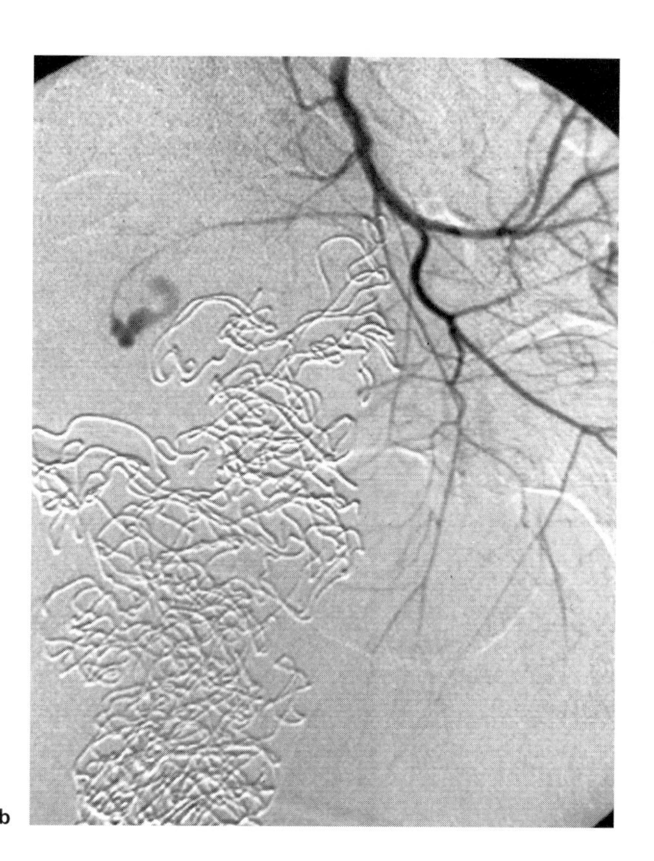

c

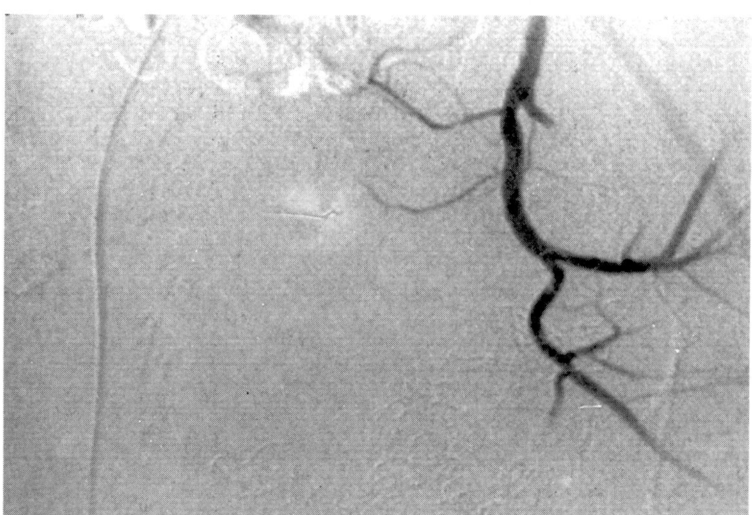

Fig. 6.17 Severe postpartum haemorrhage in a patient who had been explored twice vaginally and who continued to bleed in spite of vaginal packing.
a Control film showing a large pack in pelvis.
b Selective internal iliac arteriogram demonstrates brisk extravasation of contrast from a branch of the anterior division. This was selectively catheterized and occluded with polyvinyl alcohol particles.
c Postembolization arteriogram demonstrates occlusion of the bleeding vessel with no further extravasation of contrast.

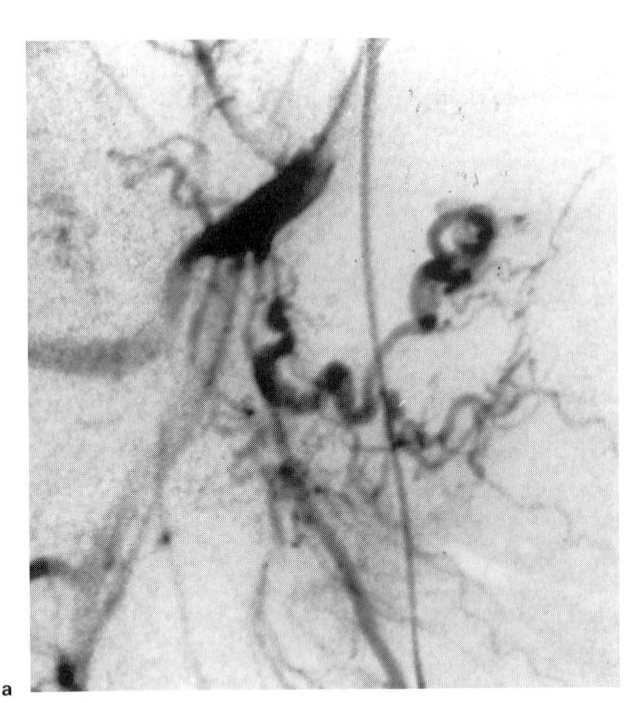

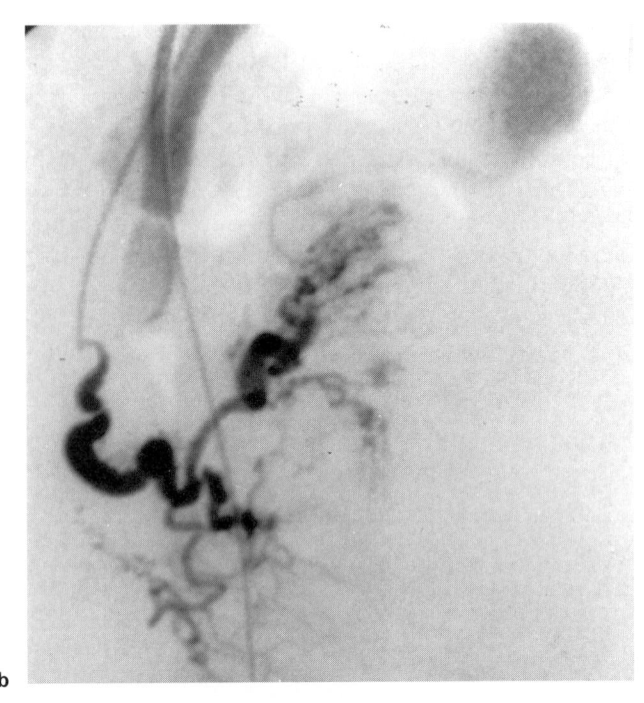

Fig. 6.18 Embolization of an area of neovascularity in the right side of the pelvis due to recurrent carcinoma of the cervix in a patient with persistent bleeding. **a** Selective right internal iliac arteriogram using digital subtraction shows encasement of the origin of the right uterine artery which supplies an extensive area of neovascularity. **b** The right uterine artery has been selectively catheterized prior to embolization. Note the marked irregularity of this vessel due to involvement by tumour. Embolization performed with polyvinyl alcohol particles gave excellent control of bleeding.

Cervical carcinoma

The cervix

In cervical carcinoma, precise staging of the primary disease provides a prognosis, allows the institution of correct treatment and permits comparison of different treatment protocols. Clinical staging, applied according to the system of the International Federation of Gynaecology and Obstetrics (FIGO), is subjective and is notoriously poor, so that some centres use pretreatment laparotomy as the staging method of choice (Levenback et al 1992). Imaging with ultrasound does not improve the accuracy of clinical staging (Levenback et al 1992), thus transabdominal ultrasound is of little value in the assessment of patients with cervical cancer. Poor image quality and difficulty in interpretation are the major problems. Transrectal ultrasound produces clearer views of the cervix but definition of tumour from normal cervix is still poor. The same difficulty limits the value of CT, since both the normal cervix and cervical carcinoma have similar attenuation values, so that the primary tumour can only be recognized if it alters the contour or size of the normal cervix (Subak et al 1995).

Several studies have now confirmed the accuracy of MRI in the staging of early cervical cancer in comparison to the surgical stage (Powell et al 1986b, Togashi et al 1987). Patients are best assessed using T_2-weighted MRI of the primary tumour which is superior to CT in tumour detection (sensitivity 75 vs. 51%, $p < 0.005$) and in overall tumour staging (accuracy 75–77 vs. 32–69%, $p < 0.025$) (Ho et al 1992, Kim et al 1993).

The resolution of MRI of the primary tumour may be further improved by using intracavitary receiver coils. Endorectal coils give high resolution images of the posterior cervix, but the anterior margin of the tumour and its relation to the bladder base is often difficult to define because of drop-off of signal. Endovaginal coils give very high resolution images of the cervix and adjacent parametrium (deSouza et al 1996). The distortion of the low signal ring of inner stroma may be apparent and any breaks in the ring representing tumour extension may be identified (Fig. 6.19a,b).

With MRI, the invasion of cervical cancer may be assessed in three planes: the coronal and axial planes may be used for determining parametrial invasion, the axial plane for determining extension into the bladder and rectum and the sagittal plane for extension into the uterine body, bladder and rectum (Goto et al 1990). Using newly developed sequences improves the quality of the images still further (Fig. 6.20). The use of 3-D volume imaging also provides the information necessary to calculate tumour volumes, which is of prognostic significance. Volumes obtained with MRI correlate well with those obtained by histomorphometric methods but only weakly with clinical stage (Burghardt et al 1989). The volumetry of the tumour also gives a more accurate prediction of parametri-

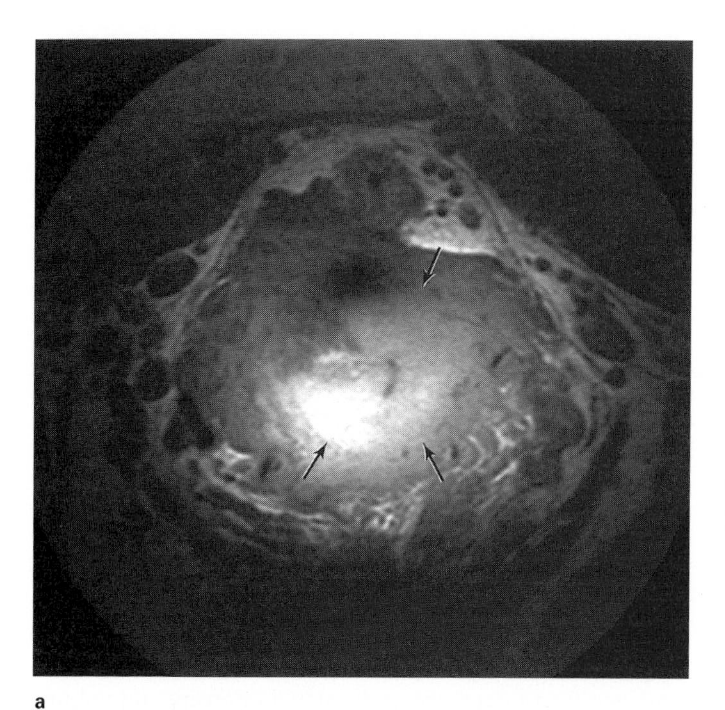

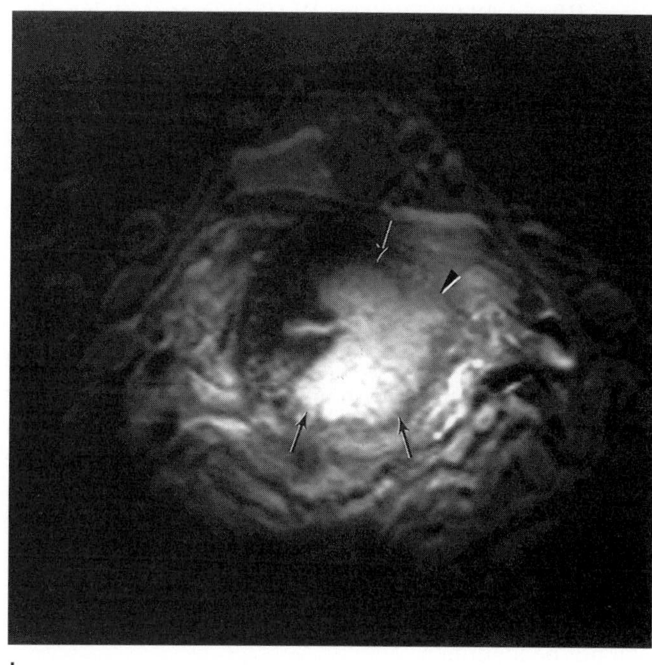

a b

Fig. 6.19 Carcinoma of the cervix. **a** T_1-weighted (SE 780/20), and **b** T_2-weighted (SE 2500/80) transverse spin echo through the cervix showing a large intermediate signal intensity mass mainly on the left. There is distortion and displacement of the normal low signal band of inner stroma (arrows). A break in this stromal ring indicating parametrial extension is seen on the T_2-weighted images (arrowhead in **b**).

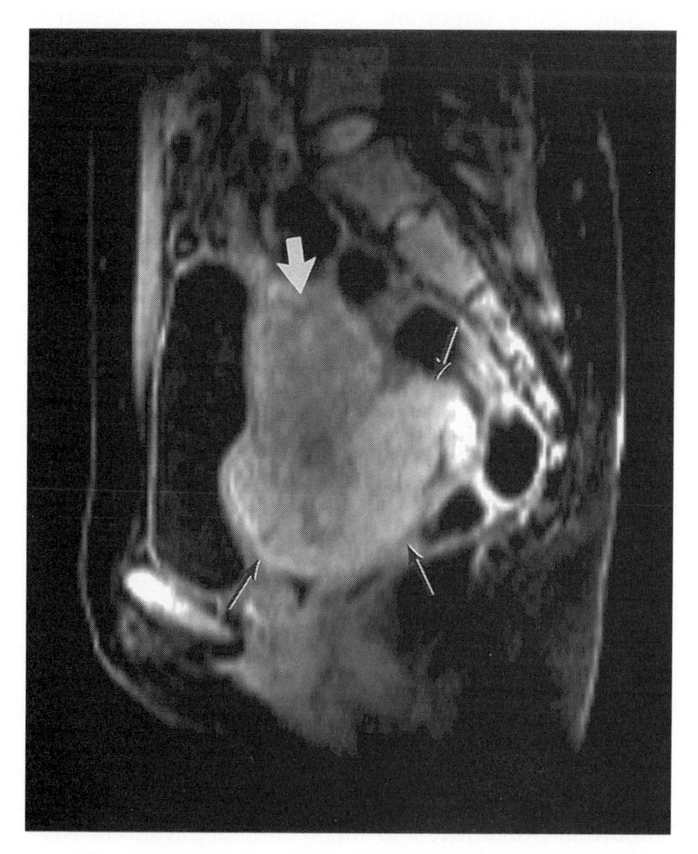

Fig. 6.20 Carcinoma of the cervix: a sagittal MRI image using a newly developed double inversion recovery sequence through the pelvis. A large carcinoma is seen (arrows) abutting but not invading the bladder base anteriorly and the rectal wall posteriorly. The uterus lies immediately cranial (large arrow).

al invasion and lymph node involvement (Burghardt et al 1992).

Parametrium

Transrectal ultrasound, CT and MRI have all been used to assess parametrial spread. In a series of 180 patients, good correlation was found between the ultrasound and surgical findings, but significant problems arose in distinguishing between inflammatory or fibrotic change and tumour invasion (Yuhara et al 1987). Similarly, false-positive diagnoses may arise from misinterpreting normal inflammatory parametrial soft tissue strands as tumour invasion, on both CT and MRI. A comparison of the assessment by these modalities with histological findings after radical hysterectomy showed an accuracy rate for parametrial involvement of 87–90% for MRI, 55–80% for CT and 82.5% for examination under anaesthesia (Kim et al 1993, Ho et al 1992). Extracervical extension on MRI is best defined using contrast enhancement and varied pulse sequences. MR therefore yields valuable information for treatment planning (Sironi et al 1991) and should be used routinely in conjunction with clinical staging to determine the appropriate therapy in patients with cervical carcinoma.

An intravenous urogram (IVU) is an essential part of the staging process and may sometimes demonstrate partial or complete ureteric obstruction or displacement and distortion of the bladder outline. The IVU is abnormal in 2.1% of apparent Stage I cases, 5.1% in Stage II, 26.8% in

Stage III and 48.9% in Stage IV (Griffin et al 1976). The presence of a hydronephrosis or non-functioning kidney due to stenosis from tumour invasion of the ureter puts the patient into Stage III, even if according to the other findings the case should be allotted to an earlier stage.

Barium enema abnormalities are rare in cervical cancer and proctoscopy is also positive if an abnormality is observed on the enema.

Nodal involvement

The role of lymphangiography in the staging of cervical cancer is controversial, with up to 71% false-positives and 16% false-negatives. Percutaneous fine-needle aspiration biopsy of nodes may improve the results that can be obtained with pelvic lymphangiography. CT has proved to be a reliable method for staging and following lymph node disease in patients with lymphoma, but the major drawback for epithelial tumours is that the nodes require to be enlarged to be detected. Thus metastases less than 2 cm will not be identified.

MRI is superior to CT in pelvic lymph node evaluation (accuracy 88 vs. 83%, $p < 0.01$) (Kim et al 1993). However, like CT it relies on changes in the size of the lymph nodes (Fig. 6.21) since the tumour deposits themselves are not highlighted. Although an in vitro study has shown that lymph nodes containing metastases have a significantly longer T_2 than do normal or hyperplastic nodes (Weiner et al 1986), in vivo tissue characterization based on relaxation times or signal intensities does not support this data.

A small clinical study suggested that ^{123}I-labelled epidermal growth factor may be used to recognize cervical cancer lymph node metastases because these tumours express high levels of the receptor (Schatten et al 1992).

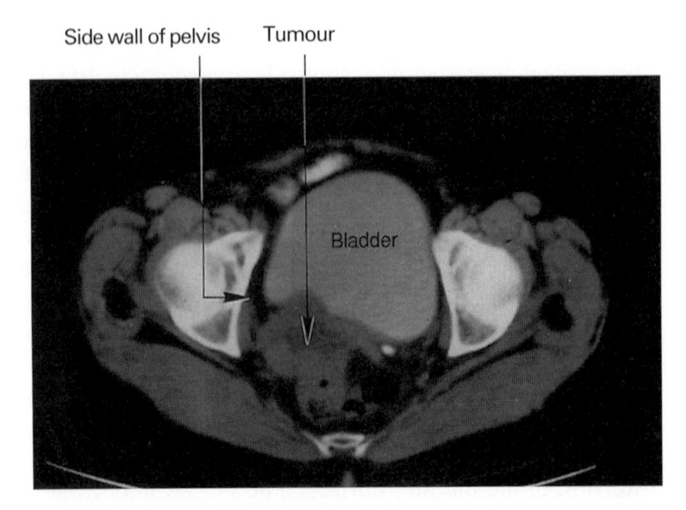

Fig. 6.21 CT scan of stage IIIb cervical carcinoma.

Distant spread

Even with advanced pelvic spread, involvement of distant sites is the exception rather than the rule. In only one of 160 patients was a bone scan positive and this patient had stage IV disease with liver metastases (Hirnle et al 1990). Patients with stage I and II cervical cancer do not need to have bone scans.

A chest X-ray is a routine pretreatment investigation but the yield of lung metastases at first presentation is likely to be no more than 2%.

Assessing response and recurrence

In conjunction with clinical examination, MRI may provide an objective assessment of the effects of surgery or radiotherapy. Serial MRI may be used before and after primary radiation therapy to assess tumour response (Flueckiger et al 1992). Primary tumours with a volume of >50 cm^3 are likely to have no response or a delayed response (Flueckiger et al 1992). An early (2–3 months) and significant decrease in the signal intensity and volume of tumour indicates a favourable response.

With the increased use of new cytotoxic regimes for primary and recurrent tumour, accurate imaging techniques become more important. Early detection of recurrent cervical cancer in order to institute cytotoxic therapy may be of value. CT and ultrasound have limited ability to differentiate between fibrosis and tumour. While some say that infiltration of the parametrium may be easily recognizable, it is difficult to differentiate fibrosis after treatment from tumour recurrence. Although isolated reports promote MRI in distinguishing post-treatment fibrosis and recurrent pelvic neoplasm by measuring signal intensities from the different tissues on T_2-weighted pulse sequences (Ebner et al 1988), in individual cases fibrosis is often impossible to differentiate from recurrence.

Endometrial carcinoma

Primary tumour

Thickening of the endometrium is characteristic of endometrial carcinoma and is well demonstrated on transvaginal ultrasound (Fig. 6.22). However specificity is low and Doppler has been suggested as a way to distinguish hormonal causes of thickening (weak signals) and malignancy which gives marked colour and spectral Doppler signals.

In patients already proven to have an endometrial cancer, the presence and depth of myometrial extension has important prognostic and therapeutic implications. Myometrial invasion may be classified as absent, superficial or deep. It may be possible to assess the depth of myometrial invasion with high-resolution ultrasound probes. In a study of 20 patients 70% of the ultrasound estimations of inva-

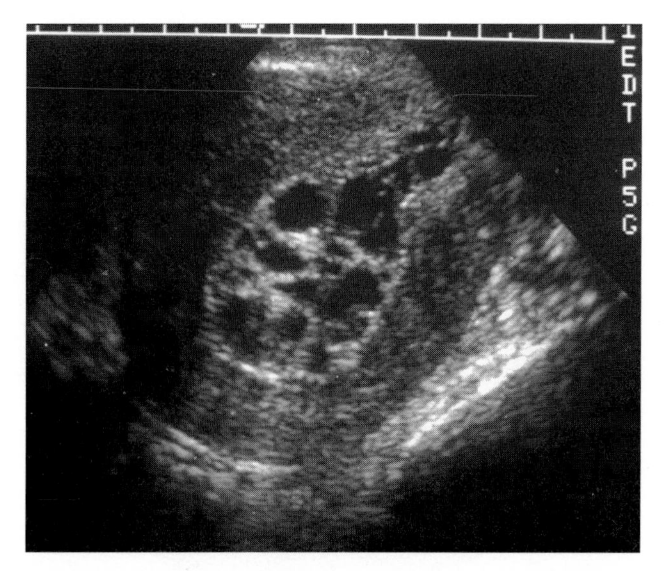

Fig. 6.22 Transvaginal ultrasound image of cystic hyperplasia of the endometrium: the grossly thickened endometrium is clearly seen, together with the cystic spaces, in this patient on Tamoxifen.

sion depth were within 10% of the actual pathological measurement (Fleischer et al 1987). Errors of estimation occurred when the tumour was exophytic and had significant extension into the uterine cavity. False positives also occur if the uterine cavity is overdistended with pus or blood when a subendometrial hypoechoic halo may be seen. Ultrasound assessment of the integrity of the hypoechoic layer can be improved by the use of transvaginal or transrectal sonography.

Changes in uterine blood flow have been used to detect endometrial cancer using endometrial thickness (including tumour) and the pulsatility index (PI) derived from flow velocity waveforms recorded from both uterine arteries and from within the tumour. Bourne et al (1991) found an overlap in endometrial thickness between women with endometrial cancer and those without, but the PI was invariably lower in women with postmenopausal bleeding due to endometrial cancer than in those with other reasons for bleeding. Blood flow impedance is inversely related to the stage of the cancer. However, although PI values in healthy women increase slightly with age, they decrease with oestrogen replacement therapy, so although Doppler studies may be helpful in the detection of endometrial cancer, allowance must be made for oestrogen replacement therapy.

Computerized tomography may also be used to stage endometrial cancer. CT depicts endometrial cancer as a hypodense lesion in the uterine parenchyma (Suzuki 1989), or as a fluid-filled uterus due to tumour obstruction of the endocervical canal or vagina. These findings, however, are non-specific and are easily confused with leiomyomata, intrauterine fluid collections and extension of a cervical carcinoma into the uterine body. In addition, a central lucency may occur in normal postmenopausal women.

MRI appears to represent a unique method of assessing a patient with an endometrial cancer, possessing advantages over other radiological techniques in stage I and II disease, but probably equal to CT in usefulness in the patient with a more advanced tumour (Powell et al 1986a). Figure 6.23 is a series of MRI scans of patients with endometrial cancer. On a T_2-weighted pulse sequence, endometrial cancer has an intermediate high signal intensity, similar to that of normal endometrium, but showing some degree of variability. The high signal makes the tumour quite distinct from the surrounding myometrium, which possesses an intermediate signal intensity. In a premenopausal uterus, however, it may be difficult to differentiate tumour from adenomatous hyperplasia or indeed from the high signal of normal endometrium. Contrast-enhanced T_1-weighted MR imaging improves the ability to assess the depth of myometrial invasion by endometrial tumour (Sironi et al 1992a). MR imaging has been found to have a sensitivity of 57% and a specificity of 96% for tumour confined to the endometrium, a sensitivity and specificity of 74% for superficial invasion and a sensitivity and specificity of 88 and 85% respectively for deep penetration (Sironi et al 1992b). However the degree of invasiveness may be overestimated for exophytic polypoid tumours with significant extraluminal extension (Gordon et al 1989, Lien et al 1991). Powell et al (1986a) found the low-signal band of inner myometrium to be thinned or absent in those patients with deeply invasive tumours, and this correlated well with the pathological measurement of myometrial invasion.

The sagittal plane is the most appropriate for examination of a patient with primary endometrial cancer, as this provides a longitudinal view of the uterus which will include both corpus and cervix. Using the sagittal plane also provides the opportunity to assess anterior invasion of the tumour into the bladder and posteriorly to the rectum.

Recurrent disease

Transrectal sonography has been investigated in cases where recurrent endometrial cancer is suspected (Squillaci et al 1988). Physical examination may be difficult because of postsurgical fibrosis. Infiltration into the surrounding connective tissues and organs such as the rectum and bladder can be identified and transrectal ultrasound can be used to guide transvaginal or transperineal fine-needle biopsy. CT (Balfe et al 1986) or MRI may also be used to detect recurrent disease and metastatic carcinoma to omentum or lymph nodes.

Ovarian carcinoma

In patients with ovarian cancer, the dramatic difference in

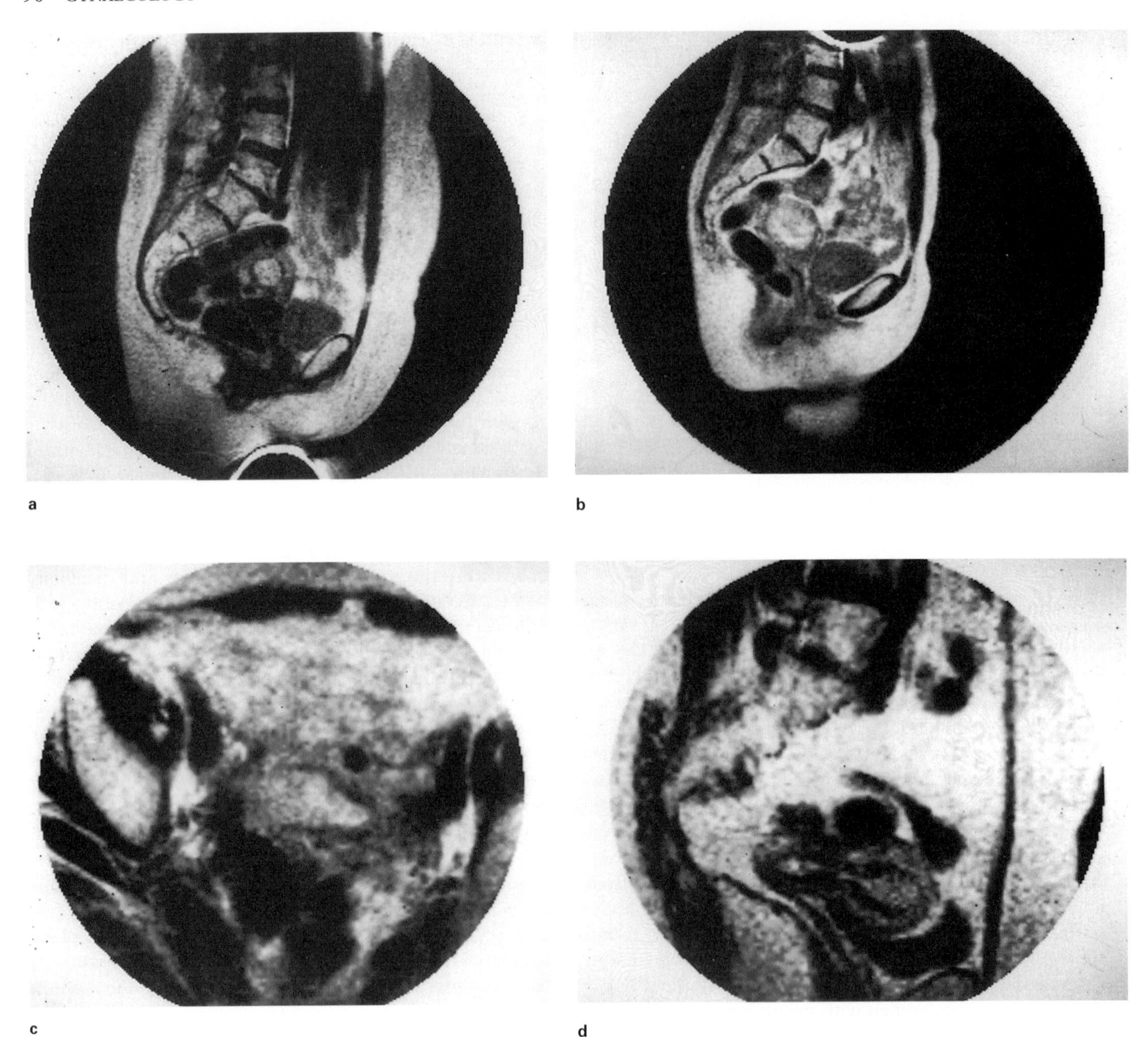

Fig. 6.23 MRI scans (T_2) of four patients with endometrial cancer. **a,b** The sagittal views show the low intensity band intact. **c** Transverse view: the low intensity band is breached laterally on the figure. **d** Sagittal view of an acutely anteverted uterus. The low intensity band is breached at the uterine fundus.

cure between patients with local disease (80–90%) and those with distant disease (15–25%), means that imaging to detect ovarian cancer early is desirable.

The ovary

Ultrasound is being explored as a screening method for carcinoma of the ovary, in the attempt to detect early disease. Out of 5479 women screened in one study (Campbell et al 1989), five women with primary stage I cancer and four with metastatic disease to the ovary were diagnosed. The overall rate of false positives was 2.3% and the likelihood of a positive scan being a primary ovarian cancer was 1 in 67. The improved resolution of transvaginal scanning permits a more detailed morphological examination (Fig. 6.24a,b). A scoring system has been evolved which reduces the number of false positives which otherwise result from confusion with unusual-appearing corpora lutea and with benign tumours (Bourne et al 1993). Benign lesions are unilocular or multilocular with

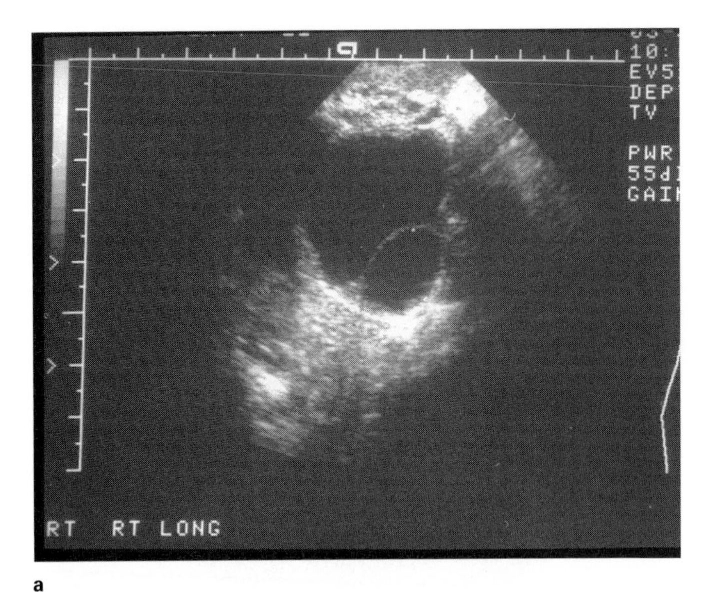

a

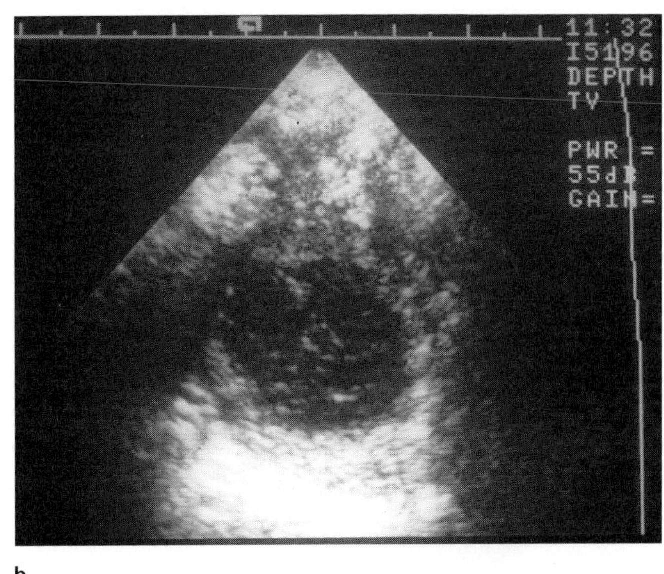

b

Fig. 6.24 Ultrasound scan of ovarian tumours. The smooth walls and echo-free contents of the benign cystic mass in **a** are very different from the complex appearance of the carcinoma in **b**.

thin septae and no nodules, whereas malignant lesions are often multilocular with thick septae and nodules. Uniformly echogenic lesions are less likely to be malignant than those of mixed echogenicity. In postmenopausal women, anechoic lesions less than 5 cm in diameter are unlikely to be malignant but those greater than 5 cm in diameter carry a one in ten chance of malignancy (Andolf & Jorgenson 1989). Campbell et al (1989) were unable to identify any morphological characteristics to differentiate reliably between ovarian tumour-like conditions, benign ovarian tumours and early malignant tumours.

Bourne et al (1989) proposed that the false-positive rate may be reduced by the use of transvaginal colour flow imaging, but these studies have been variously reported as disappointing (Hata et al 1992) or useful (Kawai et al 1992). Initially a low resistance index (less than 0.4) was advocated as the best discriminator but this has proved unreliable and a high peak velocity may be a better feature. At present the role of ultrasound in screening, though attractive, remains unvalidated and the results of larger trials are awaited (Taylor et al 1994). Despite these reservations, a transvaginal scan is accepted as a reasonable way to monitor the ovaries in patients with a high risk of ovarian carcinoma, such as those with a family history of the disease. Because of the risk of interval cancers, the screening interval should be less than 2 years (Bourne et al 1993).

As a tumour arising from a non-essential organ that remains primarily confined to the peritoneal cavity, ovarian cancer makes an attractive target for monoclonal antibodies. In the last decade, progressive improvement in tumour imaging has been observed when one compares the best examples of early studies, performed with ^{131}I heterosera to the best of modern images obtained with ^{123}I-, ^{99m}Tc- or ^{111}In-labelled monosera. Several monoclonal antibodies have been developed that have actual or potential clinical use for monitoring the course of disease. An antibody to CA125 has been widely assessed in monitoring the course of the disease (Fayers et al 1993). However, these antibodies are limited by problems that include antibody specificity, stability and immunoreactivity as well as patient reaction to the antibodies used.

Methods have therefore been developed to label with ^{198}Au a human monoclonal antibody (TC5) developed against an ovarian cell surface antigen (Chaudhuri 1994) which has a high sensitivity and specificity for detecting ovarian cancer. Antibodies coupled to drugs or biological toxins are also under investigation. Some antibodies may have direct anti-tumour effects through binding to biologically active receptors or through immune receptor functions. The use of antibody fragments, chimeric antibodies, and genetically engineered antibodies is also under active investigation (Rubin 1993). Monoclonal antibodies therefore have enormous potential for improving the diagnosis and monitoring the response to therapy in the treatment of ovarian cancer.

The potential of positron emission tomography (PET) to distinguish benign from malignant tumours is being evaluated by comparing the results of F^{18}-fluro-2-deoxyglucose (F^{18}-FDG) PET scans with surgical findings. The positive predictive value from one such study was 86% and, more importantly, the negative predictive

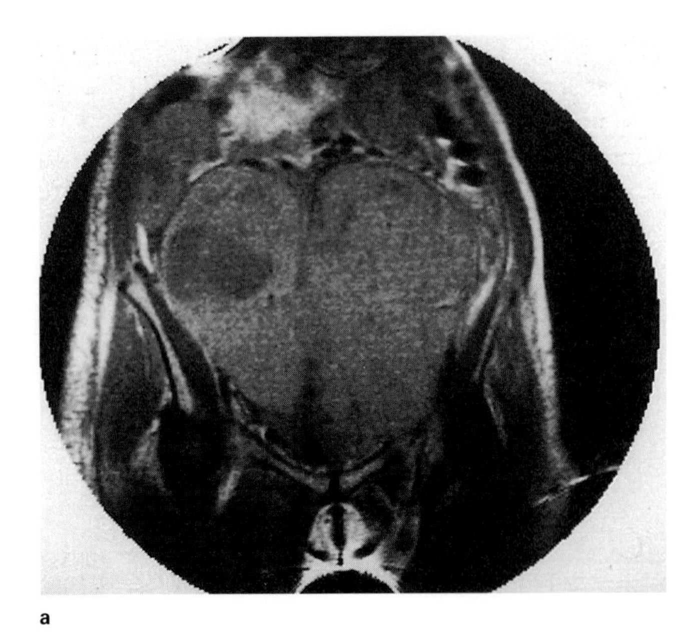

a

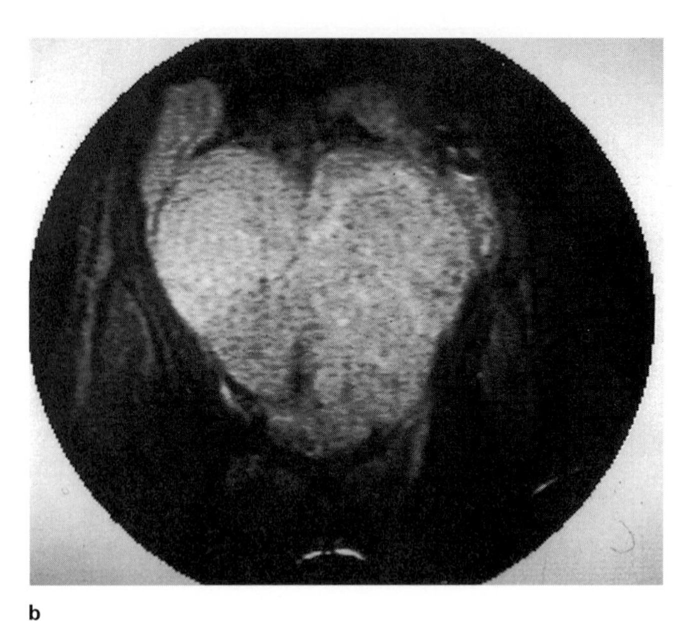

b

Fig. 6.25 MRI scan: coronal view showing a primary ovarian cancer with a predominantly solid element. An element of necrosis is visible. **a** T_1/T_2. **b** Short inversion recovery (STIR).

value was 76% (Hubner et al 1993). It may be possible, using such techniques, to identify metabolically active tumours that do not appear on morphological studies.

Pelvic and abdominal spread

Computed tomography is the most useful imaging modality for demonstrating macroscopic recurrence, and can spare patients a second-look laparotomy. A variety of manifestations can be seen with CT, each of which can have a spectrum of appearances including ascites, peritoneal seeding and visceral and nodal metastases (Lee et al 1994). Ultrasound may also be used to detect ascites and liver metastases. MRI should be performed in women with questionable macroscopic recurrent tumour and negative CT examination. In a small study MRI was at least as good as and may be superior to CT in the evaluation of ovarian malignancy (Semelka et al 1993) (Fig. 6.25) Neither CT nor MRI can exclude microscopic disease (Prayer et al 1993).

Fab′2 fragments of ^{111}In-labelled monoclonal antibody to CA125 gave immunoscintigrams, even with a negative CT and ultrasound, which were highly suggestive of recurrence in the abdomen and pelvis (Peltier et al 1992). ^{111}In CYT103 immunoscintigraphy detected occult disease in 20 of 71 patients with surgically documented ovarian adenocarcinoma (Surwit et al 1993), and this approach may be a valuable addition to presurgical evaluation in patients with suspected, persistent or recurrent pelvic tumour.

SAFETY ISSUES

Although the majority of imaging procedures described are largely non-invasive, some modalities involve exposing the patient to ionizing radiation. This is one of the reasons why techniques such as ultrasound and MRI have received so much attention in obstetrics and gynaecology. Nevertheless, ultrasound necessitates irradiation of the patient with sound waves (mechanical vibrations) and MRI involves the application of strong and rapidly changing magnetic fields combined with radio waves. Careful studies have shown that no harmful effects result from the clinical use of ultrasound or MRI investigations but each modality has an associated risk which must be appreciated.

In the case of ultrasound and MRI the main biological effect is of the conversion of the interrogating source of energy (sound, magnetic flux, radio waves) into heat. The American Institute for Ultrasound in Medicine has issued the following guidelines: ‘In the low megahertz frequency range there have been no demonstrated significant biological effects of ultrasound in mammalian tissues exposed in vivo to intensities below 100 mW/cm^2’. Higher powers do damage tissue mainly by heating, a feature used in physiotherapy, but, at diagnostic levels the heating is minimal and continuously removed by the blood circulation. Spectral Doppler delivers the highest intensity, and this is compounded by the fact that the beam is trained onto a target for longer periods of time than in imaging. It seems prudent to restrict scanning, especially spectral Doppler, to genuine clinical indications and to use it for the shortest time and at the lowest intensity needed to make the diagnosis.

As early as 1896 reports were made of a visual sensation of light flashes induced by exposure to changing magnetic fields. However the main hazards associated with rapidly changing magnetic fields are those of electroconvulsion and atrial fibrillation, hence caution should be exercised with epileptic patients and those who have recently suffered from myocardial infarction. Guidelines for the use of MRI are laid down by the National British Radiological Protection Board (1984).

Before deciding to carry out any imaging investigation however a clinical decision has to be made concerning whether the benefits accrued from the results of the investigation outweigh any possible risk to the patient from the procedure to be undertaken.

CONCLUSION

Advances in medical imaging are occurring at a rapid rate, mainly due to development of sophisticated imaging techniques, computer software and display systems. Ultrasound, due to its greater flexibility and relatively low cost, will retain an integral diagnostic role in gynaecology with transvaginal sonography a routine adjunct to a bimanual pelvic examination. MRI provides superior soft tissue contrast of the pelvic organs and will lead to an increase in detection, improved staging and assessment of a range of disease processes including cancer. The technology needed to overcome the major disadvantages of long scanning times and claustrophobic scanners is well advanced. Magnetic resonance spectroscopy remains largely unexplored in gynaecology, but is an exciting prospect for the future. The various imaging modalities are complementary to each other and the appropriate choice to produce the greatest diagnostic return while minimizing the risk to the patient should be sought.

KEY POINTS

1. Ultrasound examination is dependent upon both the technical expertise of the ultrasonographer and an understanding of the patient's history and clinical findings.
2. Ultrasound is the technique of choice for imaging the endometrial cavity and the ovaries, but it cannot yet distinguish reliably between benign and malignant disease.
3. Ultrasound is very valuable in monitoring ovulation induction and is used in directing egg collection for in vitro fertilization.
4. Ultrasound can be valuable in identifying an ectopic gestation.
5. MRI gives the best images of endometrial carcinoma and of adenomyosis. It may identify endometriosis that cannot be visualized in any other way.
6. MRI is the best method for imaging cervical carcinoma, especially when an endovaginal receiver coil is used. Imaging of pelvic lymph nodes is still not reliable.
7. CT scanning is of limited value in assessing the pelvic organs and should probably not be used if MRI is available.
8. Radionuclide imaging can be of value in identifying and locating ovarian carcinoma.
9. Angiographic embolization is probably the treatment of first choice for postoperative pelvic haemorrhage.

REFERENCES

Andolf E, Jorgensen C 1989 Cystic lesions in elderly women, diagnosed by ultrasound. British Journal of Obstetrics and Gynaecology 96: 1076–1079

Ascher S M, Arnold L L, Patt R H et al 1994 Adenomyosis: prospective comparison of MR imaging and transvaginal sonography. Radiology 190: 803–806

Balfe D M, Heiken J P, McClennan B L 1986 Oncologic imaging of carcinoma of the cervix, ovary and endometrium. In: Bragg D G, Rubin P, Youker J E (eds) Oncologic imaging. Pergamon, Oxford, pp 437–477

Barber R J, McSweeney M B, Gill R W et al 1988 Transvaginal pulsed Doppler ultrasound assessment of blood flow to the corpus luteum in IVF patients following embryo transfer. British Journal of Obstetrics and Gynaecology 95: 1226–1230

Bourne T, Campbell S, Steer C, Whitehead M I, Collins W P 1989 Transvaginal colour flow imaging: a possible new screening technique for ovarian cancer. British Medical Journal 299: 1367–1370

Bourne T H, Campbell S, Steer C V, Royston P, Whitehead M I, Collins W P 1991 Detection of endometrial cancer by transvaginal ultrasonography with colour flow imaging and blood flow analysis: a preliminary report. Gynecologic Oncology 40: 253–259

Bourne T H, Campbell S, Reynolds K M et al 1993 Screening for early familial ovarian cancer with transvaginal ultrasonography and colour blood flow imaging. British Medical Journal 306: 1025–1029

Bourne T H, Campbell S, Reynolds K et al 1994 The potential role of serum CA 125 in an ultrasound based screening programme for familial ovarian cancer. Gynecologic Oncology 52: 379–385

Brosens I A 1993 Classification of endometriosis revisited. Lancet 341: 630

Bryce R L, Shuter B, Sinosich M J 1982 The value of ultrasound, gonadotrophin and oestradiol measurements for precise ovulation prediction. Fertility and Sterility 37: 42–45

Burghardt E, Hofmann H M, Ebner F, Haas J, Tamussino K, Justich E 1989 Magnetic resonance imaging in cervical cancer: a basis for objective classification. Gynecologic Oncology 33: 61–67

Burghardt E, Baltzer J, Tulusan A H, Haas J 1992 Results of surgical treatment on 1028 cervical cancers studied with volumetry. Cancer 70: 648–655

Campbell S, Bhan V, Royston P, Whitehead M I, Collins W P 1989 Transabdominal ultrasound screening for early ovarian cancer. British Medical Journal 299: 1363–1366

Chaudhuri T R, Zinn K R, Morris J S, McDonald G A, Llorens A S, Chaudhuri T K 1994 Detection of ovarian cancer by 198Au-labelled human monoclonal antibody. Cancer 73: 878–883

Clark S L, Phelan J P, Yeh S Y, Bruce S R, Paul R H 1985 Hypogastric artery ligation for obstetric haemorrhage. Obstetrics and Gynecology 66: 353–356

Collins C D, Jackson J E 1995 Pelvic arterial embolization following hysterectomy and bilateral internal iliac artery ligation for intractable

primary post partum haemorrhage: case report and review of the literature. Clinical Radiology 50: 710–714
deSouza N M, Brosens J J, Schwieso J E, Paraschos T, Winston R M L 1995 The potential value of magnetic resonance imaging in infertility. Clinical Radiology 50: 75–79
deSouza N M, Scoones D J, Krausz T, Gilderdale D J, Soutter W P 1996 High resolution MR imaging of Stage I cervical neoplasia with a dedicated transvaginal coil: MR features and correlation of imaging and pathological findings. American Journal of Roentgenology 166: 553–559
Duggan P M, Jamieson M G, Wallie W J 1991 Intractable postpartum haemorrhage managed by angiographic embolization: case report and review of the literature. Australian and New Zealand Journal of Obstetrics and Gynaecology 31: 229–234
Ebner F, Kressel H Y, Mintz M C et al 1988 Tumour recurrence versus fibrosis in the female pelvis: differentiation with MR imaging at 1.5T. Radiology 166: 333–340
Emerson D S, Cartier M S, Altieri L A et al 1992 Diagnostic efficacy of endovaginal color flow Doppler in an ectopic pregnancy screening program. Radiology 183: 413–420
Fayers P M, Rustin G, Wood R 1993 The prognostic value of serum CA 125 in patients with advanced ovarian carcinoma: an analysis of 573 patients by the Medical Research Council Working Party on Gynaecological Cancer. International Journal of Gynaecological Cancer 3: 285–292
Fedele L, Bianchi S, Dorta M, Arcaini L, Zanotti F, Carinelli S 1992 Transvaginal ultrasonography in the diagnosis of diffuse adenomyosis. Fertility and Sterility 58: 94–98
Fleischer A C, Dudley S B, Entman S S, Baxter J W, Kalemeris G E, Everette J A 1987 Myometrial invasion by endometrial carcinoma: sonographic assessment. Radiology 162: 307–310
Flueckiger F, Ebner F, Poschauko H, Tamussino K, Einspieler R, Ranner G 1992 Cervical cancer: serial MR imaging before and after primary radiation therapy – a two year follow up study. Radiology 184: 89–93
Gordon A N, Fleischer A C, Dudley B S et al 1989 Preoperative assessment of myometrial invasion of endometrial adenocarcinoma by sonography (US) and magnetic resonance imaging (MRI). Gynecologic Oncology 34: 175–179
Goto M, Okamura S, Ueki M, Sugimoto O 1990 Evaluation of magnetic resonance imaging in the diagnosis of extension in uterine cervical cancer cases with special attention to imaging planes. Nippon Sanka Fujinka Gakki Zasshi. 42:1627–1633
Griffin J W, Parker R G, Taylor W J 1976 An evaluation of procedures used in staging carcinoma of the cervix. American Journal of Roentgenology 127: 825–827
Hamlin D J, Petterson H, Fitzsimmons J, Morgan L S 1985 MR imaging of uterine leiomyomas and their complications. Journal of Computer Assisted Tomography 9: 902–907
Hata K, Hata T, Manabe A, Sugimura K, Kitao M 1992 A critical evaluation of transvaginal doppler studies, transvaginal sonography, magnetic resonance imaging, and CA 125 in detecting ovarian cancer. Obstetrics and Gynecology 80: 922–926
Hirnle P, Mittman K P, Schmidt B, Pfeiffer K H 1990 Indications for radioisotope bone scanning in staging of cervical cancer. Archives of Gynaecology and Obstetrics 248: 21–23
Ho C M, Chien T Y, Jeng C M, Tsang Y M, Shih B Y, Chang S C 1992 Staging of cervical cancer: comparison between magnetic resonance imaging, computed tomography and pelvic examination under anaesthesia. Journal of the Formosan Medical Association 91: 982–990
Hobbs J T 1990 The pelvic congestion syndrome. British Journal of Hospital Medicine 43: 200–206
Hricak H, Alpers C, Crooks L E, Sheldon P E 1983 Magnetic resonance imaging of the female pelvis: initial experience. American Journal of Roentgenology 141: 1119–1128
Hricak H, Fincks S, Honda G, Goransson H 1992 MR imaging in the evaluation of benign uterine masses: value of dimeglumine enhanced T1W images. American Journal of Roentgenology 158: 1043–1050
Hubner K F, McDonald T W, Niethammer J G, Smith G T, Gould H E, Buonocore E 1993 Assessment of primary and metastatic ovarian cancer by positron emission tomography (PET) using 2-[18F] deoxyglucose (2-[18F]FDG). Gynecologic Oncology 51: 197–204
Kawai M, Kano T, Kikkawa F, Maeda O, Ogichi H, Tomoda Y 1992 Transvaginal doppler ultrasound with colour flow imaging in the diagnosis of ovarian cancer. Obstetrics and Gynecology 79: 163–167
Kim S H, Choi B I, Han J K 1993 Preoperative staging of uterine cervical carcinoma: comparison of CT and MRI in 99 patients. Journal of Computer Assisted Tomography 17: 633–640
Lee M J, Munk P L, Poon P Y, Hassell P 1994 Ovarian cancer: computed tomography findings. Canadian Association of Radiology Journal 45: 185–192
Levenback C, Dershaw D D, Rubin S C 1992 Endoluminal ultrasound staging of cervical cancer. Gynecologic Oncology 46: 186–190
Lien H H, Blomlie V, Trope C, Kaern J, Abeler V M 1991 Cancer of the endometrium: value of MR imaging in determining depth of invasion into the myometrium. American Journal of Roentgenology 157: 1221–1223
Marshall R H, Eliasoph J 1955 The roentgen findings in adenomyosis. Radiology 64: 846–851
National British Radiological Protection Board 1984 Revised guidelines on acceptable limits of exposure during nuclear magnetic clinical imaging. British Journal of Radiology 56: 974–977
Noval E, deLima A 1948 A correlative study of adenomyosis and pelvic endometriosis with special reference to the hormonal reaction of eutopic endometrium. American Journal of Obstetrics and Gynecology 56: 634–644
Peltier P, Wiharto K, Dutin J P 1992 Correlative imaging study in the diagnosis of ovarian cancer recurrences. European Journal of Nuclear Medicine 19: 1006–1010
Powell M C, Womack C, Buckley J H, Worthington B S, Symonds E M 1986a Pre-operative magnetic resonance imaging of stage I endometrial adenocarcinoma. British Journal of Obstetrics and Gynaecology 93: 353–360
Powell M C, Buckley J H, Wasti M, Worthington B S, Sokal M, Symonds E M 1986b The application of magnetic resonance imaging to cervical carcinoma. British Journal of Obstetrics and Gynaecology 93: 1276–1285
Prayer L, Kainz C, Kramer J et al 1993 CT and MR accuracy in the detection of tumor recurrence in patients treatment for ovarian cancer. Journal of Computer Assisted Tomography 17: 626–632
Randall J M, Fisk N M, McTavish A 1989 Transvaginal ultrasonic assessment of endometrial growth in spontaneous and hyperstimulated menstrual cycles. British Journal of Obstetrics and Gynaecology 96: 954–959
Rubin S C 1993 Monoclonal antibodies in the management of ovarian cancer. A clinical perspective. Cancer 71: 1602–1612
Schatten C, Pateisky N, Vavra N et al 1992 Lymphoscintigraphy with (123) I-marked epidermal growth factor in cervix cancer. Gynakol Geburtshilfliche Rundsch 32: 17–21
Semelka R C, Lawrence P H, Shoenut J P, Heywood M, Kroeker M A, Lotocki R 1993 Primary ovarian cancer: prospective comparison of contrast enhanced CT and pre- and post-contrast, fat suppressed MR imaging, with histological correlation. Journal of Magnetic Resonance Imaging 3: 99–106
Shingawa S 1964 Extraperitoneal ligation of the internal iliac arteries as a life and uterus saving procedure for uncontrollable post partum haemorrhage. American Journal of Obstetrics and Gynecology 88: 130–134
Sichlau M J, Yao J S, Vogelzang R L 1994 Transcatheter embolotherapy for the treatment of pelvic congestion syndrome. Obstetrics and Gynecology 83: 892–896
Sironi S, Belloni C, Taccagni G L, DelMaschio A 1991 Carcinoma of the cervix: value of MR imaging in detecting parametrial involvement. American Journal of Roentgenology 156: 753–756
Sironi S, Taccagni G, Garancini P, Belloni C, DelMaschio A 1992 Myometrial invasion by endometrial carcinoma: assessment by MR imaging. American Journal of Roentgenology 158: 565–569
Sironi S, Colombo E, Villa G 1992 Myometrial invasion by endometrial carcinoma: assessment with plain and gadolinium-enhanced MR imaging. Radiology 185: 207–212
Squillaci E, Salzani M C, Grandireth M L et al 1988 Recurrence of

ovarian and uterine neoplasms: diagnosis with transrectal US. Radiology 169: 355–358
Subak L L, Hricak H, Powell C B, Azizi L, Stern J L 1995 Cervical carcinoma computed tomography and magnetic resonance imaging for preoperative staging. Obstetrics and Gynecology 86: 43–50
Surwit E A, Childers J M, Krag D N et al 1993 Clinical assessment of 111In-CYT-103 immunoscintigraphy in ovarian cancer. Gynecologic Oncology 48: 283–284
Suzuki M 1989 Role of X-ray, CT and magnetic resonance imaging is the diagnosis of gynecological malignant tumor. Nippon Sanka Fujinka Gakkai Zasshi 41: 942–952
Taylor K J, Schwartz P E 1994 Screening for early ovarian cancer. Radiology 192: 1–10
Timor-Tritsch I E, Bar-Yam Y, Elgali S, Rotlem S 1988 The technique of transvaginal sonography with the use of a 6.5 MHz probe. American Journal of Obstetrics and Gynecology 158: 1019–1024
Togashi K, Nishimura K, Itoh K 1987 Uterine cervical cancer: assessment with high field MR imaging. Radiology 160: 431–435
Togashi K, Nishimura K, Itoh K et al 1988 Adenomyosis diagnosis with MR imaging. Radiology 166: 111–114
Weiner J L, Chako A C, Merten C W, Gross S, Coffey E L, Stein H L 1986 Breast and axillary tissue MR imaging correlation of signal intensities and relaxation times with pathologic findings. Radiology 160: 229–305
Yuhara A, Akamatsu N, Sekiba K 1987 Use of transrectal radial scan ultrasonography in evaluating the extent of uterine cervical cancer. Journal of Clinical Ultrasound 15: 507–517

7

Preoperative care: inpatient and day case management

J.–P. van Besouw J. Tidy

'Inside every adult is a child afraid of the dark.'

Anonymous

OBJECTIVES

Preoperative preparation for surgery should begin once the surgeon has placed the patient's name on the waiting list. In an ideal world this would involve close cooperation between surgeon and anaesthetist with patient assessment, relevant investigations and the appropriate modification of treatment regimens arranged prior to admission. Potentially difficult problems should be assessed in an anaesthetic or surgical outpatient clinic.

Unfortunately the more common practice in the UK in an increasingly cost-driven health service is for patients to be admitted either on the day of or day prior to surgery, and to be subjected to blanket and often inappropriate investigations with insufficient time to act on results or to change therapies, where necessary, prior to surgery. It is therefore of paramount importance that the gynaecologist is aware of the precepts of preoperative assessment and the relevant course of action to take in order to improve the efficiency and safety of the system. Preoperative preparation revolves around the following objectives:

1. the evaluation of physical status;
2. investigations relevant to the course of surgery and anaesthesia;
3. the evaluation of current medication and the modification of therapy where indicated;
4. consent and counselling prior to surgery.

EVALUATION OF PHYSICAL STATUS

The assignment of a physical status category to patients, based upon history and examination, can act as a useful language when conveying information to anaesthetists on their preoperative visit. The most widely used system at present is that recommended by the American Society of Anesthesiologists (ASA 1963; Table 7.1). In this system, patients are placed into one of five categories. Although this is a good indicator of the physical status of the patient prior to surgery, because the nature of the intended surgery is not taken into consideration it is not a good prognosticator of postoperative morbidity.

Table 7.1 Classification of physical status

Status	Definition
ASA 1	Normal healthy patient: no known organic, biochemical or psychiatric disease
ASA 2	Patient with mild to moderate systemic disease
ASA 3	Patient with severe systemic disease that limits normal activity
ASA 4	Patient with severe systemic disease that is a consistent threat to life
ASA 5	Patient who is moribund and unlikely to survive 24 h

The addition of the letter E indicates those patients in whom emergency surgery is undertaken (e.g. ASA 4E). After The American Society of Anesthesiologists (1963).

History

It is important in the preoperative preparation to take a detailed history, with particular emphasis on those points relevant to the course of surgery and anaesthesia. This should include details of the presenting complaint, current medication and past medical and surgical history. The anaesthetist will be interested in any cardiorespiratory problems as well as any adverse reactions to anaesthesia that the patient may have suffered during previous surgery. Some of the more important questions are outlined in Table 7.2 and their relevance to the course of surgery and anaesthesia is detailed in subsequent sections.

Examination

The importance of a full examination documented in the notes by the house surgeon cannot be overemphasized. The anaesthetist will be interested in signs of respiratory disease including the nature and pattern of respiration, the presence of abnormal breath sounds plus additional signs of respiratory incapacity, e.g. tracheal deviation or cyanosis. Simple bedside tests of respiratory function, such as peak expiratory flow measurements, may be useful indicators of respiratory reserve.

Cardiovascular examination should include assessment of heart rate and rhythm, and auscultation for cardiac murmurs with particular emphasis on diastolic murmurs or the presence of a third or fourth heart sound. The measurement of arterial blood pressure is essential and should be repeated at least twice at intervals if it is found to be elevated.

The gynaecologist will obviously be interested in examination pertinent to the presenting complaint. More detailed examination of other systems is dictated by the presence of intercurrent disease. For example, neurological assessment of the patient with multiple sclerosis, or assessment of joint mobility in the patient with rheumatoid arthritis is of particular importance if leg stirrups are to be employed.

Table 7.2 Important questions in an anaesthetic preoperative assessment

System or organ	Condition
Cardiovascular	Angina pectoris Myocardial infarction Rheumatic fever Systemic vascular disease
Respiratory	Acute coryza Exercise tolerance Dyspnoea and orthopnoea Asthma and allergic lung disease Bronchitis; cough and sputum production Pulmonary infection Pulmonary surgery Smoking
Nervous system	Epilepsy Neuromuscular disease Neuropathy Psychiatric disease and treatment
Liver	Alcohol consumption Hepatitis
Endocrine	Diabetes mellitus Thyroid disease Adrenal disease
Genitourinary	Renal disease Sexually transmitted disease Menstrual history: ? pregnant
Previous anaesthesia	Nausea and vomiting Adverse reactions Postspinal headache Familial problems with anaesthesia

Intercurrent medical disease

It is not possible or intended to give a comprehensive account of the effects of medical conditions on the course of surgery and anaesthesia, but rather to give an overview of problems which are commonly found in patients presenting for surgery and the measures which can be taken in order to ensure that perioperative morbidity is kept to a minimum.

Cardiovascular disease (Treasure & van Besouw 1993)

The presence of cardiovascular disease is associated with increased morbidity and mortality following anaesthesia. Evaluation of the severity of the condition and instigation of measures to reduce the incidence of complications is therefore an essential part of preoperative assessment.

A number of attempts have been made to identify perioperative risk factors in order to try and improve perioperative morbidity. The most widely known is the cardiac risk index score (Goldman et al 1977; Table 7.3). Patients with a score greater than 13 should receive further medical treatment prior to surgery.

Table 7.3 Preoperative factors predisposing to the development of postoperative cardiac complications

Factors	Points
Gallop rhythm or elevated jugular venous pressure	11
Myocardial infarction in preceding 6 months	10
Abnormal rhythm other than premature atrial contractions on preoperative ECG	7
> 5 premature ventricular contractions per minute	7
Age > 70 years	5
Emergency surgery	4
Intraperitoneal, intrathoracic or aortic operation	3
Poor general physical status	3
Significant aortic stenosis	3

After Goldman et al (1977).

Coronary artery disease (Mangano 1990)

The incidence of coronary artery disease in this country is high and patients may present with a spectrum of conditions from angina pectoris to myocardial infarction. The presence of coronary artery disease is associated with a significant increase in perioperative morbidity and mortality, including an increased incident risk of postoperative reinfarction in individuals presenting for surgery within 3 months of myocardial infarction.

The development of angina is indicative of an imbalance between the oxygen demands of the myocardium and the oxygen supply, not necessarily the severity of coronary arteriosclerosis. It is aggravated by perioperative hypertension or hypotension and tachycardia. Hypertension and tachycardia increase heart work whilst hypotension and tachycardia reduce myocardial perfusion. In the preoperative assessment of these patients it is therefore essential to assess the nature, frequency and duration of the anginal attacks, the efficacy of current medication and, where control of symptoms is inadequate, a cardiological opinion should be sought. If possible, elective surgery is best postponed for at least 3 months in individuals who have suffered recent myocardial infarction.

Hypertension

Hypertension has been defined by the World Health Organization as a persistently elevated systolic pressure > 160 mmHg and/or a diastolic pressure > 95 mmHg. Severe hypertension is present when blood pressure exceeds 180/100 mmHg and is found in 11% of patients presenting for surgery. Anaesthesia in the presence of uncontrolled hypertension has a significant morbidity and mortality. Therefore preoperative assessment should determine the adequacy of blood pressure control, the nature of current therapy and assessment of any major organ dysfunction associated with sustained hypertensive disease, notably coronary artery disease, renal disease and cerebrovascular disease. Instigation of appropriate treatment is indicated. Where patients have diastolic blood pressure in excess of 120 mmHg, surgery should be postponed as, untreated, they have extreme lability of blood pressure perioperatively (Prys-Roberts 1984).

Valvular heart disease

Valvular heart disease may be congenital or acquired. It more commonly affects the left side of the heart, resulting in haemodynamic disturbances in left ventricular function producing pressure-related disorders secondary to stenotic lesions of the aortic or mitral valves, or volume-related disorders secondary to regurgitant lesions of the same valves.

In the preoperative assessment, the degree of cardiac reserve must be ascertained by evaluating patient exercise tolerance. The degree of compensatory mechanisms, such as increased sympathetic activity and myocardial hypertrophy, in the maintenance of normal cardiac output should be noted. Non-invasive assessment of valvular function by the use of echocardiography is most informative.

At-risk patients (Table 7.4) undergoing high risk procedures (Table 7.5) should have prophylactic antibiotics before surgery in order to prevent the development of bacterial endocarditis, although proof of the efficacy of such treatment is not available. The current recommendations (Dajani et al 1991) for gynaecological surgery are gentamicin 1.5 mg/kg intravenously and ampicillin 1 g intravenously 30 min prior to surgery, followed by two further doses at 8 and 16 h postoperatively. In those individuals who are penicillin-sensitive, erythromycin 500 mg intravenously is given by infusion over 30 min before the induction of anaesthesia.

Dysrhythmias

The presence of dysrhythmias may be associated with cardiovascular, renal, pulmonary or metabolic disease, or

Table 7.4 Conditions requiring antibiotic prophylaxis against endocarditis

Prosthetic cardiac valves
Congenital cardiac abnormalities
Previous history of endocarditis
Acquired valvular dysfunction, including rheumatic fever
Hypertrophic cardiomyopathy

Table 7.5 Gynaecological procedures for which antibiotic prophylaxis against endocarditis is recommended

Vaginal hysterectomy
Urethral dilatation
Drainage of perineal infection
In the presence of infection during the following procedures:
Urethral catheterization
Urinary tract surgery
Vaginal delivery

they may occur secondarily to drug therapy such as digoxin. If untreated they may result in marked haemodynamic disturbance. The frequency of dysrhythmia is increased by perioperative events, such as hypoxia, hypercarbia, alterations in acid–base status or potassium homeostasis.

Preoperative assessment should focus on the nature and frequency, whether supraventricular or ventricular, of the dysrhythmia, the correction of any exacerbating conditions and the initiation of appropriate therapy. Heart block of any kind is always due to organic damage to the conducting system, and if it is third-degree or second-degree Mobitz type 2 should be treated with transvenous pacing prior to surgery.

Respiratory disease

The primary function of the lungs is to provide an interface for the exchange of oxygen and carbon dioxide between blood and the atmosphere, a necessary part of the metabolic process. Pulmonary disease has the effect of decreasing the efficiency of this exchange which, in combination with the respiratory depressant effects of anaesthesia and surgery on pulmonary function, results in an increase in postoperative morbidity and mortality. Preoperative pulmonary evaluation is mandatory for all patients scheduled for surgery. Preoperative tests of respiratory reserve are dictated by the severity of the presenting symptoms.

Upper respiratory tract infections

It is seldom necessary for patients with upper respiratory tract infections to undergo elective surgery. The infection, combined with the immunosuppressive effects of anaesthesia, the postoperative inhibition of coughing and the sedative effects of narcotic agents used to relieve postoperative pain, increases the risk of developing postoperative viral pneumonia. It is therefore advisable to withhold surgery for at least 2 weeks until recovery is complete.

Obstructive lung disease

This is a heterogeneous group of conditions, ranging from bronchitis to asthma, which may be chronic or acute, reversible or irreversible, and which together constitute the largest single group of respiratory diseases. Preoperative preparation should aim to assess the severity of the condition using a combination of clinical judgement, simple spirometry such as the measurement of vital capacity, forced expiratory volume in one second (FEV1) and blood gas analysis where indicated.

From the results of those tests, appropriate therapy may be instigated. This should include advice on stopping smoking, preoperative physiotherapy, and breathing exercises, the use of bronchodilators in those cases where reversibility is demonstrated and antibiotics for the treatment of any acute exacerbations of chronic bronchitis. It is advisable to repeat these tests following treatment and, if necessary, to delay surgery until the patient is in an optimal condition. In those patients with severe pulmonary disease, where the FEV is $< 25\%$ of that predicted and arterial oxygen tensions are < 7.3 kPa in air, the possibility of surgery under regional or local anaesthesia should be considered.

Restrictive lung disease

This group of pulmonary diseases includes fibrosing alveolitis, sarcoidosis, asbestosis and the pulmonary manifestations of systemic disease such as rheumatoid arthritis and systemic lupus erythematosus. They are characterized by a decreased transfer capacity with a restrictive lung volume. The clinical features are of dyspnoea and hypoxia on mild exertion with a normal sensitivity to carbon dioxide. Patients are frequently on steroid therapy. Most cases will not be a problem to the anaesthetist; however, any chest infection should be treated before surgery and postoperative oxygen therapy may be necessary.

Diseases of the nervous system

Although there are a large number of neurological diseases, few are of consequence to the course of surgery and anaesthesia; however, problems may be encountered with the following conditions.

Epilepsy

It is advisable for patients to continue with anticonvulsant therapy in the perioperative period and for the anaesthetist to be informed of the epilepsy, as a number of anaesthetic agents predispose to seizure activity.

Multiple sclerosis

It is important to document the degree of neurological impairment before surgery and to explain to the patient that the stress associated with surgery has been shown to exacerbate the condition in the postoperative period.

Renal disease

The most important feature in the preoperative preparation of patients with renal disease is the assessment of the biochemical abnormality relative to the therapeutic manoeuvres taken to correct it. Patients on dialysis with established renal failure presenting for elective surgery should be dialysed 12–24 h prior to surgery to correct any hyperkalaemia or acid–base abnormality.

In patients with chronic anaemia, correction by preoperative transfusion is generally unnecessary. However, it is worth remembering that it will be difficult to detect cyanosis when the patient is anaemic. Drugs excreted by routes other than the kidneys should be used where possible. Infusions of morphine should be used cautiously as its active metabolite, morphine-6-glucuronide, is excreted by the kidneys and may accumulate in sufficient concentrations to produce respiratory depression.

Hepatic disease

Patients with moderate to severe hepatic disease are at considerable risk of developing perioperative problems. Hepatic failure is associated with alterations of renal, pulmonary and cardiovascular physiology, impaired metabolic and haematological homeostasis and altered pharmacokinetics. Preoperative assessment is aimed at identifying the severity of the hepatic disease both clinically and biochemically.

In the preoperative preparation it is necessary to give prophylactic antibiotics, vitamin K and possibly diuretics for ascites. Clotting abnormalities should be corrected with the appropriate blood products. There is a high risk of developing renal failure postoperatively. This is frequently fatal.

Endocrine disease and obesity

Perioperative problems in patients with endocrine diseases tend to arise as a result of mismanagement of replacement therapy. As such they are dealt with in the section on the influence of pre-existing medication.

One important condition to consider however is the effect of obesity on the course of surgery and anaesthesia. Obesity can be defined as body fat content in excess of 30% in the female or where the ratio of weight over height^2 is greater than 30 kg/m^2. Patients in this category have a considerable risk because of abnormalities of respiratory and cardiovascular physiology. There are also technical problems with access for surgery and problems with postoperative mobilization. Appropriate dietary advice in the outpatient clinic with regular follow-up by a dietician, prior to surgery, may reduce some of these problems.

Haematological disorders

Anaemia

Anaemia is an acute or chronic reduction in the number of circulating erythrocytes manifest by a decrease in the concentration of haemoglobin and a concomitant reduction in the oxygen-carrying capacity of the blood. In most cases the cause may be known, for example menorrhagia. However where this is unclear, relevant investigations to elucidate the cause are essential before surgery. In patients with chronic anaemia (for example, chronic renal failure) compensatory changes include a shift to the right of the oxyhaemoglobin dissociation curve (thus increasing oxygen release at a tissue level) and an increase in cardiac output to maintain oxygen availability.

The necessity for a minimum preoperative haemoglobin of 10 g/dl is based on the physiological necessity for a minimum oxygen availability of 250 ml of oxygen per minute. Oxygen availability is the product of the cardiac output, the haemoglobin concentration, the haemoglobin saturation and ability to carry oxygen. Therefore in patients with a normal cardiac output and a normal haemoglobin, the oxygen availability is in the region of 1000 ml oxygen/min. A reduction of the haemoglobin to 10 g/dl decreases this to around 650 ml oxygen/min. If during the course of surgery, hypovolaemia or myocardial depression because of anaesthesia occurs, oxygen availability will fall further and approach a level where tissue oxygen availability will be impaired. If it is not possible to delay surgery while anaemia is corrected, or if there is no other practicable means of increasing the haemoglobin concentration, blood transfusion 48 h before surgery may be required.

Sickle cell disease

Described by Herrick in 1910, sickle cell disease is an inherited group of disorders ranging from benign sickle cell trait to a severe form of sickle cell anaemia characterized by the substitution of normal haemoglobin A by abnormal haemoglobin S. The symptoms of the disease are related to the inability of haemoglobin S to withstand hypoxia, which results in the reduced haemoglobin forming tactoids which cause disruption and eventual rupture of the red cell. This leads to microvascular occlusion with infarction and organ damage. Sickle cell trait, the heterozygous form of the condition, generally presents few problems as far as surgery and anaesthesia are concerned.

Sickle cell anaemia presents a grave threat to the patient in the perioperative period and preoperative exchange transfusion is indicated in those individuals with a haemoglobin of < 8 g/dl, preferably with freshly donated blood. It is desirable to achieve $> 70\%$ normal red cells in a peripheral blood film.

Thalassaemia

This is a collective term for a group of inherited disorders associated with a reduction in α globulin production (α thalassaemia) or β globulin production (β thalassaemia). Patients should be treated in a similar way to those who have sickle cell disease.

RELEVANT INVESTIGATIONS PRIOR TO SURGERY

All patients scheduled for major surgery should have basic

haematological and biochemical screening beforehand. In ASA grade 1 patients, without evidence of intercurrent disease, who are undergoing minor surgery, the value of such tests is contentious.

Haematological tests

A full blood count is a minimum requirement prior to surgery, supplemented in patients of negroid or Mediterranean extraction by a sickle cell test and, if necessary, haemoglobin electrophoresis. Where perioperative transfusion is envisaged, blood should be sent for grouping, including Rhesus group and cross-match, preferably 24 h before surgery. In those patients with abnormalities of clotting, such as those on anticoagulant therapy or with liver disease, full clotting profiles should be sent and appropriate corrective therapy instituted prior to surgery.

Biochemical tests

Biochemical analysis of a patient's urine is generally performed by the nursing staff on admission, or in the outpatient clinic, using one of the many multitest dipstick kits. These can detect glycosuria, proteinuria etc. and if results are abnormal, further investigation is warranted.

Serum analysis for abnormalities of urea, electrolytes and liver function are indicated in the following circumstances:

1. if renal function is impaired by virtue of the primary gynaecological pathology, such as late-stage carcinoma of the cervix, or secondarily to systemic disease;
2. if current medication includes drugs likely to affect serum electrolytes, e.g. diuretic therapy or corticosteroids;
3. if hepatic or bony secondaries are suspected;
4. if postoperative nephrotoxic cytotoxic therapy is contemplated;
5. if postoperative enteral or parenteral nutrition is envisaged.

Microbiology

A mid-stream urine specimen should be sent for microscopic examination and culture to exclude urinary tract infection before any gynaecological procedure is carried out. In those patients in whom pelvic inflammatory disease is suspected or where tubal surgery is to be undertaken with a known previous history of pelvic inflammatory disease, swabs from the vagina, cervix and urethra should be sent for microscopic culture and sensitivity studies.

Virology

In those individuals where hepatitis B virus infection is suspected, such as drug abusers or those with a previous history of hepatitis, testing for hepatitis surface antigen is necessary.

Human immunodeficiency virus (HIV) is a lente virus and the aetiological agent responsible for causing the acquired immune deficiency syndrome. The screening of at-risk individuals for HIV antibodies, e.g. prostitutes, intravenous drug abusers and partners of bisexual males, can only be undertaken with a patient's permission and following counselling. At-risk individuals should be managed according to local hospital policy following the Department of Health guidelines (DHSS 1985a,b, 1986, HMSO Circular 1990).

Imaging and electrocardiography

Many of these procedures are indicated by the nature of the presenting complaint and the anticipated surgery: for example lymphangiography and pelvic carcinoma, or ultrasound of the liver where hepatic secondaries are suspected. Preoperative chest X-ray is only necessary in those patients where underlying pulmonary or cardiac disease is present, or in those individuals such as immigrants where exposure to chest diseases such as tuberculosis is suspected. Routine electrocardiographic examination is only necessary in the elderly or if cardiovascular disease is present. An abnormal electrocardiogram is associated with an increased perioperative risk.

INFLUENCE OF PRE-EXISTING MEDICATION, SMOKING AND ALCOHOL

Corticosteroids

Patients treated with systemic corticosteroids may develop suppression of the hypothalamic–pituitary–adrenal axis. The degree of suppression is dependent on the dosage and duration of treatment but some adrenal suppression can occur within 1 week of starting corticosteroids. Following the cessation of corticosteroid therapy it may be some months before complete recovery in the hypothalamic–pituitary axis occurs.

A surgical operation promotes a stress response leading to an increased output of corticosteroids. It has been estimated that a major surgical operation results in an increase of around 200–400 mg cortisol. Therefore additional corticosteroids should be given to avoid the risk of adrenal cortical insufficiency. Patients undergoing minor surgery can be managed by a small increase in the daily dose of corticosteroids or by monitoring vital signs and treating with incremental hydrocortisone if features suggestive of adrenal cortical insufficiency arise.

For major surgery it is usual to give increased cover in the form of hydrocortisone 100–200 mg intramuscularly with the premedication, and then 50–100 mg four times daily, reducing to a daily maintenance dose after several days. Patients treated with topical steroids (e.g. to the skin or rectum) occasionally absorb sufficient quantities to cause adrenal suppression and those patients who use high-dose beclomethasone inhalers to treat their asthma have may have a degree of adrenocortical insufficiency.

Oral contraceptives and hormone replacement therapy

Women taking the older formulations of the combined oral contraceptive pill have a higher incidence of deep venous thrombosis than non-pill users. This risk is increased by anaesthesia and surgery with its accompanying immobilization. It has been estimated that among pill takers undergoing major surgery, the relative risk of deep vein thrombosis was twice that of non-users (0.96 vs. 0.5%; Vessey et al 1986). With the reduction in the dosage of the oestrogen component of modern pills, that risk may now be less. At 6 weeks after discontinuation of the pill, changes in the coagulation and fibrinolytic systems have reverted to normal, but epidemiological evidence suggests that the excess risk of deep vein thrombosis reverts to normal in less than a month.

The risk of deep vein thrombosis following minor surgery, including laparoscopy, is extremely small and any risk from the oral contraceptive pill is more than outweighed by the risk of pregnancy. In the absence of other risk factors, there is insufficient evidence to support a policy of routinely stopping the oral contraceptive pill prior to major surgery (Royal College of Obstetricians and Gynaecologists 1995). When patients continue to take the pill up until the time of surgery, prophylactic low-dose heparin should be considered if there are other risk factors such as obesity and smoking.

These recommendations do not apply to those individuals taking the progestogen-only pill because there is no evidence of any increased risk of thrombosis with this method of contraception. Similarly, there is insufficient evidence to suggest that hormone replacement therapy (HRT) is associated with a high risk of thromboembolic disease. Thus, there is no indication for stopping HRT prior to surgery (Royal College of Obstetricians and Gynaecologists 1995).

Insulin and oral hypoglycaemic agents

Anaesthesia and surgery lead to a stress reaction resulting in an outpouring of catabolic hormones such as catecholamines, corticosteroids, glucagon and thyroxin. One of the metabolic effects of these is to stimulate glycogenolysis and gluconeogenesis, resulting in increased glucose liberation. These hormones also promote an increase in lipolysis which under normal circumstances is offset by the antilipolytic effect of the increased secretion of insulin which occurs as a result of the hypoglycaemia. The result is a depletion of liver glycogen and protein catabolism. In patients with untreated type 1 insulin-dependent diabetes, hyperglycaemia and ketoacidosis results. In type 2 diabetics where some residual insulin secretion is retained, these effects may be less profound and the tendency to ketoacidosis is less marked. The perioperative management of diabetic patients aims to avoid these problems by control of glucose homeostasis.

Type 1 diabetics

For all surgery involving general anaesthesia, the patients should be admitted prior to the operation and stabilized on short-acting insulins. Numerous different regimens for perioperative management have been advocated; however, the simplest consists of omission of the insulin dose on the day of operation and an infusion of 10% glucose with potassium and soluble insulin. Alternatively an infusion of glucose and potassium may be supplemented by soluble insulin administered separately, intravenously by a pump or by regular small subcutaneous injections. These are continued until the patient is reestablished on her normal diet and insulin regimen. All such regimens require regular and careful monitoring of glucose and potassium. Suitable regimens are suggested by Alberti & Hockaday (1983).

Type 2 diabetes

For minor surgery it is often sufficient to omit the oral hypoglycaemic agent on the morning of the operation with perioperative measurement of the blood sugar using dextrosticks. The hyperglycaemic effect of the operation is usually counteracted by the residual effect of the previous day's dose of hypoglycaemic agents. If there are problems, or the operation becomes prolonged, the patient may be managed as for type 1 diabetes. For major surgery patients should be treated as for type 1 diabetes.

Drugs acting on the cardiovascular system

Patients whose cardiovascular disease is controlled with drugs should, in general, continue on their medication in the perioperative period. Many patients with cardiovascular disease will be on various permutations of beta-adrenergic blocking drugs, calcium channel-blocking agents and nitrates. In general all cardiac medication should be continued through the perioperative period, as abrupt withdrawal may precipitate myocardial infarction. The myocardial depressant nature of these agents is of importance to the anaesthetist as some volatile anaesthetic agents may synergise with these drugs with adverse effects on cardiovascular haemodynamics. Patients with coronary artery disease, and those with a recent history of myocardial infarction in particular, will be on low dose aspirin therapy to reduce platelet coagulability. Although these patients are at increased risk of perioperative bleeding, this is less than the risk of perioperative myocardial infarction.

Patients on potassium-losing diuretics, whether or not being given potassium supplements, should have their plasma potassium estimated and hypokalaemia corrected preoperatively, particularly in the presence of concurrent digoxin therapy.

Patients on short-term anticoagulation treatment, e.g. for deep vein thrombosis, should have surgery postponed until full anticoagulation is reversed. When the need for coagulation is long-term, for example for those with prosthetic heart valves, it is important to liaise with the supervising physician. In general the patient should be admitted several days before surgery to allow the degree of anticoagulation to be adjusted. A British corrected ratio in the range of 2 to 3 is considered suitable for surgery, and stabilization on intravenous heparin is advocated. Postoperatively, anticoagulation should be maintained with intravenous heparin until the patient is once again able to take the oral agent. Where an anticoagulated patient requires emergency surgery, the British corrected ratio is adjusted to the suitable range by the administration of fresh frozen plasma or a small amount of vitamin K (1 mg).

Drugs acting on the nervous system

Monoamine oxidase inhibitors

These drugs are used in the treatment of resistant depression. Their therapeutic effects are believed to result from the inhibition of monoamine oxidase in the brain, leading to an increase in the concentrations of catecholamine and 5-hydroxytriptamine. Their peripheral effects include monoamine oxidase inhibition, inhibition of hepatic drug oxygenation and a variable degree of sympathetic blockade. Sympathomimetic agents may promote a hypertensive crisis, opiates (in particular pethidine) may cause profound hypotension, and barbiturates are metabolized at a variable and unpredictable rate. Although these problems can be overcome by withdrawing the drug at least 2 weeks before surgery, this can only be done in liaison with the prescribing psychiatrist.

Tricyclic, quadricyclic antidepressants and major tranquillizers

It is generally safe for patients to continue on these drugs, provided that the anaesthetist is made aware that they are being given so that the anaesthetic may be varied appropriately. The sudden cessation of administration of these agents may result in an acute exacerbation of the psychiatric illness. In the case of patients suffering from a psychotic illness stabilized on an oral major tranquillizer, it may be worth considering giving it parenterally over the operative period.

Lithium

It is the usual practice to withdraw lithium 1 week before major surgery because of the risk of toxicity should there be an electrolyte imbalance or a deterioration in renal function. This risk however must be balanced against the possible relapse of the affective disorder for which the drug is being prescribed, and again liaison with the psychiatrist is important.

Anticonvulsants

It is vital that patients continue to receive anticonvulsant medication over the operative period. It is usual to give the dose orally on the day of surgery and then parenterally until such time as the patient is able once again to take oral tablets.

Sodium valproate deserves particular mention because in addition to its anticonvulsant properties it interferes with haemostasis. This drug causes depression of platelet count, including frank thrombocytopenia, in a dose-related fashion, and it has been reported on occasions to cause impairment of platelet aggregation and minor defects of coagulation, including hypofibrinogenaemia. It is therefore recommended that patients taking this agent who require surgery should have a platelet and coagulation screen beforehand.

Smoking

Although not strictly medication, the effects of smoking on perioperative events and the necessity to encourage patients to stop smoking before surgery is important in the preoperative preparation of the patient. Cigarettes have a number of deleterious effects, including:

1. reduction in oxygen availability secondary to carbon monoxide binding to haemoglobin;
2. impairment of mucociliary clearance and hyperreactivity of small airways increasing the predisposition to postoperative chest infections;
3. reduction in neutrophil chemotaxis and immunoglobin concentration;
4. increase in platelet aggregatibility.

Patients should be encouraged to stop smoking at least 6 weeks before surgery in order to improve pulmonary function. They should at the very least, stop 48 h prior to surgery in order to eliminate carbon monoxide and thereby improve oxygen availability.

Alcohol

The heavy drinker is at greater risk because of diminution of the stress response, an impaired immunity and abnormalities of electrolyte control. The development of withdrawal symptoms can occur within 8 h of abstention, and treatment with infusions of alcohol is sometimes necessary. In the alcoholic with symptoms of severe hepatic disease (e.g. bleeding diathesis), pretreatment with parenteral vitamins and the correction of clotting abnormalities are essential. The preoperative administration of steroids may also be necessary for alcoholics with severe impairment of the stress response.

COUNSELLING AND CONSENT

The objective of preoperative counselling is to present the patient with sufficient information to enable her to make a reasoned choice regarding her treatment. It is necessary for the doctor to inform the patient of the nature of her medical condition, the available treatment regimens, including the necessity for surgery, and the success or prognosis associated with these options. In doing so, the nature and extent of potential complications must be outlined and any patient anxiety or apprehension should be discussed and allayed where appropriate. Armed with this information the patient will then be in a position to give her expressed rather than implied consent.

Counselling is very much a procedure with several stages, allowing constant reinforcement and giving the patient ample opportunity to voice any concern. It begins the moment the patient is told that treatment is necessary and is continued in the preoperative period: both medical and nursing staff have important roles to play. The value of counselling in allaying preoperative anxiety is well known. It is constantly being reviewed, as new techniques emerge to cope with the influences of personality variations on behavioural responses in the postoperative period. The value of such techniques (for example, cognitive coping) which encourage patients to focus on positive aspects of their treatment is well recognized.

The role of the patient is also important. Factors such as her physical and mental state, intellectual capacity, prior knowledge and expectations of the treatment will dictate the extent and the nature of the counselling process. The extent to which treatment procedures, complications and side-effects are explained is also influenced by the society in which she lives. In the highly litigation-conscious American society, counselling may be protracted and patient anxiety increased by the discussion of every conceivable complication. Coupled with this there may be very defensive medical practice, associated with inappropriate investigations and monitoring with their inherent risks. Within the UK there is an increasing level of compensation for medical negligence; however there is as yet no statutory medical requirement for doctors to discuss every potential complication or side-effect associated with a procedure. The legal precedent (Sidaway 1985) regarding the degree of disclosure of risk allows for doctors to make an assessment of the information they should disclose to the patient and limit it to that amount which will allow the patient to make a rational choice about treatment. The level of information should not deter the patient from undergoing treatment to the ultimate detriment of her health.

It may be pertinent to involve the patient's relatives in counselling, provided she consents, particularly where the elderly or mentally ill are concerned or where malignancy is present and where special provisions need to be made for terminal care. In addition to patient–doctor communication, information can also be imparted by the use of pamphlets and videos. It should be presented in a lucid fashion, in clear language, and should not be patronizing. It is advisable to include a disclaimer, such as the one used by the American College of Obstetricians and Gynecologists: 'The information in this pamphlet does not indicate an exclusive course of treatment or procedure to be followed and should not be considered as excluding other acceptable methods of practice'. The Royal College of Obstetricians and Gynaecologists' 14th Study Group on litigation in obstetrics and gynaecology (1985) made the following recommendations.

1. Communication between doctors and patients must be adequate.
2. Preoperative discussion with the patient should be full and noted in the hospital records.
3. The patient should be informed of likely operative complications. Not every conceivable complication should be discussed but the patient's questions should be answered truthfully.
4. A postoperative appointment should be offered to discuss any problems which may have arisen.
5. The opinions of senior staff and operative notes, including details of any complications, must be fully documented.

Informed consent

Failure to obtain consent may result in a doctor's facing a criminal prosecution for assault or a civil claim for damages. The way in which consent is obtained is also of importance: failure to give the patient sufficient information about the possible complications of a given procedure leaves the doctor open to a potential claim for damages for negligence. UK law allows the doctor to set that level of information, although it must be one which is acceptable to the majority of practitioners within the field. It is also imperative that consent be obtained for all aspects of perioperative management, e.g. the use of regional anaesthesia, vaginal or rectal examination under anaesthesia by medical students and the use of suppositories administered whilst the patient is anaesthetized.

However the ultimate decision as to whether or not the patient was sufficiently well informed lies with the courts. In England anyone of sound mind and over 16 years of age can give legally valid consent for surgical or medical treatment, provided that at the time it was obtained the patient was not under the influence of alcohol or drugs, including premedication. Under the age of 16 years, a parent, guardian or local authority (for children in care) or High Court (for children who are wards of court) can give consent provided the necessary explanations have been given.

Consent in relation to a child only allows for diagnostic or therapeutic procedures which will benefit the child. Therefore consent to non-therapeutic sterilization or experimentation without benefit is unlawful. In the case of contraception and termination of pregnancy, the General Medical Council advise that parental consent should be obtained. However patient confidentiality must be respected, and the doctor should use his or her judgement prior to agreeing to contraception or termination in a minor, if necessary following discussion with a colleague. Where a doctor feels it necessary to obtain parental consent against a patient's expressed wish, he or she should inform the patient accordingly.

Consent from mentally handicapped people is more complex and is governed by the provisions of the Mental Health Act 1983. However, this Act only provides statutory powers covering formal consent for treatment in respect of mental illness, and does not allow the undertaking of elective surgery for any other condition unless it is a threat to the patient's life. Therefore the consent of a mentally handicapped person should be sought as for a normal individual. The validity of the consent will however be determined by the underlying degree of mental handicap, and should involve a full discussion with all the interested parties. In those who are severely handicapped a guardianship order should be obtained, although a guardian may not give consent to medical treatment without the patient's permission. It is therefore wise to seek legal advice in situations involving mentally handicapped patients where informed consent is unobtainable.

A ruling by the Court of Appeal in 1989 has clarified some of the points regarding sterilization in mentally handicapped women. In an extreme emergency where the patient's condition renders it impossible to obtain consent, then a doctor may proceed to carry out treatment in order to protect the patient's life without her prior consent. It is advisable to discuss the situation with the next of kin but they have no legal right to consent or to withhold consent for treatment for the patient. Consent may be implied by a patient's conduct or may be given expressly in conversation. Ideally however it should be in writing, in order that it can be maintained as primary evidence. Consent forms should be simple, stating the nature of the procedure intended, including the consent for further or alternative procedures as deemed necessary at the time of operation; that the procedure has been fully explained, and (where applicable) no specific individual will perform the surgery or anaesthesia. The form is then signed by the patient and the doctor who explained the procedure and placed in the patient's notes. Forms for sterilization procedures should carry a disclaimer stating that there is a possibility of failure.

DAY CASE SURGERY

Day surgery represents an important facet of modern gynaecological practice. Both patients and hospitals benefit from the provision of a properly run service. With the ever increasing demands for improvement in patient care and the financial restraints that now affect all health care provision, expansion of day care will continue. In the report *Guidelines for day case surgery* (1985) the Royal College of Surgeons suggested that about 50% of all elective procedures could be performed as day surgery. This figure has already been achieved in North America and is likely to increase further. In the UK only 20% of elective surgery is performed on a day care basis.

Establishing a good day surgery service is not the same as admitting all minor surgical cases for the day. Forethought, communication and discussion between administrators, anaesthetic, nursing and surgical staff are prerequisites for a successful and safe service. Ideally day surgery should be performed in a dedicated unit. These units should be self-contained with their own operating suites and wards. To ease access they should be located on the lower floor of the building and with their own reception area. Only 30% of UK hospitals had such units in 1991 (Audit Commission 1992). Much day surgery is still performed as part of an inpatient operating list. This is thought to be less effective, but a perfectly adequate service can be achieved. Many of the procedural and nursing functions of day surgery are not compatible with the successful management of a general gynaecological inpatient ward, and the provision of a dedicated day surgery ward to be used in conjunction with the other surgical specialities will improve patient and nursing satisfaction whilst also increasing throughput. The ward should be as near to the operating suite as possible to reduce transit time, and modern trolleys suitable for preoperative examination, transportation, surgery and postoperative recovery facilitate patient throughput. Success of a day surgery unit is dependent on the appointment of a clinical director with responsibility for unit policy.

Selection of procedures and patients

The nature and the extent of day surgery offered should be agreed by both surgical and anaesthetic staff. Operations should not be unduly complex and should last less than one hour. Postoperative analgesia should be achievable with simple analgesics (Table 7.6).

The nature of modern gynaecological practice, with an increasing demand and use of hysteroscopy and laparo-

Table 7.6 Gynaecological procedures suitable for day surgery

Examination under anaesthesia
Dilatation and curettage
Hysteroscopy
Loop or laser conization
Cystoscopy
Excision or ablation of small vulval lesions
Marsupialization of Bartholin's gland cysts
Termination of pregnancy
Evacuation of retained products of conception (ERCP)
Laparosopic procedures:
- Diagnostic, including dye insufflation
- Division of adhesions
- Treatment of endometriosis by laser
- Ovarian diathermy
- Ovarian surgery
- Sterilization

Transcervical resection or ablation of endometrium or fibroids

scopy, requires the presence of more senior surgeons in day care theatres. Such a strategy should achieve a higher turnover of patients and a reduced complication rate.

Correct selection of patients is essential and local guidelines should be established. In general, patients need to be of ASA 1 or ASA 2 status, non-obese and have an appropriate carer to support and help in the first 24 h after surgery. Where social support is inadequate, an on-site patient hotel facility may be used.

Assessment of suitability for day case surgery is similar to that for inpatients. The majority of modern units adopt a preadmission clinic where patients are seen, assessed, relevant investigations ordered, consent taken and information pertaining to the perioperative course of the proposed surgery discussed. Such clinics are run by a combination of medical and nursing staff, conforming to local policies as dictated by individual circumstances.

After the operation, patients should be seen by both surgeon and anaesthetist. Prior to discharge, future plans for treatment, analgesia and emergency procedures should be communicated to the patient. It is essential that the patient's family doctor is informed.

Table 7.7 Risk assessment and prophylaxis for thromboembolism in gynaecological surgery

Degree of risk	Risk factors	Prophylactic measures
Low risk	Minor surgery (< 30 min) with no other risk factors Major surgery (> 30 min), less than 40 years old and no other risk factors	Early mobilization and hydration
Moderate risk	Minor surgery (< 30 min) in patients with a personal or family history of thromboembolic disease or thrombophilia Major surgery (> 30 min) Extended laparoscopic surgery Obesity (> 80 kg) Gross varicose veins Current infection Immobility prior to surgery for more than 4 days Heart failure or recent myocardial infarction Major current illness, e.g. heart or lung disease, inflammatory bowel disease, nephrotic syndrome, non-gynaecological malignancy	Unfractionated heparin, 5000 iu 12-hourly, subcutaneously Begin heparin 2–8 h before surgery Plus graduated elastic compression stockings
High risk	Three or more of the moderate risk factors above Major pelvic or abdominal surgery for gynaecological cancer Major surgery (> 30 min) in patients with: A personal or family history of thromboembolic disease Paralysis or immobilization of lower limbs	Unfractionated heparin, 5000 iu **8-hourly,** subcutaneously **or** Low molecular weight heparin (e.g. enoxaparin, 40 mg/day) subcutaneously Begin heparin at least **12 h** before surgery Plus graduated compression stockings

Modified from the Report of the Royal College of Obstetricians and Gynaecologists Working Party on prophylaxis against Thromboembolism in Gynaecology and Obstetrics (1995)

PREOPERATIVE PREPARATION

Thromboembolism prophylaxis

Thromboembolism is a major cause of postoperative death but a significant proportion of gynaecologists have yet to realize the perioperative need for prophylactic measures (NCEPOD 1993). The risk of deep vein thrombosis (DVT) following gynaecological surgery is comparable to that for general surgery. For example, there is a 12% prevalence of DVT after abdominal hysterectomy, and this is increased in the presence of old age, obesity and malignancy. The Thromboembolic Risk Factors Consensus Group (THRIFT 1992) and the Royal College of Obstetricians and Gynaecologists Working Party on Prophylaxis against Thromboembolism (1995) both recommended that all patients be individually assessed as to risk of thromboembolism and treated appropriately (Table 7.7).

Most gynaecological surgery is associated with a moderate risk of thromboembolism; there is a 10–40% risk of DVT and 0.1–1% risk of fatal pulmonary embolism. In major pelvic surgery this rises to a 40–80% risk of DVT and a 1–10% risk of fatal pulmonary embolism. Mechanical measures such as the use of antiembolism stockings or the intraoperative use of pneumatic compression devices should be used in addition to perioperative low dose heparin. A regimen of 5000 U of heparin given subcutaneously every 12 h from 2–8 h prior to surgery is recom-

Table 7.8 Administration of prophylactic subcutaneous heparin

1. Begin 2–24 h before surgery depending on degree of risk.
2. Administer at a site well away from the wound: flank or thigh.
3. Introduce full length of needle vertically into a skin fold which should be held throughout the procedure.
4. Continue heparin for 5 days or until fully mobilized.
5. Check platelet count daily if continued more than 5 days.

mended for moderate risk patients. An 8-hourly regimen, beginning at least 12 h before the operation, is suggested for high-risk women (Table 7.8) (Clarke-Pearson et al 1990). These regimens will reduce the incidence of thromboembolic events by two-thirds. There is an increase in the use of low molecular weight heparin fractions in DVT prophylaxis, although no improved efficacy over conventional treatments has been reported in gynaecological patients. A filter may be inserted transcutaneously into the inferior vena cava to prevent pulmonary embolism in women at particularly high risk (see Ch. 6). Such patients might include those who already have lower limb or pelvic thrombosis distal to a pelvic mass due to be removed surgically.

The increasing requirement for prophylaxis against thromboembolism, coupled with the widespread use of low dose aspirin in the treatment of coronary artery disease and cerebrovascular disease, and the increasing use of non-steroidal anti-inflammatory drugs for pain relief, has focused interest on the place of regional anaesthesia in patients where platelet and clotting abnormalities may be present. A comprehensive review of the subject (Vandermeulan et al 1993) concluded that there was no universal answer to the problem and that each case should be judged on its merits.

Antibiotics

All major gynaecological surgery, either vaginal or abdominal, carries a significant risk of infectious morbidity (20%), and the prophylactic use of antibiotics is strongly recommended since they will reduce the incidence by 50% (Mittendorf et al 1993). The antibiotic regimen chosen should have appropriate activity against likely infective agents, be easily administered and be cost-effective. The bacteria commonly associated with postoperative wound or pelvic infection arise from the normal vaginal flora: a combination of aerobic and anaerobic bacteria consisting of coliforms, streptococci and bacteroides.

While the UK has concentrated on metronidazole as a single agent, cephalosporins are more popular in North America. Both agents are effective although their spectrum activity is different. Combination therapy increases the spectrum of cover and may further reduce the incidence of postoperative infections. Augmentin is more effective than metronidazole in reducing postoperative infections (13.8 vs. 33.1%) and shortening hospital stay (Brown et al 1988). There are no comparisons of augmentin with the combination of metronidazole and a cephalosporin but they are probably equally effective. The final choice may rest on the issues of cost and local preference.

Intravenous agents should be given on induction of anaesthesia while oral and rectally administered drugs must be given at least 90 min prior to surgery. A single dose will provide cover for surgery that lasts for up to 1 h but if surgery takes longer it is advisable to give two further doses postoperatively. In prolonged surgical cases where there is a high risk of bacterial infection, a second intravenous dose may be repeated after 2 h.

Bowel preparation

Most gynaecological procedures do not require a rigorous bowel preparation unless bowel surgery is expected. However, it is useful in pelvic surgery to try to ensure that a loaded colon does not limit access. A disposable enema or two suppositories given the night before surgery helps to avoid this in most patients. More radical measures may be required for patients known to be constipated! In circumstances where bowel resection is anticipated, mechanical agents such as sodium picosulphate are effective in preparing the bowel and are easier to give than an electrolyte and antibiotic regimen.

JEHOVAH'S WITNESSES

The Jehovah's Witnesses are a fundamentalist sect formed in the USA in the 1870s. There are now more than 80 000 members in the UK. A minor part of their doctrine is taken to imply that blood transfusion should be forbidden as violating God's law. Jehovah's Witnesses accept medical treatment in all other respects and make no attempt to argue against the medical indications for blood transfusion. They are willing to take responsibility for their lives and accept that the constraints they place on their medical attendants may lead to their death. Health authorities have produced forms, with the help and guidance of the medical defence societies, in which the patient consents to treatment but states that blood transfusion is unacceptable and that the doctor will be absolved of any consequence of its omission. The legal value of these documents has been questioned. Each individual doctor must decide if he or she is willing to treat such a patient given the constraints placed on management. Techniques of haemodilution and autotransfusion are acceptable to some Jehovah's Witnesses and have been developed to facilitate surgery. It must be remembered that to administer blood against the wishes of the patient constitutes assault. The situation with regard to children is different by virtue of the Children and Young Persons Act 1933.

The Medical Defence Union and the Medical Protection Society stress that they are always happy to offer advice in such circumstances, and that whatever decision is taken, they will give full support to the individual doctor if that decision is subsequently challenged.

KEY POINTS

1. Assignment of physical status category to a patient is based on history and examination but should take account of the intended surgery as well.
2. Cooperation between surgeon and anaesthetist for preoperative patient assessment is of particular value in difficult cases.
3. Preoperative stabilization of patients with intercurrent medical disease is important.
4. Prompt and adequate communication is vital in preventing litigation.
5. Day case surgery requires both skilled anaesthesia and skilled surgery.
6. An effective day surgery unit benefits patients, hospitals and staff.
7. Thromboembolic prophylaxis is an important part of preoperative management and should be tailored to the patient's risk status.
8. Antibiotic prophylaxis will reduce infective morbidity and the duration of hospital stay.
9. Regional anaesthesia requires individual patient risk–benefit analysis if prophylactic heparin is used.

REFERENCES

Alberti K G M M, Hockaday T D R 1983 Diabetes mellitus. In: Weatherall D J, Ledingham J G, Warrell D A (eds) Oxford textbook of medicine, vol 1. Oxford University Press, Oxford, pp 5–48

American Society of Anesthesiologists 1963 New classification of physical status. Anesthesiology 24: 111

Audit Commission 1992 All in a day's work: an audit of day surgery in England and Wales. HMSO, London

Brown E J, Depares J, Robertson A A, Jones S, Hugher A B, Coles E C, Morgan J R 1988 Amoxycillin-clavulanic acid (Augmentin) versus metronidazole as prophylaxis in hysterectomy: a prospective, randomised clinical trial. British Journal of Obstetrics and Gynaecology 95: 286–293

Clarke-Pearson D L, DeLong E R, Synan I S et al 1990 A controlled trial of two low-dose heparin regimens for the prevention of deep vein thrombosis. Obstetrics and Gynecology 75: 684–689

Dajani A S, Biani A L, Chung K J et al 1991 Prevention of bacterial endocarditis. Circulation 83: 1174–1178

DHSS 1985a Acquired immune deficiency syndrome booklet 1: AIDS General information for doctors; CMO(85)7. Department of Health and Social Security, London

DHSS 1985b Acquired immune deficiency syndrome booklet 2: Information for doctors concerning the introduction of HTLV III antibody tests; CMO(85)12. Department of Health and Social Security, London

DHSS 1986 Acquired immune deficiency syndrome booklet 3: Guidance for surgeons, anaesthetists, dentists and their teams in dealing with patients infected with HTLV III; CMO(86)7. Department of Health and Social Security, London

Goldman L, Caldera D, Nussbaum S R et al 1977 Multifactorial index of cardiac risk in non-cardiac surgical procedures. New England Journal of Medicine 297: 845–850

HMSO Circular 1990 Guidance for clinical health care workers: protection against infection with HIV and hepatitis viruses. HMSO, London

Mangano D T 1990 Perioperative cardiac morbidity. Anesthesiology 72: 153–184

Mittendorf R, Aronson M P, Berry R E 1993 Avoiding serious infections associated with abdominal hysterectomy: a meta-analysis of antibiotic prophylaxis. American Journal of Obstetrics and Gynecology 169: 1119–1124

NCEPOD 1993 The report of the National Confidential Enquiry into Perioperative Deaths 1991/2 National Confidential Enquiry into Perioperative Deaths, London

Prys-Roberts C 1984 Anaesthesia and hypertension. British Journal of Anaesthesia 56: 711–724

Royal College of Obstetricians and Gynaecologists 14th Study Group 1985 Litigation and obstetrics and gynaecology. Chamberlain G, Orr C, Sharp F (eds) Royal College of Obstetricians and Gynaecologists, London, p 311

Royal College of Obstetricians and Gynaecologists 1995 Report of the Working Party on Prophylaxis against Thromboembolism in Gynaecology and Obstetrics. Royal College of Obstetricians and Gynaecologists, London

Royal College of Surgeons 1985 Commission on the provision of surgical services. Guidelines for day case surgery. Royal College of Surgeons in England, London

Sidaway v. Board of Governors of Bethlem Royal and Maudsley Hospital 1985. Weekly Law Rep 2: 480

Treasure T, van Besouw J P 1993 The surgical patient with cardiac disease. In: Hobsley M, Johnson A, Treasure T (eds) Current Surgical Practice. Edward Arnold, London, pp 39–55

Thromboembolic Risk Factors (THRIFT) Consensus Group 1992 Risk of and prophylaxis for venous thromboembolism in hospital patients. British Medical Journal 305: 567–574

Vandermeulan E P E, Vermylen J, van Aken H 1993 Epidural and spinal anaesthesia in patients receiving anticoagulant therapy. In: van Aken H (ed) Clinical Anaesthesiology 7:3. New developments in spinal and epidural drug administration. W B Saunders, London, pp 663–690

Vessey M P, Mant D, Smith A, Yeates D 1986 Oral contraceptives and venous thromboembolism: findings in a large prospective study. British Medical Journal 292: 526–528

FURTHER READING

Healey T E J (ed) 1990 Anaesthesia for day case surgery. Clinical Anaesthesiology 4. Baillière Tindall, London

Stoelting R K, Dierdorf F F 1993 Anaesthesia and coexisting disease, 3rd edn. Churchill Livingstone, Edinburgh

8

Intraoperative complications and their management

G. A. J. McIndoe

INTRODUCTION

In major surgery, occasional damage to vital structures is unavoidable but with good training, appropriate experience, and careful application such damage should be rare. Timely recognition of potential problems has a major impact on the long-term outcome for patients. The request for appropriate assistance from a more experienced colleague either within the speciality or from another speciality, and early repair, preferably during the original operation, can make the difference between complete and rapid recovery, and long-term morbidity and further surgery.

To minimize complications, a surgical technique should be developed that involves careful and accurate identification of tissue planes, preferably with sharp dissection, with the aim of causing the minimum of damage to tissues and structures that are to be preserved. A gentle approach should be used and tissues handled in such a way as to maintain optimum viability.

Operate under direct vision at all times. Avoid the temptation to push an instrument deep into a plane of dissection since inadvertent damage may be caused and bleeding down a deep hole is more difficult to control. Allow enough time for each operation and do not hurry surgery. Particularly when in training, greater speed will develop by a methodical attention to detail of technique, rather than by hurrying individual cases, and outcome is always more important than operative time.

Every case undertaken should be seen as a training opportunity to improve technique. Straightforward cases are particularly useful for the practice of sharp dissection to the correct tissue planes. When tissue planes are more difficult to identify, this practice will be invaluable.

Aim to keep the operation under control at all times; it is much better to spend a little time controlling bleeding so that the operation can proceed unhurriedly and with good visibility, than to rush on hoping to stop the bleeding as the operation progresses.

In this chapter I will discuss the common intraoperative complications, and the aspects of technique that reduce the likelihood of these complications occurring. I will also highlight the range of methods used to repair damage, although for the most part, detailed descriptions are not appropriate in a textbook of this type.

URETERIC DAMAGE

Ureters are the organs most respected by gynaecologists. They lie close to the genital tract, and repair of a damaged ureter is technically demanding with results that are not always satisfactory. By recognizing when and where the ureters are most at risk, and by adopting a safe technique, the risk of damage to the ureter should be minimized.

Anatomical relations

The urinary and genital tracts are closely related in embryological development, and their anatomy and physiology, not surprisingly, are intertwined. The ureter develops from a bud on the posterolateral border of the mesonephric duct near the cloaca, which elongates and eventually fuses with the developing kidney. The ventral portion of the cloaca develops into the urethra, bladder and lower portion of the vagina.

The ureters enter the pelvis by crossing the common iliac arteries in the region of their bifurcation. They descend on the pelvic side wall, medial to the branches of the internal iliac arteries and lateral to the ovarian fossae. From there, they run on the anterior surface of the levator ani muscles lateral to the uterosacral ligaments to pass beneath the uterine arteries, 1–1.5 cm lateral to the cervix and vagina. The ureters then swing medially around the vagina, to enter the bladder 2–3 cm below the anterior vaginal fornix.

The ureter is accompanied by a plexus of freely anastomosing fine vessels running in the loose tissue surrounding it. The blood supply in the upper portion is derived from the renal and ovarian vessels, in the middle third from branches of the aorta, common iliac and internal iliac arteries, and in the lower part from branches of the uterine, vaginal, middle haemorrhoidal and vesical arteries. The ureter may be mobilized extensively provided this plexus of vessels is preserved.

The ureter is at risk during gynaecological surgery in four regions: at the pelvic brim where it can be confused with the infundibulopelvic ligament; lateral to the ovarian fossa where it can be adherent to an ovarian mass; in the ureteric tunnel beneath the uterine artery, and anterior to the vagina where it runs into the bladder (Table 8.1).

Table 8.1 Areas where the ureter is vulnerable to surgical trauma

Locations at which the ureter is at risk	Reason for risk
Pelvic brim	Lies very close to ovarian vessels
Ovarian fossa	May become adherent to an ovarian mass
Ureteric tunnel	Lies immediately posterior to uterine artery
Anterior to vagina at entry into bladder	May not be mobilized during bladder dissection

The ureter at the pelvic brim and ovarian fossa

At the pelvic brim, the infundibulopelvic ligament with the ovarian vessels also crosses the iliac vascular bundle, usually 1–2 cm distal to the bifurcation of the common iliac artery and the ureter (Fig. 8.1). At this point the ureter and the ovarian vessels are running in parallel in a similar plane and may be confused if care is not taken. Occasionally the ureter may be duplex. Where the ureter runs lateral to the ovary, it will almost inevitably be associated with any inflammatory or malignant mass. Happily, it will lie on the lateral aspect of the mass where it can be identified and dissected free, usually without difficulty, although in patients with endometriosis the ureter may be fixed in dense fibrosis.

The key to the safe identification of the ureter on the pelvic side wall is to open the peritoneum and dissect in the retroperitoneal space. This is most easily done by dividing the round ligament between two clips, dividing the peritoneum in a cranial direction 1.5 cm lateral to the ovarian vessels, and in a caudal direction down towards the uterovesical fold. The loose areolar tissue then encountered should be separated by blunt dissection with careful diathermy of any small vessels. The ureter will lie on the lateral aspect of the leaf of peritoneum reflected by this manoeuvre. At this stage the infundibulopelvic ligament can be safely divided with the ureter under direct

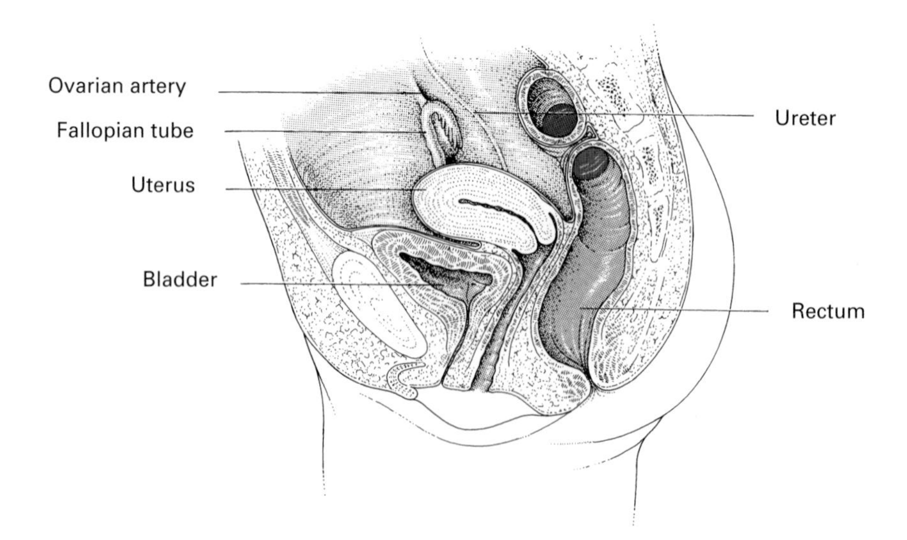

Fig. 8.1 Relationship of ureter to ovarian vessels in the infundibulopelvic ligament. Note how close the ureter lies to the ovarian vessels at the pelvic brim.

vision. If the anatomy of the pelvic side-wall has been distorted, this technique will almost always allow the ureter to be identified and followed within the pelvis. If an ovarian mass is present the ureter may be dissected free from the mass in this retroperitoneal plane.

The lower ureter

The third position where the ureter is at risk is in the ureteric tunnel, where the ureter crosses beneath the uterine artery but superior to the cardinal ligament and about 1–1.5 cm lateral to the angle of the vagina (Fig. 8.2). It is possible to palpate the ureter in this position by gripping the paracervical tissue between one finger in the pouch of Douglas and the thumb placed laterally in front of the uterine pedicle. The ureter, which is felt as a firm cord running across the cardinal ligament, is surprisingly well lateral to the cervix if the bladder has been properly reflected and the anatomy is normal. However, adhesions, fibrosis or inadequate dissection may disrupt these relationships, causing the ureter to remain fixed near the lateral margin of the cervix.

Damage to the ureter in this site is prevented by carefully reflecting the bladder, and by not taking a large pedicle which includes both the uterine artery and the paracervical tissue. I prefer to take the uterine artery relatively high, at the level of the internal os, which allows the parametrium to fall laterally taking the ureter with it. The ureter can then be palpated again and a second pedicle taken medial to the first, to include the cardinal ligament.

In most cases, damage to the ureter occurs at this site because the pedicle slips or the original ligature is not adequate. Avoid this by preparing the pedicle carefully before clamping it. Use modern clamps such as Roget's or Zeppelin's parametrial clamps which rarely slip, and place ties accurately. If bleeding does occur, palpate the ureter again after replacing the clamp to ensure that it has not been included.

The ureter is occasionally damaged in its course across the anterior surface of the vagina. This may occur when taking a cuff of vagina, during a vaginal hysterectomy or colposuspension. When dissecting the upper vagina it is important to keep in the correct plane close to the vaginal wall. Stitches placed either vaginally or abdominally in this area must be in tissue that has been accurately identified.

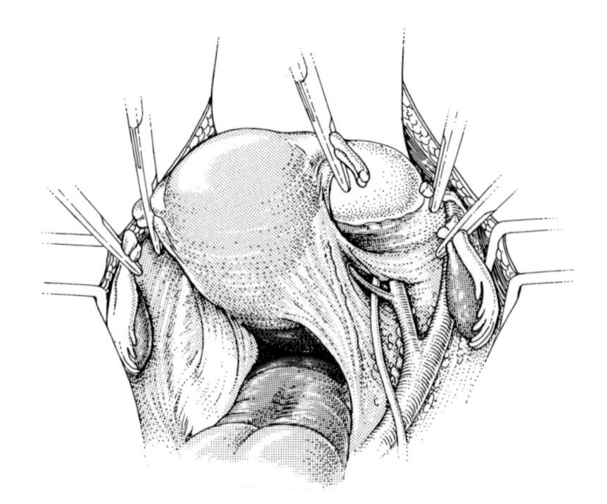

Fig. 8.2 Relationship of ureter to the uterine artery. This diagram shows the dissection performed for a radical hysterectomy, but illustrates the close relationship between the ureter and the uterine artery.

Repairing ureteric damage

If a ureter is damaged, the presence of the contralateral kidney should be checked. If the ureter has not been cut across, but merely crushed or ligated in error, and this is recognized on the table, it is acceptable to remove the ligature and insert a stent into the ureter in the hope that a stenosis will not result. If the ureter is divided, repair will be necessary. In the past, gynaecologists have resorted to simply tying off the divided ureter but this is rarely justifiable now.

Repair of the ureter is technically demanding and may lead to long-term complications. It is not appropriate for a gynaecologist without urological training or extensive urological experience to undertake this. In principle, an end-to-end anastomosis can be performed for ureteric damage at the pelvic brim or above. The ureter is mobilized so that the ends can be brought together without tension. They are spatulated and the anastomosis performed using fine interrupted sutures over a silastic stent. This is removed several weeks later (Fig. 8.3). An alternative for damage at this level is to perform a uretero-ureteric anastomosis.

If the damage has occurred at the level of the ureteric tunnel or lower, the safest method of repair is to reimplant the ureter into the bladder. The bladder is opened between stay sutures. A submucosal tunnel is fashioned taking care to avoid the other ureter. The distal end of the ureter is brought through the tunnel and, after spatulating the end, it is sutured to the bladder mucosa. A couple of sutures into the serosal surface anchor the ureter to the outer layer of the bladder (Fig. 8.4).

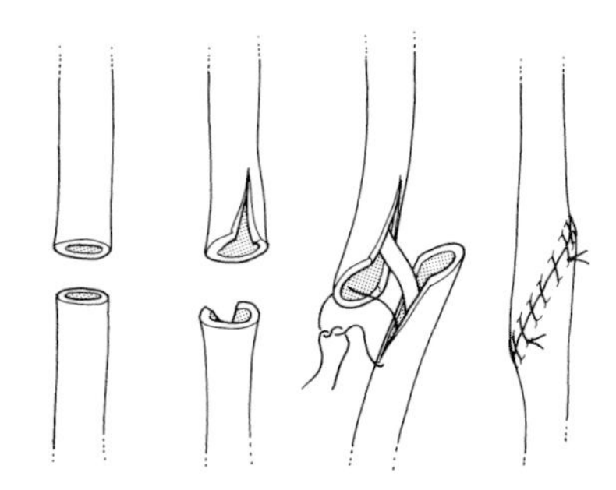

Fig. 8.3 Reanastomosis of a divided ureter. A cleanly cut ureter may be reanastomosed by spatulating the ends and repairing it with fine sutures over a suitable splint. The splint is withdrawn from the bladder at a later date.

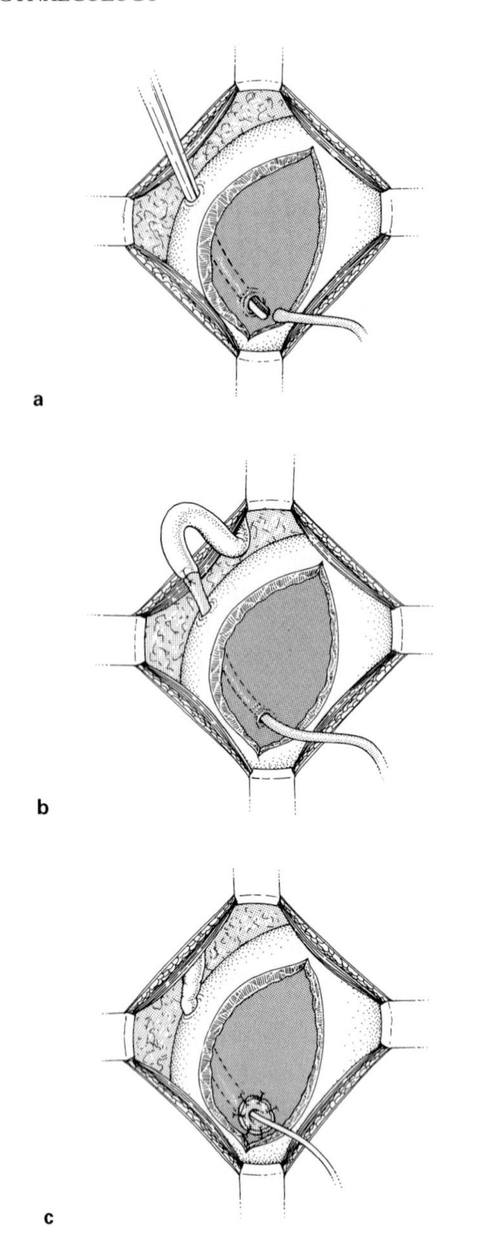

Fig. 8.4 Reimplantation of the ureter. **a** After opening the bladder, a submucosal tunnel is made along the lateral posterior wall of the bladder. A thin rubber tube is slipped over the ends of the scissors. **b** The ureter is drawn through the tunnel with the rubber tube. **c** The end of the ureter is spatulated and sutured to the bladder mucosa with fine sutures. An indwelling stent may be left in place, although this is not usually necessary.

When damage has occurred higher on the pelvic sidewall, the bladder can be elevated to the cut end of the ureter to allow reimplantation without tension, using either a psoas hitch or a Boari flap. In the former, an appropriate part of the bladder is elevated towards the end of the ureter. To facilitate this, the cystotomy is performed across the direction of elevation and is closed in the opposite direction to elongate the bladder. In addition, the contralateral superior vesical pedicle may be divided. The ureter is reimplanted as previously described, and the

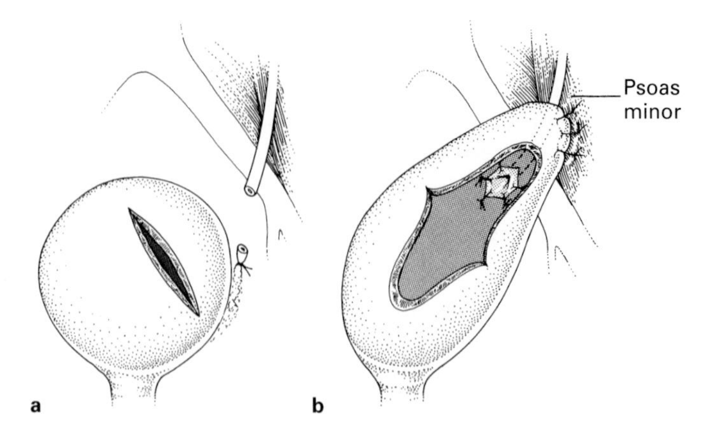

Fig. 8.5 The psoas hitch procedure. **a** The bladder is incised in the transverse axis. **b** The bladder is fixed to the psoas minor tendon to relieve tension and the ureter is reimplanted as described. The bladder is closed in the longitudinal axis.

bladder is fixed to the psoas muscle to relieve any tension. This technique will allow a ureter divided at any level in the pelvis up to the pelvic brim to be safely reimplanted (Fig. 8.5).

The Boari flap is an alternative to the psoas hitch. A flap of bladder is elevated, the ureter is reimplanted into this and the flap is closed as a tube (Fig. 8.6). This allows good elevation of the bladder at the expense of a reduced bladder capacity.

Alternatively a uretero-ureteric anastomosis to the opposite ureter can be performed. This has the disadvantage that both ureters may be compromised but may be the only method if access to the bladder is difficult.

BLADDER DAMAGE

Anatomical relations

The bladder, like the ureters, is intimately related to the genital tract by virtue of its embryological development. Repair of the bladder, however, is more straightforward and the results are very good. It is an extraperitoneal organ that is located behind the symphysis pubis and rests on the anterior part of the levator diaphragm, the anterior vaginal wall and the cervix. The trigone is at the level of the upper vagina, with the base of the bladder related to the anterior vaginal fornix and cervix. When full, the bladder rises out of the pelvis reaching towards the level of the umbilicus, and presents a hazard during abdominal incision. The bladder is also at risk in this position if it is adherent after previous surgery or during caesarean section in labour, when the lower segment of the uterus is lifted out of the pelvis, elevating the bladder with it.

Avoiding damage

The bladder must always be emptied prior to pelvic

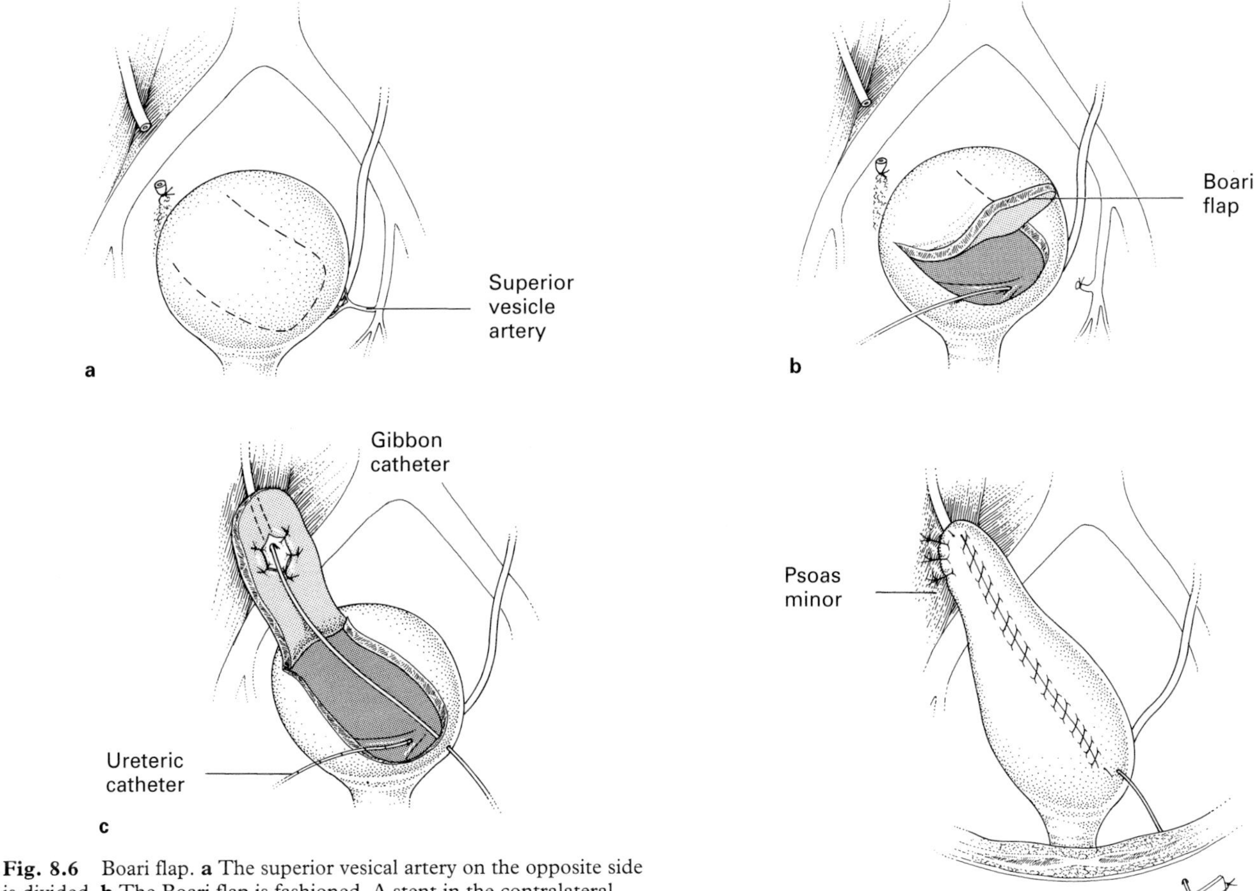

Fig. 8.6 Boari flap. **a** The superior vesical artery on the opposite side is divided. **b** The Boari flap is fashioned. A stent in the contralateral ureter may be helpful. **c** The ureter is reimplanted through a submucosal tunnel in the flap. **d** The Boari flap is closed and fixed to the psoas muscle to relieve tension.

surgery, and the peritoneum should be opened superiorly, away from the bladder, when making a transverse incision. It can be palpated as a thickening in the peritoneum, and if there is any doubt about its position, careful dissection should allow the detrusor muscle to be recognized before the mucosa is opened. Opening the peritoneum by blunt dissection with fingers will not necessarily protect the bladder, as it is possible to dissect bluntly into it. Similarly, the technique of tearing the parietal peritoneum open by 'stretching' the wound once the abdominal cavity has been opened, can lead to damage to the top of the bladder, particularly after previous surgery.

An essential part of any hysterectomy is separation of the bladder from the cervix and upper vagina. This plane can be found after division of the uterovesical fold of peritoneum merely by pushing caudally with a swab applied firmly to the anterior surface of the cervix cranial to the bladder. This is very quick, but inevitably leaves a few small bleeding points on the back of the bladder which may be difficult to find. In addition, the bladder is occasionally damaged by this manoeuvre, particularly after previous surgery.

An alternative approach is to use a combination of sharp and blunt dissection. After dividing the uterovesical fold of peritoneum, the scissors are held slightly opened to begin separation in this plane by pushing the bladder off the cervix. Small blood vessels can be recognized and diathermied before cutting, to maintain haemostasis at all times. Once the correct plane has been identified in the midline, the dissection is extended laterally to mobilize the ureters and can be continued as far as necessary down the vagina. Although a little more time-consuming, this technique is safe, and can be used on simple cases to gain experience for more difficult situations.

When performing the operation vaginally, the same plane needs to be defined and dissected. If the plane does not develop easily, it is important to use sharp dissection, as merely pushing on the bladder may tear a hole. A sound in the bladder may help to define the correct plane. Alternatively, a finger over the fundus of the uterus or over the broad ligament to the side, once the pouch of Douglas is opened, can define the uterovesical fold of peritoneum and clarify the correct plane for dissection.

The bladder can also be damaged during closure of the

vaginal vault, particularly if it has not been sufficiently mobilized. Sutures may be placed through the detrusor muscle or even into the bladder itself, although this rarely causes problems. However, if this is recognized at the time of surgery, such stitches should be removed, and the bladder mobilized to allow closure of the vault without including the bladder. If damage to the bladder has occurred, this should be repaired and the bladder drained as discussed below.

Repair of the bladder

Should a hole be made in the bladder, this can be repaired after the dissection of the bladder is complete. A stay stitch is usually placed at either end of the hole, and the incision is repaired in two layers using either chromic catgut or vicryl. Care is taken that the ureters are well away from the sutures, and if there is any doubt, ureteral stents should be inserted. After repair, the bladder is drained with an indwelling catheter for 7–10 days. Provided the bladder is well mobilized and repaired without tension, an excellent result should be achieved.

Repair of the bladder is less likely to be successful after radical radiotherapy, and a high incidence of fistulae is seen in this situation. An additional blood supply is provided by interposing a flap of omentum.

BOWEL DAMAGE

Inadvertent damage to the bowel should be unusual, unless adhesions are present. The occasions where damage is most likely to occur are during opening of the peritoneal cavity, or when dissecting dense intra-abdominal adhesions. In addition, the rectum lies close to the uterosacral ligaments and posterior wall of the vagina, and may be at risk during extensive pelvic dissection for cervical or vaginal carcinoma.

When reopening a previous incision, it is preferable to enter the peritoneal cavity away from the previous closure. If that is not possible, great caution should be used when approaching the peritoneum. Very occasionally, the peritoneal cavity is almost obliterated and it may be necessary to dissect extraperitoneally around the adhesions to enter the peritoneal cavity.

When dense intraperitoneal adhesions are encountered, with care and patience the adhesions can usually be divided safely. Occasionally, the bowel is so matted together that resection of a small portion may be necessary. Particular care must be used in a patient who has been treated with radiotherapy, as the bowel is more friable and often densely adherent.

When dividing the uterosacral ligaments close to the pelvic side-wall during a radical hysterectomy, the rectum is at risk of being included in the clamps. The rectovaginal space must be opened widely and the rectum dissected free. Care is necessary when entering this space to avoid direct damage to the rectum.

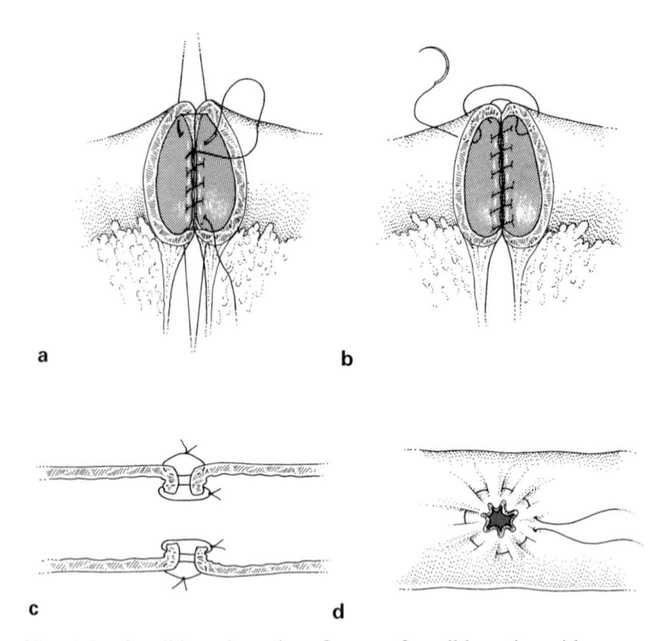

Fig. 8.7 Small bowel repair. **a** Suture of small intestine with continuous all-layers suture. **b** Connell inverting suture. **c** Full thickness sutures reinforced with inverting Lembert suture. **d** Purse-string suture of small intestinal perforation.

Repair of bowel

Repair of damaged bowel either may involve primary closure of a small hole or may be facilitated by the excision of a portion of unhealthy bowel and reanastomosis (Fig. 8.7). Consideration should be given to a defunctioning colostomy proximal to anastomosis of large bowel, particularly if the blood supply to the bowel wall is compromised in any way. Factors that have bearing on this decision are previous radiotherapy, bowel obstruction, gross infection of the operative field, or other medical factors such as diabetes, steroid therapy, malignancy and advanced age. If no adverse factors are present, a colostomy may not be necessary. Small bowel usually heals without the need for defunctioning. If there is any doubt about the safety of a repair, a surgeon who specializes in bowel should be involved to help with the repair.

VASCULAR DAMAGE

Damage to large vessels is uncommon during routine gynaecological surgery, but can occur during radical surgery. If the blood supply to the leg is compromised by damage to the external or common iliac vessels, serious morbidity can result, and it is vital that repair is carried out to the highest standard. Usually a vascular surgeon should be involved.

The internal iliac vessels may be safely ligated if damage occurs, but bleeding from the thin-walled veins on the pelvic side-wall can be very difficult to control. Initially bleeding should be controlled by direct pressure, either by a well-placed finger or using a swab. This allows time to assemble the necessary instruments, a fine sucker and fine sutures on small needles to repair the laceration or ligate the vessel, and also a chance to take a deep breath so that the subsequent suturing is not carried out in a panic. Great care should be taken as the situation can be made worse by rough handling of the vessels. If in doubt, more experienced help should be obtained.

The often quoted technique of tying off the internal iliac artery in cases of troublesome bleeding is not without its own hazards. The origin of the artery lies over the bifurcation of the common iliac vein, and great care is needed to avoid damaging the internal iliac vein while dissecting behind the artery to pass the ligature. This technique is often less effective than might be hoped in controlling pelvic haemorrhage because such bleeding is often venous.

UTERINE PERFORATION AND FALSE PASSAGE

During dilatation of the cervix, a false passage may be created by pushing an instrument through the substance of the cervix rather than following the canal. Instruments may also be pushed through the fundus of the uterus into the peritoneal cavity.

When learning to dilate the cervix one must develop a gentleness of touch which combines pressure with a sensitivity or 'feel' for the tissues. It is important to avoid using force with instruments, but rather to feel for the path of least resistance. Because of the barrel-shaped contour of the endocervical canal, an exploring instrument can deviate from the axis of the cervix and not engage the internal os. The size of instrument chosen for this exploration is important as a fine probe will more easily create its own passage, and therefore less pressure should be used. It is said that right-handed people are more likely to perforate towards the right side of the cervical canal although a false passage can be created in any direction. It then becomes very difficult to identify the true cervical canal and gain access to the uterine cavity.

If a false passage is suspected, one helpful manoeuvre is to perform a bimanual examination with the vulsellum and sound still within the passage. It is often possible to feel where the sound is in relation to the axis of the cervix, and in which direction the true passage is likely to be found.

When a false passage has been created, provided damage to other organs is not suspected, and the patient is not pregnant, the situation can usually be managed conservatively. In most cases it is best to desist from further attempts at dilatation. In the pregnant patient, however, significant haemorrhage may occur, particularly following lateral perforation into the broad ligament and damage to the uterine vessels. If vaginal bleeding continues or the patient's general condition deteriorates, laparotomy will be necessary. The broad ligament will be full of blood if the uterine vessels have been damaged, and hysterectomy may be necessary to control the blood loss, although ligation of the uterine artery and repair of the perforation may be an option. In some cases, bleeding into the retroperitoneal space may not become apparent for several hours. Careful postoperative observation is necessary to detect this at an early stage.

The consequences of fundal perforation depend on whether the patient is pregnant and what instrument has created the perforation. In a non-pregnant uterus, a dilator through the fundus is very unlikely to cause any problems. Probably most perforations are not recognized by the surgeon at all. The patient should be observed for a period after recovery but is unlikely to need further intervention. In a pregnant patient, perforation is said to be more likely to cause haemorrhage, but in general a simple perforation can be managed conservatively. Avoid the temptation to 'confirm' the perforation by repeatedly reintroducing instruments into the uterus as this may make matters worse.

If there is significant risk of damage to intra-abdominal organs, a laparotomy is indicated because laparoscopy cannot be relied upon to exclude damage to bowel. For example, if a suction catheter has been inserted through a perforation with suction connected, laparotomy and careful examination of the bowel is mandatory.

LAPAROSCOPY

The incidence of complications in laparoscopic surgery relates very closely to the experience of the surgeon and the training they have received. Gynaecologists have built up an extensive experience in the speciality with simple procedures over the last generation. Most SHOs and junior registrars are trained at diagnostic laparoscopy as one of their earliest procedures. Nevertheless, the adoption of the more advanced operative techniques has been slow, and experience in these areas is still very limited. If a high incidence of complications is to be avoided, it is essential that individual surgeons are well trained in the procedures they undertake. General complications of laparoscopy will be discussed, but consideration of complications encountered in advanced laparoscopic surgery is outside the scope of this chapter. (See Ch. 4, Laparoscopy.)

Damage to bowel

Blind insertion of the Veress needle and first trocar may lead to perforation of intra-abdominal and retroperitoneal structures. Bowel is rarely damaged unless it is adherent to the anterior abdominal wall, but great care must be taken if the patient has had a previous operation or intra-abdominal sepsis. In these cases, the initial trocar may be placed away from the site of the previous incision in an attempt to avoid fixed bowel. Alternatively, the abdomen may be entered using an open minilaparotomy technique and then the incision sealed around a blunt-ended trocar. Difficulty may be encountered in maintaining a good seal using this technique, but specially designed trocars reduce this problem. A new device is available now that incises the tissue in front of a blunt-ended trocar 1 mm at a time and allows visualization of the end of the instrument as it is being inserted. This may prove to be useful in the small number of cases where difficulty is anticipated.

Minor damage to the bowel may be repaired laparoscopically by a surgeon experienced in laparoscopic suturing. In most cases it is much safer to perform a laparotomy to allow careful inspection of the whole bowel and open repair of any damage. Because it can be difficult to find the hole in the bowel subsequently, it is wise to leave the offending instrument in place until the abdomen is open.

Damage to blood vessels

When inserting the Veress needle and the first trocar it is vital that these instruments are kept away from the major vessels. The position of the sacral promontory can be palpated and the instruments angled in such a way that they pass below the promontory and into the free space in the midline of the pelvis. While damage to a major blood vessel may be all too obvious, the bleeding may be predominantly retroperitoneal and difficult to see laparoscopically. If the patient's blood pressure has dropped and pulse rate risen sufficiently to suggest the possibility of vascular damage, a laparotomy should be performed immediately. If the abdomen has to be opened in a hurry, one technique is to lift the laparoscope up to the anterior abdominal wall, and cut down onto it, allowing immediate access.

Blood vessels in the abdominal wall may also be damaged. To reduce this risk, the abdominal wall is usually transilluminated to visualize vessels prior to insertion of secondary trocars. The location of the inferior epigastric vessels should be recognized, as they will bleed profusely and this may be difficult to control. Minor bleeding around a trocar may be controlled either by leaving the trocar in place to tamponade the vessel, or by inserting a Foley catheter through the trocar, inflating the balloon with 30–50 ml of saline, and withdrawing the trocar and balloon to apply pressure to the bleeding point. If the vessel requires suturing, this is facilitated by a long J-shaped needle.

Diathermy damage

Problems with laparoscopic use of diathermy stem either from the heat generated at the site of tissue destruction, or from current finding an alternative path to earth through an adjacent organ. Tissue coagulated by diathermy becomes very hot and may retain its heat for several minutes. This heat will spread to underlying structures and adjacent organs and may cause damage. Diathermied tissue must be allowed to cool before coming in contact with adjacent structures. A further problem is the rising impedance in desiccated, diathermied tissue. This may result in the current arcing to a nearby organ that offers a low resistance path to earth. In a similar way, current may arc to nearby organs if the current is activated before the electrode is in contact with the tissue to be treated.

ACKNOWLEDGEMENT

Figures 8.3, 8.4, 8.5 and 8.6 have been redrawn from Blandey J 1986 Operative urology, 2nd edn with permission of the publishers, Blackwell Science Ltd.

KEY POINTS

1. Accurate identification of tissue planes and careful dissection will reduce intraoperative complications.
2. The ureter should always be identified on the pelvic side wall before the infundibulopelvic ligament is divided.
3. Identify and free the ureter from ovarian masses by opening the retroperitoneal space.
4. If the ureter is damaged, repair should usually be undertaken by a urologist.
5. The bladder may be repaired using two layers of absorbable sutures. Ensure that the ureters are not included in this repair.
6. Repair of bowel or great vessels, apart from minor damage, should usually be undertaken by a specialist surgeon.
7. Uterine perforation may often be managed conservatively.
8. Repair of laparoscopic damage to bowel will usually require a laparotomy.
9. If laparoscopic damage to major pelvic vessels is suspected, a laparotomy must be performed without delay.
10. Diathermy should be applied only when the electrodes are securely applied to the target tissue and the target and surrounding tissues are in clear view.

9

Postoperative care

John Tidy

INTRODUCTION

The postoperative management of women undergoing surgery is an area of care that sometimes receives less attention than preoperative and perioperative management. This is unfortunate, since if it is performed well there should be an associated reduction in morbidity leading to shorter and less costly hospital admissions and an increase in patient satisfaction.

Gynaecologists benefit, in general, from operating on fit and relatively young patients, with the majority of procedures undertaken having a low surgical morbidity. The prevention of postoperative complications rather than their diagnosis and treatment should therefore be our goal. The use of protocols such as those for thromboembolic disease prophylaxis should reduce the morbidity and mortality from deep vein thrombosis and pulmonary embolism. Infective complications can be reduced by the use of prophylactic antibiotics, and by observing high standards of surgical aseptic technique. Adherence to good surgical technique will reduce the incidence of haematoma formation and wound dehiscence. The development of local surgical audit should help in identifying areas of concern and lead to reduced morbidity. In an attempt to prevent postoperative complications, known risk factors such as obesity and smoking should be identified at the time of preoperative assessment, and the postoperative care planned so as to minimize the potential complications.

POSTOPERATIVE CARE

Fluid replacement

Most gynaecological procedures do not require the patient to be 'nil by mouth' for any considerable length of time. Oral fluids and food can often be reintroduced by the end of the first postoperative day and even earlier when vaginal surgery is performed. The average gynaecological patient will require between 2 and 2.5 l of water per 24 h and have a minimum requirement of 75–100 mEq per day for sodium and 60 mEq per day for potassium. Potassium supplementation is required only after 24 h because cell death and a mild renal acidosis will maintain potassium levels during the acute postoperative phase.

These basic requirements may need further supplementation in certain situations (Table 9.1). There may be a high volume loss through a drain, as may occur after lymphadenectomy. During a long abdominal procedure, insensible loss from the viscera may be as high as 1 l per hour. There is also an increased fluid requirement when a patient is pyrexial and 15% more fluid should be given for each 1 degree C rise in body temperature. The movement of water into the third 'space' in the form of pleural fluid, ascites or intestinal secretions is not usually a problem; however, the reaccumulation of pleural effusions and ascites drained at the time of surgery may result in the depletion of intravascular fluid. Without adequate replacement, hypotension and reduced urine output may occur.

While young, fit patients will tolerate minor changes in fluid and electrolyte balance without difficulty, elderly patients require careful monitoring of fluid and electrolyte

Table 9.1 Circumstances in which additional fluid supplementation will be needed

High fluid loss through a drain
A long abdominal operation, 1 l lost per hour
Pyrexia; 15% extra per 1 degree C rise in body temperature
Loss into the 'third space', e.g. ascites or pleural effusion

balance. The rate of fluid replacement in the elderly should be reduced because of a 10% fall in total body water by the age of 60. The release of antidiuretic hormone after surgery leads to fluid retention which further reduces fluid requirements in elderly women. Fluid overload will result in the development of peripheral and pulmonary oedema with cardiac failure if not recognized.

Postoperative analgesia

The management of postoperative pain is often a neglected area of care. This was highlighted by a joint commission of the Royal College of Surgeons in England and the College of Anaesthetists (1990) which found that postoperative pain was often inadequately recognized, monitored and treated. This situation is changing with the increasing recognition of the benefits of effective analgesia (Table 9.2). The effect of pain in reducing deep breathing impairs oxgenation and compounds the process of atelectasis which starts as a result of general anaesthesia. Patient mobility is reduced and hospitalization may be prolonged. Effective management of postoperative pain will reduce these complications and reduce postoperative morbidity and mortality.

The requirement for analgesia may be reduced by advice and information provided at the consultation. Elsass et al (1987) demonstrated that concise explanations are as effective in reducing anxiety as more detailed descriptions. Provision of postoperative analgesia has focused on the use of regional techniques such as spinal analgesia and patient-controlled analgesia (PCA).

The use of opioids in spinal analgesia gives effective pain relief without the loss of mobility and hypotension associated with local anaesthetic agents. However, the opioids may lead to respiratory depression. This risk is reduced by using more lipid-soluble agents such as fentanyl and giving the drug as a continuous infusion rather than as a repeated bolus injection. A combination of opioids and local anaesthetic agents is effective and appears to potentiate the effect and duration of action of both drugs. The dose of opioid may be reduced, but the risk of hypotension remains a potential problem. The routine use of this technique should be confined to wards where the nursing staff are trained in monitoring the side-effects of these agents and supported by an 'on call' pain relief service.

Patient-controlled analgesia (PCA) systems allow the patient to control the rate and level of analgesia. The patient is instructed on how to use the 'trigger' to release a bolus of drug but, by pre-setting the minimum delay between boluses, overdosage is prevented. The patient must be totally pain-free before they take over control of their own analgesia if this method is to be effective. A constant background infusion may be used but this does not proportionately reduce the number of boluses required, and it increases the risk of respiratory depression. The major side-effects are nausea and vomiting. This problem may be reduced by regular antiemetic injections or inclusion of the antiemetic in the infusion. Because the maximum delivery rate of the opioids is limited, the risk of respiratory depression is reduced and so this technique may be used on wards with less intensive nursing levels.

Non-steroidal analgesics are useful once the acute pain has started to subside. Long-acting agents or preparations such as diclofenac and ketoprofen, given as a suppository, provide effective analgesia and are less traumatic than repeated intramuscular injection. Breakthrough pain can be controlled with agents such as co-proxamol. The use of these agents after minor gynaecological procedures reduces the need for intramuscular injections of opioids. These drugs, however, should not be used in women with a history of asthma or upper gastrointestinal haemorrhage or ulceration.

Table 9.2 Effects of inadequate analgesia

Impaired oxygenation
Reduced deep breathing
Increased risk of atelectasis
Longer hospitalization

The management of urinary catheters

Most obstetricians and gynaecologists will electively catheterize patients before abdominal surgery (Hilton 1988). This is done to reduce the risk of bladder damage at the time of surgery and for patient comfort in the acute recovery phase.

After suprapubic surgery for incontinence or radical surgery involving significant dissection of the bladder base, suprapubic catheterization has several advantages over the urethral route. As well as reducing discomfort this allows a more accurate assessment of the ability to void and reduces the time interval before resumption of spontaneous voiding (Bonanno et al 1970). In women who have poorly compliant bladders, such as after radical surgery, it is important to ensure that postvoiding residuals are low, to prevent the development of bladder atony. A suprapubic catheter is of value in this situation in that the woman may be discharged home with the catheter in situ and asked to continue to measure residuals until they are satisfactory.

Intermittent self-catheterization, taught to the woman before discharge from hospital, is an alternative technique which appears to be less favoured by gynaecologists.

The routine use of prophylactic antibiotics to prevent urinary tract infection in women with short-term bladder catheters is not justified.

The management of surgical drains

When to use a drain and what sort of drain to use are

questions that perplex many gynaecologists. Drains are used either therapeutically, to remove pus, infected material and products from an abscess, or they may be used to prevent an accumulation of blood, pus, urine, lymph, bile or intestinal secretions. There is little evidence to support the use of prophylactic drains. Drained incisions are more likely to become infected (Cruise & Foord 1973), and pelvic drains do not seem to reduce infection following radical pelvic surgery (Orr et al 1987).

Drains may either be passive or active. Active drains are closed suction drains which are linked to either a high (300–500 mmHg) or low (100–150 mmHg) vacuum system. Active drains should be used to remove fluid from a potential space created following surgery, such as the pelvic side wall or inguinal region after lymphadenectomy. However, the high vacuum will encourage soft tissues to enter the fenestrations in the tube and create blockages. These types of drains are therefore best avoided in the peritoneal cavity and where a passive drain is preferred. The drain may be removed if less than 100 ml per day is being collected. Drains should be avoided when ascites is present since it may be difficult to decide when to remove the drain and a sinus may develop. After long-term use, the drain is withdrawn 2–3 cm each day until completely removed. This allows the drainage tract to heal from below to prevent the formation of a persistent tract.

POSTOPERATIVE COMPLICATIONS

Infection

Postoperative pyrexia is common after gynaecological surgery but the incidence can be reduced from 20 to 10% with the routine use of prophylactic antibiotics (Mittendorf et al 1993). Many patients with fever in the first 48 h do not have an identifiable infection and the temperature settles without active treatment (Table 9.3).

Pyrexia within the first 48–72 h is usually caused by pulmonary atelectasis developing during general anaesthesia. The risk of atelectasis is increased by age, obesity, a history of smoking, poor postoperative analgesia and upper abdominal surgery. Patients may be asymptomatic but crepitations and reduced air entry will be found. This condition is best treated with physiotherapy, incentive spirometry and adequate analgesia. Antibiotic therapy may be required if atelectasis persists.

Table 9.3 Common causes of postoperative pyrexia

Early pyrexia, < 36 h	Late pyrexia, > 36 h
Unexplained fever	Any of the early causes
Atelectasis	Urinary tract infection
Peritoneal soiling	Pneumonia
Occult bowel injury	Haematoma
Anastomotic leak	Pelvic
Urinoma	Wound
Occult ureteric or bladder injury	Deep venous thrombosis
Ureteric obstruction	Septic thrombophlebitis
Wound infection	
Streptococcal	
Clostridial	

After 72 h the most likely cause of a pyrexia is a urinary tract infection, especially if the patient has been catheterized. Many patients are asymptomatic so urine should be sent for microscopy and culture in any suspected cases. Antibiotic therapy may be started empirically if the patient is unwell. The routine use of prophylactic antibiotics at the time of surgery does not reduce the incidence of urinary tract infection but may alter the pattern of bacterial isolates (Brown et al 1988).

Wound infections present on about the 5th postoperative day and are usually preceded by induration and erythema around the incision. Sutures should be removed and the wound opened in the infected area if there are signs of a collection. The wound should be probed to break down any loculations of pus and necrotic material should be removed. A moist pack soaked in honey helps to clean the wound and reduce the oedema. The defect should be allowed to heal by secondary intention. Antibiotic therapy is only indicated if there is significant cellulitis, systemic signs of bacteraemia or evidence of necrotizing infection. A swab should be taken before starting antibiotic treatment. Flucloxacillin or erythromycin are suitable antibiotics while sensitivities are awaited.

Necrotizing fasciitis is a rare, rapidly progressive and often fatal infection of the superficial fascia and subcutaneous tissues (Addison et al 1984). Diabetic patients are especially vulnerable but any chronic illness may predispose to this condition. It is seen most commonly on the vulva or perineum, and it is often not related to surgery but it can be seen in the region of a recent surgical wound. There is extensive tissue necrosis and a moderate or severe systemic toxic reaction. Very radical excision is essential with antibiotics and supportive therapy.

Haematomas

Large pelvic or subrectus sheath haematomas may be the cause of a low grade undulating pyrexia. Transvaginal ultrasound will reveal a pelvic fluid collection after hysterectomy in about one-third of cases and two-thirds of the latter will develop postoperative pyrexia (Toglia & Pearlman 1994). Patients may feel generally unwell in addition to having local symptoms and signs.

Subcutaneous haematomas are usually self-limiting and will discharge through the incision often with symptomatic improvement. Pelvic and subrectus sheath haematomas may need drainage if they fail to resolve spontaneously and continue to cause systemic symptoms. Pelvic haematomas may be drained transvaginally under ultrasound guidance or by culdotomy if ultrasound is not available. If the haematoma becomes infected, intravenous antibiotics may help in controlling symptoms but will not affect the resolution of the haematoma.

Wound dehiscence and incisional hernias

This complication may range from a small defect in the skin to a burst abdomen. A small dehiscence does not require active management and will heal by secondary intention. Provided any infection has been adequately treated and the edges can be brought together easily, without tension, larger skin defects can be closed using sutures or skin tapes under local or general anaesthesia. Any necrotic tissue should be debrided before this is undertaken. If the wound is not clean or cannot be closed easily, it is better to pack it with gauze soaked in honey and allow it to heal by secondary intention. It is surprising how rapidly this can occur.

Complete wound dehiscence is a rare event. It is very exceptional after a Pfannensteil incision and can be largely prevented in vertical incisions by mass closure (Bucknall et al 1982). There may be problems with the surgical technique or the use of incorrect suture material, but factors such as wound infection, abdominal distension and postoperative coughing are also contributory. Dehiscence is more common in patients who are infected, malnourished or have an underlying malignancy. The first line of management is replacement of the bowel and resuturing of the wound. The high mortality (15–24%) associated with this condition is largely due to the coexisting medical problems.

Incisional herniation occurs in 7–8% of patients with midline incisions, and the incidence after lower transverse incisions is believed to be much lower (Bucknall et al 1982). Several studies have reported a high incidence (16–22%) of incisional hernias following gynaecological surgery (Devlin & Nicholson 1994). Many hernias do not present until 1 year after surgery. Primary closure of the defect may be feasible, but the use of synthetic prolene grafts will aid repair of larger hernias. It is advisable that the repair should be undertaken by a surgeon experienced in the technique.

Paralytic ileus

After manipulation of the bowel during surgery, normal peristaltic activity of the small bowel will return within 16 h. Its failure to recommence will result in the development of a paralytic ileus. The patient will complain of nausea, abdominal distension and a failure to pass flatus. Vomiting will occur as fluid collects in the stomach and upper gut. On examination, the abdomen will be distended and bowel sounds will be absent or 'tinkling' due to the movement of intestinal contents between loops of dilated bowel.

Table 9.4 The effect of peritoneal closure on wound infection and adhesion formation (% incidences)

	Closed	Not closed
Wound infection	3.6	2.4
Adhesions	22.2	15.8
Obstruction	1.6	0

After Tulandi et al (1988)

Any abdominal sepsis should be treated and hypokalaemia corrected, as both will contribute to ileus. Intravenous fluids should be given and the bowel decompressed by inserting a nasogastric tube and aspirating gastric contents regularly. Most patients will respond to these conservative measures but some will require surgical intervention to establish if there is any pathological cause.

Bowel obstruction

Bowel obstruction in the immediate postoperative period is rare following gynaecological surgery and usually does not become apparent before the 5th postoperative day. In parenthesis, it is worth noting that closure of the pelvic peritoneum does not reduce the incidence of postoperative adhesions or obstruction (Table 9.4; Tulandi et al 1988).

In the absence of peritonism, the initial treatment should be conservative with nasogastric suction and intravenous fluids. This will usually resolve the problem within 48–72 h. Persistent vomiting or pain or high volumes of nasogastric aspirate and minimal passage of flatus after this length of time will usually mean that surgery will be required. Large amounts of aspirate from a woman who otherwise appears to have improved may be due to the end of the catheter having migrated into the duodenum! If abdominal tenderness increases or if pyrexia or tachycardia develop suggesting peritonitis, immediate surgery is required.

Surgical damage to the bowel

Damage to the bowel is an uncommon event. The incidence is reported to be between 0.3 and 0.8% with the majority (70%) being minor lacerations. The small bowel is the site for injury in approximately 75% of cases. Abdominal surgery, rather than vaginal or laparoscopic surgery, is associated with a higher rate of damage and the majority (72%) follow uncomplicated gynaecological procedures. Risk factors for bowel damage include the presence of abdominal adhesions from malignancy, endometriosis or sepsis (Krebs 1986). Women who have received abdominal or pelvic radiotherapy are also at increased risk of bowel damage at the time of surgery. The incidence of bowel damage after laparoscopy is reported to be under 0.3% (Chamberlain & Brown 1978, Franks et al 1987). The risk of bowel perforation increases 10–20-fold after previous abdominal or pelvic surgery. Obesity or a history of pelvic inflammatory disease may increase the risk twofold (Brill et al 1995, Franks et al 1987).

The presentation, management and outcome of any injury to the bowel are dependent on the site and extent of the injury and the delay between injury and repair. Injuries that are recognized and repaired at the time of damage are associated with good outcomes; high morbidity and occasional mortality occurs in the group presenting late with peritonitis. Patients who have received more than a minor laceration, such as puncture with a Veress needle at the time of laparoscopy, will normally present after 48–72 h with the signs and symptoms of peritonitis: nausea which may proceed to vomiting; anorexia; lower abdominal pain, and fever. On examination they may be dehydrated and have general abdominal tenderness with guarding, and bowel sounds will be decreased or absent. Abdominal X-ray may show signs of gas under the diaphragm or distended loops of small bowel but, in general, plain films are not helpful.

The patient will need rehydration with intravenous fluids and placement of a nasogastric tube if vomiting or an ileus are significant factors. Intravenous antibiotics should be commenced using a combination of a cephalosporin, metronidazole and gentamicin if the patient is particularly unwell. Repair of any significant bowel injury is best performed by a general surgeon with experience in the field. The low incidence of bowel injury means that the general gynaecologist will not have enough experience to undertake such surgery. The method of repair of a small bowel injury will depend on its extent. Small lacerations with no devitalized bowel may be repaired with a simple one- or two-layer closure parallel to the mesentery, using absorbable sutures on the inner layer. Larger lacerations or where the bowel is not viable require resection with either an end-to-end or side-to-side anastomosis. The bowel is closed in two layers with absorbable sutures and the edges of the mesentery approximated.

The techniques used to repair defects in the large bowel will depend on the site of injury. The ascending colon may be repaired as described for small bowel injuries. Injury to the descending and sigmoid colon produces faecal peritonitis, and requires the creation of a temporary defunctioning colostomy to reduce the risk of leakage from the repair. The operation performed will depend on the site of damage and the extent of abdominal contamination. When the transverse colon or upper part of the descending colon are damaged, a loop colostomy may be performed proximal to the repair. Damage to the lower portion of the descending colon and rectum above the peritoneal reflection may be repaired by Hartman's procedure. If the injury is below the reflection, reanastomosis by a two-layer closure or stapler is appropriate. The temporary colostomy may be reversed after 4–6 weeks, but if irradiated bowel is involved the closure should be delayed and the adequacy of the anastomosis confirmed radiologically.

Postoperative enterocutaneous fistulae usually result from damage to the bowel which may or may not have been recognized. They are more common in women with malignant disease or prior radiotherapy. Many are associated with intra-abdominal sepsis and antibiotic therapy may be required. Conservative therapy with measures to protect the skin, nasogastric suction, and total parenteral nutrition is most likely to be successful in women with no previous risk factors and a low output fistula. Surgery will have to be considered if no improvement is obvious after 4 weeks, but in women with malignancies, further surgery may not be appropriate.

Surgical damage to the urinary tract

The incidence of ureteric injury in gynaecological surgery is between 0.5 and 2.5%. Damage which is recognized at the time of surgery and repaired correctly will have low morbidity. Damage to the urinary tract occurs at three sites. The most common injury is to the bladder, particularly if there has been previous surgery. The other sites of injury are the ureter at the angle of the vagina and near the pelvic brim close to the ovarian blood supply. Conditions such as endometriosis and ovarian cancer are associated with distortion of the normal course of the ureter, which increases the likelihood of damage. A higher incidence of injury and fistula formation is associated with surgery following pelvic radiotherapy because the dissection is more difficult and irradiated tissue does not heal well. Preoperative intravenous urography (IVU) is very unlikely to reduce the risk of ureteric injury.

Damage to the urinary tract may become apparent within a few days of surgery or may not present for several weeks. Sometimes, postoperative ureteric obstruction is only discovered many years later as an incidental finding. A vesicovaginal fistula developing in the first postoperative week is more likely to be due to trauma to the bladder at surgery. The aetiology of fistulae presenting later is shrouded in uncertainty but often they may be the end result of a pelvic haematoma.

The signs and symptoms will result from extravasation of urine or ureteric obstruction. Urine may leak from the abdominal or vaginal incision or collect in a pelvic drain. A collection of urine may develop in the pelvis, causing discomfort and pyrexia. Loin pain and pyrexia may occur following ureteric obstruction. Delayed ureteric injury may present with persistent vaginal discharge from a fistula or abdominal wound.

If a fistula is suspected in the immediate postoperative phase, the patient should be catheterized to assess urine output. This will often reduce the amount of urine leaking through a bladder fistula. Fluid from any abdominal drain may be analysed for urea or creatinine content. It is often difficult to see a small fistula in the vagina and the 'three swab test' is helpful in confirming the presence of such a fistula. Three swabs are placed in the vagina and the patient is given a preparation which colours the urine. Pyridium (phenazopyridine) 100 mg orally was often used as it gives a strong orange colour to the urine. However, it is now difficult to obtain and intravenous indigo carmine may be used instead. When the urine in the bladder is strongly coloured, the swabs are removed. The lower swab is often coloured by urine from the urethra, but staining of the upper two swabs indicates a fistula. The same strategy can be used to confirm the nature of fluid leaking from abdominal wounds or drains. Alternatively, dilute methylene blue can be instilled into the bladder. However, this will not help to identify a ureteric fistula.

Imaging of the renal tract by intravenous urography will help in locating the site of damage but small fistulae may be difficult to see. Percutaneous nephrostomy should be performed when there is evidence of hydronephrosis. This relieves the obstruction and allows antegrade pyleo-ureterography to locate the site of injury. Cystoscopy and retrograde insertion ureteric stents is an alternative but often less satisfactory approach.

Repair of the damaged bladder is dependent upon the extent of urinary leakage. Women who are voiding spontaneously and troubled only by a small volume leak may be managed satisfactorily by catheterization for 7–10 days. If this fails or if the leakage is more significant, surgical repair of the defect will be required. The fistula must be fully mobilized and the edges debrided (see Ch. 8 for details). The repair should be performed using absorbable sutures in one or two layers. An omental flap should be placed between the suture lines in the bladder and the vault of the vagina to improve the blood supply and to prevent apposition of the suture lines. The patient should remain catheterized for 7–10 days. Repair of the ureter should only be undertaken by a urologist with expertise in the area. Injury near the brim of the pelvis is managed by end-to-end anastomosis or, more commonly, by end-to-side anastomosis to the opposite ureter. Damage near to the bladder is better repaired with ureteric reimplantation into the bladder, using either a psoas hitch or bladder flap to relieve tension on the repair.

Postoperative bleeding

Monitoring

The normal clinical monitoring of postoperative patients with pulse and blood pressure recordings is adequate for most gynaecological patients. In high risk cases, the hourly urine output is a sensitive measure of peripheral circulation. However, a fall in urine volume may occur because of relative dehydration and an increased volume will result in the diuretic phase of recovery from renal failure. Measurement of the difference between the core temperature, measured rectally, and the peripheral temperature, measured on the toe, is a very sensitive indication of peripheral perfusion and, by inference, blood volume and cardiac output. It is widely used in intensive care units, and deserves more frequent use in monitoring high risk patients. Oximetry, measuring the oxygenated haemoglobin content in peripheral vessels is also dependent in part on peripheral perfusion.

The central venous pressure is a less useful indicator than the above, it is invasive, requires constant supervision and is much more prone to measurement errors. However, it is particularly valuable in warning of fluid overload during resuscitation. This is more important in older women or patients with cardiac or renal disease, whose ability to cope with excess fluid is limited.

When massive blood loss occurs, a consumptive coagulopathy may develop as all the coagulation factors are exhausted. It is therefore important to monitor the coagulation status of the patient repeatedly during resuscitation, and if an abnormality develops expert advice from a haematologist should be sought (Fig. 9.1).

Volume replacement

There is much debate over the value of colloid preparations compared with crystalloids when a patient requires volume replacement because of haemorrhage. In the immediate management, crystalloids will maintain the cardiac output and renal function as effectively as colloids although twice the volume is required. Crystalloids are more effective than colloids in replacing the deficit in the extracellular fluid compartment. The mobilization of this extra fluid during the recovery phase leads to a diuresis which may protect against renal failure (Shires et al 1983, Virgilio et al 1979). However, if more than 1000 ml of fluid are required, synthetic colloid replacement fluids such as haemacell are generally recommended until blood becomes available. It is wise not to use more than 1000–1500 ml of haemacell in 24 h. It may cause clotting in giving sets if mixed with citrated blood or fresh frozen plasma (FFP). A 4.5% human albumin solution (HAS) is very expensive. Its role in replacing blood loss is described in Figure 9.1. FFP contains all the protein constituents of plasma, including the coagulation factors. It is used to replace coagulation factors, and should not be used for plasma expansion. Cryoprecipitate contains a high concentration of fibrinogen. This may be required in massive blood transfusion (Fig. 9.1).

Red blood cell products are required to correct the loss of oxygen-carrying capacity. Whole blood is seldom available now because transfusion centres remove the plasma and other components to prepare products required for other purposes. Supplemented red cell concentrate (SAG-M) is generally supplied in the UK. All the plasma has been removed from these cells and replaced by a supplement of adenine, glucose and mannitol. This product

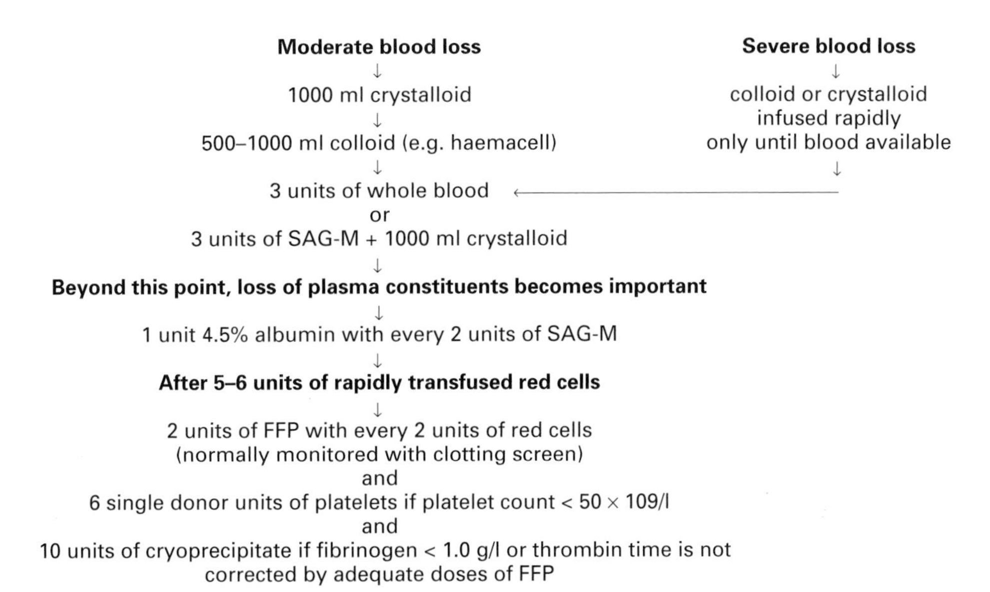
Moderate blood loss
1000 ml crystalloid
500–1000 ml colloid (e.g. haemacell)
3 units of whole blood
or
3 units of SAG-M + 1000 ml crystalloid
Severe blood loss
colloid or crystalloid
infused rapidly
only until blood available
Beyond this point, loss of plasma constituents becomes important
1 unit 4.5% albumin with every 2 units of SAG-M
After 5–6 units of rapidly transfused red cells
2 units of FFP with every 2 units of red cells
(normally monitored with clotting screen)
and
6 single donor units of platelets if platelet count < 50 × 109/l
and
10 units of cryoprecipitate if fibrinogen < 1.0 g/l or thrombin time is not
corrected by adequate doses of FFP
The blood transfusion registrar can give advice on the products required and can facilitate their
rapid delivery.

Fig. 9.1 Correction of acute blood loss: suggested procedure. The first priority is to replace the volume lost. This may be done initially with crystalloid. It should be noted that oxygen delivery is not impaired at haematocrit values down to 22% (Hb 7 g/dl), even in patients with multisystem disease. (Modified from Guidelines on the Use of Blood and Blood Products, Hammersmith Hospital Blood Audit Committee, 1992; SAG-M, supplemented red cell concentrate; FFP, fresh frozen plasma.)

flows just as well as whole blood. If more than three units of SAG-M are given to patients with a previously normal serum albumin, the plasma deficit should be made up with 4.5% albumin (Fig. 9.1).

Re-exploration

Deciding when to re-explore a patient who is bleeding postoperatively can be one of the most difficult decisions a gynaecologist has to face. The advice and help of the most experienced person available should be sought. If at all possible, the patient should be stabilized by transfusion first. The sooner after surgery the bleeding presents, the more likely it is that re-exploration will identify a single obvious bleeding vessel. If the patient presents with an obvious haematoma more than 24 h after surgery, it can be very difficult to identify a single bleeding vessel. More often a generalized ooze is encountered and adequate haemostasis is difficult to achieve. In this situation, it may be better to continue the transfusion and correct any coagulation defect rather than to re-explore. Angiographic embolization is probably the management of choice if it is available (see below, and Ch. 6).

It is important to avoid hypothermia in any patient who requires further surgery because this will tend to worsen any coagulation abnormalities. If the patient is bleeding vaginally after a hysterectomy, it is often worth examining her vaginally under anaesthesia in the hope of identifying a bleeding point that can be sutured from below. The vaginal branch of the uterine artery is often the culprit. If relaparotomy is required, the clot must be removed gently to avoid provoking more bleeding and the operation site explored carefully. Do not close up without examining all the pedicles even after a bleeding vessel has been identified – there are often multiple bleeding sites! Intra-abdominal bleeding frequently originates from the ovarian vessels. These must be clearly identified and separated from the ureter, which lies very close at this point. Bleeding in the pelvis is often difficult to localize and may be venous rather than arterial. It is often necessary to extend the dissection substantially in order to visualize the source of the problem. Sutures can be placed medial to the uterine pedicles without fear of ureteric damage but, if in doubt after careful palpation, dissect out the ureter so that it can be seen or ask for help.

Ligation of the internal iliac artery is often advocated when bleeding cannot be controlled by other means. The effect of this is often disappointing. The technique is simple if the surgeon has experience of the method but there is the potential for damaging the underlying vein and compounding the problem. If in doubt, do not do it! Large, hot packs pressed firmly into the pelvis for a full 5 min will often be effective, or will at least reduce the general ooze so that the main bleeding sites can be seen. If it proves impossible to achieve satisfactory haemostasis, the omentum may be brought into the pelvis and several large packs placed firmly over it. The abdomen is then closed loosely over the packs with the tapes gathered together and brought through the wound. These may be removed under general anaesthesia 24–48 h later.

Angiographic embolization of bleeding vessels in the pelvis

Embolization of actively bleeding blood vessels using interventional radiological techniques is a highly effective alternative to surgery in the management of surgical haemorrhage in the pelvis. It requires a skilled team of intervention radiologists who are able to provide an emergency service. Percutaneous angiography is performed via the femoral artery to identify the source of the bleeding and then the offending arteries are selectively embolized using materials such as gelatin sponge or metal coils, or adhesive agents like iso-butyl-2-cyanocrylate (Allison et al 1992, see Ch. 6). This avoids what is often very difficult surgery in very sick patients. It is often the more reliable and faster method of controlling the bleeding.

Deep vein thrombosis

The development of a deep vein thrombosis (DVT) is a common postoperative event with 30% of patients developing a DVT after moderate and major surgical procedures. The most common site for the thrombosis is the calf (Kakkar et al 1969). The level of risk is dependent on various factors, some patient-, some disease- and some procedure-related. The summation of these factors allows each patient to be assigned a risk level for developing a DVT (Thromboembolic Risk Factors (THRIFT) Consensus Group 1992). Although less well studied than general surgery, there is no evidence to suggest that the incidence of DVT is lower after gynaecological surgery. It is therefore prudent to offer appropriate prophylaxis against thromboembolic disease to all gynaecology patients undergoing surgery. (See Ch. 7 on Preoperative care).

Unfortunately the majority of patients with acute deep venous thrombosis are asymptomatic and in patients with fatal pulmonary embolism the preceding DVT goes unrecognized (Karwinski & Svendsen 1989). It is the extension of the clot into the proximal veins that causes the majority of significant pulmonary embolisms and most of the fatal ones. The symptoms associated with DVT are pain, swelling and erythema of the affected calf. On examination, there may be a low grade pyrexia, the leg may be warmer and larger in circumference, the peripheral veins distal to the occlusion may be dilated and the calf may be tender to palpation over the site of the thrombosis. Eliciting Homan's sign, pain on forced dorsiflexion of the foot, should be avoided as it may inadvertently lead to embolization of clot. In symptomatic patients the investigation of choice is compression ultrasonography. The vein is visualized using B mode ultrasound and the vein compressed with the transducer. If the vein fails to collapse an intraluminal clot is present even if it cannot be visualized. Venography is occasionally necessary, but it is associated with the risk of embolism.

Once the diagnosis has been made the patient must receive anticoagulation therapy to prevent pulmonary embolism and to restore venous patency. Heparin is equally effective intravenously (28 000–40 000 units/24 h by continuous infusion) or subcutaneously (15 000–17 500 units, 12-hourly) (Drug and Therapeutics Bulletin 1992). It should be administered with the goal of achieving full anticoagulation within 24 h, and the treatment should be continued at a level to maintain the activated partial thromboplastin time (APTT) at 1.5–2.5 times the control. Low molecular weight heparin given subcutaneously once daily is as effective as standard heparin regimens in preventing further thromboembolic events without increasing the risk of major bleeding (Hull et al 1992). Although more expensive it may well be cost-effective because it can be given as an outpatient procedure without monitoring coagulation, and there are savings in labour and disposables.

Conversion to oral anticoagulation therapy with warfarin should commence after 5 days of heparin therapy and the heparin discontinued once oral anticoagulation is within the therapeutic range. The dosage of warfarin should be adjusted to maintain the international normalized ratio (INR) at between 2.0 and 3.0 (Hyers et al 1993). The duration of warfarin therapy has been the subject of a randomized trial, comparing 4 weeks against 3 months of treatment, and 4 weeks anticoagulation appears adequate for postoperative DVT (Research Committee of the British Thoracic Society 1992). Although this treatment is very effective it should be remembered that the risk of pulmonary embolism or further DVT is not zero.

Pulmonary embolism

The true incidence of pulmonary embolism after surgery is unknown. In patients not receiving prophylactic treatment the incidence of recognized pulmonary embolism is about 4% with about 25–50% of these being fatal (Kakkar et al 1969). Despite previous calls for routine prophylaxis against thromboembolic disease, pulmonary embolism accounted for 20% of fatalities after hysterectomy in 1991/2 (Report of the National Confidential Enquiry into Perioperative Deaths, 1993). The low usage of perfusion/ventilation scanning and postmortems suggests that this figure is probably an underestimation.

Minor pulmonary embolism is associated with a history of pleuritic chest pain, haemoptysis, a pleural rub and fine crepitations at the base of the lungs. At least 50% of the pulmonary tree must be involved to cause any haemodynamic disturbance. In this situation the patient may complain of central chest pain, dyspnoea or have collapsed. The ECG may show signs of right-sided strain with an S wave in lead 1, a Q wave in lead 3 and T-wave inversion in lead 3 (S_1,Q_3,T_3). The chest X-ray after a massive pulmonary embolism may show areas of reduced vascular shadowing due to oligaemia, enlarged pulmonary arteries and abrupt ending of pulmonary arteries. Arterial blood gas analysis may show a reduced oxygen tension in the presence of a normal carbon dioxide tension. A ventilation/perfusion scan is probably the investigation of choice, an area of hypoperfusion in the presence of normal ventilation confirming the diagnosis. In an emergency, a perfusion scan alone with a chest X-ray will also aid diagnosis. Pulmonary angiography may be required in cases of uncertainty, but requires a degree of expertise not always available.

Resuscitation of a patient with a massive pulmonary embolism should ensure that venous return to the heart is maintained to help with right ventricular function. Having stabilized the patient, thrombolysis of the clot may be performed although this is contraindicated within 5 days of surgery. Pulmonary embolectomy with cardiac bypass may be life-saving but is associated with a high mortality.

Cardiovascular complications

Cardiovascular disease is a common coexisting medical condition in women undergoing gynaecological surgery. Any patient receiving a general anaesthetic is at increased risk of myocardial ischaemia but this is greatly increased when there is pre-existing cardiac disease. Eliciting a good preoperative history of cardiac disease is generally more predictive than screening tests such as ECG stress testing, which are associated with a high false-positive rate. Elective surgery should be delayed in patients with a history of myocardial infarction within the preceding 6 months.

Patients with chest pain postoperatively should be investigated with serial cardiac enzymes and ECG. If patients have received postoperative analgesia, pain may not be a profound symptom. In a patient with tachycardia and hypotension, myocardial infarction must come into the differential diagnosis once haemorrhage has been excluded. Women with pulmonary oedema or a new heart murmur should also be investigated for evidence of myocardial infarction. The association of acute pulmonary oedema and myocardial infarction implies a poor prognosis. Referral to a cardiologist is warranted but thrombolytic therapy is contraindicated within 5 days of surgery.

SUMMARY

In general, gynaecological surgery is associated with low morbidity and mortality rates. Preoperative assessment of patients for risk factors linked to postoperative complications will allow for care plans to be instigated to prevent or reduce these complications. With measures to ensure good postoperative analgesia, appropriate surgical technique and infection control and with the use of prophylactic measures against thromboembolic disease and infection, postoperative morbidity and mortality can be reduced. Good postoperative care benefits not only the patient but also the surgeon and the hospital.

KEY POINTS

1. All patients should be assessed for risk factors associated with postoperative complications.
2. Effective postoperative analgesia should be the norm and will reduce the incidence of atelectasis and allow early mobilization.
3. Atelectasis and urinary tract infection are the commonest causes of postoperative pyrexia.
4. Pelvic haematomas are common after hysterectomy.
5. Angiographic embolization is a rapid, effective and safe way of arresting postoperative pelvic haemorrhage.
6. There is a significant risk of DVT after moderate or major gynaecological procedures.
7. The majority of DVTs which precede pulmonary embolism are not recognized clinically.
8. Elective surgery should be delayed for 6 months after a myocardial infarction.
9. Early recognition of bowel and urinary tract damage reduces the risk of serious morbidity.
10. Damage to bowel and urinary tract should be repaired only by experienced practitioners.
11. Local audit will identify areas of concern in surgical technique and infection control.

REFERENCES

Addison W A, Livengood C H, Hill G B, Sutton G P, Fortier K J 1984 Necrotizing fasciitis of vulvar origin in diabetic patients. Obstetrics and Gynecology 63: 473–479

Allison D, Wallace S, Machan L S 1992 Interventional radiology. In: Grainger R G, Allison D J (eds) Diagnostic radiology, 2nd edn. Churchill Livingstone, Edinburgh, pp 2329–2390

Bonanno P J, Landers D E, Rock D E 1970 Bladder drainage with the suprapubic needle. Obstetrics and Gynecology 35: 807–813

Brill A I, Nezhat F, Nezhat C H, Nezhat C 1995 The incidence of adhesions after prior laparotomy, a laparoscopic appraisal. Obstetrics and Gynecology 85: 269–272

Brown E M, Depares J, Robertson A A et al 1988 Amoxycillin – clavulanic acid (Augmentin) versus metronidazole as prophylaxis in hysterectomy: a prospective, randomised clinical trial. British Journal of Obstetrics and Gynaecology 95: 286–293

Bucknall T E, Cox P J, Ellis H 1982 Burst abdomen and incisional hernia: a prospective study of 1129 major laparotomies. British Medical Journal 284: 931–933

Chamberlain G, Brown J C (eds) 1978 Gynaecological laparoscopy: report on the confidential enquiry into gynaecological laparoscopy. Royal College of Obstetricians and Gynaecologists, London

Cruise P J E, Foord R 1973 A 5-year prospective study of 23,649 surgical wounds. Archives of Surgery 107: 206

Devlin H B, Nicholson S 1994 Hernias of the abdominal wall and pelvis, incisional hernias and parastomal hernias. In: Keen G, Farndon J (eds) Operative surgery and management. Butterworth Heinemann, Oxford, pp 41–54

Drug and Therapeutics Bulletin 1992 How to anticoagulate. 30: 77–80

Elsass P, Eikad B, Junge J et al 1987 Pyschological effect of detailed pre-anesthetic information. Acta Anaesthesiologica Scandinavica 31: 579–583

Franks A L, Kendrick J S, Peterson H B 1987 Unintended laparotomy associated with laparoscopic tubal sterilisation. American Journal of Obstetrics and Gynecology 157: 1102–1105

Hilton P 1988 Bladder drainage: a survey of practices among gynaecologists in the British Isles. British Journal of Obstetrics and Gynaecology 95: 1178–1189

Hull R D, Raskob G E, Pineo G F et al 1992 Subcutaneous low-molecular-weight heparin compared with continuous intravenous heparin in the treatment of proximal vein thrombosis. New England Journal of Medicine 326: 975–982

Hyers T M, Hull R D, Weg J G 1993 Antithrombotic therapy for venous thromboembolic disease. Chest 102 (suppl): 408S–425S

Kakkar V V, Howe C T, Flanc C, Clarke M B 1969 Natural history of postoperative deep-vein thrombosis. Lancet 2: 230–232

Karwinski B, Svendsen E 1989 Comparisons of clinical and post mortem diagnosis of pulmonary embolism. Journal of Clinical Pathology 42: 135–139

Krebs H B 1986 Intestinal injury in gynecologic surgery: a ten-year experience. American Journal of Obstetrics and Gynecology 155: 509–514

Mittendorf R, Aronson M P, Berry RE et al 1993 Avoiding serious infections associated with abdominal hysterectomy: a meta-analysis of antibiotic prophylaxis. American Journal of Obstetrics and Gynecology 169: 1119–1124

Orr J W Jr, Garter J F, Kilgore L C et al 1987 Closed suction pelvic drainage following radical pelvic surgery. American Journal of Obstetrics and Gynecology 155: 867

Report of the National Confidential Enquiry into Perioperative Deaths 1991/2 (1993) National Confidential Enquiry into Perioperative Deaths, London

Research Committee of the British Thoracic Society 1992 Optimum duration of anticoagulation for deep vein thrombosis and pulmonary embolism. Lancet 340: 873–876

Royal College of Surgeons in England 1990 Pain after surgery. Report of the Working Party of the Commission on the Provision of Surgical Services of the Royal College of Surgeons in England and the College of Anaesthetists, London

Shires G T III, Pettzman A B, Albert S A et al 1983 Response of extravascular lung water to intraoperative fluids. Annals of Surgery 197: 515–518

Thromboembolic Risk Factors (THRIFT) Consensus Group 1992 Risk of and prophylaxis for venous thromboembolism in hospital patients. British Medical Journal 305: 567–574

Toglia M R, Pearlman M D 1994 Pelvic fluid collections following hysterectomy and their relation to febrile morbidity. Obstetrics and Gynecology 83: 766–770

Tulandi T, Hum H S, Gelfand M M 1988 Closure of laparotomy incisions with or without peritoneal suturing and second look laparoscopy. American Journal of Obstetrics and Gynecology 158: 536

Virgilio R W, Rice C L, Smith D E et al 1979 Crystalloid vs. colloid resuscitation: is one better? Surgery 85: 129–139

SECTION 2

Reproductive medicine

10

Hormones: their action and measurement in gynaecological practice

J. G. Grudzinskas

INTRODUCTION

Hormones are one of the important means by which cells communicate with each other. They ensure that the body's physiological systems are coordinated appropriately. Impaired communication leads to abnormal function. Classically, hormones are secreted by a gland and transported through the circulation to a distant site of action. However, as cellular communication also occurs at a local level, it is evident that several factors can combine to modulate and coordinate function. The types of communication to be considered are endocrine, paracrine and autocrine.

1. *Endocrine.* Intergland or structure communication involves secretion from a gland into the circulatory system (blood or lymph) of a regulatory substance that has a specific effect on another gland or structure, e.g. pituitary secretion of follicle-stimulating hormone (FSH) stimulating ovarian activity (Fig. 10.1).
2. *Paracrine.* Intercellular communication involves the local diffusion of regulating substances from a cell to contiguous cells, e.g. insulin-like growth factor (IGF-1) secretion by granulosa cells in the ovary (Fig. 10.1).
3. *Autocrine.* Intracellular communication involves the production of regulating substances by a single cell which binds to receptors on or within the same cell, e.g. oestradiol, modulating granulosa cell action (Fig. 10.1).

Hormones comprise two chemical groups – steroid hormones and trophic hormones. Steroid hormones include oestrogens, progestogens and androgens. Trophic hormones include the releasing hormones originating in the

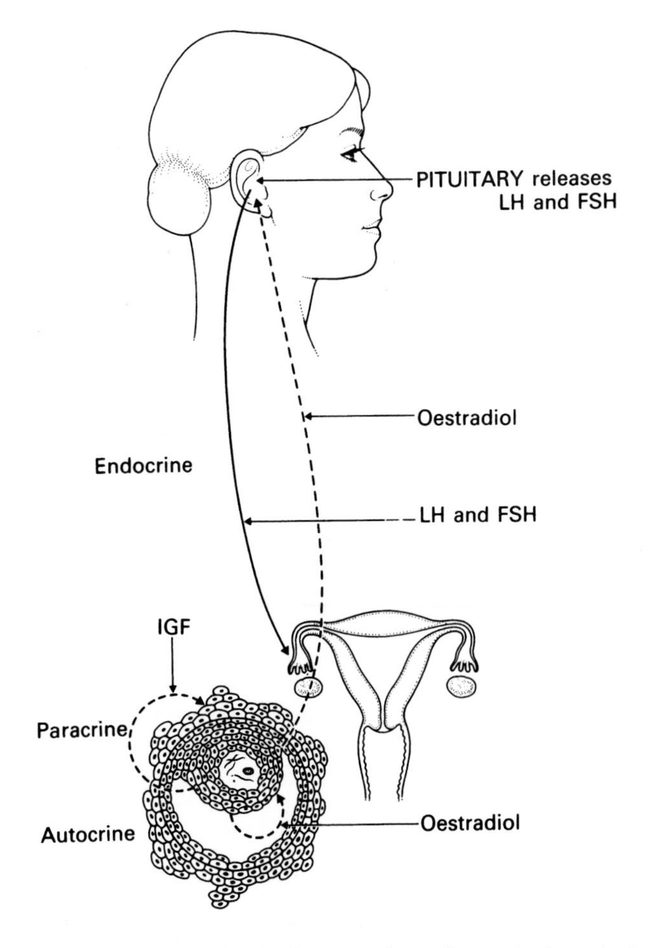

Fig. 10.1 Examples of endocrine, paracrine and autocrine hormonal communication. LH, luteinizing hormone: FSH, follicle-stimulating hormone; IGF, insulin-like growth factor.

hypothalamus, and a variety of hormones released by the pituitary gland and trophoblast. The composition of these substances is summarized here.

Steroids

Steroids are a group of lipids composed of four linked carbon rings (hydrogenated cyclopentophenanthrene ring system). Steroid hormones, which are derived from cholesterol, can be classified according to the number of carbon atoms they possess: C-21 (progestogens, cortisol, aldosterone), C-19 (androgens) and C-18 (oestrogens).

Peptides

Peptides are compounds which yield two or more amino acids on hydrolysis. Linked together they form polypeptide hormones, e.g. gonadotrophin-releasing hormone (GnRH).

Glycoproteins

Glycoproteins consist of a protein (combination of amino acids in peptide linkages) to which carbohydrate groups (CHO-) are bound, e.g. luteinizing hormone (LH).

Hormones often circulate in extremely low concentrations and, in order to respond in a specific manner, target cells require specific receptors which recognize and bind the hormone and thereby alter cell function. Hormones act at the cellular level in two ways. Steroid hormones enter the cell and mediate action via receptors within the nucleus (King 1988). By contrast trophic hormones bind to receptors on the cell membrane which then activate 'second messenger' systems within the cell (Segaloff & Ascoli 1988). It is the affinity, specificity and concentration of receptors for a particular hormone which allow a small amount of hormone to produce a biological response.

MECHANISM OF ACTION OF STEROID HORMONES

The specificity of the tissue reaction to steroid hormones is due to the presence of specific intracellular receptor proteins for each hormone. The mechanism, illustrated in Figure 10.2, is common to the five main classes of steroid hormone: oestrogens, progestogens, androgens, glucocorticoids and mineralocorticoids (Speroff et al 1989).

Stage 1. Transfer across the cell membrane

Circulating free (unbound) hormone is able to diffuse across cell membranes. However, most steroid hormone is bound with low affinity to albumin, or with high affinity to a specific binding globulin: sex hormone-binding globulin (SHBG) or cortisol-binding globulin (CBG). The concentration of free (unbound) hormone in the blood stream seems to be an important determinant of the rate of diffusion but there may be specific membrane-bound receptors which transport the hormone into the cell.

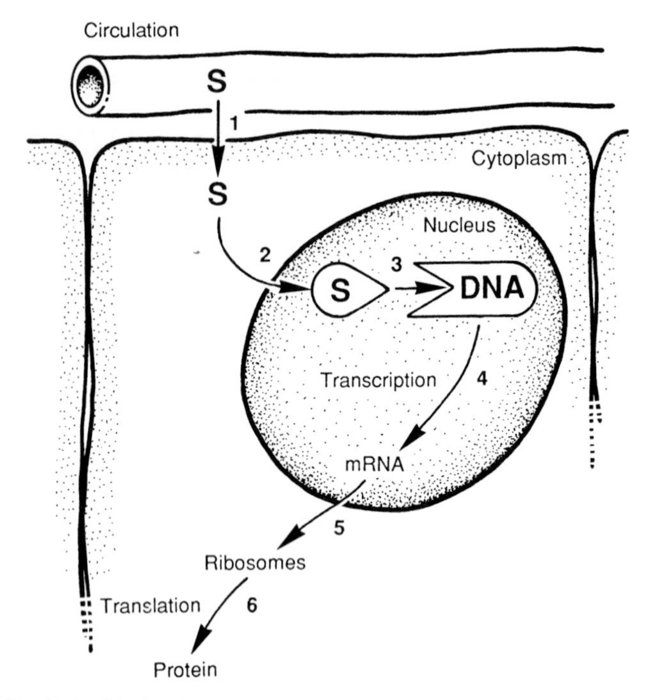

Fig. 10.2 Mechanism of action of steroid hormones. See text for details.

Stages 2 and 3. Transfer into the nucleus and binding to receptor protein

Once in the cell, the hormone dissociates from the binding globulin and is transported across the nuclear membrane. The hormone binds with the receptor causing a conformational change that allows the receptor to bind directly with DNA (activation).

Stages 4 and 5. Synthesis of messenger RNA (mRNA)

Once bound to the nuclear receptor, the hormone–receptor complex then moves down the DNA molecule, binding with a specific gene. The mechanism by which hormone–receptor binding activates a gene is poorly understood but leads to a modification of mRNA synthesis (transcription). The RNA is synthesized and then transported to the ribosome.

Stage 6. Protein synthesis

Transfer of mRNA to the cytoplasmic ribosome results in the synthesis of protein (translation). The proteins produced, e.g. enzymes, have specific intracellular effects, the endpoint of the hormone action. For example, high midcycle levels of oestradiol from the ovary lead to the increase in LH synthesis and secretion by the anterior pituitary that results in ovulation (Yen & Lein 1976).

Regulation of steroid hormone action

Regulation of hormone action is required to enhance or reduce target tissue response and is used in clinical therapy. There are six major components:

1. availability of hormone to cell;
2. hormone specificity of receptor;
3. availability of receptor;
4. binding of hormone–receptor complex;
5. protein synthesis;
6. agonism/antagonism.

Availability of hormone to cell

Even if a cell has multiple receptors it will not be active in the absence of its specific hormone. For example, uterine epithelial cells have receptors for oestrogen, androgen, glucocorticoid and progestogen but because progesterone is not produced in the first half of the menstrual cycle, there is no progestational response (Robertson 1982).

In addition, a hormone can be present in the blood stream but unavailable to the target cell. A hormone circulating in the blood stream, not attached to a binding protein, readily enters cells by diffusion. However, most of a circulating hormone is bound to protein carriers, such as SHBG, and therefore unavailable (King 1988). Consequently, alterations in the amount of circulating binding globulins can modulate the biological activities of their respective hormones. For example, about 80% of circulating testosterone is bound to SHBG, approximately 19% is loosely bound to albumin, and about 1% is unbound. Androgenicity is mainly dependent upon the unbound fraction and partly upon the fraction associated with albumin (Siiteri 1986). SHBG production in the liver is decreased by androgens, hence the binding capacity in men is lower than in normal women. In a hirsute woman, the SHBG level is depressed by the excess androgen, and the percentage of free and therefore active testosterone is elevated (Rosenfeld 1971).

Hormone specificity of receptor

This is the most important factor which determines specificity of action and occurs at two levels (King 1988). Presence or absence of a given receptor determines whether a cell will respond to a given class of steroids whilst hormone specificity controls which particular compound is active. For example, the oestrogen receptor which has the greatest specificity binds oestradiol 10 times more efficiently than oestrone and about 1000 times more than the androgen, testosterone; progesterone and cortisol are not recognized at all (Garcia & Rochefort 1977). This recognition specificity is a reflection of the different affinities the receptor has for the different hormone structures (Fig. 10.3). In biological terms, this means that oestradiol is more active than oestrone whilst testosterone can have oestrogenic effects but only at pharmacological concentrations (Fig. 10.4).

Androgen, glucocorticoid, progestogen and mineralocorticoid receptors are less precise in their binding requirements than the oestrogen receptor (Raynaud et al

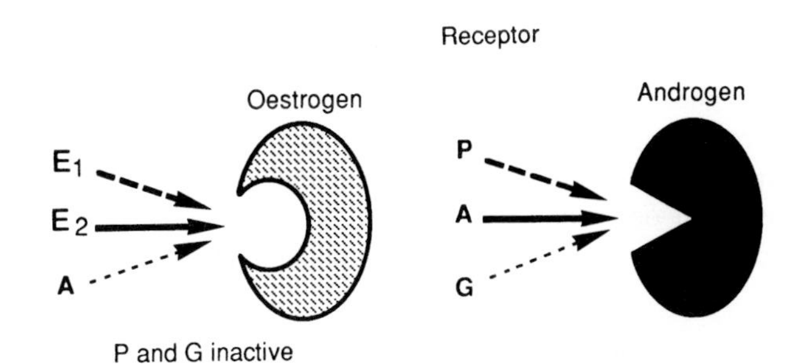

Fig. 10.3 Specificity determined by structural specificity of receptor. The oestradiol receptor has a higher affinity for oestradiol (E_2) than oestrone (E_1); androgens (A) such as testosterone have very low affinity while progestogens (P) and glucocorticoids (G) are inactive. The androgen receptor has less precise specificity, recognizing both P and G, albeit with less affinity than androgens.

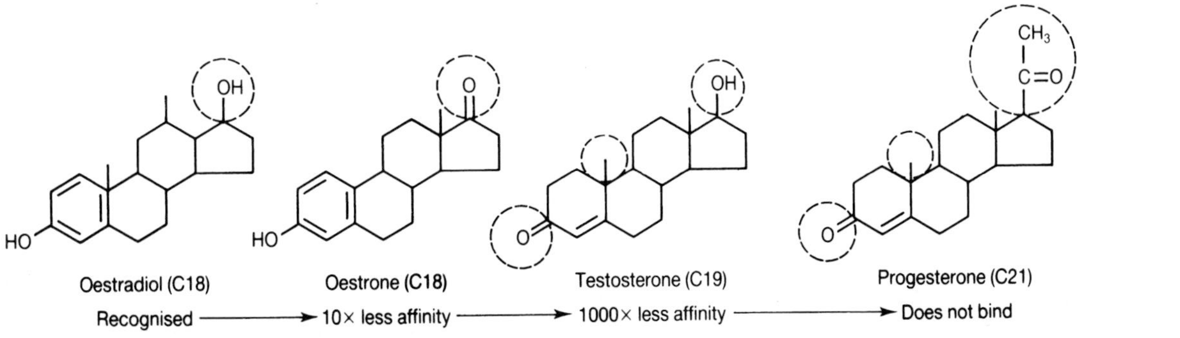

Oestradiol (C18) — Recognised → Oestrone (C18) — 10× less affinity → Testosterone (C19) — 1000× less affinity → Progesterone (C21) — Does not bind

Fig. 10.4 Oestrogen receptor recognition is influenced by the differing side chains of hormones, e.g. oestrogens, testosterone and progesterone.

1981). For example, many progestogens, especially the synthetic ones, bind to both progestogen and androgen receptors when present in pharmacological concentrations. This dual specificity is reflected in the biological activities of the compounds. For example, the practice of giving synthetic progestogens to pregnant women to prevent miscarriage resulted in some of their offspring having clinical features associated with androgen exposure (Aarskog 1979). The androgenic side-effects of the synthetic progestogens used in the oral contraceptive pill are another example.

Availability of receptor

A hormone can modify its own and/or another steroid hormone's activity by regulating the concentration of receptors in a cell. This has the biological effect of increasing tissue response to the hormone if the receptor number is increased, and vice versa if the receptor number is decreased. Oestrogen, for example, increases target tissue responsiveness to itself by increasing the concentration of FSH receptors in granulosa cells (Hillier et al 1981). This process is important in the selection and maintenance of the dominant ovarian follicle in the menstrual cycle. In order to respond to the ovulatory surge and become a 'successful' corpus luteum, the granulosa cells must acquire LH receptors. FSH induces LH receptor development on the granulosa cells of large antral follicles with oestrogen acting as chief coordinator (Erikson 1986).

Progesterone, on the other hand, limits the tissue response to oestrogen by reducing over time the concentration of oestrogen receptors (Tseng & Gurpide 1975), hence its use in the prevention of endometrial hyperplasia.

Binding of hormone–receptor complex

Biological activity is maintained only while the nuclear site is occupied with the hormone–receptor complex (King 1988, Scholl & Lippman 1984). The dissociation rate of the hormone and its receptor is therefore an important component of the biological response. Only low circulating levels of oestrogen are necessary for biological activity because of the long half-life of the oestrogen hormone–receptor complex (Sutherland et al 1988). As a consequence of a lower affinity for the oestrogen receptor, the less potent oestrogens (oestrone, oestriol) also have higher rates of dissociation from the receptor and therefore the oestrogen–receptor complex occupies the nucleus for a short period of time (Katzenellenbogen 1984).

The higher rates of dissociation with a weak oestrogen can be compensated for by continuous application to allow prolonged nuclear-binding activity. Cortisol and progesterone circulate in higher concentrations because their receptor complexes have short half-lives in the nucleus. This regulatory mechanism is used clinically in the induction of ovulation with clomiphene citrate (Adashi 1986). The structural similarity between clomiphene citrate and oestrogen is sufficient to achieve uptake and binding of clomiphene citrate by oestrogen receptors. It has a very weak oestrogenic effect but occupies the nuclear receptor for long periods of time – weeks rather than hours (Mickkelson et al 1986).

Protein synthesis

The limited ability of the receptors for progestogens, glucocorticoids and mineralocorticoids to discriminate between these hormones reduces their biological specificity. However, this effect could be counteracted if a gene's response to a hormone could be determined by specificity requirements in the DNA. Multiple regulatory units are present in the DNA proximal to the site when RNA transcription is initiated and interactions between these units and hormone–receptor complexes occur (Yamamoto 1985). It is generally agreed that these interactions are involved in the regulation of protein synthesis by steroids.

Agonism/antagonism

When a compound binds to a receptor, it can act as an agonist or antagonist. An agonist is a substance that has affinity for cell receptors of a naturally occurring substance and stimulates the same type of physiological activity. An antagonist tends to nullify the action of another substance, binding to its receptor without eliciting a biological response. In the case of the steroid hormones these activities do not necessarily require the compound to have the four-ring steroid structure. For example, diethylstilboestrol is a non-steroidal oestrogen agonist, while tamoxifen is a non-steroidal oestrogen antagonist (Fig. 10.5). Cyproterone acetate and RU486 (Mifepristone; Roussel) are the steroidal antagonists of testosterone and progesterone, respectively (Fig. 10.6). In these cases the conversion of agonists to antagonists is achieved by the addition of side chains. Each of these compounds blocks hormone action at the receptor level. Some clinical uses of steroid antagonists are listed in Table 10.1.

There are problems, however, in the clinical application of antagonists, related to the regulatory mechanisms described above. Firstly, because of the relative lack of receptor specificity, an antagonist for one class of hormone can have antagonistic effects on another class of hormone (Wakeling 1988). For example, the progesterone antagonist RU486 has affinity for the glucocorticoid receptor as well as the progesterone receptor and therefore is a potent antiglucocorticoid. Secondly, hormones have central and peripheral actions, mediated by specific receptors. Therefore an antagonist may have adverse effects apart from the intended use. Cyproterone acetate, for example, an androgen antagonist, illustrates this diversity.

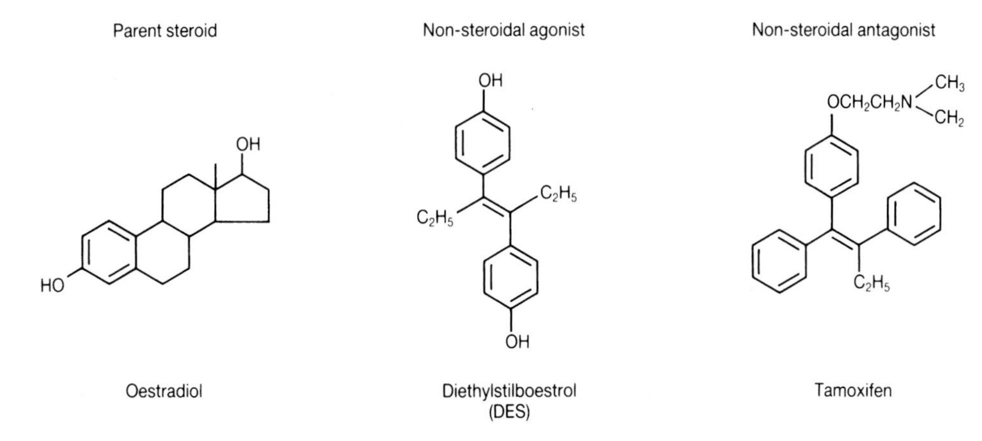

Fig. 10.5 Oestradiol with examples of a non-steroidal agonist (diethylstilboestrol) and antagonist (tamoxifen).

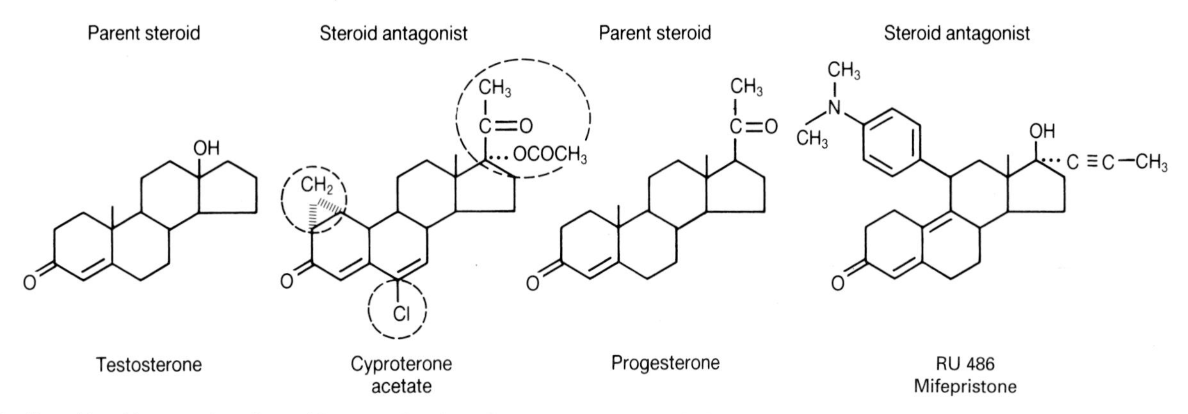

Fig. 10.6 Steroids with examples of steroid antagonists (e.g. Cyproterone acetate, Mifepristone).

It has effects as diverse as suppression of libido and regression of the prostate gland. In addition cyproterone acetate may act as agonist for other chemically related hormones. It acts as a potent progestogen having agonist effects on the progesterone receptor. Hence it is used as a contraceptive agent in combination with ethinyl oestradiol.

Table 10.1 Clinical uses of steroid hormone antagonists

Drug	Clinical use
Antiprogestogens	Contraception Termination of pregnancy
Antiandrogens	Acne Benign prostatic hypertrophy Hirsutism Prostate cancer
Antioestrogens	Breast cancer Benign breast disease Endometriosis Uterine disease
Antiglucocorticoids	Adrenocortical carcinoma Cushing's syndrome
Antimineralocorticoids	Essential hypertension Oedema/ascites

MECHANISM OF ACTION OF TROPHIC HORMONES

As trophic hormones cannot enter the cell, they stimulate physiological events by uniting with a receptor on the surface of the cell and activating a sequence of communications using a second messenger system within the cell. The most widely studied and best understood of these systems is adenylate cyclase/cyclic adenosine monophosphate (cAMP) (Fig. 10.7; Rodbell 1980).

Stage 1. Binding to the cell membrane

The hormone, sometimes called the 'first messenger', binds to a receptor on the cell surface.

Stage 2. Activation of adenyl cyclase in the cell membrane

Binding of the hormone to the receptor activates the enzyme, adenylate cyclase, within the membrane wall which catalyses the conversion of adenosine 5′-triphosphate (ATP) within the cell to cyclic AMP, the second messenger. Some hormones, such as GnRH, use other second messengers, such as calcium.

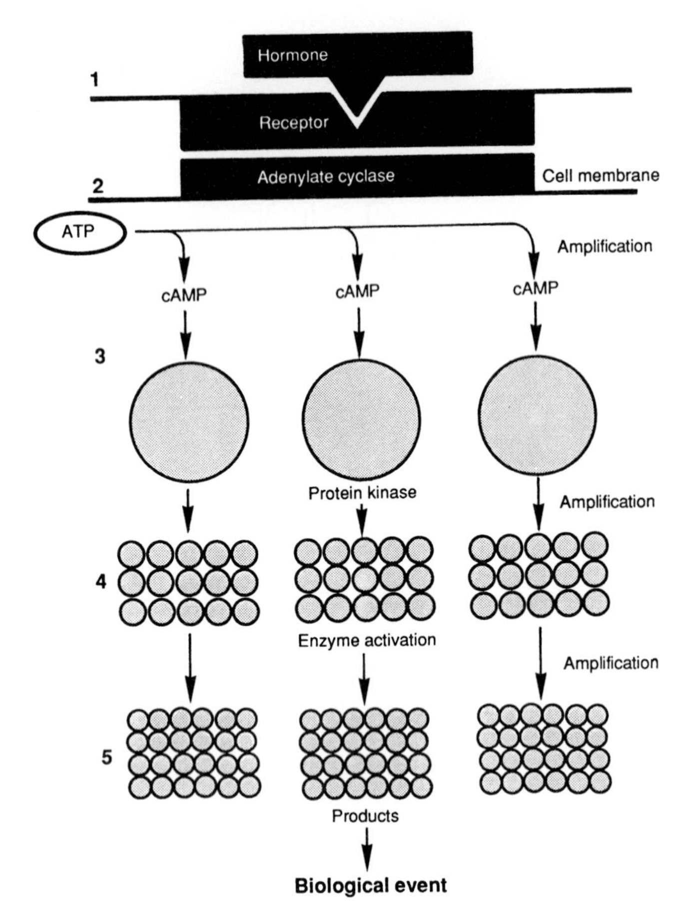

Fig. 10.7 Mechanism of action of trophic hormones. ATP, adenosine triphosphate; cAMP, cyclic adenosine monophosphate. See text for details of stages 1–5.

Stage 3. Activation of protein kinase

The cAMP is bound to a cytoplasmic receptor protein which activates a protein kinase.

Stages 4 and 5. Activation of enzymes

The protein kinase causes phosphorylation and thereby activation of specific enzymes. These enzymes catalyse specific intracellular processes which give rise to the observed physiological effect of the hormone. The cAMP system provides a method for amplification of the hormonal signal in the circulation. Each cyclase molecule produces a lot of cAMP; the protein kinases activate a large number of molecules which in turn lead to the production of an even greater number of cellular products.

Regulation of trophic hormone action

Regulation of hormone action is required for enhancing or reducing target tissue response, and is used in clinical therapy. There are five major components:

1. availability of the hormone to the cell;
2. hormone specificity of the receptor;
3. availability of the receptor (up- and down-regulation);
4. regulation of second messengers;
5. agonism/antagonism.

Availability of hormone to cell

An effect can only occur if a cell carries a receptor for that hormone and the hormone is available to the cell receptor.

Hormone specificity of receptor

The specificity of a hormone's action and/or intensity of stimulation are dependent upon the configuration of the cell membrane receptor (Hwang & Menon 1984). It can be altered by changes in the structure or concentration of the receptor in the cell membrane. Similarly, changes in the molecular structure of a trophic hormone can interfere with cellular binding and therefore physiological action. Hormones that are structurally similar may have some overlap in biological activity. For example, the similarity in structure between growth hormone and prolactin means that growth hormone has a lactogenic action whilst prolactin has some growth-promoting activity and stimulates somatomedin production (Speroff et al 1989).

The glycoprotein hormones (LH, FSH, thyroid-stimulating hormone (TSH) and human chorionic gonadotrophin (hCG)) share an identical alpha-chain and require another portion, the beta-chain, to confer the specificity inherent in the relationship between hormones and their receptors. The beta subunits differ in both amino acid and carbohydrate content and the chemical composition may be altered under certain conditions, thereby affecting the affinity of the hormone and its receptor.

Availability of the receptor (up- and downregulation)

The cell's mechanism for sensing the low concentrations of circulating trophic hormone is to have an extremely large number of receptors but to require only a very small percentage (as little as 1%) to be occupied by the hormone for its action to be evident (Sairam & Bhargavi 1985). Positive and negative modulation of receptor numbers by hormones is known as up- and downregulation. The mechanism of upregulation is unclear, but prolactin and GnRH, for example, can increase the concentration of their own receptors in the cell membrane (Katt et al 1985).

In downregulation, an excess concentration of a trophic hormone such as LH or GnRH results in a loss of receptors on the cell membrane and therefore a decrease in biological response. This process occurs by internalization of the receptors, and is the main biological mechanism by which the activity of polypeptide hormones is

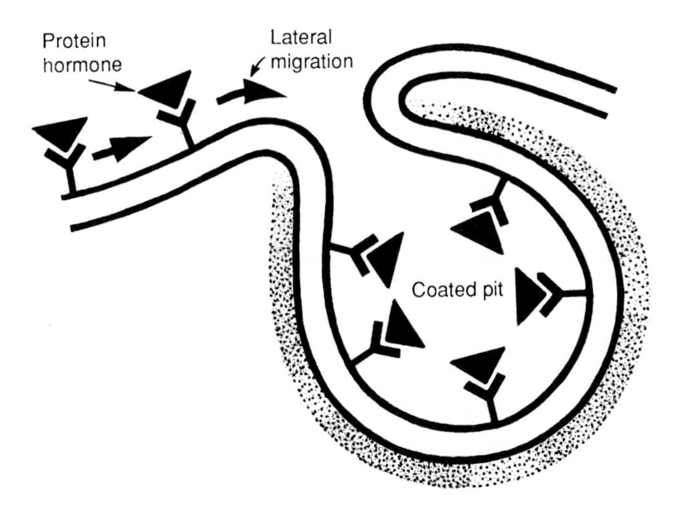

Fig. 10.8 Structure of a coated pit, illustrating lateral migration.

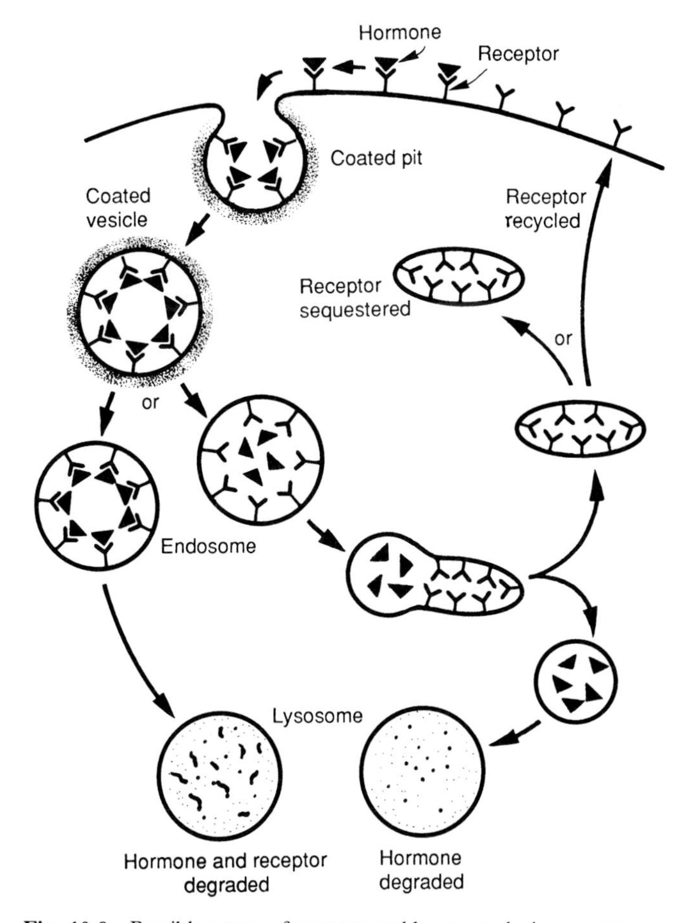

Fig. 10.9 Possible routes of receptor and hormone during receptor-mediated endocytosis.

limited (Segaloff & Ascoli 1988). Thus the formation of the hormone–receptor complex on the cell surface initiates the cellular response, and the internalization of the complex (with eventual degradation of the hormone) terminates the response. It therefore appears that the principal reason for the pulsatile, secretion of trophic hormones is to avoid downregulation and to maintain adequate receptor numbers. The pulse frequency, therefore, is a key factor in regulating receptor number .

It is believed that receptors are randomly inserted into the cell membrane after intracellular synthesis. They have two important sites – an external binding site which is specific for a polypeptide hormone, and an internal site which plays a role in the process of internalization (Kaplan 1981, Segaloff & Ascoli 1988). When a hormone binds to the receptor and high concentrations of the hormone are present in the circulation, the hormone–receptor complex moves laterally in the cell membrane in a process called lateral migration to a specialized area, the coated pit, the internal margin of which has a brush border (Goldstein et al 1979). Lateral migration, which takes minutes rather than seconds, thus concentrates hormone–receptor complexes in the coated pit, a process referred to as 'clustering' (Fig. 10.8). When fully occupied, the coated pit invaginates, pinches off, and enters the cell as a vesicle. The coated vesicle is delivered to the lysosomes where it undergoes degradation, releasing the hormones and receptors. The receptor may be recycled to the cell membranes and used again or the receptor and hormone may be metabolized, thus decreasing the hormone's biological activity. This process is called receptor-mediated endocytosis (Goldstein et al 1979; Fig. 10.9).

Besides downregulation of polypeptide hormone-receptors, the process of internalization can be utilized for other cellular metabolic events, including the transfer into the cell of vital substances such as iron and vitamins. Hence, cell membrane receptors can be separated into two classes. The class I receptors are distributed in the cell membrane and transmit information to modify cell behaviour for these receptors. Internalization is a method for downregulation and recycling is not usually a feature. Hormones which utilize this category of receptor include FSH, LH, hCG, GnRH, TSH and insulin (Kaplan 1981). The class II receptors are located in the coated pits. Binding leads to internalization which provides the cell with required facts or removes noxious agents from the biological fluid bathing the cell. These receptors are spared from degradation and can be recycled. Examples of this category include low-density lipoproteins which supply cholesterol to steroid-producing cells (Parinaud et al 1987) and transfer of immunoglobulins across the placenta to provide fetal immunity.

Regulation of second messengers

The second messenger system provides amplification of a small hormone signal in the blood stream and only a small percentage of the cell membrane receptors need to be occupied in order to generate a response. The regulation of adenylate cyclase and cyclic AMP production is important in regulating intracellular metabolic activity (Gilman

1984). Prostaglandins, guanine nucleotides, calmodulin and calcium all appear to participate in controlling the second messenger cascade (Segaloff & Ascoli 1988). The ability of the hormone–receptor complex to work through a common messenger (cAMP) and produce contrasting actions (stimulation and inhibition) is thought to be due to the presence of both stimulatory and inhibitory regulatory units (Gilman 1984, Rodbell 1980). For example, LH stimulates steroidogenesis in the corpus luteum through the coupling of stimulatory regulatory units to adenylate cyclase, stimulating the production of cAMP. Prostaglandin $F_{2\alpha}$ is directly luteolytic, inhibiting luteal steroidogenesis, and this action may be exerted via inhibitory units that block the production of cAMP (Rojas & Asch 1985).

Increasing concentrations of trophic hormones, such as gonadotrophins, are directly associated with desensitization of adenylate cyclase. There are some exceptions, namely the trophic hormones which do not utilize the adenylate cyclase mechanism (oxytocin, insulin, growth hormone, prolactin and human placental lactogen). The message of these hormones is passed directly to nuclear and cytoplasmic metabolic sites (Rasmussen 1986, Speroff et al 1989). GnRH is calcium-dependent in its mechanism of action (Jennes & Conn 1988).

Agonism/antagonism

In common with the steroid hormones, compounds can have agonist or antagonist effects. So far, only synthetic peptide agonists have come into clinical usage, analogues to GnRH being those most commonly known. The potency of the analogues is up to 200 times greater than GnRH, due to an increased affinity for pituitary GnRH receptors and a prolonged association with the receptor compared to GnRH. Though the analogues act as agonists, chronic administration stops the normal pulsatile pattern of GnRH, leading to a loss of pituitary GnRH receptors and, therefore, downregulation. This has profound effects on the pituitary, leading to a fall in serum LH and FSH and consequently gonadal steroid secretion.

The mode of action of GnRH antagonists at the GnRH receptor is quite different from that of the agonists. Although the antagonists bind to the receptor, the downregulation characteristic of agonist action does not occur (Clayton 1984). Rather, there is continuous occupancy of a large proportion of the receptors. Clinical application of antagonists has been delayed by the occurrence of significant toxicity.

CLINICAL ASSAYS

This section considers assay methodology for the endocrinological investigations commonly used in gynaecological practice. An understanding of basic methodology permits the clinician to have confidence in the selection of specific laboratory tests, and leads to a greater understanding of the assay for better interpretation of results (Chard 1987).

An assay determines the amount of a particular constituent of a mixture. The three types of analytical procedure commonly available in clinical practice are physicochemical assays, bioassays and binding assays.

Physicochemical assays

Some aspect of the physicochemical properties of a compound is utilized for its quantification. These are the assays used to measure electrolytes.

Bioassays

Detection or quantification is dependent on the biological actions of the compound. This was the original method of hormone assay. For example, human pregnancy could be diagnosed by the injection of maternal urine into the Black African Toad. If a high concentration of hCG was present in the urine, the toad would lay eggs.

Very recently, bioassays have stimulated interest with the development of very sensitive systems. For example, in the bioassay of prolactin, when neural tumour cells grown in culture are exposed to prolactin, they replicate.

Binding assays

These assays involve the combination of the compound, for example, an antigen, with a binding substance, for example, an antibody, which is added in a fixed amount to the solution. The distribution of the antigen between the bound and free phases is directly related to the total amount of antigen present and provides a means for quantifying the latter (Fig. 10.10). Binding assays can be further subdivided into three groups: receptor assays, competitive protein-binding assays and immunoassays.

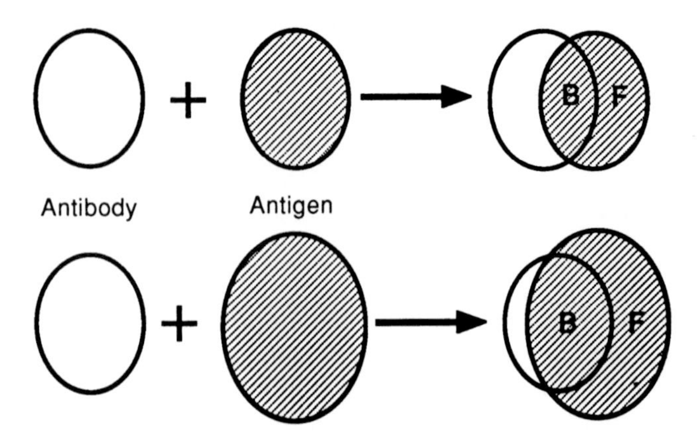

Fig. 10.10 Distribution of free (F) and bound (B) antigen in the presence of a fixed amount of antibody.

Receptor assays

A specific site on the surface of a tissue acts as the binding agent for a particular hormone, for example oestrogen receptors in breast tissue.

Competitive protein-binding assays

A naturally occurring binding protein, for example, SHBG, is used as the binder to quantify the amount of hormone present.

Immunoassays

A reaction which reaches equilibrium occurs between the hormone to be measured (antigen) and an antibody to monitor the reaction. A 'tracer' is attached to either the antigen or antibody. This tracer can be isotopic (radioactive), e.g. ^{125}I, or non-isotopic, e.g. based on fluorescence, or enzymatic action.

The basic principle of an immunoassay and how a result is obtained is described below:

1. A tracer such as a radioactive-labelled antigen (*Ag) is added to a fixed but *limited* quantity of antibody (Ab);

   Ab + *Ag

   When the reaction commences the two reagents react quickly to form a complex. The reverse action is slow. This is the basis of a radioimmunoassay.

   $$\text{Ab} + {}^{*}\text{Ag} \rightleftharpoons \text{Ab}{}^{*}\text{Ag}$$

   If the amount of antibody (Ab) is kept constant and a known amount of tracer (e.g. *Ag 10 000 u) is added, by leaving the reaction long enough to reach equilibrium 100% binding is reached.

   $$\text{Ab} + \underset{10\,000\text{ u}}{{}^{*}\text{Ag}} \rightleftharpoons \underset{10\,000\text{ u}}{\text{Ab}{}^{*}\text{Ag}}$$

2. If a small quantity of the antigen (Ag) we wish to measure is added to the same quantity of antibody (Ab) and tracer (*Ag) then labelled antigen (*Ag) and unlabelled antigen (Ag) will compete for the same limited number of binding sites offered by the antibody (Ab). Consequently, at equilibrium not all the labelled antigen (*Ag) will be bound by the antibody (Ab). Some will be displaced by the antigen (Ag) to be measured.

   $$\text{Ab} + \underset{10\,000\text{ u}}{\overset{\text{Ag}}{{}^{*}\text{Ag}}} \rightleftharpoons \underset{8000\text{ u}}{\left[\text{Ab} \angle \begin{matrix}\text{Ag}\\ {}^{*}\text{Ag}\end{matrix}\right]} + \underset{2000\text{ u}}{{}^{*}\text{Ag}}$$

   Now only 80% of the *Ag is antibody-bound, while 20% is 'free' and can be separated from the bound antibody by quantification.

3. If we now introduce more unlabelled antigen (Ag) to the reaction:

   $$\left.\begin{matrix}\text{AgAg}\\ \text{Ab} + {}^{*}\text{AgAb}\end{matrix}\right\}_{10\,000\text{ u}} \rightleftharpoons \underset{5000\text{ u}}{\left[\text{Ab} < \begin{matrix}\text{Ag}\\ {}^{*}\text{Ag}\end{matrix}\right]} + \underset{5000\text{ u}}{{}^{*}\text{Ag}}$$

   there is even greater competition for the limited number of binding sites, so now only 50% of the added tracer is antibody-bound. This can be repeated for differing amounts of unlabelled antigen. The percentage of bound labelled antigen (*Ag) is progressively reduced with increasing concentrations of added unlabelled antigen (Ag).

   If it is known how much unlabelled antigen is added each time to the fixed quantities of antibody (Ab) and labelled antigen (*Ag) then a standard curve can be derived (Fig. 10.11).

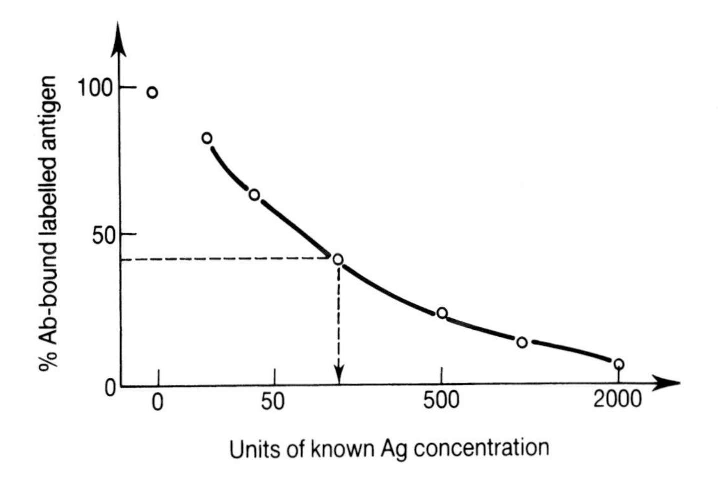

Fig. 10.11 Relationship between bound radiolabelled antigen and concentration of antigen in a dose–response curve.

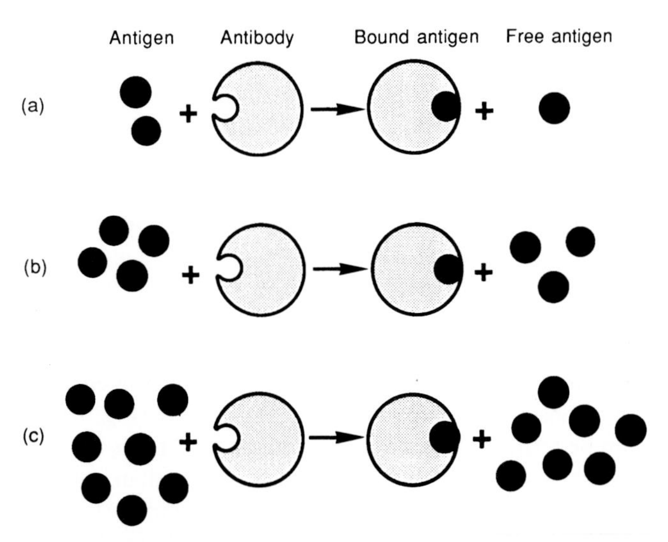

Fig. 10.12 Immunoassay: with a 'limited' concentration of antibody, varying concentrations of antigen give rise to increasing proportions of antigen in the free fraction.

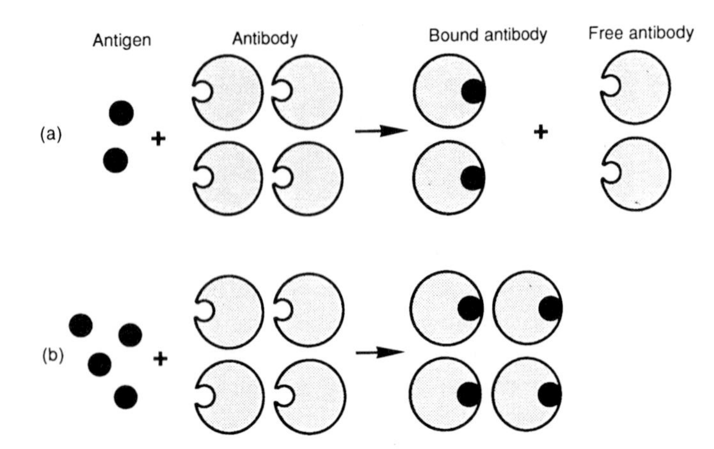

Fig. 10.13 Immunometric assay: with an 'excess' of antibody, increasing concentrations of antigen give rise to a corresponding increase in bound antibody.

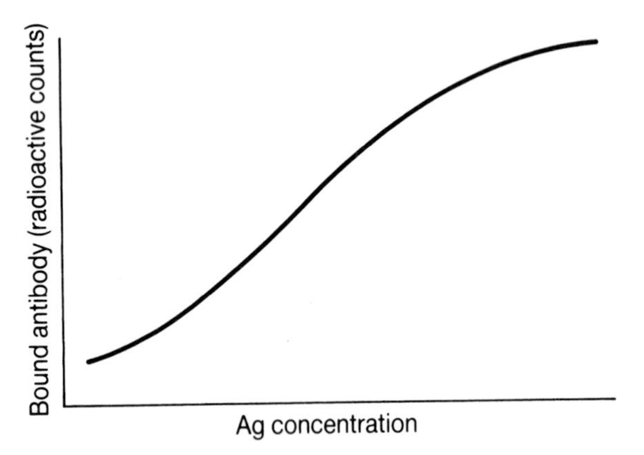

Fig. 10.14 Relationship between bound radiolabelled antibody and concentration of antigen in the immunoradiometric assay.

Hence, when a patient specimen containing an unknown amount of antigen is to be measured, the percentage of bound labelled antigen (shown by the dashed line in Fig. 10.11) left after equilibrium with the sample will then relate to the unknown amount of antigen in the sample.

This basic binding reaction can be subdivided into two categories, based on whether the antibody is present in a limited concentration or whether it is present in excess. When labelled antigen acts as the tracer, as in radioimmunoassay, the amount of antibody is constant but limited (Fig. 10.12).

If varying concentrations of the labelled antigen react with a constant but excess amount of antibody (Fig. 10.13) it can be termed an 'immunometric assay'. This is the type of assay used when labelled antibody, rather than antigen, acts as the tracer. In this case, the standard curve slopes in the reverse direction (Fig. 10.14) to that above, because the amount of antigen is measured by the binding of the labelled antibody. As the concentration of antigen increases, so does the amount of complexed labelled antibody. Many factors can influence the construction of the standard curve, hence every time a sample analysis is performed, a standard curve is also constructed. The acceptance of the results on the patient sample is dictated by quality control specimens containing known amounts of the antigen to be measured.

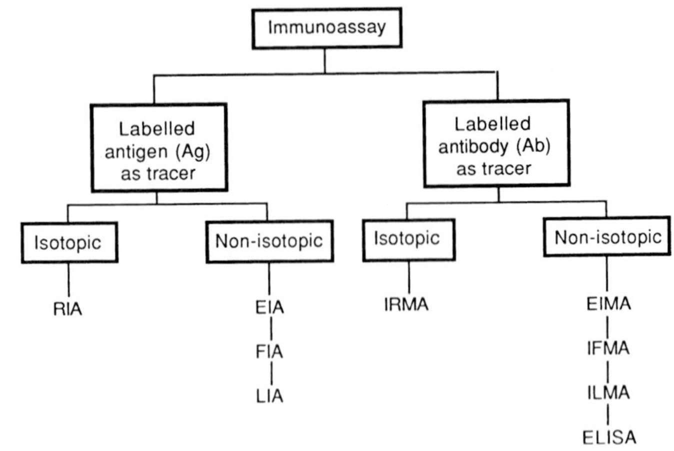

Fig. 10.15 Types of immunoassay used in clinical practice. RIA, radioimmunoassay; EIA, enzymoimmunoassay; FIA, fluoroimmunoassay; LIA, luminoimmunoassay; IRMA, immunometric assay; EIMA, enzymoimmunometric assay; IFMA, ILMA, immunofluorometric assay; ELISA, enzyme-labelled immunosorbent assay.

TYPES OF IMMUNOASSAY

Immunoassays are divided into two basic groups: those that use a radioactive label (isotopic assays) and those that use a non-radioactive label (non-isotopic assays). They can also be divided on the basis of whether the tracer or label is on the antigen or the antibody, as indicated in Figure 10.15.

Isotopic assays

Isotopic tracers can be divided into two types: those with an internal label and those with an external label. With an internal label, an existing atom in the molecule is replaced by a radioactive isotope of that atom (e.g. ^3H for ^1H — called a tritiated sample) and the tracer should be identical with that of the unlabelled molecule. With an external label, an atom or atoms of a radioactive isotope (e.g. ^{125}I) is covalently linked to an existing atom on the molecule. A tracer with an external label, by definition, is not identical to the unlabelled ligand though in practice its behaviour may not be distinguishable from the latter. Tracers with an internal label are commonly used in the case of small molecules such as steroid hormones and drugs. Tracers with an external label are commonly used in the case of larger peptide and protein hormones.

Radioimmunoassay (RIA)

This was the earliest form of immunoassay to be developed. The tracer is a radioactive antigen, originally ^{3}H but superseded by ^{125}I. The antibody used in the reaction tube is polyclonal (derived from different cells) and is present in a restricted amount.

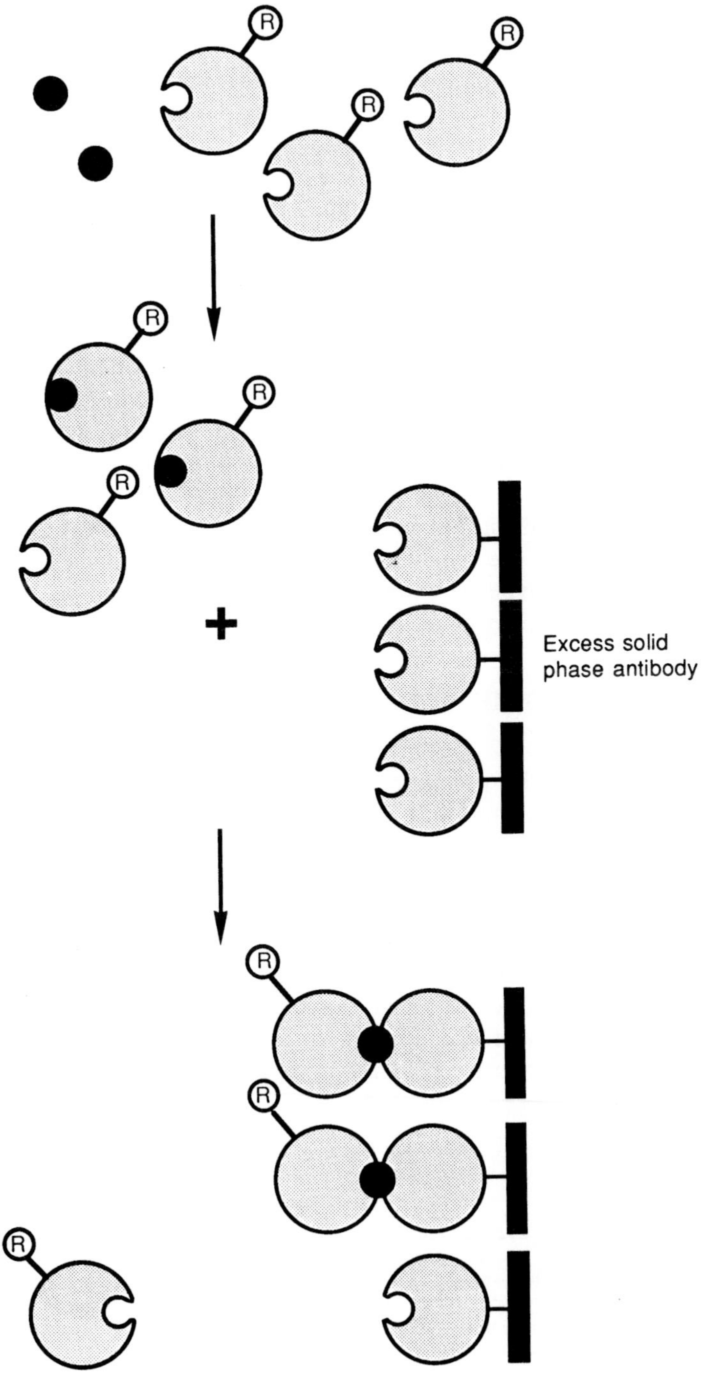

Fig. 10.16 'Two-site' immunoradiometric assay technique: the antigen is bound by two antibodies, therefore two binding sites on the antigen are involved. This technique is also referred to as a 'sandwich' assay.

Immunometric assay (IRMA)

This is now an important immunoassay with distinct advantages over RIA. The major application of IRMA has been in the quantification of proteins and peptides. The radioactive label is attached to the antibody, which is present in excess, and is a highly specific monoclonal antibody. The production technique of these antibodies results in a virtually limitless uniform supply of the reagent. One advantage of an IRMA is that the excess amount of radioactive antibody enables a wider range of antigen concentrations to be measured. Another advantage is that it may be performed by the 'two-site' immunometric method. This procedure is illustrated in Figure 10.16. It is also referred to as the 'sandwich' assay. The complex of the radiolabelled antibody and antigen is precipitated from the reaction mixture by the addition of another antibody directed against a second antigenic site on the antigen. This sandwich technique increases the accuracy of the assay compared to RIA.

Non-isotopic assays

In this group, the second marker antibody has an enzymatic, fluorescent or chemiluminescent tag. Assay systems that require separation of bound and free phases after incubation are referred to as heterogeneous and are more sensitive than those that do not require separation (homogeneous).

Enzyme

Enzymoimmunoassay (EIA), enzymoimmunometric assay (EIMA), enzyme-labelled immunosorbent assy (ELISA). These are currently the most widely used non-isotopic labels. Small quantities of antigen can be quantified by studying enzymatic substrate conversion that leads to a colour change. The colour formation can be a simple yes/no answer (Fig. 10.17) as in a rapid pregnancy test, or the intensity of colour can be used

Porous white cellulose with coupled Ab against hCG

↓

Urine/blood containing hCG from patient

↓

2nd Ab coupled to an enzyme

↓

Cellulose solid-phase reagent washed

↓

Add enzyme substrate to generate colour on white background

Fig. 10.17 Principle of rapid pregnancy test (tube test) using non-isotopic reagents; hCG, human chorionic gonadotrophin.

to quantify the patient sample. The second marker antibody will not be bound, so following the wash-step will not be present to react with its substrate.

Fluorescence

Fluoroimmunoassay (FIA), immunofluorometric assay (IFMA). Fluorescence is the property of certain molecules to absorb light at one wavelength and emit light at a longer wavelength. The incident light excites the molecule to a higher level of vibrational energy: as the molecule returns to the ground state it emits a photon which is the fluorescence emission. The potential sensitivity of fluorescence determination is very high, but in practice it is often limited by background noise. As with EIA, FIA can be divided, according to whether a separation step is required, into heterogeneous and homogeneous assays.

Chemiluminescence

Luminoimmunoassay (LIA), immunofluorometric assay (ILMA). Luminescence is a very similar phenomenon to fluorescence. Whereas the exciting energy in fluorescence is in the form of light, in luminescence it is provided by a chemical reaction. Chemiluminescent reactions produce light from simple chemical reactions, involving the action of oxygen or a peroxide on certain oxidation organic substances. Because there is high sensitivity inherent in the techniques, and the instrumentation is potentially simple, the application of luminescent labels in immunoassays should increase dramatically.

Agglutination assays

Agglutination assays are another type of immunoassay, using the principle that if the antigen–antibody reaction is coupled with visible compounds, such as red blood cells (haemagglutination) or latex particles (latex particle immunoassay), the presence or absence of a specific antigen or antibody can be detected in a patient sample by the presence or absence of agglutination of the cells or particles. As these assays lack the sensitivity of the assays described above, they have been largely superseded, but they can be used without any sophisticated instrumentation. The results are evaluated by eye, although the endpoint is subjective.

The future

Since the advent of RIA, immunoassays have played a major role in the quantification of many compounds and enabled the development of endocrinology as a medical science. As the number and variety of applications increase, the goal of assay technology remains the development of assays that give a high degree of sensitivity and specificity with ease, speed, and without the hazards of radioactivity. The new breed of non-isotopic assays, which utilize enzymes, fluorescence and chemiluminescence, are fulfilling these hopes. As budgeting continues to be a problem for all institutions, cost, which is related to personnel, reagents and equipment required for an assay, will also play a part in determining the assay of choice in the future.

Table 10.2 illustrates some of the advantages and disadvantages of the types of assay currently available, including the type of equipment and time required to obtain a result.

ACTION AND MEASUREMENT OF INDIVIDUAL HORMONES

In any assay, the precision and accuracy of the results depend upon the antibody and reference standard for the antigen used, so the results on the same sample can vary from laboratory to laboratory depending upon the reagent used. When interpreting results on a patient sample, the normal ranges for the laboratory must be consulted. The chemical composition and assay methods of the hormones measured in endocrinological practice are summarized in Table 10.3. Only those hormones most relevant to gynaecological practice are considered in detail below.

Table 10.2 Advantages and disadvantages of assays

Type of immunoassay	Degree of instrumentation	Time needed to do assay	Uses radiolabel
Latex agglutination	None necessary	2–30 min	No
ELISA (semiquantitative)	None necessary	10 min–4 h	No
Enzyme-labelled assay	Colorimeter ± centrifuge*	6–12 h	No
Radiolabelled assay	Counter and centrifuge*	1–24 h	Yes
Fluoroimmunoassay	Fluorimeter ± centrifuge*	1–3 h	No
Chemiluminescent assay	Luminometer and centrifuge*	1–3 h	No

* Alternatively, other method of separation, e.g. magnets or filtration. ELISA, enzyme-labelled immunosorbent assay.

Table 10.3 Chemical composition and assay methods of hormones

Site	Hormone	Steroid	Peptide	Assay
Hypothalamus	GnRH		Decapeptide	RIA
	TRH		Tripeptide	RIA
Anterior pituitary	FSH		Glycoprotein	RIA, IRMA
	LH		Glycoprotein	RIA, IRMA, IFMA
	ACTH		Polypeptide	RIA, IRMA
	TSH		Glycoprotein	RIA, IRMA, LIA
	Growth hormone		Protein	IFMA, RIA, IRMA
	Prolactin		Protein	RIA, IRMA, bioassay
Posterior pituitary	Oxytocin		Nonapeptide	RIA
	Vasopressin (ADH)		Nonapeptide	RIA
Thyroid	T_3		Iodinated amino acid (tyrosine)	RIA, IRMA, bioassay
	T_4		Iodinated amino acid (tyrosine)	RIA, IRMA
Pancreas	Glucagon		Polypeptide	RIA
	Insulin		Polypeptide	RIA
Adrenal	Cortisol	Steroid		RIA, FIA
	Aldosterone	Steroid		RIA
	Androgens	Steroid		RIA
Ovary/testis	Oestradiol	Steroid		RIA, LIA (plasma)
	Oestrone	Steroid		LIA (urine)
	Progesterone	Steroid		RIA, LIA, FIA
	Testosterone	Steroid		RIA, LIA
	Inhibin		Peptide	RIA, bioassay
Endometrium	IGF-1, PP12		Glycoprotein	RIA
	PEP, PP14		Glycoprotein	RIA
Trophoblast	hCG		Glycoprotein	RIA, IRMA, ELISA, latex agglutination, FIA, IFMA
	PAPP-A		Glycoprotein	RIA, IRMA, EIA
	Oestriol	Steroid		RIA
	hPL		Glycoprotein	RIA, FIA
	SP1		Protein	RIA, EIA
Fetus	AFP		Glycoprotein	RIA, EIA, IFMA

GnRH, gonadotrophin-releasing hormone; TRH, thyrotrophin-releasing hormone; FSH, follicle-stimulating hormone; LH, luteinizing hormone; ACTH, adrenocorticotrophic hormone; TSH, thyroid-stimulating hormone; ADH, antidiuretic hormone; T_3, triiodothyronine; T_4, tetraiodothyronine; IGF-1, insulin-like growth factor 1; PP12, placental protein 12; PEP, progesterone-dependent endometrial protein; PP14, placental protein 14; hCG, human chorionic gonadotrophin; PAPP-A, pregnancy-associated plasma protein A; hPL, human placental lactogen; SP1, Schwangerschaft's protein 1; AFP, alphafetoprotein. RIA, radioimmunoassay; IRMA, immunometric assay; IFMA, immunofluorometric hormone; LIA, luminoimmunoassay; FIA, fluoroimmunoassay. ELISA, enzyme-linked immunosorbent assay; EIA, enzymoimmunoassay.

Table 10.4 Normal levels for follicle-stimulating hormone (FSH) and luteinizing hormone (LH)

Clinical state	Serum FSH	Serum LH
Normal adult female	5–20 iu/l with the ovulatory mid-cycle peak about twice the base level	5–20 iu/l with the ovulatory mid-cycle peak about three times the base level
Hypogonadotrophic state: Prepubertal, hypothalamic and pituitary dysfunction	< 5 iu/l	< 5 iu/l
Hypergonadotrophic state: Postmenopausal, castrate and ovarian failure	> 40 iu/l	> 40 iu/l

Anterior pituitary hormones

Follicle-stimulating hormone

Normal levels of FSH are shown in Table 10.4.

Because of the marked fluctuations in levels in a normal ovulatory cycle, timing of the blood sample in relation to ovulation is required to interpret results. The level can be as low as 0.5 iu/l at the luteal phase nadir and as high as 20 iu/1 at the midcycle peak. However, values below 1 iu/1 are associated with hypothalamic pituitary failure and values of 20 iu/l or above indicate ovarian failure, as in the menopause.

In addition, FSH values within the wide range of normal can be associated with absent ovarian function if the production is below the threshold of follicular development for that patient, i.e. a normal result does not guarantee a normal endocrinological pattern in an individual patient. Fluctuating FSH levels mean the investigation might need to be repeated in the follicular phase, in particular in a perimenopausal patient.

Luteinizing hormone

As for FSH, timing the sample in relation to the phase of the ovulatory cycle is vital. For example, the ovulatory surge is taken as above 20 iu/l. However, in polycystic ovarian disease, a raised LH (13-25 iu/l) with normal FSH values is characteristic. Therefore, a raised LH in the early to midfollicular phase is of more significance than a midcycle raised LH. The LH level is within the normal range in a significant number of women with polycystic ovarian disease and the diagnosis requires the use of other tests.

The prospective timing of ovulation using the LH peak presents the difficulty that the peak cannot be identified until the next value significantly lower than the peak is observed. Thus, although rapid assays for LH are now available, it is still necessary to plan the action to be taken on the basis of the first definite rise in LH values rather than on the peak, which usually occurs a day later.

As discussed earlier, unless the assay uses an antibody that is specific for the beta subunit of LH, cross-reaction can occur in the assay with the other glycoproteins of the anterior pituitary (FSH, TSH) and hCG.

Prolactin

Prolactin levels are influenced by the time of day when blood is collected and are increased by stress (including venepuncture). Transient rises can occur at ovulation. Therefore a small elevation above the normal range can occur in normal women. Such a rise should be judged in the clinical setting. If a woman has a normal menstrual cycle, the result is unlikely to be significant. However, if she is amenorrhoeic she should be investigated further.

Growth hormone

Growth hormone is secreted in short bursts, most of which occur in the first part of the night. These bursts are more frequent in children, so the results vary depending upon timing and age. Secretion is also stimulated by stress and hypoglycaemia and is inhibited by glucose and corticosteroids.

Thyrotrophin-stimulating hormone

Normal levels of TSH range from 0.4 to 5 mmol/l. The measurement of tetraiodothyronine (T_4) and TSH provides the most accurate assessment of thyroid function. When using thyroid hormone replacement therapy, both TSH and T_4 should be measured because TSH alone cannot detect overdosage.

Thyroid gland hormones

Deficiency of thyroid hormones triiodothyronine (T_3) and T_4 leads to anovulation associated with increased gonadotrophin levels. Therefore, it is important to assess thyroid function prior to diagnosing premature ovarian failure.

Normal levels are as follows: free T_4, 10–25 pmol/l; T_3, 1.1–2.3 nmol/l (non-pregnant, no OCP), 1.4–4.3 nmol/l (pregnant/OCP) (OCP = oral contraceptive pill).

Circulating thyroid hormone is tightly bound to a group of proteins, chiefly thyroxine-binding globulin. Oestrogen produces a rise in thyroxine-binding capacity and, therefore, thyroid function tests are affected by pregnancy and oestrogen-containing medications such as the contraceptive pill. Consequently, a raised thyroxine level does not mean that the free thyroxine concentration (the unbound and metabolically active hormone) is above the normal range.

Because of the peripheral source of T_3, its levels are not a direct reflection of thyroid secretion. In addition T_3 levels may be normal despite the presence of a goitre with elevated TSH and depressed T_4 concentrations, as T_4 plays the instrumental role in TSH regulation. Therefore, measurement of free T_4 and TSH provides the most accurate assessment of thyroid function. RIA of T_3 is important for the occasional case of hyperthyroidism due to excessive production of T_3 with normal T_4 levels (T_3 toxicosis). Drugs taken orally for cholecystograms inhibit the peripheral conversion of T_4 to T_3, and can disrupt normal thyroid levels (giving elevated T_4) for up to 30 days after administration.

Adrenal cortex

The adrenal cortex comprises three morphologically and functionally distinct regions. The outmost region (zona glomerulosa) secretes aldosterone. The zona fasciculata is the intermediate region and produces cortisol, which will be dealt with here. The zona reticularis encircles the medulla and synthesizes oestrogens and androgens.

Cortisol

Normal levels of cortisol in adults at 09.00 hours range from 300 to 700 nmo/l.

If a 24-h urine collection is used, it is necessary to ensure that a complete collection has been obtained. The measurement of creatinine excretion will identify whether a collection is incomplete. As blood levels of cortisol vary greatly throughout a 24-h period, sample timing is important. Blood levels are highest in the morning and lowest in the evening. Most laboratories' normal values are based on sampling at 09.00 hours.

Ovarian hormones

Oestradiol

Normal levels of oestradiol are shown in Table 10.5.

There is a variation in oestradiol levels throughout the menstrual cycle. Results, therefore, need to be interpreted in relation to the timing of the sample in the cycle.

Progesterone

Levels in the mother during pregnancy increase in parallel with the growth of the placenta (Table 10.5). Maternal progesterone levels are related to the weight of the fetus and placenta at term.

Variations throughout the menstrual cycle can lead to difficulties in interpretation if the result is taken at an unidentified time in the cycle, particularly if a single progesterone level is taken as a marker of ovulation. Normally results taken 5–8 days prior to the next menstruation are suitable for the detection of ovulation, so the patient should be asked to keep a record of the timing of the blood sample and her next last menstrual period. A result >30 nmol/l indicates ovulation, even if timing is not known.

Testosterone

The normal levels of testosterone in females are shown in Table 10.5. Testosterone levels in females are lower than in males (females 0.5–3.0 nmol/1, males 9–35 nmol/1). The reverse is the case for SHBG (females 38–103 nmol/1, males 17–50 nmol/1.

Testosterone arises from a variety of sources in the female. Approximately 50% is derived from peripheral conversion of androstenedione (secreted by the adrenal cortex), while the adrenal gland and ovary contribute approximately equal amounts (25%) to the circulating levels of testosterone, except at midcycle when the ovarian contribution increases by 10-15%. About 80% of circulating testosterone is bound to SHBG.

Placenta

Human chorionic gonadotrophin (hCG)

This is secreted by the blastocyst and appears in maternal blood shortly after implantation and then rises rapidly until 8 weeks' gestation. Levels show little change at 8–12 weeks, then decline to 18 weeks and remain fairly constant until term. There is some short-term variation in blood hCG levels but no circadian rhythm. At term, the levels in the female fetus are substantially higher than those in the male (Obiekwe & Chard 1983). The mechanisms which determine the levels of hCG in maternal blood are unknown.

In structure hCG is similar to LH, and thus antibodies to one cross-react with the other unless an assay for the beta subunit of hCG is used. The sensitivity of most commercial assays in the past had to be limited in order to avoid false-positive tests due to LH cross-reaction. Peak levels of hCG (approximately 100 000 iu/l) occur at 10 weeks' gestation. A patient can continue to have a positive pregnancy test for at least a week after a spontaneous or therapeutic abortion due to the prolonged half-life of hCG; hCG may be detected up to 20 weeks later if sensitive assays are used.

The range of serum hCG levels in ectopic pregnancy is very wide (Stabile et al 1989) so that a negative result does not rule out an ectopic pregnancy, or distinguish it from a missed abortion. Quantification of hCG is used to monitor postoperative progress in trophoblastic disease.

Table 10.5 Normal ranges for oestradiol, progesterone and testosterone

	Oestradiol	Progesterone (nmol/l)	Testosterone (nmol/l)
Follicular phase	200–400 pmol/l	<4	0.5–3.0
Mid-cycle peak	400–1200 pmol/l	4–10	0.5–3.0
Luteal phase	2–10 nmol/l	30–45	0.5–3.0
Pregnancy			
First trimester	2–10 nmol/l	30–45	
Second trimester	10–30 nmol/l	70–150	
Third trimester	20–80 nmol/l	150–600	
Postmenopause	<100 pmol/l	<4	0.5–1.5

Measurements of free βhCG are used for screening for Down's syndrome (Grudzinskas et al 1994).

Fetus

Alphafetoprotein (AFP)

AFP is synthesized by yolk sac, fetal liver and gastrointestinal tract. Its function is unknown. It is used as a marker in clinical practice for the identification of congenital abnormalities.

Neural tube defects are associated with raised midtrimester levels of AFP while Down's syndrome is associated with reduced midtrimester AFP levels.

Normal levels. The value of AFP varies with gestation and number of fetuses present. The concentration of AFP in fetal serum rises rapidly to reach a peak at 12–14 weeks' gestation, at which time the levels are 2–3 g/l. Thereafter it falls until term with a sharp drop at 32–34 weeks. In the mother, circulating AFP levels rise progressively to reach a peak at 32 weeks, then decrease towards term. Check with the local laboratory as levels also vary from one type of assay to another.

The interpretation of normality of levels depends upon gestation. Therefore incorrect assessment of gestation could lead to an erroneous conclusion on the normality of the fetus. Levels are also raised in obstetric problems (threatened miscarriage, intrauterine growth retardation, perinatal death and antepartum haemorrhage) and some congenital abnormalities (exomphalos, nephrosis, Turner's syndrome, trisomy 13), but depressed in trisomy 21 (Grudzinskas et al 1994).

KEY POINTS

1. Steroids exert their action through intracellular receptors whereas trophic hormones act through receptors located on the cell membrane, then through a second messenger system within the cell.
2. Androgen, progesterone and glucocorticoid receptors are less precise than oestrogen receptors in their binding affinity.
3. Synthetic progestogens can bind to both androgen and progesterone receptors reflecting the dual biological activities of progestogens.
4. Hormone potency is directly related to the length of time the hormone–receptor complex occupies the nucleus.
5. Due to structural similarity with oestrogen, clomiphene citrate binds to oestrogen receptors and occupies the nucleus for long periods.
6. Agonists are substances that occupy cell receptors and stimulate natural physiological activities.
7. Antagonists are substances that can occupy receptors without being internalized, hence blocking the cell function.
8. An antagonist may block different classes of hormones due to the lack of receptor specificity.
9. Due to amplification of hormone signals by the second messenger system, only 1% of the cell receptors need to be occupied by the hormone for its action to be evident.
10. Downregulation by internalization of hormone receptors is a unique mechanism for limiting polypeptide hormone activity.
11. Depending upon the reagent used, hormone analysis results vary from one laboratory to another.
12. Endocrine investigations should be timed early in the follicular phase and repeated testing may be necessary to guard against false results.
13. The use of TSH estimation only cannot detect overdosage and T_4 should be measured as well in women receiving thyroxine replacement therapy.
14. T_3 measurement is necessary only in patients suspected to be thyrotoxic yet with normal T_4 values.
15. Due to its long half-life, hCG can be detected in blood or urine for a few weeks after a miscarriage using a sensitive assay method.
16. Oestrogen increases target tissue responsiveness to itself by increasing FSH receptors in granulosa cells whereas progesterone limits the tissue response to oestrogen by reducing the concentrations of oestrogen receptors.

REFERENCES

Aarskog D 1979 Maternal progestins as a possible cause of hypospadias. New England Journal of Medicine 300: 75

Adashi E Y 1986 Clomiphene citrate-initiated ovulation: a clinical update. Seminars in Reproductive Endocrinology 4: 255

Chard T 1987 An introduction to radioimmunoassay and related techniques. Elsevier, Amsterdam

Clayton R N 1984 LH-RH and its analogs. In: Vickery B H, Nestor J J, Hafez E S E (eds) MTP Press, Lancaster, p 35

Erikson G F 1986 An analysis of follicle development and ovum maturation. Seminars in Reproductive Endocrinology 4: 233

Garcia M, Rochefort H 1977 Androgens on the oestrogen receptor. II. Correlation between nuclear translocation and uterine protein synthesis. Steroids 29: 11

Gilman A G 1984 Guanine nucleotide-binding regulatory proteins and dual control of adenylate cyclase. Journal of Clinical Investigation 73: 1

Goldstein J L, Anderson R G W, Brown M S 1979 Coated pits, coated vesicles, and receptor-mediated endocytosis. Nature 279: 679

Grudzinskas J G, Chard T, Chapman M, Cuckle H (eds) 1994 Screening for Down's syndrome. Cambridge University Press, Cambridge

Hillier S G, Reichert L E, Van Hall E V 1981 Control of preovulatory follicular estrogen biosynthesis in the human ovary. Journal of Clinical Endocrinology and Metabolism 52: 847

Hwang J, Menon K M J 1984 Spatial relationships of the human chorionic gonadotropin (hCG) subunits in the assembly of the hCG-receptor complex in the luteinized ovary. Proceedings of the National Academy of Science 81: 4667

Jennes L, Conn P M 1988 Mechanism of gonadotrophin releasing hormone action. In: Cooke B A, King R J B, van der Molen H J (eds) Hormones and their action part II. Elsevier Science, Amsterdam, p 135

Kaplan J 1981 Polypeptide-binding membrane receptors: analysis and classification. Science 212: 14
Katt J A, Duncan J A, Herbon L et al 1985 The frequency of gonadotrophin-releasing hormone stimulation determines the number of pituitary gonadotrophin-releasing hormone receptors. Endocrinology 116: 2113
Katzenellenbogen G S 1984 Biology and receptor interactions of estriol and estriol derivatives in vitro and in vivo. Journal of Steroid Biochemistry 20: 1033
King R J B 1988 An overview of molecular aspects of steroid hormone action. In: Cooke B A, King R J B, van der Molen J G J (eds) Hormones and their actions. Elsevier Science, Amsterdam, p 29
Mickkelson T J, Kroboth P D, Cameron W J et al 1986 Single-dose pharmacokinetics of clomiphene citrate in normal volunteers. Fertility and Sterility 46: 392
Obiekwe B C, Chard T 1983 Placental proteins in late pregnancy: relation to fetal sex. Journal of Obstetrics and Gynaecology 3: 163
Parinaud J, Perret B, Ribbes H et al 1987 High density lipoprotein and low density lipoprotein utilization by human granulosa cells for progesterone synthesis in serum-free culture: respective contributions of free and esterified cholesterol. Journal of Clinical Endocrinology and Metabolism 64: 409
Rasmussen H 1986 The calcium messenger system. New England Journal of Medicine 314: 1094
Raynaud J P, Ojasso T, Labrie F 1981 Steroid receptors. In: Lewis G P, Ginsburg M (eds) Mechanisms of steroid action. Macmillan, London, p 145
Robertson W B 1982 The endometrium. Butterworths, London
Rodbell M 1980 The role of hormone receptors and GTP-regulatory proteins in membrane transduction. Nature 284: 17
Rojas R J, Asch R H 1985 Effects of luteinizing hormone-releasing hormone agonist and calcium upon adenyl cyclase activity of human corpus luteum membranes. Life Sciences 36: 841
Rosenfeld R L 1971 Plasma testosterone binding globulin and indexes of the concentration of unbound plasma androgens in normal and hirsute subjects. Journal of Clinical Endocrinology and Metabolism 32: 717
Sairam M R, Bhargavi G N 1985 A role for glycosylation of the alpha subunit in transduction of biological signal in glycoprotein hormones. Science 229: 65
Scholl S, Lippman M E 1984 The estrogen receptor in MCF-7 cells: evidence from dense amino acid labelling for rapid turnover and a dimeric model of activated nucleic receptor. Endocrinology 115: 1295
Segaloff D L, Ascoli M 1988 Internalization of peptide hormones and hormone receptors. In: Cooke B A, King R J B, van der Molen J G J (eds) Hormones and their actions. Elsevier Science, Amsterdam, p 133
Siiteri P K 1986 Androgen binding proteins. In: Foret M G. Pugeat M (eds) Binding proteins of steroid hormones. John Libbey, London, p 593
Speroff L, Glass R H, Kase N G (eds) 1989 Clinical gynecologic endocrinology and fertility. Williams & Wilkins, Baltimore
Stabile I, Campbell S, Grudzinskas J G 1989 Ultrasound and circulating placental protein measurements in complications of early pregnancy. British Journal of Obstetrics and Gynaecology 96: 1182–1191
Sutherland R L, Watts C K W, Clarke C L 1988 Oestrogen actions. In: Cooke B A, King R J B, van der Molen H J (eds) Hormones and their actions. Elsevier Science, Amsterdam, p 193
Tseng L, Gurpide E 1975 Effects of progestins on estradiol receptor levels in human endometrium. Journal of Clinical Endocrinology and Metabolism 41: 402
Wakeling A E 1988 Physiological aspects of luteinizing hormone releasing factor and sex steroid actions: the interrelationship of agonist and antagonist activities. In: Cooke B A, King R J B, van der Molen H J (eds) Hormones and their actions. Elsevier Science, Amsterdam, p 151
Yamamoto K R 1985 Steroid receptor regulated transcription of specific genes and gene networks. Annual Review of Genetics 19: 209
Yen S C, Lein A 1976 The apparent paradox of the negative and positive feedback control system on gonadotrophin secretion. American Journal of Obstetrics and Gynecology 126: 942

FURTHER READING

Chard T 1987 An introduction to radioimmunoassay and related techniques. Elsevier/North Holland Biomedical Press, Amsterdam
Edwards R 1985 Immunoassay: an introduction. Heinemann Medical Books, London
Grudzinskas J G, Chard T, Chapman M, Cuckle H 1994 Screening for Down's syndrome. Cambridge University Press, Cambridge
Lagone J J, Van Vunakis H (eds) 1982 Methods in enzymology, vol 84: Immunochemical techniques. Academic Press, London
Voller A, Bartlett A, Bidwell D (eds) 1981 Immunoassays for the 80s. MTP Press, Lancaster

11

Sexual differentiation – normal and abnormal

D. K. Edmonds

INTRODUCTION

Sexual differentiation and its control is fundamental to the continuation of most species. The understanding of this process has advanced greatly in recent years and before abnormalities of intersex can be discussed, an understanding of normal sexual development is important. At fertilization, the haploid gametes unite and the conceptus contains 46 chromosomes, 22 autosomes derived from each of the sperm and ovum, the ovum donating one X chromosome and the sperm either one X or a Y. The axiom of mammalian reproduction is that 46XX embryo will differentiate into a female whereas a 46XY embryo becomes a male. However, it is the presence or absence of the Y chromosome which determines whether the undifferentiated gonad becomes a testis or an ovary.

Genetic control of testicular differentiation

A factor must exist on the Y chromosome which is responsible for testicular differentiation. Localization of the testicular-determining factor (TDF) was finally discovered when individuals with 46X,i(Yq) were found to be phenotypically female with streak gonads. The lack of the short arm of the Y chromosome (Yp) in those individuals localized TDF to this area.

Recent work (Page et al 1987), using DNA probes for the gene copies in XX males, has localized a segment of the short arm of the Y chromosome that contains the gene for TDF, confirming that the position of DXYS5 is the most likely sequence. This gene is known as the SRY (sex-determining region on Y) gene.

The mechanism by which differentiation occurs seems to depend on a cell surface antigen (histocompatibility antigen Y or H-Y antigen). The evidence for this is based on the work summarized by Wachtel (1983):

1. H-Y antigen is present in all individuals containing the Y chromosomes.
2. H-Y antigen is found in XY females.
3. Sex-reversed males (46XX) and true hermaphrodites have H-Y antigen.
4. H-Y antigen is present in the testicular portion of ovotestes but not the ovarian part.

Wachtel also suggests that the locus for the H-Y antigen is near that of TDF, and it may be that TDF regulates H-Y antigen expression (Wolf 1981).

Although H-Y antigen plays an integral part in testicular

development, other autosomally located genes must also be involved, as evidenced by the hereditary disorder of testicular regression syndrome. Here, the testes atrophy in late gestation – although normally functional during differentiation – and the familial nature of the condition makes autosomal genetic control most likely. Cryptorchidism is also hereditary and is associated with other genetically determined syndromes.

Genetic control of ovarian differentiation

The presence of two X chromosomes results in ovarian development, but some females with deletions of either the short or long arms of the X chromosome have variable ovarian development, or even streak ovaries alone. With regard to the short arm of X, ovarian determinants seem to be located in the region p11.2 to p21 as loss of this region results in ovarian agenesis (Simpson 1987). Deletions of the long arm in the region of Xq13 are usually associated with ovarian failure, but distal deletions may be of less importance, although X926 deletion seems to be associated with premature menopause (Fitch et al 1982). Autosomal loci are certainly involved in ovarian maintenance as gonadal dysgenesis in 46XX females is often a familial autosomal recessive disorder (Simpson 1979).

The development of müllerian and wolffian structures must also be under genetic control. The inheritance is probably polygenic multifactorial although autosomal recessive genes may be involved.

Normal embryological development of the reproductive system (Fig. 11.1)

Although the chromosomal sex is determined at the time of fertilization, gonadal sex results from differentiation of the indifferent gonad to become either a testis or an ovary. This begins during the 5th week of development. At this time, an area of coelemic epithelium develops on the medial aspect of the urogenital ridge and proliferation leads to the establishment of the gonadal ridge. Epithelial cords then grow into the mesenchyme (primary sex cords) and the gonad now possesses an outer cortex and inner medulla. In XY individuals, the medulla becomes the testis and the cortex regresses, and in embryos with an XX complement, the cortex differentiates to become the ovary and the medulla regresses. The primordial germ cells develop by the 4th week in the endodermal cells of the yolk sac and during the 5th week they migrate along the dorsal mesentery of the hindgut to the gonadal ridges, eventually becoming incorporated into the mesenchyme and the primary sex cords by the end of the 6th week.

Development of the testis

The primary sex cords become concentrated on the medulla of the gonad and proliferate and their ends anastomose to form the rete testis. The sex cords become isolated by the development of a capsule called the tunica albuginea, and the developing sex cords become the seminiferous tubules; mesenchyme grows between the tubules to separate them (Leydig cells). The seminiferous tubules are composed of two layers of cells, supporting cells (Sertoli cells) derived from the germinal epithelium and spermatogonia derived from the primordial germ cells.

Development of the ovary

The development of the ovary is much slower than that of the testis, and the ovary is not evident until the 10th week. Now the primary sex cords regress and finally disappear. Around 12 weeks, secondary sex cords arise from the germinal epithelium and the primordial germ cells become incorporated into these cortical cords. At 16 weeks, these cortical cords break up to form isolated groups of cells called primordial follicles; each cell contains an oogonium derived from a primordial germ cell, surrounded by follicular cells arising from the cortical cords. These oogonia undergo rapid mitosis to increase the numbers to thousands of germ cells called primary oocytes. Each oocyte is surrounded by a layer of follicular cells, the whole structure being called a primary follicle. The surrounding mesenchyme becomes the stroma.

Development of the genitalia

Both sexes develop two pairs of genital ducts, known as wolffian ducts (mesonephric ducts) and the müllerian ducts (paramesonephric ducts; Fig. 11.2). The wolffian ducts arise in the mesonephros on either side and run caudally to enter the urogenital sinus near the müllerian tubercle. The müllerian duct develops laterally to the wolffian duct and has an open upper end into the peritoneal cavity. It runs inferiorly and parallel to the wolffian duct, but as it reaches the caudal region, it crosses the wolffian duct anteriorly and meets it opposite, to fuse in the midline and enter the urogenital sinus, forming the müllerian tubercle.

Male development

Development of the male internal structures requires regression of the müllerian ducts by müllerian inhibitor secreted by the testis, primarily by Sertoli cells. This seems to be mediated through the release of hyaluronidase by the müllerian duct cells and thus local destruction, and also inhibition of growth factor stimulation, presumably through a specific cell membrane-associated receptor as the regression is tissue-specific. The wolffian ducts develop under the stimulation of testosterone and result in the epididymis and vas deferens, and the seminal vesicles. The

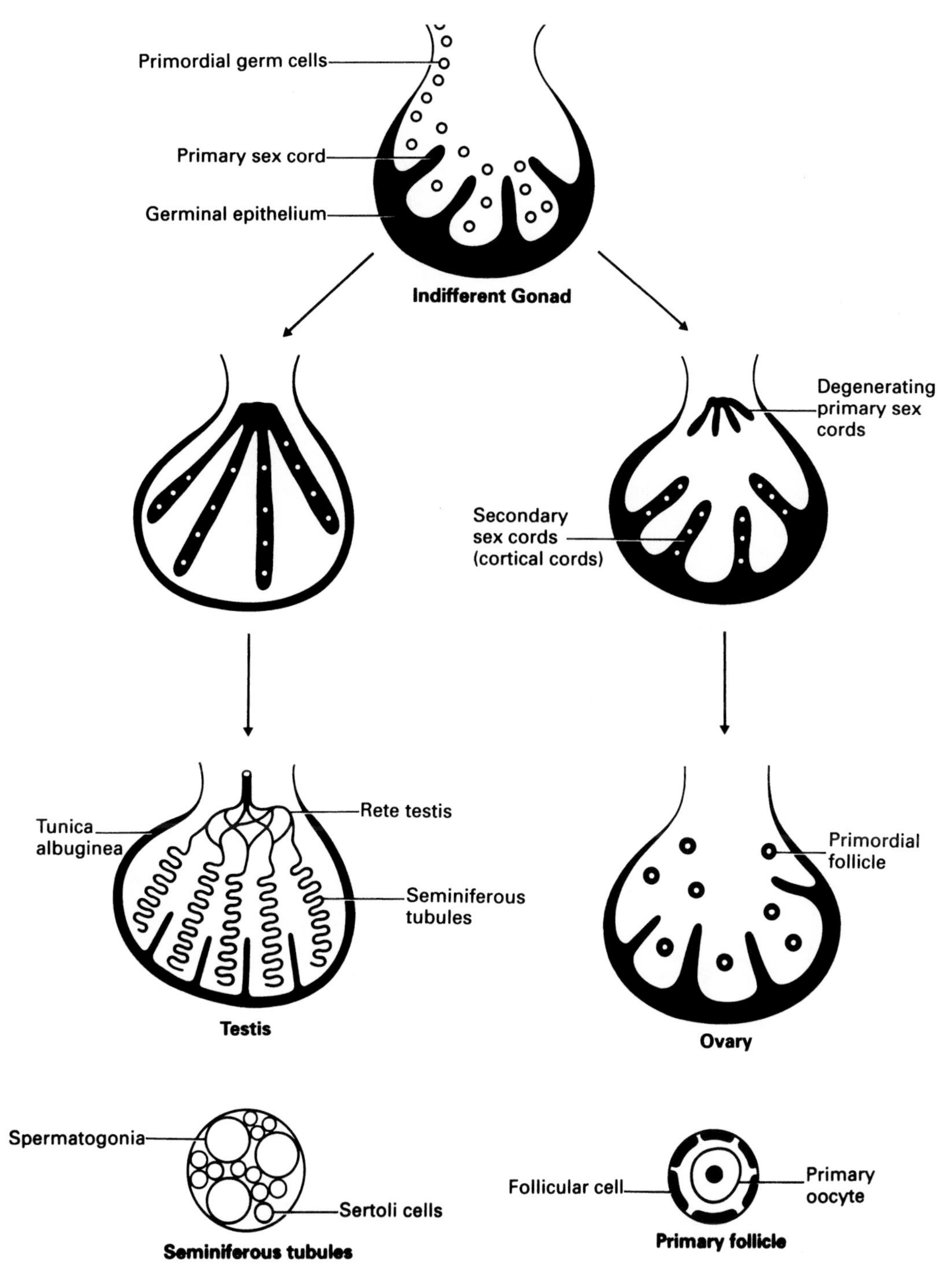

Fig. 11.1 Normal gonadal differentiation.

urogenital sinus undergoes masculinization; the penis forms from the müllerian tubercle, and the urethra forms as a result of elongation of the urogenital folds which fuse with each other along the ventral surface. The scrotum forms from fusion of the labioscrotal swellings.

Female development

The open cranial ends of the müllerian ducts become the fallopian tubes and the fused portion gives rise to the epithelium and glands of the uterus; the myometrium is derived from surrounding mesenchyme. At the point of fusion, a uterine septum is present for a short time before regressing to form a single cavity. The fusion of the müllerian ducts brings two peritoneal folds towards the midline, forming the broad ligaments. The vagina develops from two sources – the vaginal plate which arises from the sinovaginal bulbs, in the urogenital sinus, and the

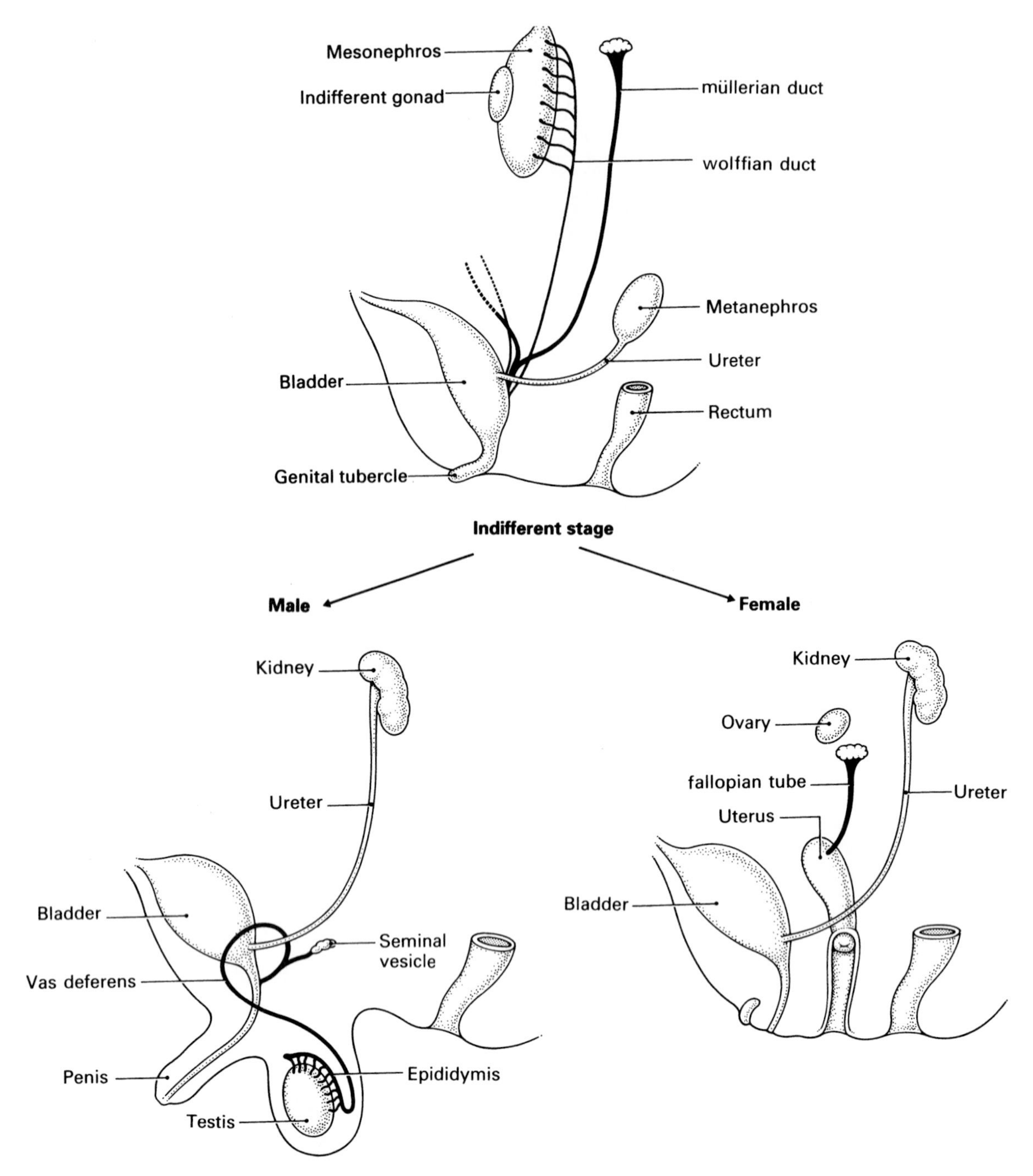

Fig. 11.2 Development of internal genitalia.

uterovaginal canal. As the uterovaginal canal reaches the pelvic portion of the urogenital sinus, there is stimulation of two endodermal autogrowths which are called the sino-vaginal bulbs. These fuse to form a solid vaginal plate and this grows rapidly in a cranial direction giving the vaginal plate length. It eventually cavitates, beginning caudally, and by 20 weeks the vagina is fully formed (Fig. 11.3). The hymen represents the remains of the müllerian tubercle. The wolffian structures regress due to lack of testosterone stimulation, although occasional remnants may persist, i.e. hydatid cyst of Morgagni, Gartner's duct cysts.

The external genitalia in the female result from feminization of the urogenital sinus. The müllerian tubercle grows initially before ceasing and becoming the clitoris. The unfused urogenital folds form the labia minora; the labioscrotal folds form the labia majora.

FEMALE INTERSEX DISORDERS

Definition

This group of disorders comprises conditions in which masculinization of the external genitalia occurs in patients

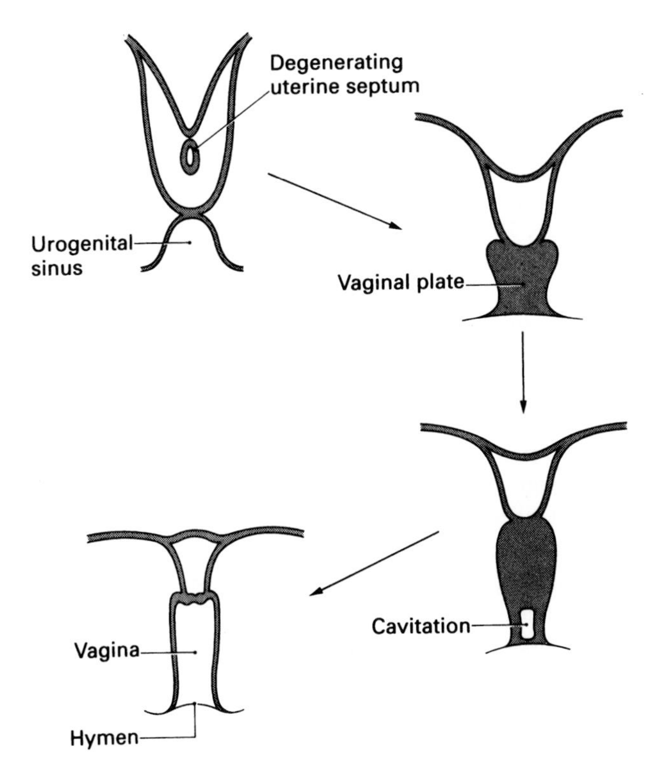

Fig. 11.3 Development of uterus and vagina.

with a normal 46XX karyotype. The degree of masculinization is variable, ranging from mild clitoromegaly to complete fusion of the labial folds with a penile urethra.

Pathophysiology

The abnormalities occur when a female fetus is exposed to elevated levels of androgens. As the differentiation of the external genitalia to male or female depends on the conversion of testosterone to dihydrotestosterone (DHT) in the tissues of the cloaca, the presence of DHT leads to male-type development. If the female fetus is exposed to low levels of androgen, partial masculinization may occur, leading to ambiguous genitalia, but if the levels are high enough, then complete male external genital development may occur, although the testes are naturally absent. If androgen exposure is delayed until after 12 weeks, then virilizaton is limited to clitoral enlargement with no effect on the already differentiated labia. Androgens have no effect on internal sexual development and therefore the ovaries, uterus and upper vagina are normally formed and functional.

Aetiology

The causes of the androgenization are due to excessive androgens either:

1. arising in a fetus, e.g. congenital adrenal hyperplasia;
2. arising in the mother, e.g. androgen-secreting tumour;
3. ingested by the mother, e.g. progestogens, danazol.

There are also cases which are associated with other congenital abnormalities or which are idiopathic.

Congenital adrenal hyperplasia

Pathophysiology

This is the most common cause of female pseudohermaphroditism and is an autosomal recessive disorder resulting in enzyme deficiency in the biosynthesis of cortisol in the adrenal. Cortisol production occurs in the zona fasciculata and zona reticularis (Fig. 11.4) and is con-

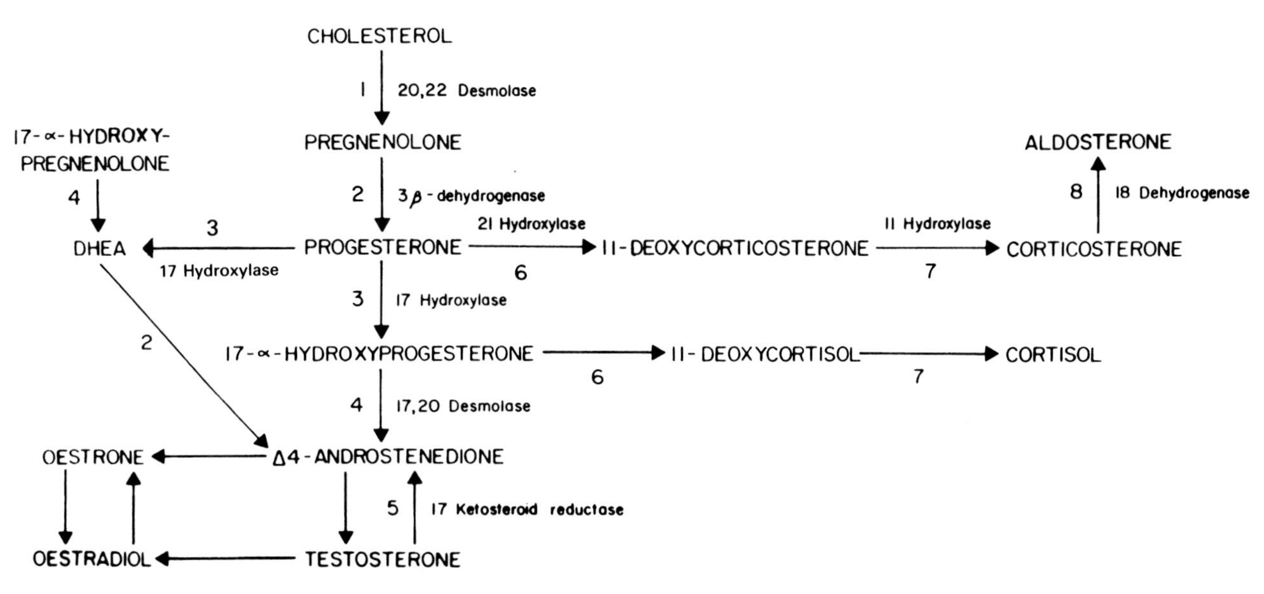

Fig. 11.4 Adrenal synthesis of steroids.

trolled by adrenocorticotrophic hormone (ACTH) secreted by the pituitary gland. Adrenal androgen production occurs in the same area and is influenced by ACTH. A deficiency in any enzyme in the pathway results in decreased production of cortisol with resultant elevated levels of ACTH. This leads to increased steroid production by the adrenal reticularis and consequent hyperplasia. The stimulation by ACTH elevates the levels of circulating androgens and this results in the virilization of the female fetus.

There are three adrenal enzyme deficiencies which result in masculinization: 21-hydroxylase, 11-hydroxylase and 3β-dehydrogenase deficiency.

21-Hydroxylase deficiency

This accounts for 90% of all cases of congenital adrenal hyperplasia. The deficiency results in an increase in progesterone and 17α-hydroxyprogesterone and this substrate is therefore converted to androstenedione and subsequently to testosterone.

Failure of 21-hydroxylase to convert progesterone to 11-deoxycorticosterone may result in aldosterone deficiency; this occurs in about two-thirds of cases. This is the so-called 'salt-losing' type of CAH.

Aetiology. Deficiency of 21-hydroxylase is an autosomal recessive disorder. The link between human leukocyte antigen (HLA) type and 21-hydroxylase deficiency was established by Dupont et al (1977) and this allowed mapping of the gene which was located on the short arm of chromosome 6. It is located between the HLA-B and HLA-DR loci, and subgroups of HLA-B have been closely linked to congenital adrenal hyperplasia types; HLA-BW47 is linked to salt-losing congenital adrenal hyperplasia, and HLA-BW51 to the simple virilizing form. Studies by Donohoue et al (1986), have shown that there are two 21-hydroxylase genes, i.e. 21-OHA and 21-OHB. Only one is active (21-OHB) and they both lie between the fourth components of complement C4A and C4B. A variety of mutations have been reported, including gene deletions of 21-OHB, gene conversions and point mutations.

Epidemiology. The incidence of 21-hydroxylase deficiency is between 1/5000 and 1/15 000, based on neonatal screening programmes (Cacciari et al 1983), although a higher incidence (1/700) has been reported in specific populations of Eskimos (Pang et al 1982). The incidence of the non-classic form of the disease, when androgenization fails to appear before late childhood or puberty, is much more common, about 1/300 in the white population and 1/30 in European Jews (Pang et al 1988).

Presentation. Affected females are born with an enlarged clitoris, fused labioscrotal folds and a urogenital sinus which may become a phallic urethra. There is often a great variation of the degree of masculinization of the external genitalia; this is classified according to Prader (1958).

The internal genitalia develop normally as they are not influenced by androgens.

In the salt-losing form, the infants develop dehydration, hypotension and hyponatraemia between 7 and 28 days of age, known as a salt-losing crisis. The non-salt-losing form tends to cause less severe masculinization than the salt-losing type. In general, all children born with ambiguous genitalia, including cryptorchidism and hypospadias, should be screened for congenitial adrenal hyperplasia. Without treatment, severe salt-losing disease is fatal.

When an infant is born with ambiguous genitalia, the management of the parents is very important. It is helpful to reassure them that the infant is healthy and that there is a developmental anomaly of the genitalia. If the initial examination of the child fails to identify palpable gonads, it is most likely that the child is female, and the parents should be informed as such and the likelihood of congenital adrenal hyperplasia may be raised. The diagnosis must then be made with as much haste as possible to alleviate parental anxiety.

Investigation. The initial investigations are karyotyping, pelvic ultrasound and then endocrine studies. The karyotype may be performed on a sample of cord blood or on a venous sample and rapid results obtained. Pelvic ultrasound to discover the presence of a uterus and vagina will confirm the diagnosis. The specific diagnosis is made by measuring 17α-hydroxyprogesterone in serum, although a 24-hour urinary estimate of 17-ketosteroids will also confirm the diagnosis.

Treatment. This is divided into four parts:

1. *Acute salt-losing crisis.* This involves correcting the electrolyte imbalance and replacing the cortisol deficiency with desoxycorticosterone acetate (DOCA), 1 mg/24 h For the majority of cases (9α-fludrocortisol is used in a dose of 0.1–0.2 mg/day added to the oral feed, and the dosage of DOCA or fludrocortisol adjusted against the electrolyte levels.
2. *Long-term cortisol replacement therapy.* Although previous reports suggested that mineralocorticoid therapy could be discontinued after infancy (Newns 1974), more recent data suggest that it is essential to continue therapy for life (Hughes et al 1979).
3. *Surgical correction.* Once the sex of rearing has been established as female, some attempt to feminize the genitalia may be made, usually within the first 18 months of life. If the clitoris is enlarged, a reduction clitoridectomy can be performed, and the perineal region modified (Edmonds 1989). There are major surgical problems associated with severe virilization in congenital adrenal hyperplasia. The urogenital sinus has been formed by labial fold fusion and the folds are usually thin, but may be thick with associated narrowing of the lower vagina, especially in salt-losers. If the labial folds are thin, division by a simple

posterior incision may be performed around age 3 or 4 years. However, thick perineal tissue should be left until after puberty and no attempt at surgery should be made until the girl is physically and mentally sexually mature. The operation, when it is performed, involves a flap vaginoplasty with a pedicle graft of labia used to recreate the vagina. Alternatively, a Williams vaginoplasty may be used.

Mulaikal et al (1987) reviewed the fertility rates in 80 women with 21-hydroxylase deficiency: of 25 with the simple form who attempted pregnancy, 15 were successful, whereas of the salt-losers who tried to become pregnant, only one succeeded. There is no doubt that a major reason for the failure of the salt-loser group is the disappointing results of surgery and subsequent lack of adequate sexual function.

4. *Psychological support.* As the child grows, long-term psychological guidance and support will be required for the parents initially, and then the child.

Prenatal diagnosis. If the parents are heterozygous carriers of 21-hydroxylase deficiency, the fetus has a 1 in 4 chance of being affected. Thus, prenatal diagnosis is important, either by amniocentesis to measure amniotic fluid 17-hydroxyprogesterone levels or by HLA typing of amniotic cells, or chorionic villus sampling and the use of specific DNA probes. Once the diagnosis has been made, the option is available to treat the pregnant woman with oral dexamethasone, which crosses the placenta and suppresses the secretion of ACTH and thus the circulating androgen levels.

11-Hydroxylase deficiency

This is the hypertensive form of congenital adrenal hyperplasia which accounts for about 5–8% of all cases (Zachmann et al 1983). The absence of 11-hydroxylase leads to elevated levels of 11-deoxycorticosterone (DOC) and although this means a decreased amount of aldosterone, DOC has salt-retaining properties, leading to hypertension. Androstenedione levels are also elevated and this can result in ambiguous genitalia.

The diagnosis is made by measuring elevated levels of urinary 17-hydroxycorticosteroids, and raised serum androstenedione. Treatment is similar to 21-hydroxylase deficiency, with glucocorticoid replacement therapy.

The genetics, however, are rather different. There is no HLA association with 11-hydroxylase deficiency, but the use of a DNA probe has located the gene on the long arm of chromosome 8 (White et al 1985).

3β-Dehydrogenase deficiency

This rare form of congenital adrenal hyperplasia results in a block of steroidogenesis very early in the pathway, giving rise to a severe salt-losing adrenal hyperplasia. The androgen most elevated is dehydroepiandrosterone, an androgen which causes mild virilization. The diagnosis rests on the measurement of elevated dehydroepiandrosterone. The gene encoding 3β-dehydrogenase has not yet been cloned but it is not linked to HLA.

Androgen-secreting tumours

Androgen-secreting tumours are rare in pregnancy, but may arise in the ovary or the adrenal. They cause fetal virilization. When they occur in the non-pregnant woman, anovulation is induced.

Ovary

A number of androgen-secreting tumours have been reported including luteoma (Cohen et al 1982, Hensleigh & Woodruff 1978), polycystic ovaries (Fayez et al 1974), mucinous cystadenoma (Novak et al 1970, Post et al 1978), arrhenoblastoma (Barkan et al 1984) and Krukenberg tumours (Connor et al 1968, Forest et al 1978). Not all female fetuses will be affected and there is no association with gestation and exposure. The fetus may be partly protected by the conversion of the maternally derived androgen to oestrogen in the placenta, and thus the degree of virilization is variable.

Adrenal

There are only two reports of adrenal adenomas causing fetal masculinization (Fuller et al 1983, Murset et al 1970). These tumours may be human chorionic gonadotrophin-responsive, and thus levels of androgen may be higher in pregnancy than in the non-pregnant state, leading to androgenization of the fetus.

Drugs

The association between the use of progestogens and masculinization of the female fetus has received much publicity, but the only progestogen proven to have such an effect is 17-ethinyl testosterone (Ishizuka et al 1962). These infants had clitoromegaly and in some cases labioscrotal fusion, but the risk is very small (1/50). Gestogens which are derived from testosterone should be avoided in the pregnant woman. There have been two case reports of androgenization of female fetuses from exposure to danazol during pregnancy (Castro-Magana et al 1981, Duck & Katamaya 1981) and both babies were born with external genitalia similar to those with adrenogenital syndrome.

Associated multiple congenital abnormalities

Female intersex has been described in association with a

number of multiple abnormality states, most commonly those associated with the urinary and gastrointestinal tracts. It has also been described in association with VATER syndrome (Say & Carpentier 1979).

The management of these children with masculinized genitalia is to ensure the assignation of a sex of rearing and modify the genitalia appropriately. In all of these rare cases, the female role has been chosen and reduction clitoroplasty performed.

XY FEMALE

The normal differentiation of the gonad to become a testis has been described above, and its subsequent secretion of testosterone leads to development of the wolffian duct and the urogenital sinus to produce the normal male internal and external genitalia. Testosterone is the predominant male sex hormone secreted by the testis but two other processes are necessary for normal development: the conversion of testosterone to DHT by 5α-reductase, and the presence of androgen receptors in the target cell which bind with the DHT or testosterone and produce appropriate nuclear function. Thus, normal male genotype, i.e. XY, with a female phenotype will occur if there is:

1. failure of testicular development,
2. error(s) in testosterone biosynthesis, or
3. androgen insensitivity at the target site.

Failure of testicular development

This group of disorders includes true gonadal dysgenesis, Leydig cell hypoplasia and the persistent müllerian duct syndrome.

True gonadal agenesis

True gonadal agenesis is characterized by the complete absence of any gonadal tissue and therefore the development of female internal and external genitalia. The karyotype can be either 46XY or 46XX. These patients present in the teenage years with failure of pubertal development (Ch. 13).

Leydig cell hypoplasia

Leydig cell hypoplasia is an uncommon condition, of which the aetiology remains speculative. The role of fetal luteinizing hormone in normal testicular development is unknown, but it may be necessary for maturation of the interstitial cells into Leydig cells. Failure of luteinizing hormone production in the first trimester will result in Leydig cell hypoplasia and male pseudohermaphroditism (or an autosomal recessive disorder resulting in absent luteinizing hormone receptors will cause absence of Leydig cells). This manifests as ambiguous genitalia, in both circumstances due to some androgen production by Sertoli cells. Clinically, Leydig cell hypoplasia usually presents as a phenotypical female with primary amenorrhoea and sexual infantilism (see Ch. 1) but ambiguity at birth may result in diagnosis in infancy.

Errors in testosterone biosynthesis

This type of disorder accounts for only 4% of XY females, and results from deficiency of an enzyme involved in testosterone synthesis (see Fig. 11.4).

20–22 Desmolase deficiency

Absence of this enzyme results in failure to convert cholesterol to pregnenolone and a failure of subsequent steroid production. Most of the reported cases have died in early life due to adrenal insufficiency, but the XY individuals are all partially virilized with a small blind vaginal pouch. It is considered to be an autosomal recessive disorder.

3β-Hydroxysteroid dehydrogenase deficiency

This is a rare disorder which affects both adrenal and gonadal function, and is again autosomally recessive. The deficiency may be complete or incomplete and thus the degree of virilization is variable, to various degrees of hypospadias, or a small blind vagina with normal internal male genitalia and absent müllerian structures. Those individuals who have survived and reached puberty have developed gynaecomastia, presumably because the absence of testosterone during fetal life has allowed breast bud development. The diagnosis is made by elevated levels of pregnenolone and 17-hydroxy-pregnenolone and low levels of corticosteroids and testosterone.

17α-Hydroxylase deficiency

This syndrome produces a phenotype in XY individuals, varying from normal female external genitalia and a blind vaginal pouch to hypospadias with a small phallus. The diagnosis is usually only made in adulthood with failure to develop secondary sexual characteristics. The impaired adrenal production of cortisol is not associated with clinical symptoms as the elevated levels of corticosterone compensate. The gonads should be removed if the patient is assigned a female gender and hormone replacement therapy instituted.

17–20 Desmolase deficiency

This enzyme defect primarily affects testosterone production and there is no adrenal insufficiency. The clinical findings range from normal female to undervirilized male genitalia, and the endocrine findings are of very low serum levels of testosterone with normal corticosteroids. Again, diagnosis may not be made until failure of pubertal development.

17-Ketosteroid reductase deficiency

This enzyme is responsible for the reversible conversion of androstenedione to testosterone and oestrone to oestradiol. These patients almost always present at birth with female external genitalia and testes in the inguinal canal, and undergo masculinization at puberty. Those individuals to be raised as females should have their gonads removed before puberty, and oestrogen therapy begun at puberty.

Androgen insensitivity at the target site (Table 11.1)

In this group of patients testicular function is normal and circulating levels of androgen are consistent with normal male development. The majority of patients present at puberty with primary amenorrhoea, but some will present with ambiguous genitalia. The defect may be 5α-reductase deficiency, or complete or partial androgen insensitivity.

5α-Reductase deficiency

This results in the failure of the conversion of testosterone to DHT in target tissues and thus a failure of masculinization of the site. In infancy, there is usually a small phallus, some degree of hypospadias, a bifid scrotum and a blind vaginal pouch. The testes are found either in the inguinal canal or in the labioscrotal folds, and müllerian structures are absent. At puberty, elevated levels of androgen lead to masculinization, including an increase in phallic growth, although this remains smaller than normal. Seminal production has been reported (Petersen et al 1977).

It is an autosomal recessive trait, and the resulting enzyme defect gives predictable hormone profiles with normal levels of testosterone, but low levels of DHT. The diagnosis is important in individuals born with ambiguous genitalia in order to assign the sex of rearing, and this should be based on the potential for normal sexual function in adult life. The gonads should be removed if the sex of rearing is to be female, and at puberty oestrogen replacement therapy instituted.

Table 11.1 Types of androgen insensitivity and their abnormalities

Defect	External genitalia	Internal genitalia	Gonad	Phenotype at puberty
5α-Reductase deficiency	Female or ambiguous	Male	Testis	Masculine
Complete androgen insensitivity	Female	Male	Testis	Infantile and breast growth
Partial androgen insensitivity	Ambiguous	Male	Testis	Partial masculine and breast growth

Complete androgen insensitivity

This is an X-linked recessive disorder characterized by the clinical features of normal female external genitalia, a blind vaginal pouch and absent müllerian and wolffian structures. The testes are found either in the labial folds or inguinal canal or they may be intra-abdominal.

These patients may lack the presence of the androgen receptor, and may be shown to lack the gene located on the X chromosome between Xp11 and Xq13. Work by Brown et al (1982) however suggests that there may be a variety of defects, ranging from absence of receptors to presence of a normal number of receptors which are inactive. The exact mechanism of the defects in patients with androgen receptors awaits definition.

The hormonal levels of testosterone which are elevated above normal due to increased luteinizing hormone production and the associated increase in testicular oestradiol and peripheral conversion of androgens to oestradiol promotes some breast development. Pubic hair growth depends on the degree of insensitivity but is usually rather scanty.

Patients either present with a hernial mass or with primary amenorrhoea despite secondary sexual characteristics; karyotyping makes the diagnosis. The gonads should be removed because of the malignant potential. The vagina may be of variable length and may be adequate, but those with a short vaginal pouch may need manual dilatation.

Partial androgen insensitivity

This is a complex condition which has been found to be due to a reduced binding affinity of DHT to the receptor, or because the receptor binds the DHT but there are defects in the transcription to the nucleus. It is an X-linked recessive disorder and the partial expression means inevitable ambiguous genitalia with a blind vaginal pouch and phallic enlargement. The penis can be normal. The wolffian ducts can be rudimentary or normal, but the testes are azoospermic. The most common presentation in infancy is hypospadias with the urethra opening at the base of the phallus, and there may be cryptorchidism. At puberty, male secondary sexual characteristics develop poorly, but there is usually gynaecomastia. The management is dependent on the degree of ambiguity and subsequent choice of sex of rearing, with gonadectomy and hormone replacement therapy for those assigned the female role.

ANOMALOUS VAGINAL DEVELOPMENT

When the vagina does not develop normally, a number of abnormalities have been described. The vagina may be partially maldeveloped, leading to a vaginal obstruction which may be complete or incomplete, or there may be total maldevelopment of the müllerian ducts leading to various disorders.

Classification

Vaginal anomalies may be categorized as follows:

1. congenital absence of the müllerian ducts (the Mayer–Rokitansky–Kuster-Hauser syndrome),
2. disorders of vertical fusion,
3 failure of lateral fusion.

Aetiology

There are three mechanisms which may explain most vaginal anomalies. They may be familial, for example XY females who have a hereditary disorder as described previously. Congenital absence of the vagina has been very rarely reported in XX siblings (Jones & Mermut 1974) and also in monozygotic twins with only one child affected (Lischke et al 1973).

The case of a female limited autosomal dominant trait was first reported by Shokeir (1978) who studied 16 Saskatchewan families in which there was a proband with vaginal agenesis. However Carson et al (1983), in a study of 23 probands, disputed the Shokeir theory. The previous evidence with regard to monozygotic twins also makes this mode of inheritance unlikely. Polygenic or multifactorial inheritance does, however, offer some explanation that families may exhibit the trait as reported. The recurrence risk of a polygenic multifactorial trait in first-degree relatives is reported to be between 1 and 5%.

Finally, it is possible that müllerian duct defects could be secondary to teratogens or other environmental factors but no definite association has been demonstrated.

Epidemiology

The incidence of vaginal malformations has been variously estimated between 1/4000 and 1/10 000 female births (Evans et al 1981). The infrequency of this anomaly makes accurate estimates of the true incidence very difficult to obtain but when considered as a cause of primary amenorrhoea, vaginal malformation ranks second to gonadal dysgenesis.

Pathophysiology

The pathophysiology of vaginal absence may be either as a result of failure of the vaginal plate to form, or failure of

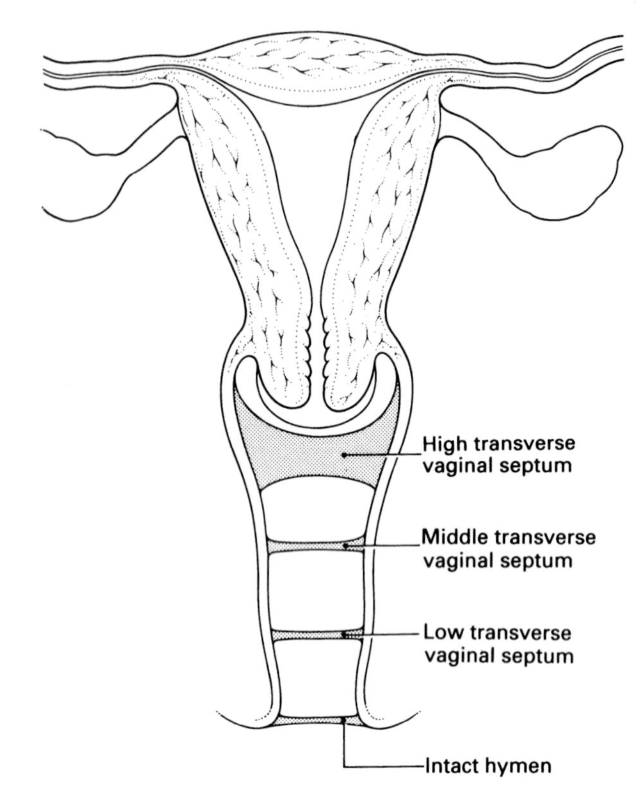

Fig. 11.5 Disorders of vertical fusion.

cavitation. Absence of the uterus and fallopian tubes indicates total failure of müllerian duct development but in the Rokitansky syndrome, the uterus is often present although rudimentary, and therefore it must be failure of vaginal plate formation and subsequent vaginal development which leads to the absent vagina. Vertical fusion defects (Fig. 11.5) may result from failure of fusion of the müllerian system with the urogenital sinus, or it may be due to incomplete canalization of the vagina, Disorders of lateral fusion are due to the failure of the müllerian ducts to unite and may create a duplicated uterovaginal septum which may be obstructive or non-obstructive, depending on the mode of development (Fig. 11.6).

Presentation

Vaginal atresia

Vaginal atresia presents at puberty with complicated or uncomplicated primary amenorrhoea. In the majority who have an absent or rudimentary uterus, uncomplicated primary amenorrhoea is the presenting symptom, but those women who have a functional uterus may develop an associated haematometra and present with cyclical abdominal pain. If a haematometra does develop, there will be uterine distension and an abdominal mass may be palpable but more commonly is felt on rectal examination.

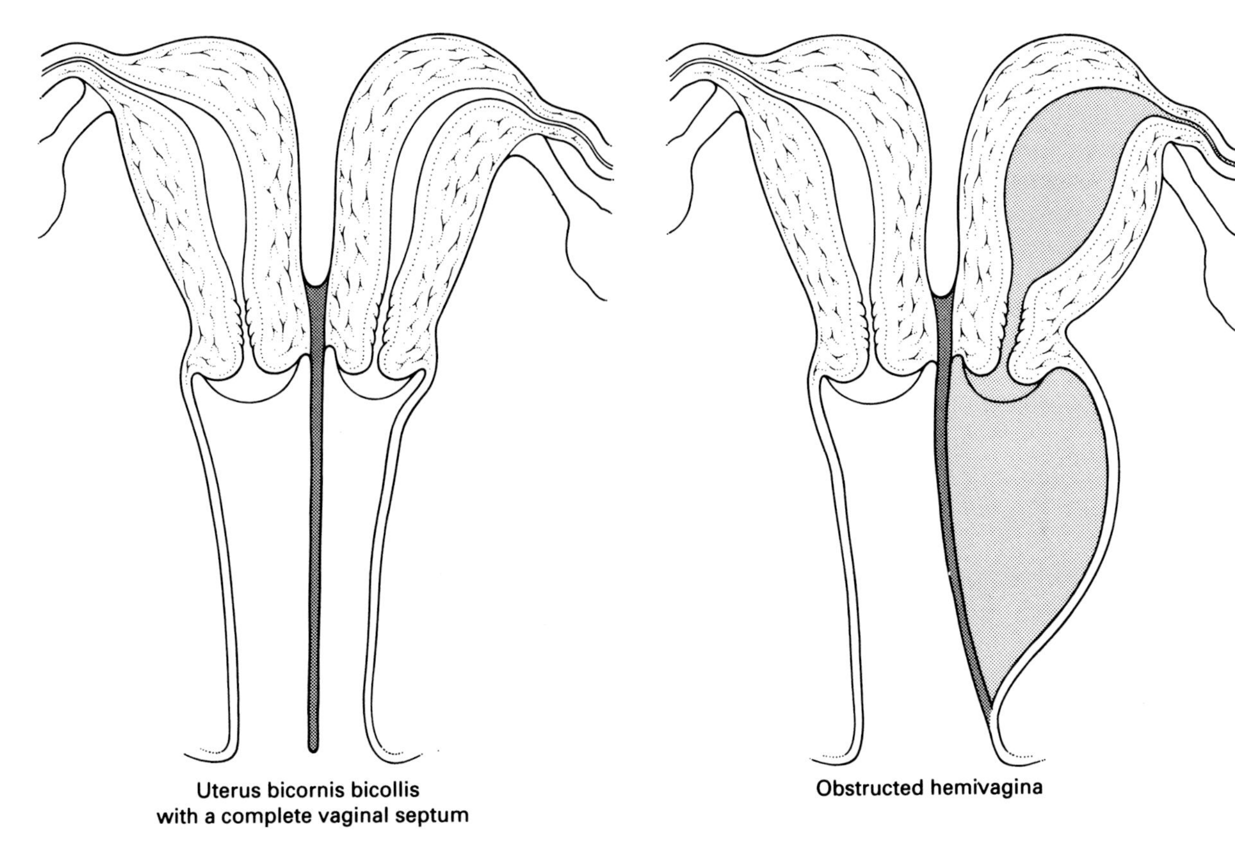

Fig. 11.6 Lateral fusion defects.

Vertical fusion defects

Here, the transverse vaginal septum prevents loss of menstrual blood and therefore cryptomenorrhoea results. Most patients present as teenagers with cyclical abdominal pain and a haematocolpos will be palpable within the pelvis on rectal examination. The patient may also present from associated pressure symptoms of urinary frequency and/or retention. The incidence of vertical fusion defects is reported as 46% high, 35% mid, and 19% low septae in the vagina (Rock et al 1982).

Disorders of lateral fusion

These patients usually present with the incidental finding of a vaginal septum which is usually asymptomatic. It may well first be diagnosed during pregnancy at which time excision will be necessary to ensure a vaginal delivery. However, these patients may present with dyspareunia caused by the septum and in most cases one vagina is larger than the other and intercourse may have occurred partially successfully in the larger side. In the unilateral vaginal obstruction group, presentation is usually with abdominal pain and the associated symptoms of a haematometra and haematocolpos. The confusing clinical sign is the associated menstruation from the other side and the diagnosis may be missed if careful examination is not performed in these teenagers.

Investigation

Vaginal atresia

A patient presenting with a clinically absent vagina and no cyclical abdominal pain requires an ultrasound examination of the pelvis to determine the presence or absence of a uterus and/or a haematometra. Laparoscopy in these patients is unnecessary. Some 15% of patients with the Rokitansky syndrome suffer major defects of the urinary system, including congenital absence of a kidney; 40% of patients also have trivial urinary abnormalities (D'Alberton et al 1981). It is therefore important to perform an intravenous urogram in order to establish any abnormalities in the renal system or the presence of a pelvic kidney which may alert the surgeon to take extra care if abdominal operation becomes necessary.

Anomalies of the bony skeleton occur in about 12% of patients. These include abnormalities of the lumbar spine, the cervical vertebrae and also limb abnormalities. However, it may be that the incidence of bony abnormalities is higher than this, as investigation of the skeletal system is rarely performed.

Transverse vaginal septum

Investigations in these patients is limited to ultrasound assessment of the uterus for the detection of a haematometra and haematocolpos, and this may also be used to assess the level of the septal defect. Again, investigation of the urinary tract is pertinent.

Lateral fusion defects

Investigations in this group are only important if there is an obstructed outflow problem and should follow those outlined for vertical fusion defects.

Treatment

Vaginal atresia

The patient with müllerian agenesis requires careful psychological counselling and associated therapy. The psychological impact of being informed that there is an absent vagina comes as an immense shock to both patient and parents. It is almost always followed by a period of depression in which many patients question their femininity and look upon themselves as abnormal females. They very much doubt their ability to enter a heterosexual relationship which will be lasting, and feel worthless both sexually and certainly as regards being a reproductive partner. In some patients the depression can be very profound and suicide may be threatened. There is also great maternal anxiety over the aetiology as most mothers feel that they are responsible for the abnormality. Reassurance of the mother is as important as that of the daughter in the management of the patient.

Occasionally cultural problems arise which make management much more difficult, especially in ethnic groups where the ability to procreate is fundamental to marriage and social acceptance. These patients and their parents can be very difficult to console and often refuse to accept the situation, questioning the diagnosis of their sterility over a number of years. The immediate reaction of most patients is to request surgical correction of the abnormality to return them to 'normal'. Unfortunately, opting for surgical treatment without adequate psychological and physical preparation inevitably leads to disaster. We recommend a minimum of 6 months of preparation before any surgical procedure is performed, and during this time psychological support can be implemented for the patient and her parents. There are two major areas of support required: firstly, the correction of the loss of esteem and inevitable depression, and repeated counselling sessions by trained personnel are required if these symptoms are to be overcome. The second problem involves the psychological aspect, and again prolonged counselling sessions will be required if an adequate and fulfilling sex life is going to be possible in the future. The sexual life achieved by well managed patients can be excellent and has been reported as comparable to that of the normal population (Poland & Evans 1985, Raboch & Horejsi 1982).

Management of the absent vagina with a non-functioning uterus

In a patient with an absent or rudimentary uterus, the creation of a vaginal passage may be non-surgical or surgical. The non-surgical technique involves the repeated use of graduated vaginal dilators over a period of 6–12 months. A minimum of 1 cm of vaginal dimple is necessary for this technique to succeed and patients require support and encouragement during this time. Patients are instructed to begin with a small vaginal dilator which is pressed firmly against the vaginal dimple for a period of some 20 minutes twice a day. Pressure is exerted but pain should be avoided and repeated use of these vaginal dilators will be met with success in about 90% of cases with appropriate selection (Broadbent et al 1984). This technique was first described by Frank in 1938 and in view of the undoubted success of the technique with no complications, this method must be attempted in all girls with an absent vagina and a 1 cm dimple before any surgical procedure be considered.

In those girls with a vagina of less than 1 cm or those in whom Frank's procedure fails, vaginoplasty will be required. There are currently three techniques in popular usage: the McIndoe–Reed operation, the amnion vaginoplasty and the Williams vulvovaginoplasty.

The *McIndoe–Reed* procedure was first described in 1938 (McIndoe & Banister 1938) and involved the use of a split-thickness skin graft over a solid mould; this mould is placed in a surgically created space between the urethra and the rectum. This space is created digitally following a transverse incision in the vaginal dimple. Digital exploration of the space must be performed with great care as damage to the bladder or the rectum may occur. The space created must reach the peritoneum of the pouch of Douglas if an adequate length of vagina is to be created. A split-thickness skin graft is then taken from a donor site and an appropriately sized mould is chosen. The skin graft is then fashioned over the mould with the external skin surface in apposition to the mould. The skin-covered mould is then placed in the neovaginal space and the labia are sutured together to hold the mould in situ. McIndoe reported his own series of 105 patients in 1959 and had a satisfactory outcome in 80% of patients. Cali & Pratt (1968) reported on their series of 123 patients; 90% had good sexual function. However, 6% had major complications which were primarily fistulae; subsequent reconstructive surgery was necessary in 8%. These complications resulted in modifications of the technique and the use of a soft material for the mould to prevent fistula formation due to pressure necrosis.

The search for an alternative material to line the neovagina and avoid the scarring of the donor skin site led to the use of *amnion* for the vaginoplasty procedure (Ashworth et al 1986). The technique involves the creation of a neovaginal space in the same way as described for the McIndoe–Reed procedure but amnion obtained at the time of elective caesarean section is used to line the neovagina. The mesenchymal surface of the amnion is placed against the new vaginal surface to promote epithelialization and the mould is kept in situ for 7 days and then replaced with a new amnion graft for a further 7 days. Subsequently patients are encouraged in the frequent use of dilators to maintain the vaginal passage. Again, reported success of around 90% has been achieved by these authors.

The *Williams vulvovaginoplasty* (Williams 1976) still has an important place in the management of these disorders, but is much less frequently used than in the past. In patients in whom dissection of a neovagina is impossible but the labia majora are normal, this technique is invaluable. The principle of the operation is to create a vaginal pouch from the full-thickness skin flaps created from the labia majora, which are united in the midline. Following surgery and adequate healing, the patient is taught to use vaginal dilators in the same way as described in the Frank technique. There is no doubt that this does allow the patient and her partner to enjoy a sex life with mutual orgasm but the angle of the vagina is unnatural and unsatisfactory for some patients. Although the operation is simple to perform, the psychological problems of the distorted external genitalia can be considerable.

The absent vagina with a coexistent functional uterus

This situation presents major problems as the release of menstrual blood and the relief of associated pain are the primary aims; the creation of a normal vagina is an equally important yet secondary role. The functional uterus may be normal and a cervix may be present or absent. This situation is very rare; an operation to create a neovagina in an attempt to reanastomose a uterus which has been drained of its haematometra is highly specialized and will not be discussed further.

Complications

Some 25% of women will have some degree of dyspareunia following a vaginoplasty (Smith 1983). This is most commonly due to scarring at the upper margin of the vagina, involving the peritoneum. Similar incidences of dyspareunia occur in nearly all series and it is difficult to know how best to avoid this. It seems to occur regardless of technique, but contraction of the upper part of the vagina is difficult to avoid. The artificial vagina created in these ways acquires all the characteristics of normal vaginal epithelium and the exposure of the grafted epithelium to a new environment means that care has to be taken to ensure it remains healthy. Four cases of intraepithelial neoplasia in neovaginas have been reported (Duckler 1972, Imrie et al 1986, Jackson 1959, Rotmensch et al 1983).

Management of disorders of vertical fusion

In these abnormalities, the type of procedure is governed by the type of abnormality. In the obstructed hymen the procedure is extremely simple and a cruciate incision through the hymen will release the accumulated menstrual blood and resolve the problem. In obstructing transverse vaginal septae in the lower and middle thirds, surgical removal of the septum can almost always be performed transvaginally and a reanastomosis of the upper and lower vaginal segments may be performed. Great care must be taken to ensure that the excision is adequate or a vaginal stenosis at the site of the septum will remain a problem. The high vaginal septum is the most difficult abnormality to manage and it is almost always necessary to perform a laparotomy in order to expose the haematometra. The passage of a probe through the uterine cavity and cervix into the short upper vagina allows a second vaginal surgeon to explore the vagina from below and excise the septum. It is usual that the absent portion of vagina is so great that reanastomosis of the vaginal mucosa cannot be achieved and either a soft mould is inserted and granulation allowed to occur, or an amnion-covered soft mould should be inserted to promote epithelialization. Vaginal dilatation following removal of the mould must be encouraged in order to prevent constriction of the new vaginal area.

Results. The results of surgery are extremely good when judged by sexual satisfaction. However, Rock et al (1982) reported pregnancy success following surgical correction of transverse vaginal septa and noted that patients with a transverse vaginal septum had only a 47% pregnancy rate when the site of the septum was taken into account. If the obstruction was in the lower third, then all patients achieved a pregnancy; in the middle third 43% and in the upper third 25% of patients became pregnant. It is suggested that the difficulties in conceiving may be secondary to the development of endometriosis and the higher the site of the septum, the more likely the development of this disorder may be. Thus prompt diagnosis and surgical correction is important in an attempt to preserve the maximum reproductive capacity in these patients.

Complications. Complications are primarily those of dyspareunia and failure of pregnancy, as described above.

Disorders of lateral fusion

The treatment of this condition depends on the abnormality. In patients with a midline septum and no other abnormality, excision of the septum should be performed and care must be taken as these septa can be very thick and removal can be rather difficult. When resecting the septum, generous pedicles should be taken to ensure haemostasis and the results are extremely good as the remaining tissue usually retracts and causes no problem. In patients in whom there is an incomplete vaginal obstruction, again the septum needs to be removed and care must be taken to remove as much of it as possible. Failure to do this will result in healing of an ostium and repeat obstruction of the hemivagina. The results and outlook for these patients are extremely good.

MALFORMATIONS OF THE UTERUS

Classification and pathophysiology

There have been numerous classification systems for uterine malformations varying between those based on embryological development to those based on obstetric performance. However, the most widely used classification in current use is that of Buttram & Gibbons (1979) which is based upon the degree of failure of normal development. There are six categories described.

Class I: Müllerian agenesis or hypoplasia.
Class II: Unicornuate uterus.
Class III: Uterus didelphis.
Class IV: Uterus bicornuate.
Class V: Septate uterus.
Class VI: Diethylstilboestrol (DES) anomalies.

A separate class of uterine malformations has been identified in the presence of communication between two separate uterocervical cavities.

The pathophysiology of failure of normal union of the müllerian ducts is not clear. As proposed in the section on vaginal agenesis, the hypothesis of teratogens has been suggested but again evidence is unsupported. It is most likely that this is a polygenic or multifactorial inheritance which slightly increases the risk of a uterovaginal abnormality arising in a family with no anomalies.

Incidence

The incidence of uterine anomalies is difficult to define as it depends entirely upon the interest of the investigator and the diligence to which investigation will be pursued. Obstetric series show an incidence of uterine abnormalities ranging from 1/100 to 1/1000 (Semmens 1962). In an infertile population, the incidence increases to around 3% (Sanfillippo et al 1978). It is likely that the incidence of uterine malformations is greatly underestimated, as in the vast majority of patients no gynaecological or reproductive problems are ever experienced.

Presentation

Abnormal uterine development may be symptomatic or asymptomatic. The most common clinical situations that will lead to a diagnosis of malformation of the uterus are recurrent pregnancy loss, primary infertility, urological abnormalities, menstrual disorders and DES exposure.

Recurrent pregnancy loss

Recurrent pregnancy wastage in the form of abortion or premature labour is a common way in which uterine anomalies will be discovered. The role of uterine anomalies in pregnancy wastage is discussed in Chapter 20.

Primary infertility

Uterine abnormalities may be discovered during investigation of an infertile woman. However, the relationship between infertility and uterine abnormalities remains controversial.

Urological abnormalities

Not uncommonly, urologists who discover malformations of the urinary system investigate the genital system and find abnormalities. Thompson & Lynn (1966) reported that 66% of patients with a maldevelopment of the renal tract had an associated müllerian duct abnormality. However only 13.5% of women with anomalous renal development had anomalous uterine development. In patients with a single kidney, the most common uterine abnormality is uterus didelphus with a vaginal septum which is associated with unilateral occlusion.

Menstrual disorders

Uterine abnormalities may be responsible for a number of menstrual disorders including oligomenorrhoea, dysmenorrhoea and menorrhagia. The specific menstrual symptoms will depend on the anomaly. In an interesting study by Sorensen (1981), investigating infertile women with oligomenorrhoea, 56% of patients were found to have mild uterine abnormalities. The author suggested that this oligomenorrhoea might be due to poor vascularization or steroid receptor development in the malformed uterus. With regard to dysmenorrhoea, uterine abnormalities seem to be associated with a higher incidence of primary dysmenorrhoea, although this may also be associated with obstructed outflow problems. Rudimentary hemiuteri may be also the cause of dysmenorrhoea in some women.

DES exposure

The malformations associated with DES exposure have

been well described (Kaufman et al 1980). These abnormalities include the classic T-shaped uterus with a widening of the interstitial and isthmic portions of the fallopian tubes and narrowing of the lower two-thirds of the uterus, as well as non-specific uterine abnormalities with changes of cavity seen on hysterosalpingography. These patients may present with impaired reproductive function and pregnancy wastage may be as high as 50–60%.

Investigations

It is obvious that investigation of patients with suspected uterine abnormalities must be done with the aid of hysterosalpingography. This radiographic demonstration of the intrauterine shape is the most appropriate procedure, although care must be taken to ensure that if a double cervix is present, both cervical canals are cannulated and contrast medium is injected. A wide range of uterine abnormalities has been described and this has led to the classification system of Buttram & Gibbons (1979).

Treatment

A number of uterine malformations are suitable for surgical repair and the types of treatment and results are described in Chapter 20.

KEY POINTS

1. Gonadal differentiation into a testicle or ovary depends on the presence or absence of a Y chromosome.
2. The testis develops from the medulla whereas the ovary originates from the cortex of the primitive gonad.
3. Development of normal ovaries depends on the presence of two X chromosomes.
4. Deletion of either the short or long arms of the X chromosome may result in variable ovarian development or dysgenesis.
5. Development of the testis depends on the testicular determining factor which controls the expression of the H-Y antigen, but other autosomally located genes are also involved.
6. Female intersex disorders denote external genitalia masculinization in patients with 46XX karyotype.
7. Differentiation of internal female sexual organs is not androgen dependent and unlike the clitoris, the labia are adversely affected only if exposed to androgens before the 12th week of intrauterine life.
8. 21-Hydroxylase deficiency is an autosomal recessive disorder and accounts for 90% of cases of congenital adrenal hyperplasia (CAH).
9. 21-Hydroxylase deficiency is the only adrenal enzymatic deficiency associated to the HLA gene located in chromosome 6.
10. Female fetus defeminization may follow maternal use of testosterone related progestogens.
11. Prenatal diagnosis of CAH in heterozygous carriers is necessary and treatment with dexamethasone prevents fetal infliction.
12. Successful pregnancy following resection of vaginal septa is inversely related to the level of the septa in the vagina.
13. Intrauterine diethylstilboestrol (DES) exposure may lead to T-shaped uterus with impaired reproductive function.

REFERENCES

Ashworth M F, Morton K E, Dewhurst C J et al 1986 Vaginoplasty using amnion. Obstetrics and Gynecology 67: 443–444

Barkan A, Cassorla F, Loriaux D, Marshall J C 1984 Pregnancy in a patient with virilising arrhenoblastoma. American Journal of Obstetrics and Gynecology 149: 909–910

Broadbent R T, Woolf R M, Herbertson R 1984 Non-operative construction of the vagina. Plastic and Reconstructive Surgery 73: 117–122

Brown T R, Maes M, Rothwell S W, Migeon C J 1982 Human complete androgen insensitivity with normal dihydrotestosterone receptor binding capacity in cultured genital skin biopsies. Journal of Clinical Endocrinology and Metabolism 55: 61–69

Buttram V S, Gibbons W E 1979 Mullerian anomalies — a proposed classification. Fertility and Sterility 32: 40–48

Cacciari E, Balsamo A, Cassio A et al 1983 Neonatal screening for congenital adrenal hyperplasia. Archives of Disease in Childhood 58: 803–806

Cali R W, Pratt J H 1968 Congenital absence of the vagina. American Journal of Obstetrics and Gynecology 100: 752–754

Carson S A, Simpson J L, Malinak L R et al 1983 Heritable aspects of uterine anomalies II. Genetic analysis of mullerian aplasia. Fertility and Sterility 40: 86–91

Castro-Magana M, Chervanky T, Collipp P J, Ghavami-Maibadi Z, Angulo M, Stewart C 1981 Transient adrenogenital syndrome due to exposure to danazol in utero. American Journal of Diseases of Childhood 135: 1032–1034

Cohen V A, Daughaday W H, Weldon V 1982 Fetal and maternal virilization association with pregnancy. American Journal of Diseases of Childhood 136: 353–356

Connor T B, Ganis F M, Levin H S, Migeon C J, Martin L G 1968 Gonadotrophin dependent Krukenberg tumour causing virilization during pregnancy. Journal of Clinical Endocrinology and Metabolism 28: 198–201

D'Alberton A, Reschini E, Ferrari N, Candiani P 1981 Prevalence of urinary tract abnormalities in a large series of patients with uterovaginal atresia. Journal of Urology 126: 623–627

Donohoue P A, Van Dop C, McLean R H et al 1986 Gene conversion in salt-losing congenital adrenal hyperplasia with absent complement C4B protein. Journal of Clinical Endocrinology and Metabolism 62: 995–1002

Duck S C, Katamaya K P 1981 Danazol may cause female pseudohermaphroditism. Fertility and Sterility 35: 230–231

Duckler L 1972 Squamous cell carcinoma developing in an artificial vagina. Obstetrics and Gynecology 40: 35

Dupont B, Oberfield S E, Smithwick E M et al 1977 Close genetic linkage between HLA and congenital adrenal hyperplasia. Lancet ii: 1309–1312

Edmonds D K 1989 Intersexuality. In: Dewhurst's practical paediatric

and adolescent gynaecology, 2nd edn. Butterworths, London, pp 6–26
Evans T N, Poland M L, Boving R L 1981 Vaginal malformations. American Journal of Obstetrics and Gynecology 141: 910–916
Fayez J A, Bunch T R, Miller G L 1974 Virilization in pregnancy associated with polycystic ovary disease. Obstetrics and Gynecology 44: 511–521
Fitch N, de Saint Victor J, Richer C L et al 1982 Premature menopause due to a small deletion in the long arm of the X chromosome. American Journal of Obstetrics and Gynecology 142: 968–971
Forest M G, Orgiazzi J, Tranchant D, Mornex R, Bertrand J 1978 Approach to the mechanism of androgen production in a case of Krukenberg tumor responsible for virilization during pregnancy. Journal of Clinical Endocrinology and Metabolism 47: 428–434
Frank R T 1938 The formation of an artificial vagina without operation. American Journal of Obstetrics and Gynecology 35: 1053–1055
Fuller P J, Pettigrew I G, Pike J W, Stockigt J R 1983 An adrenal adenoma causing virilization of mother and infant. Clinical Endocrinology 18: 143–153
Hensleigh P A, Woodruff D A 1978 Differential maternal fetal response to androgenizing luteoma or hyperreactio luteinalis. Obstetrical and Gynecological Surgery 33: 262–271
Hughes I A, Wilton A, Lole C A, Glay O P 1979 Continuing need for mineralocorticoid therapy in salt-losing congenital adrenal hyperplasia. Archives of Disease in Childhood 54: 350–358
Imrie J E A, Kennedy J H, Holmes J D et al 1986 Intraepithelial neoplasia arising in an artificial vagina. British Journal of Obstetrics and Gynaecology 93: 886–887
Ishizuka S C, Kawashima Y, Nakanishi T et al 1962 Statistical observations on genital anomalies of newborns following the administration of progestins to their mothers. Journal of the Japanese Obstetrical and Gynaecological Society 9: 271–282
Jackson G W 1959 Primary carcinoma of an artifical vagina. Obstetrics and Gynaecology 14: 534
Jones H W, Mermut S 1974 Familial occurrence of congenital absence of the vagina. Obstetrics and Gynecology 42: 38–40
Kaufman R H, Adam E, Binder G L, Gerthoffer E 1980 Upper genital tract changes and pregnancy outcome in offspring exposed in utero to DES. American Journal of Obstetrics and Gynecology 137: 299–306
Lischke J H, Curtis C H, Lamb E J 1973 Discordance of vaginal agenesis in monozygotic twins. Obstetrics and Gynecology 41: 920–922
McIndoe A H 1959 Discussion on treatment of congenital absence of the vagina with emphasis on long term results. Proceedings of the Royal Society of Medicine 52: 952–953
McIndoe A H, Banister J B 1938 An operation for the cure of congenital absence of the vagina. Journal of Obstetrics and Gynaecology of British Commonwealth 45: 490–495
Mulaikal R M, Migeon C J, Rock J A 1987 Fertility rates in female patients with congenital adrenal hyperplasia due to 21-hydroxylase deficiency. New England Journal of Medicine 316: 178–181
Murset G, Zachmann M, Prader A, Fischer J, Labhart A 1970 Male external genitalia of a girl caused by a virilizing adrenal tumour in the mother. Acta Endocrinologica 65: 627–638
Newns G H 1974 Congenital adrenal hyperplasia. Archives of Disease in Childhood 49: 716–724
Novak D J, Lauchlan S C, McCauley J C 1970 Virilization during pregnancy: case report and review of literature. American Journal of Medicine 49: 281–286
Page D C, Mosher R, Simpson E M et al 1987 The sex determining region of the human Y chromosome. Cell 51: 1091–1104
Pang S, Murphey W, Levine L S et al 1982 A pilot newborn screening for congenital adrenal hyperplasia in Alaska. Journal of Clinical Endocrinology and Metabolism 55: 413–420
Pang S Y, Wallace M A, Hofman L et al 1988 Worldwide experience in newborn screening for congenital adrenal hyperplasia. Pediatrics 81: 866–874
Petersen R E, Imperato-McGinley J, Gautier T, Sturla E 1977 Male pseudohermaphroditism due to 5αreductase deficiency. American Journal of Medicine 62: 170–191
Poland M L, Evans T N 1985 Psychologic aspects of vaginal agenesis. Journal of Reproductive Medicine 30: 340–348
Post W D, Steele H D, Gorwill H 1978 Mucinous cystadenoma and virilization during pregnancy. Canadian Medical Association Journal 118: 948–953
Prader A 1958 Vollkommen männlichie aussere Genitalentwicklung und Salzverlustsyndrom bei Mädchen mit kongenitalem adrenogenitalem Syndrom. Helvetica Paediatrica Acta 13: 5–14
Raboch J, Horejsi J 1982 Sexual life of women with Kuster–Rokitansky syndrome. Archives of Sexual Behavior 11: 215–219
Rock J A, Zacur H A, Dlugi A M et al 1982 Pregnancy success following surgical correction of imperforate hymen and complete transverse vaginal septum. Obstetrics and Gynecology 59: 448–454
Rotmensch J, Rosenheim N, Dillon M et al 1983 Carcinoma arising in a neovagina. Obstetrics and Gynecology 61: 534
Sanfillippo J S, Yussman M A, Smith O 1978 Hysterosalpingography in the evaluation of infertility. Fertility and Sterility 30: 636–639
Say B, Carpentier N J 1979 Genital malformations in a child with VATER association. American Journal of Diseases of Childhood 133: 438–439
Semmens J P 1962 Congenital anomalies of the female genital tract. Obstretrics and Gynecology 19: 328–333
Shokeir M H K 1978 Aplasia of the mullerian system. Evidence of probable sex limited autosomal dominant inheritance. Birth Defects 14: 147–151
Simpson J L 1979 Gonadal dysgenesis and sex chromosome abnormalities. In: Vallet H L, Porter I H (eds) Genetic mechanism of sexual development. Academic Press, New York, p 365
Simpson J L 1987 Genetic control of sex determination. Seminars in Reproductive Medicine 5: 209–220
Smith M R 1983 Vaginal aplasia: therapeutic options. American Journal of Obstetrics and Gynecology 146: 534–538
Sorensen S S 1981 Minor mullerian anomalies and oligomenorrhoea in infertile women. American Journal of Obstetrics and Gynecology 140: 636–640
Thompson D P, Lynn H B 1966 Genital abnormalities associated with solitary kidney. Mayo Clinic Proceedings 41: 438–442
Wachtel S S 1983 H-Y antigen and the biology of sexual differentiation. Grune & Stratton, New York
White R, Leppert M, Bishop D T et al 1985 Construction of linkage maps with DNA markers for human chromosomes. Nature 313: 101–105
Williams E A 1976 Uterovaginal agenesis. Annals of the Royal College of Surgeons of England 58: 266–277
Wolf U 1981 Genetic aspects of H-Y antigen. Human Genetics 58: 25–34
Zachmann M, Tassinari D, Prader A 1983 Clinical and biochemical variability of congenital adrenal hyperplasia due to 11-hydroxylase deficiency. Journal of Clinical Endocrinology and Metabolism 56: 222–229

12

Control of hypothalamic-pituitary ovarian function

R. W. Shaw

INTRODUCTION

Over the last 50 years it has become increasingly apparent that a major component of endocrine regulation is a function of the brain and of the hypothalamus in particular (Hohlweg & Junkmann 1932, Moore & Price 1932).

The hypothalamus lies at the base of the brain between the anterior margin of the optic chiasma anteriorly and the posterior margin of the mammillary bodies posteriorly. Precise boundaries are difficult to define but it extends from the hypothalamic sulcus above to the tuber cinereum below, which itself connects the hypothalamus with the pituitary gland via its extension distally into the pituitary stalk.

The hypothalamus is the important final pathway between the brain and the pituitary gland. Secretion of hormones from the anterior pituitary is under the control of hypothalamic releasing or inhibiting factors. In turn the pituitary hormones regulate cellular growth and differentiation and functional activity in their separate target organs. Internal environmental maintenance results in multiple biochemical signals converging upon neurons within the hypothalamus whose response in turn leads to the release of the pituitary hormones which coordinate appropriate metabolic responses.

ANATOMY OF THE HYPOTHALAMIC–PITUITARY AXIS

The portion of the hypothalamus of special interest in the control of reproductive function is the neurohypophysis, which can be divided into three regions:

1. the infundibulum, which constitutes the floor of the third ventricle (often termed the median eminence) and parts of the wall of the third ventricle, which is continuous with
2. the infundibular stem, or pituitary stalk, which is continuous distally with
3. the infundibular process or posterior pituitary gland (Fig. 12.1).

The adenohypophysis consists of:

1. the pars distalis or anterior lobe of the pituitary;
2. the pars intermedia, the intermediate lobe;
3. the pars tuberalis, which is a thin layer of adenohypophyseal cells lying on the surface of the infundibular stem and infundibulum.

The anterior pituitary does not normally receive an arterial vasculature but it receives blood through portal vessels. The arteries supplying the median eminence and infundibular stalk empty into a dense network of capillaries, which are heavily innervated and drain into the portal venous plexus. In the human these are present on all sides of the infundibular stalk, particularly posteriorly. These lead to the anterior pituitary formed by vessels from the median eminence and upper stalk joined ventrally by the short portal vessels arising in the lower infundibular stalk.

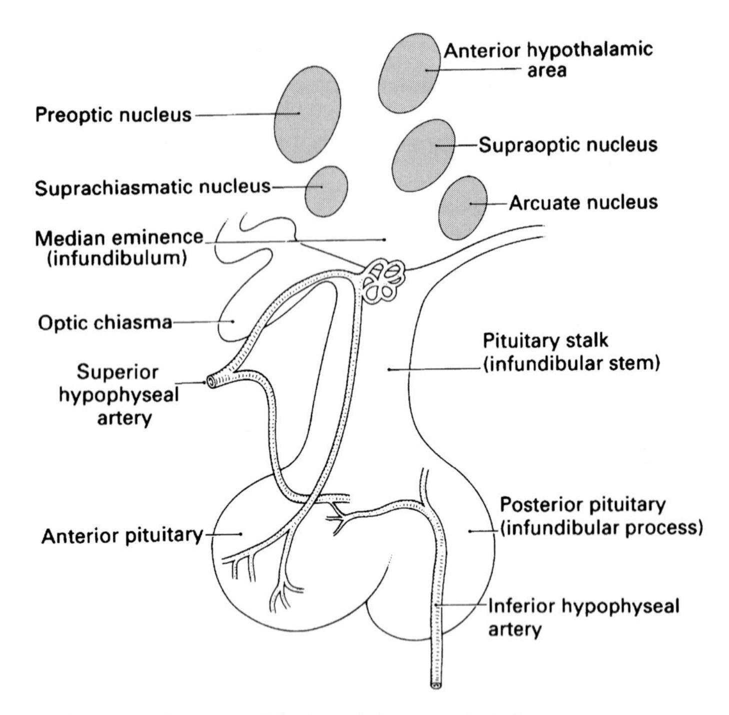

Fig. 12.1 Anatomy of the hypothalamus and pituitary.

Some 80–90% of the blood supply to the anterior pituitary is provided by the long portal vessels; the remainder comes from the short portal veins. The sinusoids of the adenohypophysis thus receive blood that has first traversed capillaries residing in the neurohypophyseal complex, and this unique relationship provides the basis for the view that the hypothalamus regulates the secretion of adenohypophyseal hormones through neurohormonal mechanisms involving hypothalamic releasing and inhibiting factors.

Neural connections

There are numerous and extensive neural pathways connecting the hypothalamus with the rest of the brain. The majority of afferent hypothalamic nerve fibres run in the lateral hypothalamic areas whilst efferent pathways are more medially placed. One important efferent connection is the supraopticohypophyseal nerve tract carrying fibres from the supraoptic and paraventricular nuclei to the infundibular process of the pituitary, whilst other fibres carry hypothalamic releasing or inhibiting factors from the medial and basal parts of the hypothalamus to the anterior pituitary (Fig. 12.2).

The gonadotrophin-releasing hormone (GnRH) secreting neurons appear in the medial olfactory placode and enter the brain with the nervus terminalis, a cranial nerve that projects from the nose to the septal preoptic nuclei in the brain. The cells that produce GnRH thus originate from the olfactory area and migrate to their final positions. Failure of this migration has now been shown to occur in Kallmann's syndrome, resulting in both a failure of GnRH

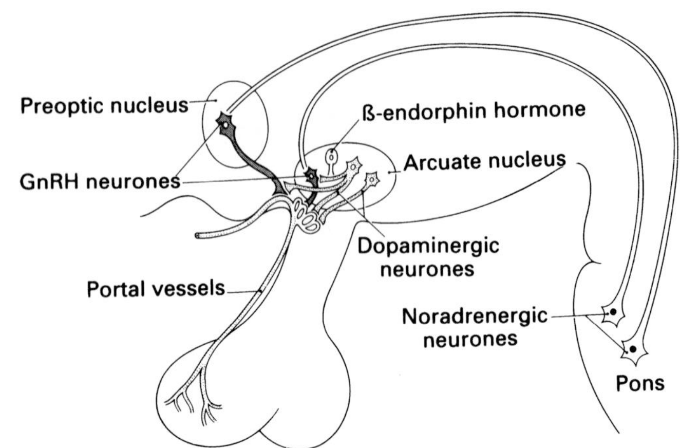

Fig. 12.2 Representation of neurochemical interactions which are important in the control of gonadotrophin-releasing hormone (GnRH) secretion.

secretions and of smell, i.e. anosmia (Schwanzel-Fukunda et al 1989).

HYPOTHALAMIC REGULATION OF PITUITARY SECRETION

Considerable efforts have been made in the past two decades to identify, characterize and synthesize the substances thought to be produced in the neural elements of the infundibulum. Several substances which can either stimulate or suppress the rate of release of one or more hormones from the pituitary gland have been found in the infundibular complex. These can be classified into hypophysiotrophic, neurohypophyseal and pituitary peptide hormones, and are listed in Table 12.1. Other substances will probably be added to this list in the future

Further discussion in this chapter will be restricted to

Table 12.1 Hypothalamic and pituitary hormones

Hypophysiotrophic hormones	
Gonadotrophin-releasing hormone	GnRH
Thyrotrophin-releasing hormone	TRH
Corticotrophin-releasing hormone	CRH
Growth hormone-releasing hormone	GHRH
Somatostatin	
Prolactin-inhibiting factor	PIF
Neurohypophyseal products	
Vasopressin	
Oxytocin	
Neurophysin I and II	
Pituitary peptide hormones	
Adrenocorticotrophic hormone	ACTH
Beta-endorphin	
Alpha-melanocyte-stimulating hormone	
Prolactin	PRL
Luteinizing hormone	LH
Follicle-stimulating hormone	FSH
Growth hormone	GH
Thyroid-stimulating hormone	TSH

the roles played by GnRH, dopamine and other neurotransmitters controlling the rates of release and synthesis of the gonadotrophins.

GnRH

In 1971 Schally and co-workers isolated pure preparations of porcine luteinizing hormone-releasing hormone (LHRH) from hypothalamic extracts and subsequently its structure was discovered and synthesis was achieved (Matsuo et al 1971a,b). The finding of follicle-stimulating hormone (FSH)-releasing activity of this LHRH led to the hypothesis of a single hypothalamic releasing hormone, gonadotrophin-releasing hormone (GnRH), controlling secretion of both luteinizing hormone (LH) and FSH from the pituitary gland, with the suggestion that sex steroids might play a role in modulating the proportions of LH and FSH released. The amino acid sequence of GnRH is shown in Figure 12.3.

GnRH neuron system

The GnRH neuron system has been mapped in detail, using primarily immunocytochemical methods. The GnRH neurons are not grouped into specific nuclei but form a loose network in several anatomical divisions. However GnRH neurone bodies are found principally in two areas: the preoptic anterior hypothalamic area and the tuberal hypothalamus, particularly the arcuate nucleus and periventricular nucleus. Axons from GnRH neurons project to many sites in the brain; the most distinct tract is from the medial basal hypothalamus to the median eminence where extensive plexuses of boutons are found on the primary portal vessels. GnRH, then, has ready and direct access to the anterior pituitary gonadotroph cells via the portal capillary plexus (see Fig. 12.2). There are also numerous projections of GnRH secreting neurons to the limbic system and the circumventricular organ, other than the median eminence. The role of these connections is currently unknown. The GnRH terminals in the median eminence remain outside the 'blood–brain' barrier and thus can be exposed to chemical agents within the general circulation.

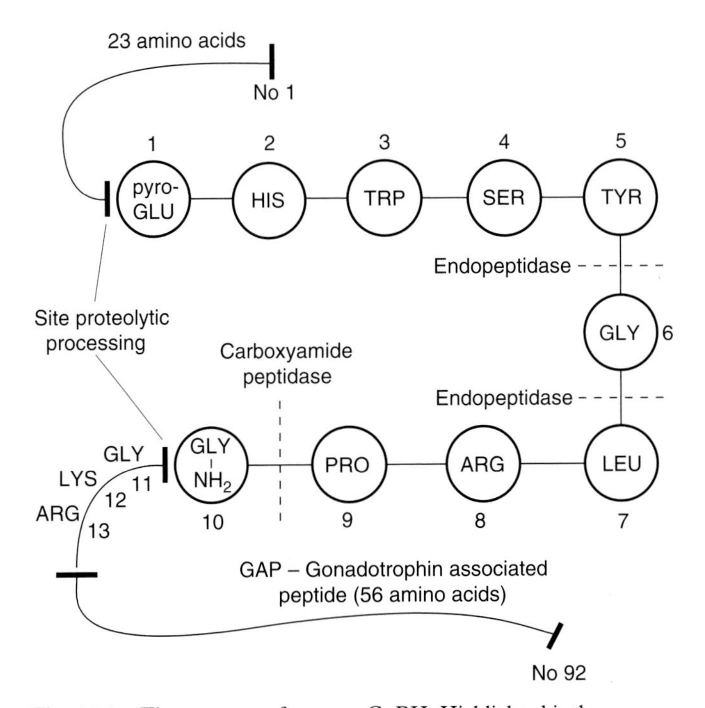

Fig. 12.3 The structure of pre-pro-GnRH. Highlighted is the decapeptide of the active molecule GnRH (mol wt. 1181). Sites of cleavage from the gonadotrophin-associated peptide (GAP) are shown, as well as the main sites of enzymatic degradation of GnRH by endo- and carboxyamide-peptidases in the pituitary.

Regulation of gonadotrophin secretion by GnRH

The GnRH gene sequence was first isolated by Seeburg & Adelman in 1984. The GnRH decapeptide is derived from the post-translational processing of a larger precursor molecule that has been termed pre-pro-GnRH. This appears to be a tripartite structure with a preceding 23-amino acid sequence, joined to the decapeptide GnRH, which is then attached via a 3-amino acid sequence, glycine ((GLY)-lycine (LYS)-arginine (ARG)), to a 56-amino acid terminal peptide, which is termed the gonadotrophin-associated peptide (GAP). The post-GnRH-decapeptide GLY-LYS-ARG 3-amino acid section is an important site for proteolytic processing. GAP itself is thought to have some prolactin-inhibiting properties (Fig. 12.3). GnRH genes are encoded from a single gene located on the shorter arm of chromosome 8.

Using radioimmunoassays, GnRH has been demonstrated in the hypophyseal portal blood from a number of animal species (Carmel et al 1976). Electrical stimulation of the preoptic area of the brain in female rats on the day of pro-oestrus increases the GnRH concentration in portal blood and the stimulus induces a marked release of LH from the anterior pituitary. In contrast, administration of antibodies against GnRH prevents this electrically stimulated LH release. These data provide evidence favouring a cause-and-effect relationship between GnRH release by the hypothalamus and LH release by the anterior pituitary.

It is now firmly established that GnRH can stimulate the secretion of both LH and FSH in animals and humans. Following intravenous administration of synthetic GnRH a significant rise in serum LH will be seen within 5 min, and sometimes of FSH, reaching a peak within about 30 min, but FSH peaks are often delayed further. LH release has a linear log-dose relationship, up to doses of 250 μg but no such relationship can be found for FSH.

In the female the magnitude of gonadotrophin release,

particularly LH, in individuals, varies with the stage of the menstrual cycle, being greatest in the preovulatory phase, less marked in the luteal phase and least in the follicular phase of any individual cycle (Shaw et al 1974, Yen et al 1972) (Fig. 12.4).

GnRH is thus the humoral link between the neural and endocrine components controlling LH and FSH release.

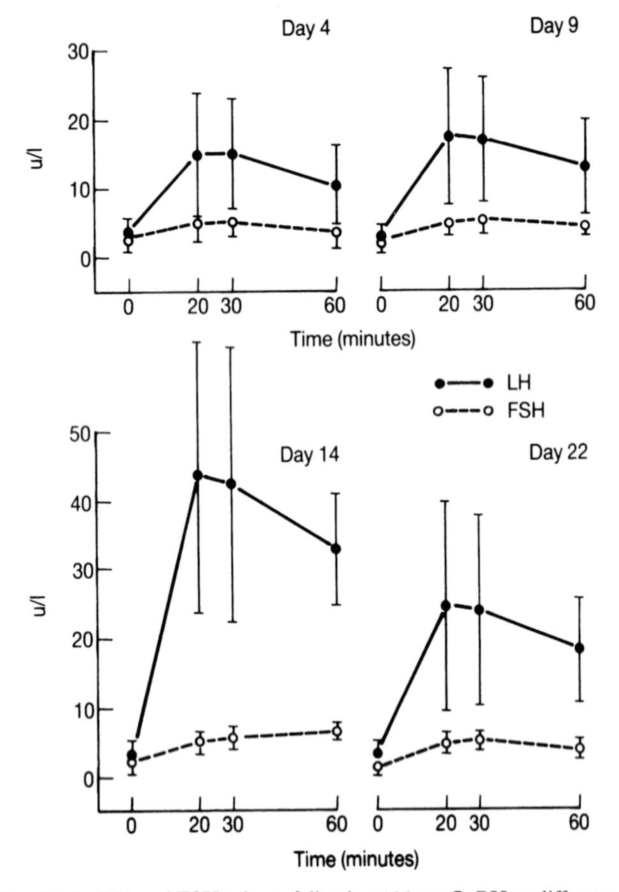

Fig. 12.4 LH and FSH release following 100 μg GnRH at different phases of the same menstrual cycle in 6 normal women (mean ± SD). From Shaw et al (1974).

Mechanism of action of GnRH on pituitary cells

The first step in the action of GnRH on the pituitary gonadotroph is recognition of a specific receptor. The GnRH receptor complexes often form clusters and become internalized, then undergo degradation in the lysosomes. The receptor fragments then pass back rapidly to the surface of the cell. This recycling process is causally related to *up-regulation* of the receptor by GnRH. GnRH receptors tend to be of 60 kDa, to be a glycoprotein and to have a transmembrane character of a complex nature with seven transmembrane domains. A negatively charged domain interacts predominantly with arginine (ARG) in position 8 of the GnRH molecule.

Prolonged exposure to GnRH produces suppression of LH release, which is called *down-regulation*, which is associated with reduced numbers of GnRH receptors. This phenomenon is vitally important in understanding the mechanism of action of the gonadotrophin-releasing hormone analogues.

The current generation of GnRH analogues are agonistic analogues, and when administered initially produce supraphysiological levels of LH and FSH from multiple receptor activation. The analogues are predominantly modified in position 6, with replacement of the glycine with a number of D-amino acids. The structures of some of the commoner analogues are shown in Table 12.2. The replacement of glycine in position 6 introduces a foreign amino acid which the endopeptidases in the pituitary are less able to degrade. In addition, many current GnRH agonistic analogues have a substitution in amino acid position 10 ($GLY-NH_2$), or the replacement of amino acid 10 by an NH-ethylamide group, thus interrupting the action of the carboxyaminopeptidase in degradation. Such changes result in an increased 'half-life' of the GnRH agonists to between 2 and 6 h.

The binding of GnRH to its receptor induces a complex series of intracellular responses, which result in hormone secretion and biosynthesis of the alpha and beta subunits of LH and FSH.

Table 12.2 Some of the commoner GnRH agonists now used in clinical practice and their amino acid sequence compared to native GnRH

	Amino acid position number									
	1	2	3	4	5	6	7	8	9	10
Native GnRH	pGLU	HIS	TRP	SER	TYR	GLY	LEU	ARG	PRO	$GLY-NH_2$
Decapeptide analogues										
Nafarelin						$(D-NAL)_2$				
Tryptorelin						D-TRP				
Goserelin						D-SER (BU^t)			$AzaGLY-NH_2$	
Nonapeptide analogues										
Buserelin						D-SER (BU^t)			PRO-N-Et	
Leuprorelin						D-LEU			PRO-NEt	
Histrelin						D-HIS (Imbzl)			PRO-NEt	

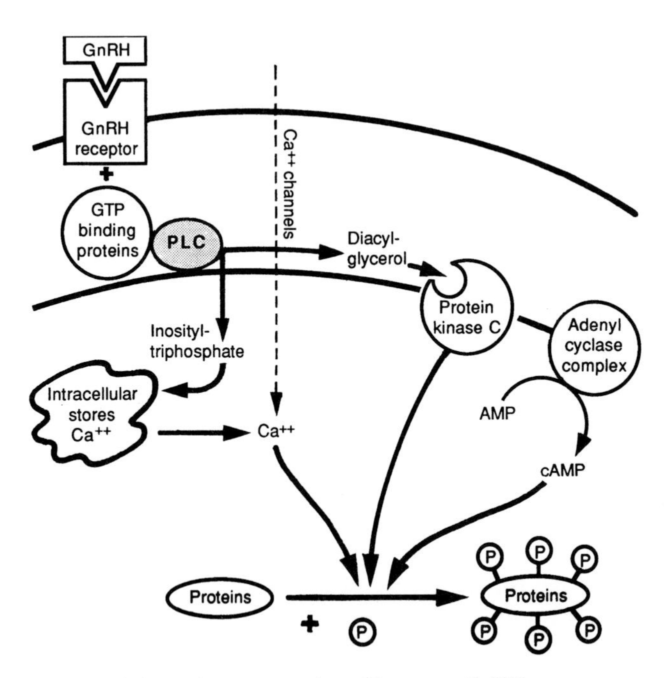

Fig. 12.5 Schematic representation of hormone GnRH-receptor signal activation. GTP, guanosine triphosphate; PLC, phospholipase-C enzyme; AMP, adenosine monophosphate; cAMP, cyclic AMP; P, phosphate group.

In addition, dimerization of alpha and beta subunits and the glycosylation processes are induced. The mechanism of action of GnRH is depicted in Figure 12.5. Within seconds of GnRH binding to and activating GnRH receptors on the pituitary gonadotrophs, intracellular free Ca^{2+} concentrations increase. This Ca^{2+} is initially mobilized from intracellular stores (e.g. endoplasmic reticulum) but also, to maintain sustained LH release, extracellular Ca^{2+} enters the gonadotroph through receptor-regulated voltage-dependent Ca^{2+} channels.

The initial mobilization of intracellular Ca^{2+} is induced by inositol triphosphate, released as a consequence of receptor activation of the membrane-bound phospholipase-C enzyme. Diacylglycerol is also released by the action of phospholipase-C, and in turn activates the phosphorylating enzyme protein kinase C. The adenyl cyclase complex is also stimulated and cyclic adenosine monophosphate (cAMP) is generated. Ca^{2+}, protein kinase C and cAMP all then interact to stimulate release of stored LH and FSH and subsequent biosynthesis (for review, see Clayton 1989).

MODULATORY ROLE OF MONOAMINES, OTHER NEUROTRANSMITTERS AND SECOND MESSENGERS ON GnRH SECRETION

Past studies indicated that LH release and ovulation were dependent upon drug-affected neural stimuli of both cholinergic and adrenergic origins. The infundibulum contains large stores of noradrenaline (norepinephrine), a lesser quantity of dopamine and a small amount of adrenaline (Fig. 12.6).

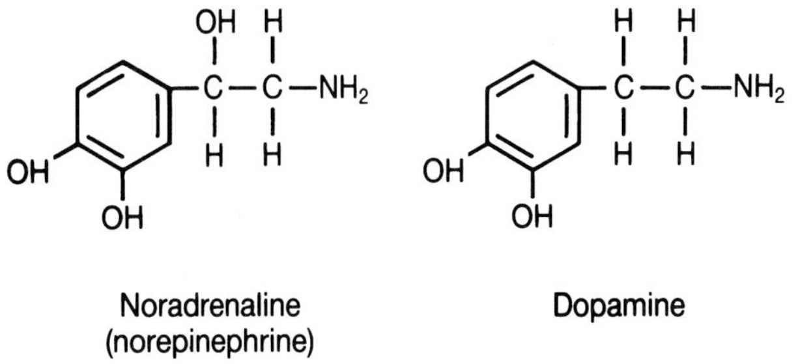

Noradrenaline (norepinephrine) | Dopamine

Fig. 12.6 Chemical structure of biogenic amines.

Dopamine and norepinephrine are synthesized in nerve terminals by decarboxylation of dihydroxyphenylalanine (DOPA), itself derived from hydroxylation from tyrosine.

Dopamine

The hypothalamic tuberoinfundibular dopaminergic pathway is formed by neurons, with cell bodies located in the arcuate nucleus and axons which project to the external layer of the median eminence in close juxtaposition to portal vessels. The coexistence of dopamine- and GnRH-containing axons in the same region of the median eminence suggests the possibility of dopaminergic involvement in the control of gonadotrophin secretion.

The addition of dopamine to pituitaries coincubated with hypothalamic fragments increases the release of LH, while the addition of phentolamine, an alpha-receptor blocker, prevents dopamine-induced LH release. These early in vitro experiments suggested that the hormonal background was capable of modifying the response to dopamine, since it seemed ineffective in ovariectomized animals or during oestrus or dioestrus day 1 of the oestrous cycle. Dopamine was more effective at pro-oestrus or in oestrogen- and progesterone-primed rats (McCann et al 1974, Ojeda & McCann 1978).

In humans the inhibitory role of dopamine and its agonists on LH, as well as that of prolactin release, has been demonstrated (Lachelin et al 1977, LeBlanc et al 1976). Elevated levels of prolactin can also stimulate dopamine turnover in the hypothalamus and it is postulated that the stimulated dopamine secretion in turn alters GnRH secretion and hence reduces FSH and LH release. Hence dopamine in the human may principally have an inhibitory effect on GnRH secretion.

The contradictory roles played by dopamine in GnRH release are, in all likelihood, the consequence of more than one action of dopamine on the GnRH-secreting neuron. The steroid environment appears to modify the components involved in the dopaminergic control of GnRH secretion, with oestrogen appearing to affect the population of excitatory or inhibitory dopamine receptors, and suggesting that the feedback control of GnRH output by oestrogen is partly exerted at a hypothalamic level by reducing dopamine neuronal activity.

Noradrenaline

Most experimental evidence supports a stimulatory role for noradrenaline in the control of gonadotrophin release. Turnover of hypothalamic noradrenaline is increased during the preovulatory surge of gonadotrophins at pro-oestrus, and noradrenaline synthesis in the anterior hypothalamus is enhanced in ovariectomized rats. These effects on GnRH secretion appear to be mediated by alpha receptors, since phenoxybenzamine, an alpha-blocker, suppresses the postcastration rise in gonadotrophins in male rats, and phentolamine blocks the pulsatile release of LH in ovariectomized monkeys (for review, see McCann & Ojeda 1976).

Selective blockade of noradrenaline synthesis prevents the preovulatory LH surge and that induced by gonadal steroids; the above data suggest that noradrenergic terminals in the preoptic or anterior hypothalamic area synapse with GnRH neurons involved in the control of the preovulatory surge of gonadotrophins.

Serotonin

High concentrations of serotonin are found in the median eminence, with most of the serotonin-containing neurons originating from the raphe nucleus in the midbrain–pons area. Present evidence shows that serotonin plays a predominantly inhibitory role in gonadotrophin release (see McCann & Ojeda 1976).

Endogenous opioids

Endogenous opioids play a central role in the neural control of gonadotrophin secretion, by way of an inhibitory effect on hypothalamic GnRH secretion. These are a fascinating group of peptides, endorphins being the name coined to denote a substance with morphine-like action, of endogenous origin, in the brain. Endorphin production is regulated by gene transcription and since these are precursor peptides, all opioids are derived from three precursor peptides:

- pro-opiomelanocortin (POMC) is the source of endorphins;
- pro-enkephalin A and B are the source of enkephalins;
- pro-dynorphin yields dynorphins.

A single injection of morphine, administered to oophorectomized monkeys, brings about immediate cessation of GnRH pulse generation (Yen et al 1985). Hypothalamic opioidergic neurons are found in the actuate nucleus of the medial basal hypothalamus, in close contact with GnRH neurons. The administration of an opioid antagonist, naloxone, produces an increased frequency and amplitude of GnRH and LH secretion. These changes are most marked in the luteal phase of the cycle, and it is thought that the negative feedback of oestrogen may partly be effected through opioid-induced inhibition of GnRH secretion (Ropert et al 1981).

OTHER TRANSMITTERS AND SECOND MESSENGERS

Other neurotransmitters may play a less important role in the regulation of GnRH neurons. Acetylcholine and gamma-aminobutyric acid stimulate LH release. Both these agents are far commoner as neurotransmitting agents than dopamine or noradrenaline in central nervous system nerve terminals in general, but their importance in GnRH neuronal activity seems to be less than that of dopamine and noradrenaline.

Prostaglandins

The role of prostaglandins in brain function is not clear, but the brain can synthesize and release prostaglandins and they do modify the adenyl cyclase-AMP system in central and peripheral neurons. Prostaglandins, particularly those of the E series, can induce gonadotrophin release in several species and prostaglandin synthetase inhibitors, e.g. indomethacin, block steroid-induced LH release (Ojeda & McCann 1978). Prostaglandin E is found in the median eminence in greater quantity than the rest of the medial basal hypothalamus; this distribution is consistent with the concept of its physiological role in the neural control of pituitary function.

The role played by prostaglandin E in GnRH release from hypothalamic secretory neurons appears to be an intracellular one. Activation of noradrenaline release from nerve terminals synapsing with GnRH neurons stimulates postsynaptic production of prostaglandin E which in turn enhances the release of GnRH. The prostaglandin E effect may either be a direct one or be mediated by a cyclic nucleotide.

Inhibins and activins

A group of compounds recently isolated from developing follicles, termed inhibins and activins, are now thought to be important in the control of FSH secretion from the pituitary. In addition they play an important role in the paracrine regulation of androgen production in the ovary, with activins having an effect on granulosa cells. The nature of these gonadal inhibins has recently been clarified and they are shown to be composed of alpha and beta subunits derived from separate genes. FSH secretion is suppressed by the alpha-beta heterodimer, and stimulated by

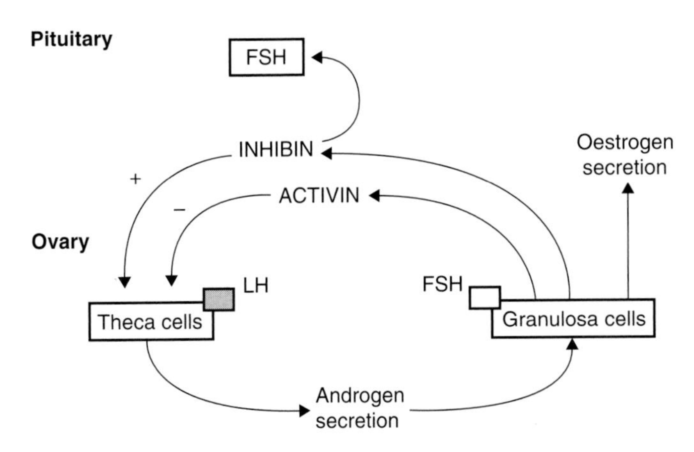

Fig. 12.7 Presumed interactions of INHIBIN and ACTIVIN in the control of pituitary and ovarian hormone production.

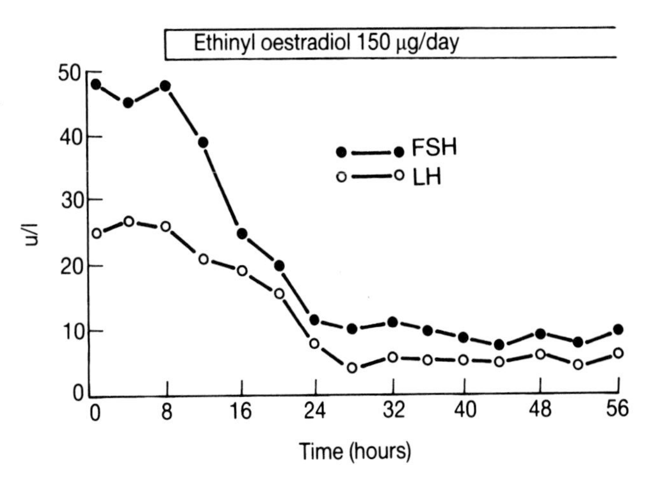

Fig. 12.8 The negative feedback effect of oestrogen on serum LH and FSH in a postmenopausal woman (Shaw 1975, unpublished data).

the beta homodimer, activin (Vale et al 1990). The molecular weight of the alpha subunit is approximately 18 000 Da, and that of the beta A and beta B subunits is 14 000 Da. The secretory patterns and the role of inhibins and activins throughout the menstrual cycle in the human have yet to be precisely elucidated (Fig. 12.7).

The control of GnRH secretion is thus highly complex and dependent upon a number of inhibitory and excitatory pathways involving various neurotransmitters. The control mechanisms are further complicated by the role of ovarian steroids in altering GnRH release and in modifying pituitary responsiveness to GnRH.

MODULATORY EFFECT OF OVARIAN STEROIDS

Negative feedback

Negative feedback control or inhibition of pituitary LH and FSH release has been postulated since 1932, when Moore & Price considered that the ovary and adenohypophysis were linked in a rigid system of hormonal interactions. The quantitative relationship between ovarian steroids and gonadotrophin release can be demonstrated by disturbing the negative feedback loop by oophorectomy which produces, over a period of days, an increase in circulating LH and FSH; this reaches a plateau at about 3 weeks with levels which are some 10 times preoperative values. Alternatively the administration of exogenous oestrogens to oophorectomized or postmenopausal women will result in rapid suppression of elevated circulating gonadotrophin levels (Fig. 12.8).

The negative feedback changes result from both a direct pituitary site of action of oestradiol, with a decrease in sensitivity of the gonadotroph to GnRH (McCann et al 1974), and an action within the hypothalamus and a decrease in GnRH secretion, possibly via increased inhibitory dopaminergic and opiate activity.

The threshold for the negative feedback action of oestrogen is set to bring about suppression of gonadotrophin release with relatively small increases in oestradiol-17β in the normal female. This negative feedback loop is the main factor which maintains the relatively low basal concentrations of plasma LH and FSH in the normal female. Circulating levels of oestradiol-17β within the range of 100–200 pmol/l will suppress the early follicular phase gonadotrophin rise which initiates follicular development.

A negative feedback effect of progesterone on gonadotrophin secretion is now well established. Whilst progesterone, even in large doses, has little effect on baseline LH release, it can suppress the ovulatory surge of LH, as demonstrated in human females administered synthetic progestogens (Larsson-Cohn et al 1972), and oestrogen-induced positive feedback surges cannot be produced during the luteal phase in women (Shaw 1975). The principal negative feedback action of progesterone is thus upon the midcycle gonadotrophin surge and it may be responsible for its short 24-h duration. It also seems likely that progesterone is an important factor in the reduced frequency of gonadotrophin pulses observed during the luteal phase of the cycle when compared to their frequency in the follicular phase (see below).

Positive feedback

The fact that under certain circumstances oestrogen may stimulate (positive feedback) rather than inhibit gonadotrophin release was first proposed by Hohlweg & Junkmann (1932). Their proposal has since been substantiated by numerous experimental reports in animals and humans. Under physiological conditions the positive feedback operates only in females; it is brought about by oestrogen and appears to be an essential component in producing the midcycle ovulatory surge of gonadotrophins. Administration of oestradiol-17β to females

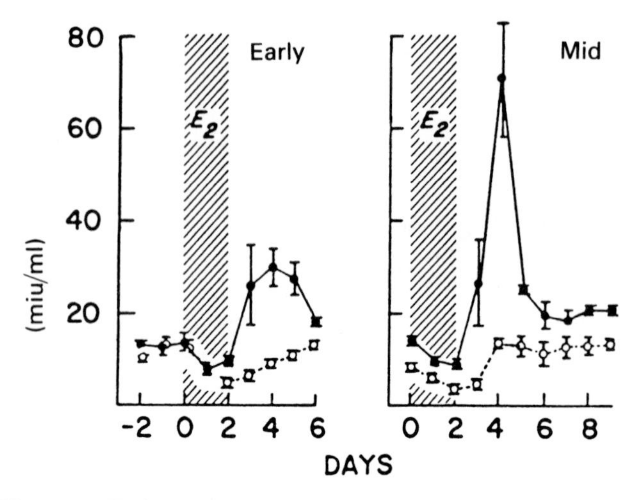

Fig. 12.9 The positive feedback effect of exogenous oestrogen (E_2 = 200 μg ethinyl oestradiol/day) on gonadotrophin release; qualitative differences in the early and midfollicular phase of the cycle. ●, LH; ○, FSH. From Yen et al (1974) with permission.

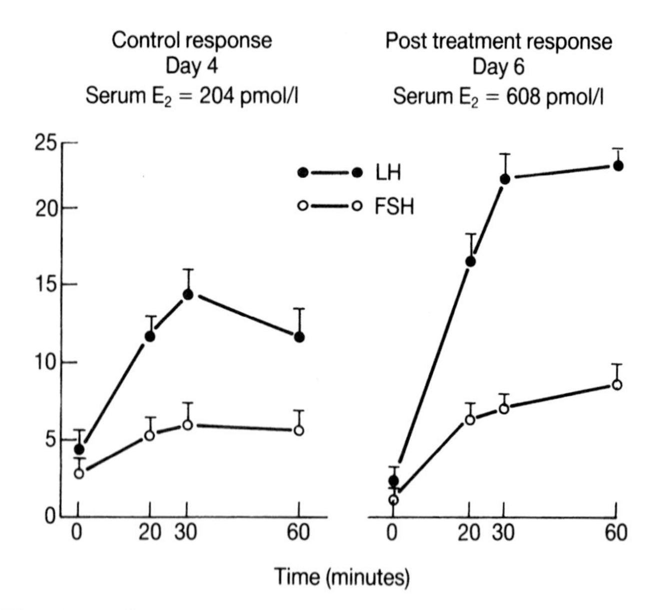

Fig. 12.10 Oestrogen augmentation of pituitary response to 100 μg LHRH bolus in 4 women receiving 2.5 mg oestradiol benzoate i.m., 2 h after initial control response on day 4 of cycle and retested 48 h later on day 6 of cycle. From Shaw (1975).

during the early or midfollicular phase of the cycle will induce a surge of gonadotrophins (Shaw 1975, Yen et al 1974) (Fig. 12.9), but treatment with the same doses of oestrogen during the midfollicular phase induces a far greater release of LH than during the early follicular phase (Yen et al 1974), (Fig. 12.9). Studies on the dynamics of this positive feedback response to oestrogen, observed in greatest detail in the rhesus monkey, demonstrate an activation delay of some 32–48 h from the commencement of oestrogen administration until the onset of the positive feedback-induced gonadotrophin surge; a minimum threshold level to be exceeded, and a strength–duration aspect of the stimulus (Karsch et al 1973).

Oestrogen elicits gonadotrophin release by increasing pituitary responsiveness to GnRH and possibly by stimulating increased GnRH secretion by the hypothalamus. In the normally menstruating female, oestrogen pretreatment produces an initial suppressive action on pituitary responsiveness (Shaw et al 1975a) followed by a later augmenting action which is both concentration- and duration-dependent (Shaw et al 1975a, Young & Jaffe 1976). The augmenting effect of oestrogen on GnRH pituitary responsiveness is demonstrated in Figure 12.10.

These data and others suggest that the midcycle oestrogen-induced surge of gonadotrophins may occur without any increased output of hypothalamic GnRH being necessary, and indeed this occurs in patients with endogenous GnRH deficiency receiving pulsatile GnRH treatment at a constant rate.

Progesterone by itself does not appear to exert a positive feedback effect. However, when administered to females in whom the pituitary has undergone either endogenously induced or exogenously administered oestrogen priming, progesterone can induce increased pituitary responsiveness to GnRH (Shaw et al 1975b, Fig. 12.11). Since

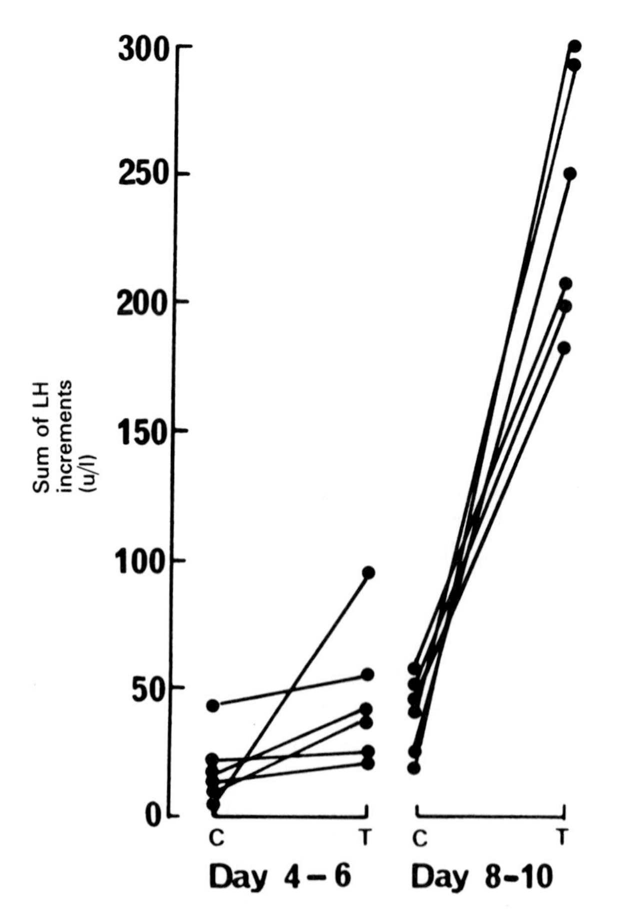

Fig. 12.11 Effect of progesterone pretreatment (12.5 mg i.m.) on LH response to 100 μg GnRH i.v., during the early and midfollicular phases of the cycle, showing the increased priming effect of oestrogen. C, control; T, after progesterone. Modified from Shaw et al (1975b).

circulating progesterone levels are increasing significantly during the periovulatory period, this action may be of importance in determining the magnitude and duration of the midcycle gonadotrophin surge.

SELF-PRIMING OF THE PITUITARY GONADOTROPH BY GnRH

Results from in vitro experiments with pituitary cells in culture indicate that GnRH is involved not only in the release of stored LH and FSH, but is of importance in maintaining the synthesis of gonadotrophins within the gonadotroph. Hence repeated exposure to GnRH of the gonadotrophin-producing cells seems essential for the maintenance of adequate pituitary stores.

Rommler & Hammerstein (1974) first demonstrated that the response to a second injection of GnRH was greater than the initial response in females, when they were retested 1–4 h following the first exposure. This response has been termed 'self-priming'.

Wang and co-workers (1976) published more intensive studies, carried out throughout the menstrual cycle, and were able to demonstrate that self-priming had a definite cycle relationship which was greatest in the late follicular phase and around midcycle, i.e. at times of increased circulating oestrogen levels, and that oestrogen preferentially induces LH rather than FSH release (Fig. 12.12).

This self-priming effect of GnRH is of importance in understanding the physiological control mechanism of gonadotrophin release. It suggests that there are two pools of gonadotrophins, one readily releasable by initial exposure to GnRH and a second reserve pool. The exposure of this larger reserve pool to GnRH allows it to be more readily released by a subsequent exposure to GnRH and is suggestive of a transfer of gonadotrophins from one pool to the other. The stage of the cycle, i.e. the prevailing environment of endogenous sex steroids, which are the modulators, and the degree of GnRH stimulation which is the prime controller, together influence these transfer capabilities and sensitivity of the pituitary in its response to GnRH.

PULSATILE NATURE OF GONADOTROPHIN RELEASE

The pulsatile nature of hypothalamic GnRH release is now known to determine episodic pituitary gonadotrophin secretion.

This pulsatile pattern of GnRH concentration has been reported in the pituitary stalk effluent of the rhesus monkey (Carmel et al 1976). This suggests that the pulsatile pattern of gonadotrophin release from the anterior pituitary is probably causally related to the periodic increase in the hypothalamic GnRH system.

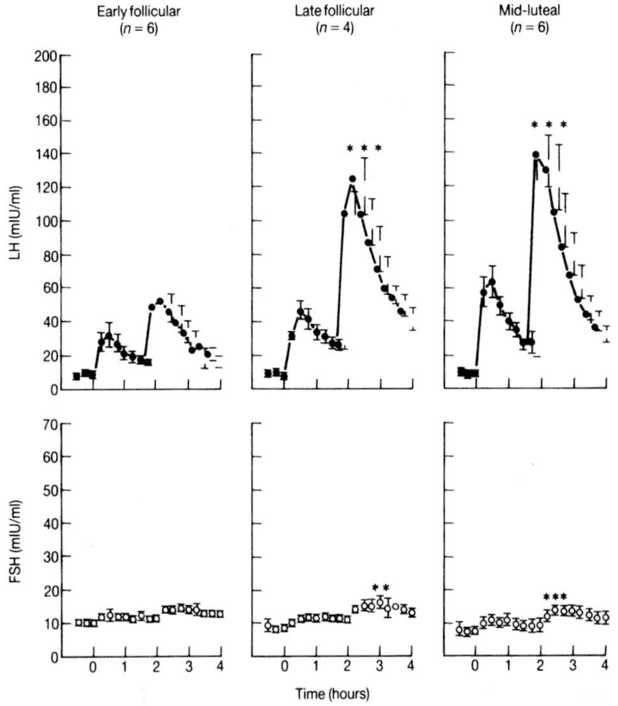

Fig. 12.12 Self-priming effect of bolus injection of GnRH: differing responses at different phases of the menstrual cycle. From Wang et al (1976), with permission.

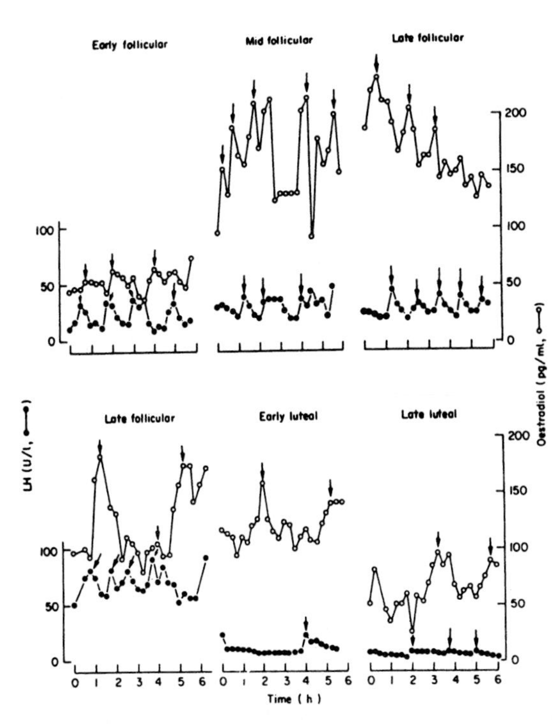

Fig. 12.13 Concentrations of LH and oestradiol at different phases of the menstrual cycle, demonstrating different pulse frequency and amplitude. From Backstrom et al (1982), with permission.

Further support for this hypothesis is obtained from the facts that antisera to GnRH abolish the pulsatile release of gonadotrophins and that pulsatile LH release can only be reinstated by pulsed delivery of GnRH, and not by constant infusion.

Comparison of the pulsatile pattern of gonadotrophin release at different phases of the menstrual cycle demonstrates profound modulation by ovarian steroids (Fig. 12.13).

In hypogonadal subjects, pulses exhibit high amplitude and high frequency with reversal of the LH:FSH ratio. However, the higher circulating level of FSH is probably not due to a higher FSH secretory rate, but rather to an accumulation related to its slower clearance rate (longer half-life).

In females with normal cycles, a characteristic low-amplitude, high-frequency pulse pattern is observed during the follicular phase. This suggests that oestrogen appears to be most effective in reducing the amplitude of gonadotrophin pulses, more markedly in FSH than LH. In contrast the pulse pattern during the luteal phase is one of high amplitude and low frequency, probably modified by progesterone effects, on the catecholaminergic and GnRH neuron systems (Fig. 12.13).

INTEGRATIVE CONTROL OF THE HYPOTHALAMIC–PITUITARY UNIT DURING THE MENSTRUAL CYCLE

How can the complex interrelated changes in ovarian steroids and pituitary gonadotrophins that occur within each menstrual cycle be explained on the basis of our present understanding of the control of the hypothalamic pituitary unit (Fig. 12.14).

LH and FSH are released from the anterior pituitary in an episodic, pulsatile manner and the available evidence supports a hypothalamic mechanism for this pulsatile release. Both oestradiol-17β and progesterone can induce a positive feedback release of gonadotrophins, in many respects comparable to that seen at midcycle, but progesterone can only produce its effect on a previously oestrogen-primed pituitary gland. There is presumptive evidence that these positive feedback stimuli also involve a direct pituitary action, with alteration in sensitivity to GnRH preceding an induced increase in hypothalamic release of GnRH.

The pattern of gonadotrophin release from the pituitary in response to repeated pulses of submaximal dose of GnRH or constant low-dose infusion over several hours suggests the presence of two functionally related pools of gonadotrophins. The first primary pool is immediately releasable, while the secondary pool requires a continued stimulus input and represents the effect of GnRH on synthesis and storage of gonadotrophins within the pituitary cell. The sizes or activity of these two pools represent pituitary sensitivity and reserve respectively which vary throughout the cycle and are regulated by the feedback action of ovarian steroids and by the self-priming action of GnRH itself. Oestradiol preferentially induces the augmentation of reserve and impedes sensitivity to GnRH, with a differential effect apparent for LH release. This oestradiol effect is both dose- and time-related.

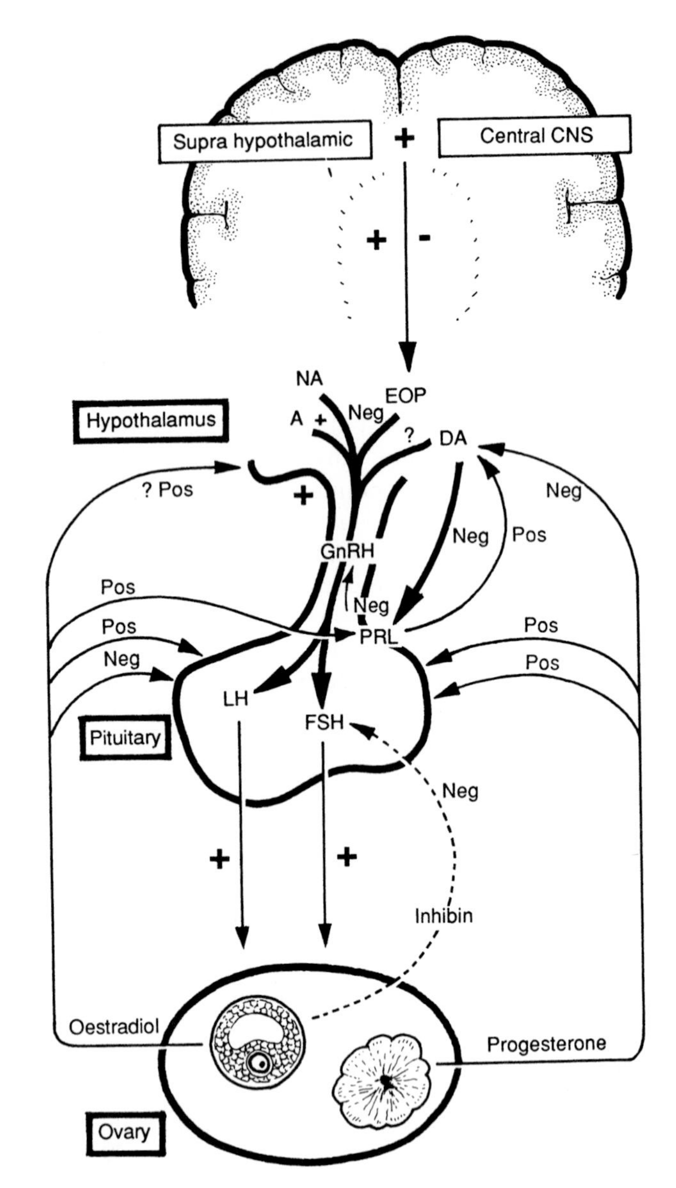

Fig. 12.14 Feedback control mechanisms in the hypothalamic–pituitary–ovarian axis. CNS, central nervous system; NA, noradrenaline; A, adrenaline; EOP, endogenous opioids; PRL, prolactin; DA, dopamine; GnRH, gonadotrophin-releasing hormone; LH, luteinizing hormone; FSH, follicle-stimulating hormone.

Follicular phase

In the early follicular phase, both the immediately releasable and the reserve pool of gonadotrophins are at a minimum. The increased FSH release, responsible for initiating follicle development, must indicate an increased output of GnRH, with the lowering of negative feedback action in the presence of low levels of oestrogen and progestogen. As follicles develop oestrogen levels rise, and the negative feedback action of oestrogen on GnRH increases, suppressing FSH levels.

With these progressive increases in oestradiol throughout the midfollicular phase, the quantitative estimates of the primary, immediately releasable, pool of gonadotrophins increase slightly, whilst the reserve pool increases greatly, thus demonstrating the augmentation action of oestradiol primarily upon the reserve pool. Since there is no marked increase in circulating gonadotrophin levels during this phase, secretion of GnRH must be minimal or else there is evidence of impedance of GnRH sensitivity by oestrogen.

Mechanism for preovulatory gonadotrophin surge

During the late follicular phase there is an increase in the amount of oestradiol secreted by the ovary. Under this influence, the sensitivity of the gonadotroph to GnRH eventually reaches a phase when GnRH can exert its full self-priming action. The consequence is the transference of gonadotrophins from the secondary reserve pool to the releasable pool. The increased pituitary responsiveness to GnRH may be further enhanced by the slight progesterone rise which can affect its action on a fully oestrogen-primed anterior pituitary. These changes culminate in the production of the ovulatory gonadotrophin surge. It is possible that these events could occur even if the gonadotrophs were exposed to a constant level of GnRH. However, an increased secretion of GnRH, as reported in rhesus monkeys and rats (Sarker et al 1976), at midcycle, which would act synergistically with the changes in pituitary sensitivity seems likely also in the human.

The LH and FSH surges begin abruptly (LH levels doubling over 2 h), and are temporarily associated with attainment of peak oestradiol-17β levels. The mean duration of the LH surge is 48 h, with an ascending limb of 14 h which is accompanied by a decline in oestradiol-17β and 17-hydroxyprogesterone concentrations but a sustained rise in inhibin levels.

The ascending limb of LH is followed by a peak plateau of gonadotrophin levels lasting some 14 h and a transient levelling of progesterone concentrations. The descending limb is long, lasting about 20 h, and accompanying this is a second rise in progesterone, a further decline in oestradiol-17β and 17-hydroxyprogesterone and a rise in inhibin levels.

The concentration of inhibin during the periovulatory interval is not correlated with oestradiol-17β or progesterone changes. It may merely reflect the release from follicular fluid of stored inhibin.

Ovulation occurs 1–2 h before the final phase of progesterone rise or 35–44 h from the onset of the LH surge.

Luteal phase

The significantly lower basal gonadotrophin secretion in the face of high pituitary capacity during the midluteal phase suggests that endogenous GnRH should be very low.

A progressive decrease in sensitivity and reserve characterizes pituitary function during the late luteal phase and into the early follicular phase of the next cycle. This is probably due to a progressive decline in oestrogen and progesterone on which sensitivity and reserve are dependent. The role played by the proposed ovarian inhibin on preferentially controlling FSH secretion has still to be determined.

It is therefore apparent that the functional state of the pituitary gonadotroph as a target cell is ultimately determined by the modulating effect of ovarian steroid hormones via their influence on the gonadotroph's sensitivity and reserves and upon the hypophysiotrophic effect of GnRH.

With such a complex interrelated control mechanism, it is perhaps not surprising that many drugs which affect neurotransmitters, or ill health or associated endocrine disorders can disrupt normal hypothalamic–pituitary–ovarian function, resulting in disordered follicular growth and suppression of ovulation.

KEY POINTS

1. The unique portal blood supply to the pituitary gland provides the basis of hypothalamic regulation of the pituitary secretion. It also explains the vulnerability of the gland to hypotension.
2. GnRH, secreted by neurons of the hypothalamus into the portal system, controls the release of both FSH and LH, with ovarian sex steroids playing the role in modulating the proportions of each hormone secreted.
3. The final step in the release of stored LH and FSH, and subsequent induction of further biosynthesis of both hormones following GnRH stimulation, involves Ca^{2+}, protein Kinase C and cAMP.
4. The control of GnRH secretion is highly complex and depends upon a number of inhibitory (dopamine, endorphins) and excitatory (noradrenaline, prostaglandins) neurotransmitters, modulated by stimulation.
5. The response of the pituitary gland to exogenous GnRH depends upon the ovarian sex steroid environment prevailing and the degree of GnRH stimulation. Prolonged exposure to GnRH produces down-regulation of LH release.

6. Ovarian steroids modulate the pattern of gonadotrophin pulse secretion. Oestrogens are more effective in reducing the pulse amplitude (more so of FSH than LH) whereas progesterone reduces the pulse frequency of LH as shown during the luteal phase.
7. The positive feedback of oestradiol and progesterone on gonadotrophin secretion may involve a direct pituitary action with alteration in sensitivity to GnRH preceding an induced increase in hypothalamic release of GnRH.
8. Follicular inhibins and activins are also important in the control of FSH secretion as well as regulation of androgen production in the ovary. The role of these compounds on the menstrual cycle is gradually becoming clear but has yet to be fully elucidated.
9. GnRH is not only necessary for the release of gonadotrophins (primary or release pool), but repeated exposure of the pituitary gland to GnRH is essential for adequate synthesis and storage of these hormones (secondary or reserve pool).
10. The size or activity of these primary and secondary pools and accordingly the pituitary response to GnRH varies throughout the menstrual cycle. It is regulated by the feedback of ovarian steroids and the level of GnRH itself. Oestrogen preferentially augments the secondary while it impedes the primary pool, especially for LH release.
11. The final modulation of pituitary sensitivity as a target organ to GnRH is ultimately determined by the effect of ovarian steroids.
12. Progesterone can induce an LH surge by increasing the gonadotroph's responsiveness to GnRH, only in women previously primed by endogenous or exogenous oestrogen.
13. The role of prostaglandin E in GnRH release may be an intracellular one. Activation of noradrenaline release from nerve terminals stimulates postsynaptic production of prostaglandin E which enhances GnRH release.

REFERENCES

Backstrom C T, McNeilly A S, Leask R M, Baird DT 1982 Pulsatile secretion of LH, FSH, prolactin, oestradiol and progesterone during the human menstrual cycle. Clinical Endocrinology 17: 29–42

Carmel P D, Araki S, Ferin M 1976 Prolonged stalk portal blood collection in rhesus monkeys. Pulsatile release of gonadotrophin-releasing hormone (GnRH). Endocrinology 99: 243–248

Clayton R N 1989 Cellular actions of gonadotrophin-releasing hormone: the receptor and beyond. In: Shaw R W, Marshall J C (eds) LHRH and its analogues – their use in gynaecological practice. Wright, London, pp 19–34

Hohlweg W, Junkmann K 1932 Die hormonal-nervosae Regulierung der Funktion des Hypophysenvorderlappens. Klinische Wochenschrift II: 321–323

Karsch F J, Weick R F, Butler W R et al 1973 Induced LH surges in the rhesus monkey: strength–duration characteristics of the oestrogen stimulus. Endocrinology 92: 1740–1747

Lachelin G C L, LeBlanc H, Yen S S C 1977 The inhibitory effect of dopamine agonists on LH release in women. Journal of Clinical Endocrinology and Metabolism 44: 728–732

Larsson-Cohn V, Johansson E D B, Wide L, Gemzell C 1972 Effects of continuous daily administration of 0.1 mg of norethindrone on the plasma levels of progesterone and on the urinary excretion of luteinizing hormone and total oestrogens. Acta Endocrinologica (Copenhagen) 71: 551–556

LeBlanc H, Lachelin G C L, Abu-Fadil S, Yen S S C 1976 Effects of dopamine infusion on pituitary hormone secretion in humans. Journal of Clinical Endocrinology and Metabolism 43: 668–674

Matsuo H, Arimura A, Nair R M G, Schally A V 1971a Synthesis of the porcine LH- and FSH-releasing hormone by the solid phase method. Biochemical and Biophysical Research Communications 45: 822–827

Matsuo H, Baba Y, Nair R M G, Arimura A, Schally A V 1971b Structure of porcine LH- and FSH-releasing hormone. I The proposed amino acid sequence. Biochemical and Biophysical Research Communications 43: 1334–1339

McCann S M, Ojeda S R 1976 Synaptic transmitters involved in the release of hypothalamic releasing and inhibiting hormones. In: Ehrenpreis S, Kopin I J (eds) Reviews of Neuroscience, vol 2. Raven Press, New York, pp 91–110

McCann S M, Ojeda S R, Fawcett C P, Krulich L 1974 Catecholaminergic control of gonadotrophin and prolactin secretion with particular reference to the possible participation of dopamine. Advances in Neurology 5: 435

Moore C R, Price D 1932 Gonad hormone function and the reciprocal influence between gonads and hypophysis. American Journal of Anatomy 50: 13–72

Ojeda S R, McCann S M 1978 Control of LH and FSH release by LHRH: influence of putative neurotransmitters. Clinics in Obstetrics and Gyaecology 5: 283–303

Rommler A, Hammerstein J 1974 Time-dependent alterations in pituitary responsiveness caused by LH-RH stimulations in man. Acta Endocrinologica (Copenhagen) 21 (suppl): 184

Ropert J R, Quigley M E, Yen S S C 1981 Endogenous opiates modulate pulsatile LH release in humans. Journal of Clinical Endocrinology and Metabolism 52: 584–585

Sarker D K, Chiappa S A, Fink G 1976 Gonadotrophin releasing hormone surge in proestrus rats. Nature 264: 461–463

Schally A V, Arimura A, Kastin A 1971 Gonadotrophin releasing hormone – one polypeptide regulates secretion of LH and FSH. Science 173: 1036–1038

Schwanzel-Fukunda M, Bick D, Pfaff D W 1989 Luteinizing hormone-releasing hormone (LHRH) – expressing cells do not migrate normally in an inherited hypogonadal (Kallmann) syndrome. Molecular Brain Research 6: 311–315

Seeburg P H, Adelman J P 1984 Characterisation of CDNA for precursor of human luteinizing hormone-releasing hormone. Nature 311: 611

Shaw R W 1975 A study of hypothalamic–pituitary–gonadal relationships I the female. MD thesis, Birmingham University, Birmingham, UK

Shaw R W, Butt W R, London D R, Marshall J C 1974 Variation in response to synthetic luteinizing hormone-releasing hormone (LHRH) at different phases of the same menstrual cycle in normal women. Journal of Obstetrics and Gynaecology of the British Commonwealth 81: 632–639

Shaw R W, Butt W R, London D R 1975a Effect of oestrogen pretreatment on subsequent response to luteinizing hormone-releasing hormone (LH-RH) in normal women. Clinical Endocrinology 4: 297–304

Shaw R W, Butt W R, London D R 1975b The effect of progesterone on FSH and LH response to LH-RH in normal women. Clinical Endocrinology 4: 543–550

Vale W, Hsueh A, Rivier C, Yu J 1990 The inhibin, activin family of hormones and growth factors. In: Sporn M B, Roberts A B (eds)

Peptide growth factors and their receptors II. New York, Springer-Verlag, pp 211–248
Wang C F, Lasley B L, Lein A, Yen S S C 1976 The functional changes of the pituitary gonadotrophs during the menstrual cycle. Journal of Clinical Endocrinology and Metabolism 42: 718–724
Yen S S C, Van den Berg G, Rebar R, Ehara Y 1972 Variations of pituitary responsiveness to synthetic LRF during different phases of the menstrual cycle. Journal of Clinical Endocrinology and Metabolism 35: 931–934
Yen S S C, Van den Berg G, Tsai C C, Siler T 1974 Causal relationship between the hormonal variables in the menstrual cycle. In: Ferin M et al (eds) Biorhythms and human reproduction. John Wiley, New York, pp 219–238
Yen S S C, Quigley M E, Reid R L, Cetel N S 1985 Neuroendocrinology of opioid peptides and their role in the control of gonadotrophin and prolactin secretion. American Journal of Obstetrics and Gynecology 152: 485–493
Young J R, Jaffe R B 1976 Strength duration characteristics of estrogen effects on gonadotrophin response to gonadotrophin-releasing hormone in women. II Effects of varying concentrations of estradiol. Journal of Clinical Endocrinology and Metabolism 42: 432–442

13

Disorders of puberty

S. L. B. Duncan

INTRODUCTION

Puberty in girls is the first phase of transition from child to mature woman. Normally, it is a coherent process involving oestrogen production, increased somatic growth and the development of secondary sexual characteristics. Most of the changes are gradual, though menarche is a single event that can be dated. Normal puberty involves a fairly regular sequence of events between the ages of 10 and 16 years and abnormal puberty can be defined as any disturbance in this. However, the range of normality is wide and can tax clinical acumen.

In this chapter, puberty is defined as the first phase of the changes of the development of secondary sex characteristics and the onset of menstruation. Full sexual maturity involves completion of breast development, the occurrence of regular ovulation and especially psychological maturity related to sexuality; it takes longer and occupies the mid and later teens.

Some gynaecological conditions are liable to occur for the first time in the early teenage girl. These include vaginitis, genital warts, or problems of menstrual hygiene (e.g. retained tampon). At this age they have special importance in diagnosis and management but are outside the scope of this chapter. Likewise, causes of secondary amenorrhoea will not be considered. However, pubertal menorrhagia and dysmenorrhoea, when associated with the first menstrual year, have important implications and will be referred to.

PATHOPHYSIOLOGY AND CLASSIFICATION

Normal puberty

The key events of puberty development are well described (Dewhurst 1984, Rosenfield & Barnes 1993) and all doctors, nurses and health care personnel who deal with this very sensitive age group should understand the normal sequence of events.

Longitudinal studies of pubertal girls have been conducted as part of more comprehensive studies of human growth (auxology) and our understanding of this area owes much to the pioneering work of Marshall & Tanner (for references see Tanner 1981, Brook 1982). The first external signs are the onset of the growth spurt then breast budding and, almost simultaneously, the appearance of pubic hair; all being consequences of oestrogen production (Figs 13.1–13.3; Marshall & Tanner 1969).

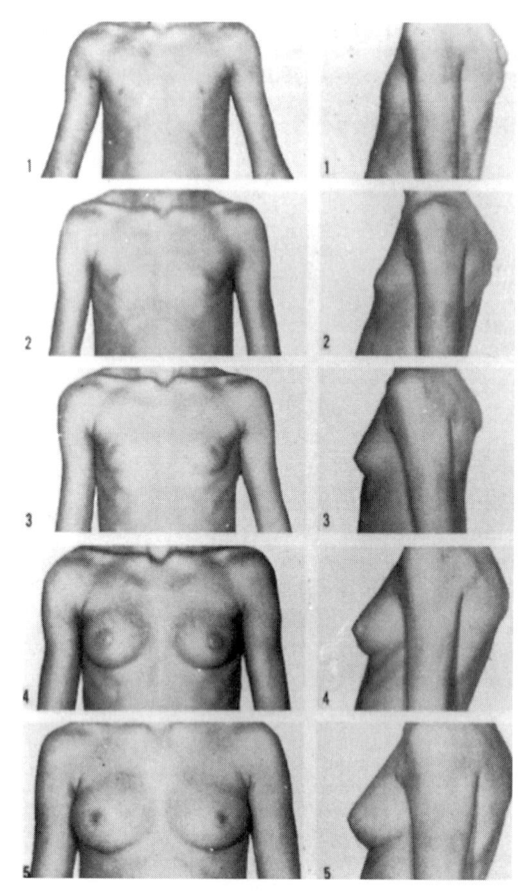

Fig. 13.1 Stages of breast development at puberty. **Stage 1** This is the infantile stage, which persists from the time the effect of maternal oestrogen on the breasts disappears, shortly after birth, until the changes of puberty begin. **Stage 2** The bud stage. The breasts and papillae are elevated as a small mound and there is an increase in the diameter of the areola. This stage represents the first indication of pubertal change in the breast. **Stage 3** The breasts and areola are further enlarged to create an appearance similar to that of a small adult breast, with a continuous rounded contour. **Stage 4** The areola and papilla enlarge further to form a secondary mound projecting above the contour of the remainder of the breast. **Stage 5** The typical adult breast with smooth rounded contour. The secondary mound present in stage 4 has disappeared.

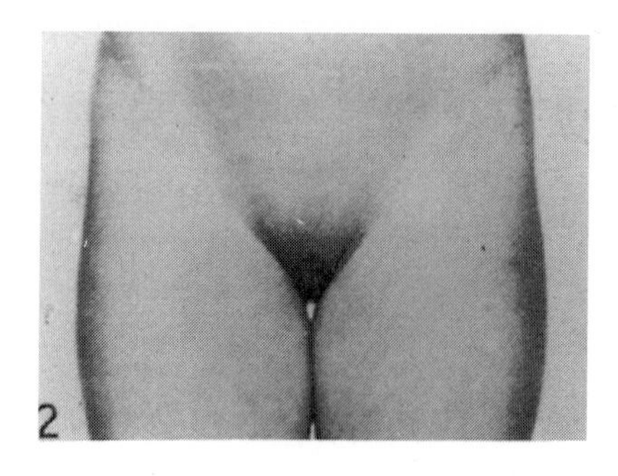

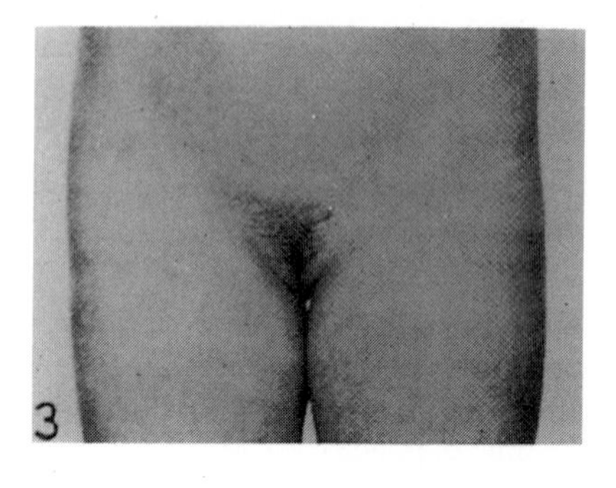

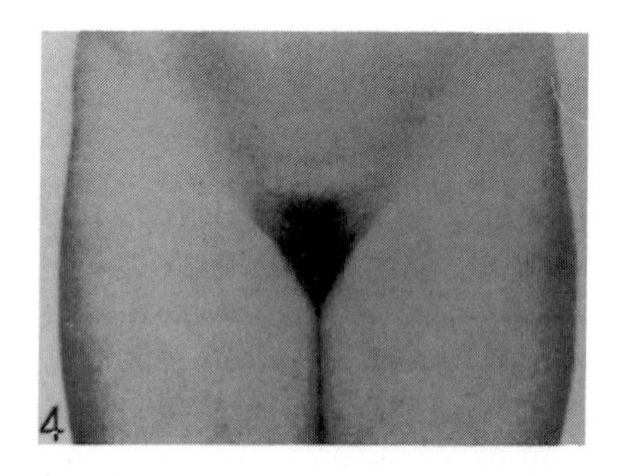

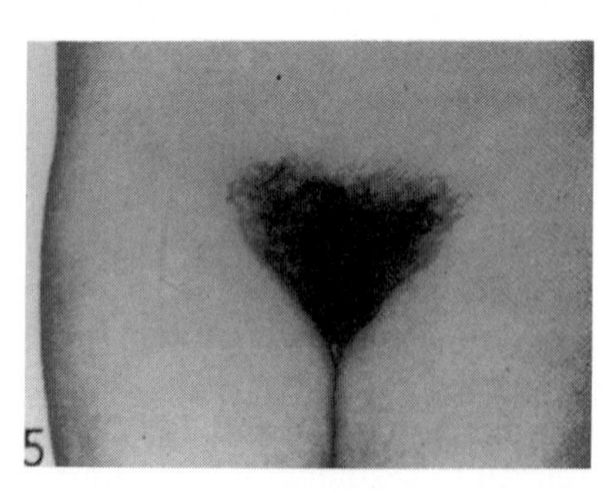

Fig. 13.2 Stages of pubic hair development at puberty. **Stage 2** Sparse growth of slightly pigmented hairs on either the labia or the mons pubis. **Stage 3** The hair is darker and coarser and spreads sparsely over and on either side of the midline of the mons pubis. **Stage 4** The hair is adult in character but covers a smaller area than in most adults and has not spread to the medial surface of the thighs. **Stage 5** Hair distributed as an inverse triangle and spreading to the medial surfaces of the thighs. It does not spread to the linea alba or elsewhere above the base of the triangle.

Hormonal events

The hormonal secretions are an essential element. This involves the hypothalamus, the pituitary and the ovaries and is a coordinated evolution of the behaviour of the relevant endocrine glands. The process is capable of promoting ovarian function very much earlier, even in utero, and the events of puberty result from maturation of dynamic processes rather than acquisition of new functions. Much study has gone into understanding these interrelationships from early childhood to teens (Reindollar & McDonough 1987, Rosenfield 1991) and with progressive refinement of measurement of hormones our concepts have required constant fine-tuning. Only a brief summary is given here.

After fetal and neonatal life, the gonadotrophin functions of the hypothalamus and pituitary are heavily sup-

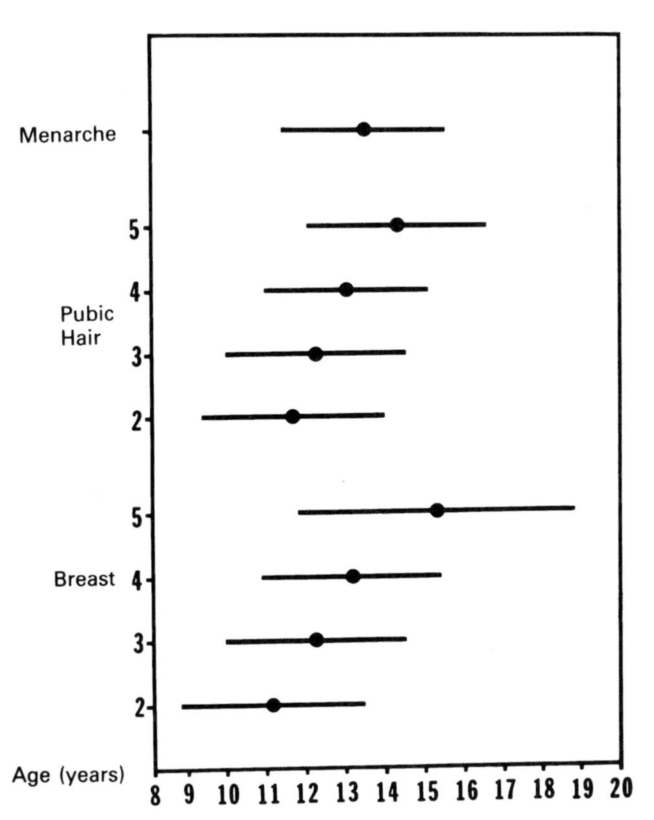

Fig. 13.3 Timing of pubic hair and breast changes and menarche. Horizontal line represents mean ± 2SD.

pressed, although both FSH and LH are released in childhood and there is a little ovarian activity.

The essential hormonal event of puberty is augmentation of pulsatile gonadotrophin secretion. This gonadotrophin release is controlled by the releasing hormones of the hypothalamus which, in turn, receives stimuli from the central nervous system and from other endocrine glands (see Ch. 12). The complex events of pubertal maturation specifically involve adrenal and thyroid glands, and are also influenced by nutritional and psychological factors. The magnitude of the early pubertal pulses is greater for LH than FSH, and they are initially mainly nocturnal and are very variable. Thus, measurements on different days may vary widely. The net effect is of intermittent bursts of stimuli to the ovaries and uterus. Differences in measured levels of oestrogen can be detected between girls and boys from about age 8 years. Thereafter, in the girl, oestrogen levels gradually increase. Despite this increase, gonadotrophin activity is greater. The former notion that the negative feedback system of ovarian suppression of pituitary activity is especially sensitive in the child, and becomes less so, is widely doubted (Reindollar & McDonough 1987). The system is much more complex than this, and is almost certainly controlled from more central mechanisms. The final event of pubertal maturation of this system is the development of the positive feedback system which requires pulsatile secretion and eventually leads to regular LH surges and ovulation.

The role of the thyroid gland is ill defined. The adrenal glands also increase their activity involving sex steroids from about 7 years of age in girls. Increased sebum formation, pubic and axillary hair, erectility of the clitoris and change in voice timbre are attributed primarily to the production of adrenal androgens but these differential roles are not clear cut and both adrenal and ovarian hormone levels are rising at the same time.

The role, if any, of the pineal gland in influencing gonadal function in the human is obscure. In subprimates, a suppressive effect on gonadotrophin release is influenced by exposure to light. Such a regulatory mechanism is of importance in seasonal mating behaviour but has no exact parallel in the human. Nevertheless, it is of interest that girls who are blind to light perception (as well as vision) tend to have an earlier menarche (Zacharis & Wurtman 1964). Without some light there may be release of inhibitory effect.

Ovarian and uterine development

Development of primordial follicles and secretion of oestrogens may be regarded as the final common path in all this hormonal activity, and there is a close correlation between oestrogen levels and sexual maturation.

In recent years pelvic ultrasonography has refined the description of the hitherto known anatomical changes. The ovaries often contain microcysts in the child, and increase very little in size until the pubertal changes actually begin. The uterus grows in concordance with somatic growth, with differential increased growth of the corpus starting from about the age of 7 years. However, the main differential increase of uterine size compared with somatic growth is obvious only after oestradiol secretion is measurably increased and tends to occur between breast stage 3 and 4 (Salardi et al 1985). Awareness of this comparatively late relative increase in uterine size has clinical relevance in the differentiation of arrested puberty and müllerian agenesis and also in the diagnosis of cause of precocious puberty. Blood oestrogen levels rise before and during puberty and continue to do so for about 3 years after menarche before the normal adult follicular levels of oestrogen are seen. This gradual maturation is a reflection of the finding that many of the early cycles are not ovulatory, and of the observation that the early postmenarchial years are relatively infertile, even in populations where sexual activity without contraception is usual in these years.

Menarche. The first period occurs because there has been sufficient endometrial stimulation to result in a withdrawal bleed when there is a temporary fall in the oestrogen level. It can be associated with an ovulatory/corpus luteum sequence but this is not usual. Although it really only indicates that a particular threshold has been reached in an already oscillating system, it is an obvious outward sign and of significance. In so far as it denotes an intact hypothalamic–pituitary–ovarian axis, functioning ovaries, presence of a uterus and patency of the genital tract it is indeed a notable event.

It may occur anywhere between 10 and 16 years (peak time is 13 years). The exact age is of less importance in diagnosis than its place in a girl's developmental process. Menarche generally occurs within 2 years of the earliest sign of breast development and within 1 year of peak growth velocity and close to breast stage 4. It tends to occur earlier in girls who are taller and heavier for their age. Bone age is generally about 13 years.

Disorders of timing of puberty

The gynaecologist is most likely to be consulted where there is delay or arrest of puberty or anomalous development.

Delay and arrest

Delay and arrest can overlap but include:

1. no thelarche by age 13;
2. abnormalities in the sequence and tempo of pubertal development;
3. amenorrhoea.

Any classification of delay in the onset of puberty depends on the diagnostic techniques available, and these have evolved over recent years. A useful aetiological classification is given in Table 13.1. Girls with ovarian failure, more than half of whom have chromosome anomalies, constitute the largest single group. Arrest of development involves initial changes, with incomplete development of secondary sex characters and/or failure of menarche.

Precocious puberty

Breast development before 8 years of age or menarche before 10 years, both of which are more than 2 standard deviations before the mean ages, are regarded as sexual precocity (Kulin 1987). There may or may not be accompanying presence of pubic hair and sebaceous secretion (adrenarche). Basic reasons are central (gonadotrophin production driving the ovaries) or peripheral (autonomous adrenal or ovary production). The commonest cause is constitutional early development (Table 13.2).

When precocious puberty occurs, there is disturbance of the normal sequence of changes and evidence of dissociation between adrenarche and gonadarche (Sklar et al 1980). Thus, where precocious puberty is evident under the age of 6 years, some important disturbance driving ovarian development is usually operating, and (except in primary adrenal disorders) the adrenal status is not affected and is in accordance with chronological age. However, when precocious features occur closer to the normal time of puberty onset, it is more likely that the problem is one of general advance of maturational processes and the adrenal status is more likely to be part of this and be advanced for age. Bone maturation is accelerated in precocious puberty, leading to premature epiphyseal closure and curtailed stature. If menstrual cycles occur, they may be ovulatory.

If a girl has primary hypothyroidism, there is elevation of thyroid-stimulating hormone levels, maintained by production and release of thyrotropin-releasing hormone and this also causes some release of prolactin.

Table 13.1 Causes of delayed onset of puberty

With little or no evidence of gonadal function		
Hypergonadotrophic		
Chromosomal, e.g. 45X, mosaic cell lines	27%	43%
Normal chromosomes but ovarian failure (includes 46XY, gonadal failure)	16%	
Hypogonadotrophic		
Reversible causes – constitutional delay, weight loss, adrenal disease, thyroid disorder	19%	31%
Irreversible causes – pituitary deficiency, cerebral tumours, congenital central nervous system defects	12%	
With definite evidence of gonadal function		
Anatomical causes, e.g. müllerian agenesis, genital tract obstruction	18%	26%
Inappropriate feedback anovulation Androgen insensitivity	8%	

From Reindollar et al 1981.

Table 13.2 Causes of precocious puberty

Basic drive	Origin	Example
Central	Constitutional	More likely when approaching the time of normal onset, i.e. 6 years upwards.
	Hypothyroidism	Autoimmune thyroiditis
	Specific central nervous system lesion	Craniopharyngioma Hydrocephaly Postinfective encephalitis Neurofibromatosis Congenital brain defects Cysts of third ventricle Hamartomas McCune–Albright syndrome
Peripheral	Ovary Adrenal Rare tumour	Tumour Tumour Chorion epithelioma
Extraneous	Exogenous oestrogens	

Anomalous puberty

This arises when there is inappropriate hormonal secretion with virilization. Causes include:

1. partial androgen insensitivity;
2. 5α-reductase deficiency;
3. gonadal dysgenesis with formation of functioning tumour;
4. congenital adrenal hyperplasia;
5. adrenal tumours.

Pubertal menorrhagia

This is usually associated with anovulation and attributed to impaired positive feedback. There may be endometrial hyperplasia (see Ch. 28).

Pubertal dysmenorrhoea

This can be caused by:

1. early ovulatory cycles;
2. congenital anomaly of genital tract causing obstruction (can be partial or unilateral);
3. endometriosis;
4. other pelvic disease.

AETIOLOGY

Delay

Essentially, delay or arrest of pubertal development happens because:

1. the ovary is not stimulated;
2. the ovary cannot respond;
3. the hormones produced are inappropriate;
4. there is no uterus to respond to hormonal stimulation;
5. there is obstruction.

These causes are set out in Table 13.1; differentiation between them depends on the outcome of investigation. Precocious or anomalous puberty may be due to tumour or inappropriate hormonal release. Menorrhagia is usually due to unopposed oestrogen action but may be associated with hypothyroidism or, rarely, a clotting disorder. Dysmenorrhoea may be obstructive or due to adnexal disease.

EPIDEMIOLOGY

Earlier menarche

Much interest has been shown in recent years in the tendency for menarche to occur at progressively earlier ages, thus tending to shorten childhood and prolong the interval between physiological and psychosocial maturity. There are many reviews of this trend (Dewhurst 1984). The essential conclusion from the study of many facets is that this change has coincided with a period of dramatic improvement in social conditions and nutrition. Children progress through childhood with comparatively accelerated growth, with fewer impediments and are, on average, taller and heavier than children of comparable age in previous generations. Girls are reaching their physiological maturity and genetic potential unimpeded by malnutrition and illness. Within a population, age of menarche is mainly correlated with socioeconomic factors including education, nutrition and urbanization. Adverse factors include poor nutrition and increasing size of family. Climate, season and race are not, of themselves, important. There is a strong genetic component and correlations in the time of menarche between uniovular twins, binovular twins, sisters and mother/daughter pairs (Huffman et al 1981).

There are important associations between low body weight, especially a low proportion of fat in delayed pubertal development including menarche, although the concept of a critical weight or weight-for-height (Frisch 1985) is a matter for debate. Menarche certainly tends to occur earlier in taller, heavier girls (Maclure et al 1991) but this, of course, is partly a reflection of the effect of the oestrogen production. Delay occurs in athletes as well as in girls of low absolute weight for height. The association is not necessarily causal (Baxter-Jones et al 1994). In well nourished girls, genetic influences seem to matter more (for discussion and references, see Stark et al 1989).

Incidence of pubertal disorders

The incidence of many of the conditions affecting puberty is not known because systematic surveys have not been carried out on a firm geographic base. Many valuable series (Reindollar et al 1981) have been from tertiary centres where there has been high selectivity for referral and treatment. Thus, a girl with Turner's syndrome or with an imperforate hymen is more likely to be treated locally, whereas a girl with precocious puberty or anomalous development is more likely to be referred to an expert in a more limited field. Some very important conditions are quite rare but there is a large number of them and the combined clinical effect is of significance. Most early teenage girls have normal pubertal development, and the few with a significant underlying anomaly are easily overlooked among many comparatively minor problems. Thus, most girls with an unusual problem of development are likely to be seen first by a doctor who has never encountered that problem before.

For example, if an average family practice cares for 2000 people, this would include about 70 girls between 10–15 years at any one time. This number will obviously vary with the age distribution of the practice. Even if one allows for 30 years of practice with 15 girls/year growing up, a family doctor would care for about 500 girls in a professional lifetime. Conditions rarer than 1 in 500 are likely never to be seen, and even for commoner conditions random chance will affect the number.

A gynaecologist might be expected to see referred problems from about 350 girls of any one age at a time (assuming one gynaecologist per 50 000 total population). In a professional lifetime this represents the problems of about 10 000 girls passing through puberty. On average, a gynaecologist may see a fair selection of commoner anomalies, e.g. uterine abnormalities, but only about four girls with Turner's syndrome (incidence about 1 in 2500) and only two or three girls with an imperforate hymen (incidence about 1 in 4000). Subspecialization will tend to distort these figures, but is necessary to provide expertise in this field.

PRESENTATION

Initial consultation

Handling the initial approach is crucial to the doctor's future relationship with the girl. The exact circumstances and age will determine the best way to proceed. Extreme sensitivity about burgeoning sexuality or its failure can be assumed even if not overtly expressed. The occasional important deviation from normal pubertal development has to be distinguished from the much commoner minor variations within the normal, but it is better to err on the side of excessive rather than too little concern. Apart from a few urgent conditions, study of the problem can be stepwise and based on observations of dynamic changes. When a mother brings a girl (or she comes of her own accord) there is a problem, no matter how trivial it may appear to be. A dismissive approach may be disastrous and inhibit correct diagnosis for years. Correct diagnosis is most likely to be achieved by interested acceptance of the presenting feature.

The prepubertal girl

Some problems of puberty will have been foreseen since infancy, e.g. imperforate vagina or congenital adrenal hyperplasia. Problems of genital anatomy may come to notice at any stage of childhood. Differentiation will be that appropriate to age. In the prepubertal child an unusual appearance may be associated with:

1. labial adhesions;
2. vaginal agenesis;
3. vaginal cyst;
4. unusual anomalies;
5. uterovaginal prolapse.

Any bleeding before secondary sexual development should be investigated further.

Precocious puberty will present with the untimely appearance of breast development together with pubic hair and/or vaginal bleeding.

Around the time of puberty

The main presenting features include:

1. lack of breast development;
2. amenorrhoea;
3. an unusual genital feature, e.g. enlarged clitoris or enlarged labia;
4. abdominal swelling;
5. inability to insert a tampon;
6. abdominal pain;
7. heavy or irregular bleeding;
8. dysmenorrhoea.

An important aspect of presentation is the combination of features. Short stature has not been included in the above list, but it is a very important accompanying feature and is sometimes present, yet has often been overlooked when a girl presents with delay of puberty (Fig. 13.4). It is easy to screen for, but if it is the primary presenting feature it is more likely to be noted in childhood and the patient referred to a paediatric endocrinology clinic (Fig. 13.5).

In considering the history at the presenting consultation, it should be appreciated that a girl at this age (10–16 years) will often seem to have little awareness of the timescale of her body development and of previous events. Her mother may be helpful over early childhood illnesses but may have limited awareness of the puberty changes so far.

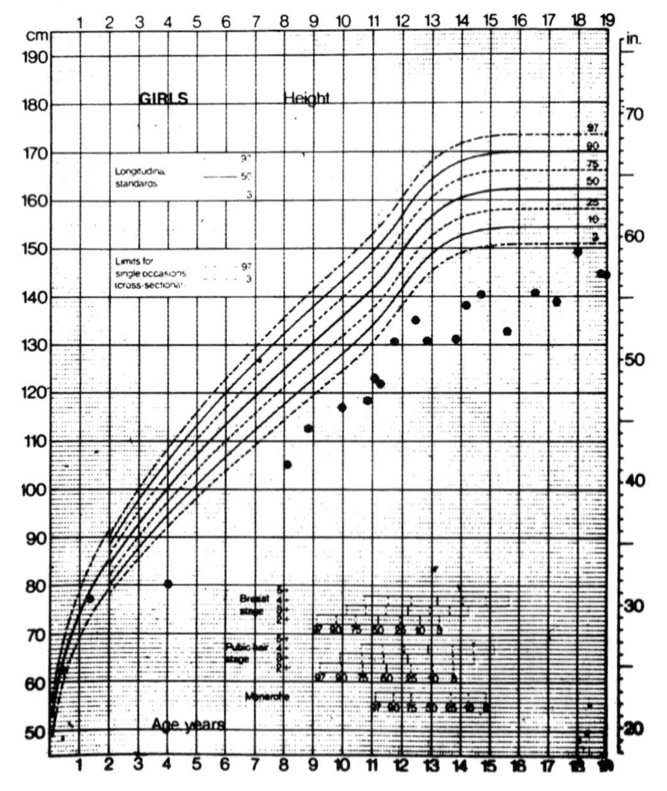

Fig. 13.4 Height of 21 girls with Turner's syndrome at the time of first diagnosis. Several were over 14 years of age before the diagnosis was made, despite the short stature which was a feature in all.

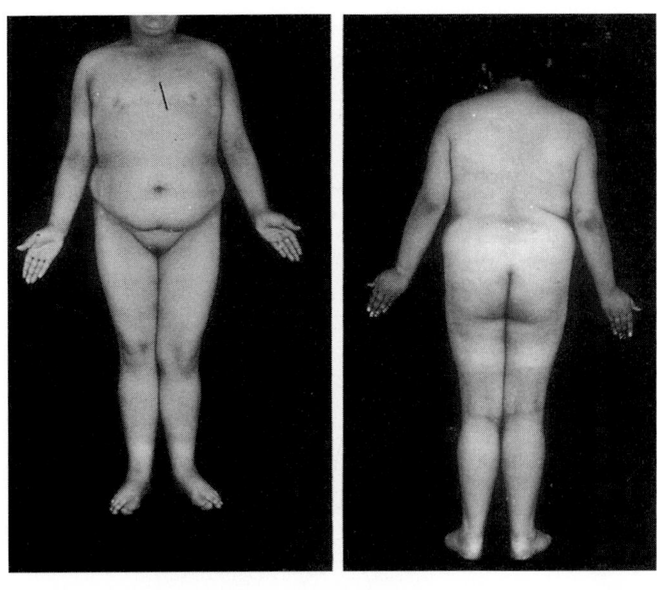

Fig. 13.5 Characteristic phenotype of Turner's syndrome.

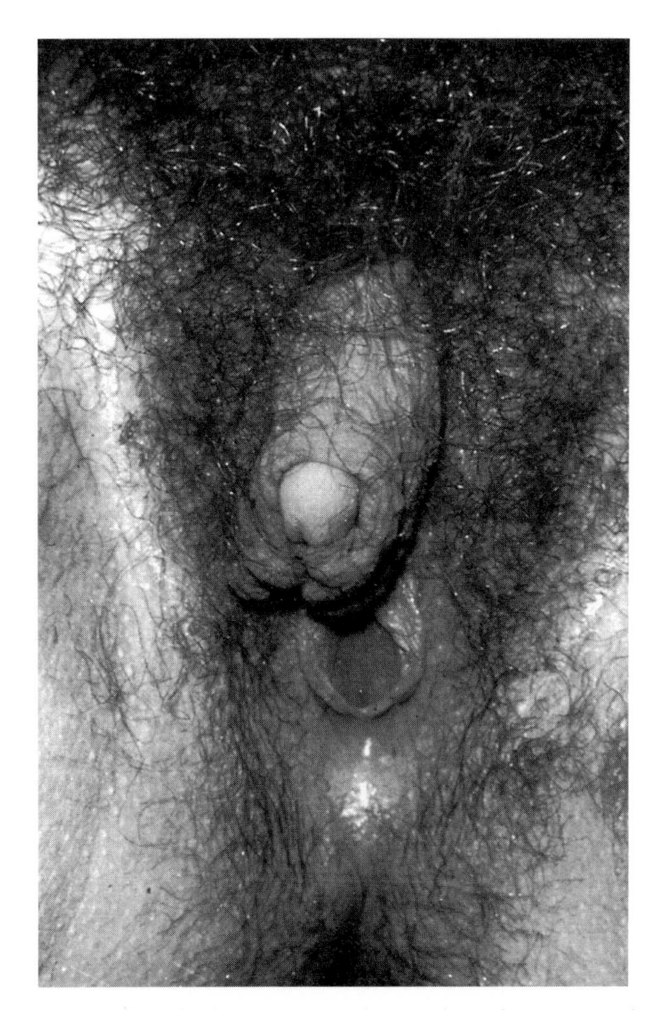

Fig. 13.7 Clitoral enlargement occurring at puberty due to tumour in an abdominal testis.

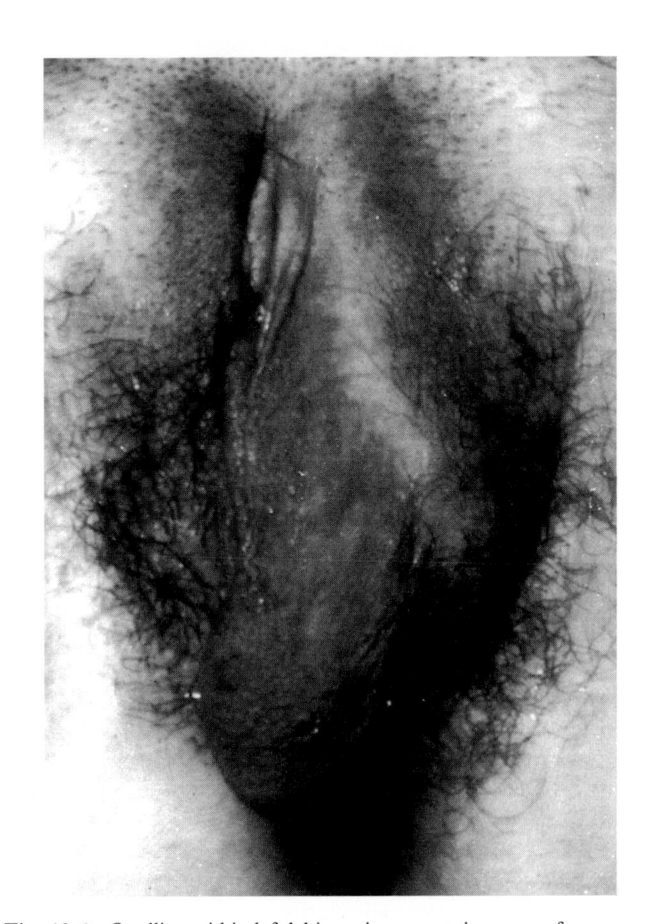

Fig. 13.6 Swelling within left labia majora occurring soon after puberty. Although alarming to a teenage girl, this proved to be a simple cyst.

Particular attention should be paid to some associations.

1. Heart disorders or operations – chromosome anomalies.
2. Bowel or urinary investigations – anatomical anomalies of the genital tract.
3. Hernia repair – gonadal disorder.
4. Hip or leg problems – apt to be blamed for short stature.
5. Slow general development – hypothyroidism, hypothalamic disorder.
6. Anorexia – hypothalamic delay.

Where the presenting features include abdominal swelling, with or without a history of amenorrhoea, pregnancy as well as ovarian swellings and menstrual obstruction should be remembered.

If primary amenorrhoea is the presenting feature, the following differential approach can streamline the possibilities.

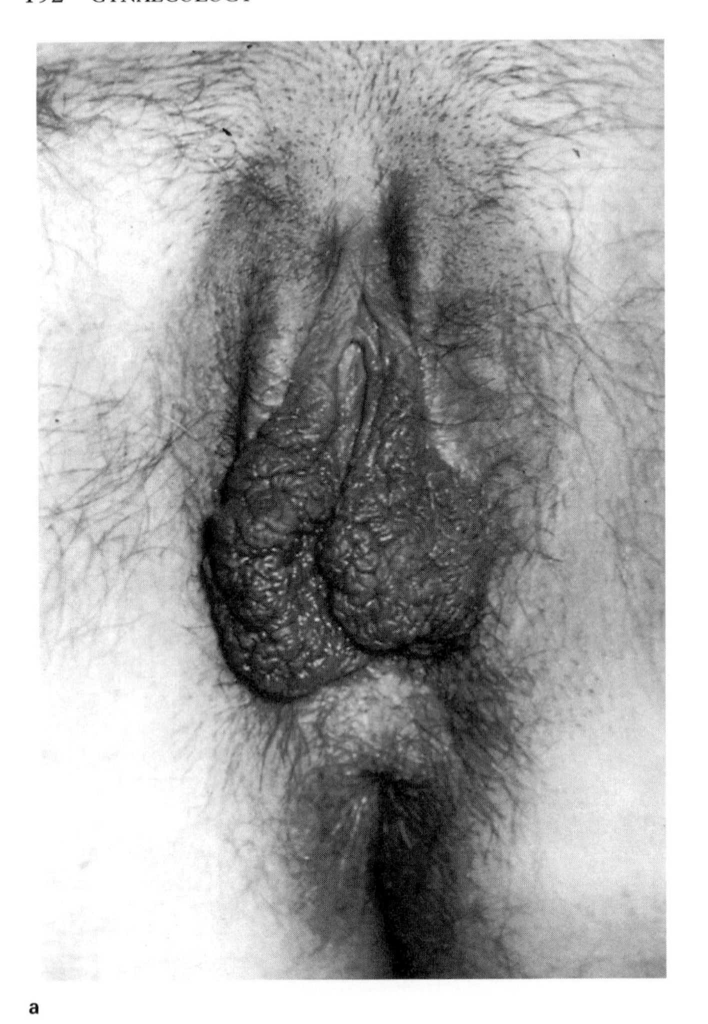

a

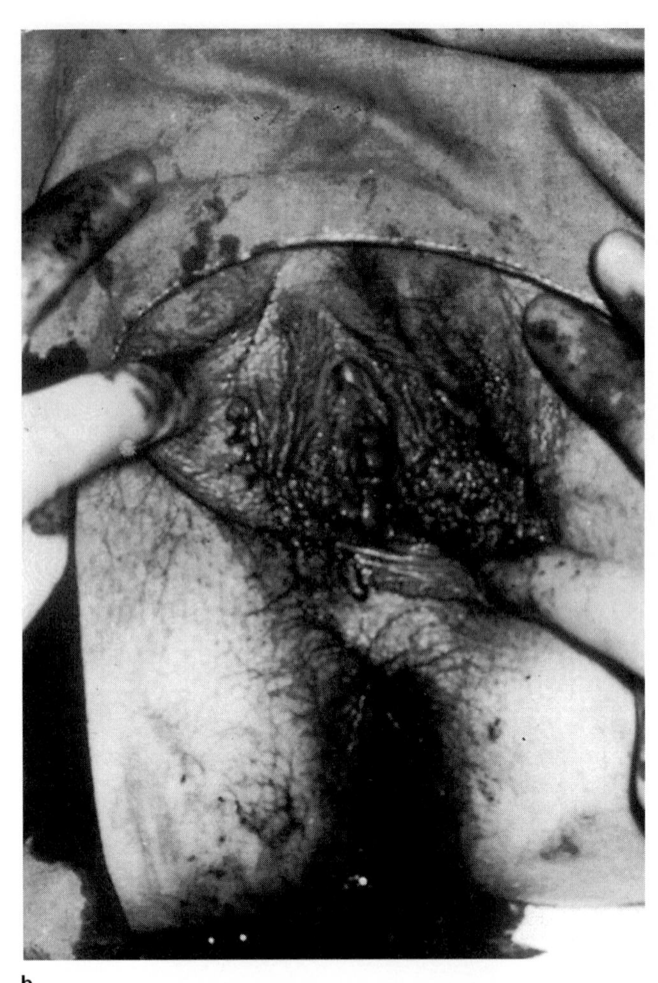

b

Fig. 13.8 **a** Unduly large pigmented labia causing discomfort. **b** Reduction in progress; right side completed, the left is still intact.

If secondary sex characteristics are:

1. Good
   a. Haematocolpos.
   b. No vagina or uterus.
   c. Polycystic ovary disorder.
   d. (Pregnancy.)
2. Poor or absent
   a. Constitutional delay.
   b. Primary gonadal failure.
   c. Hypothalamic or pituitary failure (includes weight-related arrest of development).

Heavy, prolonged bleeding may be a feature of early cycles. There may be dramatic exsanguination.

Awareness of anomalous development by the girl or her mother is an unusual presentation and is likely to be associated with secondary sex characteristics since it is the gonadal function that has probably caused the change (Fig. 13.6). Clitoral enlargement (Fig. 13.7), unduly large labia (Fig. 13.8) or awareness of a septum or blockage may be the presenting event.

INVESTIGATION AND DIAGNOSIS

The history, clinical examination, assessment of stature and stage of pubertal development are fundamental, and will often lead to identification of the category of problem if not the exact diagnosis (Duncan 1995).

The range and sophistication of investigations have developed in recent years. Some are basic and others are best reserved for interpretation at specialized centres.

Karyotype

This is particularly relevant where there is short stature and/or suspicion of ovarian failure. A buccal smear for Barr bodies is of very limited value since some of the girls with a mosaic pattern will be positive (see Ch. 1).

Banding techniques will clarify some of the more complex X chromosome patterns. Where there is deletion of X material, cardiac screening should be performed.

Endocrine

Measurement of gonadotrophin levels (FSH and LH) is important where there is amenorrhoea and lack of secondary sex development. This distinguishes between hypo- and hypergonadotrophic causes, and enables rationalization of further testing. Where levels are low, then testing of the pituitary response to gonadotrophin-releasing hormone will help to distinguish primary pituitary from hypothalamic causes.

Measurement of thyroxine and prolactin levels may be useful in amenorrhoea.

Measurement of oestrogen levels is of little value if there is no clinical evidence of ovarian activity, but is useful where there is apparent arrest of early development or where there are secondary sex characteristics and when menstrual obstruction has been excluded. In the latter event, normal or even above normal levels may be associated with polycystic ovarian disorder or congenital adrenal hyperplasia, even with primary amenorrhoea.

Measurement of blood testosterone level is essential where there is suspicion of testicular or Leydig cell tissue.

Where congenital adrenal hyperplasia is due to 21-hydroxylase deficiency 17-αOH-progesterone will be raised.

X-ray

Bone age is an extremely useful indicator where there is delay or acceleration of pubertal development. It permits a biological rather than chronological age to frame other observations.

Intravenous pyelography has largely been superseded by ultrasound for examination of the renal tract, which should always be investigated where there are anatomical abnormalities of the genital tract. Where hypogonadotrophic hypopituitarism is diagnosed, studies of the pituitary fossa by X-ray or computerized tomography scan are indicated. Anosmia (Kallman's syndrome) is an unusual accompaniment.

Ultrasound

Pelvic ultrasound scanning has extended diagnostic possibilities in recent years. It is particularly useful where there is menstrual obstruction (see Ch. 1, Fig. 1.16) and polycystic ovaries (e.g. in pubertal menorrhagia), abdominal swelling and for identification of kidneys. It is an essential early step when there is good secondary sex development and no menarche. It is of some use in girls with delayed puberty in that the presence of ovaries and uterus can generally be established.

However, there are pitfalls. The prepubertal ovary may not be seen. The gonad without a müllerian system may be very high and lateral and is easily missed. Recognition of an unstimulated uterus (e.g. in primary ovarian failure) may be difficult and presence of a rudimentary, but uncanalized, uterus may deceive. Awareness and better technical resolution will hopefully reduce these misinterpretations.

Scanning of the premenarchial pelvis has proved particularly useful in surveillance of ovarian or uterine development during spontaneous or therapeutic progress towards menarche. The steep increase in uterine size between about 10 and 13 years can be measured (Ivarsson et al 1983). The mean volume of the ovary is 3.30 cm^3 at menarche. Girls with precocious puberty tend to have ovaries greater than the mean plus 2SD for their age, while those in girls with Turner's syndrome are less than the mean minus 2SD (Ivarsson et al 1983). Normally, as menarche approaches, there is a 'megalocystic' appearance indicative of multiple follicular development without ovulation (Stanhope et al 1985).

Where precocious puberty is being investigated, abdominal ultrasound and hormonal investigation are basic. The diagnostic challenge in this condition is to establish whether the abnormal presenting feature(s) is isolated or part of a coordinated disturbance. Thus ultrasound examination of the ovaries and uterus may distinguish between absence of stimulation, a physiological response to abnormally early oestrogen stimulation or local pathology. If peripheral causes are excluded, cerebral investigation by computerized tomography scan and nuclear magnetic resonance investigation will require specialized referral.

Where pubertal menorrhagia is the problem, a balance has to be struck between reluctance to interfere and concern lest there is a pathological cause. An ultrasound scan may reveal unusual intrauterine contents: the possibility of an incomplete abortion should be remembered. The multicystic ovaries associated with anovulation and endometrial hyperplasia are an exaggeration of the normal findings, and the condition is self-limiting but may require treatment.

Magnetic resonance imaging

This will certainly demonstrate anatomy but there is limited experience of its use in diagnosing abnormalities.

Laparoscopy

Where there is doubt about the internal anatomy, obstruction that cannot be effectively drained vaginally or severe dysmenorrhoea in the early cycles, this is a useful investigation.

It is of very limited value if there is primary gonadal failure. If there are raised gonadotrophins, it is possible to establish whether there are streak gonads or ovaries with primordial follicles which cannot be stimulated (resistant ovary syndrome). However, this differentiation can be deferred since there appear, at present, to be no useful therapeutic options (Ledger et al 1989).

Special situations

Assessment of growth, especially a growth spurt, stage of puberty development and identification of discrepancies provide the important diagnostic clues. If a girl is well grown, has had a growth spurt but no menarche, there is likely to be a significant cause and investigation must be pursued. Precocious puberty may be accepted to be constitutional once important pathological causes have been excluded. However, there are times when a systematic sequence of investigation does not enable diagnosis, and observation over a period of weeks or months may be helpful.

A particular difficulty is to distinguish between constitutional delay, hypothalamic causes and weight-related delay.

Where there is hypogonadotrophic hypogonadism, normal chromosomes, normal anatomy and delayed bone age, an increase in weight, increased growth velocity and onset of breast development, on successive examinations, would be important clues.

TREATMENT

This follows from the cause. Therapeutically, there may be several possible outcomes.

Cure

Surgical

1. Imperforate hymen: adequate cruciate incision may suffice (Fig. 13.9).
2. Vaginal atresia with a functioning uterus: this may be difficult and prolonged, but the aim is the restoration of normal function (where there is cervical atresia this would still be the primary objective; see Ch. 1 for discussion and references and Ch. 11).
3. Unduly enlarged labia.
4. Removal of ovarian or adrenal cyst or tumour.
5. Some cerebral tumours.

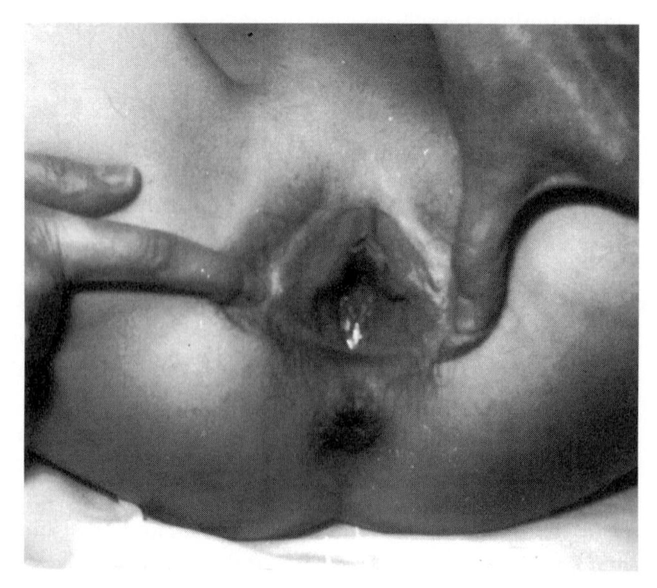

Fig. 13.9 Imperforate hymen, presenting with amenorrhoea and requiring excision and drainage.

Medical

1. Hypothyroidism: treatment of this may normalize the development of puberty.
2. Hyperprolactinaemia.
3. Constitutional delay: self-limiting but pubertal development can be expedited.

Management with irremediable cause

1. Primary ovarian failure, e.g. Turner's: replacement therapy possibly with GH, certainly with oestrogens. If there is Y chromosome material gonadectomy is necessary.
2. Androgen insensitivity: gonadectomy strongly advisable, oestrogen replacement.
3. Müllerian agenesis: consideration of vaginal enlargement and its timing.
4. Pituitary deficiency (with or without cerebral tumour): replacement treatment.
5. Hypothalamic deficiency: LH-releasing hormone may enable pubertal development. Alternative is oestrogen replacement.

Treatment of cause

When treatment is possible but may not cure the puberty problem:

1. Polycystic ovarian disorder: treatment may suppress the condition and the problem may be self-limiting.
2. Congenital adrenal hyperplasia: steroid treatment or adjustment may enable menarche to occur.
3. Weight-related amenorrhoea: this is apt to persist or recur.
4. Some pituitary/hypothalamic disorders may be treatable.

Primary ovarian failure

Replacement oestrogen is the basis of treatment. In most circumstances of primary ovarian failure there is a uterus and vagina, and in the long term oestrogen/progestogen in an oral contraceptive type of pill is advisable for endometrial protection. Initial replacement with oestrogen alone is reasonable, especially if the girl is young, as this simulates nature. In girls of average stature a starting dose of 0.02 mg ethinyloestradiol or equivalent is reasonable.

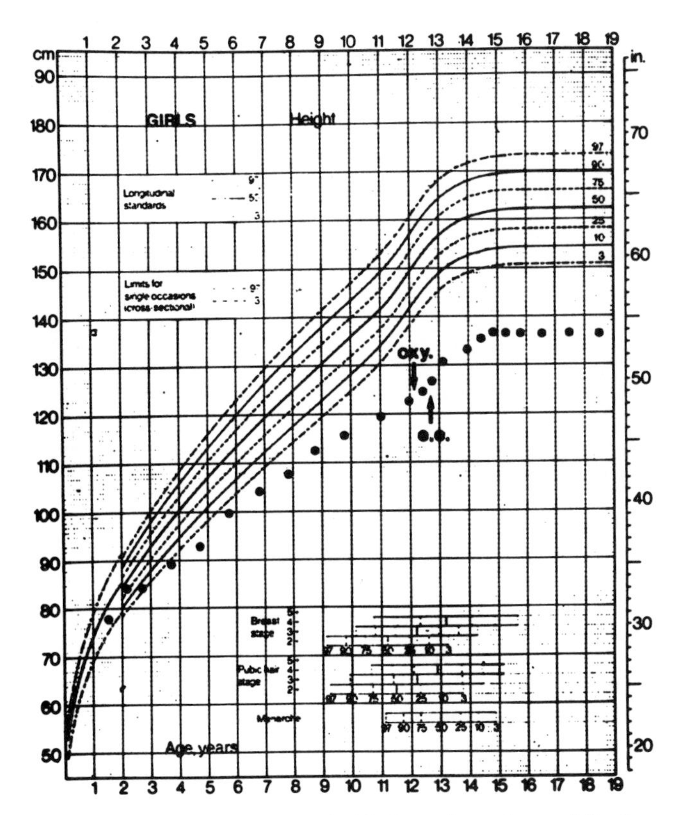

Fig. 13.10 Growth spurt in a girl with Turner's syndrome, following oxymetholone and later oestrogen administration.

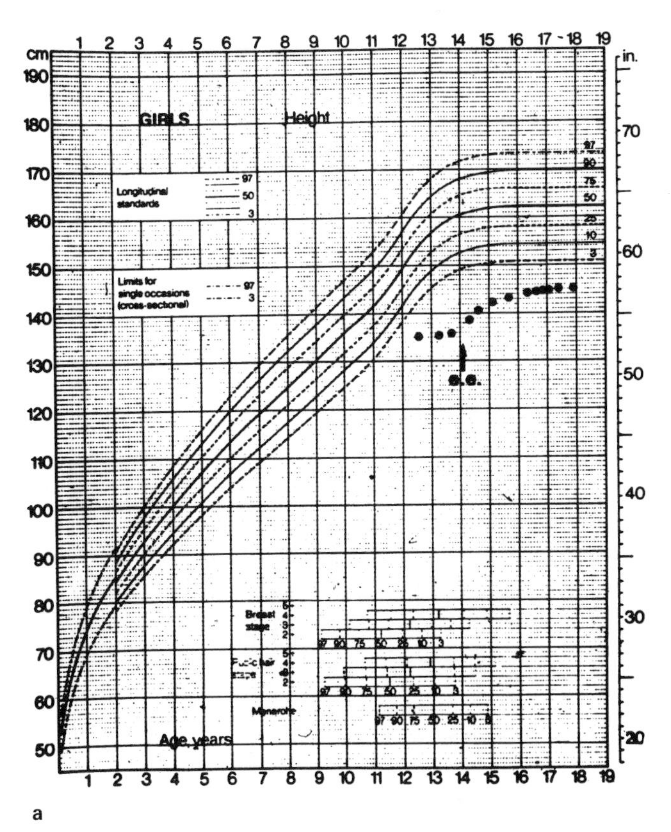

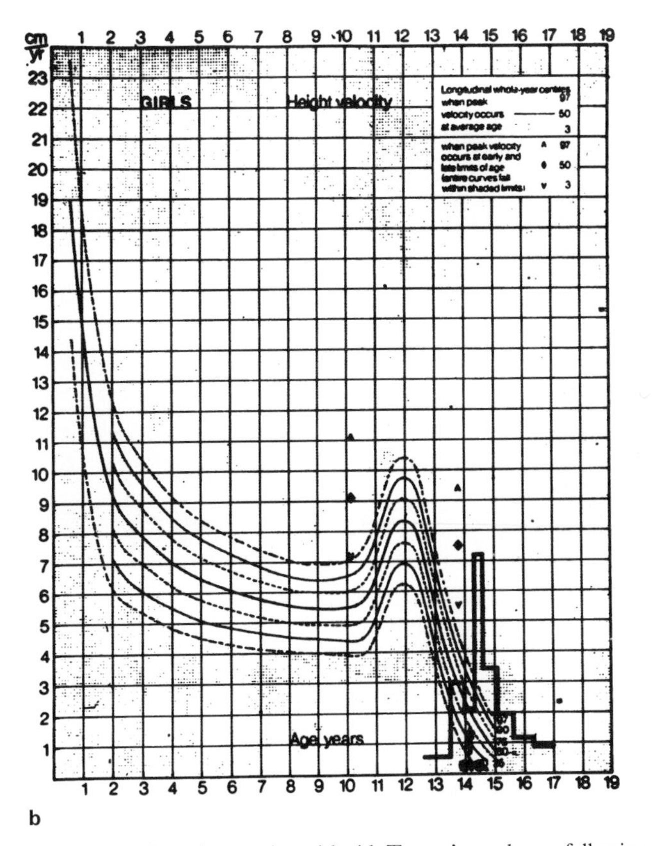

Fig. 13.11 Growth spurt in a girl with Turner's syndrome following oestrogen administration. **a** Although there is a clear growth spurt with increased height velocity, **b** the spurt is short-lived and makes little impact on the deficit in stature.

This will usually produce a growth spurt and then hasten epiphyseal closure as well as encourage breast and pubic hair development. If the girl is eunuchoid and considerably above average height, increased dosage may be used to accelerate the growth spurt and close the epiphyses quickly.

Where gonadal failure accompanies short stature (Turner's syndrome and its variants), special considerations apply and treatment depends on age. Hopefully the diagnosis will increasingly be made before the age of puberty and treatment started in a paediatric clinic. Without treatment there is no growth spurt (Ranke et al 1983) but there is prolonged continued growth. Final height, on average, is 150 cm. Oestrogen and oxymetholone each cause a growth spurt but this is of short duration and magnitude (Figs 13.10–13.12). The therapeutic aim in girls with Turner's syndrome involves both prepubertal increase in growth and a more sustained growth spurt. The former can be assisted by growth hormone (GH) and the latter by very low, physiological levels of oestrogen. The addition of oxymetholone seems to add little. Early trials of biological GH were halted before full evaluation because of Creutzfeldt–Jakob disease but more recent reports of synthetic GH are encouraging (Rosenfield et al 1992).

Maximum growth rate occurs in the first 2 years of

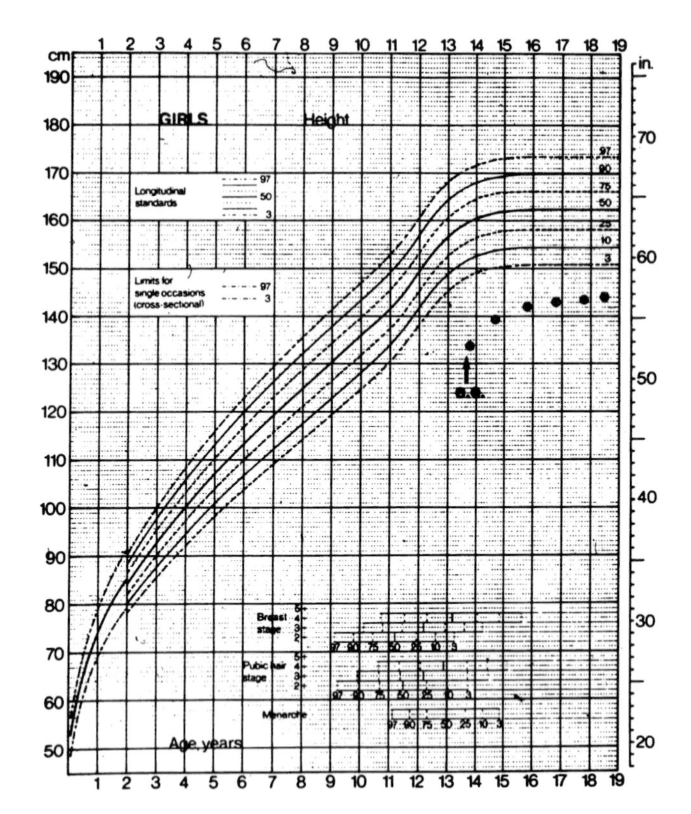

Fig. 13.12 Mean growth spurt in 7 girls with Turner's syndrome, treated with oestrogens at a mean age of just under 14 years, and followed annually for 5 years. There was continuing slow growth.

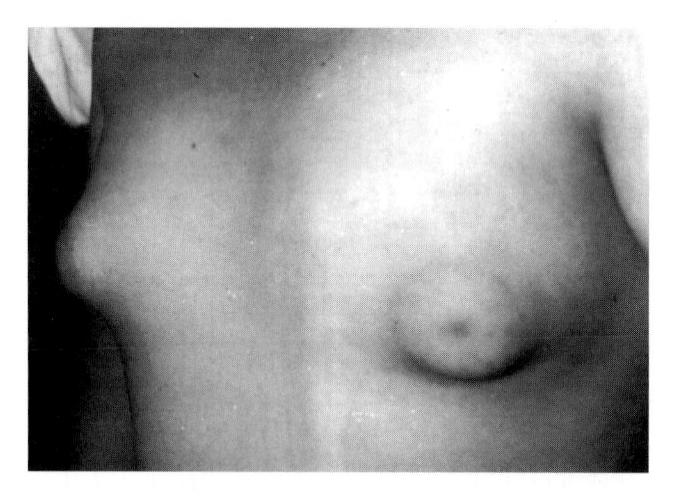

Fig. 13.13 Breast development in Turner's syndrome following oestrogen administration. There is good areolar development but little breast tissue after several years of hormone replacement.

treatment with GH, with sustained growth for as much as 6 years resulting in a net gain in height compared with previous standards. If treatment is started early enough in childhood, the prepubertal growth deficit can be reduced and a growth spurt by the addition of oestrogens brought in at a physiological time. In normal girls peak height velocity occurs before the menarche at very low oestrogen levels and the therapeutic regime in Turner's attempts to mimic this (Ross et al 1986). Thus, a current regime is to start ethinyl oestradiol at about age 10 at a dose of 2 to 5 μg/day (50–100 ng/kg/day) increasing after about a year to 5–10 μg/day (100–200 ng/kg/day) and after another year to 10–20 μg/day, achieving these increments according to the growth spurt and pubertal development, and aiming to reach withdrawal bleeds by cyclical administration by about 13 years. A combined oestrogen–progestogen preparation can then be introduced for long-term use.

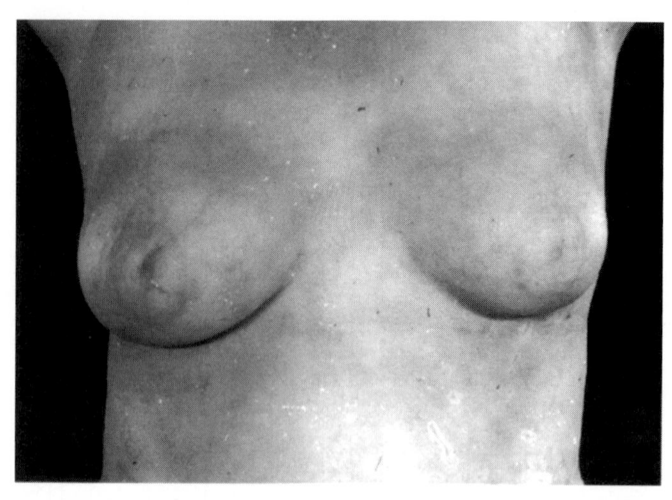

Fig. 13.14 In this girl with Turner's syndrome, hormone replacement resulted in good breast but poor nipple development.

It is not yet certain that final height will be increased by combined use of GH and slow increment of oestrogens but the attainment earlier than before of some height increase, of pubertal development and 'periods' closer to the age of her peer group are great benefits to girls with Turner's syndrome. The quality of breast development appears to be very variable and it is uncertain whether dosage or timing of oestrogens affects this critically (Figs 13.13 and 13.14).

Girls who look younger than their years tend to be treated accordingly, and advice should be offered to counteract this. Ensuring that the girl and her mother understand about infertility, despite apparent puberty development, requires tact with clarity. Long-term considerations include the addition of progestogens to the oestrogen replacement, advice concerning the value of continuing replacement treatment throughout the reproductive years and the possibility of donor egg pregnancies. Where there is a Y chromosome (e.g. 45X/46XY) the streak gonads should be removed (see below).

Androgen insensitivity

Management must include advice concerning removal of gonads and then replacement oestrogens (see Ch. 11). There is longer than usual prepubertal growth and a growth spurt at the mean age for boys, and final stature, therefore, is usually above the female mean. Breast development tends to be less than usual and there is poor vulvar development with almost no pubic hair. The build is generally slim and boyish. The exact incidence of gonadoblastoma or dysgerminoma formation in XY individuals is uncertain since there may be biased reporting from positive cases, but it is estimated at about 30% (for discussion, see Verp & Simpson 1987). There is no advantage in retaining the gonads and removal is advised when the diagnosis is made (Batch et al 1992). Teenagers may be reluctant to have their gonads removed in this condition as it seems unphysiological and the miracles of modern reproductive technology appear to offer hope. It remains to be seen whether ultrasound scanning (e.g. at 6-monthly intervals) offers sufficient reliability in this situation at least to defer gonadectomy. Laparoscopic removal might be more appealing.

After gonadectomy, long-term oestrogens should be prescribed for their effect on vaginal epithelium, osteoporosis and cardiovascular system. There seems no point in recommending progestogens as well unless there is shown to be a protective effect on breast disease. Where incomplete androgen insensitivity or 5α-reductase deficiency is diagnosed, there is concomitant virilization and, assuming the female gender is to be reinforced, gonadectomy becomes a matter of greater urgency. Clitoral reduction or recession may be required.

Hypogonadotrophic hypogonadism

Where the cause is treatable, this should be effected first.

Where the basic cause is hypogonadotrophic, options are available. Replacement oestrogens (later, with progestogens) can be offered, and the effect should be similar to that in girls with ovarian failure. Gonadotrophin therapy should be reserved for induction of ovulation and prior achievement of secondary sex characteristics is preferable. A more physiological approach is the use of pulsatile LH-releasing hormone (GnRH) but this is difficult to sustain in the teenage girl (Stanhope et al 1987).

Anorexia nervosa and weight-related amenorrhoea

Management is notoriously difficult, and is essentially similar whether there is delay in onset of puberty, arrest of development or secondary amenorrhoea. Use of oestrogens to promote development of puberty may be associated with slight weight gain and may help over a difficult patch.

Precocious puberty

Treatment depends on the cause and should, where possible, remove the gonadotrophic or oestrogen stimulus. This may require neurosurgery or radiotherapy. Where the diagnosis is constitutional precocious puberty, the treatment of choice nowadays is a GnRH analogue (Swaenepoel et al 1991). This usually results in regression of the breast, uterine and ovarian development and cessation of menses. It seems promising that there will also be delay of bone maturation and an increase in final height.

Other therapies include cyproterone acetate, which suppresses gonadotrophin secretion (Lorini et al 1981) and medroxyprogesterone acetate (Grumbach 1985). These will delay the progression of puberty and diminish some of the effects, but tend to have side-effects. Danazol can also be used but side-effects are a disadvantage.

Psychological aspects of treatment are important. Management should usually be according to age, despite the physical appearance.

Pubertal menorrhagia

If rare pathological causes are excluded, use of oestrogen/progestogen as in the combined pill will usually permit acceptable withdrawal bleeds. If not, then continuous administration to achieve complete amenorrhoea may be more acceptable. Treatment should be discontinued after, say, 6 months and the natural cycle reviewed. Alternative hormonal treatment includes dihydrogesterone, which is less likely to inhibit ovulation, or depot injections of a progestogen.

Dysmenorrhoea

If this is due to a rudimentary horn which may be obstructed, then removal may be indicated. Occasionally endometriosis may be present, starting at, or soon after menarche, and if diagnosed should be appropriately treated. Otherwise the use of prostaglandin synthetase inhibitors, e.g. mefenamic acid or suppression of ovulation by a combined oestrogen–progestogen pill are the main therapeutic strategies.

RESULTS

Where the cause of the pubertal problem is reversible, the outcome is usually good.

There are, however, situations with continuing problems.

Following obstruction

Vaginal or cervical atresia. Maintenance of patency for menstrual function may be difficult or impossible (see Ch. 11). Endometriosis may be a severe problem resulting from obstruction.

Müllerian agenesis

Available techniques usually enable an adequate vagina.

Gonadal failure or removal

Results in terms of maintenance of secondary sex characteristics are usually good. Long-term replacement treatment, especially the addition of progestogens, where indicated, may be difficult to sustain. Sexual function is usually good.

Weight-related amenorrhoea

Despite achievement of normal weight for height, amenorrhoea may persist or recur.

Congenital adrenal hyperplasia

Good adrenal control may not necessarily result in normal ovarian function. Inappropriate feedback with hypergonadotrophin and polycystic ovarian disorder may occur. Fertility is reduced and early ovarian failure appears to be common.

Precocious puberty

The long-term outlook for girls with precocious puberty in terms of menstrual function and subsequent fertility is good, provided there was no serious pathology in the first instance (Murram et al 1984). Long-term follow up after GnRH analogues is still limited but, encouragingly a high rate of ovulation (about 90%) in treated girls studied 2 years after menarche has been found (Jay et al 1992).

Pubertal menorrhagia

The condition is generally self-limiting but if acceptable ovulatory cycles do not become established after the first 2 years, long-term menstrual problems are likely in about 50% of such girls (Rosenfield & Barnes 1993).

Dysmenorrhoea

Teenage endometriosis, arising either spontaneously or as a result of premenarchial obstruction, may have a very variable outcome. Treatment should aim for eradication.

Primary dysmenorrhoea has a very variable long-term outlook.

COMPLICATIONS

Normal menstrual function and fertility are not always achieved. Conditions resulting in positive complications are referred to here.

Cervical or vaginal atresia

Despite surgical endeavours there may be severe pelvic infection with pyosalpinx or peritonitis. Hysterectomy may be necessary.

Vaginal agenesis

Despite surgery, apareunia may result.

Hypo-oestrogenism

If oestrogen status is low in teenage life, there is an association with reduced bone mass (Emans et al 1990).

Psychological aspects

In many of the conditions causing disordered puberty there may be a substantial psychological aftermath, for example in learning about ovarian failure or müllerian agenesis. Even in constitutional delay in puberty, where the long-term outcome is good, there is evidence of considerable recollected distress and social disadvantage relating to the time of delayed puberty (Crowne et al 1991).

CONCLUSIONS

There is overlap between normal and abnormal pubertal development. Anatomical abnormalities of the genitalia are often complex. Short stature or the presence of other disorders may provide important diagnostic clues when pubertal development seems to be disordered.

It is important to avoid false reassurance concerning abnormal features, such as short stature, unexpected bleeding, failure to develop secondary sex characteristics or failure to menstruate. It is wise to seek another opinion if there are unresolved or unusual features.

It is extremely important to avoid undermining a girl's confidence in her own observations or her sexuality. A poor prognosis with respect to fertility must be conveyed tactfully.

KEY POINTS

1. Puberty is a coherent process involving oestrogen production, increased somatic growth and the development of secondary sexual characteristics.
2. The essential hormonal event of puberty is the augmentation of pulsatile gonadotrophin secretion, which is affected by endocrine, nutritional and psychological factors.
3. Menarche occurs after sufficient endometrium has developed to result in a withdrawal bleed when the oestrogen level temporarily falls. It usually occurs within 2 years of the earliest sign of breast development.
4. Appropriate investigation of abnormal events surrounding puberty must be based upon detailed history and examination of the patient.
5. The commonest cause of delayed puberty is ovarian failure.

More than half of the girls with delayed puberty have chromosome anomalies.

6. Serum gonadotrophin levels are important in distinguishing hypo- and hypergonadotrophic causes of delayed puberty.
7. Oestrogen and progesterone replacement are used in primary ovarian failure to induce pubertal growth and secondary sexual characteristics.
8. Precocious puberty, where breast development occurs before the age of 8 years, is most commonly due to constitutional early development.
9. Precocious puberty requires prompt investigation and treatment in order to avoid short stature from premature closure of the epiphyses.
10. Anorexia nervosa and acute weight loss are associated with amenorrhoea.
11. The psychological stress of pubertal disorders must be recognized and dealt with sympathetically in order to avoid excessive undermining of the patient's self-confidence.
12. Oocyte donation has been successfully used to allow patients with primary ovarian failure to achieve pregnancy and have their own children.

REFERENCES

Batch J A, Patterson N M, Hughes I A 1992 Androgen insensitivity syndrome. Reproductive Medicine Review 1: 131–150

Baxter-Jones A D G, Helms P, Baines-Preece J, Preece M 1994 Menarche in intensively trained gymnasts, swimmers and tennis players. Annals of Human Biology 21: 407–415

Brook C G D 1982 Growth assessment in childhood and adolescence. Blackwell Scientific, Oxford

Crowne E C, Shalet S M, Wallace W H B et al 1991 Final height in girls with untreated constitutional delay in growth and puberty. European Journal of Paediatrics 150: 708–712

Dewhurst C J 1984 Female puberty and its abnormalities. Churchill Livingstone, Edinburgh, pp 57–81

Duncan S L B 1995 Delayed puberty. Current Obstetrics and Gynaecology 5: 85–90

Emans S J, Grace E, Hoffer E A et al 1990 Estrogen deficiency in adolescents and young adults: impact on bone mineral content and effects of estrogen replacement therapy. Obstetrics and Gynecology 76: 585–592

Frisch R E 1985 Body fat, menarche and reproductive ability. Seminars in Reproductive Endocrinology 3: 45

Grumbach M M 1985 True or central precocious puberty. In: Krieger D T, Bardin C W (eds) Current therapy in endocrinology and metabolism. Dekker, Toronto

Huffman J W, Dewhurst C J, Capraro V D 1981 The gynaecology of childhood and adolescence. W B Saunders, Philadelphia

Ivarsson S A, Nilsson K O, Persson P-H 1983 Ultrasonography of the pelvic organs in pre-pubertal and post pubertal girls. Archives of Disease in Childhood 58: 352–354

Jay N, Mansfield J, Blizzard R M et al 1992 Ovulation and menstrual function of adolescent girls with central precocious puberty after therapy with gonadotrophin-releasing hormone agonists. Journal of Clinical Endocrinology and Metabolism 75: 890–894

Kulin H E 1987 Precocious puberty. Clinical Obstetrics and Gynecology 30: 714

Ledger W L, Thomas E J, Browning D, Lenton E A, Cooke I D 1989 Suppression of gonadotrophin secretion does not reverse premature ovarian failure. British Journal of Obstetrics and Gynaecology 96: 196–199

Lorini R, Colombo A, Ugazio A G et al 1981 Cyproterone acetate in precocious puberty. Journal of Endocrinological Investigation 4: 263

Maclure K M, Travis L B, Willett W, MacMahon B 1991 Prospective cohort study of nutrient intake and age at menarche. American Journal of Clinical Nutrition 54: 649–656

Marshall W A, Tanner J M 1969 Variations in the pattern of pubertal changes in girls. Archives of Disease in Childhood 44: 291–303

Murram D, Dewhurst J, Grant D B 1984 Precocious puberty: a follow up study. Archives of Disease in Childhood 59: 77–78

Ranke M B, Pfluger H, Rosendahl W et al 1983 Turner syndrome: spontaneous growth in 150 cases and review of the literature. European Journal of Pediatrics 141: 81–88

Reindollar R H, McDonough P G 1987 Neuroendocrine processes relevant to the childhood years. Clinical Obstetrics and Gynecology 30: 633

Reindollar R H, Byrd J R, McDonough P G 1981 Delayed sexual development: a study of 252 patients. American Journal of Obstetrics and Gynecology 140: 371–380

Rosenfeld R G, Frane J, Attie K M et al 1992 Six-year results of a randomised, prospective trial of human growth hormone and oxandrolone in Turner syndrome. Journal of Pediatrics 121: 49–55

Rosenfield R L 1991 Puberty and its disorders in girls. Endocrinology and Metabolism Clinics in North America 20:15-41

Rosenfield R L, Barnes R B 1993 Menstrual disorders in adolescence. Endocrinology and Metabolism Clinics in North America 22: 491–505

Ross J L, Long L M, Skerda M et al 1986 Effects of low doses of oestradiol on 6-month growth rates and predicted height in patients with Turner syndrome. Journal of Pediatrics 109: 950–953

Salardi S, Orsini L F, Cacciari E et al 1985 Pelvic ultrasonography in pre-menarchial girls: relation to puberty and sex hormone concentrations. Archives of Disease in Childhood 60: 120–125

Sklar C A, Kaplan S L, Grumbach M M 1980 Evidence for dissociation between adrenarche and gonadarche. Journal of Clinical Endocrinology and Metabolism 51: 548–556

Stanhope R, Adams J, Jacobs H S, Brook C G D 1985 Ovarian ultrasound assessment in normal children, idiopathic precocious puberty, and during low dose pulsatile gonadotrophin releasing hormone treatment of hypogonadotrophic hypogonadism. Archives of Disease in Childhood 60: 116–119

Stanhope R, Brook C G D, Pringle P J, Adams J, Jacobs H S 1987 Induction of puberty by pulsatile gonadotrophin releasing hormone. Lancet ii: 552–555

Stark O, Peckham C S, Moynihan C 1989 Weight and age at menarche. Archives of Disease in Childhood 64: 383–387

Swaenepoel C, Chaussain J L, Roger M 1991 Long-term results of long-acting luteinizing-hormone-releasing hormone in central precocious puberty. Hormone Research 36: 126–130

Tanner J M 1981 A history of the study of human growth. Cambridge University Press, Cambridge

Verp M S, Simpson J L 1987 Abnormal sexual differentiation and neoplasia. Cancer Genetics and Cytogenetics 25: 191–218

Zacharis L, Wurtman R 1964 Blindness: its relation to age of menarche. Science 144: 1154

14

Amenorrhoea and oligomenorrhoea, and hypothalamic–pituitary dysfunction

M. G. R. Hull M. I. M. Abuzeid

INTRODUCTION

This chapter focuses attention on the understanding and practical management of amenorrhoea and oligomenorrhoea due to endocrine disorders involving the hypothalamus and anterior pituitary, as they usually present to a gynaecologist, i.e. because of consequent ovarian endocrine and reproductive failure. Therefore discussion will be limited in the case of, for example, disorders of the thyroid or adrenal axis, and of primary ovarian failure, to what is needed for essential awareness and basic diagnosis. Some aspects are only touched on here because they are detailed in other chapters in this book.

Amenorrhoea and oligomenorrhoea are of course not diagnoses but the common presenting symptoms of a wide range of different causes. Each cause will therefore be separately discussed as a whole.

DEFINITIONS

Pathological amenorrhoea

Pathological amenorrhoea is usually defined as the absence of menstruation for at least 6 months, not due to pregnancy, in a woman of childbearing age. The usual age limits are 16 and 40 years, for menarche and menopause respectively. On the other hand, amenorrhoea may be recognized and specific treatment required before 16 years of age in a girl who has previously menstruated, or after 40 years if a cause is established other than primary ovarian failure.

Primary amenorrhoea

Primary amenorrhoea is defined as failure even to have menstruated by the age of 16 years, as the normal upper age limit for menarche is 15 years. It therefore means the same as delayed menarche, but may or may not be associated with delayed puberty. Puberty strictly means procreative ability but is generally used to mean secondary sexual development. Secondary sexual development begins before menarche with the onset of breast development (thelarche), normally by 13 years of age. Delayed puberty can therefore be recognized at 14 years, and its definition need not wait to include delayed menarche at 16 years.

Oligomenorrhoea

Oligomenorrhoea is usually defined by menstrual intervals between 6 weeks and 6 months. Those definitions are, however, arbitrary and do not necessarily reflect important distinctions; indeed they can be misleading. Oligomenorrhoea is so defined because the upper normal limit of the menstrual cycle length is 5 weeks. On the other hand, cycles of around 6 weeks' length are usually indistinguishable from normal in terms of follicular growth and hormonal development, apart from the delay in onset (Aksel 1981). Therefore oligomenorrhoea is likely to include a spectrum of conditions ranging from virtual normality at one end to the same causes as of amenorrhoea at the other. The main difference appears to be in the frequency of polycystic ovaries, which ultrasound and endocrine studies show account for about 90% of cases of oligomenorrhoea and 33% of amenorrhoea (although often without the classical syndrome, including hirsutism and obesity: Adams et al 1986, Hull 1987, 1989).

Some authors take 4 or 12 months as the criterion for amenorrhoea. Absence of menstruation for only 4 months after sudden cessation of previously normal cycles is undoubtedly appropriately treated as amenorrhoea; oligomenorrhoea implies repeated occurrence of prolonged menstrual intervals.

The distinction between primary and secondary amenorrhoea can also be misleading. Menstrual periods are sometimes described as having occurred once or twice at the expected age by patients who could not possibly have menstruated, for example with male pseudohermaphroditism and vaginal atresia, presumably from self-examination and wishful thinking! Primary and secondary amenorrhoea cannot be distinguished by any tests of endocrine function. The only endocrine disorder presenting specifically in either way is congenital hypothalamic failure; it presents of course with primary amenorrhoea and lack of pubertal development. By contrast, ovarian dysgenesis if partial can present with secondary amenorrhoea, whilst anorexia nervosa or hyperprolactinaemia can occur before puberty.

For all those reasons, primary and secondary amenorrhoea and oligomenorrhoea should be considered in the same way clinically and within a unified classification of causes as described later.

The definitions of individual conditions accounting for oligomenorrhoea will be considered where they are described. The reader first needs to appreciate that different authors employ inconsistent or ill-defined terminologies, for example hypothalamic–pituitary 'failure' versus 'disorder', and 'polycystic ovarian syndrome', 'polycystic ovarian disease' and 'polycystic ovaries'. These distinctions must be made within the context of a particular classification.

Physiological amenorrhoea

Physiological amenorrhoea occurs, of course, as normal before menarche and after the menopause. It is important never to overlook the possibility of pregnancy as the cause, even after years of amenorrhoea. Some conditions can resolve spontaneously, such as weight loss-related hypothalamic disorder, whilst in others, such as polycystic ovarian disease, ovulation may occur sporadically at long intervals; when ovulation occurs it does so unheralded by any warning menstruation.

CLASSIFICATION OF CAUSES

Anatomical abnormalities of the genital tract account for only about 1% of cases of amenorrhoea. The usual causes, affecting endocrine function, used to be classified nosologically (e.g. psychological, tumour, autoimmune disease) but this has given way to a systematic endocrinological approach:

1. Disorders of the hypothalamic – (anterior) pituitary–ovarian (H–P–O) axis
    a. hypothalamic
    b. pituitary
    c. ovarian
2. Disorders of other endocrine systems, e.g. thyroid, adrenal.

Disorders of the H–P–O axis

The disorders of the H–P–O axis can be further classified into primary failures and functional disorders. We now run into difficulties due to inconsistent use of such terms by different authors. Some use the term 'hypothalamic–pituitary failure' to mean any condition affecting the hypothalamus or pituitary resulting in impaired gonadotrophin secretion (hypogonadotrophism), while others simply refer to 'hypothalamic amenorrhoea'. Another common term is 'functional amenorrhoea', which is generally used to mean disorders not due to any evident lesion such as a tumour. We do not hold with the use of these terms and must make our own views clear.

We use *primary failure* to mean inherent failure of an endocrine organ, or at least of a specific cellular component, e.g. the gonadotrophin-releasing hormone (GnRH) neurons of the hypothalamus, or gonadotrophs of the pituitary, which may be affected selectively. This could result for example from a congenital malformation, compression by a tumour, or surgical destruction. This will lead to secondary (or tertiary) failure further down the axis; for example, a tumour compressing the hypothalamus can cause secondary pituitary failure and consequent (tertiary) ovarian failure.

By contrast, we use the term *functional disorder* to imply a reversible functional failure in which the affected func-

Table 14.1 Disorders of the H–P–O axis

Hypothalamic
Primary failures
  Compression by tumours
  Kallmann syndrome
Functional disorders
  Psychological disturbances
  Weight loss
  Extreme exercise

Pituitary
Primary failures
  Compression by tumours
  Damage by surgery, radiotherapy
  Infarction (e.g. Sheehan syndrome)
Hyperprolactinaemia
Functional failure secondary to hypothalamic failure or disorder

Ovarian
Primary failures
  Dysgenesis
  Damage by surgery, radiotherapy, chemotherapy
  Autoimmune disease
  Premature menopause
  Resistant ovary syndrome
Functional failure secondary to hypothalamic–pituitary failure or disorder
Polycystic ovarian disease

tional elements are structurally undamaged. Thus psychological disturbance can lead to hypothalamic disorder. An interesting example is a prolactin-secreting adenoma of the pituitary (prolactinoma). It is the commonest tumour disturbing reproductive function, but it rarely compresses the pituitary sufficiently to cause primary pituitary failure. It acts by short-loop feedback of the excess prolactin on hypothalamic GnRH secretion, i.e. causing secondary hypothalamic disorder and consequent (tertiary) pituitary hypogonadotrophism and (quaternary) ovarian failure.

There are anomalies in any classification. Pubertal failure, for example, may be due to primary hypothalamic failure, which can be permanent (e.g. Kallmann syndrome) or temporary (delayed puberty). It is often not possible, however, to predict whether puberty will merely be delayed, and all cases are treated in the same way.

Another odd example for classification is polycystic ovarian disease. There is a genetically determined primary defect in the ovary (increased enzymic capacity to secrete androgens), but its full expression depends on effects of hyperinsulinaemia (one of which is to stimulate hypersecretion of luteinizing hormone, LH), occurring incidentally due to a separate genetic defect causing insulin resistance. We therefore classify polycystic ovarian disease as an ovarian functional disorder in the system concerning the H–P–O axis (Table 14.1).

Unclassified disorders

Conditions are commonly described, such as 'post-pill amenorrhoea' and 'pseudocyesis', which are not proven entities. The particular historical features have been taken

Table 14.2 Anatomical causes of amenorrhoea

Simple developmental defects
Absent ovaries (extremely rare)
Absent uterus
  With or without absent vagina
Imperforate hymen (lower vaginal aplasia)

Developmental defects of endocrine origin
Androgen-resistant syndrome (testicular feminization) in male pseudohermaphrodites (genetic and gonadal males) including inhibition of uterovaginal development

Acquired conditions
Endometrial fibrosis
  Traumatic (Asherman syndrome)
  Infective (tuberculosis)
Cervical stenosis (extremely rare)
  Surgical trauma
  Infective
Vaginal stenosis (extremely rare)
  Chemical inflammation

as distinctive, but the conditions appear to be no more than one or other of the functional disorders mentioned above.

Anatomical causes of amenorrhoea

These are summarized in Table 14.2. Note that incomplete endometrial fibrosis will present with hypomenorrhoea, not oligomenorrhoea.

KALLMANN SYNDROME

Absent or impaired olfactory sensation (anosmia or hyposmia, respectively) is the characteristic feature of the syndrome described by Kallmann and colleagues in 1944, associated with delayed pubertal development and occurring in one in 50 000 girls. The impairment of olfactory sensation is often subtle. Special standardized tests can be done, but the classic test is to distinguish between the smell (not the taste) of coffee and tea. Failure is diagnostic in a girl with delayed pubertal development and serum follicle-stimulating hormone (FSH) and prolactin levels which are not raised.

The link with olfactory impairment is interesting, and has been recently explained embryologically and genetically. The GnRH and olfactory neurons have a common origin in the ectodermal olfactory placode (which forms the olfactory epithelium). The olfactory axons grow towards the brain and form synaptic links (which comprise the olfactory bulb) with cells of the olfactory tracts in the brain. The GnRH neurons migrate along the olfactory axons to reach their final site in the hypothalamus. In Kallmann syndrome there is failure of the olfactory axons and accompanying GnRH neurons to penetrate the brain (Rugarli & Ballabio 1993). The resulting absence or reduction of the olfactory bulbs and tracts — the latter being indicated by lack of depth of the olfactory sulcus,

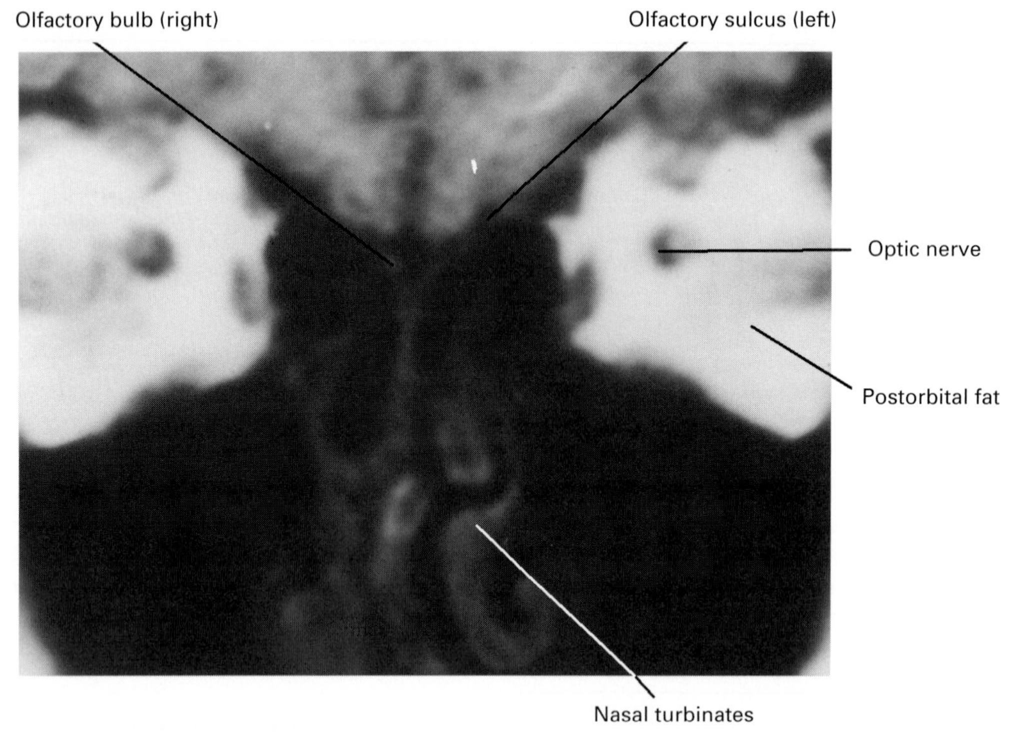

Fig. 14.1 Magnetic resonance image in coronal section of the preoptic area of the brain. The small image at lower left shows the section being just behind the eyes; the optic nerve is seen passing through the bright postorbital fat on each side. The left olfactory bulb is absent (right of picture), the left olfactory sulcus is shallow, and the right olfactory sulcus is absent. (Picture kindly provided by Dr Pierre-Marc Bouloux of the Royal Free Hospital, London.)

can usually be clearly recognized on magnetic resonance imaging (Vogl et al 1994), as illustrated in Figure 14.1. Such imaging is not routinely needed in practice, however, given the distinct history. Other causes of damage to the olfactory nerves are extremely rare.

The mode of genetic transmission is variable and the condition can occur sporadically by mutation or in families. It is worth reflecting that induction of ovulation may lead to inheritance of a condition which would not otherwise be transmitted. Other abnormalities can happen in association with Kallmann syndrome but occur mainly in boys, in whom it is much more frequent, all presumably being X-linked in those cases. In girls, major uterine abnormalities have occasionally been described but whether there is a true association is not known.

Failure of pubertal development is permanent, and treatment is needed without delay. The theoretical choice is pulsed GnRH but this is unnecessarily complicated and oestrogen therapy is employed until ovulation induction is eventually required to achieve pregnancy. Oestrogen dosage and combination with progestogen will depend primarily on skeletal development as discussed later.

IDIOPATHIC DELAYED PUBERTY

As discussed earlier, delayed puberty can be recognized by the age of 14 years in girls if breast development has still not started. Idiopathic hypothalamic failure, which usually resolves spontaneously, accounts for most cases of delayed puberty in boys but only for a minority in girls. There is often a family history of delayed puberty. If there is no history of hyposmia, obsessive dieting or ill health, other causes of amenorrhoea with oestrogen deficiency must be excluded by lateral skull X-ray (non-endocrine tumours, e.g. craniopharyngioma) and serum prolactin (prolactinoma) and FSH measurement (ovarian dysgenesis).

It is not reliably possible to distinguish between primary hypothalamic and primary pituitary failure by measuring the gonadotrophin response to an acute stimulus with GnRH, because that only tests the releasable pool of LH and FSH; in either condition positive or negative results can be obtained. The secretory capacity of the pituitary can be properly tested only by prolonged repeated stimulation, preferably using relatively physiological pulses about every 90 min.

Thus, a diagnosis of idiopathic delayed puberty due to hypothalamic failure can be made after relatively simple exclusion of other causes. It only remains to distinguish whether the failure is permanent or whether puberty will only be delayed. The distinction is impossible, however, although suggested by a familial association. Treatment should begin anyway without delay as for Kallmann syndrome. The only difference is that when secondary sexual maturation is complete, treatment might be interrupted from time to time in order to test for spontaneous H–P–O activity.

HYPOTHALAMIC LESIONS

Congenital aplasia

Congenital aplasia can occur in association with other rare midline malformations of the head and central nervous system, including pituitary aplasia and cleft palate.

Traumatic lesions

Traumatic lesions include accidental injury, surgical damage and postradiotherapy fibrosis. Forward whiplash injuries are more likely to transect the pituitary stalk than damage the hypothalamus. However, hypothalamic infarction can occur in association with hypophyseal portal vein thrombosis, after prolonged hypovolaemia, hypotension and coma.

Inflammatory lesions

Inflammatory lesions include, particularly, tuberculous meningitis, granulomas and abscess. They also include sarcoidosis, giant cell granulomas in middle-aged women, and hystiocytosis-X in children causing delayed growth and puberty (Hand–Schüller–Christian disease).

Tumours

The most likely cause to present to a gynaecologist is a tumour, particularly a craniopharyngioma, compressing the hypothalamus and suppressing GnRH secretion or interrupting portal flow of GnRH in the pituitary stalk. Craniopharyngiomas arise from remnants of Rathke's pouch and commonly present clinically around the age of onset of puberty. They are usually cystic and calcification is common and is readily recognizable on a lateral skull radiograph. Other tumours of the hypothalamus include gliomas (which may arise in the optic tract), meningiomas, endodermal sinus tumour (or yolk sac carcinoma) which secretes alpha-fetoprotein, and congenital hamartomas composed of GnRH neurosecretory cells which can lead to precocious puberty.

Pineal tumours can affect hypothalamic function in different ways. Melatonin secretion by the pineal, which is increased during darkness, suppresses reproductive function. Non-parenchymal pineal tumours (gliomas, teratomas) thus tend to cause sexual infantilism presumably by secreting excessive melatonin. By contrast, parenchymal tumours (e.g. germinomas, which are similar to ovarian dysgerminomas and testicular seminomas, and were previously called pinealomas) can cause sexual precocity, presumably by suppressing pineal function; however, this is rare in girls compared with boys.

PSYCHONEUROENDOCRINE DISORDERS

The modulatory influence of extrahypothalamic brain centres on hypothalamic pulsatile secretion of GnRH was discussed in Chapter 12 to explain the possible mechanisms whereby psychological disorders cause amenorrhoea. They are the commonest cause, accounting for about a third of all cases of amenorrhoea.

Weight loss by associated dietary restriction is a common accompaniment of psychological disorder, and weight loss alone may contribute to neuroendocrine disturbance. Fat tissue is an important extragonadal source of oestrogens by conversion from adrenal androgen precursors. Lack of oestrogen appears to withdraw the normal oestrogenic inhibition of endogenous opioid peptide production; opioids normally inhibit pulsatile GnRH secretion (Bhanot & Wilkinson 1983). Another effect of weight loss is disturbance of the metabolism of oestrogens both in the liver and brain in favour of catechol oestrogens (e.g. 2-alpha-hydroxy- and 4-hydroxy-metabolites of oestrone, oestradiol and oestriol). Catechol oestrogens appear to have contrasting effects to the classical oestrogens in the hypothalamus and pituitary on gonadotrophin secretion, amplifying the negative rather than positive effects (Fishman 1980).

Psychological and weight disturbances take various forms, which may explain the variety of neuroendocrine and clinical features. Weight loss may result from true anorexia (loss of appetite) in response to stress, or from obsessional starvation as a primary psychological feature of anorexia nervosa. Extreme exercise is obviously stressful in other ways, but amenorrhoea is common only in competitive long-distance runners, unlike swimmers (Sanborn et al 1982), and in ballet dancers. Inadequate caloric intake to meet the energy demands of the physical activity seems to be an important factor (Meyer et al 1994).

The hypothalamus is the focus of neuroendocrine disturbance; in particular there is functional impairment of the GnRH pulse generator in the arcuate nucleus. Excessive hypothalamic beta-endorphin and dopamine have been implicated as a cause in some but not all cases (Quigley et al 1980), and naloxone infusion has been shown to increase pulsatile secretion of LH (Laatikainen et al 1986). It is also possible that augmentation of opioid secretion is the mechanism whereby corticotrophin-releasing factor (CRF) has been shown to inhibit gonadotrophin secretion experimentally in monkeys. Stress-induced stimulation of CRF secretion is suggested by the unique pattern of hypersecretion of cortisol, characterized by increased amplitude of secretory episodes during the daytime, in women with functional amenorrhoea (Suh et al 1988).

However, recent clinical and experimental animal studies have drawn attention to caloric restriction as a key factor (Cameron et al 1993, Meyer et al 1994). Pulsatile LH secretion is impaired within 4 h of missing a meal and the effect cannot be reversed by naloxone infusion (excluding an opioid mechanism) or dexamethasone (excluding a CRF-mediated stress effect) (Cameron et al 1993).

The pineal may play a part in suppressing hypothalamic GnRH secretion, as suggested by raised plasma melatonin levels in women with hypothalamic amenorrhoea (Berga et al 1988, Brzezinski et al 1988). This may be associated with disturbance of sleep patterns, as occurs in chronic anorexia, or with acute effects of exercise, as discussed later.

Indirect evidence of hypothalamic impairment is provided by the normal pituitary responsiveness to administration of exogenous releasing hormones, in particular by restoration of normal pituitary–ovarian cyclicity and ovulation in response to prolonged physiological pulsed treatment with GnRH. Direct evidence of other specific hypothalamic disturbances is provided by abnormal body heat production in response to changes in environmental temperature, demonstrable at least in women with weight loss-related amenorrhoea (Vigersky 1981).

Weight loss-related amenorrhoea

According to the critical weight hypothesis of Frisch & McArthur, the onset of female puberty and the maintenance of regular menstrual cycles depend on reaching a critical body weight (47 kg) and ratio of fat to lean mass. It is estimated that body fat should reach at least 17% to achieve menarche, and at least 22% to sustain the adult menstrual pattern (Frisch 1984). Loss of 10–15% of body weight, equivalent to a loss of about one-third of body fat, commonly results in amenorrhoea. There is, however, marked individual variation. The rate of loss of weight seems to be important, and rapid loss is frequently associated with psychological disturbance.

There are different patterns of dieting to lose weight, as originally emphasized by Fries et al (1974). There is dieting for straightforward cosmetic reasons; loss of appetite (true anorexia) in response to stress, as often occurs when young women are taking examinations, or leave home for the first time to travel abroad or take up institutional training; and anorexia nervosa, a specific psychiatric disorder which, after the obvious acute phase, commonly persists in a partly recovered chronic phase that is easily overlooked. A more subtle variation of anorexia nervosa, or at least related to it, is bulimia nervosa. ('Bulimia' means self-induced vomiting.) These conditions will be discussed in more detail later.

Dieting in adolescence. It is important to appreciate how widespread dieting is in adolescent girls and that simple cosmetic dieting can lead directly to anorexia nervosa. In Sweden, where the prevalence of anorexia nervosa seems to be the same as in the UK (about 0.5–1.0% of teenage girls), it has been found that about half of all teenage girls feel fat, and most diet to lose weight although many are below average weight at the start. About 1% lose more than 10 kg and half of those have anorexia nervosa. It is clear that such weight loss due to cosmetic dieting in adolescence is a warning of serious danger. Other particular warning signs are faddishness about the preparation and eating of food (often in isolation), combined with one or more of the following: signs of anxiety, depression, feeling cold, constipation, mental sluggishness, loss of interest in previous activities, and of course amenorrhoea.

Anorexia nervosa

Anorexia nervosa is a misnomer. 'Nervous' the patients may be, but there is no loss of appetite. The starvation is self-imposed; hunger could not be admitted when refusing to eat. The condition is more readily recognized in its acute phase than its chronic phase when some of the lost weight has been regained, as when a woman commonly presents to the gynaecologist some years later with a complaint only of amenorrhoea. Amenorrhoea is an invariable feature of anorexia, not only in its acute phase but also if it continues chronically.

Then, as the patient walks into the consulting room, she seems unremarkable; perhaps only modishly slim and a little reserved in her manner. She will usually admit on direct questioning to an episode of rapid weight loss associated with the onset of amenorrhoea. It can require skilful questioning, however, and usually only at subsequent visits, to uncover the typical, bizarre features of chronic anorexia nervosa: whilst at first claiming to eat normally, she takes irregular and often lonely meals, carefully avoiding carbohydrate; so faddish that she may have ostracized herself rather than dine socially; sometimes giving in to her appetite by gargantuan but secret binges, immediately followed by self-induced vomiting so as to enjoy feeling empty again, or purging habitually to achieve the same end.

At the first consultation few clues are likely to be revealed apart from the history of the original acute weight loss. Constipation is commonly admitted, and often used to explain the need for purgatives. While claiming unconcern about weight, when encouraged to increase her weight she could not bear to do so as she would feel too fat. Yet such patients are usually markedly underweight, and to demonstrate that, it is particularly useful to have a weight/height charge available for reference, as shown in Figure 14.2. That has a more effective impact than calculating the body mass index (weight (kg)/height $(m)^2$), which should be greater than about 19.

Anorexia nervosa does not seem to be a specific psychological disease as once believed. The self-imposed starvation is now thought to be a response to the psychosexual pressures of adolescence, the response in these particular individuals being conditioned by their constitution and family environment, in which there is often marked weight consciousness including obesity and sometimes anorexia

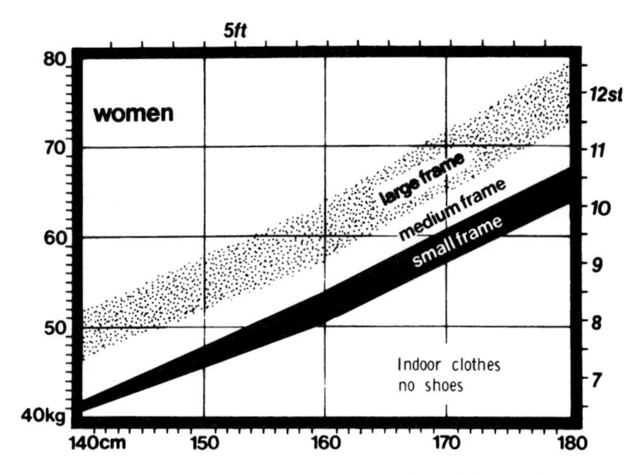

Fig. 14.2 Normal weight of women for height and frame size. Modified from Fletcher (1974).

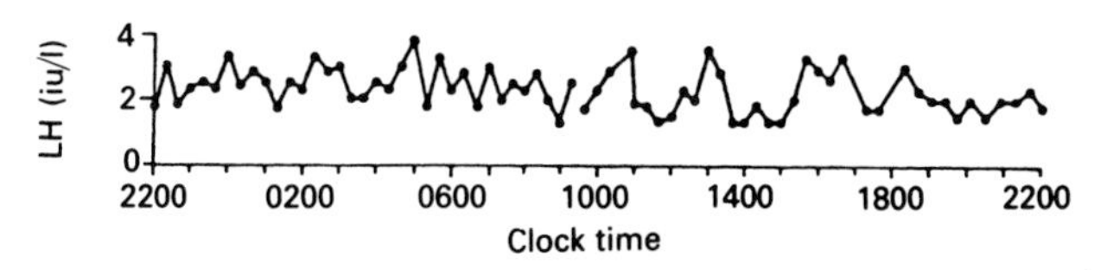

Fig. 14.3 Plasma luteinizing hormone (LH) concentration every 20 min for 24 h in a case of acute anorexia nervosa. Modified from Boyar et al (1974).

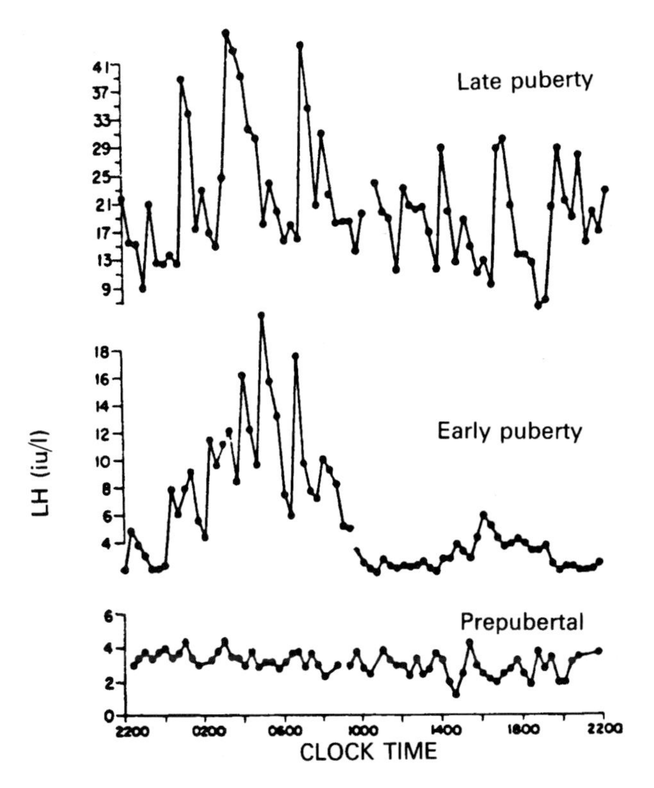

Fig. 14.4 Plasma luteinizing hormone (LH) concentration every 20 min for 24 h in individual girls at different stages around the onset of puberty. Modified from Boyar et al (1974).

nervosa in other members. There are usually greater family problems than weight consciousness, however, and the parents' own anxieties are easily conveyed to their daughter.

One particular characteristic is the patient's illusion of her body size and shape, which is grossly overestimated and distorted in her mind, particularly after meals. Although this may be part of her strategy of denying her abnormality, it is probably a genuine distortion effected by the memory of her premorbid obesity, as this same phenomenon is observed in previously obese but otherwise normal women.

Management of weight loss-related amenorrhoea

Weight loss accounts for about a third of all cases of amenorrhoea presenting to gynaecologists, and chronic anorexia nervosa accounts for half of those. Anorexia nervosa tends to be a lifelong condition and acute exacerbations can be life-threatening. Chronic anorexia nervosa is difficult to treat, because patients deny their problem, an attitude that hardens with time, and they reject formal psychiatry. Gynaecologists can be faced with an ethical dilemma when very disturbed patients want help to become pregnant because the risk of psychological disturbance in their children is high. That may be difficult to argue, but the physical risks for the fetus associated with an underweight mother are clearly defined, and the patients should be encouraged to restore themselves to normal reproductive function by dietary measures to increase their weight rather than resort to pharmacological stimulation of ovulation.

Increasing their weight can be too difficult for some patients with anorexia nervosa, however. It is essential strategy to set a target weight, which usually needs to be the premorbid weight. If reached, ovulation induction should be promised then if necessary. The patient can often be helped to accept the importance of weight by appreciating the serious endocrinological and other physical consequences of her being underweight.

Endocrinopathy of weight loss-related amenorrhoea

The distinct effects of weight loss and psychological disorder on central neuroendocrine processes have been discussed. In the acute phase of anorexia nervosa there is almost complete suppression of gonadotrophin secretion and pulsatility, evident peripherally, as shown in Fig. 14.3. As weight is restored FSH secretion returns ahead of LH as in prepuberty, and LH pulsatility returns in association with sleep (or improved sleep in the case of anorexia nervosa) as initially occurs through the stages of puberty (Fig. 14.4). LH pulsatility is entrained particularly with rapid eye movement sleep, which is only restored when weight has returned to within 15% below the normal mean for height and age (Lacey et al 1975).

As weight is gradually regained, there is gradual restoration of pituitary LH production even before normal pulsatility is achieved, as indicated by the differential basal levels and responses to acute stimulation with GnRH,

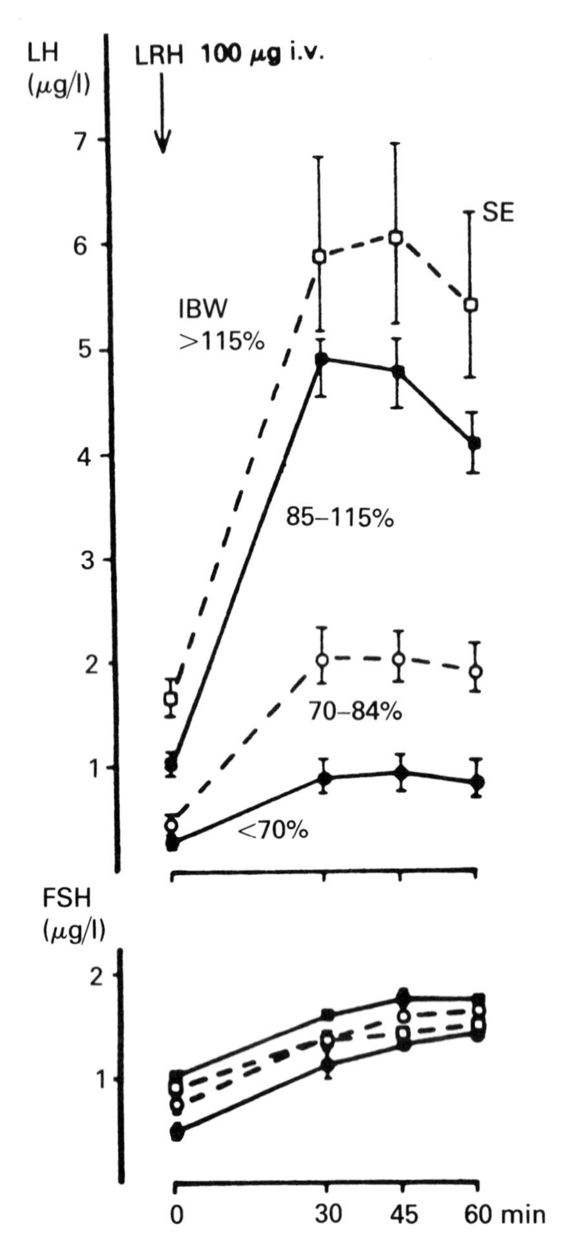

Fig. 14.5 Plasma luteinizing hormone (LH) and follicle-stimulating hormone (FSH) responses to intravenous luteinizing hormone-releasing hormone (LRH = GnRH) in women with amenorrhoea, related to their ideal (normal mean) body weight (IBW). Modified from Bergh et al (1974).

shown in Figure 14.5, of patients remaining amenorrhoeic. This partial but still incomplete return of LH secretion may explain the ultrasound evidence of early ovarian follicular development described as 'multicystic ovaries'. These are the typical appearances of prepubertal ovaries, with a few small or medium-sized follicles in ovaries that are not enlarged (distinct from polycystic ovaries), representing at most feeble activity associated with infrequent LH pulses (Mason et al 1988). The patients are still demonstrably oestrogen-deficient.

There is also continuing evidence of impaired negative and positive feedback by oestrogen on the hypothalamus and pituitary. There is a lack of gonadotrophin and consequent ovulatory response to clomiphene, and a lack of differential LH response to acute GnRH stimulation after priming with oestrogen. Responsiveness to clomiphene may return in the final stage of weight recovery before menstrual cycles are restored, however, and if the target weight has been reached but amenorrhoea continues, it is worth trying clomiphene therapy again, before resorting to pulsed GnRH or gonadotrophin therapy to achieve pregnancy.

Serum oestradiol levels are reduced on average, the endometrium appears thin (⩽ 4 mm double layer) on ultrasonography, and the menstrual response to a progestogen challenge is almost invariably lacking or at least impaired.

One consequence of oestrogen deficiency, the importance of which is becoming increasingly recognized, is osteoporosis. Osteoporotic fractures occur even in young women (Fahy et al 1994). Loss of bone mineral content particularly affects weight-bearing vertebral trabecular bone (Cann et al 1984), and crush fractures sometimes occur without specific injury (Fahy et al 1994).

Another effect of oestrogen deficiency, of minor diagnostic importance, is reduction in certain hormone-binding proteins in plasma, notably thyroxine-binding protein. This leads to misleadingly reduced thyroxine levels but the free thyroxine index is normal, like thyroid-stimulating hormone.

In clinical practice, to define the endocrinopathy of weight loss-related amenorrhoea it is sufficient to detect normal or low basal FSH and LH levels, oestrogen deficiency by ultrasonography of the endometrium or a progestogen challenge test, and if pregnancy is desired, failure to ovulate normally or usually even to menstruate in response to a single course of clomiphene. The history of weight fluctuation and psychological disturbance is the critical diagnostic feature.

Other causes of weight loss

Physical illness, famine and chronic undernutrition can all cause amenorrhoea, but are of little relevance to gynaecologists. It is of passing interest, however, that chronic undernutrition may be an important regulator of general fertility: the onset of puberty is delayed; skeletal growth although delayed is protected until reproductive maturity is reached, and the effects of physiological (lactational) hyperprolactinaemia may be accentuated, so extending birth intervals.

Other psychological disorders

In the absence of a distinct history of weight loss related to the onset of amenorrhoea, the cause can be ascribed confidently to psychological disorder only if there is an obvious condition like chronic depression or if there had been unusual emotional disturbance or anxiety, such as commonly leads to amenorrhoea when young women commence institutional life. The latter should not be taken as a simple explanation and consequently dismissed as unimportant.

Patients with serious psychiatric disorders are unlikely to present to a gynaecologist. It should be remembered, however, that psychotropic drug therapy could be the direct cause of amenorrhoea by inducing hyperprolactinaemia (see later).

Bulimia nervosa. This is becoming increasingly recognized as a common psychological disorder, characterized by covert self-induced vomiting to achieve weight control while overeating in response to normal appetite, associated with morbid fear of fatness (Fairburn & Cooper 1982). It is difficult to diagnose because weight is usually normal and bulimia is not readily admitted. The psychological disorder seems to be related to anorexia nervosa and is therefore interesting, demonstrating that it can lead to amenorrhoea independent of weight loss. Only a minority of bulimic women develop amenorrhoea but many have menstrual irregularity.

Exercise-related amenorrhoea

An uncommon cause of amenorrhoea is extreme exercise involving endurance, as occurs in up to half of top-class competitive long-distance runners and in professional ballet dancers. World-class gymnasts also seem to be at their best during the early teenage years and their pubertal development is commonly delayed. The exact aetiology and endocrine mechanisms are unclear but there is growing evidence that inadequate caloric intake, relative to the energy needs of the physical activity undertaken, is a key factor (Meyer et al 1994), suppressing LH pulsatility (Cameron et al 1993).

There appear to be anomalies; for instance, in swimmers amenorrhoea is relatively infrequent and unrelated to distance training (Sanborn et al 1982). This has been thought to be due to greater redistribution of fat to lean weight in the runners, combined with general loss of weight. Psychological factors associated with extreme competitiveness are important determinants (Gadpaille et al 1987), and ballet dancers are also especially concerned about their weight and many admit to having had anorexia nervosa. Physical stress has been considered to be a key factor as indicated by the rapid return of menstruation when rest is enforced by injury without any increase in weight. However, return to caloric adequacy due to reduced energy requirements is an explanation supported by animal experiments (Meyer et al 1994).

Acute exercise is known to lead to rapid increases in stress hormones including adrenocorticotrophic hormone, cortisol, beta-endorphin, beta-lipoprotein, growth hormone, prolactin and catecholamines; it is also known to cause an increase in melatonin. Acute exercise in already amenorrhoeic runners, however, does not increase prolactin levels, which suggests that it is not the mechanism by which GnRH secretion is suppressed.

In patients who develop amenorrhoea, the clinical endocrine picture is that of hypothalamic disorder and secondary ovarian failure, as already described for psychogenic and weight loss-related amenorrhoea. The secretion and control of prolactin are normal (Chang et al 1984). It is perhaps specially important to appreciate that even in such physically fit athletes there is reduction in mineral density of weight-bearing (vertebral) bones associated with oestrogen deficiency (Drinkwater et al 1984).

Obesity

In contrast to weight loss-related amenorrhoea, from which recovery can be confidently predicted if weight is restored, there is no clear relationship to obesity or therapeutic certainty from shedding excess weight.

Obesity may be associated with polycystic ovarian disease and Cushing's syndromes, but those conditions involve specific endocrine disorders that can cause oligo- or amenorrhoea. Otherwise obesity, even when gross, is associated with menstrual disturbance in only about one-third of cases, and there are no endocrine features to distinguish those from non-obese patients with similar menstrual disturbances. Only in the massively obese is there any convincing evidence that weight reduction (when massive) leads to improvement in endocrine state and menstrual function (Kopelman et al 1981).

CONGENITAL PITUITARY ENDOCRINE FAILURES

Congenital absence of the anterior pituitary in association with other midline structural developmental defects is extremely rare, and in the presence of the gland primary deficiencies of pituitary hormone secretion are very uncommon. Growth hormone deficiency is the commonest, in isolation or with panhypopituitary dwarfism. Reproductive capacity is potentially intact, usually together with lactation. Isolated deficiencies of prolactin and thyroid-stimulating hormone have been reported, but not of adrenocorticotrophic hormone, as this is incompatible with life.

Gonadotrophin deficiency is usually secondary to hypothalamic failure of GnRH secretion as previously described and rarely primary. Isolated LH deficiency in a man gives rise to a 'fertile eunuch'. Isolated FSH deficiency has been reported in men and in one case in a woman; it was successfully treated using exogenous gonadotrophins.

Other genetic syndromes involving hypogonadotrophic

hypogonadism and various congenital defects include the Laurence–Moon–Biedl syndrome (with obesity, retinitis pigmentosa, mental retardation and polydactyly), and various syndromes with cerebellar ataxia that are thought to be inherited as X-linked recessive conditions.

A not uncommon congenital defect that may present in adult life is the (presumably gradual) herniation of the arachnoid through the dura roofing the pituitary fossa. The fossa becomes filled with cerebrospinal fluid within the hernia which can compress the pituitary stalk and gland. The fossa may be enlarged, giving the appearance of an intrasellar tumour on ordinary radiography, and giving rise to the so-called empty sella syndrome including hyperprolactinaemia (see below).

PITUITARY LESIONS

Congenital absence, in association with other midline structural developmental defects, has been mentioned above as an extremely rare occurrence. Haemochromatosis of the pituitary is the consequence of a hereditary disorder of iron metabolism but functional damage from the iron deposition presents relatively late in life.

Traumatic lesions include accidental injury such as whiplash transection of the pituitary stalk, surgical damage and postradiotherapy fibrosis. Infarction can occur as a result of hypovolaemic shock, notably as a result of massive postpartum haemorrhage (Sheehan syndrome), presumably because of increased vascularity and growth of the pituitary (specifically of the lactotrophes) that occur in pregnancy in response to the massive increase in oestrogens from the placenta. Tuberculous and other granulomas can affect the pituitary as well as the hypothalamus (see above).

Tumours arising in the hypothalamic area or from the integuments of the pituitary fossa can compress the pituitary stalk or the gland itself, as in the case of the hypothalamus (see above). Tumours arising in the anterior pituitary gland are common, usually benign and small in women, and often of no functional relevance. Macroadenomas are more common in men. Amongst normal women about one-third can be found to have a tumour on radiological or subsequent postmortem examination. Some may be trophic tumours representing nodal hypertrophy of the secretory cells in response to their respective hypothalamic stimulatory hormones (although classically only when the stimulation is excessive, as for example in primary hypothyroidism).

About a quarter of all pituitary adenomas appear to be non-secretory and present a clinical problem only by compression of the normal pituitary tissue or the pituitary stalk. FSH- and/or LH-secreting tumours are extremely rare, and then usually occur in men rather than women. Prolactin secretion is commonest, but is sometimes combined with growth hormone or adrenocorticotrophic hormone secretion, which may not be clinically evident at first. Non-secretory tumours can present with hyperprolactinaemia, usually of only modest degree, by compressing the pituitary stalk and interrupting hypothalamic dopamine inhibition of normal pituitary secretion of prolactin.

HYPERPROLACTINAEMIA

Unlike the other trophic hormones secreted by the anterior pituitary, prolactin is controlled primarily by inhibition from the hypothalamus (by dopamine, and to a minor extent, gamma-aminobutyric acid) and, in common only with growth hormone, is not subject directly or indirectly to negative feedback by peripheral hormones. It exercises inhibitory self-regulation via short-loop feedback on hypothalamic dopamine by means of counter-current flow in the hypophyseal portal system (as well as inhibition of GnRH pulsatile secretion). Hypothalamic stimulatory factors appear to be of minor importance normally; they include serotonin, opioids and notably thyrotrophin-releasing hormone (TRH). Prolactin secretion is stimulated by peripheral oestrogen, particularly in pregnancy from the placenta, and by a thoracic sensory nerve pathway from the nipple in reflex response to suckling.

Thus pathological hyperprolactinaemia can be caused by drugs that inhibit dopamine production or action; by primary hypothyroidism via excessive TRH; by tumours or granulomas compressing the pituitary stalk or hypothalamus, and rarely, by traumatic or neoplastic lesions of the thorax or spine affecting the suckling sensory nerve pathway. An additional rare cause is ectopic production of prolactin by a distant extrapituitary tumour. Chronic renal failure is also often associated with hyperprolactinaemia, both due to reduced excretion of the hormone and probably by central mechanisms affecting dopamine action. By far the commonest causes of hyperprolactinaemia, however, are pituitary prolactinomas and idiopathic hypersecretion. Amongst patients presenting to a gynaecologist the key diagnostic considerations are a tumour (found in 40–50% of cases), primary hypothyroidism (3–5%) and pharmacological causes (1–2%). First, however, it is necessary to confirm hyperprolactinaemia as the cause of oligo- or amenorrhoea.

Diagnosis of hyperprolactinaemia

Galactorrhoea, the typical symptom of hyperprolactinaemia, is not a reliable index. It occurs in less than half the patients with hyperprolactinaemia amenorrhoea. Conversely, only about half the patients with galactorrhoea and normal menstrual cycles have hyperprolactinaemia.

Serum prolactin measurement is therefore critical, and always needs to be undertaken in cases of ovulatory failure. Spurious hyperprolactinaemia was commonly attributed to the stress of clinical procedures, examination of the breasts, or normal episodic secretion of prolactin, but these explanations are now generally discounted. It now seems necessary to repeat prolactin measurement in a second blood sample only if the first is raised, and again if the second is discrepant, accepting normal values and excluding an isolated raised value.

The commonest problem has been simple misinterpretation of the upper normal limit by assuming an arithmetic instead of the actual geometric (skewed) distribution of normal values. The upper limit should be taken at about 800 mu/1. There is of course overlap between normal and abnormal ranges, and there are anomalies to mislead the unwary diagnostician. Unfortunately there is no endocrine test to distinguish the functional relevance of borderline hyperprolactinaemia. What really matters, it seems, is how well distinguished the ovulatory disorder is for which hyperprolactinaemia is being considered as a possible cause: true hyperprolactinaemia nearly always causes amenorrhoea or severe oligomenorrhoea.

One anomaly is the association of mild hyperprolactinaemia with some cases of polycystic ovarian disease (see Ch. 23). Although there is some evidence that excessive prolactin might stimulate adrenal androgen precursor secretion, it appears more likely to be the consequence rather than the cause of polycystic ovarian disease, due to stimulation by oestrogen which is produced in substantial amounts both by the polycystic ovaries and by peripheral conversion in fat tissue from androgens. By contrast, prolactin levels tend to be subnormal in amenorrhoea due to hypothalamic disorder, presumably because of lack of oestrogenic stimulation.

Another uncommon anomaly is the occurrence of molecular forms (notably 'big-big' prolactin) that are biologically inactive but detected by radioimmunoassay for prolactin. This may explain many of the cases of very high prolactin levels sometimes found in normally ovulating women. It is worth repeating: it is the distinctiveness of ovulatory disorder that determines the pathological relevance of raised prolactin levels.

Endocrine effects of hyperprolactinaemia

Hyperprolactinaemia interferes with ovarian function by indirectly suppressing gonadotrophin secretion, by means of short-loop feedback via the hypophyseal portal system on hypothalamic GnRH pulsatile release. Whilst basal gonadotrophin levels and release remain normal there is suppression of LH pulsatility (Moult et al 1982) and loss of positive and negative feedback by oestrogen.

Early in vitro studies suggesting a direct inhibitory effect of excess prolactin on human granulosa cell function were clearly misleading, and there is now much indirect evidence to disprove that idea. Both the pituitary and ovary respond as normal to pulsed GnRH therapy in arcuate-lesioned and pituitary stalk-sectioned monkeys despite accompanying hyperprolactinaemia (Knobil 1980), and also in women with pathological hyperprolactinaemic amenorrhoea (Polson et al 1986).

There appears to be a relationship between the degree of hyperprolactinaemia and that of secondary ovarian dysfunction, but there is usually progression to amenorrhoea or severe oligomenorrhoea and associated oestrogen deficiency. Hyperprolactinaemia accounts for about 15% of patients with amenorrhoea and 2% with oligomenorrhoea. It is very unconvincing as a cause of persistent follicular/luteal dysfunction and infertility in normally menstruating women. The only convincing association with such dysfunction is in temporary situations as after stopping bromocriptine therapy before amenorrhoea supervenes again; or after incomplete surgical excision of a prolactinoma; or in women during prolonged lactation. Generally in normally menstruating women there is no relation between prolactin levels and midluteal progesterone levels or pregnancy rates (Glazener et al 1987).

In women with hyperprolactinaemic amenorrhoea one important consequence of oestrogen deficiency is osteoporosis, which deserves specific therapeutic consideration (Klibanski & Greenspan 1986, Schlecte et al 1987). Some women may also be troubled by atrophic changes in the vulva and vagina.

Pharmacological causes of hyperprolactinaemia

Drugs are an uncommon but easily identified cause of hyperprolactinaemia. They are all dopamine antagonists, but have a wide range of therapeutic uses, as shown in Table 14.3. Oestrogens, as in contraceptive pills, also increase prolactin levels but only slightly, i.e. within the nomal range. The usual drug to cause hyperprolactinaemia in a young woman is a phenothiazine or metoclopramide.

Table 14.3 Pharmacological agents associated with hyperprolactinaemia

Phenothiazines
Perphenazine (Fentazin)
Chlorpromazine (Largactil)
Thioridazine (Melleril)
Trifluoperazine (Stelazine)
Prochlorperazine (Stemetil)
Butyrophenones
Haloperidol (Haldol, Serenace)
Pimozide (Orap)
Benzamides
Metoclopramide (Maxolon)
Clebopride (Cleboril)
Cimetidine (Tagamet)
Rauwolfia alkaloids
Reserpine (Serpasil)
Methyldopa (Aldomet)

Prolactinomas

Prolactinomas are benign prolactin-secreting adenomas that arise in the lower lateral wings of the anterior pituitary from lactotrophes (the prolactin-secreting cells), which are normally sited there and make up about one-third of the functioning cells of the pituitary gland. The tumours are usually soft and discrete, sometimes partly degenerated and cystic, surrounded by a pseudocapsule of compressed

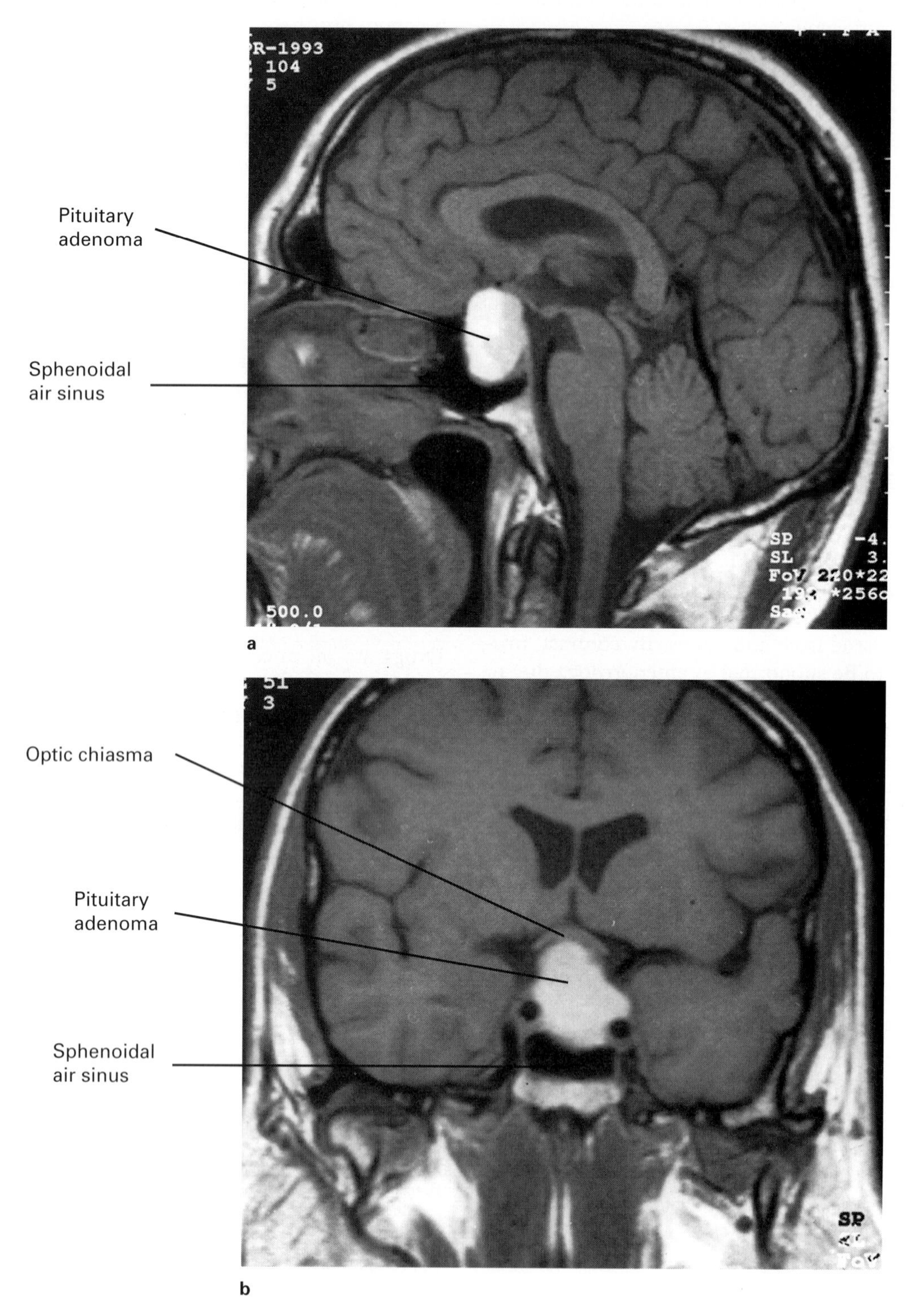

Fig. 14.6 **a** Sagittal and **b** coronal views of the head by magnetic resonance imaging showing a large pituitary adenoma, its appearances enhanced by bleeding, extending upwards and compressing the optic chiasma, as seen in **b**. Pictures kindly provided by Dr Julian Kabala of the Bristol Royal Infirmary.

pituitary tissue. Infrequently, the tumour may be diffuse and locally invasive, but rarely malignant. The bony fossa of the pituitary often becomes remodelled in response to a large tumour but is seldom eroded by it. Extension mostly occurs upwards and can compress the optic tracts (Fig. 14.6). Compression of the hypothalamus and pituitary stalk can lead to panhypopituitarism. When the tumour is less than 10 mm in diameter it is called a microadenoma; otherwise it is a macroadenoma.

Diagnosis

Diagnostic confirmation requires special immunohistochemical staining of the tissue, but surgical extirpation is seldom undertaken except in the case of particularly large tumours with suprasellar extension. Most prolactinomas (in women) are microadenomas. Unfortunately the radiological appearances of a microprolactinoma are unreliable. Standard radiology may show downward distortion of one side of the fossa floor (reflecting the usual site of origin of a prolactinoma) but is easily misinterpreted. Computerized tomographic (CT) scanning shows a rounded area of inhomogeneity in the pituitary gland, which is usually taken as diagnostic in combination with hyperprolactinaemia. That is an unreliable conclusion, however, given the high frequency of adenomas to be found in women without endocrine disease. Therefore the main diagnostic value of a CT scan is to detect a macroadenoma, whether prolactin-secreting or not, and not to make a diagnosis of a microprolactinoma. Magnetic resonance imaging offers even better resolution to detect very small microprolactinomas, but in the light of the previous discussion there is little practical relevance in that.

Non-secreting macroadenomas can lead to hyperprolactinaemia by compressing the pituitary stalk, but the prolactin levels are usually much lower than with a prolactinoma of the same size. Prolactin levels correlate roughly with the size of prolactin-secreting adenomas, and a macroprolactinoma is to be expected when serum prolactin levels are greater than 2500–3000 mu/l. However, because lower levels may be due to a non-secreting macroadenoma, or occasionally a subarachnoid hernia expanding the fossa (empty sella syndrome; see earlier), CT scanning of the pituitary region is always advisable in addition to a lateral radiograph, which is mainly intended as a simple crude screening method for gross abnormality of the pituitary fossa or calcification in a craniopharyngioma. Radiology is of no value in oligomenorrhoeic or amenorrhoeic patients who are not hyperprolactinaemic and do not have clinical evidence of other distinct pituitary endocrine disorders.

Pathogenesis and natural history

The aetiology and pathogenesis of prolactinomas are unknown, indeed it is arguable whether a microprolactinoma is a true neoplasm. Adenoma cells behave like normal lactotrophes and are normally receptive to dopamine.

Studies over the course of several years have shown that microprolactinomas generally show little or no enlargement (Schlecte et al 1989, Sisam et al 1987). However, because enlargement can occur, annual monitoring by prolactin measurement is advisable. Prolactin levels reflect the functional size of a tumour. Up to a third of patients with apparent prolactinomas experience spontaneous resolution (Schlecte et al 1989), which may be encouraged by pregnancy, possibly by inducing infarction of the tumour (Crosignani et al 1989).

Treatment

Transnasal–transsphenoidal microsurgical excision of a microadenoma is a fairly straightforward, safe procedure. Unfortunately excision is often incomplete, and therefore fails to cure the condition although prolactin levels are lower than before. Furthermore, even after apparent cure later relapse often occurs. Interestingly, when hyperprolactinaemia then recurs, it is usually not associated with any evidence of tumour, suggesting there may be an inherent functional disturbance of the pituitary or hypothalamus–pituitary affecting prolactin secretion and underlying the pathogenesis of prolactinomas (Ciccarelli et al 1990). Surgery and radiotherapy are therefore usually reserved for very large tumours with suprasellar and frontal extension.

The treatment of choice is a dopamine agonist such as bromocriptine. Shrinkage of the tumour usually occurs rapidly, with concomitant improvement of any associated visual field defects. Although prolactin levels may not be fully suppressed at first, steady improvement can be achieved by prolonged treatment, which can often be reduced gradually to quite low maintenance doses, but should be continued indefinitely. Tumour regrowth usually occurs again quickly after treatment is stopped.

In pregnancy, after bromocriptine has been used to induce ovulation but then discontinued, the possibility of serious enlargement of a tumour can be monitored by visual field perimetry every 2 months, and bromocriptine therapy can be effectively reintroduced if necessary. Alternative urgent treatment including surgery needs specialist consideration. The reader is referred to a review of the management of prolactinomas by Molitch (1989).

Idiopathic hyperprolactinaemia

This diagnosis is made by exclusion of identifiable causes and will apply to about half the cases of hyperprolactinaemic amenorrhoea or oligomenorrhoea. The aetiology and pathogenesis are unknown, as for prolactinomas. Serum prolactin levels are usually only modestly raised (to less than 2500 mu/l) and some authors consider, although speculatively, that idiopathic hyperprolactinaemia may be an entity distinct from a prolactinoma, partly because there appears to be a greater chance (about 20%) of eventual spontaneous recovery (Schlecte et al 1989).

Treatment

Spontaneous recovery is unlikely and unpredictable, therefore treatment is specifically needed to achieve pregnancy, suppress galactorrhoea, or relieve symptoms associated with vulvovaginal atrophy. Furthermore, greater liveliness and libido, previously forgotten, are often distinct benefits to be gained from restoration of ovarian function. In the long term, however, the main considerations are choice of contraceptive method and protection from osteoporosis, and these apply along with specific management of a prolactinoma as described above.

Dopamine receptor agonists like bromocriptine are very effective inhibitors of prolactin secretion by the normal pituitary, and in cases of idiopathic hyperprolactinaemia. Fertility is not restored in cases of (apparent) hyperprolactinaemia without associated ovulatory failure.

Bromocriptine is also very effective in suppressing galactorrhoea, although that is not of inherent concern, only in so far as it is a nuisance. Oestrogen deficiency symptoms are overcome by restoration of normal ovarian hormone production. Fertility is of course also restored, and contraceptive measures need to be taken if required. The choice can be made from the full range, including oral oestrogenic preparations, which have no adverse effect on prolactin secretion during bromocriptine therapy.

Osteoporosis

Perhaps most important of all, oestrogen therapy can be used to protect against osteoporosis which results from the lack of ovarian oestrogen production (Klibanski & Greenspan 1986, Schlecte et al 1987). The use of a simple contraceptive preparation is therefore particularly attractive for that purpose in the long term. It needs to be used with special caution if there is a macroadenoma, because of the limited experience with it (Fahy et al 1992). On the other hand, the risk of osteoporosis is also of serious concern and deserves effective treatment.

A reasonable compromise with oestrogen therapy, particularly when there is intolerance of bromocriptine, might be to combine it with only a small dose of bromocriptine, sufficient to be protective without aiming to suppress prolactin levels substantially.

Control of bromocriptine therapy

The aim should be to suppress serum prolactin levels to around mid-normal values (200–300 mu/l), not to very low levels. The dose should therefore be titrated accordingly. When attempting to induce ovulation there is usually scarcely time to optimize the dose before pregnancy is achieved. A daily dose of 5.0 mg is effective in about two-thirds of cases, but to save time we usually commence with 7.5 mg. Only about 10% of patients will need a higher dose than that but it is usually ineffective to raise the dose above 20–30 mg/day if prolactin levels are still not adequately suppressed. Side-effects are discussed in Chapter 15.

Alternative drug treatments

Bromocriptine remains the first choice because of its long established effectiveness and safety, particularly in pregnancy. Other dopamine receptor agonists with fewer side-effects would be valuable, and for long-term usage there may be advantages from long-acting alternatives. Cabergoline and quinagolide appear to be beneficial (Bevan & Davis 1994) and are licensed in the UK for the treatment of hyperprolactinaemic ovarian failure. Other dopamine agonists include lysuride, pergolide, terguride and metergoline, all ergot/ergoline derivatives. At present, however, the main reason for choosing an alternative to bromocriptine is in cases of apparent idiosyncratic intolerance.

OTHER HYPOTHALAMIC–PITUITARY DISORDERS

The hypothalamic–pituitary failures and disorders described so far, which are mostly related to weight loss and psychological disorders, and hyperprolactinaemia, account for about 50% of cases of amenorrhoea and 10% of oligomenorrhoea. In addition, primary ovarian failure accounts for about 10 and 2% respectively. What about the remainder?

It is notable that the foregoing disorders are all associated with secondary ovarian failure, and consequent oestrogen deficiency is evident in nearly all cases. By contrast, the remainder are nearly all oestrogenized. Polycystic ovarian syndrome, typified by hirsutism, accounts for about 8% of the amenorrhoea cases and 20% of oligomenorrhoea. The few cases of polycystic ovarian syndrome that appear to be oestrogen-deficient do not so much have low serum oestrogen levels as exceptionally high androgen levels, often with specific evidence of adrenal origin (because of raised dehydroepiandrosterone sulphate levels).

The rest, about a quarter of all patients with amenorrhoea and two-thirds of those with oligomenorrhoea, are oestrogenized and present no unusual features in their histories or physical make-up. For want of an explanation these patients are sometimes said to have 'euestrogenic oligo- or amenorrhoea'. Some authors have assumed a diagnosis of hypothalamic disorder, to distinguish the condition from hypothalamic failure which they use to describe the patients with oestrogen deficiency, inferring more profound disturbance (failure) of the H-P-O axis. However, patients with euestrogenic oligo- or amenorrhoea nearly all respond fully to treatment with clomiphene, which clearly indicates intact responsiveness of the hypothalamus–pituitary to negative and positive feedback signals. For that reason the condition has also been called 'cycle initiation defect', implying a simple but unexplained inability to trigger a H-P-O cycle in response to the usual decline in luteal hormone levels, although otherwise normal.

Some patients with euestrogenic oligo- or amenorrhoea have raised serum LH levels but normal FSH, which has led some authors for many years to assume a diagnosis of polycystic ovarian disease even in the absence of hirsutism or obesity. It has now become clear by the use of refined vaginal ultrasonography that the ovaries are in fact polycystic in nearly all the oestrogenized patients (Fox et al 1991a,b, Hull 1989, Shulman et al 1989). The specific ultrasound features are at least 15 follicles of 2–10 mm diameter per ovary (scanned vaginally, or 10 scanned abdominally, the smallest follicles not being seen), usually but not invariably arranged around the cortex, and in particular a prominent expanded, echogenic stroma (Fox & Hull 1993). These ultrasound appearances of polycystic ovarian disease have been confirmed histologically (Saxton et al 1990).

Thus it is now clear that polycystic ovarian disease, with or without hirsutism, accounts for about a third of all cases of amenorrhoea and nearly 90% of oligomenorrhoea (Adams et al 1986, Hull 1987), and the most consistent endocrine feature is an oestrogenized state. The reader should appreciate that this view of polycystic ovarian disease as the essential cause of euestrogenic oligo-amenorrhoea or cycle initiation defect is new, and not universally accepted yet. A seemingly semantic debate continues about the distinction between polycystic ovaries, disease and syndrome. There seems no doubt, however, about the common underlying condition of the ovaries; only its dysfunctional degree and symptomatic expression vary.

Feedback mechanisms in the hypothalamus–pituitary are intact, and the primary disorder appears to be usually in the ovary, although incidental critical factors, such as hyperinsulinism usually and adrenal hyperandrogenism in a few cases, may be involved (see Ch. 23). We therefore classify polycystic ovarian disease as an ovarian, not a hypothalamic–pituitary, disorder.

UNCLASSIFIED CAUSES OF OLIGO/AMENORRHOEA

Post-pill amenorrhoea and pseudocyesis are two conditions in particular that need discussion here because they are reported as though they were specific entities, usually along with the assumption that the underlying mechanism is hypothalamic–pituitary dysfunction in response to a particular pharmacological or psychological stimulus. It seems clear to us, however, that they are not specific entities, bearing only coincidental not causal relations to the factors suggested by their names; they encompass any and many of the conditions discussed earlier in this chapter.

Post-pill amenorrhoea

A causal relation to combined oestrogen–progestogen oral contraception was assumed for several reasons: the coincidental timing of onset with cessation of treatment; the common association with previous menstrual disorder, which was presumed to represent special susceptibility; the common delay in first menstruation after cessation of oral contraceptive treatment, and apparent reduced fertility subsequently.

Post-pill amenorrhoea occurs in about 0.5% of oral contraceptive users, not significantly more than the incidence in non-users as suggested by the prospective study (at least up to 3 months' duration) by Berger et al (1977). Also, previous menstrual disturbance was as common in women whose amenorrhoea was unrelated to oral contraceptive usage as in those with post-pill amenorrhoea (Hull et al 1981, Sherman et al 1984). Endocrine studies have revealed no consistent mechanism. Prospective and case–control studies have specifically shown no relationship of hyperprolactinaemia and prolactinomas to oral contraceptive usage, which had once been of particular concern (Sherman et al 1984). It seems that the coincidental timing of post-pill amenorrhoea is to be expected, the underlying cause having been masked by oral contraceptive-induced menstruation.

The usually brief initial impairment of fertility after oral contraceptive use may not be entirely due to biological effects, but may be at least partly behavioural. Spira et al (1985) noted that amongst women in Paris giving up contraception to conceive, 60% delayed their attempts, after using oral contraceptives, by nearly 4 months on average, and 30% did so after using an intrauterine contraceptive device (IUCD) by nearly 3 months. After correction for these delayed attempts the differences in observed conception rates disappeared completely (Fig. 14.7).

Conclusions

The H–P–O system is remarkably robust, predictable in its response to contraceptive steroids, and in its return to normal function and fertility. There is no evidence that oral contraceptives cause subsequent amenorrhoea. Therefore in practice post-pill amenorrhoea should not be treated as an entity. It should not be dismissed, but investigated and treated as any case of amenorrhoea. If reliable contraception is required again, standard oestrogen/progestogen preparations can be safely recommended. Hyperprolactin-

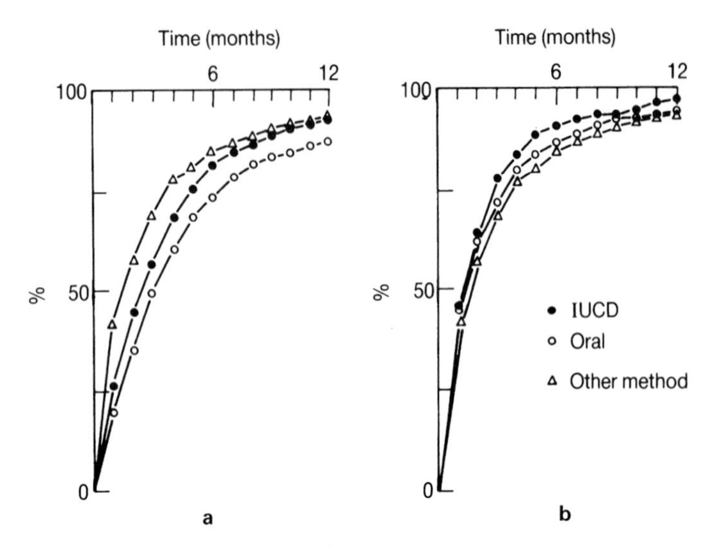

Fig. 14.7 Cumulative conception rates in fertile women after discontinuing contraception, related to the method used. **a** From the time of discontinuing contraception; **b** after correcting for those who delayed their attempts to conceive. IUCD, intrauterine contraceptive device; Oral, oral contraceptive. Modified from Spira et al (1985).

aemia is a possible exception because of oestrogenic stimulation, as discussed earlier.

Pseudocyesis

Phantom pregnancy and its psychological origin have been recognized since ancient times but the condition is now rare. It is still relatively common in some parts of the world, probably because of the overwhelming importance attached to fecundity in certain cultures, even amongst older women. The menopause accounts for many cases reported from West Africa, for example (Osotimehin et al 1981). Although a persistent corpus luteum occurs in some non-primates it does not explain human pseudocyesis. A wide range of disparate endocrinopathies have been reported (e.g. DeVane et al 1985, Osotimehin et al 1981, Starkman et al 1985, Tulandi et al 1985) including primary ovarian failure, hyperprolactinaemia, polycystic ovarian disease and psychogenic hypothalamic disorders.

The only sensible conclusion is that pseudocyesis is usually nothing more than an exaggerated emotional misinterpretation of amenorrhoea of different origin as being due to pregnancy; whilst in some cases the overwhelming desire for pregnancy can lead to typical psychogenic hypothalamic disorder. Pseudocyesis is not an entity and should be managed as any case of amenorrhoea, attending, of course, to the particular emotional problems of each patient.

PRIMARY OVARIAN FAILURE

There is space here for only an outline of the subject to fit into the context of management of oligo/amenorrhoea. There are numerous possible causes, briefly listed in the introductory classification given at the beginning of this chapter, and reviewed by Friedman et al (1983). The essential questions are whether primary ovarian failure can resolve, whether resolution is predictable, and whether any treatment can help recovery. In fact recovery is very uncommon and unpredictable, and treatment seems ineffective.

The key diagnostic feature is postmenopausal levels of FSH. Laparoscopic visualization alone is sufficient in the case of 'streak' ovaries, but in other cases laparoscopic and even laparotomy ovarian biopsy is unreliable. The typical inflammatory cell infiltration of autoimmune disease in the presence of plentiful follicles provides a little more optimism for recovery, but the diagnosis could be made equally by serology and other autoimmune endocrine disorders should be considered.

Immunosuppressive therapy for autoimmune ovarian failure even with high dosage of glucocorticoids is ineffective, but spontaneous recovery occurs occasionally and then sometimes intermittently. In the general type of case, claims for successful treatment with exogenous oestrogen, sometimes followed by gonadotrophins, are unconvincing. Any chance of recovery seems to be entirely fortuitous, the only optimistic hints being in those women with some menstrual activity, without extremely low oestrogen or extremely high FSH values, and with histological evidence of primordial follicles. None of those features discriminate between outcome completely, however. Up to 10% of women with primary ovarian failure recover and conceive. What is clear is that recovery is impossible while FSH levels remain raised.

A rare alternative possibility is a genetic defect of the β-subunit of FSH, rendering it biologically inactive although detected by immunoassays. The ovaries should be responsive to exogenous gonadotrophins but this is rarely the case in women who appear to have classical hypergonadotrophic ovarian failure.

Advice to individual patients is a matter of practical philosophy. Those who do not want to conceive need to be aware of the small chance of recovery and consider contraception if reliability is essential. Oestrogen replacement therapy will usually be necessary and a contraceptive preparation would do well. Those who want to conceive should interrupt the replacement therapy from time to time to reassess symptoms and FSH levels. Egg donation with in vitro fertilization is a more realistic alternative.

Resistant ovary syndrome

This diagnosis implies the presence of ovarian follicles that are temporarily unresponsive to the usual gonadotrophic stimuli. The reasons for that are not clear except in the case of autoimmune disease. Also, the diagnosis and prognosis are unreliable because recovery can occur even when there were insufficient follicles to have been found on biopsy, as already discussed. The diagnosis can only be made in retrospect, when recovery has occurred, and is of no practical importance.

ENDOCRINE DISORDERS ARISING OUTSIDE THE H–P–O AXIS

It is beyond the scope of this chapter to review in detail other specific endocrine disorders. They seldom present simply with oligo/amenorrhoea to a gynaecologist. Routine attention in the history to involuntary weight changes, true anorexia, weakness, or heat or cold intolerance should point to Cushing's or Addison's adrenal disorder or thyroid disorder. The latter can also be easily screened by serum thyroid-stimulating hormone measurement (using the new assays with improved sensitivity to detect reduced levels) or the free thyroxine index. Routine testing for glycosuria is sufficient for diabetes mellitus, although it is not clear whether that can cause oligo/amenorrhoea. Acromegaly should be recognized by the typical clinical features, particularly if hyperprolactinaemia is found by routine assay, being commonly associated with excessive growth hormone secretion.

A common effect of these disorders on the H–P–O axis is modulation of circulating levels of sex hormone-binding globulin, which is increased in thyrotoxicosis and reduced in hypothyroidism, hyperadrenalism and acromegaly. Other specific mechanisms also occur. In hyperadrenalism excess cortisol may directly suppress gonadotrophin secretion. Addison's disease does not seem to interfere with ovarian function except by association with polyendocrine autoimmune disease. Most notably, primary hypothyroidism often leads to hyperprolactinaemia, essentially by excess TRH stimulation of prolactin secretion. A prolactinoma may be induced, which may explain why the degree of hyperprolactinaemia is usually related to the duration of hypothyroidism. Otherwise there is plentiful evidence that appropriate treatment of specific underlying endocrine disorders restores normal reproductive function.

GENERAL MANAGEMENT OF OLIGO/AMENORRHOEA

The prevalence of pathological amenorrhoea in young women is 1–2% and that of oligomenorrhoea is about the same. They are common conditions with a wide range of causes. Specific diagnosis and treatment may in some cases need referral to other specialists by a gynaecologist but most can be managed along common lines within a simplified diagnostic framework as follows.

Apart from wanting a diagnosis, patients have different requirements which include advice about future fertility and its possible protection, about contraception, hirsutism (see Ch. 23), secondary sexual development, protection against osteoporosis, and protection against endometrial cancer.

Basic diagnosis of endocrine disorder

After simply excluding an unlikely anatomical cause of amenorrhoea, the first step in diagnosis is to classify the type of endocrine disorder in a systematic way, as shown in Table 14.4. Then more detailed investigations can be undertaken to define the specific underlying cause if necessary. The diagnosis of hypothalamic–pituitary failure or disorder requires routine exclusion of primary ovarian failure (raised serum FSH), hyperprolactinaemia (raised serum prolactin) and thyroid disorder (raised or low thyroid-stimulating hormone or free thyroxine index). Because dynamic gonadotrophin-releasing tests are unhelpful, distinction between hypothalamic failure and

Table 14.4 Basic diagnostic classification and frequencies of endocrine disorders causing amenorrhoea or oligomenorrhoea

Class	Percentage of cases of		Criterion	Oestrogen state
	Amenorrhoea	Oligomenorrhoea		
Primary failures (H–P–O axis)				
Hypothalamic	2	0	History	Deficient
Pituitary	<1	0	History	Deficient
Ovarian	12	2	Raised FSH	Deficient
Functional disorders (H–P–O axis)				
Hypothalamic	30	5	History	Deficient
Hyperprolactinaemia	20	2	Raised PRL	Deficient
Polycystic ovaries	33	88	(Hirsutism if present)	Oestrogenized
Other endocrine disorders				
Thyroid	1	2	TSH (or FTI)	Variable
Adrenal	<1	<1	History (cortisol if indicated)	Variable

FSH, follicle-stimulating hormone; PRL, prolactin; TSH, thyroid-stimulating hormone; FTI, free thyroxine index.

hypothalamic disorder then depends primarily on the history, e.g. of hyposmia, a known treated pituitary tumour, or weight fluctuation or psychological disorder.

In the diagnosis of polycystic ovarian disease, hirsutism is virtually specific (see summary of investigations below) but occurs in only about 25% of cases. The remainder, usually identifiable by high-resolution vaginal ultrasonography, are distinguished endocrinologically by their oestrogenized state, in contrast to the oestrogen deficiency which characterizes ovarian failure both primary and secondary to hypothalamic–pituitary failure or disorder. LH and androgen measurements are less reliable. Ultrasound diagnosis is also limited in some ways: it is not always possible to define the ovaries well enough, or to use a vaginal probe; on the other hand, polycystic ovaries can be found misleadingly (because of their common occurrence in apparently normal women; Polson et al 1988) in some women with amenorrhoea due to some other overriding cause.

From an ovarian viewpoint the classification of oligomenorrhoea can be simply reduced to the following, and whether failure is primary or secondary there is consequent oestrogen deficiency.

1. Primary ovarian failure.
2. Secondary ovarian failure: due to hypothalamic or pituitary failure or disorders, including hyperprolactinaemia which acts by hypothalamic disorder of GnRH secretion.
3. Polycystic ovarian disease: essentially a primary ovarian disorder although modulated by extraneous influences like hyperinsulinaemia.

Assessment of oestrogen state

Assessment of oestrogen state provides 90% diagnostic reliability in distinguishing between polycystic ovarian disease and other causes of oligo/amenorrhoea (Fox et al 1991a,b, Hull 1989). It also provides a reliable index of responsiveness to clomiphene when ovulation induction is needed. In addition, it indicates the need for long-term therapy to protect the endometrium from overstimulation with endogenous oestrogen, or the bones from lack of it.

Assessment of oestrogen state is therefore of central importance in the management of oligo/amenorrhoea. Some use oestrogen measurements in blood or urine, whilst others favour biological methods, including simple examination of the lower genital tract, particularly the cervix, vaginal cytology, and ultrasound measurement of uterine size and endometrial thickness (Shulman et al 1989), and the menstrual (endometrial) response to administered progestogen (the progestogen challenge test). Various progestogen regimens are used, by injection or tablet, but the one that has been systematically studied is a 5-day oral course of medroxyprogesterone acetate, in a daily dose of 5 mg (Hull et al 1979) or 15 mg (Shulman et al 1989).

The menstrual response to a progestogen challenge test is assessed in the following week: a normal menstrual loss indicates oestrogenized state (of the endometrium) and failure to menstruate indicates oestrogen deficiency. In only a small proportion of cases an impaired response occurs, defined by only scanty menstrual bleeding for no more than 2 days, and this also indicates oestrogen deficiency by correlation with other indices of oestrogen state (Hull et al 1979) including ultrasound measurement of double endometrial thickness of 4 mm or less (Shulman et al 1989).

By contrast, serum oestradiol levels range too widely, overlapping to a large extent between oestrogenized and oestrogen-deficient groups of patients, to be diagnostically useful (Shulman et al 1989) except when the level is distinctly low, below 100 pmol/l (Hull et al 1979) as illustrated in Figure 14.8.

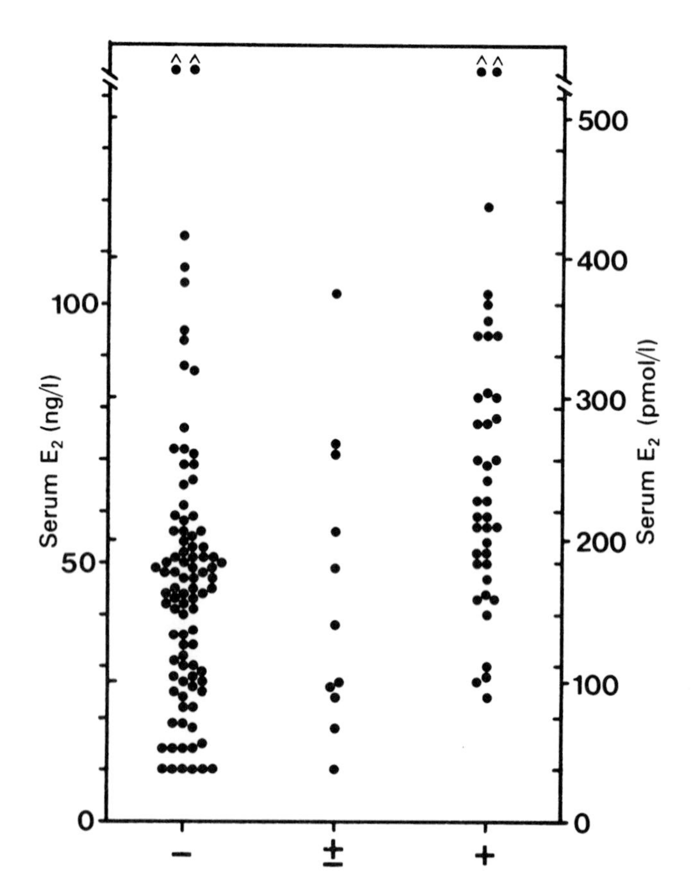

Fig. 14.8 Serum oestradiol (E_2) concentrations in women with amenorrhoea, related to their menstrual response to a progestogen challenge. Menstrual bleeding: +, normal; ±, scanty loss; –, nil loss. From Hull et al (1979) with permission of Blackwell Science Ltd.

Summary of primary investigations

1. History
   a. Previous weight loss.
   b. Psychological disorder.
   c. Prolactinergic drugs.
   d. Thyroid symptoms.
   e. Hirsutism.
2. Examination
   a. Hirsutism.
   b. Vaginal atresia.
3. Serum
   a. FSH.
   b. Prolactin
   c. Testosterone (if hirsutism is present: to screen for very high levels suggesting androgenic tumour).
   d. Thyroid-stimulating hormone (or free thyroxine index).
4. Progestogen challenge test (oestrogen state); or endometrial measurement
5. Clomiphene test (only if pregnancy is desired).

Future fertility

Patients can be reassured about their future fertility. Given appropriate treatment, those with amenorrhoea have been shown to have a completely normal chance of conceiving and delivering a baby, excluding those with primary ovarian failure, while those with oligomenorrhoea have only a slightly reduced chance overall (Hull et al 1982). In fact the majority have a better chance than average because the overall success rates are reduced by the subgroup with overt polycystic ovarian syndrome (Hull 1987).

Patients with clinically 'occult' polycystic ovarian disease, i.e. as indicated only by evident oestrogen production and ultrasound appearance of the ovaries, are mostly successfully responsive to clomiphene treatment (Hull 1987). Those with overt polycystic ovarian syndrome have a more severe disorder as indicated for example by higher levels of androgens and insulin; they are much less likely to respond adequately to clomiphene, whilst their response to gonadotrophin therapy is particularly difficult to control.

Contraceptive advice

Nulliparous patients with oligo/amenorrhoea may be concerned about contraceptive need, while protecting their future fertility. Others need advice, having had a baby after successful ovulation induction therapy. An unexpected pregnancy is likely to be as unwelcome to such a woman as to any other new mother. Advice will depend on knowing their chance of spontaneous ovulation and recognizing that oral contraception does not affect their underlying condition.

Oligomenorrhoeic women may ovulate normally in association with menstruation, albeit infrequently, and even amenorrhoea can resolve spontaneously and unpredictably. Virtually only Kallmann syndrome and ovarian failure with streak ovaries are certain not to resolve. The chance of conception is reduced, however, sometimes severely so, and this must be balanced against the degree of contraceptive reliability required. A married amenorrhoeic patient may be happy to do without any contraceptive protection.

The usual range of contraceptives can be considered, but with certain limitations. An IUCD should of course be avoided if possible in nulliparous women as usual. It should also be avoided, however, in all oligo/amenorrhoeic patients who are oestrogen-deficient because of uterine atrophy, which occurs even in parous women to such a degree as to prevent proper containment of the IUCD.

The choice of oestrogen/progestogen oral contraception depends partly on the evidence for any possible association with subsequent amenorrhoea or subfertility following its use generally. Those fears are unfounded, as discussed earlier, therefore such contraception can be safely considered. It may also carry other advantages (see below). In women with polycystic ovarian disease, androgenic progestogens should be avoided. A preparation containing an antiandrogenic progestogen like cyproterone acetate would seem particularly appropriate.

One concern about oestrogenic contraceptives is possible worsening of hyperprolactinaemia and in particular critical enlargement of a prolactinoma. Protective combination with low-dose bromocriptine could be considered but needs studying, and progestogen-only therapy may be a reasonable compromise (Fahy et al 1992).

Endometrial protection

Cystic hyperplasia of the endometrium is a well recognized association with prolonged anovulatory intervals between menstruation, as typically occurs with polycystic ovarian disease, and polycystic ovarian syndrome has been clearly linked with an increased risk of endometrial carcinoma in relatively young women, under 40 years of age (Lucas 1974, Nisker et al 1978). It therefore seems important to offer protective therapy to oligo/amenorrhoeic patients who are oestrogenized. Progestogen courses of at least 12 days are required, although in low dose, sufficient to induce menstrual bleeding only in young oligo/amenorrhoeic women. How often such cyclical therapy needs to be given is unclear, but every 1–2 months would seem appropriate and timing will depend partly on the personal wishes of each patient. An alternative approach combining endometrial protection with menstrual cycle control and reliable contraception would of course be a standard combined oestrogen/progestogen contraceptive preparation.

Oestrogen deficiency

Oestrogen deficiency is a consequence of all the hypothalamic–pituitary disorders leading to secondary ovarian failure associated with oligo- or usually amenorrhoea, as well as primary ovarian failure. This may result in acute symptoms, or chronic but often unrecognized impairment of well-being, and osteoporosis. Osteoporotic fractures including vertebral crush fractures can occur in young women (Fahy et al 1994). Oestrogen replacement therapy is therefore a major prophylactic requirement, particularly because of the young age of the patients. Points of practical concern are: possible risks of adverse stimulation in cases of hyperprolactinaemia (Fahy et al 1992); unwelcome return of menstruation in some patients with particular psychological disorders, and the dosage required.

Low-dose oestrogen therapy as for postmenopausal hormone replacement therapy (HRT) is sufficient to protect the bones. It cannot be relied on for contraception, however, should that be needed, because recovery from hypothalamic disorder is unpredictable. On the other hand, combination with continuous low-dose progestogen should be sufficient, although imperfect control of bleeding may be a nuisance. Alternatively a standard combined oral contraceptive preparation provides for all requirements.

When should HRT be started? Experience with treatment to induce oestrogen deficiency by pituitary desensitization (e.g. for endometriosis) demonstrates significant bone loss within 6 months. That would be too soon to start, however, in cases of hypothalamic amenorrhoea. Even when the patient presents with more prolonged amenorrhoea effort should first be concentrated on restoring normal function. When that seems unlikely to occur soon is the time to start HRT. It should then be continued indefinitely, or perhaps with short breaks to see if spontaneous menstruation occurs.

Delayed puberty

The particular therapeutic needs of young patients with primary amenorrhoea and lack of secondary sexual development are early recognition of their need, low-dose oestrogen therapy to stimulate skeletal growth, and warning that full secondary development requires patience. Delayed pubertal development should be recognized and treatment started for its psychological benefit by the age of 14 years, if breast development has not started by then. Full breast development takes 4–5 years to complete and cannot be hurried by increasing the dose of oestrogen; indeed the shape of the breasts, in particular the areolae, can become distorted.

In general, without allowing for variation in body weight, it requires a dose of ethinyl oestradiol of only 5 μg daily to stimulate bone growth maximally, and any stimulant effect is lost at about 20 μg/day. Breast development, by contrast, is less sensitive to oestrogen and needs about 10 μg/day (Ross et al 1983). Continuous oestrogen alone seems appropriate at first, later combining with progestogen only if any irregular vaginal bleeding occurs or when breast development is well advanced.

KEY POINTS

1. Delayed puberty is diagnosed if breast development does not start by 14 years of age. Diagnosis and management should not be postponed waiting for delayed menarche.
2. Primary and secondary amenorrhoea and oligomenorrhoea should be considered in the same way clinically, as distinction may be misleading. In addition oligomenorrhoea is likely to include a spectrum of conditions ranging from virtual normality at one end to the same causes as those of amenorrhoea at the other.
3. It is not possible to distinguish between primary hypothalamic or pituitary failure by measuring the gonadotrophin responses to an acute GnRH stimulus. The secretory capacity of the pituitary gland can only properly be tested by prolonged pulsed stimulation with GnRH.
4. Weight loss, usually accompanied by psychological disorder, accounts for about one-third of all cases of amenorrhoea, and anorexia nervosa accounts for half of those. It usually presents to the gynaecologist in a chronic state and much of the original weight loss has been restored and is no longer obvious. The history must always be sought.
5. Cosmetic dieting to lose weight in adolescent girls may become obsessional, leading to anorexia nervosa. Warning signs include faddishness about the preparation and eating of food (often in isolation) combined with anxiety, depression, feeling cold, constipation and behavioural changes.
6. Anorexia nervosa may not be a specific psychological disease as once believed. Starvation may be a response to the psychosexual pressure of adolescence conditioned by the individual's constitutional and family environment (parents' own anxieties).
7. Women with weight loss-related amenorrhoea wanting to become pregnant should not be treated with drugs to induce ovulation if avoidable. They should rather be encouraged to first gain weight and psychological well-being to avoid adverse fetal and long-term effects.
8. The most common causes of hyperprolactinaemia are pituitary adenomas (40–50%) and idiopathic hypersecretion (50%). Primary hypothyroidism and pharmacological causes account for 3–5% and 1–2% respectively.
9. Prolactin levels and symptoms like headache are usually good guides to a large tumour. Detailed radiology to discover a microadenoma is of no practical value. Amongst normal women, one-third can be found to have a pituitary microadenoma on radiological or postmortem examination.
10. True hyperprolactinaemia nearly always causes amenorrhoea or severe oligomenorrhoea, with no convincing evidence of

its causing persistent follicular or luteal dysfunction and infertility in normally menstruating women.

11. Treatment of hyperprolactinaemia is necessary, even if pregnancy is not desired, to reduce tumour size and relieve symptoms of oestrogen deficiency and galactorrhoea.
12. Hyperprolactinaemia causes amenorrhoea by negative feedback on hypothalamic pulsatile secretion of GnRH, leading to gonadotrophin deficiency and consequent secondary ovarian failure.
13. Hypothalamic and pituitary failure and disorders are thus all associated with oestrogen deficiency. Osteoporosis is a major risk, sometimes causing fractures even in young women, and needing long-term oestrogen replacement therapy.
14. Polycystic ovarian disease (PCOD) accounts for about one-third of all cases of amenorrhoea and nearly 90% of oligomenorrhoea, often without the classical symptoms of obesity or hirsutism.
15. Women with PCOD are well oestrogenized and should receive cyclic progestogen treatment (or oestrogen/progestogen) to guard against endometrial hyperplasia and increased risk of carcinoma.
16. Menstrual dysfunction associated with obesity may be a reflection of an associated endocrine dysfunction (e.g. PCO) rather than being due to obesity itself. Only in massive obesity is there any convincing evidence that weight reduction may lead to improvement in the endocrine state and menstrual function.

REFERENCES

Adams J, Polson D W, Franks S 1986 Prevalence of polycystic ovaries in women with anovulation and idiopathic hirsutism. British Medical Journal 292: 355–359

Aksel S 1981 Hormonal characteristics of long cycles in fertile women. Fertility and Sterility 36: 521–523

Berga S L, Mortola J F, Yen S S 1988 Amplification of nocturnal melatonin secretion in women with functional hypothalamic amenorrhea. Journal of Clinical Endocrinology and Metabolism 66: 242–244

Berger G S, Taylor R N, Treloar A E 1977 The risk of post-pill amenorrhea: a preliminary report from the menstruation and reproduction history research program. International Journal of Gynaecology and Obstetrics 15: 125–127

Bergh T, Nillius S J, Wide L 1978 Serum prolactin and gonadotrophin levels before and after luteinizing hormone-releasing hormone in the investigation of amenorrhoea. British Journal of Obstetrics and Gynaecology 85: 945–956

Bevan J S, Davis J R E 1994 Cabergoline: an advance in dopaminergic therapy. Clinical Endocrinology 41: 709–712

Bhanot R, Wilkinson M 1983 Opiatergic control of gonadotrophin secretion during puberty in the rat: a neurochemical basis for the hypothalamic 'gonadostat'? Endocrinology 113: 596–603

Boyar R M, Katz J, Finkelstein J W et al 1974 Anorexia nervosa. New England Journal of Medicine 291: 861–865

Brzezinski A, Lynch H J, Seibel M M, Deng M H, Nader T M, Wurtman R J 1988 The circadian rhythm of plasma melatonin during the normal menstrual cycle and in amenorrheic women. Journal of Clinical Endocrinology and Metabolism 66: 891–895

Cameron J L, Helmreich D L, Schreihofer D A 1993 Modulation of reproductive hormone secretion by nutritional intake: stress signals versus metabolic signals. Human Reproduction 8: 162–167

Cann C E, Martin M C, Genant H K, Jaffe R B 1984 Decreased spinal mineral content in amenorrhoeic women. Journal of the American Medical Association 251: 626–629

Chang F E, Richards S R, Kim M H, Malarkey W B 1984 Twenty four-hour prolactin profiles and prolactin responses to dopamine in long distance running women. Journal of Clinical Endocrinology and Metabolism 59: 631–635

Ciccarelli E, Ghigo E, Miola C, Gandini G, Muller E E, Camanni F 1990 Long-term follow-up of 'cured' prolactinoma patients after successful adenomectomy. Clinical Endocrinology 32: 583–592

Crosignani P G, Mattei A M, Scarduelli C, Cavioni V, Boracchi P 1989 Is pregnancy the best treatment for hyperprolactinaemia? Human Reproduction 4: 910–912

DeVane G W, Vera M I, Buhi W C, Kalra P S 1985 Opioid peptides in pseudocyesis. Obstetrics and Gynecology 65: 183–188

Drinkwater B L, Nilson K, Chesnut C H, Bremner W J, Shainholtz S, Southworth M B 1984 Bone mineral content of amenorrheic and eumenorrheic athletes. New England Journal of Medicine 311: 277–281

Fahy U M, Foster P A, Torode H W, Hartog M, Hull M G R 1992 The effect of combined estrogen/progestogen treatment in women with hyperprolactinemic amenorrhea. Gynecological Endocrinology 6: 183–188.

Fahy U M, Cahill D J, Wardle P G, Hull M G R 1994 Osteoporotic fractures in young amenorrheic women. Acta Obstetrica et Gynecologica Scandinavica 73: 417–419

Fairburn C G, Cooper P J 1982 Self induced vomiting and bulimia nervosa: an undetected problem. British Medical Journal 284: 1153–1155

Fishman J 1980 Fatness, puberty and ovulation. New England Journal of Medicine 303: 42–43

Fletcher R 1974 Assessment of nutritional status. Medicine Series 1 28: 1650–1666

Fox R, Hull M G R 1993 Ultrasound diagnosis of polycystic ovaries. Annals of the New York Academy of Sciences 687: 217–223

Fox R, Corrigan E, Thomas P, Hull M G R 1991a Oestrogen and androgen states in oligo-amenorrhoeic women with polycystic ovaries. British Journal of Obstetrics and Gynaecology 98: 294–299

Fox R, Corrigan E, Thomas P, Hull M G R 1991b The diagnosis of polycystic ovaries in women with oligo-amenorrhoea: predictive power of endocrine tests. Clinical Endocrinology 34: 127–131

Friedman C I, Barrows H, Kim M H 1983 Hypergonadotropic hypogonadism. American Journal of Obstetrics and Gynecology 145: 360–372

Fries H, Nillius S J, Petterson F 1974 Epidemiology of secondary amenorrhea. 11. A retrospective evaluation of etiology with special regard to psychogenic factors and weight loss. American Journal of Obstetrics and Gynecology 118: 473–479

Frisch R E 1984 Body fat, puberty and fertility. Biological Reviews 59: 161–188

Gadpaille W J, Sanborn C F, Wagner W W 1987 Athletic amenorrhoea, major affective disorders, and eating disorders. American Journal of Psychiatry 144: 939–942

Glazener C M A, Kelly N J, Hull M G R 1987 Prolactin measurement in the investigation of infertility in women with a normal menstrual cycle. British Journal of Obstetrics and Gynaecology 94: 535–538

Hull M G R 1987 Epidemiology of infertility and polycystic ovarian disease: endocrinological and demographic studies. Gynecological Endocrinology 1: 235–245

Hull M G R 1989 Polycystic ovarian disease: clinical aspects and prevalence. Research and Clinical Forums 11: 21–30

Hull M G R, Knuth U A, Murray M A F, Jacobs H S 1979 The practical value of the progestogen challenge test, serum oestradiol estimation or clinical examination in assessment of the oestrogen

state and response to clomiphene in amenorrhoea. British Journal of Obstetrics and Gynaecology 86: 799–805
Hull M G R, Bromham D R, Savage P E, Barlow T M, Hughes A O, Jacobs H S 1981 Post-pill amenorrhoea: a causal study. Fertility and Sterility 36: 472–476
Hull M G R, Savage P E, Bromham D R 1982 Anovulatory and ovulatory infertility: results with simplified management. British Medical Journal 284: 1681–1685
Klibanski A, Greenspan S L 1986 Increase in bone mass after treatment of hyperprolactinemic amenorrhea. New England Journal of Medicine 315: 542–546
Knobil E 1980 The neuroendocrine control of the menstrual cycle. Recent Progress in Hormone Research 36: 53–88
Kopelman P G, White N, Pilkington T R E, Jeffcoate S L 1981 The effect of weight loss on sex steroid secretion and binding in massively obese women. Clinical Endocrinology 15: 113–116
Laatikainen T, Virtanen T, Apter D 1986 Plasma immunoreactive beta-endorphin in exercise-associated amenorrhea. American Journal of Obstetrics and Gynecology 154: 94–97
Lacey J H, Crisp A H, Kalucy R S, Hartmann M K, Chen C N 1975 Weight gain and the sleeping electroencephalogram: study of 10 patients with anorexia nervosa. British Medical Journal iv: 556–558
Lucas W E 1974 Causal relationships between endocrine-metabolic variables in patients with endometrial carcinoma. Obstetrics and Gynecology Survey 29: 507–528
Mason H D, Sagle M, Polson D W et al 1988 Reduced frequency of luteinizing hormone pulses in women with weight loss-related amenorrhoea and multifollicular ovaries. Clinical Endocrinology 28: 611–618
Meyer W R, Pierce E F, Katz V L 1994 The effect of exercise on reproductive function and pregnancy. Current Opinion in Obstetrics and Gynaecology 6: 293–299
Molitch M E 1989 Management of prolactinomas. Annual Reviews of Medicine 40: 225–232
Moult P J A, Rees L H, Besser G M 1982 Pulsatile gonadotrophin secretion in hyperprolactinaemic amenorrhoea and the response to bromocriptine therapy. Clinical Endocrinology 16: 153–162
Nisker J A, Ramzy I, Collins J A 1978 Adenocarcinoma of the endometrium and abnormal ovarian function in young women. American Journal of Obstetrics and Gynecology 130: 546–550
Osotimehin B O, Ladipo O A, Adejuwon C A, Otolorin E O 1981 Pituitary and placental hormone levels in pseudocyesis. International Journal of Gynaecology and Obstetrics 19: 399–402
Polson D W, Sagle M, Mason H D, Adams J, Jacobs H S, Franks S 1986 Ovulation and normal luteal function during LHRH treatment of women with hyperprolactinaemic amenorrhoea. Clinical Endocrinology 24: 531–537
Polson D W, Adams J, Wadsworth J, Franks S 1988 Polycystic ovaries a normal variant? Lancet i: 870–872
Quigley M E, Sheehan K L, Casper R F, Yen S S 1980 Evidence for increased dopaminergic and opioid activity in patients with hypothalamic hypogonadotropic amenorrhea. Journal of Clinical Endocrinology and Metabolism 50: 949–954
Ross J L, Cassorla F G, Skerda M C, Valk I M, Loriaux D L, Cutler G B 1983 A preliminary study of the effect of estrogen dose on growth in Turner's syndrome. New England Journal of Medicine 309: 1104–1106
Rugarli B I, Ballabio A 1993 Kallmann syndrome from genetics to neurobiology. Journal of the American Medical Association 270: 2713–2716
Sanborn C F, Martin B J, Wagner W W 1982 Is athletic amenorrhea specific to runners? American Journal of Obstetrics and Gynecology 143: 859–861
Saxton D W, Farquhar M, Rae T, Beard R W, Anderson M C, Wadsworth J 1990 Accuracy of ultrasound measurements of female pelvic organs. British Journal of Obstetrics and Gynaecology: 95–699
Schlecte J, El-Khoury G, Kathol M, Walkner L 1987 Forearm and vertebral bone mineral in treated and untreated hyperprolactinemic amenorrhea. Journal of Clinical Endocrinology and Metabolism 64: 1021–1026
Schlecte J, Dolan K, Sherman B, Chapler F, Luciano A 1989 The natural history of untreated hyperprolactinemia: a prospective analysis. Journal of Clinical Endocrinology and Metabolism 68: 412–418
Sherman B M, Wallace R B, Chapler F K, Luciano A A, Bean J A 1984 Prolactin-secreting pituitary tumors: an epidemiologic approach. In: Cammani F, Muller E E (eds) Pituitary hyperfunction: physiopathology and clinical aspects. Raven Press, New York, pp 167–174
Shulman A, Shulman N, Weissenglass L, Bahary C 1989 Ultrasonic assessment of the endometrium as a predictor of oestrogen status in amenorrhoeic patients. Human Reproduction 4: 616–619
Sisam D A, Sheehan J P, Sheeler L R 1987 The natural history of untreated microprolactinomas. Fertility and Sterility 48: 67–71
Spira N, Spira A, Schwartz D 1985 Fertility of couples following cessation of contraception. Journal of Biosocial Science 17: 281–290
Starkman M N, Marshall J C, La Ferla J, Kelch R P 1985 Pseudocyesis: psychologic and neuroendocrine interrelationships. Psychosomatic Medicine 47: 46–57
Suh B Y, Liu J H, Berga S L, Quigley M E, Laughlin G A, Yen S S 1988 Hypercortisolism in patients with functional hypothalamic amenorrhea. Journal of Clinical Endocrinology and Metabolism 66: 733–739
Tulandi T, McInnes R A, Lal S 1983 Altered pituitary hormone secretion in patients with pseudocyesis. Fertility and Sterility 40: 637–641
Vigersky R A 1981 Functional disorders of the hypothalamic-pituitary axis. In: Beardwell C, Robertson G L (eds) The pituitary. Butterworths, London, pp 1–46
Vogl T J, Stemmler J, Heye B et al 1994 Kallman syndrome versus idiopathic hypogonadotropic hypogonadism at MR imaging. Radiology 191: 53–57

15

Ovarian function and ovulation induction

Khaldoun Sharif Masoud Afnan

INTRODUCTION

It is impossible to imagine sound gynaecological practice without an in-depth understanding of ovarian function. Proper management of menstrual disorders, fertility control and ovulatory dysfunction must be based upon an understanding of the mechanisms involved in the regulation of the normal cycle. Furthermore, ovulation induction is a fundamental part of the treatment of almost all types of infertility. Apart from being the mainstay of the treatment of ovulatory dysfunction, it is an integral component of superovulation and intrauterine insemination, and of assisted reproductive technologies (e.g. in vitro fertilization (IVF), gamete intrafallopian transfer (GIFT)) which are used in the treatment of infertility due to tubal disease, endometriosis, male factor and unexplained infertility.

OVARIAN FUNCTION

The function of the ovary is the cyclic release of oocytes and production of steroid hormones. Both these functions are integrated and finely controlled by a sequence of hypothalamic–pituitary–ovarian interactions which are orchestrated mainly by the endocrine, paracrine and autocrine products of the ovary.

Primordial follicles

The embryological origins of the oocytes are the primordial germ cells, originating in the endoderm of the yolk sac, allantois, and hindgut of the early embryo. At 6 weeks' gestation these germ cells migrate to the area of the genital ridge where the ovary is formed and, over the following 10–14 weeks, undergo rapid mitotic division and multiply to form oogonia. The oogonium is transformed into an oocyte by entering the first meiotic division which is arrested at the diplotene stage of the prophase. This oocyte is then surrounded by a single layer of spindle-shaped granulosa cells to form the primordial follicle. The first meiotic division is completed only at ovulation and the second division after fertilization, perhaps some 30–40 years later.

The maximum number of oocytes (6–7 million in both ovaries) is reached by 20 weeks' gestation (Baker 1963). From then on they undergo atresia, and their numbers decrease throughout the female's life, both intra- and extrauterine; at birth there are about 1–2 million and at puberty only 300 000.

Follicular recruitment

Each month many follicles are recruited from the pool of primordial follicles and only one of these is destined to

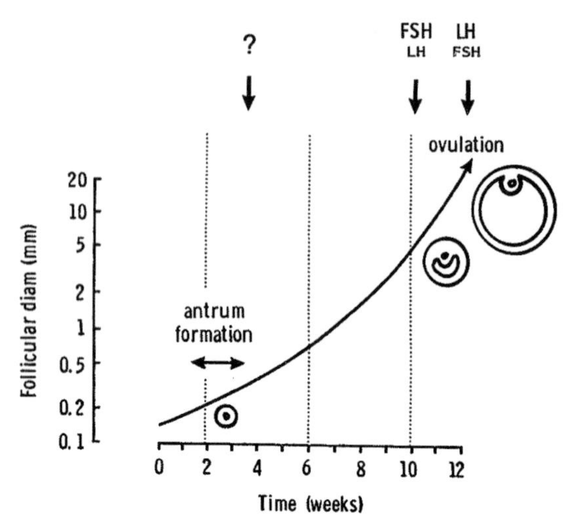

Fig. 15.1 Follicular growth from preantral phase to ovulation.

eventually ovulate (Fig. 15.1). This stage of initial growth is independent of gonadotrophin stimulation, as evidenced by the persistence of this phase of growth in gonadotrophin-deficient mutant mice. It was originally thought (based on non-primate data) that the period from the initial recruitment to reaching preovulatory stage takes about 85 days and, therefore, occurs over the previous several cycles. Recent human data, however, suggests a shorter duration of growth (Speroff et al 1994).

Growth

The regression of the corpus luteum of the previous cycle is associated with a decline in the serum levels of steroid hormones and inhibin, with a resultant increase in the follicle-stimulating hormone (FSH) levels. This increase begins about 2 days before the onset of menstruation and continues throughout the following early follicular phase. The granulosa cells of the selected follicles (now known as preantral follicles) have, by now, acquired FSH receptors and respond by cell proliferation, differentiation, and increased aromatase activity. Aromatization leads to oestrogen production (from androgen precursors) and further enhance the FSH effect on the follicles by increasing their FSH receptor content. FSH activity has been shown to be modulated by a range of paracrine factors (Table 15.1).

Under the synergistic effects of oestradiol and FSH, the granulosa cells produce fluid which first accumulates in the intercellular spaces before coalescing to form a cavity (antrum). In these antral follicles luteinizing hormone (LH) receptors are exclusive to the theca cells, while FSH receptors are present only in the granulosa cells. LH induces theca cells to produce androgen which is aromatized into oestradiol by FSH-driven granulosa cells. Ovarian steroidogenesis is, thus, LH-dependent. This is clearly

Table 15.1 Paracrine modulators of FSH action

Steroids	Oestrogens Androgens
Polypeptides	
Stimulatory	Insulin IGF I and II TGFβ
Inhibitory	TGFα EGF Inhibin?

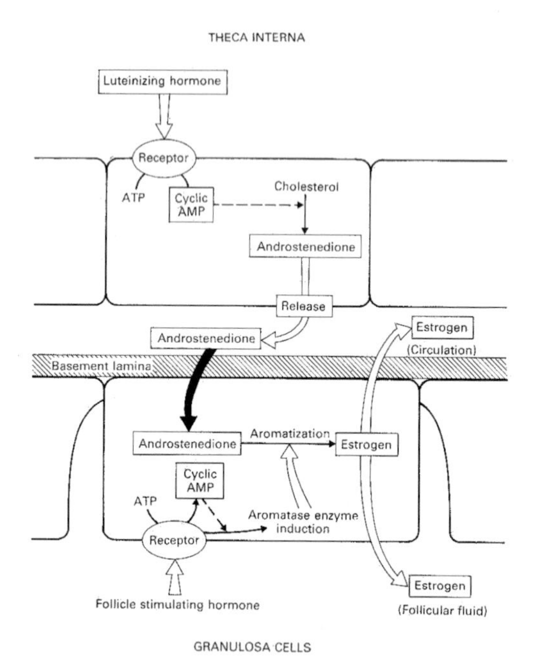

Fig. 15.2 Two-cell, two-gonadotrophin theory.

illustrated by the fact that hypogonadotrophic women need both FSH and LH for successful induction of ovulation; FSH alone will lead to folliculogenesis with no adequate steroidogenesis. This is termed the 'two-cell, two-gonadotrophin' theory (Fig. 15.2) (McNatty et al 1980).

Selection and dominance

The rising levels of oestradiol (produced by the growing follicles) exert a negative feedback effect at the hypothalamic–pituitary level and lead to a fall in FSH. This, in turn, leads to a decline in the aromatase activity in all but the largest antral follicle. This largest follicle has more granulosa cells and therefore more FSH receptors, and hence it is able to maintain its growth despite the new low FSH levels (Fig. 15.3). This dominant follicle will be selected (cycle days 5–7) for subsequent ovulation. Occasionally there is more than one follicle at this stage at

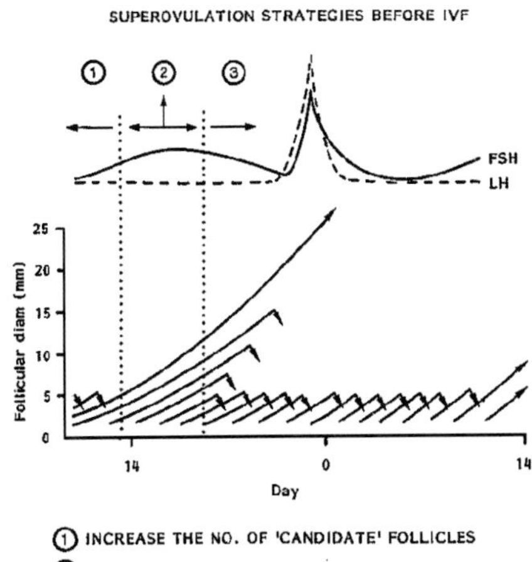

Fig. 15.3 Follicular selection in relation to endocrine changes.

the same time, with the consequent release of more than one oocyte and the potential for multizygotic multiple pregnancy. The other follicles, now deprived of adequate gonadotrophin stimulation, undergo atresia. This process of natural programmed cell death has been termed 'apoptosis'.

Preovulatory follicle

The continued oestradiol production in the dominant follicle is responsible for the rise in serum oestradiol levels in the late follicular phase and causes a positive feedback influence on LH secretion. The LH leads to more androgen production in the theca cells. The high oestrogen milieu of the dominant follicle will enhance its sensitivity to FSH and more oestradiol will be produced from the androgen precursors. A new function for FSH at this stage is the induction of LH receptors in the granulosa cells of the dominant follicle. This is an essential preovulatory step, and prepares the preovulatory follicle to respond to the LH surge. In the preovulatory follicle, LH initiates luteinization and progesterone production in the granulosa cells; a rise in progesterone levels can be detected as early as day 10 of the cycle.

Ovulation

In midcycle oestradiol levels reach a peak which initiates the LH surge. This LH surge initiates resumption of meiosis in the oocyte, luteinization of the granulosa cells and synthesis of prostaglandins. The prostaglandins stimulate the release of proteolytic enzymes within the follicular wall and play an important role in weakening an area in the ovarian capsule (stigma) from which ovulation occurs. Consequently, drugs that inhibit prostaglandin synthesis (e.g. non-steroidal anti-inflammatory drugs) can interfere with ovulation.

Ovulation (the physical release of the oocyte and its cumulus mass of granulosa cells) occurs approximately 24–36 h after the oestradiol peak, 34–36 h after the onset of the LH surge, and 10–12 h after the LH peak.

The luteal phase

The normal luteal phase (from the LH surge to menses) is between 11 and 17 days with a mean of 14 days. Soon after ovulation the stigma heals and blood capillaries penetrate into the granulosa cells which hypertrophy markedly and incorporate lipoid vacuoles within their cytoplasm (luteinization). This process of vascularization and luteinization has already started in the theca cells during the late follicular phase. The luteinized granulosa and theca cells are now termed luteal cells. Their lipoid content is responsible for the yellow colour of the corpus luteum (yellow body).

The main function of the corpus luteum is steroidogenesis; it is now the main source of oestrogen and progesterone. Oestradiol levels, which declined sharply as the LH reached its peak, start to rise again, and in the midluteal phase reach levels similar to those of the mid to late follicular phase. Progesterone levels rise steeply after ovulation and reach their peak about 8 days after the LH surge. Progesterone induces secretory changes in the endometrium in anticipation for pregnancy, and suppresses new follicular growth in the ovary during the luteal phase.

Luteal oestradiol and progesterone levels exert a negative feedback effect on FSH and LH. Steroidogenesis, however, remains LH-dependent and the normal function of the corpus luteum requires the presence of small amounts of LH.

The corpus luteum starts to decline about 9 to 11 days after ovulation, perhaps in response to yet unidentified luteolytic factors, which probably include oestradiol. This is another example of apoptosis. The resultant decrease in steroid levels releases the negative feedback on FSH, which starts to increase in preparation for the next cycle. If pregnancy occurs, the embryonic human chorionic gonadotrophin (hCG) 'rescues' the corpus luteum and maintains its steroidogenetic function until the placental 'shift' occurs at 7–10 weeks.

Ovarian morphology

As can be seen, the ovary is a dynamic organ, both functionally and morphologically. At any stage of the cycle the ovary normally contains cystic structures (Fig. 15.4). The finding of an ovarian cyst should be viewed in the context of the stage of the cycle as well as of the whole clinical picture.

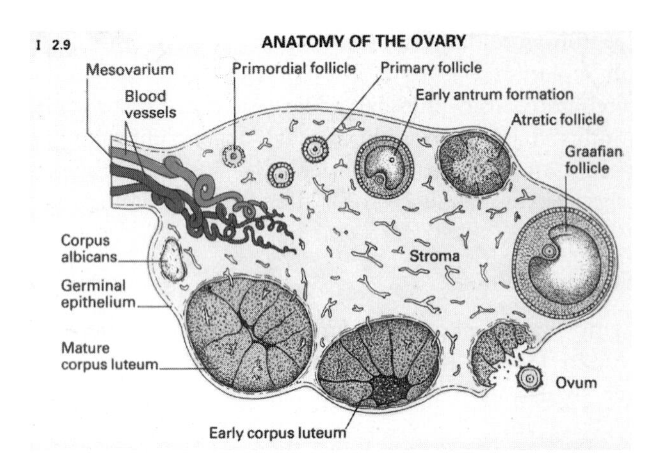

Fig. 15.4 Functional anatomy of the ovary.

OVULATORY DYSFUNCTION

Almost 30% of female infertility patients present with ovulatory dysfunction. In the majority of cases medical treatmant is effective in re-establishing fertility to near normal levels. The selection of proper treatment is heavily dependent upon reaching the right diagnosis. In all cases adequate history and physical examination are essential and, in the majority of cases, a few simple endocrine investigations will be enough to reach a meaningful diagnosis. Occasionally more detailed investigations are necessary, not only to direct treatment, but also to exclude serious progressive disorders (e.g. pituitary tumours).

History

Detailed menstrual, medical, surgical, and drug history should be taken. History of previous infertility investigations and treatment should also be elicited, so as to avoid unnecessary repetition.

Ovulatory dysfunction is usually indicated by amenorrhoea (absence of menstruation for at least 6 months), oligomenorrhoea (menses occurring less frequently than every 6 weeks), or polymenorrhoea (menses occurring more frequently than every 21 days), each reflecting either very low, low, or normal but unopposed oestrogen levels, respectively.

Ovulatory cycles are more likely to be associated with dysmenorrhoea and midcycle pain (*mittelschmerz*), which is a preovulatory (associated with the LH surge) rather than an ovulatory event.

Examination

The height and weight of the patient are of particular relevance (e.g. short stature in Turner's syndrome, obesity in polycystic ovarian syndrome). To facilitate reference to normograms, a body mass index (BMI = weight in kg/ height squared in m) should be calculated; the average adult BMI is 25 with a range of 19–28. A BMI of 30 implies 30% excess body weight.

General physical examination should be performed, with particular reference to the thyroid gland, breasts, facial and body hair. A thorough gynaecological examination should also be performed.

Investigations

Any couple presenting with infertility should be investigated for ovulation, even if the woman has a regular menstrual cycle or there is another obvious cause of infertility; 10% of normally menstruating women have ovulatory dysfunction and in up to 15% of infertile couples there is more than one infertility factor (Pepperell 1984). The extent of the investigations, however, will vary according to history and examination findings.

In the normally menstruating woman with no obvious markers for ovulatory dysfunction, midluteal (4–10 days before the onset of the next menses) serum progesterone (P) should be measured. As with all hormonal measurements, normograms for assays used in different laboratories should be consulted.

In the presence of markers in the history or examination, or after an abnormal midluteal serum progesterone is found, a more detailed hormonal profile should be obtained. This should include measurement of FSH, LH, prolactin (PRL), testosterone (T), and thyroid-stimulating hormone (TSH). The timing of the tests is important for FSH and LH; it should be in the early or midfollicular phase to avoid confusing the normal midcycle surge with abnormally high values. Obviously, in amenorrhoeic patients or those who have very infrequent periods this timing does not apply, and the tests could be taken at any time and the results interpreted with reference to the following period. The other hormonal measurements could be done at any time of the cycle.

Another investigation commonly performed in amenorrhoeic patients is the 'progestogen withdrawal test'. The aims of the test are to determine if there is endogenous oestrogen stimulation, functioning endometrium, and patent lower genital tract (uterus, cervix, vagina). Medroxyprogesterone acetate is administered in a dose of 5 mg orally twice daily for 5 days. This stimulates secretory changes in the oestrogen-primed endometrium (because oestrogen induces progesterone receptor formation). At 2–4 days after the last tablet, a withdrawal vaginal bleeding occurs (positive progestogen test). This bleeding, however, may be delayed for 8–10 days if ovulation has occurred, as the endometrium will be maintained by the progesterone produced by the corpus luteum.

With the results of the investigations performed so far, a working diagnosis can be reached in the majority of cases. In a few cases some other investigations will be required. These may include imaging studies of the skull in cases of

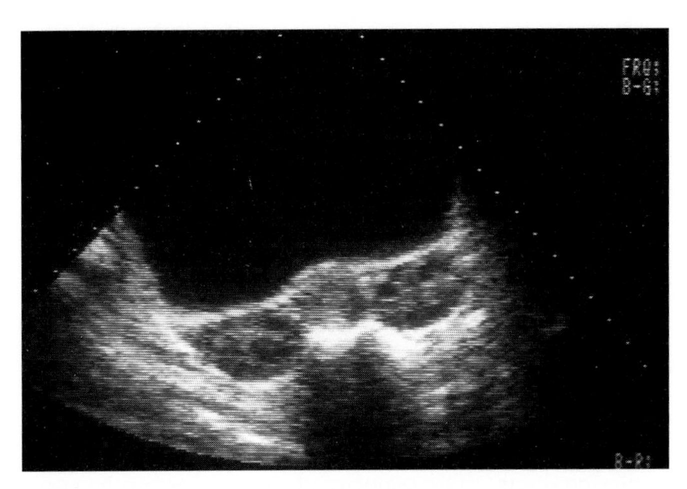

Fig. 15.5 Abdominal ultrasound of a patient with polycystic ovarian syndrome (PCOS). Note the enlarged ovaries and relatively small uterus.

high PRL or low gonadotrophins; chromosomal analysis in some cases of primary amenorrhoea or premature ovarian failure, or pelvic ultrasound scan to confirm the presence of pelvic genital organs in cases of primary amenorrhoea, or to detect polycystic ovaries and thickened ovarian stroma in cases of polycystic ovarian syndrome (PCOS) (Fig. 15.5).

Diagnosis

The World Health Organization (WHO) Scientific Group on Agents Stimulating Ovarian Function in the Human has proposed a working classification of ovarian dysfunction (WHO 1976). Despite many advances in the understanding of ovulatory pathophysiology since then, this classification has stood the test of time; it remains widely used and provides a logical approach to a diagnosis-orientated management. Ovulatory dysfunction is divided into seven main groups as described below.

Group I. Hypothalamic–pituitary failure

These patients present with a history of amenorrhoea (primary or secondary) due to inadequate (or absent) gonadotrophin release. The FSH and LH levels are low (hypogonadotrophic hypogonadism), PRL is normal, T is normal or low, and the progestogen test is negative (no endogenous oestrogen). Because of the low gonadotrophins, computerized tomography (CT) of the skull should be performed to exclude space-occupying lesions; in this group (by definition) this will be normal.

Examples of patients belonging to this group include those with anorexia nervosa, where both excessive weight loss and psychological stress (acting through neuropeptides) interfere with gonadotrophin-releasing hormone (GnRH) release. Patients with Kallmann's syndrome (isolated gonadotrophin deficiency and anosmia) also belong to group I. This congenital disorder has an incidence of 1:50 000 and is thought to be due to early degeneration of GnRH neurons, which are of the same embryological origin as olfactory neurons. Patients with postpartum pituitary necrosis (Sheehan's syndrome), and hypophysectomized patients also belong to this group.

The treatment for patients with anorexia nervosa is psychotherapy and weight gain. Other causes could be viewed as deficiency states and treated by replacement of either GnRH or gonadotrophins.

Group II. Hypothalamic–pituitary dysfunction

This includes a heterogeneous group of patients who can present either with regular cycles, oligomenorrhoea, or even amenorrhoea. The midluteal P is low, FSH and LH levels are in the normal range, PRL is normal, and the progestogen test is positive. Serum T levels may be elevated.

The classical example of this group of conditions is polycystic ovarian syndrome (PCOS), originally described by Stein & Leventhal in 1935. Classically in PCOS there is elevation of LH, the LH/FSH ratio and T. The exact aetiology is still a matter of debate, but it is thought that a state of chronic anovulation leads to an androgenic milieu and a chronic elevation of basal LH, which further enhances the state of hyperandrogenism, thus starting and maintaining a vicious circle. Commonly there are multiple small ovarian cysts, thickened ovarian capsule, hirsutism, obesity, elevated peripheral insulin levels, and increased insulin resistance (Fig. 15.6).

Other causes of this type of ovulatory dysfunction include congenital adrenal hyperplasia (CAH), classical or non-classical (Azziz et al 1994), adrenal tumours, and androgen-producing ovarian tumours. In all these conditions T levels are elevated, which should initiate more detailed investigations such as measurement of dehydro-

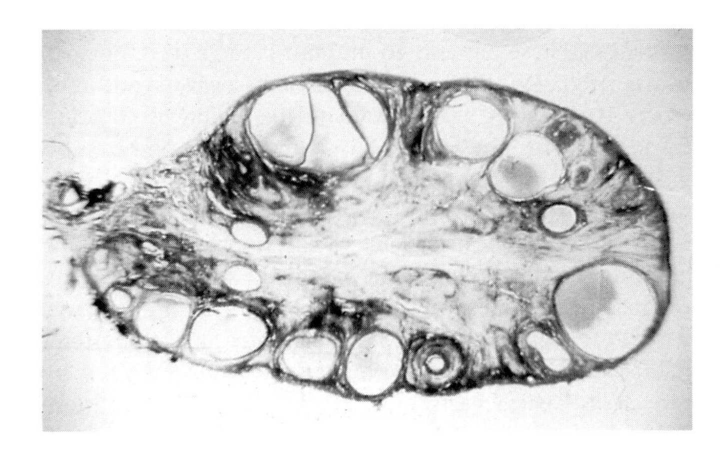

Fig. 15.6 Polycystic ovary.

epianderosterone sulphate (DHEAS) and 17-OH progesterone.

Group II patients usually respond well to clomiphene citrate or, failing that, to gonadotrophins for induction of ovulation. Specific causes, such as ovarian tumours, should be treated by removing the cause. CAH benefits from corticosteroid therapy.

Group III. Ovarian failure (OF)

These are amenorrhoeic women with no (or low) endogenous oestrogen (negative progestogen test) and elevated FSH levels (hypergonadotrophic hypogonadism), indicating primary ovarian failure. Of all women presenting with amenorrhoea, 10–15% fall into this group.

One-third of patients belonging to this group will have a genetic cause. The classical example is Turner's syndrome (45X), characterized by short stature and other variable phenotypic abnormalities such as webbed neck, shield chest, and cubitus valgus. The ovaries are 'streak'-shaped and although they contain a normal complement of oocytes during early intrauterine life, these oocytes fail to be surrounded by granulosa cells and undergo a rapid rate of degeneration, so much so that by the age of puberty no functioning follicles are left. In mosaic Turner's syndrome (45X/46XX) spontaneous menstruation may occur. Other genetic causes include pure gonadal dysgenesis (46XX) or Swyer's syndrome (46XY) where the Y chromosome is defective and does not express the testis-determining factor. As a rule, all gonads in phenotypic females containing a Y chromosome are at an increased risk of developing malignancy, and these women should undergo gonadectomy perhaps best performed once puberty is completed.

Ovarian failure before the age of 40 (premature ovarian failure (POF)) occurs in about 1% of the female population. It may be due to autoimmune disorders, genetic factors, infection (mumps oophoritis), and irradiation or cytotoxic drugs. Many cases, however, are idiopathic. Women with POF should have chromosomal analysis and autoantibody screen in addition to the other investigations. In the past, laparoscopy and ovarian biopsy was performed on these patients to find out if there were normal ovarian follicles (the so-called resistant ovary syndrome, where the follicles are resistant to the action of gonadotrophins). The rationale behind this was to find a subgroup of POF patients who might benefit from ovulation induction. This approach, however, is now obsolete, as it is invasive and does not lead to any improvement in the clinical outcome; ovulation induction with subsequent pregnancy is almost invariably unsuccessful in patients with POF. Furthermore, POF can run an intermittent course, with spontaneous pregnancies being reported in rare cases, which casts more doubt on the contribution of ovulation induction to the reported success in some cases. The only realistic treatment for patients with POF (and all others with primary OF) is IVF using donated eggs. In addition, they should be offered long-term hormone replacement therapy to protect their bones and cardiovascular systems from the deleterious effects of hypo-oestrogenism.

Group IV. Congenital or acquired genital tract disorders

These patients present with amenorrhoea due to anatomical disorders (congenital or acquired) of the genital tract. Congenital disorders present with primary amenorrhoea and can range from the simple imperforate hymen to the complex Rokitansky–Küster–Mayer syndrome (congenital absence of the vagina and failure of fusion of the two müllerian ducts). The majority of these cases can be easily diagnosed from the history and the clinical examination. They have normal secondary sexual characters and normal levels of FSH, LH, and PRL but a negative progestogen test. Pelvic ultrasonography will establish the presence of a uterus and ovaries, but laparoscopy and hysteroscopy may be needed for detailed classification. The common association between genital and urinary congenital anomalies should be remembered and looked for using renal ultrasound.

Acquired disorders present with secondary amenorrhoea; the classical example being Asherman's syndrome (intrauterine adhesions). Hysteroscopy is helpful in the diagnosis.

Group V. Hyperprolactinaemia with a space-occupying lesion in the hypothalamic–pituitary region

Hyperprolactinaemic patients can present with a variety of menstrual disorders, as raised PRL levels interfere with the normal pulsatility of GnRH; 20% of patients with menstrual irregularities will be found to have raised PRL and in 30–50% of these there will be evidence of pituitary tumour (mainly adenoma) on CT scanning. The PRL level will reflect the size of the tumours, which are divided into macro- (≥ 10 mm) and micro- (< 10 mm) adenomas.

Patients presenting with menstrual irregularities or showing anovulatory levels of luteal progesterone should have their serum PRL level measured. Hyperprolactinaemic patients should have radiological assessment of the pituitary fossa by CT scan, in addition to neurological examination and ophthalmic assessment of the visual fields. The treatments of choice are dopamine agonists such as bromocriptine or carbergoline.

Group VI. Hyperprolactinaemia without a space-occupying lesion in the hypothalamic–pituitary region

These patients are similar to those of group V except that there is no evidence of a space-occupying lesion. Recognized causes include hypothyroidism; chronic renal failure, and a variety of drugs such as oestrogens (combined oral contraceptive), dopamine-depleting agents (reserpine, methyldopa) and dopamine receptor blocking agents (phenothiazines, metoclopramide). A detailed drug history is, therefore, essential in all cases of infertility. The investigations and treatment are essentially the same as in group V.

Group VII. Amenorrhoea with a space-occupying lesion in the hypothalamic–pituitary region with normal or low PRL

These patients (by definition) have amenorrhoea, low levels of FSH and LH, normal PRL and a negative progestogen test, implying low endogenous oestrogen levels. The abnormal gonadotrophin levels indicate radiological assessment of the hypothalamic–pituitary region which shows evidence of a space-occupying lesion. The commonest tumour of the pituitary region in childhood and adolescence is craniopharyngioma, a tumour of the Rathke's pouch. Detailed neurological and ophthalmic examinations are required, and the opinion of a neurosurgeon should be sought as, depending on the symptoms, and size and location of the tumour, surgery may be required.

Treatment

The treatment of patients belonging to groups I and II (hypothalamic–pituitary failure and dysfunction, respectively) is induction of ovulation, and this will be discussed in detail below. Group III patients (OF) will not respond to induction of ovulation and should be counselled accordingly and offered ovum donation. Treatment in group IV patients should be directed towards their specific anatomical abnormality. Hyperprolactinaemic patients, whether with (group V) or without (group VI), a space-occupying lesion respond to treatment with bromocriptine, and this is fully discussed in Chapter 14. Group VII patients may need neurosurgical treatment. Obese anovulatory women (mainly those with PCOS) will benefit from weight loss, as this will not only improve their response to ovulation induction but also might lead to resumption of spontaneous ovulation.

MEDICAL INDUCTION OF OVULATION

Effective use of ovulation induction agents requires a sound understanding of their mechanism of action, proper indications, monitoring methods, and potential complications. However, it is important at the outset to have a clear grasp of two fundamental concepts. First, it should be recognized that normal fertility rates are a function of time; the peak normal fertility rate is about 30% during the first month of trying, falling quickly to about 5%. The cumulative conception rate is 50% at 6 months and 90% at 1 year. With ovulation induction, a similar timescale should be allowed (Hull 1982). Second, because of this prolonged, and often costly commitment required from both the couple and the clinician, other infertility factors should be assessed before embarking on a prolonged period of ovulation induction. To assume that an amenorrhoeic woman has no tubal pathology or to omit investigating her male partner is a recipe for later disappointment, not to mention a waste of time and money.

Clomiphene citrate

Mechanism of action

Clomiphene citrate (CC) is an orally active non-steroidal compound structurally related to diethylstilboestrol. Because of this structural similarity, it occupies the oestrogen receptors in the hypothalamic–pituitary axis, thus blinding them to the endogenous oestrogen levels. This diminishes the negative feedback and increases the pulse amplitude of the GnRH and the release of gonadotrophins. An intact hypothalamic–pituitary axis and the presence of endogenous oestrogen are, therefore, essential for the effective use of CC; this is the case in the WHO group II patients and is indicated by a positive progestogen test.

Regimen

CC is available in 50 mg tablets. Treatment should be started with a daily dose of 50 mg, taken from day 5 of the cycle for 5 days (i.e. days 5–9). Alternatively, starting the treatment on day 2, 3, or 4 of the cycle gives the same results in terms of ovulation and pregnancy (Wu & Winkel 1989). Amenorrhoeic patients need not have a withdrawal bleed before starting the treatment, as long as pregnancy is excluded. The preovulatory LH surge is expected to occur 5–10 days after the last tablet and the couple are advised to have intercourse on alternate days for 1 week starting 5 days after the last day of taking CC.

During the first cycle midluteal serum P levels should be measured to check for ovulation. If this does not occur, the dose is increased to 100 mg daily and given in a similar fashion. Increments of 50 mg are used until ovulation occurs, or a dose of 200 mg is reached. If the patient fails to ovulate on the 200-mg dose for 3 months, treatment is stepped up to human menopausal gonadotrophins.

Results

Almost 80% of properly selected patients will ovulate in response to CC treatment and 40% will conceive. The monthly fecundity in each ovulatory cycle is about 25% and the 6-month cumulative conception rate is about 60%; similar to normal fertility. Also, as with normal fertility, the majority of pregnancies will occur in the first 6 ovulatory cycles. After 6 ovulatory cycles an alternative method of ovulation induction should be considered. There is no increase in spontaneous abortion or congenital abnormalities in CC pregnancies. The rate of multiple pregnancy is 5–10%, with the great majority being twins, although higher order multiple pregnancies have been reported (Levene et al 1992).

The commonest two causes of failure to conceive in response to CC are the presence of other infertility factors, and the failure to persist with repeated attempts.

Side-effects

Due to its combined oestrogenic and antioestrogenic properties, CC can lead to hot flushes, breast discomfort, hair loss, visual symptoms, abdominal distension, headache, nausea and vomiting. All side-effects are transient. Ovarian enlargement can also occur, sometimes to a large extent, but usually disappears by the end of the cycle. Significant ovarian hyperstimulation syndrome is very rare with CC.

Human menopausal gonadotrophins

Mechanism of action

Human menopausal gonadotrophins (hMGs), as their name implies, are extracted from the urine of postmenopausal women. They are available mainly in three preparations: an FSH and LH mixture with a 1:1 ratio (e.g. Pergonal); a 3:1 ratio (e.g. Normegon), and a pure FSH preparation (e.g. Metrodin HP). A new preparation of genetically engineered recombinant FSH (rFSH) is now available with the added advantage of being free from any of the extraneous proteins which are invariably present in most urinary extracted compounds.

The classical indications for hMG are patients with hypothalamic–pituitary failure (group I), and patients with hypothalamic–pituitary dysfunction (group II) who failed to ovulate or conceive on CC. As mentioned earlier, group I patients should be given a preparation containing both FSH and LH because of the fundamental role of LH in ovarian steroidogenesis. In group II patients CC must always be tried before resorting to hMG which is more expensive, has to be administered parenterally and is associated with a higher rate of multiple pregnancy and side-effects.

Regimen

The hMG is administered by intramuscular injection (subcutaneously for purified FSH). The patient is started on day 2 of the cycle with 150 U daily and seen on cycle day 8, and every 1–3 days thereafter, for monitoring. This monitoring takes the form of serum oestradiol measurement, and pelvic ultrasonography for the number and size of ovarian follicles. The first aim of monitoring is to decide on the appropriate time to administer (intramuscularly or subcutaneously) 5000–10 000 U of hCG as a 'surrogate' LH surge to induce ovulation. This is administered when the leading follicle is 16–18 mm in mean diameter. The couple are advised to have intercourse on the day of hCG injection and on the following 2 days. As the treatment involves daily injections, many programmes have successfully adopted a policy of teaching the patient or her partner how to administer the injections.

The second aim of monitoring is to reduce the possibility of high-order multiple pregnancy and ovarian hyperstimulation; hCG is withheld and the couple advised to abstain from intercourse for 1 week if there are more than four follicles with a mean diameter of 14 mm or over (preovulatory size) with corresponding oestradiol levels. The oestradiol level per preovulatory follicle is about 300 pg/ml, but the presence of many smaller follicles can raise the level of oestradiol with no corresponding preovulatory follicles. The use of ultrasound and serum oestradiol measurements is, therefore, complementary.

Group II patients in general, and those with PCOS in particular are more sensitive to hMG than group I patients and have a higher incidence of cancelled cycles due to overstimulation. Patients with PCOS are, therefore, started on 75 U (one ampoule) daily and monitored every 5 days, when the dose is increased by half an ampoule if there is no response (Sagle et al 1991). Some programmes use a similar 'stepwise' method for all their hMG patients.

Results

Treatment with hMG is very effective in inducing ovulation, and the 6-month cumulative conception rate in group I patients is around 90%, with a spontaneous abortion rate of 21–25%. This is rather higher than the general population and perhaps reflects the higher incidence of multiple pregnancies, older age, and early recognition of pregnancy (Bohrer & Kemmann 1987).

The results of hMG treatment in group II patients are not as good. After 12 months of treatment, only 60% are pregnant, with an abortion rate of 32–40%. However, group II patients, particularly those with PCOS and raised tonic LH are known to have a high rate of spontaneous abortion whatever the method of conception. Therefore, when purified and recombinant FSH became available, it was thought that their use in PCOS patients would lead to higher success and lower abortion and hyperstimulation rates. This hope, however, was not proven in randomized studies, and careful use of low-dose hMG can lead to similar results to those with purified FSH (Sagle et al 1991).

Treatment with hMG leads to a 25% incidence of twins and to an incidence of about 5% of higher-order multiple pregnancies. Proper monitoring can reduce the chance of this happening, but not abolish it. Treated couples should be counselled accordingly.

Side-effects

The most serious complication of hMG therapy is ovarian hyperstimulation syndrome (OHSS) which occurs in its severe form in 1–2% of hMG cycles. OHSS is discussed in detail later in this chapter. Other complications include local reaction at the site of the injection, perhaps due to the protein content of the hMG. Such patients should be switched to purified FSH preparations.

CC and hMG combination

Some programmes use a combination of CC and hMG, to lessen the overall cost by reducing the amount of hMG needed. CC is used initially (100 mg daily from days 2–6) for follicular recruitment, followed by hMG (150 U daily or on alternate days) to promote follicular growth, thus reducing the hMG requirement by up to 50% (Fig. 15.7). This regimen is only of use in anovulatory patients who have endogenous gonadotrophins (group II).

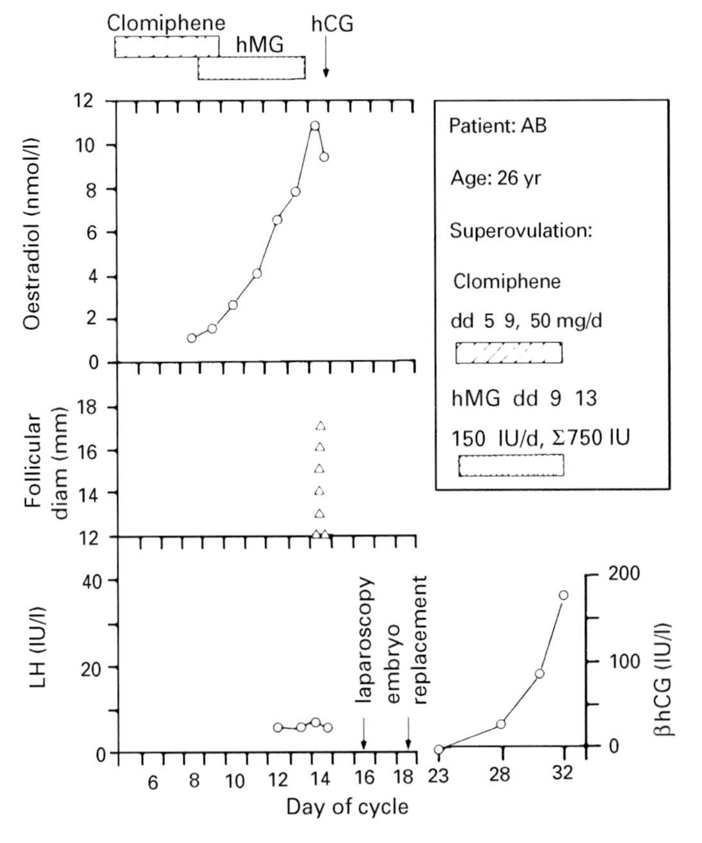

Fig. 15.7 A clomiphene citrate–human menopausal gonadotrophin (CC–hMG) cycle prior to in vitro fertilization.

GnRH agonists and hMG combination

As noted above, hypogonadotrophic patients (group I) have a better response and a more successful outcome than normogonadotrophic patients (group II). Furthermore, patients with elevated basal levels of LH (as in PCOS) are particularly prone to a lower success rate after hMG treatment and to a higher abortion rate.

This has led to the suggestion that converting those patients into a hypogonadotrophic state might improve their results. This is done by administering GnRH agonists prior to starting hMG; the so-called 'medical menopause'. It is worth noting, however, that the only similarity between this treatment and the menopause is the hypo-oestrogenic state; natural menopause is a hypergonadotrophic state while GnRH agonist treatment is a hypogonadotrophic one. The use of the GnRH agonist–hMG combination for ovulation induction in PCOS patients has been suggested to increase the pregnancy rate and reduce the abortion rate (Homburg et al 1993).

Native GnRH has a short half-life because it is rapidly cleaved between amino acids 5–6, 6–7, and 9–10. Agonists with a longer half-life are produced by substitution of amino acids at the 6 and/or 10 positions. These agonists are administered by subcutaneous injections (e.g. buserelin 500 μg once daily) or as a nasal spray (e.g. nafarelin 200 μg twice daily). They produce an initial 'flare-up' effect, increasing the release of gonadotrophins and the production of oestrogen. This is soon followed by a 'downregulation' effect on the gonadotrophs of the anterior pituitary and a hypogonadotrophic hypo-oestrogenic state. The flare-up effect is more prolonged if the agonists are started during the follicular phase, when it is accentuated by the natural rise in FSH levels at that time. Complete downregulation (serum oestradiol <50 pg/ml) takes about 3 weeks if started in the follicular phase and 10–14 days if started in the midluteal phase. The hypo-oestrogenic state is responsible for the common menopausal-like symptoms (hot flushes, headaches, vaginal dryness, irritability) experienced with GnRH agonists. Patients should be forewarned and reassured that these symptoms will disappear once they start taking the hMG. Another side-effect of GnRH agonists is the development of functional ovarian cysts (due to the flare-up effect), particularly if the treatment is started during the follicular phase.

Following downregulation, hMG is started in the usual way, but patients usually need higher doses (with increased costs). GnRH agonists are continued until the ovulating hCG dose is given. It is important to recognize that downregulation may persist for some time after stopping the agonists, and exogenous luteal support should be given to replace the reduced endogenous LH levels. This support is in the form of hCG (2000 U twice, 3 and 6 days after the ovulating dose), or progesterone by intramuscular injections (50–100 mg daily) or vaginal suppositories

(100–200 mg daily) for 14 days. The hCG has the advantage of needing less frequent administration, but increases the risk of hyperstimulation. It is important to be aware that the hCG injections will lead to a false positive pregnancy test if this is performed too early (earlier than 2 weeks after ovulation). Forgetting this fact has, not infrequently, given some patients false hope with subsequent disappointment.

Gonadotrophin-releasing hormone (GnRH)

Mechanism of action

Normally, the hypothalamic–pituitary–ovarian cycle is initiated at the level of the hypothalamus by the pulsatile release of GnRH. Induction of ovulation using hMG or CC initiates this process at a different level and can thus lead to the non-physiological effects of multiple pregnancies and hyperstimulation. Using GnRH, administered in a pulsatile fashion, for ovulation induction produces a semiphysiological response with very low rates of multiple pregnancies or hyperstimulation.

Regimen

The GnRH is given via a small battery-operated pump, delivering a dose every 90 min (mimicking the natural follicular phase pulsatility). It can be administered either subcutaneously (20 μg starting dose) or intravenously (5 μg) through a small butterfly cannula which remains in situ for the duration of the treatment. Serum oestradiol measurements and a pelvic scan are performed weekly and the dose increased accordingly, in 5-μg increments. Ovulation usually occurs after 14 days of treatment (range 10–21 days). When the leading follicle is 14 mm or over, the woman is instructed to use the urinary LH kit and when the surge is detected the couple are advised to have intercourse on the following 3 days. Luteal support is needed, either by continuing with the GnRH pump or using hCG or progesterone as described above.

Results

Hypogonadotrophic (group I) patients are the best candidates for this treatment, with a 30% conception rate per ovulatory cycle and a multiple pregnancy rate of about 5%. PCOS patients, however, have lower pregnancy rates.

Side-effects

GnRH is less expensive than hMG, requires less monitoring, is associated with a lower multiple pregnancy rate and very rarely leads to significant hyperstimulation. However, many patients and some clinicians worry about pump failure and the problems of the needle being left in situ for such a long time (e.g. displacement, local reaction, infection). As a result, it is used in very few patients for whom alternatives are available.

SUPEROVULATION

Superovulation refers to the induction of multiple ovulation in normally ovulating patients. It is used in the treatment of prolonged unexplained infertility, usually combined with intrauterine insemination (IUI). It is also a fundamental part of assisted conception programmes, such as in vitro fertilization (IVF) and gamete intrafallopian transfer (GIFT).

Superovulation for unexplained infertility

Patients with unexplained infertility of under 3 years' duration have an excellent prognosis, with a cumulative spontaneous conception rate of 80% over the following 2 years. Those with prolonged (over 3 years') unexplained infertility, however, have very little chance of spontaneous conception, with a monthly fecundity of only 1–2%. Patients with prolonged unexplained infertility are usually offered empirical treatment in the form of ovulation induction, alone or combined with IUI. This is also offered to those who have shorter periods of unexplained infertility but are in their late thirties (>35 years old). In practice, many younger patients, understandably, request treatment, and it is the clinician's duty to explain to them that the only advantage it may offer is that it may bring pregnancy a few months earlier than would have happened spontaneously, as well as having the disadvantage of a higher chance of multiple pregnancy. Infertile couples often view the chance of multiple pregnancy as an added blessing; they should be counselled about the attendant increased perinatal morbidity and mortality. If, after proper explanation and counselling, these couples still request treatment, it is usually given.

There is some evidence to suggest that CC may lead to a 3–5% pregnancy rate per cycle in patients with prolonged unexplained infertility; a 50% increase over placebo (Glazener et al 1990). This effect is limited to the first 3–4 treatment cycles only, and in practice it is not worth pursuing treatment with CC for unexplained infertility for longer than 6 months. Combining CC with IUI has been associated with an even higher pregnancy rate in some studies (Deaton et al 1990).

Treatment with hMG for prolonged unexplained infertility is usually combined with IUI and has been shown to lead to a pregnancy rate of 10–15% per cycle (Serhal et al 1988). As with CC, this effect has been limited to the first 3–5 cycles only. After that the only treatment with proven success is IVF or GIFT.

Superovulation for IVF

Although the world's first IVF baby was from a natural

unstimulated cycle, it has been shown since then that the chances of pregnancy are related to the number of embryos replaced. Furthermore, unreplaced embryos could be frozen for later transfer, which increases the overall pregnancy rate per cycle and reduces the cost per pregnancy achieved. Superovulation, therefore, is used in the majority of IVF programmes. Natural cycle IVF is still being used, but it requires three natural cycles to achieve the pregnancy rate achieved in one stimulated cycle. The aim of superovulation in IVF is to produce the maximum number of mature oocytes without producing ovarian hyperstimulation. Obviously, the limitation of a maximum of 4 preovulatory follicles does not apply here as only the desired number of embryos will be replaced. The GnRH agonist–hMG regimen is used in most programmes, with a higher hMG dose than that used in ovulation induction. This is discussed in more detail in Chapter 19.

OVARIAN HYPERSTIMULATION SYNDROME (OHSS)

Ovulation induction entails stimulating the ovaries to produce oocytes. A degree of ovarian hyperstimulation is, therefore, inherent in all patients who respond to ovulation induction. This should be distinguished from OHSS which is a pathological entity characterized by ovarian enlargement, abdominal distension, nausea, vomiting, and diarrhoea. In severe cases there is ascites, pleural effusion, hypovolaemia, hypotension, haemoconcentration and oliguria (Fig. 15.8). The symptoms start during the luteal phase of the cycle and usually resolve within 7 days. If the patient becomes pregnant, however, a more protracted course could be expected, sometimes lasting for weeks. OHSS can be life-threatening and is the most serious complication of ovulation induction.

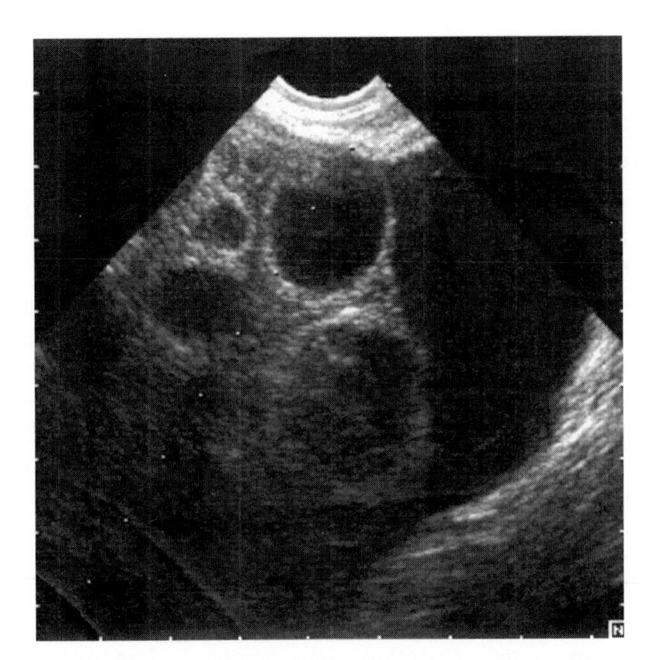

Fig. 15.8 Vaginal scan of a patient with moderate ovarian hyperstimulation syndrome (OHSS). Note the enlarged ovaries, luteal cysts and ascites.

Classification

Many classifications for OHSS have been proposed. A commonly used classification by Golan et al (1989) divides OHSS into the following categories.

Mild OHSS

Grade 1: abdominal distension and discomfort.
Grade 2: features of grade 1 plus nausea, vomiting, and/or diarrhoea; ovaries enlarged to 5–12 cm.

Moderate OHSS

Grade 3: features of mild OHSS plus ultrasonic evidence of ascites.

Severe OHSS

Grade 4: features of moderate OHSS plus clinical evidence of ascites, and/or hydrothorax and breathing difficulties.
Grade 5: all of the above plus changes in blood volume, increased blood viscosity due to haemoconcentration, coagulation abnormalities, and diminished renal perfusion and function.

Risk factors

Significant (moderate to severe) OHSS is very rare with CC. In hMG cycles the incidences of mild, moderate and severe OHSS are approximately 20%, 3–5%, and approximately 1%, respectively. PCOS patients are at a particularly higher risk of developing OHSS.

Pregnancy is a well-recognized risk factor; OHSS is four times more common in conception cycles, and pregnancy is three times more likely in cycles where OHSS develops. This is thought to be due to the effect of embryonic hCG. This is supported by the observation that OHSS is more common if exogenous hCG is used for luteal support. In high risk patients, therefore, progesterone should be used if luteal support is needed.

Some reports indicate that OHSS is more common if hMG is combined with GnRH agonists. This, however, might be due to the fact that luteal support is always needed with such a regimen. Furthermore, this combination leads to higher preovulatory serum oestradiol levels and more mature oocytes developing; both are risk factors for OHSS.

Younger patients and those who are lean are more prone to develop OHSS.

Pathophysiology

The basic pathophysiology of OHSS is fluid shift from the intravascular compartment to the third space (mainly the peritoneal cavity). The exact mechanism of this is unclear. Ovarian endocrine, paracrine, and autocrine factors may lead to angiogenesis, increased capillary permeability and leakage of protein-rich fluid into the peritoneal cavity. This leads to intravascular hypovolaemia and haemoconcentration.

In more severe conditions there is also hypotension, increased coagulability, reduced renal perfusion, and oliguria. Deranged liver function tests, venous and arterial thrombosis, renal failure and adult respiratory distress syndrome have all been reported in severe cases and some fatalities have occurred.

Prevention

Prevention of OHSS is based upon detecting those patients with high-risk factors and implementing preventive measures, i.e. starting with low dose hMG, more frequent monitoring, withholding or delaying the ovulating hCG injection, and the use of progesterone for luteal support. Whatever methods are used, OHSS is never totally predictable nor preventable. A major part of the pretreatment counselling is to discuss the possibility of OHSS with the patient.

Treatment

Treatment of OHSS is conservative and symptomatic, awaiting spontaneous resolution. These women are usually very anxious about their condition, and mainly about the effect it may have on the outcome of their treatment. Adequate explanation and reassurance should be given. They tend to think that because a complication has occurred then pregnancy is less likely; they should be reassured that pregnancy is more likely with OHSS.

Initially a critical assessment of the patient's symptoms and hydration state should be made, including a full blood picture, clotting profile, renal and liver function tests, and ultrasound examination for ovarian size, ascites, and pleural effusion. Symptomatic relief should be given: paracetamol or even opiates for pain, and metoclopramide or prochlorperazine for nausea. Avoidance or correction of reduced intravascular volume (as evidenced by a high haematocrit) is a priority (Jenkins et al 1995). Colloids are preferred to crystalloids and, in the presence of hypoproteinaemia and oliguria, albumin is the volume expander of choice. In some cases aspiration of ascites (under transvaginal ultrasound guidance to avoid the enlarged ovaries and distended bowels) can lead to rapid improvement (Aboulghar et al 1993). Management of severe OHSS should be conducted in conjunction with a clinician with experience of managing this problem. Eventually, gradual resolution is the rule. The subject of OHSS has been recently extensively reviewed by Rizk (1994).

Other conditions with similar presentation (abdominal pain, hypovolaemia, and hypotension) should be excluded. These include ruptured ectopic pregnancy and torsion and rupture of ovarian cysts. The key difference is in the full blood count; these conditions will be associated with low haematocrit and haemoglobin levels.

OVARIAN CANCER AND OVULATION INDUCTION

The possibility that ovulation induction may cause ovarian cancer has been raised by a few case reports, as well as by a recent combined analysis of three case-control studies reporting a positive association between the risk of ovarian cancer and prior treatment with infertility drugs (Whittemore et al 1992). Also, the fact that a decreased risk of developing ovarian cancer is associated with conditions in which there is less frequent ovulation (e.g. the use of oral contraception, multiparity, prolonged breast feeding) makes this possibility, at least biologically plausible. Nevertheless, the aforementioned analysis of case-control studies has been heavily criticized on epidemiological and clinical grounds (Cohen et al 1993). Furthermore, a study reporting long-term follow-up of 2632 women who received ovulation induction drugs reported no increase in the incidence of ovarian cancer (Ron-El et al 1987). At our current state of knowledge, there is no sound evidence that ovulation induction causes an increase in the incidence of ovarian cancer.

SURGICAL INDUCTION OF OVULATION

Multiple ovarian puncture

Before the availability of ovulation induction drugs, the only available method for treating anovulatory PCOS patients was ovarian wedge resection, performed via laparotomy (Stein & Leventhal 1935). This is thought to work by removing part of the hormone-producing ovarian tissue, thus reducing androgen and inhibin levels. This is usually followed by a rise in FSH, a drop in LH, and resumption of spontaneous ovulation. However, the response is variable and the operation may lead to postoperative adhesions, thus reducing the chance of conception. The availability of successful medical induction of ovulation made the classical wedge resection obsolete.

More recently, as laparoscopic surgery became part of the gynaecologist's armamentarium, a new method of 'ovarian wedge resection' has emerged. Laparoscopic multiple ovarian puncture (at 15–20 sites) using cautery, diathermy or laser vaporization (Fig. 15.9) leads to a

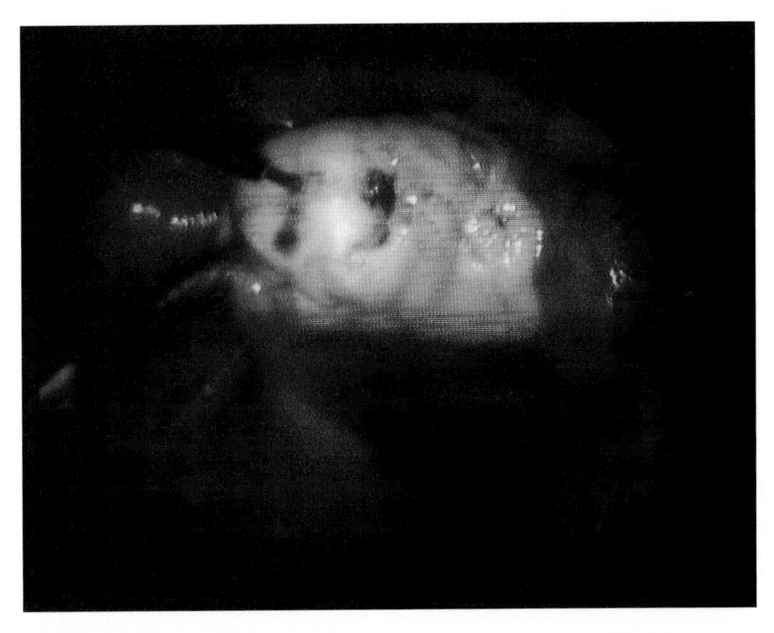

Fig. 15.9 Multiple ovarian punctures being performed laparoscopically on a polycystic ovary. (Photograph courtesy of Professor R W Shaw, Cardiff, UK.)

response similar to that with hMG in CC-resistant PCOS patients (Gadir et al 1990). Furthermore, patients who do not ovulate spontaneously following the procedure become more responsive to medical therapy, and up to 60% of them will ovulate when CC is recommenced.

The advantages of ovarian puncture over hMG are that it is a one-step treatment, no monitoring is required, and the risk of iatrogenic multiple pregnancy is eliminated. The disadvantages are that it requires an operative procedure with general anaesthesia, and postoperative adhesions can still occur, albeit at a lower rate than with laparotomy. The choice between ovarian puncture and hMG in CC-resistant patients will depend on the local availability of facilities and expertise as well as on the patient's wishes.

FUTURE DEVELOPMENTS

Genetically engineered recombinant FSH has been produced and successfully tested (Germond et al 1992). Large-scale clinical studies are underway and the product is now available for general clinical use. It has the advantages of purity, subcutaneous administration and accurate dosage. Recombinant LH is also under development.

GnRH antagonists have been synthesized by multiple amino acid substitution into native GnRH. They produce rapid downregulation without a prior flare-up effect. They have a potential use in induction of ovulation as well as in fertility control. The early compounds, however, were associated with undesirable side-effects due to histamine release and newer, more usable compounds are being developed (Rabinovici et al 1992).

KEY POINTS

1. Functioning of the ovary ensures regular folliculogenesis and ovulation during the reproductive years.
2. The cohort of growing follicles undergo a process of development and differentiation which takes about 85 days and 3 ovarian cycles.
3. Negative feedback from rising levels of oestrogen, leads to a fall in FSH in the midfollicular phase. This results in a decline in aromatase activity in all but the largest antral follicle.
4. Ovulation occurs approximately 24–36 h after the peak of oestradiol levels, 34–36 h after the onset of the LH surge and 10–12 h after the LH peak.
5. In developed countries, roughly 30% of patients who present with infertility have some form of ovulatory dysfunction.
6. The calculation of body mass index can be a useful parameter in predicting success in ovulation induction regimes and potential causation of ovulation dysfunction.
7. Appropriate investigation of the hypothalamic–pituitary–ovarian axis, thyroid and adrenal function are necessary to accurately categorize patients and choose appropriate ovulation induction regimes.
8. With hypogonadotrophic hypogonadism and low levels of endogenous gonadotrophins, pulsatile GnRH should be continued throughout the cycle to provide gonadotrophin support for the corpus luteum.
9. Despite increased vigilance during administration of exogenous gonadotrophins for induction of ovulation, there is no foolproof way to avoid ovarian hyperstimulation syndrome and multiple pregnancy. However, careful ultrasound and

endocrine monitoring are mandatory to reduce the likelihood of such complications.

10. Clomiphene citrate is usually the first line of treatment in subjects who are normoprolactinaemic and not grossly oestrogen-deficient.
11. Prior to treating patients with hyperprolactinaemia with dopamine agonists, it is essential to exclude the presence of a pituitary tumour which may enlarge quite rapidly in pregnancy.
12. In clomiphene-resistant polycystic ovary patients, multiple ovarian cautery may be an alternative treatment to exogenous gonadotrophins, and is associated with a return, albeit not permanent, to spontaneous ovulation.
13. Patients who demonstrate premature luteinization during exogenous gonadotrophin treatment may benefit from concomitant use of GnRH agonists to induce pituitary down-regulation.
14. Ovarian hyperstimulation syndrome is potentially life-threatening, and needs careful evaluation and management in a unit used to dealing with such cases.

REFERENCES

Aboulghar M A, Mansour R T, Serour G I, Sattar M A, Amin Y M, Elattar I 1993 Management of severe ovarian hyperstimulation syndrome by ascitic fluid aspiration and intensive intravenous fluid therapy. Obstetrics and Gynecology 81: 108

Azziz R, Dewailly D, Owerbach D 1994 Nonclassic adrenal hyperplasia: current concepts. Journal of Clinical Endocrinology and Metabolism 78: 810

Baker T G 1963 A quantitative and cytological study of germ cells in human ovaries. Proceedings of the Royal Society of London 158: 417

Bohrer M, Kemmann E 1987 Risk factors for spontaneous abortion in menotropin-treated women. Fertility and Sterility 48: 571

Cohen J, Forman R, Harlap S 1993 IFFS Expert Group Report on the Whittemore study related to the risk of ovarian cancer associated with the use of infertility agents. Human Reproduction 8: 996

Deaton J L, Gibson M, Blackmer K M, Nakajima S T, Badger G J, Brumsted J R 1990 A randomized controlled trial of clomiphene citrate and intrauterine insemination in couples with unexplained infertility or surgically corrected endometriosis. Fertility and Sterility 54: 1083

Gadir A, Mowafi R S, Alnaser H M I, Alrashid A H, Alonezi O M, Shaw R W 1990 Ovarian electrocautery versus human menopausal gonadotrophins and pure follicle stimulating hormone therapy in the treatment of patients with polycystic ovarian disease. Clinical Endocrinology 33: 585

Germond M, Dessole S, Senn A, Loumaye E, Howles C, Beltrami V 1992 Successful in-vitro fertilisation and embryo transfer after treatment with recombinant FSH. Lancet 339: 1170

Glazener C M A, Coulson C, Lambert P A et al 1990 Clomiphene treatment for women with unexplained infertility: placebo-controlled study of hormonal responses and conception rates. Gynecological Endocrinology 4: 75

Golan A, Ron-El R, Herman A, Soffer Y, Weinraub Z, Caspi E 1989 Ovarian hyperstimulation syndrome: an update review. Obstetric and Gynecologic Survey 44: 430

Homburg R, Levy T, Berkovitz D et al 1993 Gonadotropin-releasing hormone agonist reduces the miscarriage rate for pregnancies achieved with polycystic ovarian syndrome. Fertility and Sterility 59: 527

Hull M G R 1982 Ovulation failure and induction. In: Studd J (ed) Progress in obstetrics and gynaecology, vol 2: 208. Churchill Livingstone, Edinburgh

Jenkins J M, Mathur R S, Cooke I D 1995 The management of severe ovarian hyperstimulation syndrome. British Journal of Obstetrics and Gynaecology 102: 2

Levene M I, Wild J, Steer P 1992 Higher multiple births and the modern management of infertility in Britain. British Journal of Obstetrics and Gynaecology 99: 607

McNatty K P, Markis A, DeGrazia C, Osathanondh R, Ryan K J 1980 Steroidogenesis by recombined follicular cells from the human ovary in vitro. Journal of Clinical Endocrinology and Metabolism 51: 1286

Pepperell R 1984 The investigation of infertility. In: Studd J (ed) Progress in obstetrics and gynaecology, vol. 4: 272. Churchill Livingstone, Edinburgh

Rabinovici J, Rothman P, Monroe S E, Nerenberg C, Jaffe R B 1992 Endocrine effects and pharmacokinetic characteristics of a potent new gonadotropin-releasing hormone antagonist (Ganirelix) with minimal histamine-releasing properties: studies in postmenopausal women. Journal of Clinical Endocrinology and Metabolism 75: 1220

Rizk B 1994 Ovarian hyperstimulation syndrome. In: Studd J (ed) Progress in obstetrics and gynaecology, vol. 11: 311. Churchill Livingstone, Edinburgh

Ron-El R, Lunenfeld B, Menczer J et al 1987 Cancer incidence in a cohort of infertile women. American Journal of Epidemiology 125: 780

Sagle M A, Hamilton-Fairley D, Kiddy D S, Franks S 1991 A comparative, randomized study of low-dose human menopausal gonadotropin and follicle-stimulating hormone in women with polycystic ovarian syndrome. Fertility and Sterility 55: 56

Serhal P F, Katz M, Little V, Wooronowski H 1988 Unexplained infertility – the value of Pergonal superovulation combined with intrauterine insemination. Fertility and Sterility 49: 602

Speroff L, Glass R H, Kase N G 1994 Regulation of the menstrual cycle. In: Speroff L, Glass R H, Kase N G (eds) Clinical Gynecologic endocrinology and infertility, 5th edn, pp 183. Williams & Wilkins, Baltimore

Stein I F, Leventhal M L 1935 Amenorrhoea associated with bilateral polycystic ovaries. American Journal of Obstetrics and Gynecology 29: 181

Whittemore A S, Harris R, Itnyre J and the Collaborative Ovarian Cancer Group 1992 Characteristic relation to ovarian cancer risk: collaborative analysis of twelve US case-control studies. American Journal of Epidemiology 136: 1175

World Health Organization 1976 WHO consultation on the diagnosis and treatment of endocrine causes of infertility. WHO, Hamburg.

Wu C H, Winkel C A 1989 The effect of therapy initiation day on clomiphene citrate therapy. Fertility and Sterility 52: 564

16

Fertilization and implantation

R. W. Shaw

INTRODUCTION

The process of fertilization and implantation is highly complex. It involves a final maturation of the gametes, transport of the gametes in the female genital tract, the establishment of the diploid number of chromosomes at fertilization, transport of the fertilized ovum (zygote) from the fallopian tube to the uterine cavity, attachment of the pre-embryo to the endometrium, and finally implantation.

THE SPERMATOZOON

The testis performs two major functions: the first is the synthesis of androgens in the Leydig cells which lie between the seminiferous tubules, and the second is to produce spermatozoa which are developed within the tubules where they come in contact with the Sertoli cells. Although the process of steroid production and spermatogenesis take place in these discrete compartments, their production is an interrelated function since adequate sperm production is only possible when androgen synthesis occurs. This ensures that the mature spermatozoa are delivered into an extragonadal environment which has been suitably prepared for efficient transfer to the female genital tract. (For further details, see Ch. 18).

Differentiation of spermatozoa

A mature spermatozoon is an elaborate and highly specialized cell (Fig. 16.1). It contains the basic elements common to all cells but their organization has been highly specialized. A mature spermatozoon contains the haploid number of chromosomes (22+1).

The major changes which occur during spermiogenesis include generation of the tail for provision of motility and forward propulsion; the midpiece which contains the mitochondria or energy generators for the cell; the acrosome, necessary for penetration of the oocyte, and the residual body which contains other tail elements of the residue of superfluous cytoplasm. This is the final differentiation into the mature spermatozoon, whose complex structure is seen in Figures 16.1 and 16.2. These are highly complex structural changes and it is not surprising therefore that many cells commencing on this process of differentiation do not complete it successfully. It is not uncommon to find abnormally developed spermatozoa comprising 25–40% of the total contained in an ejaculate in normal fertile males.

Maturation of spermatozoa

The spermatozoon is a few microns in length. To reach the female gamete in the tube, it must travel a distance of some 30–40 cm through the reproductive tract. It must overcome a number of obstacles in its journey; it has been estimated that less than 1 in a million spermatozoa ever complete the journey. In addition, the spermatozoa must successfully undergo a series of changes in both the male and female genital tracts before they gain full capacity to fertilize an oocyte.

Following their release from association with the Sertoli cells, spermatozoa enter a specific fluid within seminiferous tubules which washes the spermatozoa towards the

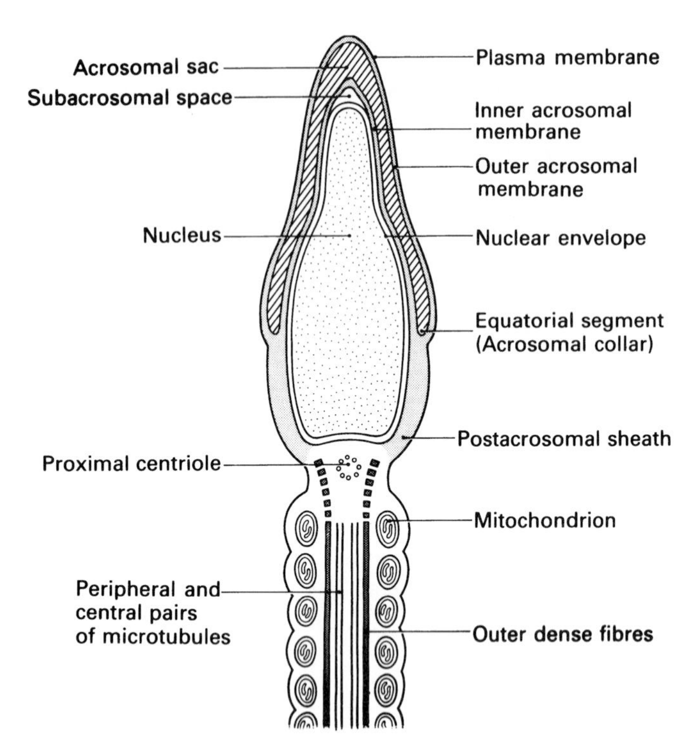

Fig. 16.1 A human spermatozoon, showing principal structures.

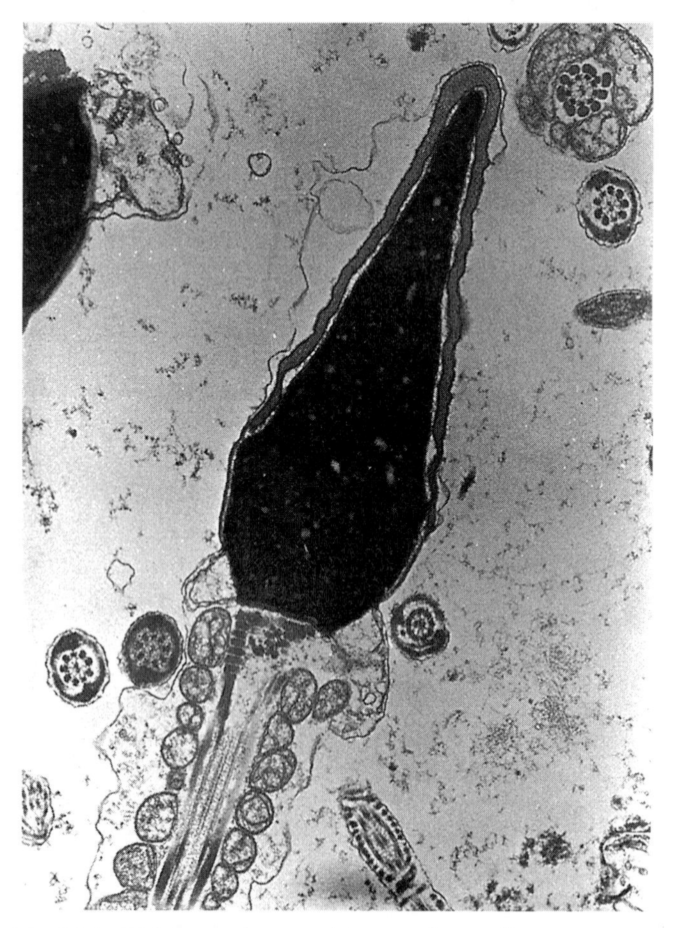

Fig. 16.2 High-power electron microscopy picture of human spermatozoon, complementing the features shown in Figure 16.1.

rete testis and then into the vasa efferentia and the epididymis. In the epididymis the composition and volume of the fluid undergoes major changes; the concentration of the spermatozoa increases by fluid absorption. In addition, specific secretory products from the epididymis, including various glycoproteins, carotene and glyceryl phosphoryl choline, are added. This passage through the vasa efferentia and epididymis takes some 12 days. During this process the spermatozoa gain the capability of movement as well as the potential to fertilize an oocyte. Other subtle structural changes also occur during this time. It is uncertain whether the biochemical morphological changes are critical for the functional maturity of the spermatozoa. Adequate stimulation by androgens of the epididymis is essential for this process of maturation.

The final passage of the spermatozoa from the tail of the epididymis to the vas deferens is no longer as a result of fluid movement, but due to muscular activity of the epididymis and vas.

The fluid which carries the spermatozoa into the female tract is largely derived from the major accessory sex glands, but its presence is not essential for sperm function. This is apparent from the evidence that spermatozoa taken directly from the vas deferens can fertilize oocytes.

At coitus, sperm are introduced into the female genital tract by ejaculation which expels the semen from the posterior urethra. This is achieved by contractions of the smooth muscles from the urethra and striated muscles of the bulbocavernosus and ischiocavernosus.

Transport of the spermatozoa in the female tract

Semen forms a gel almost immediately following ejaculation but is then liquefied in 20–30 min by enzymes derived from prostate gland secretions. The alkaline pH of semen provides protection for sperm from the acid environment of the vagina. Protection is transient and most sperm left in the vagina are immobilized by 2 h. The most fortunate sperm, by their own motility, gain entrance to the tongues of cervical mucus present on the ectocervix. Within a minute or so of ejaculation some spermatozoa can be detected in the cervix. The exact mechanism of entry is not known, but sperm swim and migrate through the pores in the cervical mucus microstructure. The pores are themselves smaller than the diameter of the sperm heads, which must therefore actively push their way through the mucus and movement is probably influenced by the interaction between the mucus and surface proteins on the sperm head. Sperm antibodies on the spermatozoa head have been shown to inhibit progress and movement in cervical mucus (Wang et al 1985).

The majority of spermatozoa (95%) from an ejaculate probably do not gain entry to the cervix and are lost by leakage from the vagina. Those that do enter the cervix successfully survive for many hours deep in the cervical crypts and are nourished by the cervical mucus and secretion. Further progress to the uterus depends on the consistency of the mucus which permits further sperm penetration only in the absence of progesterone domination.

Sperm appear to be released from the mucus and cervical crypts in batches, and uterine contractions propel the sperm upward such that they can be found in the fallopian tube within 5 min of intracervical insemination. Sperm have been shown to be released from storage in the cervix over a period up to 72 h, but do not appear to be stored in the fallopian tubes. Within the fallopian tube the sperm begin to display a new pattern of motility, i.e. hyperactivated motility, which has characteristics of greater speed and more positive direction. This change may result from an interaction between spermatozoa and tubal mucosa and/or secretions.

Cervical mucus is a complex structure which is not homogeneous. It is secreted in granular form and a networked structure of the mucus is formed within the cervical canal. Not all areas of the mucus appear to be equally penetrable. (For review, see Harper 1988).

Capacitation and activation

Immediately following ejaculation spermatozoa are unable to achieve fertilization. They only gain this capacity after a delay of several hours as they pass through the female genital tract.

The initial change of *capacitation* appears to involve the stripping from the spermatozoa of the surface coat of glycoprotein molecules, which have been adsorbed in the epididymis and from the seminal plasma. The loss of this protein coat is a result of the effects of proteolytic enzymes and the high ionic concentration found in the secretions of an oestrogen-dominated uterus.

Despite completing this process of capacitation, the sperms are still not fully ready to fertilize oocytes until the final process of *activation* has occurred. This process is calcium-dependent and involves changes throughout the spermatozoon. Before sperm are activated three accomplishments are required. They must:

1. undergo the acrosome reaction;
2. acquire the ability to bind to the zona pellucida;
3. acquire appropriate motility patterns, i.e. hyperactivated motility.

The first process or 'acrosome reaction', is one in which the acrosome swells and its membrane fuses at a number of points, with the overlying plasma membrane acquiring a vesiculated appearance (Fig. 16.3). As a result of this process, the contents of the acrosomal vesicle and the inner acrosomal membrane are exposed to the exterior. At the same time there is a change in the movement pattern of the spermatozoon. The tail movements of the spermatozoon, which previously demonstrated regular

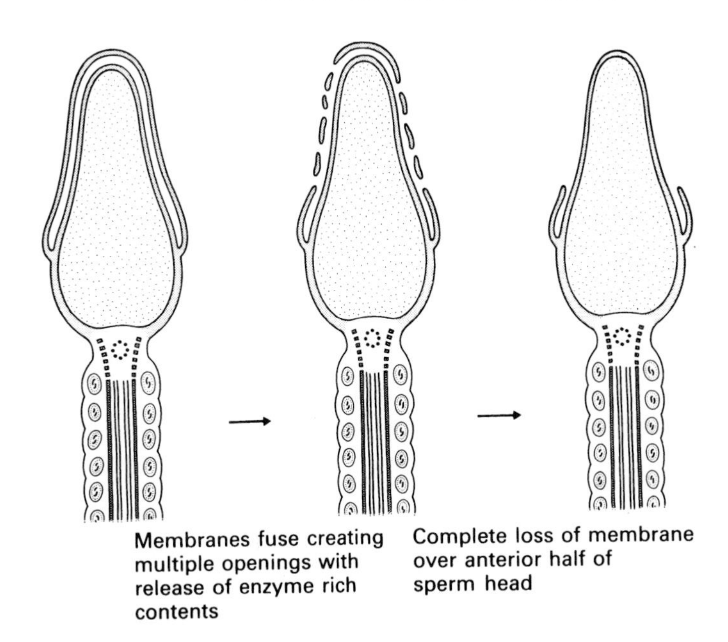
Membranes fuse creating multiple openings with release of enzyme rich contents
Complete loss of membrane over anterior half of sperm head

Fig. 16.3 Acrosome reaction.

wave-like flagellar beats, now become replaced by more episodic wide-amplitude whiplash movements which carry it forward.

The other apparent change occurs in the surface membrane overlying the middle and posterior half of the spermatozoon head. This membrane, previously incapable of fusion, now becomes capable of fusing with the surface membrane of the oocyte.

The exact mechanisms involved in this process of activation are not fully determined. However, activated spermatozoa tend only to be found in close association with the oocyte and cumulus mass. This suggests that a constituent of follicular fluid, a secretion from the cumulus mass or a product in the zona pellucida itself may be responsible for this activation which facilitates the binding of the spermatozoa to the oocyte membrane.

THE OOCYTE

Structure of the ovary

The ovary consists of stromal tissue which contains the primordial follicles, and glandular tissue consisting of interstitial cells. It is the primordial follicle, consisting of the primordial germ cell surrounded by a layer of flattened mesenchymal cells, which is the fundamental functional unit within the ovary. The process of gamete production in the female consists of the processes of cell proliferation by mitosis, the process of genetic reshuffling and reduction, i.e. meiosis, and finally the reduction to the haploid number of chromosomes during oocyte maturation. One major difference between the female and the male is the vast difference between the need for proliferation by mitosis, essential in the male to maintain a massive sperm output from the testes, but less essential in the female since only one or at most a few eggs are released during each menstrual cycle.

The primordial germ cells which enter the gonad continue mitotic proliferation well after ovarian morphology is established in utero. However, unlike the situation in the male, the mitotic phase of the primordial germ cells, or oogonia, terminates finally before birth when all oogonia enter into their first meiotic division and hence become the primary oocytes. One major consequence of this early meiosis is that by the time of birth the woman has within her ovary all the oocytes that she will ever have. In the progress through the first meiotic phase, oocytes become surrounded by ovarian mesenchymal cells to form the primordial follicles. These follicles form the oocytes which become arrested in the diplotene stage of their first meiotic phase. The chromosomes remain enclosed by a nuclear membrane in the nucleus, known as the germinal vesicle. The primordial follicle remains in this arrested state within the ovary until it receives the appropriate signals to resume development.

Selection and maturation of follicles

Regular recruitment of primordial follicles to a pool of subsequently growing developing follicles occurs first at puberty. Thereafter follicles recommence growth daily so that there is a continuing supply of developing follicles being formed. During the late luteal phase, the largest healthy follicles are between 2 and 5 millimetres in diameter. Their number and quality rise in response to the rising FSH levels during the late luteal phase and early follicular phase of the cycle. It is from amongst these follicles that the follicle destined to ovulate in a subsequent cycle will be selected (Di Zerega & Hodgen 1981, Erickson 1986).

Morphological changes

Once the primordial follicle is recruited to begin maturational changes (Fig. 16.4), the granulosa cells surrounding the oocytes start to change from squamous to cuboidal in appearance. An increase in follicular diameter occurs in the major part of growth, resulting from an increase in diameter in the primordial oocyte from 20 microns to between 60 and 100 microns. During this critical growth phase a massive synthetic activity is occurring, particularly with the synthesis of large amounts of RNA; this activity loads the oocytes' cytoplasm with essential materials for the later stages of egg maturation. During this increase in size of the oocyte an acellular glycoprotein matrix, termed the zona pellucida, is secreted by the granulosa cells and forms an envelope surrounding the oocyte. Contact with the oocyte and the granulosa cells is maintained by cytoplasmic processes which penetrate the zona and form gap junctions at the oocyte surface. Gap junctions are also formed between adjacent granulosa cells, thus providing a basis for intracellular communication. Through this network, low molecular weight substrates, some amino acids and nucleotides, can be passed to the growing oocyte. Concurrently spindle-like stromal cells come into close proximity with the basal lamina of the granulosa cells. These theca cells and cells most proximal to the basal membrane are termed theca interna cells.

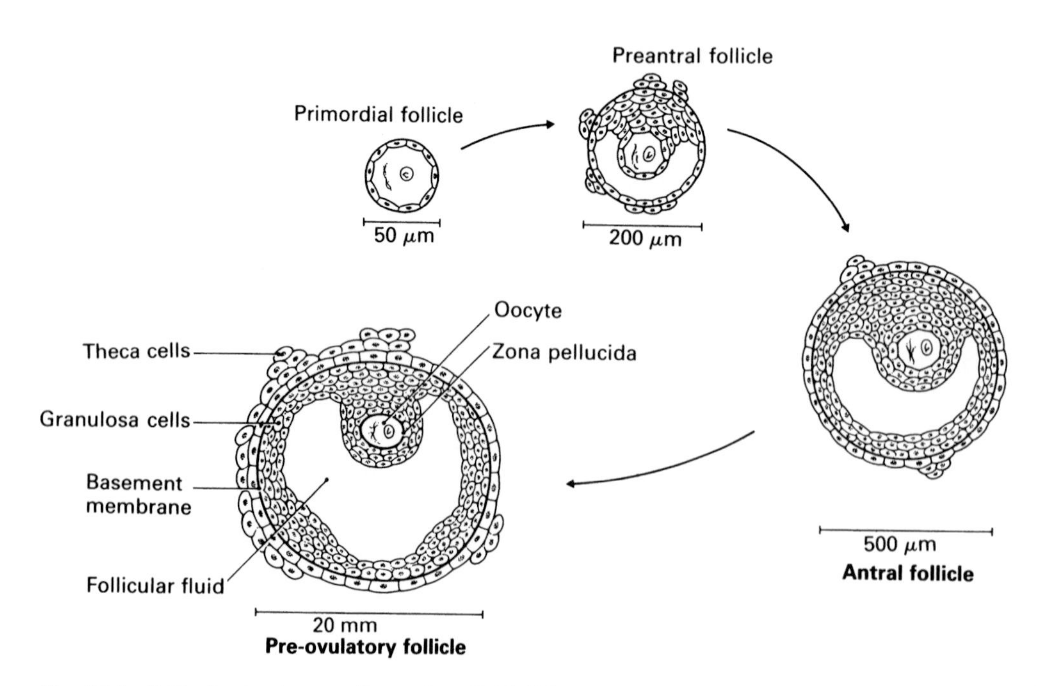

Fig. 16.4 Follicular development from primordial follicle to preovulatory stage.

Towards the end of this critical growth and reorganization phase of the follicle, cells of the granulosa layer develop receptors for oestrogen and follicle-stimulating hormone (FSH) and the theca cells develop luteinizing hormone (LH) receptors. These are essential to gain entry into the next phase of follicular development, which becomes greatly dependent upon gonadotrophin secretion patterns.

This gonadotrophin stimulation converts preantral follicles to antral follicles, and encourages further proliferation of granulosa and theca cells. However, there is little addition or increase in size of the oocyte itself, its chromosomes remain in the dictyate stage while RNA synthesis and protein production continue.

At the start of the follicular phase, the largest healthy follicles appear to be the selected follicles with diameters between 5.5 and 8 millimetres. Apart from size and granulosa cell mitotic index, there are no morphological differences apparent between the selected and other non-selected healthy follicles. Responsive follicles contain granulosa cells with high numbers of FSH receptors which lead to an increase in aromatase activity (in response to FSH stimulation). It may well also be that there is selected activation of the insulin-like growth factor 1 (IGF-1) system in the chosen follicle. As a follicle matures granulosa cells become able to bind FSH and the theca cells increase their facility to synthesize 3β-hydroxysteroid dehydrogenase which also appears in granulosa cells following ovulation.

Steroid hormone production – two-cell theory

During this second phase of growth, follicles show a steady increase in the synthesis of androgens and oestrogens. Production of these steroids is under the control of gonadotrophins; these gonadotrophins appear to facilitate effects at different locations within the follicle. Only the granulosa cells bind FSH and only the theca cells LH. LH primarily stimulates the cells of the theca interna to synthesize androgens from acetate and cholesterol. Oestrogen synthesis by these cells, is possible to only a limited degree, particularly in the early stages of growth. In contrast, the granulosa cells are unable to form androgens. However androgen supplied to the granulosa cells from the theca cells is readily aromatized to oestrogens (Fig. 16.5). Thus androgens are produced by developing follicles from the theca cells whilst oestrogens arise via two routes: primarily from thecal androgens aromatized by granulosa cells, and to a lesser degree by de novo synthesis from acetate in thecal cells.

Both the production of steroids and the increase in follicular size are interlinked. Oestrogen in conjunction with FSH plays a crucial role within the follicle towards the end of the second phase of growth. Oestrogen and FSH together stimulate the appearance of LH-binding sites in the outer layers of the granulosa cells. These LH-binding sites are crucial for the antral follicle to enter

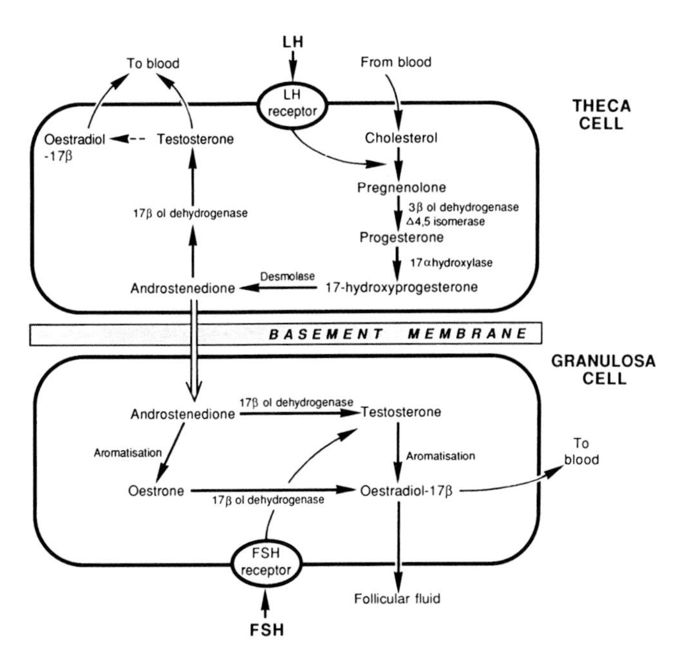

Fig. 16.5 Two-cell theory of follicular oestrogen production. LH, luteinizing hormone; FSH, follicle-stimulating hormone.

the final phase of development: the conversion to the preovulatory follicle.

Regulation of oocyte maturation

There are complex interactions between the oocyte and the follicular somatic cells (granulosa and theca cells) which are essential for the development and function of both cell types. The oocyte nucleus is called the germinal vesicle. The most obvious manifestation of reinitiation of meiosis is the disappearance or breakdown of the germinal vesicle. This appears to be initiated by the preovulatory surge of gonadotrophins. The gonadotrophins do not directly act on the oocyte since the oocyte does not contain gonadotrophin receptors. The competence to undergo germinal vesicle breakdown is a multi-step process and the apparently LH-induced germinal vesicle breakdown is by an indirect action mediated by follicular somatic cells. LH may induce a positive germinal vesicle breakdown susbtance in granulosa cells and this is passed to the oocyte. The process is thought to involve alterations in calcium ions and may also result in alterations in the level of cyclic AMP within the oocyte.

With the completion of the final stage of meiosis and extrusion of the first polar body the oocyte is then capable of undergoing fertilization.

THE FALLOPIAN TUBE

Structure of the fallopian tube

The ovulated oocyte plus attached cumulus cells is picked

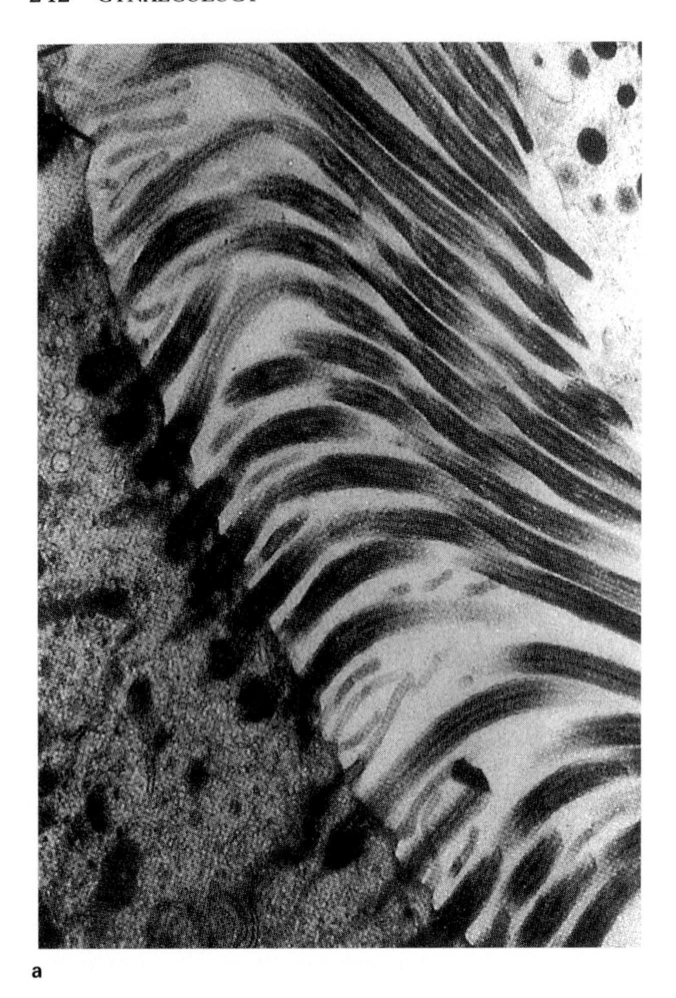

a

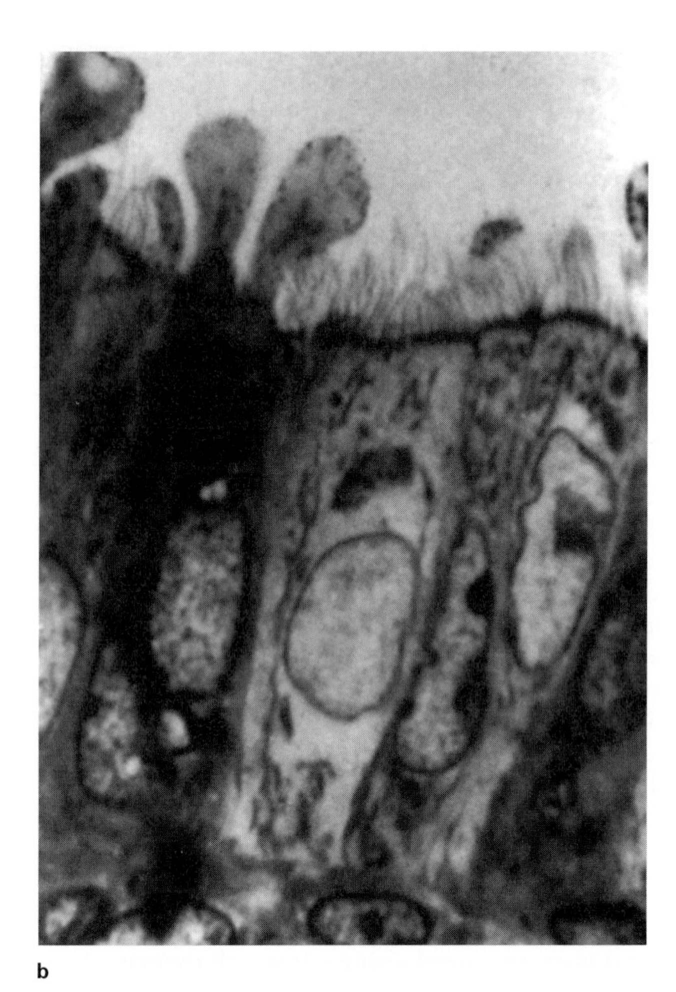

b

Fig. 16.6 Electron microscopy pictures of **a** fimbrial cilia, and **b** the postovulatory tubal mucosa demonstrating secretory and ciliated cells. From Mastroianni & Coutifaris (1990).

up from the peritoneal cavity by the fimbriated ostium of the oviduct (fallopian tube) and swept by oviductal cilia along the ampulla towards the junction with the isthmus. The fallopian tube serves a number of essential functions in the reproductive process. First, it is responsible for transferring the ovum into its lumen when discharged from the rupturing follicle. Second, it provides an environment for the ovum and spermatozoa in which fertilization can occur, and finally it transfers the fertilized, cleaving, embryo into the uterus after a timed interval of 3–4 days (Diaz et al 1980). At the distal end of the tube are the delicate finger-like projections, or fimbriae. These are lined with cilia which beat in the direction of the tubal lumen. The fimbrial cilia are capable of cyclic regeneration which occurs under the influence of oestrogen. The entire length of the fallopian tube contains cilia; ciliary beat creates a current within the tubal lumen to transport the oocyte from the peritoneal cavity into the uterus (Fig. 16.6).

Oocyte transport is affected adversely if cumulus cells are lacking and/or if oviductal cilia are malfunctional. There is no evidence that muscular activity in the tube is essential for transport of the oocyte along its course, but pharmacological doses of ovarian steroids and prostaglandin may adversely affect oocyte transport (Coutinho & Mala 1971). Oocytes and spermatozoa come together in the ampulla, and it is here that the final events of spermatozoal activation become clear as the first phase of fertilization commences.

Tubal secretory proteins in the human oviduct

During the reproductive events in the oviduct, the male gametes and the resultant embryo are antigenically different from the female host but appear not to be affected by the maternal immune system. The mechanism of protection is unknown, and at present our ability to test tubal function is limited to a simple patency test or the more recent development of visualization of the fallopian tubal mucosa with falloposcopy, the value of which is yet to be proven.

The secretory elements of the tubal mucosa are modified during a normal menstrual cycle but as ovulation approaches, under the influence of oestrogen, the secretory cells become tall and columnar and project beyond the cilial ends, discharging secretions into the tubal lumen. The production of fluid in the fallopian tube is greatest immediately before ovulation but still remains a poorly investigated area (Lippes et al 1973). What is known is that the total concentration of many constituents in oviductal fluid, is lower than in serum, and that there is selected passage of macromolecules, such that lactate is 50% and complement component C3 is 17% of serum concentrations (Oliphant et al 1978). Immunoelectrophoresis of oviduct fluid has suggested the presence of unique proteins which may be synthesized and secreted by the oviduct: a specific betaglycoprotein of molecular weight 54 000 daltons capable of binding to spermatozoa heads, PAPP-A, and placental protein 5 (PP5) have been reported (Butzow 1989). Thus the oviduct synthesizes and secretes both specific proteins and proteins of general müllerian origin. There are few results from human studies to determine the relevance or importance of these specific components to date, but further knowledge may lead to improved in vitro fertilization culture media and our increased understanding of the important role of the fallopian tubes in the process of fertilization and early development.

FERTILIZATION

Fertilization is not a single event but a continuum. The fertilization process begins when the capacitated spermatozoa come in contact with the ovum and its cellular coverings. Before a spermatazoon can achieve fertilization it must first penetrate the cellular covering of the oocyte, the cumulus oophorus, the corona radiata and the zona pellucida (Fig. 16.7). The cumulus cells are embedded in a matrix rich in hyaluronic acid and the acrosome located at the end of the spermatozoon contains the enzyme hyaluronidase. This may well be important in the dispersion of the cumulus cells. This process of dispersion is further completed by the action of the cilia of the fallopian tube.

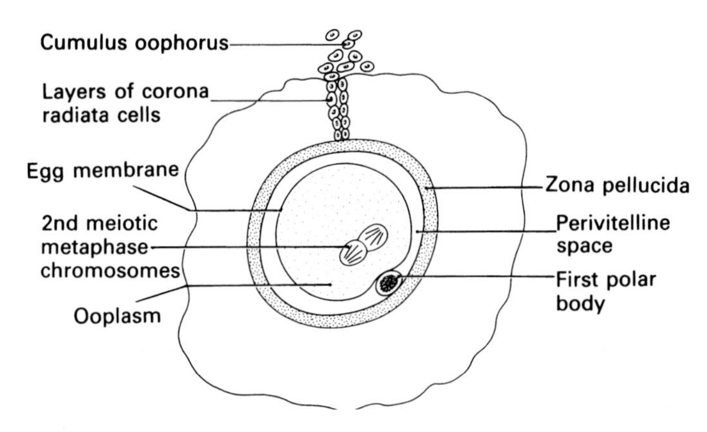

Fig. 16.7 Schematic representation of freshly ovulated oocyte.

The zona pellucida

The zona pellucida is a dense translucent protein layer immediately surrounding the oocyte. This acellular layer remains in place until implantation. It appears to have two functions. First, it contains receptors for sperm which are species-specific and second it undergoes a zonal reaction in which the zona becomes impervious to other sperm once the fertilizing sperm has penetrated the oolema, thus providing a bar to polyspermia.

Zona–sperm binding

Initial contact between sperm and oocyte is a receptor-mediated process. A number of glycoproteins have been identified in the zona, termed ZP1, ZP2, ZP3 of which ZP3 is the most abundant and expressed only in growing oocytes (Shabonowitz & O'Rand 1988).

Initial binding of sperm to the zona requires recognition on the part of the sperm of the carbohydrate component of the species-specific glycoprotein receptor molecules. Once binding is accomplished (Fig. 16.8), the acrosome reaction is triggered by the peptide chain component of the receptor glycoprotein. Formation of the enzyme–ZP3 complex therefore not only produces binding but also induces the acrosome reaction.

During the acrosome reaction, there is a release of acrosomal contents which include hyaluronidase. Granulosa cells are held together by an intracellular matrix of hyaluronic acid. This is digested by the enzyme hyaluronidase, thus allowing sperm to pass through the corona radiata cells towards the zona pellucida. Thus the sperm binds to the glycoprotein receptor on the zona, and the proteolytic proenzyme proacrosin on the exposed acrosomal membranes is activated to form acrosin. This digests through the zona, aided by the whiplash forward propulsion of the sperm. The spermatozoon, both the head and tail, is then incorporated into the cytoplasm of the oocyte, completing the penetration process. The first phase of fertilization from entry of the cumulus mass to fusion lasts between 10 and 20 min. The assumed process of fertilization lasts some 20 h or so, and results in the return

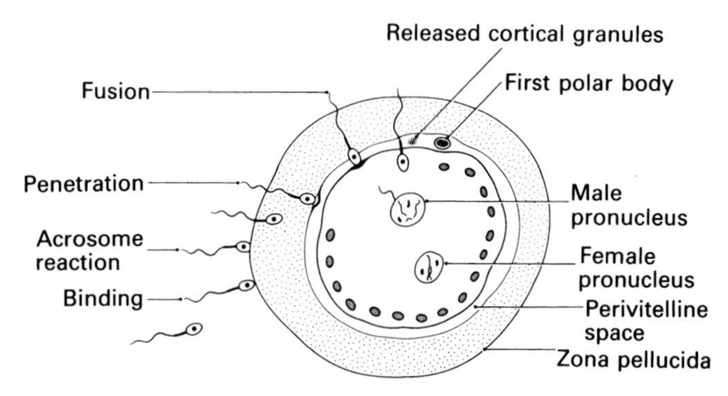

Fig. 16.8 Schematic representation of fertilization.

of the diploid genetic constitution of the embryo and the initiation of the latter's development programme.

Initiation of the block to further penetration of spermatozoa is mediated by the cortical reaction. This is a release of materials from the cortical granules, lysosome-like organelles which are found just below the egg surface (Barros & Yamagimachi 1971). The lysosomes include hydrolytic enzymes which induce the zona reaction, producing a hardening of the extracellular layers by cross-linking of proteins and inactivation of sperm receptors. As the sperm enter the perivitelline space at an angle, the postacrosomal region of the sperm makes initial contact with the vitelline membrane. First the egg membrane engulfs the sperm head, and subsequently there is fusion of the egg and sperm membranes. This fusion is mediated by specific proteins of which two have been sequenced: PH20 which is important for binding, and PH30 which is important for fusion (Blobel et al 1992). The fusion triggers the cortical reaction, metabolic activation of the oocyte and completion of meiosis, such that the second polar body is released.

Conception

Within 2 or 3 h of oocyte–sperm fusion, the second polar body has been expelled, and the remaining haploid set of female chromosomes lies in the ooplasm. When the sperm head enters the ooplasm its chromosome material is tightly packed. During the next 2–3 h these chromosomes uncoil under the influence of cytoplasm of the oocyte, and the sperm head is transformed into the male pronucleus. The male and female pronuclei increase somewhat in size and then migrate towards the centre of the egg; with the formation of the metaphase spindle, the chromosomes assume their position at its equator. This occurs 18–21 h after gamete fusion. The coming together of the gametic chromosomes, syngamy, is the final phase of fertilization. Immediately anaphase and telophase are completed, the cleavage furrow forms and the one-cell zygote becomes a two-cell embryo.

IMPLANTATION

Changes in the endometrium

The endometrium has undergone extensive proliferation under the influence of oestrogen in the days prior to ovulation. Its cells exhibit marked mitotic activity. Under the combined influence of oestrogen and progesterone following ovulation, with the increasing quantities of these hormones secreted by the corpus luteum, the endometrial stroma and glands change rapidly. The glands display a secretory pattern and the products of their secretion are discharged into the uterine lumen (for further details, see Ch. 28).

The differentiation of endometrium prior to implantation is controlled by a large variety of growth factor interactions in which epidermal growth factor (EGF) and insulin like growth factor-1 (IGF-1) are thought to be important. Receptors for both of these are expressed in the endometrium and regulated by receptor number or specific binding proteins throughout the menstrual cycle. In vitro progesterone downregulates IGF-1 binding sites in intact stromal cell culture layers. In the uterus, messages of the oestrogenic signal between the different cellular compartments have been postulated. A combination of EGF and progesterone seems necessary to fully decidualize endometrial stromal cells, thus modulating the secretion of IGF-binding proteins (Guidice et al 1992).

The implantation process

The embryo remains in the fallopian tube, the site of fertilization, for approximately 3–4 days (Diaz et al 1980). It is suspended in the tubal fluid and continues to develop into the morula. It is then transferred through the isthmus of the tube into the uterine cavity. This transfer is facilitated by the change in endocrine environment of the early luteal phase. Within the uterine cavity the embryo establishes nutritional and physical contact with the maternal tissue at the site of implantation (Fig. 16.9).

After hatching and attachment the penetration process starts.

Human implantation occurs during a period of endometrial change, preceded by intense tissue remodelling by growth factors such as cytokines and proteases, induced by embryo–maternal interactions and endocrine events. Implantation involves extensive modification of the embryo and the endometrium. This is induced by contacts between the embryo and uterus, and by extracellular signals which affect both blastocyst and uterine epithelium (For review see Denker 1983, Glasser 1986). These include:

1. the binding of invading cells to glycoproteins within the basement membranes (laminin, fibronectin) through their specific receptors (integrins);
2. activation of proteases and pericellular degregation of matrix components (matrix metalloproteinases);
3. migration of the cells into the matrix, i.e. cells progressing through the endometrial epithelium towards basement membrane, recognizing laminin and collagen type IV through their integrins.

These processes activate the expression of the gene for gelatinases A and B, which degregate the basement membrane. This allows the cytotrophoblastic cells to migrate through the basement membrane and make contact in the extracellular matrix through their fibronectin receptors. During the invasion process, the collagenolytic activity of cytotrophoblast is modulated by endometrial

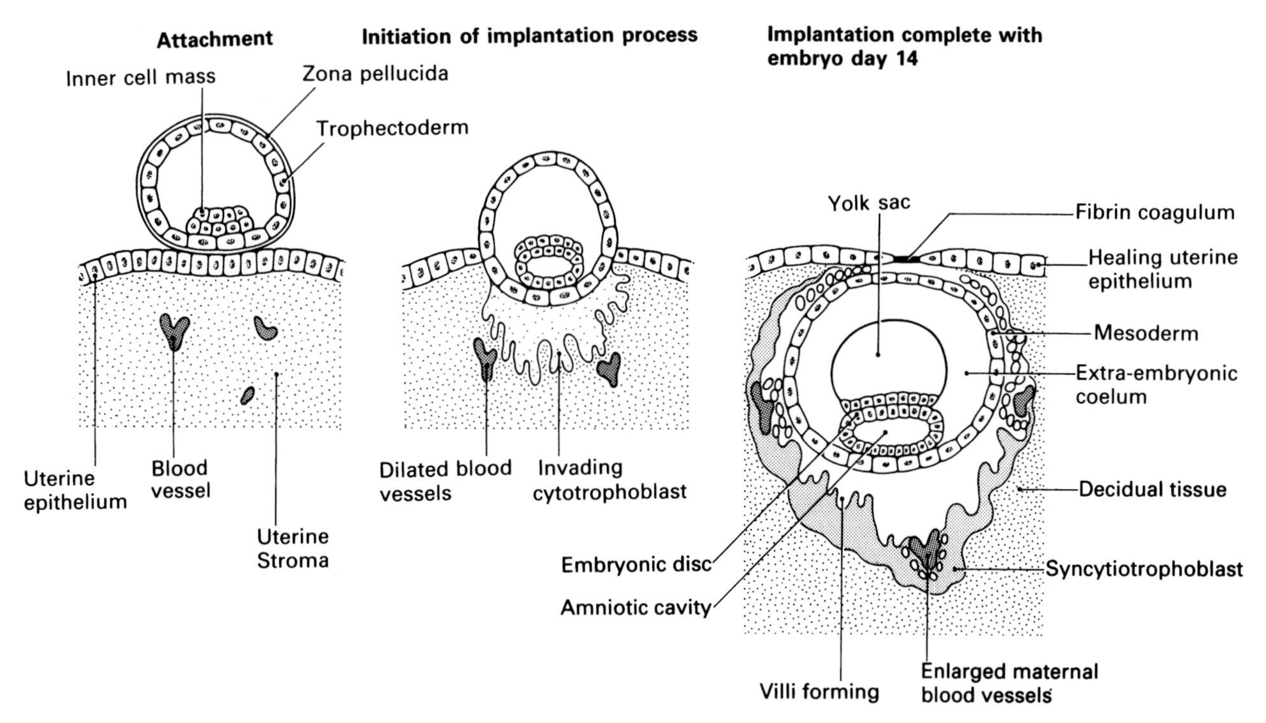

Fig. 16.9 Stages of implantation.

factors such as cytokines that inhibit trophoblastic proteolytic activity, thus controlling the depth of invasion (Liotta et al 1984). Within 3–5 days of attachment, the whole embryo is completely embedded within the uterine epithelium in the endometrial stroma. By 14–21 days after fertilization, the trophoblastic structure at the periphery of the blast cells resembles the villi of the mature placenta and the area of the inner cell mass has started to organize itself into the embryo proper.

The details of the further development undergone by the embryo are beyond the scope of this book, and readers are referred to relevant chapters in the textbook of *Obstetrics* (Chamberlain 1995).

KEY POINTS

1. The process of fertilization and implantation is highly complex. It entails the completion and coordination of a number of highly organized events which involve the gametes, the male and female genital tracts and the various components of the endocrine system.
2. A mature spermatozoon contains the haploid number of chromosomes. It possesses a head which includes the acrosome, a midpiece that contains the mitochondria, the residual body and a tail which is essential for propulsion.
3. Abnormally developed spermatozoa comprise up to 40% of the total contained in a fertile semen sample.
4. During its passage through the vasa efferentia and the epididymis, the spermatozoon gains the capability of movement and the potential to fertilize an oocyte.
5. Following entry into and storage within the cervical crypts, the intermittent release of sperm (over a period of up to 72 h after coitus) is dependent on uterine contraction and intrinsic sperm motility.
6. In order to gain full ability to fertilize, the spermatozoon undergoes the processes of capacitation and activation. The latter occurs within the fallopian tube and consists of three components: acrosome reaction, binding to the zona pellucida and attainment of hyperactivated motility.
7. The number of oocytes a woman possesses is predetermined by the number of oogonia entering into the first meiotic division which is arrested in the diplotene stage, during fetal life.
8. Following recruitment to the pool of maturing follicles, the primordial oocyte undergoes development that includes acquisition of the acellular zona pellucida which is secreted by the granulosa cells.
9. The theca cells, with specific receptors for LH, synthesize androgens in response to LH stimulation. Oestrogen synthesis is brought on by the availability of androgens to the granulosa cells which, in response to FSH stimulation, increase their aromatase activity responsible for the conversion of androgen to oestrogen. This is the 'two-cell two-gonadotrophin' hypothesis.
10. The preovulatory surge of gonadotrophins induces the breakdown of the germinal vesicle which is followed by the completion of the final stage of meiosis, such that the oocyte is capable of undergoing fertilization.

11. The fallopian tube serves as a vessel where fertilization occurs and provides an appropriate environment for the cleaving embryo prior to its transfer into the uterus 3–4 days later.
12. Hyaluronidase released from the acrosome enables the sperm to penetrate the cumulus oophorus and the corona radiata, which are held together by an intercellular matrix of hyaluronic acid.
13. Binding of a single sperm to the zona pellucida, via a species-specific receptor, leads to the zonal cortical reaction. This reaction results in hardening of the extracellular layers and inactivation of sperm receptors, thus preventing polyspermia.
14. Conception is completed when syngamy takes place some 18–21 h after gamete fusion, resulting in the return of the diploid genetic constitution of the embryo.
15. The differentiation of the endometrium, prior to implantation of the embryo, is governed by oestrogen and progesterone as well as a number of growth factors including EGF and IGF-1.
16. Implantation is induced by contacts between the embryo and the endometrium, and modified by various factors including cytokines, integrins and proteases.

REFERENCES

Barros C, Yamagimachi R 1971 Induction of zona reaction in golden hamster eggs by cortical granule material. Nature 233: 2368

Blobel C P, Wolfsberg T G, Turck C W, Myles D G, Primakoff P, White J M 1992 A potential fusion peptide and an integrin ligand domain in a protein active in sperm–egg fusion. Nature 356: 248

Butzow R 1989 The human fallopian tube contains placental protein 5. Human Reproduction 1: 17–20

Chamberlain G (ed.) 1995 Turnbull's Obstetrics, 2nd edn. Churchill Livingstone, New York

Coutinho E M, Mala H S 1971 The contractile response of the human uterus, fallopian tubes and ovary to prostaglandins in vivo. Fertility and Sterility 22: 539–543

Denker H W 1983 Basic aspects of ova implantation. Obstetrical and Gynaecological Annual Reviews 12: 15–42

Diaz S, Ortiz M E, Crozatto H B 1980 Studies on the duration of ovum transport by the human oviduct. The time interval between the luteinizing hormone peak and recovery of ova by transcervical flushing of the uterus in normal women. American Journal of Obstetrics and Gynecology 137: 116

Di Zerega G S, Hodgen G D 1981 Folliculogenesis in the primate ovarian cycle. Endocrine Reviews 2: 27

Erickson G F 1986 An analysis of follicle development in ovum maturation. Seminars in Reproductive Endocrinology 4: 233–254

Glasser S R 1986 Current concepts of implantation and decidualization. In: Hoszar G (ed) The physiology and biochemistry of the uterus in pregnancy and labor. CRC Press, Boca Raton, Florida

Guidice L C, Dsupin B A, Irwin J C 1992 Steroid and peptide regulation of insulin-like growth factor binding proteins secreted by human endometrial stromal cells is dependent on stromal differentiation. Journal of Clinical Endocrinology and Metabolism 75: 1235–1241

Harper N J K 1988 Gamete and zygote transport. In: Knobil E, Neill J (eds) The physiology of reproduction. Raven Press, New York, pp 103–134

Liotta L A, Rao C N, Terranova V P, Barksy S, Thorgeirsson U 1984 Tumour cell attachment and degradation of basement membrane. In: Nicholson G L, Milas L (eds) Cancer invasion and metastasis, biologic and therapeutic aspects. New York, Raven Press, pp 168–176

Lippes J, Enders R G, Pragay D A, Bartholomew W R 1973 The collection and analysis of human fallopian tube fluid. Contraception 5: 85–93

Mastroianni L, Coutifaris C (eds) 1990 Reproductive physiology, vol I. Parthenon, Carnforth

Oliphant G, Bowling A, Eng L A, Keen S 1978 The permeability of the rabbit oviduct to proteins present in the serum. Biology of Reproduction 18: 516–520

Shabonowitz R B, O'Rand M G 1988 Characterisation of the human zona pellucida from fertilized and unfertilized eggs. Journal of Reproductive Medicine 82: 151–161

Wang C, Baker H W G, Jennings M G, Burger H G, Lutjen P 1985 Interaction between human cervical mucus and sperm surface antibodies. Fertility and Sterility 44: 484–488

17

Investigation of the infertile couple

N. McClure W. Thompson

INTRODUCTION

This chapter is aimed at presenting a simple account of the investigation of the infertile couple. Emphasis is placed on clinical practice through an ordered scheme of basic investigations. This is supported by descriptions of more complex procedures of which the practising gynaecologist should be aware though they are only required occasionally. It is more important to perform relevant tests in their proper order and at the correct time, than to subject the couple to a large range of investigations, many of which bear little relevance to the day-to-day management of the couple's infertility.

Using life table analysis, it has been calculated that the chances of conception for a given couple having regular, unprotected intercourse are 80% after 12 and 90% after 18 months (Cooke et al 1981). Based on these figures, it is usual to wait for at least 1 year of frequent, unprotected intercourse in the presence of regular menstruation, before beginning investigations for infertility. The timescale and range of investigation should be dictated by the couple. Medically, it should be possible to complete a programme of basic tests within 6 months. However, it would be inappropriate to proceed with laparoscopy to evaluate tubal status if a significant, uncorrected male factor or a disorder of ovulation exists. Throughout the work-up a clear explanation of the indication and nature of the tests must be given to both partners. This is facilitated if they are seen together in dedicated infertility clinics. Here adequate time is available for counselling, and facilities exist to permit a proper assessment of the situation.

The causes of infertility and their relative frequency are shown in Figure 17.1. Unexplained infertility is an ill-defined entity. To some extent its frequency will depend on the extent and complexity of investigations available to a particular clinic. This explains, in part, the variation from 6 to 60% in the reported incidence of this condition (Templeton & Penney 1982).

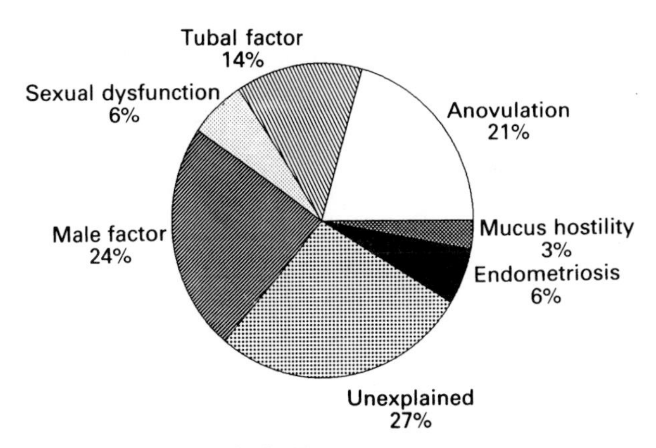

Fig. 17.1 The causes of infertility.

The approach to the infertile couple should begin with a detailed medical, sexual and social history followed by physical examination of both partners. The sequence of investigations should be ordered so that the simplest, least invasive and most productive tests are completed first. Therefore, at the initial consultation, semen analysis and a test of ovulation are arranged. At the second consultation the results are reviewed with the couple. If the results are normal and the couple so wish, they should then proceed to assessment of tubal patency and antisperm antibody status.

HISTORY AND EXAMINATION

The female history

There are three main disorders of female fertility which may be symptomatic: anovulation, tubal disease and endometriosis. However, it is essential first to establish accurately the duration of infertility. Therefore, the couple should be asked about the use of contraception and about incidents of separation through, for example, work, social activities or marital breakdown. A detailed sexual history is also vital. What is the frequency of coitus? Is dyspareunia a significant factor? Do both partners achieve orgasm? Is sexual intercourse limited to the so-called 'best time' of the month and, if so, how is this determined?

Abnormalities of ovulation are likely if the menstrual cycle is irregular. Mittelschmerz and a mid-cycle 'cascade' of cervical mucus both suggest ovulation. If the periods are irregular, historical factors associated with polycystic ovarian syndrome (acne, oily skin, hirsutism); hyperprolactinaemia (galactorrhoea); hypothalamic–pituitary axis failure (excessive weight loss or an aggressive training schedule, anorexia or bulimia nervosa), or with thyroid dysfunction may be present.

Tubal disease is the commonest cause of secondary infertility. Nevertheless, all patients should be asked about pelvic inflammatory disease, vaginal discharge and deep dyspareunia. With parous patients a history of puerperal sepsis is relevant. A general medical history must also be taken; a ruptured appendix, for instance, may result in tubal damage.

Endometriosis can be asymptomatic even when quite advanced. However, it may present with secondary (worsening) dysmenorrhoea or deep dyspareunia.

The points to be elicited in the history are summarized in Table 17.1.

The male history

The male should be asked about episodes of testicular pain, swelling, or trauma and about any history of testicular or groin surgery, including treatment of maldescent of the testes. Severe head injury, meningitis and encephalitis can affect the function of the hypothalamic–pituitary axis. Chronic general illnesses may be associated with infertility; cystic fibrosis, for example, is associated with absence of the vas deferens, whilst sulphasalazine, given for the treatment of Crohn's disease, adversely affects seminal parameters. An acute pyrexial illness can alter sperm counts for several weeks. There is evidence to suggest that the testes function most efficiently if their temperature is approximately 1 degree below normal body temperature. Therefore, jobs which are sedentary or the use of tight-fitting underwear may also be relevant. Excessive use of tobacco, alcohol or cannabis can lower sperm counts. Chronic exposure to various noxious substances, possibly at work, such as aniline dyes may also be significant.

The points to be elicited in the history are summarized in Table 17.2.

Examination

Once the history is taken both partners should be examined. In the female, height and weight are recorded and the body mass index (kg/m^2) calculated. Breasts are checked for development and secondary sexual characteristics are noted. Abdominal palpation and a pelvic examination should check for the gross normality of the pelvic organs. Tenderness or nodularity of the uterosacral ligaments often indicates endometriosis. Vaginal ultrasound is often performed at this stage to exclude the presence of ovarian cysts, especially if endometriosis is suspected.

In the male, weight and general appearance are recorded. Abdominal palpation is followed by examination of the external genitalia. The penis is inspected for hypospadias, and the testes are assessed for size (with reference

Table 17.1 Investigation of infertility: the female history

Sexual dysfunction	Dyspareunia and vaginismus Coital frequency Orgasm
Endocrine	Menstrual pattern Hirsutism/acne/oily skin Weight changes and eating disorders Galactorrhoea Thyroid symptoms
Uterine and tubal	Pelvic/abdominal surgery Pelvic infection/sexually transmitted diseases Pelvic pain Dysmenorrhoea
Cervical factor	Mucus secretion (ovulation cascade) Conization/cautery Incompetence
Previous obstetric history	Pregnancy loss Puerperal sepsis
Contraception	Hormonal Intrauterine contraceptive device

Table 17.2 Investigation of infertility: the male history

Occupation	Sedentary Toxin/irradiation
Illnesses/operations	Febrile conditions Bladder neck surgery Cryptorchidism
Infection	Venereal Orchitis/epididymitis Tuberculosis
Drugs	Sulphasalazine Chemotherapy Antimicrobials Antihypertensives Alcohol/nicotine/cannabis
Sexual function	Coital frequency Erection/orgasm Ejaculation
Trauma/stress	

to an orchidometer) and consistency. The vasa deferentia are checked, (characteristically they feel like 'whipcord'), and varicoceles and inguinal herniae excluded with the patient standing, performing a Valsalva manoeuvre. If the presence of varicocele is questioned, Doppler or ultrasound examination may be of help. Finally, rectal examination should be performed for prostatic enlargement or tenderness which might indicate prostatitis.

INVESTIGATION OF MALE FACTORS

The standard basic investigation of male infertility is the semen analysis. What constitutes a normal semen analysis remains controversial although the World Health Organization (WHO) criteria are now broadly accepted (WHO 1992). There can be considerable within- and between-laboratory variation in the analysis of the same semen sample. Therefore, it is essential that semen laboratories are subject to within- and between-laboratory quality control. Such a scheme has recently been implemented in the UK under the auspices of the British Andrology Society.

Computer-aided sperm analysis has been extensively researched. However, the presence of contaminating cells and debris in the sample can confuse the computer. Therefore, whilst counts appear to be reasonably reproducible, the analysis of morphology is unsatisfactory (Boyers et al 1989). By contrast, a number of new motility parameters have been developed including the curvilinear velocity, the straight-line velocity, and the average path velocity (Fig. 17.2). Agreement between different laboratories in the analysis of these parameters is good (Davis et al 1992), but their relationship with fertility in vivo is unknown. However, a clear association has been demonstrated between good sperm progression and the ability of sperm to penetrate cervical mucus (Mortimer et al 1986), and between good sperm progression and zona-free hamster egg penetration (Aitken et al 1985).

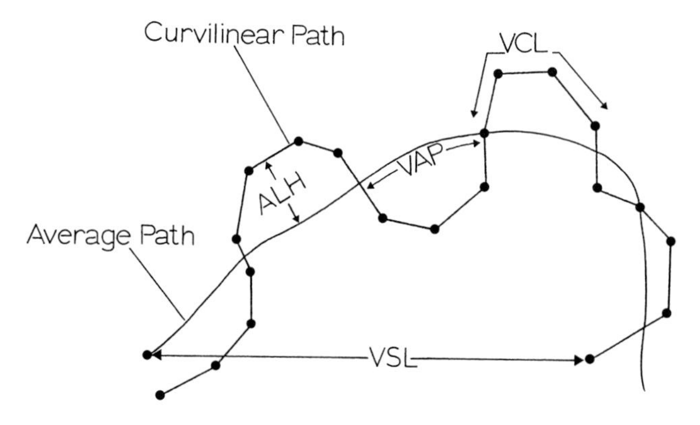

Fig. 17.2 Terminology of measurements of sperm motility in computer-assisted semen analysis: ALH, amplitude of lateral head displacement; VAP, average path velocity; VCL, curvilinear velocity; VSL, straight-line velocity (Reproduced with permission Cambridge University Press from WHO, 1992.)

In vitro fertilization has allowed a crude assessment of fertilization potential. In an attempt to rationalize and standardize the investigation of these problems, tests for the attachment and penetration by sperm for both the zona pellucida and the oolemma have been developed. However, these tests are only relevant where fertilization has failed to occur during in vitro fertilization with adequate, normal sperm.

Routine semen analysis

All semen samples should be obtained by masturbation into a clean, wide-mouthed non-toxic plastic container. It is preferable to obtain the sample within the hospital and a special room should be identified for this. However, some patients will be unable to produce a sample under this 'pressure'. They should be allowed to masturbate at home, but should be given written and verbal instructions about the importance of delivering the sample at body temperature and within 1 h of collection. For some masturbation is offensive. Non-toxic condoms exist and the couple can be supplied with these in order to obtain the sample during coitus. Coitus interruptus is not recommended as the first part of the ejaculate may well be lost. This part usually contains the greatest density of sperm.

Different clinics recommend different intervals of abstinence prior to the production of semen for analysis. It is our practice to advise the male to have ejaculated at least once within the week prior to the test but not within the previous 2 days. It is perhaps more relevant to obtain a history of recent ejaculation at the time of the test. Because of the known variability in semen quality from the same individual, at least two specimens should be examined during the course of the infertility investigations.

The basic semen analysis should provide the information given in Table 17.3, as well as an analysis of the presence of antisperm antibodies. This can be done using either the mixed antiglobulin reaction test (MAR test) or, more usually now, the Immunobead test (see below).

Semen liquefaction and viscosity

Human semen forms a gel-like clot soon after ejaculation due to a fibrinogen-like substrate from the seminal vesicles. Liquefaction, which is necessary for microscopic examination, usually occurs within 30 min and depends on

Table 17.3 Routine semen analysis

Volume	2–6 ml
Liquefaction	Complete in 30 min
Count	20 million/ml or more
Motility	60% (forward progressive)
Morphology	70% or more normal forms

the liquefying enzyme, vesiculase. This is produced by the prostate gland. Whilst liquefaction is awaited, the semen sample should be stored at 37°C. Analysis should be performed as soon as possible after this.

A complete absence of the coagulum indicates an obstruction of the ejaculatory duct or congenital absence of the seminal vesicles.

The relevance of increased viscosity is unclear. It may be associated with chronic infection in the accessory glands. Sperm from hyperviscid semen usually show no difficulty in entering cervical mucus at microscopy. Further, the viscosity of the ejaculate may vary considerably between different patients and also between samples from the same individual. If the specimen of semen is excessively viscid it should be repeatedly forced through a narrow gauge hypodermic needle (no. 19) prior to microscopic examination.

A prolonged liquefaction time (more than 1–2 h) can be caused by a deficiency of vesiculase from reduced prostatic secretion. This situation, particularly if found in association with a negative postcoital test, may be a cause of infertility. Several methods can be used to liquefy the ejaculate prior to microscopic examination, for example the addition of bromelin 1 g/l, plasmin 0.35–0.50 casein units/ml or chymotrypsin 150 USP/ml.

Semen volume

The volume of the ejaculate should be measured either with a graduated cylinder or by aspirating the whole sample into a pipette. The average range is 2–5 ml. The commonest cause of low volume is spillage of the sample either at production or during transport. This should be excluded by questioning the patient and the test repeated.

A persistently low semen volume (<0.5 ml) may be due to an obstruction of the ejaculatory ducts or congenital absence of the seminal vesicles. In both cases, the low volumes are associated with reduced seminal plasma fructose levels. Absence of ejaculatory fluid, but with the sensation of orgasm, may suggest a diagnosis of retrograde ejaculation and such men will sometimes have noted a 'cloudy' urine after coitus. To confirm this diagnosis a urine sample is obtained as soon as possible after masturbation and centrifuged for 10 min at 3000 r.p.m. The residue is then resuspended in a small volume of buffer and examined for the presence of motile sperm.

An abnormally large semen volume (greater than 6 ml) may be associated with a reduced sperm concentration but this is not usually a problem.

Semen pH

A drop of semen is spread over litmus paper and the colour change read from the scale on the litmus paper dispenser. If pH is <7.0, with azoospermia, there may be dysgenesis of the vas deferens, epididymis or seminal vesicles.

Sperm count and concentration

The haemocytometer (improved Neubauer) counting chamber is the most frequently used method of assessment of sperm concentration (Fig. 17.3). The ejaculate is diluted (usually 20-fold) with a spermicidal solution and both chambers are loaded with the sample. After counting, if there is a discrepancy of >10% between the two chambers the sample should be remixed and assessed again.

Other techniques for counting sperm include the Makler chamber (Makler 1980) or a similar device such as the Howell Fertility Counting Chamber. These chambers have a depth of 10 μm and permit direct estimation of the sperm concentration without dilution. However, they are less accurate than the Neubauer chamber.

Oligozoospermia. The World Health Organization defines oligozoospermia as a sperm concentration <20 million per ml. However, for many centres 10 million per ml is an acceptable figure. It is obvious that a high count of dead sperm is of little value whilst a low count of highly progressively motile sperm may result in normal fertility. Various motility parameters have been produced to allow for this (see section on motility below).

Azoospermia. If two semen analyses show azoospermia, blood should be taken for follicle-stimulating hormone (FSH) and testosterone estimation. A high serum

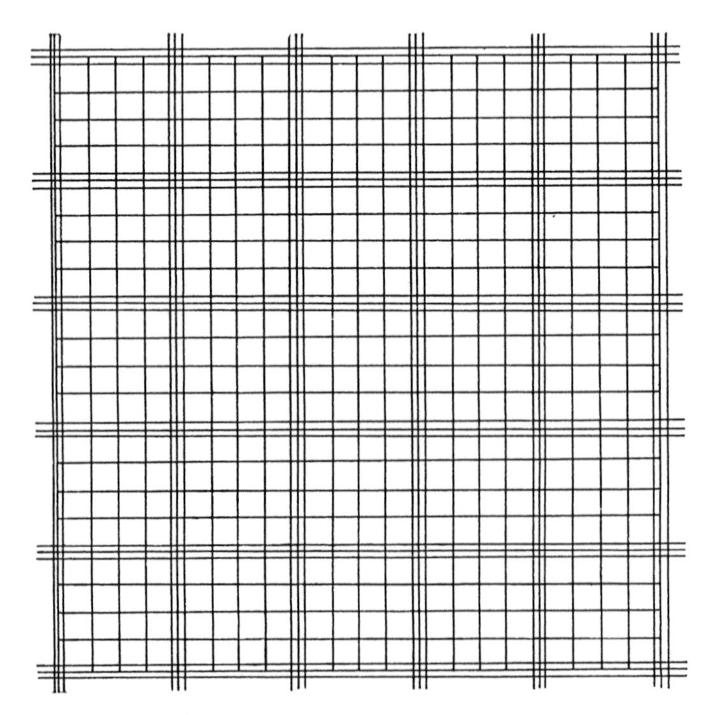

Fig. 17.3 Neubauer haemocytometer grid with 25 large squares each containing 16 small squares.

FSH with a normal or low testosterone confirms testicular failure and, usually, is not remediable. By contrast, azoospermia in the presence of testes of normal size and consistency and with a normal serum FSH level may indicate an obstructive lesion. A testicular biopsy should be performed to determine whether normal sperm maturation is occurring. Recently a technique has been described for performing this procedure under local anaesthetic (Mallidis & Baker 1994). With the advent of intracytoplasmic injection of sperm (ICSI) the outlook for patients with obstructive azoospermia has been transformed. Previously, their only option was surgery, for example to connect the vas with the epididymis, but in practice success was limited. Early reports suggest that with ICSI success rates promise to be comparable to those for men with severe oligospermia (Tournaye et al 1994).

In a few cases FSH levels are low (hypogonadotrophic hypogonadism). Here the outlook is more optimistic and fertility can be restored in more than 50% of cases by the use of exogenous gonadotrophins, typically human chorionic gonadotrophin (Finkel et al 1985).

Azoospermia in association with eunuchoid features suggests a diagnosis of Klinefelter's syndrome. This can be confirmed by chromosomal analysis.

Sperm morphology

At its worst morphology is analyzed by direct visualization of the sperm. To assess morphology properly semen should be smeared onto a slide, air-dried and stained. A variety of stains exists. The Giemsa stain is better for leucocyte than sperm morphology. The Papanicolaou is the most commonly used stain and in its modified form gives good definition to the acrosomal and postacrosomal regions of the head, the midpiece and the tail. The Bryan–Leishman stain is useful for differentiating immature sperm cells from leucocytes. However, the Shorr stain is the simplest to perform and gives good overall definition of sperm morphology.

The World Health Organization manual (1992) recommends that at least 100 and preferably 200 sperm are examined. Each one is assessed for normality of its head, neck and midpiece and tail, and for the presence of cytoplasmic droplets of more than one-third the area of a normal sperm head. Using these strict criteria at least 30% of all sperm should be of normal morphology.

Debilitating illnesses, including viral and bacterial infections, will produce an increase in the number of abnormal sperms as will certain drugs, such as nitroferans. In a long-term follow-up of patients, Bostofte et al (1982) have shown a clear relationship between a high number of abnormal sperm and reduced fertility. The increase in abnormal sperm cells usually starts occurring within 30 days of an acute illness and may be present for up to 2–3 months, even though the clinical condition of the patient has markedly improved. The presence of a large number of sperm containing cytoplasmic droplets may suggest incomplete maturation and thus epididymal pathology. Scanning and transmission electron microscopy may also be employed to identify specific structural abnormalities of the sperm, but routine evaluation of the ultrastructure is neither practical nor necessary.

Table 17.4 Sperm progression ratings

0	None = absence of forward progression
1	Poor = weak or sluggish forward progression
2	Moderate = definite forward progression
3	Good = good forward progression
4	Excellent = vigorous, rapid forward progression

Sperm motility

Traditionally motility has been expressed as the percentage of moving sperm in the sample with an accepted normal value of at least 60% at 1 h. However, a more detailed analysis of the percentages showing different degrees of forward progression is now thought to be of value. Using the scoring system in Table 17.4, a motility index can be calculated using the equation from Pandaya et al (1986):

$$\text{Motility index} = (\%\,\text{progressive} \times \text{progression ratings} \times 2.5) + \%\text{non-progressive}$$

Poor motility, particularly in the presence of normal sperm numbers, suggests that the sample may have become cold and a repeat specimen should be analyzed. Other causes of reduced motility include seminal infection and sperm autoantibodies. Most often, however, it is merely one aspect of poor semen quality, together with reduced count and increased numbers of abnormal sperm.

If sperm motility is very poor, the question may arise as to whether there is an intrinsic defect in sperm movement (as in Kartagener's syndrome) or whether the sperm are all dead. Therefore, tests for sperm vitality may be applied. These include the eosin Y (or eosin–nigrosin) test where sperm with physically intact membranes appear bluish-white, whilst dead sperm are coloured reddish-yellow. Alternatively, the H33258 fluorochrome test or the hypo-osmotic swelling tests may be used. A sample is considered abnormal if more than 50% of the sperm stain 'dead'.

The hypo-osmotic swelling test has been shown to be a reasonable predictor of semen fertilizing capacity. However, its correlation with the zona-free hamster egg penetration test (Van der Ven et al 1986) has not been confirmed.

Sperm aggregation and agglutination

Aggregation refers specifically to the situation where

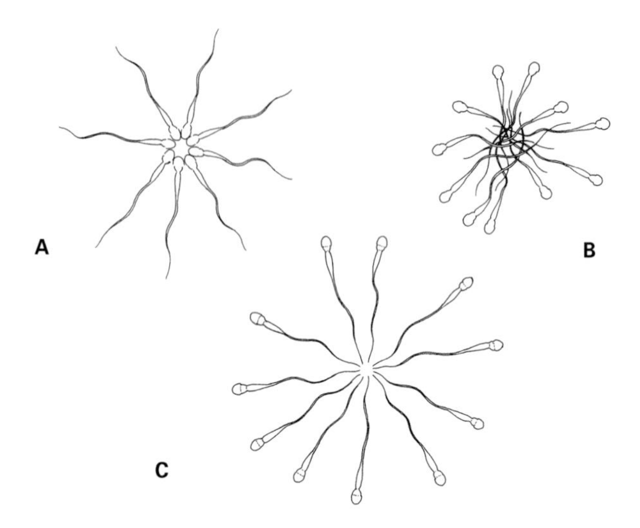

Fig. 17.4 Human sperm agglutination patterns: **A** head-to-head; **B** tail-to-tail; **C** tail tip-to-tail tip.

sperm are clumped with other particulate debris or cells. Often, in normal samples there are small aggregates, however, large aggregates are abnormal. Agglutination refers to the sticking together of sperm by antibodies. The pattern should be recorded: head-to-head, midpiece-to-midpiece, tail-to-tail or tail tip-to-tail tip. Sometimes the patterns are mixed. Agglutination, whilst indicating the presence of antisperm antibodies, is not confirmatory for antibodies and further tests are required (Fig. 17.4).

Antisperm antibodies

Sperm antibodies are typically IgA or IgG in type. Depending on the individual laboratory's set-up, it may be that these tests are reserved for samples exhibiting marked agglutination or for those couples with an abnormal cervical mucus–sperm interaction. Alternatively, some laboratories offer these tests on all semen samples. The two most commonly used tests, as mentioned above, are the immunobead and the MAR test (Fig. 17.5). However, results from these two tests do not always agree (Hellstrom et al 1989). Immunobeads are polyacrylamide spheres with covalently bound rabbit antihuman immunoglobulins directed against IgG, IgA and IgM. Sperm are washed, resuspended and mixed with the beads. If the sperm has antibodies on its membrane, the immunobeads will bind to it. If more than 20% of sperm show binding the test is positive, although usually 50% of sperm should show binding before the test is thought clinically significant as only at this level of binding is cervical mucus penetration impeded (Ayvaliotis et al 1985). Immunobead binding to the tail tip is irrelevant.

The MAR test can be performed either by mixing washed sperm with sheep red blood cells or with latex particles coated with human IgG. Antihuman IgG antiserum is then added. If the particles or red blood cells

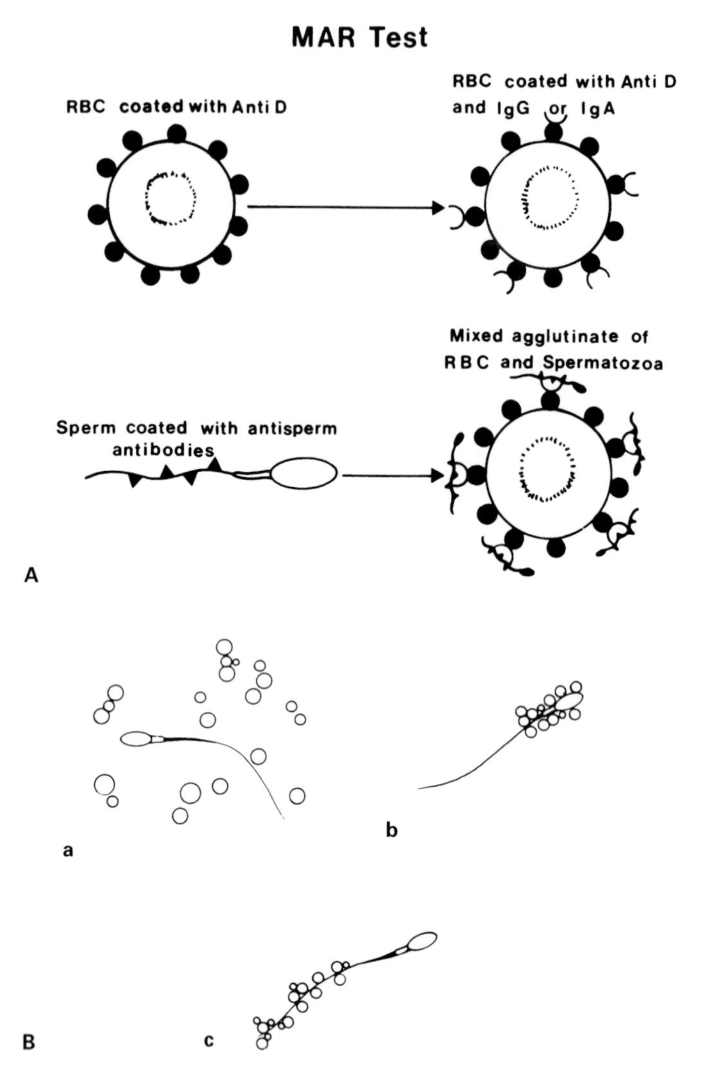

Fig. 17.5 **A** The mixed antiglobulin reaction (MAR) test. Red blood cells (RBC), coated with IgA or sensitized with IgG, are mixed with a non-specific anti-IgA or an anti-IgG and then incubated with sperm under test. Sperm with antisperm antibodies will adhere to the red blood cells. **B** The immunobead test: **a** negative test; **b** and **c** positive tests showing beads attached to sperm head and tail, respectively.

agglutinate with more than 50% of the sperm, IgG antisperm antibodies are said to be present in clinically significant amounts. The major disadvantages of this test are that it requires a ready supply of sensitized sheep erythrocytes and that it is only sensitive to the IgG class of antibody. The immunobead test has the additional advantage of being able to detect the presence of antisperm antibodies in serum or in cervical mucus if used as an indirect test.

Further tests of sperm function

If the routine semen analysis is normal it is not usually necessary to proceed with any further investigation of sperm function. However, if it is not, then some of the additional tests listed in this section may be of use.

Semen culture

Pyospermia is not necessarily an indicator of infection of the accessory glands. However, it has been associated with significant adverse effects on seminal parameters (Wolff et al 1990). Furthermore, infection of the accessory glands is often asymptomatic. In the prostate, infection may cause enlargement which in turn may produce an obstructive oligo- or azospermia. In these cases the semen volume will be slightly lowered and the zinc content will be significantly decreased. Infection of the seminal vesicles results in a substantial reduction in ejaculate volume and a low seminal fructose concentration. Therefore, both fructose and zinc content should be measured. If culture of semen is indicated, the sample should be collected aseptically after the patient has urinated and washed both hands and penis in soap and water. Chlamydia cannot be cultured from semen as it is toxic to the cell line used to culture this organism. Thus, urethral swabs should be used. Where epididymitis is suspected, L-carnitine has been used as a specific marker of epididymal function. However, this has been replaced by the measurement of the neutral isoform of alpha-glucosidase.

Tests of fertilization potential

With the introduction of in vitro fertilization techniques for the treatment of infertility, it has become obvious that sperm from some infertile couples may not have the ability to fertilize oocytes. Therefore, several tests have been developed to investigate this further. For fertilization to occur, the sperm first undergoes capacitation. This process results from a variety of influences including the release of the sperm from the inhibition of the seminal plasma and exposure to the various endocrine and anatomical environments of the female reproductive tract. Once capacitated the sperm is seen in a state of hyperactivation, that is its movement becomes highly vigorous but non-progressive. This hyperactivation appears to be necessary for both penetration of the cumulus cells and for the acrosome reaction. Previously it was thought that the acrosome reaction was essential for penetration of the cumulus. It would now appear that the acrosome reaction occurs only once the sperm has come in contact with the zona pellucida. Having passed through the zona the sperm then fuses with the oolemma, is absorbed into the oocyte, and fertilization occurs.

The zona-free hamster egg penetration test is a measure of the adsorption of the sperm into the oocyte. It depends on the fact that the hamster egg is not species-specific for sperm. However, as the zona has been removed, the acrosome reaction must occur spontaneously. This is aided by washing and incubating the sperm. It is a major drawback of the test that the acrosome reaction is left to chance. Recently, a method has been described for inducing the acrosome reaction with the divalent cation ionophore A23187 (Aitken et al 1991). It is hoped that this will improve the sensitivity of the test.

As the major weakness of the above test is the absence of an effective zona, tests have been developed to assess the zona–sperm interaction. Oocytes are obtained from in vitro fertilization programmes or from ovaries at oophorectomy. They are then either frozen or stored in high salt solutions. In order to have an effective control either the zona is split and one half exposed to test and the other to control sperm, or the test and control samples are labelled with different fluorochromes and the ratios of the two sperm populations in the zona counted. In this way an assessment of the ability of the sperm to penetrate the zona can be obtained. This test has the advantage that the acrosome reaction occurs naturally. However, its clinical value remains to be established, although reports are promising (Liu et al 1988).

FEMALE FACTORS

Ovulation detection

Symptoms and signs

Ovulation pain (mittelschmerz) and midcycle staining occur regularly in some women. Observation of midcycle mucus is the best clinical marker of ovulation and is useful in the timing of procedures such as donor insemination, although anovulatory oestrogen-dominant states may produce an apparently ovulatory mucus. Therefore, none of these symptoms or signs should be considered proof of ovulation.

Basal body temperature recording

This technique has been used for ovulation detection in infertility and natural family planning. It has also been used to diagnose luteal phase deficiency, but it is of little value in this role. The midcycle rise of 0.5–1.0 degrees C, due to the thermogenic effect of progesterone, is detected using a fertility thermometer, usually first thing in the morning. The oral route is most popular although vaginal or rectal readings approximate better to core temperature. A comparison of this technique with endocrine markers of ovulation has shown a poor correlation (Heasley & Thompson 1986). In addition, it can be confusing, stressful and inconvenient for the patient. However, from a practical point of view, it may be of some value for timing luteal phase progesterone estimation or as an adjunct to monitoring the response to clomiphene in anovulatory women.

Hormone assays

In women with regular periods the simplest and most reliable method of confirming ovulation is to measure the midluteal phase serum progesterone level. Those patients with oligomenorrhoea or amenorrhoea may have their progesterone measured weekly from day 21 of the cycle until menstruation. Alternatively, a hormone profile for polycystic ovaries, hyperprolactinaemia, hypothyroidism, premature menopause and hypothalamic hypogonadism may be taken to determine the cause of the irregular menstruation. Serum progesterone should be measured in at least two cycles to confirm the regularity of ovulation. The minimum level of serum progesterone taken to indicate ovulation (within 95% confidence limits) is 30 nmol/l. This is in keeping with the data of Hull et al (1982). Higher values have been suggested.

Detection of the preovulatory surge of luteinizing hormone (LH) may also be used to predict ovulation. The LH peak occurs between 8 and 20 h before ovulation. Levels are usually elevated for 24 h but may be detectable for only 12 h. Therefore, accurate detection requires twice daily blood or urine sampling. There are now several commercially available kits allowing women to undertake this test at home. However, the kits are expensive and, as with basal body temperature charts, they focus the couple's attention onto their infertility and away from their marriage and relationship.

Ovarian ultrasonography

Ultrasonographic visualization of developing follicles is useful in tracking follicle development in ovulation induction. However, it is also of use in detecting the luteinized, unruptured follicle syndrome (Daly et al 1985). In this condition the follicular diameter increases but the typical rupture of the follicle does not occur, even though serum progesterone levels rise into the ovulatory range.

Endometrial biopsy

Using the criteria of Noyes et al (1950), the luteal phase endometrium can be histologically dated. Biopsies should be obtained from high in the uterus, most frequently as an outpatient procedure with disposable curettes (Thompson 1995). This method is probably best for assessing inadequate luteal function. However, the Noyes criteria for endometrial dating were determined using cycle length and basal body temperature charts for cycle timing. When the LH peak was used as a reference point, the method was shown to be imprecise (Tredway et al 1973). Further, there is considerable interobserver variation in the interpretation of the histology results.

Tubal, uterine and pelvic factors

Hysterosalpingography was the traditional way to assess the uterine cavity, tubal structure and tubal patency. However, it has now been largely superseded by hysteroscopy and laparoscopy. Salpingoscopy and falloposcopy are recent developments in the assessment of the internal tubal architecture.

Hysterosalpingography

In this investigation a cannula is inserted into the cervical canal. A radio-opaque dye is injected through the uterine cavity into the fallopian tubes and out into the peritoneal cavity under fluoroscopic control. The procedure can be painful, though this is minimized if the dye is injected very slowly and under very low pressure. Tubal spasm may occur in some women, suggesting cornual blockage. There is also a risk of reactivation of previous salpingitis, and if tubal disease is discovered the patient should receive prophylactic antibiotics. To a large extent this test has been superseded by hysteroscopy (Leeton 1988) and laparoscopy. However, the latter investigations provide no information about internal tubal anatomy and therefore, where salpingitis isthmica nodosa (SIN) is suspected hysterosalpingography is indicated (Fig. 17.6). This condition cannot be diagnosed by visualization of the exterior aspects of the tubes. Salpingoscopy and falloposcopy will allow a more accurate identification of this condition in the future.

Laparoscopy

Over the last 10 years there has been an explosion in gynaecological endoscopic surgery: almost all operations which were previously performed by laparotomy can be performed by this route. However, diagnostic laparoscopy remains an essential part of the full assessment of the infertile couple. It is important to emphasize that a thorough examination of the pelvic organs cannot be per-

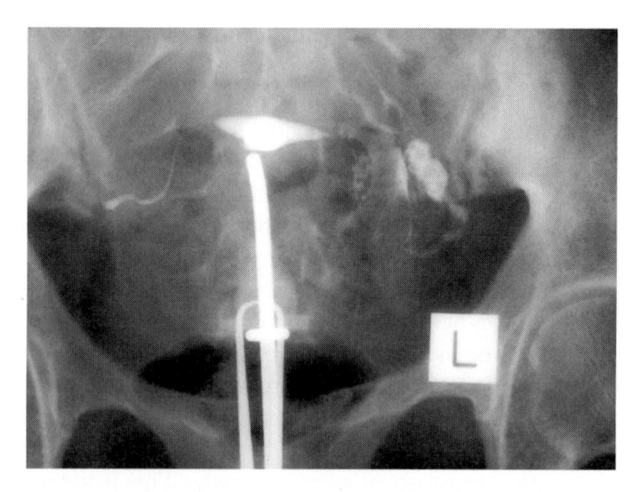

Fig. 17.6 Hysterosalpingogram showing no flow from the distal end of the right tube, a left hydrosalpynx and salpingitis isthmica nodosa (SIN), with its typical cottonwool appearance, around the isthmic portion of the left tube.

UR

Surname Given Names

Date of Birth Age Religion Sex Marital Status

R.B.U. LAPAROSCOPY REPORT

Medical Officer

Date Surgeon Assistant

Anaesthetist Theatre Scrub Nurse

Procedure

Findings

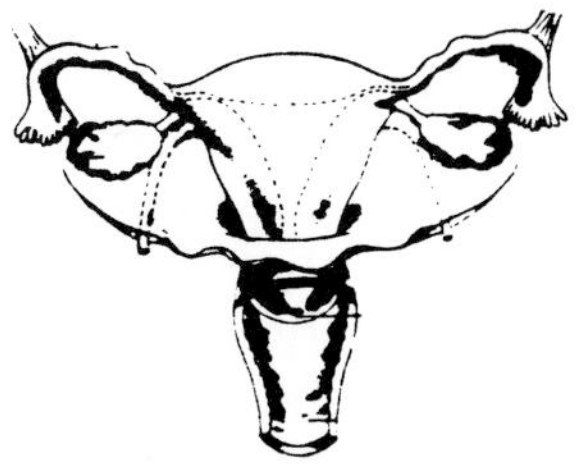

Left Tube

Normal / Abnormal

Right Tube

Normal / Abnormal

For anastomosis demonstrate tubal segments and lengths on diagram.

Left Ovary

Normal / Abnormal GRAF. FOL. /CORP. LUT. /PCOS

Right Ovary

Normal / Abnormal GRAF. FOL. /CORP. LUT. /PCOS

Uterus

Normal / Abnormal

Anterior Pouch

Normal / Abnormal

Pouch of Douglas

Normal / Abnormal

Upper Abdomen / Appendix

Normal / Abnormal

Other Findings

Summary

Management

Doctor's Signature

Fig. 17.7 An example of a standard laparoscopy report form.

formed unless a double-puncture technique is employed. This permits the introduction of a probe or grasper to manipulate the fallopian tubes and ovaries, to determine the presence of adhesions or endometriosis. A third or even fourth puncture site can be used for the introduction of scissors to divide adhesions, for diathermy or laser for the treatment of endometriosis, for graspers and suction/irrigation.

At the end of the laparoscopic examination, a detailed description of all the findings (including negative ones) should be made with the aid of simple diagrams (Fig. 17.7). The presence of a lead follicle or of a corpus luteum should also be recorded as useful information about ovulation. Accurate records ensure that others gain an accurate impression of the problems that may be present and of the prognosis for fertility. Some units now routinely provide their patients with a videorecording of their surgery. Whilst this is expensive it is particularly useful for any surgeon who is subsequently considering surgery.

Hysteroscopy

It is sensible to perform this technique, in infertile women, at the same time as laparoscopy. Whilst liquid can be used, carbon dioxide is the preferred medium for uterine distension. However, it is essential that the insufflators for the abdominal and uterine cavities are not confused: the former delivers gas at 10 times the rate of the latter, and several deaths have been reported from insufflation with the wrong machine. Hysteroscopy can also be performed as an outpatient procedure. Either way, uterine malformations, endometrial polyps, intrauterine adhesions, fibroids and other conditions can be detected. These conditions are now relatively easily treated by operative hysteroscopy.

Salpingoscopy and falloposcopy

Until recently the only method of assessment of the internal tubal structure was hysterosalpingography. If external tubal disease is identified at laparoscopy, it is important to assess the state of the lining of the tube if the patient is to be advised whether tubal surgery or in vitro fertilization would be of greater benefit. Salpingoscopy is the passage of a very fine rigid endoscope through the fimbriated end of the tube. Whilst it is performed at laparoscopy, it only allows direct visualization of the tubal lining to the isthmoampullary junction (Fig. 17.8).

Falloposcopy is a more complicated, and much more expensive procedure involving the passage of an extremely fine flexible fibreoptic device from the uterine cavity distally to the fimbriae (Kerin et al 1990) In order to pass the device a balloon surrounding the endoscope is inflated along the tube and the scope advanced, bit by bit, to minimize tubal damage. The tube is then assessed as the scope is withdrawn (Fig. 17.9). Neither of these procedures is ideal but both provide a much more detailed assessment of tubal status than was previously available.

Cervical factor

Around the time of ovulation, cervical mucus becomes both watery and stretchy. This is due to the predominance of oestrogen and to the lack of progesterone. The stretchiness of the mucus, known as *spinnbarkeit*, can be determined either whilst removing mucus from the cervix or by using two glass slides to pull the sample apart: at ovulation it should stretch at least 8 cm. Ovulatory mucus can be further identified by microscopic examination of a dried sample to identify the characteristic ferning pattern. If satisfactory mucus is not seen, previous cervical surgery and chlamydial infection should be excluded. Oral oestrogen may be given to improve cervical mucus quality. If the mucus fails to improve, intrauterine insemination of washed sperm may be of some therapeutic value.

The postcoital test

After ejaculation, sperm pass very quickly into the cervical mucus. There they are stripped of the seminal plasma as part of the process of capacitation. The most common test of the sperm–mucus interaction is the postcoital test (PCT). This test can only be performed around the time of ovulation in the ovulating patient. Perversely, in patients with anovulation due to polycystic ovarian syndrome where oestrogen is always dominant, it can be performed virtually any time. If there is difficulty in pinpointing the correct time, it is important to be certain that ovulation is occurring. It may also be necessary either to perform the test on alternate days near midcycle, or to see the patient daily until adequate cervical mucus is observed, and then perform the test the following day. There are no firm rules about a period of abstinence prior to the test though a period of 2 or 3 days is thought sufficient. There has also been disagreement about the optimum timing of the PCT in relation to coitus: intervals of 2–24 h have been reported. A 2-h interval usually means having intercourse in the early morning which can lead to temporary impotence. A more reliable approach is to perform the test 8–12 h after coitus so that intercourse can take place the previous evening.

For the test, mucus is collected from the cervix using either a tuberculin syringe or a fine plastic tube (Rocket, UK) and its amount, viscosity and cellularity recorded. In the standard PCT, the cervical mucus is placed on a slide, a coverslip applied and high-power microscopic examination performed. A more complex capillary tube method has been devised but is only employed for research purposes.

Various scoring systems have been proposed for the interpretation of results, but the scores obtained do not correlate well with future fertility. A simpler classification, based on the presence or absence of progressively motile sperm, is easier to use and correlates better with the final outcome in terms of pregnancy rates (Hull et al 1982). The actual number of progressively motile sperm per high-power field which constitutes a normal test is unclear. Usually 5 is taken as the lower limit of normal. However, Collins et al (1984) found no difference in pregnancy rates between groups with no sperm, no motile sperm, 1–5, 6–10 or >10 motile sperm per high-power field. In a study of couples with normal fertility, 20% had 0 or 1 sperm per high-power field (Kovacs et al 1978). By contrast, Hull et al (1982) found significantly higher pregnancy rates in those couples with progressively motile sperm compared with those with no motile sperm.

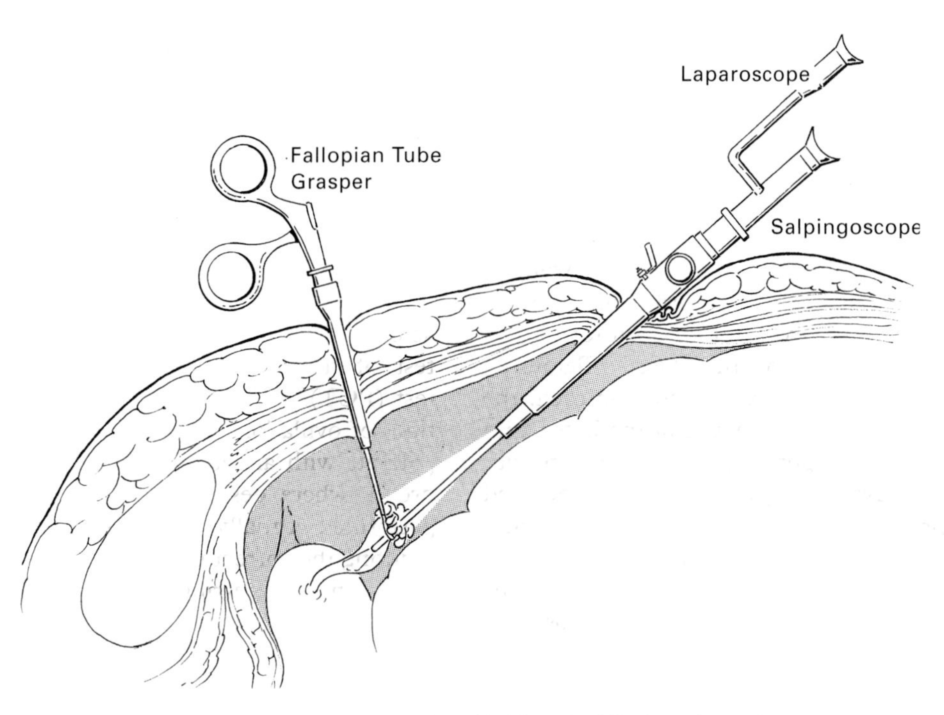

Fig. 17.8 Salpingoscopy: the salpingoscope is guided into the fallopian tube, under direct vision, from the operating channel of the laparoscope.

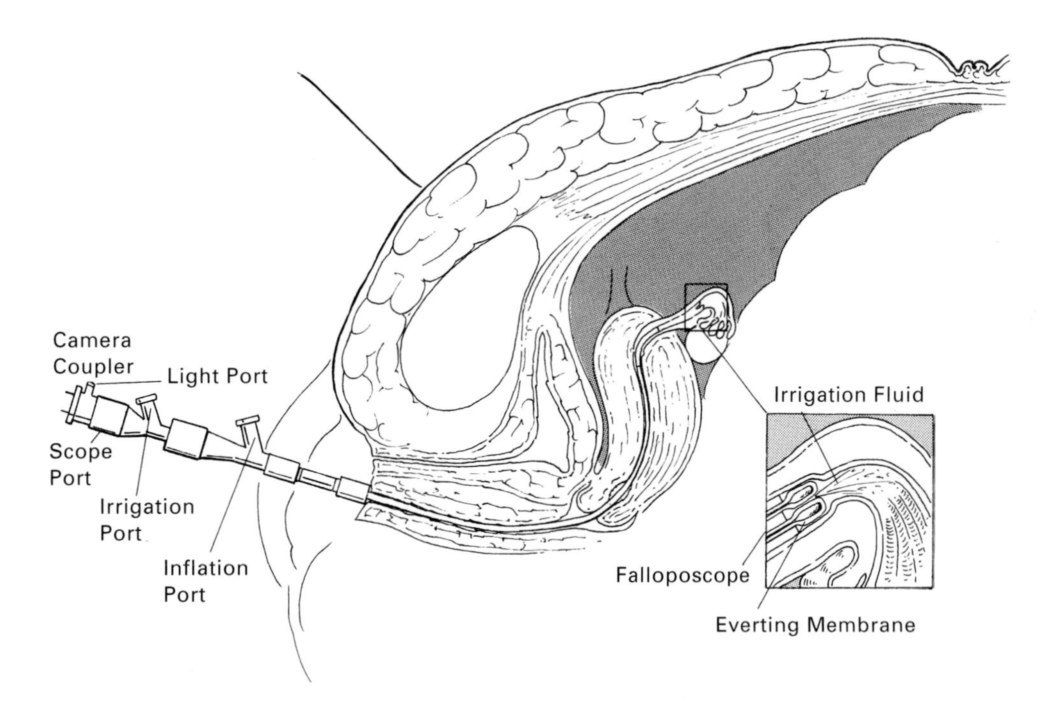

Fig. 17.9 Falloposcopy: the falloposcope is introduced through the uterine cavity into the fallopian tube. The tube is flushed, lubricated and distended by the irrigation fluid. The flexible fibreoptic scope is introduced along the tube, using the inflated membrane to protect and open the tube in advance of the scope.

If sperm are not present in repeated PCTs despite a normal semen analysis, a coital problem should be suspected. Gross asthenospermia or a very low semen volume may also give a negative test. The presence of sperm which are immotile or which exhibit the 'shaking phenomenon' (non-progressive motility) suggests the presence of antisperm antibodies. In a few instances non-progressive motility may simply be due to thick sticky cervical mucus, despite proper timing of the test. A negative test in the presence of poor cervical mucus should be repeated in a subsequent cycle.

In vitro mucus penetration tests

If the PCT is repeatedly negative despite good cervical mucus and sperm counts, an in vitro mucus penetration test should be performed. This permits a more detailed assessment of sperm–mucus interaction and allows cross-over tests with donor sperm and donor mucus to be undertaken. The two commonly used techniques are the sperm penetration test (SPT) and the sperm–cervical mucus contact test (SCMCT). The former is usually performed on a microscope slide although tube methods have also been reported. A drop of semen is placed adjacent to an equivalent amount of preovulatory mucus and a coverslip applied to form an interface (Fig. 17.10a). The donor mucus may be obtained for example from another patient attending the clinic or from a patient attending for artificial insemination. Bovine mucus and synthetic gels are both commercially available as alternatives, but the results are unsatisfactory. Penetration of the mucus by sperm is assessed by microscopic examination over the course of the next hour. A negative test is indicated by complete failure of penetration or immobilization of those sperm which have penetrated. The shaking phenomenon (see below) may also be observed.

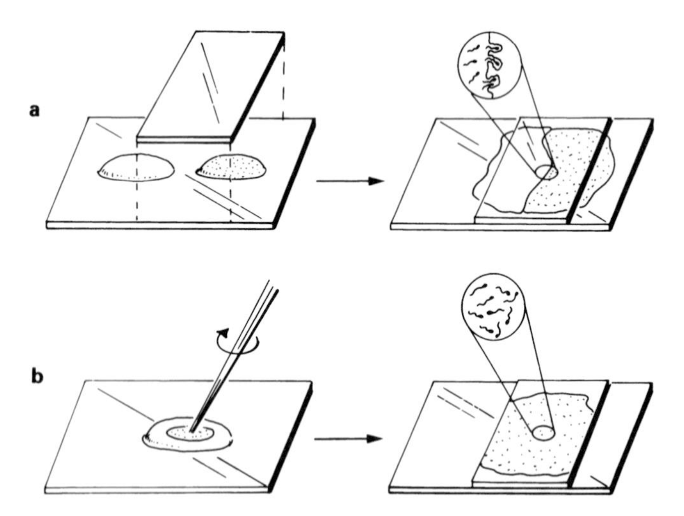

Fig. 17.10 **a** The sperm penetration test; here an interface is produced between the sperm and the cervical mucus. **b** The sperm–cervical mucus contact test (SCMCT), where there is mixing of the components.

This test is simple to perform but is less specific for the presence of sperm antibodies than the SCMCT, since non-immunological factors may lead to a negative test.

The SCMCT, devised by Kremer & Jager (1976), is reported to correlate well with the presence of antisperm antibodies in either semen or cervical mucus. It can, therefore, be used as the primary diagnostic method for local immunological factors if more complex antibody tests are not available. The test is performed by mixing a drop of cervical mucus with a similar volume of semen at one end of a microscope slide and placing a drop of semen at the other end. Both drops are covered with a coverslip. After 30 min the drops are observed (Fig. 17.10b). If more than 25% of sperm are exhibiting jerking or shaking movements rather than forward motility in the sample mixed with mucus but not in the pure sample, the presence of antibodies is presumed. In strongly positive tests the proportion of such sperm equates to the antibody titre. Cross-over testing with donor sperm and donor mucus permits an accurate assessment of whether antibodies are present in the semen or the mucus.

UNEXPLAINED INFERTILITY

If the basic investigations are normal yet there is a persistent failure to conceive, couples are said to have unexplained (idiopathic) infertility. This poorly defined entity is usually reported in 10–20% of cases although a range of 6 to 60% has been cited (Templeton & Penney 1982). It has been clearly demonstrated that the chance of conception in such couples is most closely related to the duration of their infertility, the age of the female partner and whether the infertility is primary or secondary (Hull et al 1985, Lenton et al 1977). These authors all basically agree that an eventual pregnancy rate of 60–70% will be achieved after 3 years of follow-up with no specific treatment. In view of this, counselling forms the basis of management in a situation which is frustrating for both patient and doctor.

Despite the presence of these solid epidemiological data, in some clinics couples with unexplained infertility may undergo a range of more detailed investigations in an effort to find a cause for their failure to conceive. There is no evidence that this approach is superior to waiting for spontaneous conception to occur (Haxton et al 1987). Furthermore, if treatment is undertaken on the basis of results of these tests its apparent success may be wrongfully attributed to the therapy, rather than to natural conception.

KEY POINTS

1. It is more important to perform the relevant investigations in a logical order at the correct time than to perform a battery of tests blindly.
2. Investigations should be performed only if there is at least a 1-year history of infertility, as the chances of pregnancy occurring for a given couple having regular unprotected intercourse are 80% after 1 year and 90% after 18 months.
3. The simplest, least invasive and most productive investigations should be performed first.
4. Irregular cycles are suggestive of ovulatory dysfunction; polycystic ovaries are the commonest found pathology.
5. Men with an obstructive cause for azoospermia now have a relatively good prognosis with the advent of intracytoplasmic sperm injection (ICSI). The success rates are similar to those obtained with severe oligospermia using standard in vitro fertilization procedures.
6. Hypogonadotrophic hypogonadism is manifested by a low FSH and low testosterone level, and is amenable to treatment with gonadotrophins.
7. At least two semen analyses should be carried out, because of known variability within an individual, before consistency of abnormality can be determined.
8. Midluteal progesterone is the simplest and most reliable method of ovulation assessment (progesterone measurements in excess of 30 nmol/l confirming ovulation).
9. Laparoscopy is the most useful method of assessment of the patency of fallopian tubes, and gives other information concerning pathology/normality of the pelvis. It is essential to use a double-puncture technique for adequate inspection of the pelvis, with careful inspection of all areas, especially the ovarian fossae.
10. A hysterosalpingogram is indicated if salpingitis isthmica nodosa is suspected, but it may be superseded by salpingoscopy and falloposcopy in the future.
11. A negative postcoital test may be due to poor semen quality, coital difficulty, failure to produce adequate cervical mucus or immunological factors in either partner, but is most often due to inappropriate timing. LH monitoring kits may overcome this problem.
12. Of couples with unexplained infertility, 60–70% will conceive within 3 years without any intervention. Beyond that time a number of empirical treatments have been shown to be beneficial.

REFERENCES

Aitken R J, Irvine D S, Wu F S W 1991 Prospective analysis of sperm oocyte fusion and reactive oxygen species generation as criteria for the diagnosis of infertility. American Journal of Obstetrics and Gynecology 164: 542

Aitken R J, Sutton M, Warner P, Richardson D W 1985 The relationship between the movement characteristics of human spermatozoa and their ability to penetrate cervical mucus and zona-free oocytes. Journal of Reproduction and Fertility 73: 411–449

Ayvaliotis B, Bronson R, Rosenfeld D, Cooper G 1985 Conception rates in couples where autoimmunity to sperm is detected. Fertility and Sterility 43: 739–742

Bostofte E, Serup J, Rebbe H 1982 Relation between morphologically abnormal spermatozoa and pregnancies obtained during a 20-year follow-up period. International Journal of Andrology 5: 379–386

Boyers S P, Davis R O, Katz D F 1989 Automated semen analysis. Current Problems in Obstetrics, Gynaecology and Fertility XII: 173–200, Year Book Medical Publishers, Chicago

Collins J A, So Y, Wilson E H, Wrixon W, Casper R F 1984 The post coital test as a predictor of pregnancy among 355 infertile couples. Fertility and Sterility 41: 703

Cooke I D, Sulaiman R A, Lenton E A, Parsons R J 1981 Fertility and infertility statistics: their importance and application. Clinics in Obstetrics and Gynaecology 8: 3

Daly D C, Soto-Albors C, Walters C, Ying Y, Riddick D H 1985 Ultrasonic evidence of luteinised unruptured follicle syndrome in unexplained infertility. Fertility and Sterility 43: 62–67

Davis R O, Katz D F 1992 Standardisation and comparability of CASA instruments. Journal of Andrology 13: 81–86

Finkel D M, Phillips J L, Snider P J 1985 Stimulation of spermatogenesis by gonadotrophins in men with hypogonadotrophic hypogonadism. New England Journal of Medicine 313: 651

Haxton M J, Fleming R, Hamilton M P R, Yates R W, Black W P, Coutts J R T 1987 Unexplained infertility – results of secondary investigations in 95 couples. British Journal of Obstetrics and Gynaecology 94: 539–542

Hellstrom W J G, Samuels S J, Waits A B, Overstreet J W 1989 A comparison of the usefulness of the sperm-MAR and immunobead tests for the detection of antisperm antibodies. Fertility and Sterility 36: 219–221

Hull M G R, Savage P E, Bromham D R 1982 Prognostic value of the postcoital test: prospective test based on time specific conception rates. Fertility and Sterility 38: 384

Hull M G R, Glazener C M A, Kelly N J 1985 Population study of causes, treatment and outcome of infertility. British Medical Journal 291: 1693–1697

Kerin J, Daykhovsky L, Segalowitz J et al 1990 Falloposcopy: a microendoscopic technique for visual exploration of the human fallopian tube from the uterotubal ostium to the fimbria using a transvaginal approach. Fertility and Sterility 54: 390–400

Kovacs G T, Newman G B, Henson G L 1978 The postcoital test: what is normal? British Medical Journal 1: 818

Kremer J, Jager S 1976 The sperm–cervical mucus contact test: a preliminary report. Fertility and Sterility 27: 335–340

Leeton J 1988 The investigation of pelvic lesions in infertility. Australian and New Zealand Journal of Obstetrics and Gynaecology 28: 126–127

Lenton E A, Weston G A, Coke I D 1977 Long term follow-up of the apparently normal couple with a complaint of infertility. Fertility and Sterility 28: 913–919

Liu D Y, Lopata A, Johnson W I H, Baker H G W 1988 A human sperm–zona pellucida binding test using oocytes that failed to fertilise in vitro. Fertility and Sterility 50: 782

Makler A 1980 The improved 10-micrometer chamber for rapid sperm count and motility evaluation. Fertility and Sterility 33: 337–338

Mallidis C, Baker H W G 1994 Fine needle aspiration biopsy of the testis. Fertility and Sterility 61: 367–375

Mortimer D, Pandaya I J, Sawers R S 1986 Relation between human sperm motility characteristics and sperm penetration into cervical mucus in vitro. Journal of Reproduction and Fertility 78: 93

Noyes R W, Hertig A T, Rock J 1950 Dating the endometrial biopsy. Fertility and Sterility 1: 3

Pandaya I J, Mortimer D, Sawers R S 1986 A standardized approach for evaluating the penetration of human spermatozoa into cervical mucus in vitro. Fertility and Sterility 45: 357

Paulson J D, Negro-Vilar A, Lucena E, Martini L 1986 The prediction and detection of ovulation in artificial insemination. In: Heasley R N, Thompson W 1986 Andrology. Male fertility and sterility. Academic Press, Florida, pp 491–509

Templeton A A, Penney G C 1982 The incidence, characteristics and prognosis of patients whose infertility is unexplained. Fertility and Sterility 37: 175–181

Thompson W 1995 Endometrial sampling. The Diplomate 1(4): 276–279. (Journal of the Diplomates of the Royal College of Obstetricians and Gynaecologists, London)

Tournaye H, Devroey P, Liu J, Nagy Z, Lissens W, van Steirteghem A 1994 Microsurgical epididymal sperm aspiration and intracytoplasmic sperm injection: a new effective approach to infertilty as a result of congenital bilateral absence of the vas deferens. Fertility and Sterility 61: 1045–1051

Tredway D R, Misschell D R Jr, Moyer D 1973. Correlation of endometrial dating with luteinizing hormone peak. American Journal of Obstetrics and Gynecology 117: 1030–1033

Van der Ven H H, Jeyendran R S, Al-Hasani S et al 1986 Correlation between human sperm swelling in hypoosmotic medium (hypoosmotic swelling test) and in vitro fertilization. Journal of Andrology 7: 190–196

Wolff H, Politch J A, Martinez A, Haimovici F, Hill J A, Anderson D J 1990 Leukocytospermia is associated with poor semen quality. Fertility and Sterility 53: 528–536

World Health Organization 1992 WHO laboratory manual for the examination of human semen and sperm–cervical mucus interaction, 3rd edn. Cambridge University Press, Cambridge

18

Disorders of male reproduction

John P. Pryor F. C. W. Wu

INTRODUCTION

There has been rapid progress during the past 20 years in our understanding of male reproductive physiology with wide-ranging contributions from cell and molecular biologists, urologists and endocrinologists, whose efforts have contributed to establishing the discipline of andrology. Some of these advances are beginning to be translated into clinical practice, so that the management of male reproductive disorders can be based on rational scientific principles. Males with reproductive disorders often present to the gynaecologist and family practitioner through the intermediary of their female partners. It is therefore important for both the community doctors and hospital specialists to have a high degree of awareness, in order to recognize potential problems, as well as being cognisant of the newer diagnostic techniques and treatment modalities now becoming increasingly available for male reproductive dysfunction.

This chapter aims to provide the practising gynaecologist with an overview of clinical andrology with emphasis on male infertility. A description of normal physiology is given as the foundation for explaining pathophysiological mechanisms and as a basis for formulating rational treatment where possible.

PHYSIOLOGY

Spermatogenesis

Spermatogenesis takes place in several hundred tightly coiled seminiferous tubules arranged in lobules (Fig. 18.1;

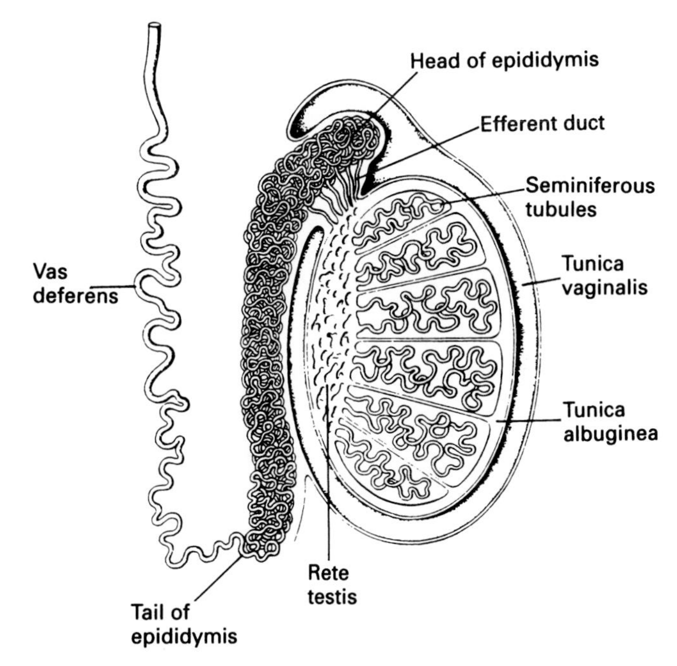

Fig. 18.1 Human testis, epididymis and vas deferens showing efferent ducts leading from the rete testis to the caput epididymis and the cauda epididymis continuing to become the vas deferens. (From Dym 1977, with permission.)

Dym 1977) which constitute some 80% of testicular volume in man. Each tubule resembles a loop draining at both ends into the rete testis, with which the head of the epididymis is connected by several efferent ducts. Seminiferous tubules are lined by germ cells and Sertoli cells around a central lumen, and surrounded by peritubular myoid cells and a basement membrane (Fig. 18.2).

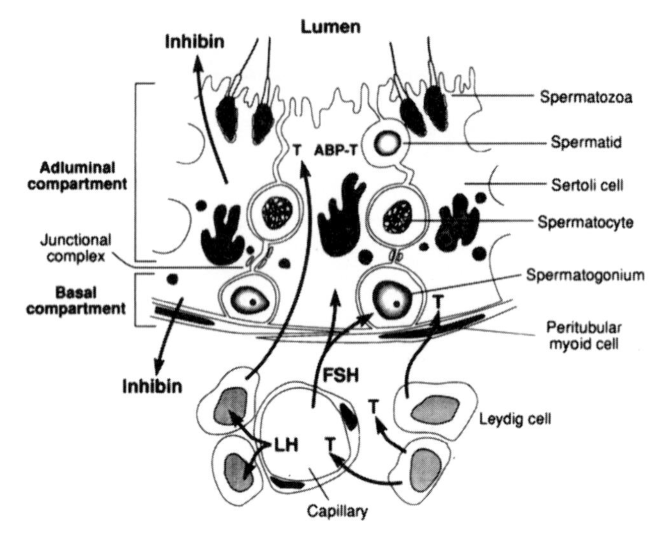

Fig. 18.2 Diagrammatic representation of the anatomical and functional relationship between germ cells, Sertoli cells and Leydig cells. Note the division of the seminiferous epithelium into adluminal and basal compartments by the tight junctions between adjacent Sertoli cells, and the bidirectional secretion of Sertoli cell products (e.g. inhibin) into the lumen and interstitial space. ABP-T, androgen-binding protein testosterone; FSH, follicle-stimulating hormone; LH, luteinizing hormone.

Within this seminiferous epithelium resides the most active and dynamic collection of cells in the body, but the complicated cellular multiplication and remodelling take place in a virtually avascular environment.

Spermatogenesis is a continuous sequence of highly organized (spatially and temporally) and closely regulated events, whereby cohorts of undifferentiated diploid germ cells (spermatogonia) multiply and are then transformed into haploid spermatozoa. The following events, occurring with a precise sequence and duration, can be observed in the seminiferous epithelium during normal spermatogenesis.

1. Mitotic division (at least four) of stem cells to form cohorts of spermatogonia which, at intervals of 16 days, differentiate into primary preleptotene spermatocytes to initiate meiosis.
2. Meiotic reduction divisions of spermatocytes to form round spermatids.
3. Continuous remodelling of Sertoli cells in order to direct the migration of germ cells from basal to luminal positions.
4. Transformation (spermiogenesis) of large spherical spermatids into compact virtually cytoplasm-free spermatozoa with condensed DNA in the head crowned by an apical acrosome cap, and a tail capable of propulsive beating movements.
5. Spermiation or release of spermatozoa from Sertoli cell cytoplasm into tubular lumen.

Cohorts of undifferentiated germ cells, joined to each other by cytoplasmic bridges, progress through these different steps in synchrony, so that several generations of developing germ cells are usually observed at any one part of the seminiferous epithelium at any one time. The total duration for a cohort of spermatogonia to develop into spermatozoa is 4 days, during which time at least three further generations of spermatogonia have also successively, at intervals of 16 days, initiated their development.

Sertoli cell function

Sertoli (sustentacular) cells have extensive cytoplasm which spans the full height of the seminiferous epithelium from basement membrane to the lumen (Fig. 18.2). Where adjacent Sertoli cells come into contact with each other near the basement membrane, special occluding junctions are formed which divide the seminiferous epithelium into a basal (outer) compartment, which interacts with the systemic circulation, and an adluminal (inner) compartment enclosed by a functional permeability barrier, the blood–testis barrier (Fig. 18.2). In the cytoplasmic scaffolding provided by the Sertoli cells, spermatogonia divide by mitosis in the basal compartment, while the two reduction divisions of the spermatocytes and spermiogenesis are confined to the unique avascular microenvironment of the adluminal compartment created by the blood–testis barrier. The developing germ cells are therefore completely dependent on Sertoli cells for metabolic support. As germ cells mature, the formation and dissolution of a variety of special junctional connections with adjacent Sertoli cell membrane suggest that functional interactions between them are highly probable. In response to appropriate trophic stimuli (follicle-stimulating hormone (FSH) and testosterone), Sertoli cells secrete a wide range of substances including androgen-binding protein (ABP), inhibin, plasminogen activator, transferrin, lactate, growth factors and a distinctive tubular fluid high in potassium and low in protein which bathes the mature spermatozoa.

Much of the Sertoli cell secretion is bidirectional, occurring either from the apex into the lumen or via the base into interstitial fluid and thence into the blood stream. The particular direction of secretion seems to be influenced by hormones and the state of the seminiferous epithelium. Whether any of these secretory products of the Sertoli cell is essential for spermatogenesis or sperm maturation, or whether there is any physiological significance of the direction of secretion, is at present unknown. Nevertheless, the fact that both apically and basally secreted products can eventually reach the systemic circulation (e.g. inhibin, the hormone that is responsible for the negative feedback mechanism controlling FSH secretion) provides the potential for detecting circulating markers of Sertoli cell function or dysfunction.

Unlike the actively dividing germ cells, Sertoli cells do not proliferate in the adult testis. However, the active cell division and morphogenesis are matched by the functional diversity and variation of Sertoli cells. Viewed from this perspective, spermatogenesis is a cyclical process, which is critically dependent on the periodic changes in Sertoli cell function associated with the constantly changing combination of germ cells in contact with its cytoplasm. Changes in the germ cell complement in contact with any one Sertoli cell occur at a fixed sequence and interval. Thus the synchronization of these repetitive cyclical changes in Sertoli cell function, associated with the variations in germ cell metabolic requirement as they divide and differentiate, has now become one of the central tenets of our conceptualization of normal spermatogenesis (Sharpe 1990). Although pituitary gonadotrophins provide obligatory trophic support for testicular function as a whole, the classical concept that luteinizing hormone (LH) stimulates Leydig cell steroidogenesis and FSH controls functions in the seminiferous tubules is far too simplistic in the light of our current understanding of spermatogenesis. There is now good evidence that the interstitial and tubular compartments are not functionally distinct but that there is a close and complex interrelationship between them (Skinner 1991). Thus testosterone from the interstitial Leydig cells stimulates Sertoli cell functions either directly or via the peritubular cells. Altered tubular/Sertoli cell function, on the other hand, can induce changes in Leydig cell steroidogenesis, although the identity of the intercompartmental regulator(s) is unknown.

Systemic gonadotrophins are not directly involved in this intricate local intratesticular cross-talking. Furthermore, the ability to prepare relatively pure populations of isolated cells from the testis, for in vitro studies, has demonstrated that individual cell types have receptors for and respond to a large variety of hormones and humoral factors. That these factors are produced within the testis, and that testicular cells respond to them in concentrations much higher than those found in peripheral plasma, provides strong circumstantial evidence to suggest that specific functional interactions between Sertoli, Leydig, peritubular and germ cells exist within the testis. One can envisage interactions in which a particular combination of germ cell types dictates the functional response in adjacent Sertoli cells, which are also under the influence of Leydig cells and peritubular cells. The Sertoli cells in turn govern or initiate the next step in the cytodifferentiation of those germ cells, via some paracrine and/or growth factors.

At present the nature of these putative paracrine mechanisms is far from clear. Testosterone is the only, and probably the most important paracrine hormone identified, and its presence in sufficient concentrations in the seminiferous tubules is an absolute requirement for spermatogenesis. How much testosterone is required and how it exerts its effects are just some of the fundamental questions that are still unanswered. Despite the large gaps in our existing knowledge, it is becoming increasingly accepted that local coordination of the multifarious functions in a variety of different cell types within the testis, orchestrated by the diverse functional capabilities of the Sertoli cells, holds the key to quantitatively normal spermatogenesis.

Hormonal control of spermatogenesis

The hormonal control of spermatogenesis requires the actions of the pituitary gonadotrophins LH and FSH. There is general agreement that both LH and FSH are needed for the initiation of spermatogenesis during puberty. However, the specific roles and relative contributions of the two gonadotrophins in maintaining spermatogenesis are unclear (Sharpe 1987).

LH stimulates Leydig cell steroidogenesis, resulting in increased production of testosterone. Normal spermatogenesis is absolutely dependent on testosterone, but its mode of action and the amount required remain uncertain. Specific androgen receptors have not been demonstrated in germ cells but are present in Sertoli and peritubular cells. This implies that the actions of androgens in spermatogenesis must be mediated by somatic cells in the seminiferous tubules. The concentration of testosterone in the testis is 50 times higher than that in the peripheral circulation. There is thus a gross overabundance of testosterone within the normal adult testis and any testosterone-related abnormalities must be due to defects in steroid utilization rather than supply. However, testosterone on its own, in hypogonadotrophic conditions, can only maintain qualitatively normal spermatogenesis when testicular weight and total sperm production remain subnormal (Matsumoto 1989).

FSH initiates function in immature Sertoli cells, prior to the onset of spermatogenesis, by stimulating the formation of the blood–testis barrier and the secretion of tubular fluid and other specific secretory products via FSH receptors which activate intracellular cyclic adenosine monophosphate (AMP). Once spermatogenesis is established in the adult testis, Sertoli cells become less responsive to FSH.

However, it can be shown in animals immunized against FSH, and in experimentally induced hypogonadotrophic men given gonadotrophin replacement, that both testosterone (depending on LH) and FSH are required for quantitatively normal spermatogenesis in the adult (testosterone-replete) testis by determining the number of spermatogonia available by meiosis. FSH therefore acts either by increasing spermatogonial mitosis or decreasing the number of cells that degenerate at each cell division. Testosterone is essential for the subsequent stages from meiosis to spermiogenesis.

Leydig cells

The adult human testis contains some 500 million Leydig

cells clustered in the interstitial spaces adjacent to the seminiferous tubules. The biosynthesis of testosterone in Leydig cells is under the control of LH which binds to specific surface membrane receptors. Steroidogenesis is stimulated through a cyclic AMP–protein kinase C mechanism which mobilizes cholesterol substrate and promotes the conversion of cholesterol to pregnenolone by splitting the C21 side chain. The subsequent steps in the biosynthetic pathway involve the weakly androgenic intermediates of dehydroepiandrosterone and androstenedione before testosterone, the principal secretory product, is obtained. Testosterone is secreted into spermatic venous system, testicular lymphatics and tubular fluid.

Testosterone is the most important circulating androgen in the adult male, since most dehydrotestosterone is formed locally in androgen-responsive target tissues. When circulating in plasma, testosterone is bound to sex hormone-binding globulin (SHBG) and albumin. The latter binds to all steroids with low affinity (testosterone 3.6×10^4 mol/l), while SHBG, a glycoprotein synthesized in the liver with a molecular weight of 80–94 kDa, has a high affinity (8×10^8 mol/l) but a low capacity ($3–5 \times 10^{-8}$ mol/l) for testosterone. In man, 60% of circulating testosterone is bound to SHBG, 38% to albumin and 2% is free. Free and albumin-bound testosterone constitute the bioavailable fractions of circulating testosterone, but recent evidence suggests that SHBG-bound testosterone may also be extractable in some tissues, namely prostate and testis.

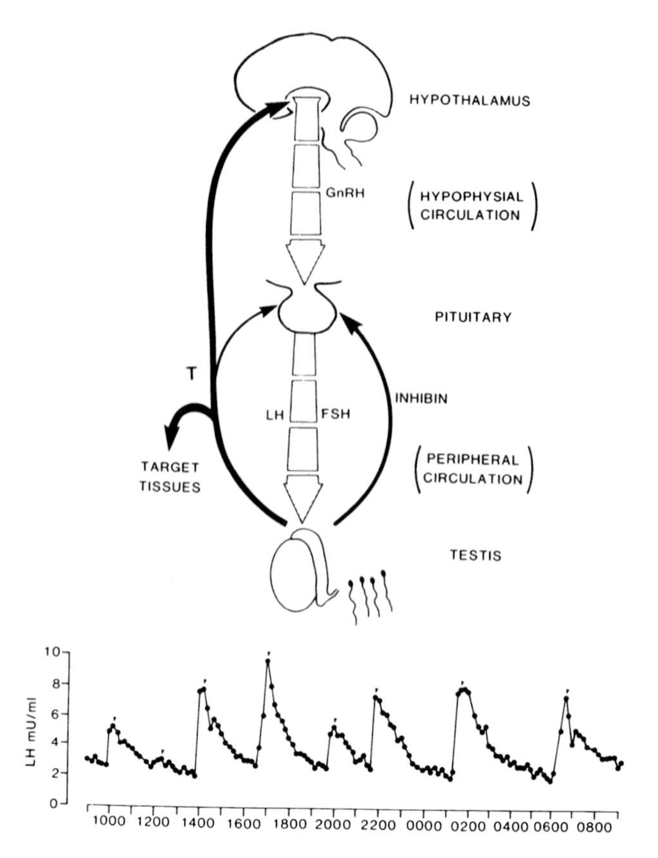

Fig. 18.3 **Top** Functional relationships in the hypothalamic–pituitary–testicular axis. Gonadotrophin-releasing hormone (GnRH) is secreted into the hypophysial circulation in an episodic manner, represented by a luteinizing hormone (LH) pulse (arrowed below) in the peripheral circulation. **Bottom** Peripheral blood LH concentration sampled in an adult male at 10-min intervals for 24 h from 0900 to 0900 h.

Hypothalamic–pituitary–testicular axis

Anterior pituitary gonadotrophin secretion is controlled by hypothalamic gonadotrophin-releasing hormone (GnRH) released into the pituitary portal circulation by axon terminals in the median eminence. The neurosecretory neurons in the medial basal hypothalamus are responsive to a wide variety of sensory inputs as well as to gonadal negative feedback. GnRH stimulates both LH and FSH secretion. The GnRH precursor gene has been identified and mapped to the chromosome 8p (Hayflick et al 1989). In the adult male, GnRH is released episodically into the pituitary portal circulation at a frequency of about every 140 min; each volley of GnRH elicits an immediate release of LH producing the typical pulsatile pattern of LH in the systemic circulation (Fig. 18.3; Wu et al 1989). Though also secreted episodically, FSH and testosterone pulses are not apparent in normal men, because of the slower secretion of newly synthesized rather than stored hormone, and the longer circulating half-lives. The intermittent mode of GnRH stimulation, within a narrow physiological range of frequency, is obligatory for sustaining the normal pattern of gonadotrophin secretion. Continuous or high-frequency GnRH stimulation paradoxically desensitizes the pituitary gonadotrophin response, because of depletion of receptors and refractoriness of postreceptor response mechanisms.

Testosterone exerts the major negative feedback action on gonadotrophin secretion. Its effect is predominantly to restrict the frequency of GnRH pulses from the hypothalamus to within the physiological range. Testosterone also acts on the pituitary to reduce the amplitude of LH response to GnRH; this may require the local conversion of testosterone to oestradiol in the pituitary. These inhibitory actions are best seen in agonadal or castrated males where high-frequency and high-amplitude LH pulsatile secretion prevail. Feedback inhibition of pituitary FSH synthesis is also affected by testosterone, particularly at high concentrations, as well as by the recently purified glycoprotein Sertoli cell product, inhibin (McLachlan et al 1987). It is believed that tubular damage associated with Sertoli cell dysfunction, and a consequently reduced capacity for inhibin secretion, is the cause for the FSH rise, with normal LH, commonly found in infertile men.

The spermatozoon

The spermatozoon has a dense oval head capped by

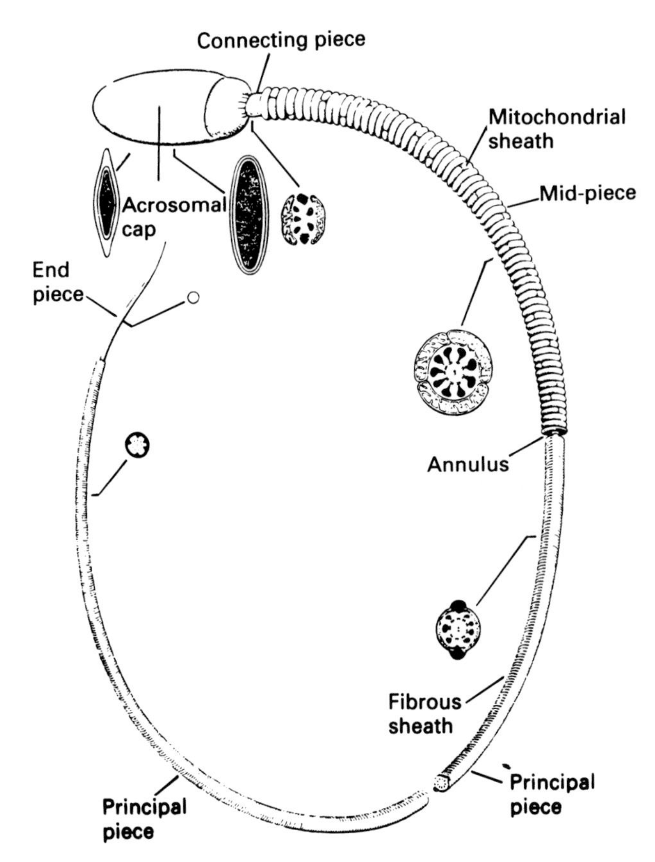

Fig. 18.4 The internal structure of a spermatozoon with the cell membrane removed (from Fawcett 1975).

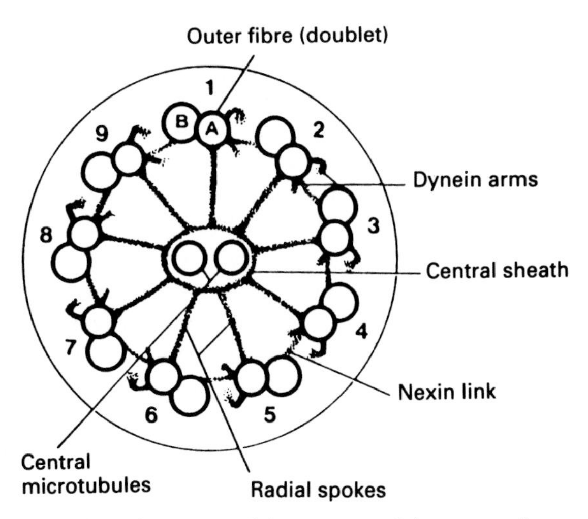

Fig. 18.5 Typical structure of the axoneme of the sperm tail.

an acrosome granule and is propelled by a motile tail (Fig. 18.4; Fawcett 1975). These highly specialized structural features reflect the unique functional activities of the spermatozoon. The acrosome contains enzymes essential for fertilization; the tail contains the energy course and machinery for motility, these combine to deliver the paternal contribution of genetic information in the nucleus to the egg, to initiate development of a new individual.

The head is made up largely of highly condensed nuclear chromatin, constituting the haploid chromosome complement, and it is covered in its anterior half by a membrane-enclosed sac of enzymes, the acrosome. The area of the sperm head immediately behind the acrosome is important as it is this part which attaches and fuses with the egg.

The tail is usually further divided into the midpiece, principal piece and endpiece. The motor apparatus of the tail is the axoneme which consists of a central pair (doublets) of microtubules of non-contractile tubulin protein enclosed in a sheath linked radially to nine outer pairs of microtubules (Fig. 18.5). Each doublet is also joined by nexin bridges to its neighbour via two adenosine triphosphatase-rich dynein protein arms. The axonemal complex is surrounded by columns of dense fibres, which are in turn covered by a helix of mitochondria in the midpiece, and a fibrous sheath in the principal piece. The dense fibres and the fibrous sheath form the cytoskeleton of the flagellum. Through the hydrolysis of adenosine triphosphate, the dynein arms undergo a series of conformational changes resulting in adjacent doublets sliding over one another. Synchronized movement of groups of microtubules propagating waves of bending motions of the tail is the key to the various modes of coordinated sperm motility. Energy for sperm motility is provided by the sheath of mitochondria in the midpiece of the tail through a second-messenger system, involving the calcium-mediated calmodulin-dependent conversion of adenosine triphosphate to cAMP and interaction with the adenosine triphosphatase of the dynein.

Sperm transport and maturation

Spermatozoa are functionally immature and immotile when they pass from the testis into the caput epididymis, and the maturation process continues as they pass through the epididymis. The epididymis is a 3–4 m long single coiled tube whose function is under androgen and neural (adrenergic) control. The epididymal epithelium actively reabsorbs testicular fluid but also secretes a hyperosmolar fluid rich in glycerophosphorylocholine, inositol and carnitine. The specific transport of these compounds across the epithelium creates a favourable fluid environment where progressive motility and fertilizing capacity of the spermatozoa are normally acquired. Thus the cytoplasmic droplets decrease in size and move distally along the midpiece, the acrosome membrane swells, the epididymal glycoproteins are incorporated into the plasma membrane, s–s bonds are formed in the sperm tail cytoskeleton and the cyclic AMP content increases.

Secretions of the accessory glands form over 90% of the volume of semen and mix with spermatozoa at emission. The seminal vesicles contribute the largest volume of alkaline fluid to the ejaculate and are also the source of seminal fructose, prostaglandins and coagulating proteins. Prostatic secretion contains proteolytic enzymes (which normally liquefy the coagulated proteins in semen within 20–30 min) and are rich in citric acid and zinc. Seminal plasma provides a support medium for transporting male gametes out of the body and for buffering the acidic pH (<5) of the vagina so that a reservoir of functional sperm can be established after ejaculation. Additionally, seminal plasma–sperm interaction at ejaculation may contribute to the continuing process of sperm maturation. The normal storage site of sperm in the male genital tract is in the cauda epididymis and ampulla of the vasa.

Just as testicular germ cells are subjected to constant attrition, ejaculated spermatozoa have to traverse the cervix, uterus and uterotubal junction before reaching the middle third of the oviduct, which is the site of fertilization, and at each barrier the sperm population is further reduced so that eventually only 200 or so of the most robust spermatozoa have the opportunity to fertilize the ovum. It is the number of these functionally complete sperm that is more important than the total number ejaculated.

The cervical canal is the first selective filtering barrier to meet the ejaculated sperm. This barrier is virtually complete except during midcycle when oestrogenized cervical mucus glycoprotein fibrils form parallel chains called micelles which permit spermatozoa with active progressive motility to swim through at a rate of 2–3 mm/min. It is believed that crypts of the cervical glands are colonized by migrating spermatozoa, forming sanctuaries from where sperm can be gradually released over a prolonged period. Sperm is transported rapidly through the uterus by uterine myometrium contraction.

The uterotubal junction is the second of the major physical barriers for spermatozoa. The mechanism for selectivity is not clear, but may depend on factors other than sperm motility since inert particles can pass through. Once the uterotubular junction has been successfully negotiated, a minority of sperm immediately traverse the oviduct to the ampulla but the majority congregate in the isthmus until ovulation has occurred. At this time, capacitated sperm showing hyperactivated movements of the tail gradually progress towards the fimbriated end, helped on by the muscular contraction of the oviduct wall and the flow of fluid in the oviduct.

MALE INFERTILITY

Definition and epidemiology

The currently accepted definition of infertility is the inability to produce a pregnancy after 12 months of unprotected intercourse. However, it should be remembered that only 86% of normal fertile couples achieve a pregnancy in the first year so that some patients being investigated for infertility merely need more time to realize their goal. It should also be appreciated that there is a spontaneous pregnancy rate, albeit decreased, in those with reduced semen quality. It follows that most patients are subfertile rather than sterile, and this has important implications in patient management strategies as well as the critical assessment of treatment results.

General population surveys in developed countries have indicated that some 8–15% of married couples experience involuntary subfertility (Hull et al 1985). Of these, male factors alone are estimated to be responsible in 30% and contributory in a further 20% of subfertile couples. Thus, male subfertility may affect 5% of men of reproductive age.

Pathophysiology

In the simplest terms, male infertility is a failure to fertilize the normal ovum arising from a deficiency of functionally competent sperm at the site of fertilization. Since less than 0.1% of ejaculated sperm actually reach the fallopian tube, it is defective sperm function rather than inadequate numbers of sperm ejaculated that constitutes the most important pathophysiological mechanism in male infertility. Specific lesions leading to defective sperm motility or transport and abnormal sperm–egg interaction are probably the key factors responsible for loss of fertilizing capacity in the gametes. In most instances however, inadequate sperm function is usually but not invariably accompanied by reduced sperm production, suggesting that specific defects in spermatozoa could have arisen from disturbances in regulatory mechanisms which interfere with both germ cell multiplication and maturation in the seminiferous tubules. There is rarely any clinical evidence of systemic gonadotrophin or androgen deficiency in men with male infertility; indeed circulating gonadotrophins are frequently raised. By inference therefore, disturbances in paracrine regulation within the testis could lead to low sperm output (oligozoospermia), from an increased rate of degeneration in the differentiating spermatogonia at successive mitotic divisions, as well as abnormal spermiogenesis giving rise to spermatozoa with poor motility (asthenozoospermia) and/or abnormal morphology (teratozoospermia).

The nature of these putative defects in paracrine control remains to be identified but the current hypothesis provides a useful conceptual framework in directing research efforts and planning patient management. Abnormal epididymal function may lead to defective sperm maturation, impairment of sperm transport or even cell death. Interruption of the transport of normal sperm may be due to mechanical barriers between the epididymis and fallopian tube or abnormal coitus and/or ejaculation.

Aetiologies

One of the central problems in male infertility is the dif-

Table 18.1 Aetiologies of male infertility (percentages)

Diagnosis	Edinburgh 1979–1982	WHO 1979–1882 (Cates et al 1985)	Melbourne 1979–1980 (Baker 1989)
Unrecognized	56.3	48.3	47.9
Idiopathic azoo-, oligozoospermia	8.4	16.1	7.3
Idiopathic astheno-teratozoospermia	19.5	16.8	
Varicocele	7.2	17.2	25.0
Genital tract infection	2.1	4.0	
Sperm autoimmunity	1.8	1.6	5.0
Congenital (cryptorchidism) chromosomal disorders	1.2	2.1	1.9
Genital tract obstruction	0.6	1.8	10.8
Systemic/iatrogenic	0.6	1.3	1.0
Coital disorders	1.8	1.0	0.5
Gonadotrophin deficiency	0	0.6	0.6

ficulty in identifying genuine rather than presumptive aetiological factors. In the World Health Organization survey on the pattern of infertility in 25 countries (Cates et al 1985), 66.6% of males either have no demonstrable cause for their infertility or the aetiology of abnormal semen quality is unidentifiable (Table 18.1). This was confirmed in specialist referral clinics in Edinburgh (for couples) and Melbourne (Baker 1989) (mainly for males), emphasizing the point that a minority of infertile men have specific recognizable aetiologies and only a small proportion of these are treatable.

Chromosome disorders

Normal spermatogenesis is critically dependent on the ordered arrangement of chromosome pairing during cell division. Certain abnormalities of chromosomes may therefore be expected to interfere with spermatogenesis. In over 2000 men attending the male subfertility clinic in Edinburgh over 10 years, the incidence of chromosome abnormalities was 2.2% (Chandley 1979). The frequency of chromosomal abnormalities increased as sperm concentration declined. Abnormal chromosome karyotypes were found in 15% of azoospermic patients, 90% of whom had Klinefelter's syndrome (47XXY), which accounted for half of the entire chromosomally abnormal group. In oligozoospermic patients, the incidence of chromosome abnormalities was 4%.

Other chromosomal abnormalities encountered more commonly in the infertile male population than in newborns included reciprocal X or Y autosomal translocations, XYY and XX males, reciprocal and Robertsonian autosomal translocations, supernumerary autosomes and inversion autosomes. Absence of the long arm of the Y chromosome is known to be associated with azoospermia and the 'azoospermia factor' or AZF gene would appear to be located at this site (Ma et al 1993).

Chromosomal studies of meiotic germ cells afford an opportunity to study the mechanism by which chromosomal aberrations interfere with spermatogenesis. However this rarely reveals chromosomal abnormalities involving the germ line exclusively without any detectable changes in somatic karyotype. Though useful as a research tool, meiotic chromosome studies in germ cells require tissues obtained at testicular biopsy and are therefore rarely indicated in routine diagnostic investigation.

Cryptorchidism

The testis which is not in a low scrotal position by the age of 2 years has been found to be histologically abnormal; spontaneous descent rarely occurs after 1 year. It is generally believed that the lower temperature in the scrotum is a prerequisite for normal spermatogenesis. There is little evidence that surgical orchidopexy for an undescended testis after 2 years of age improves fertility. For these reasons, treatment should ideally be undertaken between 1 and 2 years of age. Evidence suggests that fertility may also be impaired in boys with retractile testis who experience spontaneous descent during puberty.

Apart from the association with infertility, cryptorchidism is a well established risk factor for testicular malignancy. Some 10% of cases have a history of cryptorchidism. The risk of testicular tumour in a patient with a history of undescended testis, whether successfully treated or not, is 4 to 10-fold higher than in the general population. Other risks of cryptorchidism such as testicular torsion and psychological morbidity also argue for an aggressive approach to treatment in early childhood.

Testicular toxins

The actively dividing male germ cells are one of the most sensitive cell types in the body with regard to the toxic effects of radiation, cytotoxic drugs and an increasing number of chemicals. Indeed, male gonadal function is probably the most sensitive index for overexposure to potential toxins (in the workplace, environment, foods, cosmetics and medicines). The classic example is lead, which the ancient Romans used to sweeten their food and wine, contributing to a decline in fertility. The best documented modern example is the pesticide dibromochloropropane (DBCP), which was responsible for azoospermic infertility in half of the male workers in a factory (Whorton et al 1977). The most common example in clinical practice today is sulphasalazine for the treatment of inflammatory bowel diseases. The carrier moiety, sulphapyridine, reversibly impairs sperm motility and sperm function in some patients (Bonnie et al 1981). There has been concern that environmental toxins, possibly in the form of oestrogens, have led to a reduction in the number of sperm and an increased incidence of testicular maldescent and cryptorchidism (Sharpe 1994).

Cytotoxic treatment regimes for Hodgkin's disease, lymphoma, leukaemia and other malignancies damage the differentiating spermatogonia, so that most patients become azoospermic after 8 weeks. The degree of stem cell killing governs whether there is recovery of spermatogenesis or not after treatment. This is dependent on the cumulative dose of the drug combination used. Long-term follow up has shown that following six or more courses of MOPP (mustine, vincristine, procarbazine and prednisolone), over 85% of patients remained azoospermic, and recovery is unlikely after 4 years. Similarly, radiation exposure of over 6 Gy destroys germ cells with no chance of recovery. While 1–4 Gy produces complete cessation of spermatogenesis with only some stem spermatogonia surviving, there may be recovery after 12–36 months and spermatogenesis may continue to improve for several years but even then it may not be complete. Diagnostic procedures and therapeutic irradiation to other organs such as the thyroid usually expose the testis to 1 Gy.

A number of other drugs are also associated with detrimental effects on spermatogenesis. These include nitrofurantoin, anabolic steroids, sex steroids and anticonvulsants. Recreational drugs such as cigarettes, alcohol and cannabis have all been linked with lower semen quality.

Testicular function is impaired in chronic renal failure; improvement may occur after successful transplantation but not dialysis. Pyrexial illness may non-specifically depress spermatogenesis for some weeks but recovery is complete.

Orchitis

Symptomatic orchitis occurs as a complication in 27–30% of males over the age of 10–11 years who suffer from mumps. In 17% of cases, orchitis is bilateral. Seminiferous tubular atrophy is a common sequela of mumps orchitis but recovery of spermatogenesis even after persistent azoospermia for 1 year has been reported (Sandler 1954). The prevalence of infertility after mumps orchitis is unknown but fertility should only be significantly impaired if the orchitis is bilateral and occurs after puberty.

Gonadotrophin deficiency

Secondary testicular failure due to gonadotrophin deficiency is a rare but important condition to recognize, because it is the only category of male infertility that is consistently treatable by hormone replacement. The diagnosis is prompted by clinical evidence of androgen deficiency, and confirmed by low or undetectable levels of gonadotrophin associated with subnormal testosterone. Depending on severity, cause and the time of onset, the clinical features and responsiveness to treatment are variable.

The spectrum includes patients with complete congenital deficiency in LH-releasing hormone (GnRH), which results in total failure of testicular and secondary sexual development. Other patients with the so-called fertile eunuch syndrome have less severe or partial GnRH deficiency, so that they have larger (4–10 ml) but still underdeveloped testes with more evidence of germ cell activity. There is also the rare form with an isolated deficiency of FSH where the man is androgenized but with absent sperm production. In three-quarters of these patients, anosmia or hyposmia and a variety of midline defects can be detected; this is the association known as Kallmann's syndrome.

In contrast to these congenital varieties of isolated hypogonadotrophic hypogonadism, postnatally or postpubertally acquired gonadotrophin deficiency may arise from tumours, chronic inflammatory lesions, iron overload or injuries of the hypothalamus and pituitary, so that deficits in other pituitary hormones usually coexist. These patients have developed seminiferous tubules which regressed through lack of trophic hormone support. Their testes volumes are larger (10–15 ml) than in the former two groups.

Varicocele

The significance of varicocele in male infertility is controversial (see review by Hargreave 1995), but in adolescents a varicocele leads to reduced testicular size and reduced semen quality (Laven et al 1992). Reflux of blood in the internal spermatic vein gives rise to distension of the pampiniform venous plexus and reduction in ipsilateral testicular volume. In infertile patients with unilateral varicocele, varying degrees of non-specific histological abnormalities can be detected in both testes. Increased scrotal temperature, hypoxia and exposure of the testes to adrenal metabolites have been postulated as possible mechanisms by which spermatic vein reflux can induce seminiferous tubular damage. Since varicoceles can be detected clinically in 15% of young males and semen quality is not different in fertile men presenting for vasectomy with or without varicoceles (de Castro & Mastorocco 1994), it must be emphasized that the condition is not invariably associated with reduced fertility. Therefore the clinician should not automatically assume that the varicocele is directly responsible for infertility without actively excluding other possible aetiologies in a full assessment.

The diagnosis of visible (grade 3) and palpable (grade 2) varicoceles is not difficult when the patient is examined in a standing position. The detection of subclinical (grade 1) varicoceles, where spermatic vein reflux can only be detected during the Valsalva manoeuvre, requires more experience and has been aided by the use of Doppler or scrotal thermography.

Idiopathic testicular failure

Failure of seminiferous tubular function to the extent of producing azoospermia or severe oligozoospermia (<5 million) is usually associated with small (under 15 ml) and soft testes and elevated FSH. Histologically, the tubules may show completely absent or reduced numbers of germ cells, narrow tubular diameter and thickening and hyalinization of peritubular tissue. These changes are non-specific and are not always uniformly distributed throughout the testes. Although the Leydig cells appear normal, there is evidence of malfunction in that near-normal testosterone is maintained only by higher amplitudes of LH pulsatile secretion in these patients (Wu et al 1989). It is however unlikely that testosterone deficiency is the primary cause of defective spermatogenesis.

There is also no evidence to support the contention that abnormalities in pulse frequency of GnRH may be the underlying cause of idiopathic hypospermatogenesis. According to our current view these structural and functional abnormalities are the end-results of the most extreme degrees of disruptions in the paracrine regulation in the testis. These patients usually remain infertile and there is no treatment available. Less severe degrees of oligozoospermia are commonly associated with abnormal morphology and reduced motility.

Asthenozoospermia

Absent or extremely low sperm motility of only 1–2% may result from absence of dynein arms, radial spokes or nexin bridges and dysplasia of fibrous sheath. This is associated with similar defects in respiratory cilia and therefore frequently a history of chronic respiratory infection, bronchiectasis and sinusitis: the immotile cilia syndrome. In addition, some of these patients have situs inversus (Kartagener's syndrome). Based on this classic but extremely rare example, it is now becoming clear that more common but less severe degrees of asthenozoospermia may also be associated with more subtle structural malformations in the axonemal complex, recognizable only with ultrastructural examination and functionally evident as suboptimal sperm movements.

Teratozoospermia

Surface morphology directly reflects the maturity and functional integrity of the spermatozoa so that morphological analysis of ejaculated sperm is an important means of assessing spermatogenesis in the testis. Indeed, some workers believe that sperm morphology is the best predictor of spontaneous fertility or the outcome of in vitro fertilization (Kruger et al 1988, 1995). It has been reported that morphology in the individual spermatozoon is positively related to movement characteristics (swimming velocity, sperm head trajectories, flagellar beat frequency) which reflect the vigour of the cell (Morales et al 1988) and its ability to exhibit hyperactivation. Similarly, the ability to undergo the acrosome reaction has also been shown to be significantly higher in sperm with morphologically normal, compared with abnormal, sperm heads (Fukuda et al 1989). Ultrastructural studies have also revealed a variety of structural malformations of the acrosome complex, the most extreme example being the round-headed sperm where the acrosome is completely missing, but lesser degrees of acrosomal defects are increasingly being identified.

Fertilization blocks in these developmental (morphological) abnormalities, i.e. teratozoospermia, are unlikely to be amenable to treatment by assisted reproductive procedures.

These attempts to relate specific functional defects to recognizable structural malformations in individual spermatozoa provide evidence that morphologically abnormal sperm are also functionally impaired. If the information extrapolates to morphologically abnormal sperm in the semen of infertile men, then this could be one reason why teratozoospermia is associated with subfertility. Functional differences between subpopulations of morphologically normal and abnormal sperm may be accentuated after the spermatozoa are separated from seminal plasma. This may be an important reason for the success of in vitro fertilization in treating cases of male infertility with good morphology, using sperm subpopulations harvested into artificial media (Kruger et al 1988).

Androgen insensitivity

Low androgen receptor levels in cultured fibroblasts from genital or pubic skin were reported to be present in 40% of oligozoospermic men with normal male phenotypes (Aiman & Griffen 1982) but this has not been confirmed. Testosterone and LH are usually normal in these patients, and the defect has been regarded as the least severe manifestation of the spectrum of phenotypic abnormalities associated with defects in androgen receptor function. Because of the low concentration and instability during isolation, our understanding of the role of the androgen receptor in regulating spermatogenesis is poor. The recent cloning of the human androgen receptor cDNA has cleared the way for studying possible alterations in androgen receptor expression, structure and function in relation to abnormal spermatogenesis.

Sperm autoimmunity

The significance of immunological infertility due to antibodies against spermatozoa has been a matter for dispute but has now gained acceptance. Much of this controversy arose because of the inadequacies in differentiating specific antibodies which suppress sperm function from those that are of doubtful clinical relevance. The realization that immunological infertility is a specific disorder caused by sperm membrane-bound immunoglobulin gamma A has resolved some of the discrepancies from earlier data, based mainly on sperm agglutination or immobilization tests, which correlated with circulating immunoglobulin gamma G or M antibodies and had little direct pathophysiological significance. The newer methods of detecting specific classes of antibody on the sperm surface membrane or seminal plasma have therefore greatly refined the accuracy of this diagnosis and brought it into the realms of potentially treatable infertility.

The incidence of sperm autoimmunity has been reported to be between 2.7 and 23% of men presenting for infertility. This obviously depends on patient selection and the method of testing, but the true incidence of significant sperm antibody is unlikely to be higher than 5%. Conditions predisposing to sperm autoimmunity include vasectomy, testicular injury or inflammation, genital tract obstruction and family history of autoimmune disease. The incidence of sperm antibody in female partners is not well documented but is believed to be much less common than in males. This however should be regarded as an open issue and more attention should be focused on antibodies in cervical mucus in women with unexplained infertility. It is now the practice of most clinics to screen for sperm antibodies in all male patients except those with testicular failure due to chromosomal abnormalities.

Male patients with significant sperm antibody usually have severely suppressed fertility potential (<0.5%/month pregnancy rate). The major identifiable defect is interference with sperm passage through cervical mucus but there is evidence that fertilization may also be impeded (Clarke et al 1985, Dom et al 1981).

Genital tract infection

Infection in the lower genital tract is a treatable cause of male infertility and the incidence varies in different communities. Gram-negative enterococci, chlamydia and gonococcus are established pathogenic organisms which usually produce unequivocal clinical evidence of infection (adnexitis), such as painful ejaculation, pelvic or sacral pain, urethral discharge, haematospermia, dysuria, irregular tender epididymides and tender boggy prostate. This can be confirmed by semen culture, urethral swabs, and the presence of more than 1 million peroxidase-positive polymorphonuclear neutrophils per millilitre of semen or in expressed prostatic fluid. Inflammation of the accessory glands and excurrent ducts may give rise to disturbed function, formation of sperm antibody and permanent structural damage with obstruction in the outflow tract.

The entity of asymptomatic prostatitis is poorly defined and there is little evidence to support a genuine role for occult infections in male infertility. There is thus no place for microbiological screening investigations unless there is clinical suspicion of adnexitis. Furthermore, the isolation of non-pathogenic organisms such as staphylococcus, streptococcus, diptheroids, *Ureaplasma urealyticum* and *Mycoplasma hominis*, which are commensals in the normal urethra, does not warrant the indiscriminate use of antibiotics in the hope of correcting any abnormalities in the semen parameters.

Genital tract obstruction

The combination of azoospermia, normal testicular volume and normal FSH bears the hallmarks of genital tract obstruction. The incidence and relative importance of individual causes of obstruction differ according to geographic locality. The relative frequency of the different sites of obstruction, as presented in England, is shown in Table 18.2 (Hendry et al 1990b, Pryor 1994b). Post-congenital and postvasectomy obstructions are the most common, but in some parts of the world infectious causes, particularly gonorrhea, tuberculosis and smallpox, are of greater importance.

Three specific congenital abnormalities are recognized. The commonest is agenesis or malformations of the wolffian duct-derived structures: the corpus/cauda epididymis, vas deferens and seminal vesicles. Diagnosis is usually quite easy: the scrotal vasa are not palpable and the ejaculate consists of low volumes (<1 ml) of acidic non-coagulating prostatic fluid devoid of fructose and sperm. Virtually all males with cystic fibrosis are sterile because of this congenital bilateral absence of the vas deferens (CBAVD). It is of interest that 10% of healthy men with CBAVD are homozygous for the cystic fibrosis genes and 40% are heterozygous (Oates & Amos 1995).

In Young's syndrome the obstruction is at the junction of the caput and body of the epididymis and there is marked inspissation of amorphous secretion in the lumen. In these patients, the high incidence of chronic sino-pulmonary infection and bronchiectasis is presumably the consequence of the same abnormality in the respiratory tract and may be the result of mercury poisoning (Hendry et al 1990).

Table 18.2 Site of obstruction in azoospermia (excluding vasectomy)

	Hendry et al (1990b)		Pryor (1994)		Total	
	n	%	*n*	%	*n*	%
Intratesticular	4	1.2	47	16	51	8
Epididymal	176	55	163	51	349	54
Vasal	40	13	39	12	79	12
Bilateral absent vasa	67	21	58	18	125	20
Unilateral absent vas	19	6	11	3	30	5
Ejaculatory duct	14	4	3	1	17	3
Total number	320		321		641	

Table 18.3 Classification of ejaculatory duct obstruction

Congenital	
Midline (müllerian)	23
Lateral (wolffian)	28
Traumatic	17
Inflammatory	30
Neurogenic	22
Neoplastic	2
Total	122

Obstruction of the ejaculatory duct is an uncommon cause of obstructive azoospermia with semen abnormality as in CBAVD, but it may be distinguished by palpation of the scrotal vasa. The causes of ejaculatory duct obstruction are shown in Table 18.3.

Coital disorders

Inadequate coital technique (including the use of vaginal lubricants with spermicidal properties) and frequency and faulty timing of intercourse may contribute to continuing infertility, but are rarely the only aetiological factor in the infertile couple. Erectile and ejaculatory failure may be caused by psychosexual dysfunction, depression, spinal cord injuries, retroperitoneal and bladder neck surgery, diabetes mellitus, multiple sclerosis, vascular insufficiency, adrenergic blocking antihypertensive agents, psychotropic drugs, alcohol abuse and chronic renal failure. Primary endocrine pathologies such as androgen deficiency, hyperprolactinaemia and hypothyroidism seldom present with infertility without diminished libido and clinical features specific to the hormonal disturbance, e.g. hypogonadism, loss of visual fields and myxoedema. Retrograde ejaculation must be differentiated from aspermia or anejaculation by examination of postejaculatory urine for the presence of spermatozoa.

CLINICAL MANAGEMENT

The essence of clinical management is to assess the prognosis (chances of conception per year or per cycle of assisted conception) and to advise the couple as to those treatment options that should improve the prognosis. This advice is based upon a sound knowledge of the causes of infertility and the treatment options available. It is also necessary to take account of the age of the female partner and the duration of fertility. It is important to obtain a full history and examination and basic investigations of the man.

History

A thorough history is essential for identifying underlying aetiologies and devising individual management strategies. Particular attention should be paid to the following aspects. Previous surgery such as herniorrhaphy in childhood, trauma or torsion suggests possible damage to the vas or testis. Cryptorchidism, especially if bilateral, is associated with severe impairment of fertility and carries an increased risk of testicular malignancy. Although most patients presenting in infertility clinics with a history of cryptorchidism have generally received treatment when younger, orchidopexy is seldom carried out so early as to completely avoid testicular damage. Previous genitourinary infections in the form of orchitis (mumps, syphilis, leprosy, tuberculosis, schistosomiasis) are serious causes of infertility in a global context. Painful ejaculation, haematospermia and pain in the perineum are symptoms, suggestive of chronic infection in the prostate and seminal vesicles. Delayed onset of puberty may suggest the possibility of gonadotrophin deficiency. A history of recurrent chest infection, sinusitis or bronchiectasis may be obtained in patients with epididymal obstruction (Young's syndrome), or those with absent sperm motility (immotile cilia syndrome) and agenesis of the vasa (cystic fibrosis). Chronic disorders such as renal failure, liver disease, malignancy, diabetes and multiple sclerosis are associated with a variety of testicular and sexual dysfunctions. Because feverish illness can transiently suppress spermatogenesis, the patient should be asked about episodes of pyrexia within the past 6 weeks. Careful enquiry should also be made about occupational or environmental exposure to testicular toxins (herbicides, pesticides, lead, cadmium), radiation, or the use of medications (cytotoxic agents, sulphasalazine, nitrofurantoin, anabolic steroids, sex steroids, anticonvulsants, psychotropic and antihypertensive drugs and cimetidine) or recreational drugs (alcohol, tobacco, cannabis).

It is important to establish that vaginal intercourse takes place with appropriate frequency and timing, without the use of vaginal lubricants which may have spermicidal properties. With experience, it is not difficult to detect the presence of psychosexual dysfunction and varying degrees of more general psychiatric symptoms not uncommonly associated with the stigma and stress of continuing infertility.

Examination

The general physical assessment of height, weight, body habitus and secondary sexual development should be carried out in all patients. If androgen deficiency is suspected look for gynaecomastia, a female distribution of hair, cryptorchidism, hypospadias, anosmia and visual field defects. Measurement of testicular volumes by comparison with a series of standard ellipsoids known as the Prader orchidometer (Fig. 18.6) provides a convenient clinical index of seminiferous tubular mass. The length of the testes may be measured and used as a guide to spermatogenesis in azoospermia (Table 18.4) and is useful in

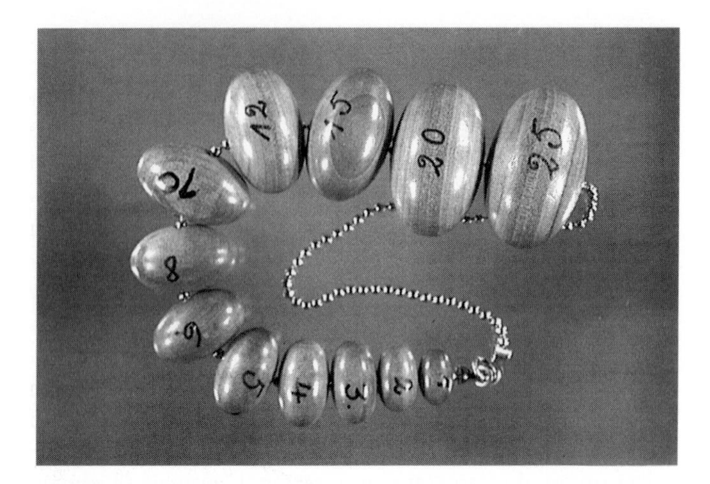

Fig. 18.6 Prader orchidometer for the assessment of testicular volume.

Table 18.4 Relationship between testicular size and spermatogenesis in azoospermic men

Testicular size		Biopsies, number and (%)	Mean Johnsen (1970) score, number and (%)		
Length, cm	Volume, ml		≤2.0	2.1–7.9	≥8.0
2	3	11 (100)	11(100)		
3	8	71 (100)	36 (51)	34(48)	1 (1)
4	15	118 (100)	39 (33)	35(30)	44 (37)
5	30	198 (100)	11 (6)	35(18)	152 (77)

differentiating between azoospermia due to seminiferous tubular failure (reduced volumes) and that arising from excurrent duct obstruction (normal volume). Testicular size is also a useful indicator of the degree of testicular development in hypogonadotrophic patients.

Special attention should also be paid to the palpation of the epididymis and scrotal vas. An enlarged and tense caput epididymis may be palpable in obstructive azoospermia and absence of the vas deferens should always be detected. The scrotal contents should also be examined with the patient standing so that varioceles become visible (grade 3) or palpable (grade 2) or are detected as a venous impulse in the spermatic cord during the Valsalva manoeuvre (grade 1). Rectal examination may show irregular contour or consistency and tenderness in the prostate in the presence of chronic prostatitis.

Investigations

Semen analysis

Traditionally, the most important starting point for investigating the male contribution to a couple's infertility is the semen analysis (World Health Organization (WHO) 1992) but it must be emphasized that conventional parameters of semen analysis such as sperm concentration, percentage of motile sperm, quality of sperm movements and sperm morphology (Table 18.5) are predominantly subjective, and at best are semiquantitative evaluations with poor reproducibility. It must be realized that these values refer to normal men rather than to normal fertility. Hargreave & Elton (1983) found that the chances of conception did not improve once there were more than 2 million motile sperm per millilitre (Table 18.6) and this figure is similar to the finding of Hull and colleagues (1985). The total number of sperm is of less importance than the number of sperm with fertilizing capacity.

Table 18.5 Normal values of semen variables (WHO 1992)

Volume	2.0 ml or more
pH	7.2–7.8
Sperm concentration	20×10^6 spermatozoa/ml or more
Total sperm count	40×10^6 spermatozoa or more
Motility	50% or more with forward progression 25% or more with rapid linear progression within 60 min after collection
Morphology	30% or more with normal morphology
Viability	75% or more live, i.e. excluding dye
White blood cells	Fewer than 1×10^6/ml
Fructose (total)	13 μmol or more per ejaculate
MAR test	Fewer than 10% spermatozoa with adherent particles

Table 18.6 Percentage chance of spontaneous conception during the subsequent 12 months for couples attending an infertility clinic (Hargreave & Elton 1983)

Motile sperm concentration, million/ml	Duration of infertility, years			
	1	2	4	8
0	0	0	0	0
0.5	16	12	9	6
1	25	19	14	9
2	34	26	19	13
5	36	28	21	14
>10	37	28	21	14

Sperm function tests

The need for sperm function tests arises from the apparent failure of the standard semen analysis to discriminate between the fertile and the infertile. The semen analysis should be performed according to the guidelines established by the World Health Organization (WHO 1992) and with adequate quality controls (Mortimer 1994). Fertilization requires the correct sequence of many distinct processes, and a variety of biological tests have been developed to identify abnormalities of these processes.

The swim-up test. Assisted conception techniques aim to resuspend spermatozoa and the 'swim-up' technique used to be the one most commonly used. The seminal sample is overlaid with a well buffered sperm medium, and incubated for 1 h at 37°C in a carbon dioxide incubator and with the incubation tubes inclined at an angle of 30 degrees. The motile sperm swim into the upper layer and are then used for in vitro fertilization. In some patients the initial semen sample has appeared to be normal but there was repeated failure to find spermatozoa in the upper layer of fluid. It is also customary to maintain the spermatozoa in culture for 24–48 h and a decrease in sperm motility is associated with decreased fertilizing capacity.

In many laboratories the standard swim-up technique has been replaced by one using Percoll filtration (silica gel particles coated with polyvinylpyrolidone in colloidal solution, marketed by Pharmacia). The results of swim-up techniques have not been systematically analysed, but they were frequently used as a guideline before embarking upon in vitro fertilization.

Computer-assisted seminal analysis (CASA). This technique should be more reproducible and independent of observer error, and its great advantage is that it is capable of analysing the amplitude, frequency and velocity of spermatozoa. It is of less value for measuring sperm concentration and the number of motile sperm. It may be adapted for assessing sperm morphology, using the strict criteria of Kruger and colleagues (1993).

The results of such analyses have been applied to the outcomes of donor insemination and in vitro fertilization programmes but in general terms they have proved disappointing in predicting fertilization (Irvine & Aitken 1987, Liu et al 1991) and there is still variation in the results obtained (Holt 1994).

Capacitation. This is characterized by the development in spermatozoa of the hyperactive motility that is necessary in order for penetration of the oocyte to occur. Hyperactivated sperm may be recognized by CASA and show an increase in sperm beat amplitude, increased asymmetrical movement of the sperm head and a loss of forward progressive motility. Although such hyperactivated movement may be identified using CASA, particularly with a video attachment, it does not correlate well with the outcome of penetration of zona-free hamster oocytes (Wang et al 1991).

Hypo-osmotic swelling assay (HOS). This assay (WHO 1992) determines the functional integrity of the sperm's plasma membrane, which is assessed by observing curling of the tail under hypo-osmotic conditions. It was described in 1984 and its role was reviewed in 1992 (Jeyendran et al 1992, Van der Suffele et al 1992), but it does not seem to be of great value in predicting fertility (Biljan et al 1994).

Hemizona assay (HZA). It is necessary for the spermatozoa to bind to the zona pellucida in order for fertilization to occur. This may be tested in ova stored in a high salt solution, but as zona binding is dependent on oocyte maturity it is necessary to have a control. The oocyte must then be divided in two with a micropipette so that each half acts as its own control with a fertile sample. The hemizona test is a useful means of assessing human zona binding and gives some correlation with fertility (Burkman et al 1988, Franken et al 1993, Oehminger 1992). Difficulties in obtaining human oocytes, and the frequent failure of the test to identify the cause of failed fertilization, has limited the clinical usefulness of this test.

Acrosome reaction. Spermatozoa undergo the acrosome reaction as they bind to the surface of the zona pellucida with liberation of proteases from the acrosome vesicle. This process facilitates the passage of spermatozoa through the zona pellucida. Unfortunately the acrosome vesicle is too small to be seen by light microscopy and it is necessary to use monoclonal antibodies labelled with fluorolein to identify non-acrosome-reacted spermatozoa. These staining tests of acrosome reaction (Cross et al 1986, Cummings et al 1991, De Jonge 1994, Mendoza et al 1992) are complemented by biochemical assays for acrosin (Francavilla et al 1992), semen adenosine triphosphate (ATP) (WHO Task Force 1992) and sperm creatine kinase (Huszar et al 1992). The acrosome reaction identifies one of the many causes for failure of fertilization, but although it has been suggested that it may be used to identify those patients who might benefit from the use of sperm stimulants (Yovich et al 1994), this has not found popular acceptance.

Biochemical aspects of sperm function. The possibility of using a biological chemical substance as a marker of sperm function is attractive. Human spermatozoa can generate reactive oxygen species such as superoxide anion and hydrogen peroxide. The former may be measured and increased levels may be associated with impaired sperm function (Aitken et al 1991, Kraus et al 1994).

Creatine phosphokinase is another marker of defective sperm function. The enzyme is essential in the synthesis, transport and dephosphorylation of creatinine phosphate and there is some correlation of its level with fertility (Huszar 1994). The results are independent of sperm number and, whilst promising, it is unlikely that they will have sufficient predictive value to be more than a research tool.

Sperm penetration tests. A good result from an in vivo postcoital test is sometimes considered to be the best single test of sperm function (Hull et al 1982) but a poorly performed test, often at the wrong time in the woman's cycle, is a waste of time. In an attempt to overcome some of the difficulties of in vivo testing, attempts have been made to replace human ovulatory cervical mucus with hyaluronic acid polymers or bovine cervical mucus. The outcome of these tests would appear to depend upon sperm motility (Aitken et al 1992, Mortimer et al 1990), and they have less to offer than a proper postcoital test.

The hamster oocyte penetration assay (HOP). In 1976 Yanagimachi and colleagues discovered that spermatozoa from man, and other mammalian species, would penetrate zona-free oocytes from the golden hamster (Yanagimachi et al 1976). The possibility of a real test of sperm function offered exciting possibilities, and two negative tests in semen of otherwise normal quality indicated a cause for infertility, as was shown in a reported study when eight out of 10 wives rapidly conceived when inseminated with donor sperm (Sutherland et al 1985). It should be noted that when the result was compared to the results of in vitro fertilization a false-negative result occurred in 44% of instances and a false-positive result in 11% (Sutherland et al 1985). Enthusiasm for the test soared and a conference was organized to standardize the conditions under which the test was performed (Aitken 1986, WHO 1992).

The test gives some correlation with fertility (Margalioth et al 1989, Soffer et al 1992), but Aitken and colleagues found that there was a 24% pregnancy rate in men with zero penetration (Aitken et al 1991) and it would therefore seem to remain as a research tool rather than of clinical significance (Aitken 1994).

Application of sperm function tests. The realization that the definition of normal quality semen (WHO 1992) has little predictive value with regard to fertility has led many authors to seek better predictive tests of sperm function. In reality it is the definition that is false and it is important to recognize that normal fertility is associated with lesser quality semen. When the definition of normality is changed, then the results of the standardized semen test offer good predictive values of fertility.

Many of the advanced sperm function tests that have been described are difficult to perform and also have poor predictive values. They are useful research tools and capable of identifying some of the specific causes for infertility. In clinical practice, in vitro fertilization remains the best test of sperm function, and failed fertilization is best treated by intracytoplasmic sperm injection.

Hormone measurements

The measurement of plasma FSH is useful in distinguishing primary from secondary testicular failure and in identifying patients with obstructive azoospermia. In the presence of azoospermia or oligozoospermia, an elevated FSH, particularly with reduced testicular volume, is presumptive evidence of severe and usually irreversible seminiferous tubular damage. Low or undetectable FSH (usually associated with low LH and testosterone, with clinical evidence of androgen deficiency) is suggestive of hypogonadotrophism. Conversely, azoospermia with normal FSH and normal testicular volume usually indicates the presence of bilateral genital tract obstruction. Occasional exceptions to these general rules occur from time to time, as azoospermic men with the Sertoli cell-only syndrome may be associated with normal FSH levels while some men with high FSH may have normal spermatogenesis.

Testosterone and LH measurements are indicated in the assessment of the infertile male when there is clinical suspicion of androgen deficiency, sex steroid abuse or steroid-secreting lesions such as congenital adrenal hyperplasia or functioning adrenal/testicular tumours. In men presenting with infertility, testosterone is usually within the normal range although some degree of Leydig cell dysfunction, as evidenced by statistically lower testosterone and higher LH compared to normal, is not uncommon. This may identify those who may be considered for androgen replacement, although this has no bearing on fertility. High LH and testosterone should raise the possibility of abnormalities in androgen receptors while low LH and testosterone suggest hypogonadotrophism.

Hyperprolactinaemia is not a frequent cause of male infertility, but prolactin measurement should be undertaken if there is clinical evidence of sexual dysfunction (particularly diminished libido) or pituitary disease leading to secondary testicular failure. Oestradiol measurement is rarely indicated except in the presence of gynaecomastia.

Dynamic tests of pituitary–testicular function such as GnRH, thyrotrophin-releasing hormone and human chorionic gonadotrophin stimulation generally do not add to the basal measurements already described. Bearing in mind the episodic nature of LH secretion, the diurnal variation in testosterone and the stress-related secretion of prolactin, it is usually sufficient to repeat their measurements in the morning under resting conditions if necessary.

Chromosome analysis

Buccal smear and/or chromosome karyotyping may be carried out in patients with azoospermia or severe oligospermia with testicular atrophy and elevated FSH. Cytogenetic abnormalities, by far the commonest being Klinefelter's syndrome, may be detected in about 10% of this group.

Testicular biopsy

With the use of plasma FSH in recent years to differentiate between primary testicular failure and obstructive lesions, the need for testicular biopsy in the investigation of male infertility has largely been superseded. However, when genital tract obstruction is suspected, testicular biopsy is still useful in confirming normal spermatogenesis and excluding spermatogenic arrest. When the clinical differentiation between spermatogenic failure and obstruction is uncertain (e.g. asymmetrical findings on examination between right and left testes or adnexae), scrotal exploration with testicular biopsy may be helpful. Vasography during scrotal exploration is required to confirm the diagnosis of obstructed ejaculatory ducts. Some would also advocate testicular biopsy, with or without scrotal exploration, to diagnose partial epididymal obstruction in patients with severe oligozoospermia and normal FSH. It is important to remember that even in primary testicular failure with small testes, elevated levels of FSH and a testicular biopsy showing Sertoli cell-only syndrome, some areas of spermatogenesis may be present in the testis (Silber et al 1995).

There are many techniques for describing the appearances of a testicular biopsy but the combination of words and a qualitative assessment, using Johnsen scoring (Johnsen 1970) is useful. In the Johnsen score the histological features of spermatogenesis are scored from 1 to 10 (2, Sertoli cell only; 3, spermatogonia; 4, 5, spermatocytes; 6, 7, spermatids; 8, 9, 10, spermatozoa).

Antisperm antibodies

The mixed agglutination reaction (MAR test) uses sheep red blood cells coated with rabbit antibodies to specific classes of human immunoglobulins, which will attach to motile sperm carrying immunoglobulins of the same class on their surface membrane (Bronsen et al 1984). This permits the detection of immunoglobulin gamma A, G or M on the surface of the sperm head or tail. The direct test uses washed sperm from the patient, and the presence of surface-bound antibody, indicated by particulate binding in over 10% of spermatozoa, is considered to be a positive result. It depends on the availability of sufficient numbers of motile sperm in the patient's fresh semen sample and is currently the standard screening test in most laboratories.

The indirect test uses decomplemented patient serum or seminal plasma which is incubated with motile donor sperm and is known as the tray agglutination test. Antisperm antibodies will bind to donor sperm and their presence is detected by attachment of particles to the sperm surface. The indirect test is therefore more convenient for screening larger numbers of patients.

A positive screening test, however, must be substantiated by investigations to assess the biological significance of sperm antibody. This is usually a test to determine the ability of sperm to penetrate normal midcycle cervical mucus.

MANAGEMENT

The management of male infertility often remains a difficult and somewhat unsatisfactory experience for patients as well as doctors. Many patients present no recognizable or reversible aetiological factors for treatment, and the doctor frequently fails to appreciate that normal semen values do not relate to fertility. In recent years there have been a number of advances which have made a significant impact on our therapeutic capabilities. It is important to improve semen quality and to treat those factors that impair fertility.

General measures

The man should be encouraged to improve his lifestyle: avoiding stress, having a healthy diet and taking exercise. Recreational drugs such as cigarettes, alcohol and cannabis should be withdrawn if possible. Medications that interfere with fertility, such as nitrofurantoin, anabolic steroids, sex steroids and anticonvulsants, should be avoided if possible. In patients with inflammatory bowel disease treated by sulphasalazine, changing treatment to 5-aminosalicylic acid removes the toxic agent, sulphapyridine, and leads to a rapid recovery of fertility without deterioration in disease activity. Although testicular function may improve in patients with chronic renal failure after successful transplantation, fertility impairment may be perpetuated by the continued use of immunosuppressive agents.

The merits of a positive approach are undoubted, particularly when the partner is young and the duration of infertility short.

Medical treatment

Management of gonadotrophin deficiency

Patients with gonadotrophin deficiency due to acquired conditions and, to a lesser extent, those with partial GnRH deficiency, usually respond to human chorionic gonadotrophin (Profasi 2000 iu i.m. once or twice weekly) alone for 6–12 months (Burger & Baker 1982). During this time the rise in testosterone will virilize the patient and the testes will usually increase in size. If there is no sperm in the ejaculate at the end of 12 months, human menopausal gonadotrophin (Pergonal) which contains both FSH and LH should be added, 37.5 iu i.m. thrice weekly initially, increasing to 75 iu thrice-weekly if necessary after 6 months. This graded approach may take up to 2 years before one can ascertain if spermatogenesis is established or not.

The treatment outcome of gonadotrophin induction of spermatogenesis is variable but in general, 64–76% should show some degree of spermatogenesis and 54–60% could be expected to achieve pregnancies. Previous treatment with testosterone does not appear to compromise the response to subsequent exogenous gonadotrophin (Burger & Baker 1982).

In patients with more profound degrees of GnRH deficiency, it might be anticipated that the most suitable form of replacement to induce maximal testicular growth and development is to emulate the physiological mode of pulsatile GnRH stimulation of the pituitary and in turn, the testes. This has been made possible by the development of battery-driven portable infusion minipumps which can automatically deliver a desired dose of GnRH at a set time interval.

Management of genital tract infection

The presence of organisms in the ejaculate is a potent cause of poor sperm function and may lead to obstructive lesions of the genital tract. Symptomatic urethritis is readily diagnosed and responds to treatment with the appropriate antibiotics.

Chronic infection of the male genital tract is more difficult to diagnose and the presence of pus cells in the semen only indicates an infection in some patients. An alkaline pH (greater than 8.0) may occur in prostatitis due to decreased secretion of acid phosphatase by the prostate. Repeated growth on culture of the same organisms is probably of significance as is the finding of organisms during a modified Stamey test (Meares & Stamey 1972) where the semen culture replaces the culture of expressed prostatic secretions.

The antibiotics chosen to treat prostatoseminal vesiculitis (such as doxycycline, erythromycins, cephalosporins or oflaxacin) should be secreted by the male accessory glands, and treatment should be continued for 4–12 weeks depending on the chronicity of the infection. In longer courses of treatment it is customary to rotate the antibiotics, but overall the current tendency is towards a shorter duration (6 weeks) of treatment consisting of two antibiotics each of which is taken for 3 weeks.

Culture of mycoplasma and of chlamydia is difficult and this makes diagnoses of the prevalence and importance of chronic male genital tract infection controversial. There is a wide variation of infection in different communities and for this reason many clinicians opt for a brief (4–6 week) course of empirical treatment with antibiotics if there is any suspicion of infection.

Management of antisperm antibodies

The presence of antisperm antibodies is a common cause of unexplained male factor infertility. It should be suspected when there is a poor postcoital test and in these circumstances the MAR test will usually be positive. Antisperm antibodies may be associated with decreased sperm motility. The diagnosis should be confirmed by finding a significant titre of antibody (greater than 1:32) in the blood, and before commencing treatment it is necessary to exclude any biochemical abnormality in the man and to check for a history of indigestion, bone pain or a family history of diabetes. Alcohol intake should be low during treatment with high doses of steroids, and the wife should have been fully investigated to exclude any other cause of infertility. The treatment regimen, with 20 mg twice daily doses of methyl prednisolone on days 1–10 of the wife's cycle and half the dose on days 11–12 is given for 3 months. The steroids are usually well tolerated although the man may gain a little weight, develop acne and become irritable. The dose of steroids is increased after 3 and 6 months if the wife has not conceived and I usually suggest that the couple proceed to standard IVF in the ninth cycle.

Treatment with methyl prednisolone was successful in 40% of couples in a double-blind controlled trial, where the female partner was fully assessed (Hendry et al 1990). There is also a small group of men with azoospermia, or even extreme oligozoospermia, normal spermatogenesis and no extratesticular obstruction where there may be an immunological cause for obstruction, as in some of these men there is a round cell infiltrate on the testicular biopsy (Hendry et al 1990b). It is worthwhile treating men with obstructive azoospermia with prednisolone, 5 mg three times daily, when there is no evidence of extratesticular obstruction, even when round cells are not seen on testicular biopsy.

Erectile failure

The inability of the man to obtain vaginal penetration may be overcome by the intracavernous injection of a vasoactive agent. Such a strategy is particularly useful in men with neurological problems or with performance anxiety. The physician should be familiar with the technique and avoid the tragedy of a priapism. Papaverine was for many years the drug of choice but this has been superseded by the licencing of alprostadil (Caverject) a prostaglandin E_1 preparation. In those men with organic impotence, the implantation of a penile prosthesis is a satisfactory solution to the problem.

Ejaculatory failure

Absent emission or retrograde ejaculation due to sympathetic denervation may respond to sympathomimetic drugs. The first choice is desipramine (50 mg on alternate days) for its noradrenaline reuptake blocking action. Ephedrine, 30 mg twice daily, brompheniramine maleate, 8 mg twice daily, or Imipramine, 25 mg three times daily may also be tried. It is always worthwhile trying desipramine in those men with a diabetic autonomic neuropathy. Urine inhibits sperm motility and for this reason spermatozoa should be separated from the urine as soon as possible and used for artificial insemination or assisted conception. Surgical reconstruction of the bladder neck is rarely required (Pryor 1994a).

Miscellaneous treatments

Free radicals undoubtedly have a role to play in male infertility (Aitken et al 1989) but few centres measure

Table 18.7 Categories of oligozoospermia

Intrinsic testicular failure	Sertoli cell-only Klinefelter's syndrome
Testicular failure	
(a) Secondary to hormone abnormalities	Hypogonadotrophic hypogonadism Hyperprolactinaemia
(b) Secondary to testicular damage	Maldescent Torsion Mumps/smallpox orchitis Devascularization Epididymitis Hernia repair Carcinoma-in-situ and tumour Radiotherapy Varicocele
Obstructions	
(a) Intratesticular	Congenital Immunological Infective
(b) Epididymal	Congenital dysplasia Pink disease Infective Iatrogenic
(c) Vasal	Congenital Infective Iatrogenic
(d) Ejaculatory duct	Congenital Infective Iatrogenic Adynamic

them as a routine. It is for this reason that ascorbic acid (1 g four times daily) and/or vitamin E (200 mg three times daily) are used on an empirical basis.

No drugs have been consistently shown to improve in vivo sperm motility but the elimination of infection or an antibody problem may be associated with improved motility. Ascorbic acid has been used empirically for poor motility and there has been some evidence to suggest that low levels of vitamin C are associated with auto-agglutination and poor motility.

There is good evidence to suggest that fertility is only reduced when there are less than 1–5 million motile sperms per ejaculate (Hargreave & Elton 1983, Hull et al 1985). This is reflected in the British Fertility Society guidelines and only extreme oligozoospermia (less than 1 million sperm per ejaculate) or severe oligozoospermia (up to 2.5 million/ml or up to 5 million/ejaculate) require investigation and treatment.

There are many causes for oligozoospermia (Table 18.7) and few are amenable to medical therapy (e.g. hormonal deficiency, infection or antibody). Over the years, a wide variety of essentially empirical treatments have been used in attempts to improve fertility in subfertile men. These include testosterone suppression and rebound, gonadotrophins, GnRH, clomiphene, tamoxifen, testolactone, antibiotics, bromocriptine, pentoxiphylline, pancreatic kallikrein, vitamin C, zinc and homologous artificial insemination.

Any new form of treatment has a strong placebo effect, not only on semen quality but also on conception rates. There is no evidence to suggest that androgens ever achieve more than this, and the inappropriate use of hCG or hMG may be detrimental and inhibit spermatogenesis.

Surgical treatments

Relief of obstruction

Obstructive lesions of the seminal tract should be suspected in azoospermia or severe oligozoospermia with normally sized testes (greater than 4 cm in length or 15–20 ml in volume), and with normal plasma follicle stimulating hormone levels. It is convenient to explore and biopsy the testes, perform vasography and correct any obstruction that is identified, under the same general anaesthetic. A fuller account of the indications, techniques and outcomes of surgical treatments of male infertility may be found elsewhere (Hull et al 1985, Pryor 1994).

Epididymal obstruction. The results of reconstructive surgery on the epididymis are varied and depend upon the cause and duration of obstruction and the expertise of the surgeon. Congenital blockages, and those that might be due to pink disease (Hendry et al 1990b) have a poor outcome, as do blockages resulting from tuberculous or chlamydial infections. The overall patency rate would appear to be about 10–15% of operations, as in many patients there is a great deal of scarring and the epididymis is filled with inspissated material. The best results are achieved when there is localized postgonococcal obstruction in the cauda epididymis, and in these instances sperm may appear in 50% of ejaculates after surgery. A microsurgical technique would appear to give a 10% improvement in patency rates. Spermatozoa acquire motility as they pass through the epididymis and higher pregnancy rates occur when the blockage is in the distal part of the epididymis (Schoysman & Bedford 1986).

Vasal obstruction. Vasal obstruction is less common in infertility practice and is treated by vasovasostomy. Many techniques are described but an end-to-end one-layer anastomosis with 6–0 sutures is simple and effective. Vasal obstruction most commonly occurs following vasectomy, and after vasovasostomy patency is to be expected in 80–90% of men with a conception rate of 40–50% in 1 year. Magnification is desirable and the use of an operating microscope for vasovasostomy is excellent training for the more difficult tubulovasostomy that is necessary in epididymal obstruction. The prognosis is worse for those men with a long interval between the vasectomy and reversal, but time does not prohibit any attempt to operate. The age of the female partner is of importance with regard to conception rates.

Ejaculatory duct obstruction. This is an uncommon cause of obstruction and is readily diagnosed by a low volume of semen, azoospermia or extreme oligozoospermia and an acid pH in a man with palpable vasa. Müllerian duct cysts are amenable to treatment (Pryor 1993) with sperm appearing in the ejaculate of 80% of men and conception in 33% of wives. Other forms of ejaculatory duct obstruction do less well and are probably best treated by sperm retrieval.

Surgery to overcome sexual problems

Surgery for ejaculatory failure. Surgical means to correct ejaculatory failure are rarely required, as in men with retrograde ejaculation spermatozoa may be obtained from the bladder and used for insemination. Some men insist on the restoration of antegrade ejaculation, and this may be performed using the Young–Dees technique with good results (Pryor 1988).

Surgery for erectile failure. The implantation of a penile prosthesis enables an impotent man to impregnate his wife through normal sexual intercourse. The choice of prosthesis is a personal one and depends upon considerations of cost, reliability and the requirement for flaccidity. Most men (90%) and their partners are satisfied with the outcome, and dissatisfaction stems from poor preoperative counselling allowing the man to have false expectations or from the removal of the prosthesis due to infection or mechanical failure.

Varicocele ligation

It is difficult to assess the true benefits of varicocele ligation owing to the impracticality of performing a true double-blind controlled trial. Dubin & Amelar (1977), in a series of 986 men, found that the semen quality improved in 80% of men and 50% of the wives conceived. In contrast, Nilsson et al (1979) found no difference in semen quality or conception rates between those varicoceles operated upon and those left untreated. Infertility is multifactorial in origin and treatment of a varicocele will not improve fertility if there are other more serious causes for the problem (e.g. tubal obstruction in both male and female partners). My own practice is to recommend treatment in otherwise unexplained infertility or in those men with extreme or severe oligozoospermia. It should be remembered that embolization of the varicocele is a practicality for those men with good sperm numbers. Laparoscopic varicocelectomy may be performed for those men with bilateral varicoceles and open operation for those requiring additional testicular biopsy and vasography. Embolization of the internal spermatic vein is an effective treatment when the services of a skilled interventional radiologist are available.

An alternative to varicocele ligation is in vitro fertilization and this may be applicable in couples with an older woman.

Table 18.8 The relationship between clinical pregnancy rate per cycle, with standard in vitro fertilization, and semen quality at the Lister Hospital 1989–1990 (Pryor 1992)

Motile sperm concentration, million motile/ml	Number	Pregnancy rate
<1	22	5%
1–4	42	12%
5–9	34	21%
10–14	21	14%
15–19	11	18%
>20	30	20%
Normal	665	31%

Assisted conception for male infertility

Pregnancy rates for male factor infertility have been found to be low with standard in vitro fertilization (Table 18.8). The quality of progressive movement was found to be of even greater significance, and there was no conception when the progressive movement was less than grade 2 (WHO grades b–d; Pryor 1992). The advent of intracytoplasmic sperm injection (Palermo et al 1992) has increased the success rate and it is now the treatment of choice for men with severe oligozoospermia (see Ch. 19).

Untreatable sterility

Nowadays there are few men who fall into this category. Most patients should be informed of their prognosis and counselled regarding the options of continuing childlessness, adoption and donor insemination. It is unlikely that an orchidopexy will improve prognosis in the cryptorchidic adult presenting with infertility, but the risk of malignancy should be discussed. Placing the testis in a satisfactory position may facilitate examination and lessen the risk of malignancy, trauma and torsion. Long-term androgen replacement should be considered in those men with evidence of primary testicular failure.

KEY POINTS

1. Spermatogenesis is a continuous sequence of highly organized and closely regulated events within the seminiferous tubules. The total duration for adevelopment of spermatozoa ia 74 days.
2. The presence of testosterone in sufficient quantities in the seminiferous tubules is an absolute requirement for spermatogenesis.
3. Spermatozoa acquire motility during passage through the epididymis.

4. Secretions of the accessory glands form over 90% of the volume of semen.
5. Only 200 or so of the most robust spermatozoa reach the site of fertilization.
6. Capacitation is a series of functional changes which render sperm capable of fertilization.
7. The acrosome reaction can only take place after the sperm have undergone capacitation, and it is triggered by the binding of sperm to zona pellucida.
8. Normal parameters of semen analysis are subjective, semiquantitative and do not relate to fertility.
9. Surgical orchidopexy for undescended testis is unlikely to improve infertility after the age of 2 years.
10. Pyrexial illnesses may non-specifically depress spermatogenesis for some weeks but recovery is complete.
11. The significance of varicocele in male infertility is controversial.
12. Azoospermia, normal testicular volume and normal FSH indicates genital tract obstruction, which may be amenable to surgical correction.
13. Treatable causes of male infertility, include genital tract infection, free radicals and the presence of antisperm antibodies.
14. ICSI is of benefit for men with severe oligozoospermia/azoospermia. AID is now rarely required even for men with grossly impaired spermatogenesis.

REFERENCES

Aiman J, Griffen J E 1982 The frequency of androgen receptor deficiency in infertile men. Journal of Clinical Endocrinology and Metabolism 54: 725–732

Aitken J 1994 On the future of the hamster oocyte penetration assay. Fertility and Sterility 62: 17–19

Aitken R J 1986 The zona-free hamster oocyte penetration test and the diagnosis of male infertility. International Journal of Andrology 6(suppl): 1–19

Aitken R J, Clarkson J S, Hargreave T B, Irvine D S, Wu F C W 1989 Analysis of the relationship between defective sperm function and the generation of reactive oxygen species in cases of oligospermia. Journal of Andrology 10: 214–220

Aitken R J, Bowie H, Buckingham D, Harkiss D, Richardson R W, West K M 1992 Sperm penetration with hyaluronic acid polymer as a means of monitoring functional competence. Journal of Andrology 13: 44–54

Aitken D J, Irvine D S, Wu F C 1991 Prospective analysis of sperm–oocyte fusion and reactive oxygen species generation as criteria for the diagnosis of fertility. American Journal of Obstetrics and Gynecology 164: 542–551

Baker H W G 1989 Clinical evaluation and management of testicular disorders in the adult. In: Burger H, de Kretser D M (eds) The testis, 2nd edn. Raven Press, New York, pp 419–440

Biljan M M, Taylor C T, Manasse P R, Joughin E C, Kingsland C R, Lewis-Jones D I 1994 Evaluation of different sperm function tests as screening for male fertilisation potential – the value of sperm migration. Fertility and Sterility 62: 591–598

Bonnie G G, McLoad E I F, Watkinson G 1981 Incidence of sulphasalazine-induced male infertility. Gut 22: 452–455

Bronson R A, Cooper G W, Rosenfeld D 1984 Sperm antibodies: their role in infertility. Fertility and Sterility 42: 171–183

Burger H G, Baker H W G 1982 Therapeutic considerations and results of gonadotrophin treatment in male hypogonadotrophic hypogonadism. Annals of the New York Academy of Sciences 438: 447–453

Burkman L J, Coddington C C, Franken D R 1988 The hemizona assay (HZA): development of a diagnostic test for the binding of human spermatozoa to the human hemizona pellucida to predict fertilisation potential. Fertility and Sterility 49: 688–697

Cates W, Farley T M M, Rowe P J 1985 Worldwide patterns of infertility: is Africa different? Lancet ii: 596–598

Chandley A C 1979 The chromosomal basis of human infertility. British Medical Journal 35: 181–186

Clarke G N, Lopata A, McBain J C, Baker H W G, Johnson W I H 1985 Effects of sperm antibodies in males on human in vitro fertilization. American Journal of Immunology and Microbiology 8: 62–66

Cross N, Morales P, Overstreet J W, Hanson F W 1986 Two simple methods for detecting acrosome-reacted sperm. Gamete Research 15: 213–226

Cummings J M, Pember S M, Jequier A M, Yovich J L, Hartman P E 1991 A test of the human sperm acrosome reaction following ionophore challenge. Journal of Andrology 12: 98–103

De Castro M P P, Mastorocco D A M 1994 Reproductive history and semen analysis in prevasectomy fertile men with and without varicoceles. Journal of Andrology 5: 17

De Jonge C J 1994 The diagnostic significance of the induced acrosome reaction. Reproductive Medicine Review 3: 159–178

Dom J, Rudak E, Aitken R J 1981 Antisperm antibodies: their effect on the process of fertilisation studied in vivo. Fertility and Sterility 35: 535–541

Dubin L, Amelar R D 1977 Varicocelectomy: 986 cases in a 12-year study. Urology 10: 446–449

Dym 1977 In: Weiss L, Greep R O (eds) Histology, 4th edn. McGraw Hill, New York, p 981

Fawcett D W 1975 Developmental Biology 44: 394

Francavilla S, Palermo G, Gabrielle A, Cordeschi G, Poccia G 1992 Sperm acrosin activity and fluorescence microscopic assessment of proacrosin/acrosin in ejaculate of infertile and fertile men. Fertility and Sterility 57: 1311–1316

Franken D R, Acosta A A, Kruger T F 1993 The hemizona assay: its role in identifying male factor infertility in assisted reproduction. Fertility and Sterility 59: 1075–1080

Fukuda M, Morales P, Overstreet J W 1989 Acrosome function of human spermatozoa with normal and abnormal head morphology. Gamete Research 24: 59–65

Hargreave T B 1995 Debate on the pros and cons of varicocele treatment – in favour of varicocele treatment. Human Reproduction 10(suppl): 151–157

Hargreave T B, Elton R A 1983 Is conventional sperm analysis of any use? British Journal of Urology 55: 780–784

Hayflick J S, Adelman J P, Seeberg P H 1989 The complete sequence of human gonadotrophin releasing gene. Nucleic Acids Research 17: 6403–6404

Hendry W F, Hughes L, Scammell G, Pryor J P, Hargreave T B 1990a Comparison of prednisolone and placebo in subfertile men with antibodies to spermatozoa. Lancet 335: 85–88

Hendry W F, Levison D A, Parkinson M C, Parslow J M, Royle M G 1990b Testicular obstruction: clinicopathological studies. Annals of the Royal College of Surgeons of England 72: 396–407

Holt W 1994 Reproducibility of computer–aided semen analysis: comparison of five different systems used in a practical workshop. Fertility and Sterility 62: 1277–1282

Hull M G R, Savage P H, Bromham D R 1982 Prognostic value of the post coital test: prospective study based on time-specific conception rates. British Journal of Obstetrics and Gynaecology 89: 299–305

Hull M G R, Glazener C M A, Kelly N J et al 1985 Population study of causes, treatment and outcome of infertility. British Medical Journal 291: 1693–1697

Huszar G 1994 The role of sperm creatinine kinase in the assessment of male fertility. Reproductive Medicine Review 3: 179–197
Huszar G, Vigne L, Morshedi M 1992 Sperm creatine phosphokinase m isoferm rations and fertilising potential of men: a blinded study of 84 couples treated with in vitro fertilisation. Fertility and Sterility 57: 882–888
Irvine D S, Aitken R J 1987 Predictive value of in vitro sperm function tests in the context of an AID service. Human Reproduction 1: 539–545
Jeyendran R S, Van der Ven H H, Zanefeld L J D 1992 The hypo-osmotic swelling test: an update. Archives of Andrology 29: 105–116
Johnsen S G 1970 Testicular biopsy score count – a method for registration of spermatogenesis in human testis. Normal values and results in 335 hypogonadal males. Hormones 1: 2–25
Krausz C, Mills C, Rogers S, Tan S L, Aitken R J 1994 Stimulation of oxidant generation by human sperm suspensions using phorbol esters and formyl peptides: relationships with motility and fertilisation in vitro. Fertility and Sterility 62: 599–605
Kruger T F, Acosta A A, Simmons K F, Swanson R J, Matta J F, Oehninger S 1988 Predictive value of abnormal sperm morphology in in vitro fertilisation. Fertility and Sterility 49: 112–117
Kruger T F, Du Toit T C, Frankel D R et al 1993 A new computerized method of reading sperm morphology (strict criteria) is as efficient as technician reading. Fertility and Sterility 59: 202–209
Kruger T F, Du Toit T C, Frankel D R, Menkveld R, Lombard C J 1995 Sperm morphology: assessing the agreement of the manual method (strict criteria) and sperm morphology analyzer NOS. Fertility and Sterility 63: 134–141
Laven J S E, Haans L C F, Mali W P T M et al 1992 Effects of varicocele treatment in adolescents – a randomised study. Fertility and Sterility 58: 756–762
Liu D Y, Clarke D N, Baker H W G 1991 Relationship between sperm motility assesed with the Hamilton Thorn motility analyser and fertilisation rates in vitro. Journal of Andrology 12: 231–239
Ma K, Inglis J D, Sharkey A 1993 A Y chromosome gene family with RNA-binding protein homology: candidates for the azoospermia factor AZF controlling human spermatogenesis. Cell 75: 1287–1295
Margalioth E J, Feinmesser M, Navot D, Mordel N, Bronson R A 1989 The long-term predictive value of the zona-free hamster ova penetration assay. Fertility and Sterility 52: 490–494
Matsumoto A M 1989 Hormonal control of spermatogenesis. In: Burger H, de Kretser D (eds) The testis, 2nd edn. Raven Press, New York, pp 181–186
McClachlan R I, Robertson D M, de Kretser D M, Burger H G 1987 Inhibin – a non-steroidal regulator of pituitary follicle stimulating hormone. Baillière's Clinical Endocrinology and Metabolism 1: 89–112
Meares E M, Stamey T A 1972 The diagnosis and management of bacterial prostatitis. British Journal of Urology 44: 175–179
Mendoza C, Carreras A, Moos J, Tesavik J 1992 Distinction between true acrosome reaction and degenerative acrosome loss by a one-step staining method using pisum sativum agglutination. Journal of Reproduction and Fertility 95: 755–763
Morales P, Katz D F, Overstreet J W et al 1988 The relationship between the motility and morphology of spermatozoa in human semen. International Journal of Andrology 9: 241–247
Mortimer D 1994 Laboratory studies in routine clinical andrology. Reproductive Medicine Review 3: 97–111
Mortimer D, Mortimer S T, Shu M A, Swart R 1990 A simplified approach to sperm–cervical mucus interaction using a hyaluronate migration test. Human Reproduction 5: 835–841
Nilsson S, Edvinson A, Nilsson B 1979 Improvement of semen and pregnancy rate after ligation and division of internal spermatic vein. British Journal of Urology 51: 591–596
Oates R D, Amos J A 1995 The genetic basis of congenital bilateral absence of the vas deferens and cystic fibrosis. Journal of Andrology 15: 1–8
Oehninger S 1992 Diagnostic significance of sperm–zona pellucida interaction. Reproductive Medicine Review 1: 57–81
Palermo G, Joris H, Devroey P, Steirtegheim A C 1992 Pregnancies after intracytoplasmic injection of single spermatozoon into an oocyte. Lancet 340: 17–18
Pryor J P 1988 Reconstruction of bladder neck for retrograde ejaculation. In: Gingell C, Abrams P (eds) Controversies and innovations in urological surgery. Springer Verlag, London, pp 433–437
Pryor J P 1992 Simple seminal analysis is a useful predictor for the outcome of assisted conception. An update. In: Progress in reproductive biology and medicine, vol 15: Colpi G M, Pizza D (eds) treating male infertility, new possibilities and limits. Karger, Basle, pp 222–225
Pryor J P 1993 Ejaculatory duct obstruction. In: Hendry W F, Whitfield H N (eds) Rob & Smith's operative surgery, volume 2: genitourinary surgery, 5th edn. Butterworth Heinemann, London, pp 606–608
Pryor J P 1994a Erectile and ejaculatory problems in infertility. In: Hargreave T B (ed) Male infertility, 2nd edn. Springer Verlag, Berlin, pp 319–336
Pryor J P 1994b Surgery of genital tract obstruction. Epididymovasotomy and vasovasotomy. In: Krane R J, Siroky M B, Fitzpatrick J M (eds) Clinical urology. J B Lippincott, Philadelphia, pp 1131–1142
Sandler B 1954 Recovery from sterility after mumps orchitis. British Medical Journal 2: 795
Schoysman R J, Bedford J M 1986 The role of the human epididymis in sperm maturation and sperm storage as reflected in the consequences of epididymovasotomy. Fertility and Sterility 46: 293–299
Sharpe R M 1987 Testosterone and spermatogenesis. Journal of Endocrinology 113: 1–2
Sharpe R M 1990 Intratesticular control of steroidogenesis. Clinical Endocrinology 33: 1–21
Sharpe R M 1994 Could environmental oestrogenic chemicals be responsible for some disorders of human male reproductive development? Current Opinion in Urology 4: 295–301
Silber J, van Steirtegheim A C, Devroey P 1995 Sertoli cell-only revisited. Human Reproduction 10: 1031–1032
Skinner M K 1991 Cell-cell interactions in the testis. Endocrinological Review 12: 45–47
Soffer Y, Golan A, Herman A, Pansky M, Caspi E, Ron-Ei R 1992 Prediction of in vitro fertilisation outcome by sperm penetration assay with TEST yolk buffer preincubation. Fertility and Sterility 58: 556–562
Sutherland P D, Matson P L, Moore H D M et al 1985 Clinical evaluation of the heterologous oocyte penetration (HOP) test. British Journal of Urology 57: 233–236
Van der Suffele J, Vermeulen L, Schoonjans F, Comhaire F H 1992 Evaluation of the hypo-osmotic swelling test in relation with advanced methods of semen analysis. Andrology 24: 213–217
Wang C, Leung A, Tsoi W C et al 1991 Evaluation of human sperm hyperactivated motility and the relationship with zona-free hamster oocyte penetration assay. Journal of Andrology 12: 253–258
Whorton D, Knauss R M, Marshall S, Milby T H 1977 Infertility in male pesticide workers. Lancet ii: 1259–1261
World Health Organization 1992 WHO laboratory manual for the examination of human semen and sperm–mucus interaction, 3rd edn. Cambridge University Press, Cambridge
World Health Organization Task Force on the Prevention and Management of Infertility 1992 Adenosine triphosphate in semen and other sperm characteristics: their relevance for fertility prediction in men with normal sperm concentration. Fertility and Sterility 57: 877–881
Wu F C W, Taylor P L, Sellar R E 1989 Luteinising hormone–releasing hormone pulse frequency in normal and infertile men. Journal of Endocrinology 123: 149–158
Yanagimachi R, Yanagimachi H, Rogers B J 1976 The use of zona-free animal ova as a test system for the assessment of the fertilising capacity of human spermatozoa. Biology of Reproduction 15: 471–476
Yovich J M, Edirisinghe W R, Yovich J L 1994 Use of the acrosome reaction to ionophene challenge test in managing patients in an assisted reproduction programme: a prospective double-blind randomised controlled study. Fertility and Sterility 61: 902–910

19

Assisted reproduction treatments

Nazar N. Amso Robert W. Shaw

INTRODUCTION

There are now around 150 000 children worldwide born as a result of assisted reproduction techniques (ART). This reflects the true dimension of the success of these treatments in relieving today's human misery of infertility. Since the publication of the first edition of this textbook, new drugs have become available and new treatments have been introduced and become established over an incredibly short period of time, creating more ethical dilemmas and encouraging continuing debate. The provision of these treatments, both in the UK and worldwide, has unfortunately remained limited due to financial constraints, thus augmenting the distress felt by many couples. This chapter will expand on these new clinical developments and controversies, including innovations in stimulation protocols, new techniques in the treatment of male factor infertility and prenatal genetic diagnosis, as well as examining the clinical risks associated with assisted reproduction techniques.

SELECTION AND PREPARATION OF PATIENTS

Although in vitro fertilization (IVF) was initially introduced to bypass tubal blockage, it is now utilized in the treatment of infertility with various causes. The current indications are:

1. tubal disease
2. unexplained infertility
3. treated endometriosis
4. male factor infertility
5. failed artificial insemination by donor (AID)
6. cervical hostility
7. failed ovulation induction
8. absent or inappropriate ovaries
9. therapy for female cancer.

Many assisted reproduction centres are selective in entering patients on their programmes and have evolved specific inclusion criteria. Each couple should be assessed carefully prior to their enrolment on the waiting list. Factors such as female age, antisperm antibodies, and sperm dysfunction affect success rates considerably. Women with mild and treated endometriosis or unexplained infertility have a better prognosis. Prior to initiation of therapy, it is important to evaluate the couple's suitability for IVF treatment. Additionally, information-giving and decision-making aspects of counselling should be made available by a specially trained counsellor as a matter of routine, to all couples. These couples have frequently undergone extensive investigations, are under considerable stress, and their marriage is often under considerable strain. IVF treatment should not be used as a panacea for marital or psychosexual disorders, but to fulfil the wishes of a well adjusted couple to have a baby.

The male and female partner should be interviewed

Table 19.1 Tests for the female and male partners

Female	Baseline hormone profile Luteal phase progesterone Assessment of tubal patency Serum antisperm antibodies Rubella status HIV III, and Hepatitis B screening
Male	Semen analysis and microbiology Hamster egg penetration test* Serum antisperm antibodies Human immunodeficiency virus III (HIV III) and hepatitis B screening

*Where indicated in unexplained infertility and male sperm dysfunction.

together and an appropriate history and clinical examination are undertaken for both. A number of tests are carried out prior to initiation of the treatment (Table 19.1). Hepatitis B and human immunodeficiency virus (HIV) III screening is carried out to ensure the safety of the staff, to prevent spread of infection should the patient's serum be used for culture media or when oocytes are being donated. Laparoscopy should be carried out to confirm a normal pelvis if gamete intrafallopian transfer (GIFT) is to be the treatment of choice. Similarly, the male partner undergoes various tests. Semen assessment should be repeated more than once before initiation of the treatment cycle, and all semen parameters (total count, density, motility, progression, morphology, presence of white cells) should be recorded.

The couple must be well informed about the details of their treatment, the techniques involved, and the indications for the tests they have to undergo. Assisted reproduction involves four principal steps:

1. the induction and timing of ovulation;
2. egg collection;
3. fertilization (IVF);
4. the replacement of gametes/embryos.

CLINICAL MANAGEMENT OF THE TREATMENT CYCLE

The first successful birth from IVF–embryo transfer (IVF–ET) in 1978 resulted from a single oocyte obtained from the dominant follicle in a natural ovarian cycle. Success rates were found to be improved when multiple embryos were transferred; thus at present, the majority of assisted reproduction programmes undertake ovarian stimulation to induce multiple follicular development.

Normal folliculogenesis

This involves several important and interrelated steps.

1. Follicular recruitment: this occupies the first few days of the ovarian cycle and allows the follicle to continue to mature in the correct gonadotrophic environment and to progress towards ovulation.

2. Selection: the mechanism whereby a single follicle is chosen and ultimately achieves ovulation.

3. Dominance: the selected follicle maintains its pre-eminence over all other follicles, occupying days 8–12 of the primate ovarian cycle.

Follicular development beyond the antral stage depends on the concentration of follicle-stimulating hormone (FSH) in the circulation. Once a threshold level has been attained, follicular growth beyond 4 mm occurs. The interval during which FSH remains elevated above threshold level can be regarded as a gate through which a follicle must pass to avoid atresia. The width of the gate will therefore determine the number of follicles which can be selected for ovulation (Fig. 19.1). The preovulatory luteinizing hormone (LH) surge is triggered by the positive feedback of oestradiol (E_2) from the dominant follicle as well as by other follicular contributory factors. Ovulation occurs between 24 and 36 h after the onset of the LH surge.

Stimulation protocols

The pregnancy rate with natural-cycle IVF remains much lower than in stimulated cycles, achieving a delivery rate of 4% per initiated cycle and 6.3% per retrieval in women ≤40 years (Society for Assisted Reproductive Technology (SART) 1995). Although an unstimulated cycle is simpler, faster, less painful or expensive and has no risk of ovarian hyperstimulation, it requires relatively extensive monitoring which increases the cost and results in inconvenience in the timing of oocyte retrieval. Additionally, women with irregular cycles and/or hormonal imbalance, or couples with male factor infertility, where fertilization may be a problem, are not suitable for natural-cycle IVF.

The aims of superovulation regimens in assisted reproduction are: to maximize the number of follicles which mature; to minimize the degree of asynchrony amongst developing follicles, and to minimize the deleterious effects of the abnormal follicular environment on luteal function and endometrial receptivity. Multiple follicular development and ovulation can be achieved by widening the FSH gate. Several drug combinations have been used to achieve this, and are listed here:

1. clomiphene citrate plus human menopausal gonadotrophin (hMG) and/or pure FSH;
2. hMG and/or pure FSH alone;
3. gonadotrophin-releasing hormone (GnRH) analogue plus hMG and/or pure FSH.

Many centres commence ovarian stimulation with the onset of the menstrual cycle. This will lead to oocyte recoveries taking place at random according to follicular

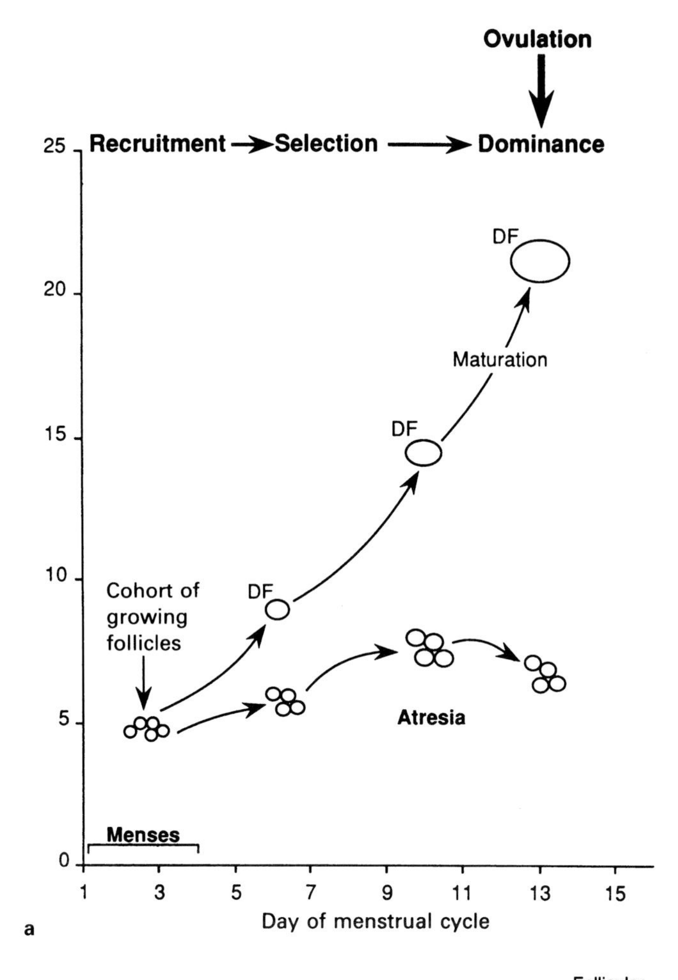

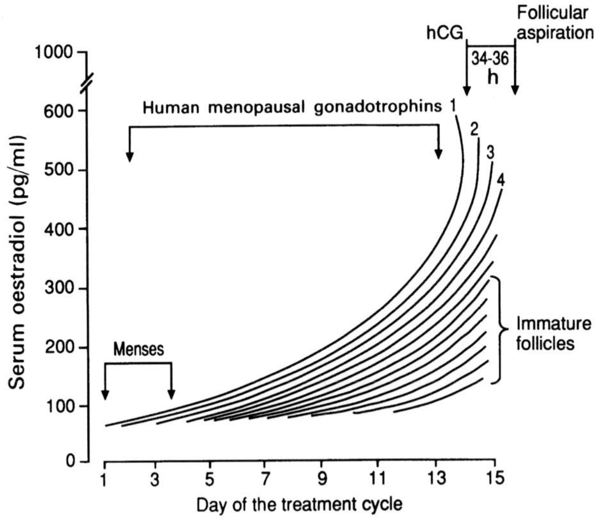

Fig. 19.1 **a** Selection and maturation of the dominant follicle (DF) during a natural cycle. **b** Induced follicular maturation with gonadotrophin therapy overriding selection of a single dominant follicle, as in the natural cycle.

development and maturation. Consequently, such units are obliged to work seven days a week which stretches human resources. Alternatively, oocyte retrieval may be programmed to coincide with a working day by manipulating the onset of the menstrual cycle using norethisterone tablets or utilizing the hypogonadotrophic effect of GnRH analogues prior to commencing gonadotrophins on a predetermined day of the week. The GnRH analogue is commenced either in the midluteal phase and continued until complete downregulation is achieved (long protocol), or started on the 1st day of the menstrual cycle (short protocol). The downregulatory phase may be prolonged to allow a fixed number of patients to be treated each week. Follicular response is monitored by ultrasound scans and serum hormone assays for oestrogen, LH, and progesterone, commencing on the 8th day of the treatment cycle. The gonadotrophin dosage is adjusted according to ovarian response. When three or more follicles are greater than 18 mm in diameter, 5000 U of human chorionic gonadotrophin (hCG) are given intramuscularly 34–36 h prior to oocyte collection. Oocyte retrieval takes place on a weekday, 13 days or more after commencing gonadotrophin stimulation.

Figure 19.2 depicts a typical ovarian response, where follicles are noted to grow at a rate of 2–3 mm/day accompanied by a steady increase in serum E_2 levels. Unfortunately, not all stimulation cycles progress in this typical pattern, and many may have to be abandoned before oocyte collection for a variety of reasons. In a retrospective analysis of 314 stimulation cycles commenced in 1988, we found that 30.9% of cycles were abandoned prior to oocyte collection (Table 19.2). While premature LH surge and preoperative ovulation have been largely eliminated by the introduction of GnRH analogues, other problems, such as poor ovarian response or the development of ovarian hyperstimulation, remain unresolved.

The use of GnRH analogues in stimulation protocols has increased steadily since their introduction into clinical practice, and appears to result in a reduction in the cancellation rates and an increase in the number of oocytes retrieved. An integrative analysis of research publications between 1987 and 1992 by Kenny (1995), reported significantly higher clinical pregnancy rates for GnRH analogue plus hMG/FSH than for clomiphene citrate plus hMG/FSH cycles. Additionally, in a meta-analysis of randomized controlled trials of GnRH analogue use prior to IVF and GIFT, Hughes et al (1992) found no significant differences for clinical pregnancy rates per cycle commenced, when the short and long protocols were compared.

Luteal phase defect in GnRH analogue cycles was reported as early as 1987 (Smitz et al) and luteal phase supplementation with either progesterone or hCG has been reported to improve pregnancy rates. A meta-analysis by Soliman et al (1994) reported that hCG was superior to progesterone, but resulted in a definite increase in the rate of moderate and severe ovarian hyperstimulation syndrome. The improved pregnancy rates in supplemented cycles may be due to beneficial effects on endo-

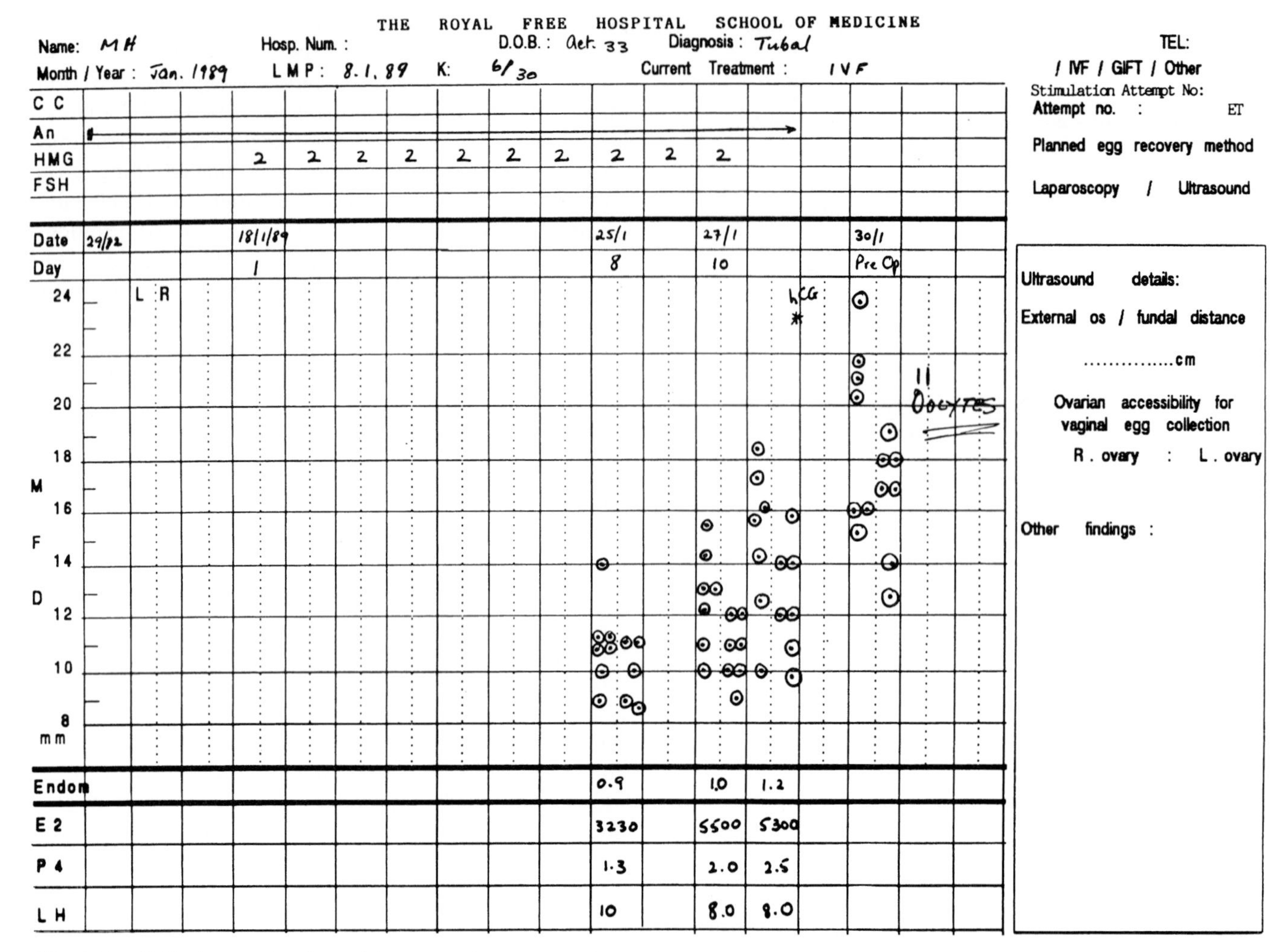

Fig. 19.2 Folliculogram showing satisfactory ovarian response after 10 days of gonadotrophin therapy.

Table 19.2 Causes of abandoned stimulation cycles in IVF/GIFT

	n	%
Total number of IVF/GIFT cycles	314	
Abandoned cycles	97	30.9
Poor/no response	56	57.7
Premature LH surge	15	15.5
Preoperative ovulation	12	12.4
Risk of hyperstimulation	11	11.3
Other	3	3.1
Number proceeding to oocyte collection	217	69.1

metrial maturation, where fine structural features and expression of steroid receptors are similar to those seen in physiological conditions.

Both FSH and hMG have been used in stimulation protocols and are effective in inducing follicular growth and maturation. However, the relative importance of FSH and LH in this process has been the subject of much debate. Excessively high levels of LH during the time of follicular development and in the periovulatory phase may have detrimental effects on fertilization, cleavage, and embryo quality. Raised LH levels may also be associated with a lower probability of conception and high rate of spontaneous abortion. A meta-analysis of FSH versus hMG for IVF cycles (Daya et al 1995) demonstrated that the use of FSH is associated with a significantly higher clinical pregnancy rate than hMG whether GnRH analogue was used or not. The benefit was higher in the former situation, as the use of GnRH analogue would be associated with a significant reduction in the endogenous LH levels.

Commercially available gonadotrophin preparations extracted from human postmenopausal urine have been shown to be of low purity, with the major protein components not being gonadotrophins! The repeated injection of non-gonadotrophin proteins may be the cause of unwanted effects, such as pain and allergic reactions. The desirability of having high purity preparations led to the development of an immunopurified FSH product with >95 % purity. However, variations in bioactivity and continued dependence on human menopausal urine collection remain as major obstacles in the production of these compounds. Recent progress in purification technology as well as genetic and molecular engineering, led to the production of recombinant human FSH (rhFSH) with high purity (>99%), high specific bioactivity (≈ 10 000 IU/mg protein) and absent intrinsic LH activity, which is suitable for intramuscular or subcutaneous administration (Mannaerts et al 1991). Early reports indicated that rhFSH successfully stimulated follicular development and steroidogenesis in anovulatory women, and for IVF, resulting in the establishment of pregnancies. Although ovarian follicles develop to preovulatory stage, there appears to be minimal serum and intrafollicular increase in oestradiol levels, confirming a dissociation between the mitogenic and steroidogenic activity of FSH. The clinical outcome of a pilot efficacy study (Devroey et al 1994) confirmed the effectiveness of rhFSH (with an ongoing pregnancy rate of 18.6% per transfer) and its safety for patients and their offspring. Larger clinical trials to determine the influence of the cell type (expression system) in which the glycoprotein is synthesized are awaited before specific solutions are tailored to fit the specific problems of individual patients.

Abnormal ovarian response

Ovarian response is poor when no or fewer than three follicles develop after 14 days of gonadotrophin treatment, and generally results in cancellation of the stimulation cycle (Fig. 19.3). This problem is frequently encountered in women over the age of 37 years and those with severe ovarian endometriosis, where few oocytes of low quality are obtained and pregnancy rates are usually poor. Increasing the starting dose of gonadotrophins may sometimes improve the response and enable recruitment of a larger number of oocytes. Excessive ovarian response (Fig. 19.4) may result in ovarian hyperstimulation syndrome (OHSS). This complication is discussed in the section on the potential health risks associated with assisted reproductive technology.

Premature LH surge or preoperative ovulation are responsible for a high proportion of abandoned cycles, especially when facilities to carry out oocyte retrieval, once the surge is detected, are not available; when endocrine monitoring is not performed, and when oocyte retrievals

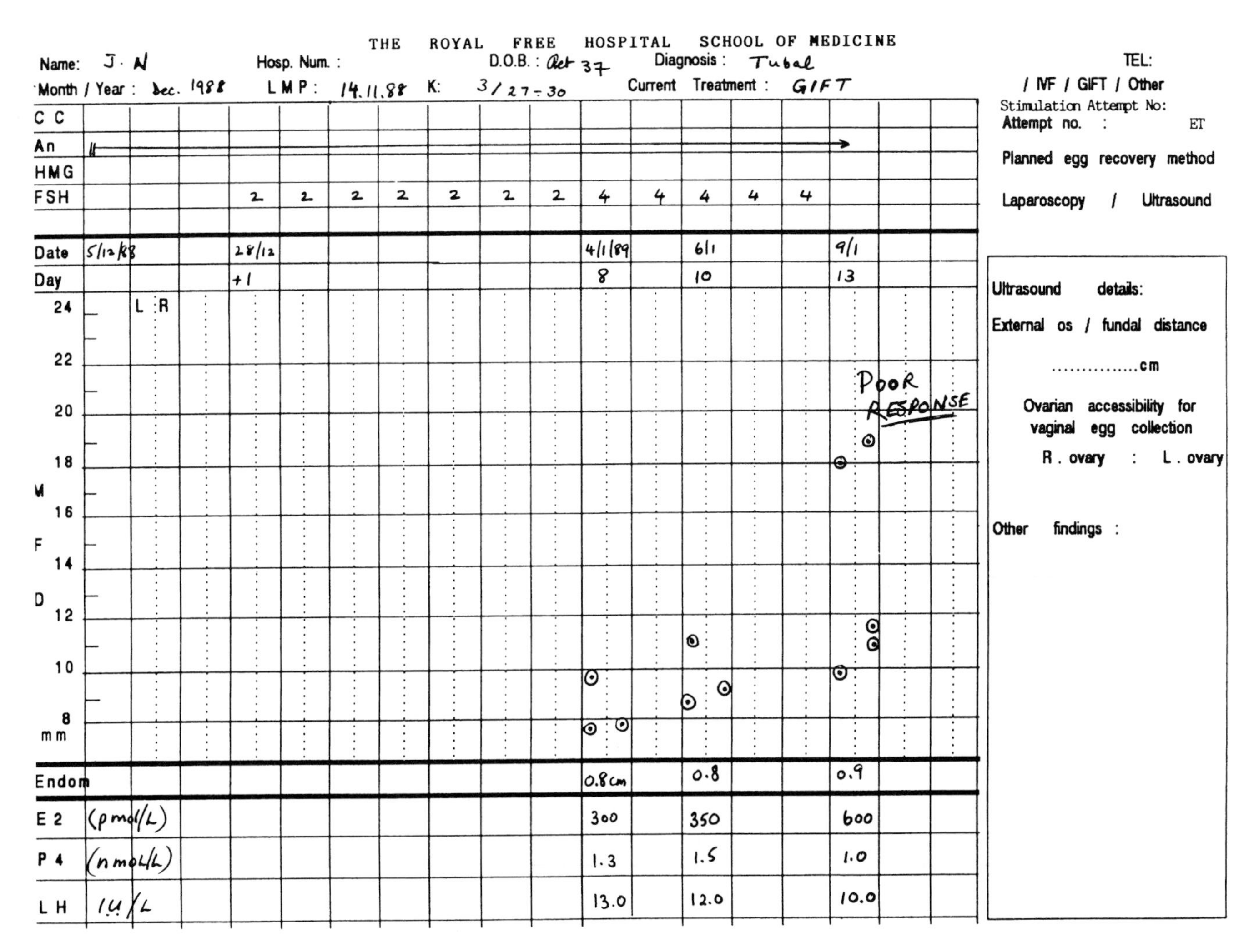

Fig. 19.3 Poor follicular response in a patient aged 37 years.

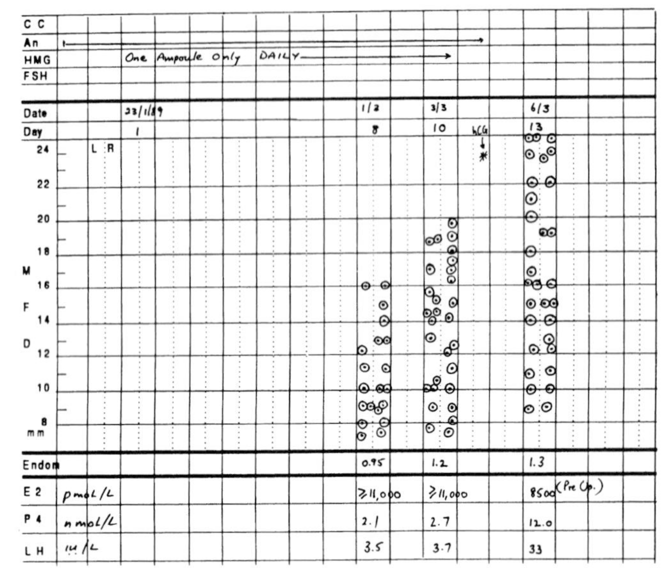

Fig. 19.4 Excessive follicular response in a patient with polycystic ovaries in spite of receiving only 1 ampoule of Pergonal daily. A total of 23 oocytes were retrieved at vaginal egg collection. The patient, however, did not develop symptoms and signs of ovarian hyperstimulation syndrome.

are programmed to take place on determined days of the week only. The introduction of GnRH analogues in superovulation protocols has largely eliminated these problems and enabled a better control of the stimulation cycle (Fig. 19.5).

OOCYTE COLLECTION

Methods of egg collection have improved considerably over the past decade. The main motivation for these technical advances was to limit the high cost of IVF treatment, which was largely due to time spent in hospital, the type of anaesthesia, and the degree of invasiveness of the procedure and its morbidity. At first, all egg collections were laparoscopic, while presently this is reserved for patients being treated with GIFT. The need for general anaesthesia and the frequently encountered limited access to adherent or covered ovaries meant that simpler ultrasound-guided techniques, such as the transvesical and transurethral methods, replaced laparoscopy as the principal methods for egg collection. They were easy to learn,

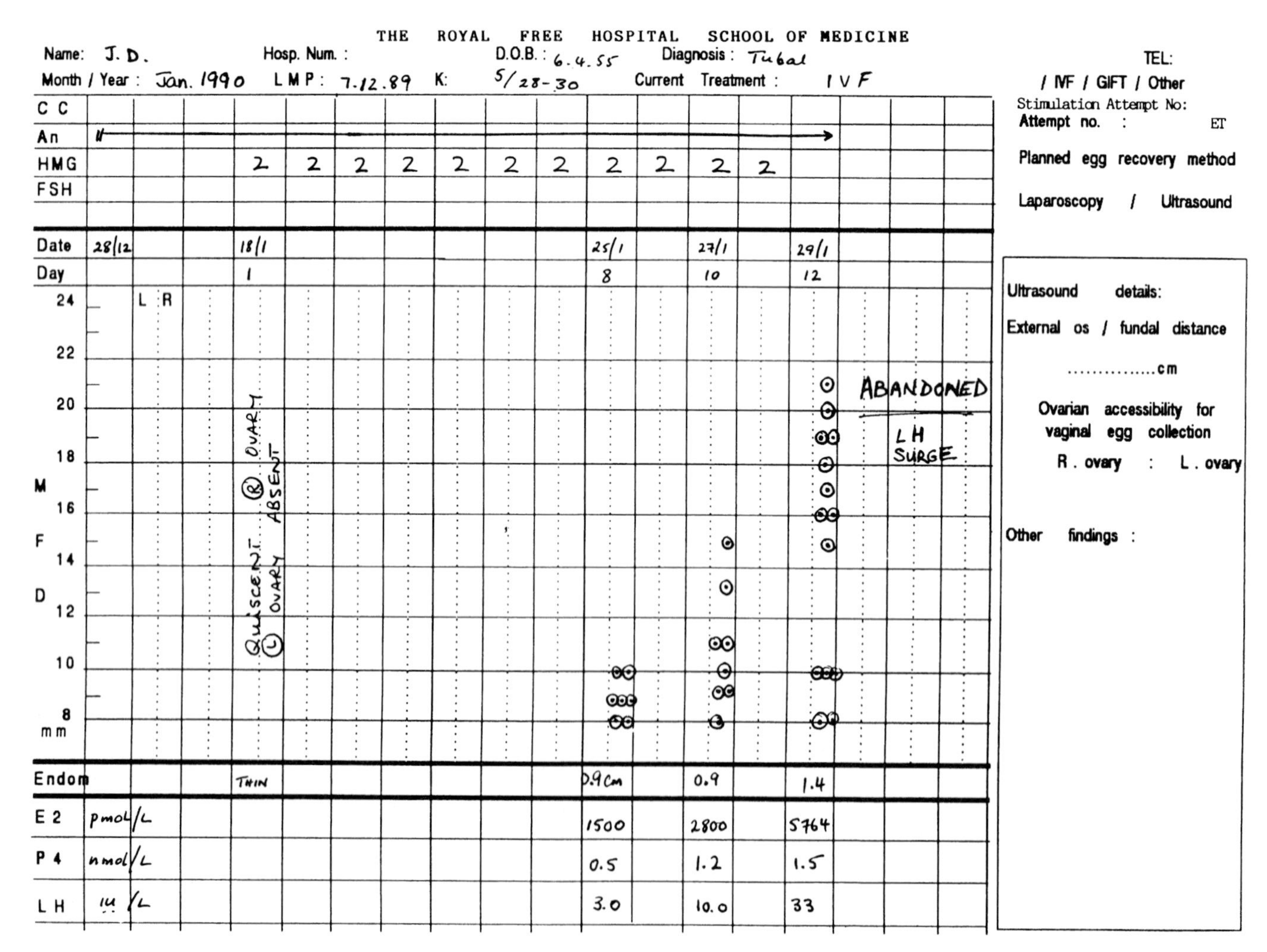

Fig. 19.5 Premature LH hormone surge prior to the hCG injection. The treatment cycle was abandoned.

quick and did not require prolonged hospitalization. However, discomfort was frequently experienced by filling the bladder and haematuria was a frequent complication of the transurethral approach.

With the introduction of endovaginal transducers, the transvaginal route became the predominant method for egg collection. In this, the specially designed transducer is used to visualize the follicles and the aspirating needle is passed along its side. This method is generally well tolerated when carried out under light intravenous sedation, can be learnt very quickly and is associated with minimal morbidity. It has almost completely replaced all previously described ultrasound methods. Ideally, both laparoscopy and ultrasound-guided techniques should be available to accommodate the anatomical needs of all patients.

Equipment and preparation

Several ultrasound machines are now equipped with slimline vaginal probes with frequencies between 6 and 7.5 MHz. The probes may have a diameter of only 1.5 cm and, together with the needle guide, occupy minimal space in the vagina, causing least discomfort.

Several designs of aspiration needles are available. They may have a single or double lumen to enable aspiration and flushing through different routes. The needle must have a very sharp tip to enable easy puncture of mobile ovaries and its distal 2 cm be roughened to enhance ultrasound visualization. The needle is connected by tubing to a test tube to which suction is applied from a foot-operated pump (Fig. 19.6).

The ultrasound transducer (Fig. 19.7) is enclosed in a special sterile condom and plastic sleeve prior to insertion into the vagina, and should be thoroughly cleaned with a damp cloth after each procedure.

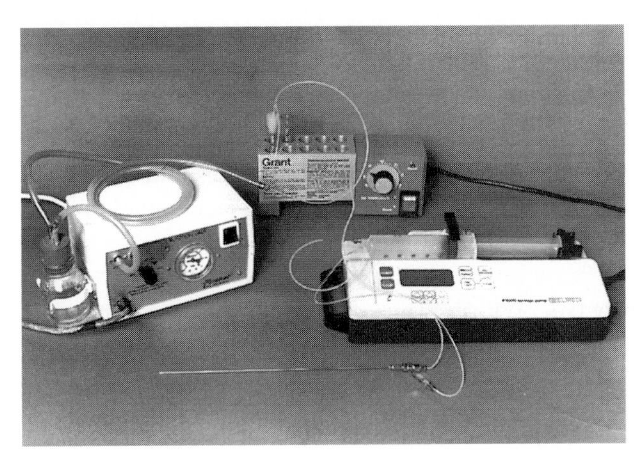

Fig. 19.6 An assembled follicle aspiration needle connected to a test tube and a flushing syringe pump. The test tube is in turn connected to a suction pump.

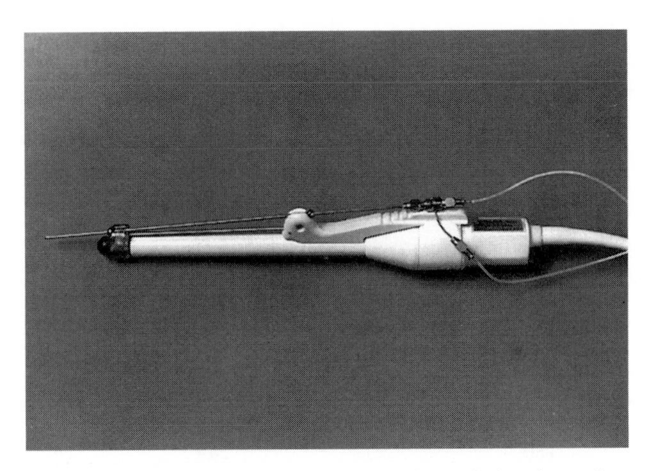

Fig. 19.7 Vaginal ultrasound transducer with needle bracket and guide. The needle tip is protruding from the proximal end of the probe.

Anaesthesia

Vaginal egg collections may be performed under general anaesthesia or intravenous/intramuscular sedation with diazepam (5–12.5 mg) and pethidine (75–125 mg). The dose given varies according to the patient's tolerance and the time taken to complete the operation.

Technique

The patient is placed in the lithotomy position and the vagina is cleaned carefully. Prior to puncture of the lateral vaginal vault, the ovaries should be carefully scanned to determine the plane which will enable the best access to the largest follicles. The needle is pushed through the vaginal wall and into the first follicle by a single, firm thrusting movement. Suction is applied as soon as the needle tip is seen to be within the follicle which will be seen to collapse as the follicular fluid is aspirated (Fig. 19.8). During aspiration, the needle is rotated and moved gently in all directions within the follicle to increase the chance of oocyte

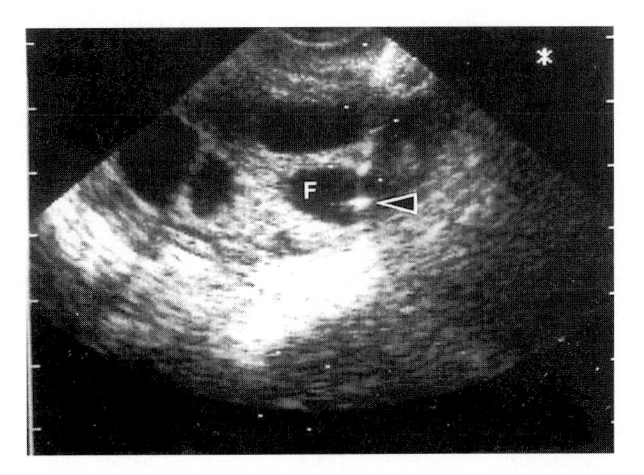

Fig. 19.8 Ultrasound picture during vaginal egg recovery. The tip of the needle (arrow) is seen within the follicle (F). The two parallel dotted lines demarcate the path of the needle. The dots are 1 cm apart.

retrieval. If the oocyte is not recovered in the first aspirate, the follicle may be flushed, either manually or using a foot pedal-controlled pump to facilitate delivery of flushing media at a steady rate. Once the egg is obtained, the needle is lined against a neighbouring follicle without removing it from the ovarian surface. Unanaesthetized patients will experience pain or discomfort when the external follicular surface is entered. However, the procedure is well tolerated and usually completed in about 30 min. At the end, the vaginal vault should be inspected to exclude bleeding from puncture sites. The patient recovers quickly, and will be able to leave the hospital after a few hours.

In our experience, very few technical difficulties have been encountered during vaginal egg collections. Mobile ovaries may be stabilized with gentle suprapubic/iliac fossa pressure and the use of sharp needles usually overcomes this difficulty. If the uterus lies between the vaginal vault and the ovary, manual suprapubic pressure or redirection of the transducer will often bring the ovary in direct line with the needle. Occasionally, the ovary will need to be accessed by passing the needle through the uterus. This is rather painful for the unanaesthetized patient but appears to have minimal risk of damage or bleeding. Complications of the procedure are discussed later.

CLINICAL DEVELOPMENTS AND CONTROVERSIES

Outcome measures and factors affecting success rate

Pregnancy and live birth rates, in national registers in North America, France and Britain, have improved by about 50% since the first annual reports were published in these countries (Tables 19.3–19.6). It is now widely accepted that when attempting to ascertain whether or not a treatment is required, it is essential that time-specific or cycle-specific conception rates are used. Crude pregnancy rates per couple are almost meaningless. Pregnancy rates per cycle can also be misleading if limited to the first cycle or two, because the rate may fall in subsequent cycles. Thus, cumulative conception rates or cumulative live birth rates, have been increasingly used in reporting conventional and assisted reproduction treatment outcomes. Cumulative conception rates for some of the commonest causes of infertility in the untreated population were compared to those in couples following treatment with conventional methods (Hull 1992). The results showed that in some conditions, such as amenorrhoea and oligomenorrhoea, or in those being treated with donor insemination, the cumulative conception rate following conventional therapy is almost the same as in normal women. However, in other circumstances, such as salpingostomy for distal tubal occlusion, or the use of high dose glucocorticosteroids for seminal antisperm antibodies, the prognosis is worse and the cumulative conception rates are lower than that which can now be expected in a single cycle of IVF treatment.

The influence of age on cumulative conception rates and cumulative live birth rates was closely analysed (Tan et al 1992) in a retrospective analysis of 5055 consecutive IVF cycles undertaken on 2735 patients. Both cumulative conception and live birth rates (after 5 treatment cycles) declined with age from 54 and 45%, respectively, at 20–34 years, to 39 and 29% at 35–39 years and further to 20 and 14% at 40 years and older. These results in the under-34 years group compared favourably with spontaneous conception rates in the natural menstrual cycle, and were in agreement with similar findings reported by others (Hull et al 1992). Additionally, the probability of pregnancy also declined with repeated treatment cycles and couples with male infertility or multiple infertility factors had the lowest cumulative conception rates.

Table 19.3 IVF clinical pregnancy and live birth rates in the United Kingdom 1985–1993 (HFEA 1995)

	Clinical pregnancy rate per treatment cycle, %	Live birth rate per treatment cycle, %	Treatment cycles
1985	11.2	8.6	4308
1986	9.9	8.6	7043
1987	12.5	10.1	8899
1988	12.9	9.1	10489
1989	15.4	11.1	10413
1990	17.3	12.5	11583
1991	17.8	13.9	6653*
1992	16.9	12.7	18224
1993	18.0	14.2	21823

*Data available for 1 August–31 December 1991 only.

Table 19.4 Annual throughput and success rates for IVF, taken from the United States and Canada Registry 1987–1993 (MRI, SART 1989–1992, SART 1993, 1995, AFS, SART 1994)

	1987	1988	1989	1990	1991	1992	1993
Cycles started	NA	NA	18 211	19 079	24 671	29 404	31 900
Retrievals	8725	13 647	15 392	16 405	21 083	24 996	27 443
Pregnancies	1367	2243	2811	3057	4017	5279	6321
(% per retrieval)	(15.7%)	(16.4%)	(18.3%)	(18.6%)	(19.1%)	(21.1%)	(23%)
Deliveries	991	1657	2104	2345	3215	4206	5103
(% per retrieval)	(11.4%)	(12.1%)	(13.7%)	(14.3%)	(15.2%)	(16.8%)	(18.6%)
Number of clinics	96	135	163	180	212	249	267

NA, data not available.

Table 19.5 Annual throughput and success rates for IVF, taken from the French Registry 1986–1990 (FIVNAT 1993)

	1986	1987	1988	1989	1990
Retrievals	7159	14 425	14 955	17 591	17 181
Pregnancies (% per retrieval)	15%	16.6%	17.4%	17.9%	18.7%
Live birth rate (% per retrieval)	12%	12.1%	12.8%	12.9%	13.6%

Table 19.6 Annual throughput and success rates for GIFT and ZIFT, taken from the USA and Canada Registry 1987–1993 (MRI, SART 1989–1992, SART 1993, 1995, AFS, SART 1994)

	1987	1988	1989	1990	1991	1992	1993
Gamete intrafallopian transfer (GIFT)							
Retrievals	1987	3080	3652	3750	4474	4837	4202
Pregnancies	492	846	1112	1093	1515	1621	1472
(% per retrieval)	(25%)	(27.5%)	(30.4%)	(29.1%)	(33.9%)	(33.5%)	(35%)
Deliveries	362	654	848	842	1188	1273	1182
(% per retrieval)	(18.4%)	(21.2%)	(23.2%)	(22.5%)	(26.6%)	(26.3%)	(28.1%)
Number of clinics	71	101	133	135	166	176	180
Zygote intrafallopian transfer (ZIFT)							
Retrievals	—	355	908	1370	1808	1696	1557
Pregnancies	—	97	190	292	442	488	466
(% per retrieval)		(27.3%)	(20.9%)	(21.3%)	(24.4%)	(28.8%)	(29.9%)
Deliveries	—	71	151	215	357	386	380
(% per retrieval)		(20%)	(16.6%)	(15.7%)	(19.7%)	(22.8%)	(24.4%)
Number of clinics	—	20	79	90	167	202	173

The duration of infertility has an adverse effect on the chance of conceiving naturally (Hull 1992). However, its effect on the success rate of assisted reproduction techniques has not been studied extensively. In a prospective study comparing uterine with tubal embryo transfers (Amso 1996), the highest pregnancy and live birth rates in both arms of the study were noted when the duration of infertility at recruitment was less than 4 years. It is thus clear that when counselling couples or deciding on treatment, clinicians should take the duration of infertility into consideration in addition to the age of the female partner and infertility factors.

Tubal or uterine embryo/gamete transfer?

The overall benefit from tubal transfer of gamete or embryos remains unproven, and there is no consensus as to the explanation for a possible increase in the overall success with tubal compared with uterine transfer. Uterine embryo replacement is a relatively simple procedure which must be carried out meticulously to ensure appropriate placement of the embryos (Fig. 19.9).

After the initial excitement of the greatly increased pregnancy rates with gamete intrafallopian transfer (GIFT) (Asch 1987, Craft et al 1988), controlled trials comparing GIFT with IVF failed to demonstrate any significant benefit (Leeton et al 1987). It is likely that the somewhat higher pregnancy rates are due to patient profiles including different age distribution, different diagnostic categories or variations in the interpretation of the diagnoses, especially that of unexplained infertility and, possibly, differences in the numbers of gametes or embryos transferred per patient. The effect of restriction of the number of gametes transferred to a maximum of four was demonstrated in a number of studies (Craft et al 1988, Yee et al 1989) and in the UK figures (HFEA 1993) where pregnancy and live birth rates declined to 16.3 and 11.3% respectively.

Similar variations were noted with zygote intrafallopian transfers (ZIFT) or tubal embryo transfers (TET) in comparison with conventional uterine transfers. The high success rate of up to a 48% pregnancy rate reported initially (Devroey et al 1989) was not reproduced subsequently in randomized studies which failed to demonstrate any significant differences in the overall results between tubal and uterine transfer of embryos (Amso 1996, Tanbo et al 1990, Tournaye et al 1992). Thus, any comparison should be made prospectively on specific groups of patients such as those with unexplained infertility, male factor or endometriosis rather than using a mixed cohort of patients. Indeed, the results of a randomized controlled study, comparing uterine with tubal transfers after IVF, found that the largest gap in pregnancy and implantation rates

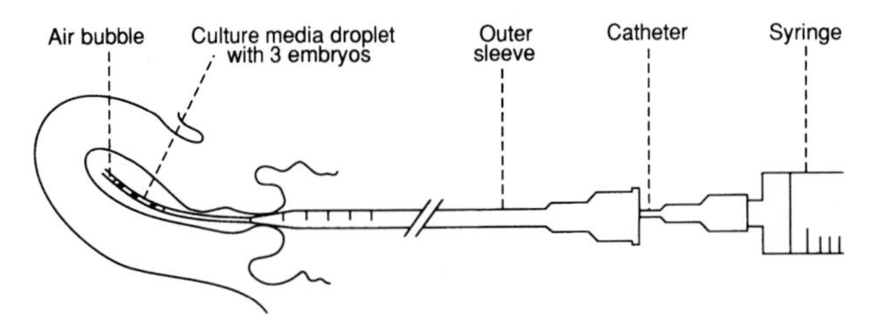

Fig. 19.9 Loaded ET catheter. Three embryos are ready to be deposited within 1 cm of the uterine fundus.

occurred in the unexplained infertility group, while in the male factor infertility group it was considerably less (Amso 1996). Similar findings for male factor infertility were reported by Tournaye et al (1992).

Perhaps an indication of the impact of both GIFT and tubal embryo transfer on assisted reproduction is derived from the US registry figures between 1987–1993. The peak numbers of retrieval cycles for ZIFT (1808) and GIFT (4837) appear to have occurred in 1991 and 1992 respectively (Table 19.6), while the IVF stimulation and retrieval cycles continued to increase, accomplishing record levels (31 900 and 27 443 respectively) in 1993 (Table 19.4). The number of centres participating in the US registry has also increased considerably during the same period and thus contributed to the overall rise in the levels of activity (Tables 19.4 and 19.6).

Assisted reproduction for endometriosis patients

Pelvic endometriosis refractory to medical or surgical therapy currently accounts for between 7 and 35% of patients undergoing IVF procedures (Damewood 1989, HFEA 1993). Several groups have reported varying degrees of success following IVF treatment in women with different stages of endometriosis, and with further expansion of IVF technology, GIFT and TET have been used as additional modalities in the treatment of these women.

All stages of endometriosis are viewed as suitable indications for assisted reproduction treatment. Its timing is dependent on the severity of the disease and previous therapy, as well as other factors, such as female age and duration of infertility. In women with severe endometriosis with mechanical blockage and where surgical therapy is inappropriate, IVF should be expedited. IVF should also be recommended 1–2 years after previous unsuccessful medical or surgical therapy, while in minimal or mild endometriosis, the balance of choice seems to be in favour of IVF or GIFT after more than 2 years of expectant management.

Early reports of IVF treatment in women with endometriosis were very encouraging and the pregnancy rate in women who had been pretreated with danazol was similar to other groups of infertile women (Mahadevan et al 1983). Prospective (Mills et al 1992) and retrospective (Sharma et al 1988) studies reported high pregnancy rates in women with minimal or mild endometriosis irrespective of prior treatment, and implantation (12%) as well as pregnancy rates (27%) per transfer compatible with tubal disease and unexplained infertility were achieved. Similarly, other parameters such as the fertilization and miscarriage rates do not appear to be different from other groups of infertile couples. Large national registers (Medical Research International (MRI, SART) 1990, 1991, HFEA 1993) have also reported similar pregnancy rates, following IVF or GIFT, for women with endometriosis in comparison with other categories. However, these figures should be interpreted with care as these registers include women with different grades of the disease, undergoing a variety of stimulation protocols, and treated in different centres. Initially, poor results were reported in women with severe disease (Matson & Yovich 1986). The introduction of ultrasound-guided techniques for oocyte collection resulted in the retrieval of larger numbers of oocytes and hence to higher pregnancy and implantation rates in advanced stage disease (Geber et al 1995, Olivennes et al 1995). The use of GnRH analogues in stimulation protocols, or as a pretreatment in women with endometriosis, has also resulted in a higher number of preovulatory oocytes retrieved and transferred, a lower cancellation rate for treatment cycles and a higher pregnancy rate especially in women with advanced stage disease.

The effect that assisted reproduction treatment may have on the progression of endometriosis has been insufficiently studied, and evidence suggests that one or repeated superovulations for IVF have minimal deleterious effects on the disease or chances of subsequent spontaneous pregnancy (Amso 1995a).

Embryo cryopreservation and its influence on IVF results

The first pregnancy following embryo cryopreservation was reported in 1983 (Trounson & Mohr 1983). Cryopreservation of embryos following IVF or GIFT procedures provides further possibilities for conception in addition to those achieved from fresh transfer. Additionally, cryopreservation has an important role when severe ovarian hyperstimulation is anticipated in the treatment cycle, allowing a delay of embryo transfer to a later cycle (Amso et al 1990).

The number of cryopreserved embryos and transfer procedures have increased considerably over the years (Table 19.7). Well over one-third of couples undergoing ovarian stimulation for IVF or GIFT have oocytes or embryos in excess of the number required for fresh transfer and it is expected that between 60–80% of embryos survive cryopreservation. Although the potential effects of currently used cryoprotectants and of the freezing or thawing processes on surviving embryos remain unclear, infants born following frozen/thawed embryo transfers have not shown increased incidence of birth defects (0.8–1.8% of total births) (SART 1993, 1995). The overall contribution of cryopreservation to the expectation of ongoing pregnancy in such couples is approximately 13% (ranging from 10.8 to 24.6%) and dependent on the number of oocytes recovered. The benefit is particularly marked for those couples who have more oocytes recovered and a greater number of embryos frozen. The implantation rates in all treatment cycles, or in pregnant cycles only, and the potential for establishing pregnancy

Table 19.7 Throughput and success rates following frozen/thawed embryo replacements, from the USA Registry 1987–1993 (MRI, SART 1989–1992, SART 1993, 1995, AFS, SART 1994) and UK in 1993 (HFEA 1995)

	USA registry							
	1987	1988	1989	1990	1991	1992	1993	UK 1993
Transfer procedures	490	1025	2124	3290	4225	5354	6194	2421
Clinical pregnancy	50	101	234	382	559	820	984	379
(% per transfer)	(10.2%)	(9.6%)	(11%)	(11.6%)	(13.2%)	(15.3%)	(15.9%)	(15.7%)
Delivery	38	73	172	291	431	619	791	304*
(% per transfer)	(7.8%)	(7.1%)	(8.1%)	(8.8%)	(10.2%)	(11.6%)	(12.8%)	(12.6%)

*Live birth and live birth rate per transfer.

differs little between the transfer of frozen/thawed or fresh embryos at IVF (Wang et al 1994).

Other factors which may affect the outcome of frozen/thawed embryo transfers include recipient age, male factor infertility, endometrial receptivity, and possibly the stimulation protocol. The overall impact may also be dependent on the original success rate for fresh embryo transfer procedures and the legal limits on the embryo storage time (Kahn et al 1993). As couples who conceive after a fresh cycle are unlikely to return for a frozen/thawed cycle within 2 years, it is crucial that this is taken into consideration when the impact on cumulative success rates, or any time limitations on embryo storage are considered.

Oocyte donation as a treatment modality

In the past decade, sociological changes have resulted in an overall delay of women's decisions to achieve pregnancy. This fact, along with a tremendous increase of the therapeutic alternatives offered to infertile couples, has resulted in a significant increase in the number of women of more advanced age seeking solutions to infertility. The majority of studies suggest that oocyte ageing is the main factor responsible for decreasing fertility, and the increasing pregnancy rates from oocyte donation strongly support this evidence. Indications for oocyte donation include: premature ovarian failure or resistant ovary syndrome, 'poor responders', abnormal, or unfertilized or degenerate oocytes during IVF treatments, surgical castration or following chemo- or radiotherapy, ovarian dysgenesis, and in women with hereditary genetic disease.

In all instances, the most critical component is the synchronization between the donor and recipient for appropriate timing of embryo replacement. In recipients with normal ovarian function, the LH surge can be monitored easily, in addition to determining serum levels of E_2 and progesterone. Recipients with ovarian failure must have oestrogen and progesterone therapy to prime the endometrium prior to ET. Hormonal replacement regimens may be either a fixed cyclical regimen, with E_2 administered in an incrementally increasing fashion in the follicular phase to mimic a natural cycle, followed by the introduction of progesterone on day 15 of E_2 replacement in a 28-day cycle. Alternatively, a constant low-dose, variable length E_2 regimen may be employed. This approach will overcome the problem of donor-recipient asynchrony by extending the follicular phase of the latter. Progesterone is commenced the day before or on the day of oocyte retrieval. Embryos at 4–8-cell stage should be available for transfer on days 17–19 of the recipient's menstrual cycle. In agonadal women, exogenous steroids must be continued for at least 10 weeks, until it is certain that the placenta will provide adequate endogenous support.

In treatments using donated eggs, the age of the woman has less of an effect on the clinical pregnancy and live birth rates. The success rates are higher following the use of donor oocytes (clinical pregnancy rate 38% and live birth rate 26% per treatment cycle) in all corresponding age groups and irrespective of using fresh or frozen/thawed embryos (HFEA 1995, SART 1995). The age of the women producing the oocytes affects the chances of implantation of an embryo in a manner that appears to be independent from other factors that contribute to the infertility of a couple (Balmaceda et al 1994).

The obstetric profile of pregnancies after oocyte donation poses special risks for the fetus and the mother. In the first trimester of pregnancy, there is a high incidence of uterine bleeding while later, the incidence of pre-eclampsia and intrauterine growth retardation is increased. The influence of maternal age as well as the high multiple pregnancy rate may contribute significantly to the above complications and increase the caesarean section rate. The long term physical and psychological development of these children is still under evaluation. Undoubtedly the inclusion of ever-older recipients of oocyte donation raises sociological and ethical questions which are discussed later.

Doppler ultrasound as a predictor of pregnancy in IVF treatment

Uterine receptivity and embryo quality are among many factors that are responsible for the establishment of pregnancy. The use of Doppler ultrasound provides an ideal non-invasive method to assess the uterine blood flow during the treatment cycle and may give an indication of the functional normality of the endometrium. Several indices have been used to interpret the flow velocity waveform (FVW) signal, and all these attempt to calculate an index of resistance or impedance to the blood flow distal to the area being examined. These indices are based on the ratio of the peak systolic flow (A) to the end-diastolic flow (B) and are independent of the angle of insonation. The most commonly used indices are the A/B ratio, the resistance index (RI)

$$RI = \frac{A - B}{B},$$

and the pulsatility index (PI)

$$PI = \frac{A - B}{\text{mean }(A + B)}.$$

Uterine perfusion and its deficiency have been hypothesized to be factors associated with subfertility and failure of implantation. It has also been suggested that the administration of exogenous oestradiol may be beneficial in reducing an abnormally elevated uterine artery resistance and hence may improve the pregnancy rate (Goswamy et al 1988). Using transvaginal colour Doppler, Steer et al (1992) reported that no pregnancy occurred in women where the PI score was ≥3 on the day of embryo transfer, while in those with a PI between 1 and 1.99, the pregnancy and implantation rates were 41 and 15.5 % respectively. The authors predicted that the PI on the day of embryo transfer may become a useful guide in the clinical management of women undergoing assisted reproduction treatment, and if it is abnormally raised, then all embryos may be cryopreserved and replaced in a subsequent hormone-regulated cycle. The same group (Steer et al 1995) reported significantly lower PI during conception cycles in women undergoing frozen embryo replacement. Other investigators (Tekay et al 1995) were either unable to detect any difference in the PI between pregnant and non-pregnant IVF cycles, or detected a tendency for higher pregnancy rates when the PI score was between 2.00–2.99. At present, the precise role of Doppler ultrasound in human reproduction remains under investigation.

POTENTIAL HEALTH RISKS ASSOCIATED WITH ASSISTED REPRODUCTION TECHNOLOGY

Potential health risks arising from assisted reproduction techniques have been the subject of important debate. Seamark & Robinson (1995) voiced concerns regarding the effect of such treatments on fetal development antenatally and the long-term postnatal outcome. They also drew our attention to 'disconcerting' results from animal research and sounded caution on the potential harmful effect on human reproduction. It is likely that more studies and several years of observation will be needed before we establish the full impact and potential health problems arising in the resultant babies. Equally pressing is the need to address the risks to couples and in particular women undergoing such treatments (Amso 1995b).

In most centres, women undergoing assisted reproduction treatments such as IVF or GIFT receive medication to induce multiple follicular development. Problems may arise due to inadvertent exposure of the developing embryo to these medications or due to side-effects resulting from their pharmacological actions. More serious complications such as ovarian hyperstimulation syndrome (OHSS), the potential risk of genital cancer, and physical/psychological health problems related to assisted reproduction therapy will be addressed in this section.

Ovarian hyperstimulation syndrome (OHSS)

OHSS with its poorly understood pathophysiology, remains the most serious and potentially lethal complication of ovulation induction. It correlates positively with conceptual cycles and is almost exclusively related to either exogenous or endogenous hCG stimulation. The risk increases with the total number of follicles in the preovulatory period including immature and intermediate follicles, and it may present 3–7 days (early presentation) or 12–17 days (late presentation) after the hCG injection. The key to prevention is proper identification of the population at risk before treatment and close monitoring of hormone levels as well as follicular response on ultrasound (Fig. 19.10). When a high risk situation is recognized, withholding the ovulatory dose of hCG injection and cancellation of the treatment cycle will almost certainly prevent OHSS. The couple should be advised to avoid intercourse as spontaneous ovulation may occur up to 11 days after discontinuing gonadotrophin treatment resulting in conception and development of severe OHSS.

Alternative strategies usually succeed at ameliorating the severity of this complication rather than its total prevention and include the following.

1. Reduction of the ovulatory hCG dose and avoiding its use in the luteal phase.
2. Triggering ovulation with GnRH analogue (intranasal or subcutaneous administration) instead of hCG in suitable subjects.
3. Reduction of the gonadotrophin dose in subsequent treatment cycles has been attempted, with varying degrees of success.
4. Delay in the administration of hCG (controlled drift period or prolonged coasting) results in rapid decline of serum E_2 levels but an increase in the size of the lead follicles. Clinical pregnancy rates of between 25–35% have been reported (Urman et al 1992), but with an unacceptably high multiple pregnancy rate (50%) and severe OHSS in 2.5% of all cases.

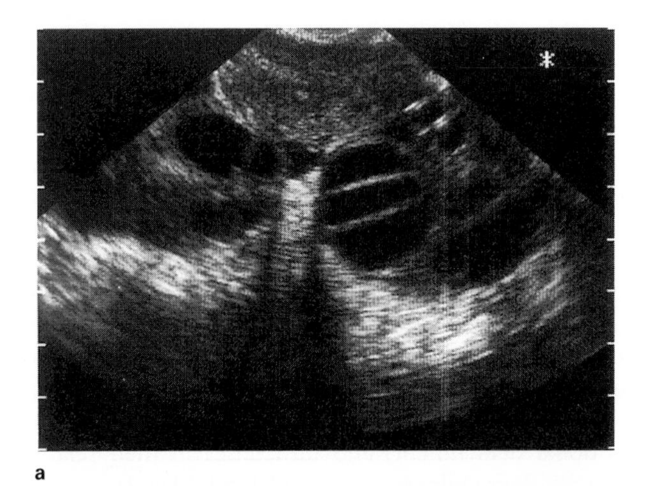

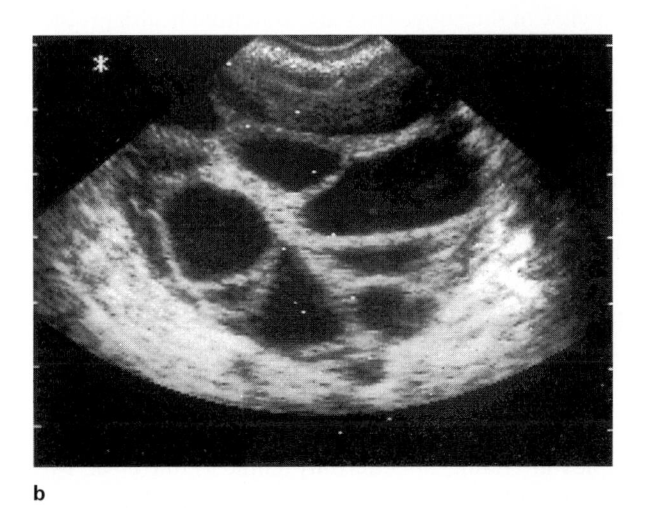

Fig. 19.10 **a** Vaginal ultrasound appearance of the hyperstimulated ovaries. The enlarged ovaries almost completely occupy the pelvis and contain an excessive number of large, intermediate and small follicles. **b** Vaginal ultrasound appearance of the mature follicles in a normal ovary prior to vaginal egg collection.

5. Conversion of superovulation with or without intrauterine insemination cycles to IVF.
6. Elimination of the endogenous pregnancy-derived hCG by aspiration of all follicles, fertilization of oocytes and cryopreservation of all embryos (Amso et al 1990). Subsequent frozen/thawed embryo replacement cycles result in pregnancy and implantation rates comparable to those with fresh embryo transfers.
7. The use of intravenous albumin infusion at the time of oocyte recovery. This has been reported to prevent the development of severe OHSS or to markedly reduce its incidence and severity (Asch et al 1993, Shoham 1994).

The use of steroids in high risk patients has also been found to be ineffective in reducing the rate of OHSS after superovulation for IVF.

Treatment of established OHSS depends on its severity, the stage at which the diagnosis is made and whether the patient is pregnant or not. In mild/moderate OHSS (haematocrit ≤44%), bed rest, increased fluid intake, and close monitoring of electrolyte balance may be sufficient. The patient's progress can be supervised daily as an outpatient procedure. Patients with severe OHSS (haematocrit ≥45%, massive ascites) should be hospitalized and if critically ill should be cared for in intensive care units. Paracentesis, for symptomatic relief or falling renal function, was reported to result in dramatic improvement in clinical symptoms with almost instantaneous diuresis, decrease in haematocrit, improved creatinine clearance, and prevention of respiratory distress (Aboulghar et al 1992). In an extreme situation, therapeutic interruption of an early pregnancy may be the only lifesaving action when other measures have failed.

Risk of genital cancer

The potential risk of genital cancer from follicular stimulation has initiated considerable debate (Cohen et al 1993, Fishel & Jackson 1989, Rossing et al 1994, Whittemore 1994). Excessive oestrogen secretion has been implicated in ovarian, endometrial and breast carcinoma, and excessive gonadotrophin secretion may have a direct carcinogenic effect as well.

Although a number of case reports of ovarian tumours (benign, borderline malignancy, carcinoma) in women undergoing infertility treatment have raised questions about the potential neoplastic effects of ovulation induction medication, none proves a causal relationship. Results of recent case–control and case–cohort studies are conflicting. Whittemore et al (1992) pooled data from case–control studies of ovarian cancer between 1956 and 1986 and reported positive associations between the use of fertility medications and the risk of invasive and borderline epithelial tumours, and a possible association between the use of such medications and the risk of nonepithelial cancers. In a case–control study, Franceschi et al (1994) analysed the relationship between fertility drugs and ovarian cancer in four areas of Italy, and the authors were able to exclude any association between the use of fertility drugs and the risk of epithelial ovarian cancer, contradicting the earlier finding by Whittemore et al (1992). Rossing et al (1994) examined the risk of ovarian tumours in a cohort of infertile women, and reported a higher risk of malignant ovarian tumours in gravid and nulligravid women treated for infertility, and in particular for those who used clomiphene citrate for 12 or more cycles.

All of the above studies had their limitations and included a relatively small number of tumours during the follow-up period. However, all authors agreed on the need for further studies, with appropriate control groups, to determine whether the link is causal and, if so, the magnitude of the risks, the treatments that are more risky, and the women who are most susceptible.

Concerns relating to the high oestrogen and progesterone levels on the potential risk for the development of breast cancer have also been expressed, but there is scarce information. In a recent report (Venn et al 1995) the incidence of breast cancer in women who have had IVF treatment with ovarian stimulation was not different from the incidence in the general population or in women referred for IVF but not treated. An interesting finding in the latter study was the significant association between unexplained infertility and both invasive ovarian and uterine corpus cancer, independent of IVF exposure.

Further studies are required to allow for a longer latency effect between exposure to fertility drugs and the later development of cancer.

Procedure-related health problems

Whilst ultrasound-guided transvaginal oocyte recovery is at present the most commonly used method, the laparoscopic approach is still used in certain circumstances and is associated with risks related to anaesthesia, pneumoperitoneum, visceral and vascular injuries and infections. In women undergoing transvaginal oocyte retrievals, intestinal, vascular, uterine, and tubal injuries with the aspiration needle have been reported. Bleeding and infections may be serious, sometimes even fatal, complications. A previous history of pelvic inflammatory disease may imply a higher risk of pelvic reinfection. Appropriate preoperative vaginal preparation and minimizing the number of repeated vaginal penetrations may serve to lower the risk of infection. The long-term effects of repeated oocyte collections on the pelvic structures have not been fully evaluated.

In one study of 15 women with endometriosis who were undergoing tubal embryo transfer, only one patient was noted to have a change, in that one fallopian tube had become tethered to the corresponding ovary. Similarly, the culture of micro-organisms in peritoneal samples obtained at the time of laparoscopic tubal embryo transfer (coagulase-negative *Staphylococcus*, β-haemolytic *Streptococcus*, and *Chlamydia trachomatis*) was not associated with the development of symptoms or signs of pelvic infection, nor were three conceptions and subsequent normal deliveries without any sequelae to the newborn prevented. Furthermore, spontaneous pregnancies were also reported up to 18 months after an unsuccessful attempt (Amso 1996). The results in this small group of women are very reassuring, but larger studies are required to determine the full impact of these techniques on the pelvic organs.

Psychological and emotional effects

The intensive monitoring that is commonly required during ovulation induction may cause undue stress and anxiety. In the immediate aftermath of a failed treatment cycle or following early pregnancy loss, the couple may experience shock, frustration and depression. Long-term effects of failed treatment(s) may lead to marital discord and breakdown of the relationship. Similarly, in addition to the increased antenatal medical risks associated with multiple pregnancy, considerable psychological difficulties are encountered by mothers after birth. The increased perinatal mortality and morbidity are well known and further increase the couples' anxiety and emotional strain. The majority of these mothers report considerable fatigue and stress, social isolation, strain on marital relationship, emotional detachment, and difficulties in their relationship with their children (Garel & Blondel 1992).

In view of the above risks and potential health problems, it is imperative that clinicians should define the risks as not only those associated with the medication itself, but also the short- and long-term effects which are either physical, emotional or pregnancy-related. As many of the long-term effects are still undetermined, clinicians must offer couples appropriate counselling and exercise extreme care and caution before and during treatment.

NEW TECHNIQUES IN THE MANAGEMENT OF MALE SUBFERTILITY

Male infertility is a very common cause of childlessness. Indeed it may be a contributing factor in nearly half of all couples attending an infertility clinic (Hull et al 1985). Male infertility may also interact with problems in the female and vice versa. The application of modern diagnostic and therapeutic reproductive technology to male infertility represents a major advance in the treatment of infertile couples.

Careful evaluation of the male with appropriate clinical examination shows that the aetiology of male subfertility can be divided into four main groups as follows.

1. Primary spermatogenic failure, a testicular disorder, resulting in a reduction in sperm numbers and abnormalities in sperm function. A number of different factors can induce this condition, including testicular maldescent, trauma, karyotype abnormalities, severe infection and antimitotic therapy, but in many patients a cause cannot be ascertained.
2. The presence of an obstructive lesion such as failure of reversal of vasectomy. This group is forming an increasing percentage of men seen in infertility clinics, and at present constitutes up to 10% of all male problems.
3. Disturbances of erection or ejaculatory disorders including those following spinal injuries.
4. Endocrine disorders such as Cushing's disease, thyroid disorders and androgen receptor abnormalities.

It should be remembered that many types of male infertility may have considerable congenital implications for the children of such patients. The recent application of advanced reproductive techniques to generate offspring from men with congenital absence of the vas deferens, and the subsequent demonstration of the presence of one or more of the cystic fibrosis genes in the majority of these men (Rigot 1991), is an example of a treatment modality preceding a full understanding of the underlying cause of one type of male infertility.

Diagnostic techniques

The descriptive assessment of semen parameters is of comparatively limited prognostic value in predicting the achievement of pregnancy, a problem which remains central to clinical andrology. Consequently, numerous additional tests of sperm function have been developed, and have recently culminated in the introduction of computer-assisted image analysis of sperm motion (also known as CASA). Sperm movement has been found to be correlated to critical aspects of sperm function, including interaction with cervical mucus and with the zona pellucida. Sperm morphology and morphometry have also been examined as possible predictors of sperm function. Several problems arise including the well known phenomena of inter-ejaculate variability, both qualitative and functional, and interobserver variability.

The introduction of computer-assisted image analysis systems has become widespread despite their yet unclear clinical usefulness. Their potential advantages over subjective assessment techniques include better objectivity, sensitivity and reliability, and thus their use should improve laboratory standardization and the implementation of quality control procedures.

Several of the conventional criteria of semen quality have been assessed by computer-assisted analysis in comparison with standard laboratory techniques (Macleod et al 1994), and similarly the reproducibility of the different systems has been reported (Holt et al 1994). Interestingly, the computer-assisted techniques did not provide data on semen quality comparable to that from the standard laboratory techniques, but the measurements obtained were more consistent. Additionally, the morphometric data generated by image analysis did not appear to be related to the conventional morphology assessment. Analysis of a single donor sample by a number of computer systems showed that all parameters examined, namely sperm concentration, percentage of motile sperm, mean average path velocity, and mean amplitude of lateral head displacement varied considerably 'within-system' rather than 'between-system'. This suggested that differences in handling of samples and operator expertise were more significant sources of variation than the computerized systems themselves, and highlight the need for a high degree of operator training, standardization of sample handling techniques and formal assessment of these systems in the clinical context.

A new therapeutic technique: intracytoplasmic sperm injection (ICSI)

Male infertility as a whole leads to a poorer outcome following in vitro fertilization than do other causes for infertility. Although efforts have been made to improve the fertilization rate of poor quality semen by varying the techniques of sperm preparation, the outcomes remain unsatisfactory. Invasive techniques such as partial zona dissection (PZD) and subzonal insemination (SUZI) have not improved these results substantially, although occasional success in well selected cases has been achieved.

A more recent breakthrough for severe male factor infertility is the successful introduction of intracytoplasmic sperm injection (ICSI) (Palermo et al 1992, Van Steirteghem et al 1993) which has led to high fertilization and implantation rates. The incorporation of ICSI technology into clinical IVF programmes worldwide has reversed the thinking that male infertility is the major stumbling block to the treatment of subfertile couples. The technique requires a high quality inverted microscope and special equipment with 'holding' and 'injection' pipettes being used to stabilize and inject the oocyte respectively. The injecting pipette is pushed almost entirely through the ooplasm before the spermatozoon is deposited inside the oocyte (Fig. 19.11).

Comparison of the results following ICSI with those of other treatments for male factor infertility, such as SUZI and PZD, indicate that ICSI is a much more efficient technique than either of the others (Tarin 1995). The overall results from SUZI and PZD were especially dis-

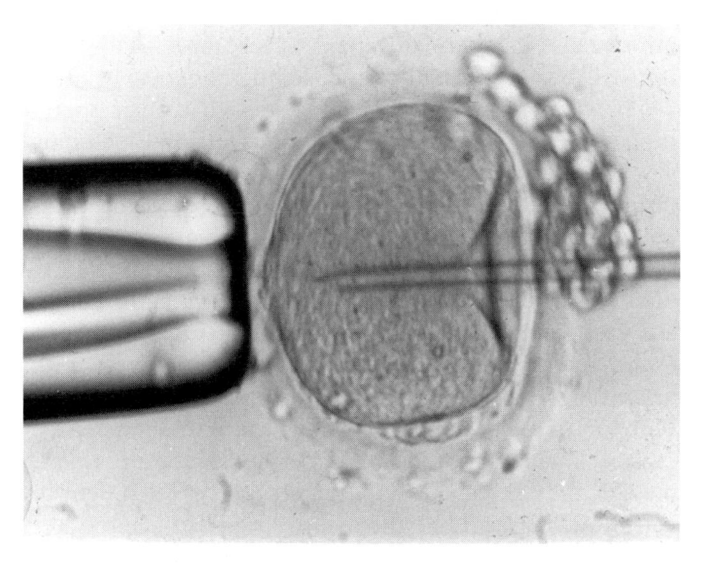

Fig. 19.11 Intracytoplasmic injection of a single sperm into the egg (courtesy of Dr Simon Fishel, Scientific Director, Nottingham University Research and Treatment Unit in Reproduction — NURTURE).

appointing as the monospermic fertilization rate was generally low, averaging only 18% and with unacceptable levels of polyspermic fertilization. Furthermore, the latter techniques appeared to be beneficial only in men with moderately abnormal semen profiles (>5 million motile spermatozoa/ml) (Cohen et al 1991). Conversely, ICSI appears to be suitable for treatment of men with severely impaired semen characteristics, does not require special treatment of the spermatozoa before injection into the oocyte, and achieves a higher fertilization rate (≈ 49%) which is not affected by sperm concentration, motility or morphology in the fresh ejaculate (Tarin 1995). Microinjection of epididymal and testicular spermatozoa have also been successfully used resulting in equally high fertilization, pregnancy and implantation rates (Tucker et al 1995).

The main indications for ICSI at present are: previous failure of fertilization with conventional IVF or where very low fertilization rates were obtained, when there are less than 5 million spermatozoa in the whole ejaculate with poor progressive motility or when sperm is obtained from testicular biopsies or the epididymis. Morphologically abnormal sperm have also been successfully utilized. A remarkable change in fertilization rate with a significant increase in the percentage of two pronuclei oocytes occurred when the technique was slightly modified by breaking the sperm tail before injection (Fishel et al 1995, Gerris et al 1995). A review of the published literature (Tarin 1995) on the early experience with ICSI showed that pregnancy rates in the order of 21–39% per embryo transfer, and implantation rates ranging from 6 to 27% have been achieved, and that the average number of embryos transferred was over 2 in the majority of studies. In several instances there were excess embryos for cryopreservation.

Concern about the use of ICSI has been expressed in view of our ignorance of the underlying cause of the impairment in spermatogenesis. More specifically, the view has been expressed that 'male infertility may be associated with germ cell mutations and that such sperm mutations transmit inheritable characteristics including susceptibility to infertility which may be expressed in future generations' (Baker et al 1993). To date, the available evidence suggests that there is no increase in chromosomal abnormalities in the fertilized oocytes after the use of SUZI in comparison with fertilized eggs after classic IVF techniques. If chromosomal anomalies have not been found to increase, other factors (e.g. fertilization with genetically or physiologically abnormal spermatozoa, fertilization of abnormal oocytes) might lead to an increased number of malformations or other congenital problems, possibly only detectable at a later stage of development or when such offspring themselves start to reproduce. Bonduelle et al (1994) prospectively followed up 55 children after subzonal insemination and intracytoplasmic sperm injection. Only one child from a singleton pregnancy presented multiple congenital malformations, one twin child presented a quadriparesis and no malformations were detected by ultrasonography. Prenatal screening with amniocentesis due to maternal age risk did not reveal any abnormal results. Although the number of children was small, the incidence of major and minor malformations was not different from the incidence in the general population and within the range expected following assisted reproduction treatment. A follow up of a larger number of children (n = 877) born after ICSI, by the same group, showed a 2.6% incidence of major malformations leading to functional impairment or necessitating surgery (Liebaers et al 1995). Six (1%) chromosomal anomalies in 585 prenatal diagnostic procedures (chorion villus sampling or amniocentesis) were reported, five of which were sex chromosome aberrations. The authors acknowledged that there might indeed be a slightly increased risk of these chromosomal aberrations and thus routinely advised all couples to have prenatal diagnosis and to participate in a prospective pregnancy and offspring follow-up study.

A study of the obstetric outcomes of 424 pregnancies resulting from ICSI for severe male factor infertility reported an early pregnancy loss of 23%, a perinatal mortality rate of 18.9 per 1000 births, and problems of prematurity and low birth weight related to multiple pregnancies (Wisanto et al 1995). The study concluded that obstetric outcome was similar to that obtained after conventional IVF and other assisted reproduction techniques. Larger studies and longer periods of follow-up are necessary before the safety and full impact of these techniques can be evaluated. Without such a strategy, professionals in this field would be open to severe criticism and risk that this practice be rejected by society.

PREIMPLANTATION GENETIC DIAGNOSIS: BREAKING THE BARRIERS

Preimplantation genetic diagnosis (PGD) is a new procedure which has been developed in the past few years as an alternative to prenatal diagnosis for carriers of chromosomal or sex-linked disorders (Handyside et al 1990). As with other forms of prenatal diagnosis, its primary aim is to avoid severe genetic disease in the offspring of a couple who have a high probability of passing on mutant genes, but with an added advantage that it avoids termination of pregnancy. The procedure involves biopsy of a single cell from the human cleavage stage embryo at around the 8-cell stage followed by the application of a sensitive diagnostic technique to that cell. At present, biopsied polar body and/or blastomeres have been used and pregnancies as well as healthy babies have resulted from such biopsied and diagnosed embryos. The diagnostic technique, specific for the disorder being tested, may be analysis of enzymes, chromosomes or specific mutation in the DNA. If the cell shows no abnormality in the course of this analysis, the embryo is judged to be normal and transferred to the mother to initiate pregnancy.

The enzyme approach has been disregarded, for the few genes studied, as it has been difficult to differentiate between maternal gene expression (mRNA inherited in the egg cytoplasm), and embryonic gene expression in the early embryo (Braude et al 1989). However, the analysis of sex chromosomes, using fluorescent in situ hybridization (FISH), and the analysis of specific gene sequences, using sensitive polymerase chain reaction (PCR), for sexing or for detection of a specific gene mutation such as cystic fibrosis have been used successfully.

Preimplantation diagnosis of single gene defects and chromosomal abnormalities by analysis of the first and second polar bodies had been proposed as an alternative to embryonic biopsy. The limitations of this approach lie in the fact that the genotype of polar bodies is not identical to that of the oocyte and that the validity of predicting chromosome abnormalities in the pre-embryo from observations of the chromosome complement of either polar body has been subject to uncertainty. The variety of combinations that may arise through random segregation of each single chromatid, either to the second polar body or oocyte, indicate that it would not be possible to predict the chromosome normality or otherwise of the female gamete (Angell 1994) and more data is needed. It has also been reported that polar bodies are more difficult to manipulate than blastomeres due to their size and that, for some reason, embryos obtained after polar body biopsy show a reduced implantation rate (Egozcue 1994). Hence, subject to the success of polar body analysis techniques, the possible application in clinical practice would be limited to those couples who, on moral grounds, reject embryo selection after preimplantation diagnosis.

Since the introduction of PGD, attempts have been made to maximize the results through simultaneous detection of more than one mutation, increase efficiencies and to be able to analyse these biopsied cells further for chromosomal abnormalities. Avner et al (1994) reported the successful development of a PCR-based method for the simultaneous detection of the two most common mutations of the cystic fibrosis gene in a single blastomere. The diagnostic system allowed the identification of affected embryos as well as phenotypically normal carriers. The completion of the multiple loci analysis with this method required about 17 h and embryo transfer was possible on the same day or within 24 h of biopsy. Thornhill et al (1994) introduced the concept of recycling the single cell to detect specific chromosome and investigate unique gene sequences. The two techniques, PCR and FISH, were carried out on the same single cell. In this system a fixed cell is used as a DNA template for PCR prior to the FISH analysis. The combination of the two techniques provides an even greater potential for the efficiency and accuracy of preimplantation diagnosis. It was also proposed that the potential of cell recycling could be extended using multiplex PCR with different sets of primers to examine between 5 and 10 specific gene sequences simultaneously. The FISH analysis can also be extended to employ up to 7 specific chromosomal DNA probes using combinatorial labelling. More recently, Muggleton-Harris et al (1995) demonstrated that dual stage biopsies are possible, where blastomeres are taken from the 8–10-cell embryos and the biopsied cleavage-stage embryo is cultured to the blastocyst stage, where the serial biopsy of 3–5 mural trophectoderm cells provides two further cell samples. Repeat or additional preimplantation diagnostic analyses were undertaken again. This approach answers to a certain extent the uncertainty as to what extent the chromosome constitution of the single blastomere is representative of the whole embryo. Equally there would be a significant advantage for genetic diagnosis studies if retrospective PCR analysis could be undertaken on stored cell samples used previously for preimplantation genetic diagnosis. Pregnancy rates have continued to improve following replacement of cleavage stage embryos and cultured blastocysts. So far, the techniques have been used to diagnose cystic fibrosis, sickle-cell disease and Duchenne muscular dystrophy, as well as the identification (using the FISH technique) of human chromosomes X, Y, 13, 18 and 21. Preimplantation diagnosis may also be achieved after natural conceptions by obtaining blastocysts through a uterine lavage procedure.

The psychological implications and acceptability of preimplantation diagnosis are areas that require further evaluation. Palomba et al (1994) examined the degree of acceptability of preimplantation diagnosis with blastocyst stage biopsy in women at risk of beta thalassaemia who were awaiting chorionic villus sampling. The authors reported that all women who had had a previous therapeutic termination of pregnancy found blastocyst biopsy acceptable, while only 30% of women who had not had a previous therapeutic abortion favoured the technique, and 25% of primigravid women also favoured blastocyst biopsy to chorionic villus sampling. In this group of women, blastocysts were anticipated to have been obtained through uterine lavage, hence the diagnosis would have been made on the 5th day after fertilization offering psychological advantages, both by reducing the waiting time of 11 weeks and by avoiding therapeutic abortion in the first trimester of pregnancy when there was an affected fetus. In women undergoing in vitro fertilization, PGD also offers the option of replacing only healthy embryos and possibly increasing the chances of implantation and pregnancy.

ETHICAL DILEMMAS IN ASSISTED REPRODUCTION

The problems related to social values and research on the human embryo were first raised by Edwards & Sharpe

(1971). The Human Fertilization and Embryology Act (1990) resulted in the establishment of a statutory body, the Human Fertilization and Embryology Authority, within the UK to regulate and monitor, by means of an inspection and licensing system, the provision of treatment and research using human gametes and embryos.

The Authority has also issued consultation documents on a number of ethical and social dimensions of the new aspects of assisted human reproduction. The use of oocytes from donated ovarian tissue for infertility treatment and embryo research has generated considerable debate, and views were obtained from a wider public before determining the Authority's position. The current opinion is that it would be acceptable to use ovarian tissue for treatment purposes only from live donors. In the case of a deceased woman over the age of 18 years there appears to be no objection in principle to the use of donated ovarian tissue for the treatment of other women; however, informed consent should be provided before death. Not unexpectedly, there was widespread and fundamental objection to the use of fetal tissue for treatment in view of the difficult psychological consequences for the offspring.

The debate in the UK has contributed to the establishment in many countries of similar public mechanisms to review clinical and ethical questions relating to assisted reproduction treatment and provide counsel. Self-regulation supported by national and/or local codes of practice appear to be the most popular means, but countries like Germany and the UK impose strict codes underlined by the power of the law. In the USA, the National Advisory Board on Ethics and Reproduction was set up in 1992 to fill the vacuum created by the lack of systematic reflection on the ethical questions raised by reproductive research and medicine. However, in parts of the United States, legislation relating to assisted reproduction has been implemented such as the State of Florida Assisted Reproduction Technology Act of 1993.

Pregnancies in postmenopausal women have been controversial. The introduction of oocyte donation with its high clinical pregnancy, implantation and live birth rates has meant that pregnancy is now possible in virtually any woman with a uterus, and no definitive physiological limitation appears to exist based solely on the age of the patient. There are arguments and counterarguments with respect to this treatment. At present, the consensus of opinion in the UK is that no category of women should automatically be denied treatment, it is not necessary nor advisable to fix an upper age limit for the treatment of infertility and each case should be considered individually. It is also required by law that the welfare of the prospective child should be considered and the implications for the couple concerned. A survey of community attitudes to maternal age and pregnancy after assisted reproduction technology reported support for the use of a woman's own eggs or embryos after the menopause, but only minority support for oocyte or embryo donation to postmenopausal women (Bowman & Saunders 1994). Public opinion may alter over time, especially if the attitudes of the younger portion of the community, as reflected in the above survey, are maintained, and furthermore, opinion expressed in one community may or may not reflect that of other communities.

The psychosocial effects of such treatment are largely unknown and the nature of obstetric complications will not be known without greater numbers being reported. Epidemiological statistics from the USA suggest that one in five mothers and one in three fathers having a child at the age of 50 years will not survive to see the child at college; if the age of delivery is 55 years, then one in three mothers and one in two fathers will not survive the same length of time (Meldrum 1993).

Other ethical controversies have also attracted worldwide debate such as the control of human sex ratios and 'sex selection', posthumous reproduction and artificial insemination of single and lesbian women with donor sperm. Posthumous reproduction can result in complex and expensive legal proceedings and generate undue anxieties for the parties involved. It has also been argued that this lacks the very values that most people find in the reproductive experience, such as interests in rearing one's child, or giving birth. Several countries (Canada, France, Germany and Sweden) have legislation that forbids posthumous reproduction on the basis of a moral commitment to fairness and respect for children, and an obligation to treat them as ends in themselves (Aziza-Shuster 1994). Whilst all these issues are brought about through advances in technology it is clear that irrespective of the current guidelines, clinicians need better understanding of the background and needs of the people involved and their views towards the resulting child and its future development. Similarly, clinicians must have the right of non-participation should their moral conscience tell them so.

WHERE ARE WE GOING?

It is clear that there is much in this field that we do not know about, and advances are taking place rapidly. However, based on recent developments, the temptation is great to highlight areas of anticipated progress over the next few years.

Perhaps the most exciting progress will be achieved with recombinant human FSH and LH. These products will permanently modify the way that ovulation induction is performed and provide control that was not previously available over dosage. The use of genetic engineering techniques and different cell types to produce these glycoproteins will permit availability of molecular variants of 'isohormones' or 'isoforms' with differential activities. A totally new philosophy of 'flexible', 'customized', and 'individualized' ovulation induction regimens will be standard practice.

The continued improvement in success rates with ICSI treatment will no doubt consolidate the role of this technique for male infertility. It will place considerable pressure on units to provide it, and may pave the way for emergence of 'transport ICSI' as a concept for smaller units unable to provide the costly investment and/or the highly skilled personnel required for this technique. Long-term monitoring is needed to ensure the safety of this treatment regarding the offspring. Perhaps the main challenge will be the need for a greater understanding of the factors involved in male infertility and how to increase fecundity.

Preimplantation genetic diagnosis is now becoming a reality in the clinical field, and new techniques are being developed to identify the presence or absence of specific genes in a short period of time, to allow biopsied pre-embryos to be evaluated before their transfer to the uterus. Additionally, these advances will permit rapid progress in gene therapy for single or multiple gene disorders where a normal cloned gene is used to replace the faulty genome. Advances in basic science should improve our understanding of the mechanisms involved in oocyte maturation, both in vivo and in vitro, in embryo implantation and in early placentation and are crucial for the improvement of pregnancy rates and outcome.

One of the major technological revolutions in our time which will have a great impact on patient care is that of the interactive information technology network. Simultaneous transfer and sharing of images and information will enable many main centres to supervise some aspects of patient care from a distance, telemonitoring, thus reducing the overall cost of treatment. Similarly, wide availability of information on the Internet and the World Wide Web would encourage IVF centres to disseminate general information, specific instructions, and up-to-date success rates of the different techniques in their units to any couple requiring such therapy.

The ethical issues involved will continue to be the focus of much attention, from ethics committees and legislators worldwide. The establishment of voluntary or statutory bodies to consult and to develop guidelines or policies and implement laws is necessary to ensure the continued trust and support of society for the scientists and clinicians working in this field. These bodies will need to evaluate continuously the moral views and position of society on the constantly evolving technologies in this field. In the UK, it is reassuring to see that such measures are in place and fulfilling their role.

KEY POINTS

1. In vitro fertilization should not be used as a panacea for marital or psychosexual disorders, but to fulfil the wishes of a well adjusted couple to have a baby.
2. The aims of superovulation regimens in assisted reproduction are to maximize the number of follicles which mature, minimize the degree of asynchrony amongst developing follicles, and minimize the deleterious effects of the abnormal follicular environment on luteal function and endometrial receptivity.
3. The use of GnRH analogues in stimulation protocols has increased steadily since their introduction into clinical practice, and appears to result in a reduction in the cancellation rates, an increase in the number of oocytes retrieved and significantly higher clinical pregnancy rates.
4. The ultrasound-guided transvaginal route is the predominant method for egg collection and has almost completely replaced all other techniques.
5. Pregnancy and live birth rates in national registers in the US, France and Britain have improved by about 50% since the first annual reports were published in these countries.
6. Crude pregnancy rates per couple are almost meaningless and cumulative conception or live birth rates should be increasingly used in reporting conventional and assisted reproduction treatment outcomes.
7. The outcome of assisted reproduction treatment depends on the age of the female partner, the duration of infertility, the multiplicity of factors responsible for the couple's subfertility and the number of treatment cycles which they have undergone.
8. Endometriosis at all stages is viewed as a suitable indication for assisted reproduction treatment.
9. The overall contribution of cryopreservation to the expectation of ongoing pregnancy to couples with excess embryos is approximately 13%, and dependent on the number of oocytes recovered.
10. In view of the potential health risks arising from assisted reproduction techniques, it is imperative that clinicians should define the risks as those associated with the medication itself as well as the short- and long-term physical, emotional and pregnancy-related effects.
11. Male infertility is a very common cause of childlessness.
12. Intracytoplasmic sperm injection (ICSI) is a major breakthrough for the treatment of severe male factor infertility but requires a long period of follow up before its safety and full impact can be evaluated.
13. Preimplantation genetic diagnosis techniques have been used to detect cystic fibrosis, sickle cell disease, Duchenne muscular dystrophy, and chromosomes X, Y, 13, 18 and 21.
14. Ethical dilemmas in assisted reproduction continue to provoke considerable debate in the community and some treatments have been controversial.
15. Clinicians must have the right of non-participation, according to their conscience.

REFERENCES

Aboulghar M A, Mansour R T, Serour G I, Riad R, Ramzi A M 1992 Autotransfusion of the ascitic fluid in the treatment of severe ovarian hyperstimulation syndrome. Fertility and Sterility 58: 1056–1059

Amso N N 1995a Role of assisted reproduction in endometriosis. In: Shaw R W (ed) Endometriosis: current understanding and management. Blackwell Science, Oxford, pp 282–295

Amso N N 1995b Potential health hazards of assisted reproduction: problems facing the clinician. Human Reproduction 10: 1628–1630

Amso N N 1996 Studies of the Fallopian tube environment and an assessment of its role in assisted reproduction. PhD thesis submitted to the Faculty of Medicine, University of London

Amso N N, Ahuja K K, Morris N, Shaw R W 1990 The management of predicted ovarian hyperstimulation involving gonadotropin-releasing hormone analog with elective cryopreservation of all pre-embryos. Fertility and Sterility 53: 1087–1090

Angell R R 1994 Polar body analysis: possible pitfalls in preimplantation diagnosis of chromosomal disorders based on polar body analysis. Human Reproduction 9: 181–182

Asch R H 1987 GIFT: a multicentric international study. In: Proceedings of VIth World Congress of Human Reproduction, Tokyo

Asch R H, Ivery G, Goldsman M, Frederick J L, Stone S C, Balmaceda J P 1993 The use of intravenous albumin in patients at high risk for severe ovarian hyperstimulation syndrome. Human Reproduction 8: 1015–1020

Avner R, Laufer N, Safran A, Karem B-S, Friedmann A, Mitrani-Rosenbaum S 1994 Preimplantation diagnosis of cystic fibrosis by simultaneous detection of the W1282X and delta F508 mutations. Human Reproduction 9: 1676–1680

Aziza-Shuster E 1994 A child at all costs posthumous reproduction and the meaning of parenthood. Human Reproduction 9: 2182–2185

Baker H W G, Liu D Y, Bourne H, Lopata A 1993 Diagnosis of sperm defects in selecting patients for assisted fertilization. Human Reproduction 8: 1779–1780

Balmaceda J P, Bernardini L, Ciuffardi I et al 1994 Oocyte donation in humans: a model to study the effect of age on embryo implantation rate. Human Reproduction 9: 2160–2163

Bonduelle M, Desmyttere S, Buysse A et al 1994 Prospective follow-up study of 55 children born after subzonal insemination and intracytoplasmic sperm injection. Human Reproduction 9: 1765–1769

Bowman M C, Saunders D M 1994 Community attitudes to maternal age and pregnancy after assisted reproductive technology: too old at 50 years? Human Reproduction 9: 167–171

Braude P R, Monk M, Pickering S J, Cant A, Johnson M H 1989 Measurement of HPRT activity in the human unfertilised oocyte and pre-embryo. Prenatal Diagnosis 9: 839–850

Cohen J, Alikani M, Malter H E, Adler A, Talansky B E, Rosenwaks Z 1991 Partial zona dissection or subzonal sperm insertion: microsurgical fertilization alternatives based on evaluation of sperm and embryo morphology. Fertility and Sterility 56: 696–706

Cohen J, Forman R, Harlap S et al 1993 IFFS Expert Group Report on the Whittemore study related to the risk of ovarian cancer associated with the use of fertility agents. Human Reproduction 8: 996–999

Craft I, Al-Shawaf T, Lewis P et al 1988 Analysis of 1071 GIFT procedures – the case for a flexible approach to treatment. Lancet 1: 1094–1097

Damewood M D 1989 The role of the new reproductive technologies including IVF and GIFT in endometriosis. Obstetric and Gynecological Clinics of North America 16: 179–191

Daya S, Gunby J, Hughes E G, Collins J A, Sagle M A 1995 Follicle-stimulating hormone versus human menopausal gonadotropin for in vitro fertilization cycles: a meta-analysis. Fertility and Sterility 64: 347–354

Devroey P, Staessen C, Camus M, De Grauwe E, Wisanto A, Van Steirteghem A C 1989 Zygote intrafallopian transfer as a successful treatment for unexplained infertility. Fertility and Sterility 52: 246–249

Devroey P, Mannaerts B, Smitz J, Coelingh Bennink H, Van Steirteghem A 1994 Clinical outcome of a pilot efficacy study on recombinant human follicle-stimulating hormone (Org 32489) combined with various gonadotrophin-releasing hormone agonist regimens. Human Reproduction 9: 1064–1069

Edwards R G, Sharpe D J 1971 Social values and research in human embryology. Nature, 231: 87–91

Egozcue J 1994 Polar body analysis: possible pitfalls in preconception diagnosis of single gene and chromosome disorders. Human Reproduction 9: 1208

Fishel S, Jackson P 1989 Follicular stimulation for high tech pregnancies: are we playing it safe? British Medical Journal 299: 309–311

Fishel S, Lisi F, Rinaldi L, Green S, Hunter A, Dowell K 1995 Systematic examination of immobilizing spermatozoa before intracytoplasmic sperm injection in the human. Human Reproduction 10: 497–500

FIVNAT (French In Vitro National) 1993 French national IVF registry: analysis of 1986–1990 data. Fertility and Sterility 59: 587–595

Franceschi S, La Vecchia C, Negri E et al 1994 Fertility drugs and risk of epithelial ovarian cancer in Italy. Human Reproduction 9: 1673–1675

Garel M, Blondel B 1992 Assessment at 1 year of the psychological consequences of having triplets. Human Reproduction 7: 729–732

Geber S, Paraschos T, Atkinson G, Margara R, Winston R M L 1995 Results of IVF in patients with endometriosis: the severity of the disease does not affect the outcome, or the incidence of miscarriage. Human Reproduction 10: 1507–1511

Gerris J, Mangelshcots K, Van Royen E, Joostens M, Eestermans W, Ryckaert G 1995 ICSI and severe male-factor infertility: breaking the sperm tail prior to injection. Human Reproduction 10: 484–486

Goswamy R, Williams G, Steptoe P 1988 Decreased uterine perfusion – a cause of infertility. Human Reproduction 3: 955–959

Handyside A H, Kontogianni E H, Hardy K, Winston R M L 1990 Pregnancies from biopsied human pre-implantation embryos sexed by Y-specific DNA amplification. Nature 344: 768–770

HFEA 1993 Human Fertilisation and Embryology Authority Second Annual Report. HFEA, London

HFEA 1995 Human Fertilisation and Embryology Authority Fourth Annual Report. HFEA London

Holt W, Watson P, Curry M, Holt C 1994 Reproducibility of computer-aided analysis: comparison of five different systems used in a practical workshop. Fertility and Sterility 62: 1277–1282

Hughes E G, Sagle M A, Fedorkow D M, van de Koppel M, Daya S, Collins J 1992 The routine use of gonadotrophin-releasing hormone agonists prior to in vitro fertilization and gamete intrafallopian transfer: a meta-analysis of randomized controlled trials. Fertility and Sterility 58: 888–896

Hull M G R 1992 Infertility treatment: relative effectiveness of conventional and assisted conception methods. Human Reproduction 7: 785–796

Hull M G R, Glazener C M A, Kelly N J et al 1985 Population study of causes, treatment and outcome of infertility. British Medical Journal 291: 1693–1697

Hull M G R, Eddowes H A, Fahy U et al 1992 Expectations of assisted conception for infertility. British Medical Journal 304: 1465–1469

Kahn J A, von During V, Sunde A, Sordal T, Molne K 1993 The efficacy and efficiency of an in-vitro fertilisation programme including embryo cryopreservation: a cohort study. Human Reproduction 8: 247–252

Kenny D T 1995 In vitro fertilisation and gamete intrafallopian transfer: an integrative analysis of research, 1987-1992. British Journal of Obstetrics and Gynaecology 102: 317–325

Leeton J, Rogers P, Caro C, Healy D, Yates C 1987 A controlled study between the use of gamete intrafallopian transfer (GIFT) and in vitro fertilization and embryo transfer in the management of idiopathic and male infertility. Fertility and Sterility 48: 605–607

Liebaers I, Bonduelle M, Van Assche E, Devroey P, Van Steirteghem 1995 Sex chromosome abnormalities after intracytoplasmic sperm injection. Lancet 346: 1095–1097

Macleod I C, Irvine D S, Masterton A, Taylor A, Templeton A A 1994 Assessment of the conventional criteria of semen quality by computer-assisted image analysis: evaluation of the Hamilton–Thorn

motility analyser in the context of a service andrology laboratory. Human Reproduction 9: 310–319
Mahadevan M M, Trouson A D, Leeton J F 1983 The relationship of tubal blockage, infertility of unknown cause, suspected male infertility, and endometriosis to success of in vitro fertilization and embryo transfer. Fertility and Sterility 40: 755–762
Mannaerts B, De Leeuw R, Geelen J et al 1991 Comparative in vitro and in vivo studies on the biological characteristics of recombinant human follicle stimulating hormone. Endocrinology 129: 2623–2630
Matson P L, Yovich J L 1986 The treatment of infertility associated with endometriosis by in vitro fertilization. Fertility and Sterility 46: 432–434
Medical Research International, the Society for Assisted Reproductive Technology, the American Fertility Society (MRI, SART) 1989 In vitro–fertilization embryo transfer (IVF–ET) in the United States: 1987 results from the National IVF–ET Registry. Fertility and Sterility 51: 13–19
Medical Research International, the Society for Assisted Reproductive Technology, the American Fertility Society (MRI, SART) 1990 In vitro fertilization–embryo transfer (IVF–ET) in the United States: 1988 results from the IVF–ET Registry. Fertility and Sterility 53: 13–20
Medical Research International, the Society for Assisted Reproductive Technology, the American Fertility Society (MRI, SART) 1991 In vitro fertilization–embryo transfer (IVF–ET) in the United States: 1989 results from the IVF–ET Registry. Fertility and Sterility 55: 14–23
Medical Research International, the Society for Assisted Reproductive Technology, the American Fertility Society (MRI, SART) 1992 In vitro fertilization–embryo transfer (IVF–ET) in the United States: 1990 results from the IVF–ET Registry. Fertility and Sterility 57: 15–24
Meldrum D R 1993 Female reproductive aging – ovarian and uterine factors. Fertility and Sterility 59: 1–5
Mills M S, Eddowes H A, Cahill D J et al 1992 A prospective controlled study of in vitro fertilization, gamete intra-Fallopian transfer and intra uterine insemination combined with superovulation. Human Reproduction 7: 490–494
Muggleton-Harris A L, Glazier A M, Pickering S, Wall M 1995 Genetic diagnosis using polymerase chain reaction and fluorescent in-situ hybridization analysis of biopsied cells from both the cleavage and blastocyst stages of individual cultured human preimplantation embryos. Human Reproduction 10: 183–192
Olivennes F, Feldberg D, Liu H-C, Cohen J, Moy F, Rosenwaks Z 1995 Endometriosis: a stage by stage analysis – the role of in vitro fertilization. Fertility and Sterility 64: 392–398
Palermo G, Joris H, Devroey P, Van Steirteghem A 1992 Pregnancies after intracytoplasmic injection of single spermatozoon into an oocyte. Lancet 340: 17–18
Palomba M L, Monni G, Lai R, Cau G, Olla G, Cao A 1994 Psychological implications and acceptability of preimplantation diagnosis. Human Reproduction 9: 360–362
Rigot J M 1991 Cystic fibrosis and congenital absence of the vas deferens. New England Journal of Medicine 325: 64–65
Rossing M A, Daling J R, Weiss N S, Moore D E, Self S G 1994 Ovarian tumors in a cohort of infertile women. New England Journal of Medicine 331: 771–776
Seamark R F, Robinson J S 1995 Potential health hazards of assisted reproduction: potential health problems stemming from assisted reproduction programmes. Human Reproduction 10: 1321–1322
Sharma V, Riddle A, Mason B A, Pampiglioni J, Campbell S 1988 An analysis of factors influencing the establishment of a clinical pregnancy in an ultrasound-based ambulatory in vitro fertilization program. Fertility and Sterility 49: 468–478
Shoham Z, Weissman A, Barash A, Borenstein R, Schachter M, Insler V 1994 Intravenous albumin for the prevention of severe ovarian hyperstimulation syndrome in an in vitro fertilization programme: a prospective, randomized, placebo-controlled study. Fertility and Sterility 62: 137–142
Smitz J, Devroey P, Braeckmans P et al 1987 Management of failed cycles in an IVF/GIFT programme with the combination of GnRH analogue and HMG. Human Reproduction 2: 309–314
Society for Assisted Reproductive Technology, the American Fertility Society (SART) 1993 Assisted reproductive technology in the United States and Canada: 1991 results from the Society for Assisted Reproductive Technology generated from The American Fertility Society Registry. Fertility and Sterility 59: 956–962.
Society for Assisted Reproductive Technology, American Society for Reproductive Medicine (SART) 1995 Assisted reproductive technology in the United States and Canada: 1993 results generated from the American Society for Reproductive Medicine/Society for Assisted Reproductive Technology Registry. Fertility and Sterility 64: 13–21
Soliman S, Daya S, Collins J, Hughes E G 1994 The role of luteal phase support in infertility treatment: a meta-analysis of randomised trials. Fertility and Sterility 61: 1068–1076
Steer C V, Campbell S, Tan S L, Mills C, Mason B 1992 The use of transvaginal colour flow imaging after in vitro fertilization to identify optimum uterine conditions before embryo transfer. Fertility and Sterility 57: 372–376
Steer C V, Tan S L, Dillon D, Mason B A, Campbell S 1995 Vaginal color Doppler assessment of uterine artery impedance correlates with immunohistochemical markers of endometrial receptivity required for the implantation of an embryo. Fertility and Sterility 63: 101–108
Tan S L, Royston P, Campbell S et al 1992 Cumulative conception and livebirth rates after in-vitro fertilisation. Lancet 339: 1390–1394
Tanbo T, Dale P O, Abyholm T 1990 Assisted fertilization in infertile women with patent fallopian tubes. A comparison of in-vitro fertilization, gamete intra-fallopian transfer and tubal embryo stage transfer. Human Reproduction 5: 266–270
Tarin J J 1995 Subzonal insemination, partial zona dissection or intracytoplasmic sperm injection? An easy decision? Human Reproduction 10: 165–170
Tekay A, Martikainen H, Jouppila P 1995 Blood flow changes in uterine and ovarian vasculature, and predictive value of transvaginal pulsed colour Doppler ultrasonography in an in-vitro fertilization programme. Human Reproduction 10: 688–693
The American Fertility Society, Society for Assisted Reproductive Technology (AFS, SART) 1994 Assisted reproductive technology in the United States and Canada: 1992 results generated from the American Fertility Society/Society for Assisted Reproductive Technology Registry. Fertility and Sterility 62: 1121–1128
Thornhill A, Holding C, Monk M 1994 Recycling the single cell to detect specific chromosomes and to investigate specific gene sequences. Human Reproduction 9: 2150–2155
Tournaye H, Devroey P, Camus M, Valkenburg M, Bollen N, Van Steirteghem A C 1992 Zygote intrafallopian transfer or in vitro fertilization and embryo transfer for the treatment of male-factor infertility: a prospective randomized trial. Fertility and Sterility 58: 344–350
Trounson A, Mohr L R 1983 Human pregnancy following cryopreservation, thawing and transfer of an eight-cell embryo. Nature 305: 707–709
Tucker M J, Morton P C, Witt M A, Wright G 1995 Intracytoplasmic injection of testicular and epididymal spermatozoa for treatment of obstructive azoospermia. Human Reproduction 10: 486–489
Urman B, Pride S M, Yuen B H 1992 Management of overstimulated gonadotrophin cycles with a controlled drift period. Human Reproduction 7: 213–217
Van Steirteghem A C, Nagy Z, Joris H et al 1993 High fertilization and implantation rates after intracytoplasmic sperm injection. Human Reproduction 8: 1061–1066
Venn A, Watson L, Lumley J, Giles G, King C, Healy D 1995 Breast and ovarian cancer incidence after infertility and in vitro fertilisation. Lancet 346: 995–1000
Wang X J, Ledger W, Payne D, Jeffrey R, Matthews C D 1994 The contribution of embryo cryopreservation to in-vitro fertilization/gamete intra-Fallopian transfer: 8 years experience. Human Reproduction 9: 103–109
Whittemore A S 1994 The risk of ovarian cancer after treatment for infertility. New England Journal of Medicine 331: 805–806
Whittemore A S, Harris R, Intyre J 1992 The collaborative ovarian cancer group. Characteristics relating to ovarian cancer risk: collaborative analysis of 12 US case control studies. II. Invasive

epithelial ovarian cancers in white women. American Journal of Epidemiology 136: 1184–1203
Wisanto A, Magnus M, Bonduelle M et al 1995 Obstetric outcome of 424 pregnancies after intracytoplasmic sperm injection. Human Reproduction 10: 2713–2718
Yee B, Rosen G F, Chacon R R, Soubra S, Stone S C 1989 Gamete intrafallopian transfer: the effect of the number of eggs used and the depth of gamete placement on pregnancy initiation. Fertility and Sterility 52: 639–644

20

Spontaneous and recurrent abortion

D. K. Edmonds

INTRODUCTION AND DEFINITION

In the United Kingdom spontaneous abortion is defined as a pregnancy loss occurring before 24 completed weeks of gestation. In 1977 the World Health Organization defined an abortion as the 'expulsion or extraction from its mother of a fetus or an embryo weighing 500 g or less'. (WHO 1977). A woman who has three or more spontaneous abortions is generally regarded to be a recurrent aborter, although the definition is complicated by the interspersion of successful pregnancies.

SPONTANEOUS ABORTION

This is a hugely traumatic emotional event in any woman's reproductive career, and greatly underestimated by medical practitioners in its impact. Great care and compassion are required in order to manage these women sympathetically so that they return to physical and mental health as soon as possible.

Pathophysiology and classification

It is evident that the process of abortion is a major route by which natural selection operates in humans. It may be considered that the abortion results either from an inherent abnormality in the conceptus or is related to outside influences leading to its elimination from the uterus. The pathophysiological processes will depend upon the aetiology and will be considered in this regard in the next section. The causes of spontaneous abortion may be classified depending on the aetiological defect which may relate to the fetus, placenta or uterus:

1. genetic factors
2. developmental problems
3. placental problems
4. infection
5. undetermined cause.

A number of these causes may result in recurrent miscarriage.

AETIOLOGY OF SPONTANEOUS ABORTION

Fetal problems may be divided into chromosomal problems and developmental abnormalities.

Chromosomal and developmental anomalies

It is generally accepted that 50% of all clinically recognized first trimester losses are chromosomally abnormal. In the second trimester the incidence falls but it is still sig-

Table 20.1 Frequency of chromosomal abnormalities from nine major studies of spontaneous abortion

Authors	No. of abortuses	No. abnormal	% abnormal
Dhadial et al 1970	547	128	23
Boué et al 1975	1498	921	61
Creasy et al 1976	986	290	29
Takahara et al 1977	505	237	47
Therkelsen et al 1977	254	139	54
Geisler & Kleinebrecht 1978	166	65	39
Hassold et al 1980	1000	463	46
Kajii et al 1980	402	215	54
Warburton et al 1980	967	312	32
	6325	3069	49

Table 20.2 Chromosomal abnormalities related to gestational age

Gestation	Chromosomal abnormalities
8–11 weeks	50%
12–15 weeks	40%
16–19 weeks	19%
20–23 weeks	12%
24–28 weeks	8%

From Warburton et al (1980).

nificant. Table 20.1 gives the combined data from nine cytogenetic surveys of spontaneous abortuses, showing an overall rate of 49% for chromosomal abnormalities. However, the prevalence of chromosome abnormalities is gestation-dependent (Table 20.2) and the variation in prevalence shown in Table 20.1 is explained by the greater proportion of abortuses in the second trimester in the studies of Dhadial et al (1970), Creasy et al (1976),

Table 20.3 Types of chromosomal abnormalities in abortions

Abnormality	%
Normal	54.5
Monosomy X	8.6
Triploidy	7.0
Tetraploidy	2.6
Trisomy	30.4
Sex chromosomal polysomy	0.6
Structural abnormalities	1.5

Geisler & Kleinebrecht (1978) and Warburton et al (1980). Some concern has been expressed with regard to the culture techniques used to derive these figures, with evidence from Simoni et al (1985) showing that 15% of abnormalities seen in chorionic villus sampling were not subsequently confirmed when fetal tissue was cultured. Thus there may be a resulting slight overestimation in the studied series.

About 30% of abortuses have an extra chromosome (trisomy) which is usually an autosome and only 6% have a sex chromosome polysomy. The other major abnormalities are monosomy X and triploidy (Table 20.3). However over 54% of all abortuses are euploid.

Trisomy has been described for all chromosomes except chromosome 1 and the Y chromosome, although the frequencies are vastly different (Fig. 20.1). Some 32% of cases are trisomy 16 whilst chromosomes 2, 13, 15, 18, 21 and 22 account for the majority of the remainder. Increasing maternal age increases the risk of trisomy conception although there is no age effect with regard to trisomy 16. Most trisomies are believed to be a consequence of non-disjunction during maternal meiosis. Trisomic pregnancies result in empty sacs ('blighted ova' or 'anem-

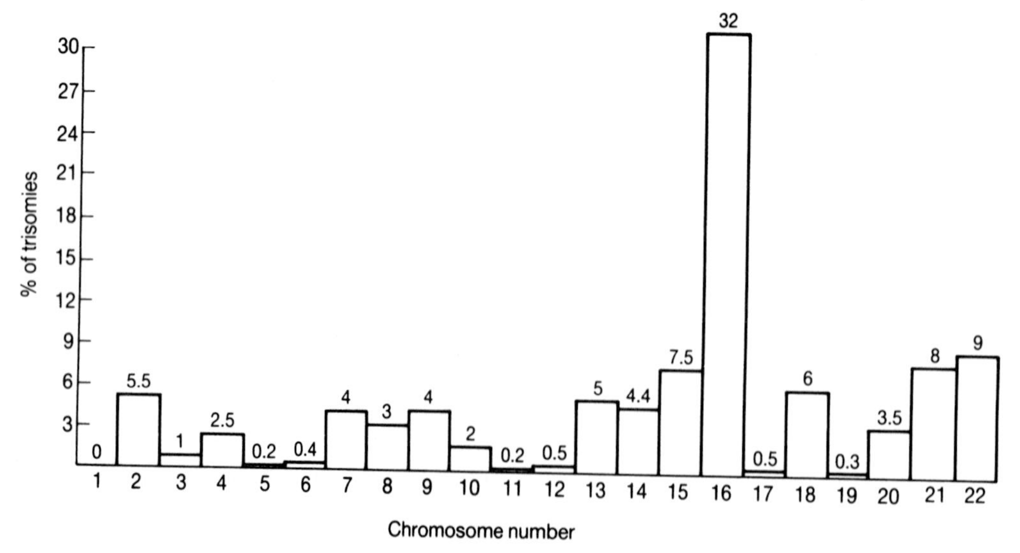

Fig. 20.1 Distribution of differing trisomies (based on Kajii et al 1973, Boué et al 1975, Hassold et al 1980, Warburton et al 1980).

bryonic pregnancies') or very stunted fetal growth, although trisomies 13 and 15 show cyclopia and facial abnormalities. Trisomy 16 gives rise to only the most rudimentary embryonic growth with an empty sac.

Monosomy X is usually associated with the presence of a fetus, although focal abnormalities may occur, e.g. encephaloceles and hygromata. It results from paternal sex chromosome loss which can be X or Y.

Polyploidy (triploidy or tetraploidy) results from the addition of complete haploid sets of chromosomes. Triploid abortions are usually 69XXY or 69XXX and usually result from dispermy. The mean duration of survival is around 5 weeks of embryonic life and polyploidy is characterized by neural tube defects, omphaloceles and placental changes including a large sac, hydropic villi and intrachorial haemorrhage. Tetraploidic pregnancies (92 chromosomes) are rare and the majority are empty sacs or grossly abnormal stunted fetuses which rarely progress beyond 3 weeks of embryonic life.

Polysomy of the sex chromosome polysomy (47XXX, 47XXY or 47XYY) occurs infrequently in abortuses and is more commonly seen in liveborn infants. It is not considered a lethal gene constitution.

Structural chromosomal abnormalities may arise de novo or may be inherited. They are rarely the cause of spontaneous abortion per se but are associated with recurrent abortion.

In a large series by Fantel & Shepherd (1987), reporting the morphological abnormalities in 1441 specimens, a wide variety of structural defects were discovered. Many were related to chromosome defects, but it is interesting to compare the defect rate in abortions and liveborns (Table 20.4). The major abnormalities are more frequently seen in the abortuses and there is little difference in the more minor abnormalities.

Placental abnormalities

There have been scant published data on placental findings in spontaneous abortions, in comparison with information about the fetus. However, the role of the placenta must be paramount in the maintenance of pregnancy and the continued growth of the fetus. Rushton (1988) has reported the largest study of placentae, considering 1426 specimens. The pregnancies were grouped into those with blighted ova, those with macerated fetuses and those with fresh fetuses.

The blighted ova group showed a mixed histological pattern with fibrotic avascular villi as well as microscopic hydropic villi. The macerated group showed a much greater variety of changes (Table 20.5). The maternal floor infarction probably reflects cessation of blood flow following fetal demise, but the uteroplacental ischaemia and retroplacental haemorrhage group also showed evidence of placental bed fibrinoid necrosis and spiral artery arterosis, as is seen in pre-eclampsia and intrauterine growth retardation. Perhaps these cases are the early end of this disease spectrum.

In the third group, associated with a fresh fetus, the placental changes were as seen in Table 20.6. In 30% of cases, chorioamnionitis was present although no specific infections were identified. As in the macerated group, the presence of ischaemia and haemorrhage were associated with vascular lesions.

Thus the role of the process of abnormal placentation may have greater importance in the aetiology of chromosomally normal and some chromosomally abnormal spontaneous abortions than previously realized; some may be amenable to treatment.

Table 20.4 Defect rate per 1000 cases

Structural abnormality	Spontaneous abortuses	Liveborn
Neural tube defect	1.38	0.6
Cleft palate	1.3	1.8
Cleft lip or palate	6.9	0
Cyclopia	2.7	0
Polydactyly	2.7	0.95
Sirenomelia and caudal regression	4.2	0
Amniotic bands	4.2	0.03

Modified from Fantel & Shepard (1987).

Table 20.5 Placental abnormalities associated with macerated abortions

Placental abnormality	%
Maternal floor infarction	22.1
Malformation	11.2
Uteroplacental haemorrhage	10.0
Chorioamnionitis	8.5
Hydrops	8.5
Retroplacental clot	5.6
Cord abnormalities	3.0
Non-specific	31.1

Adapted from Rushton (1988).

Table 20.6 Placental pathology in association with a fresh fetus

Placental abnormality	%
Chorioamnionitis	30.1
Retroplacental haemorrhage	12.6
Uteroplacental ischaemia	5.8
Malformations	5.3
Non-specific	46.2

Adapted from Rushton (1988).

Infection and spontaneous abortion

A number of organisms have been associated with spontaneous abortion (Table 20.7) and although anecdotal evidence exists for sporadic abortion, no evidence exists for a role in recurrent abortion.

Listeria monocytogenes is a notorious pregnancy-associated pathogen and spontaneous abortion clearly may result from maternal bacteraemia during early pregnancy. Cases of abortion associated with *Campylobacter* spp. have been reported although they are scant. *Brucella* spp. well known as a cause of abortion in animals and human infection can occur, but rarely cause abortion. Both *Ureaplasma urealyticum* and *Mycoplasma hominis* have been associated with spontaneous abortion. However, much emphasis has been laid on these organisms as a cause of recurrent abortion but no evidence exists for this. The confusion arises as *Ureaplasma* and *Mycoplasma* can be isolated from 40–90% of pregnant women where no evidence of chorioamnionitis exists, and a successful pregnancy results.

Syphilis is more commonly the cause of late second-trimester abortion and stillbirth, but cases have been reported in the first trimester and of course this is a treatable cause of miscarriage. *Toxoplasma gondii* has also been linked to spontaneous abortion, although there are no studies to corroborate the relationship.

Cytomegalovirus (CMV) is a common infection and known to affect the neonate prenatally but reports of CMV causing abortion are scant (Kriel et al 1970) and inconclusive. Rubella, however, has been alleged to increase the risk of spontaneous abortion and congenital abnormalities (Charles & Larsen 1987) and herpes simplex may increase the risk of abortion by threefold (Gronroos et al 1983).

It is evident, therefore, that whilst spontaneous abortion may result from isolated placental and fetal infection with various organisms, no evidence exists for their involvement in a recurrent problem.

Undetermined causes

A percentage, perhaps around 25%, of spontaneous abortions remain undetermined in their aetiology, but it is most likely that a lack of ability to investigate these cases is the reason. A greater diligence amongst clinicians and pathologists is necessary if a greater understanding of these tragic cases is to be gained.

Table 20.7 Organisms associated with spontaneous abortion

Bacteria	Parasites
Listeria monocytogenes	*Toxoplasma gondii*
Campylobacter spp.	
Brucella spp.	Viruses
Mycoplasma hominis	Cytomegalovirus
Ureaplasma urealyticum	Rubella Herpes
	Coxsackie
Spirochaetes	
Treponema pallidum	

Adapted from Watts & Eschenbach (1988).

EPIDEMIOLOGY

It is very difficult to estimate the frequency of early pregnancy loss since the advent of sophisticated biochemical assays which detect the presence of human chorionic gonadotrophin (hCG) in women. There have been five studies considering early pregnancy loss prior to 6 weeks' gestation (Table 20.8), there is considerable variation in the results, which may well be explained by the sensitivity and specificity of the methods used to detect β-hCG. It is of note, however, that the data from Walker et al (1988) is unique in not detecting any evidence of β-hCG in preclinical pregnancies, which differs from all other studies. Whilst the figure of 58% by Edmonds et al (1982) is probably an overestimate, the results of Wilcox et al (1988) using a highly specific β-hCG assay are probably the best estimate at 22%.

All these studies are based on the detection of postimplantation hCG and thus any losses of pre-embryos or blastocysts which failed to implant are undetected. In a mathematical consideration of the total loss rate, Roberts & Lowe (1975) calculated the total loss to be around 78%. The risk of spontaneous abortion of a clinically recognized pregnancy is around 15% (Warburton & Fraser 1964) and this is borne out by the longitudinal studies quoted in Table 20.8.

PRESENTATION

Spontaneous abortion may present clinically as either a threatened or inevitable abortion (Fig. 20.2).

Threatened abortion

This is said to occur when a woman bleeds through the uterus prior to 24 weeks of gestation. The bleeding is not associated with pain although there may be some backache. It is usually assumed that the bleeding is placental in origin, from some placental disruption as a result of vascular disturbance at the site of implantation or the union of the decidua capsularis and the decidua vera. Bleeding can also be due to the loss of a second non-viable twin pregnancy.

The bleeding is initially bright red and then becomes brown presumably as the primary vessel ceases bleeding and any surrounding clot breaks down. Clinical examination reveals a soft non-tender uterus of appropriate size for the gestation with a closed cervix. Whilst there may be considerable anxiety shown by the mother at the thought of being examined per vaginam, there is no evidence that this procedure precipitates miscarriage. If a mother is reluctant or refuses examination, then one should not persist.

Table 20.8 Preclinical and clinical pregnancy loss rates

Authors	Positive hCG	Clinical pregnancies	Preclinical loss rate	Clinical loss rate
Miller et al (1980)	152	102	50/152 (33%)	14/102 (14%)
Edmonds el al (1982)	118	51	67/118 (58%)	6/51 (12%)
Whittaker et al (1983)	92	85	7/92 (8%)	11/85 (13%)
Walker et al (1988)	25	25	0/0 (0%)	4/25 (16%)
Wilcox et al (1988)	198	155	44/198 (22%)	18/155 (12%)

hCG, human chorionic gonadotrophin.

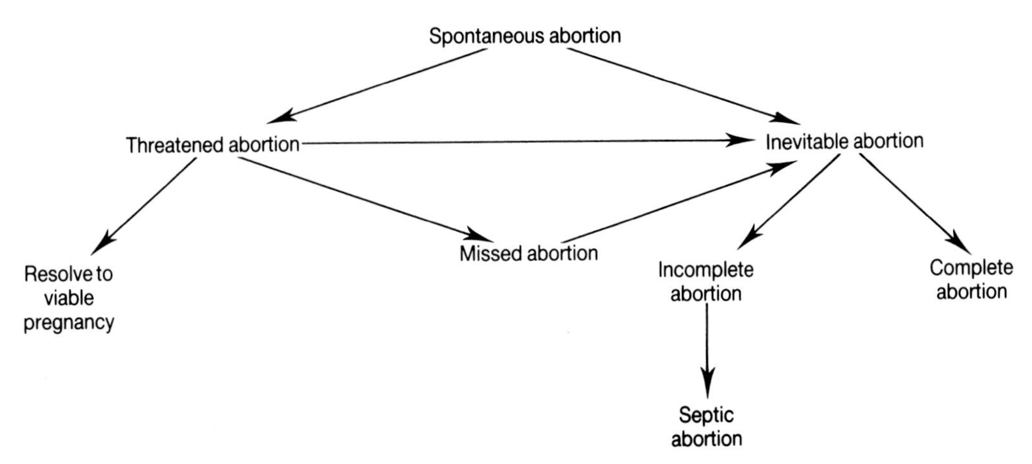

Fig. 20.2 Clinical classification of spontaneous abortion.

All cases of threatened abortion should be assessed for viability using ultrasound, and the course of the pregnancy may proceed in one of three ways from here: resolution or becoming a missed or an inevitable abortion. The management of the patient depends entirely upon ultrasound investigation.

Missed abortion

In this condition there is either failure of embryonic growth in spite of placental viability or a viable fetus dies. In the first instance, an empty amniotic sac develops and this is known as a missed abortion (i.e. there is maternal failure to recognize the non-viable pregnancy) or, incorrectly, an anembryonic pregnancy (all pregnancies develop from an embryo) or blighted ovum (the pregnancy cannot result from an ovum alone). The situation of fetal demise usually occurs before 8 weeks' gestation, although the uterus does not expel the products. In both instances, the concept of dependence of the placenta on fetus circulation for viability is undermined; much more research needs to be performed in this area to delineate the mechanisms of placental growth in the early weeks in order to define the causes of demise.

The mother usually reports a disappearance of the symptoms and signs of pregnancy and a brown vaginal loss may ensue which may result from increasingly non-viable placental tissue. When the non-viable pregnancy becomes surrounded by clot in utero, it is termed a carneous mole.

Examination of the patient reveals a uterus which is smaller than the gestation would suggest but the cervical os is closed. Further assessment of the pregnancy involves an ultrasound examination which will either confirm a missed abortion, or the possibility of a viable pregnancy at a lesser gestational age than expected. A missed abortion may proceed in time to an inevitable abortion.

Inevitable abortion

If a woman presents with vaginal bleeding in association with crampy lower abdominal pain, the abortion is said to be inevitable. The pain is due to cervical dilatation secondary to uterine contractions and this results from prostaglandin release as the placenta and membranes separate from the uterine site. Once the internal os is open, the products will be expelled either completely or, as in the vast majority, incompletely. Thus, the patient may give a history of passing products of conception. Blood loss may be considerable and care must be taken not to underestimate this fact.

Examination reveals a tender, firm uterus which may be smaller than the gestational age expected and the internal cervical os is open. Products of conception may be felt through the os.

Occasionally, the woman may present with shock, either secondary to haemorrhage which will require appropriate measures, or out of proportion to the blood loss. This is due to products of conception being held in the cervix with a resultant sympathetic stimulation, known as cervical shock syndrome. Removal of the products results in relief of the shock.

Complete and incomplete abortion

If the pregnancy is expelled intact, the abortion is said to be complete, but this is a rare event in the first trimester; in the majority of cases products of conception remain behind, and are liable to cause bleeding or become infected if untreated.

Examination reveals the os to be open and products may be palpated or discovered in the vagina.

Septic abortion

Failure of the patient to present with an incomplete abortion, or failure to diagnose the condition means that non-viable tissue remains in the uterus and may become infected. Whilst this is an unlikely event following spontaneous abortion, the risk is considerably higher following therapeutic abortion, i.e. around 3.6% (Frank 1985). The most common organisms are *Escherichia coli*, *Bacteroides* spp., streptococci (both anaerobic and, less commonly, aerobic) and *Clostridium welchii*.

The patient usually complains of abdominal suprapubic pain, malaise, some mild vaginal bleeding and pyrexia. Examination reveals abdominal rigidity and the bimanual examination reveals a tender uterus and adnexae, with the cervical os closed. Rarely, a septicaemia may ensue – bacteraemic endotoxic shock – which may result in maternal death.

INVESTIGATIONS

In threatened abortion or in patients suspected of having a missed abortion, an ultrasound scan for fetal viability is vital. The presence of a fetal heart can be reliably identified by 7 weeks' gestation and its presence or absence governs subsequent management. If a gestation sac is seen on a scan and there is no fetus visible, the diagnosis rests between a missed abortion or a pregnancy of earlier gestation than expected. Management at this stage depends on the clinical assessment, but frequently repeat ultrasound examination in 7–10 days is suggested, and failure to demonstrate the appearance of a fetus or diminution of the size of the gestation sac confirms the diagnosis of a missed abortion.

In some cases of threatened abortion, with a viable pregnancy, a second sac may be seen, indicating a non-viable twin gestation which is the cause of the symptoms and signs. These sacs usually reabsorb and the viable pregnancy proceeds unaffected. A low placental site is not a reliable ultrasound diagnosis of the aetiology of a threatened abortion in early pregnancy, although this may be the case.

The diagnosis of a hydatidiform mole on ultrasound is particularly obvious, and the 'snowstorm' appearance of earlier technologies is now superseded by the appearance of the vesicles.

Patients with an inevitable complete or incomplete abortion require no further investigations in order to manage their situation. The management is entirely based on the clinical findings, unless the patient refuses vaginal examination and then ultrasound may be performed to confirm the diagnosis. Care must be taken in managing these patients as there is an expectation amongst them that a scan is the ultimate diagnostic test. The role of the scan is very important in that the patient is able to visualize the viability or non-viability of the pregnancy, and if the latter is the case, she is able to accept the demise more readily. Thus *any* patient who requests a scan should be allowed to have that investigation.

All women who present with any degree of spontaneous abortion should have their blood group investigated so that any rhesus-negative mothers may receive anti-D immunoglobulin.

TREATMENT OF SPONTANEOUS ABORTION

This depends on the clinical presentation and the results of the ultrasound investigations performed.

Treatment of threatened abortion

The traditional management for this condition is bedrest and forbidden intercourse. However there are no studies to suggest that such management has any bearing on the outcome of the pregnancy. Having considered the aetiologies, bedrest will have no influence on a chromosomally or developmentally abnormal fetus, and neither will there be any change in abnormal placentation. If there is an infective cause, the difficulty of diagnosing the organism until the products have been expelled negates the efficacy of bedrest, although if a specific agent is identified the appropriate antibiotic can be administered.

Whilst most women may express the desire for and necessity of bedrest, the medical support of this wish merely surrounds the problem of miscarriage with a sense of desperation. Patients should be reassured and not made to feel that the threatened loss of a pregnancy is their fault by doing something they ought not to have done, or not doing something they should have done. When ultrasound has demonstrated a viable pregnancy, the chances of a spontaneous abortion occurring subsequently are only 2–3% (Christiaens & Stoutenbeck 1984) and thus reassurance and support will suffice in the vast majority.

Treatment of inevitable and missed abortions

Having established the diagnosis, the primary aim of treatment is evacuation of the retained products of conception (ERPC) from the uterus, as the only way of being certain that the abortion is complete is the demonstration of no products of conception at ERPC. All cases, whether thought to be complete or incomplete, ought to have an ERPC. If bleeding has been sufficient to result in compromise of the maternal condition, then appropriate resuscitative measures should be taken prior to surgery. Bleeding may be arrested with the aid of Syntocinon (20 i.u.) or ergometrine (0.5 mg) i.v. if the situation requires this.

Evacuation should be performed under general anaesthesia and a suction curettage should be performed. The use of sharp curettes in the uterus should be avoided in view of the risk of surgical removal of the basal endometrium by over-vigorous curettage, leading to Ascherman's syndrome and subsequent fertility problems. Whilst it is ideal to arrange histological and chromosomal analysis of the products to help reach a possible diagnosis, this service is rarely available in the UK.

In the case of missed abortion, evacuation is again required, but the cervix should be prepared preoperatively using a gemeprost 1-mg pessary inserted high in the vagina. This synthetic prostaglandin acts by softening the cervix and inducing uterine contractions to cause cervical dilation and allow easy access to the uterine cavity with the suction curette. Attempts to dilate the cervix forcibly with Hegar dilators should be avoided so that traumatic damage does not occur to the internal cervical os, with a subsequent risk of cervical incompetence.

Treatment of septic abortion

These cases present in two ways, either with a localized infection in the uterus and fallopian tubes, or with bacteraemic endotoxic shock. The management of the latter problem is outside the remit of this chapter (see Wright & Trott 1988), but the initial problem requires prompt action. If the patient is not bleeding heavily, which is usually the case, systemic antibiotics should be given for 24 h before the ERPC, because the action of curettage exposes arterioles into which bacteria enter and a bacteraemia results. Great care must be taken at the time of the ERPC as the risk of Ascherman's syndrome is highest in these patients. The most appropriate antibiotic regimen would be ampicillin 500 mg 6-hourly, combined with metronidazole 200 mg 8-hourly.

COMPLICATIONS

Spontaneous abortion is such a common phenomenon that scant attention is paid to the associated risks. There is a mortality rate of 12.5 per million pregnancies; death occurs primarily as a result of haemorrhage and/or sepsis (Reports on confidential enquiries into maternal deaths in England and Wales 1986).

There is always blood loss associated with abortion and this is often impossible to assess from the patient's history. Thus, careful attention to physicial signs of acute anaemia and anticipation of a problem by cross-matching blood, prompt use of antibiotics when appropriate, and the use of oxytocics can avoid the chance of severe problems. Rarely, a coagulopathy may develop, particularly in association with septic cases; management, with the aid of a haematologist, needs to be swift and effective. The use of fresh whole blood and fresh frozen plasma may be life-saving. Acute, prolonged hypovolaemia may result in renal cortical necrosis or renal tubular necrosis, and careful management of fluid balance is required to avoid this.

Patients who suffer a threatened abortion during the first trimester, and in whom the situation resolves, are prone to late pregnancy complications. These include an increased incidence of preterm labour, small-for-dates infants and retained placentae, and therefore a patient reporting bleeding in the first trimester must be identified as being in a higher-risk group.

PSYCHOLOGICAL ASPECTS

The emotional effect of an abortion varies greatly. Some women have reported frank happiness or had positive feelings at the loss of an 'abnormal' pregnancy, whilst almost 60% had feelings of depression and hostility (Seibel & Graves 1980). There is always associated fear and anxiety caused by the pain and bleeding and the uncertainty with regard to the cause. A sense of bereavement is the typical reaction to abortion. Around 30% of women begin to regard the fetus as a 'real person' by the 8th to 12th week of pregnancy and a miscarriage at this stage is seen as the loss of a child. There is often a loss of self-esteem with the view of a failure of womanhood and a loss of social identity, that of the 'mother-to-be'.

Often the intensity of the emotions is not appreciated by those who care for the patient, or by her friends and relatives. Interaction with other people is very important and unfortunately, many people try to avoid discussing the loss, thereby further isolating the woman and prolonging the grief. Thus, all health workers should aim to help the woman express her grief and then reinforce her self-esteem.

Giving the news to the patient that the pregnancy is lost should be done in the best possible surroundings so that the parents may express emotion without embarrassment, but patients should not be isolated. The use of sedatives is inappropriate in these circumstances. It is important to understand that these women have a deep desire for an explanation of what happened and why, and this information helps greatly in their acceptance of the tragedy of their pregnancy loss. Women who have experienced a loss will require considerable reassurance and support in a subsequent pregnancy if they are to have the confidence necessary to enjoy the hopefully successful outcome.

RECURRENT SPONTANEOUS ABORTION

There must be few conditions encountered by reproductive gynaecologists which are as distressing to the patient or frustrating to the doctor as recurrent miscarriage. A very large deficiency in our knowledge of fertilization, embryo development, implantation and the maintenance of pregnancy means that our understanding of repetitive pregnancy wastage is also limited.

AETIOLOGY OF RECURRENT SPONTANEOUS ABORTION

The causes of recurrent spontaneous abortion are summarized below.

1. Genetic factors
   a. parental chromosomal anomalies
   b. recurrent aneuploidy
   c. multifactorial problems
   d. recurrent euploidy.
2. Anatomical factors
   a. uterine problems
   b. cervical factors.
3. Endocrine factors
   a. hypersecretion of LH
   b. corpus luteum problems.
4. Immunological factors
5. Maternal chronic disease
   a. diabetes mellitus
   b. systemic lupus erythematosus (SLE)
   c. chronic systemic diseases.
6. Environmental factors
   a. smoking
   b. alcohol
   c. environmental toxins.

Genetic factors

Parental chromosomal anomalies

Recurrent genetically abnormal pregnancy may result from parental chromosomal anomalies or the parents may be euploid. The incidence of chromosome abnormalities in couples who experience recurrent pregnancy loss is 6.14%, as opposed to a 1/500 rate in the normal population. When the couples are divided into recurrent aborters or multiple reproductive losses (i.e. recurrent aborters with live or stillborn offspring), there is still an equally high incidence of parental chromosome anomaly (Warburton & Strobino 1987) and the incidence of anomalies is threefold higher in women than men (Lippman-Hand & Vekemans 1983).

Robertsonian translocations. This is a condition in which two chromosomes adhere to each other, at either the centromere or the short arms. The total chromosome number is then 45, although one chromosome represents two. The frequency in the normal population is around 1/1000 and in recurrent aborters this is 10/1000 individuals (or 2% of couples). The risk of an abnormal conceptus is 100% if the translocation involves homologous chromosomes; only those involving chromosomes 13 and 21 result in live birth (i.e. trisomy 13 and trisomy 21). Thus chromosomal analysis resulting in the recognition of a robertsonian translocation is important for the counselling of these couples.

Reciprocal translocations. Here, a portion of one chromosome is exchanged with a portion of another, resulting in two abnormal chromosomes, but a total complement of 46. This occurs in around 3% of recurrent aborters, and here the female to male ratio is 2:1. Translocations are reported for all the chromosomes and in all combinations and therefore estimating risk factors is very difficult. The risk of an unbalanced fetus is 11% in a subsequent pregnancy at amniocentesis, although 40% of chorionic villus samples demonstrate the translocation (Mikkelson 1985).

Inversions. This involves the reversal of order of genes, usually as a result of two chromosomal breaks, followed by reinsertion in reverse order of the free segment. Inversions in which the breakpoints are on either side of the centromere are known as pericentric inversions, and those on the same side are known as paracentric inversions. Inversions increase the risk of fetal loss due to abnormal combination during cross-over of the meiotic loop. The result is fetal wastage, although if a balanced situation exists the fetus may be normal. Interestingly, inversions of chromosome 9 are relatively common and are generally considered of no clinical consequence (for review, see Simpson & Bombard 1987).

X chromosome mosaicism. This has been reported on a number of occasions, associated with recurrent miscarriage. Recurrent abortion seems to depend on the ratio of 45X : 46XX cells, with the greater risk associated with a larger percentage of 45X.

Recurrent aneuploidy

The risk of a chromosomal abnormality in a second abortus depends on the chromosomal complement of the first (Table 20.9). If the complement of the first abortus is normal, the likelihood of the second being normal is 80%, whereas a repeated trisomy chance is 70%. This implies that some couples are predisposed to production of chromosomally abnormal conceptions. There are several suggested mechanisms for this phenomenon. If there is an error in gametogenesis in the oocyte, abnormal embryos may result, and increased maternal age may be associated

Table 20.9 Risks of karyotypes in successive abortuses

First abortus	Second abortus			
	Normal	Trisomy	Monosomy	Polyploidy
Normal	80%	9%	4%	7%
Trisomy	24%	70%	3%	3%
Monosomy	45%	36%	9%	9%
Polyploidy	40%	40%	10%	10%

From Hassold (1980) with permission of The University of Chicago Press.

with an increased incidence of such oocytes being selected. Ageing of the oocyte following ovulation and prior to fertilization has also been suggested as increasing the abnormalities of the embryo. Human trisomy is almost always maternal in origin whereas triploidy is male in origin, i.e. fertilization by diploid sperm in 30% of cases or dispermy in 70%.

Multifactorial problems

These situations are most commonly neural tube defects, although other syndromes, e.g. Potter's syndrome, are described. There seems to be an increased risk of subsequent abortion if a pregnancy is diagnosed as having a neural tube defect, especially anencephaly, although the exact risks are difficult to estimate.

Genetic factors in recurrent euploid abortion

Many abortuses which are examined cytogenetically turn out to be euploid (46XY or 46XX), even missed abortions, and the possibility of the presence of lethal genes seems highly likely. Much work on transgenetic mice has indicated that DNA fragments can be inserted to cause lethal mutations in recessive or dominant offspring. In the mouse, a lethal gene called the t-complex can be found on chromosome 17, but no equivalent has been found in the human, although the hypothesis that certain homologues exist on human chromosomes 6 and 19 suggests that lethal mutations could exist in these sites. Abnormal development may occur as a result of another mutation. Homeobox genes control the expression of groups of genes through transcription regulation; they regulate the development of groups of cells which become morphologically recognized. Mutation of a homeobox sequence results in inappropriate or abnormal development, and their importance is proven in mice and *Drosophila*. Whether the early findings of homeobox genes in humans on chromosome 17 (Rabin et al 1985) will lead to further discovery of homeobox genes and their mutations remains to be seen, but the potential for discovering the control of development is immense.

Another genetic possiblity in normal and abnormal development is the role of oncogenes. Oncogenes have been established as being involved in unregulated neoplastic growth and may be the origin of growth factors which are involved in embryo growth. An abnormality or absence of an oncogene may lead to failure of embryonic growth, or perhaps selective failure. Thus, whilst routine karyotyping may fail to identify a chromosomal cause for recurrent abortion, the possibility of gene mutations and deletions remains a very likely aetiology for euploid abortion.

Anatomical factors

Uterine problems

The origin of congenital uterine anomalies is not straightforward and requires an understanding of normal development. The müllerian ducts give rise to the fallopian tubes, uterus and upper two-thirds of the vagina. Each duct grows in a cephalocaudal direction, canalizing as they do so, and eventualy uniting in the midline to form the uterus and müllerian tubercle. This forms the vaginal plate which grows inferiorly to reach the urogenital sinus; canalization of this downgrowth results in the vagina. It seems that the uterus is distinguishable by 11 weeks' gestation and the vagina is complete by weeks 20–22. Defects in the process of fusion or canalization can produce numerous anomalies, from complete failure of fusion and duplication of the system (uterus didelphys), partial fusion (bicornuate uterus), failure of reabsorption (septate uteri) and failure of canalization (vaginal agenesis).

The incidence of uterine anomalies is unknown, but patients with recurrent pregnancy loss have a 10–15% incidence of uterine anomalies (Sandler 1977). The aetiology of the recurrent reproductive failure is not clear, although implantation on a septum may lead to decreased placental vascularization. Uterine anomalies also arise secondarily to intrauterine exposure to diethylstilboestrol, which results in abnormal development of the uterus and cervix, and reproductive failure is high. The existence of Ascherman's syndrome is associated with recurrent abortion, presumably due to inadequate placentation. Finally, the role of fibroids in recurrent abortion is somewhat contentious, although Buttram & Reiter (1981) suggested a reduction in recurrent abortion following myomectomy.

Cervical factors

Pregnancy loss from cervical incompetence is due to weakness in the sphincteric mechanism of the internal os. This may be congenital (rare) or acquired and the aetiology is primarily a previous pregnancy. A history of a therapeutic abortion or a dilatation and curettage prior to pregnancy are risk factors, as is a previous cone biopsy. Finally diethylstilboestrol exposure results in an incompetent cervix in about 20% of patients.

Endocrine factors

Hypersecretion of LH

The observation that miscarriage rates in women with polycystic ovaries (PCO) could be as high as 45% has been known for many years, but it was not until 1990 that Regan et al (1990) reported the association of hypersecretion of LH with infertility and miscarriage in a normal population. The incidence of polycystic ovarian syndrome in the normal population is around 22% (Polsen et al 1988), and the incidence of polycystic ovarian syndrome in recurrent aborters was reported at 82% (Sagle et al 1988). Regan et al (1990) first suggested the link between PCO and early pregnancy failure and that this was secondary to the hypersecretion of LH.

The process by which this elevated LH level in the follicular phase of the cycle induces recurrent abortion has yet to be explained. However, it is hypothesized that the LH affects the oocyte maturation, causing premature meiosis in the oocyte and thereafter interfering with normal fertilization and embryo development. The mechanism by which this genetic influence is manifest remains unclear. Other possibilities for the influence of hypersecretion of luteinizing hormone are a direct effect on endometrial function or an indirect effect of androgen production on oocyte maturation.

Corpus luteum problems

The functional corpus luteum is essential for the implantation and maintenance of early pregnancy, through the production of progesterone. A normally functional corpus luteum follows the adequate growth and maturation of the follicle, without which the corpus luteum will be inadequate. Hence, progesterone production is reduced, endometrial maturation is retarded and menstruation may occur prematurely.

Whilst measurement of luteal phase parameters, e.g. progesterone levels, may be valuable in the non-conceptual cycle, there is no method of assessing luteal phase function in a pregnant patient. In fact, the corpus luteum of pregnancy and that in the non-conceptual cycle are entirely different, both morphologically and endocrinologically. The idea, however, that 'inadequate' production of progesterone is associated with recurrent abortion seems to have persisted without any evidence to support the theory. Attempts to improve pregnancy outcome using clomiphene citrate have failed, as has the use of luteal phase progesterone. Similarly the use of hCG in the luteal phase and early pregnancy remains unsubstantiated, although studies are in progress (Harrison 1988). It would seem unlikely that inadequate luteal function is a cause of recurrent abortion.

Immunological factors

The risk of a recurrent abortion following three consecutive spontaneous miscarriages is variously reported as between 26 and 47% (Warburton & Strobino 1987). The percentage of aneuploidy in this population is small (6%) and thus another explanation for recurrent euploid losses may be immunological.

The major histocompatibility complex is located on chromosome 6 and is encoded for two classes of antigens. Class I antigens are glycoproteins, coded by the genes human leukocyte antigen (HLA) A, B and C, and are the cell surface and allograft responses. Class II antigens are also glycoproteins, are products of the gene HLA D, and are responsible for presenting antigens to immunocompetent cells, thereby regulating the immune response. The continuous layers of syncytiotrophoblast and underlying cytotrophoblast that surround the conceptus are HLA class I and II antigen-negative.

Class I antigen production seems to be inhibited at the stage of transcription. The cytotrophoblast attaching the trophoblast to the decidua certainly does express class I antigens; however the expression is incomplete. The lack of class II antigens, especially HLA DR, implies an inability to mount a cytotoxic immune response at this level, which may be important in pregnancy maintenance.

Another antigen has been found to bind to both trophoblast and leukocytes, and is referred to as the trophoblast leukocyte cross-reacting (TLX) antigen. A positive response to this antigen is considered necessary in the establishment of fetomaternal immunological coexistence. The reason for the lack of a graft–host rejection response at the site of placentation has concerned a number of investigators. It seems that local production of suppressor cells within the decidua may play a role in this phenomenon. Two types of suppressor cell have been described, one that is non-antigen-specific and suppresses all cytotoxic immune responses, and a second type that is immunosuppressive through its ability to produce prostaglandin E, which indirectly inactivates uterine T helper cells. Macrophages also accumulate in the uterus during pregnancy and they too suppress T helper cells.

Thus a major modification of the normal immune mechanism is necessary in the establishment of a successful pregnancy, and failure to achieve this may result in recurrent abortion. Why some women fail to mount this response is uncertain, although it has been suggested that HLA compatibility between couples, especially HLA B and DR, and perhaps the TLX antigens, means a failure to generate an immune response. However, if this theory were correct, couples with recurrent abortion would not benefit from immunotherapy; the HLA theory has few advocates.

Unsuccessful pregnancies may arise because of:

1. failure to mount a protective maternal immune response;
2. failure of the cytotrophoblast to express a local non-cytotoxic immune response;
3. failure of T lymphocytes to produce lymphokines which induce trophoblastic growth.

These deficiencies will result in an inappropriate immune response mounted by the mother against the pregnancy, and in its subsequent demise.

A condition known as the 'antiphospholipid syndrome' has been associated with recurrent pregnancy failure. This syndrome is characterized by recurrent pregnancy loss, thrombocytopenia, arterial or venous thrombosis, intrauterine growth retardation and a family history of cardiovascular or a cerebral thrombosis. The women exhibit raised titres of lupus anticoagulant or anticardiolipin antibody, and it is postulated that the presence of the antibodies influences thrombosis and fibrin deposition in small vessels which may lead to disruption of placentation or the uteroplacental circulation, thereby preventing normal fetal development.

Maternal chronic disease

Diabetes mellitus

There is general agreement that there is an increased risk of spontaneous abortion in uncontrolled diabetics who may become recurrent aborters. The rate of spontaneous abortion is 26–30% overall (Wright et al 1983) although the series by Crane & Wahl (1981) failed to demonstrate that the risk was increased above that of the normal population.

Systemic lupus erythematosus (SLE)

There is no doubt that pregnancies in patients with SLE have a very poor prognosis. Patients who are positive for lupus anticoagulant prior to the clinical onset of the disease have a high spontaneous abortion rate, and pregnancies of those with the clinical disease almost always result in fetal death. Lupus anticoagulant is an antiphospholipid antibody which interferes with coagulation by excluding the phospholipid surface of platelets from the generation of thrombin. The most appropriate test for the presence of lupus anticoagulant is the kaolin clotting time, although other autoantibodies are also often present, e.g. anticardiolipin antibody (100% of cases), antinuclear antibody (90% of cases).

Chronic systemic diseases

Conditions such as chronic essential hypertension and chronic renal diseases may be associated with recurrent abortion. This may be as a result of reduction of uterine blood flow due to small vessel damage.

Environmental factors

Smoking

Smoking has been implicated by Klein et al 1980 as associated with recurrent abortion, women smoking more than 14 cigarettes a day having an abortion risk that was 1.7 times greater than women who did not smoke. The abortuses of these heavy smokers were found to be chromosomally normal.

Alcohol

Alcohol has also been reported as an associated risk factor for abortion, and women who drank more than 20 units a week had a twofold increased risk of miscarriage compared with women who did not drink during pregnancy.

Environmental toxins

Spontaneous abortion is found to be increased in those women who are exposed to toluene, xylene and formalin in their workplace, and although other toxins have been suggested to be associated with spontaneous and recurrent abortion, e.g. caffeine, there are no randomized trials that have proved this association. No association with the magnetic fields of video display units has been proved.

INVESTIGATION OF RECURRENT SPONTANEOUS ABORTION

History taking is very important in cases of recurrent abortion and must include the following:

1. history of the abortions and the histological/karyotype findings;
2. family history of neural tube defects or other malformations;
3. history of chronic disease states.

Patients should all be examined, although there are rarely any abnormal physical signs. It is sometimes possible to diagnose uterine anomalies, e.g. a duplex cervix, on clinical examination. Investigations should include parental karyotype, pelvic ultrasound, serum LH, lupus

Table 20.10 Probability of a spontaneous abortion given the previous abortion history

Authors	No. of previous abortions			
	0	1	2	3+
Warburton & Fraser (1964)	12.3%			
Boué et al (1975)		13.8%		24.9%
Lauritsen (1976)		13.2%		32.5%
Harger et al (1983)			17.4%	29.2%
Total	12.3%	13.5%	17.4%	28.9%

anticoagulant, anticardiolipin antibodies and a hysterosalpingogram or hysteroscopy to investigate for uterine abnormalities. Further investigations are probably of little value in managing the patient or discovering the aetiology of their problem.

TREATMENT OF RECURRENT SPONTANEOUS ABORTION

This must be tailored towards the identified cause, although in the majority of cases the investigations will reveal no apparent abnormality.

One of the problems faced in advising patients is an understanding of the risks of recurrence. Only four prospective studies have addressed this problem (Table 20.10); and the risk of repeated abortion rises with increasing recurrence. However, it is important to note that even after three miscarriages, without any treatment, a couple may expect a 71% chance that the next pregnancy will be successful, and when evaluating treatments this must be used as the standard rate upon which improvement is based. Patients may therefore be given positive advice if the investigations discover no obvious cause.

Chromosomal problems

Genetic counselling is of paramount importance for couples who have either a chromosomal disorder themselves, or in whom there is a history of recurrent chromosomal abortions. Couples with balanced translocations can be positively advised with regard to further pregnancies and the availability of prenatal diagnosis by either chorionic villus sampling or amniocentesis. In reciprocal translocation, again counselling should be against further pregnancies in view of the absolute nature of the problem.

In certain circumstances, when the abnormal chromosome complement is traced to the male partner, artifical insemination with donor sperm may be suggested as a possible solution, but great care must be taken when introducing this concept.

Gynaecologists must be certain of the genetic basis of the disease process for which they are counselling, and if any uncertainty exists, referral to a clinical geneticist is strongly advised.

Treatment of anatomical problems

Uterine anomalies

Patients with a unicornuate uterus have a high abortion rate, but if there is evidence of cervical incompetence (which may occur in about 25% of cases), cervical cerclage should be performed in the first trimester. If a rudimentary horn also exists, serious consideration should be given to its removal, as a pregnancy in a rudimentary horn has a 90% chance of rupturing the uterus (O'Leary & O'Leary 1963). It is probably adequate to rely on ultrasound to identify the pregnancy in the rudimentary horn and remove the horn if this occurs. In uterus didelphys, there is no proven therapy to improve the obstetric performance.

Bicornuate uteri have been treated primarily by Strassman's procedure (Strassman 1966). The latter reported an 85% fetal survival rate out of 289 women. The use of cervical cerclage has also been used to improve the reproductive outcome of bicornuate uteri with similar success, but no trials to compare these two methods have been reported.

Patients with a septate uterus may be managed by abdominal (Tompkin's) or hysteroscopic metroplasty, with dramatic improvement of fetal survival, from around 6 to 80%. However, there is infertility following abdominal surgery due to adhesion formation; this may be as high as 30%. The use of the hysteroscope may improve this rate; DeCherney et al (1986) report a 7% rate of failure to conceive, and hysteroscopic resection of a septum is the preferred operative choice.

In patients who have uterine anomalies secondary to diethylstilboestrol exposure, the obstetric outlook is poor and there are no surgical procedures which improve the uterus.

Patients who have had second-trimester abortions may benefit from cervical cerclage in a subsequent pregnancy (for review, see Kaufman & Irwin 1987).

Fibroids

Women whose uterine cavity is distorted by fibroids may be advised to undergo myomectomy, but again great care must be taken as the postoperative adhesion rate is high and a significant infertility rate will ensue. However, fetal loss rate may be reduced from around 40 to 20% (Buttram & Reiter 1981).

Incompetent cervix

The incompetent cervix and its management is controversial. The role of cervical cerclage and the effect on outcome remains unresolved as there are no truly randomized trials. Two studies which have attempted this have, unfortunately, a patient selection bias (Papiernik et al 1984,

Rush et al 1984), but neither of these studies was able to support the concept that cervical cerclage is valuable in prolonging pregnancy. In view of the exclusion of patients with proven cervical incompetence by HSG, the data for these patients must be based on uncontrolled series. If a cerclage is inserted prophylactically, one can expect an 80% successful outcome, and 60% if inserted after cervical dilatation has commenced.

Whilst cervical incompetence is usually associated with midtrimester abortion, Ayres et al (1982) and Edmonds (1988) have attempted the use of cervical cerclage to prevent recurrent first-trimester losses. Both studies showed an equal improvement to other therapies, with successful outcomes in excess of 80%. However, the series were not randomized and the results must be interpreted with caution. There may well be a major effect of psychotherapy which is influencing the outcome.

Immunological therapy

Transfusions of leucocytes have been demonstrated to have a number of effects on the immune system, primarily regarding the concept of increased allograft survival. This theory led Mowbray et al (1985) to use leukocyte transfusions in women with idiopathic recurrent abortion in an attempt to modify the immune system within the uterus. Although this study did demonstrate an advantage in doing this with respect to pregnancy outcome, no other randomized trials have been able to support this theory. As the placenta does not express class II antigen, it is therefore not likely that such therapy would be successful. The use of this treatment must therefore be considered of no proven benefit.

Psychotherapy

Whether psychological factors affect the outcome of pregnancy has perplexed clinicians and patients for many years. A spontaneous abortion has, until recently, been considered a less serious emotional event than other types of bereavement, but this belief is changing. The eventual effect on subsequent reproductive performance is difficult to quantify but could be significant, and this idea has led to the use of psychotherapy in the management of recurrent abortion. The largest study was published by Stray-Pedersen & Stray-Pedersen (1988), in which 205 patients with idiopathic recurrent abortion received psychotherapy and 42 did not, and the success rates were 85 and 36% respectively. Thus, although the studies are not randomized, there is a suggestion that psychological factors may adversely affect pregnancy outcome and therapy may improve the reproductive performance.

CONCLUSIONS

The aetiology of repetitive fetal wastage is diverse and ill-understood. In the last 15 years there has been an increasing ability to diagnose the aetiology of recurrent pregnancy loss, but there has been very little in the way of treatment that has improved pregnancy outcome. If hypersecretion of LH or the antiphospholipid syndrome are aetiological to recurrent abortion, then future randomized controlled trials of therapies, including downregulation and gonadotrophin therapy or the use of heparin, may bring some hope. It is probable however, at the moment, that the idiopathic group should be offered psychotherapy rather than anything interventionist.

KEY POINTS

1. A spontaneous abortion is now defined in the UK as a pregnancy loss occurring before 24 weeks of gestation. A recurrent aborter is a woman who has had three or more successive abortions.
2. Spontaneous abortion is the main mechanism by which natural selection operates, 50% of all first-trimester losses having a chromosome abnormality.
3. Trisomy is nearly always maternal in origin and the risk increases with maternal age. Triploidy is male in origin and results from dispermy.
4. Infections may cause isolated abortions but are not implicated in recurrent abortions.
5. The overall risk of spontaneous abortion occurring in a clinically recognized pregnancy is 15%.
6. There is a small mortality rate (due usually to haemorrhage or sepsis) associated with spontaneous abortion, of 12.5 per million pregnancies.
7. The incidence of chromosomal abnormalities in couples suffering from recurrent pregnancy loss is of the order of 6.0%.
8. If ultrasound demonstrates fetal viability following a threatened abortion, the subsequent risk of pregnancy loss is only 2–3%.
9. Of women with recurrent pregnancy loss 10–15% have a uterine anomaly.
10. The prognosis for a subsequent pregnancy following three successive miscarriages is very good, the chance of normal outcome being about 70%.
11. Investigations of a recurrent abortion must include a full history (including family history), examination, FBC, karyotyping of both partners, lupus anticoagulant screening and hysterosalpingogram.
12. The emotional impact of miscarriage is often considerable and akin to a bereavement/grief reaction. Psychotherapy may not only help to overcome the grief reaction but may improve pregnancy outcome subsequently.

REFERENCES

Ayers J W, Petersen E P, Ansbacher R 1982 Early therapy for the incompetent cervix in patients with habitual abortion. Fertility and Sterility 38: 177–181

Beer A E 1988 Pregnancy outcome in couples with recurrent abortions following immunological evaluation and therapy. In: Beard R W, Sharp F (eds) Early pregnancy loss: mechanisms and treatment. Royal College of Obstetricians and Gynaecologists, London, pp 337–349

Buttram V C, Reiter R 1981 Uterine leiomyomata: etiology, symptomatology and management. Fertility and Sterility 30: 644–652

Cauchi M N, Limb D, Young D E, Kloss M, Pepperell R J 1991 Treatment of recurrent abortions by immunisation with paternal cells – controlled trial. American Journal of Reproductive Immunology 25: 16–17

Charles D, Larsen B 1987 Infectious agents as a cause of spontaneous abortion. In: Bennett M J, Edmonds D K (eds) Spontaneous and recurrent abortion. Blackwell Scientific, Oxford, pp 149–167

Christiaens G C M L, Stoutenbeck P H 1984 Spontaneous abortions in proven intact pregnancies. Lancet ii: 572–574

Crane J P, Wahl N 1981 The role of maternal diabetes in repetitive spontaneous abortion. Fertility and Sterility 36: 477–479

Creasy M R, Crolla J A, Alberman E D 1976 A cytogenetic study of human spontaneous abortions using banding techniques. Human Genetics 31: 177–196

DeCherney A H, Russell J B, Graebe R A, Polen M L 1986 Resectoscopic management of mullerian fusion defects. Fertility and Sterility 45: 726–728

Dhadial R K, Machin A M, Tait S M 1970 Chromosomal anomalies in spontaneously aborted human fetuses. Lancet ii: 20–21

Edmonds D K, 1988 Use of cervical cerclage in patients with recurrent first trimester abortion. In: Beard R W, Sharp F (eds) Early pregnancy loss: mechanisms of treatment. Royal College of Obstetricians and Gynaecologists, London, pp 411–415

Edmonds D K, Lindsay K S, Miller J F, Williamson E, Wood P J 1982 Early embryonic mortality in women. Fertility and Sterility 38: 447–453

Fantel A G, Shepard T H 1987 Morphological analysis of spontaneous abortuses. In: Bennett M J, Edmonds D K (eds) Spontaneous and recurrent abortion. Blackwell Scientific, Oxford, pp 8–28

Frank P 1985 Sequelae of induced abortion. In: Abortion: medical progress and social implications. Pitman, London, pp 67–82

Gatenby P A, Cameron K, Simes R J, Addlestein S, Bennett M J, Jansen R P 1993 Treatment of recurrent spontaneous abortion by immunisation with paternal lymphocytes – a controlled trial. American Journal of Reproductive Immunology 29: 88–94

Geisler M, Kleinebrecht J 1978 Cytogenetic and histological analysis of spontaneous abortions. Human Genetics 45: 239–251

Gronroos M, Honkonen E, Punnonen R 1983 Cervical and serum IgA and serum IgG antibodies to *Chlamydia trachomatis* and herpes simplex virus in threatened abortion. British Journal of Obstetrics and Gynaecology 90: 167–170

Harrison R F 1988 Early recurrent pregnancy failure treatment with human chorionic gonadotrophin. In: Beard R W, Sharp F (eds) Early pregnancy loss: mechanisms and treatment. Royal College of Obstetricians and Gynaecologists, London, pp 421–431

Hassold T 1980 A cytogenetic study of repeated spontaneous abortions. American Journal of Human Genetics 32: 723–731

Hassold T, Chen N, Funkhouser J et al 1980 A cytogenetic study of 1000 spontaneous abortions. Annals of Human Genetics 44: 151–178

Howe H N, Gill T J, Hsieh H J, Jaing J J, Lee T Y, Hsieh C Y 1991 Immunotherapy for recurrent spontaneous recurrent abortion in the Chinese population. American Journal of Reproductive Immunology 25: 10–15

Kajii T, Ferrier A, Niikawa N, Takahara H, Ohama K, Aviroachan S 1980 Anatomic and chromosomal anomalies in 639 spontaneous abortuses. Human Genetics 55: 87–98

Kaufman R H, Irwin J F 1987 Diethylstilboestrol exposure and reproductive performance. In: Bennett M J, Edmonds D K (eds) Spontaneous and recurrent abortion. Blackwell Scientific, Oxford, pp 130–148

Kline J, Stein Z, Susser M, Warburton D 1980 Environmental influences on early reproductive loss. In: Porter I H, Hook E B (eds) Embryonic and fetal death. Academic Press, New York, pp 225–240

Kriel R L, Gates G A, Wulff H 1970 Cytomegalovirus isolations associated with pregnancy wastage. American Journal of Obstetrics and Gynecology 106: 885–890

Lauritsen J G 1976 Aetiology of spontaneous abortion. Acta Obstetrica Gynaecologica Scandinavica 52: 1–9

Lippman-Hand A, Vekemans 1983 Balanced translocations among couples with two or more spontaneous abortions. Human Genetics 63: 252–257

Mikkelson M 1985 Cytogenetic findings in first trimester chorionic villus sampling. In: Fraccaro G, Simoni G, Brambati B (eds) First trimester fetal diagnosis. Springer-Verlag, Berlin, p 108

Miller J F, Williamson E, Glue J, Gordon Y B, Grudzinskas J G, Sykes A 1980 Fetal loss after implantation: a prospective study. Lancet ii: 554–556

Mowbray J F, Gibblings C, Liddel H, Reginald P W, Underwood J L, Beard R W 1985 Controlled trial of treatment of recurrent abortion by immunization with paternal cells. Lancet i: 941–943

O'Leary J L, O'Leary J A 1963 Rudimentary horn pregnancy. Obstetrics and Gynaecology 22: 371–375

Rabin M, Hart C P, Ferguson-Smith A et al 1985 Two homeobox loci mapped in evolutionary related mouse and human chromosome. Nature 314: 175–178

Regan L, Braude P R 1987 Is antipaternal cytotoxic antibody a valid marker in the management of recurrent abortion? Lancet ii: 1280

Regan L, Owen E J, Jacobs H S 1990 Hypersecretion of luteinising-hormone, infertility and miscarriage. Lancet ii: 1141–1144

Reports on confidential enquiries into maternal deaths in England and Wales 1979–1981 1986 HMSO, London

Roberts C J, Lowe D B 1975 Where have all the conceptions gone? Lancet i: 498

Rushton D I 1988 Placental pathology in spontaneous miscarriage. In: Beard R W, Sharp F (eds) Early pregnancy loss: mechanisms and treatment. Royal College of Obstetricians and Gynaecologists, London pp 149–157

Sagle M, Bishop K, Ridley N 1988 Recurrent early miscarriage and polycystic ovary. British Medical Journal 297: 1027–1028

Sandler S W 1977 Spontaneous abortion in perspective. South Africa Medical Journal 52: 1115–1124

Seibel M, Graves W L 1980 The psychological implications of spontaneous abortion. Journal of Reproductive Medicine 25: 161–172

Simoni G, Gimelli G, Cuoco C 1985 Discordance between prenatal cytogenetic diagnosis after chorionic villus sampling and chromosomal constitution of the fetus. In: Fraccaro M, Simoni G, Brambati B (eds) First trimester fetal losses. Springer-Verlag, Berlin, pp 108–119

Simpson J L, Bombard A 1987 Chromosomal abnormalities in spontaneous abortion. In: Bennett M J, Edmonds D K (eds) Spontaneous and recurrent abortion. Blackwell Scientific, Oxford, pp 51–76

Strassman E O 1966 Fertility and unification of the double uterus. Fertility and Sterility 17: 165–171

Stray-Pedersen B, Stray-Pedersen S 1988 Recurrent abortion: the role of psychotherapy. In: Beard R W, Sharp F (eds) Early pregnancy loss: mechanisms and treatment. Royal College of Obstetricians and Gynaecologists, London, pp 433–440

Takahara H, Ohama K, Fukiwara A 1977 Cytogenetic study in early spontaneous abortion. Hiroshima Journal of Medical Science 26: 291–296

Therkelsen A J, Grunnet N, Hjort T, Myre Jansen O, Jonasson J, Lauritsen J G 1977 Studies in spontaneous abortion. In: Boue A, Thibault C (eds) Chromosomal errors in relation to reproductive failure. INSERM, Paris, pp 81–83

Tulsen D W, Wadsworth J, Adams J, Franks S 1988 Polycystic ovaries, a common finding in normal women. Lancet ii: 870–872

Walker E M, Lewis M, Cooper W, Marnie M, Howie P W 1988 Occult biochemical pregnancy: fact or fiction? British Journal of Obstetrics and Gynaecology 95: 659–663

Warburton D, Fraser F C 1964 Spontaneous abortion risks in man: data from reproductive histories collected in a medical genetics unit. Human Genetics 16: 1–25

Warburton D A, Strobino B 1987 Recurrent spontaneous abortion. In: Bennett M J, Edmonds D K (eds) Spontaneous and recurrent abortion. Blackwell Scientific Publications, Oxford, pp 193–213

Warburton D, Stein Z, Kline J, Susser M 1980 Chromosome abnormalities in spontaneous abortions. In: Porter I H, Hook E B (eds) Human embryonic and fetal deaths. Academic Press, New York, pp 261–287

Watts D H, Eschenbach D A 1988 Reproductive tract infections as a cause of abortion and preterm birth. Seminars in Reproductive Medicine 6: 203–215

Whittaker P G, Taylor A, Lind T 1983 Unsuspected pregnancy loss in healthy women. Lancet i: 1126–1127

WHO 1977 Recommended definitions, terminology and format for statistical tables related to the perinatal period. Acta Obstetrica Gynecologica Scandinavica 56: 247–253

Wilcox A J, Weinberg C R, O'Connor J F et al 1988 Incidence of early pregnancy loss. New England Journal of Medicine 319: 189–194

Wright S W, Trott A T 1988 Toxic shock syndrome: a review. Annals of Emergency Medicine 17: 268–273

21

Tubal disease

R. A. Margara G. Trew

INTRODUCTION

Tubal disease can be defined as tubal damage caused by pelvic infection such as pelvic inflammatory disease, tuberculosis, salpingitis isthmica nodosa or iatrogenic disease with varying degrees of tubal damage or obstruction, sometimes involving the surrounding ovary or pelvic peritoneum, and adhesion formation. As a result patients with tubal damage suffer from infertility and/or pelvic pain. Tubal disease is accountable for 30–40% of cases of female infertility.

AETIOLOGY OF TUBAL DISEASE

Salpingitis

Most salpingitis is the result of an ascending infection from the lower genital tract (Fig. 21.1). The mechanisms whereby the infection ascends through the cervical canal and reaches the tubes are still unknown. It is possible that cervical resistance diminishes, allowing the bacteria to pass through, and is at its lowest during ovulation and menstruation. This theory fits with observations that in cases of cervical gonorrhoea the symptoms of salpingitis appear after menstruation, and patients on oral contraception appear to be 'protected' due to anovulation.

Salpingitis is not in general seen in women who are not sexually active and it is possible that coitus produces uterine contractions, facilitating the spread of infection into the uterus and tubes. In other cases, iatrogenic manoeuvres such as insertion of an intrauterine device, termination of pregnancy, hysterosalpingography or curettage can spread a cervical infection into the uterus and tubes.

Iatrogenic tubal disease is tubal damage caused by surgical procedures carried out in a manner damaging the peritoneum and tubes, rendering young women infertile.

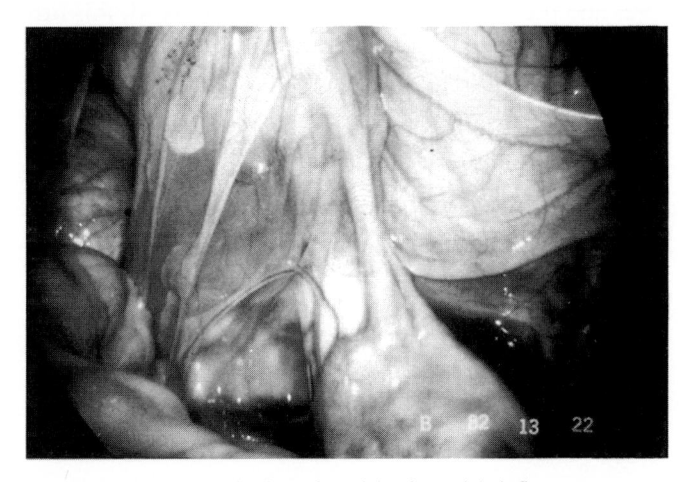

Fig. 21.1 Laparoscopic view of a pelvis after pelvic inflammatory disease. There is a 'curtain' of adhesions covering the pelvic organs.

Pelvic inflammatory disease has by tradition been associated with gonorrhoea. Improvement of microbiological techniques has allowed the identification of numerous other organisms capable of producing salpingitis, including *Chlamydia trachomatis, Mycoplasma hominis* and anaerobic bacteria.

Neisseria gonorrhoeae

Neisseria gonorrhoeae has been isolated from cervical mucus in women with salpingitis in between 10 and 70% of cases, but among those that have positive cervical cultures not all have positive peritoneal cultures. What are the reasons for the variation? There may be differences in host resistance to the organisms; the non-white population seems to be more at risk of having salpingitis with gonococcal cervicitis than others. The use of oral contraception may increase resistance towards the gonococcus and it is probably because of this that in the USA, where since 1974 the use of oral contraception has decreased, the risk of women having salpingitis has increased.

Certain autotypes of gonococcus are more sensitive to antibiotics; when they are localized in the cervix they are easily treated, thus preventing the organism spreading to the tubes.

Chlamydia trachomatis

Chlamydia trachomatis was isolated for the first time in Sweden by Eilard et al (1976) from women with salpingitis. Positive cultures from cervices have been found in up to 36% of patients, but only 6% of them have positive cultures from the tubes. There is no doubt, that *Chlamydia* is responsible for a significant amount of salpingitis but it is not possible to determine how much. There is a discordance between identification of *Chlamydia*-positive cultures and the titre of immunoglobulin gamma M; this titre does not correlate with the severity of salpingitis found at the time of laparoscopy.

There is evidence that Chlamydia is also responsible for causing postpartum endometritis with perihepatic adhesions (Fig. 21.2). Infertile women on average have higher *Chlamydia* antibody titres than pregnant women. Peritonitis following salpingitis may be the result of an immunological mechanism and it has been suggested that the perihepatic adhesions are not caused by *C. trachomatis* directly, but are more likely to be caused by a heterogeneous infection.

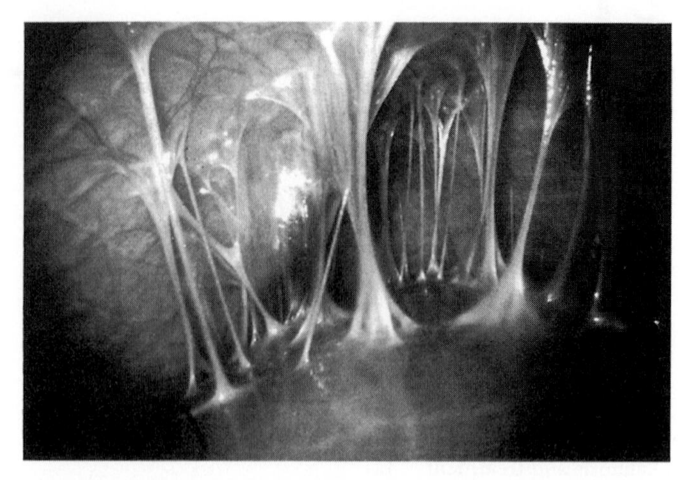

Fig. 21.2 Laparoscopic photograph of perihepatic adhesions: Fitz–hugh–Curtis syndrome.

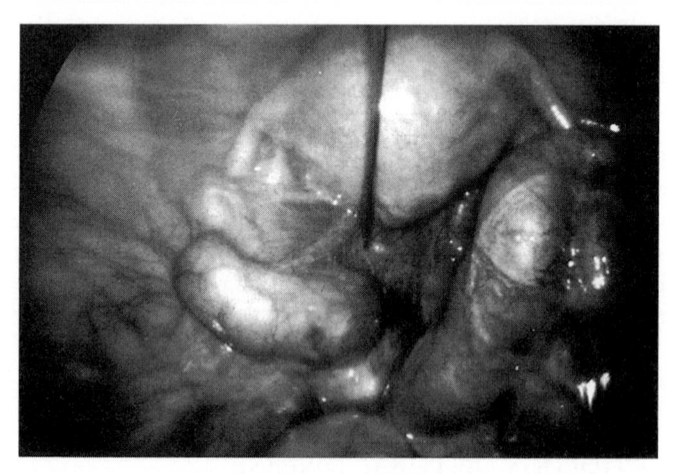

Fig. 21.3 Laparoscopic appearance of bilateral hydrosalpinges as a result of previous pelvic inflammatory disease.

Other organisms

In the general female population there are many organisms capable of producing salpingitis. Most of them are part of the vaginal flora or from the perianal region and are called polymicrobial salpingitis.

Gonococcal infection seems to pave the way for other micro-organisms to cross the cervical mucus and affect the uterus or the tubes; there may be a relation between the intensity of the symptoms, the duration of a gonococcal salpingitis and superinfection with other micro-organisms (Fig. 21.3). Gonococcal salpingitis may increase tubal susceptibility to a subsequent infection, and one attack of salpingitis may protect against the same strain of gonococcus, the subsequent salpingitis being non-gonococcal.

Mycoplasma hominis

Mycoplasma hominis has been isolated from peritoneal fluid from patients with salpingitis. Animal experiments suggest that *Mycoplasma hominis* produces parametritis as well as salpingitis, implying a source of infection other than canalicular.

Mycobacterium tuberculosis

Tubal damage of tuberculous origin is still seen in developed countries, although rarely. *Mycobacterium tuberculosis* reaches the pelvic organs from a primary focus of entry, such as lung or intestine, and then spreads to the genital organs. The most common organs affected are the endometrial cavity and the tubes. Primary genital tuberculosis has been described, as a result of infection from semen of an affected partner, this being the most common source of entry to the cervix.

The aetiology, trends, incidence and epidemiology of pelvic inflammatory disease are discussed in other chapters.

Salpingitis isthmica nodosa

Salpingitis isthmica nodosa was described by Chiari (1887) as nodular thickening of the proximal part of the fallopian tube. The aetiology of this entity is unknown but it is

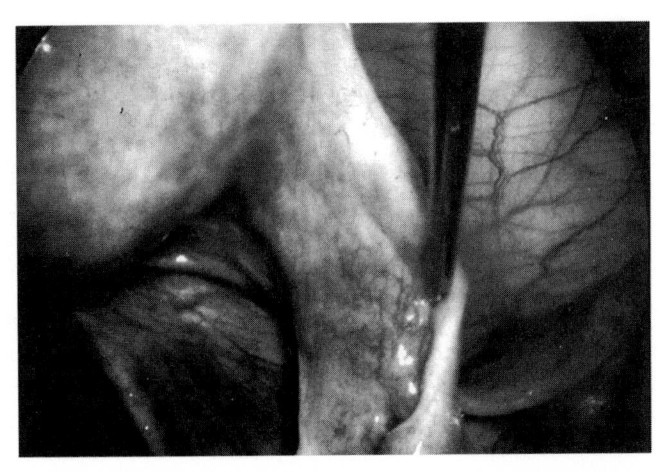

Fig. 21.4 Laparoscopic photograph of the same patient as in Figure 21.3 with salpingitis isthmica nodosa. There is extravasation of dye through the tubal wall.

probably due to a non-inflammatory process similar to adenomyosis (Benjamin & Beaver 1951) or related to diverticulosis in other organs (Burne 1973); infection may always be a secondary process (Fig. 21.4).

Salpingitis isthmica nodosa can be defined as the microscopic presence of tubal epithelium within a hypertrophied and hyperplastic myosalpinx or beneath the tubal serosa, and characterized radiologically by a small diverticulum. It has been classified into grades I–III according to the degree of invasion or depth of the tubal epithelium in the myosalpinx.

The real incidence of salpingitis isthmica nodosa is very difficult to determine. Honore (1978) reported an incidence of 0.6% in a control population who had undergone salpingectomy for sterilization. He also noted a frequency of 2.86% in patients with ectopic pregnancy. Creasy et al (1985) reported that in a large series of hysterosalpingograms of infertile women 3.9% had changes of salpingitis isthmica nodosa on their hysterosalpingograms and half of these had bilateral involvement.

Other causes

Endometriosis, endosalpingiosis, cornual polyps can be the cause of cornual obstruction or tubal damage. Endometriosis is reviewed in Chapter 30.

Cornual polyps

Cornual polyps have been described by Lisa et al (1954); they can cause infertility if they are bilateral. The exact aetiology is not known, but they seem to have two origins: infection and endometriosis.

Previous tubal/pelvic surgery

In a survey done at Hammersmith Hospital in 1980, in 100 consecutive patients referred to the unit because of a mechanical cause of their infertility, no less than 24 had had previous pelvic surgery which appeared to be the reason for the tubal damage (Winston, unpublished results). The operations that had been performed were ovarian cystectomy, wedge resection, myomectomy, salpingectomy, and shortening of round ligament.

Tubal sterilization procedures

Tubal sterilization can be done by laparotomy, culdoscopy and laparoscopy; probably the latter is the most widely used. The laparoscopic methods can be diathermy (monopolar or bipolar); tubal clips (Hulka–Clemens or Filshie) and Yoong's tubal rings. Laparotomy is most used in general at the time of a caesarean section. Methods of sterilization are reviewed in Chapter 26.

DIAGNOSIS AND TREATMENT

The diagnosis of tubal disease is made by laparoscopy and hysterosalpingography. Laparoscopy does not replace the hysterosalpingogram and vice versa. The two are complementary investigations, both offering very important information (Figs 21.5 and 21.6).

In recent years falloposcopy has been introduced as a potential method of assessing tubal damage (Kerin et al 1990). Trials are currently being carried out in different centres. There is no evidence yet that this method has a real clinical application. Selective transcervical salpingography and tubal catheterization can be done in cases where it is doubtful that there is the presence of cornual obstruction (Ataya & Thomas 1991). Mucus plug and debris can be mobilized and a tube that was apparently obstructed can be 'opened'.

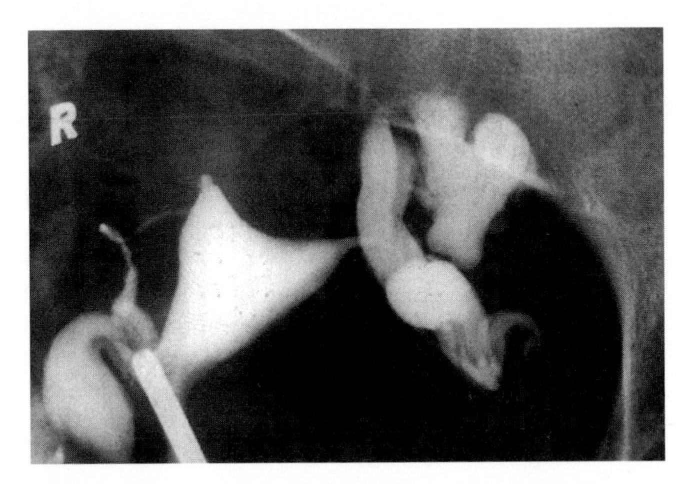

Fig. 21.5 Hysterosalpingogram of a patient with bilateral hydrosalpinges.

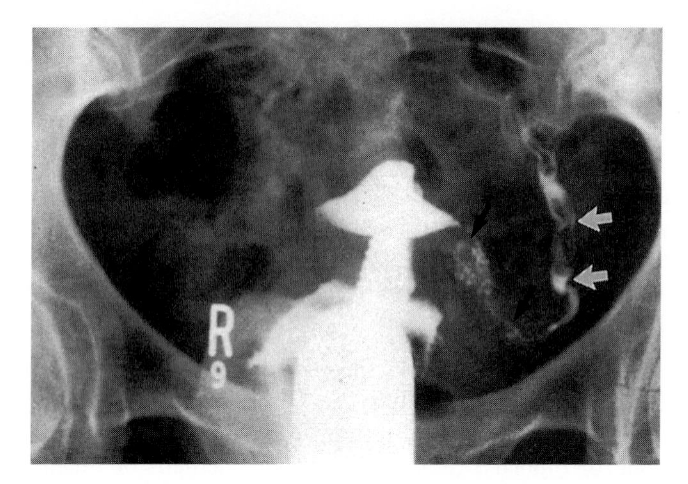

Fig. 21.6 Hysterosalpingogram of a patient with salpingitis isthmica nodosa. Arrows indicate the diverticula filled with contrast medium.

Laparoscopy

Laparoscopy should be performed by the surgeon or a member of the team who will eventually operate on the patient, if surgery is the treatment of choice, because of the variation between units in experience and approaches to varying tubal diseases.

The criteria for patient selection for treatment depend very much on the surgeon's experience and on the possibility of being able to offer alternative treatment. Other points to be considered at the time of making the decision regarding treatment are the patient's wishes about the type of treatment that she and her husband prefer, and the problem of pain. Large numbers of patients with tubal disease have pelvic pain due to adhesions. In some of them the surgical freeing of the ovaries and tubes from adhesions can give symptomatic relief.

The treatment of tubal disease in the infertile patient is surgical. The use of magnification and microsurgical techniques has been the traditional method. With the development of laparoscopic instruments the laparoscopic approach is very much favoured by many gynaecologists as a method of choice amongst patients with minor tubal disease and/or adhesions.

Microsurgical treatment

The microscope was used for tubal surgery for the first time by Walz (1959). Whilst others used delicate electrosurgery and magnification (loupes) in the treatment of hydrosalpinges, Paterson & Wood (1974) in Australia and Winston & McClure-Browne (1974) in England adapted their laboratory techniques to the human situation and operated on infertile women, under high magnification, using an operating microscope.

Microsurgery is not only the use of a microscope, it is based on gentle tissue handling, reperitonealization of raw areas, the use of non-reabsorbable suture materials and irrigation of the tissues using Ringer-lactate solution as this tends to prevent adhesion formation.

There were heated arguments about how useful the microscope was and how much its use improved pregnancy rates. Now microsurgery is well established and is a routine procedure for tubal infertility.

Coadjuvants

The use of coadjuvants can sometimes help to avoid adhesion formation, but remember that no coadjuvants will replace a lack of surgery. If a coadjuvant is used, probably steroids are the best choice (Winston 1982).

Cornual occlusion (Figs 21.7, 21.8)

Cornual occlusion due to inflammatory causes was treated by uterotubal implantation with very poor results. Ehrler (1963) described his technique and suggested that in most patients the intramural portion of the tube could be spared. Since Winston (1977) and Gomel (1977) described their methods based on the use of the microscope it has become the surgical technique of choice. Cornual implantation is now rarely used in our department except in cases of severe damage of the intramural portion of the tubes, and is reserved for cases where there is a severe degree of adenomyosis or tubal damage. We avoid tubocornual implantation whenever possible. Destroying a possible sphincter at the uterotubal junction is associated with excessive bleeding and damage to the tubal blood supply; it shortens the tube and may increase the risk of rupture of the uterus in the event of subsequent preg-

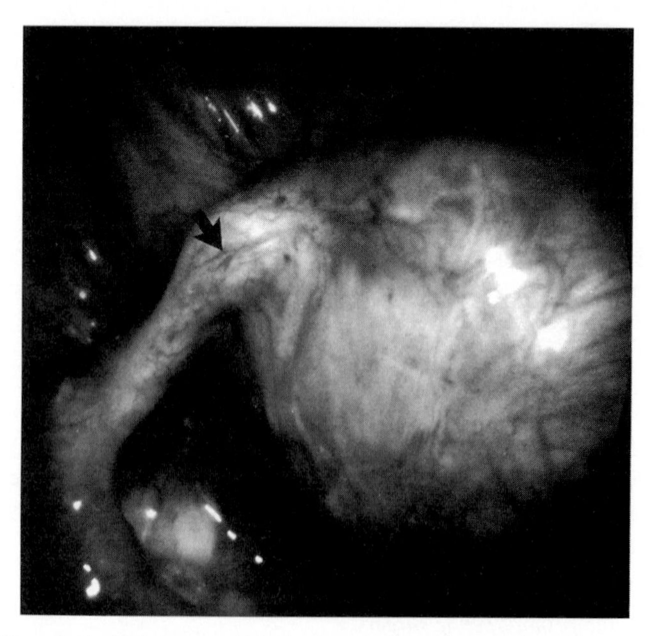

Fig. 21.7 Tubal cornual block: there are irregular vessels on the peritoneum surface as a result of previous inflammation (arrow).

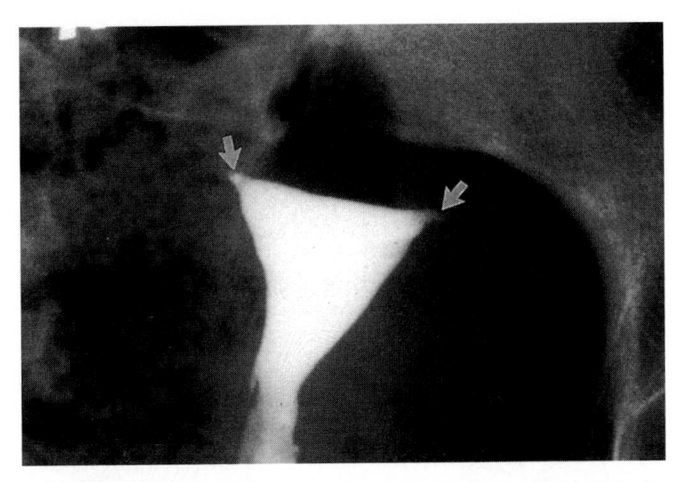

Fig. 21.8 Hysterosalpingogram of a patient with bilateral tubal block (arrows).

nancy, thus patients must be delivered by caesarean section.

The use of magnification allows the surgeon better identification of the intramural portion of the tube by careful shaving of the cornua until healthy tissue is found, permitting a more accurate tissue apposition with a watertight anastomosis between healthy tubal tissues. Once the ends are well defined the anastomosis is done in two layers, using 8/0 nylon as a suture. The suture material should not penetrate the mucosa, only the muscularis (Seki et al 1977). In some cases the use of a temporary splint gives considerable help, especially in deep cornual tubal anastomosis (Fig. 21.9), but it should be removed at the end of the surgical procedure, and if left in situ should not remain more than 48 h. Longer periods of time cause mucosal damage. Tension between the anastomosed ends must be avoided. A stitch of 6/0 prolene between both ends of the mesosalpinx should be applied as a stay suture. More details about the technique have been given elsewhere (Winston 1977, Margara 1982).

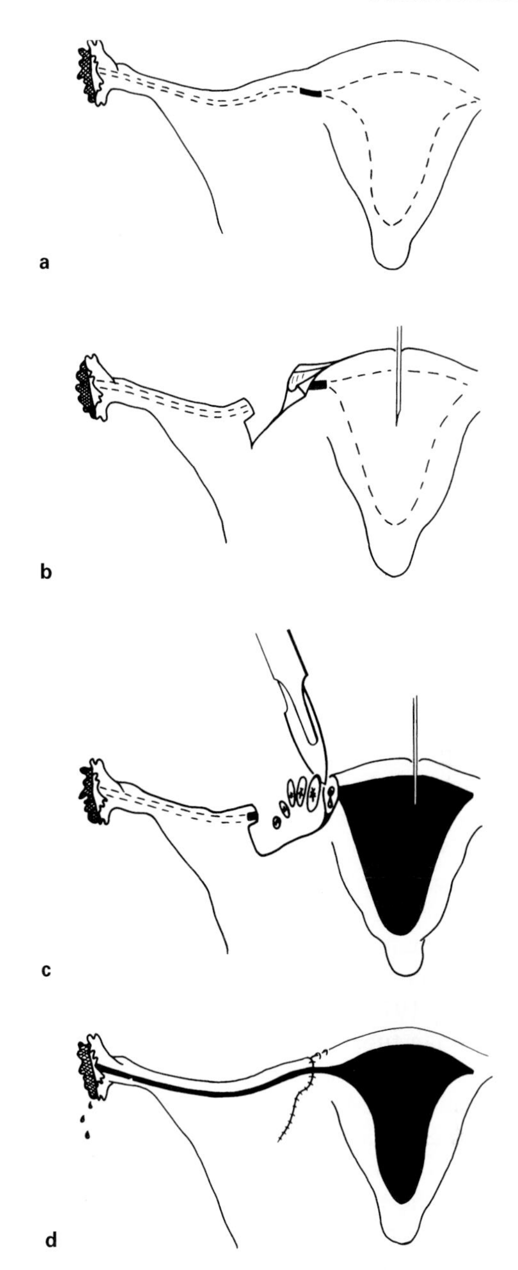

Fig. 21.9 Cornual block diagram showing a cornual anastomosis. **a** Superficial cornual block. **b** Opening of the cornua to expose the intramural part of the tube. **c** Shaving of the tube to find healthy mucosa for anastomosis. **d** Cornual anastomosis completed.

Cornual polyps

Removal of cornual polyps is still a matter of controversy. Glazener et al (1987) stated that the removal of cornual polyps does not improve fertility, and they are not a cause of infertility. We believe that large polyps present in the intramural or isthmic portion of the tube should be removed, depending on the location and size of the polyp. This can involve salpingotomy and resection of the polyp without tubal resection or the opening of the cornu, and removal of the affected portion of the tube followed by cornual–isthmic anastomosis in two layers. In some cases when a large polyp is implanted deep in the intramural portion of the tube, the anastomosis can be difficult due to disparity of the lumen of the tubal ends. The portion where the polyp was present is wider than the isthmic portion of the tube and it is not always easy to achieve a watertight anastomosis. For this reason some surgeons prefer salpingotomy whenever possible.

Tubal anastomosis

Tubal anastomosis for reversal of sterilization is the most successful technique in microsurgery for two reasons: healthy tissues are anastomosed and the localized damage is removed completely (Fig. 21.10). These patients are in general fertile.

Success depends on the length of the remaining tube.

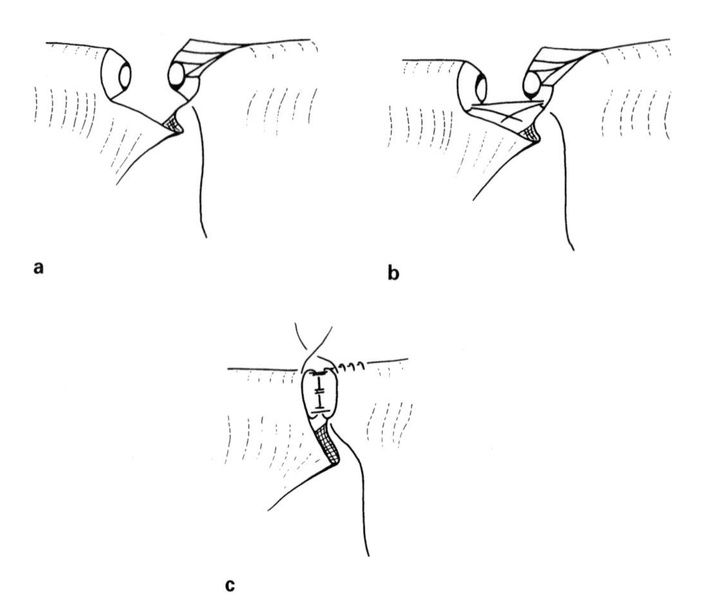

Fig. 21.10 Anastomotic procedure: **a** both tubal lumens are exposed (healthy mucosa); **b** the first stitch is at six o'clock and must be extra mucosa; **c** the anastomosis is completed in two layers. The suture material used is 8/0 nylon.

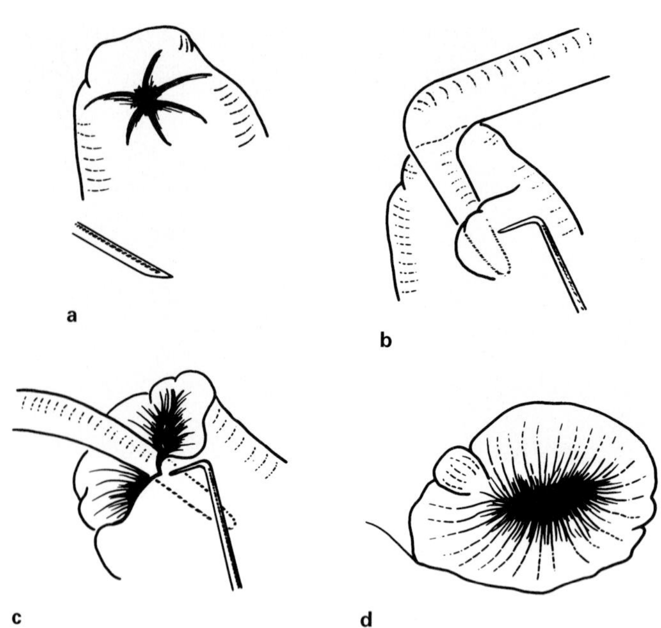

Fig. 21.11 Salpingostomy. **a** Identification of the terminal part of the hydrosalpinx where the incision must be made. **b** An incision is made using diathermy, and the tip of the glass is inserted into the hole in the tube. **c** The salpingostomy is enlarged using the diathermy needle and glass rods. **d** The salpingostomy is completed.

The minimum length of tube necessary to maintain fertility in women is not known. Winston & Boeckx (unpublished data), studied its importance in rabbits. Fertility diminished in a linear fashion depending on the length of the ampulla resected; when more than 70% was missing, none of the animals became pregnant. Resection of the ampullary–isthmic junction did not appear to alter fertility (Winston et al 1977). The rabbit is far from an ideal model for human tubal physiology, but these results emphasize the fact that the ampulla seems to be important to maintain fertility. We have found that women with very short tubes occasionally conceive but patients with very short ampullary segments are less fertile, and when the total length of the tube following anastomosis is shorter than 4 cm the pregnancy rate decreases markedly.

The length of time between sterilization and reversal is important and has a prognostic value. Vasquez et al (1980), demonstrated that after 5 years of sterilization the proximal portion of the tube had a severely damaged mucosa with flattening of the epithelium and polyp formation. The surgical technique of reversal of sterilization has been described elsewhere (Winston 1977, Margara 1982).

Hydrosalpinges

The value of microsurgery varies in the treatment of hydrosalpinges. In some cases where the tube is completely free of adhesions the use of loupes suffices. Where complex adhesions are present, the use of the microscope is mandatory. When performing a salpingostomy the following points should be borne in mind. Before starting the salpingostomy, mobilization of the tube must be completed. Division of adhesions between tube and ovary or other pelvic organs is very important in order to leave the tube fully mobile, with the possibility of the new ostium being able to cover the whole ovarian surface and make egg pick-up more likely.

While dividing adhesions, special care must be taken to avoid damage to the fimbrial blood supply. These vessels are in the area of the connecting ligament between the ovary and the tube at the outer margin of the mesosalpinx. The hydrosalpinx must be opened at the most terminal part, the 'pucker point'. This is where the fimbrial end has closed; it is clearly seen under the microscope as a thin fibrous line, often with an H-shaped configuration, and is not always the thinnest part of the tube. Linear salpingostomy has a high chance of healing over. Using fine diathermy, the tube is then opened and a glass probe introduced, following the fibrous tracts parallel to the blood vessels and ensuring that the mucosal folds are not cut. Using small incisions the new tubal ostium is completed and then the mucosa can be everted (Fig. 21.11).

Two or three stitches of 8/0 nylon are used to secure the mucosal eversion. If the ovarian surface is damaged during the division of adhesions, the raw area should be repaired using fine non-absorbable suture material to avoid recurrence of adhesions.

Adhesions

Omental adhesions are not infrequent and when they are more than minimal, a partial omentectomy is performed.

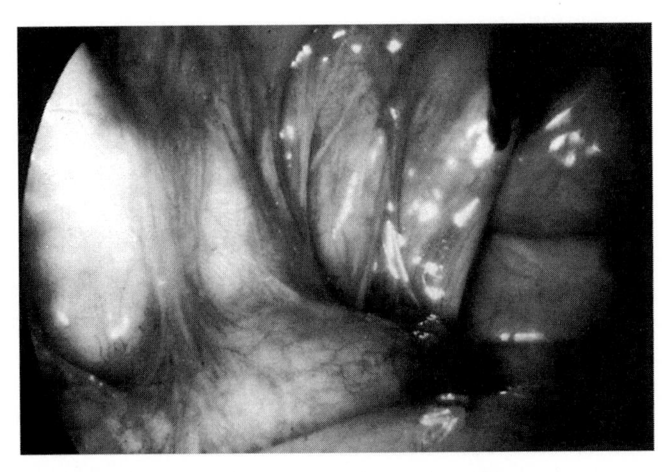

Fig. 21.12 Laparoscopic appearance in a patient with severe periovarian adhesions after pelvic inflammatory disease.

It is best done at the beginning of the operation. Fine 2/0 linen is used to secure the pedicles. We do not use this as a routine procedure, but it seems to be a very effective way of avoiding recurrent adhesion in the pelvis (Fig. 21.12).

The most frequent adhesions are between the ampulla, the ovary and the mesosalpinx. It is easy to work from the isthmus towards the fimbrial end. Using a glass probe the adhesions are hooked and with monopolar diathermy they are incised. Care should be taken not to damage the tubal peritoneum. The use of the microscope simplifies the process because the peritoneal edges can be easily seen. If the tubal peritoneum is incised it must be repaired using 8/0 nylon as a suture material.

Ovarian adhesions should be removed from the ovarian capsule using diathermy or scissors, leaving the ovarian capsule as free as possible. Ovulation and egg release seem to improve after careful ovariolysis, and may depend on the amount of the ovarian surface left free.

Special attention must be paid to raw areas. The uterine surface and the surrounding peritoneum must be carefully inspected. Peritonealization is very important and all raw areas must be covered. If the ovarian fossa has been damaged in order to free or liberate a firmly adherent ovary, the raw area should be closed using a linear suture of 4/0 prolene. If the raw area cannot be peritonealized using the surrounding peritoneum, a peritoneal graft can be applied. The peritoneum should be thin and without fatty tissue. It is attached to the raw area using 8/0 nylon or 6/0 prolene. The donor areas can be the peritoneum layer of the anterior abdominal wall, the peritoneal space between the round ligament and the bladder, and in some cases the peritoneum of the mesentery of the small or large bowel. This technique has proved very effective in experimental animals and the results with humans are very encouraging. Synthetic materials are available to replace peritoneum (Hunter et al 1988, Haney et al 1992). They can be applied during open surgery as well as laparoscopic procedures and can remain in situ, apparently without side-effects, but if removal is necessary, this can be done through a laparoscope.

Special mention should be made of the treatment of tubal damage due to tuberculosis. The treatment is always medical and the tubal damage cannot be repaired by surgery. In this group of patients if the uterine cavity remains unaffected or without damage, in vitro fertilization is the only option.

Laparoscopic surgery

With the development of endoscopic techniques in the last two decades, gynaecologists, using the laparoscope, have been able to perform numerous operations in the field of infertility as in general gynaecology.

Since the use of the first endoscope in medicine in the 1800s as a diagnostic tool, developments in optics and related technology have revolutionized the use of the laparoscope. In the 1940s Palmer in France promoted the laparoscope as a diagnostic instrument. In the 1970s Gomel published the first results of laparoscopic surgery. He performed salpingo-ovariolysis and fimbrioplasties using this approach with results comparable to those he achieved using magnification in open procedures. At the same time Semm in Germany also developed the technique, and a large number of new instruments were available for laparoscopic surgery.

The development of laser beams for medical use had an impact in laparoscopic surgery too. The use of video-laparoscopy is favoured by most surgeons. It is less tiring, the assistant has a more active role during surgical procedures and facilitates training and teaching. There are excellent publications regarding this technique (Nezhat et al 1987, Reich 1987). Surgeons have discussed different methods of dissection using laser diathermy (Donnez et al 1989) or cold cutting (Serour et al 1989). There is no evidence that one is better than the other.

After the initial experiences, procedures that can now be performed safely using operative laparoscopy include salpingo-ovariolysis, fimbrioplasty, salpingostomies, management of ectopic pregnancy and endometriosis and other gynaecological operations such as ventrosuspension, adnexectomies and hysterectomies.

One of the most important attributions of this method is that it apparently has a low rate of adhesion formation, although there are currently no controlled randomized trials to prove this.

There is no doubt that laparoscopic adhesiolysis is very effective for pain (Kolmorgen et al 1991), and open surgery may cause more adhesion formation (Lundford et al 1991). The question still remains whether patients with severe tubal damage, not suitable for open procedures, should be operated upon using the laparoscopic approach when the prognosis is very poor anyway and there are alternative methods available to them.

Great financial advantages are offered by this method. This procedure can be done as a day case or overnight stay. The patient resumes her normal activities in a very short period of time. Laparoscopic surgery, as with any other surgical procedure, has its risks and therefore intensive training is fundamental in order to diminish complications and achieve good results.

Nevertheless, some microsurgeons have difficulties in accepting the method, but there is no doubt that using strict criteria for patient selection, laparoscopic surgery has a lot to offer to the infertile patient.

RESULTS

Results of cornual anastomosis

Cornual anastomosis offers very good results in selected groups of patients; 50% of our patients with inflammatory cornual block have conceived providing the isthmic portion resected was 1 cm or less. With greater degrees of damage, the results are not so good. The miscarriage rate was high (five among 14 patients) but all of them managed to deliver one full-term pregnancy (Table 21.1). In all, 85% of the patients who conceived did so during the first 6 months after surgery.

Postoperative laparoscopies show a high patency rate amongst those patients who have not conceived. The major limiting factors seem to be the recrudescence of the disease or extension of the original inflammation into the anastomotic site, rather than lack of patency. Gomel (1980) has reported similar results: 53% of his patients conceived and had at least one term pregnancy. Only 9% of his patients had abortions. At Hammersmith Hospital we have found abortion to be very common after cornual anastomosis whilst ectopic pregnancy has not been a major problem.

Table 21.1 Cornual anastomosis after inflammatory damage

	Patients	Pregnancies	Miscarriages	Ectopic pregnancies
Isolated cornual block	29	14	5	1
Salpingitis isthmica nodosa	15	4	1	0
Total	44	18	6	1

Data from Hammersmith Hospital, London

Salpingitis isthmica nodosa: treatment results

The surgical treatment of salpingitis isthmica nodosa in the infertile patient is similar to that of cornual block. In nearly half of the patients the tubes are open, and the diagnosis is made on the basis of the typical images of diverticula on the hysterosalpingogram and at laparoscopy. The anastomotic procedure is in general much easier but the length of isthmic portion that must be removed can be difficult to assess. The prognosis depends on the length of tube removed, but if we do not remove enough tissue the surgical procedure will probably fail.

The use of the microscope and the experience of the surgeon are very important in the evaluation of the amount or length of tissue that must be resected. In general we must accept that this condition involves most of the isthmic portion of the tube, so the anastomosis is between the cornu and the ampullary–isthmic junction.

Where the intramural portion of the tube is extensively involved in the process, the patient probably should not be treated surgically. The surgical procedure itself does not vary from that of tubocornual anastomosis. When the whole of the isthmus is removed, the problem of tension at the anastomotic level can be solved using stay sutures of 6/0 prolene between the uterus and the mesosalpinx in order to approximate the tubal ends. Conception rates in this group of patients are approximately 35%.

Reversal of sterilization

Reversal of tubal sterilization is the most successful procedure in tubal microsurgery. At Hammersmith Hospital, in a series of 126 patients 58% conceived; the pregnancy rates varied according to the site of the anastomosis (Table 21.2). Results with reversal of sterilization are very much influenced by the length of tube remaining (Table 21.3).

Table 21.2 Reversal of sterilization according to the site of the anastomosis

Site of anastomosis	Number of patients	Number of pregnant patients	Number of ectopic pregnancies	Percentage of pregnancies
Cornu–isthmus	17	12	0	71
Cornu–ampulla	26	14	1	54
Isthmus–isthmus	16	12	0	75
Isthmus–ampulla	27	17	2	63
Ampulla–ampulla	19	8	0	42
Others	21	10	0	48
Total	126	73	3	58

Data from Hammersmith Hospital, London

Table 21.3 Reversal of sterilization in 95 patients: pregnancy rates according to the length of the longer tube

Length of tube, cm	Patients	Number of pregnancies	Percentage
<2.5	7	2	28
2.5–4	15	4	30
4.1–6	30	14	46
6.1–8	25	16	64
>8	20	18	90

Data from Hammersmith Hospital, London

Salpingostomy

In general it is difficult to assess the results of salpingostomy because a very heterogeneous group of patients is involved. Patient selection varies widely between units, and there is no agreement regarding classification, especially where salpingostomy and fimbrioplasty are concerned.

Salpingostomy is a surgical procedure that many gynaecologists think is obsolete, because in vitro fertilization techniques offer comparable or better results in some cases. As in any other surgical procedure, if we select the patients well, good results will be achieved.

Boer-Meisel et al (1986) in a prospective study classified hydrosalpinges as grades I, II and III, based on the nature and extent of the adhesions, the microscopic aspect of the endosalpinx, the thickness of the tubal wall and the diameter of the hydrosalpinx. In their series, 77% of patients with grade I hydrosalpinx had the possibility of conception, 21% with grade II, and only 3% with grade III. Thus surgery is the obvious treatment for patients with grade I hydrosalpinges. Patients with grade III should avoid surgery and be treated using in vitro fertilization techniques. The difficult group is that of grade II hydrosalpinx, where treatments with in vitro fertilization or tubal surgery have the same prognosis. Age, social and religious background, the possibility of alternative treatment, and the patient's wishes must be considered very carefully.

In a series of 323 patients from Hammersmith Hospital, 81 (25%) of the patients conceived, most of them during the first 8 months following surgery or after the second year. After the second year the ectopic pregnancy rate seemed to be higher. Of these patients, 20 have more than one child, and one has already had four (Table 21.4).

Table 21.4 Results of salpingostomies (1971–1985)

Patients	Pregnancies	Miscarriages	Ectopic pregnancies
323	81 (25%)	54 (16.7%)	32 (10%)

Data from Hammersmith Hospital, London

In our hands laparoscopic salpingostomy has shown poorer results than those achieved using the microsurgical approach. It is possible that laparoscopic surgery was performed in patients with more severe tubal damage, with the open procedures being used for the less complicated cases (Table 21.5).

Table 21.5 Results of laparoscopic salpingostomy

		Pregnancies		
	Patients	Term	Intrauterine	Ectopic
Primary	33	4	6 (18%)	2
Repeat	45	2	4 (8%)	4
Total	78	6	10 (13%)	6

Data from Hammersmith Hospital, London

CONCLUSIONS

There is no doubt that we can treat a large group of patients with tubal disease using in vitro fertilization techniques. In a well selected group of infertile patients with tubal damage, surgical procedures, performed using laparoscopy or open surgery (microsurgery), offer a very good prognosis, and many patients can conceive more than once after only one treatment. In a highly specialized reproductive unit these methods should be available and the choice of procedure adapted to each individual case.

KEY POINTS

1. Tubal disease is tubal damage caused by pelvic infection or iatrogenic disease with varying degrees of damage, and sometimes involving surrounding structures.
2. Tubal disease is accountable for 30–40% of cases of female infertility.
3. Salpingitis most commonly results from ascending infection from the lower genital tract.
4. Cervical resistance diminishes during ovulation and menstruation, possibly allowing bacteria to ascend.
5. Salpingitis is not generally seen in women who are not sexually active.
6. The non-white population seems to be more at risk of salpingitis with gonococci cervicitis. Host resistance is important and resistance to gonococci may be increased by use of the oral contraceptive pill.
7. *Chlamydia trachomatis* is responsible for a significant amount of salpingitis, postpartum endometriosis and perihepatic adhesions.
8. Many organisms are capable of producing salpingitis. Gonococcal infection seems to pave the way for other micro-organisms to cross the cervical mucus and affect the uterus or tubes.
9. Tubal damage of tuberculous origin is rare in developed countries. *Mycobacterium tuberculosis* reaches pelvic organs

either by spreading from a primary focus or, occasionally, as the primary disease resulting from infection with infected semen.

10. The treatment of tubal disease in the infertile patient is surgical. Two methods are available. One is based on the principles of microsurgery: gentle tissue handling; reperitonealization of raw areas; use of non-absorbable sutures, and irrigation with Ringer's solution. The other method is laparoscopic surgery, for patients with minor tubal disease and pain due to pelvic adhesions.
11. Tubocornual implantation is avoided where possible since destroying a possible sphincter at the uterotubal junction is associated with excessive bleeding and may increase the risk of rupture.
12. Tubal anastomosis for reversal of sterilization is the most successful technique of microsurgery, and success depends upon the length of the remaining tube and the time elapsed since the sterilization.
13. Laparoscopic surgery offers important advantages. Less invasive procedures are done as day cases or overnight and allow the patient to reassume normal activities in a very short period of time.

REFERENCES

Ataya K, Thomas M 1991 New techniques for selective transcervical osteal salpingography and catheterisation in the diagnosis and treatment of proximal tubal obstruction. Fertility and Sterility 56(5): 980–983

Benjamin C L, Beaver D C 1951 The pathogenesis of salpingitis isthmica nodosa. American Journal of Clinical Pathology 21: 212–222

Boer-Meisel M E, te Velde E R, Habbena J D F, Kardaun J W P F 1986 Predicting the pregnancy outcome in patients treated for hydrosalpinx; a prospective study. Fertility and Sterility 45: 23–29

Burne J C 1973 Salpingitis isthmica nodosa. In: Fox H, Langley F A (eds) Postgraduate obstetrical and gynaecological pathology. Pergamon Press, Oxford, p 269

Chiari H 1887 Zur pathologischen Anatomic des Eileiter-Catrrhs. Zeitschrift fur Heilkunde 8: 457–473

Creasy J L, Clarke R L, Cuttino J T, Groff T R 1985 Salpingitis isthmica nodosa: radiologic and clinical correlates. Radiology 154: 597–600

Donnez J, Nisolle M 1989 CO_2 laser laparoscopy surgery. Adhesiolysis, salpingostomy, laser uterine nerve ablation and tubal pregnancy. Baillères Clinics in Obstetrics and Gynaecology 3: 525–543

Eilard T, Brorsson J E, Hamark B, Forssman L 1976 Isolation of chlamidya in acute salpingitis. Scandinavian Journal of Infectious Diseases (suppl): 82–84

Ehrler P 1963 Die intramurale tubenanastomoze (ein Beitrag zur Uberwindung der Tubaren Steritat). Zentralblatt für Gynaekologie 85: 393–400

Eschenbach D A, Holmes K K 1979 The etiology of acute pelvic inflammatory disease. Sexually Transmitted Diseases 6: 224–227

Glazener C M A, Loveden L M, Richardson S J, Jeans W D, Hull M G R 1987 Tubocornual polyps: their relevance in subfertility. Human Reproduction 2: 59–65

Gomel V 1977 Tubal reanastomosis by microsurgery. Fertility and Sterility 28: 59

Gomel V 1980 Clinical results of infertility microsurgery. In: Crosignani P G, Rubin B L (eds) Microsurgery in female infertility. Academic Press, New York, pp 77–94

Haney A F, Dotty E 1992 Murine peritoneal injury and de novo adhesion formation caused by oxidized-regenerated cellulose (Interceed TC7) but not expanded polytetrafluoroethylene (Gore-Tex surgical membrane). Fertility and Sterility 57: 202–208

Honore L H 1978 Salpingitis isthmica nodosa in female infertility and ectopic pregnancy. Fertility and Sterility 29: 164–168

Hunter S K, Scott J R, Hull D, Urry R L 1988 The gamete and embryo compatibility of various synthetic polymers. Fertility and Sterility 50(1): 110–116

Kerin J, Daykhovsky L, Grundfest W, Surrey E 1990 Falloposcopy: a micro-endoscopic transvaginal technique for diagnosis and treating endotubal disease incorporating guide wire cannulation and direct balloon tuboplasty. Journal of Reproductive Medicine 35: 606–612

Kolmorgen et al 1991 Ergebnisse nach per laparoscopiam ausgefulnten Adhäsiolysen bei Patientinnen mit draneschen Unterbauchen-beschwerden. Zentrobe Gynekol 113(6): 291–295

Lisa J R, Gioia J D, Rubin I C 1954 Observations on interstitial portion of the fallopian tube. Surgery, Gynecology and Obstetrics 99: 159–169

Lundford P, Hahlin M, Kallfelt B, Thourburn J, Lindblon B 1991 Adhesion formation after laparoscopic surgery in tubal pregnancy: a randomised trial versus laparotomy. Fertility and Sterility 55: 911–915

Margara R A 1982 Tubal reanastomosis. In: Chamberlain G, Winston R M L (eds) Tubal infertility. Blackwell Scientific, Oxford, pp 106–119

Nezhat C, Hood J, Winer F, Nezhat F, Crowgey S R, Garrison C P 1987 Video-laparoscopy and laser laparoscopy in gynaecology. British Journal of Hospital Medicine 38: 219–224

Paterson P, Wood C 1974 The use of microsurgery in the reanastomosis of the rabbit fallopian tube. Fertility and Sterility 25: 757–761

Reich H 1987 Laparoscopic treatment of extensive pelvic adhesions including hydrosalpinx. Journal of Reproductive Medicine 32: 736–742

Seki K, Eddy C A, Smith N K, Pauerstein C J 1977 Comparison of two techniques of suturing in microsurgical anastomosis of the rabbit oviduct. Fertility and Sterility 28: 1215–1219

Serour G I, Bandroui M H, Agizi H M, Hamed A F, Abdel-Aziz F 1989 Laparoscopic adhesiolysis for infertile patients with pelvic adhesive disease. International Journal of Gynaecology and Obstetrics 30: 249–252

Vasquez G, Winston R M L, Boeckx W, Brosens I 1980 Tubal lesions subsequent to sterilisation and their relation to fertility after attempts at reversal. American Journal of Obstetrics and Gynecology 138: 86–92

Walz W 1959 Fertilitäts Operationen mit Hilfe eines Operationemkroscopes. Geburtshilfe und Gynaekologe 153: 49–53

Winston R M L 1977 Microsurgical tubocornual anastomosis for reversal of sterilisation. Lancet i: 284–285

Winston R M L 1982 Reconstructive microsurgery of the lateral end of the fallopian tube. In: Chamberlain G, Winston R M L (eds) Tubal infertility. Blackwell Scientific, Oxford, pp 79–104

Winston R M L, McClure-Browne J C 1974 Pregnancy following autograph transplantation of the fallopian tube and ovary in the rabbit. Lancet i: 494–497

Winston R M L, Frantzen C, Oberti C 1977 Oviduct function following resection of the ampullary–isthmic junction. Fertility and Sterility 28: 284–289

22

Ectopic pregnancy

R. A. Margara, G. H. Trew

INTRODUCTION

Ectopic pregnancy can be defined as the implantation of a fertilized ovum outside the uterine cavity. It was first described in the literature in 936 AD by Abulcasis. Parry & Lea in 1876 reported a mortality of nearly 70%, and it was Tait who in 1884 published the first cases of surgical management of ectopic pregnancy.

PATHOPHYSIOLOGY

The reason why a fertilized ovum can implant in an apparently normal fallopian tube is still unknown but abnormalities of the mechanisms involved in ovum transport may be a predisposing factor. Ovum transport from when the ovum is released by the ovary until it reaches the uterine cavity takes 3–4 days with the ovum being retained in the ampulla for most of that time. Passage through the isthmus is very rapid.

Innervation

The adrenergic innervation of the myosalpinx is important; the nerve fibres are concentrated in the isthmus. This suggests that a sphincter mechanism might influence ovum transport but adrenergic or antiadrenergic drugs do not seem to disrupt transport to any great extent in primates.

Muscular contractions

The contribution of contractions of the tubal muscle to tubal transport varies according to the portion of the tube and the time from when the ovum was released. Measurement of tubal contractility without interference with tubal function is practically impossible. One of the methods used for assessment is electrical activity: electrical stimuli to the circular muscle of the ampulla increase intraluminal pressure and movement of the ovum. In rabbits this mechanism is complicated by the flow of fluid in the tubal lumen.

The muscle has longitudinal and circular layers, making the interpretation of measurements difficult as there may be functional independence between layers.

Ovarian hormones

Tubal transport is influenced by hormone levels; oestrogens stimulate tubal contractility but progesterone causes decreased activity. Progesterone also decreases local prostaglandin secretion and causes relaxation of the isthmic portion of the tube, which may allow the fertilized ovum to progress into the uterus.

Cilial action

Beating of the cilia is also involved in transporting the egg towards the uterus. At the ampulla the cilia beat towards the isthmus, assisting transport. In animals, tubal contractions can be stopped pharmacologically but the egg still progresses. Surgical reversal of 1 cm of the isthmus in rabbits does not prevent pregnancy, but if the segment reversed is from the ampulla no pregnancy occurs (Eddy et al 1977). Cilia beating continues, but after the reversal it is in the opposite direction to that in the remaining portion of the ampulla. If ova are placed in the fimbrial end of these tubes they are transported until they reach the reversed segment; if they are placed on the surface of the reversed segments, transport is back towards the ovary. In contrast, in oviducts in which 1 cm segments were transected but not reversed, ovum transport was normal. These observations suggest an important role for the cilia in transporting the ova though the ampulla but not through the isthmus.

Loss of ciliated cells due to pelvic inflammatory disease may decrease the quality of ovum transport and delay the ovum in reaching the isthmus and the uterine cavity (Brosens & Vasquez 1976). Cilia do not seem to be strictly necessary for ovum transport as patients with Kartagener's syndrome, where the cilia are immobile, are able to conceive and have intrauterine pregnancies.

Changes at site of implantation

Exactly where the blastocyst implants in the tube is still a matter of speculation, as it is difficult to observe very early tubal implantation. It seems likely that the blastocyst implants on the tips of the papillary fronds.

It has been assumed that when an ectopic pregnancy implants and grows in the tubal lumen, placentation involves the endosalpinx with obliteration of the tubal epithelium without trophoblastic invasion into the muscularis. The trophoblast does not differ histologically from that normally formed in the uterus; as it penetrates the tubal wall and invades the muscularis it becomes extraluminal although retroperitoneal. When blood vessels are involved bleeding occurs and a retroperitoneal haematoma is formed with tubal dilatation. The haematoma, with dilation of the retroperitoneal space, may explain the pain that patients observe well before the occurrence of tubal rupture and complications of ectopic pregnancy.

CLASSIFICATION

Tubal ectopic pregnancy can be classified in order of frequency according to the site of implantation. It can be ampullary, isthmic, fimbrial or in the interstitial portion of the tube (Fig. 22.1). These sites account for 95% of ectopic pregnancies.

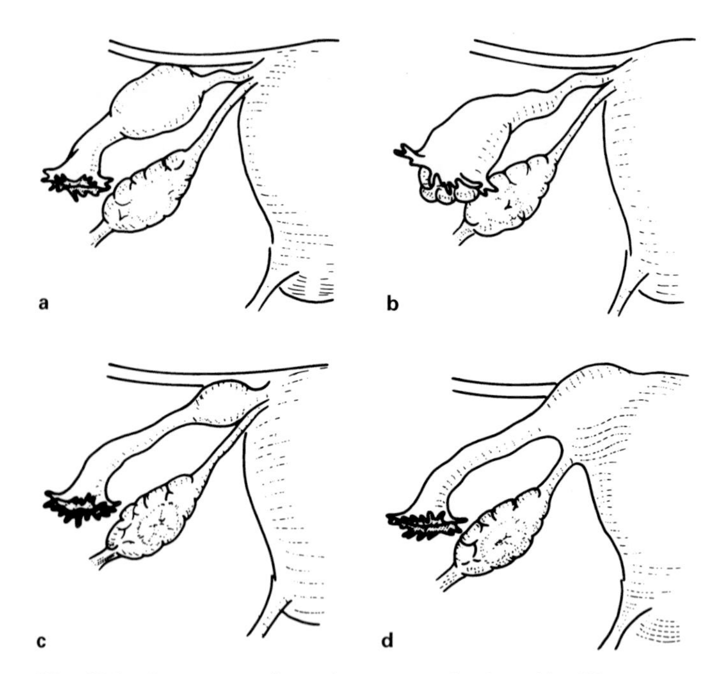

Fig. 22.1 Appearance of ectopic pregnancy implanted in different parts of the tube: **a** ampulla; **b** infundibulum/fimbria; **c** isthmus; **d** cornual or interstitial.

Table 22.1 Implantation sites of 417 tubal ectopic pregnancies

Site	*n*	%
Fimbrial	29	7.0
Ampullary	176	42.0
Isthmic	117	28.0
Interstitial	54	13.0
In stump of tube	9	2.0
Unrecorded	32	8.0

From Douglas (1963) with permission of BMJ Publishing Group.

Douglas in 1963 reviewed 438 ectopic pregnancies; 417 were tubal and the implantation sites were as shown in Table 22.1.

Ovarian ectopic

Ovarian ectopic pregnancies can be primary or secondary, depending upon whether the implantation was directly on the ovary or the result of a tubal abortion and reimplantation on the ovary. The incidence is reported as being in between 1/2000 and 1/8500 deliveries. The identification of the type of ectopic pregnancy can be difficult. To classify an ectopic pregnancy as a primary ovarian implantation, the fallopian tube should be normal and the gestational sac have ovarian tissue in its wall.

Abdominal ectopic

Similarly, abdominal implantation of an ectopic pregnancy can be primary or secondary, depending on whether the pregnancy implants directly in the abdominal cavity or implantation occurs as a result of a tubal abortion or ruptured tubal ectopic pregnancy without major clinical symptoms. In primary implantation the tubes and ovaries are intact and the pregnancy is associated with peritoneal tissue only. The frequency of abdominal pregnancies varies between 1/3400 and 1/8000 deliveries.

Cervical ectopic

Cervical ectopic pregnancy is a rare event with a frequency varying between 1/10 000 and 1/16 000 deliveries. To identify a cervical ectopic pregnancy, cervical glands must be attached to the placenta, the placenta must be implanted below the place where the uterine vessels reach the uterus, and the attachment between the placenta and the cervix should be intimate.

Other sites

A case of vaginal ectopic pregnancy presenting as a suburethral cyst has been described by Duckman et al (1984). After removal of the cyst the presence of trophoblastic tissue was confirmed histopathologically.

Intraligamentous ectopic pregnancy has been defined by Kobak et al (1955) as a pregnancy below the tube bordered by the broad ligament, the levator ani muscle, laterally by the pelvic side wall, and medially by the uterus. It is extremely uncommon.

Ectopic pregnancy in a rudimentary uterine horn has also been reported and live births have been confirmed as resulting from such an implantation site.

Heterotopic pregnancy is the combination of an intrauterine and an ectopic pregnancy, generally tubal. Heterotopic pregnancy used to be a very rare eventuality with an incidence of 1/30 000 deliveries. Since in vitro fertilization and multiple embryo transfers have become common practice, the incidence of heterotopic pregnancy has increased, but at the moment it is not possible to confirm by how much.

AETIOLOGY

Many factors are known to contribute to the occurrence of ectopic pregnancy or can put patients at risk of having an ectopic pregnancy. Any mechanism, infectious, surgical or hormonal, that can alter tubal transport or the quality of the egg may contribute directly or indirectly to the aetiology of ectopic pregnancy.

Causes related to tubal function

Pelvic inflammatory disease

Ectopic pregnancies associated with pelvic inflammatory disease have increased dramatically in the last 15 or 20 years. Endosalpingitis may damage the tubal endothelium and cause adhesion formation, creating gland-like spaces and pockets where the fertilized ovum may be trapped and implant. Westrom et al (1981) found that in Sweden the likelihood of ectopic pregnancy is correlated with the age of the woman. The incidence was 4.1/1000 in teenagers, 6.9/1000 in women 20–29 years old and 12.9/1000 in the age group of 30–39 years. The risk of an ectopic pregnancy increased sevenfold after acute salpingitis and was associated with the use of intrauterine contraceptive devices.

Clark & Baranyai (1987) found a 38% increase in ectopic pregnancy in New Zealand over 15 years (1970–1984) and histological evidence of tubal infection in patients with ectopic pregnancy increased from 40% in 1970 to 61% in 1984.

There is an association between ectopic pregnancy and *Chlamydia trachomatis* infection and in general the infection has been subclinical. Brunham et al (1986) reported that only 10% of women with ectopic pregnancy and 6% with serology positive for *Chlamydia trachomatis* had a history of clinical pelvic inflammatory disease.

Salpingitis isthmica nodosa

Salpingitis isthmica nodosa was first described by Chiari in 1887 and its incidence, aetiology and clinical significance are still a matter of controversy. It seems to have an effect on the reproductive performance of the infertile woman and is often associated with ectopic pregnancy, but to what degree is very difficult to establish. Persaud (1970) found diverticula which occur in salpingitis isthmica nodosa in 49% of specimens of ectopic pregnancies and Majmudar et al (1983) found that 57% of specimens of their cases of ectopic pregnancies had signs of salpingitis isthmica nodosa.

A possible reason why ectopic pregnancy occurs in the tubes damaged by this condition is that the embryo is trapped in extensions of the tubal mucosa into the myosalpinx, with subsequent nidation. One of the major problems in accepting this mechanical theory is that in the majority of patients ectopic pregnancies are implanted on the distal part of the tube, where salpingitis isthmica nodosa is less common. It might be that, due to the thickness of the muscular layer of the tube in patients with the condition, the women may have spasmodic contractions of the tubes and obstruction or dysfunction of the mechanism of tubal transport without a real mechanical obstruction.

Tubal reconstruction

Tubal reconstruction is associated with an increased incidence of ectopic pregnancy. The success of tubal surgery is measured by a high intrauterine and low extrauterine pregnancy rate. The fact that microsurgery can achieve tubal patency in severely damaged tubes with abnormal function may predispose to or increase the risk of ectopic pregnancy.

In a large series of 653 patients from 14 different centres, 54% of patients had ectopic pregnancies when the microsurgical approach was used (Winston 1981). In his first series after magnification and electrocautery were introduced for tubal surgery, Swolin (1975) had 18% of ectopic pregnancies after salpingostomy.

The ectopic pregnancy rate is less among patients who have had tubal anastomosis due to tubal damage. Reversal of sterilization is the most successful of the anastomotic surgical procedures and carries a lower risk of ectopic pregnancy.

Conservative surgery for ectopics

Conservative surgery in ectopic pregnancies may increase the chances of having another ectopic pregnancy, but it will depend very much on any pre-existing conditions in the tube where the first ectopic originated, the localization of the ectopic and whether the contralateral tube is healthy or damaged.

Intrauterine contraceptive devices

The use of intrauterine contraceptive devices has been associated with an increase in ectopic pregnancy. Although Ory (1981) in a multicentre study concluded that women who had never had an intrauterine device had the same chances of having an ectopic pregnancy as those who had, Erkkola & Liukko (1977) found that in Finland there is an increase with time in the number of ectopic pregnancies in patients who had had a device: 59% of their patients with ectopic pregnancy had had devices inserted. Contraceptive users of any kind have less chance of having an ectopic pregnancy than non-users, but long term device users were 2.5 times more likely to have an ectopic pregnancy than those who had the device for a shorter period of time (less than 25 months).

Ovarian pregnancy appears to have an increased incidence amongst intrauterine device users and it has been postulated that deciliation of the endosalpinx might be the cause, or that increased secretion of prostaglandins by mast cells of the mesosalpinx can alter tubal transport.

Tubal sterilization procedures

A high risk of ectopic pregnancy has been reported in patients who conceive after sterilization, as there has been major destruction of tube. When a tuboperitoneal fistula results, there is a higher chance of pregnancy and also a higher chance that it will be an ectopic pregnancy. Patients who are sterilized and have had a previous illegal abortion are at higher risk of having an ectopic pregnancy than those who have had an induced abortion, but previous intrauterine device usage is not a factor. No differences were found in cases of old pelvic infection or device users before sterilization.

The chances of conceiving after sterilization are very low, i.e. approximately 1/1000, and the chances of that pregnancy being an ectopic range between 15.6 and 63.3%.

Exposure to diethylstilboestrol

Women who were exposed to diethylstilboestrol in utero have an increased chance of ectopic pregnancy. De Cherney et al (1981) reported that 16 such patients had unique findings at laparoscopy with 'withered' tubes, described as a 'foreshortened, sacculated, convoluted tube with a pinpoint os and constricted fimbria' and all had the classic T-shaped uterus. There were no significant findings with respect to the tubal lumen or any other pathology in the hysterosalpingogram. The effect of diethylstilboestrol was said to be related to the dose used but no specific evidence was given.

Previous termination of pregnancy

Controversy still exists regarding the incidence of ectopic pregnancy related to termination of pregnancy. In 1948 Sawar & Roth suggested a relationship between the increase in ectopic pregnancy and termination of pregnancy.

Induced abortion may be one of the factors that increases the risk of having an ectopic pregnancy; the risk increases among those who have had two or more terminations of pregnancy.

Causes related to the embryo

Ovulation induction

Gemzell et al in 1982 showed that in women who have had ovarian stimulation with gonadotrophins there is an increased chance of having an ectopic pregnancy. The theory is that hyperstimulation produces higher oestrogen levels, affecting tubal transport and that oocytes of different degrees of maturity are released at the same time, with possible delay of fertilization. High levels of oestrogen before human chorionic gonadotrophin (hCG) is released might increase this risk.

In vitro fertilization

In vitro fertilization has been associated with increased chances of ectopic pregnancy. The reasons are not very clear, but the possible explanations are that the embryo might be injected directly into the tube; that it migrates spontaneously, or that it is moved by uterine contractions. It is possible that some such embryos are expelled back into the uterine cavity by the tube, but the largest group of patients in an in vitro fertilization programme have tubal disease. Tubal function is impaired so that re-expulsion of embryos may not always be possible. In vitro fertilization patients have high oestrogen levels and this could contribute to altered tubal transport by affecting the beating of the cilia.

Direct placement of gametes, as in gamete intrafallopian transfer (GIFT) or zygote intrafallopian transfer (ZIFT), may well increase the risk further.

Gamete transmigration

Many series have reported the finding of the corpus luteum in the contralateral ovary to the side of the ectopic, suggesting ovum transmigration.

In theory the fimbria may aspirate the oocyte or a fertilized egg from the pouch of Douglas. If an embryo has been aspirated it can then implant in the ampulla, or because of its size cannot go through the intramural portion of the tube-ending as in an interstitial implantation. The hormonal background with high levels of progesterone may influence tubal transport.

Transmigration of spermatozoa has been described as a possible cause of ectopic pregnancy. There are cases where the tubal lumen has been interrupted by sterilization, or conservative surgery in a previous ectopic pregnancy. It has also been suggested that in cases of reversal of sterilization where only one oviduct could be repaired, the remaining portion of the other tube should be removed, especially the fimbrial end.

EPIDEMIOLOGY

The increased number of ectopic pregnancies is well documented, but it is in some way related to the fact that an early diagnosis of pregnancy can be made with the use of β-hCG and the ability to locate the site of implantation at an early stage. The gynaecologist feels it is urgent to confirm the diagnosis, which always involves in one way or another a surgical procedure. Possibly a proportion of ectopic pregnancies with abnormal implantation or abnormal embryos would resolve on their own without any consequences.

Race and socioeconomic factors influence the risk of ectopic pregnancy. In the USA ectopic pregnancy is twice as high in non-white than in white populations (Erkkola & Liukko 1977, Lehfeldt et al 1970). In England and Wales, there was little change in the incidence of ectopic pregnancy or death due to ectopic pregnancy between 1970 and 1981, but from 1982 to 1985 the number of ectopic pregnancies increased by 19%.

Until 1981 ectopic pregnancy had been the leading cause of maternal mortality in the first trimester. The decrease in the subsequent 3 years may be due to chance, but the incidence of non-fatal cases has increased, so the decrease of mortality is due to earlier diagnosis and better treatment. Similar trends have been seen in the USA.

The availability of early diagnosis and treatment, and the degree of awareness of doctors and patients of the possibility of ectopic pregnancy, are very important factors which contribute to the decrease in maternal deaths.

PRESENTATION

Ectopic pregnancy can present in different ways. Probably the most important factor in detection and making an early diagnosis is always to think about that possibility in patients at high risk, such as infertile patients or those who have had previous tubal surgery; those with a history of pelvic inflammatory disease, and those who have been sterilized or are using intrauterine contraceptive devices.

The signs and symptoms of ectopic pregnancy vary according to whether the presentation is acute or subacute.

Acute presentation

Acute presentation is associated with rupture of the ectopic pregnancy and massive intraperitoneal bleeding, with acute abdominal pain and cardiovascular collapse. Some patients have a history of menstrual irregularity, local pain and shoulder pain. Abdominal rigidity and rebound tenderness are in general present. Vaginal examination is not necessary: it does not add any specific information except that there may be some localized tenderness in one of the fornices and it can be dangerous, producing the total rupture of the ectopic gestation and increasing intraperitoneal bleeding.

Subacute presentation

Subacute presentation occurs in the majority of cases. The patient complains of abdominal pain which may be localized to one iliac fossa, vaginal bleeding and a delayed menstrual period. Some may report shoulder pain if free blood is in the peritoneal cavity, due to the irritation of the peritoneum. On bimanual examination there may be localized tenderness in one of the fornices, cervical excitation pain, and sometimes a very tender posterior fornix, due to the presence of the affected tube in the pouch of Douglas. The examination has to be very gentle due to the possibility of rupture of an unruptured ectopic pregnancy with severe intraperitoneal bleeding and collapse. In some cases the patients are referred by the family doctor due to the symptoms of pregnancy and a positive urine pregnancy test.

Since the availability of β-hCG subunit assay, the early diagnosis of ectopic pregnancy can be made in most cases, and with the help of ultrasound to exclude intrauterine pregnancy the diagnosis is often made even before the patient has symptoms. With other than tubal ectopic pregnancies, the diagnosis is sometimes made late due to lack of symptoms.

Non-tubal ectopics

The diagnosis of abdominal pregnancy can be very difficult. Abdominal tenderness in a pregnant woman with a mass separated from the uterus and cervical displacement can be present. Some patients have bowel or urinary symptoms related to the implantation of the ectopic placenta. Ultrasound scan and β-hCG can confirm the absence of an intrauterine pregnancy, but routine diagnostic ultrasound scans are usually done in patients who are between 12 and 14 weeks pregnant.

The symptoms of an ovarian ectopic pregnancy do not differ from those of a tubal pregnancy, which in general are abdominal pain, vaginal bleeding and menstrual irregularity.

Cervical pregnancy in general has the manifestations of a threatened or incomplete abortion. Uterine bleeding in a pregnant woman, with a partially open cervix which is enlarged and sometimes bigger than the uterus, is suggestive of a cervical pregnancy. The products of conception are attached to and confined to the cervix.

Implantation of pregnancies in a rudimentary horn, whether connected to the main uterine cavity or vagina or not, is very infrequent and does not have specific signs. In a pregnant woman with a known uterine abnormality, a pregnancy identified by ultrasound outside the main uterine cavity but still surrounded by myometrium, should suggest the presence of an anomalous implantation.

Patients with an intrauterine pregnancy and an ectopic pregnancy, i.e. a heterotopic pregnancy, have often had multiple embryos transferred during an in vitro fertilization–embryo transfer (IVF–ET) treatment cycle. They do not have special signs or symptoms except of abdominal pain and, if complicated, those of the ectopic pregnancy as well as those of a normal pregnancy. The in vitro fertilization practitioner must bear the possibility of heterotopic pregnancy in mind and arrange careful ultrasound scans on patients with pain until he or she is completely certain that a heterotopic pregnancy has not been missed.

INVESTIGATION AND DIAGNOSIS

Laparoscopy

The early diagnosis of ectopic pregnancy depends very much on the environment in which the practitioner is working and the facilities available. Years ago a patient with the symptoms of early pregnancy complaining of irregular bleeding, abdominal pain or adnexal mass with excitation pain would have proceeded directly to emergency laparotomy. Laparoscopy as a method of diagnosis of ectopic pregnancy has been used since 1937, when Hope reported the first 10 cases. The development of laparoscopy and its wide use have facilitated the diagnosis and treatment of ectopic pregnancy, thereby decreasing its mortality. When laparoscopy became a routine procedure, up to 40% of laparotomies were avoided and definitive diagnosis was possible early, with less morbidity and mortality. The development of a very sensitive radioimmunoassay capable of detecting β-hCG subunits at an early stage of pregnancy, together with the use of ultrasound, has again changed the diagnosis and management of suspected ectopic pregnancy.

Measurement of β-hCG

Detection of β-hCG in serum confirms the presence of trophoblastic tissue in 99–100% of cases. In normal pregnancy, gonadotrophins have a pattern of regular increase in the first weeks of pregnancy. Variation or abnormalities in the rate of increase can indicate the presence of an abnormal implantation.

When fertilization and implantation occur, hCG can be detected in serum as early as 7–10 days after ovulation or embryo transfer and it increases exponentially, following the development of trophoblastic tissue, but with daily spasmodic variations. The increase in hCG level in a normal pregnancy has a doubling time of 48 h and can be predicted using a formula or normogram. The normal range of the doubling time is from 1.2 to 3.5 days, depending on the age of the pregnancy. In a normal pregnancy the doubling time is 1.2–1.4 days during the first week after conception, before menstruation, and it is 3.3–3.5 days 6–8 weeks after conception.

Abnormal hCG rises can be compatible with both normal and abnormal pregnancies. However, when doubling time is less than 85% or the level starts reaching a plateau or decreasing, it is most likely that there is an abnormal pregnancy of undetermined site of implantation which needs to be confirmed by ultrasound or laparoscopy.

Ultrasound

Ultrasound has been widely used in the diagnosis of ectopic pregnancy since the time of Donald (1965), but to rely on ultrasound scans to diagnose the presence of an ectopic pregnancy can be dangerous, because a tubal pregnancy can be missed. The role of ultrasound scanning is to exclude an intrauterine pregnancy (Figs 22.2 and 22.3). The presence of an intrauterine gestational sac in general excludes an ectopic pregnancy, but it is possible in the presence of a heterotopic pregnancy.

The use of β-hCG and ultrasound in combination is the safe way of making a really early diagnosis, although serum β-hCG is detected very early in pregnancy whereas

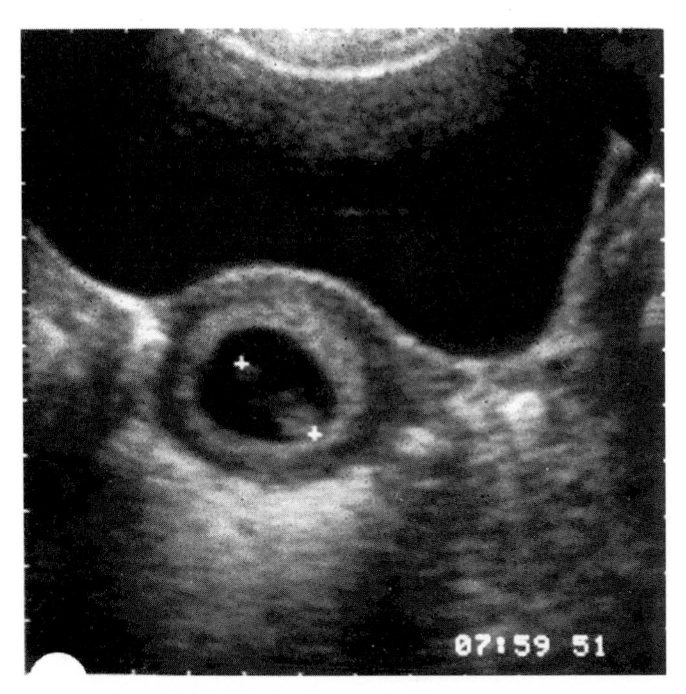

Fig. 22.2 Abdominal scan of pelvis. Transverse section of uterus showing a normal intrauterine pregnancy (fetal pole 1.77 cm).

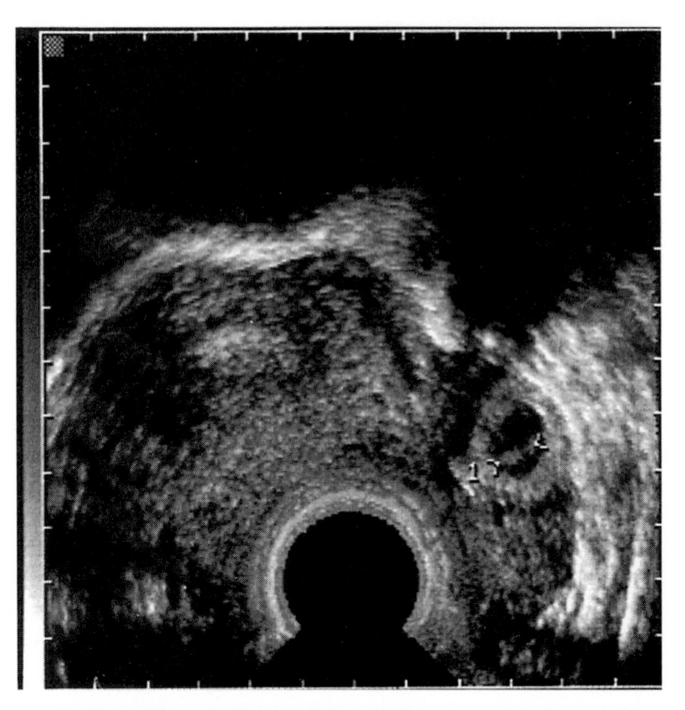

Fig. 22.3 Vaginal scan of pelvis. Transverse view of the pelvis. Arrow shows an empty uterine cavity. Dots show an ectopic pregnancy of the left tube lying on the ovary.

an intrauterine gestational sac cannot be visualized by ultrasound until 28 days after conception.

Confirmation of the presence of an ectopic pregnancy in the tube can eventually be made by ultrasound but this may be too late. An intrauterine sac can be detected in normally ovulating women at $5\frac{1}{2}$ weeks after the last menstrual period, when the β-hCG titre is above 6500 IU/l. Kadar et al (1981) demonstrated that the presence of an intrauterine sac and β-hCG below 6500 IU/l carry a poor prognosis and it is very probable that it is an ectopic pregnancy or a pregnancy that will miscarry. The visualization by ultrasound of an image like a gestational sac has been observed in suspected ectopic pregnancies, but it may be the endometrial cavity with a decidualized endometrium.

The presence of a 'double ring' image has been proposed to differentiate between a healthy intrauterine sac and a pseudouterine sac with an ectopic pregnancy. These images are produced by the presence of decidua capsularis and parietalis, with a double ring in a normal pregnancy and only a single ring in a sac of an abnormal one.

Ultrasound diagnosis of abdominal pregnancy can sometimes be made at an early stage with an empty cavity, fetal parts outside of the uterine cavity, and the identification of an ectopic placenta. In some patients it can be very difficult to identify the uterus or the placenta due to their displacement in the abdominal cavity.

Arias–Stella phenomenon

The Arias–Stella phenomenon consists of marked secretory and proliferative activity, often on the same endometrial gland lumen, forming syncytial masses with very tall and vacuolated cells which have hypertrophic and hyperchromatic nuclei with different shapes and bizarre forms. The phenomenon has been said to be important in the diagnosis of ectopic pregnancy, but its incidence in ectopic pregnancies varies from 3 to 100%. The exact nature of the Arias–Stella phenomenon is still obscure; it may be due to the response of the stimulation produced by oestrogens and chorionic gonadotrophins. This process is not typical of ectopic pregnancy but can be associated with normal pregnancy, abortion, chorioepithelioma, endometriosis and patients treated with oestrogens and progestogens for a long time.

Abdominal X-rays

In advanced abdominal pregnancies X-ray of the abdominal and pelvic cavities can be very useful. A lateral view can show fetal parts lying on the maternal spine and this is a sign of abdominal pregnancy. Hysterosalpingography can be of use as a diagnostic tool but carries the risk of irradiation of a viable pregnancy.

The widespread availability and use of ultrasound has displaced the use of X-rays in the diagnosis of abdominal pregnancy.

TREATMENT

There are many ways to treat an ectopic pregnancy. The

treatment may be completely expectant, medical or surgical. Surgically either an open or a laparoscopic procedure may be used. The decision as to which modality is the most appropriate will depend on many factors; the clinical situation of the patient, the site of the ectopic pregnancy, the past history of the patient, the desire for further pregnancies, future options for treatment, (such as in vitro fertilization), the skills of the surgeon as well as the equipment available. In principle the procedure should be as conservative as possible taking into account the overall safety of the patient.

Expectant management

A proportion of ectopic pregnancies will not progress from an early implantation stage to tubal rupture, but will die in the tube and be slowly reabsorbed. The difficulty is in trying to decide which ectopic pregnancies will progress and which can safely be treated by expectant management. The patients where expectant management may be a possibility are those diagnosed as having an ectopic pregnancy when they are completely asymptomatic. These are normally patients who are undergoing fertility treatment where they are closely monitored and where a high index of suspicion already exists. Expectant management should only be performed in centres where there is easy access to quantitative β-hCG assays whose results are quickly available, and 24-hour access to an operating theatre. The patient should be kept in hospital until the β-hCG levels have been seen to consistently fall. Exclusions to this form of management include any symptoms of pain, haemodynamic instability, β-hCG levels greater than 2000 IU/l, previously failed conservative treatment and patient desire for active management.

Medical

Several chemotherapeutic agents have been tried as a systemic treatment for ectopic pregnancies but the most promising has always been methotrexate. This has been tried as a single-dose alternative to surgical intervention, in a dose of 50 mg/m^2 given intramuscularly. Unfortunately not only have the results been generally disappointing but the majority of patients have suffered side-effects from the methotrexate given in this way.

Open surgical techniques

Salpingectomy

Salpingectomy, as first described by Tait (1884), is still the method mostly used as a treatment for ectopic pregnancy, with or without an ipsilateral oophorectomy. For a large number of authors salpingectomy is still an orthodox management of ectopic pregnancy in patients with a normal contralateral tube. Salpingectomy is particularly indicated in patients with a second ectopic pregnancy in a tube already treated conservatively, patients who have been sterilized and do not desire further pregnancy, ruptured ectopic pregnancy with severe destruction of tubal tissue or severe haemorrhage, and patients with a frozen pelvis, in whom the severity of the tubal damage is pre-existing and does not justify conservative treatment. For many clinicians salpingectomy would still be the orthodox management of ectopic pregnancy in patients with a normal contralateral tube, although this should be questioned.

The removal of the ipsilateral ovary is very rarely indicated these days. The only indication is when the ectopic pregnancy has involved the ovarian tissue to a great extent and the remaining ovarian tissue is badly damaged by a previous disease such as endometriosis, severe pelvic inflammatory disease or previous ovarian surgery.

Open conservative procedures

Conservative procedures for ectopic pregnancies were probably attempted at the end of the last century, but it was Stromme (1953) who published the first case of salpingotomy in an unruptured ectopic pregnancy. Partial salpingectomy with removal of the site of implantation is performed in cases of early isthmic ectopic implantation, followed by reanastomosis of the remaining segments, allowing the patient to conceive again spontaneously (Figs 22.4 and 22.5). The reanastomosis can be done immediately after the removal of the ectopic pregnancy during the same procedure or at a later stage in a separate or second procedure.

Based on the fact that the ectopic trophoblast invades the muscularis leaving the tubal lumen undamaged, conservative procedures such as salpingotomy without removing the segment of the tube have become widely used by many authors with good results.

At the time of the laparotomy, the tube is opened in the antemesenteric border on the site of the tubal implantation, using scalpel or electrosurgery, and once the embryonic sac has been exposed and removed using gentle pressure, haemostasis is completed using electrocoagulation. The salpingotomy can then be closed or not. If the salpingotomy is closed a fine non-absorbable suture material such as 6/0 prolene should be used. If the bleeding does not stop, some sutures can be placed in the mesosalpinx in the base of the tube in the area where the ectopic pregnancy implanted, and good haemostasis will be accomplished. In cases where the ectopic pregnancy is situated in the ampulla very close to the fimbrial end or on the fimbria, 'milking' of the ectopic pregnancy can be the method of choice. Once the pregnancy has been milked out, gentle pressure on the site of implantation is sometimes necessary to complete haemostasis.

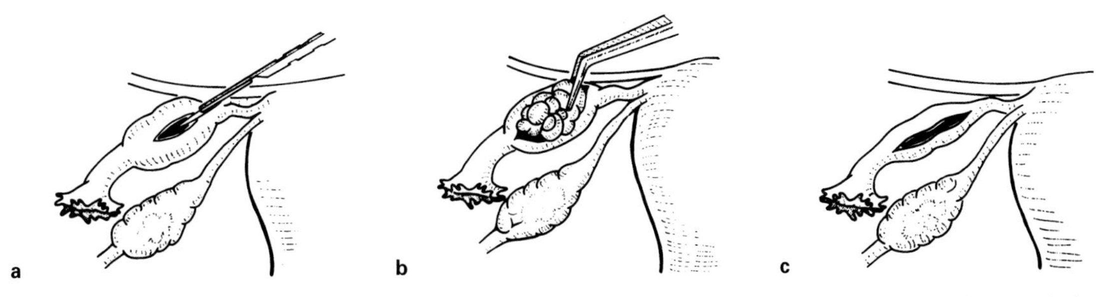

Fig. 22.4 Conservative surgical management of an ampullary ectopic pregnancy: **a** linear salpingotomy; **b** removal of the gestational sac; **c** salpingotomy left open to heal without closure.

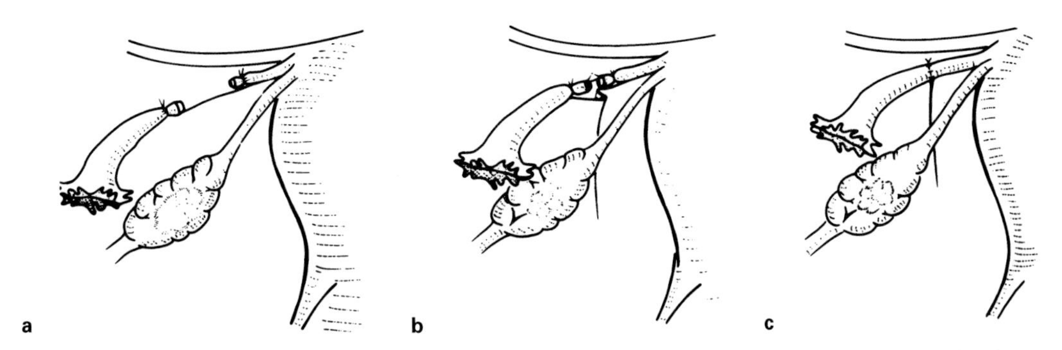

Fig. 22.5 Conservative surgical management of an isthmic ectopic pregnancy: **a** resection of the gestational sac; **b** blind ends left tied in order to perform a reanastomosis as a second procedure; **c** reanastomosis done during the same procedure.

Whatever the surgical procedure, radical or conservative, it must always be based on microsurgical principles: gentle handling of the tissues, avoidance of peritoneal damage, peritonealization of the raw areas, and the use of fine and non-resorbable suture material (prolene 5/0 or 6/0) which will prevent further damage and adhesion formation. If the tube is to be removed, it should be done so that the ovary is not displaced from its anatomical position, leaving it available for egg retrieval should the patient wish to be included in an in vitro fertilization programme. The use of drugs in order to diminish adhesion formation is debatable, but always remember that no drug or coadjuvant will compensate for a lack of surgical technique, and if the decision is made to use one, probably the best choice is steroids with local effect.

Open procedures have the benefit of being the most widely used and established treatment and can be performed in almost all hospitals. They do, however, tend to require a hospital stay of approximately 4 days and a more prolonged postoperative recovery period.

Laparoscopic techniques

The early diagnosis of ectopic pregnancy and the improvement of laparoscopic surgical methods and instruments, allowing the surgeon to perform laparoscopic surgery, have opened a new chapter in the treatment of ectopic pregnancy. Semm was the pioneer of laparoscopic surgery for ectopic pregnancy, and his first series of cases was published in 1980. The same principles of conservation should be applied with laparoscopic surgery as with open operations. For successful laparoscopic surgery, selection of patients is important and this depends to a large extent on the laparoscopic skills of the surgeon. For the average laparoscopist the patient should be haemodynamically stable; the ectopic pregnancy should be less than 6 cm in diameter; the hCG level less than 6000 IU/l; the pelvis should have only a minor amount of adhesions, and the pregnancy should be implanted in the tube. For the advanced laparoscopist, though, even adhesions, haemoperitoneum or tubal rupture are not absolute contraindications (Dubuisson et al 1987, Pouly et al 1986, Reich et al 1987). Apart from the surgeon's skill, the next most important prerequisite for safe laparoscopic surgery is good equipment. Essential equipment includes: a 10-mm 0° laparoscope, a light source of 250 watts or greater, TV camera and monitor, suction/irrigation probe, monopolar needlepoint diathermy and a selection of grasping forceps. Additional equipment including bipolar coagulation forceps, scissors and pre-tied ligature loops will facilitate most procedures. Some centres use lasers but this is not necessary for the majority of cases.

Most of the procedures that are performed at open operations can be performed laparoscopically. These include direct injection of cytotoxic agents, linear salpingostomy and salpingectomy.

Direct injection

Many different agents have been tried over the last 20 years; these include:

20% potassium chloride
vasopressin
actinomycin
mifepristone
hyperosmolar glucose
prostaglandins
methotrexate

Only the last two have shown any reasonable results, and even these have a significant failure rate. The patients have to be carefully monitored by serial quantitative β-hCG for several weeks afterwards to ensure that there is no persistent trophoblastic tissue. The advantage of this form of treatment is that it is easy to learn and that you do not need to have the full range of laparoscopic equipment available.

Methotrexate is the agent most commonly used and the dose used varies between 50 and 100 mg. There has been no evidence, though, that the higher dose has a better success rate. The dose of 50 mg is in 2 ml of solution. This is injected directly into the gestational sac, after aspirating from the sac if possible, and to ensure that a blood vessel has not been penetrated. Direct injection is of particular use in cases of interstitial or cornual ectopic pregnancies where other forms of surgery are more difficult and bloody.

Relative contraindications to injection include haemoperitoneum, a gestational sac >3 cm and β-hCG >2000 IU/l. Even following these guidelines, however, Kooi & Kock (1992) stated that the absence of a parameter that reveals the threat of tubal rupture is the major problem for these forms of treatment.

Salpingotomy

Pouly et al (1993) wrote that laparoscopic linear salpingotomy was the surgical management of choice for the unruptured tubal ectopic and nearly all gynaecologists would agree with this. Since the publication of the papers of Pouly et al (1986) and DeCherney & Diamond (1987), this form of conservative treatment has become more widespread and the techniques involved are now taught to gynaecologists worldwide.

The linear salpingotomy can be performed with laser, scissors or microscalpel, but the most commonly used technique is needlepoint monopolar cutting diathermy. This gives an excellent incision with a reasonable amount of haemostasis from the coagulation element of the diathermy, and is also easy to learn and does not require very expensive equipment such as a laser generator. The incision is performed as at open operation, that is along the antemesenteric border. The ectopic is then either removed with grasping forceps or aqua-dissected out with the use of the suction irrigation probe. The resultant incision is not closed after evacuation of the ectopic and this does not seem to cause any major postoperative problems. Any significant bleeding from the implantation site in the tube can easily be controlled using bipolar coagulation forceps. As with all laparoscopic procedures the pelvis is thoroughly irrigated after completion of the procedure.

The subsequent intrauterine pregnancy results from this technique are very good. Pouly et al (1986), in a series of 321 ectopic pregnancies treated in this way, reported a rate of 64% and a subsequent ectopic rate of 22%. DeCherney et al (1987) reported a 52% intrauterine pregnancy rate and a 10% ectopic rate after the same procedure.

Salpingectomy

Laparoscopic salpingectomy, in most circumstances, is a straightforward procedure. With the introduction of pretied loop ligatures the fallopian tube can be 'lassooed' by the ligature, then cut and removed. Bipolar diathermy can also be used safely to perform the salpingectomy, and is more commonly used if the tube is adherent to other structures and is not free enough for correct placement of loop ligatures. Recent methods using disposable stapling devices have also been tried but have not met with universal acceptance because of their prohibitive cost.

Salpingectomy is generally performed for the same indications as at open procedure, and can be performed laparoscopically even if there is tubal rupture *as long as the patient is haemodynamically stable.* An excellent suction/irrigation device is obligatory to keep the visual field clear of blood, and a fast flow insufflator is also required in these procedures to ensure that an adequate pneumoperitoneum is maintained with the rapid suction of peritoneal contents. One of the main problems with this technique is how to remove the tube and ectopic from the peritoneal cavity. Several methods are used: it can be morcellated and removed piecemeal by 10-mm grasping forceps; it can be removed intact through a posterior colpotomy, or it can be placed in a specially designed plastic bag introduced through a 10-mm port, the bag being sealed at its neck and then removed intact through the port. The advantage of the latter technique is that a posterior colpotomy is not necessary, the specimen is intact and there is a much reduced chance of trophoblastic tissue being left in the cavity or in the skin incision.

Ovarian ectopic surgery

Ovarian ectopic pregnancy is a rare event, and in general treatment depends on how early the diagnosis is made and how much the ovary and the tube, bowel or other pelvic organs are involved. The experience of the surgeon and the circumstances determine the type of operation necessary, but in general oophorectomy or salpingo-oophorectomy are the most common options. Historically this has always been performed at laparotomy, but it can also be performed laparoscopically using techniques similar to those employed in laparoscopic salpingectomy.

Abdominal pregnancy

Abdominal pregnancy is a completely different problem, and fortunately a very rare one. The mortality is not negligible. The fetus can be removed or delivered without major problem. The main difficulty is presented by the ectopic placenta, sometimes inserted in the bowel or overlarge vessels. In these cases the removal of the placenta should not be attempted because it can cause major bleeding, and sometimes even ligation of the internal iliac artery may not save the patient's life. In general placental function disappears over several weeks. Resorption of the placenta can be a very slow process and in some cases can last years. Methotrexate has been used to manage residual placenta, but can accelerate necrosis of the tissue, causing severe infections and adding another morbidity factor.

RESULTS

Analysis of long-term results of treatment of ectopic pregnancy is rather difficult due to the diversity of surgeons and procedures involved. It is even more difficult to compare or draw conclusions when treatment has been conservative. Due to the frequency of ampullary ectopic pregnancy; the major published series are related to this site of ectopic implantation.

There does not seem to be a great difference in long-term results, whether radical or conservative methods are used, in the treatment of ectopic pregnancy in patients in whom both fallopian tubes are present. Oelsner et al (1987) collected a series of 1630 patients from the literature, and found that 40.9% had intrauterine and 14.2% repeated ectopic pregnancy when radical surgery (salpingectomy) was the treatment of choice; with a conservative approach 45.5% had an intrauterine and 11.5% repeated extra uterine pregnancy. When analysing their results of salpingostomy DeCherney et al (1982) reported that among 15 patients with only one functional tube, 53% subsequently had an intrauterine pregnancy and 20% a recurrent extrauterine pregnancy.

The results of treatment of isthmic ectopic pregnancy are very scarce because of the low frequency of implantation of pregnancy in this site. Stangel & Gomel (1980) reported on seven patients: only two desired further pregnancies and both achieved intrauterine pregnancy. Gomel (1983) in another series of nine patients with delayed reanastomosis found that six subsequently conceived with only one repeat ectopic pregnancy. DeCherney & Boyers (1985) found that among six patients with segmental resection and delayed reanastomosis, four conceived and only one had a recurrent ectopic pregnancy.

Since the wider application of laparoscopic treatment of ectopic pregnancies, larger series have been published, but most have been concentrated on the success of the technique, overall cost and duration of hospital stay rather than the reproductive outcome for the patient. Vermesh et al (1989) comparing patency and pregnancy rates in a prospective, randomized trial showed patency rates of 80 and 89% and pregnancy rates of 56 and 58% for laparoscopy and laparotomy respectively.

LAPAROSCOPIC OR OPEN PROCEDURE?

As with all surgical techniques there are advantages and disadvantages to each one. When laparoscopic treatment was first used in the late 1970s (mainly on the Continent) there were more intra- and postoperative problems. With the advent of better equipment, training and more refined techniques, these problems have become far less common, and as Bruhat et al (1991) commented, laparoscopic treatment is now the treatment of choice.

The benefits of laparoscopic treatment are many. Murphy et al (1992), Vermesh et al (1989) and many others have all shown a significant reduction in hospital stay, postoperative analgesia requirements and a shorter recovery period. All of these benefits have major financial implications, not only for the hospital but also for the patient. The patient also prefers the cosmetic result of laparoscopic techniques. DeCherney & Diamond (1987) also confirmed that blood loss at laparoscopic treatment is significantly less than at laparotomy, and in the present climate of possibly contaminated blood products, any reduction in the amount of blood transfusions required is not only economically sensible but also safer for the patient.

The disadvantages of laparoscopic treatment are few. It requires more capital expenditure on equipment, but this can then also be used in general gynaecological procedures to make them safer and easier. It also allows other procedures to be performed laparoscopically, with the resultant cost–benefit savings from these. It requires more training for the surgeon, but with the increasing use of minimal access surgery (MAS) this also should be part of general gynaecological training for junior staff. Initially, as surgeons hone their skills, the operation, as will all surgical procedures, will take longer, but after 10 or so cases the operative time will come down to, or even be less than the time taken to perform a laparoscopy followed by a laparotomy to treat the ectopic.

The final decision as to which procedure to use will ultimately be decided by the patient's condition and the skills and preference of the surgeon.

COMPLICATIONS

The major complication of ectopic pregnancy is death and ectopic pregnancy is still an important cause of maternal mortality in the first trimester of pregnancy.

One of the complications of treatment of ectopic pregnancy is iatrogenic disease. It is quite common and very disappointing to laparoscope patients complaining of infertility and to find the pelvis covered by adhesions following ectopic pregnancy, although the remaining fallopian tube is reasonably healthy. The fact that ectopic pregnancy operations are in general emergency procedures is not a justification for not taking maximum precautions and so avoiding this common problem. Gentle handling of the tissues and the use of wet swabs and fine sutures, aspiration of the free blood in the abdominal cavity, and washing the peritoneal cavity using Ringer's lactate are all that is required. Hopefully the increasing treatment of ectopics laparoscopically will decrease the severity of postsurgical adhesions. Lundorff et al (1991), in a randomized prospective study, found that laparoscopic treatment of ectopic pregnancy resulted in less postoperative adhesion formation than ectopics treated by laparotomy.

Since the early diagnosis of pregnancy became possible, with the use of β-hCG and ultrasound, doctors can perform a laparoscopy on a patient too early and miss seeing an ectopic gestation, especially in a patient with distorted anatomy due to pelvic adhesions, although as Doo et al (1987) reported, laparoscopy still has the highest positive predictive value for the diagnosis of ectopic pregnancy. Ewen et al (1994) reiterated the necessity of close follow-up with β-hCG measurements and ultrasound in order to avoid fatal consequences.

Persistent ectopic trophoblast can remain in the implantation site after conservative surgery. Chapron et al (1991) reported an incidence of 5% in their series. In some cases this is asymptomatic, the only finding being a persistent β-hCG which slowly resolves. In other patients persistent trophoblast can cause intra-abdominal haemorrhage requiring an emergency laparotomy. Severe intra-abdominal bleeding can be a complication after conservative laparoscopy, but with the injection of vasopressin in the mesosalpinx of the affected tube, the occurrence of this has decreased greatly.

A new problem occurs in those patients who have successfully been through an IVF–ET programme when multiple embryo transfer has been performed. An intrauterine pregnancy may be confirmed by ultrasound, without follow-up in later weeks to exclude the possibility of a heterotopic pregnancy. The latter used to be a rare event, but is not so now, and the doctor should always be aware of it as a possibility.

There are some complications that are more prevalent with, or unique to, laparoscopic treatment. Collateral damage to other organs by the careless use of electrosurgery is well documented and can be prevented by fanatical care when electrosurgical techniques are used and awareness of the problems, such as capacitative coupling, that may occur with certain combinations of equipment.

Pouly et al (1986), in their series of 321 ectopic pregnancies, performed conservative surgery, using laparoscopic linear salpingostomy only. Of these 321, 5.9% needed a laparotomy after laparoscopic surgery due to bleeding, and 4.8% needed a secondary procedure because of retention of trophoblastic tissue. Dubuisson et al (1987) found laparotomy necessary in only 2% of 100 consecutive cases managed by laparoscopic salpingectomy.

De Waart et al (1994) and Ewen et al (1994) reported an increase in the reintervention rate compared with laparotomy, mainly for failed diagnosis. This tends to happen more frequently with very early gestation ectopics and they can be missed at laparotomy as well, but are missed more frequently at laparoscopy because of the inability to palpate the fallopian tube. De Waart et al (1994) also reported a 3% pelvic infection rate in their group. They had not prescribed prophylactic antibiotics, but in conclusion they did recommend them for future attempts.

KEY POINTS

1. Ectopic pregnancy occurs when there is implantation of the fertilized ovum outside the uterine cavity.
2. Abnormalities of the mechanisms involved in ovum transport may be a predisposing factor.
3. Tubal transport is influenced by hormone levels. Oestrogens stimulate tubal contractility but progesterone decreases the activity. Progesterone also decreases local prostaglandin secretion and causes relaxation of the isthmic portion of the tube, which may allow the fertilized ovum to progress into the uterus.
4. Cilia are important in transporting the ovum through the ampulla but not through the isthmus.
5. The most common site for tubal implantation is the ampulla.
6. Ovarian or abdominal ectopics may be primary or secondary depending on whether the pregnancy implants directly or as a result of tubal abortion.
7. A cervical ectopic is rare. To identify it, cervical glands must be attached to the placenta, and the placenta must be implanted below where the uterine vessels reach the uterus.
8. Heterotopic pregnancy is the combination of an intrauterine pregnancy and an ectopic (generally tubal) pregnancy. It occurred in 1:30 000 pregnancies, although this rate has risen with the use of IVF techniques.
9. The risk of an ectopic increases sevenfold following an attack of salpingitis, and is associated with the use of the IUCD.

10. Tubal reconstruction is associated with an increased incidence of ectopic pregnancy.
11. The likehood of conceiving after a sterilization procedure is between 1/600 and 1/1000.
12. Race and socioeconomic factors influence the risk of ectopic pregnancy. In the USA, ectopic pregnancy is twice as high in non-white than in white populations.
13. The decrease in mortality rate is due to earlier diagnosis and better and more prompt treatment.
14. When laparoscopies became a routine procedure, up to 40% of laparotomies were avoided and an early diagnosis was possible with less morbidity and mortality.
15. Serum β-hCG is detectable 7–10 days after ovulation. The role of ultrasound scanning is to exclude an intrauterine sac after $5\frac{1}{2}$ weeks.
16. For laparoscopic treatment, patient selection, surgical skill and the facilities available are extremely important.
17. Laparoscopic treatment, either by salpingotomy or salpingectomy, is the treatment of choice as long as the patient is haemodynamically stable.

REFERENCES

Abulcasis (Abul Qasimi) 936–1013, De chirurgia, arabice et latine cura Johannis Channing, vol 3, Oxonii, e typ, Clarendoniano, 1778. M S H Spink, G L Lewis, London, 1973 Wellcome Institute for the History of Medicine

Brosens I A, Vasquez G 1976 Fimbrial microbiopsy. Journal of Reproductive Medicine 16: 171–178

Bruhat M A, Mage G, Pouly J L, Manhes H, Canis M, Wattiez A, 1991 Operative Laparoscopy. McGraw Hill, New York

Brunham R C, Binns B, McDowell J, Paraskevas M 1986 Chlamydia trachomatis infection in women with ectopic pregnancy. Obstetrics and Gynecology 67: 722–726

Chapron C, Querleu D, Crepin G 1991 Laparoscopic treatment of ectopic pregnancies: a 100 case study. European Journal of Obstetrics and Gynaecology and Reproductive Biology 41: 187–190

Chiari H 1887 Zur pathologischen Anatomie des Eileiter-Catrrhs. Zeitschrift für Heilkunde 8: 457–473

Clark K, Baranyai J 1987 Pelvic infection and the pathogenesis of tubal ectopic pregnancy. Australian and New Zealand Journal of Obstetrics and Gynaecology 27: 57–60

DeCherney A H, Boyers S P 1985 Isthmic ectopic pregnancy: segmental resection as the treatment of choice. Fertility and Sterility 44: 307–312

DeCherney A H, Diamond M P 1987 Laparoscopic salpingostomy for ectopic pregnancy. Obstetrics and Gynecology 70: 948–950

DeCherney A H, Cholst I, Naftolin F 1981 Structure and function of the fallopian tubes following exposure to diethylstibestrol (DES) during gestation. Fertility and Sterility 36: 741–745

DeCherney A H, Maheux R, Naftolin F 1982 Salpingostomy for ectopic pregnancy in the sole patient oviduct: reproductive outcome. Fertility and Sterility 37: 619–622

De Waart M J, de Blok S, Hemrika D J 1994 Complications of laparoscopic treatment of tubal ectopic pregnancies. Gynaecological Endoscopy 3: 173–175

Donald I 1965 Diagnostic uses of sonar in obstetrics and gynaecology. Journal of Obstetrics and Gynaecology of the British Commonwealth 72: 907–919

Doo S K, Sung R C, Moon I L P, Young P K 1987 Comparative review of diagnostic accuracy in tubal pregnancy: a 14 year survey of 1040 cases. Obstetrics and Gynecology 70: 547–554

Douglas C P 1963 Tubal ectopic pregnancy. British Medical Journal 2: 838–841

Dubuisson J B, Aubriot F X, Cardone V 1987 Laparoscopic salpingectomy for tubal pregnancy. Fertility and Sterility 47: 225

Duckman S, Suarez J, Spitaleri J 1984 Vaginal pregnancy presenting as a suburethral cyst. American Journal of Obstetrics and Gynecology 149: 572–573

Eddy C A, Antonini R Jr, Pauertein C L 1977 Fertility following microsurgical removal of the ampullary–isthmic junction in rabbits. Fertility and Sterility 28: 1090–1093

Erkkola R, Liukko P 1977 Intrauterine devices and ectopic pregnancy. Contraception 16: 569–580

Ewen S, Nair S, Henderson A, Sutton C 1994 Problems in the management of ectopic pregnancy: laparoscopy versus laparotomy in diagnosis and treatment. Gynaecological Endoscopy 3: 105–107

Gemzell L, Guillome J, Wang F C 1982 Ectopic pregnancy following treatment with human gonadotrophins. Americal Journal of Obstetrics and Gynecology 143: 761–765

Gomel V 1983 Conservative surgical treatment of tubal pregnancy. In: Gomel V (ed) Microsurgery in female infertility. Little, Brown, Boston, p 53

Hope R B 1937 The differential diagnosis of ectopic gestation by peritoneoscopy. Surgery, Gynecology and Obstetrics 64: 229–233

Kadar N, DeVore G, Romero R 1981 Discriminatory HCG zone: its use in the sonographic evaluation for ectopic pregnancy. Obstetrics and Gynecology 58: 156–161

Kobak A J, Fields C, Pollack S L 1955 Intraligamentary pregnancy: the extraperitoneal type of abdominal pregnancy. American Journal of Obstetrics and Gynecology 70: 175–184

Kooi S, Kock H C 1992 A review of the literature on non-surgical treatment in tubal pregnancies. Obstetrics and Gynaecology Surveys 47: 739–749

Lehfelft H, Tietze C, Gorstein F 1970 Ovarian pregnancy and the intrauterine device. Americal Journal of Obstetrics and Gynecology 108: 1005–1009

Lundorff P, Hahlin M, Kallfelt B, Thornburn J, Lindblom B 1991 Adhesion formation after laparoscopic surgery in tubal pregnancy: a randomised trial versus laparotomy. Fertility and Sterility 55: 91–115

Majmudar B, Henderson P H III, Semple E 1983 Salpingitis isthmica nodosa: a high risk factor for tubal pregnancy. Obstetrics and Gynecology 62: 73–78

Murphy A A, Nager C W, Wujek J J et all 1992 Operative laparoscopy versus laparotomy for the management of ectopic pregnancy: a prospective trial. Fertility and Sterility 576: 1180–1185

Oelsner G, Morad J, Carp H, Mashiach S, Serr D M 1987 Reproductive performance following conservative microsurgical management of tubal pregnancy. British Journal of Obstetrics and Gynaecology 94: 1078–1083

Ory H W and The Women's Health Study 1981 Ectopic pregnancy and intrauterine contraception devices: new perspectives. Obstetrics and Gynaecology 57: 137–144

Parry J S, Lea H C 1876 Extrauterine pregnancy. Americal Journal of Obstetrics and Gynaecology 9: 169–170

Persaud V 1970 Etiology of tubal ectopic pregnancy. Obstetrics and Gynecology 36: 257–263

Pouly J L, Manhes H, Mage G, Canis M, Bruhat M A 1986 Conservative laparoscopic treatment of 321 ectopic pregnancies. Fertility and Sterility 46: 1093–1097

Pouly J L, Chapron C, Wattiez A 1993 Endoscopic surgery for gynaecologists. W B Saunders, London

Reich H, Freifeld M L, McGlynn F et al 1987 Laparoscopic treatment of tubal pregnancy. Fertility and Sterility 47: 275

Semm K, Mettlesr L 1980 Technical progress in pelvic surgery via operative laparoscopy. American Journal of Obstetrics and Gynecology 138: 121–127

Stangel J J, Gomel V 1980 Techniques in conservative surgery for tubal gestation. Clinical Obstetrics and Gynaecology 23: 1221–1228

Stromme W B 1953 Salpingotomy for tubal pregnancy. Obstetrics and Gynecology 1: 472–476
Swolin K 1975 Electromicrosurgery and salpingostomy long term results. American Journal of Obstetrics and Gynecology 121: 418–419
Tait T 1884 Five cases of extrauterine pregnancy operated upon at the time of rupture. British Medical Journal 1: 1250–1251
Vermesh M, Silva P D, Rosen G F et al 1989 Management of unruptured ectopic gestation by linear salpingostomy: a prospective randomised trial of laparoscopy and laparotomy. Obstetrics and Gynecology 73: 400
Westrom L, Bengtsson L P H, Mardh P A 1981 Incidence, trends and risks of ectopic pregnancy in a population of women. British Medical Journal 282: 15–18
Winston R L M 1981 Is microsurgery necessary for salpingostomy? The evaluation of results. Australian and New Zealand Journal of Obstetrics and Gynaecology 21: 143–152

23

Hirsutism and virilization

Carole Gilling-Smith   Stephen Franks

INTRODUCTION

Hirsutism is defined as the excessive growth of terminal hair in a typical male pattern distribution. Virilization refers to more severe effects of hyperandrogenism in a female including male hair pattern and body habitus, clitoromegaly, increased libido, deepening of the voice and increased muscle mass. Since androgens are the principal endocrine regulators of terminal hair growth, hirsutism may be caused by increased androgen production by the ovaries and/or adrenal glands, increased target tissue sensitivity to androgens or an increase in the level of biologically active free circulating androgens. Virilization usually results from a rapidly growing, androgen-producing tumour or use of certain androgenic drugs.

The key to successful diagnosis and treatment of any problem depends on understanding the pathogenesis of the condition. This chapter first reviews the biology of hair growth and androgen metabolism in the female before presenting a systematic approach to diagnosis and therapeutic management.

BIOLOGY OF HAIR GROWTH

Hair follicles start to develop from the epidermis between 8 and 10 weeks of intrauterine life and the total complement of hair follicles is reached by 22 weeks. Hair cells are formed from the dermal papilla at the base of the hair follicle. The column of dead, keratinized cells so formed, elongates to form a hair shaft consisting of a central medulla of loosely connected cells surrounded by a cortex of compressed cells and a hard external cuticle. Sebaceous glands are connected to the hair follicle. Hair colour is provided by the pigment, melanin, produced in the medulla. If the dermal papilla is damaged or degenerates, there will be no further hair growth from that follicle.

The hair cycle

Hair grows in cyclical fashion with alternate growing and resting phases, as shown in Figure 23.1. In telogen, the resting phase, the hair is short and the follicle inactive. Anagen, the active growing phase, involves rapid division of the basal matrix cells and upward extension of the hair shaft. During catagen, the bulb shrivels and the hair is shed. Final hair length on different parts of the body is determined by the relative duration of each phase. Scalp hair has a relatively long anagen of 3 years and only a short telogen. Conversely, on other parts of the body, the hair has a long telogen and short anagen phase resulting in much shorter hair.

Normally, hair growth is asynchronous. Pregnancy and

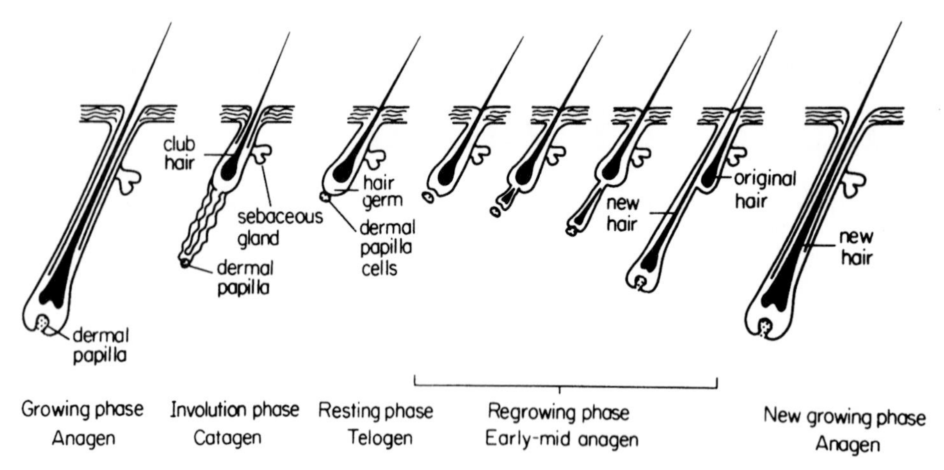

Fig. 23.1 Stages in the hair cycle. (Reproduced with permission of Blackwell Science Ltd and the author from Randall 1994.)

certain drugs can increase the synchrony of hair growth, resulting in periodic growth and shedding.

Types of hair

1. Lanugo hair is lightly pigmented, short, fine hair which covers the fetal body until about 7 months of intrauterine life.
2. Vellus hair is fine downy hair which covers most of the body during the prepubertal period.
3. Terminal hair is coarse, pigmented hair which grows on certain parts of the body, primarily during adult years.
4. Sexual hair is terminal hair which responds specifically to sex steroids and characteristically grows on the face, chest, axillae, pubic area, lower abdomen and anterior thighs.

Hirsutism is characterized by the conversion of vellus to sexual hair, primarily under the influence of androgens, in a male pattern distribution. This is in contrast to hypertrichosis in which there is excessive growth of fine lanugo hair in a nonandrogenic pattern, a condition often resulting from the use of certain drugs, starvation (anorexia) or malignancy.

Genetic and ethnic influences on hair growth

The number of hair follicles per unit area of skin is genetically predetermined. Significant differences exist between races, e.g. caucasian women have significantly more hair follicles than their oriental counterparts. More importantly, with respect to management, body hair which may be socially acceptable to a mediterranean woman may be a source of great distress to a woman of nordic descent.

Hormonal influences on hair growth

1. Androgens are the principal hormonal regulators of hair growth. They initiate growth and increase the diameter and pigmentation of the hair column of facial, axillary and pubic hair. Conversely, on the scalp, they cause regression of terminal hair to vellus hair to produce androgenic alopecia or male pattern balding in genetically susceptible individuals (Randall 1994).

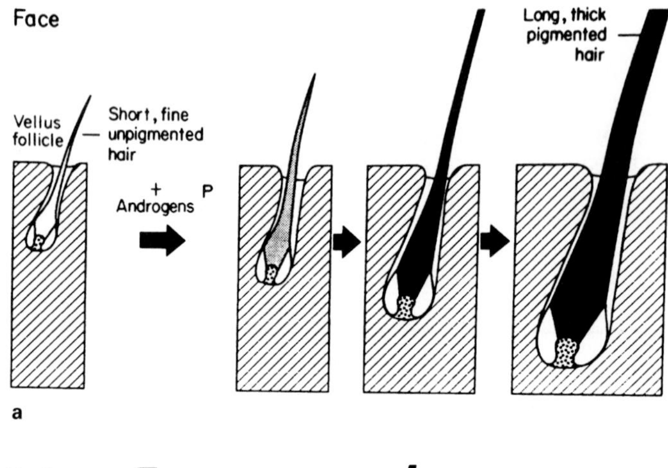

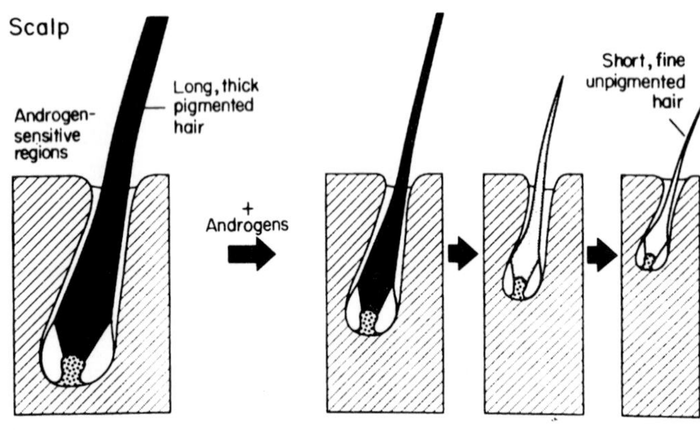

Fig. 23.2 Effect of androgens on hair follicles. **a** In areas stimulated by androgens, e.g. face. **b** On scalp of genetically predisposed individuals. (Reproduced with permission of Blackwell Science Ltd and the author from Randall 1994.)

These two opposing actions of androgens are illustrated in Figure 23.2.

2. Oestrogens reduce the rate of hair growth resulting in finer, less pigmented hair.
3. Progestogens have a variable effect on hair growth depending on their androgenic potency.

During pregnancy the combined effect of high oestrogen and progesterone can increase the synchrony of hair growth such that some women experience increased hair growth whilst others notice loss of hair.

Generalized endocrine disturbances can affect hair growth through an indirect effect on either adrenal or ovarian hormone secretion. In hypopituitarism, hair growth may slow down; conversely hirsutism develops in 15% of acromegalics and is also associated with Cushing's disease and hyperprolactinaemia.

Nonhormonal influences on hair growth

Hair growth is affected by skin temperature and blood flow and therefore is faster during the summer months. Central nervous system lesions such as cranial trauma or encephalitis may enhance hair growth. Certain nonhormonal drugs e.g. phenytoin may produce hirsutism.

ANDROGEN BIOSYNTHESIS AND METABOLISM IN THE FEMALE

The principal circulating androgens are testosterone and its metabolite dihydrotestosterone (DHT), androstenedione, dehydroepiandrosterone (DHA) and dehydroepiandrosterone sulphate (DHAS). All are C19 steroids derived from the conversion of cholesterol in either the ovaries or adrenals. DHT is the most biologically potent, followed by testosterone. Androstenedione, DHA and DHAS are comparatively weak androgens, with minimal effect on skin and hair growth under normal circumstances.

In the normal female, 25% of the circulating testosterone is produced by the ovary and 25% by the adrenal cortex. The remainder is derived from peripheral conversion of androstenedione. Of the circulating androstenedione, 50% is produced by the ovary and 50% by the adrenal. In contrast the adrenal secretes 90% of the DHA and virtually all the DHAS (Fig. 23.3). DHT is derived exclusively from the peripheral conversion of circulating testosterone and androstenedione in target tissues, principally in the liver and skin, in a reaction catalysed by the enzyme 5α-reductase.

Factors affecting the concentration of circulating androgens

Both testosterone and DHT circulate partly in a free state and partly bound to either albumin or to a β globulin called sex hormone-binding globulin (SHBG) (Anderson 1974). DHA, DHAS and androstenedione are not significantly protein-bound. In the case of testosterone, 80% is bound to SHBG, 19% is weakly bound to albumin and 1% is unbound. Since the biological effect of circulating androgens depends primarily on the unbound fraction, care needs to be taken when interpreting the results of serum testosterone concentration tests as these will measure both protein-bound and free hormone. It is not unusual therefore to find a normal total testosterone concentration in a hirsute woman. Nevertheless, it is not helpful, clinically, to measure non-SHBG testosterone or free testosterone, both of which may also be normal in hirsute subjects.

Liver SHBG production is decreased by both androgens and insulin. In hyperandrogenic, hirsute women, SHBG levels are depressed and the percentage of free testosterone is increased to about 2% (in men the level of free testosterone is about 3%). Hyperinsulinaemia enhances this effect and can exacerbate the degree of hirsutism. Conversely, oestrogens increase SHBG production so that binding is increased in women on oral contraceptives and during pregnancy, often resulting in a reduction of hirsutism.

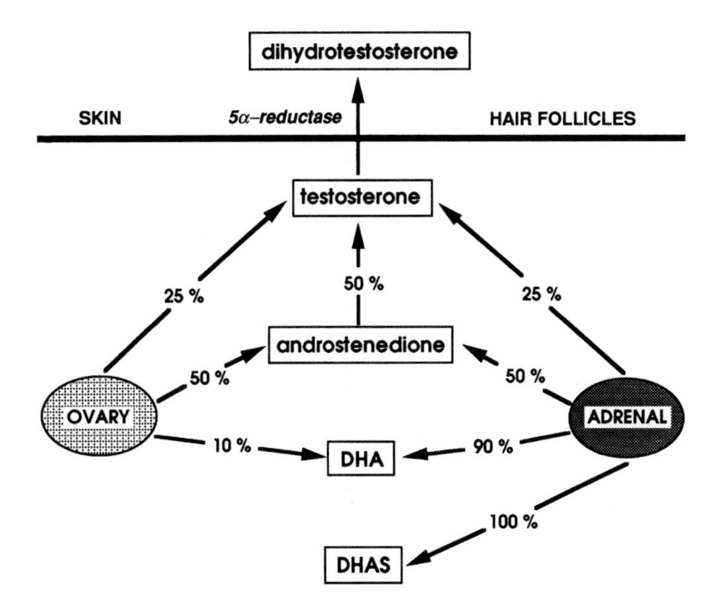

Fig. 23.3 Ovarian and adrenal contributions to circulating androgens. (DHA, dehydroepiandrosterone; DHAS, dehydroepiandrosterone sulphate.)

Androgen action in target tissues

Androgen action in target tissues depends on the interaction of the steroid with specific intracellular cytoplasmic receptors. The androgen–receptor complex is then transported into the nucleus where it interacts with specific receptor sites on the DNA, thereby influencing protein synthesis. The binding affinity of DHT to the androgen receptor is about 10 times that of testosterone. Hence the conversion of testosterone to DHT by the enzyme 5α-reductase is a key step in androgen action.

There is poor correlation between the presence or severity of hirsutism and serum levels of either testosterone or DHT (Franks 1989). This has prompted considerable interest in the measurement of DHT metabolites such as 3α-androstenediol-glucuronide (Adiol-G) and other androgen conjugates. These reflect 5α-reductase activity and in theory should be more sensitive biochemical markers for cutaneous androgen action (Greep et al 1986, Horton et al 1982). Although early studies showed an excellent correlation between serum levels of Adiol-G and hirsutism (Horton at al 1982, Serafini et al 1985), more recent studies have shown marked overlap in levels between normal and hirsute women (Matteri et al 1989, Thompson et al 1990). Furthermore studies performed during medical therapy are controversial, some showing no change in Adiol-G levels in response to treatment (Lobo et al 1985, Marcondes et al 1992) and others showing good correlation with clinical response (Kirschner et al 1987). These discrepancies are thought, in part, to be related to the fact that circulating Adiol-G is not derived exclusively from peripheral DHT metabolism but also reflects both hepatic and adrenal metabolism.

Thus, in practice, androgen conjugates are of little additional benefit over serum testosterone or DHT levels in the clinical evaluation or management of hyperandrogenism (Rittmaster 1993).

Ovarian androgen production

The specialized steroid-secreting cells of the ovary are the theca and granulosa cells. Theca cells convert cholesterol to androstenedione under the stimulation of pituitary luteinizing hormone (LH). Androstenedione crosses the basement membrane to the avascular granulosa layer where follicle-stimulating hormone (FSH) and, in the preovulatory follicle both FSH and LH, stimulate aromatization of androgens to oestrogens. This is referred to as the two-cell two-gonadotrophin theory of steroidogenesis (Fig. 23.4). Theca cell androgen production varies during the ovarian cycle in parallel with development of the dominant follicle and corpus luteum, but cyclical changes of androstenedione and testosterone in the peripheral circulation are not very great, showing a small midcycle increment only.

Adrenal androgen production

Adrenal androgens are secreted by the zona fasciculata and zona reticularis under ACTH stimulation. During prepubertal life, adrenal androgen secretion remains low until adrenarche, during which there is a selective increase in secretion of androgenic steroids leading to pubic and axillary hair development. This heralds the onset of puberty which is associated with the growth spurt, breast devel-

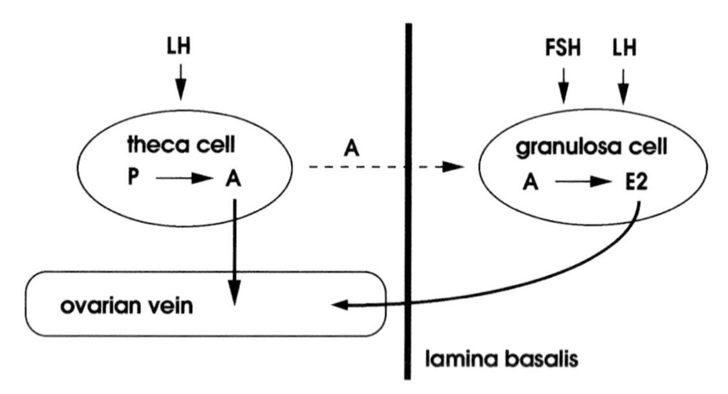

Fig. 23.4 Two-cell two-gonadotrophin theory of steroidogenesis. (P, progesterone; A, androstenedione; E2, oestradiol.)

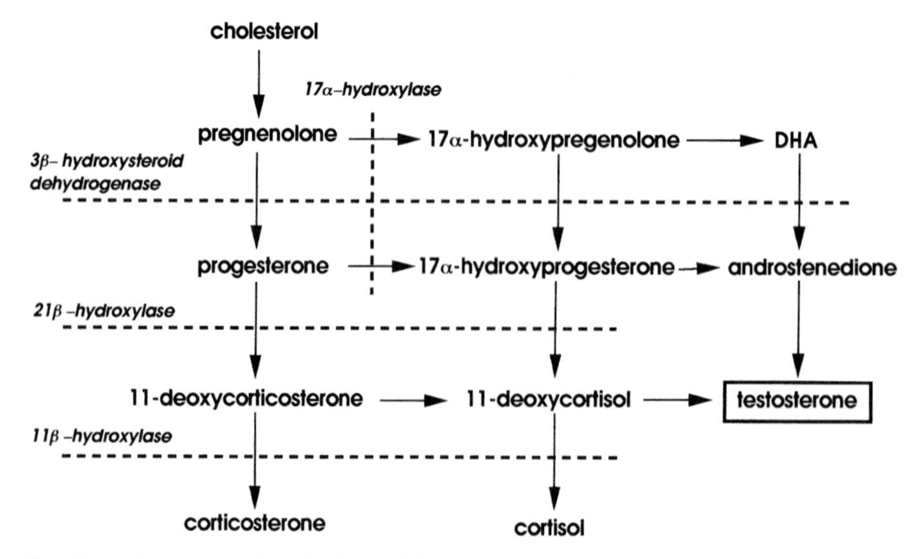

Fig. 23.5 Ovarian and adrenal androgen biosynthesis.

opment and finally menarche. Adrenal androgen secretion continues to rise for a short while after puberty but then plateaus until the menopause, when it declines slowly. In contrast to ovarian androgen production, which is minimal, the adrenal gland becomes the main source of both androgen and oestrogen production in the postmenopausal woman.

The biosynthetic pathways of ovarian and adrenal androgen metabolism are summarized in Figure 23.5.

In summary, hirsutism may result from any one or a combination of these factors:

1. increased circulating androgens derived from the ovaries or adrenals;
2. increased percentage of unbound testosterone reflecting decreased levels of SHBG;
3. increased peripheral conversion of testosterone to DHT reflecting increased 5α-reductase activity;
4. genetic or racial predisposition for an increased number of hair follicles per unit skin area.

Table 23.1 Principal causes of hirsutism

1. *Ovarian*	Polycystic ovary syndrome (PCOS) Tumour —Sex-cord stromal cell —Adrenal-like
2. *Adrenal*	Congenital adrenal hyperplasia Tumour —Adenoma —Adenocarcinoma
3. *Pituitary*	Tumour —ACTH secreting → Cushing's disease —Prolactin secreting —Growth hormone-secreting → acromegaly
4. *Ectopic ACTH*	Tumour —Bronchus —Pancreas —Thyroid —Thymus
5. *Iatrogenic*	Androgenic drugs —Testosterone —Danazol —Glucocorticoids
6. *Idiopathic*	

OTHER CUTANEOUS SIGNS OF HYPERANDROGENAEMIA

Although hirsutism is the commonest cutaneous manifestation of hyperandrogenaemia, increased circulating androgens affect the entire pilosebaceous unit, and acne and increased oiliness of the skin are commonly reported. Up to 60% of women with acne have increased peripheral 5α-reductase activity (Carmina & Lobo 1993).

As previously discussed, in some women the principal effect of androgenization is to decrease scalp hair resulting in temporal recession and, in severe cases, frontal balding. This is refered to as male pattern, or androgen-dependent, alopecia. Although alopecia may be due to a period of synchronous hair growth and shedding or even drugs, its persistence beyond 6 months to a year warrants investigation for underlying hyperandrogenaemia.

Acanthosis nigricans is a grey-brown velvety discoloration of the skin usually found in the axillae, neck and groin. It is a characteristic cutaneous manifestation of hyperinsulinaemia, often found in association with obesity (Dunaif et al 1991).

CAUSES OF HIRSUTISM

The principal causes of hirsutism are listed in Table 23.1.

Polycystic ovary syndrome (PCOS)

This syndrome, first described by Stein & Leventhal (Stein & Leventhal 1935), is a heterogeneous disorder, both clinically and biochemically (Conway et al 1989, Franks 1989). Classic features of anovulation, hirsutism and obesity are variably expressed, and serum levels of LH and testosterone are elevated in only 50% of cases. Recent advances in ultrasound imaging have provided a reliable means of identifying polycystic ovaries (PCO) (Adams et al 1986), and this is now used in preference to endocrine indices alone in making the diagnosis of PCOS (Gilling-Smith & Franks 1993). Using pelvic ultrasound, the prevalence of PCO in different populations of women has been extensively studied. Although PCO are found in up to 20% of normal women (Polson et al 1988), they have a much higher prevalence in women with androgen-related disorders such as acne, hirsutism and alopecia (Adams et al 1986, Conway et al 1989, O'Driscoll et al 1994) as well as being the commonest cause of anovulation (Adams 1986). However many women presenting with hirsutism have regular menstrual cycles, while those with cycle disturbance often show no clinical signs of hyperandrogenaemia.

The relative importance of PCOS in the differential diagnosis of hirsutism has, until recently, remained controversial. In the largest prospective study to date, of 350 women presenting with hirsutism and/or androgenic alopecia, 60% (170/350) had PCO on ultrasound. By comparison, only eight women had other clear-cut causes (mainly adrenal) for their hyperandrogenaemia, of whom three coincidentally had PCO. The remainder had normal ovaries and were therefore classified as having idiopathic hirsutism (O'Driscoll et al 1994). Jahanfar & Eden reported an even higher incidence of ultrasound PCO in their series of 173 women presenting with hirsutism, ranging from 86% in the ovulatory group to 97% in the nonovulatory group, casting doubt on the existence of the condition 'idiopathic hirsutism' (Jahanfar & Eden 1993). In a similar study, 83% of women presenting with acne vulgaris were found to have ultrasound polycystic ovaries (Bunker et al

1989). These data clearly identify PCOS as the single most common cause of hirsutism, acne or alopecia, in contrast to adrenal, pituitary or other ovarian causes, which are relatively rare.

Source of androgen excess in PCOS

The relative role of ovarian and adrenal androgens in the pathogenesis of PCOS remains a subject of considerable debate. Selective venous catheterization of ovarian and adrenal veins has produced controversial results, primarily due to methodological difficulties (Azziz 1993). Adrenal androgen secretion is episodic, and sampling should ideally be serial. Furthermore, the stress induced by such invasive techniques necessarily tends to increase adrenal secretion. Similarly, selective adrenal suppression by glucocorticoids has not yielded useful information (Azziz 1993). Conversely, studies measuring serum androgens, following either ovarian wedge resection (Katz et al 1978) or laparoscopic ovarian diathermy (Aakvaag & Gjonnaess 1985, Greenblatt & Casper 1987), in hyperandrogenic women with PCOS have provided more direct evidence for an ovarian role. Both treatments produce a significant fall in both androstenedione and testosterone within 3–4 days of ovarian tissue reduction. More recently, Barnes has demonstrated an exaggerated ovarian androgen response to the acute administration of a long-acting gonadotrophin hormone-releasing hormone analogue (GnRH-A) in women with PCO compared to normal controls. On the basis of these data, this group has proposed that PCOS results from dysregulation of the key enzyme involved in theca cell androgen biosynthesis, P450c17α (Barnes et al 1989).

In some series, up to 50% of women with hirsutism in association with PCOS have been shown to have elevated DHAS levels, suggesting an adrenal component to their hyperandrogenaemia. However obesity may have an independent effect on elevating serum levels of DHAS and thus the prevalence of raised DHAS concentration is likely to reflect the proportion of obese subjects in these series. In our own series of subjects with PCOS, 35% of whom were overweight, fewer than 10% had higher than normal serum levels of DHAS. Furthermore, ACTH levels are within the normal range in PCOS (Horrocks et al 1983) and, in the absence of coexisting adrenal pathology such as CAH or Cushing's syndrome, the adrenal response to ACTH stimulation is not significantly different to that in control populations (Hudson et al 1990).

If, as is suggested by the above data, the underlying cause of PCOS is an abnormality of ovarian androgen production, the obvious question must be, is this a primary event or one which is secondary to the increased pituitary LH secretion? Several investigators have addressed this issue by studying the effect of stimulating the ovary with human chorionic gonadotrophin (hCG), the bioequivalent of LH. Most studies show no significant increase in androgenic responsiveness to hCG in PCO women (Abraham et al 1975, Rosenfield et al 1972, Story et al 1993). More importantly, if hCG is administered after endogenous LH levels have first been suppressed by GnRH-A, androstenedione and testosterone levels remain significantly higher in the PCO women, while DHAS levels, unaltered by the effect of the GnRH-A, remain similar in both groups (Story et al 1993) suggesting a primary ovarian disturbance in androgen secretion.

In view of the ovarian morphology, hyperandrogenaemia in PCOS could be due simply to increased follicle number or theca cell hyperplasia. However, in vitro studies have found that human theca cells isolated from polycystic ovaries produce significantly more androstenedione per cell than theca cells from normal ovaries, although the magnitude of response to LH is similar as shown in Figure 23.6 (Gilling-Smith et al 1994). These data are consistent with the hypothesis that PCOS results from a primary abnormality of androgen biosynthesis and hence, effective therapy should be directed primarily against ovarian, not adrenal, androgen production.

The role of insulin and insulin-like growth factors (IGFs)

Both insulin and the IGFs have been shown to potentiate the actions of LH on theca cell androgen production in vitro (Bergh et al 1993). However there appears to be no difference between PCO and normal ovaries in the response to these factors, either in vitro or in vivo

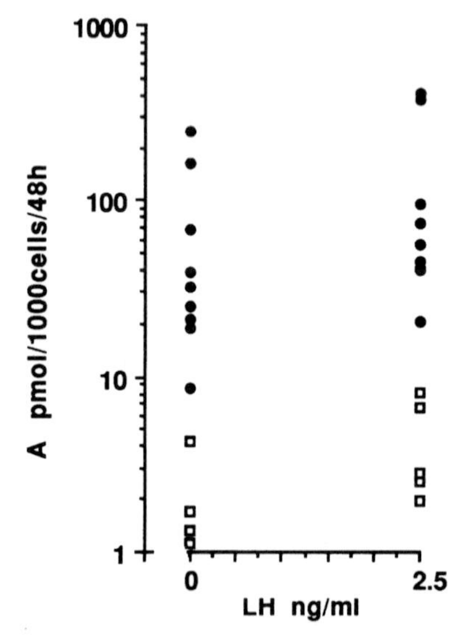

Fig. 23.6 Comparison of androstenedione (A) accumulation from five normal (□) and nine polycystic (●) ovaries under basal and LH-stimulated conditions during the first 48 h of culture. Each data point is the average of duplicate or triplicate experiments. The plating density range was 10–15 × 10^4 cells/well. (Reproduced with permission from Gilling-Smith et al 1994. Journal of Clinical Endocrinology & Metabolism 79: 1158–1165.)

(Gilling-Smith et al 1993; Franks et al 1994). Hyperinsulinaemia and insulin resistance are features of anovulatory women with PCOS and both are exacerbated in the presence of obesity (Sharp et al 1991). Body mass index (BMI) is positively correlated to serum insulin and testosterone levels and inversely correlated to SHBG levels. Weight loss results in a fall in circulating insulin and testosterone levels and a significant improvement in symptoms (Kiddy et al 1990, 1992).

Idiopathic hirsutism

This is defined as hirsutism in women with regular cycles, normal ovaries on ultrasound and no identifiable pathology to account for the symptoms. A recent report would suggest the true incidence of this condition to be far lower than previously described (Jahanfar & Eden 1993). Both free and total serum testosterone levels are often elevated and SHBG levels suppressed.

As with PCOS, there is controversy over whether the source of excess circulating androgens is adrenal or ovarian. In contrast to PCOS, LH levels are within the normal range and the response to GnRH-A is normal.

The most likely explanation for excessive hair growth in these women is increased end-organ sensitivity to normal androgen levels, possibly secondary to increased 5α-reductase activity. In support of this argument is the observation that there is an inverse correlation between Adiol-G levels and clinical response to medical therapy (Kirschner et al 1987).

Late-onset congenital adrenal hyperplasia

Congenital adrenal hyperplasia (CAH) is caused by an enzyme deficiency resulting in an inability or reduced capacity to synthesize glucocorticoids. In response to the low cortisol levels, ACTH levels rise, increasing secretion of both androgens and glucocorticoid precursors and producing hyperplasia of the adrenal cortex. In the majority of cases, the condition is inherited in an autosomal recessive mode and presents, in its most severe form, at birth with virilization of the female external genitalia. Late-onset CAH represents a milder form, which often does not present until childhood or early adult life and is thought to affect up to 5% of women with hirsutism (Kuttenn et al 1985). The majority of cases are characterized by partial 21-hydroxylase deficiency, although other enzyme defects can occur. Features suggestive of late onset CAH worth noting are onset of hirsutism at, or shortly after, puberty, a strong family history of hirsutism, and serum testosterone levels greater than 5 nmol/l. Diagnosis is based on the short synacthen test in which 17α-hydroxyprogesterone and cortisol levels are measured before, and 1 h after, the administration of a single dose (250 μg i.m. or i.v.) of synthetic ACTH.

The coexistence of PCO on ultrasound has been reported to be as high as 83% in adult females with CAH (Hague et al 1990). As in Cushing's syndrome, it is likely that the ovarian changes occur secondarily to the elevation in adrenal androgens, but these figures emphasize the importance of ACTH testing in women with PCOS with markedly elevated testosterone levels.

Cushing's syndrome

This is due to overproduction of cortisol by the adrenal and may result from the following conditions:

1. overproduction of ACTH by the pituitary (Cushing's disease);
2. ectopic ACTH secretion by a nonpituitary tumour;
3. autonomous secretion of cortisol by an adrenal or ovarian tumour;
4. ectopic corticotrophin-secreting hormone production (very rare).

Hyperstimulation of the adrenal by ACTH invariably results in varying degrees of hirsutism or alopecia, acne and occasionally virilization. The most useful screening tests for suspected Cushing's syndrome are 24-h urine free cortisol or an overnight, low-dose (1 mg) dexamethasone suppression test. If these tests prove positive, further investigations should be undertaken, including diurnal serum cortisol and ACTH measurements and a high-dose dexamethasone suppression test (2 mg at night for 5 days). Pituitary-dependent Cushing's disease is characterized by normal or elevated serum levels of ACTH in the face of an elevated diurnal serum level of cortisol, although cortisol is typically suppressed by high-dose dexamethasone. If ACTH levels are undetectable and cortisol not suppressed, this strongly suggests an autonomous adrenal or ovarian tumour, whilst high ACTH levels with failure of cortisol to suppress are consistent with an ectopic source of ACTH.

Further evaluation of the ACTH-producing tumour involves computed tomography (CT) or magnetic resonance imaging (MRI) of the adrenals, chest or pituitary, which is by far the most accurate means of detecting the site of ACTH production. An ectopic ACTH-producing tumour is found in up to 15% of cases, typically located in the thorax or abdomen and associated with bilateral adrenal enlargement. In the absence of an adrenal or ectopic tumour on imaging, inferior petrosal sinus sampling of the blood draining the pituitary is recommended. In contrast to patients with an ectopic tumour, those with Cushing's disease show a significant rise in ACTH levels after CRH stimulation (Findling et al 1991).

Androgen-producing tumours of the ovary or adrenal

These are extremely rare but should always be excluded in

a woman who develops hirsutism or virilization over a short time course, particularly if there are coexisting features of Cushing's syndrome.

Adrenal tumours are divided into the benign adenoma and malignant adenocarcinoma. Typically these are small and impalpable and, in half the reported cases, occur in premenopausal women.

Androgen-secreting ovarian tumours comprise less than 1% of all ovarian tumours. Previously these tumours were classified according to their supposed cell of origin. The currently accepted classification has been simplified and divides the tumours into two groups: sex-cord stromal cell tumours, formerly known as androblastomas, arrhenoblastomas or gynandroblastomas, and adrenal-like tumours of the ovary which include luteomas, virilizing lipoid cell tumours, hypernephromas and adrenal rest tumours. The latter are associated with cushingoid features in 50% of cases. Most androgen-secreting ovarian tumours are benign and they present in young women, typically under the age of 30 (Young & Scully 1985).

Unlike PCOS, in which the hirsutism develops over a period of years and is associated with relatively low testosterone levels (< 5 nmol/l), androgen-secreting tumours grow rapidly, resulting in relatively fast onset and progression of both hirsutism and menstrual cycle disturbance. Serum testosterone is usually > 5 nmol/l, which is more than twice the upper limit of the normal range (0.5–2.6 nmol/l). Virilization together with serum testosterone concentrations in the male range (> 10 nmol/l) are particularly ominous signs. Although androgen production is increased overall, different steroid pathways can be involved, which limits the value of endocrine studies as a method of delineating whether the source of excess androgen production is ovarian or adrenal. The most useful screening tests are serum DHAS and 17α-hydroxyprogesterone levels. Adrenal or adrenal-like ovarian tumours are often associated with elevated DHAS levels (> 20 nmol/l), while 17α-hydroxyprogesterone production is specifically increased in CAH, particularly in response to ACTH stimulation. In the presence of elevated DHAS levels, dexamethasone suppression tests are advisable, as described for the investigation of Cushing's syndrome, to exclude ACTH-dependent tumours.

Further evaluation of androgen-producing tumours relies on imaging. Although functional ovarian tumours are often palpable on pelvic examination, ultrasound imaging is always indicated, and when an ovarian mass is not present on clinical examination or ultrasound, CT or MRI imaging of both adrenals and ovaries must be carried out (see above). Selective adrenal or ovarian vein sampling is technically demanding and should be restricted to those few cases in which the source of excess androgen secretion remains equivocal after imaging.

Virilization presenting during pregnancy may be associated with a luteoma in which the ovarian stroma shows an exaggerated response to the high levels of hCG. These regress spontaneously postpartum and pose little threat to the pregnancy (Garcia-Bunuel et al 1975). The risk of masculinization of a female fetus is very small since the fetus is protected from excess androgen secretion by the high SHBG levels in the maternal circulation and by the ability of the placenta to metabolize androgens. True androgen-secreting tumours are extremely rare in pregnancy (McClamrock et al 1992).

Acromegaly

This condition arises from the excessive secretion of growth hormone by a pituitary adenoma and may occasionally present with hirsutism. Clinical suspicion should be raised if associated symptoms include headaches, arthropathy and carpal tunnel syndrome. Classic signs are an increase in the size of the skull, supraorbital ridges and jaw, vertebral enlargement often with kyphosis and spade-shaped hands and feet. Hypertension and diabetes mellitus are present in 10–15% of cases. Investigations, which should be carried out in conjunction with an endocrinologist, include growth hormone (GH) measurements during a standard glucose tolerance test (which, normally, is associated with complete suppression of serum GH), skull X-ray and, where indicated, a CT or MRI scan of the pituitary.

Iatrogenic hirsutism

A number of drugs may produce hirsutism in susceptible individuals. It is a commonly reported side-effect of danazol, testosterone and glucocorticoids. Drugs which interfere with the hair cycle, such as chemotherapy agents or interferons will result in hair loss. In either case, there should be a prompt return to normal hair growth once the drug is withdrawn (Tosi et al 1994).

CLINICAL ASSESSMENT

Attention to the patient's general body habitus (height, weight and muscle distribution) is important. This will identify obesity and signs of virilism and, in some cases, classic features of general endocrine disorders such as Cushing's syndrome or acromegaly. If there is coexisting cycle disturbance, careful examination of the breasts (for galactorrhoea) and thyroid should be performed. Care should be taken to exclude any abdominal or pelvic masses and, on pelvic examination, note taken of clitoromegaly. Acanthosis nigricans, typically found in the neck and axillae, is also commonly seen in the vulval region (Grasinger et al 1993).

In the case of patients presenting with hirsutism, a semi-quantitative assessment of the degree of hirsutism using the Ferriman–Gallwey chart (Ferriman & Gallwey 1961)

Table 23.2 The Ferriman–Gallwey scoring system

Site	Grade	Definition
Upper lip	1	A few hairs at outer margin
	2	Small moustache at outer margin
	3	Moustache extending halfway from outer margin
	4	Moustache extending to midline
Chin	1	A few scattered hairs
	2	Small concentrations of scattered hairs
	3	Light complete cover
	4	Heavy complete cover
Chest	1	Circumareolar hairs
	2	Additional midline hairs
	3	Fusion of these areas with three-quarter cover
	4	Complete cover
Upper back	1	A few scattered hairs
	2	Rather more, still scattered
	3	Light complete cover
	4	Heavy complete cover
Lower back	1	A sacral tuft of hair
	2	With some lateral extension
	3	Three-quarter cover
	4	Complete cover
Upper abdomen	1	A few midline hairs
	2	Rather more, still midline
	3	Half-cover
	4	Full cover
Lower abdomen	1	A few midline hairs
	2	A midline streak of hair
	3	A midline band of hair
	4	An inverted V-shaped growth
Upper arm	1	Sparse growth affecting not more than a quarter of the limb surfaces
	2	More than this, cover still incomplete
	3	Light complete cover
	4	Heavy complete cover
Forearm	1–4	Complete cover of dorsal surface: very light (1) to very heavy (4) growth
Thigh	1–4	As for arm
Leg	1–4	As for arm

is helpful both as a baseline and in subsequent assessment of response to treatment, particularly if follow-up is to be carried out by different clinicians (Table 23.2). Measurements of hair thickness or growth rate require complex equipment and are limited to research trials. Another useful index of growth rate is to ask the patient how frequently various cosmetic measures, such as shaving or waxing, are being carried out and to look for a fall once treatment has been initiated.

INVESTIGATIONS

The two most useful initial investigations are a pelvic ultrasound scan, best performed in the early follicular phase in an ovulatory patient, and a serum testosterone, taken at any time in the cycle.

The purpose of ultrasound is to define ovarian morphology and, at the same time, exclude rare androgen-secreting ovarian tumours. The typical features of the polycystic ovary on ultrasound are shown in Figure 23.7.

Total serum testosterone is elevated in only 40% of women with hirsutism and there is considerable variation in levels between individuals. The levels do not correlate well with severity of hirsutism or acne (Conway et al 1989, Franks 1989). Indeed, as previously discussed, serum testosterone may be within the normal range in markedly hirsute women due to the suppressive effect of androgens and insulin on SHBG levels. However, in such cases, androgen production rate is always increased along with the percentage unbound, free testosterone. There is no additional benefit to be gained by measuring free testosterone, as women with cutaneous signs of hyperandrogenaemia of sufficient severity to seek medical advice, warrant treatment, irrespective of their serum testosterone levels.

The main reason for measuring serum testosterone levels at initial assessment is to exclude more serious disorders of androgen secretion such as CAH, Cushing's or adrenal or ovarian tumours. In women with normal ovaries and idiopathic hirsutism, testosterone levels are usually less than 3 nmol/l while in those with polycystic ovaries, levels greater than 5 nmol/l are rare. If a testosterone level of greater than 5 nmol/l is found, further tests of adrenal function should be performed, along with ultrasound, CT or MRI imaging as summarized in Figure 23.8. If a benign cause for the hirsutism is found and medical

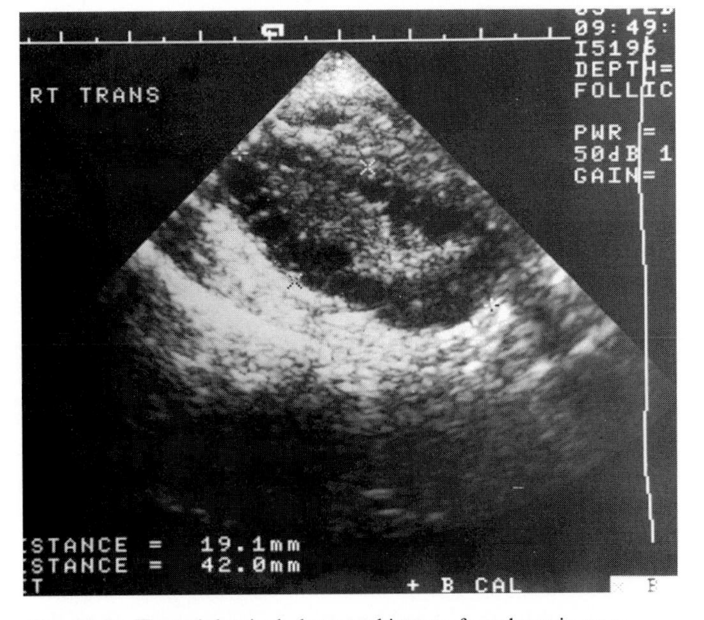

Fig. 23.7 Transabdominal ultrasound image of a polycystic ovary (courtesy of Miss D. Kiddy). To make the diagnosis of PCO at least three of the following four features should be present: (i) peripheral distribution of follicles; (ii) 10 or more follicles, typically 2–8 mm in diameter; (iii) increased stroma; (iv) increased ovarian volume (Adams et al 1986).

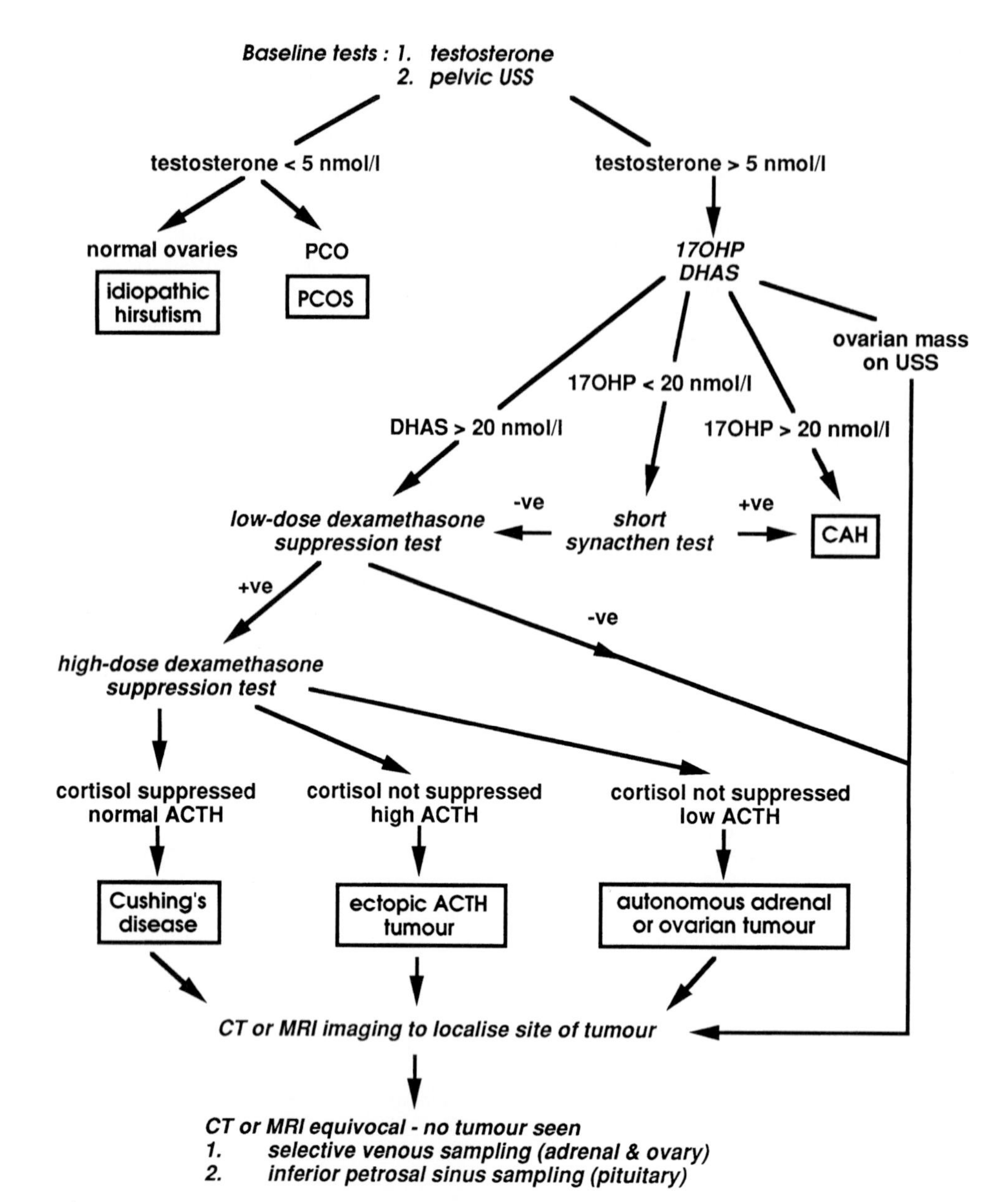

Fig. 23.8 Investigation of women presenting with hirsutism or virilization. (USS, ultrasound scan; DHAS, dehydroepiandrosterone sulphate; 17OHP, 17α-hydroxyprogesterone; CAH, congenital adrenal hyperplasia.)

treatment initiated, testosterone levels need only be checked in those patients in whom the clinical response is poor. The initial diagnosis should be reviewed and, if appropriate, an alternative treatment offered.

TREATMENT

When possible, this should be directed at treatment of the underlying pathology e.g. adrenal or ovarian tumours should be surgically removed and congenital adrenal hyperplasia treated with corticosteroids. If the cause is iatrogenic, the drug should be stopped.

Table 23.3 Steps in the management of hirsutism due to benign causes, i.e. polycystic ovary syndrome (PCOS) or idiopathic

1. Cosmetic measures	
2. Weight reduction (BMI > 25 kg/m²)	
3. Antiandrogens	• Cyproterone acetate or dianette • Spironolactone • Flutamide
4. Ovarian suppression	• Combined oral contraceptives • GnRH analogues
5. Bilateral oophorectomy	

For the remainder of patients, who will have either PCOS or idiopathic hirsutism, the treatment plan outlined in Table 23.3 should be adopted. First and foremost, it is important to reassure the patient that the underlying cause is benign and self-limiting. In cases of mild hirsutism, cosmetic measures alone are often sufficient but if these fail, or the degree of hirsutism is more severe, medical and, in certain cases, surgical treatment should be offered.

Obesity significantly exacerbates the severity of hirsutism and weight loss should therefore be encouraged in subjects who are overweight, preferably prior to therapy but certainly in addition to medical treatment.

Cosmetic treatments

The value of waxing, shaving, electrolysis, the use of depilatory creams and bleaching is often underestimated. With either medical or surgical therapy, androgen levels usually decline rapidly, but the effect on hair growth typically takes between 3–6 months to become apparent, and often an acceptable improvement is not achieved until a year of therapy. It is important to forewarn patients of this so that cosmetic measures are continued during this time.

Women concerned that shaving increases the rate of hair growth, should be reassured that this is not the case. Electrolysis is the only permanent way of removing hair and gives the best cosmetic result, but it is costly and needs to be performed by an experienced operator to minimize the risk of scarring or infection (Schriock & Schriock 1991).

Antiandrogens

These drugs inhibit androgen action primarily by competing with the androgen receptor in target tissues. They are usually prescribed in combination with oestradiol which has the additional effects of suppressing gonadotrophin production and consequently ovarian androgen production, inhibiting 5α-reductase and stimulating SHBG levels.

Cyproterone acetate (CPA)

This is the most widely prescribed antiandrogen in the UK. It is also a potent progestogen, and when prescribed in a 'reverse sequential' regimen for the first 10 days of a 21-day treatment cycle, combined with either a low-dose birth control pill or 30 μg ethinyl oestradiol taken daily, it suppresses ovulation and, in the majority of women, produces regular withdrawal bleeds. The dosage of CPA in the preparation can be varied according to the severity of hirsutism.

In mild to moderate hirsutism Dianette (35 μg ethinyl oestradiol plus 2 mg CPA daily for 21 days) should be prescribed. It is effective in improving symptoms in up to 50% of cases (Prelevic et al 1989) and is a useful 'maintenance' preparation once a response has been achieved with higher doses. If there is no response to Dianette, or the hirsutism is more severe (Ferriman–Gallwey score > 10), CPA (25 – 100 mg) should be given for 10 days in each Dianette cycle in a reverse sequential regimen. Over 70% of women treated in this way report a significant improvement in symptoms within 1 year (McKenna 1991). Side-effects of CPA include depression, weight gain and breast tenderness, and limit the time for which the higher dose regimens can be tolerated. A review of the literature would suggest that there is no overall benefit to be gained from using higher doses of CPA in preference to Dianette, although the rate of response appears to be faster at higher doses (Jeffcoate 1993). These data are, however, not necessarily consistent with the clinical experience in many centres, and most practitioners advocate using higher doses of CPA in more severe cases.

CPA should always be prescribed with either a combined oral contraceptive or an antioestrogen in order to suppress ovulation since feminization of a male fetus could occur if a woman conceived when on antiandrogen therapy. If for any reason this is not feasible, alternative contraceptive measures should be taken.

Spironolactone

This is an aldosterone antagonist which also has androgen-receptor blocking activity. Like CPA, it is usually administered with oestrogen or a combined oral contraceptive. It is widely used in the United States, as CPA is not available there, and has been shown to be effective in reducing hair growth and androgen levels (Barth et al 1989, Chapman et al 1985). In the UK the Committee on the Safety of Medicines has not approved its use in the treatment of hirsutism. In the only trial to date comparing spironolactone with CPA, there was no significant difference in response between the two groups (O'Brien et al 1991).

Flutamide

This is a nonsteroidal antiandrogen acting on peripheral target tissues which has been used successfully in the treatment of prostatic cancer. There have been few trials evaluating its use in hirsutism but those to date would suggest that, at a daily dose of 500 mg in combination with an oral contraceptive, results are comparable to those with spironolactone (Cusan et al 1994, Erenus et al 1994).

Athough, in theory, it may be effective in cases where CPA or spironolactone treatment has proved unsuccessful, our own clinical experience suggests that it is no more efficacious than these, more commonly used, antiandrogens.

Ketoconazole

This is a synthetic imidazole derivative which blocks gonadal and adrenal steroidogenesis by inhibiting key enzymatic steps in androgen biosynthesis. Data on its role in the management of hirsutism remain controversial. Most trials express concern over marked side-effects (nausea, asthenia and alopecia) which necessitate close monitoring and produce a high drop-out rate (Martikainen et al 1988, Venturoli et al 1990). In addition, clinical response is relatively poor and, in the light of the available data, few would advocate its routine clinical use.

Ovarian suppression

Combined oral contraceptives

The combined low-dose pill provides the simplest means of suppressing pituitary FSH and LH and hence ovarian androgen production. In addition oestrogen stimulates SHBG production by the liver and inhibits 5α-reductase. The choice of progestogen in the preparation is critical. Most progestogens have some androgenic activity and suppress the synthesis of SHBG. For this reason desogestrel- (Porcile & Gallardo 1991) and gestodene-based pills are favoured and should still be considered, despite recent data suggesting a higher risk of thromboembolism with these progestogens. Nevertheless, only 30% of patients will notice an improvement with such formulations, which is why we would only recommend these preparations as second-line in cases where Dianette is not tolerated.

GnRH analogues

These have been used to suppress ovarian steroid production in moderate to severe hirsutism and results are comparable to those achieved with CPA. Side-effects of vasomotor symptoms and bone loss limit the duration for which these drugs can be prescribed. However, recent trials would suggest that low-dose oestrogen replacement therapy may enhance the antiandrogenic effect of the GnRH-A, as well as minimizing the side-effects (Carmina et al 1994).

Adrenal suppression

Glucocorticoids only have a place in the treatment of hirsutism when there is an underlying adrenal component such as late onset CAH. Dexamethasone (0.25–5.0 mg) taken at night suppresses the morning ACTH surge and hence adrenal androgen production. The dose of glucocorticoid given needs to be monitored carefully, and particular care should be taken with obese subjects due to the appetite-stimulating effect of the glucocorticoid.

Interestingly, a recent randomized trial comparing the use of CPA with hydrocortisone in women with late-onset CAH found that CPA produced a significantly better clinical response: 54% responded in the CPA arm vs. 26% in the hydrocortisone arm (Spritzer et al 1990).

5α-reductase inhibitors

Finasteride is a nonsteroidal specific competitive inhibitor of 5α-reductase which has been used with success in the treatment of prostatic hyperplasia. The incidence of side-effects is low and therefore it has potential therapeutic application in the treatment of cutaneous hyperandrogenaemia, particularly in those cases where the predominant feature appears to be end-organ sensitivity to androgens (Sudduth & Koronkowski 1993). Trials to evaluate this compound are awaited, but it should be noted that finasteride is predominantly an inhibitor of type 2 5α-reductase, whereas the enzyme thought to be active in hair follicles is type 1 5α-reductase.

Surgical methods

Surgery has a limited place in the management of hyperandrogenaemia. It should be reserved for those women who have completed their families and in whom long-term steroid therapy is either unacceptable or contraindicated (due to age or cardiovascular risk).

Traditionally, ovarian wedge resection was the only treatment available for PCOS and was found to effectively lower LH and testosterone levels, restore ovarian cyclicity and produce an improvement in hirsutism (Katz et al 1978). Newer, less invasive laparoscopic techniques have to a large extent replaced wedge resection since they achieve the same end result but theoretically pose less risk of producing pelvic adhesions. Although they have been shown to be effective in the management of anovulatory subfertility (Armar et al 1990, Gadir et al 1990) the effect on serum androgens appears to be short-lived which limits their application to the management of hirsutism. Bilateral oophorectomy (usually combined with hysterectomy) may, in some cases, be a more appropriate option. The numbers of patients treated in this way, and hence follow-up data, are limited. In our centre, we have performed bilateral oophorectomy in three cases of severe hirsutism and obtained a satisfactory clinical response in two. A short trial of GnRH analogues may be useful in predicting those cases likely to benefit from surgery.

HIRSUTISM IN THE MENOPAUSAL WOMAN

Hirsutism arising de novo in the menopause should be fully investigated as described earlier, and particular care taken to exclude a tumour. CPA remains the therapy of choice for postmenopausal women with PCOS or idiopathic hirsutism and is best prescribed in a reverse sequential regimen with physiological doses of oestrogen (i.e. hormone replacement therapy). A small proportion of women will be found to have ovarian hyperthecosis and their response to antiandrogen treatment is usually poor. The high LH levels associated with ovarian failure may play a role, and some benefit may be gained by a course of GnRH-A. Oophorectomy is often the only real long-term solution if the hirsutism is severe.

PSYCHOLOGICAL CONSIDERATIONS

Hirsutism can be an extremely distressing condition, both cosmetically and psychosexually. For this reason, women requesting medical help should always be investigated, counselled as to the underlying cause and offered medical treatment if response to cosmetic measures alone has been inadequate. In more severe cases additional psychotherapy sessions may be beneficial (Sonino et al 1993).

ACNE AND ALOPECIA

The treatment principles outlined above are equally applicable to women with other cutaneous signs of hyperandrogenaemia. Alopecia is best treated with CPA, as described above. In contrast to the significant improvement reported in women with hirsutism, results with alopecia are often poor. GnRH analogues have been used in difficult cases, but again response is poor. Hair loss is usually limited although some women may get full restoration of hair growth.

Acne responds well to Dianette. Higher doses of CPA are often used when there is coexisting hirsutism or alopecia. Antibiotics (tetracycline derivatives) or retinol derivatives can be used when Dianette is not tolerated, contraception is not required and there is no associated hirsutism or alopecia.

KEY POINTS

1. Hirsutism is the excessive growth of facial and body hair in a male pattern distribution.
2. It may result from increased androgen production by the ovaries and/or adrenal glands, increased target tissue sensitivity to androgens or an increase in biologically active circulating androgens.
3. Virilization involves more severe features of hyperandrogenism including male body habitus, clitoromegaly, voice deepening and increased libido, and is characteristically associated with androgen-stimulating or -producing tumours or use of androgenic drugs.
4. The commonest cause of hirsutism is PCOS. Diagnosis is based on ultrasound appearance. Serum testosterone is usually elevated (>2.5 nmol/l but < 5 nmol/l).
5. All women with a serum testosterone > 5 nmol/l should be further investigated to exclude CAH or an androgen-secreting tumour. Investigations should include pelvic ultrasound scan, measurement of serum DHAS and 17α-hydroxyprogesterone levels and, where indicated, CT or MRI imaging of the abdomen and pelvis.
6. The diagnosis of idiopathic hirsutism should be limited to those cases in which there is no identifiable pathology to account for the symptoms; the menstrual cycle is regular, the ovaries normal on ultrasound scan and serum testosterone < 5 nmol/l.
7. Medical treatment should be offered to all women with hirsutism due to benign causes in whom cosmetic measures alone have failed.
8. Weight reduction should be encouraged in women with a BMI > 25 kg/m^2 prior to starting medical treatment.
9. Cyproterone acetate is the antiandrogen of choice in the management of benign hirsutism, given either in low dose form as Dianette or at higher doses (25–100 mg) in more severe cases.
10. Ovarian suppression with GnRH analogues should be considered in all cases resistant to cyproterone acetate therapy.

REFERENCES

Aakvaag A, Gjonnaess H 1985 Hormonal response to electrocautery of the ovary in patients with polycystic ovarian disease. British Journal of Obstetrics and Gynaecology 92: 1258–1264

Abraham G E, Chakmakjian Z H, Buster J E, Marshall J R 1975 Ovarian and adrenal contributions to peripheral androgens in hirsute women. Obstetrics and Gynecology 46: 169–173

Adams J, Polson D W, Franks S 1986 Prevalence of polycystic ovaries in women with anovulation and idiopathic hirsutism. British Medical Journal 293: 355–359

Anderson D C 1974 Sex hormone binding globulin. Clinical Endocrinology 3: 69–73

Armar N A, McGarrigle H H, Honour J, Holownia P, Jacobs H S, Lachelin G C 1990 Laparoscopic ovarian diathermy in the management of anovulatory infertility in women with polycystic ovaries: endocrine changes and clinical outcome. Fertility and Sterility 53: 45–49

Azziz R 1993 The role of the ovary in the genesis of hyperandrogenism. In: Adashi E Y, Leung P C K (eds) The ovary. Raven Press, New York, pp 581–605

Barnes R B, Rosenfield R L, Burstein S, Ehrmann D A 1989 Pituitary–ovarian responses to nafarelin testing in the polycystic ovary syndrome. New England Journal of Medicine 320: 559–565

Barth J H, Cherry C A, Wojnarowski F, Dawber R P R 1989 Spironolactone is an effective and well tolerated systemic antiandrogen therapy for hirsute women. Journal of Clinical Endocrinology and Metabolism 68: 966–970

Bergh C, Carlsson B, Olsson J-H, Selleskog U, Hillensjo T 1993 Regulation of androgen production in cultured human thecal cells by insulin-like growth factor 1 and insulin. Fertility and Sterility 59: 323–331

Bunker C B, Newton J A, Kilborn J et al 1989 Most women with acne have polycystic ovaries. British Journal of Dermatology 121: 675–680

Carmina E, Lobo R A 1993 Evidence for increased androsterone metabolism in some normoandrogenic women with acne. Journal of Clinical Endocrinology and Metabolism 76: 1111–1114

Carmina E, Janni A, Lobo R A 1994 Physiological estrogen replacement may enhance the effectiveness of the gonadotrophin-releasing

hormone agonist in the treatment of hirsutism. Journal of Clinical Endocrinology and Metabolism 78: 126–130
Chapman M G, Dowsett M, Dewhurst C G, Jeffcoate S L 1985 Spironolactone in combination with an oral contraceptive: an alternative treatment for hirsutism. British Journal of Obstetrics and Gynaecology 92: 983–985
Conway G S, Honour J W, Jacobs H S 1989 Heterogeneity of the polycystic ovary syndrome: clinical, endocrine and ultrasound features in 556 patients. Clinical Endocrinology 30: 459–470
Cusan L, Dupont A, Gomez J L, Tremblay R R, Labrie F 1994 Comparison of flutamide and spironolactone in the treatment of hirsutism: a randomized controlled trial. Fertility and Sterility 61: 281–287
Dunaif A, Green G, Phelps R G, Lebwohl M, Futterweit W, Lewy L 1991 Acanthosis nigricans, insulin action, and hyperandrogenism: clinical, histological, and biochemical findings. Journal of Clinical Endocrinology and Metabolism 73: 590–595
Erenus M, Gurbuz O, Durmusoglu F, Demircay Z, Pekin S 1994 Comparison of the efficacy of spironolactone versus flutamide in the treatment of hirsutism. Fertility and Sterility 61: 613–616
Ferriman D, Gallwey J D 1961 Clinical measurement of body hair growth in women. Journal of Clinical Endocrinology and Metabolism 21: 1440–1447
Franks S 1989 Polycystic ovary syndrome: a changing perspective. Clinical Endocrinology 31: 87–120
Franks S, Willis D, Hamilton-Fairley D, White D M, Mason H D 1994 The evidence against a role for the growth hormone/insulin-like growth factor system in the polycystic ovary syndrome. In: Adashi E Y, Thorner M O (eds) The somatotrophic axis of the reproductive process in health and disease. Springer-Verlag, New York, 220–228
Findling J W, Kehoe M E, Shaker J L, Raff H 1991 Routine inferior petrosal sinus sampling in the differential diagnosis of adrenocorticotropin (ACTH) dependent Cushing's syndrome: early recognition of the occult ectopic ACTH syndrome. Journal of Clinical Endocrinology and Metabolism 73: 408–413
Gadir A A, Mowafi R S, Alnaser H M I, Alrashid A H, Alonezi O M, Shaw R W 1990 Ovarian electrocautery versus human menopausal gonadotrophins and pure follicle stimulating hormone therapy in the treatment of patients with polycystic ovarian disease. Clinical Endocrinology 33: 585–592
Garcia-Bunuel R, Berek J S, Woodruff J D 1975 Luteomas of pregnancy. Obstetrics and Gynecology 45: 407
Gilling-Smith C, Franks S 1993 Polycystic ovary syndrome. In: Smith S (ed) Reproductive medicine review. Edward Arnold, London, pp 15–32
Gilling-Smith C, Willis D, Mason H D, Franks S 1993 Comparison of androgen production by theca cells from normal and polycystic ovaries. Human Reproduction 8: Abstract 207
Gilling-Smith C, Willis D S, Beard R W, Franks S 1994 Hypersecretion of androstenedione by isolated thecal cells from polycystic ovaries. Journal of Clinical Endocrinology and Metabolism 79: 1158–1165
Grasinger C C, Wild R A, Parker I J 1993 Vulvar acanthosis nigricans: a marker for insulin resistance in hirsute women. Fertility and Sterility 59: 583–586
Greenblatt E, Casper R F 1987 Endocrine changes after laparoscopic ovarian cautery in polycystic ovarian syndrome. American Journal of Obstetrics and Gynecology 156: 279–285
Greep N, Hoopes M, Horton R 1986 Androstenediol glucuronide plasma clearance and production rates in normal and hirsute women. Journal of Clinical Endocrinology and Metabolism 62: 22–27
Hague W M, Adams J, Rodda C et al 1990 The prevalence of polycystic ovaries in patients with congenital adrenal hyperplasia and their close relatives. Clinical Endocrinology 33: 501–510
Horrocks P M, Kandeel F R, London D R et al 1983 ACTH function in women with the polycystic ovary syndrome. Clinical Endocrinology 19: 143–150
Horton R, Lobo R A, Hawks D 1982 Androstenediol glucuronide in plasma: a marker of androgen action. Journal of Clinical Investigation 69: 1203–1206
Hudson R W, Lochnan H A, Danby F W, Margesson L J, Strang B K, Kimmett S M 1990 11 beta-hydroxyandrostenedione: a marker of adrenal function in hirsutism. Fertility and Sterility 54: 1065–1071
Jahanfar S, Eden J A 1993 Idiopathic hirsutism or polycystic ovary syndrome? Australian and New Zealand Journal of Obstetrics and Gynaecology 33: 414–416
Jeffcoate W 1993 The treatment of women with hirsutism. Clinical Endocrinology 39: 143–150
Katz M, Carr P J, Cohen B M, Millar R P 1978 Hormonal effects of wedge resection of polycystic ovaries. Obstetrics and Gynecology 52: 437–443
Kiddy D S, Sharp P S, White D M et al 1990 Differences in clinical and endocrine features between obese and non-obese subjects with polycystic ovary syndrome: an analysis of 263 consecutive cases. Clinical Endocrinology 32: 213–220
Kiddy D S, Hamilton-Fairley D, Bush A et al 1992 Improvement in endocrine and ovarian function during dietary treatment of obese women with polycystic ovary syndrome. Clinical Endocrinology 36: 105–111
Kirschner M A, Samojlik E, Szmal E 1987 Clinical usefulness of plasma androstenediol glucuronide measurements in women with idiopathic hirsutism. Journal of Clinical Endocrinology and Metabolism 65: 597–601
Kuttenn F, Couillin P, Girard F et al 1985 Late-onset adrenal hyperplasia in hirsutism. New England Journal of Medicine 313: 224–231
Lobo R A, Shoupe D, Serafini P, Brinton D, Horton R 1985 The effects of two doses of spironolactone on serum androgens and anagen hair in hirsute women. Fertility and Sterility 43: 200–205
McClamrock H D, Adashi E Y 1992 Gestational hyperandrogenism. Fertility and Sterility 57: 257
Martikainen H, Heikkinen J, Ruokonen A, Kauppila A 1988 Hormonal and clinical effects of ketoconazole in hirsute women. Journal of Clinical Endocrinology and Metabolism 66: 987–991
Marcondes J A M, Minnani S L, Luthold W W, Wajchenberg B L, Samojlik E, Kirschner M A 1992 Treatment of hirsutism in women with flutamide. Fertility and Sterility 57: 543–547
Matteri R K, Stanczyk F Z, Gentzschein E E, Delgado C, Lobo R A 1989 Androgen sulfate and glucuronide conjugates in nonhirsute and hirsute women with polycystic ovary syndrome. American Journal of Obstetrics and Gynecology 161: 1704–1709
McKenna T J 1991 Cyproterone acetate in the treatment of hirsutism. Clinical Endocrinology 35: 5–10
O'Brien R C, Cooper M E, Murray R M, Seeman E, Thomas A K, Jerums G 1991 Comparison of sequential cyproterone acetate/estrogen versus spironolactone/oral contraceptive in the treatment of hirsutism. Journal of Clinical Endocrinology and Metabolism 72: 1008–1013
O'Driscoll J B, Mamtora H, Higginson J, Pollock A, Kane J, Anderson D C 1994 A prospective study of the prevalence of clear-cut endocrine disorders and polycystic ovaries in 350 patients presenting with hirsutism or androgenic alopecia. Clinical Endocrinology 41: 231–236
Polson D W, Adams J, Wadsworth J, Franks S 1988 Polycystic ovaries – a common finding in normal women. Lancet 1: 870–872
Porcile A, Gallardo E 1991 Oral contraceptives containing desogestrel in the maintenance of the remission of hirsutism: monthly versus bimonthly treatment. Contraception 44: 533–539
Prelevic G M, Wurzburger M I, Balint P L, Puzigaca Z 1989 Effects of a low-dose estrogen antiandrogen combination (Diane-35) on clinical signs of androgenization, hormone profile and ovarian size in patients with polycystic ovary syndrome. Gynecological Endocrinology 3: 269–280
Randall V A 1994 Androgens and human hair growth. Clinical Endocrinology 40: 439–457
Rittmaster R S, Thompson D L 1990 Effect of leuprolide and dexamethasone on hair growth and hormone levels in hirsute women: the relative importance of the ovary and the adrenal in pathogenesis of hirsutism. Journal of Clinical Endocrinology and Metabolism 70: 1096–1102
Rittmaster R S 1993 Androgen conjugates: physiology and clinical significance. Endocrine Reviews 14: 121–132
Rosenfield R L, Ehrlich E N, Clearly R E 1972 Adrenal and ovarian contributions to the elevated free plasma androgen levels in hirsute women. Journal of Clinical Endocrinology 34: 92–98

Schriock E A, Schriock E D 1991 Treatment of hirsutism. Clinical Obstetrics and Gynecology 34: 852–863
Serafini P, Ablan F, Lobo R A 1985 5α-reductase activity in the genital skin of hirsute women. Journal of Clinical Endocrinology and Metabolism 60: 349–355
Sharp P S, Kiddy D S, Reed M J, Anyaoku V, Johnston D G, Franks S 1991 Correlation of plasma insulin and insulin-like growth factor-I with indices of androgen transport and metabolism in women with polycystic ovary syndrome. Clinical Endocrinology 35: 253–257
Sonino N, Fava G A, Mani E, Belluardo P, Boscaro M 1993 Quality of life of hirsute women. Postgraduate Medical Journal 69: 186–189
Spritzer P, Billaud L, Thalabard J-C et al 1990 Cyproterone acetate versus hydrocortisone treatment in late-onset adrenal hyperplasia. Journal of Clinical Endocrinology and Metabolism 70: 642–646
Stein I F, Leventhal M L 1935 Amenorrhea associated with bilateral polycystic ovaries. American Journal of Obstetrics and Gynecology 29: 181–191
Story E H, Gilling-Smith C, Short F, Franks S 1993 Comparison of ovarian androgen secretion in women with normal and polycystic ovaries. Journal of Endocrinology 139 (suppl): O30
Sudduth S L, Koronkowski M J 1993 Finasteride: the first 5 alpha-reductase inhibitor. Pharmacotherapy 13: 309–325
Thompson D L, Horton N, Rittmaster R S 1990 Androsterone glucuronide is a marker of adrenal hyperandrogenism in hirsute women. Clinical Endocrinology 32: 283–292
Tosi A, Misciali C, Piraccini B M, Peluso A M, Bardazzi F 1994 Drug-induced hair loss and hair growth. Incidence, management and avoidance. Drug Safety 10: 310–317
Venturoli S, Fabbri R, Dal P L et al 1990 Ketoconazole therapy for women with acne and/or hirsutism. Journal of Clinical Endocrinology and Metabolism 71: 335–339
White F E, White M C, Drury P L, Fry I K, Besser G M 1982 Value of computed tomography of the abdomen and chest in investigation of Cushing's syndrome. British Medical Journal 284: 771
Young R H, Scully R E 1985 Ovarian Sertoli–Leydig cell tumours. A clinicopathological analysis of 207 cases. American Journal of Surgical Pathology 9: 543–569

24

Premenstrual syndrome

P. M. S. O'Brien   R. Chenoy

INTRODUCTION

Premenstrual syndrome (PMS) is a psychological and somatic disorder of unknown aetiology. It is not proven to be of endocrine origin, or to depend on the menstrual cycle. It seems likely, however, that PMS is the consequence of the hormonal events of the normal ovarian cycle, since bilateral oophorectomy and medical suppression of the cycle eliminates PMS completely. Additionally, oestrogen with cyclical progestogen given postmenopausally gives rise to PMS-like symptoms in susceptible women. Most menstruating women exhibit some premenstrual symptomatology but hormonal differences do not account for the range of severity of the symptoms. PMS probably represents an exaggerated end-organ response to the physiological changes of ovarian hormones. This probably has a biochemical and neuroendocrine basis.

THE SYNDROME

Premenstrual syndrome was traditionally thought to affect multiparous middle class articulate women in their late 30s and 40s, the symptoms beginning after childbirth and often following postnatal depression. It is probable, however, that this group of women report their symptoms, whilst younger and less educated women experience equally severe problems, but do not recognize them as such.

The classical symptoms of irritability, aggression, depression, tension, bloatedness and mastalgia are well-known; there are many other symptoms (Table 24.1).

Behavioural changes are also recognized and include suicide, child abuse, examination failures, absence from and poor performance at work, alcohol abuse and criminal acts. Indeed, there have been several legal cases where PMS has been cited in defence of severe crime such as murder. It also appears that medical disorders such as epilepsy, cardiac disease and asthma worsen premenstrually, though few of these assumptions have been borne out by adequate scientific studies.

The prevalence of PMS has been reported to range from 5 to 95%; this probably reflects the imprecision of diagnostic criteria rather than any biological factor.

PMS is unusual in that women usually present themselves with the presumed diagnosis of PMS and it is the clinician's role to determine the validity of this. It may be confused with many other disorders (see Differential diagnosis, p. 364), and the diagnosis of PMS itself may be difficult. The classification in Figure 24.1 may provide some assistance (O'Brien 1987). Hypothetical representation of the components of PMS is set out in Figure 24.2. Women may be asymptomatic, have only physiological symptoms or may have true primary or secondary PMS. A significant proportion of so-called PMS patients have a psychiatric problem which has been wrongly attributed to PMS.

Asymptomatic women

Only 5% of women are completely free from symptoms premenstrually.

Table 24.1 Reported symptoms of PMS

Psychological	Physical
* Aggression	Accident-prone
Agitation	Asthma
Acne	Bloatedness (actual)
Anorexia	Blurred vision
* Anxiety	* Breast swelling
Argumentative	* Breast tenderness
* Bloatedness (feeling of)	Clumsiness
Confusion	Constipation
* Crying bouts	Diarrhoea
Decreased alertness	Diminished activity
Decreased libido	Diminished efficiency
* Depression	Diminished performance
Diminished self-esteem	Dizziness
Drowsiness	Epilepsy
Emotional lability	Finger swelling
Energetic	Flushes
Fatigue	Formication
Food craving	Headache
Hopelessness	Joint pain
Housebound	Mastodynia
Hunger	Migraine
Hypersomnia	Muscle pain
Impulsive behaviour	Nausea
Increased libido	Oedema
Insomnia	Oliguria
* Irritability	Pain: iliac fossa
Lack of inspiration	Pain: lower abdomen
Lack of volition	Pain: pelvic
Lethargy	Polyuria
Listlessness	Poor coordination
Loss of attention to appearance	Premenstrual dysmenorrhoea
* Loss of concentration	Pruritus
Loss of confidence	Puffiness
Loss of judgement	Sinusitis
Loss of self-control	Skin lesions
Malaise	Sore eyes
Mood swings	Sweating
Sadness	Vaginal discharge
Social isolation	Vertigo
Suicidal tendency	Weight increase (true)
* Tension	
Thirst	
Violence	
Vomiting	
Weakness	
Weight increased (perceived)	

* Commonest symptoms

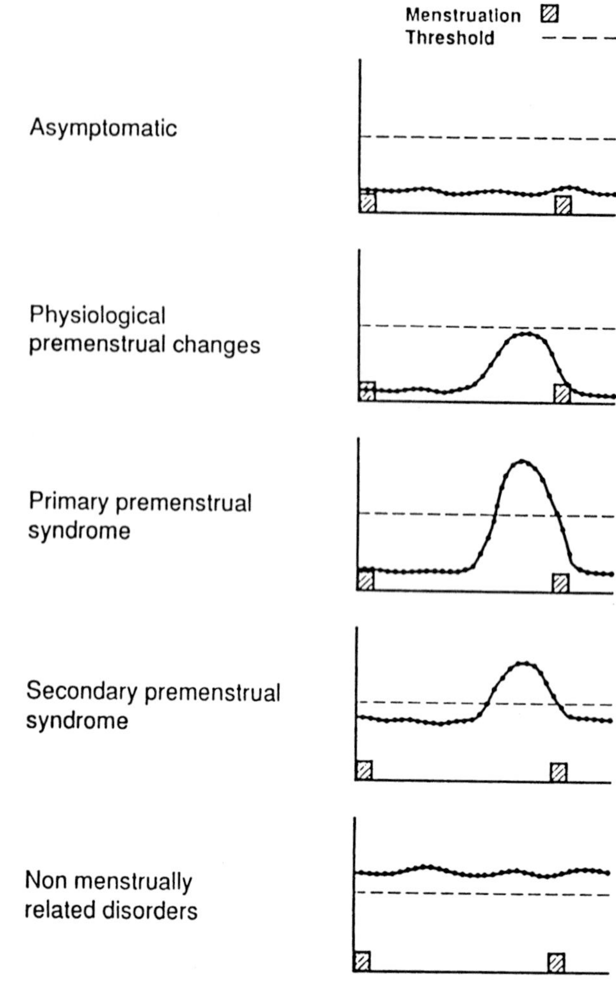

Fig. 24.1 Classification of premenstrual symptomatology.

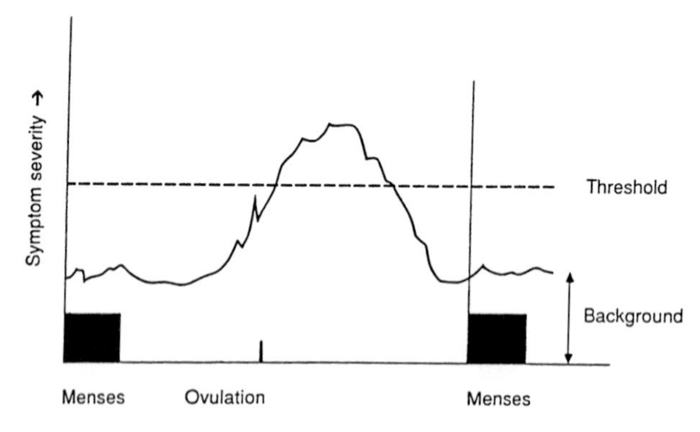

Fig. 24.2 Hypothetical representation of the components of PMS.

Physiological premenstrual change

Up to 95% of women experience at least one premenstrual symptom. In the majority, these are tolerated and there is no interference with normal functioning. When symptoms do interfere with such functioning then a woman can be considered to have PMS. It is difficult to quantify this disruption of life and hence the problem in discriminating between physiological and pathological symptoms.

PMS may be primary or secondary, depending on the degree of underlying psychopathology.

Primary and secondary PMS

In primary PMS somatic, psychological or behavioural symptoms recur in the premenstrual phase of the cycle. Symptoms resolve completely by the end of menstruation, leaving a symptom-free week. The symptoms are of sufficient severity to produce social, family or occupational disruption. Symptoms must have occurred in at least four of the six previous cycles.

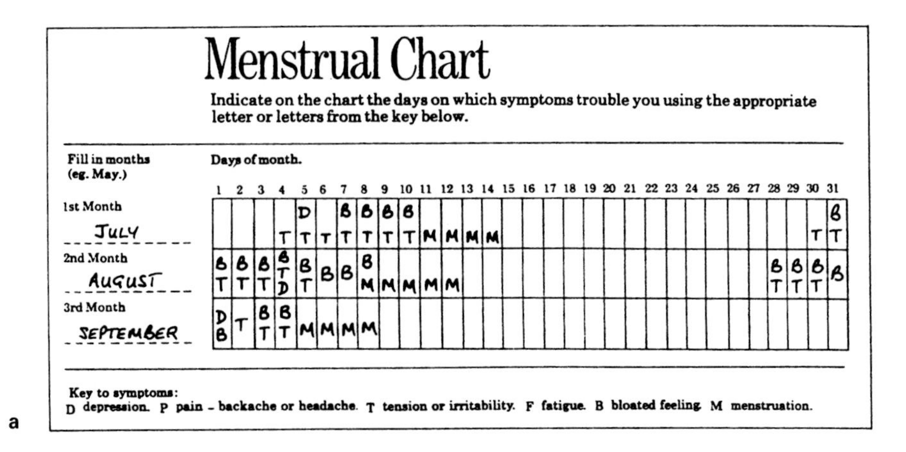

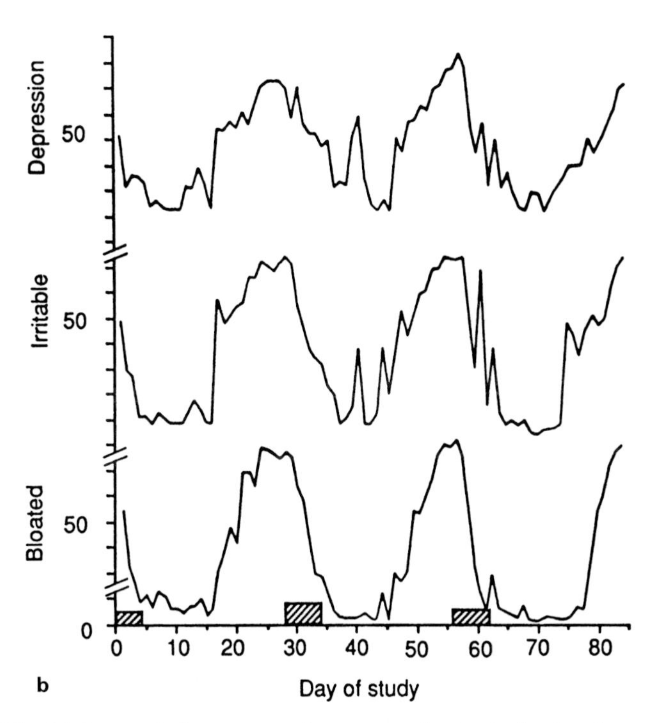

Fig. 24.3 a typical premenstrual symptom calendar; **b** visual analogue scores of typical PMS symptoms. Hatched box, menstruation.

In secondary PMS somatic, psychological or behavioural symptoms recur in the premenstrual phase of the cycle, and remain following menstruation but should significantly improve by the end of menstruation and this improvement should be sustained for at least 1 week. The symptoms are of sufficient severity to produce social, familial or occupational disruption and should have occurred in at least four of the six previous cycles.

It is implicit in these definitions that in secondary PMS there is an underlying psychological disorder whose aetiology is similar to that of common psychiatric disorders such as depression or anxiety. Both primary PMS and the cyclical component of secondary PMS are related to the ovarian cycle.

Psychological disorder wrongly attributed to PMS

A group of women encountered in the gynaecology clinic have continuous, noncyclical psychological problems wrongly attributed (by patient or doctor) to PMS. Such patients should not receive PMS therapy but psychiatric evaluation and treatment.

SYMPTOMS

Measurement and diagnosis

Quantification of PMS is difficult and ideally we would wish to measure:

1. the severity of cyclical symptoms;
2. the degree of underlying psychological dysfunction;
3. the degree of disruption of that patient's normal functioning.

It is possible to quantify underlying psychopathology using established psychiatric questionnaires such as the General Health Questionnaire (GHQ) (Goldberg & Hillier 1979). This must be completed only in the follicular phase. The cyclical symptoms are most precisely measured using visual analogue scales (Faratian et al 1984). Many other methods exist (Budeiri et al 1994), but the Moos' Menstrual Distress Questionnaire is most commonly used despite its limitations (Moos 1985).

Figure 24.3 demonstrates a typical record of symptoms obtained from specific visual analogue scales.

To measure the degree to which the patient's life is disrupted is less simple. Recently, quality of life health surveys have been introduced, for example the SF-36 quality of life questionnaire (Ware & Sherbourne 1992). These have not been used extensively in PMS.

A user-friendly hand-held PMS Symptometrics computer device has recently been developed by the author at Keele University. The instrument incorporates validated visual analogue scales, the GHQ and SF-36. This is capable of measuring, recording, calculating and transferring to a computer database all of these measures of PMS and

Table 24.2 Value of blood tests in PMS

Test	Value of diagnosis
Progesterone, day 21	No value
Oestrogen	No proven value
Sex hormone-binding globulin	Marked differences between symptomatic patients shown in one study, not confirmed by others
Prolactin	No value
Follicle-stimulating hormone (FSH)	Excludes perimenopausal
Luteinizing hormone (LH)	May diagnose polycystic ovaries (ovarian scan more appropriate)
Thyroid function tests	Exclusion of hypo- and hyperthyroidism
Electrolytes	No diagnostic value
Haemoglobin	Excludes anaemia as a cause of lethargy

producing 'clinician-friendly' graphic displays (O'Brien, unpublished data).

Blood tests

There are no objective measures such as biochemical tests for PMS. Blood tests may be useful to exclude other disorders such as the menopause, polycystic ovary syndrome, hyper- and hypothyroidism and anaemia (Table 24.2).

Clinical tests

In difficult cases it is of value to use a GnRH depot for 3 months to distinguish to what degree the ovarian cycle contributes to symptoms, i.e. to carry out the goserelin test. Those symptoms persisting after suppression of the cycle must be the consequence of the underlying psychological disorder and not related to ovarian activity.

AETIOLOGY

The aetiology of PMS is unknown though it appears to be directly related to the ovarian cycle trigger. The range of proposed theories is enormous (Fig. 24.4). The recent and most plausible explanations are psychoneuroendocrine theories, particularly in relation to the endogenous opioid peptides and serotonin.

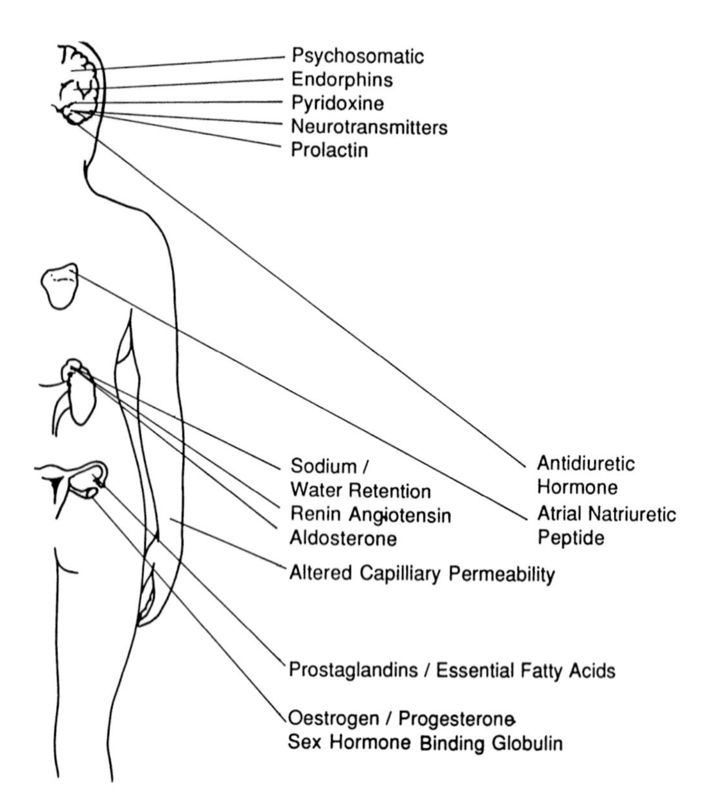

Fig. 24.4 Aetiological theories for PMS.

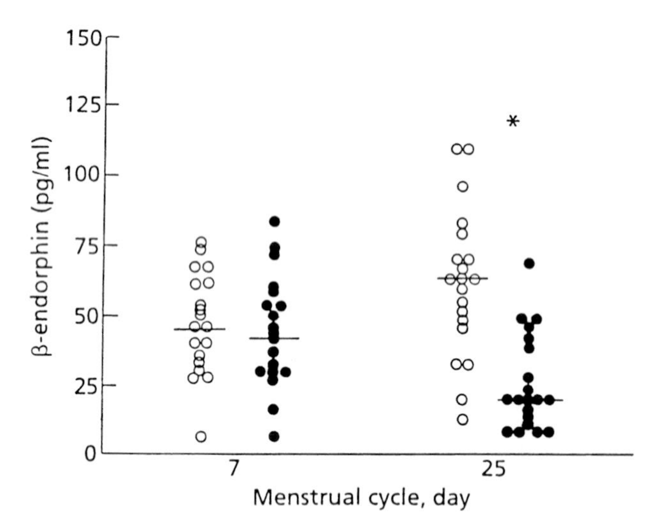

Fig. 24.5 β-endorphin levels in PMS (●) compared with controls (O). The PMS group is significantly different from controls on day 25 ($p < 0.0001$). Bars indicate the median. From Chuong et al (1985) with permission of the publisher, the American Society for Reproductive Medicine (formerly The American Fertility Society).

Neurotransmitters, endorphins, serotonin and vitamin B6

Neurotransmitters probably have a modulatory or mediatory role on neuronal function in PMS. Biogenic amines such as serotonin, dopamine, the endorphins and their synthetic pathway cofactor, vitamin B6, have been considered. Vitamin B6 (pyridoxine) is a cofactor in the final step in the synthesis of serotonin and dopamine from tryptophan. No convincing data have yet demonstrated abnormalities either of brain amine synthesis or deficiency of cofactors such as vitamin B6.

Chuong and colleagues (1985) have demonstrated diminished luteal phase levels of β-endorphin in women with PMS (Fig. 24.5). Symptoms such as anxiety, food craving and physical discomfort have been associated with a significant premenstrual decline in β-endorphin levels (Giannini et al 1994).

Recent interest in the role of serotonin in depression has extended into PMS research. Low serotonin levels in red cells and platelets (Rapkin 1992) have been demonstrated in PMS patients and treatment with selective serotonin reuptake inhibitors such as fluoxetine results in significant improvement in symptoms (Menkes et al 1992).

Prolactin

Prolactin promotes retention of sodium, potassium and water, stimulates the breast and is a so-called stress hormone. Consequently many researchers have investigated its role in PMS. However prolactin does not undergo change during the cycle, PMS patients have normal levels of prolactin and women with hyperprolactinaemia do not report PMS. Therapeutic studies of bromocriptine show no effect on the symptoms, with the notable exception of cyclical mastalgia, and its general role in PMS therapy seems in doubt (O'Brien & Symonds 1982).

Prostaglandins and essential fatty acids

The ubiquitous nature of the prostaglandins makes them candidates for an aetiological role in PMS. Inhibition of synthesis and enhancement using precursors (essential fatty acids) have been claimed to relieve PMS. The underlying theory on which essential fatty acid supplementation is based is unconvincing. In the absence of a demonstrable endocrine abnormality in PMS a differential sensitivity to the endocrine changes of the ovarian cycle has been suggested. In in vitro studies, interactions at a cellular and receptor level have been demonstrated between polyunsaturated essential fatty acids and the activity of oestrogen and progesterone. Defective essential fatty acid/prostaglandin metabolism may give rise to a breakdown in the normal balance or a change in steroid receptor status, allowing an exaggerated response to normal circulating levels of these different hormone systems (Kosikawa et al 1992).

Investigation of essential fatty acid levels in PMS has produced interesting but as yet inconclusive information. Abnormalities in essential fatty acid synthesis have been demonstrated in one study by Brush and colleagues (1984). These findings have not been replicated by others (Menden-Vrtovec & Vujic 1992, O'Brien & Massil 1990).

Sodium and water retention

There can be few articles on PMS which do not refer to premenstrual sodium and water retention. It is surprising, then, to find little scientific data which demonstrates the phenomenon. Women demonstrate an extremely severe subjective sensation of premenstrual bloatedness in the absence of weight increase, changes in abdominal dimensions or any true water or sodium retention (Faratian et al 1984, Hussain 1994). It seems that bloatedness is either perceived or due to gut distension as a result of progesterone-induced relaxation of the gut muscle. One study has demonstrated delay in intestinal transit during the luteal phase of the cycle (Wald et al 1981).

Endocrine effects on fluid and electrolytes

Lack of premenstrual water and electrolyte shift is paralleled by a similar lack of difference in those hormones which control sodium and water transport. The factors which could promote water retention include oestrogen, prolactin, antidiuretic hormone, oxytocin, renin, angiotensin, aldosterone and corticosteroids. Deficiencies of progesterone, atrial natriuretic peptide or renal prostaglandins could also permit water retention by the lack of a natriuretic effect. No clear differences have been demonstrated in any of these, with the exception of atrial natriuretic peptide which appears to be low in the luteal phase in PMS patients (Hussain et al 1990).

Ovarian hormones

It has long been suggested that fluctuation in mood may be related to ovarian hormone imbalance (Dalton 1977). Research has produced data which could support theories of oestrogen excess, progesterone deficiency, oestrogen/progesterone imbalance and progesterone excess. None of these has been confirmed and thus, factors other than differences in the levels of individual hormones must be important. Interactions with other endocrine or biochemical systems may operate, or differences in receptor status may be relevant.

A link with ovarian hormone changes, particularly progesterone, seems likely however, since the temporal relationship between progesterone secretion and symptoms is so close. There is good evidence to suggest that symptoms are directly linked to ovarian hormone changes. Ablation of the menstrual cycle by oophorectomy or more conveniently by the administration of analogues of GnRH is associated with the parallel elimination of PMS symptoms (Hussain et al 1992) (Fig. 24.6). Furthermore, in women whose ovarian cycles have ceased (due to the menopause or bilateral oophorectomy) and who subsequently receive HRT, a significant percentage develop PMS symptoms during the progesterone phase of therapy (Hammarback et al 1985).

In a recent pilot study, women with severe PMS who had undergone hysterectomy and bilateral salpingo-oophorectomy were recruited to assess the effects of hormone replacement on their PMS symptoms (Henshaw et

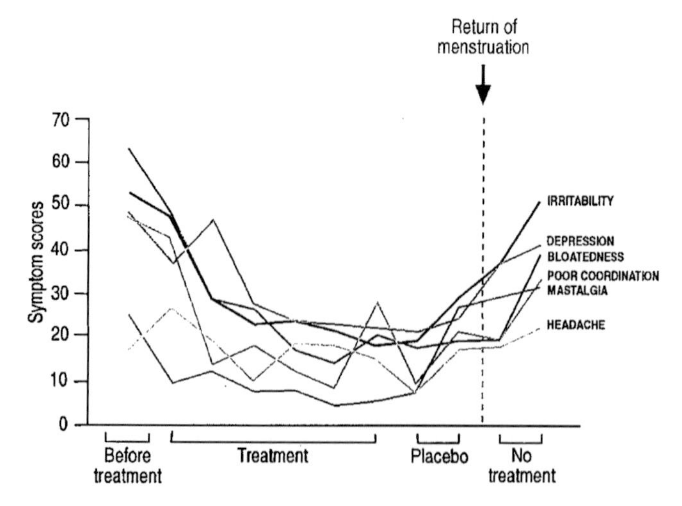

Fig. 24.6 Effect of GnRH analogue on premenstrual symptoms, showing elimination of symptoms whilst ovarian function is suppressed with return of symptoms prior to the return of menstruation during placebo. Adapted from Hussain et al (1992).

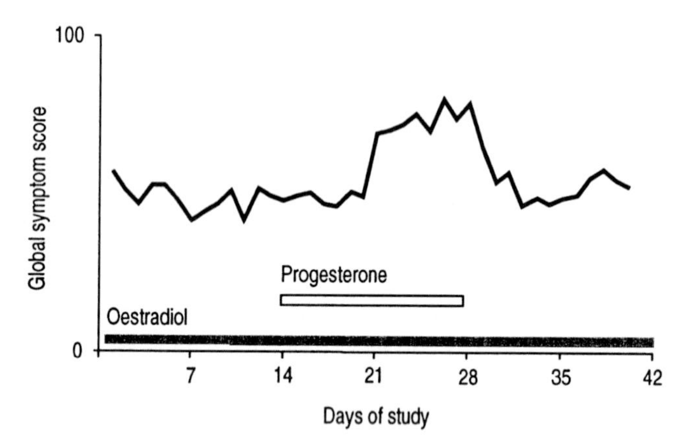

Fig. 24.7 Simulation of PMS symptoms in PMS patients after bilateral oophorectomy and hysterectomy. PMS symptoms recur during progesterone treatment but not during unopposed oestrogen. Adapted from Henshaw et al (1993).

al 1993). During oestrogen-only replacement therapy they remained asymptomatic; when progesterone was administered PMS symptoms recurred (Fig. 24.7), demonstrating fairly clearly that patients remained sensitive to the effects of ovarian hormones and that the ovarian hormones are directly responsible for the PMS.

MANAGEMENT

Diagnosis

We have seen that there is no objective method of identifying or quantifying PMS. For practical clinical purposes, reliance is placed on the history, questionnaires, exclusion of certain specific disorders and the use of prospectively administered symptom-rating methods. The simpler charts indicate only the timing and character of the symptoms; the degree to which they disrupt the patient's and her family's life is not easily quantifiable. These precise and sensitive charts are too cumbersome for routine clinical use.

The availability of the hand-held PMS Symptometrics device will simplify the measurement of PMS quite significantly.

Differential diagnosis

Unlike most medical problems, the majority of patients with PMS present self-diagnosed to the gynaecologist. The doctor's task is to confirm or exclude this diagnosis. Many disorders have been wrongly attributed to PMS (Table 24.3). We have already suggested that physiological premenstrual changes often cause patients to seek advice although the symptoms are not particularly severe. Women with psychiatric disorders unrelated to the menstrual cycle often find it more acceptable to label their problem as PMS.

The essence of diagnosis is the cyclicity of the symptoms. If they are not relieved by the end of menstruation, then an alternative explanation must be sought. This is equally true for somatic problems. Noncyclical breast pain

Table 24.3 Differential diagnosis of PMS

Psychiatric disorders
- May be confused because of the similarity in symptoms and because of the bipolar and periodic nature of some psychiatric disorders.
- Many women prefer to 'label' their psychological inadequacies as gynaecological rather than psychiatric.
- There are no objective tests but there are many questionnaires. The General Health Questionnaire may help (Goldberg & Hillier 1979).

Intrafamilial and psychosexual problems
- Distinguish between cause and effect.

Other causes of breast symptoms
- Cyclical breast pain may be considered part of PMS. Can be distinguished from noncyclical breast disease by history.
- Noncyclical disease includes severe disorders requiring breast examination and maybe mammography, ultrasonography, aspiration and biopsy.
- Breast cancer must, of course, be excluded.

Other causes of abdominal bloatedness and water retention
- Only a few women exhibit significant water retention in PMS.
- More women have idiopathic oedema which is also cyclical but only occasionally coincides by chance with the menstrual cycle.
- Some women call progressive obesity 'PMS bloatedness'.
- These can all be distinguished by twice daily weighing.

Endometriosis, pelvic infection and dysmenorrhoea
- Primary dysmenorrhoea occurs with period.
- Secondary dysmenorrhoea is related to pelvic pathology.
- Laparoscopy will exclude endometriosis or pelvic infection.

Medical causes of lethargy/tiredness and anxiety/irritability
- Occasionally anaemia; haemoglobin estimation.
- Rarely hypothyroidism or hyperthyroidism; thyroid function tests.

Menopause
- May be confused in patients over 40.
- Flushes may occur in PMS.
- Usually distinguished from history.
- Raised follicle-stimulating hormone level.

may well be due to noncyclical underlying breast pathology. Cyclical mastalgia is a part of PMS and responds to similar therapeutic measures.

Premenstrual pelvic pain must be distinguished from that due to endometriosis, by laparoscopy if necessary.

Cyclical or idiopathic oedema is a separate problem from PMS though its cyclical nature and frequent association with psychological symptoms may cause confusion. There is nearly always a history of diuretic abuse. The original reason for the diuretic use may have been for the treatment of premenstrual bloatedness or as an adjunct to diet for weight reduction; both are inappropriate indications for diuretics.

Lethargy due to hypothyroidism or anaemia may rarely be confused with PMS. Anxiety and irritability may result from hyperthyroidism. The presence of other characteristic symptoms will usually distinguish these and the diagnosis can be excluded by the appropriate blood tests.

Two gynaecological problems which are confused with PMS are dysmenorrhoea and the menopause; these are distinctly different problems. The latter is frequently confused in older menstruating women but this may be identified by measuring gonadotrophin levels.

Examination

Though the physical examination of the PMS patient will make little contribution to her diagnosis, the importance of opportunistic screening and the exclusion of disorders which may mimic somatic symptoms (i.e. pelvic pain, abdominal bloatedness) must be stressed. Reassurance that there is no breast, cervical or pelvic cancer is of particular value and, of course, patients should not receive hormonal therapy without such an examination.

A definitive test for PMS?

When doubt exists this is usually because there are coincident problems and the patient suffers from secondary PMS. It is now possible to identify what proportion of the disorder is due to the ovarian hormone change by administering a depot preparation of a GnRH agonist analogue, such as goserelin, for 3 months. There may be an exacerbation of symptoms in the first month of evaluation. These should be ignored. By the third month of amenorrhoea, persisting symptoms cannot be due to PMS. Thus, if no symptoms remain at all her diagnosis is primary PMS. If symptoms persist with equal intensity her problem is not due to the ovarian cycle. The relative cyclical and noncyclical components of secondary PMS can thus be separated.

TREATMENT

Currently treatment is offered in the absence of an aetiological explanation and must therefore be empirical, with little scientific foundation on which to base the techniques used.

Treatment depends on the diagnosis and classification. For secondary PMS, treatment of the underlying psychological component should be related directly to its nature. Severe depression should be treated by antidepressants.

Alteration of a patient's threshold to the cyclical events of the menstrual cycle may be achieved less invasively by psychotherapy, counselling or stress management and less conventional methods like hypnosis and, possibly, acupuncture. Improvement in the patient's general health and well-being through diet and exercise has also been claimed to achieve these goals. It is probable that measures like these will reduce mild underlying psychological problems, and raise the patient's tolerance to the challenge of her premenstrual changes. The informal psychotherapeutic effect of discussion, counselling and education should not be overlooked.

When considering claims for drug efficacy it must be remembered that placebo responses in excess of 90% have been reported in some studies (Magos et al 1986). Studies of PMS therapy can only be interpreted if adequate placebo controls are included in the study design.

The range of therapy

The range of proposed therapeutic regimes has been very wide and varied (Table 24.4). This may result partly from the high but short-lived placebo effect in that an apparently good response is readily observed on most therapy.

Table 24.4 Range of treatment approaches for PMS for which success has been claimed

Nonpharmacological	Nonhormonal	Hormonal
Rest	Pyridoxine	Progestogens
Isolation	Essential fatty acids	Progesterone
Psychotherapy	Vitamins	Oral contraception
Education	Diuretics	Testosterone
Yoga	Aldosterone antagonists	Danazol
Self-help groups	Clonidine	Bromocriptine
Counselling	Non-steroidal anti-inflammatories	Hormone implants
Intravaginal electrical stimulation	Beta-blockers	GnRH analogues
Diet	Vitamins	Mifepristone
Music therapy	Zinc	
Hypnosis	Tranquillizers	
Homeopathy	Antidepressants	
Acupuncture	Phenobarbitone	
Stress management	Lithium	
Nutritional manipulation	Immune complexes	
Salt restriction	Antifungals	
Irradiation of ovaries	Naltrexone	
Bilateral oophorectomy	Selective serotonin reuptake inhibitors (SSRIs)	
Endometrial ablation		
Hysterectomy		

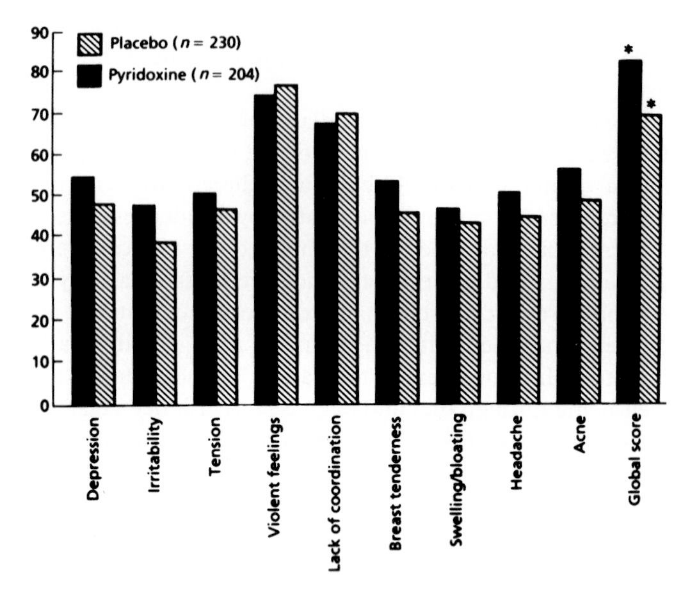

Fig. 24.8 Effect of vitamin B6 (pyridoxine) and placebo on premenstrual symptoms; *p < 0.02 for global symptoms. From Williams et al (1985).

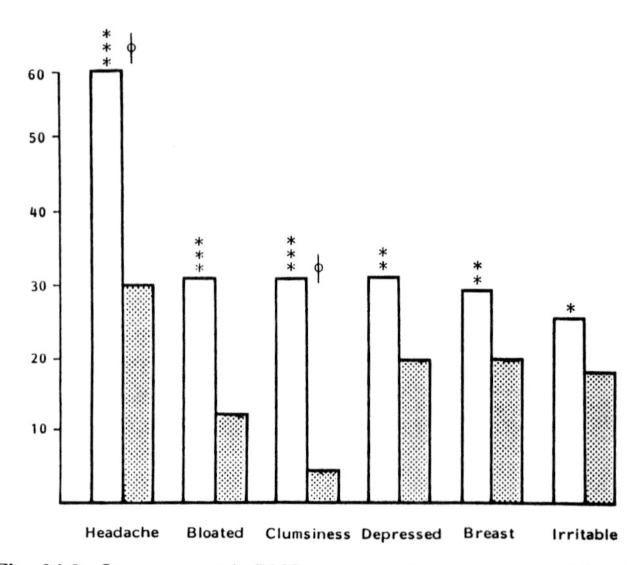

Fig. 24.9 Improvement in PMS symptoms during treatment following supplementation with linoleic and gammalinolenic acid. Although significant improvements are seen when the effect is compared to baseline placebo(*), differences in favour of active therapy (ϕ) are not statistically strong. From O'Brien & Massil (1990).

Secondly, the lack of long-term benefit leads to the quest for new methods.

Vitamin B6

Vitamin B6 is a cofactor in the final stages of neurotransmitter synthesis, particularly of serotonin and dopamine, from tryptophan. No abnormalities of these neurotransmitters or vitamin B6 have been identified. The results of trials are contradictory and it is difficult to ascertain how much improvement is attributable to placebo effect and to what extent there is a true pharmacotherapeutic response. In the trial of Williams et al (1985), which was possibly the largest, global symptom assessment showed significant improvement in 82% of patients compared with 70% on placebo (Fig. 24.8).

There has been concern about side-effects (reversible peripheral neuropathy) at high doses of vitamin B6. In practice, many patients will have self-prescribed vitamin B6 before consulting their doctor.

Oil of evening primrose

Oil of evening primrose contains the polyunsaturated essential fatty acids linoleic and gammalinolenic acids. These are the dietary precursors of several prostaglandins, mainly E_2 and E_1. It has been postulated that deficiency of E series prostaglandins and polyunsaturated fatty acids allows an enhanced response to physiological levels of the ovarian hormones. There is one study demonstrating limited benefit over placebo for certain symptoms (Fig. 24.9; O'Brien & Massil 1990).

Diuretics

The majority of women who experience bloatedness and a feeling of weight increase have no objectively demonstrable premenstrual weight increase, sodium or water retention (Hussain, 1994). There is a small group of women who experience true premenstrual water retention. Those with clearly demonstrable oedema or measured weight increase (and not simply bloatedness) may benefit from treatment with an aldosterone antagonist. Spironolactone has been shown to be effective for PMS symptoms, particularly those of swelling (Vellacott & O'Brien 1987).

Selective serotonin reuptake inhibitors (SSRIs)

Significant improvement of premenstrual symptoms has been shown in patients treated with this group of drugs. Altered serotonergic function has been reported in patients with premenstrual syndrome (Rapkin 1992). Serotonin deficiency possibly makes women with severe PMS more sensitive to their endogenous ovarian steroid cycle than women with physiological premenstrual symptoms. Boosting serotonin should improve symptoms, and several SSRI drugs, including clomipramine and fluoxetine, appear to be effective (Menkes et al 1992).

Hormonal therapy

Oral contraceptive pill

There are no conclusive recent therapeutic studies of lower oestrogen dose preparations nor of the progestogen-only pills. In the majority of studies women who had taken higher dose combined pills were compared with non-pill users. It is likely that the control groups comprised non-responders and those whose worsening of symptoms caused them to discontinue the pill. Results would thus be inherently biased. It would appear that pill users report less PMS than those using barrier contraception. In the earliest studies of the higher dose preparations Cullberg (1972) reported that oestrogen-dominant pills exacerbated symptoms, whilst those which were strongly progestogenic were associated with a reduction in PMS.

The response in an individual woman cannot be predicted. In a review of PMS in users of the combined oral contraceptive pill, Smith (1975) concluded that any of the following results could be expected:

1. complete relief of symptoms;
2. continuation of symptoms but limited to 1 or 2 days premenstrually;
3. intolerance of the pill;
4. no change.

More recent studies have not changed these conclusions.

Using the pill empirically and assessing the effect in suitable women is thus worthwhile. No evaluation of the continuous combined pill has yet been conducted, though such an approach would be logical.

Progestogens

Dydrogesterone and many other progestogens have been advocated on the basis of the unproven progesterone-deficiency theory for PMS. There are many uncontrolled studies of these preparations. One double-blind controlled study of dydrogesterone suggested trends in favour of the active drug. A later study by Dennerstein et al (1986) failed to demonstrate such improvement.

Progesterone

Progesterone as pessaries, injections and the oral micronized form have been advocated as replacement of so-called progesterone deficiency. To date no study of progesterone pessaries has demonstrated benefit superior to that of placebo (Fig. 24.10). At least 10 such studies have now been conducted. The data of Dennerstein et al (1985) suggest that oral micronized progesterone is more effective than identical placebo; however, this conclusion has been criticized on statistical grounds. In a study which most closely evaluates Dalton's regimen (Freeman et al 1990) no differences between progesterone pessaries and placebo were shown.

Progesterone and progestogen continue to be prescribed because of the large number of anecdotal reports of efficacy. If these hormones are effective it is unlikely that progesterone deficiency is being corrected but more

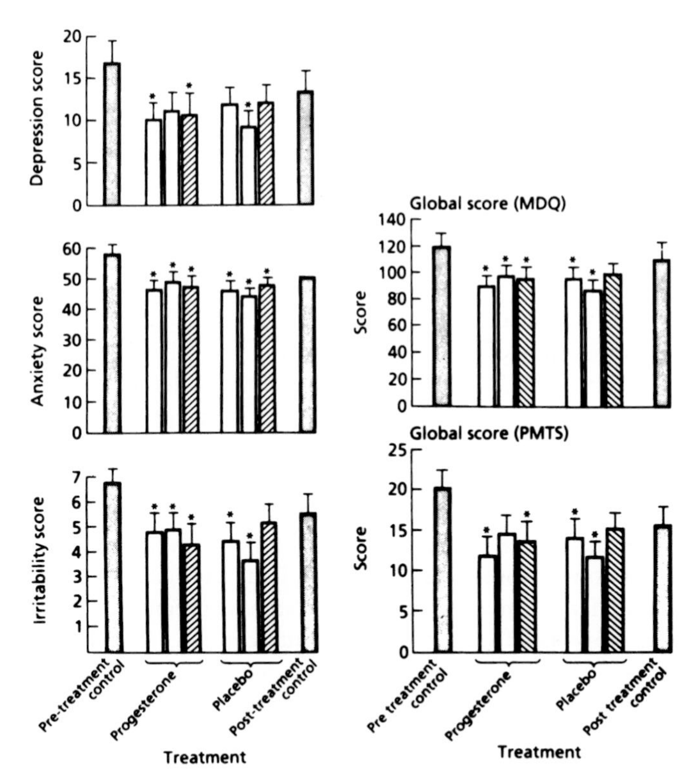

Fig. 24.10 Effect of progesterone suppositories and placebo on irritability, depression, anxiety and global score over 3 months. Although improvement is significant compared with baseline control for both placebo and active therapy, no differences are demonstrable between the two treatments. No abatement of placebo or enhancement of progesterone effect is seen with time. MDQ, menstrual distress questionnaire; PMTS, premenstrual tension symptoms. From Maddocks et al (1986).

likely that the endogenous hormone milieu is being disturbed or progesterone is acting as a 'minor tranquillizer'.

Bromocriptine

Although prolactin had originally been considered a potential candidate as the pathogenic agent in PMS, no studies have demonstrated differences in PMS nor have cyclical changes been clearly shown. Several workers have assessed the efficacy of bromocriptine in PMS treatment. The data of the study by Andersen and colleagues (1977) encompass the relevant conclusions to be drawn. Bromocriptine 5 mg daily from days 10 to 26 of the menstrual cycle effectively relieves cyclical breast symptoms but has little effect on the remaining symptoms of PMS.

Suppression of the menstrual cycle

If PMS is the direct or indirect consequence of the ovarian endocrine cycle then elimination of this cycle should be the definitive treatment of PMS. Frank (1931) advocated irradiation of the ovaries and claimed a marked benefit. Bilateral oophorectomy (but of course not hysterectomy alone) cures the ovarian component of PMS. Less invasive means of suppressing the endogenous ovarian cycle include the use of continuous combined oral contraception, continuous progestogen, danazol, oestradiol implants and transcutaneous patches and GnRH analogues. The first two of these have not been formally studied.

Danazol

Mansel & Wisbey (1980) assessed the effect of danazol on PMS symptoms as part of a study primarily aimed at treating breast pain. No convincing benefit was demonstrated except for the good response for breast symptoms. Subsequent studies have demonstrated benefit for several symptoms in doses of 400, 200 and 100 mg daily (Watts et al 1987).

Serious side-effects of masculinization are largely avoided at lower doses, but the risk of masculinization of a female fetus remains a possibility should pregnancy arise and appropriate mechanical contraception should be advised. In an attempt to avoid side-effects, a placebo-controlled study of 106 patients was conducted where luteal phase-only danazol was administered (Abukhalil & O'Brien, unpublished data). Whilst effective treatment was achieved for mastalgia no significant improvement was demonstrated for other PMS symptoms.

Oestradiol implants and transdermal patches

Suppression of the cycle can be achieved by transdermal oestradiol patches or by implants, with relief of PMS symptoms (Fig. 24.11; Magos et al 1986, Watson et al 1989).

In practice a significant number of patients withdraw from treatment because of the regeneration of symptoms by the progestogen which is necessary to prevent endometrial neoplasia. Levonorgestrel IUCDs have the potential to provide endometrial protection; the low blood progestogen levels attained avoid the regeneration of PMS.

Testosterone implants have also been given when diminished libido is a significant symptom. Most gynaecologists would reserve oestradiol implants for severe cases and in those for whom the menopause is imminent.

GnRH analogues

Agonist analogues of GnRH have been used in several clinical disorders where it is necessary to suppress the gonadal production of steroids. These include prostatic and breast cancer, endometriosis and fibroids, and recently the value of GnRH analogues in PMS has been assessed. In early trials an unclear picture emerged which was probably related to incomplete suppression of ovarian function. Muse et al (1984) demonstrated a clearer result. Adequate suppression of the cycle was associated with elimination of symptoms on active therapy but not with placebo. Similar results have been obtained using buserelin (Hussain et al 1992) and monthly depot preparations of goserelin. Unfortunately, symptoms return with ovarian function in all patients (Hussain et al 1992) (Fig. 24.6).

Thus GnRH analogues do not provide a permanent 'cure' for PMS and this is not surprising. To provide effective therapy the analogue treatment would need to be given indefinitely. Such treatment will be precluded by the genesis of menopausal side-effects, the most worrying of

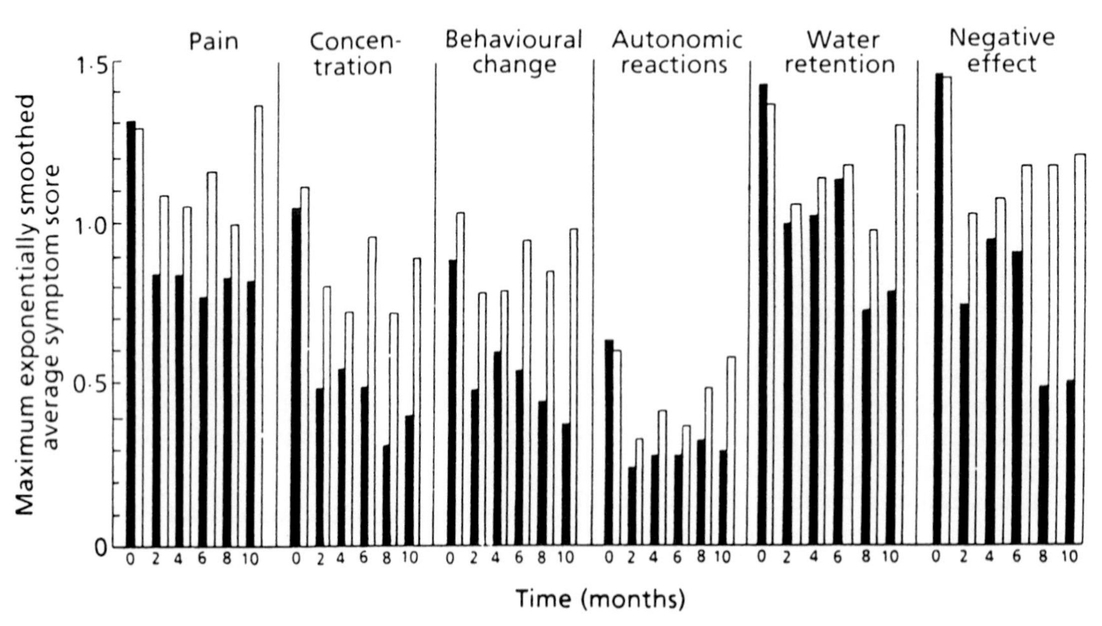

Fig. 24.11 Effect of oestradiol implant and norethisterone on PMS symptoms compared to placebo. The marked placebo effect is seen initially but the continued response is only seen during active therapy. From Magos et al (1986) with permission of BMJ Publishing Group.

which is osteoporosis. It has been well documented (see Ch. 30) that significant trabecular bone loss occurs after only 6 months of analogue treatment. Mortola et al (1991) have shown that 'add back' therapy with oestrogen replacement is successful; whether GnRH analogue plus 'add back' has anything to offer over and above oestrogen replacement alone remains to be determined.

The use of GnRH analogues in PMS serves the following purposes.

1. It allows us to determine what proportion of symptoms are of ovarian endocrine origin.
2. It pinpoints which patients with severe PMS would benefit from bilateral oophorectomy.
3. It offers short-term therapy of 6 months in particular circumstances.
4. It may be useful for women in whom oestrogens are contraindicated and who are shortly to reach the menopause.

Surgery

The role of surgery in the treatment of PMS is controversial. Endometrial ablation and hysterectomy have been advocated but of course these are illogical as ovarian function persists. Symptoms persist after hysterectomy alone, but total hysterectomy with bilateral salpingo-oophorectomy is curative (Casson et al 1990). Patients must first be identified as being treatable in this fashion following a positive goserelin test. Surgery must be followed by oestrogen replacement therapy which should be unopposed; cyclical progestogen is unnecessary and could result in the return of premenstrual symptoms. This treatment approach is the only lasting cure for PMS but it can rarely be justified except in severely affected women. Laparoscopic oophorectomy has been suggested as a less invasive alternative, but this would require opposed HRT to protect the uterus. One uncontrolled study supports the use of endometrial ablation in the treatment of PMS (Lefler & Lefler 1992).

There are two important points to make in relation to surgery for severe unresponsive PMS. First, it would seem wise to perform a goserelin test before embarking on surgery. Second, it is appropriate for all women undergoing hysterectomy to be assessed with respect to PMS prior to any discussions of ovarian conservation or removal.

CONCLUSIONS

If we were to treat PMS symptoms only with regimes which have conclusively been shown to be superior to placebo we would have little to offer PMS patients. Any treatment we do offer will scientifically contradict the majority of statements we have already made and will be essentially empirical and hierarchical (Fig. 24.12). All women with PMS cannot be treated with danazol, oestrogen implants, GnRH analogues or oophorectomy. However, only patients with a severity of PMS which warrants major intervention should be referred for gynaecological evaluation.

In the absence of a clearly identifiable endocrine abnormality it is possible that PMS should not be considered a gynaecological disorder, as it is likely that it represents a psychological or biochemical predisposition to the normal physiological endocrine events of the ovarian cycle. Although women would prefer to label their problem as gynaecological rather than psychiatric or psychological, gynaecologists, who are often accused of being unsympathetic to women's needs, should not be coerced into dealing with a problem which is not necessarily gynaecological and frequently has a large psychological component.

PMS is a disorder which should be dealt with primarily by the general practitioner, family planning and women's health care units or, for patients with severe secondary PMS, by the psychiatrist. If treatment cannot be achieved by these measures then the gynaecologist may be called upon to manipulate or suppress normal ovarian function either endocrinologically or surgically.

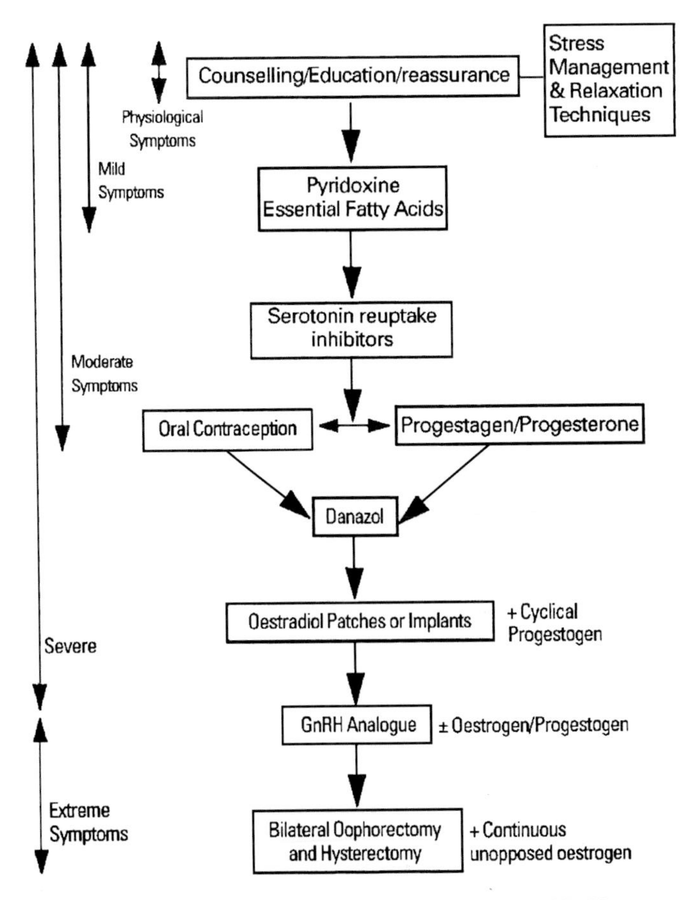

Fig. 24.12 Hierarchical approach to the management of PMS.

KEY POINTS

1. Premenstrual syndrome is a disorder of unknown aetiology.
2. The prevalence of premenstrual syndrome has been reported as ranging from 5 to 95% which probably reflects the imprecision of diagnostic criteria rather than any biological factor.
3. The diagnosis is often confusing and many other disorders may be confused with it.
4. The symptoms are numerous, producing social, familial or occupational disruption. They should have occurred in at least four of the six previous cycles before a firm diagnosis can be made.
5. There are no objective means of identifying or quantifying PMS, and for practical purposes reliance is placed on the history, questionnaires, computer-aided assessment devices and the exclusion of other specific disorders.
6. Only 5% of women are completely symptom-free premenstrually.
7. Up to 95% of women experience at least one premenstrual symptom but many of these are tolerated with no interference with a woman's normal functioning.
8. Primary PMS is a disorder of nonspecific somatic psychological or behavioural symptoms, recurring in the premenstrual phase and being resolved completely by the end of menstruation.
9. Secondary PMS is a disorder of nonspecific somatic psychological or behavioural symptoms, recurring in the premenstrual phase of the menstrual cycle and improving but not completely resolving by the end of menstruation.
10. It is implied that in secondary PMS there is an underlying psychological disorder.
11. Treatment is offered in the absence of a specific aetiological explanation and must therefore be empirical and hierarchical; an accurate diagnosis is paramount in directing therapy.
12. The placebo response is high.
13. If PMS is the direct or indirect consequence of the ovarian endocrine cycle, then elimination of this cycle should confirm the diagnosis and also offer the definitive means of treatment.

REFERENCES

Anderson A N, Larsen J G, Steenstrup O R, Svendstrup B, Nielsen J 1977 Effect of bromocriptine on the premenstrual syndrome. A double-blind clinical trial. British Journal of Obstetrics and Gynaecology 84: 370–374

Brush M G, Watson S J, Horrobin D F, Manku M S 1984 Abnormal essential fatty acid levels in plasma of women with premenstrual syndrome. American Journal of Obstetrics and Gynecology 150: 262–266

Budeiri D J, Li Wan Po A, Dornan J C 1994 Clinical trials of treatments of premenstrual syndrome: entry criteria and scales for measuring treatment outcomes. British Journal of Obstetrics and Gynaecology 101: 689–695

Casson P, Hahn P M, Van Vugt D A, Reid R L 1990 Lasting response to ovariectomy in severe intractable premenstrual syndrome. American Journal of Obstetrics and Gynecology 162: 99–105

Chuong C J, Coulam C B, Kao P C, Bergstrahl E J, Go V L W 1985 Neuropeptide levels in premenstrual syndrome. Fertility and Sterility 44: 760–765

Cullberg J 1972 Mood changes and menstrual symptoms with different gestagen/oestrogen combinations. Acta Psychiatrica Scandinavica 236(suppl): 1–86

Dalton K 1977 The premenstrual syndrome and progesterone therapy. Heinemann, London

Dennerstein L, Spencer-Gardner C, Gotts G, Brown J B, Smith M A, Burrows G D 1985 Progesterone and the premenstrual syndrome: a double-blind crossover trial. British Medical Journal 290: 1617–1621

Dennerstein L, Morse C, Gotts G et al 1986 The treatment of premenstrual syndrome. A double-blind trial of dydrogesterone. Journal of Affective Disorders 11: 199–205

Faratian B, Gaspar A, O'Brien P M S, Filshie G M, Johnson I R, Prescott P 1984 Premenstrual syndrome: weight, abdominal size and perceived body image. American Journal of Obstetrics and Gynecology 150: 200–204

Frank R T 1931 The hormonal causes of premenstrual tension. Archives of Neurology and Psychiatry 26: 1053–1057

Freeman E, Rickel K, Sondheimer S J, Polansky M 1990 Ineffectiveness of progesterone suppository treatment for premenstrual syndrome. Journal of the American Medical Association 264: 349–353

Giannini A J, Melemis S M, Martin D M, Folts D J 1994 Symptoms of premenstrual syndrome as a function of beta-endorphin: two subtypes. Progress in Neuro-Psychopharmacology and Biological Psychiatry 18(2): 321–327

Goldberg D P, Hillier B 1979 A scaled version of the general health questionnaire. Psychological Medicine 9: 139–145

Hammarback S, Backstrom T, Hoist J, von Schoultz B, Lyrenas S 1985 Cyclical mood changes as in the premenstrual tension syndrome using sequential oestrogen–progestagen postmenopausal replacement therapy. Acta Obstetrica et Gynecologica Scandinavica 64: 393–397

Henshaw C, O'Brien P M S, Foreman D, Belcher J, Cox J 1993 An experimental model for PMS. Neuropsychopharmacology 9(25): 713

Hussain S Y 1994 The compartmental distribution of fluid and electrolytes in relation to the symptomatology of the ovarian cycle and premenstrual cycle. PhD thesis. University of London

Hussain S Y, O'Brien P M S, De Souza V F, Okonofua F, Dandona P 1990 Reduced artial natriuretic peptide concentrations in premenstrual syndrome. British Journal of Obstetrics and Gynaecology 97: 397–401

Hussain S Y, Massil J H, Matta W H, Shaw R W, O'Brien P M S 1992 Buserelin in premenstrual syndrome. Gynaecological Endocrinology 6: 57–64

Kosikawa N, Tatsunuma T, Furuya K, Seki K 1992 Prostaglandins and premenstrual syndrome. Prostaglandins, Leukotrienes and Essential Fatty Acids 45(1): 33–36

Lefler H T, Lefler C F 1992 Endometrial ablation. Improvement in PMS related to improvement in bleeding. Journal of Reproductive Medicine 37: 596–598

Maddocks S, Hahn P, Moller F, Reid R L 1986 A double-blind placebo-controlled trial of progesterone vaginal suppositories in the treatment of premenstrual syndrome. American Journal of Obstetrics and Gynecology 154: 573–581

Magos A L, Brincat M, Studd J W 1986 Treatment of premenstrual syndrome by subcutaneous oestradiol implants and cyclical oral norethisterone: placebo controlled study. British Medical Journal 292: 1629–1633

Mansel R E, Wisbey J R 1980 The effect of gonadotrophin suppression by danazol on symptomatic breast disease. British Journal of Surgery 67: 827

Menden-Vrtovec H, Vujic D 1992 Bromocriptine (Bromergon, Lek) in the management of premenstrual syndrome. Clinical and Experimental Obstetrics and Gynecology 19(4): 242–249

Menkes D B, Ebrahim T, Mason P A, Spears G F S, Howard R C 1992 Fluoxetine treatment for severe premenstrual syndrome. British Medical Journal 305: 346–347
Moos R 1985 Premenstrual symptoms: a manual and overview of research with the menstrual distress questionnaire. Department of Psychiatry and Behavioural Sciences, Stanford University School of Medicine, Palo Alto, California, USA
Mortola J F, Girton L, Fischer U 1991 Successful treatment of premenstrual syndrome by combined use of gonadotrophin releasing hormone agonist and estrogen/progestin. Journal of Endocrinology and Metabolism 72: 252A–252F
Muse K, Cete N, Futterman L, Yen S 1984 The premenstrual syndrome. Effects of 'medical ovariectomy'. New England Journal of Medicine 311: 1345–1349
O'Brien P M S 1987 Premenstrual syndrome. Blackwell Scientific, Oxford
O'Brien P M S, Massil H 1990 Premenstrual syndrome: clinical studies on essential fatty acids. In: Horrobin D F (ed) Omega-6-essential fatty acids: pathology and role in clinical medicine. Wiley/Liss, New York, pp 523–545
O'Brien P M S, Symonds E M 1982 Prolactin levels in the premenstrual syndrome. British Journal of Obstetrics and Gynaecology 89: 306–308
Rapkin A J 1992 The role of serotonin in premenstrual syndrome. Clinical Obstetrics and Gynaecology 35: 658–666
Smith S L 1975 Mood and the menstrual cycle. In: Sachar E J (ed) Topics in psychoendocrinology. Grune & Stratton, New York, pp 19–58
Vellacott I D, O'Brien P M S 1987 Effects of spironolactone on premenstrual symptoms. Journal of Reproductive Medicine 32: 429–434
Wald A, Van Thiel D H, Hoechsletter I et al 1981 Gastrointestinal transit: the effect of the menstrual cycle. Gastroenterology 80: 1497–1500
Ware J E, Sherbourne C D 1992 The MOS 36-item short-form health survey (SF-36): I Conceptual framework and item selection. Medical Care 30: 473–483
Watson N R, Studd J W W, Savvas M, Garnett T, Baber R J 1989 Treatment of severe PMS with oestradiol patches and cyclical norethisterone. Lancet 2: 730–732
Watts J F, Butt W R, Logan Edwards R 1987 A clinical trial using danazol for the treatment of premenstrual tension. British Journal of Obstetrics and Gynaecology 94: 30–34
Williams M J, Harris R I, Dean B C 1985 Controlled trial of pyridoxine in the premenstrual syndrome. Journal of International Medical Research 13: 174–179

25

The menopause

Mark Brincat   Yves Muscat Baron   Ray Galea

INTRODUCTION

The menopause constitutes a watershed in a woman's life that leads to profound changes in several systems. As the realization of the multisystem nature of these changes ranging from psychological to bone to cardiovascular has developed, so also has the awareness that many of these changes can be prevented or completely modified with therapy. The mainstay of this therapy continues to be the appropriate use of oestrogen.

The population is ageing as the total lifespan of women has gradually increased. At the time of the Roman Empire, the average life expectancy of women was only 23 years (Schneider 1986). From the Middle Ages until the late 19th century, fewer than 30% of women reached the menopause. Today with the average life expectancy of women being 78 years, there are just under 10 million postmenopausal women in the United States. This constitutes 17% of the total population.

Women can now spend up to one third of their lives after the menopause in a state of profound oestrogen deprivation. The realization of the profound changes that occur as a result of this ovarian failure and the relatively simple treatments that are available for the condition make it imperative that more effort should be dedicated to the study of the postmenopausal years with specialist clinics being more widely available to women.

AGE OF ONSET

The average age of the menopause has not changed over the centuries. Amudsen & Diers (1973) quote several authors who all give the average age of the menopause at around 50 years. Amongst them are Aristotle (50 years; sixth century AD), Paulus Aegineta (50 years; seventh century AD), Hildegard (50 years; 12th century AD), Gilbertus Anglicus (50 years; 13th century AD). Currently, the average age of the menopause has been estimated as being 51 years.

Thus the age of the menopause does not appear to be related to the age of menarche, socioeconomic factors, race, poverty, weight or height. The only factor that apparently may influence the age of onset of the menopause is cigarette smoking which lowers it (Frie 1980, Wilson et al 1985). Race does not seem to influence the real age of the menopause. McKinlay et al 1972) report the same menopausal age in caucasians as Frere (1971) does in South African black women.

DEFINITIONS

The climacteric is commonly referred to as that period of time around the menopause when ovarian function is erratic, with partial gonadal failure occurring in the 2–3 year transitional phase during which reproduction ceases. This is a time of decreasing fertility, decreasing plasma oestrogen levels and the appearance of the typical symptoms of the menopausal syndrome, although of course the menstrual periods will still be present.

The menopause is the one fixed event of the climacteric. This refers to the last menstrual bleed, and subsequent unscheduled vaginal bleeding must be regarded as an abnormality which requires investigation. The menopause is generally considered to have occurred retrospectively after one year of amenorrhoea.

PATHOPHYSIOLOGY

The ageing of the ovary with a progressive decrease in the number of follicles begins even before birth (Baker 1963). The percentage of growing follicles markedly increases at puberty and is maintained through most of the reproductive life but decreases at the menopause.

The mean weight of the ovary begins to decrease at the age of 30 years (Nikko, 1986). Table 25.1 gives a summary of the endocrine changes that occur at the climacteric. A detailed description is beyond the scope of this chapter.

CONSEQUENCES OF OVARIAN FAILURE

The primary causative deficiency that leads to the clinical consequences of ovarian failure is that of oestrogen deficiency. The high levels of follicle-stimulating hormone (FSH) and luteinizing hormone (LH) are irrelevant to the production of symptoms but a single plasma FSH level of >15 IU/l would be diagnostic of the menopausal state (Chakravati et al 1976).

The well recognized reduction in bone mass, the development of what are currently regarded as adverse changes in serum lipoprotein level, the generalized atrophy of all connective tissues, (after several years after the onset of the menopause) can be directly attributed to oestrogen deficiency. In addition, evidence is also emerging that the increased incidence in dementia in older women could also be related to a lack of oestrogens.

There are other more immediate symptoms associated with the climacteric referred to collectively as the 'menopausal syndrome'. This term describes various physical and psychological symptoms which certain women develop, and once again it would seem that it is ovarian failure that contributes to this condition. This syndrome can predate the menopause. The various associated symptoms which are described can also be attributed to fluctuating levels of sex hormones and gonadotrophins but the exact relationship between the two remains unclear.

Table 25.1 Summary of endocrine changes at the climacteric

Phase I. Hypothalamic–pituitary hyperactivity
Starts 10–15 years before menopause
Compensatory for increased resistance of ovarian follicles and decreased follicular hormone secretion
Evidence by raised FSH and, later LH; pituitary may become exhausted, late postmenopause

Phase II. Ovulation and corpus luteum failure
Occurs in most women with increasing frequency as menopause approaches; anovulatory cycles or shortened luteal phase
Deficient dysfunctional uterine bleeding, endometrial hyperplasia and carcinoma

Phase III. Ovarian follicular failure
Failure of follicular development causes fall in oestradiol secretion and cessation of menses
Ovarian stroma remains active; with adrenal cortex, produces androstenedione and testosterone
Oestrone, produced by extraglandular conversion of androgens, is the main postmenopausal oestrogen; only 10–50% of postmenopausal women are truly oestrogen-deficient

SHORT-TERM CONSEQUENCES

Numerous short-term symptoms of the menopause have been documented. Table 25.2 indicates the commonest ones presenting in the immediate postmenopausal period. Many of these short-term (immediate) symptoms were shown to be present in a group of young women following hysterectomy and bilateral oophorectomy (Chakravati et al 1976) and in another group who had been subjected to radiation menopause of their ovaries as a result of radiotherapy for acute myeloid leukaemia (Whitehead & Crust 1987).

The short-term consequences of the menopause are divided for convenience into sympathetic or vasomotor symptoms, end-organ atrophy and psychological symptoms.

Short-term consequences should perhaps be more appropriately referred to as immediate consequences, as there is no evidence that peripheral vascular control gets any better with increasing age, even though flushes might subside. Likewise end-organ atrophy and to some extent psychological disturbances that are due to ovarian failure are not limiting. Women learn to live with their handicap!

Vasomotor instability

The hot flush is the most characteristic, but not necessarily the most common, symptom of the menopause with 50–70% of women in the climacteric and in their postmenopausal years complaining of the symptom,

Table 25.2 Frequency of symptoms in menopausal women, ages 45–54 years

Complaint	Percentage of women
Irritability	92
Lethargy/fatigue	88
Depression	78
Headaches	71
Hot flushes	68
Forgetfulness	64
Weight gain	61
Insomnia	51
Joint pain/backache	48
Palpitations	44
Crying spells	42
Constipation	37
Dysuria	20
Decreased libido	20

(McKinlay & Jeffreys, 1974) and 20–25% of women still complaining of these symptoms 5 years later (Thompson et al 1973).

Hot flushes may occur at any time of the day or night and can be triggered by a variety of common situations, such as sleeping or dozing, work activities, recreation and relaxation or housework. In a survey of 20 subjects with frequent flushes, Voda (1981) found that out of 974 events that were recorded as preceding a hot flush, sleep related activities showed the highest incidence and 'emotions' the lowest. Prodromal symptoms are common and for many can include a feeling of increasing pressure in the head, though most women have difficulty in describing the sensation (Tataryn et al 1980). During the night, a decrease of rapid eye movement (REM) sleep and waking often precedes a hot flush (Erlik et al 1981).

With most women, a flush starts in the face, neck, head or chest and the initial focal point may be very specific, e.g. earlobe, forehead, or between the breasts. Subsequent spread of the sensation to the head may be in any direction. The duration of a flush can last from a few seconds up to an hour and there is a large variation in the frequency of flushes (Sturdee et al 1978, Voda 1981). The more intense and severe flushing episodes may be followed by sweating, although some also will sweat without an apparent initial flush. When these episodes occur during the night they may lead to insomnia. These episodes may also be coupled with irritability and general lethargy. All these associated symptoms have been shown repeatedly to respond to successful treatment of flushes (Brincat et al 1984a,b, Campbell & Whitehead 1977).

Aetiology

Although flushes are the most characteristic symptom of the menopause, very little is known about their aetiology. The precise role that oestrogens play has yet to be established, but explanations proposing a mechanism whereby raised gonadotrophins alone cause flushes are almost certainly wrong, because flushes occur with great severity in women who have had a hypophysectomy or who are on luteinizing hormone-releasing hormone (LHRH) agonists (Lightman et al 1982).

All the major sex steroids, androgens, oestrogens and progestogens seem to play a part. Flushes have been reported in orchidectomized men, and testosterone replacement by i.m. injections every 2–4 weeks eliminates flushes in such men and restores libido and potency (De Fazio et al 1984, Fieldman et al 1976, Hendy & Burge 1983). These flushes are indistinguishable from those in hypo-oestrogenaemic women. Flushes respond well to treatment with gestogens (Appleby 1962, Patterson 1982, Schiff et al 1980).

Flushes do not seem to be isolated events. Peripheral vascular control is poor after the menopause and reactions to stimuli are altered (Fig. 25.1). This peripheral vascular control can be restored by the use of oestrogens (Brincat et al 1984a). Poor peripheral vascular control occurs in hypo-oestrogenaemic women regardless of whether flushes are present or not and thus, flushes appear to be the result of a total breakdown in peripheral vascular control leading to a massive vasodilatation, followed by a vasoconstriction, on response to some stimulus (Brincat et al 1984a).

The vasomotor symptoms have a particular importance in older women. The night sweats produce insomnia with lethargy and loss of concentration during the day. They are often manifested by giddiness and falling attacks, which may have the disastrous consequence of femoral neck fractures in women with osteoporosis. Thus oestrogens are of great importance not only in the prevention of

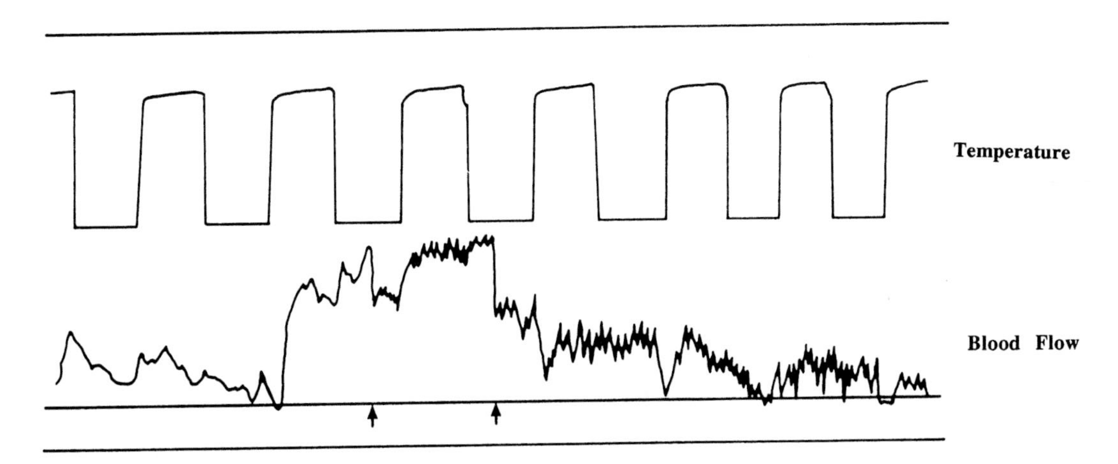

Fig. 25.1 A hot flush occurring in an untreated patient during thermal entrainment testing whilst applying a hot and cold stimulus alternating every 40 s (top trace). The first part of the bottom trace shows poor peripheral vascular control as measured by photoplatysmography. The hot flush begins coincident with a hot stimulus (elevation and thicker trace, bottom line). The baseline has to be changed twice (arrows) so as to keep the trace within the confines of the recording paper. (From Brincat et al 1984.)

osteoporosis but in the prevention of the minor falls which lead to major pathology.

End-organ atrophy

Patients can present with vaginal dryness leading to dyspareunia, apareunia and recurrent vaginal infections.

The genital tract and the urethra have a common embryological origin and oestrogen deficiency thus will affect both systems. Recurrent urinary infections may occur. Atrophy of the urethra and the trigone of the bladder may be the cause in the elderly woman of the common symptoms of dysuria, frequency and urgency, i.e. the urethral syndrome (Smith 1972).

Psychological changes

Anxiety, irritability and depression arising in association with vasomotor and atrophic symptoms are common around the time of the menopause (Brincat et al 1984b, Campbell 1975, Dennerstein & Burrows 1978, Studd et al 1977, Studd & Parsons 1977), and are often at their most severe in the year or two before periods cease.

Although vasomotor and atrophic symptoms are generally attributed to hormonal changes and can be treated with oestrogen therapy, no such agreement exists about the frequency and aetiology of psychiatric disturbances. Double-blind trials have shown the beneficial effects of oestrogen therapy on psychiatric disturbances (Campbell 1975, Thomson & Oswald 1977), but these studies have been criticized for their poor definition of postmenopausal status and the use of nonstandardized psychological tests (Dennerstein & Burrows 1978).

Montgomery et al (1987) published an important work on the subject, using a standardized method of psychiatric assessment. The women analysed were attending the Dulwich Menopause Clinic, and results must therefore be interpreted as applying to a select group. Nevertheless, it was an unexpected finding that even though most women were not attending the clinic for primary psychological symptoms, 86% had clinical psychiatric illness. This was a much greater proportion than other reports of 29% of women aged 40–55 years with clinical psychiatric illness in a general population sample (Ballinger 1975) and 52% of women of a similar age, referred to a gynaecological clinic largely due to menstrual abnormalities (Ballinger 1977).

As yet no clinical link between the menopause and depression has been established. The highest incidence of depression in middle life arises in the few years before the cessation of periods (Jazsman 1973). The suggestion has been made therefore that it is not a low level of oestrogens, but changes in hormone concentration, such as those in the cyclical depression of premenstrual syndrome (Magos et al 1986), that predispose to depression during the menopause. There is evidence that women who are depressed are those who are most anxious about the menopause and attribute their low mood to it.

A possible mechanism for the increase in psychological problems around the time of the menopause could be the interaction that exists between oestrogens and various control neurotransmitters, either by reducing available tryptophan for serotonin synthesis or by reducing dopamine receptor sensitivity (Aylward 1975).

The physical symptoms of the menopause may cause a secondary depression in some susceptible women. Alternatively, the loss of reproductive potential may be seen as a loss of femininity and result in low esteem. This loss of femininity, as described by women, is not unique to late postmenopausal women but has also been described in women with premature menopause, such as those studied by Whitehead & Crust (1987).

Depression is at least twice as common in women than in men; as this difference only begins with puberty and is associated with the premenstrual and the postnatal state as well as the postmenopausal years, it is believed by many to be the result of either deficiency or sudden change in plasma oestradiol levels. An alternative point of view is that the excess of depression in women is an environmental factor related to the middle-aged woman's role in society and not in any way related to gonadal hormones. The sad sequel to this is that approximately 40% of women in this age group are taking tranquillizers and antidepressants instead of replacement oestrogens. This results in more depression, addiction to psychoactive drugs and yet more dizziness and falls, which might lead to further postmenopausal osteoporotic fractures.

Libido and lethargy

Loss of libido and lethargy are two other common psychological symptoms attributed to the menopause (Neugarten & Kraines 1965). A distinction needs to be made between dyspareunia and loss of libido. Accurate diagnosis is essential because symptoms resulting from domestic problems are best treated by psychiatrists, marriage guidance counsellors or social workers. The loss of libido that is associated with the menopause is characteristically a loss of interest in normal sexual relations in the context of an otherwise happy marriage (Sarrel 1988, Studd & Parsons 1977, Studd et al 1977).

Psychosexual symptoms have proved very difficult to study because of the lack of objective analysis for carrying out libido studies. Montgomery et al (1987, and personal communication) have looked at the problem using an objective assessment and have established that loss of libido is indeed a feature of the postmenopausal years.

As with lethargy (Brincat et al 1984b) they have found that good responses can be achieved with adequate hormone replacement, although the role of additional testosterone is still debatable.

LONG-TERM CONSEQUENCES

The long-term consequences of ovarian failure carry a high morbidity and mortality. There is increasing evidence that with appropriate hormone replacement these can be prevented to varying degrees. New insights are being obtained into the protective influence of the female sex hormone against cardiovascular disease. The other long-term consequences that will be dealt with here are different facets of a general decrease and derangement in connective tissue after the menopause. The most important manifestations of this connective tissue disorder are in bones (osteoporosis), skin and bladder. It is also becoming apparent that dementia is commoner in women than in men and the possible association of this with oestrogen deficiency will be discussed.

Cardiovascular disease

Prior to the menopause, ischaemic heart disease is uncommon in women who do not smoke, or who do not have chronic diseases such as hypertension or diabetes mellitus. Heart disease is five times more common in men than in premenopausal women. Following the menopause, however, there is an increase in the incidence of this condition so that by the age of 70 there is no longer any sex difference. The timing of this increase in heart disease in women strongly suggests that the oestrogen deficiency of the menopause is responsible. The precise mechanism by which this is brought about remains unclear. Although it is widely believed that the menopause results in the adverse effect on the cardiovascular system through the lipoprotein metabolism, there is convincing evidence that increased low density lipoprotein (LDL) concentrations will result in increased heart disease and that increased high density lipoprotein (HDL) concentrations are cardioprotective (Gordon et al 1977). The risk factor is expressed as the HDL/LDL ratio. Prior to the menopause the serum levels of LDL cholesterol are lower in women than in men and serum HDL is higher in premenopausal women as compared to men. After the menopause there is an increase in the serum LDL level in women although this does not exceed the levels in age-matched men.

It appears, therefore, that in premenopausal women ovarian oestrogens have a protective effect against cardiovascular disease mediated to some extent by the effect on lipoprotein metabolism. It is possible that other mechanisms may also affect the role of the menopause in heart disease. Oestrogens may have a direct effect on the blood vessels and may stimulate the release of nitric oxide and peptides some of which are important vasodilators. Stress may be a risk factor in heart disease, so the various symptoms of menopause such as irritability, depression and sleeplessness may be relevant in the increased incidence of heart disease.

The effects of hormone replacement therapy on cardiovascular disease

A number of studies have demonstrated a reduction in incidence of ischaemic heart disease following the use of hormone replacement therapy (Bush et al 1987, Hammond et al 1979, Ross et al 1981, Stampfer et al 1985). However, one smaller study by Wilson et al (1985) has disagreed with this.

Oestrogen replacement therapy causes an increase in HDL and a lowering of LDL concentrations (Fig. 25.2) (Crook et al 1988, Tikkannen et al 1986). The changes in HDL and LDL levels by oestrogens appear to be effected by influencing both hepatic and endothelial metabolism. The synthetic oestrogens such as those used in the oral contraceptive pill are known to have a marked effect on the clotting system and lead to an increased risk of thromboembolic phenomena. However, the natural oestrogens used for hormone replacement therapy do not suffer from this disadvantage. Neither do natural oestrogens affect blood pressure or carbohydrate metabolism (Thom et al 1977, 1978). Cyclical administration of progestogens of between 7 and 13 days, in conjunction with continuous oestrogen, is essential for the prevention of endometrial hyperplasia (Studd et al 1980). However, the progestogens may have an adverse effect on lipoprotein and carbohydrate metabolism as well as on mood (Magos et al 1985). See below for a further discussion of this.

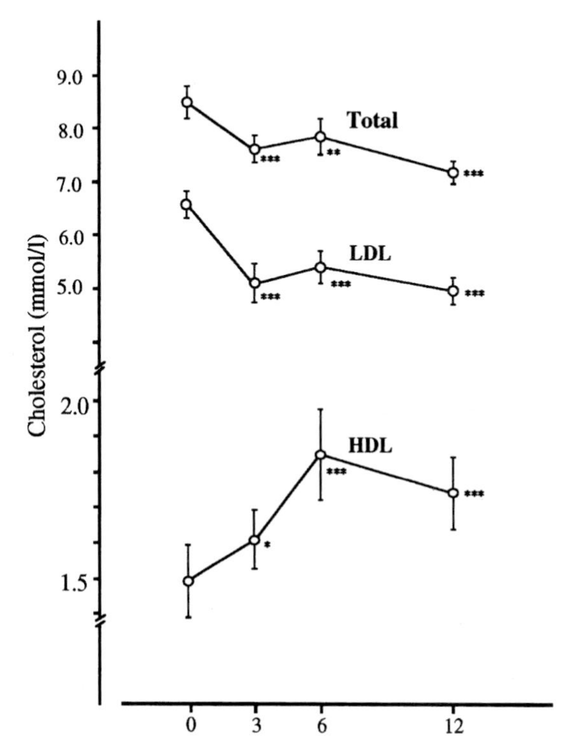

Fig. 25.2 Effect of oestradiol valerate, 2 mg/day, on serum lipoprotein lipids in postmenopausal women; mean ± SD; $n = 30$, * $p < 0.02$, ** $p < 0.005$, *** $p < 0.001$. (From Tikkannen et al 1986.)

Oestrogens and the central nervous system

Oestrogen administration has been reported to alter extrapyramidal motor control (Van Hartesveldt & Joyce 1986), mood (Sherwin 1988, Sherwin & Gelfund 1989), depression (Ditkoff et al 1991, Klaiber et al 1979) and memory (Campbell & Whitehead 1977, Sherwin & Gelfund 1989). Effects on memory are difficult to interpret because either subjective measures of memory have been used or the changes occurred in the context of relief from other menopausal symptoms. In the latter situation, memory improvement cannot be distinguished from the affective changes. In asymptomatic postmenopausal women no effect of oestrogen replacement on memory was found in one double-blind, placebo-controlled trial (Ditkoff et al 1991).

Several groups have attempted to look at the effects of oestrogen on cognitive function in patients with Alzheimer's disease, with divergent results (Fillit et al 1986, Honjo et al 1989, Weiss 1987). In all three of these uncontrolled studies, the duration of oestrogen treatment was 6 weeks or less and the number of subjects seven or less. These were too few to draw any conclusions (Birge 1994).

Oestrogen deficiency and the epidemiology of falls, fractures and Alzheimer's disease

A more compelling case for a role of oestrogen deficiency in the expression of Alzheimer's disease can be made by examining the epidemiology of Alzheimer's disease. The incidence of Alzheimer's disease increases preferentially in women after the age of 65 (Molsa et al 1982; Fig. 25.3) so that age-specific incidence rates vary from 1.5 to 3.0 times those of men (Aronson et al 1990, Jorm et al 1987) — Table 25.3. Women who have experienced a myocardial infarction are five times more likely to develop dementia (Aronson et al 1990). Since cardiovascular disease in women is considered to be an expression of oestrogen deficiency, the associated dementia may be an expression of the oestrogen deficiency state. It may also be relevant that obese women are less likely to develop Alzheimer's disease than nonobese women (Berlinger & Potter 1991). Is it possible that the apparent protection afforded by an increased body weight is due to greater endogenous oestrogen production by the adipose tissue? A recent study (Tang et al 1996) seems to suggest that oestrogens may significantly delay the onset and reduce the risk of developing Alzheimer's disease.

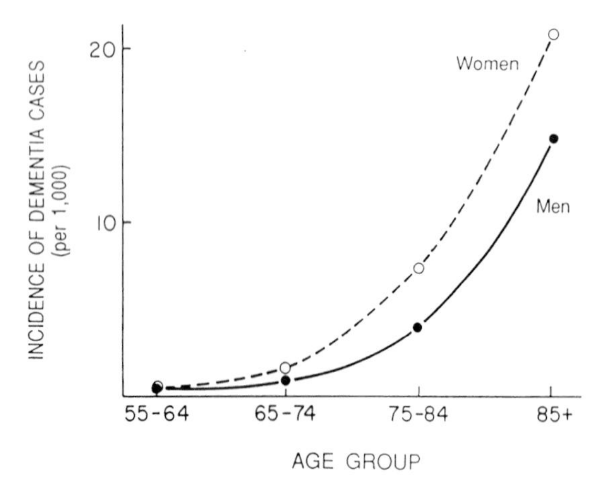

Fig. 25.3 Annual age-specific incidence rates of dementia per 1000 men (●-●) and women (O-O). (From Molsa et al 1982.)

Table 25.3 The incidence of dementia in men and women in different populations

Country	Number of studies	Male	Female	Ratio
Japan	4	0.8	1.5	1.9
Russia	1	1.1	3.8	3.5
Scandinavia	3	1.6	2.2	1.4
Britain	3	3.0	4.9	1.6
United States	3	0.7	2.1	3.0

Data from Aronson et al 1990, Jorm et al 1987

Obesity and the current use of oestrogen also protect women from hip fracture. Although this protection can be attributed at least in part to effects on skeletal strength, epidemiological data suggest that this protection may be mediated through effects on the central nervous system. Melton and colleagues (1988) developed a model to predict lifetime fracture risk based on age and bone density. Prior to age 70, bone density accurately predicts a woman's risk of hip fracture. After age 70, the age-related decline in bone density fails to account for the observed exponential increase in the rates of hip fracture. They conclude that some other age-related factor or factors become the dominant cause of hip fracture after age 70. The threefold greater age-specific incidence of hip fracture in women has been attributed to the greater degree of osteoporosis in women than in men. However, the difference in bone mass between elderly women and men is less than 1.25-fold. Although falls increase with age, this increase is also not sufficient to account for the observed rates of fracture nor the differences in fracture rates between women and men. On the other hand, the exponential increase in dementia with age closely parallels the increases in hip fracture for both men and women (Fig. 25.4). Indeed, dementia and a slowing of psychomotor speed or a slowing of the central integration of sensory input appear to be the most potent risk factors for hip fracture (Bachner & Larson 1987, Cummings et al 1985, Grisso et al 1991, Muscat Baron et al 1994, Porter et al 1990).

Osteoporosis

Peak bone mass is reached in the fourth decade of life, after which there is an age-related bone loss in both sexes. However, in women there is an acceleration in the rate of

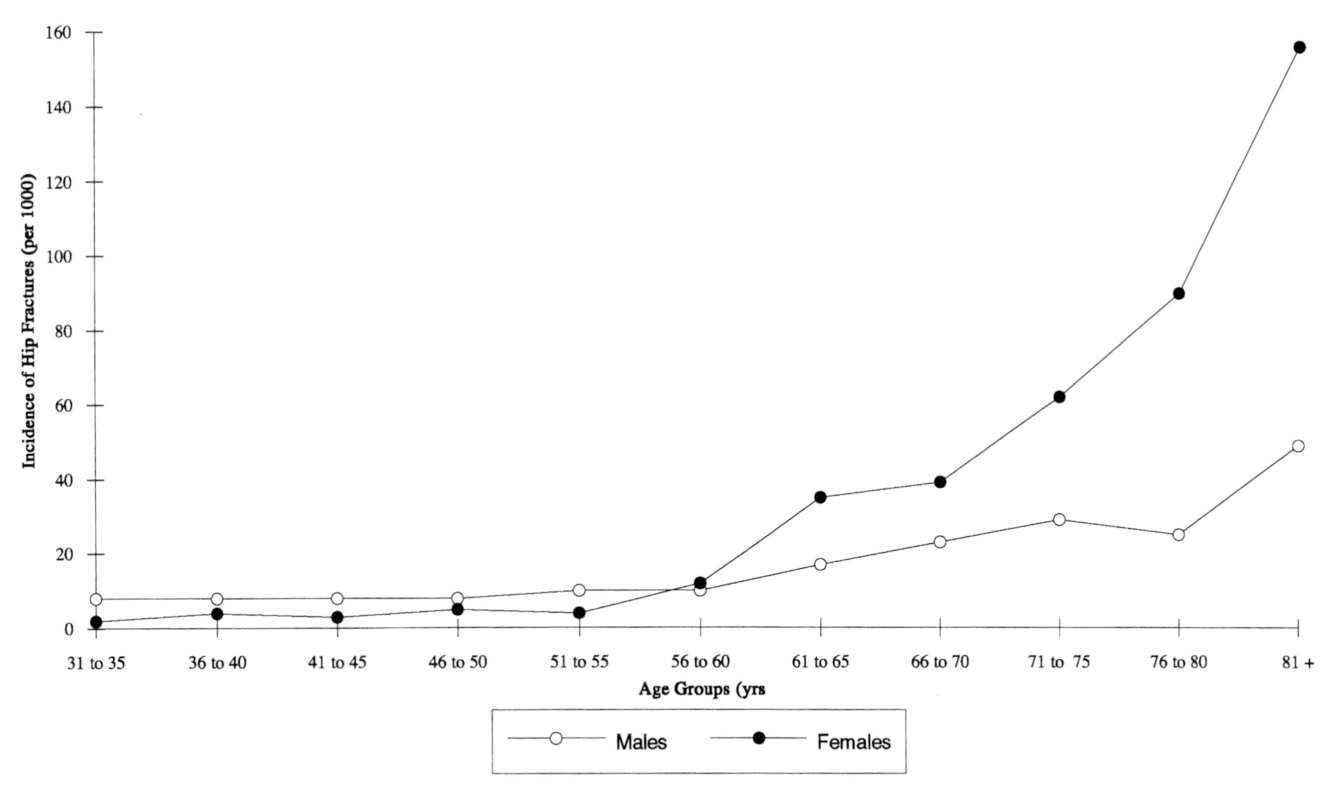

Fig. 25.4 Age-specific incidence rates of hip fractures per 1000 women in Malta from 1987 to 1989. (From: Muscat Baron et al 1994.)

bone loss following the menopause: by the age of 70 years a woman loses 50% of her bone mass while a man loses only 25% by the age of 90 (Gordan, 1984). As a result of postmenopausal osteoporosis, the fracture rate in postmenopausal women is greater than in age-matched men. This was first recognized by Bruns (1882) who showed that in those over the age of 50, fractures of the forearm and hip were more frequent in women than in men. Albright et al (1941) first demonstrated a clear relationship between the menopause and oestrogen deficiency, and osteoporosis. With an ageing population, postmenopausal osteoporosis now represents an enormous public health problem. It has been estimated by the National Osteoporosis Society that the cost of nonfatal hip fractures in the United Kingdom is about £180 million annually. Albright (1941) first postulated that a reduction in gonadal function leads to osteoporosis and demonstrated that treatment with stilboestrol could reverse the negative calcium balance in a postmenopausal osteoporotic woman. Furthermore he recognized that osteoporosis was accompanied by thin skin, and suggested that postmenopausal osteoporosis may be a disease of protein metabolism. Albright also assumed that postmenopausal osteoporosis resulted from a decrease in osteoblastic activity, but Nordin et al (1981) demonstrated that in fact it is an increase in osteoclastic activity which is responsible.

It is possible that both osteoblastic and osteoclastic activity might be responsible, with the entire bone remodelling unit functioning at a different level. Studies in the excretion of procollagen I and terminal peptides, representing bone formation, and pyridinium cross-links, representing breakdown, have been carried out. Our own series, comparing early postmenopausal women with women who had been on hormone replacement therapy (HRT), indicated that osteoclastic activity seemed to be decreased by a mean of 27% and osteoblastic activity was also decreased by a mean of 11.3% in the women on HRT (Fig. 25.5). All differences were however highly significant, indicating that bone remodelling had readjusted. The women on hormone replacement therapy in our series had only been on therapy for a short time (mean 6 months), implying that these changes occur rapidly. It is interesting to note that if the above calculations hold, then a mean change of 16% is occurring in bone remodelling and this is the mean figure of bone mineral density change that we observed at the L2–L4 vertebral region on these women.

The mechanism whereby diminished ovarian function leads to a decrease in osteoblast activity remains unclear. It has been suggested that oestrogen deficiency results in malabsorption of dietary calcium (Nordin 1960). Oestrogens are known to increase the intestinal absorption of calcium (Heaney 1978). Moreover the renal excretion of calcium is decreased, probably due to improved renal function in postmenopausal women on oestrogen therapy. It has been suggested that calcitonin plays a central role in the aetiology of postmenopausal osteoporosis. This is a

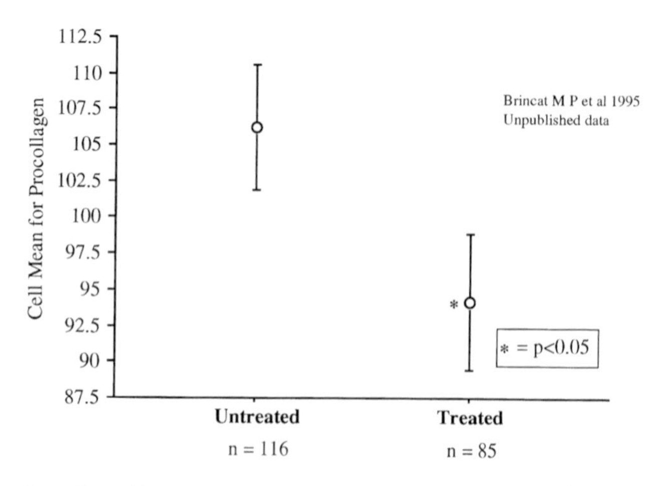

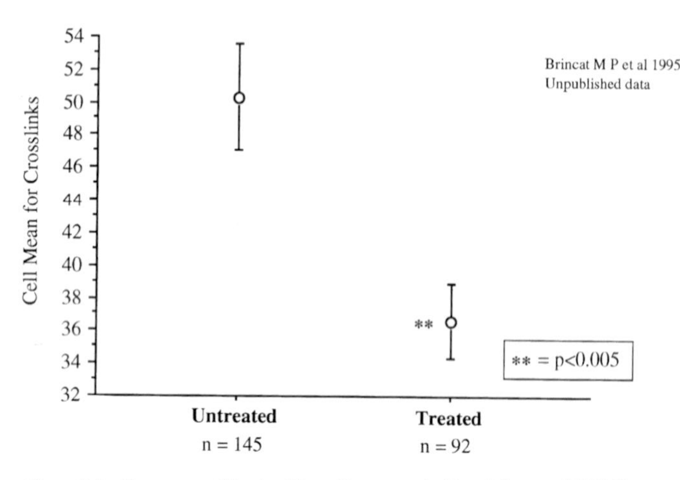

Fig. 25.5 Plot of mean levels of procollagen I and pyridinium crosslinks excretion in patients on hormone replacement therapy and in a group of early postmenopausal women not on hormone treatment.

peptide hormone released by the parafollicular cells of the thyroid gland. Calcitonin reduces both the number and activity of osteoclastic cells. Stevenson & Whitehead (1982) showed a decrease in calcitonin levels after the menopause and concluded that oestrogen deficiency may lead to a reduced level of calcitonin and thus less inhibition of osteoclastic activity, therefore causing osteoporosis. Subsequent studies have failed to confirm this, however (Chestnut 1984, Tiegs et al 1984).

Post-menopausal osteoporosis studies in the past have mostly concentrated on calcium and calcium-related hormones, ignoring the organic matrix. The latter is largely collagen and makes up approximately 35% of dry defatted bone mass. The organic matrix of bone acts rather like internal girders and confers on bone its tensile strength, and it has been suggested that it is a decline in this organic matrix that is the primary pathological event leading to osteoporosis (Brincat et al 1987a,d). The association of thin skin, low in collagen, with osteoporosis, and thin skin with such conditions as osteogenesis imperfecta and steroid-induced osteoporosis provides some evidence for the suggestion that postmenopausal osteoporosis is also a generalized connective tissue disorder, thus confirming Albright's original impressions (Albright 1941). Regardless of age, women who sustain fractures do so because their bone mass is significantly reduced when compared with that of women who do not fracture. Interestingly these women have significantly thinner skin when compared to a nonosteoporotic fracture population of controls (Fig. 25.6) (Brincat et al 1994a). Naturally more women sustain osteoporotic fractures, the older they are, but the basic message that women fracture because they have thinner skin, reflecting thinner bone, remains. Oestrogens have complex effects on the skeleton and most probably prevent osteoporosis by affecting both calcium homeostasis and the connective tissue component of bone.

Clinical implications

As a result of osteoporosis, bones are more liable to fracture spontaneously or as a result of minimal trauma. The three most common types of fracture are distal, radial and ulnar (Colles'), vertebral body and the neck of femur. These have a combined incidence of 40% in white women over the age of 65 (Crilly et al 1978). Colles' fractures frequently occur as result of falls. Approximately 0.5% of women over the age of 70 will sustain this fracture each year: 12 times the incidence in age-matched men (Alffram & Bauer 1962). The crush fractures of the vertebra typically involve T8–L4 and may occur spontaneously with normal activity such as sitting up from a chair or bed. They often cause severe pain and disability can result in a loss up to 5 inches in height, or produce marked kyphosis (dowager's hump). Of women over 65, 25% will have either clinical or radiological evidence of such a fracture.

Fracture of the neck of the femur is the most significant traumatic consequence of postmenopausal osteoporosis. The affected population tends to be older and the associated mortality and morbidity greater than with any other fracture. Approximately 27% of women who sustain such a fracture die within 1 year (Miller 1978). The death rate from osteoporotic hip fractures is greater than that of carcinoma of the breast and endometrium combined. At least 20% of those injured suffer from considerable loss of mobility 1 year after the fracture.

A number of risk factors for the development of postmenopausal osteoporosis have been identified.

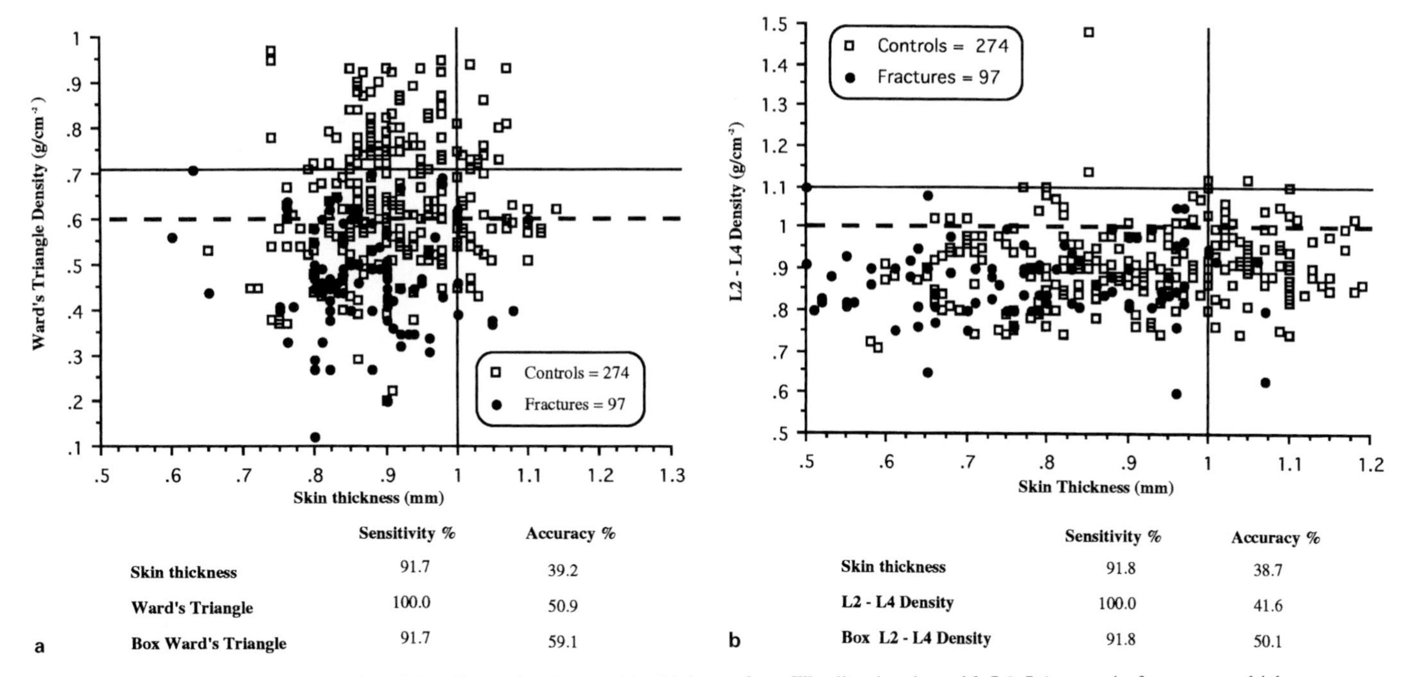

a

	Sensitivity %	Accuracy %
Skin thickness	91.7	39.2
Ward's Triangle	100.0	50.9
Box Ward's Triangle	91.7	59.1

b

	Sensitivity %	Accuracy %
Skin thickness	91.8	38.7
L2 - L4 Density	100.0	41.6
Box L2 - L4 Density	91.8	50.1

Fig. 25.6 These three-dimensional models of bone density vs. skin thickness for **a** Ward's triangle and **b** L2–L4, contain four zones which categorize women into very high risk groups, low risk groups and intermediate low risk groups. These predictive zones have different sensitivities and accuracies. A total of 274 controls were compared to some 97 women who had sustained osteoporotic fractures. (From Brincat et al 1994a.)

1. White (Caucasian) women are at greater risk of developing osteoporosis than black women because they start off with a lesser peak bone mass and may lose bone at a faster rate.
2. Underweight women, or women with a small build, may be at a greater risk because of reduced peripheral conversion of adrenal androgens to oestrogen.
3. Anorexia leading to amenorrhoea and hypoestrogenism leads to severe osteoporosis.
4. A sedentary lifestyle encourages bone loss.
5. Although exercise may have a beneficial effect on the skeleton, strenuous exercise producing amenorrhoea will lead to significant bone loss. Warren et al (1986) have shown that young ballet dancers have a high incidence of late menarche and secondary amenorrhoea resulting in an increased incidence of skeleton fractures.
6. Corticosteroid therapy causes osteoporosis, but the mechanism for this is unclear.
7. Excessive alcohol and caffeine consumption and smoking are known to increase bone loss.
8. A high protein diet is also thought to lead to increased bone loss, indicated by an increase in calcium excretion by the kidneys.
9. Nulliparity is a risk factor. It is possible that during pregnancy some of the age-related bone losses are arrested so that a woman who has had repeated pregnancies will have a greater bone mass at the time of her menopause.

A number of prospective studies have confirmed Albright's findings that oestrogen can prevent postmenopausal osteoporosis (Christiansen et al 1980, Lindsay et al 1978, Natchigall et al 1980) and epidemiological studies have shown that this will lead to a reduction in the incidence of fractures. Ross et al (1984) have estimated that 5 years of oestrogen replacement therapy will halve a woman's risk of developing osteoporotic fractures. Lindsay et al (1984) have suggested that 0.625 mg of conjugated equine oestrogens is sufficient for protection of the skeleton. Recent studies have shown, however, that the higher oestradiol levels achieved with a subcutaneous oestradiol/testosterone implant will lead to a reversal of earlier postmenopausal bone loss (Savvas et al 1988) (Fig. 25.7). There is also some evidence that progestogens may be effective in preventing osteoporosis due to stimulation of new bone formation (Lindsay et al 1978).

Skin

The skin is the largest organ of the body and also undergoes changes after the menopause. Many of these changes have formerly been attributed to the 'ageing' process but are in reality due to oestrogen deficiency. The skin of postmenopausal women who are on sex hormone replacement therapy has been shown to contain more collagen than women of the same age who are on no treatment (Brincat et al 1983).

Skin thickness declines after the menopause in a rapid fashion at a rate very similar to the decline in bone mass. This decline cannot be explained by age alone; skin colla-

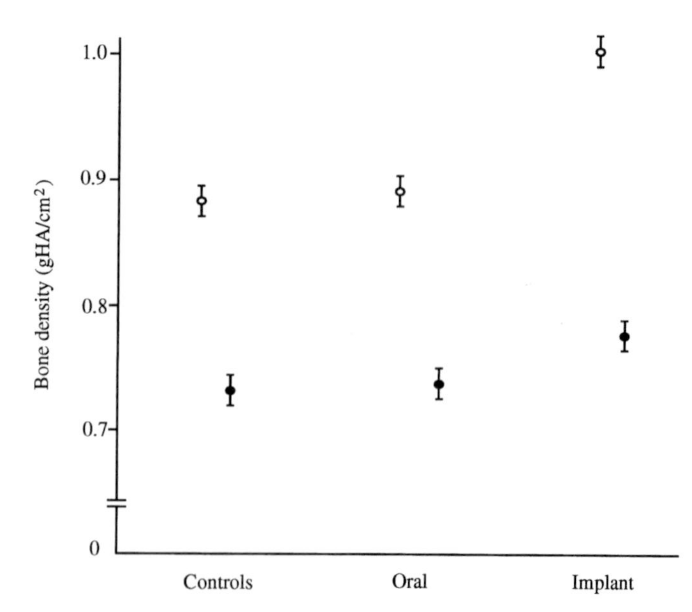

Fig. 25.7 Mean (±SEM) spine and femoral neck bone density in postmenopausal women, untreated and on oral and implant therapy; ○, spine ●, proximal femur. (Modified from Savvas et al 1988.)

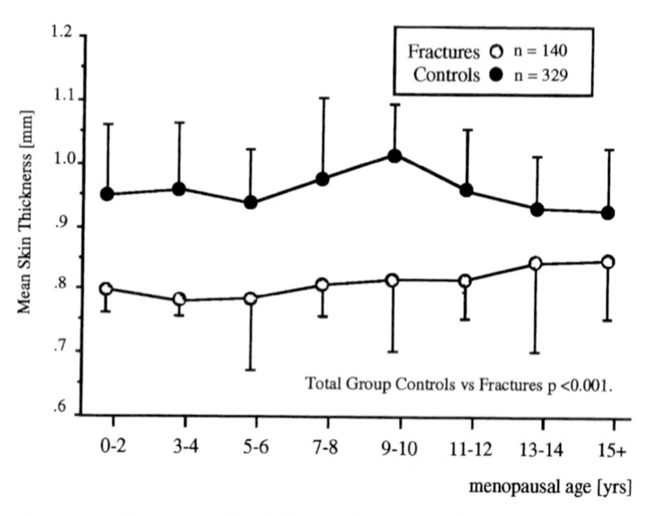

Fig. 25.8 The mean skin thickness of a group of postmenopausal women who had sustained an osteoporotic fracture and of another group who were on no treatment, plotted against menopausal age in 10-year cohorts. There was a significant statistical difference when the groups were compared to each other. (Brincat et al 1994b)

gen declines by some 30% in the first 10 years after the menopause, an amount that is comparable to bone loss over the same period (Brincat et al 1985, 1987a,c) (Fig. 25.8).

Prospective studies on skin collagen have shown that even though collagen was lost as a result of duration of ovarian failure, it was possible to restore collagen to premenopausal levels within 6 months of initiating hormone replacement therapy (Brincat 1987a,b,c,e). If hormone replacement therapy was initiated early there was no decline in the level of skin collagen or in skin thickness. (Brincat 1987a,b,c,e, Meschia 1994).

It is our belief that sex hormone deprivation after the menopause, in particular oestrogen deficiency, leads to a generalized connective tissue loss. This would therefore be the initial pathology in osteoporotic bone loss, with reduced mineral content of bone following the breakdown of the organic collagenous matrix (Brincat & Studd 1988).

Both oestrogen and androgen receptors have been identified in the fibroblasts of the skin (Black et al 1970, Stumpf et al 1976). More recently, oestrogen receptors have finally been identified on osteoblasts (Kaplan 1987), giving weight to the argument that sex steroids have a direct action on osteoblasts. In addition, the possibility of oestrogens working on both fibroblasts and osteoblasts indirectly, through an intermediary hormone such as growth hormone, must be considered (Vashinav et al 1984).

The epidermis has not been studied extensively although oestradiol receptors do exist in its basal cell layer (Shahrad & Marks 1977). Punnonen (1973) claimed significantly higher mitotic activity in the epidermis in in vitro studies exposing epidermal cells to oestrogen. He also showed that the epidermis became thinner, the longer the time interval between castration and investigation in studies that he carried out on women.

Genitourinary system

The mucosal linings of the vagina and urethra have the highest concentrations of oestrogen receptors in the body and are therefore, not surprisingly, extremely sensitive to alternations in the oestrogen levels. The trigone of the bladder, derived embryologically from the urogenital sinus, also appears to undergo atrophic changes after the menopause.

The vaginal epithelium of postmenopausal women becomes attenuated, pale and almost transparent as a result of a decrease in vascularity. Marked atrophic changes in the vagina can result in atrophic vaginitis, with the vaginal epithelium becoming thin, inflamed and ulcerated.

The cervix, instead of protruding into the vagina, atrophies, retracts and becomes flush with the apex of the vault. The uterine corpus itself becomes smaller with a return to the 1:2 corpus:cervix ratio of childhood.

The endometrium becomes thin and atrophic, although cystic glands may persist for many years. In some women with a higher endogenous oestrogen production, the endometrium may be active and proliferative and even hyperplastic. Such women tend to be obese since after the menopause the chief source of oestrogens is derived from peripheral conversion of androgens in adipose tissue.

Atrophy of both the vagina and the urethra have symptomatic sequelae which can continue to be troublesome. These include dyspareunia, apareunia and recurrent bacterial infections. In the urethra, repeated infections may lead to fibrosis which predisposes to the frequency, dysuria and urgency referred to as the 'urethral syndrome'

(Smith 1972). The submucosal vascular plexus of the urethra contributes to sphincteric function and is oestrogen-dependent (Versi & Cardozo 1985), as may be the collagen content of the urethral submucosal connective tissue (Versi et al 1988). Oestrogen receptors have been detected in the human female urethra (Iosif et al 1981), suggesting a direct action of the hormone. It would appear, therefore, that both the genital and the lower urinary tract are influenced by oestrogens.

Incontinence

Osborne (1976) studied 600 women aged between 35 and 60 and was unable to show an increased prevalence of incontinence at the time of the menopause. Iosif & Bekassy (1984), on the other hand, in a survey of 902 Swedish women aged 61 found a 29.2% incidence of urinary incontinence. The debate as to whether ovarian failure leads to incontinence still rages.

Versi (1986) reported a high incidence of stress incontinence, frequency, nocturia and urgency in peri- and postmenopausal women. Stanton et al (1983) found the incidence of pain on micturition in a similar group of women to be 30%. Tables 25.4 and 25.5 (Versi 1986) indicate symptomatology elicited by history alone, and urodynamically proven diagnosis, respectively. (There was no premenopausal control group for comparison.) These results suggest that urological changes occur in the climacteric. As in the case of bone loss, analyses relying upon a sharp definition of the menopause may be unreliable since they do not make any allowance for the possibility of fluctuating to low oestrogen levels affecting urinary function some time prior to the menopause. One-third of the population looked at by Versi (1986) had abnormal urodynamic results. Genuine stress incontinence, detrusor instability, and voiding difficulties were the most commonly found abnormalities.

Urethral pressure profilometry revealed that postmenopausal women had weaker urethral sphincters under stress than the perimenopausal groups (Versi 1986). A later study by the same group demonstrated a correlation between urethral pressure measurements and skin collagen content (Versi et al 1988). Increases in urethral pressure have been noted after hormone replacement therapy. (Faber & Heidenreich 1977, Hilton & Stanton 1983, Walter et al 1978). Since increases in skin collagen with hormone replacement therapy have also been noted (Brincat et al 1987b,e) it is suggested that the beneficial effects on urethral function may be mediated by beneficial effects on collagen control (Versi et al 1988).

In summary, therefore, lower urinary tract problems are seemingly increased as a result of oestrogen deficiency after the menopause. It is still not clear, however, what are the effects of increasing age on urinary tract function. Likewise it is still not clear which symptoms are specifically due to oestrogen deficiency, although a large number of women attending a menopause clinic will complain of such symptoms and claim benefit with oestrogen therapy.

Table 25.4 A comparison of lower urinary symptomatology in peri- and postmenopausal women

	Perimenopausal	Postmenopausal
Number of women studied	54	89
Age, mean + SD	46.5 + 0.6	52.2 + 0.5
Stress incontinence, %		
Occasional	33.3	40.4
Frequent	9.3	10.1
Frequency (>8 per day), %	31.5	28.2
Nocturia (once per night), %	29.6	29.2
Urgency, %		
Occasional	16.7	33.7
Frequent	31.5	21.3
Painful micturition, %	13.9	10.3
Poor stream, %	5.6	10.1
Incomplete bladder emptying, %	11.3	13.0

Table 25.5 The prevalence of urodynamically diagnosed pathology in women undergoing the climacteric

	Perimenopausal	Postmenopausal
Total	54	89
Normal	33 (61%)	62 (70%)
Genuine stress incontinence	10 (19%)	12 (13%)
Detrusor instability	5 (10%)	10 (11%)
Voiding difficulty	3 (6%)	4 (4%)
Urethral syndrome	0 (0%)	1 (1%)

INVESTIGATION AND DIAGNOSIS

With increasing awareness, it is no longer only women with the short-term symptoms of the menopause who are presenting to specialist clinics. Increasingly women are demanding prophylaxis for the long-term consequences of the menopause even though, at presentation they may be apparently asymptomatic.

Misdiagnosis is unlikely in the women who present with the characteristic picture of acute vasomotor disturbances and symptoms of lower genital tract atrophy coupled with oligo- or amenorrhoea. Other conditions associated with flushing and sweating such as phaeochromocytoma, carcinoid disease and thyroid disease have additional signs and symptoms.

Plasma gonadotrophins and oestrogen concentrations fluctuate widely during the climacteric (Chakravati et al 1976) and detailed biochemical investigations are often of little value in diagnosis, with symptoms always being the best guide. In premature menopause, or when there is some additional doubt as to whether the menopause has occurred or not, such as in hysterectomized women, a high serum FSH should be sufficient to establish the diagnosis. It might also be useful to estimate serum oestradiol levels. Endocrine assessments cannot accurately predict the eventual severity and duration of symptoms nor the response to therapy.

Similarly, the intensity of short-term symptoms of the menopause bear no relationship to the severity of the long-term consequences. Methods for assessing bone mass accurately such as bone densitometry or quantitative computed tomography (QCT) analysis are cumbersome and have no place as routine screening tools.

It is crucial to establish whether the psychological disturbances with which a patient may present are due to oestrogen deficiency or result from coincidental but current social, domestic or economic crises. When diagnosis proves difficult, biochemical investigations may be of value because high plasma oestrogen levels exclude ovarian failure although the converse does not necessarily apply. With the latter, it has been our practice to give the patient the benefit of the doubt and embark on a course of hormone replacement therapy.

Climacteric depression responds rapidly and well to hormone replacement especially to implant therapy (Montgomery et al 1987) and therefore if, despite this therapy, the woman still has not responded, then one can assume that the woman's psychological symptoms are not due to sex hormone imbalance or deficiency and she would probably be better helped by the psychiatrists.

TREATMENT

The treatment of choice for the management of menopausal symptoms and sequelae is oestrogen therapy which should in most cases successfully correct this multisystem deficiency state. Other treatments available only serve, at best, to manage a particular symptom without striking at the root of the problem. In some cases serious side-effects occur that could be worse than any possible from properly managed hormone replacement.

Therapy is divided into nonhormonal and hormonal.

Nonhormonal

Geist & Mintz (1937) proposed irradiating the pituitary so as to suppress excess production of gonadotrophins which they believed caused flushing. Their results were not encouraging. More recently, suppression of pituitary activity using GnRH analogues has proved not only to be useless in suppressing flushes but actually to provoke such flushes (Lightman et al 1982). Vitamin E has been proposed for the treatment and the prevention of many sex-related problems but apart from one study (McLaren 1949) this has never been substantiated.

Sedatives and tranquillizers have been widely prescribed for over a century with barbiturates, diazepam and similar drugs. Such therapy only adds to the lethargy and general loss of interest in life and certainly does nothing to prevent symptoms like flushing, although surprisingly they have been prescribed for this symptom as well. It is a sad fact of contemporary life that about 40% of middle-aged and elderly women have had long courses of psychoactive drugs. At last, however, an editorial in The Lancet asks the question 'Must we poison our old patients?' (Editorial 1988).

Amongst the adrenergic agents currently used, clonidine, an adrenergic agonist, seems to have some potential. Clayden et al (1974) supervised a multicentre, placebo-controlled, cross-over study on 100 women and reported significant benefit in controlling the severity and duration of flushes with minimal side-effects. It is noted that in common with many similar studies, there was no difference in menopause symptoms until the therapy was crossed over. Lindsay & Hart (1978) failed, however, to find any difference in flushing episodes when clonidine was compared to placebo.

Propranolol has been tried with conflicting results. Alcoff et al (1981) obtained a difference in flushing episodes when compared to placebo. Methyldopa (Tulandi et al 1984) and naproxen (Haataja et al 1984) have also been suggested but once more results as regards their use in the relief of flushes are conflicting. Ethamsylate, used principally in the treatment of menorrhagia, has been tried and Harrison (1981) reported some good results.

Hormonal: progestogens and anabolic steroids

Progestogens

Progestogens can suppress flushes (Appleby 1962, Patterson 1982); both norethisterone (Patterson 1982) and medroxyprogesterone have been reported as useful (Schiff et al 1980). Progestogens have been shown to be useful in the prevention of postmenopausal bone loss and several studies have shown this. The gestogens used in these studies were medroxyprogesterone, megestrol and norethisterone (Lindsay et al 1978, Lobo et al 1984). Moreover the protective effect of gestogens against osteoporosis has been disputed.

Anabolic steroids

In women, androgens have been used in the prevention and treatment of postmenopausal osteoporosis. Stanozolol, an anabolic steroid, has been studied extensively and shown to increase total body calcium in patients with established osteoporosis (Chestnut et al 1979, Chestnut 1984); its use in the prevention of postmenopausal bone loss, however remains to be determined.

Hormonal: oestrogens

Oestrogen replacement therapy is the most appropriate overall treatment for problems caused by ovarian failure. The aim of a therapeutic regimen is to provide the most effective treatment with the least side-effects. Oestrogens may be given either orally or parenterally, e.g. percutaneously, transvaginally, as cream or more recently as skin patches. Oestrogens can also be given subcutaneously as implants. The pharmacodynamics and biochemical effects of exogenous oestrogens can vary markedly with the route of administration.

Oral oestrogens

The oral route is the most popular (Judd et al 1981). Its major difference from the parenteral route is that administered oestrogens are exposed to the gastrointestinal tract, the portal venous system and the liver. Oestradiol is preferentially converted to oestrone in the gastrointestinal tract (Ryan & Engel 1953). The portal venous system rapidly transfers the absorbed steroid, almost in the form of a 'bolus' into hepatic tissue where much of the administered oestrogen is metabolized and inactivated before the systemic circulation is reached. This is known as the 'first-pass' effect.

Glucuronidation of oestrogen occurs almost exclusively in the liver, so percutaneous and subcutaneous oestradiol administration are not associated with an increase in plasma oestrone-3-glucuronide levels (Campbell & Whitehead 1982).

Because of the first-pass effect, oral oestrogens have to be given at a higher dose than parenteral therapy to maintain relief of symptoms. Induction of liver enzymes, particularly the glucuronidase enzymes, by other drugs such as antiepileptics may result in such a rapid oestrogen inactivation that the administered steroid is not clinically effective. Also, oral oestrogens may influence the production of renin substrate, antithrombin III, and high and low density lipoproteins.

Oral oestrogens are more potent than parenterally administered oestrogens in elevating HDL-cholesterol (Brenner et al, 1982) thereby increasing the HDL/LDL ratio with the consequent beneficial implications for arterial disease (Gordon et al 1977).

Because of depression of antithrombin III activity, oral oestrogens might be contraindicated in women with a history of clotting disorder (Van der Meer et al 1973), and likewise in hypertensives due to the theoretical risk of alteration and renin substrate (Laragh et al 1967). It must be emphasized, however, that these last two contraindications and other theoretical ones generally refer to synthetic oral oestrogens, and therefore should not be extrapolated for the natural oral oestrogens that are used in hormone replacement.

By virtue of their structure, the synthetic oestrogens have a greater affinity for the oestrogen receptor and are not substrates for the intracellular enzymes which normally downgrade oestrogens (Brenner et al 1982). This leads to an enhanced hepatic potency and because of this, synthetic oestrogens should be avoided in postmenopausal women unless given in small doses.

Parenteral oestrogens

Parenteral oestrogens are particularly advantageous when oral therapy causes epigastric discomfort and flatulence, and when patients have a psychological aversion to taking tablets. They have all the beneficial effects of oral oestrogens.

Vaginal oestrogen creams

These have long been used in the treatment of atrophic vaginitis, on the assumption that they produced a local effect only. Whitehead et al (1978) however showed that the plasma levels of oestrone and oestradiol achieved using a standard regimen daily dose of 1.25 mg of conjugated oestrogen cream are the same or higher than those produced by the same dose of oral conjugated oestrogens.

Very low doses of vaginal oestrogens (0.1 mg) daily are capable of producing significant changes in vaginal cytology and do not cause a rise in plasma oestrogens (Dyer et al 1982). At this low serum level, however, there is no relief of the generalized symptoms of the climacteric, and there are as yet no long-term studies indicating that even this low dosage does not cause deleterious effects on the endometrium when given continuously for a long time. Preparations such as oestriol are available.

The rate of absorption of oestrogens from the vagina depend on the state of the vagina. As vascularity decreases, so does absorption. The rate of absorption also depends on the medium in which the oestradiol is suspended (Schiff et al 1977).

Percutaneous oestrogen creams

This mode of delivery is becoming increasingly popular. A preparation which involves the daily application of oestradiol gel on the skin (Besins) is available. The standard manufacturer's recommended dose is 5 g cream containing 3 mg of oestradiol daily. The method of administration gives a physiological serum oestradiol to oestrone ratio by bypassing the enterohepatic circulation. The avoidance of the first-pass liver effect is common to both percutaneous and subcutaneous therapy.

Various studies have shown that this method gives good relief of symptoms and is safe in postmenopausal women (Brincat et al 1984a, Sitruk-Ware et al 1980, Strecker et al 1980), in whom it has also been shown to increase skin collagen content, at the same dosage (Brincat et al 1987e).

The daily application of cream (gel) requires patient compliance since some women find it sticky. The gel dries up quickly, however, and our own experience has not shown any real problems. Percutaneous cream leads to a relatively higher increase in serum oestradiol and achieves serum levels that are maintained for longer when compared to oral preparations (Lyrenas et al 1981, Sitruk-Ware et al 1980).

Percutaneous oestrogen patches

The transdermal patch can administer oestradiol at controlled rates of 0.025, 0.05 and 0.1 mg/day, depending on the surface area of the patch. Steady concentrations can be obtained if the systems are worn for 72 h and changed twice weekly (Vickers 1980). Utian (1987) showed that the Estraderm patches currently used are as efficacious as Premarin in the relief of symptoms of the climacteric and like Premarin need to have an added progestogen if endometrial hyperplasia is to be avoided (see below). The area of application of both percutaneous and transdermal systems should be changed regularly because of the possibility of itching and skin irritation. Various preparations are now available with differing modes of delivery. These vary between matrix patches and the original reservoir ones. Combined oestrogen and progestogen patches are also available.

Subcutaneous implants

Subcutaneous implants have been used to treat the climacteric syndrome for almost 40 years (Greenblatt & Buran 1949). The technique of insertion is simple and can be done in an outpatient clinic under local anaesthesia. Gonadotrophin levels fall dramatically within 2 weeks of implantation and do not return to pretreatment levels before 6 months if a 100-mg oestradiol implant is used (Thom et al 1981). Oestradiol levels similarly rise to reach a peak at 2–3 months and are back to pretreatment levels by 6 months.

The use of subcutaneous hormone implants avoids the need for daily patient compliance. Furthermore, a testosterone pellet (100 mg) can be safely inserted and thus give the patient further relief of the symptoms of lethargy and loss of libido (Montgomery et al unpublished data, Studd et al 1977). Methyltestosterone (which might be useful for the treatment of psychosexual symptoms) is hepatotoxic when administered orally.

Implants give good symptomatic relief for up to 6 months (Brincat et al 1984b), have few side-effects and complications are rare (Cardozo et al 1984). Even more interesting is the apparent increase in bone mass that is possible in postmenopausal women using oestradiol implant regimes. In a recent study, Savvas et al (1988) showed that a population of women who had been on oestradiol and testosterone implants for between 2 and 10 years had a higher bone mass than a comparable group who had been on oral therapy, who in turn had a bone mass as high as a population of very early postmenopausal women (Fig. 25.7). Furthermore, a prospective study now underway by the same authors is showing a considerable increase in bone mass occurring in women on oestradiol-only implants. A 5% increase in vertebral bone density was found after 6 months and a 9% increase after 1 year. The increase in the proximal femoral bone density was only about 4% of the spine increase because the trabecular bone of the femur is less biologically active.

The conclusion from this and other studies is that although it is possible to maintain bone mass using oral preparations, the higher oestradiol levels achieved with a subcutaneous oestradiol/testosterone implant will lead to a gain in bone mass and a reversal in bone loss. Similar results are obtained when collagen content and thickness of skin is studied when women receive oestradiol implants (Brincat et al 1987b,c).

The oral preparations currently used can only increase bone mass in early postmenopausal women if they are combined with pharmacological doses of an antiresorptive agent such as calcitonin (Meschia et al 1992). This would entail at least two injections a week.

Studd et al (1994, personal communication) have shown that oestradiol and testosterone implants are also effective in increasing bone mass in older (over 65 years) women, and will also retain its protective properties in preventing bone loss (Naessén et al 1993).

Campbell & Whitehead (1977) showed significant relief of climacteric symptoms with the most widely used dose and preparation, 1.25 mg of conjugated oestrogens daily. Most current regimens are opposed with a fixed period of gestogens.

Alternative forms of therapy which avoid the first-pass effect on the liver are simple to use, are efficacious and have high patient acceptability.

The importance of clinical opposed therapy

It has been established that if oestrogens are given on their own and continuously, the incidence of endometrial hyperplasia and the possibility of causing a well differentiated adenocarcinoma of the endometrium is increased, whichever route of administration is used. Assessment of oestrogen concentration within the nuclei of endometrial cells has shown a higher level of oestradiol than oestrone (Whitehead et al 1981), so it is likely that oestradiol has a greater effect on cell proliferation.

Oral oestrogen may be associated with a lower incidence of endometrial hyperplasia than other methods. If, in exceptional circumstances, oestrogens need to be used alone then it would be safer to use such preparations cyclically (i.e. 21 days out of every 28). The addition of cyclical progestogen therapy for 13 days each month has been shown to be effective in preventing endometrial hyperplasia (Studd & Thom 1981, Studd & Magos 1988).

In women who do not want cyclical bleeding or who would be better managed without a monthly withdrawal bleed, it is possible to start continuous regimens of oral oestrogens and combine these with continuous progestogens. By adjusting the progestogen dose appropriately, it is possible to obtain 100% amenorrhoea within 6–9 months of therapy (Magos et al 1985). No endometrial hyperplasia occurred in one study where women were followed up for over 2 years (Magos et al 1986, Studd & Magos 1988).

There is no evidence, however, that any extra benefit or protection anywhere is achieved if gestogens are prescribed in the absence of a uterus (Studd et al 1986). Indeed the protective effect of oestrogens on the cardiovascular system might be compromised by gestogens (Lobo et al 1987). The protective effect of gestogens against breast cancer is extremely controversial (Miller & Anderson, 1988). Evidence in favour is weak and certainly there is no consensus (Lobo et al 1987). Gambrell (1986, 1988) has suggested that such a protective effect does exist but should be considered in conjunction with the evidence of Pike et al (1983) on progestogens increasing the incidence of breast cancer. Other authors have not shown any difference in the incidence of breast cancer when women on oestrogens alone were compared to those on combined preparations (Hunt et al 1987).

Oestrogen replacement therapy

Breast cancer risk

Over the last 15 years more than two dozen epidemiological studies of menopausal replacement treatment and breast cancer have been published. The overall evidence does not indicate any consistent association between the use of oestrogen replacement treatment and subsequent breast cancer risk (La Vecchia 1994). There has however been some suggestion of elevated risk in long-term use (i.e. greater than 5 years) but the studies have several uncertainties at epidemiological level, with no consistent pattern emerging for other time factors considered (Colditz et al 1990). The situation is complicated by the fact that several different types of preparation and duration of intake of multiple preparations need to be considered. Relative risk appears to be elevated by 30–70% for long-term use (La Vecchia 1994) but this range of increased risk serves for no other purpose than to illustrate how inaccurate and unsure the situation still is. Other authors suggest that although the risk with long-term use is increased, the actual survival rate once breast cancer is present is longer in women on oestrogen replacement (Grady et al 1992). The combined therapy, with progestogens, is even more complicated but there certainly seems to be no benefit as regards protection against breast cancer. Indeed there have been suggestions that the opposite might be the case (Bergkvist et al 1989).

Ischaemic heart disease risk

Oestrogen replacement treatment seems to decrease the incidence of ischaemic heart disease by 15–20%. This figure is suggested from 18 published studies incorporating just under 3500 subjects (La Vecchia 1994). Additional progestogens in combined therapy might not be so beneficial and might reduce the protective effect of oestrogens. There are a number of mechanisms whereby oestrogens may be protective, such as the well-known beneficial effects on body fat distribution, insulin resistance and direct arterial effects (Stevenson 1994), with all of these contributing to reducing the cardiovascular morbidity rate.

Undoubtedly further epidemiological data will be available when considering the cost–benefit analysis of hormone replacement therapy. The broadest epidemiological and public health perspective including cancer as well as cardiovascular disease and bone metabolism should be considered. Mortality in women from cardiovascular disease and osteoporotic fracture is far greater than that of breast cancer. The potential benefits from the reduction of cardiovascular disease and osteoporotic fracture in women on hormone replacement therapy numerically far outweigh any possible theoretical increase in the incidence of breast cancer in women on long-term hormone replacement therapy.

Contraindications to hormone replacement therapy

As with all treatment, oestrogen therapy requires consideration of the severity of the illness to be treated and the possible side-effects. Most workers would accept that breast carcinoma and endometrial carcinoma are contraindications, but scientific support for these objections is hard to find. It is not unusual to find that women with oestrogen-dependent tumours are prepared to take the risk of oestrogen therapy because their lives are made so unbearable by menopausal symptoms. There is in fact no evidence that oestrogen therapy produces a recurrence of breast or endometrial carcinoma but if a recurrence does occur it is likely that oestrogens will be blamed.

Hypertension, varicose veins, a previous thrombotic episode, diabetes, endometriosis and fibroids are classically regarded as contraindications, but once again, there is little evidence that this is so. There is no evidence that natural oestrogens (i.e. oestradiol, oestrone, or oestriol) cause any elevation of blood pressure in normotensive or hypertensive women (Hammond et al 1979). Natural progesterone taken orally seems to lower blood pressure in established hypertensives (Rylance et al 1985) in contradiction to previous belief. There is no evidence that oestrogens either affect coagulation, fibrinolysis and platelet behaviour, or cause deep vein thrombosis (Boston Collaborative Drug Surveillance Programme, 1974, Studd et al 1978, Thom et al 1978).

The avoidance of the first-pass liver effect by utilizing percutaneous or subcutaneous routes gives even less reason to indicate that synthesis of coagulation factors from liver should be stimulated. Although synthetic ethinyloestradiol and mestranol are diabetogenic, the natural oestrogens are not (Studd et al 1978, Thom et al 1977).

Endometriosis and fibroids are certainly responsive to endogenous and exogenous oestrogens. This does not in practice represent any clinical problem, because treatment can easily be discontinued. Patients who have undergone a hysterectomy with or without oophorectomy for these conditions do not have any contraindications for oestrogen therapy. This is particularly true for endometriosis when the woman may be quite young and may have suffered a surgical castration for her condition.

CONCLUSION

The changes that occur with changing ovarian function, culminating with the menopause, cause profound changes to a woman. Although not all women have the distressing short-term symptoms, all experience an endocrinological deficiency syndrome leading to multisystem problems, ranging from connective tissue loss to psychological disturbances.

The hormone deficiency state of menopausal women must be recognized. With the increasing longevity of the population and the increase in morbidity and eventual mortality as a result of sex hormone deficiency, the philosophy of whom and whom not to treat deserves reappraisal. There is a poor correlation between the short-term symptoms and the long-term consequences of the menopause, and therefore it is not possible to select women for treatment on the basis of their immediate symptomatology alone. A case can be made for the widespread use of sex hormone replacement so as to improve the quality of life and not just its quantity (Whitehead & Studd 1988).

With continuing developments, sex hormone replacement is becoming increasingly safe and its benefits are seemingly even more extensive than once supposed, especially in the prophylaxis of cardiovascular disease and osteoporosis. Depriving a woman of hormone replacement for spurious or theoretical reasons should be considered very carefully, since very often there are no real contraindications.

KEY POINTS

1. Women in the west spend 30% of their lives in this state of profound oestrogen deprivation and only a small proportion receive HRT for any length of time.
2. Postmenopausally, the incidence of ischaemic heart disease, osteoporosis, loss of collagen and psychological disorders increases dramatically.
3. Postmenopausal atrophy in the urinary and genital tracts commonly leads to urinary disorders, dyspareunia and recurrent vaginal infections.
4. The female to male sex distribution of hip fractures after the age of 51 years is 3 to 1. Osteoporosis is the main culprit, but dementia and psychomotor slowing (both also thought to be linked to the menopause) play a part after the age of 70 years.
5. HRT has been shown quite clearly to prevent (or reverse) osteoporosis and reduce the female age-related increase in the incidence of cardiovascular disease postmenopausally.
6. Women with a uterus must be given a progestogen (in addition to oestrogen) for at least 10–12 days in each cycle.
7. The stated increased relative risk (1.3–1.7) of breast carcinoma in women on HRT for greater than 5 years, even if true, is probably negated by the fact that survival time is the same in both groups.
8. Although hypertension, varicose veins, thromboembolic phenomena, diabetes mellitus, endometriosis and fibroids, are classically cited as contraindications to HRT there is little, if any, evidence that they should be so.
9. The main reasons for the poor uptake of HRT in eligible women are poor patient (and doctor) education, poor compliance, and side-effects (including withdrawal bleeds), all of which can be potentially overcome by a whole range of newer HRT preparations.

EDITOR'S ADDENDUM

Risk of venous thrombosis with hormone replacement therapy

Until very recently, there was no evidence that hormone replacement therapy increased the risk of deep venous thrombosis or pulmonary embolism. This contrast with the effects of the oral contraceptive pill was thought to be due to the lower doses of oestrogens in hormone replacement. However, in October 1996, three linked case control studies were published in *The Lancet* (Daly et al 1996, Hershel et al 1996, Grodstein et al 1996). Each study showed a twofold to fourfold increase in risk of thromboembolism associated with current use of hormone replacement therapy. Because these were rare problems, the absolute risks remained small. The additional risk of thromboembolic disease was around 1 in 5000 users per year and the extra risk of pulmonary embolism was 5 per 100 000 women years. The conclusion was that these absolute risks were low and accounted for only a modest increase in morbidity.

REFERENCES

Alcoff J M, Campbell D, Tribble D, Oldfield B, Cruess O 1981 Double blind, placebo controlled crossover trial of Propranolol as treatment for menopausal vasomotor symptoms. Clinical Therapeutics 3: 356–364
Alffram P S, Bauer G 1962 Epidemiology of fractures of the forearm. Journal of Bone and Joint Surgery 44A: 105
Albright F, Smith P H, Richardson A M 1941 Postmenopausal osteoporosis – its clinical features. Journal of the American Medical Association 116: 2465–2474
Amudsen D W, Diers C J 1973 The age of the menopause in medieval Europe. Human Biology 45: 605–608
Appleby B 1962 Norethisterone in the control of menopausal symptoms. Lancet i: 407–409
Aronson M K, Ooi W L, Morgenstern H et al 1990 Women, myocardial infarction and dementia in the very old. Neurology 40: 1102–1106
Aylward M 1975 Oestrogens, plasma, tryptophan levels in peri-menopausal patients. In: Campbell S (ed). The management of the menopause and postmenopausal years, University Parthenon Press, London, pp 135–147
Bachner D M, Larson E B 1987 Falls and fracture in patients with Alzheimer's type dementia. Journal of the American Medical Association 257: 1492–1495
Baker T G 1963 A quantitative and cytological study of germ cells in human ovaries. Proceedings of the Royal Society of London, Series B 158: 417–433
Ballinger C B 1975 Psychiatric morbidity and the menopause. Screening of the general population sample. British Medical Journal 3: 344–346
Ballinger C B 1977 Psychiatric morbidity and the menopause. Survey of gynaecological outpatient clinic. British Journal of Psychiatry 131: 83–89
Bergkvist L, Adami H O, Persson I, Hoover R, Scharier C 1989 The risk of breast cancer after oestrogen and oestrogen replacement. New England Journal of Medicine 321: 293–297
Berlinger W G, Potter J F 1991 Low body mass index in demented outpatients. Journal of the American Geriatric Society 39: 973–978
Birge S J 1994 The role of oestrogen deficiency in the aging central nervous system. In: Lobo R A (ed) Treatment of postmenopausal woman: basic and clinical aspects. Raven Press, New York, 14: 153–157
Black N M, Shuster S, Bottoms E 1970 Osteoporosis, skin collagen and androgen. British Medical Journal 4: 773–774
Boston Collaborative Drug Surveillance Programme 1974 Surgically confirmed gall bladder venous thrombo embolism and breast tumours in relation to postmenopausal oestrogen therapy. New England Journal of Medicine 290: 15–19
Brenner P M, Mashchak C A, Lobo R A et al 1982 Potency and hepato-cellular effects of oestrogen after oral, percutaneous, subcutaneous administration. In: Van Keep P A, Utian W, Vermeulen A (eds) The controversial climacteric. MTP Press, Lancaster, pp 103–125
Brincat M, Studd J W W 1988 Skin and the menopause. The Menopause 8: 85–101
Brincat M, Moniz C E, Studd J W W et al 1983 Sex hormones and skin collagen content in postmenopausal women. British Medical Journal 287: 1337–1338
Brincat T M, de Trafford J C, Lafferty K. Roberts V C, Studd J W W 1984a A role for oestrogen in peripheral vasomotor control and menopausal flushing – a preliminary report. British Journal of Obstetrics and Gynaecology 11: 1107–1110
Brincat M, Magos A L, Studd J W W et al 1984b Subcutaneous hormone implants for the control of climacteric symptoms: a prospective study. Lancet i: 16–18
Brincat M, Moniz C J, Studd J W W et al 1985 Long term effects of the menopause and sex hormones on skin thickness. British Journal of Obstetrics and Gynecology 92: 256–259
Brincat M, Moniz C F, Kabalan S et al 1987a Decline in skin collagen content and metacarpal index after the menopause and its prevention with sex hormone replacement. British Journal of Obstetrics and Gynaecology 94: 126–129
Brincat M, Versi E, Studd J W W et al 1987b Skin collagen changes in postmenopausal women receiving different regimes of oestrogen therapy. Obstetrics and Gynecology 70: 123–127
Brincat M, Wong A, Studd J W W et al 1987c The response of skin thickness and metacarpal index to oestradiol therapy in postmenopausal women. Obstetrics and Gynecology 70: 538–541
Brincat M, Kabalan S, Studd J W W et al 1987d A study of the relationship of skin collagen content, skin thickness and bone mass in the postmenopausal woman. Obstetrics and Gynecology 70: 840–845
Brincat M, Moniz C F, Kabalan S et al 1987e Skin collagen changes in postmenopausal women treated with oestradiol gel. Maturitas 9: 1–5
Brincat M et al 1994a Italian Menopause Society Keynote Lecture, Rome
Brincat M, Muscat Baron Y, Galea R 1994b Screening of osteoporotic fractures. A new model incorporating bone density, menopausal age and skin thickness. Free communication, FIGO Conference, Montreal
Bruns P 1882 Die Allgemeine Lebra von der Knochenbruchen. Deutsche Chirurgie 27: 1–400
Bush T L, Barnett-Connor E, Cowan L D et al 1987 Cardiovascular mortality and non-contraceptive use of oestrogen in women: results from the Lipid Research Clinic Programme follow-up study. Circulation 75: 1102
Campbell S 1975 Psychometric studies on the effect of natural oestrogens in postmenopausal women. In: Campbell S (ed) Management of the menopause and postmenopausal years. MTP Press, Lancaster, pp 149–158
Campbell S, Whitehead M I 1977 Oestrogen therapy and the menopausal syndrome. Clinics in Obstetrics and Gynaecology 4 (supp 1): 31–47
Campbell S, Whitehead M I 1982 Potency and hepato-cellular effects of oestrogens after oral, percutaneous and subcutaneous administration. In: Van Keep P A, Utian W, Vermeulen A (eds) The controversial climacteric, MTP Press, Lancaster, pp 103–125
Cardozo L, Gibb D, Studd J W W, Tuck S, Thom M, Cooper D 1984 The use of hormone implants for the climacteric symptoms. American Journal of Obstetrics and Gynecology 1: 336–337
Chakravati S, Collins W P, Forecart J D et al 1976 Hormonal profiles after the menopause. British Medical Journal 2: 784–786
Chestnut C H 1984 Synthetic salmon calcitonin, diphosphales and anabolic steroids in the treatment of postmenopausal osteoporosis. Osteoporosis. Proceedings of the Copenhagen International Symposium on Osteoporosis 2: 549–555
Chestnut C H III, Ivey J L, Nelp W B et al 1979 Assessment of anabolic steroids and calcitonin in the treatment of osteoporosis. In: Barzel US (ed) Osteoporosis II. Grune and Stratton, New York, pp 135–150
Christiansen C, Christiansen M S, McNain P, Hagen C, Stockland K, Transolol I 1980 Prevention of early menopausal bone loss: controlled 2-years study in 315 normal females. European Journal of Clinical Investigation 10: 273–279
Clayden J R, Bell J W, Pollard P 1974 Menopausal flushing: double blind trial of a non-hormonal preparation. British Medical Journal 1: 409–412
Colditz G A, Stampfer M J, Willett W C, Hennekens C H, Rosner B, Speizer F E 1990 Prospective study of oestrogen replacement therapy and risk of breast cancer in postmenopausal women. Journal of the American Medical Association 264: 2648–2653
Crilly R G, Horsman A, Marshall D H, Nordin B E C 1978 Bone mass in postmenopausal women after withdrawal of oestrogen/gestogen replacement therapy. Lancet i: 459–461
Crook D, Godsland I F, Wynn V 1988 Ovarian hormones and plasma lipoproteins. The Menopause 15: 168–180
Cummings S R, Kelsey J L, Nevitt M C, O'Dowd K S 1985 Epidemiology of osteoporosis and osteoporotic fractures. Epidemiological Review 7: 178–207
Daly E, Vessey M P, Hawkins M M, Carson J L, Gough P, Marsh S 1996 Risk of venous thromboembolism in users of hormone replacement therapy. Lancet 348: 977–980
De Fazio J, Meldrum D R, Winer J H, Judd H C 1984 Direct action of androgens on hot flushes in a human male. Maturitas 6: 3–8

Dennerstein L, Burrows G 1978 A review of studies of the psychological symptoms found at the menopause. Maturitas 1: 55–64
Ditkoff E C, Crary W G, Cristo M, Lobo R A 1991 Oestrogen improves psychological function in asymptomatic postmenopausal women. Obstetrics and Gynecology 78: 991–995
Dyer G, Townsend P T, Jehowitsz J, Young O, Whitehead M I 1982 Dose related changes in vaginal cytology after topical conjugated equine oestrogens. British Medical Journal 284: 789–790
Editorial 1988 Need we poison the elderly so often? Lancet ii: 20
Erlik Y, Tatayn I V, Meldrum D R et al 1981 Association of wakening episodes with menopausal hot flushes. Journal of the American Medical Association 245: 1741–1744
Faber P, Heidenreich J 1977 Treatment of stress incontinence with oestrogen in postmenopausal women. Urologia Internationalis 32: 221–223
Fieldman J M, Postlethwaite R W, Glenn J F 1976 Hot flushes and sweats in men with testicular insufficiency. Archives of Internal Medicine 136: 606–608
Fillit H, Weinreb H, Cholst I et al 1986 Observations in a preliminary open trial of oestradiol therapy for senile dementia – Alzheimer's type. Psychoneuroendocrinology 11: 337–345
Frere G 1971 Mean age at menopause and menarche in South Africa. South African Journal of Medical Science 36: 21–25
Frie J F 1980 Ageing, natural death and the compression of morbidity. New England Journal of Medicine 303: 130–135
Gambrell D 1986 Hormonal replacement therapy and breast cancer. In: Greenblatt R B (ed) A modern approach to the perimenopausal years. Gruyter, Berlin, pp 176–188
Gambrell R D 1988 Studies of endometrial and breast disease with hormone replacement therapy. The Menopause 22: 247–261
Geist S H, Mintz M 1937 Pituitary radiation for the relief of menopause symptoms. American Journal of Obstetrics and Gynecology 33: 643–645
Gordan G S 1984 Prevention of bone loss and fractures in women. Maturitas 6: 225–242
Gordon T, Castelli W P, Hjorteand M C, Kannal W O, Dauber T R 1977 High density lipoprotein as a protective factor against coronary heart disease. The Framingham Study. American Journal of Medicine 62: 707–714
Grady D, Rubin S M, Pettiti D B, Fox C S et al 1992 Hormone replacement therapy to prevent disease and prolong life in postmenopausal women. Annals of Internal Medicine 117: 1016–1037
Greenblatt R B, Buran R R 1949 Indications for hormone pellets in the therapy of endocrine and gynaecological disorders. American Journal of Obstetrics and Gynecology 47: 294–301
Grisso J A, Chire G Y, Maislin G et al 1991 Risk factors for hip fractures in men: a preliminary study. Journal of Bone and Mineral Research 6: 865–868
Grodstein F, Stampfer M J, Goldhaber S Z, Manon J E, Colditz G A, Speizer F E, Willett W C, Hennekens C H 1996 Prospective study of exogenous hormones and risk of pulmonary embolism in women. Lancet 348: 983–987
Haataja M, Paul R, Gronroos M et al 1984 Effect of prostaglandin inhibitor and oestrogen on climacteric symptoms and serum free fatty acids. Maturitas 5: 263–269
Hammond C B, Jelovsek F R, Lee K C, Creasman W T, Parker R J 1979 Effects of long term oestrogen replacement therapy. 1. Metabolic effects. American Journal of Obstetrics and Gynecology 133: 525–535
Harrison R F 1981 Ethamsylate in the treatment of climacteric flushing. Maturitas 3: 31–37
Heaney R P, Recker R R, Saville R P 1978 Menopausal changes in calcium balance performance. Journal of Laboratory and Clinical Medicine 92: 953–963
Henderson B E 1989 The cancer question. An overview of recent epidemiologic and retrospective data. American Journal of Obstetrics and Gynecology 161: 1859–1864
Hendy M S, Burge R S 1983 Climacteric flushing in a man. British Medical Journal 287: 423
Hershel J, Derby L E, Myers M W, Vasilakis C, Newton K M 1996 Risk of hospital admission for ideopathic venous thromboembolism among users of postmenopausal oestrogens. Lancets 348: 981–983
Hilton P, Stanton S L 1983 The use of intravaginal oestrogen cream in genuine stress incontinence with oestrogen in postmenopausal women. Urologia Internationalis 32: 221–223
Holland E F N, Studd J W W, Mansell J P et al 1994 Changes in collagen composition and cross-links in bone and skin of osteoporotic postmenopausal treated with percutaneous estradiol implants. Obstetrics and Gynecology 83: 180–183
Honjo H, Ogino Y, Naitoh K et al 1989 In vivo effects of oestrone sulfate on the central nervous system senile dementia (Alzheimer's type). Journal of Steroid Biochemistry 34: 521–525
Hunt K, Vessey M, McPherson K et al 1987 Long term surveillance of mortality and cancer incidence in women receiving hormone replacement therapy. British Journal of Obstetrics and Gynaecology 94: 620–626
Iosif C S, Batia S, Ed A, Astedt B 1981 Oestrogen receptors in the human female lower urinary tract. American Journal of Obstetrics and Gynecology 141: 817–820
Iosif C S, Henriksson L, Ulmsten U 1981 The frequency of disorders of the lower urinary tract, urinary incontinence in particular, as evaluated by questionnaire survey. Acta Obstetrica et Gynaecologica Scandinavica 60: 71–76
Iosif C S, Bekassy Z 1984 Prevalence of genito-urinary symptoms in the late menopause. Acta Obstetrica et Gynaecologica Scandinavica 63: 257–260
Jazsman L 1973 Epidemiology of the climacteric complaints. Frontiers of Hormone Research 2: 220–234
Jorm A F, Korten A E, Henderson A S 1987 The prevalence of dementia: a quantitative integration of the literature. Acta Psychiatrica Scandinavica 76: 465–479
Judd H L, Cleary R E, Creasman W T et al 1981 Estrogen replacement therapy. Obstetrics and Gynecology 58: 267–275
Kaplan J A 1987 Identification of oestrogen receptors on osteoblast. International Conference on Osteoporosis, Aalburg. [Unpublished abstract]
Klaiber E L, Broverman D M, Vogel W, Kobayashi Y 1979 Estrogen replacement therapy for severe persistent depressions in women. Archives of General Psychiatry 36: 550–554
Laragh J H, Sealey J E, Ledingham J G, Newton M A 1967 Oral contraceptives, renin aldosterone and high blood pressure. Journal of the American Medical Association 201: 218–222
La Vecchia C 1994 Breast cancer risk in hormone replacement therapy-treated women. In: Crosignani P G, Paoletti R, Surrell P M et al (eds) Women's health in menopause. Kluwer Academic, Boston, pp 67–73
Lightman S L, Jacobs A S, Maguire A K 1982 Down regulation of gonadotrophic secretion in post-menopausal women by a superactive LHRH analogue: lack of effect on menopausal flushing. British Journal of Obstetrics and Gynaecology 89: 977–980
Lindsay R, Hart D M 1978 Failure of response of menopausal vasomotor symptoms to clonidine. Maturitas 1: 21–25
Lindsay R, Hart D H, Purdie D, Ferguson M, Clark A S 1978 Comparative effects of oestrogen and a progestagen on bone loss in postmenopausal women. Clinical Science and Molecular Medicine 54: 193–198
Lindsay R, Hart D H, Clark A S 1984 The minimum effect of oestrogen for the prevention of postmenopausal bone loss. Obstetrics and Gynecology 63: 759–762
Lobo R A, McCormick W, Singer F et al 1984 Depo-medroxyprogesterone acetate compared with conjugated oestrogens for the treatment of post-menopausal women. Obstetrics and Gynecology 63: 1–5
Lobo R A, Wren B, Crona N et al 1987 Effects of oestrogens and progestagens on the cardiovascular system in postmenopausal women. In: Zichella L, Whitehead M, Van Keep P A (eds) The climacteric and beyond. Parthenon Publishing, New Jersey, pp 95–107
Lyrenas S, Carlstom K, Backstrom T, van Schoultz B 1981 A comparison of serum estrogen levels after percutaneous and oral administration of oestradiol-17B. British Journal of Obstetrics and Gynaecology 83: 181–187
McKinlay S M, Jeffreys M 1974 The menopausal syndrome. British Journal of Preventative and Social Medicine 2: 108–115
McKinlay S M, Jeffreys K, Thompson B 1972 An investigation of the age at the menopause. Journal of Biosocial Science 4: 161–166

McLaren H C 1949 Vitamin E in the menopause. British Medical Journal 2: 1378–1382
Magness R R, Rosefeld C R 1989 Local and systemic oestradiol-17B: effect on uterine and systemic vasodilatation. American Journal of Physiology 256: E 536–542
Magos A L, Brincat M, Studd J W W et al 1985 Amenorrhoea and endometrial atrophy with continuous oral oestrogen and progestogen therapy in postmenopausal women. Obstetrics and Gynecology 65: 496–499
Magos A L, Brewster E, Singh R, O'Dowd T, Brincat M, Studd J W W 1986 The effects of norethisterone in postmenopausal women on oestrogen replacement therapy: a model for the premenstrual syndrome. British Journal of Obstetrics and Gynecology 93: 1290–1296
Melton L J, Kan S H, Wahner H W et al 1988 Lifetime fracture risk: an approach to hip fracture risk assessment based on bone mineral density and age. Journal of Clinical Epidemiology 41: 985–994
Meschia M, Brincat M, Barbacini P, Maini M C, Marri R, Crossignani P G 1992 Effect of hormone replacement therapy and calcitonin on bone mass in menopausal women. European Journal of Obstetrics, Gynaecology and Reproductive Biology 47: 1: 53
Meschia M, Bruschi F, Anicarelli F, Barbacini P, Monza G C, Crosignani P G 1994 Transdermal hormone replacement therapy and skin in postmenopausal women. A placebo controlled study. Menopause: the Journal of the North American Menopause Society 1: 79–82
Miller C W 1978 Survival and ambulation following hip fractures. Bone and Joint Surgery 60A: 930–934
Miller W R, Anderson T J 1988 Oestrogens, progestogens and the breast. The Menopause 21: 234–246
Molsa P K, Marttila R J, Rinne U K 1982 Epidemiology of dementia in a Finnish population. Acta Neurologica Scandinavica 65: 541–552
Montgomery J C, Appleby L, Brincat M et al 1987 Effect of oestrogen and testosterone implants on psychological disorders of the climacteric. Lancet i: 297–299
Muscat Baron Y, Brincat M, Galea R, Muscat Baron A 1994 The epidemiology of osteoporotic fractures in a mediterranean country. Calcified Tissue International 54: 365–369
Natchigall L E, Natchigall R H, Natchigall R D, Bechman E 1980 Estrogen replacement therapy: a 10 year prospective study in the response to osteoporosis. Obstetrics and Gynecology 53: 277–281
Naessén T, Persson I, Thor L, Mallmin H, Ljunghall S, Bergstrom R 1993 Maintained bone density at advanced ages after long term treatment with low dose oestradiol implants. British Journal of Obstetrics and Gynaecology 100: 5: 454–459
Neugarten B C, Kraines R J 1965 'Menopause symptoms' in women of various ages. Psychosomatic Medicine 27: 270–284
Nikko W 1986 Some aspects of oogenesis, follicular growth and endocrine involution. In: Greenblatt R B (ed) A modern approach to the perimenopausal years. Walter de Gruyter, Berlin, pp 11–38
Nordin B E C 1960 Osteomalacia, osteoporosis and calcium deficiency. Clinical Orthopaedics and Related Research 17: 235–258
Nordin B E C, Aaron J, Speed R, Crilly R G 1981 Bone formation and resorption as the determinants of trabecular bone volume in postmenopausal osteoporosis. Lancet ii: 227–295
Osborne J C 1976 Postmenopausal changes in micturition habits and in urine flow and urethral pressure studies. In: Campbell S (ed) The management of the menopause and postmenopausal years. MTP Press, Lancaster, pp 285–289
Patterson M E L 1982 A randomized double-blind cross-over trial into the effect of norethisterone on climacteric symptoms and biochemical profiles. British Journal of Obstetrics and Gynaecology 89: 464–472
Pike H C, Henderson B E, Krailo M D, Duke A, Roy S 1983 Breast cancer in young women and use of oral contraceptives: possible modifying effect of formulation and age of use. Lancet ii: 926–929
Pines A, Fisman E Z, Lev Y et al 1991 The effect of hormone replacement therapy in normal postmenopausal women: measurements of Doppler-derived parameters of aortic flow. American Journal of Obstetrics and Gynecology 164: 806–812
Porter R W, Miller C G, Grainger O, Palmer S B 1990 Prediction of hip fracture in elderly women: a prospective study. British Medical Journal 301: 638–641
Punnonen R 1973 Effect of castration and peroral therapy on the skin. Acta Obstetrica et Gynaecologica Scandinavica 21 (suppl): 1–44
Ross R K, Paganini-Hill A, Mack T N et al 1981 Menopausal estrogen therapy and protection from death from ischaemic heart disease. Lancet i: 858–861
Ross R K, Paganini-Hill A, Mack J M 1984 Reduction in fractures and other effects of oestrogen replacement therapy in human population. Osteoporosis. Proceedings of the Copenhagen International Symposium on Osteoporosis 1: 289–297
Ryan K J, Engel L L 1953 The interconversion of oestrone and estradiol by human tissue slices. Endocrinology 52: 287–291
Rylance P B, Brincat M, Lafferty K et al 1985 Natural progesterone and antihypertensive action. British Medical Journal 290: 13–14
Sarrel P M 1988 Sexuality. The Menopause 6: 65–75
Savvas M, Studd J W W, Fogelman I, Dooley M, Montgomery J, Murby B 1988 Skeletal effects of oral oestrogen compared with subcutaneous oestrogen and testosterone in postmenopausal women. British Journal of Medicine 297: 331–333
Schiff I, Tulchinsky D, Ryan K J 1977 Vaginal absorption of estrone and 17B-oestradiol. Fertility and Sterility 28: 1063–1065
Schiff I, Tulchinsky D, Cramer D, Ryan K J 1980 Oral medroxyprogesterone in treatment of postmenopausal symptoms. Journal of the American Medical Association 244: 1443–1445
Schneider H P G 1986 The climacteric syndrome. In: Greenblatt R D (ed) A modern approach to the perimenopausal years. Walter de Gruyter, Berlin, pp 39–55
Shahrad D P, Marks R 1977 A pharmacological effect of oestrone on human epidermis. British Journal of Dermatology 97: 383–386
Sherwin B B 1988 Affective changes with oestrogen and androgen replacement therapy in surgically menopausal women. Journal of Affective Disorders 14: 177–187
Sherwin B B, Gelfund M M 1989 A prospective one year study of oestrogen and progestin in postmenopausal women: effects on clinical symptoms and lipoprotein lipids. Obstetrics and Gynecology 73: 759–766
Sitruk-Ware R, de Lignieres B, Basdevant A et al 1980 Absorption of percutaneous oestradiol in postmenopausal women. Maturitas 2: 202–211
Smith P 1972 Age changes in the female urethra. British Journal of Urology 44: 667–676
Stampfer M J, Willett W C, Colditz J A et al 1985 A prospective study of postmenopausal estrogen therapy and coronary heart disease. New England Journal of Medicine 313: 1044
Stanton S L, Oszoy A, Hilton P 1983 Voiding difficulties in the female: prevalence, clinical and urodynamic review. Obstetrics and Gynecology 61: 144–147
Stevenson J C 1994 Effects of hormone replacement therapy on metabolic risk factors for cardiovascular disease. In: Crosignani P G, Paoletti R, Sarrel P M et al (eds) Women's health in menopause. Kluwer Academic, Boston, pp 19–26
Stevenson J C, Whitehead M I 1982 Postmenopausal osteoporosis. British Medical Journal 285: 585–588
Strecker J B, Lauritzen C H, Nebelung J, Musch K 1980 Climacteric symptoms, estrogens and gonadotrophins in plasma and urine after application of estradiol ointment on the abdominal skin of oophorectomized women. In: Mauvais-Jarvis P, Vickers C F H, Wepierre J (eds) Percutaneous absorption of steroids. Academic Press, London, pp 267–272
Studd J W W, Magos A 1988 Oestrogen therapy and endometrial pathology. The Menopause 18: 197–212
Studd J W W, Parsons A 1977 Sexual dysfunction: the climacteric. British Journal of Sexual Medicine 1: 11–12
Studd J W W, Thom M 1981 Oestrogens and endometrial cancer. In: Studd J W W (ed) Progress in obstetrics and gynaecology. Churchill Livingstone, London, pp 182–188
Studd J W W, Collins W P, Chakravarti S, Newton J R, Oram D, Parsons A 1977 Oestradiol and testosterone implants in the treatment of psychosexual problems in the postmenopausal woman. British Journal of Obstetrics and Gynaecology 84: 314–316
Studd J W W, Dubiel M, Kakkar W, Thom M, White P J 1978 The effect of hormone replacement therapy on glucose tolerance, clotting

factors, fibrinolysis and platelet behaviour in post-menopausal women. In: Cook I D (ed) The role of oestrogen/progestogen in the management of the menopause. MTP Press, Lancaster, pp 41–59
Studd J W W, Thom M H, Paterson N E L, Wade-Evans T 1980 The prevention and treatment of endometrial pathology in postmenopausal women receiving exogenous estrogens. In: Pasetto N, Paoletti R, Ambros J L (ed) The menopause and postmenopause. MTP Press, Lancaster, pp 127–139
Studd J W W, Anderson H M, Montgomery J C 1986 Selection of patients – kind and duration of treatment. In: Greenblatt R B (ed) A modern approach to the postmenopausal years. Walter de Gruyter, Berlin, pp 129–140
Stumpf W E, Sur M, Joshi S E 1976 Estrogen target cells in the skin. Experientia 30: 196–199
Sturdee D W, Wilson K A, Pipilli E, Crocker A D 1978 Physiological aspects of the menopausal hot flush. British Medical Journal 2: 79–80
Tang M X, Jacobs D, Stern Y et al 1996 Effects of oestrogens on risk and age at onset of Alzheimer's disease. Lancet 348: 429–432
Tataryn I V, Lomax P, Bajonek J G, Chesarek W, Meldrum D R, Judd H L 1980 Postmenopausal hot flushes: a disorder of thermoregulation. Maturitas 2: 101–107
Thom M, Chakravarti S, Oram D H, Studd J W W 1977 Effect of hormone replacement therapy on glucose tolerance in postmenopausal women. British Journal of Obstetrics and Gynaecology 84: 776–784
Thom M, Dubiel M, Kakkar V V, Studd J W W 1978 The effects of different regimes of oestrogen on the clotting and fibrinolysis system of the postmenopausal women. Oestrogen Therapy. Frontiers of Hormone Research 5: 192–202
Thom M H, Collins W P, Studd J W W 1981 Hormone profiles in postmenopausal women after therapy with subcutaneous implants. British Journal of Obstetrics and Gynaecology 88: 426–433
Thomson J, Oswald I 1977 Effect of oestrogen on sleep, mood and anxiety of menopausal women. British Medical Journal 2:1317–1319
Thompson B, Hart S A, Durno D 1973 Menopausal age and symptomatology in a general practice. Journal of Biosocial Science 5: 71–82
Tiegs R D, Body J J, Warner H W, Barta J, Riggs B L, Heath H I 1984 Calcitonin secretion in postmenopausal osteoporosis. New England Journal of Medicine 312: 1097–1100
Tikkannen M J, Nikkila E A, Kunsi T 1986 Lipids, hormonal status and the cardiovascular system in the menopause. In: Greenblatt R B (ed) A modern approach to the perimenopausal years. Walter de Gruyter, Berlin, pp 77–86
Tulandi T, Kinch R A, Guyda H, Mazella L, Lal S 1984 Effect of methyldopa on menopausal flushes, skin temperature and luteinizing hormone secretion. American Journal of Obstetrics and Gynecology 150: 709–712
Utian W H 1987 Alternative delivery systems for steroid hormones. In: Zichella L, Whitehead M I, Van Keep P A (eds) The climacteric and beyond. Parthenon Publishing, New Jersey, pp 169–183
Van der Meer J, Stoepman van Dalen E A, Jensen J M S 1973 Antithrombin III deficiency in a Dutch family. Journal of Clinical Pathology 26: 532–538
Van Hartesveldt C, Joyce J N 1986 Effects of oestrogen on the basal ganglia. Neuroscience and Biobehavioural Review 10: 1–14
Vashinav R, Gallagher J A, Beresford N N, Russell R G G 1984 Proliferative effects of oestrogens on bone derived cells. Calcified Tissue International 36 (suppl): S59
Versi E 1986 The bladder in the menopausal woman. In: Greenblatt R B (ed) A modern approach to the perimenopausal years. Walter de Gruyter, Berlin, pp 93–102
Versi E, Cardozo L D 1985 Urethral vascular pulsations. Proceedings of the International Continence Society, London, pp 503–594
Versi E, Cardozo L D, Brincat M, Cooper D, Montgomery J C, Studd J W W 1988 Correlation of urethral physiology and skin collagen in postmenopausal women. British Journal of Obstetrics and Gynaecology 95: 147–152
Vickers C F H 1980 Reservoir effect of human skin: pharmacological speculation. In: Mauvais Jarvis P, Vickers C F H, WePierre J (eds) Percutaneous absorption of steroids. Academic Press, London, pp 19–20
Voda A M 1981 Climacteric hot flush. Maturitas 3: 73–90
Walter S, Wolf I, Barlebo H, Jensen H K 1978 Urinary incontinence in postmenopausal women treated with oestrogens. A double blind clinical trial. Urologia Internationalis 33: 136–143
Warren M P, Brooks-Gunn J, Hamilton L H, Warren F, Hamilton J 1986 Scoliosis and fractures in young ballet dancers. New England Journal of Medicine 314: 1348–1353
Weiss B L 1987 Failure of nalmefene and oestrogen to improve memory in Alzheimer's disease. American Journal of Psychiatry 144: 386–387
Whitehead M I, Crust M 1987 Consequences and treatment of early loss of ovarian function. In: Zichella C, Whitehead M, Van Keep P A (eds) The climacteric and beyond. Parthenon Publishing, New Jersey, pp 63–68
Whitehead M I, Studd J W W 1988 Selection of patients for treatment. Which therapy and for how long? The Menopause 10: 116–129
Whitehead M I, Mirandi J, Kitchin Y, Sharples M J 1978 Systemic absorption of estrogen from Premarin vaginal cream. In: Cooke I D (ed) The role of estrogen/progestagen in the management of the menopause. MTP Press, Lancaster, pp 63–71
Whitehead M I, Lane G, Dyer G, Townsend P T, Collins W P, King R J B 1981 Estradiol: the predominant intranuclear estrogen in the endometrium of estrogen-treated postmenopausal women. British Journal of Obstetrics and Gynaecology 88: 914–918
Wilson P W F, Garrison R J, Castelli W P 1985 Postmenopausal estrogen use, cigarette smoking and cardiovascular morbidity in women over 50. The Framingham study. New England Journal of Medicine 313: 1038

26

Contraception, sterilization and abortion

A. Glasier

INTRODUCTION

Over the last 30 years there has been a significant rise in the use of contraception worldwide. The prevalence of contraceptive use remains low, however, in many less developed countries: only 14% of couples use contraception in some African countries. It has been estimated (World Health Organization (WHO) 1994) that some 120 million women in developing countries who do not wish to become pregnant are unable, for a variety of reasons, to use contraception. If the world is to achieve the United Nations medium-variant predicted population of 6.2 billion, the number of contraceptive users in developing countries must increase from the figure of 381 million in 1990 to 567 million by the year 2000.

A recent survey in Great Britain (Oddens et al 1994) reported that over 95% of sexually active women who wished to avoid pregnancy were using a method of contraception. The highest percentages of women not using contraception despite being sexually active and not wanting to get pregnant, were among adolescents (9%), women over 40 (9%), women with lower educational standards and those with occasional sexual partners (13%).

Despite the apparently high prevalence of contraceptive use in the UK, it has been estimated that 30% of babies delivered are the result of unplanned pregnancies. Moreover large numbers of unplanned pregnancies are terminated. Scotland has an abortion rate which is one of the lowest in countries in which abortion is legal, yet for every six babies born, one pregnancy is terminated. Although abortion is a safe procedure in Western countries, it has been estimated that almost half of the annual figure of 50 million abortions performed around the world are unsafe (WHO 1994).

Different methods of contraception are prevalent in different countries. The intrauterine device (IUD) is the commonest method in China, while the vast majority of couples in Japan, where the combined oral contraceptive pill is not licensed, use the condom. In some of the less developed parts of the world breastfeeding is still the most

Table 26.1 Use of contraceptive methods in the UK. From Oddens et al (1994)

Method	%
Oral contraceptives (OC)	36
Barrier methods	20.8
Vasectomy	16
Female sterilization	10.1
Intrauterine devices (IUD)	7.3
OC with barrier	3.3
Natural family planning (NFP)	1.5
Coitus interruptus	1.1
No method	3.6

important method of birth spacing. The prevalence of method-use in the UK is shown in Table 26.1.

CONTRACEPTION

COMBINED ORAL CONTRACEPTIVES

The combined oral contraceptive pill (COC) was developed during the 1950s and approved for use in Britain in 1961. The first preparations were thought to contain only progestogen but when purified preparations were tried, cycle control deteriorated. The impurity had been oestrogen, and when it was reinstated the combined pill as we know it today was created.

The COC contains oestrogen, usually ethinyl oestradiol, and a synthetic progesterone (progestogen). Most modern pills contain 20–35 μg ethinyl oestradiol with either a second-generation progestogen (norethisterone, levonorgestrel or ethynodiol diacetate), or a so-called third-generation progestogen (gestodene, norgestimate or desogestrel). The 20 μg-containing pills are as effective as 30 μg pills but not surprisingly are associated with poorer cycle control (Akerlund et al 1993).

Third-generation progestogens have a higher affinity for the progesterone receptor, thereby binding more strongly to it and are probably more effective in inhibiting ovulation. They also have a lower affinity for androgen receptors and are therefore less androgenic than the older progestogens. For this reason they are associated with a less adverse effect on serum lipids (Rebar & Zeserson 1991). Women taking pills containing modern progestogens have higher circulating concentrations of high density lipoproteins (HDL) and lower concentrations of low density lipoproteins (LDL). Since this profile of lipoproteins, at least in men, appears to be associated with a lower risk of cardiovascular disease, it was thought that the risk of myocardial infarction and perhaps stroke would be lower among women using third- as compared with second-generation progestogen-containing pills. As myocardial infarction is fortunately a very rare event among young women it has not been possible to establish whether this theoretical benefit is of clinical relevance.

Nevertheless the third-generation pills had been increasing in popularity since their introduction in the early 1980s, and in 1995 were the market leaders in the UK. In October 1995, however, the UK Committee on Safety of Medicines (CSM) considered evidence from three studies, two of which were published in December 1995 (Jick et al 1995, WHO 1995) which suggested that the risk of venous thromboembolic disease was significantly increased among women taking pills containing either gestodene or desogestrel compared with those taking pills containing levonorgestrel or norethisterone. In the WHO study the risk was more than doubled, although the risk of VTE was still half that associated with pregnancy. The CSM subsequently advised that women with an increased risk of thrombosis (risk factors identified were obesity, varicose veins, a family history of thrombosis and a personal history of pregnancy-induced hypertension) should change to a second-generation pill and that women taking third-generation pills should seriously consider their position. Women who experienced unwanted side-effects on second-generation pills and who were prepared to accept an increased risk of thrombosis could continue to use third-generation pills. With the exception of Germany, no other European country, or the USA has issued warnings about third-generation pills and many people believe that the CSM acted hastily (Weiss 1995). It is not clear through what mechanism third-generation pills may act to increase the risk of thromboembolism, and it is possible that preferential prescribing of these types of pills (which were thought to be safer) to women who have risk factors may account for some of the difference between pill types. A third study from the Netherlands (Bloemenkamp et al 1995) has confirmed the findings of those data considered by the CSM.

Combined pills are available in monophasic, biphasic and triphasic preparations. Phasic pills were developed in order to reduce the total dose of progestogen and, by mimicking the fluctuating pattern of steroid concentrations in the normal ovarian cycle, in an attempt to produce better cycle control. There is no good evidence that cycle control is superior compared with that achieved by monophasic pills. Moreover while the older triphasic pills do expose the user to a lower total dose of progestogen than their monophasic equivalent, the newer third-generation brands do not.

Mode of action

The COC works primarily by inhibiting ovulation. Exogenous oestrogen inhibits FSH secretion, while progestogens inhibit the development of the LH surge. The COC also alters cervical mucus rendering it hostile to the passage of sperm, and causes endometrial atrophy.

The COC is a highly effective method of contraception (Table 26.2). The failure rates associated with all forms of contraception depend on the inherent efficacy of the

Table 26.2 Method failure rates (per 100 women-years) of contraceptive methods

Method	Failure rate
Combined pill	0.1–1.0
Progestogen-only pill	1.0–3.0
Depo-Provera	0.1–1.2
Norplant	0.2–1.0
Intrauterine device	1.0–2.0
Diaphragm	1.0–5.5
Male condom	4.0–5.5
Female condom	5.0
Vasectomy	0.02
Female sterilization	0.13
Natural family planning (NFP)	2.8
Lactational amenorrhoea method (LAM)	2.0

method but also on the potential for incorrect or inappropriate use. Since ovulation is inhibited in most women who use the combined pill, failure rates of the method itself are low. However as inhibition of ovulation depends on reliable pill-taking, the overall failure rate of the COC, which includes user failures, is higher.

Contraindications

Absolute contraindications to its use are listed in Table 26.3. They include a past history of, or existing cardiovascular disease, including migraine, and most liver diseases. Women often describe headaches as migraine. The COC is contraindicated in migraine which is or may be associated with transient cerebral ischaemia; this includes crescendo migraine and focal migraine with asymmetric symptoms. Symmetrical blurring of vision, generalized flashing lights or photophobia associated with unilateral headache are not features which are regarded as absolute contraindications. It is important therefore to take a clear and detailed history before refusing to prescribe the COC because the woman has an occasional migraine.

Relative contraindications to COC use

These include the following:

1. factors which increase the risk of cardiovascular disease or venous thrombosis such as obesity, smoking, hypertension and family history;
2. sex steroid-dependent conditions including cancer e.g. breast cancer;
3. factors which adversely affect liver function;
4. factors which predispose to arterial wall disease.

Comprehensive discussions and lists of contraindications are available in most text books of contraception.

Side-effects of combined oral contraception

Oestrogen and progestogens are both metabolized by the

Table 26.3 Absolute contraindications to the combined oral contraceptive pill

Arterial or venous thrombosis
Ischaemic heart disease including myopathy
Most valvular heart disease
Past cerebral haemorrhage
Hypercholesterolaemia
Conditions predisposing to thrombosis, e.g. polycythaemia
Migraine
Pulmonary hypertension
Active liver disease
Porphyria
History of a serious condition affected by sex steroids, e.g. trophoblastic disease

liver and as such alter the metabolism of most substances including carbohydrates and lipids. Oestrogens also alter coagulation factors. A reduction in antithrombin III and alteration in platelet function increases the risk of venous thromboembolism by up to sevenfold. The risk is even greater in women who smoke. A clear history of thromboembolism is a contraindication to the COC. A possible history or a very strong family history, are indications for investigating haemostasis, particularly circulating concentrations of antithrombin III and the factor V Leiden thrombogenic mutation.

Arterial disease, including myocardial infarction and cerebrovascular accident, results from the (mainly) progestogen-related alteration to lipid profiles together with the oestrogen associated changes in blood coagulation. The risk of myocardial infarction is almost certainly related to oestrogen dose and a recent case-control study from the USA suggests a relative risk of only 1.1 (Rosenberg et al 1990a) among women using lower dose pills. Smoking and age are potent risk factors for myocardial infarction, and women who smoke should still be advised to stop the COC after the age of 35 years or give up smoking. Women with no other risk factors can continue using low-dose COC until they reach the menopause. The incidence of nonhaemorrhagic stroke is increased by two- to threefold among COC users. In contrast, the risk of subarachnoid haemorrhage is probably not significantly increased.

Around 2% of women become clinically hypertensive after starting the pill. The incidence increases with age and duration of use, obesity and family history. It does not however appear to be increased in women with a history of pregnancy-induced hypertension.

There have long been concerns that long-term use of the COC might increase the risk of breast cancer. A large number of studies published during the 1980s were analyzed by WHO in 1992. In a comprehensive review of the pill and all neoplasia, WHO concluded that while there appears to be no overall association between oral contraceptive use and breast cancer, there is a weak association between long-term use and breast cancer diagnosed in young (<36 years) women. A recent case-control study from the Netherlands (Rookus et al 1994) gives weight to this conclusion, reporting a relative risk (RR) of developing breast cancer before the age of 36 of 2.1 (1.0–4.5) for 4 or more years of COC use compared with shorter use. The risk was significantly increased in women who had started the pill before the age of 20 (1.44). It is not clear whether the increased risk continues into the menopause, but if so it should emerge in incidence and mortality data for women born around 1950 (Chilvers 1994a).

The WHO meta-analysis also reports a modest increase in the risk of squamous carcinoma of the cervix (RR 1.3–1.8) but draws attention to a number of confounding factors such as patterns of sexual behaviour and the likelihood of having cervical smears. A recent study from the USA (Ursin et al 1994) also suggested an increased risk of the much less common cervical adenocarcinoma (RR 2.1, and increasing to 4.4 after 12 years of use); no additional risk was found with early age of starting COC use.

An increased risk of gallstones is significant only during the early years of pill use.

A few women develop chloasma on the COC and it appears that both oestrogen and progestogens contribute to this. The chloasma may be slow to fade after the pill is stopped.

Minor side-effects are commonest during the first 3 months of use and often lead to discontinuation of the method. More common problems include breakthrough bleeding or spotting, nausea, breast tenderness, acne and loss of libido. Many of these resolve with time. If side-effects persist after 4 months it is often worth changing the brand of pill, opting for a lower dose of oestrogen or a different type of progestogen. Pills containing antiandrogens (Dianette) are particularly useful for acne.

While the combined pill, in general, improves menstrual bleeding patterns one common reason for presentation to a gynaecologist is breakthrough bleeding (BTB). BTB is common during the first three cycles of use. Persistence beyond 3 months may be a result of poor compliance or a coexisting gynaecological disorder such as cervical ectropion (probably more common among COC users), cervical or uterine polyp. If pelvic examination is normal, it is worth trying a formulation containing a higher dose of oestrogen or different type of progestogen. After 3 months use of a pill containing 50 μg ethinyl oestradiol the bleeding will often settle and the woman can then resume a lower dose pill. If bleeding persists, try stopping hormonal contraception altogether and if it does not resolve it should be investigated as intermenstrual bleeding, i.e. by endometrial biopsy and hysteroscopy.

Benefits of combined oral contraception

In addition to being an effective and acceptable method of contraception, the pill confers a number of health benefits. Withdrawal bleeds are usually more regular, lighter and less painful and the COC is often the treatment of choice for women with irregular heavy periods (resulting from anovulatory dysfunctional uterine bleeding) and for dysmenorrhoea. COC use is associated with a decreased incidence of benign breast disease and functional ovarian cysts, and is often used as the first line in the management of premenstrual syndrome. Inhibition of ovarian activity for the treatment of endometriosis can be achieved without the need for additional contraception (in contrast to danazol).

COC use is associated with a reduction in the risk of endometrial cancer which is related to the duration of use and reaches 50% after 4 years. The protective effect may be maintained for up to 15 years after discontinuation (WHO 1992). There is a similar duration-dependent reduction in the risk of ovarian cancer, which probably acts through the inhibition of ovulation. Protection is apparent after as little as 6 months of use and lasts at least 10 years after discontinuation. After 10 years non-users are five times more likely to develop ovarian cancer than women who have used the COC. It is interesting to note that the incidence of ovarian cancer is declining in all developed countries except Japan where the COC is not approved.

Significant numbers of unplanned pregnancies are a result of women stopping the pill for ‘a break’. There is no evidence that breaks in pill-taking reduce the long-term risks. There is also no evidence that it is necessary to stop the COC before planning a pregnancy. There is no evidence of any adverse effect on the fetus of COC use prior to conception, neither is exposure during pregnancy associated with increased risk of fetal malformation.

Fertility is restored after a delay of 1–3 months although some women take longer to resume normal cycles. So-called post-pill amenorrhoea is almost always associated with cycle irregularity before starting the pill or with coincidental factors associated with secondary amenorrhoea such as weight loss or stress.

PROGESTOGEN-ONLY CONTRACEPTION

The progestogen-only pill (POP or mini-pill) is a useful alternative for women who like the convenience of the COC but for whom oestrogen is contraindicated. It should be emphasized that not only does the POP not contain oestrogen, but the dose of progestogen is significantly lower than in equivalent combined preparations. Until the development of the very low dose (20 μg) oestrogen-containing pills, the POP was commonly advocated for women over the age of 35 who wished to continue oral contraception. The POP is still a good alternative for women with medical contraindications to the COC such as migraine and hypertension. It is often advocated for women with diabetes who are at increased risk of cardiovascular disease and who may find that insulin requirements fluctuate with COC cycles. It should be said however that the COC is not absolutely contraindicated for diabetic women without long-term complications, whose diabetes is well controlled and for whom pregnancy would be a disaster. The commonest indication for POP use in the UK is probably for women who are breastfeeding since the POP (unlike the COC) does not interfere with either the quantity or constituents of breast milk.

Mode of action

Around 50% of POP users continue to ovulate and menstruate regularly. In these women the POP works by altering cervical mucus and probably by interfering with implantation. In some 10–20% of women, follicular development is completely inhibited with resultant amenorrhoea. The remainder will experience irregular bleeding associated with follicular growth without ovulation or with inadequate luteal phase cycles.

Side-effects

The mode of action of the POP explains its side-effects. Erratic bleeding is the commonest cause for discontinuation of the pill; around 20% of women will stop using it for this reason.

Follicular growth without ovulation is associated with an increased incidence of functional ovarian cysts. Up to 20% of women using the POP will have a cyst identifiable by ultrasound. Most are symptomless and nearly all resolve spontaneously. A woman found to have a symptomless ovarian cyst should be reviewed after her next menstrual period.

POP use is associated with a slightly increased risk of ectopic pregnancy. Some 2% of pregnancies among POP failures will be ectopic, perhaps as a result of an effect of the progestogen on tubal motility.

Because of its mechanism of action (50% of women continue to ovulate) and its relatively short half-life (around 19 h) the POP has a higher failure rate than the COC (see Table 26.2). This failure rate is dependent on age and is almost as low as the COC in women over 35 years.

As relatively small numbers of women use the POP, in contrast to the COC there are very little long-term safety data. However since most of the concerns about long-term use of the COC relate to oestrogen, it seems reasonable to assume that the POP is not associated with any significant long term risks.

Injectable progestogens

Long-acting injectable progestogens are available in two forms: depomedroxyprogesterone acetate (DMPA or Depo-provera, 150 mg i.m. every 12 weeks) and norethisterone oenanthate (NET-EN, 200 mg i.m. every 8 weeks). NET-EN is seldom used in the UK.

Worldwide, DMPA is a popular method of contraception used by some 9 million women in over 90 countries. Early reports of mammary tumours in beagle dogs and endometrial cancer in rhesus monkeys led to reluctance on the part of some governments, notably the USA, to approve its use, and data on the risk of cancer and DMPA in women were scarce until the 1990s. A WHO expert group was convened in 1993 to review a number of recently published large epidemiological studies. DMPA appears to exert a powerful protective effect against endometrial cancer with a relative risk of 0.2. No association has been described between DMPA use and the risk of ovarian cancer which is surprising if the protective effect of the COC is due to the inhibition of ovulation. Nor is there any association with cervical cancer which is reassuring. Moreover there is no overall increased risk of breast cancer, although some concern remains over women using DMPA from a very young age and for many years (Chilvers 1994b).

Depo-provera was licensed for use in the UK in 1984 for women as a short-term method of contraception – one injection covered the period of infertility required after rubella vaccination for example – or as a long-term method for women who were unable to use any existing methods. These conditions were removed in 1994.

Depo-provera is a highly effective (Table 26.2) long-acting method which only requires the user to attend for injection four times a year. It inhibits ovulation and after one year of use 80% of women are either amenorrhoeic (40%) or have very scanty, infrequent periods (40%). The remaining 20% will have prolonged regular or more usually irregular bleeding episodes and around 2% of women will present, often to a gynaecologist, with troublesome menorrhagia. After excluding any pathology the most effective treatment of menorrhagia is oestrogen (Fraser 1983), and it is most easily given as one packet of the COC. If bleeding problems persist, an alternative method of contraception should be considered.

Other significant long-term side-effects include the following.

1. Weight gain; many women will gain up to six pounds during the first year of use.
2. A delay in the resumption of fertility of up to 1 year or more after cessation of use.
3. A possible reduction in bone mineral density. Recent studies from New Zealand (Cundy et al 1993) have demonstrated a small but reversible loss of bone mineral density in women using Depo-provera for 5 years or more. Although MPA has been shown in some circumstances to protect bone after the menopause, most women using

Depo-provera become relatively hypo-oestrogenic. The loss in bone density is almost certainly not sufficient to cause an increased risk of fracture in premenopausal women. It has been suggested that long-term users of Depo-provera should be managed by measuring serum oestradiol and, if it is low, by treating with oestrogen patches in addition to the DMPA. This seems to make it a complicated and relatively expensive method of contraception. A more pragmatic approach may be to suggest that women stop using Depo-provera at the age of 45 to allow for recovery of bone mineral density before postmenopausal bone loss ensues. Depo-provera was licensed in the USA in 1992 on condition that the effect on bone mineral density of long-term use was investigated; thus there should be more data available during the next decade.

Progestogen-only implants

The progestogen only implant known as Norplant was licensed for use in the UK in 1993. Comprising six silastic rods containing a total of 216 mg of crystallized levonorgestrel, Norplant is inserted subdermally on the inner aspect of the upper arm. Circulating levels of levonorgestrel are around 80 μg/day during the first 8 weeks and decline slowly to around 50 μg at the end of the first year and 25–30 μg at 60 months (see Sivin 1994 for review). The implants must be inserted and removed using local anaesthetic and the contraceptive effect lasts for 5 years. Failure rates are extremely low (Table 26.2) and obviously comprise only method failures as implants do not depend on compliance. Ovulation is inhibited in many cycles, particularly in the first years of use, and when it does occur it is associated with an inadequate luteal phase. Cervical mucus is scanty and allows poor sperm penetration.

The dose of progestogen is similar to that of the POP and the mode of action is therefore similar. Erratic bleeding occurs in around 70% of users and some 10% of women become amenorrhoeic. Fertility resumes as soon as the implants are removed. Bleeding irregularity is the commonest side-effect and reason for removal, but others include acne, hirsutism, headache, mood change and weight gain or bloating (i.e. the metabolic side-effects of progestogens).

Although many women in the UK find the long action of Norplant and the lack of a need for compliance very attractive, they should be carefully counselled before insertion. Norplant is currently significantly more costly than the most expensive combined pill, even if used for the full 5 years, and of course the real cost of the method depends on the duration of use. In the USA the average duration of use of Norplant is around 3 years.

Although the implants are not difficult to insert, removal can be troublesome particularly if the rods are inserted subcutaneously rather than subdermally.

Norplant is likely to be superseded within the next few years by newer implants. An equivalent implant consisting of only two rods (Norplant 2) has been extensively tested and a single rod (Implanon) containing the third-generation progestogen 3-keto-desogestrel and lasting for 3 years should become available in the UK in 1996.

INTRAUTERINE DEVICES

The intrauterine device (IUD) is an effective long-acting method of contraception which is perhaps underrated in the developed world. It exerts a local inflammatory reaction within the cavity of the uterus which probably interferes with the viability of both sperm and eggs as well as inhibiting implantation. Modern copper-containing devices are effective for long periods and it is now recommended that they need be changed only after every 5 years, and not at all if inserted after a woman reaches 40. For women who are happy to continue using the method indefinitely, the usual advice is that the IUD be removed 1 year after the last menstrual period.

Occasionally the string snaps off during removal. It is sometimes possible to remove the device with a pair of artery forceps or a specially designed IUD remover but some IUDs, particularly the old inert devices, appear to become deeply embedded in the endometrium and may only be removed under a general anaesthetic. Whether an IUD without its tails can be left in the cavity of the uterus for a woman's lifetime without causing any problems is not known. There is a small risk of actinomycosis but the inconvenience of admission to hospital for a general anaesthetic may outweigh this. It is probably best discussed with the individual concerned.

A recent review of the literature (Chi 1993) concluded that with modern IUDs the rates for perforation and expulsion are 4–9 and 0.2 per 100 users, respectively. The incidence of both complications is increased with postpartum insertions which should be delayed until 6 weeks among bottle-feeding women and 8 weeks among breastfeeders. If perforation is recognized early, it may be possible to remove the IUD via the laparoscope before adhesions form. For this reason it is probably wise to check the tails within 4–6 weeks of insertion.

Chi also reviewed the risk of pelvic infection among IUD users. In countries where IUDs are inserted under appropriate sterile conditions the risk of pelvic infection is only increased for 20 days after insertion. Chi concludes that PID is probably not increased among IUD users compared with noncontraceptors.

Contrary to popular belief there is no increased risk of infertility among past or current IUD users. However if an IUD user becomes pregnant the probability of that pregnancy being ectopic is greater than for women using no contraception or another method.

The commonest reason for discontinuation of the

method is menorrhagia. The local inflammatory response together with an increased production of prostaglandins causes both menorrhagia and dysmenorrhoea. In an attempt to overcome these problems new IUDs which are flexible (the frameless IUD) are being developed. Copper beads threaded onto a polypropylene string, one end of which is buried in the myometrium while the other passes through the cervical os, may be effective in reducing the incidence of menorrhagia and dysmenorrhoea (Rivera et al 1993). Some are suitable for insertion immediately after childbirth.

An alternative approach is the hormone-releasing IUD. Early trials with an IUD which released progesterone (Progestasert) were disappointing because of an increased rate of ectopic pregnancy. The levonorgestrel-releasing IUD (Lng-IUD) developed by the Population Council releases 20 μg levonorgestrel/day. With a 7-year cumulative pregnancy rate of only 0.5 per 100 women and a life-span of 5 years, the Lng-IUD appears to protect against PID (Rivera et al 1993). Moreover menstrual bleeding is significantly reduced. Women complaining of menorrhagia experienced a reduction in blood loss of 86% at 3 and 97% at 12 months after Lng-IUD insertion (Andersson & Rybo 1990). Likely to be marketed in the UK in 1995, the Lng-IUD will almost certainly have a significant role in the management of menorrhagia in addition to its attractions as a contraceptive.

NATURAL FAMILY PLANNING

Although few couples in the UK use so-called natural methods of family planning (NFP), nevertheless in some parts of the world these methods are common. All involve 'periodic abstinence', that is avoidance of intercourse during the fertile period of the cycle. Methods differ in the way in which they recognize the fertile period. The simplest is the calendar or rhythm method in which the woman calculates the fertile period according to the length of her normal menstrual cycle. Others use symptoms which reflect fluctuating concentrations of circulating oestrogen and progesterone. The mucus or Billings method relies on identifying changes in the quantity and quality of cervical and vaginal mucus. As circulating oestrogens increase with follicle growth the mucus becomes clear and stretchy allowing the passage of sperm. With ovulation, and in the presence of progesterone, mucus becomes opaque, sticky and much less stretchy or disappears altogether. Intercourse must stop when fertile-type mucus is identified and can start again when infertile type mucus is recognized. Progesterone secretion is also associated with a rise in basal body temperature (BBT) of about 0.5°C. The BBT method is thus able to identify the end of the fertile period. Other signs and symptoms such as ovulation pain, position of cervix and degree of dilatation of the cervical os can be used additionally to help define the fertile period.

Whatever method is used all rely on a period of abstinence and many couples find this difficult. Failure rates are high (Table 26.2) and most of the failures are due to conscious rule breaking. Perfect use of the mucus method is in fact associated with a failure rate of only 3.4%. There is no evidence that accidental pregnancies occurring among NFP users, which are conceived with ageing gametes, are associated with a higher risk of congenital malformations.

LACTATIONAL AMENORRHOEA METHOD (LAM)

Breastfeeding delays the resumption of fertility, and in developing countries it still has a major impact on fertility. It has been calculated that breastfeeding provides more than 98% protection from pregnancy during the first 6 months postpartum, if the mother is fully or nearly fully breastfeeding and has not yet experienced vaginal bleeding after the 56th day postpartum. On the basis of this statement, guidelines (Labbok et al 1990) have been developed for women who wish to use lactational amenorrhoea as a means of fertility regulation. The guidelines advise that as long as the baby is less than 6 months old a woman can rely on breastfeeding alone until she menstruates or until she starts to give her baby significant amounts of food other than breast milk. Prospective studies of the LAM confirm its effectiveness (Perez et al 1992). In societies where women breastfeed for prolonged periods the guidelines can probably be extended beyond 6 months.

BARRIER METHODS

The male condom remains one of the most popular methods of contraception in the UK. It is cheap, widely available over the counter and, with the exception of the occasional allergic reaction, is free from side-effects. Use of the condom has increased significantly during the last decade as a result of concern over the spread of HIV and AIDS.

In addition to protection against sexually transmitted diseases, use of the condom – and diaphragm – is associated with a significant reduction in cervical disease (Celentano et al 1987). Female barrier methods are less popular. The diaphragm and cervical cap must be fitted by a doctor or nurse and do not confer the same degree of protection from HIV. The female condom by virtue of covering the mucus membranes of the vagina and vulva is more effective in preventing sexually transmitted diseases, but has a high failure rate and low acceptability (Bounds et al 1992).

Spermicides alone are not a very effective method of contraception, but are particularly useful for women in the perimenopause who have intercourse infrequently and who are at a very low risk of pregnancy. They do reduce the risk of reinfection by some sexually transmitted diseases but there are little data to support any virucidal action in vivo.

EMERGENCY CONTRACEPTION

Hormonal preparations and the IUD can be used to prevent pregnancy after intercourse has taken place. Ethinyl oestradiol, 100 µg in combination with levonorgestrel, 1 mg, (the combined oestrogen–progestogen or CEP regimen) given twice, with the two doses separated by12 h is about 95% effective if started within 72 h of unprotected intercourse.

IUD insertion is even more effective, and can be used up to 5 days after the estimated day of ovulation which may be significantly longer than 5 days after the act of intercourse.

Although less effective, hormonal emergency contraception is usually preferred, as most women presenting for emergency contraception are young and nulliparous. Only one preparation is marketed (PC4), but equivalent doses of steroids are available in common formulations of the combined oral contraceptive pill. The relatively high dose of oestrogen is associated with nausea (up to 50%) and vomiting (up to 20%) and some doctors routinely prescribe antiemetics.

Recent efforts to find a more effective, orally active emergency contraceptive with fewer side-effects have resulted in trials of progestogen alone, danazol and the antiprogesterone RU486 (see Glasier 1993, for review). RU486 appears to be as effective if not more effective than the CEP regimen with significantly fewer side-effects, and further trials are continuing.

FUTURE PROSPECTS

Steroidal contraception

Steroid hormones remain the most successful approach to modern methods of contraception, and in addition to adjusting pill formulations, the research efforts of both pharmaceutical companies and international organizations have centred round new delivery systems for steroids.

Combined oestrogen–progestogen once-a-month injectables (Cyclofem and Mesigyna) have been developed by WHO. With failure rates of less than 0.5% they are associated with a significant reduction in menstrual irregularities compared with DMPA. These preparations are particularly useful in societies where injectables are popular and easy to deliver but where amenorrhoea is unacceptable.

Soft silastic rings have also been developed, releasing either progestogen or oestrogen and progestogen. Steroids are absorbed vaginally, avoiding the first pass through the liver, and thus the dose can be reduced. In most studies, around 8% of women are unable to use rings because of expulsion or local side-effects such as vaginal discharge. The levonorgestrel ring has a daily release rate of 20 µg and is designed to be worn continuously. Efficacy, ectopic pregnancy rates and the incidence of bleeding irregularities are equivalent to those of the mini-pill (WHO 1990a). Progestogen-only rings releasing doses of hormone sufficient to inhibit ovulation would be used in the same way as the combination ring: 3 weeks in and 1 week out. Combination rings have been developed by the Population Council in the USA and by Organon. The Organon ring releases desogestrel and only 15 µg of ethinyl oestradiol per day thus significantly reducing the dose of oestrogen.

Transdermal delivery of contraceptive steroids, strangely, lags far behind the development of this route of administration of ovarian steroids for postmenopausal hormone replacement therapy. Research in this area continues.

Vaccines

The development of contraceptive vaccines has been disappointingly slow. A vaccine against part of the β-subunit of hCG is being tested by WHO. It appears to be capable of inducing a level of antibodies sufficient to prevent pregnancy for 6–12 months but is associated with troublesome local allergic reactions. In India a vaccine against the whole β-subunit is effective and, despite cross-reacting with LH, appears to be associated with little menstrual disturbance. Individual variability in response and long-term safety however still need to be addressed.

Vaccines directed towards the zona pellucida have been developed and produce reversible contraception in monkeys. Disappointingly antizona vaccines appear to lead ultimately to irreversible interference with ovarian function, permanent sterility and premature menopause. Antisperm vaccines are proving difficult to develop despite the existence of apparently nontoxic antisperm antibodies in vivo.

Hormone agonists and antagonists

Hormone agonists and antagonists offer perhaps the most promising lead for reversible nonsteroidal contraception.

Ovulation is inhibited during chronic intranasal administration of the gonadotropin-releasing hormone agonist buserelin. If ovarian activity is completely suppressed, however, the deleterious effects of a prolonged hypoestrogenic state on bone and the cardiovascular system would probably necessitate some form of replacement therapy. In contrast incomplete suppression, with residual ovarian activity, might lead to an increased risk of endometrial hyperplasia and cancer, due to the effects of unopposed oestrogen. GnRH agonists may nevertheless have a place where there is a need for short-term contraception, and indeed have been shown to be effective during breastfeeding when minimal quantities of agonist pass into the milk (Fraser 1993).

Antagonists of progesterone offer considerable potential for the regulation of fertility. Progesterone is essential for the establishment and maintenance of pregnancy. Antagonists of progesterone, such as mifepristone, block the action of progesterone on the endometrium and hence produce an environment hostile to pregnancy. Antiprogesterones have been shown to be effective when used as emergency postcoital contraceptives (Glasier 1993). Administration of daily doses as low as 2 mg, and weekly doses of 100 mg are effective in inhibiting ovulation. Given in combination with prostaglandins, these compounds would probably be effective as a late luteal-phase contraceptive, and a single dose of 200 mg administered at the time of the LH surge has promise as a once-a-month pill (see Baird 1993, for review).

MALE CONTRACEPTION

The development of reliable methods of hormonal contraception has proved much more difficult for men than for women. The regulation of spermatogenesis is poorly understood, and the link between sexual activity and hormones is much more direct in men than in women. Any method that compromises the endocrine activity of the testes must also involve testosterone replacement if sexual function is to be maintained. Testosterone must be given by injection because orally active synthetic androgens may cause liver damage. WHO undertook a trial of testosterone enanthate, at 200 mg once per week. Complete azoospermia occurred in only 58% of 271 men, although it was more likely to occur in Asian men than in white men. In men who achieved azoospermia the method had a failure rate of <1%. WHO has since demonstrated that oligozoospermia (counts of <3.0 million/ml) induced in this way is associated with a failure rate of 1.5/100 person-years (Waites 1994).

The combination of a potent antagonist of gonadotropin-releasing hormone and testosterone causes azoospermia more reliably, but the need for daily injections of antagonist, the cost and the high incidence of local allergic reactions makes this regimen impractical.

STERILIZATION

More than 138 million women of reproductive age have chosen sterilization as their method of contraception, a 45% increase over the last decade. Over 42 million couples worldwide, the majority of whom live in developing countries (particularly China and India), rely on vasectomy. In Britain almost 50% of couples aged 35–44 are using either female or male sterilization as their method of contraception.

FEMALE STERILIZATION

Female sterilization usually involves the blocking of both fallopian tubes either by laparotomy or minilaparotomy, or more commonly by laparoscopy. It may also be achieved by bilateral salpingectomy or by hysterectomy when there is coexistent gynaecological pathology such as hydrosalpinx or fibroids.

Minilaparotomy and laparoscopic female sterilization are probably equally safe and effective; however the latter is more common in the UK because it allows sterilization to be done as a day-case procedure. Minilaparotomy is most commonly used when sterilization is performed immediately postpartum as at that time the uterus is large, the pelvis very vascular, and the risks of laparoscopy are increased. An incision in the posterior fornix allows an alternative approach to the tube (culdotomy) but has largely been abandoned because of higher complication rates.

A variety of techniques exists for occluding the tube.

1. Ligation. This is used when laparotomy or minilaparotomy are performed. The tubes can be tied with absorbable or nonabsorbable sutures and the ends left free or buried in the broad ligament or uterine cornu. Postpartum sterilization is associated with a higher failure rate.

2. Electrocautery. With this technique one or more areas of the tube are cauterized by diathermy. Bipolar diathermy allows only the tissue held between the jaws of the forceps to be cauterized. The temperature of the cauterized tube may reach 300–400°C and if allowed to touch adjacent structures can cause local burns. Failure to cauterize all the layers of the tube results in a relatively high failure rate (2–5/1000) and cautery close to the cornual portion of the tube is thought to increase the risk of ectopic pregnancy.

3. Falope ring. A ring of silicone rubber is placed over a loop of tube with a specially designed applicator. The ring destroys 2–3 cm of tube and may be difficult to apply if the tube is fat or rigid. Ischaemia of the loop causes significant post operative pain.

4. Clips. A variety of clips are available. They destroy a much smaller length of tube allowing easier reversal, but special care must be taken to ensure that the whole width of the tube is occluded; some surgeons routinely apply two clips to each tube. The Hulka–Clemens clip (stainless steel and a polycarbonate) and the smaller Filshie clip (titanium lined with silicone rubber) are probably the most commonly used in the UK.

5. Laser. Laser vaporization can be used to divide the tubes; however the carbon dioxide laser divides them very cleanly and may allow a high incidence of recanalization. The Nd:Yag laser although probably more effective, is extremely expensive.

6. Efficacy. The failure rate of clips and rings is

1–3/1000. Ligation, when the cut ends are buried, has a very low failure rate. In the Oxford FPA study (Vessey et al 1982), after 7 years follow up 1% of women who had been sterilized (by a variety of techniques) had become pregnant.

New developments

A number of chemical agents have been tested for their ability to occlude the fallopian tube when instilled into the tube either directly or transcervically into the uterus. The quinacrine pellet is the only one ready for large-scale use. The method involves insertion of a 252 mg quinacrine pellet into the uterine cavity through a modified IUD inserter passed through the cervical canal. Two insertions, 1 month apart, are made during the follicular phase of the cycle. Occlusion is caused by inflammation and fibrosis of the intramural segment of the tube. Efficacy can be increased by adding adjuvants such as antiprostaglandins or by increasing the number of quinacrine insertions. A recent trial in Vietnam reported a failure rate of 2.6% after 1 year of follow up (Hieu 1993).

The method is cheaper than surgical sterilization, avoids the use of any anaesthesia and can be performed by non-medical personnel. Large numbers of women in Asia and Pakistan have been sterilized using this method. However although quinacrine is widely use for malaria prophylaxis, the safety of quinacrine sterilization has not yet been determined, and some question the ethics of using a technique which has not been approved in developed countries.

Counselling for sterilization

Most couples seeking sterilization have been thinking about the operation for some considerable time. The initial consultation should include a discussion of:

1. the procedure involved;
2. the failure rate;
3. the risks and side-effects;
4. the possibility of wanting more children;
5. which partner should be sterilized;
6. the issue of reversibility. Despite careful counselling, a few couples will inevitably request reversal of sterilization. This is most likely to happen with remarriage. Immediate postpartum or postabortion sterilization is more likely to be regretted and should be avoided if possible. Although as many as 10% of couples regret being sterilized only 1% of these will request reversal.

Reversal of female sterilization is more likely to be successful after occlusion with clips which have been applied to the isthmic portion of the tube since only a small section of tube will have been damaged. Patients should realize that reversal involves laparotomy, does not always work (microsurgical techniques are associated with around 70% success), and carries a significant risk of ectopic pregnancy (up to 5%). Ovulation should be confirmed and a normal semen analysis obtained from the partner before reversal is undertaken. Reversal is unlikely to be available on the NHS in most parts of the UK.

The history should include the following.

1. The reason for the request; some women seek sterilization as a cure for menstrual dysfunction, sexual problems or abdominal pain.
2. Gynaecological and obstetric history and relevant medical histories of both partners.
3. Ages, occupations and social circumstances of both partners.
4. Numbers, ages and health of their children.
5. Previous and current contraception and any problems experienced. Some women request sterilization because they are unable to find any other acceptable method of contraception, this is not a good reason for sterilization.
6. The stability of the marriage and the possibility of its breakdown.
7. The quality of the couple's sex life.

It is seldom possible to arrange sterilization for a particular time of the cycle and women should be told to continue using their current method of contraception until their operation. It is not necessary to stop the combined pill before sterilization as the risk of thromboembolic complications is negligible.

If an IUD is in situ it should be removed at the time of sterilization, unless the operation is being done at mid-cycle and intercourse has taken placed within the previous few days in which case it can be removed after the next menstrual period.

Complications

Immediate complications

1. The operation carries a small operative mortality of <8 per 100 000 operations. In a large series from the USA (Petersen et al 1983) the commonest cause of death was anaesthesia.
2. Vascular damage or damage to bowel or other internal organs may occur during the procedure and is usually recognized at the time of operation. Nevertheless patients should be aware that the rare possibility of a laparotomy and longer stay in hospital does exist.
3. Gas embolism.
4. Thromboembolic disease is rare, but more likely if the procedure is done immediately postpartum.
5. Wound infection.

Long-term complications

These include the following.

1. Menstrual disorders: women who stop using the combined pill will almost certainly notice that their periods become heavier, perhaps more painful and less predictable, and they should be warned of this. In contrast, women whose previous method of contraception was an IUD will notice an improvement in their bleeding patterns. Kasonde & Bonnar (1976) were unable to demonstrate a measurable change in menstrual blood loss following sterilization in women who had been using barrier methods of contraception. Despite this there have been a number of studies which have demonstrated an increased incidence of gynaecological consultation and an increased incidence of hysterectomy among women who have been sterilized (Templeton & Cole 1982). Bearing in mind the inevitable changes in menstrual bleeding patterns associated with advancing age and with stopping the combined pill (the most commonly used method of reversible contraception) it may be that women who have been sterilized are more likely to seek hysterectomy or more willing to accept it if they are already incapable of further childbearing.
2. Abdominal pain and dyspareunia may occur after sterilization and are said to be more common after cautery. Repeat laparoscopy usually fails to demonstrate any pathology and the symptoms may sometimes be a manifestation of regret.
3. Psychological and psychosexual problems are rare and when they do arise tend to do so in those who have had problems before sterilization. Many studies in fact report a better mental state after sterilization.
4. Bowel obstruction from adhesions is a very rare complication.
5. Ectopic pregnancy has been reported in up to 50% of failures following cautery and 4% following mechanical occlusive methods. Women should be advised that if they miss a period and have symptoms of pregnancy they should seek medical advice urgently.

VASECTOMY

Vasectomy involves the division or occlusion of the vas deferens to prevent the passage of sperm. The vas is exposed through a small skin incision and ligated or occluded with small silver clips or by unipolar diathermy with a specially designed probe which can be passed into the cut end of the vas.

Excising a small portion of vas makes reversal more difficult and probably does not increase the effectiveness unless at least 4 cm is removed. It does allow histological confirmation of a correct procedure which may help in any subsequent litigation but adds to the expense. Interposing the fascial sheath between the cut ends or looping the cut ends of the vas back on itself may increase effectiveness.

The 'no-scalpel' vasectomy (NSV), developed in China in 1974, is now quite widely used. It makes use of specially designed instruments for isolating and delivering the vas through the scrotal skin and substitutes a small puncture for the skin incision. Any of the standard methods of occlusion may be used. NSV is quick and associated with a lower incidence of infection and haematoma. A comparison between NSV and conventional vasectomy in Thailand reported a complication rate of 0.4% versus 3.1% (Nirapathpongporn et al 1990).

No large randomized controlled studies have been done to determine whether one technique of occlusion is any more effective than another, and efficacy probably depends most on the skill of the surgeon.

Percutaneous injection of sclerosing agents such as polyurethane elastomers or occlusive substances such as silicone is also being used in China. The technique avoids any skin incision, the silicone plug is said to be easily removed, and pregnancy rates of 100% up to 5 years after vasectomy reversal have been claimed (Waites 1993).

The rate at which azoospermia is achieved depends on the frequency of ejaculation. In the UK seminal fluid is examined after 12 and 16 weeks and, if sperm are still present, usually monthly thereafter. When sperm are absent from two consecutive samples the vasectomy can be considered complete; until then an alternative method of contraception must be used. Around 3% of men do not become azoospermic and the vasectomy has to be redone.

Complications of vasectomy

Complications include the following:

1. Local complications. Wound infection will occur in up to 5% of men and scrotal bruising is unavoidable. Postoperative bleeding will be sufficient in 1–2% of men to cause a haematoma and perhaps 1% of these will require admission to hospital.
2. Sperm granulomas. Small lumps may form at the cut ends of the vas as a result of a local inflammatory response to leaked sperm. They can be painful and may need excising. Their presence may also increase the chance of failure.
3. Late recanalization. Failure can occur up to 10 years after vasectomy despite two negative samples of seminal fluid following the procedure. It is rare (1 in 1000).
4. Antisperm antibodies. Most men develop detectable concentrations of autoantibodies, presumably as a result of leakage of sperm, some time after vasectomy. Their presence may compromise fertility if reversal is attempted.
5. Cardiovascular and auto immune disease. Concerns about a possible link between vasectomy and cardiovascular disease were raised in the 1970s following reports

that vasectomy increased atherosclerosis in monkeys, perhaps as a consequence of increased levels of autoantibodies. Several large studies, including a cohort study in the USA of over 10 000 vasectomized men, failed to substantiate increased rates of 98 diseases (Massey et al 1984).

6. Cancer. Two studies from the USA and Scotland suggested an increased risk of testicular cancer following vasectomy. However a recent large cohort study of over 73 000 men in Denmark (Moller et al 1994) demonstrated no increase in the incidence of testicular cancer among men who had a vasectomy.

A number of reports from the USA have also suggested an increased risk of prostate cancer following vasectomy (Rosenberg et al 1990b). No known biological mechanism can account for any association or causal relationship between vasectomy and prostate cancer. Both the National Institute of Health in the USA and the WHO concluded that there was insufficient basis to change policies regarding vasectomy but both recommended further studies.

Reversal

Reversal of vasectomy is technically feasible in many cases with patency rates of almost 90% being reported in some series. Pregnancy rates are much less (up to 60%) perhaps as a result of the presence of antisperm antibodies.

ABORTION

After the Abortion Act was passed in 1967 there was a rapid rise in the number of abortions, which reached a plateau in the late 1980s. Since then there has been a gradual rise in the numbers each year with 172 063 abortions being performed in England and Wales in 1992 and 10 209 in Scotland. The abortion rate in Britain (9–14 per 1000 women aged 15–45 years) is relatively low compared to many other developed countries. However in the UK a woman's lifetime chance of having an abortion is around 1 in 40.

LEGAL ASPECTS

It is illegal in the UK to induce an abortion except under specific indications as defined by law. The conditions of the 1967 Abortion Act state that abortion can be performed if two registered medical practitioners acting in good faith, agree that the pregnancy should be terminated on one or more of the following grounds.

1. The continuance of the pregnancy would involve risk to the life of the pregnant woman greater than if the pregnancy were terminated.
2. The termination is necessary to prevent grave permanent injury to the physical or mental health of the pregnant woman.
3. The pregnancy has NOT exceeded its 24th week and the continuance of the pregnancy would involve risk, greater than if the pregnancy were terminated, of injury to the physical or mental health of the pregnant woman.
4. The pregnancy has NOT exceeded its 24th week and the continuance of the pregnancy would involve risk, greater than if the pregnancy were terminated, of injury to the physical or mental health of the existing child(ren) of the family of the pregnant woman.
5. There is a substantial risk that if the child were born it would suffer from such physical or mental abnormalities as to be seriously handicapped.

In 1990 the law was amended to reduce the upper limit from 28 to 24 weeks' gestation reflecting the lowering of the limits of fetal viability resulting from advances in neonatal care. An exception was made in the case of a fetus with severe congenital abnormality incompatible with life (e.g. anencephaly) in which case there is no upper limit.

The 1967 Abortion Act does not apply to Northern Ireland where abortion is only legal under exceptional circumstances e.g. to save the life of the mother.

The law recognizes that some doctors have ethical objections to abortion. Doctors who do have objections are obliged to refer women to another colleague who does not hold similar views.

PROVISION OF SERVICES

In Scotland and north-east England over 90% of abortions are performed in NHS hospitals while in other areas of England, the majority are carried out in private clinics or by charities. In Scotland abortion accounts for over 12% of the gynaecological workload. With the growth of NHS trusts, business managers in England are recognizing the financial benefits of providing an efficient abortion service and the situation is improving. Some hospitals are setting up dedicated clinics staffed by experts who are more sensitive and sympathetic. While it has obvious advantages for individual patients, this approach risks separating abortion from other aspects of reproductive health care and removing it from general gynaecological training. Without exposure during their training to the issue and to women who are seeking abortion, doctors may become increasingly reluctant to be involved with the provision of services as they are in the USA.

COUNSELLING

Faced with the news of an unintended pregnancy, many women are emotionally devastated and the decision to have a pregnancy terminated is never an easy one. In the UK the Committee on the Working of the Abortion Act (The Lane Committee) reporting in 1974, recommended that every woman should have the opportunity to have adequate counselling before deciding to have her pregnancy terminated. Abortion counselling should provide opportunities for discussion, information, explanation and advice in a manner which is nonjudgemental and nondirectional.

By the time most women see a gynaecologist they have already seen one doctor (usually their GP) and are certain of their decision. However in order to satisfy themselves that there are grounds for termination, gynaecologists should nonethelesss discuss the reasons why the pregnancy is unwanted and whether the woman is absolutely certain about her decision since uncertainty may be more likely to lead to regret . The woman should be encouraged to think of the practical and emotional consequences of all the possible options of abortion, continuing with the pregnancy and adoption.

Not all doctors are sympathetic and women who are seen to have conceived because of a true method failure are more likely to get a sympathetic hearing. Many women feel that they have to 'make the case' to the gynaecologist for having their pregnancy terminated and some will claim method failure even when they have not been using contraception. One in five women who have had an abortion will present for another at some time in their lives. Women who seem to use abortion as a method of contraception and present again and again probably need psychiatric help and not a punitive approach from the gynaecologist.

In the UK around 1% of women will present too late for legal abortion. These, and some of those who choose to have the baby, will need information about adoption and benefits and sometimes referral to social services.

The gynaecologist should provide information about the procedure involved, offering where available and appropriate a choice of surgical or medical methods to women below 9 weeks' gestation. The likely complications and long-term side-effects of the abortion should also be discussed, together with the implications for future pregnancies.

Future contraceptive plans are usually discussed before the abortion is carried out. Although this may not be the best time, it may be one of the few opportunities to discuss contraception as many patients do not attend for follow-up.

ASSESSMENT

After it has been decided that there are grounds for abortion, it is important to make a careful medical assessment of the woman.

1. The medical history should pay particular attention to conditions such as asthma which may influence the choice of method of abortion.
2. The stage of gestation should be determined by menstrual history and pelvic examination. A pelvic ultrasound scan is unnecessary unless there is real doubt about the gestation or if ectopic pregnancy is suspected.
3. Whether the service chooses to screen for genital tract infection, particularly chlamydia, or simply to treat everyone with prophylactic antibiotics, will depend on the background incidence of infection in the local population. If screening is chosen, it is emphasized that antibiotic therapy should be started before abortion is performed.
4. Women considered to be at high risk of hepatitis B or HIV should be offered screening with appropriate counselling. Women who refuse screening should be treated as high risk during the abortion procedure.
5. Cervical screening should be offered in accordance with national screening policies.
6. Blood should be collected for measurement of haemoglobin concentration and the group determined. All women who are rhesus negative should be injected with anti-D immunoglobulin prior to or within 48 h of the abortion to prevent the development of rhesus isoimmunization.

TECHNIQUES OF ABORTION

In general the earlier the abortion is done, the safer it is. Mortality and morbidity associated with the procedure increase with the gestation of the pregnancy at the time of termination. The risk of major complications doubles when termination is carried out at 15 as compared with 8 weeks' gestation.

The method of choice depends on gestation, parity, medical history and the woman's wishes.

Early first trimester (up to 9 weeks)

Surgical

Vacuum aspiration has been the method of choice for early surgical termination of pregnancy in industrialized countries for over 20 years. Dilatation and curettage requires more cervical dilatation and is associated with a significantly higher complication rate, including uterine injury, and a higher incidence of retained products of conception and adverse future reproductive outcome (Henshaw & Templeton 1993).

Vacuum aspiration can be performed under either local paracervical block or general anaesthesia. Some evidence suggests that the use of general anaesthesia increases the risk of the procedure. In the USA the mortality rate is two to four times greater when general rather than local anaesthesia is used for first trimester abortion. Preoperative treatment with a cervical priming agent has been shown to reduce the risk of haemorrhage and genital tract trauma associated with vacuum aspiration. Prostaglandins, bougies and the antiprogesterone RU486 are all effective but prostaglandins are probably quicker to have their effect. Pretreatment of the cervix adds to the cost of the procedure and may be difficult to organize when abortion is performed as a day case. As cervical trauma is commoner in women under the age of 17 years and uterine perforation is associated with increasing parity and increasing gestation, efforts to arrange cervical ripening should be concentrated on very young women, highly parous women and those presenting at later gestation.

A curette of up to 10 mm internal diameter is passed through the cervix and the contents of the uterus aspirated using negative pressure created by a pump. It is advisable to use the smallest diameter curette which is adequate for the gestation; most gynaecologists use an 8 mm curette at 8 weeks, 10 mm at 10 weeks and so on.

Vacuum aspiration at this stage of pregnancy is extremely safe and effective. Failure is more likely to occur before 7 weeks' gestation when it is possible to miss the fetus with the curette. For this reason it may be better to defer the operation until after this time or to use medical methods. The mortality from vacuum aspiration in the first trimester is less than about 1 per 100 000, considerably less than the maternal mortality from continuing pregnancy.

Medical

Medical abortion is available to women in the UK up to 63 days of amenorrhoea (9 weeks' gestation). Although a number of substances which could induce abortion have been known for many years, it was the discovery of the antiprogesterone mifepristone or RU486 in 1980 which made medical abortion a practical reality (Baird 1992). Mifepristone is a synthetic steroid which blocks the action of progesterone by binding to its receptor. It also binds to the glucocorticoid receptor and blocks the action of cortisol.

When mifepristone is used alone, complete abortion only occurs in around 60% of pregnancies. The rate of complete abortion rises to over 95% if a prostaglandin is given 36 or 48 h after the administration of mifepristone. In the UK currently mifepristone is given as a single oral dose of 600 mg (3 × 200 mg tablets) followed 48 h later by a 1-mg vaginal pessary of the prostaglandin cervagem (gemeprost). The antiprogesterone itself stimulates some uterine contractility but also greatly enhances the sensitivity of the myometrium to prostaglandins.

Offered the choice of method, in France and in the UK around 20–25% prefer medical abortion. Women often choose the medical method because it avoids an anaesthetic in most cases and because they feel more in control of the situation. It is however a two-stage procedure which other women find a disadvantage. The incidence of serious complications is probably similar to that associated with surgical abortion, but because 95% of women need neither anaesthesia nor instrumentation of the uterus, large randomized trials may eventually show medical abortion to be safer. Not all women are suitable for medical abortion; the contraindications are shown in Table 26.4.

Table 26.4 Contraindications to medical abortion

Absolute contraindications	Adrenal insufficiency
	Ectopic pregnancy
	>9 weeks' gestation
	Asthma
	Cardiac disease
	Heavy smoker, older than 35 years
	On anticoagulants or bleeding disorder
Relative contraindications	Heavy smoker
	>35 years
	Obesity
	Hypertension (diastolic >100 mmHg)

There are very few side-effects following administration of mifepristone. Although for legal reasons the tablets must be taken in the presence of a doctor or nurse in a hospital or approved place, it is only necessary to observe the woman for about 10 min after swallowing the tablets before she goes home. She returns to hospital 48 h later for the gemeprost prostaglandin. The fetus is usually aborted in the next 4 h and this is accompanied by bleeding and pain. The bleeding is usually described as being like a very heavy period although rarely (<1%) there may be very heavy bleeding requiring resuscitation. Nulliparous women and those with a history of dysmenorrhea are more likely to experience severe pain and 10–20% of women may need opiate analgesia. The rest will cope with paracetamol. Prostaglandin synthetase inhibitors, such as aspirin or mefanamic acid, should be avoided for obvious reasons.

Bleeding can continue for up to 20 days after the abortion although most women have usually stopped after 10 days. The total amount of blood lost is similar to that occurring at the time of vacuum aspiration.

All women should be given an appointment for follow up about 2 weeks after administration of the prostaglandin. This visit is absolutely essential for those (about 30%) who have not passed an identifiable fetus and/or placental tissue while in hospital. Although ongoing pregnancy occurs in only 1% of cases, evacuation of the uterus will be necessary in about 2–5% because of incomplete or missed abortion. These figures are no different from those associated with surgical abortion.

The risk of fetal malformation following RU486 alone or in combination with prostaglandins is not known. Women should be clearly advised that medical abortion is a two-stage procedure and that it is not possible to have a change of heart after taking RU486 and before prostaglandin administration. Women who seem even remotely uncertain about abortion should certainly not be offered the medical method. In the event of failed medical abortion and therefore ongoing pregnancy the patient must be strongly advised to have vacuum aspiration, although babies born to the few women who have chosen to continue with the pregnancy after medical abortion has failed, have been normal.

Late first trimester (9 to 14 weeks)

At this stage of pregnancy the method of choice is vacuum aspiration. Although abortion can be induced by antigestagens and prostaglandins, the incidence of incomplete abortion is high and, hence, many women require surgical evacuation of the uterus. The cervix should be pretreated.

Although vacuum aspiration is an extremely safe operation, blood loss and other complications rise as gestation advances. It is important, therefore, to refer the women for abortion promptly after the decision to terminate the pregnancy has been made.

Midtrimester abortion

Second trimester abortion accounts for 10–15% of all legal abortions in the UK. While many are done because of fetal malformation, it is often the women who are least able to cope with an unwanted pregnancy, particularly the very young, who first present at this time.

It is possible to induce abortion at this stage of pregnancy either medically or surgically. Surgical dilatation and evacuation (D&E) is the method of choice in the USA but in the UK its use is confined largely to gynaecologists in private practice. It may be necessary to dilate the cervix up to a diameter of 20 mm before the fetal parts can be extracted.

In skilled hands, D&E is a safe procedure, but if complications such as haemorrhage and perforation of the uterus are to be avoided surgeons should be adequately trained.

The alternative medical methods involve inducing uterine contractions so that the fetus is expelled from the uterus. In the past a variety of substances such as hypertonic saline, urea, and rivanol, together with a prostaglandin were either injected directly into the amniotic sac or instilled through the cervix into the extra-amniotic space using a Foley catheter connected to a pump. Often they were combined with the intravenous infusion of oxytocin to induce uterine contractions. These methods were relatively inefficient and labour was prolonged, in some cases for more than 48 h, with a substantial increase in the risk of infection. There was also a risk of cardiovascular collapse due to inadvertent injection of prostaglandin or hypertonic solution directly into the bloodstream. Instillation has largely been replaced by vaginal prostaglandins in combination with pretreatment with mifepristone.

Pretreatment with mifepristone significantly shortens the interval between administration of the prostaglandin and abortion of the fetus to 6–8 h. Thus, 600 mg mifepristone is given 36 h before insertion of a 1-mg gemeprost pessary in the vagina, repeated at intervals of 3 and 6 h until expulsion of the fetus occurs. Infusion of prostaglandin E_2 into the extra-amniotic space can be used if pessaries are not available.

Most women find the procedure painful and distressing and require opiate analgesia. Evacuation of the uterus is necessary in around 30% of women who retain all or part of the placenta.

In spite of these disadvantages, induction of abortion by medical means with prostaglandins alone or preferably in combination with mifepristone is a very effective method of abortion associated with a very low incidence of complications. Because it requires less surgical experience, the potential for serious complications is probably less than for D&E and, hence, it will continue to be used in many parts of the world.

Abortion beyond 18 weeks' gestation is rare and is usually for pregnancies complicated by severe fetal malformation. Particularly distressing for both the mother and the staff, these late abortions are often effectively managed with vaginal prostaglandins in combination with RU486 with intra-amniotic urea or fetal intracardiac injection of potassium to minimize the chances of a live birth.

FOLLOW UP

All women should receive contraceptive advice and, if appropriate, supplies before going home. Ovulation can return within 20 days following abortion, and contraception should be started early. All should be given a follow-up appointment within 3 weeks, either with the clinic which carried out the abortion or with a suitable alternative doctor. At follow up, a pelvic examination should confirm complete abortion and the absence of infection. Discussion should include contraceptive advice and post-abortion counselling if required.

COMPLICATIONS

Although maternal mortality is fortunately extremely rare following abortion, the incidence of major complications, haemorrhage, thromboembolism, operative trauma and infection is around 2%. The main factors affecting the incidence of complications in the RCGP study (Frank 1985) undertaken in the early 1980s were the place of operation (complications were less common when the abortion was done in a private hospital), gestation, method of abortion, sterilization at the time of operation and smoking habits.

Incomplete abortion

The commonest complication following abortion is the persistence of placental and/or fetal tissue. Up to 5% of women undergoing first trimester medical abortion will require surgical evacuation of the uterus within the first month. The incidence of incomplete abortion and ongoing pregnancy after vacuum aspiration rise as the gestation increases.

The occurrence of bleeding at 2 weeks after a medical or surgical abortion is not in itself an indication to evacuate the uterus. Ultrasound scans often show residual trophoblastic tissue even in women who have stopped bleeding. Although an ultrasound scan of the uterus and the measurement of human chorionic gonadotrophin (hCG) in plasma may be helpful in diagnosing an ongoing pregnancy, the decision to evacuate the uterus should be made on clinical grounds i.e. continued heavy or persistent bleeding from a bulky uterus in which the cervix is still dilated. The majority of women with an incomplete or missed abortion will pass the residual tissue with time if they are prepared to be patient. The belief that all women with an incomplete abortion had a high risk of intrauterine infection until the uterus was evacuated, probably stemmed from the time when illegal abortion was common.

Minor complications

In the RCGP study, 10% of over 6000 women undergoing abortion presented to their GP during the 3 weeks following the procedure with a variety of complaints which were felt to be related to the abortion. Lower abdominal pain, vaginal bleeding and passage of clots or trophoblastic tissue are relatively common and usually only require reassurance. It is however important to exclude infection. Established pelvic inflammatory disease with pyrexia, abdominal pain and offensive vaginal discharge occurs in around 1% of women whatever method of abortion is used.

Cervical and vaginal lacerations

Lacerations to the vagina and cervix are rare and the risk of the latter can be reduced by pretreatment of the cervix in selected cases, as discussed earlier.

Late complications

There are very few late complications from abortion if the women have been carefully counselled.

Psychological sequelae

Many women feel tearful and emotional for a few days following the abortion. However many studies have demonstrated a significant improvement in psychological well-being by 3 months after compared with before abortion (Adler et al 1990). There is no evidence of an increase in the incidence of serious psychiatric disease following abortion although relapse can occur in those with preexisting psychiatric disease. In contrast, the incidence of depression, suicide and child abuse is higher in women who have continued with the pregnancy because abortion was refused (Matejcek et al 1985).

Infertility

Postabortion infection is a significant cause of tubal disease and infertility following illegal abortion; however with modern methods performed under optimal conditions, the incidence of infection is very low particularly where preoperative screening and treatment of infection is routine.

Subsequent pregnancy

Damage to the cervix or perforation of the uterus can predispose to cervical incompetence, preterm delivery and/or uterine rupture. However, the RCGP study found no significant increase in adverse outcome of subsequent pregnancy, and this has been confirmed by many other studies from developed countries.

KEY POINTS

1. Lack of contraceptive use continues to be a major problem in many developing countries.
2. The combined oral contraceptive pill is still the most widely used method in the United Kingdom.
3. The combined oral contraceptive pill is associated with minimal increased risk of heart attack, stroke or venous thromboembolism in women without other risk factors.
4. The combined pill is associated with a highly significant reduction in the risk of ovarian and endometrial cancer but may accelerate the development of breast cancer in women who start taking it before the age of 20.
5. Long-acting progestogen-only methods are highly effective contraceptives with few long-term risks.
6. Norplant is not comparable with Depo-provera in terms of side-effects or mode of action.
7. The new levonorgestrel-releasing IUDs significantly reduce menstrual blood loss and will increase the popularity of the IUD as a method of contraception.
8. Antihormones, particularly antigestogens, show great promise for the development of new contraceptives.
9. New reversible methods for men will not be available for some considerable time and more research needs to be done on the long-term risks of vasectomy, particularly in relation to prostate cancer.
10. Medical methods of early first and second trimester abortion represent a significant advance in the management of unwanted pregnancy.

REFERENCES

Adler N E, David H P, Major B N, Roth S H, Russo N F, Wyatt G E 1990 Psychological responses after abortion. Science 268: 41–44

Akerlund M, Rode A, Westergaard J 1993 Comparative profiles of reliability, cycle control and side effects of two oral contraceptive formulations containing 150 μg desorgestrel and either 30 μg or 20 μg ethinyl oestradiol. British Journal of Obstetrics and Gynaecology 100: 832–838

Andersson J K, Rybo G 1990 Levonorgestrel-releasing intrauterine device in the treatment of menorrhagia. British Journal of Obstetrics and Gynaecology 97: 690–694

Baird D T 1992 Medical termination of pregnancy. In: Edwards C R, Lincoln D W (eds) Recent advances in clinical endocrinology and metabolism 14. Churchill Livingstone, Edinburgh, pp 83–94

Baird D T 1993 Antigestogens. British Medical Bulletin 49: 73–87

Bounds W, Guillebaud J, Newman G B 1992 Female condom (Femidom). A clinical study of its use effectiveness and patient acceptability. British Journal of Family Planning 18: 36–41

Bloemenkamp K W M, Rosendaal F R, Helerhorst F M, Buller H R, Vandenbroucke J P 1995 Enhancement by factor V Leiden mutation of risk of deep-vein thrombosis associated with oral contraceptives containing a third-generation progestagen. Lancet 364: 1593–1596

Celentano D D, Klassen A C, Weisman C S, Rosenheim N B 1987 Role of contraceptive use in cervical cancer. American Journal of Epidemiology 126: 592–604

Chi I C 1993 What we have learned from recent IUD studies: a researcher's perspective. Contraception 48: 81–108

Chilvers C 1994a Oral contraceptives and cancer. Lancet 344: 1378–1379

Chilvers C 1994b Breast cancer and depot-medroxyprogesterone acetate: a review. Contraception 49: 211–222

Cundy T, Cornish J, Evans M C, Roberts H, Reid I R 1994 Recovery of bone density in women who stop using medroxyprogesterone acetate. British Medical Journal 308: 247–249

Frank P I 1985 Sequelae of induced abortion. In: Porter R, O'Connor M (eds) Abortion: medical progress and social implications. Ciba Foundation Symposium 115. Pitman, London, pp 67–79

Fraser I S 1983 A survey of different approaches to the management of menstrual disturbances in women using injectable contraceptives. Contraception 28: 385–397

Fraser H M 1993 GnRH analogues for contraception. British Medical Bulletin 49: 62–72

Glasier A 1993 Postcoital contraception. Reproductive Medicine Review 2: 75–84

Henshaw R C, Templeton A A 1993 Methods used in first trimester abortion. Current Obstetrics and Gynaecology 3: 11–16

Hieu D T, Tan T T, Tan D N, Nguyet P T, Than P, Vinh D Q 1993 31 781 cases of non- surgical female sterilization with quinacrine pellets in Vietnam. Lancet 342: 213–217

Jick H, Jick S S, Gurewich V, Wald Myers M, Vasilakis C 1995 Risk of idiopathic cardiovascular death and nonfatal thromboembolism in women using oral contraceptives with differing progestagen components. Lancet 346: 1589–1593

Kasonde J M, Bonnar J 1976 Effect of sterilization on menstrual blood loss. British Journal of Obstetrics and Gynaecology 83: 572–577

Labbok M, Koniz-Booher P, Cooney K, Shelton J, Krasovec K 1990 Guidelines for breastfeeding in family planning and child survival programs. Institute for Studies in Natural Family Planning, Washington DC

Matejcek Z, Dytrych Z, Schüller V 1985 Follow up study of children born to women denied abortion. In: Porter R, O'Connor M (eds) Abortion: medical progress and social implications. Ciba Foundation Symposium 115. Pitman, London, pp 136–146

Massey F J, Bernstein G S, O'Fallon W M et al 1984 Vasectomy and health. Results from a large cohort study. Journal of the American Medical Association 252: 1023–1029

Moller H, Knudsen L B, Lynge E 1994 Risk of testicular cancer after vasectomy: cohort study of over 73 000 men. British Medical Journal 309: 295–299

Nirapathpongporn A, Huber D H, Krieger J N 1990 No-scalpel vasectomy at the King's birthday vasectomy festival. Lancet 335: 894–895

Oddens B J, Visser A P, Vermer H M, Everaerd W, Lehart P 1994 Contraceptive use and attitudes in Great Britain. Contraception 49: 73–86

Petersen H B, DeStefano F, Rubin G L, Greenspan J R, Lee N C, Ory H W 1983 Deaths attributable to tubal sterilisation in the United States 1977–1981. American Journal of Obstetrics and Gynecology 146: 131–136

Perez A, Labbok M, Queenan J 1992 Clinical study of the lactational amenorrhoea method for family planning. Lancet 339: 968–969

Rebar A W, Zeserson K 1991 Characteristics of the new progestogens in combination oral contraceptives. Contraception 44: 1–10

Rivera R, Chi I, Farr G 1993 The intrauterine device in the present and future. Current Opinion in Obstetrics and Gynaecology 5: 829–832

Rookus M A, van Leeuwen F E, for the Netherlands Oral Contraceptives and Breast Cancer Study Group 1994 Oral contraceptives and risk of breast cancer in women aged 20–54 years. Lancet 344: 844–851

Rosenberg L, Palmer J R, Lesko S M, Shapiro S 1990a Oral contraceptive use and the risk of myocardial infarction. American Journal of Epidemiology 131: 1009–1016

Rosenberg L, Palmer J R, Zauber A G, Warshauer M E, Stolley P D, Shapiro S 1990b Vasectomy and the risk of prostate cancer. American Journal of Epidemiology 132: 1051–1055

Sivin I 1994 Contraception with Norplant implants. Human Reproduction 9: 1818–1826

Templeton A A, Cole S 1982 Hysterectomy following sterilization. British Journal of Obstetrics and Gynaecology 89: 845–848

Ursin G, Peters R K, Henderson B E, d'Ablaing III G, Monroe K R, Pike M C 1994 Oral contraceptive use and adenocarcinoma of cervix. Lancet 344: 1390–1394

Vessey M P, Lawless M, Yeates D 1982 Efficacy of different contraceptive methods. Lancet i: 841–842

Waites G M H 1994 Male fertility regulation: the challenges for the year 2000. British Medical Bulletin 49: 210–221

Weiss N 1995 Third-generation oral contraceptives: how risky? Lancet 346: 1570

World Health Organization Task Force on Long-Acting Systemic Agents for Fertility Regulation 1990a Microdose intravaginal levonorgestrel contraception: a multicentre trial I. Contraceptive efficacy and side effects. Contraception 41: 105–124

World Health Organization Task Force on Methods for the Regulation of Male Fertility 1990b Contraceptive efficacy of testosterone-induced azoospermia in normal men. Lancet 336: 955–959

World Health Organization 1992 Oral contraceptives and neoplasia. WHO Technical Report Series 817: 1–46

World Health Organization 1994 Challenges in reproductive health research. UNDP/UNFPA/WHO/ World Bank Special Programme of Research, Development and research training in Human Reproduction. Biennial report 1992–1993. WHO, Geneva

World Health Organization Collaborative Study of Cardiovascular Disease and Steroid Hormone Contraception 1995 Effect of different progestagens in low oestrogen oral contraceptives on venous thromboembolic disease. Lancet 346: 1582–1588

27

Psychosexual disorders

A. Parsons

INTRODUCTION

The management of psychosexual disorders is an area in which only a minority of gynaecologists will be able to develop a special interest. However, all gynaecologists should be able to recognize such problems, assess them sufficiently to distinguish the organic components and guide couples about their management. The conditions which we describe as psychosexual disorders show a number of fundamental differences from other conditions described in this book. Firstly, they are not disorders in the same sense as cancer of the cervix, for example. Although there may be an underlying organic basis, the presentation and prognosis are usually highly dependent on the expectations of both the individual and the society in which she lives. Recognition of a sexual difficulty may depend heavily on the sensitivity of the professionals concerned, but each individual or couple has to define for themselves what should be perceived as a problem.

Secondly, sexual difficulties are, par excellence, a psychosomatic problem (Bancroft 1989). Whilst an enjoyable sexual experience will normally require intact pelvic organs with functioning vascular and neurological mechanisms, the pelvic changes of sexual arousal are welded to the sensations and emotions which determine their sexual meaning for the individual.

Thirdly, disorders may be situational; that is to say, they may occur within the context of one relationship, but not another. Alternatively, they may occur in two different relationships, but be interpreted as a problem in one and not the other.

Clearly then, the recognition of a problem as a psychosexual disorder will be influenced by the expectations of society and of the individual or couples concerned, as well as by those of their professional advisers. This chapter concerns what are commonly referred to as sexual dysfunctions. These are those cases where the sexual response does not appear to be working to the satisfaction of the individuals concerned. Sexual 'deviations' or 'variations' are forms of sexual behaviour or methods of sexual arousal which fall beyond the bounds of what most people consider to be normal and are to some degree culturally determined. These need to be dealt with by people with the expertise to understand the mechanisms underlying abnormal sexual behaviour. They will not be considered further in this chapter.

PATHOPHYSIOLOGY AND CLASSIFICATION

Whilst no two people or couples will ever present with exactly the same difficulties, a classification is possible based on an understanding of the physiology and anatomy of sexual response. Most of the present conventional wisdom about human sexual response is based on the research findings of Masters & Johnson (1966). It is important to remember that their observations were largely based on 2500 cycles of sexual response in approximately 600 men and women. Their subjects were volunteers who were willing to have their sexual response studied under laboratory conditions. Our assumption is that the nature of sexual response for the rest of the population is the same as it was for this group of highly responsive individuals. Masters & Johnson's classification divides human sexual response into four phases: excitement, plateau, orgasm and resolution. Each phase represents an incremental increase in sexual excitement and each is a necessary precursor for the following phase.

Excitement phase

The excitement or arousal phase is the initial response to sexual stimulation, either physical or psychological. In both men and women this has genital and systemic components.

A reflex vasodilation of blood vessels in the genitalia is mediated through two centres in the spinal cord (one at the level of segments T11–L2, the other at S2–S4), and through specific receptors in the pelvic smooth muscle. In the male, this vasodilation fills the corpora cavernosa of the penis to produce an erection, while in the female, increased vaginal wall blood flow produces a transudate which appears like beads of perspiration on the walls of the vagina and which is the main source of vaginal lubrication. This lubrication is also associated with the ballooning out of the inner two-thirds of the vagina and with varying degrees of engorgement of the vulva.

The systemic component of the excitement phase includes changes in pulse and respiratory rates and blood pressure, as well as general vasocongestion, especially over the upper torso and neck.

During this phase, arousal increases, but remains vulnerable to interruption. Fatigue, worry or alcohol may all affect the arousal phase, while distracting thoughts or the sounds of other people in the house may easily cause a reversal of the excitement changes, especially in women.

Plateau phase

The plateau phase is included by some authorities (e.g. Kaplan 1974) as part of arousal. It represents a consolidation of the changes which occur during the excitement phase which inevitably precedes it. During this phase, congestion in the outer third of the vagina reaches a maximum. This produces a firm area of engorged tissue around the vaginal introitus, which Masters & Johnson described as the 'orgasmic platform'. Breast changes are also maximal at this time with an increase in breast size of 20–25% in many women who have not previously breastfed. As the plateau phase proceeds, congestion of the areolae gives the impression of loss of erection of the nipple and finally, just prior to orgasm, the clitoris is retracted firmly against the pubic bone, often seeming to disappear. Although this phase is described as a plateau, continuing stimulation may build up sexual excitement to the intensity required for orgasm.

Orgasm

Orgasm represents a peak of pleasurable sensation associated with the discharge of the sexual tension which is built up during the preceding phases. Physiological changes during orgasm are remarkably similar in both sexes, with the subjective feeling of pleasure being associated with involuntary rhythmic contraction of the genital muscles (at 0.8/s intervals). In women the pelvic floor muscles, including the orgasmic platform, are involved, while in the male the muscles at the base of the penis and in the penile urethra contract to produce ejaculation. In the male, this part of orgasm is preceded by emission in which the seminal fluid passes into the base of the urethra.

After ejaculation, the male experiences a refractory period. During this time, further stimulation will not produce further response and may even cause feelings of discomfort. The length of this refractory period increases with age (from a few minutes in the teenager to many hours in the elderly). Many women, and some men, do not have a refractory period, and further stimulation can cause further orgasms in this group.

Many of the more important myths of human sexuality surround the orgasm. One of the more damaging of these, from a clinical point of view, is the myth of the vaginal orgasm. Freud, in particular, promoted the idea that the psychologically more mature woman would be capable of achieving an orgasm in response to vaginal stimulation alone, and that this vaginal orgasm provided a higher level of experience than a climax produced by other forms of stimulation. It is now clear that the nature of an orgasm is not affected by the type of stimulation needed to produce it, although masturbatory orgasms may be somewhat more intense. Only about 30% of women can achieve orgasm from coitus alone, and stimulation of the clitoris and other erogenous zones is a normal pathway to orgasm.

Resolution

Following orgasm, the body gradually returns to the non-aroused state, unless effective stimulation is continued. The speed of the resolution phase is related to age in men, and probably in women too. In older parous women impairment of the resolution phase, especially if associated with orgasmic failure, may lead to pelvic congestion and nonspecific symptoms of pelvic and low backache.

Sexual desire

Masters & Johnson's original four-phase cycle of excitement, plateau, orgasm and resolution is clearly quite mechanistic, and completely ignores the associated feelings. Thus, Kaplan's (1979) triphasic model of desire, arousal and orgasm fits better with the sexual difficulties people experience. Sexual desire is probably the least understood component of sexuality, and yet lack of sexual desire is one of the commonest sexual difficulties presented to the gynaecologist.

The more common categories of sexual dysfunction presenting among women are dyspareunia, vaginismus, orgasmic dysfunction and general sexual dysfunction, while the corresponding problems in the male are those of erectile difficulty, premature ejaculation, retarded ejaculation and dyspareunia. The relatively uncommon problem of retrograde ejaculation is also relevant to the gynaecologist because of its implications for fertility.

Female sexual dysfunction

Dyspareunia

Dyspareunia is defined as pain on intercourse and is perhaps one of the most common sexual difficulties presented to the gynaecologist, partly because of the assumption that there may be an underlying organic reason.

Dyspareunia is traditionally described as being superficial when the pain is solely at the vaginal introitus or deep when the pain is felt within the pelvis. As with all other sexual dysfunctions, dyspareunia may be primary (i.e. having been present since the first attempts at intercourse) or secondary (i.e. a problem which has arisen after previously pain-free intercourse). Other features which are of importance in dyspareunia are whether the pain is sufficient to prevent intercourse, whether it is continuous or intermittent, and whether it continues after attempts at intercourse have ceased.

Vaginismus

Vaginismus is characterized by the involuntary spasm of the pubococcygeus muscle, leading to an effective closure of the vaginal introitus. Attempts at penetration produce pain in the clenched muscle, thus aggravating the situation. Vaginismus may generalize to the point where any attempt at vaginal examination is impossible and the patient may take up the position of opisthotonos on the examination couch.

Contrary to many people's belief, there is no association between vaginismus and an individual's ability to become aroused or to be orgasmic. Nor does vaginismus imply any particular personality or sexual attitudes on the part of the sufferer.

Orgasmic dysfunction

Orgasmic dysfunction is the inability to achieve an orgasm or climax. This may be associated with a general inability to become aroused. Alternatively, a woman may be able to achieve normal arousal and reach a plateau phase, but be unable to climax. Masters & Johnson (1970) divided the inability to achieve an orgasm according to whether this was only a problem during intercourse or whether the individual was also unable to achieve a climax by masturbation. Inability to reach orgasm by intercourse alone is a sufficiently common problem that most women would probably not regard it as a dysfunction.

General sexual dysfunction

General sexual dysfunction is the more common term used for an inability to become aroused and has a large overlap with 'hypoactive sexual desire'. The most severe form of this is the woman who experiences no sexual interest, either spontaneously or in response to her partner. It seems unusual for such women to report mere indifference to sexual activity and they are most likely to present with a degree of aversion to any sexual advance. Milder presentations overlap with the orgasmic dysfunctions described above.

The underlying basis for sexual desire in the human is poorly understood. Clearly the psychic and endocrine components are important but, particularly in the female, there is no clear consensus on the importance of hormonal changes.

Male sexual dysfunction

Erectile difficulty

Erectile difficulty is difficulty in achieving or inability to maintain an erection. It may be primary or secondary. It may also be situational, i.e. an individual who can achieve an erection with one partner may not be able to do so with another. It may or may not be associated with a low level of sexual interest. Paraphilias are those conditions where an individual responds to an unusual sexual object or an unusual form of stimulation. Most paraphilias hide an underlying low sexual drive and erectile difficulty.

Premature ejaculation

Premature ejaculation is a relative term and may be defined as the tendency for an individual to ejaculate appreciably more quickly than a man or his partner would like. This is clearly heavily influenced by expectations. Kinsey et al (1948), for instance, found that the average American male at that time would ejaculate within 2 min of penetration.

Extreme cases of premature ejaculation, where the man ejaculates before he can approach or penetrate his partner, can be more readily accepted as a problem.

Other ejaculatory dysfunctions

Retarded ejaculation involves normal arousal and plateau phases, but ejaculation either fails to occur or requires prolonged stimulation (more than is acceptable to the couple) to trigger it. Retrograde ejaculation also occurs where the man experiences normal feelings but the seminal fluid, instead of being passed forward through the penile urethra, is forced backwards into the bladder. Men are not always aware that this phenomenon is occurring, and in some individuals it may be situational. Conditions which alter the anatomy of the bladder neck (e.g. prostatectomy or spinal cord injury) will also produce retrograde ejaculation.

Dyspareunia

Dyspareunia in the male is less common than in the female and may be divided into pain on achieving an erection and pain on actual intercourse. These complaints are usually physical in origin.

Lack of sexual desire

Loss or lack of libido is a problem which men find more difficult to present to the medical profession, perhaps partly because of society's myths about male sexual performance.

AETIOLOGY

Like many problems in gynaecology, sexual difficulties were originally regarded as being almost exclusively psychological in origin. More recently, it has been suggested that up to 60% of erectile difficulties may have at least a partly organic cause. There are no obvious reasons why this should not also apply to arousal difficulties in women, though as yet there is little substantiating evidence for this. While recognizing that there is always some overlap between the two, it may be useful to look at organic and psychological factors in sexual dysfunction separately.

Organic factors

Although most sexual problems other than dyspareunia may have no organic basis, it is important to establish the organic elements, if any, of the problem. The distinction between organic and psychological will often be clear from the history. Otherwise physical examination of the relevant partner is mandatory. General physical examination should look for signs of genetic abnormality or systemic illness and where pain is part of the presenting complaint an attempt should be made to reproduce this on examination.

Normal sexual response assumes normal genitalia with an unimpaired blood supply and an intact innervation. Any changes in these obviously modify or prevent response.

Neurological

A variety of neurological conditions will have an impact on sexual functioning. Autonomic neuropathy in diabetes mellitus or demyelination in multiple sclerosis may impair one or other phase of the sexual response cycle. Spinal cord injuries will have a variable effect depending on the level at which the cord is damaged and whether the damage is full or partial. Relatively little is known about the effect of spinal cord injury in women. In men the vast majority with upper motor neuron lesions are able to achieve reflex erections in response to tactile stimulation, though orgasmic and ejaculatory capacity are more variable.

Gynaecological cancer/surgery

Gynaecological or other cancers may cause sexual disability in a number of ways. Libido, particularly in women, is often closely linked to mood and can be suppressed by even mild levels of depression occurring either as part of the illness process or as a reaction to the diagnosis. Cancer surgery can often be mutilating and appreciably alter an individual's body image. Studies of women who have undergone radical surgery for gynaecological cancers have shown a significant deterioration both in body image and in sexual relationships. Radiotherapy, particularly for cervical cancer, may produce a degree of vaginal stenosis with reduced lubrication and soreness.

Posthysterectomy

While a total hysterectomy normally leaves the length of the vagina unchanged, deep dyspareunia becomes relatively common when a vaginal cuff has been removed, and in this case the discomfort seems to be related to thrusting against a scarred vault in a vagina which no longer has the same capacity to balloon out on arousal. Prospective studies (Helström 1994, Garth et al 1981, Martin et al 1980) all suggest that for the majority of women for whom hysterectomy is indicated, sexual relationships will be subsequently unchanged or even improve.

There is no evidence that removal or conservation of the ovaries influences this, but it should be remembered that a proportion of women with ovaries conserved at the time of hysterectomy will experience early ovarian failure (Siddle et al 1987), and continued sexual enjoyment may be dependent on oestrogen replacement.

While there may be no physical necessity for the presence of the uterus for sexual enjoyment, there is anecdotal evidence that some women gain important erotic sensation from their uterus or cervix, and because of publicity about this, some women may now elect for a subtotal hysterectomy.

Drugs

A wide variety of drugs have an impact on sexual function,

either directly or indirectly. In general, the effects of drugs on male sexuality are far better documented than those effects on the female, partly because the male response is more easily studied. However, any drugs with a central stimulatory or sedative action may be expected to have an effect either on libido or arousal. Most hypotensive agents are associated with some sexual side-effects. Alcohol, often used to enhance sexual enjoyment, will produce sexual dysfunction when abused. The aetiology of this is complex and is only partly organic.

Hormones

Whilst testosterone is clearly the hormone responsible for both libido and sexual response in the male, the situation in the female is less clear. Testosterone does seem to play a role, but oestrogen also seems to be important.

EPIDEMIOLOGY

Because many people with sexual problems never present to any source of help, the main sources of information about the incidence of such problems come either from general population studies or from surveys carried out by women's magazines, etc. The latter source tends to be biased towards those experiencing difficulties. The issue is further complicated by our poor understanding of how sexual dysfunction, sexual difficulties and sexual dissatisfaction may be linked.

Population studies

Kinsey et al's (1953) study of sexual behaviour in the human female remains one of the most important in this area. They found that of the 5900 women interviewed, 50% had not experienced orgasm in their late teens. This figure decreased to 10% by the mid thirties. In their previous study (1948) on male sexual behaviour, the Kinsey team had found that male sexual function tended to deteriorate with age. In all, 1.6% of men had more or less permanent problems achieving an erection and this figure rose to 27% by the age of 70. A further 35% reported erectile difficulties on occasions, while 6% complained of premature ejaculation.

However, orgasmic dysfunction does not necessarily correlate with sexual dissatisfaction, while a normal physiological response does not necessarily rule out sexual problems. Dissatisfaction for men and women is more likely to be associated with sexual difficulties such as difficulty in relaxing or a general lack of interest. A British population survey (Osborne et al 1988) showed 19% of women to be sexually dysfunctional in the age group 35–40 years, and 32% between 40–45 years. In a Swedish study (Fugl-Meyer et al 1987) among women aged 40–54, 24% experienced insufficient lubrication and 65% a lack of desire.

Social and cultural factors in sexual enjoyment have been poorly studied, but there is a general agreement in the literature that positive attitudes to sexual relationships and the ability to respond are positively associated in women with both social class and educational attainment.

Gynaecological clinic attendees

The incidence of sexual dysfunction in clinic populations has been the subject of only a limited number of studies. Clearly there will be a number of biasing factors in these, including the nature of the clinic and the attitude of the clinicians involved. Routine direct questioning about sexual problems will double the number presented to the clinician, yet in most clinics this approach is still not used. Nonetheless, a Dutch study (Frenken & Van Tol 1987), interviewing a sample of Dutch gynaecologists, found that during the preceding week, 1 patient in 14 presented with a sexual problem, most commonly dyspareunia or loss of sexual interest.

Clinics specifically for sexual difficulties clearly see a very selected population. However, overall, men presenting to such clinics tend to complain of problems with their genital responses while women are more likely to complain of a lack of interest or enjoyment, and there is some evidence that this trend is becoming more marked. It is important to note that in up to one-third of couples where one partner presents with a sexual dysfunction, a sexual problem will also be found in the other partner.

PRESENTATION

Patients' ability to share their sexual problems depends heavily on the attitude of the clinician. The majority of couples with sexual problems first present these to their general practitioner. In general, if these couples are referred on for specialist advice it is not usually to the gynaecologist. Others may prefer to present to a nonmedical setting, such as Relate.

Bancroft (1989) has emphasized the value of having a coordinated range of services to meet the needs of couples with sexual problems, partly in order to offer an appropriate range of helping skills, and partly to allow for different patterns of presentation.

Sexual dysfunction frequently presents in the gynaecologist's clinic as a secondary rather than a main presenting problem. Despite the apparent increase in freedom in our society to talk about sex, particularly in the media, one should not underestimate the levels of naivety and ignorance which still exist. Couples who have never managed to achieve intravaginal intercourse, yet are unaware of this, may still be seen in infertility clinics.

Other problems may be more easily presented in certain contexts; for instance, a lack of sexual interest may be presented by the gynaecological patient who is asking whether it might be related to her hormones. This is particularly common in family planning clinics where the contraceptive pill may be blamed for reduced libido or in the woman presenting with the premenstrual syndrome or with menopausal problems. Over 40% of patients attending a London menopausal clinic acknowledged either loss of libido or dyspareunia when questioned directly (Studd et al 1977).

Sexual problems in some gynaecological patients will only be discovered at the time of physical examination. Here spasm of the pubococcygeus muscle may be apparent, leading to a possible diagnosis of vaginismus. Alternatively, deep pelvic pain may be elicited on bimanual examination and it is always appropriate to ask whether similar discomfort is experienced on intercourse.

INVESTIGATIONS

Sexual dysfunction is frequently better dealt with within a context other than the gynaecology outpatient clinic. However, the clinician has three clear duties. First is the detection of the problem, and this has already been dealt with. The second is the taking of a careful sexual problem history and the third is the elucidation of underlying organic factors.

Taking a sexual problem history

The main barriers to taking a sexual problem history are usually embarrassment and discomfort, often both on the part of the patient and the clinician. In order to be able to carry out a sensitive interview in this area the clinician at least must be comfortable. This comfort can be based on a combination of a good fundamental knowledge of human sexual functioning, and experience in developing general interviewing and counselling skills.

Specific information requires specific questioning, and if the patient is indicating that she has a psychosexual dysfunction the questioning needs to be directed towards establishing the nature of the *current problem*. Focusing on the presenting complaint rather than proceeding directly to taking a more general sexual history has a number of advantages. Firstly, it reassures the patient that her complaint is being taken seriously. Secondly, it often provides the necessary information for distinguishing possible organic components.

When a clear picture of the problem as it exists has been obtained, a history of this problem should then be taken. This will include some information about the first time the problem occurred; whether it developed abruptly or has come on gradually; how long the patient has been aware of it; whether it is getting better or worse; whether it is situational (e.g. occurring with one partner and not another or in one sexual position and not another), and any obvious aggravating or ameliorating factors. In the case of deep dyspareunia, the standard eight questions which are asked about any complaint of pain should be included.

Finally, it is worth trying to get some idea of the patient's own views of the cause of the problem and her partner's reaction to it. Attempts are often made to distinguish between sexual and 'marital' problems but unless the relationship is obviously grossly unsatisfactory there tends to be little advantage in this approach.

General physical examination

Careful inspection of the external and internal genitalia will exclude developmental abnormalities such as vaginal atresia or imperforate hymen in the female, and hypospadias or undescended testes in the male. Normal secondary characteristics should also be present. A careful check of the vulva and vagina should be made, especially when there is a complaint of dyspareunia. It is important to rule out acute infections such as monilia, trichomonas or genital herpes. As well as chronic conditions such as cysts of Bartholin's gland, manual pelvic examination should look for evidence of pelvic inflammatory disease or endometriosis. A retroverted uterus can also be a source of deep dyspareunia, either because of the effect of thrusting the uterus against the base of the spine or because of direct thrusting against the ovaries which tend to prolapse into the pouch of Douglas. The important iatrogenic cause for superficial pain can be the presence of an episiotomy scar.

Kolodny et al (1979) list 37 possible causes of dyspareunia. Of these, 35 are organic and two are psychological, so the importance of careful examination cannot be over-emphasized. Laparoscopy will also be appropriate in some cases of deep dyspareunia.

A hormone profile may be appropriate if there is any evidence of gonadal failure.

TREATMENT

It is clear from what has been noted earlier in this chapter that there is no possibility of offering treatment for everyone experiencing sexual difficulties or dissatisfaction. Fortunately this is neither necessary nor is it the expectation of patients. Jack Annon (1976a,b) has devised a model by means of which the appropriate level of response can be selected for each problem presented to the clinician. This model, also known by the acronym PLISSIT, assumes that problems with an organic basis have already been filtered out, though this approach may still be appropriate for some organic problems. The term PLISSIT refers to the four levels of response: Permission, Limited Information, Specific Suggestions and Intensive Therapy.

Permission

Patients often want to check with their doctor that certain aspects of their sexual life are acceptable. They may seek permission to be less sexually active, for example, in the puerperium or postmenopausally. They may have particular aspects of their behaviour or their partner's which concern them and about which they seek the approval of a professional. This brings us again to the clinician's comfort with his or her own sexuality. Clearly, it is very difficult to give permission to other people if you do not have that permission yourself.

Limited information

Limited information may need to be given to women about normal sexual response and about the times when it may change. Most women achieve orgasm more reliably by masturbation, partner manipulation, or oral sex than by intercourse, yet many are unaware of or feel uncomfortable with this. Since the work of Masters & Johnson, demonstrating the ability of some women to be multiply orgasmic, many women now feel that this is an expectation of them. They may need to know that this is an idiosyncratic response which only some women experience.

Women in their first pregnancy may need to know about the normal changes in libido and in the sensitivity of the erogenous zones during pregnancy and in the puerperium. Those women approaching the menopause may need to know about the physiological and anatomical changes in the vagina and the possible role for oestrogen replacement in preventing urogenital aging.

Specific suggestions

Often the most useful specific suggestion, particularly for the gynaecologist whose time or experience is limited, is some appropriate reading for the patient. There are a variety of useful books varying from the general (Brown & Faulder 1979, Yaffe & Fenwick 1986a,b) to those designed for specific problems (e.g. Heiman et al 1986, Valins 1988).

Several specific suggestions are frequently offered in gynaecological clinics. If a couple are deriving less pleasure from intercourse following childbirth and there is evidence that this is related to looseness of the pubococcygeus muscle, then reteaching of Kegel's (pelvic floor) exercises may be helpful, as may the female superior position.

Suggestions about alternative positions or new stimulatory techniques may be helpful where there is an organic cause for dyspareunia which is untreatable.

Intensive therapy

Dyspareunia (without a discernible organic cause), the orgasmic dysfunctions and the male dysfunctions all need a structured form of therapy and unfortunately, because of the structure of provision of gynaecological services in the UK, this cannot normally be considered to be the province of the gynaecologist.

Modern intensive therapy usually involves some level of compromise between the psychoanalytic and the behavioural approach and most clinics now offer a form of treatment which is based loosely on the work of Masters & Johnson (1970), Annon (1976a,b) and Kaplan (1974, 1979). The features which these therapies have in common are that they are client- and couple-centred. After varying levels of assessment of both the sexual problem and the couple's relationship, a behavioural framework is adopted. Any attempt at intercourse is usually 'banned' at this stage and sexual experiences are prescribed in very small steps. 'Progress', or lack of it, in taking these steps can then be examined in the context of the couple and their relationship, while trying to tackle those factors which are commonly involved in the maintenance of chronic sexual difficulties. These include a lack of information, a failure to communicate (especially on matters with a sexual or emotional content), goal orientation, sexual anxiety and spectatoring.

These factors have been well described by Masters & Johnson (1970) and Kaplan (1974, 1979) and are a common response to continuing sexual difficulties. Repeated sexual 'failure' leads to anxiety at every sexual encounter. This in turn leads to the individuals carefully watching their bodies' responses rather than allowing arousal to happen spontaneously. Couples who previously enjoyed a varied and imaginative sexual life often restrict the expressions of their sexuality further and further when a problem arises until their behaviour is highly stereotyped and geared only to achieving the 'goal' of sexual experience which by then has become the erection or the orgasm.

This type of sex therapy has been developed to try to produce a relatively brief but effective intervention for couples with sexual problems. Treatment sessions may typically be held at fortnightly intervals with a standard initial contract of up to 12 sessions.

Sex therapy alone may not be successful even where there is no obvious organic cause for the problem, and physical treatments may also be appropriate. For erectile dysfunction, self-administered injection of papaverine into the corpora cavernosa (which should be initiated and monitored by a clinician with experience in this treatment) may enable a man to gain an erection at will, and for many this will provide a more acceptable alternative to penile prosthesis.

RESULTS

Assessment of the outcome of treatment for sexual dysfunction is fraught with difficulties. Diagnostic classifications, based as they are on the physiological sexual response cycle, are problematic and often contain heterogeneous groups. Prognoses are also clearly likely to be affected by general health, age, and the state of the relationship when help is sought. Sexual difficulties may act as a guise for marital difficulties and these underlying relationship problems may have a major effect on the prognosis. If one individual in the couple is labelled as 'the patient' he or she may be under considerable pressure to seek help, yet there may be covert reasons for avoiding a successful resolution of the problem.

The second area of difficulty in assessing outcome is the uncertainty about what constitutes success. One couple may experience only slight alterations in coital or orgasmic frequency, yet may consider that therapy has produced a substantial improvement in their sexual health and the quality of their relationship. Others may have been assisted to achieve a 'Masters & Johnson-style' physiological sexual response but still find their partner unexciting and sex unrewarding.

These difficulties in measuring outcome are aggravated further by different ways of reporting results. Masters & Johnson (1970), for instance, report the proportion of failures on the grounds that failure is easier to measure than success.

If 'complete success' and 'much improvement' are taken together, then a number of studies, (e.g. Bancroft & Coles 1976, Hawton 1982, Heisler 1983, Warner & Bancroft 1986) all show 60–65% falling into one of these groups. However, drop-out rates vary and some results (e.g. Heisler 1983) account only for those who stayed in therapy. Long-term follow-up is in more doubt. Masters & Johnson reported a 5% relapse rate among their 'non-failures' at 5 years, but both recurrence of sexual difficulties and relationship breakdown are worryingly common in most other studies.

KEY POINTS

1. Although a psychosexual disorder may have an underlying organic basis, its presentation and prognosis are usually dependent on the expectations of both the individual and the society in which she lives.
2. Psychosexual disorders may be situational; that is to say, they may occur within the context of one relationship, but not another.
3. An enjoyable sexual experience will normally require intact pelvic organs with functioning vascular and neurological mechanisms.
4. Dyspareunia is perhaps one of the most common sexual difficulties presented to the gynaecologist.
5. Vaginismus is not necessarily related to a woman's ability to become aroused or be orgasmic.
6. Inability to reach orgasm by intercourse alone is a sufficiently common problem that most women would probably not regard it as dysfunction.
7. Premature ejaculation is a relative term and may be defined as the tendency for an individual to ejaculate appreciably more quickly than he or his partner would wish.
8. Loss of libido following either a hysterectomy or sterilization is unlikely to be organic.
9. Patients' ability to share their sexual problems depends heavily on the attitude of the clinician.
10. Sexual dysfunction is frequently better dealt with in a context other than the gynaecology outpatient clinic.
11. Modern intensive therapy usually involves some level of compromise between the psychoanalytic and the behavioural approach.

REFERENCES

Annon J S 1976a The behavioural treatment of sexual problems. Volume 1: Brief therapy. Enabling Systems, Honolulu

Annon J S 1976b The behavioural treatment of sexual problems. Volume 2: Intensive therapy. Enabling Systems, Honolulu

Bancroft J 1989 Human sexuality and its problems. Churchill Livingstone, Edinburgh

Bancroft J, Coles L 1976 Three years' experience in a sexual problem clinic. British Medical Journal 1: 1575–1577

Brown P, Faulder C 1979 Treat yourself to sex: a guide for good loving. Penguin, Harmondsworth

Frenken J, Van Tol P 1987 Sexual problems in gynaecological practice. Journal of Psychosomatic Obstetrics and Gynaecology 6: 143–155

Fugl-Meyer A, Fugl-Meyer K, Gerdle B 1987 Sexuellt Valbefinnande I En Nordsvensk Stad. Socialmedicinsk Tidskrift 7: 322–325

Garth D, Cooper P, Day A 1981 Hysterectomy and psychiatric disorder: levels of psychiatric morbidity before and after hysterectomy. British Journal of Psychiatry 140: 335–342

Hawton K 1982 The behavioural treatment of sexual dysfunction. British Journal of Psychiatry 140: 94–101

Heiman J, Lo Piccolo L, Lo Piccolo J 1986 Becoming orgasmic: a sexual growth program for women. Prentice-Hall International, London

Heisler J 1983 Sexual therapy in the National Marriage Guidance Council. NMGC, Rugby

Helström L 1994 Sexuality after hysterectomy: a model based on quantitative and qualitative analysis of 104 women before and after subtotal hysterectomy. Journal of Psychosomatic Obstetrics and Gynaecology 15: 219–229

Kaplan H S 1974 The new sex therapy. Baillière Tindall, London

Kaplan H S 1979 Disorders of sexual-desire and other new concepts and techniques in sex therapy. Brunner/Mazel, New York

Kinsey A C, Pomeroy W B, Martin C F 1948 Sexual behaviour in the human male. Saunders, Philadelphia

Kinsey A C, Pomeroy W B, Martin C F, Gebhard P H 1953 Sexual behaviour in the human female. Saunders, Philadelphia

Kolodny R C, Masters W H, Johnson V E 1979 Textbook of sexual medicine. Little, Brown, Boston

Martin R L, Roberts W V, Clayton P J 1980 Psychiatric status after

hysterectomy – a one-year prospective follow-up. Journal of the American Medical Association 244: 350–353
Masters W H, Johnson V E 1966 Human sexual response. Little, Brown, Boston
Masters W H, Johnson V E 1970 Human sexual inadequacy. Little, Brown, Boston
Osborne M, Hawton K, Gath D 1988 Sexual dysfunction among middle-aged women in the community. British Medical Journal 296: 959–962
Siddle N, Sarrel P, Whitehead M 1987 The effect of hysterectomy on the age at ovarian failure: identification of a subgroup of women with premature loss of ovarian function. Fertility and Sterility 47 (1): 94–100
Studd J, Chakravarti S, Oram D 1977 The climacteric. Clinics in Obstetrics and Gynaecology 4: 3–29
Valins L 1988 Vaginismus: understanding and overcoming the blocks to intercourse. Ashgrove Press, Bath
Warner P, Bancroft J 1986 Sex therapy outcome research: a reappraisal of methodology. 2. Methodological considerations – the importance of prognostic variability. Psychological Medicine 16: 855–863
Yaffe M, Fenwick E 1986a Sexual happiness for men. A practical approach. Dorling Kindersley, London
Yaffe M, Fenwick E 1986b Sexual happiness for women. A practical approach. Dorling Kindersley, London

FURTHER READING

Comfort A 1978 Sexual consequences of disability. George F. Stickley, Philadelphia
Gillan P 1987 Sex therapy manual. Blackwell, Oxford
Wagner G, Green R 1981 Impotence, physiological, psychological, surgical diagnosis and treatment. Plenum, New York

28

Menstruation and menstrual abnormality

M. Lumsden J. Norman

INTRODUCTION

Menstrual abnormality is a frequent reason for women to present at gynaecological outpatient clinics and menorrhagia is one of the commonest causes of iron-deficiency anaemia in western women (Cohen & Gibor 1980). However before discussing the aetiology of menstrual abnormality, the mechanism of normal menstruation will be reviewed.

MENSTRUATION

At the end of the ovarian cycle, a major portion of the endometrium in primates undergoes periodic necrosis and sloughing associated with blood loss. This is at a time when the gonadal steroids reach their lowest levels. The nature of the supportive effect on the endometrium is unknown, although possible mechanisms will be discussed later.

The mechanism of menstruation

The uterine wall consists of three layers: the serous coat, the myometrium and the endometrium. The serous coat is firmly adherent to the myometrium which consists of smooth muscle fibres, the main branches of the blood vessels and the nerves of the uterus and connective tissue. The endometrium consists principally of glandular and stromal cells, although its structure does vary with the position in the uterus and the stage of the menstrual cycle.

The blood supply of the uterus

This is illustrated in Figure 28.1. The arcuate and radial arteries which supply the myometrium and basal endometrium have vascular fields which overlap. On approaching the surface epithelium, the radial arteries develop a corkscrew appearance and are known as spiral arterioles, These are present only in species which menstruate and are end arterioles, each supplying an area of 4–7 mm^2. They are sensitive to changes in gonadal steroid levels and the capillaries are lost with the glands and stroma at menstruation. There is an irregular network of venous vessels with the veins frequently intersecting, forming venous lakes. The radial and arcuate veins drain via the uterine vein into the iliac vein.

The histology of the uterus

The histology of the uterus is illustrated in Figure 28.2a. The zona compacta, which is adjacent to the uterine cavity, and the zona functionalis are sensitive to changes in gonadal steroids whereas the basal layer, which joins the myometrium, is not. The myometrium, which consists principally of smooth muscle cells, is connected by gap

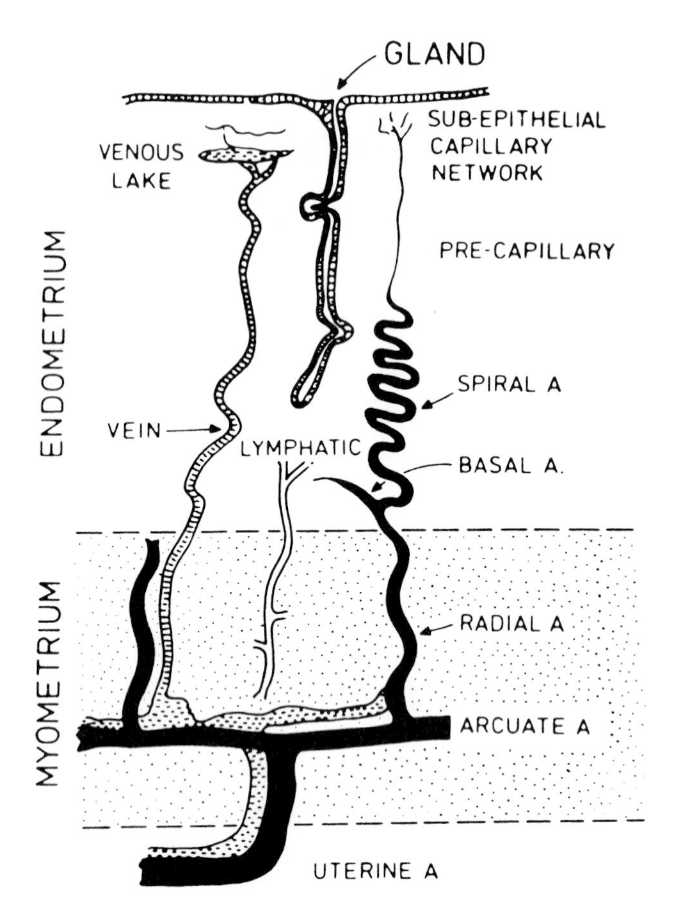

Fig. 28.1 Schematic representation of the blood supply of the uterus. A, artery.

junctions allowing free movement of ions; it offers low electrical resistance. There is a functional resemblance to cardiac muscle although there is no conclusive evidence for a pacemaker within the uterus. The endometrium responds to the cyclical changes in the gonadal steroid levels described elsewhere (see Ch. 14); these changes are probably in preparation for blastocyst implantation, as menstruation only happens when this fails to occur.

The first half of the cycle involves tissue growth and proliferation and the second, epithelial and stromal differentiation. During the proliferative phase, the short, straight, epithelial glands elongate and become tortuous (Fig. 28.2a). Changes occur in the position of the nuclei and the number of mitoses (Fig. 28.2a). During the secretory phase, the glands increase in diameter and tortuosity and vacuoles appear in the cellular cytoplasm (Fig. 28.2c). The tissue also becomes markedly more oedematous.

The spiral arterioles also undergo cyclical change. Following the cessation of menstruation they are simple in form, extending just into the endometrium. The secretory phase is characterized by growth of arterioles. In the late secretory phase coiling occurs due to proliferation and extension of the arterioles as well as the resorption of the stromal oedema (Fig. 28.2d). With the fall in steroid concentrations, menstrual shedding of the endometrium occurs (Fig. 28.2g). Cell injury becomes increasingly evident, and infiltration of macrophages occurs.

Endometrial shedding varies remarkably from one woman to another and from one area of the uterus to another in the same woman.

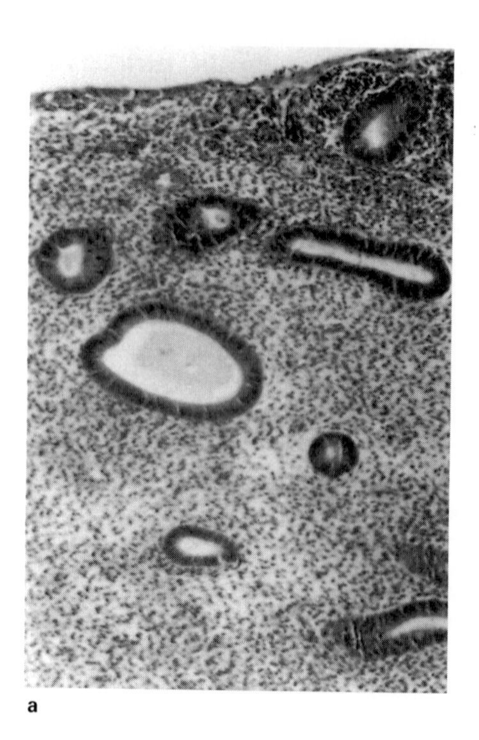
a

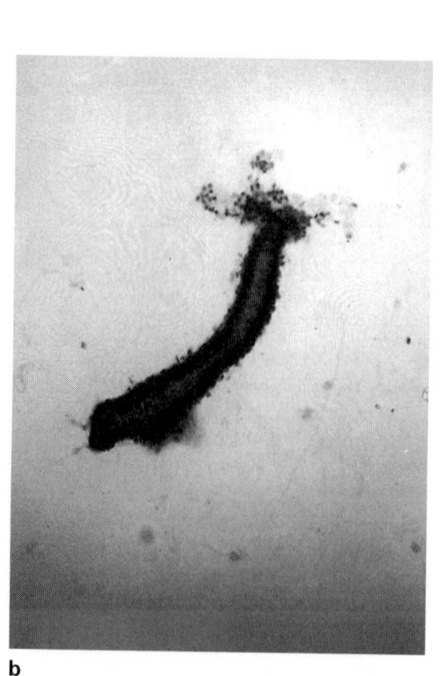
b

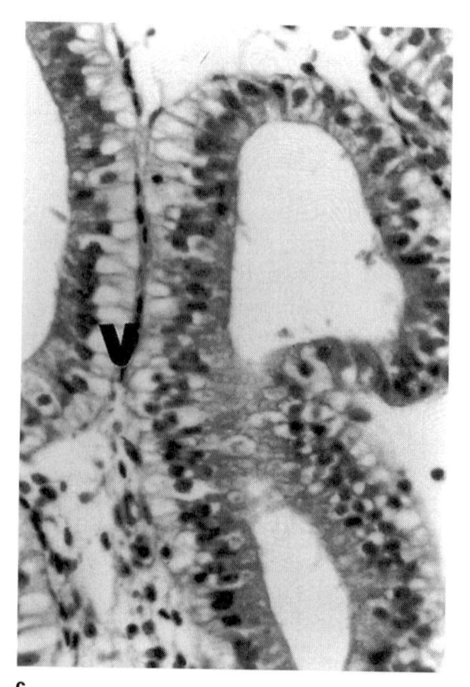
c

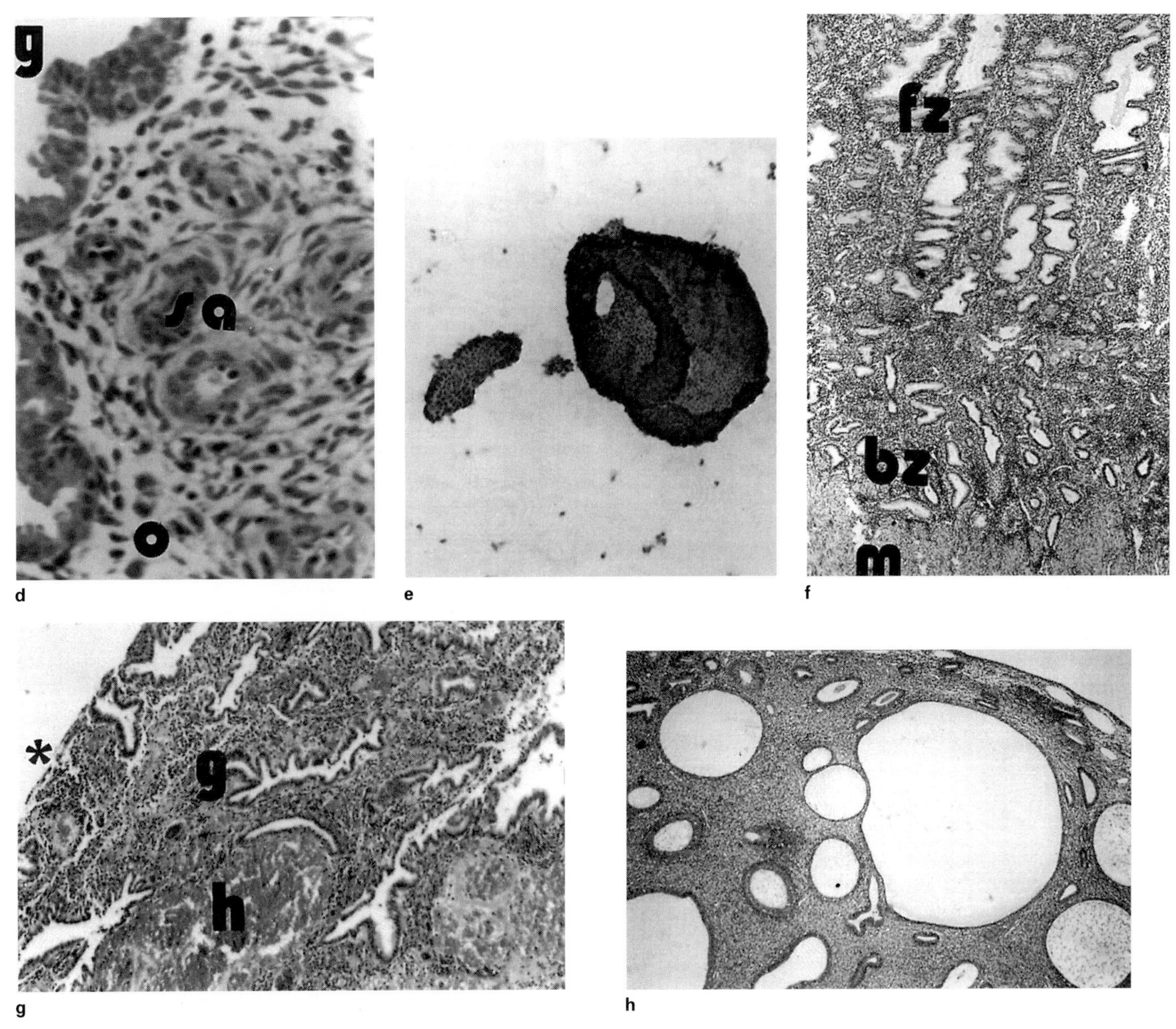

Fig. 28.2 **a** Proliferative endometrium showing tubular glands. Mitoses are present in glands and stroma (×10). **b** A proliferative gland (×63) separated from endometrium by collagenase digestion. **c** Early secretory endometrium showing subnuclear vacuolation (v) and the presence of secretions. There are now few mitoses (×40). **d** Midsecretory endometrium (day 23) characterized by 'saw-toothed' glands (g), convoluted spiral arterioles (sa) and stromal oedema (o) (×40). **e** Midsecretory gland illustrating the coiled shape (compare with **b**) (× 40). **f** Late secretory endometrium showing the functional zone (fz), basal zone (bz) and myometrium (m). **g** Menstruating endometrium. The glands (**g**) are now thin and show little secretory activity. There are lakes of haemorrhage (h) and the endometrium is beginning to break up (*). There is infiltration with white blood cells (×10). **h** Cystic glandular hyperplasia (×4).

Dramatic changes occur in the spiral arterioles at menstruation. These changes were described by Markee (1948) after experiments involving the transplantation of endometrium into the anterior chamber of the eye of the rhesus monkey. This work was the cornerstone of current concepts of menstruation. On observing the bleeding process, Markee suggested that the arteriolar coiling caused constriction of the vessel lumen with vascular stasis and leukocytic infiltration. About 24 h premenstrually, intense vasoconstriction led to ischaemic damage which was then followed by vasodilatation with haemorrhages from both arterial and venous vessels: 75% of the loss was arteriolar, 15% venous and 10% diapedesis of erythrocytes. This work has never been repeated although some support comes from experiments where endometrium was implanted into the hamster cheek pouch (an immunologically privileged site) and changes observed through a plastic window. Bleeding was observed although no hormonally induced changes in the blood vessels occurred.

The myometrium

There is no evidence for a structural change in the myometrium during the menstrual cycle. However, it is

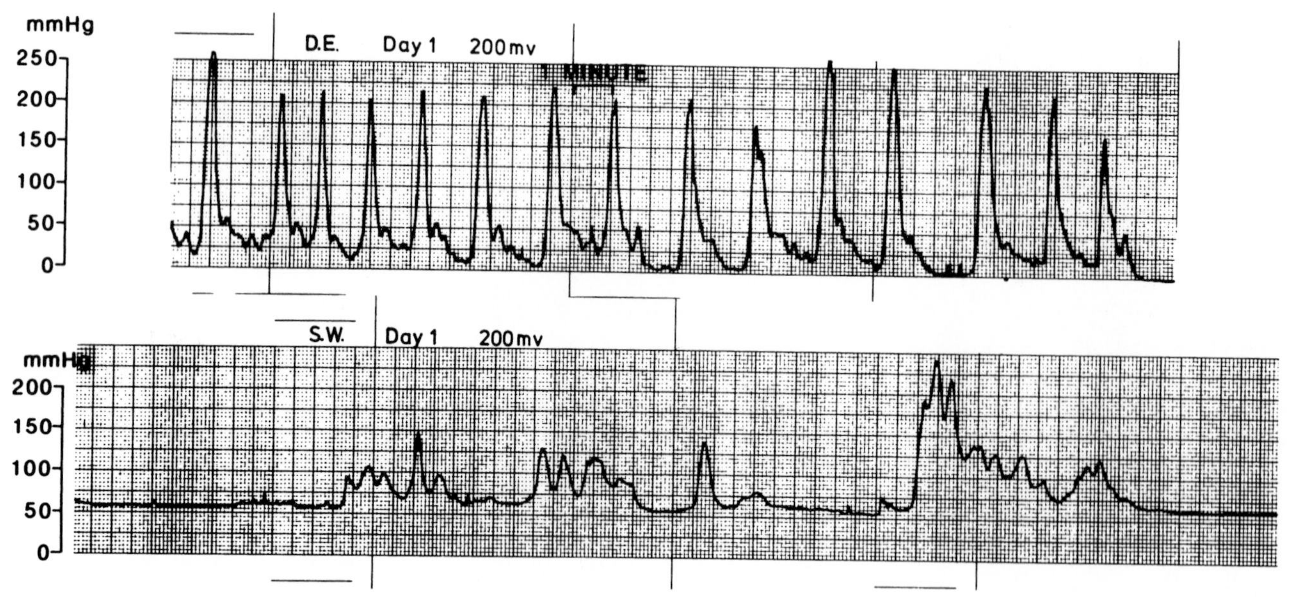

Fig. 28.3 Uterine contractility on day 1 of the menses as assessed by measuring the intrauterine pressure using a microtransducer catheter. Subject DE suffered from dysmenorrhoea whereas subject SW did not.

well known that changes occur in the pattern of contractility. This can be assessed by measuring intrauterine pressure, which demonstrates maximum activity during the first days of the menses, when a labour-like activity is observed which may or may not lead to pain (Fig. 28.3).

CONTROL OF MENSTRUAL BLOOD LOSS

The endometrial surface area is large (10–45 cm^2), indicating that haemostasis during menstruation is usually very efficient. Possible factors in the control of blood loss are:

1. platelet plug formation
2. vasoconstriction
3. endometrial repair.

Derangement of any of these mechanisms is likely to lead to excessive menstrual blood loss. This section details some of the agents derived from the endometrium (either from glandular epithelial cells, stromal cells, invading leucocytes or blood vessels) which can affect the processes described above, although the relative importance of each of these agents in controlling menstrual blood loss is currently poorly understood.

Platelet plug formation

Menstrual blood was thought not to clot and to be free of platelets and fibrin. However it is now thought that once clinical bleeding and tissue shedding has started, haemostatic plug formation occurs, but less rapidly and less completely than is observed in human skin wounds (Christiaens et al 1982). Certain haemorrhagic conditions (e.g. thrombocytopenic purpura) are associated with an increased incidence of menorrhagia suggesting that abnormalities of platelet structure may be important.

The coagulation cascade operates in the uterus and endometrium as in other tissues. Platelet accumulation, platelet degranulation and fibrin deposition occur within hours of the onset of menstruation, sealing endometrial vessels. An important difference in the uterus is the prevention of clot formation, which is necessary to deter scarring and obliteration of the endometrial cavity. Fibrinolysis is initiated in the endometrium by two types of plasminogen activator: tissue-type and urokinase-type, both of which are released by disintegrating endometrium. The hormonal control of plasminogen activator production is such that oestradiol stimulates and progesterone inhibits urokinase plasminogen activator (Casslen et al 1986). Further, progesterone inhibits production of tissue plasminogen activator, and this effect is amplified by production of plasminogen activator inhibitor. These mechanisms ensure that during menstruation, as progesterone falls and oestradiol rises, plasminogen activator levels increase to prevent uterine adhesions.

The endometrium also generates factors which inhibit platelet aggregation and platelet adhesion. Such factors include prostacyclin (PGI_2), nitric oxide (NO) and platelet activating factor (PAF) all of which are produced by human endometrium (Alecozay et al 1991, Kelly et al 1984).

Although derangements of fibrinolysis, PGI_2 concentrations or NO have not been demonstrated in women with menorrhagia, increases in endometrial plasminogen activator have been found in women with a copper-containing intrauterine contraceptive device (Shaw et al 1983), and suppression of plasminogen activator has been demonstrated during treatment with the oral contraceptive pill (Casslen & Astedt 1983). Since these agents tend to induce and prevent menorrhagia respectively, this suggests the importance of plasminogen activators in menstrual blood loss.

Vasoconstriction

At the onset of menstruation, damaged blood vessels are sealed by intravascular thrombi of platelets and fibrin. However, as menstruation progresses, the functional endometrium is shed, thus these haemostatic thrombi are lost. By 20 h after the start of menstruation, blood loss is controlled by intense vasoconstriction of the spiral arteries (Christiaens et al 1980).

The role of the prostaglandin $PGF_{2\alpha}$ in vasoconstriction is well established. The effects of the vasoconstricting $PGF_{2\alpha}$ are balanced by those of the vasodilating PGE_2. Concentrations of both these prostaglandins are increased in the luteal phase. Overproduction of vasodilatory prostaglandins, or reduced production of vasoconstrictors is likely to lead to excessive blood loss at the time of menstruation. This is confirmed by work showing an elevated $PGE_2/PGF_{2\alpha}$ ratio, increased endometrial PGE_2 or increased PGE_2 receptor concentrations in women with menorrhagia (Adalantado et al 1988, Cameron et al 1987, Smith et al 1981a,b, Smith et al 1982). The synthesis of prostaglandins by endometrium is influenced by steroid hormones and the highest levels are found during the menses. This is particularly true for prostaglandin $F_{2\alpha}$, the synthesis of which rises significantly during the secretory phase of the menstrual cycle under the influence of progesterone.

Other vasoconstrictors which have attracted recent interest are endothelin and platelet-activating factor (PAF). Endothelin is an extremely powerful vasoconstrictor which is found in various tissues including human endometrium (O'Reilly et al 1992). It has been proposed that as endometrial glandular epithelium breaks down during menstruation, stored endothelin gains access to the spiral arterioles causing long-lasting vasoconstriction. PAF is present in the endometrium in the luteal phase and has an ambiguous effect on spiral arteriolar tone: PAF itself is a vasoconstrictor but stimulates production of the vasodilator PGE_2 (Bjork & Smedegard 1983, Smith & Kelly 1988). The precise roles for PAF and endothelin in menstruation are not yet clear.

Endometrial repair

Menstruation is finally curtailed by endometrial repair. This process is stimulated physiologically by increasing levels of oestrogen released into the circulation by the developing ovarian follicle. There is increasing evidence that oestrogen-induced endometrial proliferation is mediated by epidermal growth factor (EGF). EGF is produced by the endometrium with maximal production in the late proliferative phase of the cycle (Ishihara et al 1990). It seems likely that endometrial EGF contributes to repair of both glandular and stromal tissue, although the glandular effects are predominant (Haining et al 1991).

Developing tissues need a blood supply, and thus angiogenesis is an important part of endometrial repair. Vascular endothelial growth factor (VEGF) is a highly potent endothelial mitogen produced by the endometrium (Charnock-Jones et al 1993). Production of VEGF is stimulated both by oestrogen (Charnock-Jones et al 1993) and by hypoxia (Shweiki et al 1993). These data suggest a role for VEGF in endometrial repair at the start of the menstrual cycle.

In the pregnant uterus myometrial contraction is an important mechanism for achieving haemostasis. However this is not thought to be the case in the nonpregnant uterus. Drugs which inhibit uterine contraction, such as prostaglandin synthetase inhibitors (see p. 434), and which are used to treat dysmenorrhoea, do not increase menstrual blood loss whereas ergot alkaloids which cause muscle contractions are of no use in treating menorrhagia. Myometrial activity is therefore not considered to be the principal mechanism.

Understanding of the mechanism of the control of menstrual blood loss is steadily increasing (Fig. 28.4). Further information about these mechanisms and their

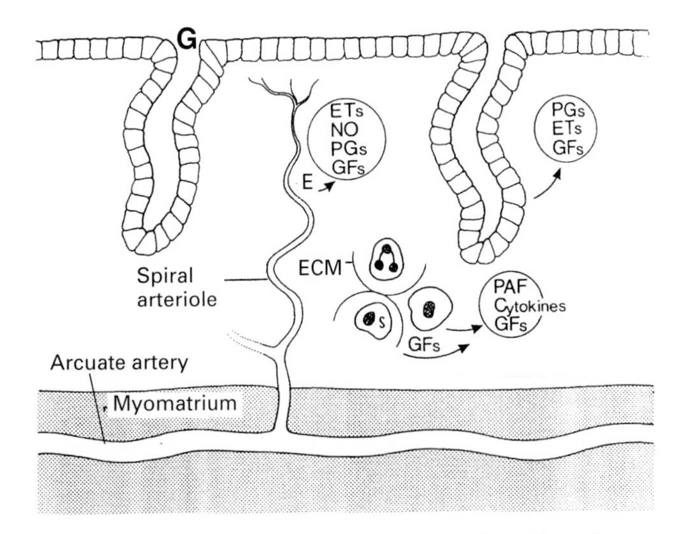

Fig. 28.4 Paracrine interactions in the endometrium. The major cellular components for the endometrium, glandular epithelium, stroma and vascular epithelium, synthesize a wide range of locally acting factors which are thought to play a fundamental role in the initiation and maintenance of menstrual bleeding, and the subsequent repair process. G, gland; S, stroma; E, endothelium; ECM, extracellular matrix; ET, endothelin; GF, growth factor; NO, nitric oxide; PAF, platelet-activating factor; PG, prostaglandin. Reproduced with permission from Cameron I T, Irvine G, Norman J E (in press) Menstruation. In: Hillier et al (eds) Scientific essentials of reproductive medicine. W B Saunders, Philadelphia.

abnormalities during menstruation will enable effective medical treatments to be developed, and reduce the need for surgical treatment.

THE NORMAL MENSTRUAL CYCLE

A majority of cycles are between 24 and 32 days and a normal cycle is considered to be 28 days. Menstrual cycle length varies during reproductive life, being most regular between the ages of 20 and 40 years. It tends to be longer after the menarche and shorter as the menopause approaches. The mean menstrual blood loss per menstruation in a healthy west European population ranges between 37 and 43 ml; 70% of the loss occurs in the first 48 h. Despite the large interpatient variability, loss between consecutive menses in the same woman does not vary to a great extent (Fig. 28.5). Only 9–14% of women lose more than 80 ml per period and 60% of these women are actually anaemic. The upper limit of normal menstruation is thus taken as 80 ml per menses (Rybo 1966). However, actual fluid loss (mucus, tissue etc.) may be considerably more than the blood loss alone and amounts vary considerably.

During the first day or two of the menses, uterine contractility is at its greatest. This may possibly aid expulsion of the degenerating endometrium from the uterus. Activity is extremely variable between women although it is remarkably constant between menses in the same women. There is no objective method of separating normal and abnormal contractility; normal contractility is considered to be that which causes no debility to a woman although mild discomfort may occur.

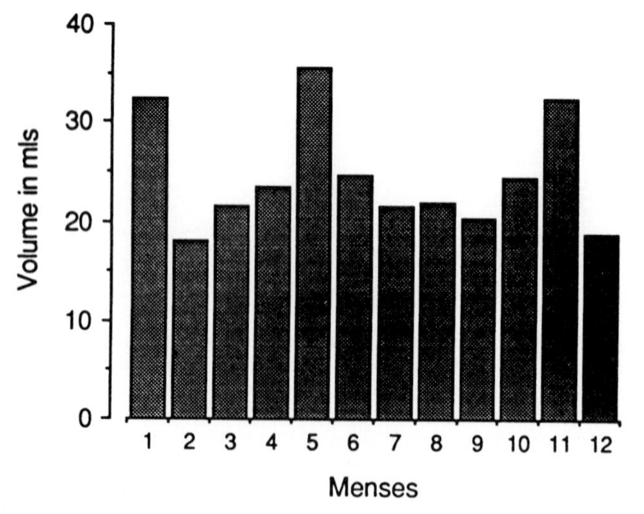

Fig. 28.5 The variability in menstrual blood loss in a single individual: values for 12 consecutive periods (adapted from Hallberg & Nilsson 1964).

ABNORMAL MENSTRUATION

During this century, widespread use of contraception and sterilization with reduction in family size has resulted in a significant increase in the number of menstrual periods experienced by women. As a result, menstrual problems have become increasingly important. The defects considered here will be menorrhagia with particular reference to dysfunctional uterine bleeding (DUB), and dysmenorrhoea. Those defects particularly associated with infertility, e.g. oligo- or amenorrhoea, will not be discussed further.

Menorrhagia

The causes of menorrhagia fall into four categories:

1. clotting defects
2. DUB
3. pelvic pathology
4. medical disorders.

Clotting defects

Certain haemorrhagic conditions, e.g. thrombocytopenic purpura and Von Willebrand's disease, are associated with an increased incidence of menorrhagia. However there is no impairment of blood coagulation in those with excess menstrual loss, nor are fibrin degradation products elevated in the menstrual fluid of those with heavy menstrual loss (Bonnar et at 1983). Patients with platelet and coagulation disorders frequently suffer from excessive menstrual blood loss, necessitating hormonal or surgical therapy and sometimes multiple transfusions. In women with thrombocytopenia, menstrual blood loss correlates broadly with platelet count at the time of the menses. Splenectomy has been known to reduce dramatically the menstrual blood loss in these patients.

Dysfunctional uterine bleeding

Disturbances in the pattern of menstruation are a common clinical presentation for abnormalities of the hypophyseal–pituitary–ovarian axis. DUB is defined as heavy and/or irregular menses in the absence of recognizable pelvic pathology, pregnancy or general bleeding disorder. It commonly occurs at the extremes of reproductive life (adolescence and perimenopausally). The abnormalities of ovarian activity may be classified as follows:

1. Anovulatory
   a. inadequate signal, e.g. in polycystic ovarian disease or premenopausally
   b. impaired positive feedback, e.g. in adolescence.
2. Ovulatory
   a. inadequate luteal phase
   b. idiopathic.

Anovulatory DUB. Occasionally anovulatory cycles occur in all women. Chronic anovulation, however, is associated with an irregular and unpredictable pattern of bleeding ranging from short cycles with scanty bleeding to prolonged periods of irregular heavy loss. Normal bleeding occurs in response to withdrawal of both progesterone and oestradiol. If ovulation does not occur then the absence of progesterone results in an absence of secretory changes in the endometrium, accompanied by abnormalities in the production of steroid receptors, prostaglandins and other locally active endometrial products. Unopposed oestrogen gives rise to persistent proliferative or hyperplastic endometrium and oestrogen withdrawal bleeding is characteristically painless and irregular. It tends to occur at the extremes of reproductive life but is rare at other times. Only 20% of those cycles with excessive menstrual blood loss are anovulatory (Haynes et al 1979); this same study fails to demonstrate any abnormalities in gonadotrophin or circulating steroid concentrations. In anovulatory cycles, the endometrium is unable to produce factors whose synthesis is controlled by progesterone, e.g. prostaglandin $F_{2\alpha}$ (Smith et al 1982). This may account for the painless nature of the bleeds.

Ovulation occurs in response to the midcycle surge of luteinizing hormone. If this fails to occur due to insufficient oestradiol secretion or impaired positive feedback, ovulation will not occur.

Failure of follicular development. Follicular development which is insufficient to produce an oestrogen signal strong enough to induce a luteinizing hormone surge is one of the common reasons for the irregularities in menstrual cycle pattern in premenopausal women. This occurs perimenopausally and in the polycystic ovarian syndrome. (The aetiology and treatment of the latter are dealt with elsewhere; Ch. 23).

Anovulatory bleeding may be associated with cystic glandular hyperplasia of the endometrium (Fig. 28.2h). This occurs in some older women and also in prepubertal girls where unopposed oestrogen secretion occurs. The first few cycles after the menarche are commonly anovulatory. However, if anovulation persists, a long period of amenorrhoea is accompanied by endometrial hyperplasia. This is probably a result of multiple follicular development (multicystic ovaries) with failure of antral follicle formation. Endometrial hyperplasia may cause excessive bleeding, anaemia, infertility and even cancer of the endometrium.

Ovulatory DUB: inadequate luteal phase. The luteal phase is usually over 10 days, with a serum progesterone peak on at least 1 day in excess of 20 nmol/l. Anything less is inadequate. The short luteal phase arises from inadequate follicular development, possibly due to a lower than normal secretion of follicle-stimulating hormone. This syndrome may be associated with irregular bleeding and infertility.

Ovulatory DUB: idiopathic bleeding. As described above, an important factor in the control of menstrual blood loss is vasoconstriction. It appears that there are a number of endometrial products which alter the degree of vasoconstriction and thus may affect the volume of menstrual blood lost. In the mid 1970s, a relationship between prostaglandin production and menorrhagia was suggested by work showing a relationship between total endometrial prostaglandin content and the degree of menstrual loss. It appears that there may be a shift in endometrial conversion of endoperoxide from the vasoconstrictor prostaglandins, ($PGF_{2\alpha}$) to the vasodilator prostaglandins, (PGE_2 or prostacyclin). However it is likely that it is not only prostaglandins which are of importance and work is now being performed on the role of endothelins in heavy menstrual loss. Endothelins are very potent vasoconstrictors which are produced within the endometrial vessels; their receptors are also present although it is not as yet clear as to whether either of these two factors differ in those with heavy menstrual loss. This is a rapidly changing area of knowledge and it is likely that other elements will come to light which will be significant.

It is still uncertain as to why there is a difference in production of local factors in those with heavy menstrual loss compared with those with normal loss. Interest has centred on the role of steroid hormones, but it has been impossible to demonstrate either a difference in the circulating levels of oestradiol and progesterone or in the receptor concentration within the endometrium, (Critchley et al 1994). It is possible that there is a genetic difference altering the production of local hormones and growth factors, or that there is a multifactorial aetiology.

Menorrhagia in the presence of pathology

Menorrhagia is thought to be associated with uterine fibroids, adenomyosis, pelvic infection, endometrial polyps and the presence of a foreign body such as an intrauterine contraceptive device (IUCD). Also the rare conditions of myometrial hypertrophy and vascular abnormality may be associated with severe, even life-threatening, menorrhagia. However, objective evidence of menorrhagia in most of these situations is remarkably limited. In women with menstrual blood loss greater than 200 ml, over half will have fibroids, although only 40% of those with adenomyosis actually have menstrual blood loss in excess of 80 ml per menses. Whether chronic pelvic inflammatory disease or endometrial polyps are associated with above average loss is unclear.

There is evidence for a role for prostaglandins in the menorrhagia associated with adenomyosis, uterine leiomyomata and the presence of an IUCD (Fraser et al 1986). Endometrial production of vasodilator prostaglandins are raised in the presence of adenomyosis, and prostaglandin production is also increased in the presence of an IUCD.

However, the nonsteroidal anti-inflammatory agents are less effective in menorrhagia associated with IUCD presence than in DUB, making it likely that other factors are also important.

Medical problems

Menorrhagia is associated with various endocrine disorders such as thyrotoxicosis and Cushing's disease, although the mechanism is unknown.

DYSMENORRHOEA

Dysmenorrhoea comes from Greek and means 'difficult monthly flow' but is now taken to mean painful menstruation. It is a symptom complex, with cramping lower abdominal pain radiating to the back and legs, often accompanied by gastrointestinal and neurological symptoms as well as general malaise. As with menorrhagia, it may be associated with pathology or may be idiopathic in origin.

Idiopathic (primary dysmenorrhoea)

There are many different theories as to why women suffer from dysmenorrhoea. The following factors may be of importance.

Uterine hyperactivity

The significance of uterine hyperactivity in women with dysmenorrhoea was first proposed in 1932. Since this time there has been much research which suggests that those with dysmenorrhoea have increased uterine activity during menstruation, (Filler & Hall 1970, Novak & Reynolds 1932). Patients often describe the pain as 'labour-like' and an increase in uterine contractility can be demonstrated by measuring the intrauterine pressure in those with dysmenorrhoea compared with women without (Lumsden & Baird 1985). The increased uterine contractility also appears to be related to uterine blood flow and the presence of pain, (Åkerlund et al 1976).

Prostaglandins

There is good evidence that prostaglandins are involved in the aetiology of primary dysmenorrhoea. Both prostaglandin $F_{2\alpha}$, and E_2 are found in higher concentrations in the menstrual fluid of those with dysmenorrhoea. Prostaglandin $F_{2\alpha}$ is a potent oxytocic and vasoconstrictor. When administered into the uterus it will give rise to dysmenorrhoea-like pain and occasionally menstrual bleeding. Menstrual fluid prostaglandin $F_{2\alpha}$ concentrations also correlate with uterine work during the menses in those with dysmenorrhoea (Lumsden et al 1983). These properties of prostaglandin $F_{2\alpha}$ could thus lead to 'angina' of the myometrium (Fig. 28.6). The role of prostaglandin E_2 is less clear, although its administration may increase the sensitivity of nerve endings.

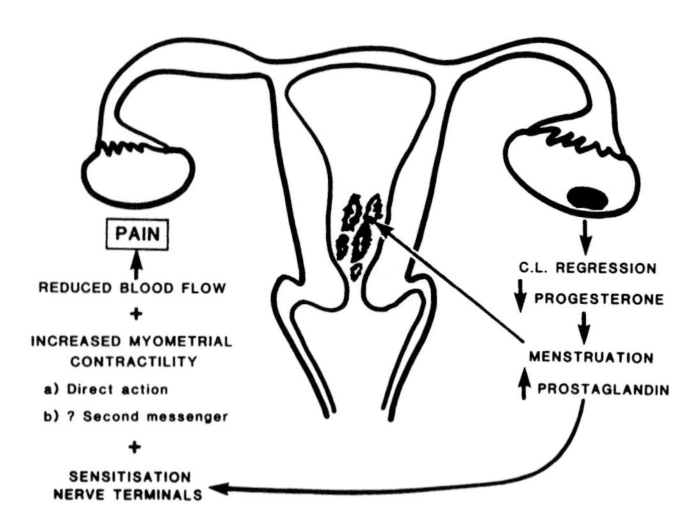

Fig. 28.6 A possible mechanism whereby prostaglandins could produce dysmenorrhea.

The reason for the abnormal prostaglandin levels is unknown. Primary dysmenorrhoea occurs almost exclusively in ovulatory cycles and steroid hormones affect both uterine prostaglandin concentration and myometrial contractility. However, no consistent abnormality of the hormone levels has been demonstrated in those with dysmenorrhoea.

Treatment with prostaglandin synthetase inhibitors reduces uterine $PGF_{2\alpha}$ production, uterine activity and dysmenorrhoea.

Leukotrienes

Leukotrienes are also produced by the endometrium; they cause increased myometrial contractility and their receptor sites are present in myometrium, although evidence for a role in dysmenorrhoea is still preliminary (Rees et al 1987).

Vasopressin

There are also other stimulants of the nonpregnant uterus such as vasopressin, a vasoconstrictor which also stimulates uterine contractility. On the first day of menstruation, circulating vasopressin levels are higher in those with dysmenorrhea than those without (Åkerlund et al 1979). Infusion of hypertonic saline results in increased uterine contactility and pain in women with dysmenorrhoea as a result of stimulation of endogenous vasopressin release, as well as a reduction in concentrations of $PGF_{2\alpha}$ metabolites.

Preliminary studies also indicate that vasopressin analogues may have a place in treating dysmenorrhoea.

Other factors

The endothelins stimulate myometrial contractions and are also potent vasoconstrictors but their role in dysmenorrhoea has yet to be evaluated (Cameron & Davenport 1992). Platelet-activating factor (PAF) is present in greater concentration in women with dysmenorrhoea (Migram et al 1991). This is somewhat surprising as PAF inhibits $PGF_{2\alpha}$ production, although it does stimulate overall phospholipid metabolism and other factors which have not been measured may be elevated.

Another factor of potential importance is the destruction of nerve endings in the myometrium and cervix by pregnancy. This may explain the observation that primary dysmenorrhoea is relieved by the birth of a baby. The literature suggests that psychological and physical causes for dysmenorrhoea are mutually exclusive. The evidence for physical factors is strong, treatment is very effective and it is unlikely that psychological problems would be removed simply by tablet-taking. However, a recurring, debilitating pain may well cause depression and anxiety in women of any age.

Secondary dysmenorrhoea

As with menorrhagia, this may be associated with uterine and pelvic pathology such as fibroids, the presence of an IUCD, pelvic inflammatory disease, adenomyosis, endometriosis or cervical stenosis. The cause of the pain is not always clear. Abnormal uterine contractility has been observed in those with fibroids, and prostaglandins may be involved when dysmenorrhoea is associated with an IUCD, pelvic inflammatory disease, adenomyosis and possibly endometriosis. However, the use of prostaglandin synthetase inhibitors is less effective in the presence of pathology, making it likely that there are also other factors.

THE EPIDEMIOLOGY OF MENSTRUAL ABNORMALITY

The distribution of blood loss for a normal population shows a positively skewed distribution, as mentioned above (Cole et al 1971). Age per se does not influence the menstrual blood loss until the sixth decade. This may be due to an increased incidence of pathology (e.g. fibroids or perimenopausal endocrine abnormalities). A hereditary influence has been demonstrated, following twin studies, and parity is also thought to be an important factor: parous women have a greater menstrual blood loss than nulliparous women. Uterine pathology, particularly fibroids, is a well documented cause for menorrhagia, although endometrial pathology is rather uncommon in menorrhagic women; it

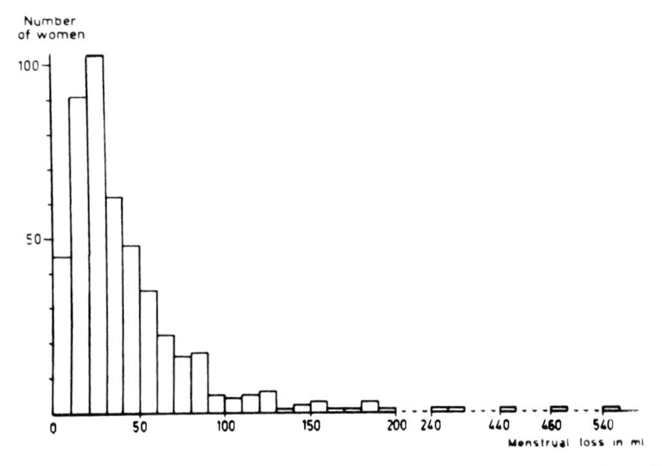

Fig. 28.7 The distribution of menstrual blood loss for a population of women who did not consider they had any menstrual abnormality. (From Hallberg et al with permission.)

is found as a reasonable cause for menorrhagia in only about 6%.

The variation between menses for an individual (intramenses) is between 20 and 40% (Fig. 28.7). The reason for this variation is unknown. About 90% of blood is lost during the first 3 days of the menses in both normal and menorrhagic women. These studies are based on objective measurement of menstrual blood loss, which is rarely done except for research purposes. The measurement of menstrual blood loss is very straightforward and perfectly safe for the patient. The most commonly used method is the alkaline haematin technique in which used menstrual pads are soaked in sodium hydroxide and haemoglobin is converted to alkaline haematin, causing a characteristic change in the colour of the solution. Blood loss is calculated after spectrophotometry (Hallberg & Nilsson 1964).

There is a poor correlation between subjective and objective assessment of loss (Chimbira et al 1980), which means that most gynaecologists treat patients without carrying out any objective tests, apart from measuring haemoglobin. This is important, as medical treatment for menorrhagia is unlikely to be effective in those with normal loss and surgical treatment carries a risk. Only about 50% of women presenting with menorrhagia actually have a loss outside the normal range (> 80 ml), which indicates that the changes which occur in the cycle are often perceived erroneously as abnormal.

The results of epidemiological studies performed over the last 50 years give a variable incidence for dysmenorrhoea. This is due to the fact that pain is a subjective symptom and cannot be assessed accurately by an outsider. Different women will react to the same pain in different ways, and how each women perceives the pain will vary with altered circumstances. Also, the definition and diagnosis allow different interpretations by different workers. Severe dysmenorrhoea which causes disruption of daily routine with time off work or study occurs in 3–10% of 19-year-olds (Andersch & Milsom 1982), while mild discomfort occurs in a majority of women. The relative risk of dysmenorrhoea in those who have smoked for 10–20 years is up to six times the risk in nonsmokers (Parazzini et al 1994). Its incidence is inversely correlated with age and parous women are less likely to report the condition. There is no correlation between the incidence of emotional stress factors and dysmenorrhoea.

PRESENTATION

Menstrual problems are a common cause for presentation to both the general practitioner and the gynaecological outpatient clinic. The bleeding pattern may be cyclical or irregular and is often accompanied by dysmenorrhoea. It is less common for dysmenorrhoea to be the major complaint. Patients complain of 'clots' and 'flooding' and the severity is often assessed only by asking the degree of disability experienced, e.g. the time lost from work. As stated above, the amount of protection used does not correlate with blood loss. Other gynaecological problems may also be present, such as intermenstrual bleeding, vaginal discharge or premenstrual syndrome.

Clinical examination seldom reveals significant observation. An enlarged uterus suggests uterine leiomyomata or a cervical polyp may cause intermenstrual bleeding. Anaemia may also be present since menorrhagia is the commonest cause of iron-deficiency anaemia in the western world. Menorrhagia may arise as a consequence of disorders of the haemopoietic system, as described above.

INVESTIGATION

Investigation of women with menstrual problems is useful only when this is performed to exclude sinister pathology or to aid in planning treatment. Concern has recently focused on the frequency with which dilatation and curettage is performed in the UK, often without a clear indication (Coulter et al 1993). In women in whom investigation is appropriate, hysteroscopy appears to be more sensitive than dilatation and curettage in the diagnosis of endometrial abnormality.

In all women presenting with menstrual problems a full history and clinical examination should be performed. If these suggest systemic disease, further investigation for this may be warranted. Abnormalities on pelvic examination should be investigated by ultrasound, with laparoscopy if required. Irregular menstrual bleeding, or menorrhagia at the extremes of reproductive life may be secondary to anovulatory cycles, and these conditions may be improved by cyclical gestogen therapy. Frequently there are no abnormalities on history or clinical examination, and a strategy for investigation of these women is outlined below. The reader is referred to Chapter 14 for the investigation of amenorrhoea.

Blood tests

Haemoglobin concentration should be determined in all women with menorrhagia, and iron supplementation given if required. Although thyroid disease is a cause of menstrual derangement in some women, screening TSH and T_4 measurements are not justified unless there are other features in the history suggestive of thyroid disease (Fraser et al 1986). Similarly, routine screening for bleeding diatheses is not appropriate.

Endometrial pathology

The main indication for the investigation of endometrial pathology is to exclude endometrial carcinoma. Until recently, dilatation and curettage has been the method of choice and is still widely used in many units.

Dilatation and curettage and other techniques

Dilatation and curettage (D&C) has been advocated to exclude the diagnosis of endometrial malignancy. The incidence of this diagnosis in women under the age of 40 is of the order of one in 10 000–100 000 and is probably not indicated in women below this age (Grimes 1982). Towards the menopause the incidence increases to around 1%.

Recently thin plastic cell samplers have been developed which provide a histological sample without the need for dilation and anaesthetic. Several makes are now available. If the initial analyses are substantiated by larger scale studies, these techniques are likely to supersede D&C as the main means of endometrial sampling.

The Vabra aspirator usually provides a greater amount of tissue for analysis, but may not be tolerated by some patients as an outpatient procedure.

Hysteroscopy

With the realization that hysteroscopy facilitated intrauterine surgical procedures such as endometrial ablation, hysteroscopy has now been accepted into UK gynaecological practice for diagnostic purposes. Given that dilatation and curettage rarely samples the entire uterine cavity (Stock & Kanbour 1975) it is not surprising that hysteroscopy and directed biopsy appear to be superior in identifying *benign* endometrial pathology (Gimpleson & Rappold 1988, Loffer 1989). More pertinently, in a significant minority of women with endometrial carcinoma, the diagnosis is missed when conventional curettage is used (Stovall et al 1989), and although large randomized studies are yet to be performed, it appears that hysteroscopy and directed biopsy is more sensitive in the diagnosis of this condition. Several authorities have suggested therefore that hysteroscopy and directed biopsy should replace dilatation and curettage for the investigation of endometrial pathology (Lewis 1990, 1993). Where appropriate equipment is available, hysteroscopy can be performed as an outpatient procedure in selected patients under local anaesthetic, using gas to dilate the uterine cavity.

Alternative methods of assessing the uterine cavity have attracted interest, including ultrasound, Doppler and endometrial aspirators. However none of these techniques has yet proved sufficiently sensitive in the detection of endometrial carcinoma to warrant their introduction into routine clinical practice.

Since the main indication for endometrial sampling is to exclude endometrial carcinoma, it is not required in women under the age of 40 with regular cycles (RCOG 1994). However older women with menstrual disturbance, young women with irregular bleeding, or young women who fail to respond to treatment should undergo some form of endometrial assessment.

Quantification of menstrual blood loss

The measurement of menstrual blood loss should be the cornerstone of the diagnosis of menorrhagia, since 50% of those complaining of menorrhagia have a blood loss within the normal range. However, this measurement is rarely performed except for research purposes.

Menstrual blood loss can be assessed either in a semi-quantitative manner relying on the patient's assessment of the bleeding, or by the use of pictorial aids (Higham et al 1990). Quantitative methods are available (see above) but are normally available on a research basis only.

Clearly, objective confirmation of normal menstrual blood loss does not mean that the patient complaining of menorrhagia should be dismissed. However it may be useful in reassurance and in choosing therapy. Those without objective menorrhagia are unlikely to respond to most medical treatments with a reduction in blood loss, and should be counselled, and then perhaps be offered surgery such as transcervical resection of the endometrium (TCRE) or hysterectomy if they find their menses problematic.

Laparoscopy

Women presenting with dysmenorrhoea who have no other complaints or abnormalities on examination, can be safely treated without further investigation. In those women in whom a therapeutic trial is unsuccessful, laparoscopy may be helpful in excluding pathology such as endometriosis.

Anovulatory menorrhagia

In the younger patient (< 40 years of age) assessment of the hypothalamic–pituitary–ovarian axis is indicated. The diagnosis of polycystic ovarian disease has increased over recent years with the finding of altered luteinizing hormone/follicle-stimulating hormone ratios in the follicular phase of the cycle and the identification of micro- and macrocystic disease by vaginal ultrasound.

Dysmenorrhoea

Those with normal pelvic examination require no further investigation initially. Laparoscopy is indicated for those with a provisional diagnosis of endometriosis or pelvic inflammatory disease. D&C and examination under anaesthetic are required only if uterine abnormality is suspected. The standard treatment for dysmenorrhoea (prostaglandin synthetase inhibitors and the oral contraceptive pill) is so effective that laparoscopy in treatment failures will often demonstrate previously unsuspected abnormalities such as mild endometriosis, even in teenage girls.

TREATMENT

Women require rapid, safe and effective treatment for their menstrual problems. There are three main categories of treatment: surgical, medical and the newer hysteroscopic techniques. In Scotland during 1987, 2300 women had a hysterectomy and 30 000 'bed-days' were occupied by women presenting primarily with heavy menses, giving some indication of the extent of the problem (data from the Common Services Agency, Scottish Home and Health Department).

Surgical treatment

Hysterectomy

Hysterectomy is certainly an effective treatment for menstrual problems. However, it is a major operation and is not without risk in terms of both mortality and morbidity. The incidence of hysterectomy is gradually increasing in the western world as a whole. The number performed in Scotland with menorrhagia as the primary indication appears to be static over the last 5 years, as shown in Figure 28.8. However, the incidence varies considerably from one country to another (Fig. 28.9), reflecting differences in the attitude of both patients and gynaecologists rather than a variation in pathology. Women in Scotland have a 20% chance of losing their uterus before the age of 60 years whereas in California this figure is 50% (Bunker & Brown 1974).

Hysterectomy may be performed by the abdominal or vaginal route. Abdominal hysterectomy involves a laparo-

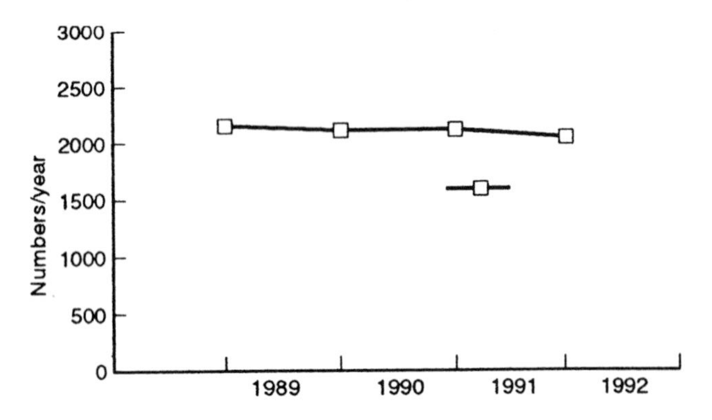

Fig. 28.8 The number of hysterectomies performed to treat menorrhagia in Scotland between the years 1989 and 1992.

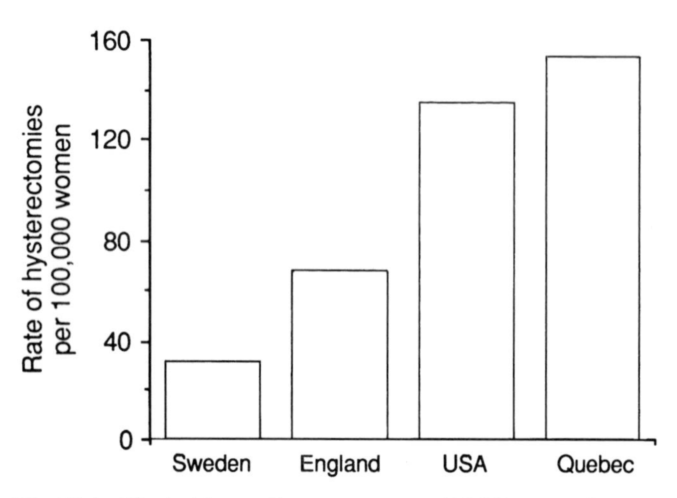

Fig. 28.9 The incidence of hysterectomy per 100 000 women for Sweden, England, the USA and Quebec. (From Domenighetti et al 1989, with permission.)

tomy incision which is transverse or longitudinal. A vaginal hysterectomy involves an incision through the vaginal wall. For many surgeons, vaginal hysterectomy is only performed on women with some degree of uterine descent and where the uterus is not excessively large. Abdominal hysterectomy allows better visualization of the pelvic cavity should there be pathology or where difficulty is anticipated. Nonrandomized studies indicate that the complication rate for abdominal hysterectomy is greater than that for vaginal hysterectomy and women having vaginal procedures are able to go home quicker than those having abdominal operations (Clinch 1994, Dicker et al 1982).

Recently it has become possible to convert an abdominal to a vaginal hysterectomy using endoscopic techniques. The laparoscope allows visualization of the pelvic cavity, and all or part of the hysterectomy may be performed using specially designed laparoscopic instruments. A laparoscopically assisted vaginal hysterectomy (LAVH) allows tissues accessible through the vagina to be ligated and the uterus to be removed by the vaginal route. This method facilitates the removal of ovaries and also aids the operation when there is no uterine descent. It allows for dissection of adhesions and the treatment of pelvic pathology, such as endometriosis, prior to the hysterectomy. Published complication rates are low at 12% (Boike et al 1993). Ureteric injury has been recorded although it is uncertain as to whether the incidence is higher than when the operation is performed in the traditional way. However, there is sometimes difficulty in removing an enlarged uterus from the body. These techniques are still being evaluated, and randomized studies are underway. The increased cost of the operation will need to be balanced against the shortened length of hospital stay.

Endometrial ablation techniques

Attempts at endometrial destruction in cases of abnormal menstruation, with the aim of producing a therapeutic Asherman's syndrome, have been made by a variety of techniques. Early trials involved the intrauterine application of cytotoxic chemicals, intracavity radium, steam and cryosurgery. However these were either ineffective or had unacceptable side-effects. They were also carried out blindly and since the endometrium has remarkable powers of regeneration, any missed areas resulted in failure.

More recently hysteroscopic techniques have been developed. These allow visualization of the uterine cavity, allowing the endometrium to be ablated under direct vision. Since regeneration of the endometrium occurs from the basal layer it is essential to destroy all the endometrium, and as the endometrial–myometrial border is irregular, the superficial layer of myometrium must also be included (Fig. 28.10). There are a number of methods or achieving this, including vaporization of the tissue using laser, removal of the tissue using a cutting loop or coagulation. Resection is illustrated in Figure 28.11.

Laser ablation. Laser beams may be produced from a variety of sources, although currently neodymium: yttrium–aluminium–garnet, (Nd:YAG) is optimal for intrauterine surgery since it can be delivered along a flexible fibre through a liquid medium and the depth of tissue penetration can be controlled. The beam produces warming, coagulation, evaporation and carbonization. Tissue destruction typically occurs to a depth of 4–5 mm. Heat

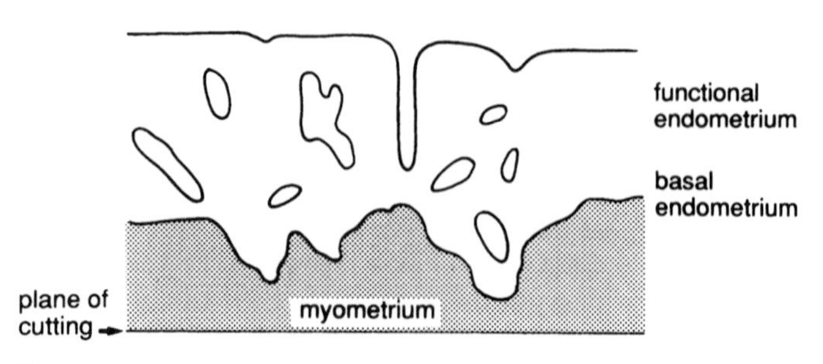

Fig. 28.10 A diagram of the uterine wall.

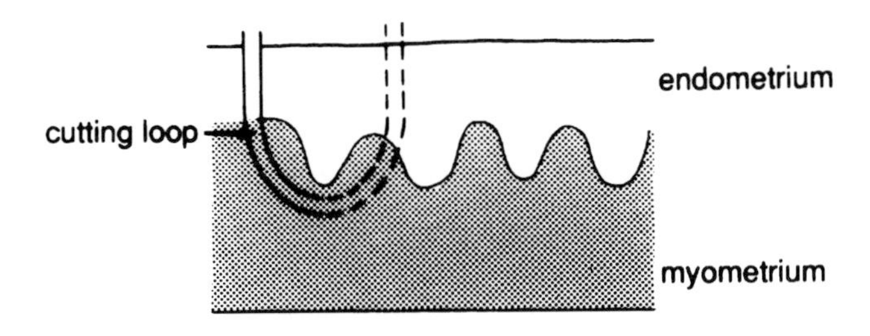

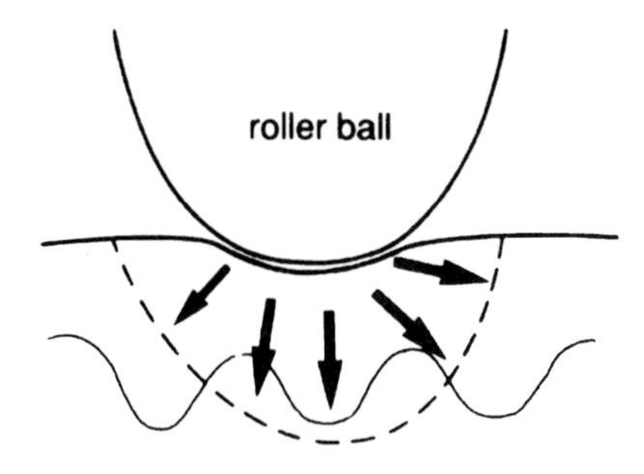

Fig. 28.11 **a** The loop of the resectoscope must cut beneath the endometrial–myometrial junction and include the superficial layer of myometrium. **b** The rollerball coagulates to a depth of approximately 4 mm.

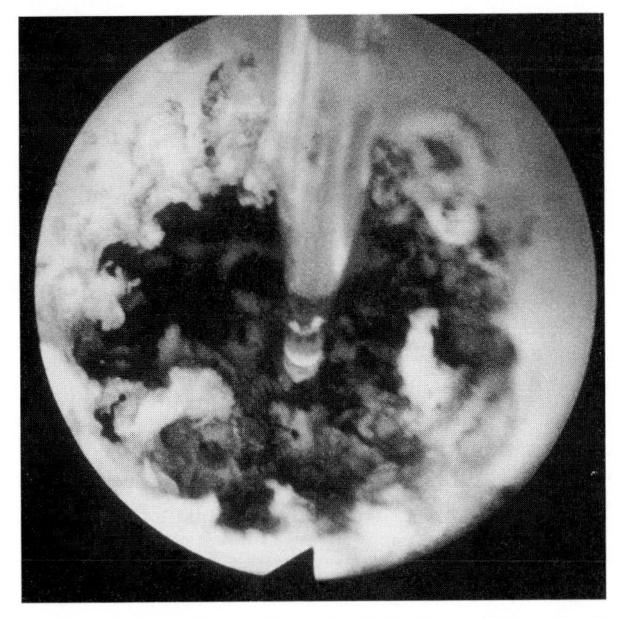

Fig. 28.12 A view of the uterine cavity during laser ablation. (By kind permission of Dr J. Davis.)

transmission through the myometrium is minimized by the continuous flow of cold irrigation fluid (Fig. 28.12).

Endometrial resection. This is one of the most commonly used methods for carrying out endometrial ablation. The technique of performing transcervical resection of the endometrium is essentially similar to that of transurethral prostatectomy in men and is performed through a continuous flow resectoscope. The endometrium is systematically excised throughout the uterine cavity (Fig. 28.13). It is important to destroy all the endometrium, otherwise regeneration will occur and the operation will fail.

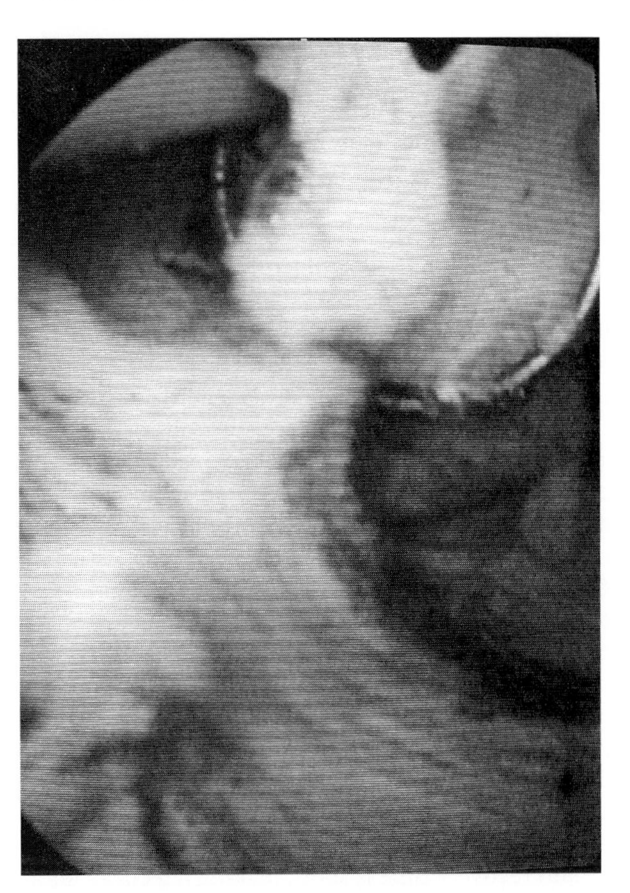

Fig. 28.13 A hysteroscopic view of the uterine cavity during an endometrial resection. Note the 'criss-cross' fibres of myometrium, indicating that the correct depth has been reached. (By kind permission of Dr R. Hawthorn.)

Other methods. One of the earliest methods of destroying the endometrium was the use of rollerball coagulation (Fig. 28.11b). Both microwave and ultrasound methods have been tried although they have not received general acceptance.

Success rates. There is little variation in success rates between the different methods. Overall approximately 30% of women will be amenorrhoiec and a further 45–50% will have significantly decreased loss giving a satisfaction rate of approximately 75% (Garry et al 1991, Magos et al 1991, Scottish Hysteroscopy Audit Group 1994). Careful counselling is essential in that if a woman is keen to have amenorrhoea then this may not be the treatment of choice for her. Success rates vary between individual surgeons but do not seem to be related to the level of experience. Endometrial ablation can also be useful in treating dysmenorrhoea although in some instances this problem will be worsened as will be described below.

Some women experience relief from symptoms of premenstrual tension.

Complications. The most significant complications are that of uterine perforation and fluid absorption. Uterine perforation occurs in less than 1%, and is not usually associated with major problems unless the electrode is activated within the abdominal cavity when bowel or blood vessels may be damaged. Some studies suggest that a majority of perforations occur when surgeons are still on their learning curve and lessen with increased expertise. Fluid absorption results in hyponatraemia, neurological symptoms, haemolysis and death. However, the incidence has decreased since surgeons became aware of this risk and stop the operation if absorption becomes excessive and symptomatic absorption is unusual. Other complications are infection, and prophylactic antibiotics are given routinely by most surgeons.

Comparison of endometrial resection with hysterectomy. Endometrial resection was developed as an alternative to hysterectomy. However, it appears that the number of hysterectomies being performed is continuing to rise, suggesting it is not serving this purpose. There have been a number of randomized comparisons between endometrial ablation and hysterectomy which show that satisfaction with both procedures is high (Pinion et al 1994). Also, the operation can be performed on a day-case basis and recovery time is short, making it a cheap alternative to hysterectomy. However, it does appear that 20% of patients will require further surgical treatment, and there is still uncertainty as to whether the number of failures will increase with time.

Guidelines. The operation is most likely to be successful in women over 40 who have a normal-sized uterus and no intrauterine pathology. Its use in dysmenorrhoea is equivocable since it appears to make women worse in approximately 12% of cases, which may be due to the formation of haematometra. However, approximately 40% will improve so the presence of dysmenorrhoea is not an absolute contraindication. The menstrual cycle length will not be changed by the procedure and in women with very irregular bleeding, hysterectomy may be an appropriate alternative (Lewis 1994).

Medical treatment

Drugs are now commonly prescribed by general practitioners for the treatment of menorrhagia and dysmenorrhoea. About 1 200 000 prescriptions for drugs to treat menstrual problems are written each year. The commonly prescribed drugs for menorrhagia are shown in Table 28.1. The acceptability of each treatment depends on the balance between effectiveness and side-effects. Menorrhagia is very rarely life-threatening and the aim of treatment is to improve the quality of life. Side-effects may therefore make an effective drug unacceptable.

Table 28.1 Drugs commonly used in the treatment of menorrhagia as a percentage of the total number of prescriptions written for menorrhagia in the UK during 1988

Drug	Proportion of prescriptions
Non-steroidal anti-inflammatory agents	13.8%
Gestogens, e.g. norethisterone	31.6%
Antigonadotrophins, e.g. danazol	9.8%
Antifibrinolytics, e.g. tranexamic acid	Unknown
Ethamsylate	10.8%
Anti-anaemics	13.0%
Other	21%

Total number of patients with primary indication of menorrhagia = 646 000.

Prostaglandin synthetase inhibitors

The role of prostaglandins in abnormal menstruation has already been discussed. Prostaglandin synthetase inhibitors, of which the different types are shown in Table 28.2 are thus a logical treatment (Anderson 1981). The fenamates not only inhibit the synthesis of prostaglandins but also interfere with the binding of prostaglandin E_2 to its receptor. The mean decrease in blood loss varies between 20 and 44.5%, and there is a suggestion that there is a correlation between the pretreatment menstrual blood loss and the volume reduction in menstrual blood loss during therapy. A decrease in the number of days of bleeding has also been reported.

The percentage decrease in menstrual blood loss in 13 women taking mefenamic acid is shown in Figure 28.14 and illustrates the variable results obtained with this treatment. IUCD-associated menorrhagia also responds to prostaglandin synthetase inhibitors although there is little evidence that they are as effective in the presence of pathology such as fibroids. About 80% of women with primary dysmenorrhoea can be successfully treated with this group of drugs although, once again, they are less effective in the presence of pathology.

Side-effects. Gastrointestinal symptoms occur in up to 50% of those taking these drugs although they are often

Table 28.2 The nonsteroidal anti-inflammatory agents

Parent compound	Example
Salicylate	Aspirin Aloxiprin
Indole	Indomethacin
*Propionic acid	Ketoprofen Ibuprofen
*Fenamates	Mefenamic acid
Pyrazone	Phenylbutazone
Indene	Sulindac
Alkanone	Nabumetone
Benzotriazine	Azapropazone
Phenylacetic acid	Diclofenac sodium

*Most commonly used for menstrual problems.

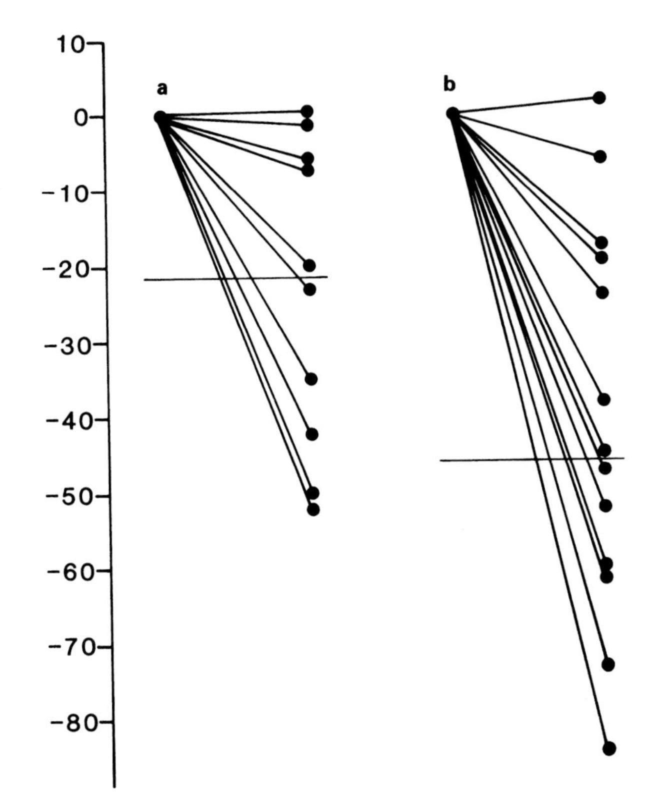

Fig. 28.14 Percentage change in menstrual blood loss (mean of two cycles) of women receiving: **a** norethisterone (5 mg b.d., days 19–25), and **b** mefenamic acid (250 mg t.d.s., days 1–5).

very mild and may be decreased by taking the drug with food. Patient response may be idiosyncratic, making the prescription of different members of the group worthwhile if symptoms occur. Central nervous system symptoms such as dizziness and headache occur in around 20%. Although significant changes in liver function have been reported, the indices have remained within the normal range. Potential serious side-effects such as blood dyscrasias and nephropathy have not been reported in any study, possibly because of the intermittent nature of drug administration.

Hormonal treatment

Progestogens

Hormonal treatments for menorrhagia have been available for at least 25 years. The most widely prescribed are the synthetic progestogens although there have been few objective studies to validate their use. There is histological evidence that in women with metropathia haemorrhagica, progestogen administration will cause secretory change in the endometrium accompanied by subjective decrease in blood loss; however in those with ovulatory DUB the effect is unpredictable and the overall median decreased menstrual blood loss is less than 25%.

Progestogens may be given by the following routes.

Oral route. The oral route is a long established method and accounts for the majority of prescriptions written for menstrual problems. The progestogen is given for 10–14 days during the luteal phase of the cycle. Although there is little decrease in blood loss, the duration of bleeding is shorter and the bleeding pattern becomes more regular. This may account for the apparent subjective success of the treatment. However, if the progestogen is administered for 21 out of 28 days, as with the oral contraceptive pill, this leads to inhibition of ovulation and a significant decrease in blood loss (Fraser et al 1986). Problems with minor side-effects are discussed below.

Depot preparation. Depots of norethisterone and medroxyprogesterone acetate have been used for contraceptive purposes for a long time. If used for long enough they induce amenorrhoea, but unfortunately during the early months bleeding tends to be unpredictable and can be heavy. This results in many women discontinuing treatment. Also, because the circulating levels of hormones are high, systemic side-effects are a problem (Faundes et al 1978).

Intrauterine device. An intrauterine device (IUD), which releases levonorgestrel, has been used recently both for contraception and also for the treatment of menstrual problems. It leads to a profound reduction in menstrual blood loss with systemic absorption of hormone in only a small proportion of cases (Andersson & Rybo 1990). The progestogen is secreted continuously from the coil and induces endometrial atrophy, the coil remaining active for about 5 years. As with all progestogen-only contraceptives, breakthrough bleeding is a problem and accounts for a large proportion of those who discontinue treatment. This coil has the advantage of also being an excellent contraceptive, and is not associated with an increase in pelvic inflammatory disease and ectopic pregnancies as are other coils (Cheng Chi 1991).

Side-effects. The side-effects associated with the administration of progestogens are generally minor, such as nausea, headache, bloating, weight gain and skin rashes. However if administered in the long-term the progestogens with a structure based on that of testosterone (e.g. norethisterone) may produce alterations in blood lipid profiles, with an increase in low density lipoprotein and a decrease in high density lipoprotein, which has the potential to increase cardiovascular disease risk. However, overall the progestogens are very safe and oral progestogens should be considered for all those with an irregular menstrual cycle. The levonorgestrel IUD is currently being developed and is not available for general prescription but is likely to become so in the near future.

Combined oestrogen/progesterone formulations

The combined oral contraceptive pill gives a significant decrease in menstrual blood loss, although use is often accompanied by oestrogen-related side-effects. Although the use of the low dose oestrogen pill in the management of menorrhagia has been affected by adverse publicity associated with their use in older women, it is now felt to be quite safe in women up to and over the age of 40 who are not obese, do not smoke and are not hypertensive. It has the added advantage of providing a regular menstrual cycle and also being effective in the treatment of dysmenorrhoea (Ekstrom et al 1989). The limiting factor is that many of the women will have been sterilized and are therefore reluctant to continue with something they see as a contraceptive agent. Also, the oral contraceptive pill may be associated with side-effects as is detailed elsewhere in this book.

Antifibrinolytic drugs

Fibrinolytic inhibitors act by inhibiting plasminogen activator, reducing the accelerated fibrinolytic activity found in menorrhagic women. Tranexamic acid is of value in the treatment of excessive menstrual bleeding, giving around a 50% decrease in those with DUB- as well as IUCD-associated menorrhagia (Milsom et al 1991). They are very widely used in Scandinavia although they have achieved less acceptance in the UK.

Side-effects. The commonest side-effects reported include nausea, dizziness, tinnitus, rash and abdominal cramps. Oral administration does give rise to low systemic levels of tranexamic acid, and cases of serious thromboembolic disorders following administration have been reported, although the underlying incidence of these disorders in women of reproductive age must always be borne in mind.

Danazol

Danazol is the isoxazole derivative of 17α-ethinyl testosterone. Its mechanism of action is not clear, but it is thought to act both directly and indirectly. The direct mechanisms are the inhibition of endometrial proliferation causing endometrial atrophy, and the displacement of endometrial oestrogen receptors. It also has an indirect action, reducing pituitary gonadotrophin secretion and inhibiting the enzymes involved in ovarian steroidogenesis.

It is an effective treatment for menorrhagia even at low doses although it must be given continuously, as it is ineffective when administered cyclically. At moderate or high doses (400 mg daily), danazol induces amenorrhoea in a majority of women, but at low doses (200 mg daily), although it reduces loss, it has no effect on cycle length. Dosage of 100 mg daily has no effect on the duration of bleeding and the mean cycle length is significantly shorter (Dockeray et al 1989).

Side-effects. The side-effects of danazol have been extensively documented and include weight gain, acne, hirsutism, muscle cramps, headaches and in severe cases, breast atrophy.

Ethamsylate

Ethamsylate is thought to act by inhibiting the increase in capillary fragility measurable in premenopausal women by reducing the rate of breakdown in mucopolysaccharide ground substance in the capillary wall. Its effectiveness has not been well documented by objective study but a significant decrease in menstrual loss in women with DUB and IUCD-associated menorrhagia is reported. Side-effects appear to be minor.

Gonadotrophin-releasing hormone (GnRH) agonists

GnRH agonists are derived from the GnRH decapeptide with a 140-fold more potent action than endogenous GnRH. They induce downregulation of the pituitary with an initial agonist phase followed by hypo-oestrogenism which results in amenorrhoea in 90% of cases. However, the menstrual problems are likely to recur on stopping treatment, although there is often a decrease in the duration of bleeding for some months (Shaw & Fraser 1984).

Side-effects due to hypo-oestrogenism occur, which could lead to bone mineral loss in the long term. Either the agonists must be used for short periods only or they must be used in combination with bone-sparing agents, e.g. hormone replacement therapy. The use of these drugs in the treatment of DUB is confined largely to women with severe problems who are unsuitable for surgery.

Other treatments for dysmenorrhoea

In young women dysmenorrhoea is frequently the only menstrual abnormality. Prostaglandin synthetase inhibitors and the oral contraceptive pill are very effective, but in some women, even in the absence of disease, these measures are insufficient. Calcium channel blockers (e.g. nifedipine) have been used in Scandinavia and are effective, although their use is limited by cardiovascular side-effects.

In the past, presacral neurectomy was performed but this involved major abdominal surgery and was effective in only about 50% of cases. Recently neurectomy has been performed using intra-abdominal lasers. The long-term effect of this treatment has not been reported and it is only available in a few centres in the UK.

In older women where childbearing is completed, hysterectomy is often the solution since dysmenorrhoea in this group is frequently associated with other menstrual problems.

RESULTS

The results of the treatment of menstrual problems are

difficult to determine. Hysterectomy is undoubtedly effective in curing menstrual problems but its effect on the quality of life of the woman is largely unknown. This is a difficult parameter to measure but the information is vital when considering patient acceptability.

Drug treatments are very effective in some women, although the response tends to be variable. In the main they are safe and reported serious side-effects are unusual. However acceptability must be questioned since it has been demonstrated that side-effects may make a very effective drug (in terms of reduction in menstrual blood loss) unacceptable (Dockeray et al 1989). Many women also find the prospect of long-term drug therapy unappealing. Endometrial destruction by laser or electrocautery is an attractive alternative to both long-term drug therapy and hysterectomy for the common gynaecological complaint of abnormal menstruation. It is associated with a shorter hospital stay and a faster recovery. Clinical improvement occurs in a majority of women, although its long-term efficacy is still uncertain.

CONCLUSIONS

Menstrual dysfunction remains one of the commonest reasons for women to seek medical advice, yet the process of menstruation is poorly understood. Strategies to improve the investigation and management of this problem are likely to arise from two directions. Firstly, a thorough investigation of the medicosociological factors is required. Secondly, the role of vasoactive substances in the endometrium needs to be further investigated, as well as determination of the factors which control endometrial proliferation. At present, the diagnosis of menorrhagia is inadequate and medical treatment is disappointing. Gynaecologists need to address these problems before significant improvements in management will arise.

KEY POINTS

1. Menorrhagia is the commonest cause of iron deficiency anaemia in western women.
2. The menstrual cycle consists of a proliferative and a secretory phase.
3. Menstruation is initiated by a withdrawal of progesterone and oestrogen support to the endometrium.
4. Menstrual loss is dependent upon the degree of platelet plug formation, vasoconstriction and endometrial repair. Abnormality in these mechanisms can result in menstrual dysfunction. Paracrine factors are also thought to play a role in control of menstruation.
5. The mean menstrual blood loss is 37–43 ml per menses. Loss in excess of 80 ml per menses is considered to be menorrhagia.
6. Abnormal menstrual loss may arise from pelvic pathology, clotting disorders, medical disorders or dysfunctional uterine bleeding.
7. Dysfunctional uterine bleeding is defined as heavy or irregular bleeding in the absence of pelvic pathology, pregnancy or clotting disorder.
8. Anovulatory cycles may be associated with cystic glandular hyperplasia. This can occur in both older women and prepubertal girls and may result in excessive menstrual loss.
9. Primary dysmenorrhoea occurs almost exclusively in ovulatory cycles and prostaglandin secretion is strongly implicated in its aetiology.
10. Subjective and objective assessments of menstrual loss are poorly correlated. Medical treatment of menorrhagia is less effective if the blood loss is, in fact, within normal limits.
11. Hysteroscopy may be more sensitive than endometrial curettage in the diagnosis of endometrial abnormality.
12. Hysterectomy is the most effective remedy for menstrual dysfunction but is associated with postoperative morbidity and mortality.
13. Laparoscopically assisted vaginal hysterectomy allows conversion of an abdominal to a vaginal hysterectomy, the latter being associated with lower postoperative morbidity. The gynaecologist requires appropriate training in order to perform such procedures.
14. Endometrial ablation is a useful alternative to medical treatment or hysterectomy in cases of dysfunctional uterine bleeding.
15. Medical treatment of menorrhagia may result in symptomatic relief but does not result in long term cure.

REFERENCES

Adalantado J M, Rees M C P, Bernal A L, Turnbull A C 1988 Increased intrauterine prostaglandin E receptors in menorrhagic women. British Journal of Obstetrics and Gynaecology 95: 162

Åkerlund M, Anderssen K E 1976 Vasopressin response and Turbutaline inhibition of the uterus. Obstetrics and Gynecology 48: 528–536

Åkerlund M, Stromberg P, Forsling M L 1979 Primary dysmenorrhoea and vasopressin. British Journal of Obstetrics and Gynaecology 86: 484–487

Alecozay A A, Harper M J K, Schenken R S, Hanahan D J 1991 Paracrine interactions between platelet-activating factor and prostaglandins in hormonally-treated human luteal phase endometrium in vitro. Journal of Reproduction and Fertility 91: 301–312

Andersch B, Milsom I 1982 An epidemiologic study of young women with dysmenorrhoea. American Journal of Obstetrics and Gynecology 144: 655–660

Anderson A 1981 The role of prostaglandin synthetase inhibitors in gynaecology. Practitioner 225: 1460–1470

Andersson K, Rybo G 1990 Levonorgestrel-releasing intrauterine device in the treatment of menorrhagia. British Journal of Obstetrics and Gynaecology 97: 690–694
Bjork J, Smedegard G 1983 Acute microvascular effects of PAF-acether, as studied by intravital microscopy. European Journal of Pharmacology 96: 87
Boike G M, Elfstrand E P, DelPriore G, Schumock D, Steele Holley H, Lurain J R 1993 Laparoscopically assisted vaginal hysterectomy in a university hospital: report of 82 cases and comparison with abdominal and vaginal hysterectomy. American Journal of Obstetrics and Gynecology 168: 1690–1701
Bonnar J, Sheppard B L, Dockeray C J 1983 The haemostatic system and dysfunctional uterine bleeding. Research and Clinical Forums 5: 27–36
Bunker J P, Brown B W 1974 The physician-patient as an informed consumer of surgical services. New England Journal of Medicine 290: 1051–1055
Cameron I T, Davenport A P 1992 Endothelins in reproduction. Reproductive Medicine Review 1: 99–113
Cameron I T, Irvine G, Norman J E. Menstruation. In: Hillier et al (eds) Scientific essentials of reproductive medicine. W B Saunders, Philadelphia. In press
Cameron I T, Leask R, Kelly R W, Baird D T 1987 Endometrial prostaglandins in women with abnormal menstrual bleeding. Prostaglandins, Leukotrienes and Medicine 29: 249–257
Cameron I T C, Haining R, Lumsden M A, Reid-Thomas V, Smith S K 1990 The effects of mefanamic acid and norethisterone on measured menstrual blood loss. Obstetrics and Gynecology 76: 85–88
Casslen B, Astedt B 1983 Reduced plasminogen activator content of the endometrium in oral contraceptive users. Contraception 28: 181–188
Casslen B, Andersson A, Nilsson I M, Astedt B 1986 Hormonal regulation of the release of plasminogen activators and of a specific activator inhibitor from endometrial tissue in culture (42360). Proceedings of the Society for Experimental Biology and Medicine 182: 419–424
Charnock-Jones D S, Sharkey A M, Rajput-Williams J et al 1993 Identification and localization of alternately spliced mRNAs for vascular endothelial growth factor in human uterus and estrogen regulation in endometrial carcinoma cell lines. Biology of Reproduction 48: 1120–1128
Cheng Chi I 1991 An evaluation of the levonorgestrel-releasing IUD: its advantages and disadvantages when compared to the copper-releasing IUDs. Contraception 44: 573–587
Chimbira T H, Anderson A B M, Turnbull A C 1980 Relation between measured menstrual blood loss and patients' subjective assessment of loss, duration of bleeding, number of sanitary towels used, uterine weight and endometrial surface area. British Journal of Obstetrics and Gynaecology 87: 603–609
Christiaens G C M L, Sixma J J, Haspels A A 1980 Morphology of haemostasis in menstrual endometrium. British Journal of Obstetrics and Gynaecology 87: 425–439
Christiaens G C, Sixma J J, Haspels A A 1982 Haemostasis in menstrual endometrium: a review. Obstetrical and Gynecological Survey 37: 281–303
Clinch J 1994 Length of hospital stay after vaginal hysterectomy. British Journal of Obstetrics and Gynaecology 101: 253–254
Cohen B J B, Gibor Y 1980 Anaemia and menstrual blood loss. Obstetrical and Gynecological Survey 35: 597–618
Cole S K, Billewicz W Z, Thomson A M 1971 Sources of variation in menstrual blood loss. Journal of Obstetrics and Gynaecology of the British Commonwealth 78: 933–939
Coulter A, Klassen A, MacKenzie I Z, McPherson K 1993 Diagnostic dilatation and curettage: is it used appropriately? British Medical Journal 306: 236–239
Critchley H, Abberton K M, Taylor N H, Healy D L, Rogers A W 1994 Endometrial sex steroid receptor expression in women with menorrhagia. British Journal of Obstetrics and Gynaecology 101: 428–434
Dicker R C, Greenspan J R, Strauss L T et al 1982 Complications of abdominal and vaginal hysterectomy among women of reproductive age in the United States. American Journal of Obstetrics and Gynecology 144: 841–848
Dockeray C J, Sheppard B L, Bonnar J 1989 Comparison between mefenamic acid and danazol in the treatment of established menorrhagia. British Journal of Obstetrics and Gynaecology 96: 840–844
Ekstrom P, Juchnicka E, Laudanski T, Åkerlund M 1989 Effect of an oral contraceptive in primary dysmenorrhoea – changes in uterine activity and reactivity to agonists. Contraception 40: 39–47
Faundes A, Sivin A, Sivin J 1978 Long acting contraceptive implants. An analysis of menstrual bleeding patterns. Contraception 18: 335–365
Filler W W, Hall W C 1970 Dysmenorrhoea and its therapy: A uterine contractility study. American Journal of Obstetrics and Gynecology 106: 104–109
Fraser I 1990 Treatment of ovulatory and anovulatory dysfunctional uterine bleeding with oral progestogens. Australian and New Zealand Journal of Obstetrics and Gynaecology 30: 353–356
Fraser I S, McCarron G, Markham R, Resta T, Watts A 1986 Measured menstrual blood loss in women with menorrhagia associated with pelvic disease or coagulation disorder. Obstetrics and Gynecology 68: 630–633
Garry R, Erian J, Grochmal S 1991 A multicentre collaborative study into the treatment of menorrhagia by Nd-YAG laser ablation of the endometrium. British Journal of Obstetrics and Gynecology 98 : 357–362
Gimpleson R J, Rappold H O 1988 A comparative study between panoramic hysteroscopy with directed biopsies and dilatation and curettage. American Journal of Obstetrics and Gynecology 158: 489–492
Goldrath M H, Fuller T A, Segal S 1981 Laser photovaporisation of endometrium for treatment of menorrhagia. American Journal of Obstetrics and Gynecology 140: 14–19
Grimes D A 1982 Diagnostic dilatation and curettage: a reappraisal. American Journal of Obstetrics and Gynecology 142: 1–6
Haining R E B, Cameron I T, van Papendorp C L et al 1991 Epidermal growth factor in human endometrium: proliferative effects in culture and immunocytochemical localisation in normal and endometriotic tissues. Human Reproduction 6: 1200
Hallberg L, Nilsson L 1964 Consistency of individual menstrual blood loss. Acta Obstetrica et Gynecologica Scandinavica 43: 352–359
Hallberg L, Hogdahl A, Nilsson L, Rybo G 1966 Menstrual blood loss and iron deficiency. Acta Medica Scandinavica 190: 639–655
Haynes P J, Anderson A B M, Turnbull A C 1979 Patterns of menstrual blood loss in menorrhagia. Research and Clinical Forums 1: 73–78
Higham J M, O'Brien P M S, Shaw R W 1990 Assessment of menstrual blood loss using a pictorial chart. British Journal of Obstetrics and Gynaecology 97: 734–739
Ishihara S, Tetetani Y, Mizuno M 1990 Epidermal growth factor-like immunoreactivity in human endometrium. Asia-Oceania Journal of Obstetrics and Gynaecology 16: 165–168
Kelly R W, Lumdsen M A, Abel M H, Baird D T 1984 The relationship between menstrual blood loss and prostaglandin production in the human: evidence for increased availability of arachidonic acid in women suffering from menorrhagia. Prostaglandins, Leukotrienes and Medicine 16: 69–78
Lewis B V 1990 Hysteroscopy for the investigation of abnormal uterine bleeding. British Journal of Obstetrics and Gynaecology 97: 283–284
Lewis B V 1993 Diagnostic dilatation and curettage in young women. British Medical Journal 306: 225-226
Lewis B V 1994 Guidelines for endometrial ablation. British Journal of Obstetrics and Gynaecology 101: 470
Loffer F D 1987 Hysteroscopic endometrial ablation with the Nd:YAG laser using a nontouch technique. Obstetrics and Gynecology 69: 679–682
Loffer F D 1989 Hysteroscopy with selective endometrial sampling compared with D&C for abnormal uterine bleeding: the value of a negative hysteroscopic view. Obstetrics and Gynecology 73: 16–20
Lumsden M A, Baird D T 1985 Intrauterine pressure in dysmenorrhoea. Acta Obstetrica et Gynecologica Scandinavica 64: 183–186
Lumsden M A, Kelly R W, Baird D T 1983 Is prostaglandin F_2

involved in the increased myometrial contractility of primary dysmenorrhoea? Prostaglandins 25: 683–692
Lundstrom V 1981 Uterine activity during the normal menstrual cycle and dysmenorrhoea. In: Darwood M Y (ed) Dysmenorrhoea. Williams and Wilkins, Baltimore, pp 53–74
Magos A L, Baumann R, Lockwood G M, Turnbull A C 1991 Experience with the first 250 endometrial resections for menorrhagia. Lancet 337: 1074–1078
Markee J E 1948 Morphological basis for menstrual bleeding. Relation of regression to the initiation of bleeding. Bulletin of the New York Academy of Medicine 24: 253–270
Migram S, Benedetto C, Zonka M, Leo Rosscerg I, Lubbert H, Hammerstein J 1991 Increased concentrations of eicosanoids and platelet-activating factor in menstrual fluid in women with primary dysmenorrhoea. Eicosanoids 4: 137–141
Milsom I, Andersson K, Andersch B, Rybo G 1991 A comparison of flurbiprofen, tranexamic acid, and a levonorgestrel-releasing intrauterine contraceptive device in the treatment of ideopathic menorrhagia. American Journal of Obstetrics and Gynecology 164: 879–883
Novak E, Reynolds S R M 1932. The cause of primary dysmenorrhoea with special reference to hormonal factors. Journal of the American Medical Association 99: 1466–1472
O'Reilly G, Charnock-Jones D S, Davenport A P, Cameron I T, Smith S K 1992 Presence of mRNA for endothelin-1, endothelin-2 and endothelin-3 in human endometrium, and a change in the ratio of ET_A and ET_B receptor subtype across the menstrual cycle. Journal of Clinical Endocrinology and Metabolism 75: 1545
Parazzini F, Tozzi L, Mezzopane R, Luchini L, Marchini M, Fedele L 1994 Cigarette smoking, alcohol consumption, and risk of primary dysmenorrhoea. Epidemiology 5: 469–472
Pinion S B, Parkin D E, Abramovich D R et al 1994 Randomised trial of hysterectomy, endometrial laser ablation and transcervical endometrial resection for dysfunctional uterine bleeding. British Medical Journal 309: 979–983
Rees M C, DiMarzo V, Tipping J R, Morris H R, Turnbull A C 1987 Leukotriene release by endometrium and myometrium throughout the menstrual cycle in dysmenorrhoea and menorrhagia. Journal of Endocrinology 113: 291–295
Rybo G 1966 Clinical and experimental studies on menstrual blood loss. Acta Obstetrica et Gynecologica Scandinavica 45(suppl): 1–23
Scottish Hysteroscopy Audit Group 1995 A Scottish audit of hysteroscopic surgery for menorrhagia – complications and follow up. British Journal of Obstetrics and Gynaecology. In press
Shaw R W, Fraser H M 1984 Use of a superactive luteinizing hormone-releasing hormone (LHRH) agonist in the treatment of menorrhagia. British Journal of Obstetrics and Gynaecology 91: 913–916
Shaw S T, Macauley L K, Sun N C, Tanaka M S, Roche P C 1983 Changes of plasminogen activator in human uterine tissue induced by intrauterine contraceptive devices. Contraception 27: 131–140
Shweiki D, Itin A, Neufeld G, Gitay Goren H, Keshet E 1993 Patterns of expression of vascular endothelial growth factor (VEGF) and VEGF receptors in mice suggest a role in hormonally regulated angiogenesis. Journal of Clinical Investigation 91: 2235–2243
Smith S K, Kelly R W 1988 Effect of platelet-activating factor on the release of PGF_{2a} and PGE_2 by separated cells of human endometrium. Journal of Reproduction and Fertility 82 : 271–276
Smith S K, Kelly R W, Abel M H, Baird D T 1981a A role for prostacyclin (PGI_2) in excessive menstrual bleeding. Lancet i: 522–524
Smith S K, Abel M H, Kelly R W, Baird D T 1981b Prostaglandin synthesis in the endometrium of women with ovular dysfunctional uterine bleeding. British Journal of Obstetrics and Gynaecology 88: 434–442
Smith S K, Abel M H, Kelly R W, Baird D T 1982 The synthesis of prostaglandins from persistent proliferative endometrium. Journal of Clinical Endocrinology and Metabolism 55: 284–289
Stock R J, Kanbour A 1975 Prehysterectomy curettage. Obstetrics and Gynecology 45: 537–541
Stovall T G, Solomon S K, Ling F W 1989 Endometrial sampling prior to hysterectomy. Obstetrics and Gynecology 73: 405–408

FURTHER READING

Cameron I T 1993 Medical treatment of menorrhagia. In: Yearbook of the RCOG 1993. RCOG Press, London, pp 55–64
Drife J O (ed) 1989 Dysfunctional uterine bleeding and menorrhagia. Clinical obstetrics and gynaecology, vol 3. Baillière Tindall, London
Lumsden M A 1993 Dysmenorrhoea and endometriosis. In: Yearbook of the RCOG 1993, RCOG Press, London, pp 77–90
Shaw R W (ed) 1990 Dysfunctional uterine bleeding. Advances in Reproductive Endocrinology vol 2. Parthenon, Carnforth, UK

29

Uterine fibroids

C. P. West

INTRODUCTION

Uterine fibroids are common benign tumours which arise from the uterine myometrium or, less commonly, from the cervix. They are composed of smooth muscle with a variable amount of connective tissue but are of smooth muscle origin, and thus classified as leiomyomata and also known as myomas. Although inaccurate by histological criteria, the term 'fibroid' is used almost universally to describe these nodular outgrowths which cause enlargement of the uterus and distortion of its normal structure with resulting implications for menstrual and reproductive function.

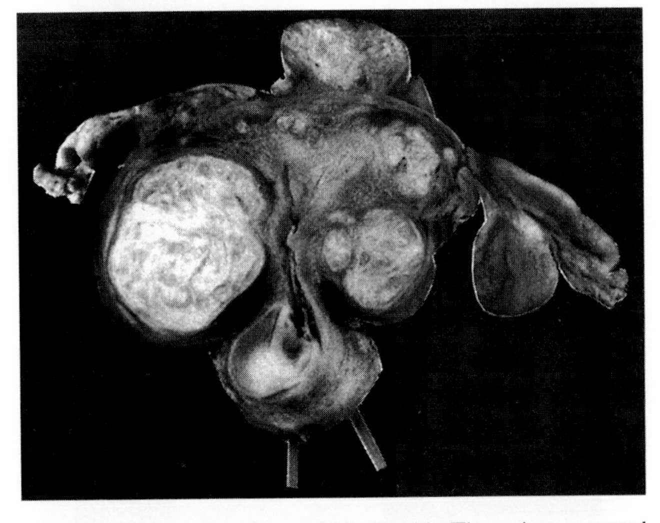

Fig. 29.1 Uterus enlarged by multiple fibroids. The patient presented at 43 years with menorrhagia; she had a 13-year history of primary infertility. Septate vagina and double cervix (marked with rods).

CLASSIFICATION AND PATHOPHYSIOLOGY

Macroscopically, fibroids are round or oval-shaped tumours, usually firm in consistency, with a characteristic white whorled appearance on cross-section. They may be single but are more commonly multiple and of varying sites and sizes (Fig. 29.1). Tiny 'seedling' fibroids are commonly seen in association with larger tumours and surgical removal of over 120 individual fibroids has been recorded in the literature. Four clinical subgroups are recognized: intramural, subserosal, submucous and cervical.

Intramural fibroids. These lie within the uterine wall, separated from the adjacent normal myometrium by a thin layer of connective tissue which forms the so-called false capsule. Small nutrient arteries penetrate this capsule although a single larger artery usually provides the major blood supply. Enlargement of a single intramural fibroid gives a globular outline to the uterus (see Fig. 29.10); the increased vascularity gives an appearance similar to that of pregnancy. Large intramural fibroids enlarge and distort the uterine cavity (Fig. 29.1), increasing its surface area, although they do not encroach upon the cavity directly.

Subserosal fibroids. These project outward from the uterine surface, covered with peritoneum. As growth is unrestricted by surrounding myometrium they may attain a very large size. Many fibroids in this site become pedun-

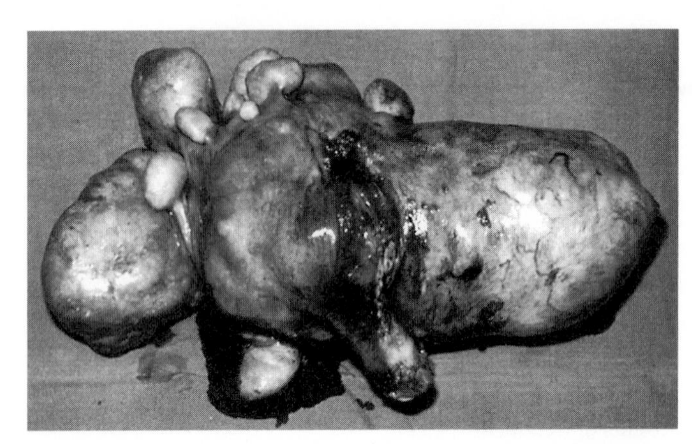

Fig. 29.2 Multiple subserous fibroids, some pedunculated. Specimen width 350 mm.

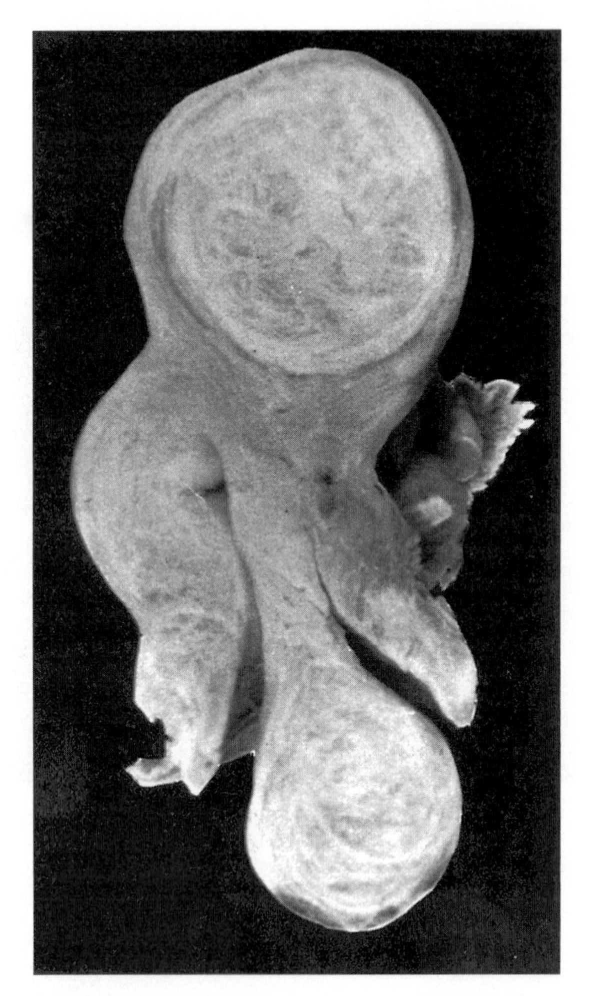

Fig. 29.3 Submucous fibroid protruding through cervix. The patient, aged 44 years, presented with a 3-week history of continuous bleeding; her haemoglobin level was 6.9 g/dl.

culated (Fig. 29.2) and torsion is a potential although rare complication. Sessile subserosal fibroids projecting from the fundal region may become adherent to omentum or bowel, particularly if there has been coincidental inflammatory disease. Fibroids which become attached to the omentum may develop an alternative blood supply, and may rarely become separated from the uterus forming a so-called 'parasitic' fibroid. Subserosal fibroids arising from the lateral uterine wall may lie between the layers of the broad ligament where large tumours may displace the ureters or bulge between the layers of the sigmoid mesocolon, lifting the bowel upwards. Broad ligament fibroids arising from the lateral uterine wall differ from true broad ligament fibroids, which have no attachment to the uterus but have their origin in smooth muscle fibres within the broad ligament, for example the round ligament, ovarian ligament or perivascular connective tissue.

Submucous fibroids. These are less common, comprising around 5% of all leiomyomata. By definition they project into the uterine cavity, are covered by endometrium, and cause irregularity and distortion although uterine enlargement may not be evident. Pedunculated submucous fibroids on a long stalk may prolapse through the cervix (Fig. 29.3) where they may cause intermenstrual bleeding or become ulcerated and infected. Although they are usually small, submucous fibroids may enlarge to fill the cavity, when attempted spontaneous expulsion may result in dilation of the cervix, so that the projecting fibroid resembles a fetal head. Very rarely this has led to uterine inversion.

Cervical fibroids. These are relatively uncommon but give rise to greatest surgical difficulty by virtue of their relative inaccessibility and close proximity to the bladder and ureters. Enlargement causes upward displacement of the uterus, and the fibroid may become impacted in the pelvis, causing urinary retention and ureteric obstruction (see Fig. 29.7).

Microscopic appearances

Microscopically, fibroids are composed of smooth muscle cell bundles, also arranged in whorl-like patterns (Fig. 29.4a), admixed with a variable amount of connective tissue, although the latter rarely predominates. The relatively poor blood supply to individual fibroids (see below) may result in degenerative changes, particularly within the large tumours. Hyaline degeneration (Fig. 29.4b) is the most common, resulting in a smoother and more homogeneous consistency, and this may become cystic if liquefaction occurs. Much more rarely fatty change may develop. This is distinct from the true lipoma of the uterus, which is extremely uncommon. Calcification (Fig. 29.5) is a later consequence of degeneration secondary to circulatory impairment. It characteristically occurs after the menopause although it may occur earlier in subserosal fibroids with narrow pedicles.

Red degeneration occurs almost exclusively in pregnancy (see p. 454) causing localized pain and tenderness which may be mistaken for an acute abdomen. Macroscopically, the fibroid appears reddish on cross-section, due to the presence of thrombotic and haemolytic changes within the blood vessels. The exact mechanism involved is not entirely clear. Sarcomatous degeneration, discussed on p. 455, is a serious although uncommon complication of fibroid growth.

Fibroids are believed to have an adverse effect on reproductive function by virtue of the resulting enlargement and distortion of the uterus, in particular the endometrial

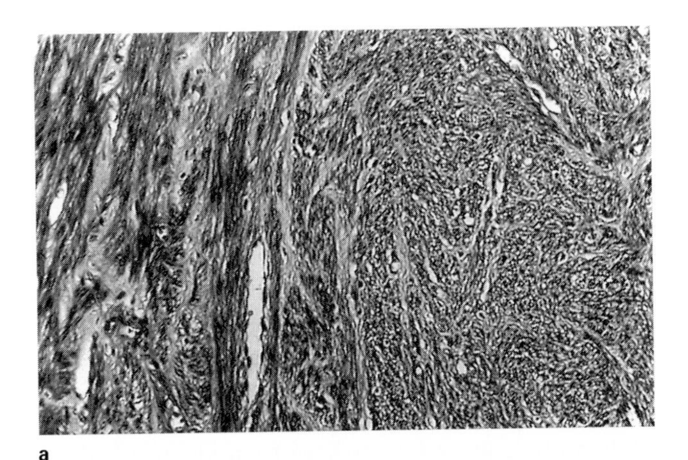

a

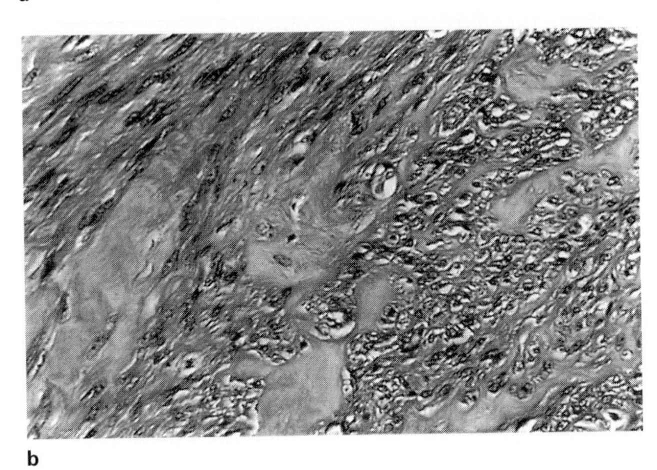

b

Fig. 29.4 Leiomyoma of uterus. **a** Bundles of elongated smooth muscle cells in both longitudinal (left) and transverse planes (×160). **b** focal hyalinization. Smooth muscle bundles are separated by dense hyalinized connective tissue (×320). (Courtesy of Dr K. Maclaren.)

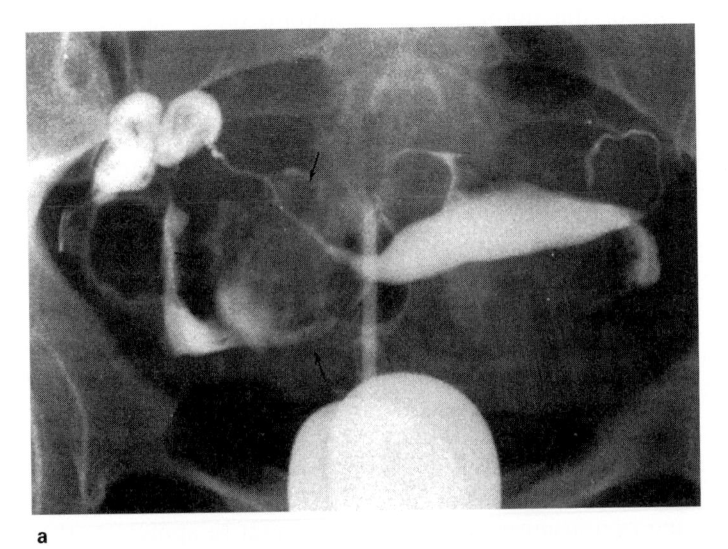

a

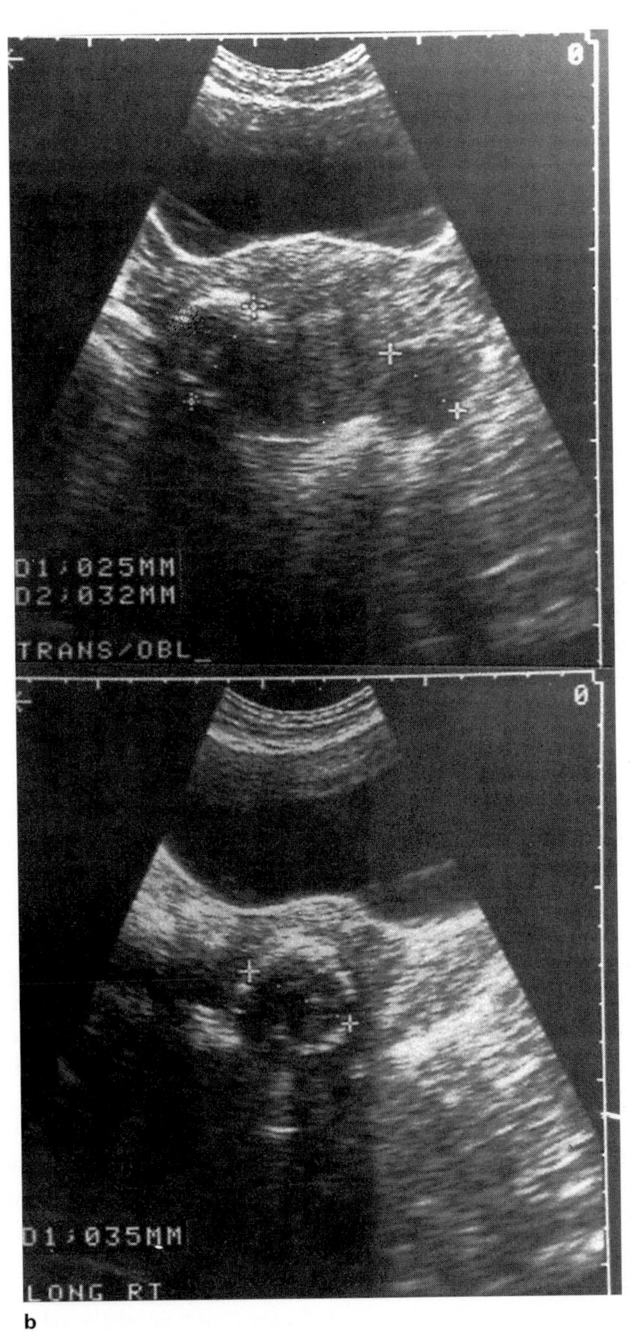

b

Fig. 29.5 **a** Calcified fibroid seen on hysterosalpingogram. (Courtesy of Dr B Muir.) **b** Ultrasound appearance of the uterus: **top**: two fibroids seen in transverse plane with calcified fibroid to left; **bottom**: calcified fibroid shown in longitudinal plane.

cavity (see Fig. 29.1). Some of the clinical features may be related to the effect of the fibroids on uterine arterial blood supply and venous drainage. Studies of blood flow using isotope clearance (Forssman 1976) and microradiographic studies of vascular patterns within fibroid uteri (Farrer-Brown et al 1971) have demonstrated that fibroids are less vascular than the surrounding myometrium, despite a rich network of surrounding arteries; hence the frequency with which degenerative changes occur. Regardless of their site, fibroids may cause mechanical obstruction to the venous drainage of both the myometrium and the endometrium, resulting in congestion and dilatation of the venous plexuses. Such congestion, if it affects the endometrium, may contribute to heavy blood loss.

AETIOLOGY

The aetiology of uterine fibroids remains unclear. Factors involved in their pathogenesis have recently been reviewed by Rein & Novak (1992) and Koutsilieris (1992). Early studies based on G-6-PD electrophoresis (Townsend et al 1970) demonstrated that fibroids are derived from single myometrial cells although the G-6-PD type may vary between individual fibroids within the same uterus. Many are chromosomally abnormal, with at least four groups of chromosomal rearrangements having been described. It is likely that such abnormalities contribute to the loss of normal growth regulation exhibited by fibroids.

It is presumed that fibroid growth is dependent on ovarian hormones since they do not occur prior to the menarche and normally show a reduction in size after the menopause. This is also supported by recent observations that regression occurs in response to the gonadal suppression induced by agonists of gonadotrophin-releasing hormone (GnRH), first reported by Filicori and co-workers in 1983 (see p. 451). However there is no evidence that women developing fibroids have any abnormality of circulating ovarian steroids. It was assumed that oestrogen was the major factor responsible for initiation and maintenance of fibroid growth but recent evidence that progestogens can inhibit GnRH agonist-induced fibroid shrinkage (see West 1993) and that fibroids shrink in response to an antiprogesterone (Murphy et al 1993) suggests that progesterone may have a major role in the control of fibroid growth.

Recent research (see Koutsilieris 1992, Rein & Novak 1992) has been directed towards elucidating the local mechanisms which may influence the initiation and growth of fibroids. Receptors for both oestrogen and progesterone are present in uterine tissues but there is evidence that the effects of circulating steroids are not exerted directly but via local growth factors: polypeptides which control cellular proliferation and have been implicated in tumour growth. Receptors for epithelial growth factor (EGF), insulin-like growth factor 1 (IGF-1) and platelet-derived growth factor (PDGF) are all present in fibroid tissue and expression of specific messenger RNA has also been demonstrated. There is also evidence that these are present to a greater extent in fibroid tissue than in surrounding myometrium and are influenced by changes in steroid exposure.

EPIDEMIOLOGY

It is estimated that around 20% of women of reproductive age have uterine fibroids although presentation occurs most commonly towards the end of their reproductive life.

While no hereditary factors have been identified, there are definite racial differences: a ninefold greater incidence has been reported among black women (Witherspoon 1935), where they also present at a younger age. Women with uterine fibroids have had fewer term pregnancies and are generally of lower parity than their contemporaries without this problem, but it is not entirely clear whether fibroids are a cause or consequence of low family size. Obesity increases the risk of developing fibroids, while cigarette smoking is associated with a reduced risk (Ross et al 1986).

Similar risk factors are associated with endometrial carcinoma but, unlike the latter, development of fibroids following the menopause has not been described, even in association with the use of hormone replacement therapy. This further supports the evidence that oestrogen alone does not provide the trigger for the initiation of fibroid growth.

PRESENTATION

The clinical presentation of uterine fibroids is dependent in part on the reproductive status of the woman and the site of the fibroids. The symptomatology has been reviewed in detail by Buttram & Reiter (1981). Many fibroids, possibly in excess of 50%, are asymptomatic and discovered at routine pelvic or abdominal examination or during pregnancy.

Menorrhagia

It is uncertain what proportion of women with fibroids have excessive menstrual loss although estimates vary between 30 and 50%. Investigation of women presenting with menorrhagia has shown the presence of fibroids in only 10% of women with moderately heavy menstrual blood loss (80–100 ml), compared with 40% of those with loss in excess of 200 ml (Rybo et al 1985). Menorrhagia attributable to fibroids may therefore be very heavy, causing significant anaemia. It is important to appreciate that fibroids are not usually a cause of irregular or intermenstrual bleeding and that any disruption of normal cyclicity

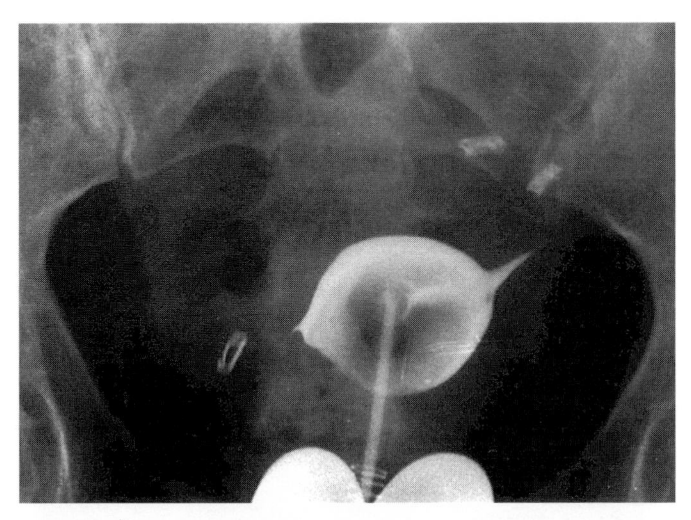

Fig. 29.6 Hysterosalpingogram showing enlargement of uterine cavity and filling defect from intramural fibroid. Extensive endometriosis had complicated laparoscopic sterilization (hence the two clips on the left tube). (Courtesy of Dr B. Muir.)

should not be attributed to the presence of fibroids without first excluding other causes.

The mechanism of the menorrhagia remains a subject of debate. Theories include ulceration and haemorrhage of the endometrium overlying submucous fibroids, enlargement of the total surface area of the endometrium due to mechanical distortion by submucous and intramural fibroids (Fig. 29.6) and stasis and dilatation of the venous plexuses draining the endometrium, due to mechanical compression of the venous drainage by fibroids at any site. All these mechanisms may be important and it is now clear that, contrary to some opinions, menorrhagia is not confined only to women with submucous fibroids and that while these may be associated with menorrhagia of greatest severity, they are sometimes asymptomatic.

Recent research has implicated disorders of prostaglandin synthesis and metabolism in the aetiology of menstrual disorders (Ch. 28) and this may also be relevant in the presence of fibroids. Fibroids are associated with disordered uterine motility but it is not clear whether this is because of mechanical factors or because of abnormalities of prostaglandin metabolism.

Pelvic pain and pressure symptoms

Fibroids do not usually give rise to pain although, exceptionally, their presentation may be acute on account of torsion or degeneration. Attempted expulsion of a large submucous fibroid through the cervix causes uterine cramp associated with bleeding and may be mistaken for spontaneous abortion, particularly with the clinical finding of a dilated cervix and a protruding mass. This situation has been described as a complication of treatment with GnRH analogues (see p. 454). Rarely it can result in uterine inversion. Torsion or painful degeneration presents with an acute abdomen and is commonly confused with complications of ovarian neoplasia. Distinction between these conditions is particularly important in pregnancy complicated by red degeneration of a fibroid, in order to avoid subjecting the woman to unnecessary laparotomy.

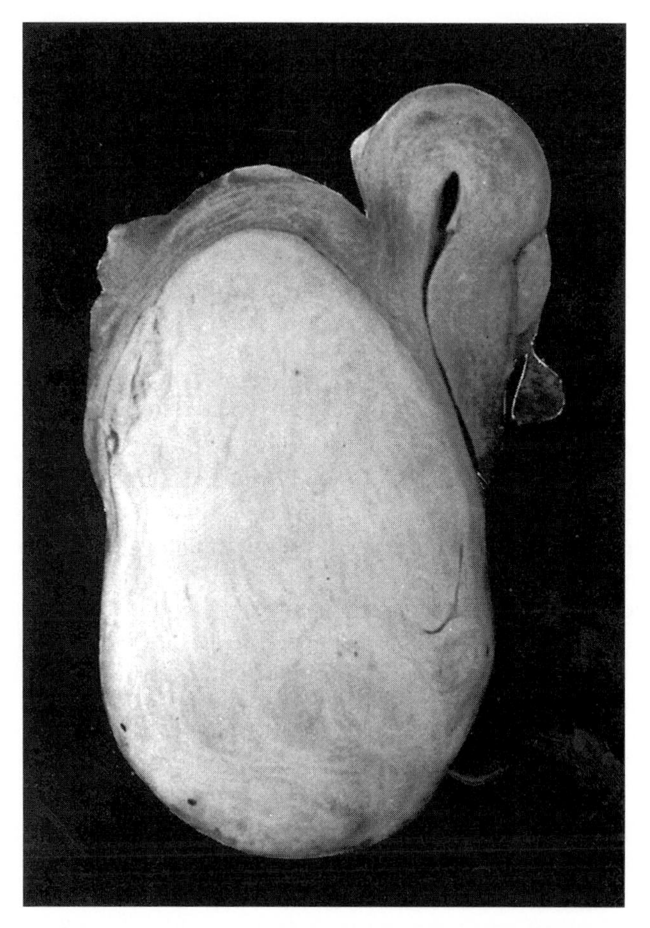

Fig. 29.7 Cervical fibroid growing anteriorly in the supravaginal cervix. Presentation was with frequency of micturition followed by acute urinary retention.

It is surprising that even in the presence of multiple fibroids menstruation may be painless. They are more often associated with pelvic discomfort and urinary symptoms, attributed to pressure from large fibroids, particularly those arising from the cervix or low down on the anterior uterine wall. Cervical fibroids may present with acute retention of urine (see Fig. 29.7), although this is a fairly uncommon complication.

Subfertility

It is estimated that infertility is the major presenting factor or a secondary feature in around 27% of women with fibroids (Buttram & Reiter 1981) and the association of fibroids with low fecundity and childlessness is well recognized. However, when compared with other causes of infertility, they are relatively uncommon, being implicated in approximately 3% of couples. This percentage is higher in negroid races where there is also a high prevalence of pelvic inflammatory disease and the two conditions often coexist.

It is probable that a delay in childbearing, whether voluntary or involuntary, may predispose towards the development of fibroids and it is thus mandatory to investigate both partners fully to exclude other factors which may be contributing towards their subfertility.

The mechanism whereby fibroids adversely affect conception is unclear, but it is likely to be mechanical, by virtue of cornual occlusion or by distortion of the cavity, preventing implantation. In addition, alterations in local blood flow and increases in the binding of steroids to fibroids, compared with myometrium, may create unfavourable factors in the local environment which prevent implantation. These mechanisms have yet to be clarified, but reports of improved pregnancy rates after myomectomy give support to the belief that in some individuals the presence of fibroids is detrimental to the chance of conception.

INVESTIGATIONS

The range of investigations appropriate to each case of fibroids will vary according to the nature of the individual problem and the proposed plan of management. General assessment must always include a full blood count, as many patients with fibroids do not complain of excessive menstruation even when this is present. Use of the available imaging techniques has been reviewed by Karasick et al (1992).

Ultrasound

Ultrasound should always be used to confirm or clarify the nature of a pelvic mass. Even in relatively unskilled hands it will diagnose pregnancy and differentiate between cystic and solid lesions (Fig. 29.8). With appropriate training and experience, the site and nature of a pelvic mass may be predicted with accuracy in over 80% of cases; difficulty mainly arises in the differentiation of pedunculated fibroids from solid ovarian lesions. Transvaginal ultrasound is particularly helpful in elucidating the nature of small lesions and in demonstrating the presence of submucosal fibroids.

Ultrasound assessment should include examination of the ovaries and kidneys and it is important to look for the presence or absence of free peritoneal fluid as well as to study the nature and consistency of the mass itself. Serial ultrasound examination is of value in monitoring fibroid size during medical or conservative treatment. The volume of individual fibroids (Fig. 29.5b) or of the whole uterus (Fig. 29.8) can be calculated by measuring the diameter in three planes at right angles, and using the formula $4/3\ \pi r^3$, where r is the radius.

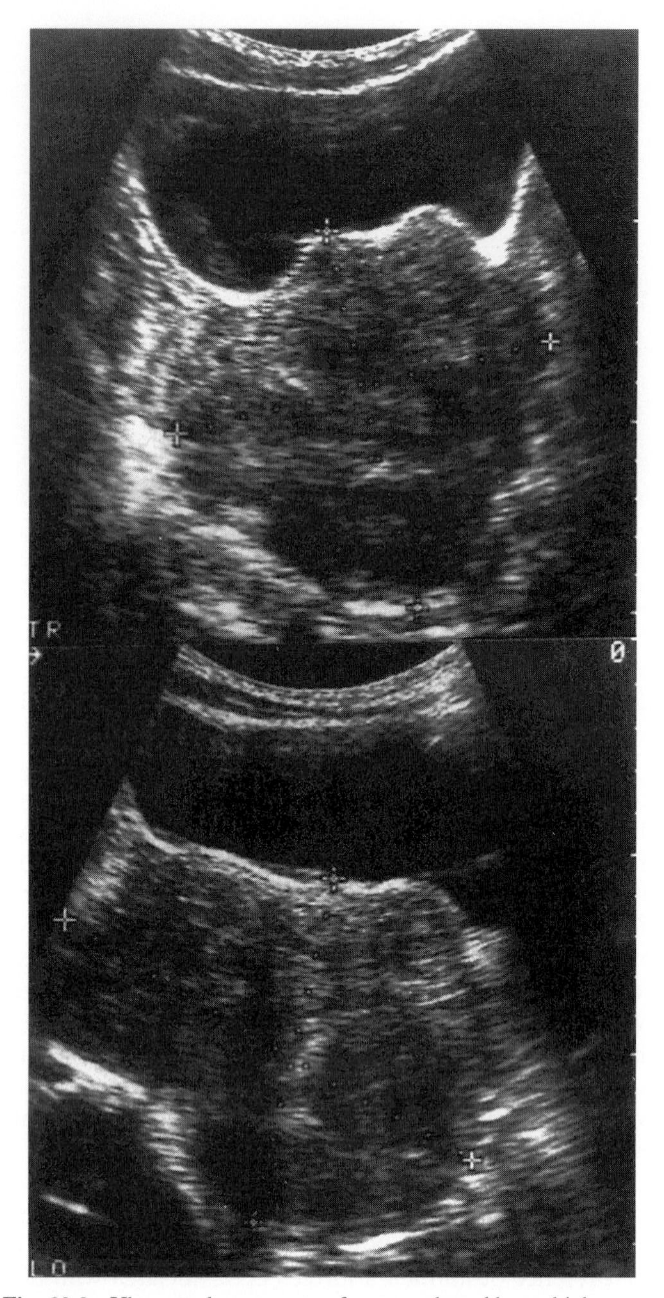

Fig. 29.8 Ultrasound appearance of uterus enlarged by multiple fibroids, showing patchy echogenicity. (Courtesy of Dr B. Muir.)

Magnetic resonance imaging

This is of considerable value in demonstrating the nature of pelvic masses although the technique is very costly and not widely available. Compared with ultrasound, it is a more accurate predictor of the histological features of a tumour (Weinreb et al 1990). While this is of value in research and in cases of diagnostic difficulty, such a high level of accuracy is not necessary for the routine management of fibroids.

Laparoscopy

Laparoscopy is of value if the uterus is not larger than a 12-week gestation size and there is associated infertility or pelvic pain. It may reveal the presence of coincidental endometriosis, pelvic adhesions or other tubal pathology.

Laparoscopy will also differentiate between a pedunculated fibroid and an ovarian neoplasm in cases where the diagnosis of an adnexal mass is unclear on the basis of clinical and ultrasound findings. It may also be possible, in some circumstances, to remove small fibroids laparoscopically (see p. 450).

Hysterosalpingography or hysteroscopy

One of these procedures should be carried out routinely in patients with a history of recurrent abortion. Examination of the uterine cavity is also important in an infertile patient with fibroids or in any patient where myomectomy is contemplated, in order to identify the presence and site of any submucous fibroids. Not only may these adversely affect implantation but they may be encroaching on to the tubal ostium causing obstruction.

Where a filling defect is evident radiologically (e.g. Fig. 29.9), direct visualization through the hysteroscope will clarify the diagnosis as well as enabling local hysteroscopic methods of treatment to be performed where appropriate.

There is also an increasing place for hysteroscopy in the investigation of menorrhagia and other menstrual abnormalities. In one study quoted by Siegler & Valle (1988), submucous fibroids were visualized hysteroscopically in 13% of patients investigated for abnormal bleeding. Hysteroscopy would not however be appropriate in cases of menorrhagia associated with large fibroids, where hysterectomy is the chosen treatment option.

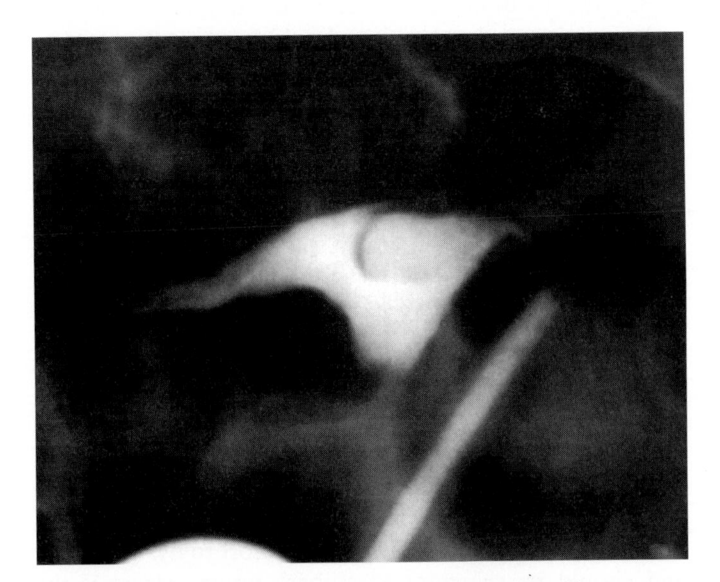

Fig. 29.9 Hysterosalpingogram of a patient presenting with recurrent abortion, showing a filling defect. (Courtesy of Dr B. Muir.)

Endometrial sampling

Endometrial sampling by biopsy or curettage is indicated in cases of irregular or intermenstrual bleeding to exclude the presence of coexisting endometrial pathology. Where heavy bleeding retains a normal cyclical pattern this is usually unnecessary, although curettage may be of diagnostic value in detecting irregularities of the uterine cavity due to submucous fibroids. Alternatively, endometrial biopsy combined with either hysteroscopy or vaginal ultrasound will identify the presence of submucous fibroids without the routine need for general anaesthesia.

TREATMENT METHODS

Recent advances in medical and surgical methods of treatment have increased the potential range of therapeutic options for women with fibroids. It is too early to assess the impact of these developments on our overall gynaecological practice and in particular on the number of hysterectomies performed annually. In decisions about management, the symptoms, reproductive status and attitude of each individual patient should be taken into consideration, and the options fully discussed. While surgery remains the treatment of choice for most symptomatic women, alternatives may be appropriate in some situations.

Expectant management

Fibroids are frequently asymptomatic, and provided that their nature can be determined with reasonable certainty using the diagnostic methods described above, active treatment is unnecessary. Surgical removal has traditionally been advocated when the uterine size exceeds that of a 12-week pregnancy but this policy has been challenged (Reiter et al 1992). Most pelvic swellings can be confidently diagnosed with the use of ultrasound. Similarly, the risk of sarcomatous change is estimated to be less than 0.1% (see p. 455) making prophylactic removal of a fibroid unjustified. Furthermore, the mere presence of a fibroid uterus is not known to carry any long-term detrimental effects and spontaneous regression after the menopause may be anticipated.

Routine hysterectomy is therefore difficult to justify in asymptomatic women. Exceptions would include very large fibroids, a rapid increase in size or where there is concern about the nature of the mass.

Hysterectomy

Hysterectomy is the definitive treatment for symptomatic uterine fibroids, although the decision to perform hysterectomy should not be undertaken without due consideration of the alternatives; for women who wish to preserve reproductive function, myomectomy or medical treatment must be considered.

The route selected for the hysterectomy will depend on the size of the uterus, the situation of the fibroids and the history of any previous surgical procedures. Abdominal hysterectomy with ovarian conservation (Fig. 29.10) will be the procedure of choice where fibroids are very large. For gynaecologists who favour the vaginal route for routine hysterectomies, consideration should be given to preoperative shrinkage with a GnRH agonist as described below. Similarly, a reduction in volume and vascularity may facilitate removal of a very large uterus by the abdominal route.

Abdominal hysterectomy is rendered difficult in the presence of large fibroids arising from the cervix or situated in the broad ligament. It is also more complicated if there are adhesions from previous myomectomies or from associated endometriosis or pelvic inflammatory disease. Difficult access to the pelvis during hysterectomy for large fibroids will be rendered easier by prior enucleation of the fibroids. The ureters may be vulnerable during an operation to remove a broad ligament fibroid and their pathway must always be identified. Regardless of the direction of displacement, they are always extracapsular. In the case of a large cervical fibroid an alternative approach is hemisection of the uterus, followed by enucleation of the fibroid in order to gain access to the uterine arteries and cervix. These techniques are described in detail by Monaghan (1988).

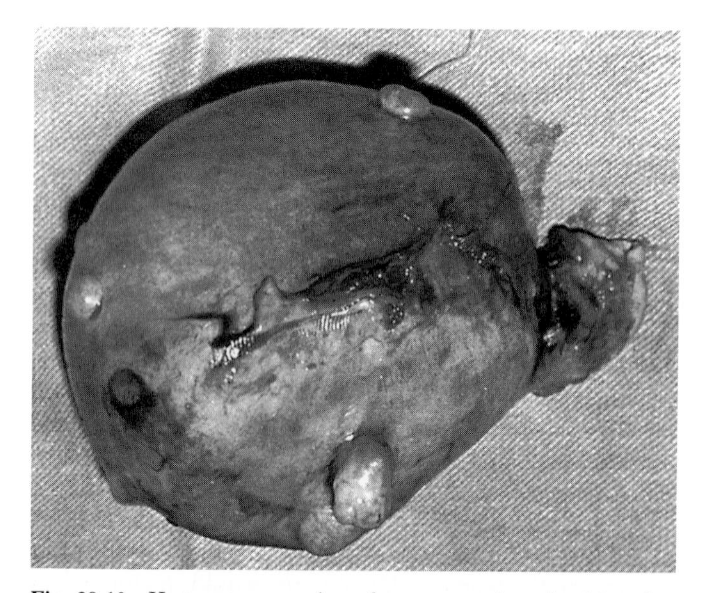

Fig. 29.10 Hysterectomy specimen from uterus enlarged to 16-week gestation size by single intramural fibroid and several small seedling fibroids. Uterine volume was 575 ml.

The increasing popularity of minimal access surgery has led to the use of laparoscopically assisted methods of vaginal hysterectomy in women with large fibroids, usually following prior shrinkage with a GnRH agonist. The role of this approach currently remains unclear although the use of the laparoscope will facilitate oophorectomy, if this is deemed to be indicated in conjunction with vaginal hysterectomy.

Myomectomy

Removal of individual fibroids was first reported in the middle of the 19th century although current surgical techniques are largely attributable to Victor Bonney who described a personal series of 403 cases. Since then there have been several large published series, reviewed in detail by Buttram & Reiter (1981) and Verkauf (1992).

Enucleation of intramural fibroids from their false capsule can be a rapid and simple procedure but may also be associated with considerable technical difficulties, major haemorrhage and a greater postoperative morbidity and mortality than hysterectomy. It is therefore an operation which should be restricted to women who have not completed childbearing. It is most satisfactory where fibroids are solitary or few in number, and although removal of as many as 125 individual tumours from one uterus was described by Bonney, such a procedure is tedious and the outcome in terms of reproductive function must be in considerable doubt. In a woman presenting with infertility, it is sometimes difficult to establish the extent to which the fibroids are interfering with conception, and full investigation of both the woman and her partner should be carried out.

Because of difficulty of access to submucous fibroids at laparotomy, consideration should be given to hysteroscopic methods of removal (see p. 450). Subserous fibroids are easily removed with minimal morbidity, particularly if pedunculated (Fig. 29.11) but such fibroids are the least likely to give rise to problems. Some authorities would advise their removal if they are large because of the risk, albeit rare, of acute torsion in pregnancy.

Potential problems with myomectomy

The major problems associated with myomectomy are heavy operative blood loss, and postoperative adhesion formation, reducing the chance of successful conception and rendering future surgery more difficult. It is therefore most important that the decision to perform a myomectomy is carefully considered. If operative haemorrhage is very heavy the surgeon may have to resort to hysterectomy and should be reluctant to embark upon surgery if the patient is not willing to consent to the latter alternative.

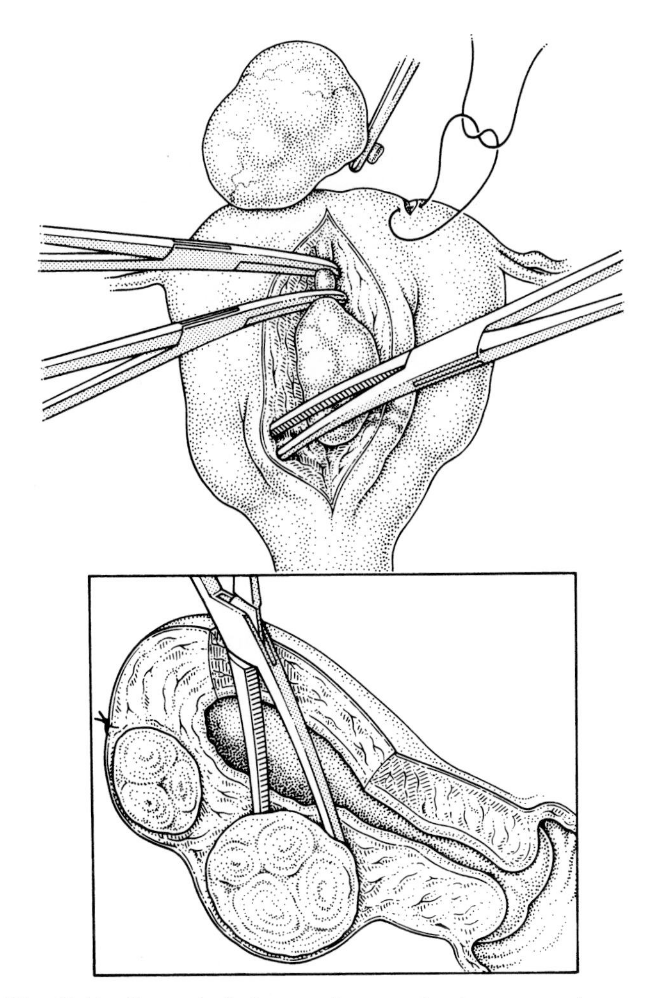

Fig. 29.11 Removal of subserous, intramural, submucous and posteriorly located intramural fibroids through a single anterior incision. (From Buttram & Reiter 1981, with permission of the publisher, the American Society for Reproductive Medicine (formerly The American Fertility Society).)

Various methods have been advocated to reduce intra- and postoperative complications. Postoperative adhesions are usually a consequence of difficulties with haemostasis and oozing from incision lines and are increased where there are multiple incisions over the uterine body. Adhesions to incisions on the posterior uterine wall are potentially more serious because of involvement of the fallopian tubes and ovaries. To minimize adhesion formation, as many fibroids as possible should be removed through a single incision (Fig. 29.11). Some authorities recommend removal of posterior wall fibroids via the uterine cavity through an incision on the anterior uterine wall. Others avoid opening the uterine cavity unless submucous fibroids are known to be present because of the risk of intrauterine adhesions. Careful obliteration of large cavities left by enucleation of fibroids is very important and opinions vary as to whether redundant myometrium should be removed or preserved. Bonney (Monaghan 1986) described a 'hood' method of closure of the cavity left after

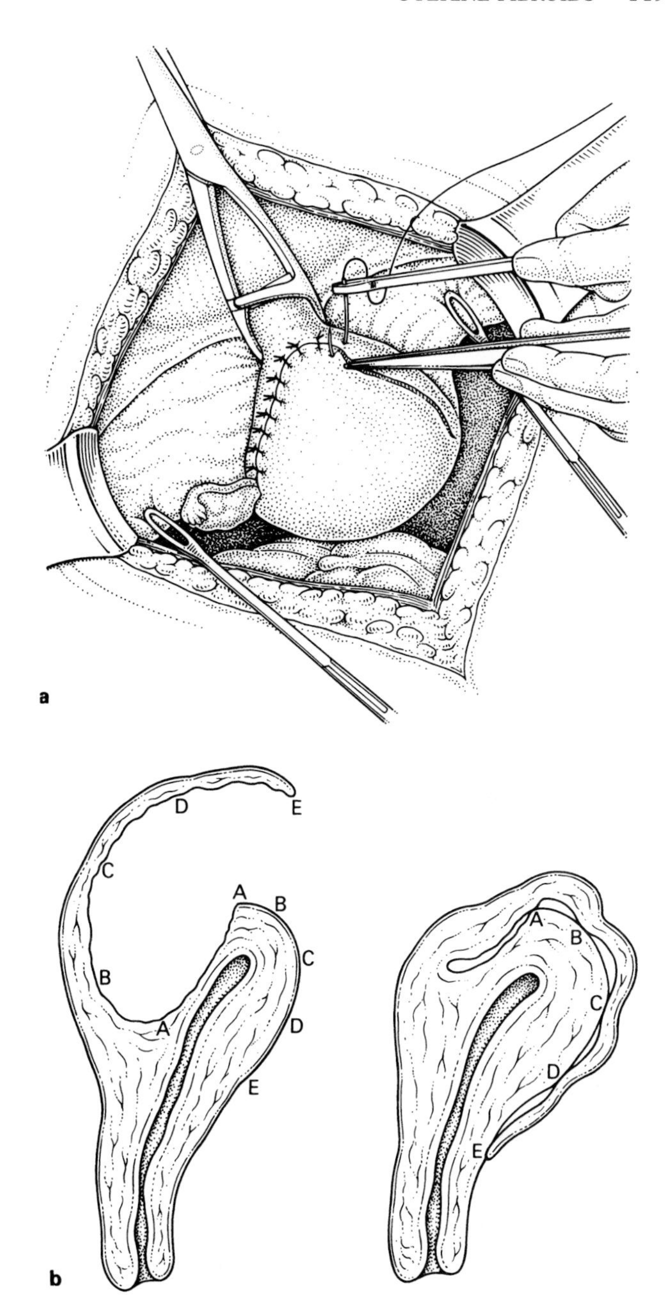

Fig. 29.12 **a** Closure of myomectomy through transverse posterior incision using Bonney's 'hood', showing final anterior suture line and Bonney's clamp in place. **b** Construction of Bonney's hood showing the capsule after enucleation (left) and the hood in place (right). (From Monaghan 1986, with permission of Chapman & Hall.)

enucleation of a very large single posterior tumour (Fig. 29.12), suturing the redundant flap of serosal-covered myometrium over the fundus and low down on to the anterior wall to avoid adhesion formation. Plication of the round ligaments at the end of the procedure to hold the uterus forward in anteversion, the instillation of concentrated solutions of dextran and the use of oxidized regenerated cellulose have also been recommended to reduce the risk of postoperative adhesions.

Both mechanical and medical methods have been

described to reduce operative blood loss. One such method is the use of the Bonney's myomectomy clamp which is placed across the lower uterus to occlude the uterine arteries (see Fig. 29.12a). It can be used in conjunction with ring forceps to occlude the ovarian blood supply. An alternative is the use of a rubber tourniquet or catheter, placed around the uterus through an incision in the broad ligament at the level of the lower segment. Occlusion of the arterial blood supply for prolonged intervals of time may cause ischaemic damage to tissues, and release of histamine-like substances into the general circulation has been reported (Monaghan 1986). During a long operation, intermittent release of the clamp or catheter at 10–20-min intervals is recommended. Such occlusive methods are unsuitable for use where there are large cervical or broad ligament fibroids, and these are the very tumours which may give rise to greatest difficulty. As an alternative or adjunct to occlusive clamps, local injection of vasopressin is recommended by some authorities, although its efficacy has been challenged. Recently, pretreatment with GnRH analogues has been used to reduce the vascularity of the uterus (see below) and this has the advantage of also reducing the size of the fibroids. However their enucleation may be rendered more difficult because the false capsule plane of cleavage between the fibroid and the surrounding myometrium becomes less well defined.

Endoscopic surgical methods

Hysteroscopy

Most submucous fibroids which are protruding through the cervix (see Fig. 29.3) can be removed vaginally with cautery or ligation of the pedicle. If the fibroid is very large, piecemeal removal has been described. Such procedures might be facilitated by preoperative treatment with a GnRH agonist (see p. 452). Diagnostic and therapeutic hysteroscopy (see review by Siegler & Valle 1988) is gaining popularity in the UK and submucous fibroids (such as those illustrated in Fig. 29.13) are amenable to hysteroscopic removal. Such procedures can be combined with endometrial ablation for the relief of menorrhagia if the woman has completed childbearing.

Techniques of hysteroscopic myomectomy are described by Drews & Reyniak (1992) and have been used for removal of lesions measuring up to 7 cm in diameter although many authorities would set a maximum of 3–4 cm. Prior shrinkage with a GnRH analogue is advantageous in this context. Small pedunculated lesions may be removed with scissors after coagulation of the base while larger broad based lesions that are predominantly submucosal are resected using electrocautery. The neodymium: YAG laser can be used for ablation of small fibroids, or alternatively larger lesions can be cut off at their base and

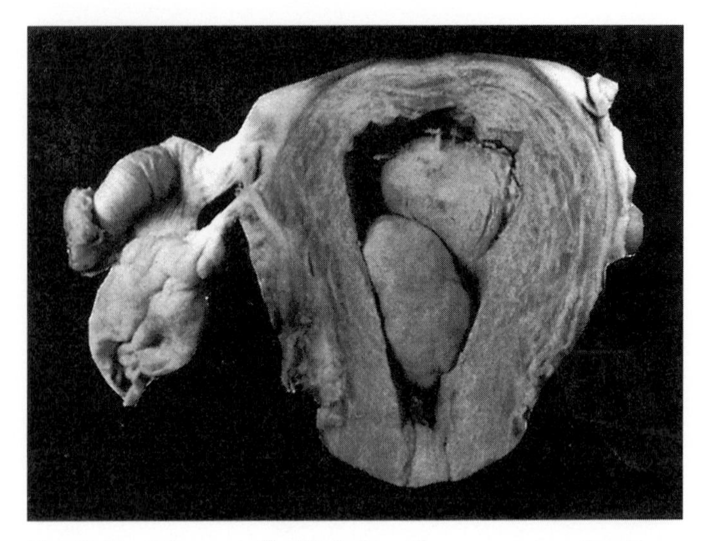

Fig. 29.13 Submucous fibroids (subtotal hysterectomy specimen).

if small, extracted whole or if larger, quartered and removed piecemeal.

Postoperative bleeding can be controlled by tamponade with the balloon of a Foley catheter.

For fibroids with an intramural extension, Donnez et al (1990) describe a two-stage removal procedure using the neodymium: YAG laser, after prior shrinkage with a GnRH analogue. They advocate leaving individual fibroids, once enucleated, in the uterine cavity where eventual expulsion during menstruation is anticipated.

Hysteroscopic surgery of this type requires considerable experience and training in order to optimize results and minimize complications, which include uterine perforation (immediate or pregnancy-related), haemorrhage, infection and excessive systemic absorption of the fluid distending medium. However these techniques have the advantage of being performed as outpatient procedures with avoidance of major surgery.

Laparoscopy

Laparoscopy is a standard investigation for infertility and inevitably many women thus investigated will be found to have small asymptomatic uterine fibroids. Laparoscopic methods of removal of both subserous and small intramural fibroids have been described (see review by Drews & Reyniak 1992), but as these are unlikely to be interfering with fertility it is not clear whether their removal will carry any long-term advantage for the patient. In theory it may prevent the growth of larger, potentially symptomatic tumours and avoid more major surgical intervention, but these advantages have yet to be proven. It is also unlikely that intramural seedlings can be removed by this method.

Recently laparoscopic techniques have been applied to the enucleation of larger intramural as well as subserosal fibroids, which are then morcellated or removed by colpotomy. Such procedures are very time-consuming and as yet there is no evidence that they offer any advantages over conventional laparotomy.

Medical management

There are two main objectives in the medical treatment of uterine fibroids, namely relief of symptoms and reduction in fibroid size. The ideal end-point of medical treatment would be their complete regression but to date this has not been described. For this reason, medical methods have in the past had a limited role in the management of fibroids. However, with recent advances in diagnostic and therapeutic techniques, enabling a more conservative approach to management, there is a greater role for medical therapies, both for symptomatic treatment of fibroids, and also as adjuncts to surgery. The role of medical therapies in the relief of fibroid-associated menorrhagia has been reviewed by West & Lumsden (1989) and Van-Eijkeren et al (1992).

Progestogens

Progestogens are widely used in the management of dysfunctional uterine bleeding but are generally regarded as ineffective in menorrhagia secondary to fibroids. However they may be specifically indicated in perimenopausal women with fibroids where bleeding is of an anovular dysfunction type rather than a direct consequence of the fibroids. There is no evidence that progestogen administration causes any alteration in the size of fibroids, although degenerative changes have been reported following the administration of high doses of medroxyprogesterone acetate.

Androgenic steroids

Androgenic steroids, such as danazol or gestrinone, are useful in reducing or abolishing menstrual blood loss in patients with menorrhagia, by virtue of direct effects on the endometrium and negative feedback inhibition of pituitary gonadotrophin release. A small reduction in the volume of uterine fibroids, of the order of 20%, has been reported during therapy with both these androgens, with relief of menstrual symptoms.

While such agents may be beneficial for the short-term relief of symptoms, their androgenic properties and side-effects make them unsuitable for long-term use. Their use should be considered in specific clinical situations where short-term symptomatic relief is required.

Prostaglandin synthetase inhibitors

While beneficial in the management of dysfunctional uterine bleeding, prostaglandin synthetase inhibitors have been shown to be ineffective in the treatment of menorrhagia secondary to fibroids. However they may be useful in the relief of pelvic pain in women with fibroids, including painful degeneration.

Antifibrinolytics

A reduction of measured menstrual blood loss of the order of 50% has been reported in women with fibroids treated with the antifibrinolytic tranexamic acid (Nilsson & Rybo 1971); a reduction equivalent to that reported for dysfunctional uterine bleeding. This agent was recently granted a licence by the CSM for unlimited use, thus making it a useful agent for the treatment of fibroid-related menorrhagia.

Oestrogen–progestogen combinations

The role of the oral contraceptive pill in women with fibroids is unclear. Since an early report of enlargement of fibroids during oral contraceptive therapy, its use has been avoided in this situation although a modest reduction in menstrual blood loss was reported by Nilsson & Rybo (1971). The relevance of early studies to modern contraceptive practice must however be questioned, as they related to much higher dose formulations than those which are in current use. In women known to have fibroids, there seems to be no clear contraindication to the use of the pill for contraceptive purposes, provided that uterine volume is monitored and there is no deterioration in its size or in any fibroid-related symptoms. For women without fibroids, long-term use of the oral contraceptive pill may be protective effect against their development (Ross et al 1986) although not all authors have reported similar findings.

The influence of the oestrogen–progestogen combinations used for hormone replacement therapy is also unclear, although re-enlargement of fibroids might be expected. This has not been confirmed in recent studies of the addition of low dose hormone replacement therapy to GnRH analogues for the shrinkage of fibroids (see below). Because of the ease of monitoring fibroid size with ultrasound, the use of low dose oral hormone replacement therapy should not be contraindicated in postmenopausal women with fibroids, particularly if these have been asymptomatic, unless there is any suspicion of coexisting endometrial pathology or sarcomatous change.

GnRH analogues

GnRH agonists

Analogues of GnRH significantly reduce the size of uterine fibroids, thus relieving pressure symptoms as well as menorrhagia. After initial transient stimulation, agonist analogues act by sustained pituitary downregulation, resulting in suppression of ovarian activity (Fig. 29.14).

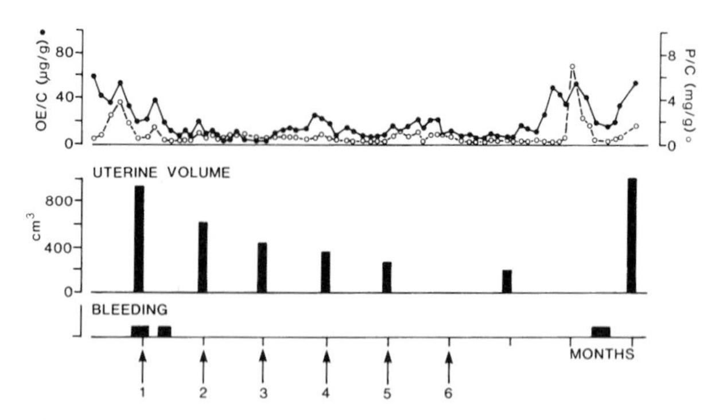

Fig. 29.14 Reversible reduction in uterine volume and amenorrhoea in a patient treated for 6 months with goserelin depot (arrows). Ovarian response was monitored by urinary oestrone glucuronide and pregnanediol excretion (expressed as steroid/creatinine ratios: OE/C and P/C).

Bleeding in response to oestrogen withdrawal occurs during the initial treatment cycle but amenorrhoea is usual thereafter. The shrinkage of fibroids is therefore a consequence of gonadal suppression and women are likely to experience side-effects, in particular vasomotor symptoms and vaginal dryness. Uterine volume, assessed by ultrasound or MRI, shrinks by an average of 35% after 3 months of administration and 50% after 6 months, with little further change thereafter. The effects of treatment persist only for the duration of administration, and cessation of therapy is usually followed by rapid regrowth of the fibroids to their pretreatment size (Fig. 29.14; see review by West 1993).

Because of the side-effects, in particular the potential risk of loss of bone mineral, the clinical applications of GnRH agonists are largely confined to short-term uses, in particular as adjuncts to surgery. Reduction of blood flow through the uterine arteries, as assessed by Doppler flow studies (Matta et al 1988), is associated with reduction in the vascularity as well as the size of fibroids. The outcomes of the use of GnRH analogues as adjuncts to hysterectomy, myomectomy and endoscopic surgical methods are discussed in the Results section below. Relief of severe menorrhagia also enables treatment of anaemia prior to surgery, when it should be used in conjunction with iron therapy.

If such treatment is to be used prior to surgery, its optimum duration is 3 months, which should be sufficient to correct any associated anaemia. Appropriate doses of currently available GnRH agonists include goserelin, 3.6 mg, or leuporelin, 3.75 mg, by monthly subcutaneous depot injection, and buserelin 900–1200 µg or nafarelin 800 µg daily in divided doses by intranasal spray. Therapy should be commenced in the early follicular phases of the cycle to avoid accidental initiation during early pregnancy. Compliance may be a problem with the nasal spray and as erratic usage may result in stimulation rather than suppression of pituitary–ovarian function, administration by subcutaneous depot may be preferable in the preoperative situation.

For women who are keen to avoid surgery, particularly those approaching the age of the natural menopause, or for those with contraindications to surgery, the use of GnRH agonists in combination with hormonal 'add-back' therapy is currently being investigated. Such therapy comprises oestrogen–progestogen combinations, equivalent to low dose hormone replacement therapy, given with the object of reducing vasomotor side-effects and protecting against bone loss. This is commenced once initial uterine shrinkage has been obtained with 3 months of GnRH agonist alone. The add-back therapy may be given cyclically or as continuous combined therapy; the latter having the potential advantage of sustained amenorrhoea. Preliminary results (see reviews by Friedman 1993, and West 1993) indicate that fibroid shrinkage and symptomatic relief can be maintained in a proportion of patients with such regimes. Use of progestogens alone as add-back therapy appears to be less effective compared with oestrogen–progestogen combinations. Regimens of this nature are very costly and some women very near the natural menopause gain sustained relief of their symptoms following 6 months of treatment with a GnRH agonist alone.

There have been reports of spontaneous pregnancy immediately following GnRH agonist-induced shrinkage of small submucous fibroids which had caused tubal obstruction. This is a relatively unusual situation and one in which hysteroscopic myomectomy may offer a more long-term solution in skilled hands. Currently, it is not clear whether medical therapies have a role in the management of younger women with larger symptomatic fibroids who wish to preserve their reproductive function but to delay childbearing. Here, early myomectomy may not be desirable because of the risk of recurrence of fibroids and the need for a second operation. In theory, interim therapy with a GnRH analogue, either alone or in combination, may control symptoms and prevent further significant enlargement of the fibroids, enabling surgery to be delayed. It is not clear whether such therapy would inhibit the initiation of new lesions or simply mask their presence, making early recurrences more prevalent.

GnRH antagonists

The antagonist analogues directly inhibit the action of GnRH on the pituitary, resulting in immediate gonadal suppression and avoidance of the stimulatory phase seen with the agonists. As yet they are not widely available for clinical use but a preliminary study (Kettel et al 1993) with one antagonist, given by daily subcutaneous injection, demonstrated a rapid reduction in uterine volume. The overall shrinkage was equivalent to that seen with agonists but was more rapidly achieved and with immediate onset of amenorrhoea.

Antiprogesterones

There have been recent reports (Reinsch et al 1994) of shrinkage of uterine fibroids in response to continuous therapy with the antiprogesterone RU486, mifepristone, given continuously at a dose of 25–50 mg daily. Shrinkage is similar to that observed during therapy with a GnRH agonist and associated with amenorrhoea but less profound oestrogen suppression, levels being maintained in the early to mid-follicular phase range. Although preliminary, these results may indicate an exciting new approach to the medical management of uterine fibroids.

RESULTS OF TREATMENT

Assessment of the results of treatment of uterine fibroids must take into consideration the effectiveness of cure of the presenting symptoms, the duration of relief, the need for further treatment, particularly surgery, and the morbidity of the treatment method itself. In particular, in those women presenting with infertility or pregnancy loss or where future fertility is desired, the results must be measured in terms of the number and the outcome of any subsequent pregnancies. While hysterectomy gives the best results in terms of symptomatic cure, this will be inappropriate for women wishing to preserve reproductive potential and thus the outcome only of the conservative methods of treatment will be considered here.

Results of myomectomy

In a comprehensive review of 18 studies, Buttram & Reiter (1981) quoted a 40% conception rate among 1202 women who were desirous of pregnancy. In a review of the subsequent literature, Verkauf (1992) reported that out of 79 women undergoing myomectomy without any other evident cause for their subfertility, 47 (59.5%) conceived, the majority within the first year. In seven studies of 1941 myomectomies reviewed by Buttram & Reiter, the spontaneous abortion rate of 19% in 405 pregnancies which followed surgery compared favourably with a rate of 41% in the same women prior to myomectomy. This is still higher than the general population rate. The consensus of opinion favours vaginal delivery rather than elective caesarean section following myomectomy, unless the procedure has been very extensive, including opening of the cavity.

Not all women undergoing myomectomy will achieve a pregnancy or even attempt to do so and it is also important to consider the degree and duration of relief of symptoms, such as menorrhagia, which may have precipitated the decision to perform surgery. Of 285 women in the review of Buttram & Reiter who complained of heavy menstrual loss, relief was reported in 230 (81%). The recurrence rate of fibroids in these series was 15% for the 2554 women for whom follow-up data were available. Overall, 10% of the women required further pelvic surgery, usually hysterectomy, for recurrent or continuing symptoms following myomectomy. In a more recent review of 622 patients by Candiani et al (1991), the 10-year recurrence rate was as high as 27%, the outcome being more favourable for those who achieved a pregnancy compared with those who did not. These figures justify a conservative approach in selected cases.

Hysteroscopic methods

Information about the outcome of treatment to date is based on a small number of specialized centres. However preliminary data are encouraging. Siegler & Valle (1988) reviewed reports of 371 women treated by hysteroscopic myomectomy for abnormal bleeding, quoting an immediate cure rate of 97% and a recurrence rate of 6%, although duration of follow up was variable and not specified. In a later series of 92 women treated by resectoscopic myomectomy and followed up for an average of 18 months (Corson & Brooks 1991), menorrhagia was relieved in 81% of 80 women. Of the women, 17% subsequently required a secondary surgical procedure. In a similar series of 94 cases, reported by Derman et al (1991), two of whom required laparotomy during the primary procedure, life-table analysis showed that the cumulative proportion requiring further surgery was 16% after 9 years of follow up; equivalent to that following open myomectomy.

Pregnancy rates reported after hysteroscopic treatment of fibroids in women desirous of fertility are encouragingly high at 60–70% (Verkauf, 1992) although there have been no comparisons with a nonintervention group. It is evident that such procedures are not without complication, and more information on outcome is required on the basis of longer term follow up and more widespread use. However evidence to date suggests that such methods have a potentially useful role in the management of women with submucous fibroids.

GnRH agonists

At present, it is only possible to comment on the results of treatment with GnRH agonist analogues although the antagonists are likely to give rise to similar or improved results in the future. Randomized controlled studies (see reviews by Friedman 1993, West 1993) have demonstrated that treatment with a GnRH analogue prior to hysterectomy results in significant improvements in preoperative haemoglobin concentrations as well as reduced operative blood loss and fewer blood transfusions. Particular benefits for the patients are greater use of low transverse rather than midline surgical incisions and of the vaginal rather than the abdominal route. Reduced blood loss at myomectomy has also been reported in cases where initial uterine volume exceeded 600 ml, but there is no evidence that pregnancy rates are improved following pretreatment. Benefits for hysteroscopic myomectomy have been confirmed in non-randomized studies (Perino et al 1993) with significant reductions in operating time, blood loss and in the volume of distension medium infused.

Specific complications may be associated with the use of GnRH agonists for fibroids (see review, West 1993). Failure of menstrual suppression, with continued irregular bleeding, occurs in 20–30% of women. This may be related to the presence of submucosal fibroids and several cases of acute prolapse associated with severe haemorrhage have been reported. Opponents of the use of GnRH agonists argue that this delays the achievement of a definitive tissue diagnosis and thus cases of uterine sarcoma (see p. 454) may be missed. Such cases are extremely rare but their reported occurrence does emphasize the need to adequately monitor the response to medical therapy of women with known fibroids, and to consider further investigation or surgical intervention should symptoms not respond adequately and promptly.

The use of GnRH analogues as adjuncts to surgery thus remains a subject of debate. Few countries have granted product licences as yet for fibroid-related indications, and there is agreement that the additional costs do not justify their routine use. Specific indications would include severe preoperative anaemia, to facilitate vaginal hysterectomy and for preoperative shrinkage of particularly large or awkwardly situated fibroids. For myomectomy, opinions vary, and in the absence of large randomized studies with long-term follow up, gynaecologists must weigh up the merits of such therapy for their individual patients. As an adjunct to endoscopic myomectomy, the current consensus is in favour of their use.

COMPLICATIONS

The complications of uterine fibroids are in part dependent on their site of origin and their size, as discussed on pp. 441–2. For example, torsion is a rare complication of pedunculated subserous fibroids while submucous fibroids may prolapse through the cervix, causing ulceration and infection. The latter is a reported complication following initiation of therapy with a GnRH analogue, where the acute withdrawal of oestrogen may cause degeneration and prolapse (see above). Large fibroids arising from the cervix may cause ureteric compression or retention of urine.

Because fibroids are so frequently asymptomatic, especially if small, most of the presenting symptoms described in detail on pp. 444–5 might be regarded as complications rather than an inevitable consequence of their presence, for example menorrhagia, infertility and pregnancy loss. Degenerative changes occur so frequently that they are not usually regarded as a complication, although degeneration occasionally presents with acute pain, particularly in pregnancy. This section will cover the other complications, although they may in most cases be the prime reason for the presentation.

Pregnancy complications

It is usually stated that fibroids increase in size during pregnancy and shrink during the puerperium, although this has not been the finding of recent studies (Aharoni et al 1988) based on serial monitoring by ultrasound (Fig. 29.15). While many pregnancies associated with fibroids proceed uneventfully, there is an increased risk of spontaneous abortion and preterm labour. Pregnancies accompanied by uterine fibroids should therefore be treated as high-risk.

These problems may be in part related to abnormalities of uterine contractility, and in particular to alterations in blood flow with the fibroids being relatively hypovascular in comparison to the surrounding myometrium. Degenerative changes appear to be very common, in particular the painful red degeneration which is typically associated with pregnancy (Fig. 29.16). Its recognition is important in order to avoid confusion with other acute intra-abdominal conditions and treatment is always conservative, with rest and analgesia. Although rare, torsion of a pedunculated subserous fibroid is more likely to occur in pregnancy and this is the only situation in which removal of a fibroid from the pregnant uterus is ever justified.

Mechanical difficulties due to the site of the fibroids may be encountered during labour and fibroids may be associated with malpresentation of the fetus. If caesarean

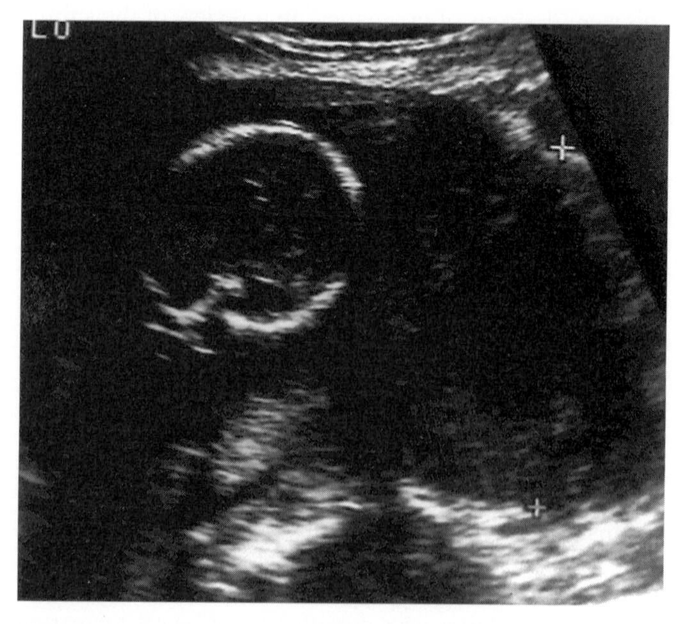

Fig. 29.15 Pregnancy (20 weeks) with lateral fibroid showing degenerative changes. Serial ultrasound measurements showed no change in volume. (Courtesy of Dr B. Muir.)

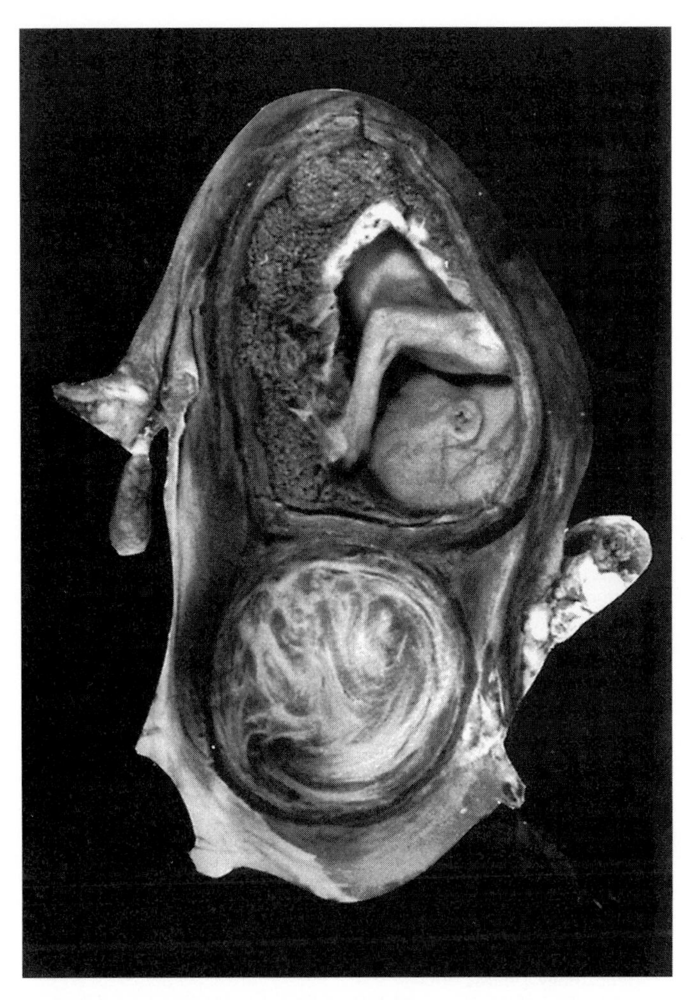

Fig. 29.16 Pregnancy (20 weeks) complicated by painful red degeneration of fibroid (museum specimen).

section is required, it is unwise to attempt myomectomy because of the associated vascularity of the procedure. Caesarean hysterectomy may be considered if there are multiple fibroids and the woman has completed her family but the operative morbidity is greatly increased and this procedure would in general be reserved for the emergency situation.

Sarcomatous change

The risk of sarcomatous degeneration is a potentially lethal but uncommon complication of uterine fibroids. Leiomyosarcoma does not inevitably originate in a fibroid uterus and must not be confused with other forms of uterine sarcoma which are totally unrelated to fibroids. Both Corscaden & Singh (1958) and Buttram & Reiter (1981) estimated the risk of sarcomatous change as being in the order of 0.1% based on the recorded incidence of fibroids in their study populations. Thus, as many cases of fibroids are not diagnosed, even this figure may be an overestimate. Recognition of this complication is nevertheless imperative. Current imaging techniques may not detect sarcomatous degeneration and thus a high index of clinical suspicion is essential. The majority of cases are symptomatic (Corscaden & Singh 1958, Schwartz et al 1993), with pain, malaise and vaginal bleeding. Rapid enlargement is another suspicious feature and any of these symptoms in a postmenopausal woman should be taken very seriously, particularly as the complication is commoner following the menopause.

Haematological complications

Anaemia secondary to menorrhagia is mentioned above, and is more commonly seen in association with fibroids than with menorrhagia due to other causes. In some cases, symptoms of anaemia may be the main presenting feature and the woman may only admit to heavy menstrual blood loss on careful questioning. Paradoxically, fibroids may be associated with polycythaemia (see Weiss et al 1975). This is attributed to erythropoietin production by the fibroids and resolves after their surgical removal.

Other unusual complications

Ascites has been described in association with parasitic fibroids which have lost their attachment to the uterus and developed an alternative blood supply from the omentum. This may be related to obstruction of omental blood vessels. Intravenous leiomyomatosis is another rare complication of apparently benign fibroids, and metastatic lesions have been described in the peritoneal cavity and also in distant sites, such as apparently benign pulmonary lesions (Clark & Weed 1977). However there is debate about the histological nature of some of these unusual lesions.

KEY POINTS

1. Uterine fibroids are common, benign tumours of the uterus affecting approximately 20% of women of reproductive age.
2. Uterine fibroids are more common in black women in whom they present at an earlier age.
3. Many cells within the fibroid are chromosomally abnormal, which may result in their abnormal cell division.
4. Uterine fibroids seem to be hormone-sensitive. They do not occur until the menarche and reduce in size at the menopause. Progesterones may play a major role in fibroid growth.
5. Fibroids may undergo hyaline or fatty degeneration, calcification, red degeneration (usually in pregnancy) and rarely sarcomatous change.
6. Fibroids may adversely affect reproductive function by

largement and distortion of the uterus and disturbance of uterine blood flow.

7. Asymptomatic fibroids may be managed conservatively without harmful effects, with regression at the time of menopause to be expected.
8. Medical management of fibroids may control patient symptoms but does not result in complete fibroid regression.
9. GnRH analogues may be used to shrink fibroids prior to surgery, be it hysterectomy or myomectomy.
10. Myomectomy is a potentially dangerous operation which should be reserved for women who need to preserve their reproductive function.
11. When using GnRH analogues to limit or shrink fibroid growth, the vasomotor and osteoporotic side-effects may be reduced by addition of hormone replacement therapy.
12. Hysteroscopic and laparoscopic management of fibroids can provide good symptomatic relief and may reduce postoperative morbidity. The gynaecologist should undergo adequate training before embarking on such procedures.
13. Myomectomy may result in conception in women who were previously infertile. The spontaneous abortion rate is reduced but remains above that of the general population.

REFERENCES

Aharoni A, Reiter A, Golan D, Paltiely Y, Sharf M 1988 Patterns of growth of uterine leiomyomas during pregnancy. A prospective longitudinal study. British Journal of Obstetrics and Gynaecology 95: 510–513

Buttram V C, Reiter R C 1981 Uterine leiomyomata: etiology, symptomatology and management. Fertility and Sterility 36: 433–445

Candiani G B, Fedele L, Parazzini F, Villa L 1991 Risk of recurrence after myomectomy. British Journal of Obstetrics and Gynaecology 98: 385–389

Clark D H, Weed J C 1977 Metastasizing leiomyomas: a case report. Americal Journal of Obstetrics and Gynecology 127: 672–673

Corscaden J A, Singh B P 1958 Leiomyosarcoma of the uterus. American Journal of Obstetrics and Gynecology 75: 149–153

Corson S L, Brooks P G 1991 Resectoscopic myomectomy. Fertility and Sterility 55: 1041–1044

Derman S G, Rehnstrom J, Neuwirth R S 1991 The long term effectiveness of hysteroscopic treatment of menorrhagia and leiomyomas. Obstetrics and Gynecology 77: 591–594

Donnez J, Gillerot S, Bougonjon D, Clerckx F, Nisolle M 1990 Neodymium:YAG laser hysteroscopy in large submucous fibroids. Fertility and Sterility 54: 999–1003

Drews M R, Reyniak J V 1992 Surgical approach to myomas: laparoscopy and hysteroscopy. Seminars in Reproductive Endocrinology 10: 367–377

Farrer-Brown G, Beilby J O W, Tarbit M H 1971 Venous changes in the endometrium of myomatous uteri. Obstetrics and Gynecology 38: 743–751

Filicori M, Hall D A, Loughlin J S, Rivier J, Vale W, Crowley W F 1983 A conservative approach to the management of uterine leiomyomata: pituitary desensitisation by a luteinizing hormone-releasing hormone analogue. American Journal of Obstetrics and Gynecology 147: 726–727

Forssman L 1976 Distribution of blood flow in myomatous uteri as measured by locally injected 133 xenon. Acta Obstetrica et Gynecologica Scandinavica 55: 101–104

Friedman A J 1993 Treatment of uterine myomas with GnRH agonists. Seminars in Reproductive Endocrinology 11: 154–161

Karasick S, Lev-Toaff A S, Toaff M E 1992 Imaging of uterine leiomyomas. American Journal of Roentgenology 158: 799–805

Kettel L M, Murphy A A, Morales A J, Rivier J, Vale W, Yen S S C 1993 Rapid regression of leiomyomas in response to daily administration of gonadotrophin releasing hormone antagonist. Fertility and Sterility 60: 642–646

Koutsilieris M 1992 Pathophysiology of uterine leiomyomas. Biochemistry and Cell Biology 70: 273–278

Matta W H, Stabile I, Shaw R W, Campbell S 1988 Doppler assessment of uterine blood flow changes in patients with fibroids receiving the gonadotrophin releasing hormone agonist buserelin. British Journal of Obstetrics and Gynaecology 96: 200–206

Monaghan J M (ed) 1986 Bonney's gynaecological surgery, 9th edn. Baillière Tindall, London

Murphy A A, Kettel L M, Morales A J, Roberts V J, Yen S S C 1993 Regression of uterine leiomyomata in response to the antiprogesterone R U 486. Journal of Clinical Endocrinology and Metabolism 76: 513–517

Nilsson L, Rybo G 1971 Treatment of menorrhagia. American Journal of Obstetrics and Gynecology 110: 713–720

Perino A, Chianchiano N, Petronio M, Cittadini E 1993 Role of leuprolide acetate depot in hysteroscopic surgery: a controlled study. Fertility and Sterility 59: 507–510

Rein M S, Novak R A 1992 Biology of uterine myomas and myometrium in vitro. Seminars in Reproductive Endocrinology 10: 310–319

Reinsch R C, Murphy A A, Morales A J, Yen S S C 1994 The effects of RU 486 and leuprolide acetate on uterine artery blood flow in the fibroid uterus: a prospective, randomised study. American Journal of Obstetrics and Gynecology 170: 1623–1628

Reiter R C, Wagner P L G, Ambone J C 1992 Routine hysterectomy for asymptomatic uterine fibroids: a reappraisal. Obstetrics and Gynecology 79: 481–484

Ross R K, Pike M C, Vessey M P, Bull D, Yeates D, Casagrande J T 1986 Risk factors for uterine fibroids: reduced risk associated with oral contraceptives. British Medical Journal 293: 359–362

Rybo G, Leman J, Tibblin R 1985 Epidemiology of menstrual blood loss. In: Baird D T, Michie E A (eds) Mechanisms of menstrual bleeding. Raven Press, New York, pp 181–193

Schwartz L B, Diamond M P, Schwartz P E 1993 Leiomyosarcoma – clinical presentation. American Journal of Obstetrics and Gynecology 168: 180–183

Siegler A M, Valle R F 1988 Therapeutic hysteroscopic procedures. Fertility and Sterility 50: 685-701

Townsend D E, Sparkes R S, Baluda M C, McClelland G 1970 Unicellular histogenesis of uterine leiomyomas as determined by electrophoresis of glucose-6-phosphate dehydrogenase. American Journal of Obstetrics and Gynecology 107: 1168–1173

Van-Eijkeren M A, Christiaens G C M L, Scholten N, Sixma J J 1992 Menorrhagia. Current concepts. Drugs 43: 201–209

Verkauf B S 1992 Myomectomy for fertility enhancement and preservation. Fertility and Sterility 58: 1–15

Weinreb J C, Barkoff N D, Megibow A, Demopoulos R 1990 The value of MR imaging in distinguishing leiomyomas from other solid pelvic masses when sonography is indeterminate. American Journal of Roentgenology 154: 295–299

Weiss D B, Aldor A, Aboulafia Y 1975 Erythrocytosis due to erythropoietin-producing uterine fibromyoma. American Journal of Obstetrics and Gynecology 122: 358–360

West C P 1993 GnRH analogues in the treatment of fibroids. Reproductive Medicine Reviews 2: 1–97

West C P, Lumsden M A 1989 Fibroids and menorrhagia. Baillière's Clinical Obstetrics and Gynaecology 3: 357–374

Witherspoon J T 1935 The hormonal origin of uterine fibroids: an hypothesis. American Journal of Cancer 24: 402–406

30

Endometriosis

R. W. Shaw

INTRODUCTION

Endometriosis is one of the commonest benign gynaecological conditions. It has been estimated that it is present in between 10 and 25% of women presenting with gynaecological symptoms in the UK and the USA (Tyson 1974). These figures are based on the findings of patients who have undergone laparoscopy for diagnostic indications, e.g. pelvic pain or infertility, or patients undergoing laparotomy. Although it is such a widespread condition, little is understood with regard to its aetiology and pathogenesis and the condition still arouses much interest and controversy with regard to its diagnosis, treatment and management.

Definition

Endometriosis may be defined as a disease characterized by the presence of functional endometrial glands and stroma in ectopic locations outside the uterine cavity. The ectopic endometrial tissue responds to hormones and drugs in a similar manner to eutopic endometrium.

Endometrial tissue deep within the myometrium, a condition termed adenomyosis, is increasingly being viewed as a separate pathological entity affecting a different population and with a probable different aetiology.

Prevalence

Continued growth of endometriotic tissue, as with that of the endometrium, is dependent upon oestrogen. Thus endometriosis is prevalent in the reproductive years with a peak incidence between 30 and 45 years of age, although it is increasingly being diagnosed in much younger women. There have been published reports of endometriosis in postmenopausal women where it has been reactivated because of hormone replacement therapy or endogenous sex hormones produced by the ovarian stroma. The apparent increase in the disorder in recent decades stems from more widespread use of laparoscopy in gynaecological practice, particularly in infertile women (in whom the disorder may otherwise be asymptomatic) or for the investigation of pelvic pain.

Endometriosis commonly affects women during their child-bearing years. In the main this is reflected in deleterious sexual, reproductive and social consequences as a result of its associated painful symptoms and often infertility. This may extend over several decades of a patient's life, because of its often late diagnosis and the recurrent nature of the disease.

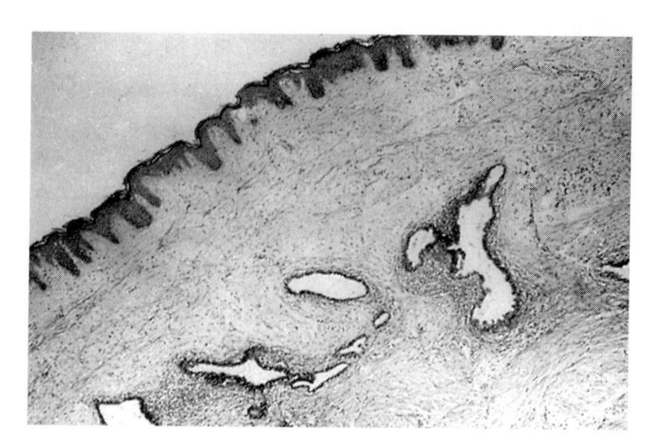

Fig. 30.1 Biopsy of deposit of endometriosis in anterior abdominal wall showing glandular elements beneath the skin (× 40). From Shaw & Marshall (1989) with permission.

PATHOGENESIS AND PATHOPHYSIOLOGY

Endometriosis can be accurately diagnosed by careful visual inspection of the pelvis. Histological confirmation is not mandatory for clinical decision-making but it is helpful if there is uncertainty about the diagnosis, and possibly where there is recurrent disease.

Histology

To make the diagnosis of endometriosis categorically, pathologists require the presence of glands, stroma and evidence of menstrual cyclicity, with tissue haemorrhage or haemosiderin-laden macrophages. The endometriotic deposits rarely have a microscopic appearance or architecture identical to normal endometrium in situ and implants can be composed of isolated scattered glandular and stromal components rather than exact replication of the eutopic uterine endometrial architecture.

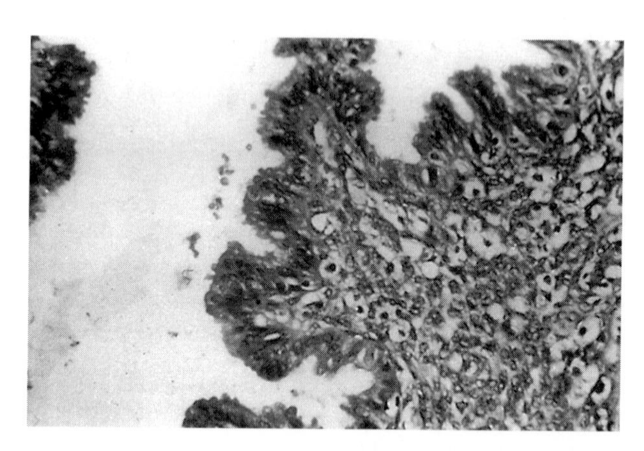

Fig. 30.2 High-power picture of biopsy from endometrial deposit demonstrating glandular structure and macrophages with lipid and haemosiderin accumulation (× 100). From Shaw & Marshall (1989) with permission.

Peritoneal deposits

The morphological characteristics of peritonal endometriosis are quite varied. The lesion is considered active when there is typical glandular epithelium and active proliferation, or if in the latter part of the menstrual cycle there is some secretory change. Some deposits have areas of oviduct-like epithelium with ciliated cells in association with endometriotic foci. Brown or black coloration of deposits is a function of the amounts of intraluminal debris and haemosiderin. The black pigmented stigmas compose the usual visual criteria for diagnosis of endometriosis and are the late consequence of the cyclical growth and regression of the lesions to the point where tissue bleeding and discoloration by blood pigment have taken place (Figs 30.1–30.3).

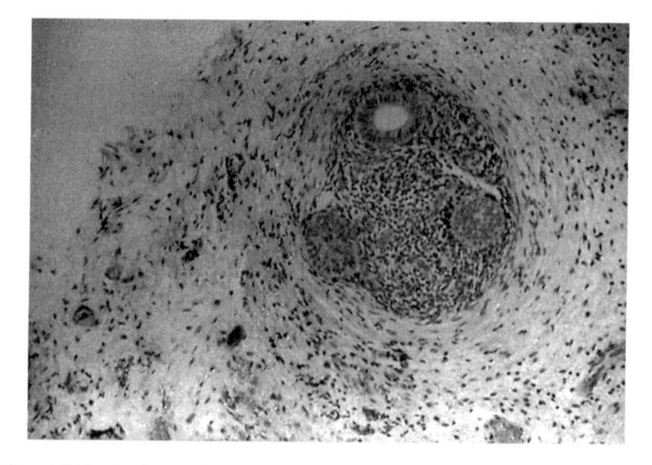

Fig. 30.3 Active endometriosis with glandular and stromal components in a biopsy specimen from a lesion on the uterosacral ligament.

Ovarian deposits

Superficial implants of endometriosis in the ovary resemble implants at other peritoneal sites; in contrast, however, the texture and structure of large endometriotic cysts or endometrial cells which have entered the ovarian stroma, are quite different.

Endometriotic cysts (endometriomas) are often termed 'chocolate cysts' and are filled with a viscous chocolate-coloured liquid, representing debris from cyclical menstruation. Such cysts usually have a well demarcated separation between the cyst wall and the normal adjacent ovarian stroma. The epithelial lining of the endometrioma may resemble the endometrium, but with continued menstrual bleeding without drainage the epithelium becomes flattened and cuboidal without specific distinguishing features, perhaps due to pressure atrophy (Fig. 30.4).

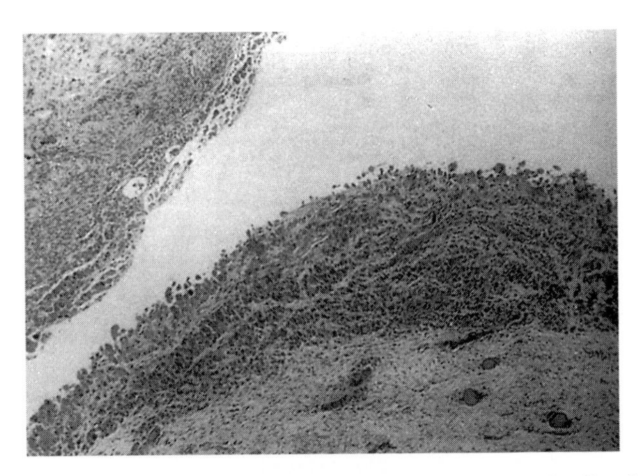

Fig. 30.4 Wall of an endometrial chocolate cyst with extensive fibrosis and haemorrhage but no recognizable endometrial glands or stroma.

Ultrastructure

Endometriotic implants do not demonstrate the characteristic ultrastructural changes of the normal endometrium, although the microscopic changes present in endometrium have been observed in ectopic implants. In some individuals there is no evidence of secretory change in deposits; even when these do develop they may not be synchronous with those of the uterine endometrium. The reasons for this probably relate to a deficiency of steroid receptors within the endometriotic tissue and the influence of surrounding scar tissue formation, pressure atrophy and the hormonal independence of the ectopic endometrial glands (Fig. 30.5a,b,c).

AETIOLOGY

The precise aetiology of endometriosis still remains un-

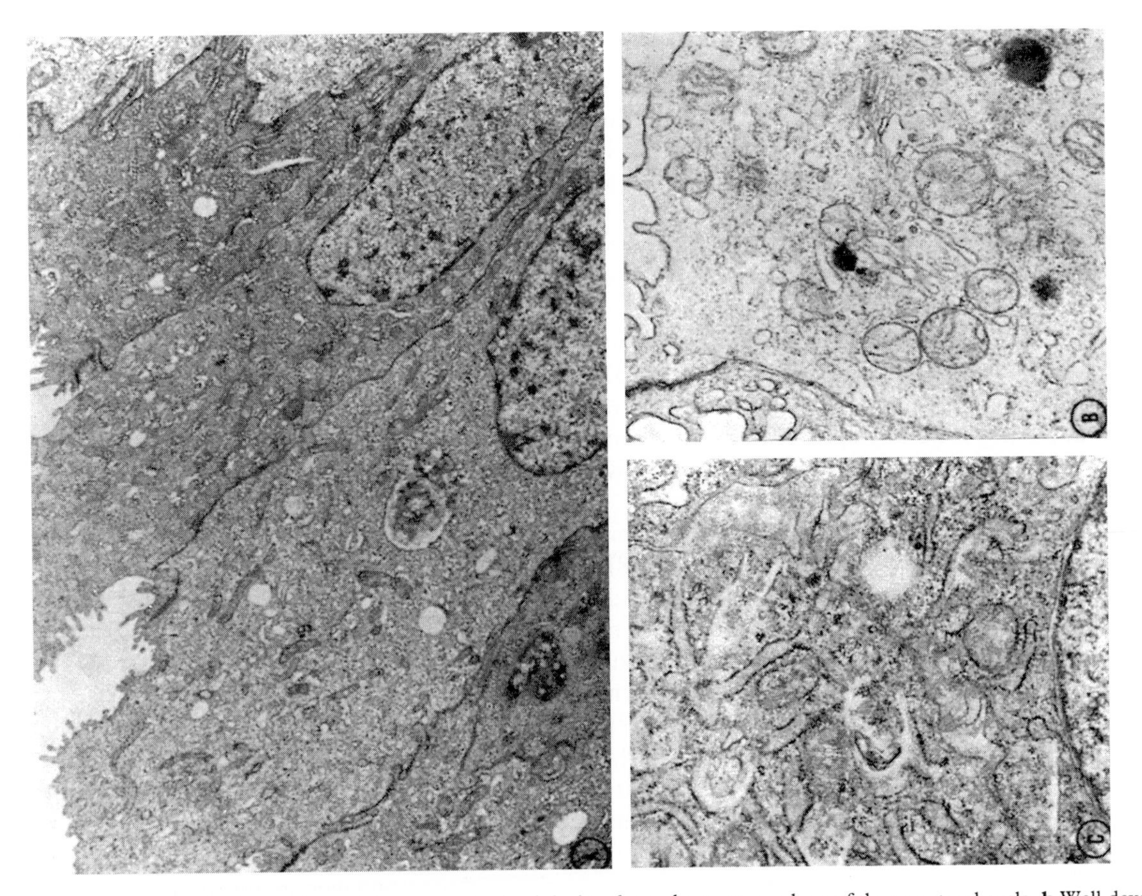

Fig. 30.5 **a** Electron micrograph of an endometrial implant obtained during the early secretory phase of the menstrual cycle. **b** Well developed mitochondria, prominent Golgi apparatus, and **c** abundant endoplasmic reticulum are apparent in the higher power views. From Schweppe et al (1984) with permission.

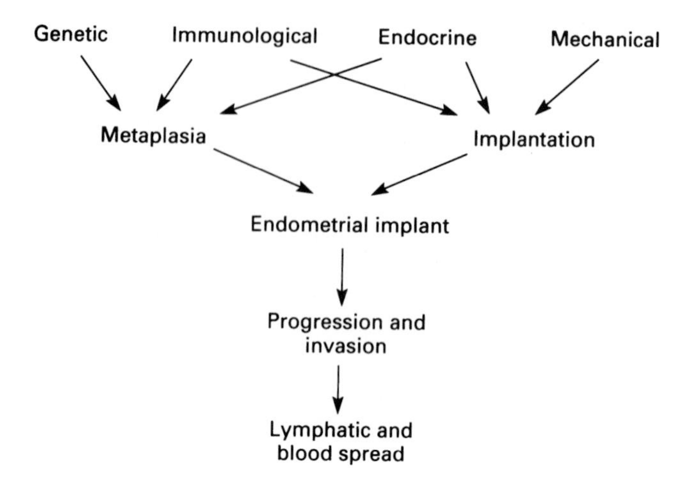

Fig. 30.6 Suggested aetiological factors in the pathogenesis of endometriotic implants.

known. Indeed it is often called the 'disease of theories' because of the many postulated mechanisms utilized to explain its pathogenesis (Fig. 30.6). It is likely that no one of these theories would explain all forms of endometriosis.

Metastatic theory

As early as 1940 Sampson proposed a metastatic theory postulating that retrograde menstrual flow transported desquamated endometrial fragments through the fallopian tubes into the peritoneal cavity. Once there the still viable cells subsequently implanted and began growth and invasion. In support of this theory experimental endometriosis has been induced in animals with the replacement of menstrual fluid or endometrial tissue in the peritoneal cavity. In young girls endometriosis has been described associated with abnormalities in the genital tract causing obstruction to the outflow of menstrual fluid (Schifrin et al 1973). Halme et al (1984) observed bloody fluid at the time of menstruation in the pelvis during laparoscopic assessment but as this occurs in up to 90% of all women in this study, it has been regarded as a physiological phenomenon.

Additional support for the metastatic theory came from the observation of Kirshon & Poindexter (1988). This showed a high risk of endometriosis in patients with an increased retrograde blood flow, in this study due to the use of intrauterine devices for contraception. On the other hand, the presence of viable glands and stroma in the peritoneal fluid does not necessarily lead to the development of endometriosis as other factors, probably in the peritoneal environment, must additionally be present to allow the tissue particles to implant and grow. Further support of the metastatic theory is the observation of endometriotic foci in laparotomy scars after caesarean section, or episiotomy scars following delivery. In addition, lymphatic vascular spread is postulated to explain the presence of endometriosis in extragenital locations such as the lung or skeletal muscle (Javert 1949).

Metaplasia theory

This theory, first described by Meyer (1919), postulated the possibility of differentiation by metaplasia of the original coelomic membrane with prolonged irritation or oestrogen stimulation towards endometrial-like tissue. It is proposed that these adult cells undergo de-differentiation back to their primitive origin and then transform to endometrial cells. This is an attractive theory which could explain the occurrence of endometriosis in nearly all the ectopic sites in the presence of aberrant müllerian cells. What induces the transformation – whether it be hormonal stimuli, inflammatory irritation or other processes – is uncertain.

Conclusion

The conclusion reached from the above theories is that pelvic endometriosis is probably a consequence of transplantation of viable endometrial cells regurgitated at the time of menstruation from the fallopian tubes into the peritoneal cavity. In addition transport of endometrial cells may occur by other routes, but some sites of endometriosis can only be explained by the metaplasia theory.

It is still unclear whether endometriotic implants are derived from in situ located pluripotential cells generated by metastatic seeding, but it is known that endocrine and immunological factors allow the growth and spread within the pelvis and neighbouring organs. It is presumed there may well be some genetic component in its formation since it has been shown that there is a statistically higher incidence of endometriosis encountered in first degree relatives of patients with this disorder compared to control groups (Simpson et al 1980).

PERITONEAL FLUID ENVIRONMENT IN ENDOMETRIOSIS

It has been suggested that peritoneal fluid volume and its contents may be adversely affected by the presence of endometriotic tissue in the pelvis, with possible consequent interference with tubo-ovarian function and/or fertilization and early implantation.

Peritoneal macrophages

The role of peritoneal macrophages in women with endometriosis has been the source of much interest in recent years. Women with endometriosis associated with infertility have been found to have significantly higher concentrations of macrophages in the peritoneal fluid than either fertile or infertile women without endometriosis (Haney et al 1981). An increased number of peritoneal fluid macrophages have also been reported in women with non-mechanical causes for infertility (Olive et al 1985). These macrophages in patients with endometriosis appear to be highly phagocytic against spermatozoa in vitro, compared with those from fertile women or infertile women without endometriosis (Muscato et al 1982). In addition they are also able to survive better in vitro than those from fertile controls (Halme et al 1986). Peritoneal fluid from patients with endometriosis has also been shown to have a cytotoxic effect on in vivo cleavage of mouse embryos. These findings on the quantitative and qualitative properties of macrophages in peritoneal fluid may explain a mechanism of infertility in patients with endometriosis.

Prostaglandins and prostanoids

The role of prostaglandins and their metabolites in peritoneal fluid in the pathogenesis and symptomatology of endometriosis is controversial. It has been reported that increased levels of prostaglandin $F_{2\alpha}$ ($PGF_{2\alpha}$) are found in peritoneal fluid of patients with endometriosis (Meldrum et al 1977); also increased peritoneal fluid volume and increased concentrations of the prostaglandin metabolites thromboxane B_2 and 6-keto $PGF_{2\alpha}$ have been noted. Other investigators have found no increase in either the volume of peritoneal fluid or its concentrations of PGE, $PGF_{2\alpha}$ or metabolites (Rock et al 1982). Conflicting reports may reflect the timing of peritoneal fluid sampling and the quality control of assay systems.

It has been appreciated in recent years that more subtle forms of endometriosis may be present with only minimal evidence of visual changes in the peritoneum. However, if there are changes in the peritoneal fluid prostaglandin content, the mechanism by which these changes influence endometriosis or its association with infertility remains unclear. Increased secretion of $PGF_{2\alpha}$ from endometriotic implants is thought to be the probable main cause of dysmenorrhoea, commonly associated with the disease, and this is supported by the fact that prostaglandin synthetase inhibitors may often be useful in alleviating this symptom.

Peritoneal environment: conclusions

Peritoneal macrophages play an important role in the intra-abdominal environment where endometrial tissue fragments often arrive within the peritoneal cavity and are likely to adhere to the mesothelial lining. The adherence may be mediated by cell adhesion molecules and other factors produced by activated macrophages. Endometrial tissue will potentially adhere if the regurgitated amount of tissue is too great or if the capacity of the intra-abdominal cells to clear the cellular debris is in any way impaired. Once adherent, endometrial tissue growth is promoted by steroids, growth factors and angiogenic factors present in peritoneal fluid in a paracrine and autocrine fashion.

SYMPTOMATOLOGY

Pain is perhaps the cardinal symptom of endometriosis. Various types of pain are associated with the disease; dysmenorrhoea, deep dyspareunia and pelvic pain unrelated to intercourse or menstruation. Infertility is another commonly associated complaint. The frequency of the more common symptoms in endometriosis patients are summarized from a number of reviews in Table 30.1. This reveals that dysmenorrhoea is the commonest presenting symptom, closely followed by pelvic pain, infertility and dyspareunia.

Atypical bleeding patterns are a leading symptom in a variety of gynaecological diseases but may also characterize endometriosis patients. Premenstrual spotting and menometrorrhagia are frequently noted (Wentz 1980). On the other hand cyclical rectal bleeding or haematuria are pathognomonic of the disease and although rarely observed (1–2% of cases), these symptoms give strong evidence for bowel or bladder involvement. Painful micturition or defecation at the time of menstruation may be the first signs of progressing disease. Symptoms of endometriosis related to the sites of implants are outlined in Table 30.2.

Table 30.1 Frequency of the more common symptoms in endometriosis patients

Symptom	Likely frequency (%)
Dysmenorrhoea	60–80
Pelvic pain	30–50
Infertility	30–40
Dyspareunia	25–40
Menstrual irregularities	10–20
Cyclical dysuria/haematuria	1–2
Dyschesia	1–2
Rectal bleeding (cyclic)	< 1

Table 30.2 Symptoms of endometriosis related to sites of implants

Symptoms	Site
Dysmenorrhoea Lower abdominal pain Pelvic pain Low back pain Menstrual irregularity Rupture/torsion endometrioma Infertility	Reproductive organs
Cyclical rectal bleeding Tenesmus Diarrhoea/cyclic constipation	Gastrointestinal tract
Cyclical haematuria Dysuria (cyclical) Ureteric obstruction	Urinary tract
Cyclical haemoptysis	Lungs
Cyclical pain and bleeding	Surgical scars/umbilicus
Cyclical pain and swelling	Limbs

Pelvic pain

Pelvic pain is arguably the symptom causing the most misery amongst endometriosis sufferers and is more distressing than infertility. Chronic pelvic pain, as with other forms of pain, often produces a serious long-term detrimental effect on the personality and affects working ability and social and marital life.

Dysmenorrhoea

Dysmenorrhoea often occurs with pelvic pain but patients commonly describe a background of constant dragging, aching pain which may be exacerbated by the menses but is often a different type of pain from the typical cramping nature of spasmodic dysmenorrhoea and often in a different site.

The basis of the pelvic pain and dysmenorrhoea is uncertain but could reflect stretching of tissues by the menstrual process and an effect of the local production of prostaglandins within the endometriotic implants. The pain also relates to tissue damage and fixity of organs from scar and adhesion formation. What is immediately clear when reviewing patients with endometriosis, is the huge variation in extent of symptomatic disease which does not correlate with the extent of the observed disease process. In addition many patients who are asymptomatic are found to have endometriosis, and in some of these patients severe disease is discovered following laparoscopy during infertility investigations. One possible explanation for this is that in these individuals the disease may have disrupted the pelvic sensation altogether.

Dyspareunia

One of the common symptoms of endometriosis is deep dyspareunia resulting from stretching at intercourse of the involved pelvic tissues such as a fixed retroverted uterus, the uterosacral ligaments or rectovaginal septum, or pressure on an involved enlarged ovary. The presence of endometriotic tissue within these areas however is not always associated with dyspareunia; perhaps less than half the patients who are coitally active admit to this symptom when deposits are found in these areas.

Whilst the symptoms of dysmenorrhoea, dyspareunia and pelvic pain can occur with other gynaecological pathologies, it is the cyclical, menstrually related component of several symptoms which should alert the clinician to the potential diagnosis of endometriosis.

Correlation between severity of endometriosis and severity of pain

There appears to be little correlation between sites involved in endometriosis and symptoms complained of. Various 'types' of symptoms can, however, to some degree be related to the system involved (see Table 30.2). However these do not always correlate with the sites of deposits, and reasons for this may be multiple and partially associated with the anatomy and type of pain innervation of the pelvis. (For review, see MacLaverty & Shaw 1995).

One reason for this apparent lack of correlation between disease severity and symptom severity is that the classification systems for endometriosis so far developed have primarily been directed towards infertility prediction rather than pain symptom severity.

Deeply infiltrating endometriosis is very strongly associated with the presence and severity of pelvic pain (Koninckx et al 1991). In addition superficial non-pigmented endometriosis has the capacity to produce more prostaglandin F (PGF) than pigmented classical powder burn lesions. PGF is implicated in pain causation (Vernon et al 1986). Thus in the early less florid stages before it has become destructive and more easily recognized, endometriosis may be producing large quantities of PGF and hence possess a greater potential to increase severity of pain. The type of pain may alter with the disease progression, with constant pain and exacerbation at the menses present initially in the disease, but pain later becoming continuous due to scar formation and organ fixity.

ENDOMETRIOSIS AND INFERTILITY

It is accepted that endometriosis resulting in structural damage to the tubes and ovaries causes infertility. However what is less clear is whether the milder forms of endometriosis are likewise the cause of infertility, often complained of by such patients even in the absence of other symptoms.

Endometriosis is one of the most frequently made diagnoses in couples undergoing infertility investigation, as routine use of laparoscopy for investigation of such couples has been employed in recent years. The assumption is made that the endometriotic implants are responsible for the patient's inability to conceive. Estimates of the incidence of endometriosis in the general population of reproductive age vary between 2 and 10% (Barbieri 1990); from retrospective studies in infertile patients the incidence has been reported as being between 20 and 40% (Mahmood & Templeton 1990). This increased incidence in infertile patients has led many clinicians to consider the endometriotic implants responsible in some way for the associated infertility. The question is how and a number of suggested mechanisms have been reported; these are summarized in Table 30.3.

Tubo-ovarian dysfunction

Increased levels of prostaglandins in peritoneal fluid have

Table 30.3 Possible mechanisms of causation of infertility with mild endometriosis

Problem area	Mechanism
Ovarian function	Endocrinopathies Anovulation LUF syndrome Altered prolactin release Altered gonadotrophin mid-cycle surge Luteolysis caused by $PGF_{2\alpha}$ Oocyte maturation defects
Coital function	Dyspareunia causing reduced penetration and coital frequency
Tubal function	Alterations in tubal and cilial motility by prostaglandins Impaired fimbrial oocyte pick-up
Sperm function	Phagocytosis by macrophages Inactivation by antibodies
Endometrium	Interference by endometrial antibodies Luteal phase deficiency
Early pregnancy failure	Increased early abortion Prostaglandin-induced or immune reaction

LUF, luteinized unruptured follicle; $PGF_{2\alpha}$, prostaglandin $F_{2\alpha}$.

been reported in infertile women with endometriosis (Drake et al 1981). It has been suggested that these prostaglandins may have an adverse impact on fertility by causing tubal dysfunction which could alter sperm, oocyte or embryo transport. However tubal transport of the oocyte in the distal tube is dependent primarily upon cilial action which is not known to be prostaglandin-dependent.

Elevated peritoneal prostaglandin levels have also been invoked to explain altered luteal function but again there is little evidence to suggest that prostaglandins are luteolytic in primates.

Subtle alterations in the pattern of LH surges with increased prolactin secretion which may alter luteal progesterone synthesis have also been suggested, but with little confirmatory evidence when comparable studies have been repeated in other centres.

More recently a variety of follicular phase defects have been observed in women with mild endometriosis including a range of abnormal follicular growth patterns, shortened follicular phases and decreased follicular size. Such changes may cause an alteration to the maturation of oocytes and result in reduced potential for fertilization following oocyte release. However, experiences of workers in in-vitro fertilization (IVF) have not added support that such features are likely to be relevant, since comparable fertilization rates are achieved in endometriosis patients as compared to other diagnostic groups (Chillik et al 1985).

Luteinized unruptured follicle (LUF) syndrome

Koninckx et al (1980), based upon the reports of altered peritoneal levels of gonadal steroids in the luteal phase, a lack of sonographic disappearance of the follicle at mid-cycle and an inability to visualize an ovulatory stigma during laparoscopy in the luteal phase, developed the hypothesis of the luteinized unruptured follicle (LUF) syndrome. More widespread investigation has shown that the LUF syndrome can occur in a wide variety of infertility cases and does not appear to be a consistent feature of consecutive cycles. At this present time it is concluded that LUF is unlikely to be an important contributing factor to either infertility in general or endometriosis-associated infertility specifically.

Autoimmunity

The presence of ectopic endometrial implants in women with endometriosis has been postulated to lead to an autoimmune response resulting in implantation failure. Autoantibodies to endometrial tissue have been identified in both the serum and peritoneal fluid of some women with endometriosis, although many studies have failed to show consistent differences between endometriosis patients, other infertile women or fertile controls. The absence of any differences in implantation rates between patients with endometriosis and other infertility causes in women undergoing IVF treatment, further suggests that the role of antibodies and the causal relationship between endometriosis and infertility is unlikely to be proven.

Habitual/recurrent abortion

A number of factors affect the rate of spontaneous abortion including the likelihood that infertile women document pregnancies earlier than the general population, and a relationship with increasing age. Such a relationship in endometriosis has been suggested, following the observation that treatment of endometriosis significantly reduced the spontaneous abortion rate. However further controlled prospective trials have failed to confirm these earlier findings (Pittaway et al 1988) thus bringing this relationship also into question.

Peritoneal environment

In addition to the reported change in peritoneal prostaglandin levels discussed above, it has been suggested that an increased number of macrophages in the peritoneum may increase the rate of sperm phagocytosis, and that other secretory products from activated macrophages may also have toxic effects on the gametes. This is supported by Curtis et al 1993, who reported a degree of sperm toxicity with reduced sperm motility in the presence of peritoneal fluid in patients with endometriosis compared with fertile controls and other infertility subgroups.

Mechanisms of infertility: conclusion

A variety of mechanisms have been postulated to try to relate infertility in the presence of mild endometriosis, but none have been shown to occur consistently and there is as much evidence to disprove as prove a relationship in any single case. When there is adhesion formation with the tube bound to the ovary, or the posterior surface of the ovary to the pelvic side wall, then in these circumstances the association between the presence of the endometriotic process and difficulty in conception can readily be explained. It is in such cases that appropriate treatment may be of value, but to date no trials of medical or surgical therapy of mild endometriosis have been proven to be beneficial by improving fecundity rates. (For review, see Ingamells & Thomas (1995).

DIAGNOSIS

The diagnosis of endometriosis still presents several problems, resulting from similarities in clinical symptoms to other benign or non-benign gynaecological diseases. These gynaecological symptoms may however be of diagnostic help in the suspicion of endometriosis, which should be a differential diagnosis in any patient presenting with worsening dysmenorrhoea, pelvic pain, dyspareunia or other cycle-associated symptoms related particularly to the bowel or bladder with, or without, infertility. In endometriosis the associated dysmenorrhoea extends to the pre- and postmenstrual phase and is typically secondary and progressive rather than primarily existent. Currently the only definitive way of confirming the diagnosis is visualization of deposits at laparoscopy, but other features and investigations may be helpful in justifying such a procedure.

General gynaecological examination

The general gynaecological examination may visualize endometriotic lesions as clear, red or bluish cysts or nodules in the vagina or on the cervix. Visual diagnosis is often misleading and cannot substitute for histological confirmation even if bleeding occurs from these lesions at the time of menstruation.

Pelvic examination often reveals induration of the uterosacral ligaments or nodules in the pouch of Douglas or the rectovaginal septum. Involvement of the ovaries can lead to the development of cysts which eventually become large enough to be palpated, and there may be fixation of the uterus in retroversion, with immobilization of the ovaries by adhesion formation and tenderness, particularly when examined in the premenstrual phase. These features may additionally add to the suspicion of the presence of endometriosis.

Pelvic endometriosis

Morphology of typical black lesions

The typical peritoneal endometriotic lesion is described as a 'powder burn' which results from tissue bleeding and retention of blood pigments, producing a brown/black discoloration of the tissue. In the early stages these lesions may appear more pink, red and haemorrhagic and develop into brown/black lesions with increasing time. Eventually, discoloration disappears altogether and a white plaque of old collagen is all that remains of the endometriotic implant.

Scarring in the peritoneum surrounding implants is also a typical finding. Apart from encapsulating an isolated implant, the scar tissue may deform the surrounding peritoneum, resulting in development of adhesions between adjacent pelvic structures. These adhesions are commonly found between the mobile pelvic structures, particularly the posterior leaf of the broad ligament and the ovary, and the dependent sigmoid colon and posterior aspect of the vagina and/or cervix.

Classification and morphology of subtle appearances

More recently more subtle laparoscopic appearances have been reported which were confirmed on biopsy as being due to endometriosis (Donnez & Nisolle 1991, Jansen & Russel 1986). The subtle forms are more common and may be more active, and more important than the puckered black lesions which represent the latter stages of the disease. These other peritoneal lesions include the following.

Red lesions

1. ***Red flame-like lesions*** on the peritoneum, with the appearance of red vascular excrescences in the broad ligament and uterosacral ligaments, largely due to the presence of active endometriosis surrounded by stroma.
2. ***Glandular excrescences*** which closely resemble the mucosa of the endometrium as seen at hysteroscopy; biopsy reveals the presence of numerous glandular elements.

White lesions

1. ***White opacification of the peritoneum.*** These lesions contain an occasional retroperitoneal glandular structure, scanty stroma surrounded by fibrotic tissue and connective tissue.
2. ***Yellow-brown peritoneal patches*** called 'cafe-au-lait spots', found in the cul-de-sac, broad ligament or over the bladder. Histologically they are similar to findings of white opacification; the yellow-brown patches indicate the presence of haemosiderin.

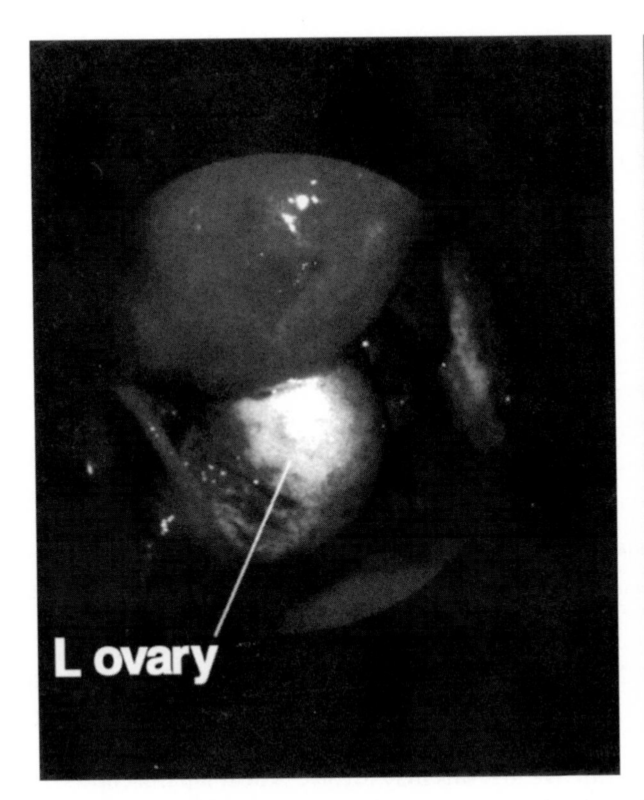

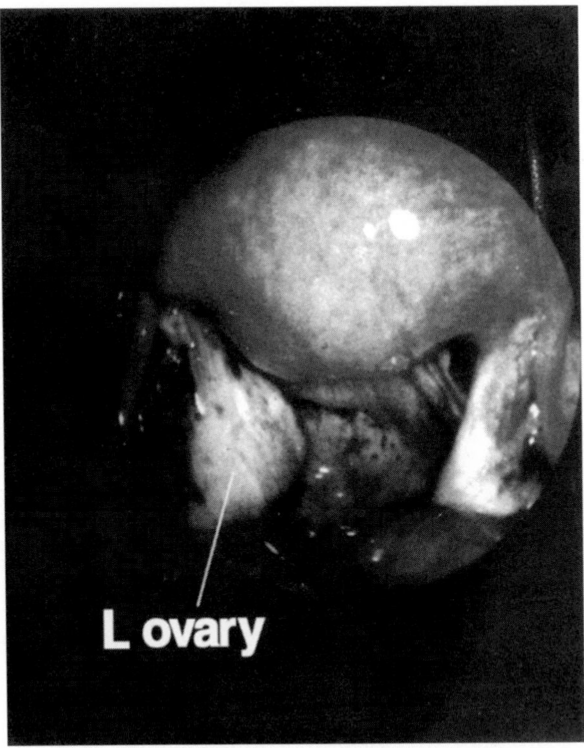

Fig. 30.7 Enlarged left ovary containing a deep-seated endometrioma **(left)** and another ovary with superficial deposits on ovarian capsule, in addition to others on the peritoneal surface in the pouch of Douglas (**right**).

3. ***Circular peritoneal defects*** of the pelvic peritoneum, uterosacral ligaments or broad ligament. Serial section has demonstrated the presence of endometrial glands in about 50% of these structures.

From the above it is clear that careful laparoscopy by an experienced surgeon is essential if cases are not to be missed. Whenever there is any doubt, the need for biopsy confirmation is apparent.

Ovarian endometriosis

The ovary represents a unique site for implantation as levels of gonadal steroids are several times higher than those in the general circulation or peritoneal cavity (see Figs 30.7 and 30.8).

Superficial endometriosis

Superficial implants on the ovary resemble implants in other peritoneal sites. Comparable features are typical black, red or white lesions as outlined above.

Subovarian adhesions

Subovarian adhesions may be condensed in the peritoneum of the ovarian fossa, which are distinctive from adhesions characteristic of previous salpingitis or peritonitis; this connective tissue often contains sparse endometrial glands.

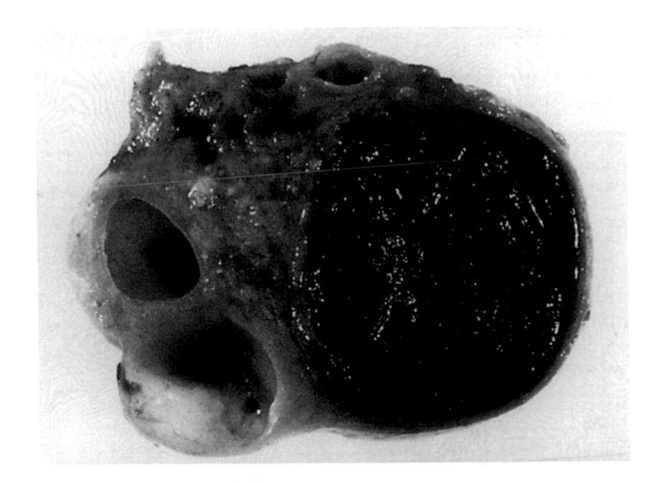

Fig. 30.8 Classical chocolate cyst of ovary (endometrioma) in an ovary containing two other fibrotic walled smaller cysts previously filled with 'chocolate' material prior to section.

Endometrioma

The pathogenesis of the typical ovarian endometrioma has now been clarified. It is a process originating from a free superficial implant which is in contact with the ovarian surface and is sealed off by adhesions. A pseudocyst

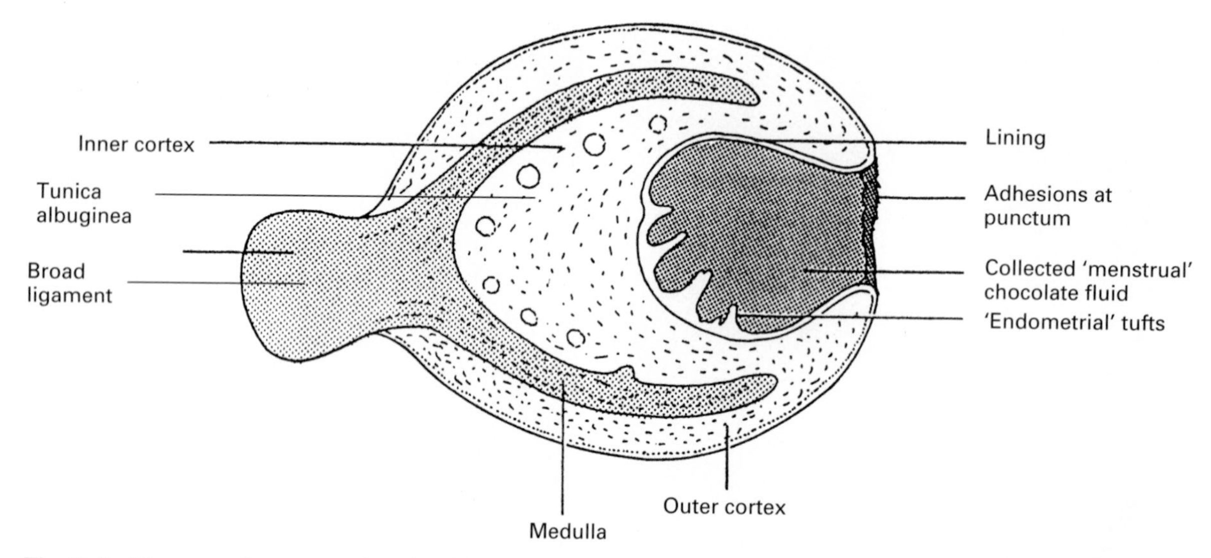

Fig. 30.9 Diagrammatic representation of endometrioma formation — beginning on serosal surface and invaginating into cortex.

is thus formed by accumulation of menstrual debris from shedding and bleeding of the small implant, resulting in fluid collection. Progressive invagination of the ovarian cortex occurs and the associated inflammatory reactive tissue progressively thickens the inverted cortex. Outgrowths through the endometrial epithelium, with or without stroma, extend over the surface or become embedded in the fibroreactive tissue covering the wall. This pathogenesis explains the typical features of an endometrium such as frequent location of the cyst, adhesions on the anterior side of the ovary opposing the posterior side of the parametrium or, when on the posterior aspect of the ovary, adhesions to the ovarian fossa. The contents of the cyst are, to a large extent, fluid which represents the debris from cyclical menstruation (Fig. 30.9).

There is usually a well defined separation between the normal adjacent ovarian stroma and the cyst wall, but whilst the epithelial lining of the cyst may initially resemble the endometrium, with increasing time and size pressure atrophy compresses the epithelium to a flat cuboidal pattern.

Ovarian endometriomas rarely occur in the adolescent but occurrence increases with age. Laparoscopic features of a typical endometrioma include ovarian cysts not greater than 12 cm in diameter; adhesions to the pelvic side wall and/or the posterior broad ligament; powder burns; minute red or blue spots with adjacent puckering on the surface, and the presence of the characteristic tarry, thick, chocolate-coloured fluid content.

Non-invasive methods of diagnosis

It is an unsatisfactory situation that in order to diagnose endometriosis with certainty an invasive, albeit minor, surgical procedure in the form of laparoscopy needs to be performed. This can readily be justified for making the initial diagnosis, but if the nature of the disease is of recurrence for the majority of patients throughout their reproductive life, this may involve repeat laparoscopies on many occasions if one is to be certain that the disease process has returned. Attempts have therefore been made to provide a non-invasive test which is highly sensitive and specific for endometriosis. Currently this has eluded investigators.

Serum markers: CA125

The most widely used serum marker for endometriosis has been the monoclonal antibody OC125, raised against a human ovarian cancer cell-line containing the antigen designated CA125 (Bast et al 1986). CA125 is a high molecular weight glycoprotein found in over 80% of cases of epithelial ovarian carcinoma. Investigation leads to the conclusion that CA125 is possessed by many tissues present in the pelvis as well as the more distant sites, including the pericardium and the pleura. Moderate elevation of serum CA125 has been observed in endometriosis, particularly in patients with severe disease (Barbieri et al 1986, Pittaway & Douglas 1989). In these studies serum levels in excess of 35 u/ml were used as a cut-off point, but sensitivity and specificity have proved inadequate for the use of CA125 as a screening test for endometriosis. However, in individuals in whom the disease has been confirmed and treated, an increase in serum levels above 35 u/ml may well be a useful marker of recurrence of the disorder.

Imaging techniques

Ultrasound. Ultrasound examination of the pelvis may be useful in delineating the presence and aetiology of ovarian cystic structures. The characteristic pictures on ultrasound are different when there is a large proportion of blood, e.g. corpus luteum cysts or endometriomas, which in a minority of cases may be echo-free. However the walls of an endometrioma are irregular as opposed to the smooth wall of the simple ovarian cyst. The commonest pattern is for the chocolate cyst to contain low-level echoes or lumps of dense high-level echoes representing blood clots. The picture may sometimes be confused if there are several cysts in different phases of evolution.

Computerized tomography (CT) scans and magnetic resonance imaging (MRI). CT provides better definition than ultrasound in many situations, but it has not established a role in the assessment of pelvic endometriosis. MRI, which is even more expensive, and currently has been used in only a limited number of patients with ovarian endometriomas, has not proved to be diagnostic since again there has been a significant overlap between endometriomas and cystic adenomas on MRI scanning appearances.

Ultrasound, CT and MRI scanning do not appear to be of any help in the diagnosis of peritoneal endometriosis, the deposits of which are too small. Currently these techniques are not sensitive enough to detect peritoneal endometriosis.

Immunoscintigraphy. Efforts have been made to use immunoscintigraphic methods to detect deposits of endometriotic tissue on the grounds that these tissue deposits do express CA125, and if an isotopic labelled OC125 (FAB) 2 fragment has been injected then binding to sites of CA125 expression could be detected (Kennedy et al 1988). Using a gamma camera the sites where binding has occurred can be detected, but whilst results from this method are encouraging, there is still great overlap with binding in other conditions, particularly pelvic inflammatory processes and to adhesions.

In summary, whilst there are promising areas of investigations currently being pursued concerning non-invasive techniques, none at present can stand in place of laparoscopy.

CLASSIFICATION SYSTEMS

Over the last three decades various classification systems have been proposed which attempt to standardize criteria from which the severity of endometriosis could be based. Such a system, if available, would help in the critical assessment of performance of various forms of treatment and hopefully provide meaningful prognostic indicators. No classification system so far devised has received uniform acceptance; all have suffered from various pitfalls which make it difficult to compare treatment results. The most recent attempt to provide a standardized classification for uniform use has been the Revised American Fertility Society Classification for Endometriosis (1985) shown in Figure 30.10. This serves to record the sites of deposits accurately and makes some effort to differentiate between superficial and deep-seated disease, as well as the presence or absence of adhesions. Whilst it offers a different weighting to the score given to different types of endometriosis, it must be appreciated that these scores are arbitrary. Classification of the extent of the disease as minimal, mild, moderate or severe is certainly helpful in explaining to the patient the problem and perhaps in determining whether a medical, surgical or combined medical and surgical approach is the most logical treatment step, at least in relation to fertility outcome.

The other major pitfall of any scoring system has been the lack of correlation between the score, or severity of the disease, and the degree of symptoms experienced.

Provided the above limitations are appreciated, the clas-

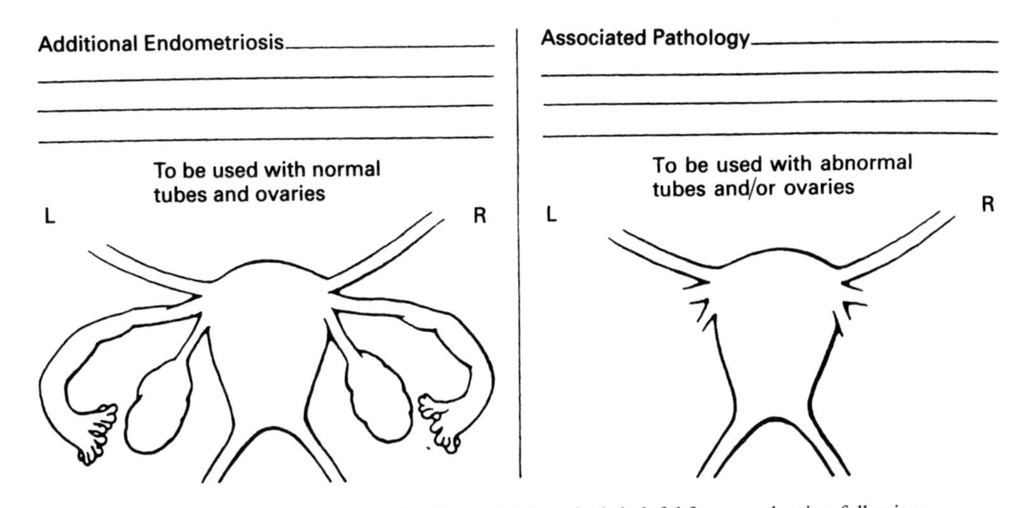

Fig. 30.10 Accurate charting of sites of endometrial deposits is helpful for re-evaluation following treatment or in suspected cases of recurrence. Modified from Revised American Fertility Society Classification of Endometriosis (1985).

sification systems do have some value and are essential in any clinical trial of a new treatment for comparison with other published series with currrently accepted therapies.

TREATMENT

Endometriosis is a particularly difficult disease to treat. Often response to therapy relies on recognition of the disease in its earliest possible stages. With most treatment modalities, there is eventual recurrence in up to 60% of cases. Thus there is no known permanent cure, and eventually clinicians have to proceed to surgical oophorectomy in selected cases; this offers the most effective available treatment to date. In addition, in minimal and mild disease (according to Revised American Fertility Society classifications), particularly in asymptomatic cases presenting only with infertility, there exists a controversy as to whether treatment should be given, since no control studies have shown a significant increase in fertility rates following such therapy. However, placebo-controlled studies in such cases have shown that endometriosis tends to be a progressive disease at least for many patients (Thomas & Cooke 1987), and hence treatment may at least arrest progression or eradicate disease for significant intervals.

When endometriosis is associated with symptoms, particularly pain, then there can be no doubt that treatment is of benefit, at least in relieving those symptoms.

The treatment should be individualized taking into account the patient's age, wish for fertility, severity of symptoms and extent of the disease. An important aspect of therapy is a sympathetic approach, with adequate counselling and explanation to the patient which will also ensure her compliance whilst on therapy.

Current treatment is essentially surgical, medical or a combination of both approaches. A combined medical and surgical treatment might utilize medical therapy before, after, or both before and following surgical intervention. This approach may be adopted in patients with moderate to severe disease in whom fertility prospects need to be improved or maintained.

SURGICAL TREATMENT

Conservative surgery

Laser ablation

With the increasing widespread availability of laparoscopic expertise and experience with laser technology, minimal access surgery is becoming a more popular treatment option for endometriosis. It is possible to destroy all visible endometriotic lesions by vaporizing these discrete areas using lasers. Laser laparoscopy appears to be an advantageous treatment for pelvic pain. One study (Sutton 1990) quoted the rates of pain relief at 1 year as being as high as 70%. However few controlled trials have been carried out and other larger trial results are awaited.

Laparoscopic uterosacral nerve ablation (LUNA). The uterosacral ligaments are a commonly affected site in patients suffering with endometriosis, and infiltration of endometriotic deposits results in invasion, inflammation and fibrosis of the anterior extension of the inferior hypogastric nerve, the uterovaginal plexus (or Lee–Frankenhauser plexus). Ablation of the uterosacral ligaments, forming two small craters, can be performed at the time of laparoscopy. The risks of the procedure are haemorrhage from a vessel within the uterosacral ligaments and damage to the ureter which needs to be identified before laser treatment commences. The results of properly conducted randomized trials are awaited to determine the value of LUNA although it does seem beneficial at reducing the severity of central dysmenorrhoea type pain.

Radical surgery

Radical surgery is reserved for those patients with severe symptoms, where there is no desired fertility potential, and especially when other forms of treatment have failed. Total abdominal hysterectomy and bilateral salpingo-oophorectomy are performed along with resection of any endometriotic lesions as completely as possible. As the majority of these patients are relatively young, hormone replacement therapy (HRT) should be commenced but kept to a minimum to control oestrogen deficiency symptoms, as a small percentage of those patients may develop a recurrence of endometriosis when on such oestrogen replacement.

Combined oestrogen–testosterone implants may minimize the risk of recurrence as well as offering the beneficial effects of the androgens in maintaining libido in young women who are sexually active, but no data exists from randomized trials to define if one particular HRT regimen is superior to others.

Surgical treatment of endometriomas

The definitive treatment of the typical endometrioma is the surgical release of the adhesions and fibrosis at the site of invagination and the eversion of the invaginated cortex. Simply puncturing and draining the endometrioma whether this is followed with GnRH agonist therapy, or not, has no beneficial effects in the long term on endometriomas (Vercellini et al 1992). Medical treatment is highly effective for the destruction of active implants located on the surface of the normal ovarian cortex. However when a definite endometrioma is present, surgery is necessary. This can be performed laparoscopically with smaller endometriomas, using laser destruction. With endometriomas larger than 3 cm diameter treatment may be facilitated to enable surgery to be performed laparoscopically if, following initial drainage, patients are pretreated for 3 months with a GnRH agonist prior to laser ablation (Donnez et al 1990).

On the other hand, fibrotic larger endometriomas have a thickened capsule which is more likely to be removed effectively by excisional techniques.

In many instances, however, because of other associated extensive adhesions and fixity of ovaries onto other structures, a laparotomy rather than laparoscopy may be necessary.

MEDICAL TREATMENT

Ectopic endometrial tissue does respond to endogenous and exogenous ovarian steroid hormones in a fashion sufficiently similar to that of normal endometrium. Thus a hormonal approach which suppresses oestrogen–progesterone levels and which prevents cyclical changes and menstruation should be beneficial in its treatment. In the hypo-oestrogenic state following the menopause, atrophy of the normal endometrium and atrophy and regression of endometriotic deposits occur. Administration of progestogens opposes the effect of oestrogen on endometrial tissue by inhibiting the replenishment of cytosolic oestrogen receptors. Progestogens also induce secretory activity in endometrial glands and decidual reaction in the endometrial stroma.

The success of various hormonal therapies depends to a large extent on the localization of the endometriotic lesions. Superficial peritoneal and ovarian serosal implants may respond better to hormone therapy than deep ovarian or deep peritoneal lesions or lesions within organs (e.g. bladder and rectum) which rapidly recur after medical therapy and require ultimate surgical excision.

Table 30.4 Various hormonal states and their effects upon normal endometrium and ectopic endometrial deposits

Hormonal state	Effects on endometrium	Effects on endometriotic implants
Oestrogenic e.g. exogenous oestrogens	Proliferative activity, hyperplasia	Proliferative activity, hyperplasia
Hypo-oestrogenic e.g. postmenopause, pseudomenopause regimens postoophorectomy GnRH analogues	Atrophic changes	Atrophy, regression, resorption
Progestational e.g. pregnancy, exogenous progestogens, pseudopregnancy treatment	Secretory activity, decidualization	Secretory activity, necrobiosis and resorption
Androgenic e.g. danazol and its metabolites Gestrinone	Atrophy	Atrophy and regression

GnRH, gonadotrophin-releasing hormone.

The treatment of endometriosis has undergone a remarkable evolution in the last 40 years. In the past, testosterone, diethylstilboestrol and high-dose combination oestrogen–progestogen pill preparations were used with some success. However, therapies which induce decidualization (pseudopregnancy regimes) or suppress ovarian function (pseudomenopausal regimes) appear to offer the best chance of inducing clinical remission of endometriosis. (See Table 30.4).

Prostaglandin synthetase inhibitors

An association with prostaglandin release and dysmenorrhoea has long been established. One might therefore expect that prostaglandin synthetase inhibitors (PGSIs) might have a beneficial effect in treating the symptoms of endometriosis. PGSIs are a heterogeneous group of non-steroidal inflammatory agents. They act mainly by inhibiting the production of prostaglandins, though some (Fenamates) also antagonize prostaglandins at the target level. These agents are perhaps beneficial in the early stages of initial or recurrence of disease but when symptoms become more severe, they are usually inadequate by themselves to control symptomatology.

Progestogen treatment

A state of pseudopregnancy can be induced effectively by the continuous administration of progestogenic preparations. The progestogens used are derivatives of progesterone (dydrogesterone or medroxyprogesterone acetate) or derivates of 19-nor-testosterone (norethisterone, norethisterone acetate, norgestrel, ethynodrel and lynoestrenol).

The use of progestogens induces a hyperprogestogenic-hypo-oestrogenic state. Treatments are available orally or injected as a depot formulation, and are administered for 6–9 months. The results achieved appear to be comparable to those achieved with combined oral oestrogen–progestogen preparations in the past. The side-effects most commonly seen with progestogen usage include breakthrough bleeding, weight gain, abdominal bloating, oedema, acne and mood changes.

The adverse effects of some progestogens on circulating levels of low- and high-density lipoproteins may determine choice of progestogen if long-term administration is planned.

Combined oestrogen–progestogen preparations

Kistner (1959) introduced the regimen of continuous combined oral contraceptives in order to reproduce the hormonal milieu of pregnancy. One of a number of the higher dose combined oral contraceptives may be administered continuously for 3 cycles. If breakthrough bleeding occurs, before planned interval bleeds, changing to another preparation with higher prostestogenic content is advocated.

Side-effects such as weight gain, headaches, breast enlargement and/or tenderness, nausea and depression may occur. The risk of thromboembolism is increased and contraindications for the use of this form of therapy are the same as those for combined oral contraception.

Danazol

Danazol is an isoxazol derivate of 17-alpha-ethinyl testosterone. Because of its base structure it has both androgenic and anabolic properties. Danazol is currently one of the most widely used medical treatments for endometriosis. Its mechanism of action is complex and includes suppression of the hypothalamic–pituitary axis with interferance in pulsatile gonadotrophin secretion and inhibition of the midcycle gonadotrophin surge, but with no change in basal gonadotrophin levels. It achieves a direct inhibition of ovarian steroidogenesis by inhibiting several enzymatic processes and by competitive blockage of androgen, oestrogen and progesterone receptors in the endometrium. An increase in free testosterone occurs because of a reduction in sex hormone-binding globulin and this explains many of danazol's androgenic side-effects. The increase in free testosterone may also contribute towards its direct action on inducing endometrial atrophy. The degree of endocrine changes described above are dose-related.

In the treatment of endometriosis, danazol is administered in a dose range of between 400 and 800 mg daily, titrated by the induction of amenorrhoea and tolerance. In the case of mild to moderate endometriosis there is a highly effective symptomatic improvement in over 85% of cases (Dmowski & Cohen 1978).

Objective resolution of endometriotic lesions has been observed at posttreatment laparoscopic evaluation in between 70 and 95% of patients, depending upon the stage of the disease (Barbieri et al 1982). However, recurrence rates of up to 40% have been reported in the 36 months after completion of a course of danazol; annual recurrences in the first, second and third years were 23, 5 and 9% respectively (Dmowski & Cohen 1978).

Danazol therapy should be commenced in the early follicular phase of the menstrual cycle. It is recommended that the patient should use additional barrier methods of contraception in order to avoid the drug being administered during early pregnancy where continued use could lead to androgenization of a developing female fetus. The drug dosage should be related to the patient's clinical staging, response and severity of side-effects, starting with a dose of 400 mg/day in mild disease and 600–800 mg/day in moderate to severe cases, for a recommended treatment course of at least 6 months.

Danazol is associated with side-effects related to its androgenic and anabolic properties. These include weight gain, acne, oily skin, fluid retention, muscle cramps, hot flushes, depression and mood changes. Less commonly, hirsutism, skin rash and deepening of voice are noted. The incidence and severity of these side-effects are dose-related. It is recommended that patients immediately discontinue treatment if they develop hirsutism, a skin rash or experience deepening of the voice.

Metabolic side-effects include elevation of low-density lipoproteins and reduction of high-density lipoproteins and cholesterol concentrations (Fahraeus et al 1984). These effects are quickly reversed after ceasing treatment. In addition, changes in liver enzymes are noted and danazol is contraindicated in patients with liver disease.

Gestrinone

Gestrinone is a synthethic trienic 19-norsteroid (13-ethyl-17-alpha-ethinyl-17-hydroxy-gona-4, 9, 11-triene-3-one). It has been shown in recent clinical trials to be another effective clinical treatment for endometriosis (Thomas & Cooke 1987). The drug exhibits mild androgenic and antigonadotrophic properties. The combined effect is to induce progressive endometrial atrophy. Gestrinone has a high binding affinity for progesterone receptors; it also binds to androgen receptors but not to oestrogen receptors (Azadian-Boulanger et al 1984). The combined endocrine effect of gestrinone therapy is similar to that of danazol in that the midcycle gonadotrophin surge is abolished, although basal gonadotrophin levels are not significantly reduced, together with inhibition of ovarian steroidogenesis and reduction of sex hormone–binding globulin levels. Gestrinone has a prolonged half-life and may be administered orally at a dosage of 2.5–5.0 mg twice weekly for a period of 6–9 months in patients with endometriosis. This dosage schedule effectively induces endometrial atrophy with 85–90% of patients becoming amenorrhoeic within 2 months.

Whilst gestrinone has only recently been introduced for the treatment of endometriosis, current controlled open studies appear to show that it compares favourably with danazol in terms of both symptomatic relief and resolution of endometrial deposits (Azadian-Boulanger et al 1984, Mettler & Semm 1984).

The side-effects, occurring in up to 50% of patients, include weight gain, breakthrough bleeding, reduced breast size, muscle cramps and, uncommonly, hirsutism, voice change and hoarseness.

Gonadotrophin-releasing hormone (GnRH) agonists

Surgical castration is known to be an effective therapy for severe endometriosis. Thus the possibility of inducing a reversible medical castration with the continued adminis-

	1	2	3	4	5	(6)	7	8	9	(10)	
	Pyro – GLU	– HIS	– TRP	– SER	– TYR	– GLY	– LEU	– ARG	– PRO	GLY – NH_2	LHRH
Nonapeptides						D – SER (Bu^t)			PRO – NET		Buserelin
						D – LEU			PRO – NET		Leuprolide
Decapeptides						D – TRP					Tryptorelin
						$(D – NAL)_2$					Nafarelin
						D – SER (Bu^t)				AZA – GLY	Goserelin

Fig. 30.11 Amino acid sequence of native luteinizing hormone-releasing hormone (LHRH) and some of the agonistic gonadotrophin-releasing hormone(GnRH) analogues used in the treatment of endometriosis.

tration of GnRH agonists has been investigated as an alternative therapy in endometriosis. Modification of the native GnRH molecule with substitution, particularly in positions 6 and 10, with alternative amino acids, produces agonistic analogues with a reduced susceptibility to degradation and hence a prolonged therapeutic half-life (Fig. 30.11). Continued administration of these analogues induces pituitary gonadotrophin desensitization via down-regulation of GnRH receptors and an eventual state of hypogonadotrophic hypogonadism. Reduced gonadotrophic stimulation of the ovaries leads to cessation of follicular growth and reduction in ovarian steroidogenesis, with circulating 17β-oestradiol levels falling to those observed in the postmenopausal range (less than 100 pmol/l, typically).

A large amount of data has now appeared in the literature, from both controlled and randomized comparative trials of GnRH analogues and danazol (for review, see Shaw 1995). These trials have all confirmed the value of GnRH analogues for the treatment of endometriosis. Rapid and effective symptomatic relief is achieved with these agents as well as a marked degree of resolution of the endometrial deposits in the majority of patients. However for both symptomatic relief and the resolution of endometrial deposits there is essentially no significant difference in comparative trials between the GnRH analogues and danazol. However, patient acceptability and the profile of side-effects may be slightly in favour of the GnRH analogues (Henzl et al 1988, Matta & Shaw 1987), (Table 30.5).

Side-effects of GnRH analogues include those which are predictable from induction of a significant degree of hypo-oestrogenism. These include hot flushes (in virtually all patients) headaches, and less commonly atrophic vaginitis, vaginal dryness and reduced libido.

Dosage varies depending on the analogue used and its formulation, but regimens include: nafarelin 200 µg twice daily intranasally; buserelin 300–400 µg three times daily intranasally; goserelin 3.6 mg subcutaneous depot monthly, and leuprorelin 3.75 mg intramuscular depot monthly.

Table 30.5 Principal side-effects experienced in patients randomized to receive buserelin or danazol for 6 months

	Buserelin	Danazol
Dose	400 µg t.d.s. intranasally	600–800 mg orally daily
Number of patients	39	18
Symptoms		
Hot flushes	74%*	22%
Breakthrough bleeding	23%	55%*
Headaches	20%	39%
Vaginal dryness	23%*	5.5%
Superficial dyspareunia	5.2%*	Nil
Weight gain (>3 kg)	Nil	66%*
Acne/oily skin	Nil	39%*

From Matta & Shaw (1987).
*$p \leq 0.05$ between treatments.

Metabolic side-effects include (as in the menopause) increased excretion of urinary calcium. Over a 6-month period there is a 3–5% loss in the vertebral trabecular bone density of the lumbar spine as assessed by dual energy X-ray absorptiometry (DEXA). In most patients, the bone density changes induced following a 6-month course of therapy with GnRH analogues are reversed after 6 months' return of ovarian function (Henzl et al 1988, Matta et al 1987). However the implications of such changes in calcium homeostasis with prolonged and repetitive treatment with GnRH analogues are being further investigated. This is likely to lead to the development of protective 'add-back' regimens, which ideally would also reduce the symptomatic effects of the GnRH agonist-induced hypoestrogenism but not result in reduced therapeutic effectiveness on symptom relief or implant resolution.

Combination of medical and surgical therapy

There is perhaps more speculation as to the value of pre- or postoperative medical therapy than hard data.

Individual gynaecologists have a 'belief' in one or the other, even though published data do not suggest advantages of one method over another.

It is the frequency of recurrent endometriosis after medical or surgical therapy, and the documentation of microscopic disease, together with differences in vascularity between various lesions, that have encouraged the use of combination therapy.

Preoperative therapy might help somewhat to reduce the size of an endometrioma prior to surgical removal, since medical therapy alone will never succeed. Preoperative treatment will also reduce vascularity and may subsequently aid dissection of implants and adhesive processes. The role of postoperative medication is to eliminate any residual macro- or microscopic disease.

The duration of such therapies is uncertain since no true randomized comparative trials exist, but most gynaecologists prescribe a 3-month treatment course preoperatively, and between 3 and 6 months postoperatively, depending upon the amount of macroscopic disease left following attempted surgical removal.

RECURRENT ENDOMETRIOSIS

The natural course of the disease remains a mystery. It has been suggested that in only one-third of cases is the disease progressive, whilst in the remainder the endometriosis remains in a steady state or eventually even resolves spontaneously.

In many instances after medical suppression of the disease or after surgical destruction of all visible deposits, residual viable (microscopic) implants can regenerate once ovarian function is re-established. In other cases new disease develops at new sites, perhaps indicating the potential for an entire 'field change' within the pelvic peritoneum. The degree of differentiation of a lesion may also correlate with persistence of disease following medical therapy. Two-thirds of those lesions which were most highly differentiated disappeared following 6 months of medical therapy, whilst three-quarters of poorly differentiated lesions persisted (Schweppe 1984).

However as far as therapeutic options are concerned, there is no essential difference between primary and recurrent endometriosis. The choice of treatment in a patient with recurrent disease is not determined by the manifestations of the disease as such but more by the extent of distortion of the pelvic anatomy and the severity of symptomatology. In many instances repeat medical therapy or repeat conservative surgery is appropriate, but when there are severe symptoms and repeated recurrence, a radical surgical approach may be the patient's best option to achieve long-standing relief of pain.

KEY POINTS

1. Endometriosis is most commonly found inside the pelvis, but rarely it has been described in sites such as the urinary tract, lungs and umbilicus.
2. Endometriosis is one of the commonest gynaecological conditions and is present in between 10 and 25% of women presenting with gynaecological symptoms.
3. The growth of endometriotic tissue depends on oestrogen, thus endometriosis occurs almost exclusively in the reproductive years, with a peak incidence between 30 and 45 years of age.
4. The theories of aetiology of endometriosis include Sampson's theory of retrograde menstruation and implantation and Meyer's theory of transformation of coelomic epithelium. Immunological factors are also thought to be important.
5. The peritoneal fluid in women with endometriosis contains higher concentrations of more active macrophages and higher concentrations of prostaglandins than in normal women. These factors may be important in explaining the link between infertility pain and endometriosis.
6. Endometriosis that is associated with tubal and ovarian damage and the formation of adhesions can compromise fertility. The link between mild endometriosis and infertility is more controversial.
7. The best means to diagnose endometriosis is by direct visualization at laparoscopy or laparotomy, with histological confirmation where uncertainty persists.
8. The typical blue-black peritoneal endometriotic lesion is described as a powder burn. Recently, non-pigmented lesions and red lesions have been described.
9. The medical treatment of endometriosis involves suppressing oestrogen–progesterone levels to prevent cyclical changes and menstruation. Treatments include progestogens, gestrinone, danazol and gonadotrophin-releasing hormone analogues
10. The surgical treatment of endometriosis is either minimally invasive, such as laparoscopic diathermy or laser vaporization, or radical, when total abdominal hysterectomy and bilateral salpingo-oophorectomy are performed.
11. The natural course of the disease is not clearly defined, but in perhaps a third of cases the disease is progressive whilst in the remainder the disease remains in a steady stage or may even resolve spontaneously.

REFERENCES

Azadian-Boulanger G, Secchi J, Tournemine C, Sakiz E, Vige P, Henrion R 1984 Hormonal activity profiles of drugs for endometriosis therapy. In: Raynaud J P, Ojasoo T, Martini L (eds) Medical management of endometriosis. Raven Press, New York, pp 125–148

Badawy S Z A, Cuenca V, Stitze A, Jacobs R D B, Tomar R H 1984 Autoimmune phenomena in infertile patients with endometriosis. Obstetrics and Gynecology 63: 271

Barbieri R L 1990 Etiology and epidemiology of endometriosis. American Journal of Obstetrics and Gynecology 162(2): 565–567

Barbieri R L, Evans S, Kistner R W 1982 Danazol in the treatment of endometriosis: analysis of 100 cases with a 4-year follow-up. Fertility and Sterility 37: 737–749

Barbieri R L, Niloff J M, Bast R C, Shaetzl E, Kistner R W, Knapp R C 1986 Elevated serum concentrations of CA-125 in patients with advanced endometriosis. Fertility and Sterility 45: 630–634

Bast R C, Feeney M, Lazarus H, Nadler L M, Colvin R B, Knapp R C 1986. Reactivity of a monoclonal antibody with human ovarian carcinoma. Journal of Clinical Investigation 68: 1331

Bayer S R, Siebel M M 1986 Endometriosis: clinical symptoms and infertility. In: Rolland R, Chandha D R, Willemsen W P (eds) Gonadotrophin down-regulation in gynecological practice. Alan R Liss, New York, pp 103–133

Brosens I A, Koninckx P R, Corvelyn P A 1978 A study of plasma progesterone, oestradiol-17_{β}, prolactin and LH levels and of the luteal phase appearance of the ovaries in patients with endometriosis and infertility. British Journal of Obstetrics and Gynaecology 85: 246–250

Cheesman K L, Ben-Nun I, Chatterton R T, Cohen M R 1982 Relationship of luteinizing hormone, pregnanediol-3-glucorinide and oestradiol-16-glucoronide in urine of infertile women with endometriosis. Fertility and Sterility 38: 542–544

Chillik C F, Acosta A A, Cardcia J E et al 1985 The role of in vitro fertilisation in infertile patients with endometriosis. Fertility and Sterility 44: 56–62

Cohen M R 1976 Endoscopy. In: Greenblatt R B (ed) Recent advances in endometriosis. Excerpta Medica, Amsterdam, pp 18–31

Curtis P, Lindsay P, Jackson A E, Shaw R W 1993 Adverse effects on sperm movement characteristics in women with minimal and mild endometriosis. British Journal of Obstetrics and Gynaecology 100: 165–169

Drake T S, O'Brien W F, Ramwell P et al 1981 Peritoneal fluid thromboxane B_2 and 6-keto prostaglandin in $F2_{\beta}$ in endometriosis. American Journal of Obstetrics and Gynecology 140: 401–404

Dmowski W P, Cohen M R 1978 Antigonadotrophin (danazol) in the treatment of endometriosis: evaluation of post-treatment fertility and 3-year follow-up data. American Journal of Obstetrics and Gynecology 130: 41–48

Dmowski W P, Steele R W, Baker G F 1981 Deficient cellular immunity in endometriosis. American Journal of Obstetrics and Gynecology 141: 377–383

Donnez J, Nisolle M, 1991 Appearance of peritoneal endometriosis. In: IIIrd Laser Surgery Symposium, Brussels

Donnez J, Nisolle M, Clerckx F et al 1990 The ovarian endometrial cyst: combined (hormonal and surgical) therapy. In: Brosens I, Jacobs H S, Runnebaum B (eds) LHRH analogues in gynaecology. Parthenon, Carnforth, pp 165–175

Fahraeus L, Larsson-Cohn U, Ljungberg S, Wallentin I 1984 Profound alterations in the lipoprotein metabolism during danazol treatment in pre-menopausal women. Fertility and Sterility 42: 52–57

Halme J, Becher S, Wing R 1984 Accentuated cyclic activation of peritoneal macrophages in patients with endometriosis. American Journal of Obstetrics and Gynecology 148: 85–90

Halme J, Becker S, Haskill S 1986 Altered life span and function of peritoneal macrophages: a new hypothesis for pathogenesis of endometriosis. Society of Gynecologic Investigation, Toronto, Abstract 48

Henzl M R, Corson S L, Moghissi K, Buttram V C, Bergquist C, Jacobson C 1988 Administration of nasal nafarelin as compared with oral danazol for endometriosis. New England Journal of Medicine 318: 485–489

Ingamells S, Thomas E J 1995 Infertility and endometriosis. In: Shaw R W (ed) Endometriosis – current understanding and management. Blackwell Science, Oxford, pp 147–167

Jansen R P S, Russel P 1986 Nonpigmented endometriosis: clinical laparoscopic and pathologic definition. American Journal of Obstetrics and Gynecology 155: 1154–1159

Javert C T 1949 Pathogenesis of endometriosis based on endometrial homeoplasia, direct extension, exfoliation and implantation, lymphatic and hematogenous metastasis. Cancer 2: 399

Kirshon B, Poindexter A N III 1988 Contraception: a risk factor for endometriosis. Obstetrics and Gynecology 71: 829

Kennedy S H, Soper N D W, Mojiminiyi O A, Shepstone B J, Barlow D H 1988 Immunoscintigraphy of ovarian endometriosis. A preliminary study. British Journal of Obstetrics and Gynaecology 95: 693–697

Kistner R W 1959 The treatment of endometriosis by inducing pseudopregnancy with ovarian hormones: a report of 58 cases. Fertility and Sterility 10: 539–545

Koninckx P R, De Moor P, Brosens I A 1980 Diagnosis of the luteinizing unruptured follicle syndrome by steroid hormone assays in peritoneal fluid. British Journal of Obstetrics and Gynaecology 87: 929–934

Koninckx P R, Meuleman C, Demeyere S, Lesaffre E, Cornillie F 1991 Suggestive evidence that pelvic endometriosis is a progressive disease whereas deeply infiltrating endometriosis is associated with pelvic pain. Fertility and Sterility 55: 759–765

MacLaverty C M, Shaw R W 1995 Pelvic pain and endometriosis. In: Shaw R W (ed) Endometriosis – current understanding and management. Blackwell Science, Oxford, pp 112–146

Mahmood T A, Templeton A 1990 The impact of treatment on the natural history of endometriosis. Human Reproduction 5: 965–970

Matta W H, Shaw R W 1987 A comparative study between buserelin and danazol in the treatment of endometriosis. British Journal of Clinical Practice 41(suppl 48): 69–73

Matta W M, Shaw R W, Hesp R, Katz D 1987 Hypogonadism induced by luteinizing hormone releasing hormone agonist analogues: effects on bone density in premenopausal women. British Medical Journal 294: 1523–1524

Meldrum D R, Shamonki I M, Clarke K E 1977 Prostaglandin content of ascitic fluid in endometriosis: a preliminary report. 25th Annual Meeting of the Pacific Coast Fertility Society, Palm Springs, California

Mettler L, Semm K 1984 Three-step therapy of genital endometriosis in cases of human infertility with lynestrenol, danazol or gestrinone administration. In: Raynaud J P, Ojasoo T, Martini L (eds) Medical management of endometriosis. Raven Press, New York, pp 233–247

Meyer R 1919 Uber den Staude der Frage der Adenomyosites Adenomyoma in Allgemeinen und Adenomyometitis Sarcomastosa. Zentralblatt für Gynäkologie 36: 745–759

Muscato J J, Haney A F, Weinberg J B 1982 Sperm phagocytosis by human peritoneal macrophages: a possible cause of infertility in endometriosis. American Journal of Obstetrics and Gynecology 144: 503–510

Olive D L, Weinberg J B, Haney A F 1985 Peritoneal macrophages infertility: the association between cell number and pelvic pathology. Fertility and Sterility 44: 772–777

Pittaway D E, Douglas J W 1989 Serum CA-125 in women with endometriosis and chronic pelvic pain. Fertility and Sterility 51: 68–70

Pittaway D E, Vernon C, Fayez J A 1988 Spontaneous abortions in women with endometriosis. Fertility and Sterility 50: 711–715

Revised American Fertility Society Classification of Endometriosis 1985 Fertility and Sterility 43: 351–352

Rock J A, Dubin N M, Ghodgaonkar R B, Bergquist C A, Erozan Y S, Kimball A W Jr 1982 Cul-de-sac fluid in women with endometriosis: fluid volume and prostanoid concentration during the proliferative phase of the cycle – days 8–12. Fertility and Sterility 37: 747–752

Sampson J A 1940 The development of the implantation theory for the origin of peritoneal endometriosis. American Journal of Obstetrics and Gynecology 40: 549

Shaw R W 1993 An Atlas of Endometriosis. Parthenon, Carnforth

Shaw R W 1995 Evaluation of treatment with gonadotrophin-releasing hormone analogues. In: Shaw R W (ed) Endometriosis – current

understanding and management. 34. Blackwell Science, Oxford, pp 206–234
Schifrin B S, Erez S, Moore J G 1973 Teenage endometriosis. American Journal of Obstetrics and Gynecology 116: 973–980
Schweppe K W 1984 Morphologie und Klinik der Endometriose. F K Schattauer Verlag, Stuttgart, pp 198–207
Schweppe K W, Wynn R M, Beller F K 1984 Ultrastructural comparison of endometriotic implants and ectopic endometrium. American Journal of Obstetrics and Gynecology 148: 1024–1039
Simpson J L, Elias S, Malinak L R, Buttram V C Jr 1980 Heritable aspects of endometriosis I: genetic studies. American Journal of Obstetrics and Gynecology 137: 327–331
Sutton C 1990 Advances in the surgical management of endometriosis. In: Shaw R W (ed) Endometriosis. Parthenon, Carnforth, pp 209–226
Thomas E J, Cooke I D 1987 Impact of gestrinone on the course of asymptomatic endometriosis. British Medical Journal 294: 272–274
Tyson J E A 1974 Surgical considerations in gynecologoic endocrine disorders. Surgical Clinics of North America 54: 425–442
Vercellini P, Vendola N, Bocciolone L et al 1992 Laparoscopic aspiration of ovarian endometriomas: effect with postoperative gonadotropin releasing hormone agonist treatment. Journal of Reproductive Medicine 37: 577–580
Vernon M, Beard J, Graves K, Wilson E A 1986 Classification of endometriotic implants in morphologic appearance and capacity to synthesize prostaglandin F. Fertility and Sterility 46: 801–805
Wentz A C 1980 Premenstrual spotting: its association with endometriosis but not luteal phase inadequacy. Fertility and Sterility 33: 605–607

SECTION 3

Benign and malignant tumours

31

Epidemiology of gynaecological cancers

N. E. Day *Eswar Krishnan*

INTRODUCTION

Epidemiological studies have contributed significantly to our understanding of the causation and risks of many common malignancies. This is particularly true in the case of gynaecological cancers, where epidemiological tools have helped to formulate and evaluate methods of efficient clinical downstaging and mortality reduction, in addition to providing leads to aetiology.

Cancer of the uterine cervix and corpus and ovarian cancer are the commonest cancers in women, excluding breast cancer. The focus of this chapter will therefore be on these three cancers.

GENERAL OVERVIEW

It has been estimated that, on a global basis, cancer of the cervix is the second most common cancer in women after breast cancer, accounting for about 15% of all cancer in women. In 1985, some 437 000 cases occurred worldwide (Parkin et al 1993). Most of these occur in the less developed nations, notably in Africa, Latin America and south Asia. In contrast, cancer of the uterine corpus and ovary have a relatively higher incidence in the industrialized countries. Table 31.1 shows an overview of incidence rates of these cancers around the world, expressed in terms of the probability (as a percentage) of developing the cancer before the age of 75, given that death has not intervened earlier. A 15–20-fold variation is seen for both cervical and endometrial cancers; ovarian cancer, in contrast, shows only a three–fourfold variation in risk. Although several convincing explanations, ranging from lifestyle and dietary factors to levels of risk behaviour and public health interventions, have been put forward to account for these patterns, the relative homogeneity of ovarian cancer risk defies elucidation. Current research promises more opportunities for pharmacological and immunological interventions to prevent cancer of the cervix.

CANCER OF THE CERVIX

Among the different histologies noted in the cervical cancers, the squamous cell type is by far the most common, followed by the adenosquamous type and adenocarcinoma. Adenocarcinoma has several features different from the squamous cancers and hence merits special consideration.

Geographical variations

The 10 highest incidence rates for cervical cancer are noted in Latin America, India and among the Maoris of New Zealand. European countries have lower incidences than others, partly owing to their mass screening programmes.

Age aspects and time trends

In a population with no mass screening programmes, and incidence rates relatively constant over time, the change in incidence with age follows a typical pattern. The incidence rises rapidly in the age span 25–40 years, reaches a plateau and even begins to fall in the sixth and seventh decades. Data from Norway (Fig. 31.1) show this pattern.

Departures from the above pattern occur when there are changes in sexual behaviour or screening policies. For example, data from Birmingham (Fig. 31.2) indicate a rapidly rising rate in the younger age group and a relatively steady

Table 31.1 Probability of developing gynaecological cancer before age 75 in selected populations across the world (from Parkin et al 1992)

	Cervix uteri (%)	Corpus uteri (%)	Ovary (%)
India			
Bangalore	3.41	0.21	0.57
Bombay	2.14	0.29	0.74
Madras	5.08	0.19	0.60
China			
Shanghai	0.56	0.33	0.52
Philippines			
Manila	2.91	0.75	1.13
Japan			
Hiroshima	2.08	0.56	0.66
Nagasaki	1.38	0.32	0.52
Singapore			
Chinese	1.89	0.72	0.93
Indian	1.49	0.37	0.93
Malay	0.91	0.43	0.71
Israel			
All Jews	0.43	1.28	1.31
Mali			
Bamako	2.45	0.08	0.09
Brazil			
Goiania	4.99	0.21	0.50
Porto Alegre	3.28	1.05	0.97
Peru			
Trujillo	5.84	0.42	0.79
Colombia			
Cali	4.68	0.80	1.01
Ecuador			
Quito	3.78	0.50	0.55
Costa Rica	2.74	0.58	0.62
USA			
SEER			
White	0.73	2.46	1.45
Black	1.23	1.25	0.87
Los Angeles			
White	0.69	2.46	1.39
Black	1.27	1.37	0.93
Japanese	0.45	1.58	1.36
Chinese	1.38	0.86	0.83
Filipino	0.84	1.07	0.79
Korean	2.17	0.25	0.50
Canada			
Saskatchewan	0.70	1.86	1.30
Cuba	2.03	0.70	0.64
Denmark	1.63	1.96	1.72
France			
Martinique	2.62	0.74	0.38
Tarn	0.78	1.32	0.82
Russia			
St Petersburg	1.18	1.27	1.29
Former GDR	2.22	1.77	1.40
Norway	1.28	1.46	1.65
Italy			
Trieste	1.13	1.38	1.06
UK			
England & Wales	1.21	0.97	1.31
Scotland	1.34	0.92	1.48
New Zealand			
Maori	3.12	2.11	1.05
Non Maori	1.16	1.13	0.52

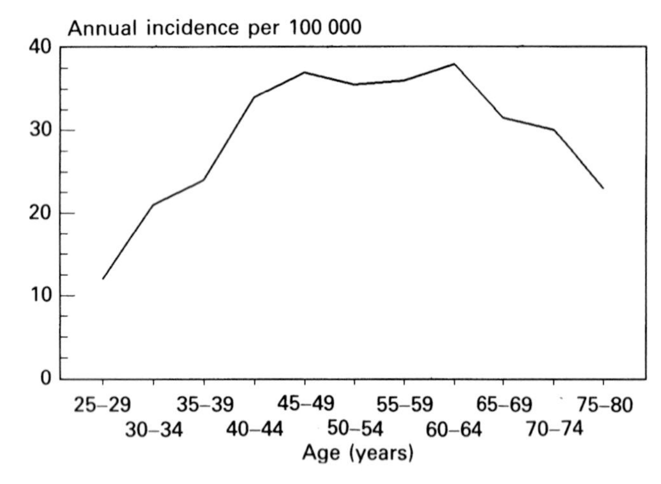

Fig. 31.1 The incidence of cervical cancer in an unscreened population in which the rate is not changing with time (data from Muir et al 1987).

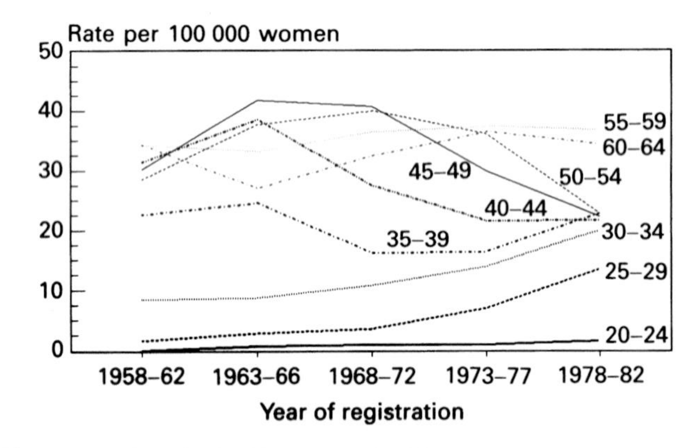

Fig. 31.2 Changing incidence rates in different age groups as a result of screening activity and changes in the underlying prevalence. Data from the Birmingham Cancer Registry.

rate over age 55 during the period 1960–1982. This is attributable to the upsurge in sexual activity among younger people and the introduction of systematic screening in the middle-aged. The variations in the rates of cervical cancer among birth cohorts could be closely related to the infection rates of sexually transmitted diseases among these cohorts (Beral 1974). In countries where cervical cancer is common, the rates in the 25–34-year group are higher than in other countries where it is less common (Muir et al 1987). This again demonstrates the extraordinary sensitivity of the cervix to oncogenic insults accompanying sexual activity. The rates plateau after age 40, meaning that either the sexual pursuits or the sensitivity of the cervix declines with advancing age.

The experience of Scandinavian countries illustrates how incidence rates fall greatly with mass screening (Hakama 1982, Laara et al 1987; Fig. 31.3). Finland, Iceland, Denmark and Sweden have had comprehensive mass

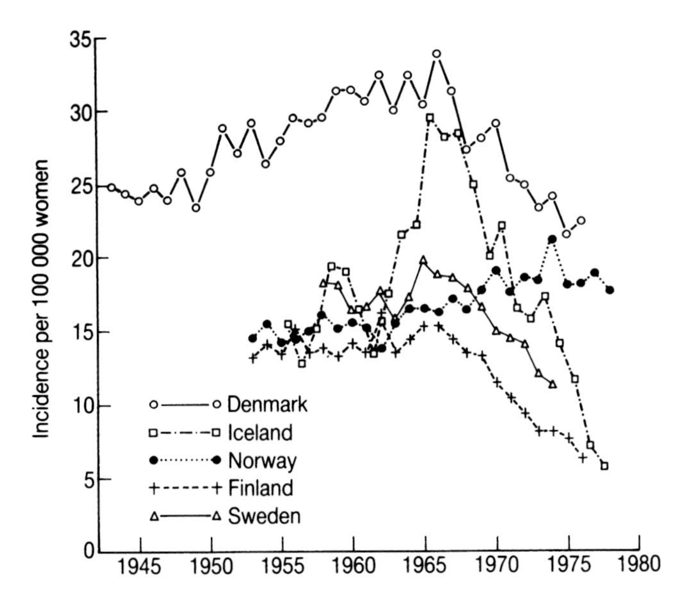

Fig. 31.3 The effect of different screening policies on changing rates of cervical cancer in the Nordic countries. (Modified from Hakama 1982)

screening since the mid to late 1960s, whereas in Norway the screening was confined to one county.

Racial and ethnic patterns

The difference in incidence rates with respect to country of origin is well illustrated in Table 31.1. This perhaps reflects the difference in the risk profiles of these population groups.

Adenosquamous and adenocarcinomas

The incidence rates of adenosquamous cancers have changed little after increasing during the early 1970s (Devesa et al 1989). Very little is known about their epidemiology. In many studies they are considered as adenocarcinoma.

Cervical adenocarcinoma resembles both endometrial carcinomas and squamous cell cancers, and shares many risk factors. It constitutes approximately 10% of all cervical cancers and its incidence in younger women has been increasing in the USA, England and Norway (Kjaer & Brinton 1993). In contrast, in older women the incidence of both adenocarcinomas and squamous cell carcinomas has been decreasing. Patients with adenocarcinoma tend to be older than those with squamous tumours (Berek et al 1981). Some clinical studies note a predilection for Asians, but the rarity of the disease allows only small studies and hence limits the validity of the conclusions.

Hysterectomy rates and cervical cancer mortality

In the US an estimated 33% of women who reach the age of 60 have had their uterus removed (Pokras & Hufnagel 1987). The corresponding figure for the UK is about 20%. Thus the reported mortality from cervical cancer is an underestimation of the actual figure. However, only 8% of the mortality reduction can be attributed to the prevalence of hysterectomy.

Aetiological factors

It has been recognized for many years that the major risk factors of cervical cancer relate to sexual activity, as exemplified by the high rates seen among commercial sex workers. Other exposures which have been proposed as risk factors include cigarette smoking, oral contraception, immunosuppression and dietary factors.

Sexual activity

The two behavioural aspects of sexual activity which modify risk for the disease are age at first intercourse and the number of sexual partners (Table 31.2). The effect of age at first intercourse has suggested to some authors that cervical tissue at a younger age might be more susceptible to oncogenic insults. An alternative and simpler explanation might be derived from the multistage model of carcinogenesis (Armitage & Doll 1954, Day 1990), which suggests that the most important variable determining the change in risk is not age but time. Many epithelial cancers exhibit a risk which increases with some high power (about 4) of either duration of exposure or time since first exposure. This behaviour would imply a difference in risk of two- to threefold between women starting sexual activity at 16 as opposed to those starting at age 21, in line with the results shown in Table 31.2. Both these observations point to the role of a sexually transmitted agent; further support is given to this hypothesis by the apparent high risk for monogamous women whose male partner has had many sexual partners (Agarwal et al 1993).

Transmissible agents

A number of studies have addressed the role of human papilloma virus (HPV) types 6, 11, 16, 18, 31, 33, 35 and 45 in the aetiology of cervical cancer. HPV DNA has been

Table 31.2 Relative risk for cervical cancer associated with factors reflecting sexual lifestyle after adjustment for other sexual factors, smoking, number of births and pap smears (modified from Brinton et al 1987)

Number of sexual partners	Relative risk	Age at first intercourse	Relative risk
1	1.0	>21	1.0
2	1.5	20–21	1.9
3–4	2.2	18–19	2.2
5+	2.8	<18	2.5

detected in 93% of invasive tumours (Bosch et al 1995). Much attention is being focused on the human papilloma viruses, particularly HPVs 16 and 18. In most studies HPV 16 DNA has been found in 40–60% of cervical cancers with HPV 18 being present in another 10–20%. HPV 18 was the commonest in Indonesia. There seems to be a significant geographical variation in the prevalence of the rarer HPV types. HPV 45 appeared to cluster in western Africa, whereas HPVs 39 and 59 are virtually confined to Latin America. In squamous cell tumours HPV 16 seems to predominate, whereas HPV 18 seems to predominate in adenosquamous tumours. It appears that the presence of HPV 16/18 DNA in cervical intraepithelial neoplasia (CIN) increases the risk of progression to more advanced CIN lesions. Women with cervical HPV infection have an 11 times higher risk to develop CIN II or III than those without HPV. (95% confidence limits 3.7–31) (Koutsky et al 1992). The population attributable risk of HPV infection on the incidence of CIN II and III is about 80%. Thus, there is convincing evidence that HPV has a causal role in cervical cancer (Munoz & Bosch 1992). The putative role of herpes simplex virus type 2 has not been experimentally or epidemiologically substantiated (Munoz et al 1995). Current research is being focused on developing a vaccine directed at the E6 and E7 oncoproteins expressed in HPV tumours. The scope for primary prevention of cervical cancer is likely to improve considerably in the near future.

Smoking

One of the basic problems in interpreting the reported association between smoking and cervical cancer is that of confounding by sexual activity. Smoking is known to be related to sexual activity and many sexually transmitted diseases are two to three times more common in smokers than in non-smokers. In order to remove the confounding effect of this, the identity of the specific aetiologic agent needs to be known. Use of surrogate variables, such as the number of sexual partners, will not be an efficient control of this confounding (Tzonou et al 1986). It is certainly plausible that, with the availability of HPV markers, the role of smoking will be unambiguously addressed. A recent report (Bosch et al 1992) suggests that the association of smoking with cervical cancer risk is largely the result of confounding with HPV infection.

Oral contraception

Oral contraception is related to the risk of sexually transmitted infection as well as to sexual activity. The increased risk for cervical cancer seen among oral contraceptive users cannot be taken to indicate a causal role for oral contraceptive use.

Immunosuppression

An increased risk of cervical cancer has been seen among women taking immunosuppressive therapy following renal transplant (Hoover 1977). A similar increase is seen in women following treatment for Hodgkin's disease (Kaldor et al 1987), where both the original malignancy and the therapy (both radiotherapy and chemotherapy) could have been immunosuppressive.

Dietary factors

There have been few studies looking into dietary factors as a possible aetiologic agent in cervical cancer. The reported association between diets low in β-carotene or vitamin C and cervical cancer suffers from serious confounding from cigarette smoking, as smoking and a diet low in fruit and vegetables are often positively associated.

Screening for cervical cancer

The use of cervical cytology to identify precancerous lesions in healthy, asymptomatic women, as opposed to its use for diagnostic purposes, was introduced in the USA and part of Scandinavia in the 1950s. Clinical enthusiasm for the discovery of early lesions outran the quality of evidence demonstrating that mass screening could reduce morbidity and mortality from the invasive disease, with the result that it was not applied within a proper epidemiological context (for example, the target population was undefined, and uptake rates were incorrectly estimated by being based on slides rather than on women screened). Consequently, population benefits were often not achieved.

In some populations, notably much of Scandinavia and parts of Scotland (Day 1984), the organization of cervical cytology services had a public health rather than a clinical orientation and the effect on disease rates was impressive. Falls of 60% or more in both death and incidence rates from the disease were seen in Finland, Iceland and the Grampian region of Scotland (Hakama 1982, McGregor et al 1986, Laara et al 1987). The basic question now with cervical cancer screening is how, using current knowledge of the natural history of the disease, population-based screening can be optimally effected within the health delivery system of the respective population.

The natural history can be represented in simplistic terms:

Normal epithelium ⟶ Atypia detectable by cervical cytology ⟶ Invasive cancer

The classification of atypia has changed frequently and depends on whether it is based on histological or cytological grounds. Carcinoma-in-situ, dysplasia and CIN are descriptions of tissue, not of individual cells, and so should refer only to a histological specimen. Much discussion has centred on the nature of CIN lesions, to what extent they progress to malignancy, how rapidly and whether CIN I or even CIN II is a genuine precursor state or simply an indicator of a high-risk individual. It appears undeniable that too many CIN lesions are found for them all to progress to malignancy, and that the rate of regression is higher for CIN I than for CIN II. The presence of HPV 16/18 may be a useful indicator of which precursor lesion will progress rapidly. It is also apparent that the great majority of squamous invasive cancers (which constitute 90% or more of invasive cancers in unscreened populations, although the introduction of the term 'adenosquamous' is a complicating factor) pass through a stage in which atypia could be detected cytologically. More work in this area is required.

The question of how long such cancers remain in this preinvasive detectable stage was investigated in an international study coordinated by the IARC (1986). A number of centralized screening centres in Europe and Canada identified women who had developed cervical cancer after at least one normal cytological smear. Incidence rates (or relative incidence rates) were calculated for invasive cancer in terms of the years that had elapsed since the last negative smear, and the number of previous negative smears. These rates were expressed as a proportion of the rate observed in the absence of screening, and so expressed the reduction in the risk produced by screening (Table 31.3). These are in fact the proportions of lesions that progress from normality to invasion in that number of years, or fewer. This study indicated clearly that screening every 3 years is virtually as effective as screening every year (Table 31.4). The only justification for annual screening is to compensate for inadequacies in the screening process, which are better rectified by direct action. The joint UICC–IARC monograph on cervical cancer concluded that: 'The main unknown question concerning cervical screening at present relates to the treatment of early atypical lesions, many of which will regress. Markers which identified the lesions which would progress would be of great utility, both in avoiding unnecessary treatment and in preventing undue delay in treatment. Use of HPV markers for this purpose appears a promising line of research'.

Table 31.3 The reduction in risk of cervical cancer among women who have had at least two cytological smears (IARC 1986)

Time since last negative smear (months)	Relative risk
<12	0.07
12–23	0.08
24–35	0.13
36–47	0.19
48–59	0.31
60–71	0.31
72–119	0.63
120+	1.00

Table 31.4 Percentage reduction in cumulative risk of invasive cervical cancer in the age range 35–64, with different screening frequencies (IARC 1986)

Screening frequency (years)	% Reduction in cumulative risk	No. of tests in 35–64 age range
1	93.3	30
2	93.3	15
3	91.4	10
5	83.9	6
10	64.2	3

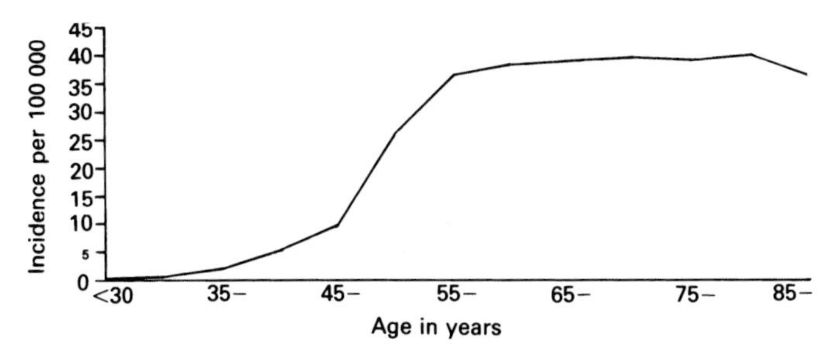

Fig. 31.4 The incidence of endometrial carcinoma in different age groups in England and Wales in 1981 (Office of Population Censuses and Surveys 1985).

ENDOMETRIAL CANCER

Cancer of the endometrium is rare before the age of 40. Thereafter, the incidence increases till the mid 50s, after which it tends to remain steady (Fig. 31.4). As seen in Table 31.1, the incidence of endometrial cancer varies widely, the lowest rates being in Asian populations and the highest among North American whites. It is noteworthy, however, that when Asian populations migrate to the USA the rates rise very markedly to approach those seen in the local white population. This rise is steeper than for almost any other cancer site.

Aetiological factors

The main risk factors identified for endometrial cancer relate to hormonal status and reproductive history. Early age at menarche and low parity increase the risk, as for breast cancer, but of greater importance are late menopause, the use of oestrogen replacement therapy and obesity. Table 31.5 presents the levels of risk that have been observed for these last factors. The major role of obesity in determining the risk for endometrial cancer is clear.

In contrast to the increase in risk associated with the above factors, a decrease in risk for endometrial cancer has been observed both for cigarette smokers and for users of the combined oral contraceptive pill (rather than

Table 31.5 Risk factors for endometrial cancer

	Daily dose (mg)	Relative risk
Oestrogen replacement therapy (unopposed)		
Mack et al (1976)	<0.625	5.0
	>0.625	9.48
Weiss et al (1979)	<1.25	6.5
	>1.25	7.6
	Weight (kg)	Relative risk
Obesity		
Premenopausal women	<59.0	1.0
Henderson et al (1983)	59.0–67.9	1.5
	68.0–77.0	2.0
	77.1–86.1	9.6
	86.2	17.7
Postmenopausal women	<52.9	1.0
La Vecchia et al (1984)	52.9–66.0	1.6
	66.1–79.2	3.3
	>79.3	7.6

sequential-type oral contraceptives). Table 31.6 indicates the degree to which the risk has been reduced.

Key and Pike (1988) hypothesize that risk for endometrial cancer is directly related to the cumulative degree of endometrial mitotic activity, and that mitotic activity of the endometrium increases directly with the levels of unopposed oestrogen up to a certain limit, beyond which oestrogen produces no further mitotic response. Progestogens greatly reduce the rate of mitotic activity. The quantitative consequences of this hypothesis are displayed in Figure 31.5, which can be considered to be a summary of the observed risk differentials associated with the different factors.

Endometrial cancer is also associated with conditions which themselves are associated with obesity, including diabetes and hypothyroidism, but the associations are through obesity.

Tamoxifen and endometrial cancer

There have been several studies that report a small excess risk for endometrial cancer among breast cancer patients treated with tamoxifen (Neven et al 1994). The weak oestrogenic effect of tamoxifen on the endometrium has been suggested to explain this effect, but the well-known doubling of the risk of endometrial cancer in women with breast cancer (Adami et al 1987) may account for the excess reported in some of the uncontrolled studies. The therapeutic benefit of tamoxifen in controlling breast cancer clearly outweighs any modest increase of endometrial cancer risk, and so there is no reason to withhold tamoxifen treatment for women with breast cancer (Fisher et al 1994). The use of tamoxifen in healthy women to prevent breast cancer is currently being investigated. These studies will allow an assessment of the reduction in breast cancer and any increase in endometrial cancer.

Table 31.6 Protective factors for endometrial cancer

		Relative risk
Cigarette smoking (ever/never)		
Levy et al (1987)	premenopausal	0.5
	postmenopausal	0.4
	Years of use	Relative risk
Combined oral contraceptive use		
Henderson et al (1983)	0	1.00
	<2	0.75
	2–3	0.79
	4–5	0.28
	>5	0.14

Conclusion

These findings suggest a major potential for primary prevention, mainly through weight loss but also through the use of combined oral contraceptives. The effect of combined oestrogen and progesterone hormone replacement therapy on endometrial cancer risk is not clear (Grady et al 1995). Given the considerable benefits in terms of osteoporosis and cardiovascular diseases resulting from hormone replacement therapy, the issue is of great importance.

Screening for endometrial cancer

There are no immediate prospects for mass screening and secondary prevention. Although a number of instruments have been developed for endometrial sampling without anaesthesia for diagnostic purposes (Iverson & Segadal 1985), none have been evaluated in an asymptomatic population.

OVARIAN CANCER

Ovarian cancer encompasses a group of histopathologically heterogeneous malignancies. In women less than 30 years old germ cell tumours are the most common. Over the age of 30 most are adenocarcinomas. The following discussion refers largely to the latter group.

Germ cell tumours

The age distribution is bimodal, with the first peak in the 15–19-year age group and a second one at 65–69 years (Fig. 31.6). Whereas the early peak consists of almost equal numbers of teratomas and dysgerminomas, the late peak consists mainly of teratomas. The incidence has not varied much in the period 1971–1984.

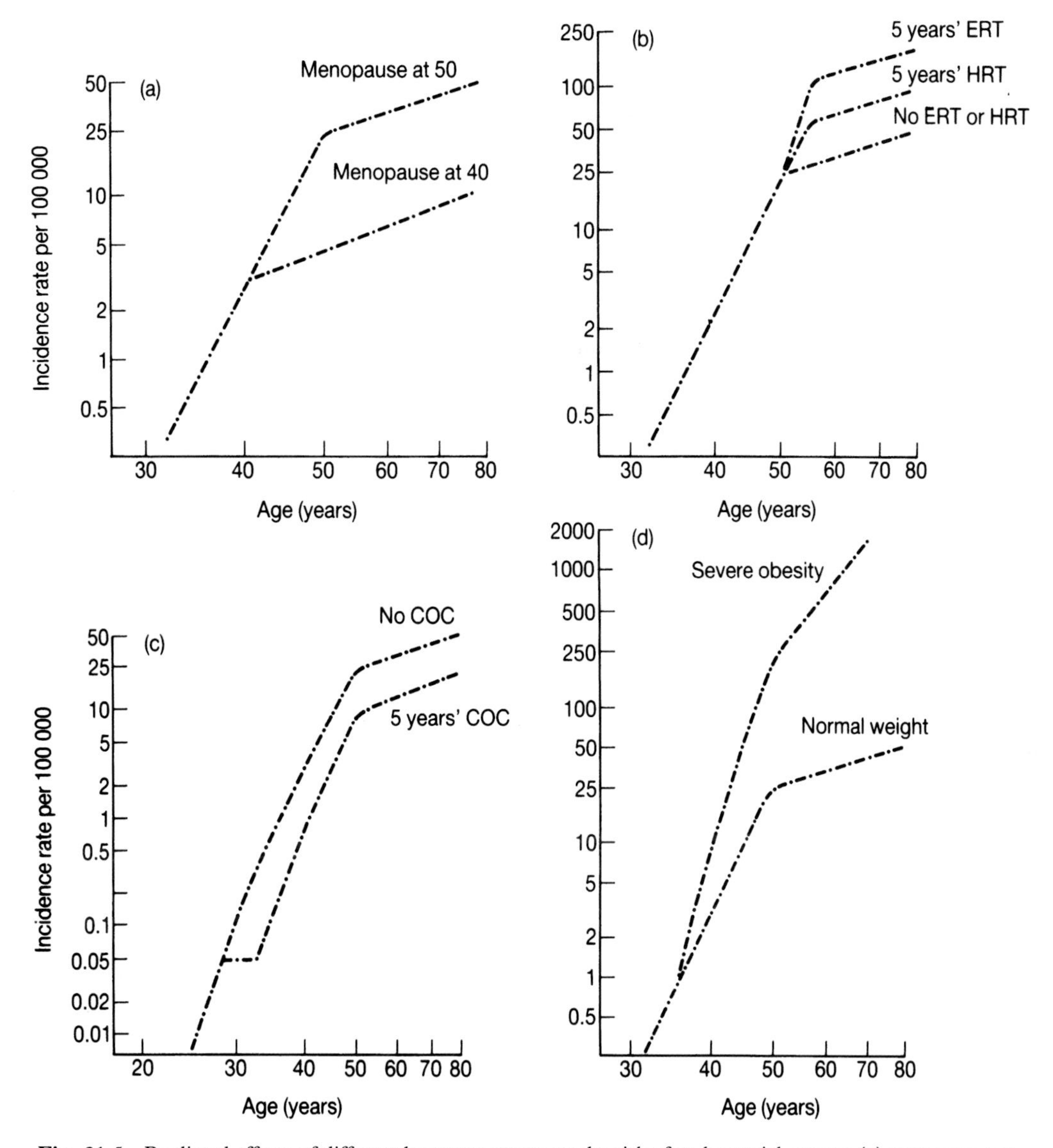

Fig. 31.5 Predicted effects of different hormone events on the risk of endometrial cancer: **(a)** menopause at age 50 years or at age 40 years; **(b)** 5 years of oestrogen replacement therapy (ERT) or combined hormone replacement therapy (HRT) starting at age 50 or no oestrogen hormone therapy; **(c)** 5 years of combined oral contraception (COC) from age 28 years or no COC; **(d)** extreme obesity (anovular from 35 years of age) or normal weight. (Modified from Key & Pike 1988)

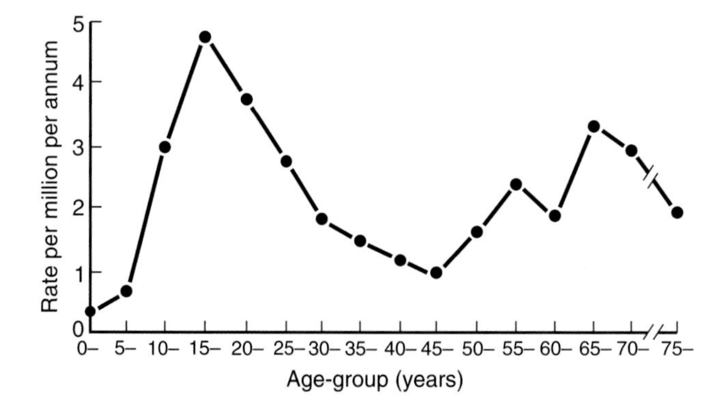

Fig. 31.6 Age distribution of ovarian germ cell cancer in England. Mean annual registration rates for 1971–1984.

Adenocarcinomas

Although there are different histological varieties of adenocarcinoma (serous, mucinous and endometrioid being the major types), there is little evidence that they have different epidemiological characteristics. Therefore, in the following discussion they are treated as a single entity.

Age aspects and time trends

Globally, among the gynaecological cancers ovarian cancer shows the least variation in incidence rates (Table 31.1). The highest rates are seen in the European countries, whereas the lowest rates are found in Asian countries. Within countries there seems to be little racial or urban/

rural variation. There has been little change in the incidence rates in European countries in the last 30 years. Analysis of Danish Cancer Registry material collected from 1943 to 1982 indicates little change in incidence by year of birth for women born in this century, but a rapid increase in the risk from the 1860–1869 decade of birth cohort to the 1900–1909 birth cohort (Ewertz & Kjaer 1988). Mortality from ovarian cancer in Denmark shows a somewhat different picture, with a decrease in risk seen over successive decades of birth from 1910 to 1950. This decrease appears to be related to survival, with an improving stage at diagnosis being seen for younger women.

Data from the Surveillance, Epidemiology and End Results (SEER) programme, which represents about 9% of the US population, indicate that the age-adjusted rate advances as age advances, peaking at 54 per 100 000 in the age group 75–79 years (Yanick 1993). Ovarian cancer is the biggest killer among gynaecological cancers in western populations.

Aetiological factors

Cancers of the ovary have been less well studied than other gynaecological cancers and only a few risk factors have been identified with any degree of certainty. The main factors affecting risk for epithelial cancers of the ovary have been reproductive: that is, parity and use of oral contraceptives, and family history. For associated factors, including age at menarche, menopause and first childbirth, the evidence is less clear. The risk factors for non-epithelial cancers are less well understood. A good discussion can be found in Horn-Ross et al (1992).

Table 31.7 Reproductive risk factors for ovarian cancer showing observed to expected (Obs:Exp) ratios from a prospective study of 425 women in Norway (Kvale et al 1988)

Factor	Obs:Exp
Parity	
0	1.50
1	1.32
2	0.89
3	0.76
4	0.73
Age at first birth	
<20	0.79
20–24	0.98
25–29	0.93
30–34	1.30
>34	0.80
Age at last birth	
<25	1.04
25–29	0.94
30–34	1.06
35–39	0.99
>39	0.97
Age at menarche	
<13	0.95
13	0.91
14	1.13
15	0.93
16	0.93
>16	1.04
Age at menopause	
<46	1.04
46–47	1.00
48–49	0.97
50–51	0.93
52–53	1.07
>53	1.08

Parity

One of the largest studies to report on parity was a retrospective study of 60 565 women in Norway (Kvale et al 1988) among whom 445 cases of ovarian cancer arose in the period 1961–1980, of which only 12 were germ cell tumours. The relative risks for parity 0 to parity 4 are given in Table 31.7, together with the relative effects of age at first birth, age at menarche and age at menopause. Each of these last four factors can be seen to have a negligible effect, a finding in agreement with most previous studies. The effect of parity is clear, however, with a smooth decreasing risk with increasing parity.

This effect of parity is seen at the population level as well. Beral et al (1978) examined changes in mortality over time for England and Wales and the USA on a birth cohort basis. Considerable variations were seen among birth cohorts, virtually all of which could be explained by the average completed family size for each birth cohort (Fig. 31.7). This elegant study suggests that the relationship with parity is primarily with the number of children a woman chooses to bear, rather than intrinsic child-bearing capacity, and also that other environmental factors which have been changing over time have little role in ovarian epithelial cancers. It should also be noted that this

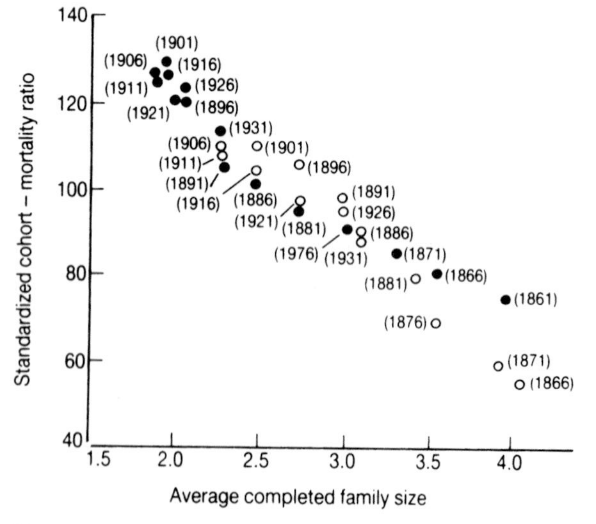

Fig. 31.7 Age-standardized mortality ratios from ovarian carcinoma are plotted against the average completed family size for different generations of women in England and Wales (●) and the USA (○). Each point represents a separate birth cohort with the mid-year of birth shown in brackets. (Modified from Beral et al 1978)

study refers to cohorts of women who would have used oral contraceptives rarely.

Oral contraception

The second factor associated with reproduction is the use of the contraceptive pill. Typical results, from a study in the USA (Wu et al 1988), are given in Table 31.8. Table 31.9 gives the results by number of full-term pregnancies. The effects of parity and of oral contraceptives are independent of each other, combining in approximately multiplicative fashion. Furthermore, the relative reduction in risk for a given number of years of oral contraceptive use does not diminish after oral contraceptive use ends, but appears to continue indefinitely. Follow-up studies over several decades have not yet been performed.

Years of ovulation

The findings on parity and oral contraceptive use support the hypothesis of Fathalla (1971) that duration of active ovulation is of major importance in determining ovarian cancer risk. The results of an American study were expressed in these terms, as shown in Table 31.10 (Whittemore et al 1992). Increasing years of ovulation have a greater effect in women under 55 years of age, as opposed to older women. The main epidemiological findings in terms of age, parity and oral contraceptive use are explicable if the ovarian epithelium is at risk during the cellular proliferation associated with ovulation, but not when the ovary is quiescent.

The lack of effect of age at menarche and age at menopause probably results from the large number of anovulatory cycles around both ages, so that data on onset and cessation are very imprecise.

Table 31.8 Risks of ovarian cancer with respect to oral contraception use, showing the results of a case-control study in San Francisco (from Wu et al 1988 with permission of Dr Whittemore and the American Journal of Epidemiology.)

Oral contraceptive use	Relative risk
Never used	1.00
Ever used	0.94
Duration of use	
1–12 months	0.97
13–36 months	0.81
>36 months	0.40

Table 31.9 Relative risk of ovarian cancer by both oral contraceptive use and parity (from Wu et al 1988 with permission of Dr Whittemore and the American Journal of Epidemiology.)

Months of oral contraceptive use	Number of pregnancies		
	0	1–2	>3
<12 months or never used	1.00	0.63	0.55
13–36 months	0.82	0.35	0.68
>36 months	0.13	0.34	0.23

Other environmental factors

Other factors which have been investigated and for which no good evidence exists for an effect on risk (in either direction) include non-contraceptive oestrogens, alcohol and tobacco. Coffee has occasionally been implicated but the data appear weak.

In Singapore the China-born Chinese have rates similar to those seen in China, whereas the rates in the Singapore-born are nearly twofold higher (Table 31.1). Similar changes are seen among Chinese and Japanese migrants to the USA (Lee et al 1988). However, in the overall epidemiological picture there are no large differences between populations to suggest that major environmental risk factors remain to be identified.

Genetic factors

Genetic factors clearly play an important role in the development of epithelial ovarian cancer. In a national study in the UK, based on the 1939 household registration, the risk was substantially elevated among women with a first-degree relative with the disease. The increase in risk was largest if the relative developed the disease under age 50, when the relative risk lay between six- and tenfold (Ponder et al 1989). If two or more close relatives were affected, the lifetime risk rises to about 40% (compared to the figures in Table 31.1), much of which occurs before the age of 50. This value of 40% is close to the 50% chance of inheriting a putative gene. It is thought that perhaps 1% of all cases in the UK may belong to this very high-risk group. Many of the families at high risk of ovarian cancer are also at high risk of breast cancer. Much of this familial risk is associated with mutation of the *BRCA1* gene on chromosome 17, but other loci may also be involved (Easton et al 1993).

Table 31.10 Odds ratios for invasive ovarian cancer by duration of ovulation – results of 12 case-control studies (modified from Whittemore et al 1992)

Years of ovulation	Odds radio	
	<55 years	>55 years
<25	1.0	1.0
25–29	1.8	1.3
30–34	2.6	1.2
>34	2.9	1.5
Overall trend per year	1.08* $P<0.001$	1.02† $P = 0.10$

* test of OR homogeneity across studies $P = 0.38$
† test of OR homogeneity across studies $P = 0.04$

Screening for ovarian cancer

A combination of carcinoembryonic antigen 125 (CA125) assay and transvaginal ultrasonography has been evaluated as a screening tool (Jacobs & Oram 1989). So far, there is no evidence that population screening reduces ovarian cancer mortality.

Conclusions

Apart from age, family history is the strongest predictor of ovarian cancer risk. Epidemiological studies have identified no major environmental causes, nor do they suggest that factors which could form the focus for intervention studies are likely to be identified in the near future. Identification of the susceptibility locus offers opportunities for identification of high-risk women, but it will take a long time to gather enough evidence for their use on a population basis. The only prospect of primary prevention appears to be in the manipulation of ovulation by judicious use of oral contraceptives. Such an approach clearly requires to balance both increased and decreased risk for a range of diseases. There is no immediate prospect of population-based mass screening.

ACKNOWLEDGEMENT

This work was undertaken during the tenure of a Research Training Fellowship awarded by the International Agency for Research on Cancer, Lyon, to Dr Eswar Krishnan.

KEY POINTS

1. On a global basis, cancer of the cervix is the second most common cancer in women after breast cancer.
2. Cancer of the ovary and endometrium are seldom more than the fifth or sixth most common cancers, in either the developed or developing nations.
3. The large variation in the incidence seen for cervical and endometrial cancer worldwide is not shown by ovarian cancer, which shows only a two- to threefold variation in risk.
4. Epidemiological evidence strongly supports a causal role for human papilloma virus 16 and 18 in cervical intraepithelial neoplasia, and is the key predictor of progression to invasive cancer. The population attributable risk of HPV infection on CIN is at least 80%, and possibly over 90%.
5. Cervical cancer epidemiology is strongly influenced by the level of sexual activity and the degree of effective mass screening.
6. In Scandinavia, the major change in incidence and mortality rates of cervical cancer since the 1950s can be closely linked to the different approaches in the five different countries to the introduction of mass screening.
7. The two main behavioural aspects of sexual activity which modify risk for the disease are age at first intercourse and the number of sexual partners.
8. Studies on the role of smoking in the aetiology of cervical cancer suffer from possible confounding by sexual activity. With the availability of HPV markers, it seems clear that most of the observed association is due to such confounding.
9. Screening for cervical cancer every 3 years is virtually as effective as screening every year. The only justification for annual cytology is to compensate for inadequacies in the screening process, which are better rectified by direct action.
10. When Asian populations migrate to the USA, the rates of endometrial cancer rise very markedly to approach those seen in the local white population.
11. Much of the data support the hypothesis that the risk of endometrial cancer is directly related to the cumulative degree of endometrial mitotic activity, which increases directly with levels of unopposed oestrogen, up to a certain limit.
12. The decreasing risk of ovarian cancer associated with increasing parity is related primarily to the number of children a woman chooses to have, rather than her intrinsic fertility. The role of environmental factors seems to be small.
13. Oral contraceptive use reduces the risk of ovarian cancer and this protective effect seems to persist even after the oral contraceptive pill is discontinued.
14. Duration of active ovulation is an important predictor of ovarian cancer risk.
15. Possibly 1% of all cases in the UK may belong to a very high-risk group with a strong family history.
16. Until large-scale randomized controlled trials are conducted, there is no justification for including ovarian screening in the national health programme.

REFERENCES

Adami H-O, Krusemo U B, Bergkvist I, Persson I, Pettersson B 1987 On the age-dependent association between cancer of the breast and of the endometrium. A nationwide cohort study. British Journal of Cancer 55: 77–80

Agarwal S S, Sehgal A, Sardana S, Kumar A, Luthra U K 1993 Role of male behaviour in cervical carcinogenesis among women with one lifetime sexual partner. Cancer 72(5): 1666–1669

Armitage P, Doll R 1954 The age distribution of cancer and a multi-stage theory of carcinogenesis. British Journal of Cancer 8: 1–5

Beral V 1974 Cancer of the cervix: a sexually transmitted infection. Lancet i: 1037–1040

Beral V, Fraser P, Chilvers C 1978 Does pregnancy protect against ovarian cancer? Lancet i: 1083–1087

Berek J S, Castaldo T W, Hacker N F et al 1981 Adenocarcinoma of the uterine cervix. Cancer 48: 2734–2741

Bosch F X, Munoz N, de Sanjose S et al 1992 Risk factors for cervical cancer in Colombia and Spain. International Journal of Cancer 52 (5): 750–758

Bosch F X, Manos M M, Munoz N et al 1995 Prevalence of human papilloma virus in cervical cancer: a worldwide perspective. Journal of the National Cancer Institute (in press)
Brinton L A, Hamman R F, Higgins G R et al 1987 Sexual and reproductive risk factors for invasive squamous cervical cancer. Journal of the National Cancer Institute 79: 23–31
Day N E 1984 The effect of cervical cancer screening in Scandinavia. Obstetrics and Gynecology 63: 714–718
Day N E 1990 The Armitage–Doll multistage model of carcinogenesis. Statistics in Medicine 9(6): 677–679
Devesa S S, Young J L Jr, Brinton L A, Fraumeni F Jr 1989 Recent trends in cervix uteri cancer. Cancer 64: 2184–2190
Easton D F, Bishop D T, Ford D, Crockford G P 1993 Genetic linkage analysis in familial breast and ovarian cancer: results from 214 families. The Breast Cancer Linkage Consortium. American Journal of Human Genetics 52(4): 678–701
Ewertz M, Kjaer S K 1988 Ovarian cancer incidence and mortality in Denmark 1943–82. International Journal of Cancer 42: 690–697
Fathalla M F 1971 Incessant ovulation – a factor in ovarian neoplasia. Lancet ii: 163
Fisher B, Constantino J P, Redmond C K, Fisher E R, Wickerham D L, Cronin W M 1994 Endometrial cancer in tamoxifen treated breast cancer patients: findings from the National Surgical Adjuvant Breast and Bowel Project (NSABP) B-14. Journal of the National Cancer Institute 86(7): 478–479
Grady D, Gebretsadik T, Kerlikowse K, Ernster V, Petitti D 1995 Hormone replacement therapy and endometrial cancer risk: a meta-analysis. Obstetrics and Gynecology 85: 304–313
Hakama M 1982 Trends in the incidence of cervical cancer in the Nordic countries. In: Magnus K (ed) Trends in cancer incidence. Hemisphere, New York
Henderson B E, Casagrande J T, Pike M C, Mack T, Rosario T, Duke A 1983 The epidemiology of endometrial cancer in younger women. British Journal of Cancer 47: 749–756
Hoover R 1977 Effects of drugs: immunosuppression. In: Hiatt H H, Watson I D, Winsten J A (eds) Origins of human cancer. Cold Spring Harbor Laboratory, New York
Horn-Ross P L, Whittemore A S, Harris R et al 1992 Characteristics relating to ovarian cancer risk: collaborative analysis of 12 US case control studies. VI Non epithelial cancers among adults. Epidemiology 3: 490–495
IARC 1986 Screening for cervical cancer – the duration of low risk following negative cervical cytology. British Medical Journal 293: 659–664
Iverson O E, Segadal E 1985 The value of endometrial cytology. A comparative study of the Gravlee jet-washer, Isaacs cell sampler and Endoscan versus curettage in 600 patients. Obstetrical and Gynaecological Survey 40: 14–20
Jacobs I J, Oram D A 1989 Potential screening tests for ovarian cancer. In: Sharp F, Leake R E (eds) Ovarian cancer: biological and therapeutic challenges. Chapman & Hall, London
Kaldor J, Day N E, Band P et al 1987 Second malignancies following testicular cancer, ovarian cancer and Hodgkin's disease: an international collaborative study among cancer registries. International Journal of Cancer 39(5): 571–585
Key T J A, Pike M C 1988 The dose–effect relationship between 'unopposed' oestrogens and endometrial mitotic rate: its central role in explaining and predicting endometrial cancer risk. British Journal of Cancer 57: 205–212
Kjaer S K, Brinton L A 1993 Adenocarcinomas of the uterine cervix: the epidemiology of an increasing problem. Epidemiologic Reviews 15(2): 486–498
Koutsky L A, Holmes H K, Critchlow C W et al 1992 A cohort study of the risk of cervical intraepithelial neoplasia grade 2 or 3 in relation to papillomavirus infection. New England Journal of Medicine 327: 1272–1278
Kvale G, Hensel I, Nilsen S, Beral V 1988 Reproductive factors and risk of ovarian cancer: a prospective study. International Journal of Cancer 42(2): 246–252
Laara E, Day N E, Hakama M 1987 Trends in mortality from cervical cancer in the Nordic countries: association with organised mass screening programmes. Lancet i: 1247–1249
La Vecchia C, Franceschi S, Decarli A, Gallus G, Tagnoni G 1984 Risk factors for endometrial cancer at different ages. Journal of the National Cancer Institute 73: 667
Lee H P, Day N E, Shanmugarathnam K 1988 Time trends in cancer incidence in Singapore 1968–82. IARC Scientific Publication no 91, IARC, Lyon
Levy F, La Vecchia C, Decarli A 1987 Cigarette smoking and the risk of endometrial cancer at different ages. European Journal of Cancer and Clinical Oncology 23: 1025–1029
McGregor J E, Moss S, Parkin D M, Day N E 1986 Cervical cancer screening in North East Scotland. British Medical Journal 290: 1543–1546
Mack T M, Pike M C, Henderson B E et al 1976 Estrogens and endometrial cancer in a retirement community. New England Journal of Medicine 294: 1262–1268
Muir C, Waterhouse J, Mack T M, Powell J, Whelan S (eds) 1987 Cancer incidence in five continents, vol. V. IARC, Lyon
Munoz N, Bosch F X 1992 HPV and cervical neoplasia: review of case-control and cohort studies. IARC Scientific publication 119: 251–261
Munoz N, Kato I, Bosch F X et al 1995 Cervical cancer and herpes simplex virus type 2: case-control studies in Spain and Colombia, with special reference to immunoglobulin sub-classes. International Journal of Cancer 60: 438–442
Neven P, De Muylder X, Van Belle Y, Campo R, Vanderick G 1994 Tamoxifen and the uterus. British Medical Journal 309: 1313–1314
Office of Population Censuses and Surveys 1985 1981 Cancer statistics – registrations. HMSO, London
Parkin D M, Muir C S, Whelan S L, Gao Y T, Ferlay J, Powell J (eds) 1992 Cancer incidence in five continents, vol. VI. IARC, Lyon
Parkin D M, Pisani P, Ferlay J 1993 Estimates of world-wide incidence of eighteen major cancers in 1985. International Journal of Cancer 54: 594–606
Pokras R, Hufnagel V G 1987 Hysterectomies in the United States, 1965–1984. Hyattesville, Maryland: US Department of Health and Human Services, Public Health Service, CDC DHHS publication no.(PHS)87-1753 (Vital and health statistics; series 13, no 92)
Ponder B A J, Easton D F, Peto J 1989 Risk of ovarian cancer associated with family history. In: Sharp F, Mason W P, Leake R E (eds) Ovarian cancer: biological and therapeutic challenges. Chapman & Hall, London
Tzonou A, Kaldor J M, Smith P G, Day N E, Trichopoulos D 1986 Misclassification in case control studies with two dichotomous risk factors. Revue d'Epidémiologie de Santé Publique 34: 10–17
Weiss N S, Szekely D R, English D R, Schweid A I 1979 Endometrial cancer in relation to patterns of menopausal estrogen use. Journal of the American Medical Association 242: 261–264
Whittemore A S, Harris R, Intyre J et al 1992 Characteristics relating to ovarian cancer risk: collaborative analysis of 12 US case control studies. IV. The pathogenesis of epithelial ovarian cancer. American Journal of Epidemiology 136: 1212–1230
Wu M L, Whittemore A S, Paffenbarger R S et al 1988 Personal and environmental factors related to epithelial ovarian cancer. I. Reproductive and menstrual events and oral contraceptive use. American Journal of Epidemiology 128: 1216–1227
Yanick R 1993 Ovarian cancer. Age contrasts in incidence, histology, disease stage at diagnosis and mortality. Cancer 71 (2 Suppl): 517–523

32

The genetics of gynaecological cancer

Ian Jacobs   Bruce Ponder

INTRODUCTION

Enormous progress has been made in understanding the molecular basis of disease during the last decade, and this has transformed our understanding of the process of carcinogenesis. In recent years these developments have begun to have an impact in gynaecological cancer. Although the details of molecular research and technology are frequently complex and of limited relevance to clinicians, the underlying principles provide a coherent and comprehensible framework of the process of carcinogenesis. The fundamental understanding achieved using molecular technology provides exciting opportunities for the prevention, early detection and treatment of cancer. Molecular knowledge has not yet had a major impact in clinical oncology but its potential is clear and likely to emerge during the next decade. It will become increasingly important for clinicians involved in the management of gynaecological malignancies to have a working knowledge of the molecular basis of carcinogenesis.

Gynaecological cancers provide examples of a number of contrasting mechanisms of carcinogenesis (Fig. 32.1). For example, ovarian and endometrial cancer can occur as components of familial cancer syndromes (familial breast/ovarian cancer and Lynch II syndrome) owing to germline inheritance of predisposing genetic abnormalities. However, most ovarian cancers are thought not to be due to inherited genetic alterations, but to result from somatic mutations occurring in ovarian cells with an initially normal genome. These somatic mutations are believed to be secondary to environmental factors associated with carcinogenesis which act to increase the opportunity for spontaneous mutation in a number of critical genes. In contrast, the genetic alteration in cervical cancer is thought to be initiated by an environmental factor (papilloma virus), and in at least some endometrial cancers from unopposed oestrogen exposure. Little is yet known about the molecular genetics of vulval, vaginal and fallopian tube cancers.

THE MOLECULAR BASIS OF CARCINOGENESIS

A fundamental characteristic of cancer cells is loss of the normal restraints controlling cell division, cell–cell interaction and cellular mobility. The fact that this characteristic is passed on to cells arising from the division of cancer cells has long been regarded as evidence for a genetic basis for carcinogenesis, and is supported by a number of other observations. First, agents which cause damage to DNA (chemical mutagens, ionizing radiation and some viruses) also increase susceptibility to cancer (Ames et al 1973). Secondly, studies of the clonal origin of tumours (Fialkow 1976) indicate that the vast majority of neoplasms arise from a single cell, which passes on its abnormality to daughter cells. An initial genetic alteration provides a selective advantage for proliferation of a clone of cells, and further genetic alterations within this expanded population of cells increases the selective proliferative advantage and eventually leads to the formation of a clinically recognizable tumour.

It has become clear that the genetic changes in cancer involve genes which control normal cell growth and pro-

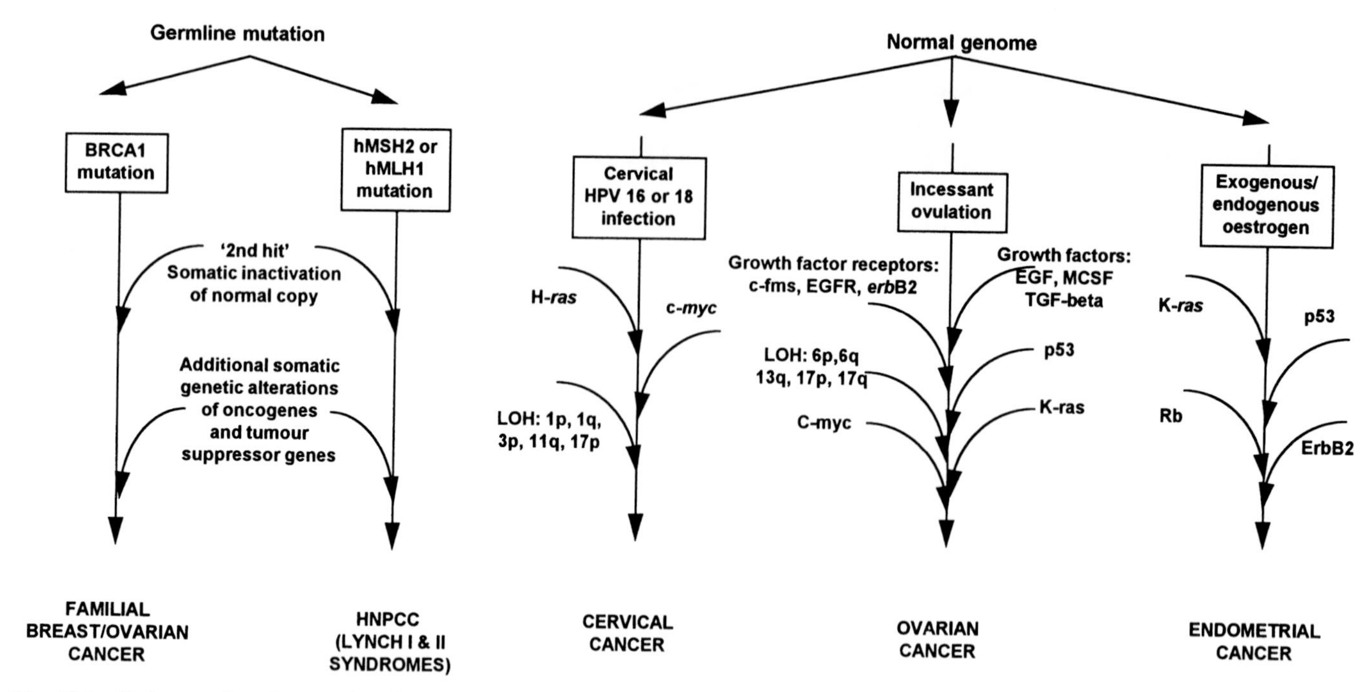

Fig. 32.1 Pathways of carcinogenesis in familial and sporadic gynaecological cancer.

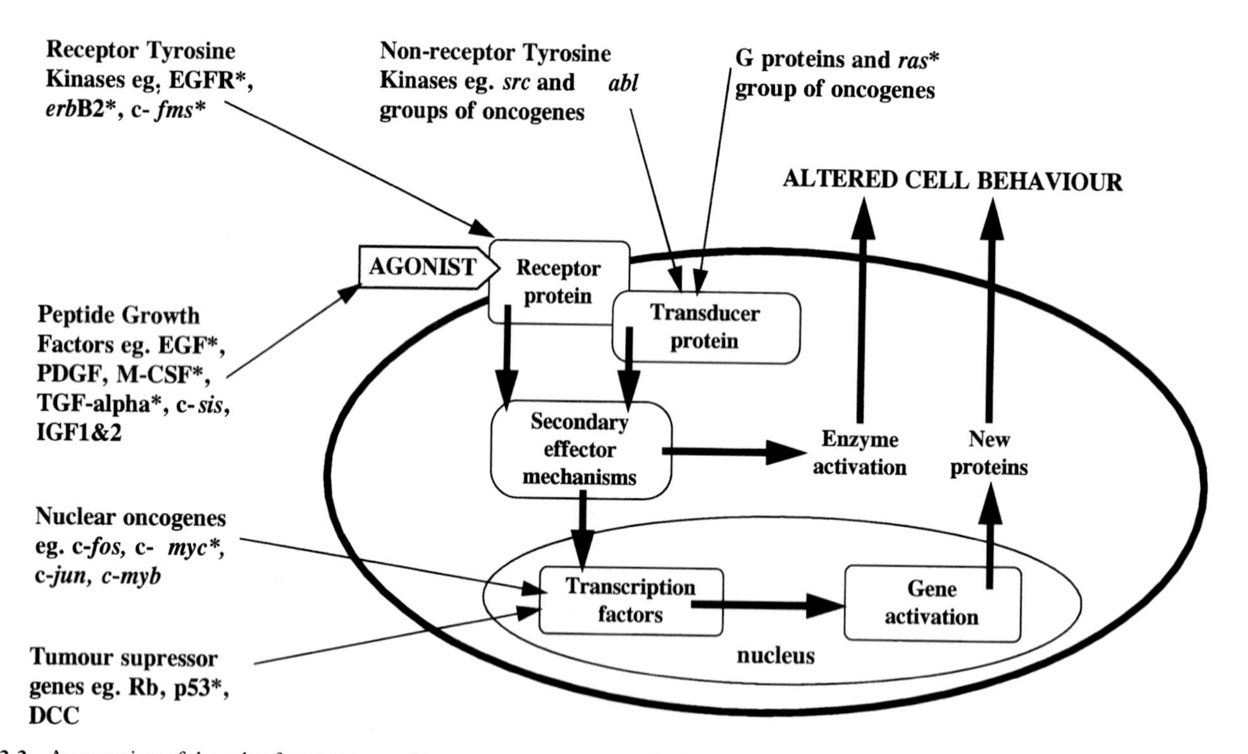

Fig. 32.2 An overview of the role of oncogenes and tumour suppressor genes in the control of cell growth and proliferation. The purpose of this figure is to emphasize that the genetic abnormalities in cancer are a result of alterations to or abnormal expression of genes which are normally involved in cell regulation. Genes which are implicated in ovarian carcinogenesis are marked*. Note that many aspects of the figure are oversimplified for clarity, e.g. although a function of *p53* and retinoblastoma is transcriptional regulation this is not true of all tumour suppressor genes.

liferation. Cells communicate via a complex interacting set of signalling pathways, the principles of which (but not the details) are well established (Alberts et al 1989) and are summarized in Figure 32.2. The best-understood mechanism of communication between cells is the release of molecules which interact as agonists with receptors, either within the cell or, more frequently, in the cell membrane. This interaction results in a further signal within

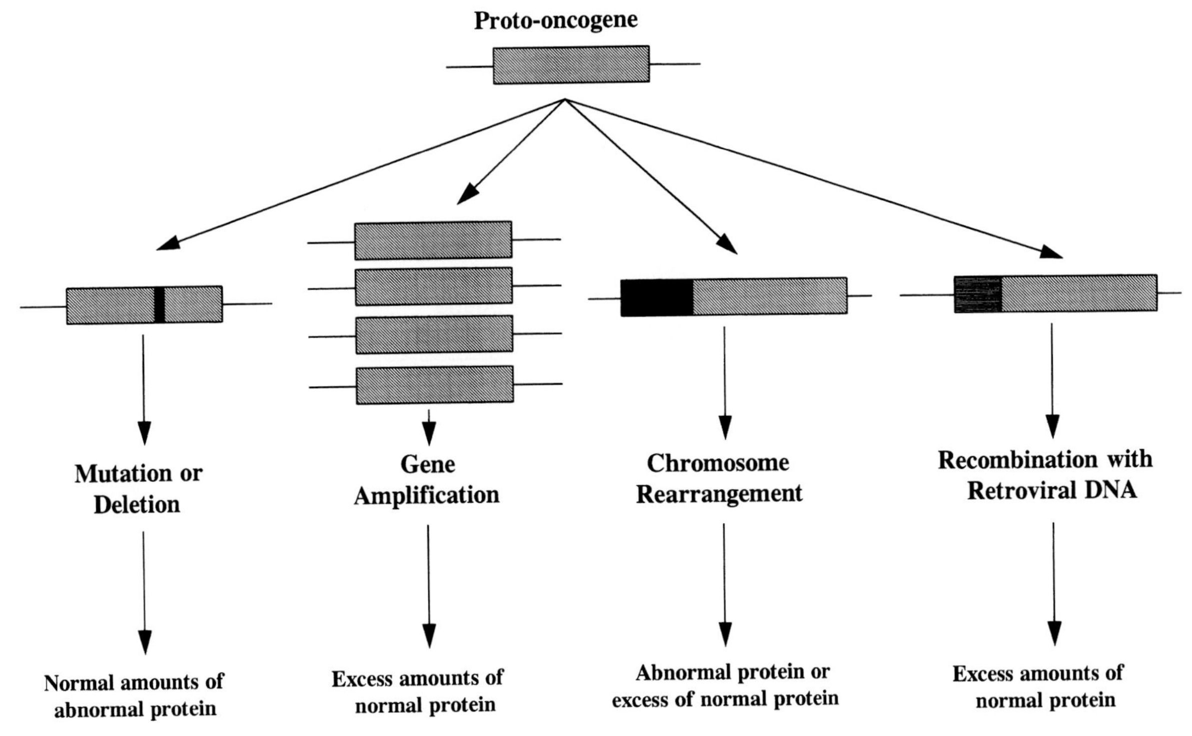

Fig. 32.3 Summary of the mechanisms of activation of oncogenes.

the cell which, via transducer proteins and secondary mechanisms, modifies cell behaviour either by activating target enzymes directly or by initiating transcription of genes and synthesis of their protein product. The genetic abnormalities observed in cancer are known to affect genes coding for all of the groups of molecules in Figure 32.2.

Oncogenes

The identification of oncogenes resulted from work with virus-induced cancers both in vitro and in animals. As the viral genome is relatively small it was possible to identify the specific genes (viral oncogenes) involved in the transforming activity of retroviruses such as the Rous sarcoma virus (Rous 1911). A number of viral oncogenes were found to have normal cellular homologues known as proto-oncogenes (Stehelin et al 1976). Other workers identified oncogenes by transfecting cell lines with DNA from human cancer cell lines (Krontiris & Cooper 1981) and found that some of the transforming oncogenes identified were mutated versions of the proto-oncogenes identified by the retroviral approach (Santos et al 1982). Subsequently it was demonstrated that chromosome translocations such as the Philadelphia chromosome in chronic myeloid leukaemia involved known oncogenes (DeKlein et al 1982). Approximately 100 proto-oncogenes have been identified and many can be assigned to the groups of functions summarized in Figure 32.2. The mutation resulting in conversion of a proto-oncogene into an oncogene may occur in several different ways (Fig. 32.3) and may result in an abnormal protein produced in normal quantity, a normal protein produced in excessive amount or a normal protein produced inappropriately owing to loss or alteration of control regions of the gene.

Tumour suppressor genes

The existence of tumour suppressor genes was suggested by cell fusion studies of transformed cells and non-transformed cells which resulted in a non-transformed hybrid cell (Harris et al 1969). The subsequent identification of the first human tumour suppressor gene followed from the study of retinoblastoma, a rare childhood cancer which may occur in a hereditary and sporadic form. On the basis of epidemiological and statistical analysis Knudson (1971) suggested that development of the cancer required two events. He postulated that in the hereditary form the first event was a germline mutation present in every cell of the individual, and that a second event in any of the many million retinoblasts could result in tumour formation. The rare, later onset and unilateral sporadic form could be attributed to the need for two events in a single retinal cell in the absence of a germline mutation. It was later confirmed that in both familial and sporadic retinoblastoma, both copies of the *Rb* gene were inactivated in tumour cells, consistent with Knudson's two-hit hypothesis (Cavenee et al 1983). Subsequently a number of other tumour suppressor genes have been identified, including *p53* (Baker

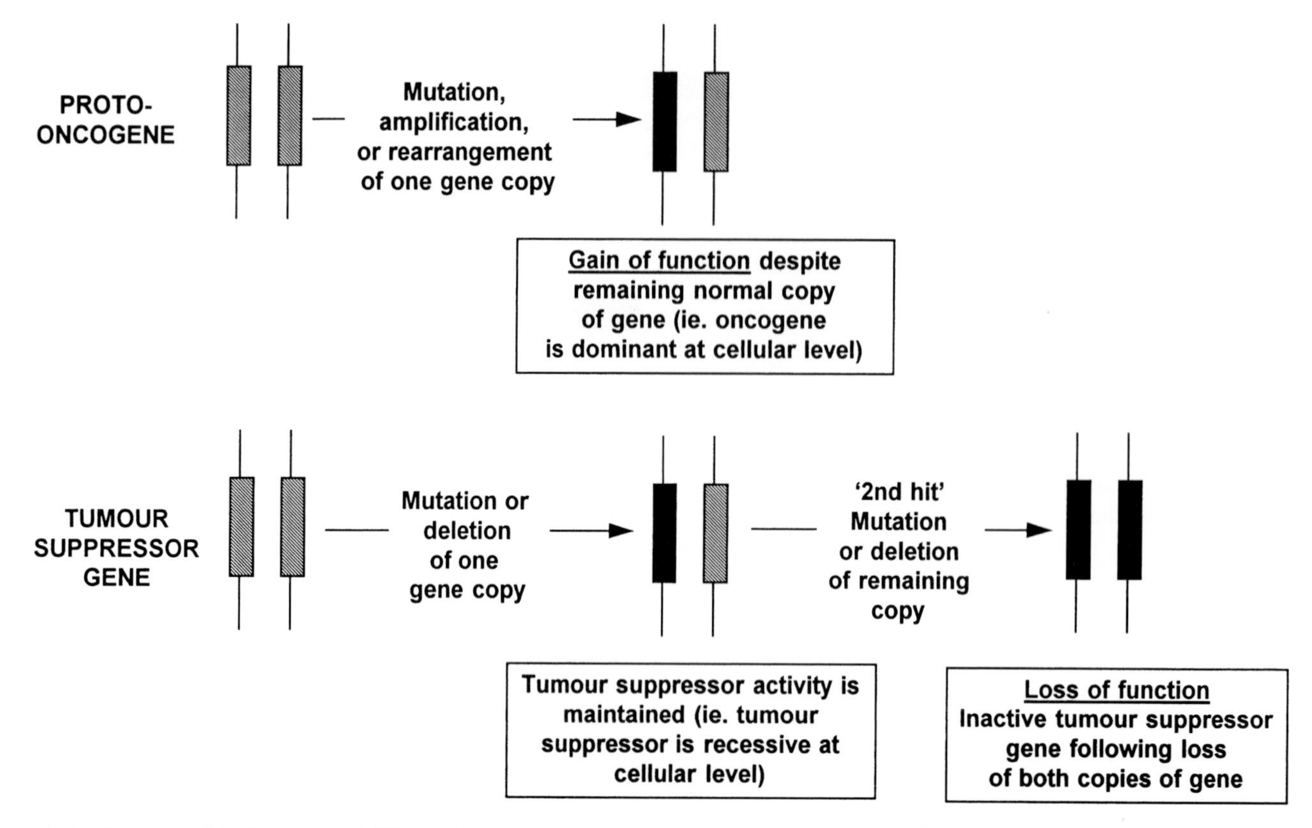

Fig. 32.4 Summary of the fundamental difference between oncogenes and tumour suppressor genes. Oncogenes are dominant at a cellular level and mutation of only one of the two gene copies is required for activation. Tumour suppressor genes are recessive at a cellular level. Both copies of the gene must usually be inactivated for loss of suppressor activity. An important exception to these general principles occurs when the product of a mutant copy of a tumour suppressor gene can interfere with the function of the product of the remaining wild-type copy of the gene. If this occurs both copies of the gene will be functionally inactive, even though a normal wild-type copy of the gene remains. This is known as a dominant-negative effect and an example is the *p53* gene. The *p53* protein functions as a dimer and dimers formed by wild-type and mutant protein are inactive. Loss of *p53* tumour suppressor activity therefore seems to occur in some tumours following mutation of just one copy of the gene.

et al 1989), *APC* (Kinzler et al 1991) and *DCC* (Fearon et al 1990).

There is a fundamental difference in the mode of action of tumour suppressor genes and oncogenes (Fig. 32.4). Mutations which create oncogenes result in a gain of function and will have an effect even in the presence of a remaining normal copy of the gene. They are dominant at a cellular level. In contrast, tumour suppressor genes involve a loss of function and act recessively at a cellular level. In general, both copies of a tumour suppressor gene must be lost or inactivated for an effect on cellular regulation to occur.

Multistep carcinogenesis

Although the spontaneous mutation rate of a gene is low (approximately 10^{-6} per gene per cell division) the total number of cell divisions in the lifetime of an individual is high (approximately 10^{16}), and consequently each gene is likely to have undergone at least 10^{10} spontaneous mutations (Cairns 1975). Mutations affecting genes involved in carcinogenesis are therefore likely to be much more frequent than the observed rates of malignancy. Clearly, a single mutation of a single gene cannot generally be sufficient to cause cancer. Several lines of evidence support the concept of carcinogenesis as a multistep process. First, the relationship of cancer incidence and age is logarithmic, and consistent with a requirement of 4–7 separate steps (Armitage & Doll 1954). Secondly, in vitro studies of fibroblasts and studies of transgenic mice indicate that transformation requires at least two complementary oncogenes, e.g. *ras* and *myc* (Land et al 1983). Thirdly, animal studies of chemical induction of tumours have revealed three stages in carcinogenesis: initiation, which is irreversible; promotion, which is reversible; and progression. Direct evidence has now been obtained in some cancers of the specific group of genetic alterations involved in carcinogenesis. One of the best examples of a genetic model of multistep carcinogenesis involving a common cancer is colorectal cancer (Fearon et al 1990) (Fig. 32.5).

Germline and somatic genetic alterations

An important distinction must be made between germline

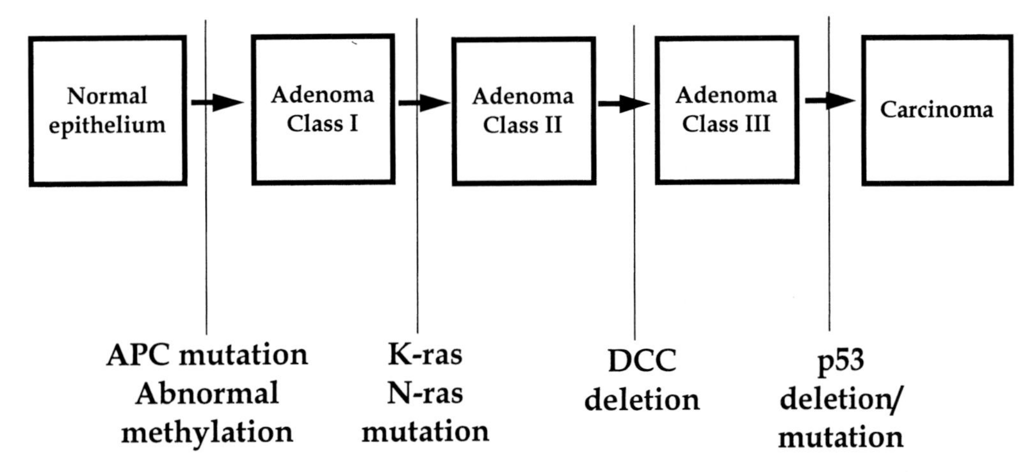

Fig. 32.5 The multistep model of carcinogenesis in colorectal cancer. (Modified from Vogelstein & Kinzler 1993)

and somatic mutations. Somatic mutations are found in the tumour cells but not the normal cells of an individual with cancer, and cannot therefore be passed on to descendants of the patient. Germline mutations predisposing to cancer involve all of the cells of the individual as well as the tumour, can be passed on to descendants of the individual and can be identified in DNA obtained from normal cells, such as a peripheral blood sample. The same genetic abnormalities frequently occur as both germline and somatic mutations in different individuals. For example, mutations of the *p53* gene are one of the commonest genetic changes found in human cancer. In most cancers mutation of *p53* occurs as a somatic event, but germline *p53* mutations have been identified in some families with the rare Li–Fraumeni syndrome, characterized by sarcomas, breast cancer and other malignancies occurring at a young age. Another example is germline mutations of the *APC* gene, which is responsible for familial adenomatous polyposis (FAP) (Kinzler et al 1991). Somatic mutations of *APC* have been detected in over 80% of sporadic colorectal cancers and appear to be one of the earliest events in colorectal carcinogenesis. Most of the familial cancer syndromes identified to date have an autosomal dominant pattern of inheritance. Individuals inheriting the germline abnormality are at high risk of developing malignancy, as the penetrance of most of these genes is of the order of 80%. It is possible that another class of genetic predispositions to cancer will be identified which increase susceptibility to cancer but with a low penetrance (i.e. a relatively small proportion of individuals with the genetic abnormality develop cancer). Such individuals would not be easy to identify by familial studies but may account for a significant proportion of cancer cases.

GENETICS OF FAMILIAL GYNAECOLOGICAL CANCER

Although there are anecdotal reports of more than one case of vulval and cervical cancer occurring in close relatives there is at present no good evidence of inherited predisposition to these cancers. Well-defined cancer family syndromes with an autosomal dominant inheritance pattern have been described for ovarian and endometrial cancers. Pedigree studies of families with a high incidence of cancer have revealed three main syndromes associated with ovarian cancer. Hereditary site-specific ovarian cancer without an excess of breast or colorectal cancer is the least common familial ovarian cancer syndrome. The most common hereditary form of ovarian cancer occurs in association with breast cancer. A large number of hereditary breast/ovarian cancer families have now been described in which there is a high frequency of both cancers and an association with an early age of onset. Less frequently, ovarian cancer occurs as part of the Lynch II syndrome. Women in Lynch II syndrome families most frequently develop colorectal or endometrial cancer. Some families have been described with an apparently high risk of site-specific endometrial cancer. It is important to recognize that all of these families combined probably account for less than 5% of cases of ovarian cancer and a smaller proportion of cases of endometrial cancer.

The *BRCA1* gene

Identification of families at high risk of breast and ovarian cancer, along with the development of polymorphic DNA markers, made it possible to perform detailed linkage analysis with the aim of locating genes involved in familial cancer. A major step forward was the report by Hall et al (1990) of the linkage of early-onset breast cancer to chromosome 17q. Subsequently, linkage to 17q was confirmed by a consortium of 13 research groups from Europe and the USA which analysed linkage data on six genetic markers on 17q in 214 families (Easton et al 1993). Almost all breast/ovarian cancer families and 40% of the families with breast cancer alone were found to have linkage to the *BRCA1* (*B*reast *C*ancer *1*) gene on chromosome 17q, and the consortium data localized the gene to a 2cM region on 17q. Intensive efforts were then made in a number of research units in Europe and the USA to further localize and clone the *BRCA1* gene. Eventually, a group in Utah described a large gene on 17q within which they had identified mutations in five affected families (Miki et al 1994). Subsequent work by other research groups has confirmed that this is the *BRCA1* gene, and over 50 mutations have now been described in breast/ovarian cancer. *BRCA1* is a large gene with 21 exons which encode a protein of 1863 amino acids. The gene has little homology to other known genes and its biological function is at present unclear. However, there is a zinc finger domain at the amino terminal portion of the protein, suggesting that *BRCA1* functions as a transcription factor. Most of the mutations of *BRCA1* are small insertions or deletions which result in the production of a truncated protein. This observation supports the concept that *BRCA1* functions as a tumour suppressor gene. In this two-hit model, although one copy of the gene is inherited as an inactive mutant form the development of cancer requires somatic mutation of the other, wild-type (normal), gene copy. Analysis of tumours from familial breast/ovarian cancer families has demonstrated that loss of heterozygosity in these tumours consistently involves the wild-type allele, thus providing further evidence that the *BRCA1* gene is a tumour suppressor (Smith et al 1992). Direct evidence of the risk of breast and ovarian cancer in *BRCA1* mutation carriers is not yet available, but evidence from linkage families indicates that the risk of breast cancer and ovarian cancer by age 70 years is 85% and 63%, respectively (Ford et al 1994, Easton et al 1995). The available data also suggest that there may be heterogeneity of ovarian cancer risk between different families, with the majority of families at 26% risk of ovarian cancer by age 70 and a minority at 89% risk. It is possible that these differences may be explained by different types of *BRCA1* mutations, but this is not clear at present. (See Addendum to this chapter.)

The Lynch II syndrome and DNA repair genes

The identification of the genetic basis of Lynch II syndrome is a notable example of the power of molecular technology. Hereditary non-polyposis colorectal cancer (HNPCC) was classified by Henry Lynch into site-specific hereditary colon cancer (Lynch I syndrome) and families with a predisposition to non-polyposis colorectal cancer in association with other cancers, including ovarian and endometrial cancer as well as stomach, pancreas and breast cancer (Lynch II syndrome) (Lynch et al 1985). The identification of the genes responsible for HNPCC was a result of several developments. First, linkage to a locus on chromosome 2p was demonstrated in affected members of two large HNPCC families (Aaltonen et al 1993, Peltomäki et al 1993). Secondly, it was observed that the tumours from HNPCC patients contained abnormalities of repeating sequences (microsatellites) at numerous loci throughout the genome, suggesting that an abnormality of a DNA mismatch repair gene may be responsible for the predisposition (Ionov et al 1993, Thibodeau et al 1993). Thirdly, it was known that inactivation of bacterial and yeast genes involved in mismatch repair (*mutS* and *mutL*) resulted in microsatellite instability similar to that observed in tumour cells. This observation provided the basis for cloning of a human homologue of *mutS* on chromosome 2p (hMSH2) and *mutL* on chromosome 3p (hMLH1), which were found to contain mutations in the germline of HNPCC patients (Fishel et al 1993, Leach et al 1993). The results indicate that HNPCC is associated with hereditary defects in mismatch repair genes. Available evidence suggests that these genes function as tumour suppressor genes in a manner consistent with Knudson's two-hit model. The inherited germline mutation inactivates one copy of the mismatch repair gene, but inactivation of the remaining wild-type copy by a second somatic mutation is required prior to tumour formation. The basis for the tumour specificity associated with the inherited mutation is unclear and an interesting issue, as the mismatch repair genes are ubiquitously expressed. Endometrial and ovarian cancers are less common in Lynch II families than colorectal cancer, but no good estimates of the degree of risk of these gynaecological malignancies are available at present.

THE MOLECULAR GENETICS OF SPORADIC GYNAECOLOGICAL CANCER

Cervical cancer

The histopathological progression of cervical neoplasia from mild to increasingly severe dysplasia and ultimately invasive cervical cancer is well described, as is the evidence for an infective aetiology for cervical cancer and the association with human papilloma virus infection. During recent years important progress has been made in understanding the mechanism of papilloma virus-induced carcinogenesis and incorporating these findings with the principles of multistep carcinogenesis outlined above.

HPV

Human papilloma viruses (HPV) are a group of more than 60 viruses, most of which give rise to benign tumours such as wart infections. The risk of cervical neoplasia is associated with particular HPV types (HPV 16 and 18) (Vousden 1989). The genomes of all HPVs have a similar organization. There are eight major regions of open reading frames (ORF) encoding early (E1–7) and late (L1–2) viral proteins. It is the early proteins E6 and E7 which are responsible for the transforming activity of the virus (Vousden 1991). The E6 and E7 proteins of high-risk HPV types (16 and 18), but not those of low-risk types, cause changes in vitro which parallel the changes in cervical intraepithelial neoplasia (CIN) (Hudson et al 1990). During normal viral infection the viral genome exists episomally without integration in the nucleus of the infected cell. In tumour cells, the viral DNA is integrated with the DNA of the host cell. Although the sites of integration of viral DNA are random in cancer cell lines, and many of the viral genes are lost, the E6 and E7 viral ORFs are always conserved and are the most abundant viral transcript in such cell lines (Shirashawa et al 1987). Furthermore, integration of E6 and E7 usually occurs in a manner which disrupts the normal viral regulation of expression of these proteins (Durst et al 1985). These observations suggest that the E6 and E7 proteins have an important role in cervical carcinogenesis.

Interaction between HPV and both p53 and Rb

This is supported by evidence that these proteins can interact with and inactivate several important cellular proteins. E7 protein binds to the product of the retinoblastoma tumour suppressor gene, interfering with normal protein complex formation and disrupting normal function. E6 protein interacts with the protein product of the *p53* tumour suppressor gene, causing rapid breakdown of the protein and loss of normal *p53* function. The overall effect of E6 and E7 expression in the cell is therefore equivalent to loss of the *Rb* and *p53* tumour suppressor genes. This is consistent with the observation that *p53* mutation is uncommon in cervical cancer but is found in HPV 16- and 18-negative cervical cancer cell lines (Crook et al 1992).

Other oncogenes

Clinical and experimental evidence suggests that, in common with other mechanisms of carcinogenesis, HPV infection alone is not sufficient to cause cervical cancer, but requires other factors which may influence local immune responses or result in other genetic alterations. First, only a small proportion of women with HPV infection develop cancer and there is a long latent period before this occurs. Secondly, epidemiological studies suggest that other factors, such as smoking and herpes simplex infection, may play a role. Thirdly, a number of genetic abnormalities have been identified in cervical cancers. These include amplification or overexpression of c-*myc*, mutation of c-H-*ras* and loss of heterozygosity at a number of chromosomal loci.

Ovarian cancer

The majority of cases of ovarian cancer are not associated with familial predisposition. There is good evidence from epidemiological studies that the risk of sporadic ovarian cancer is associated with factors that influence the frequency of ovulation (e.g. parity, breastfeeding, oral contraceptive use). Ovulation results in disruption of the ovarian epithelium, which is repaired by proliferation of ovarian epithelial cells exposed to growth factors present in follicular fluid. The proliferation of ovarian epithelium at the time of ovulation may provide the opportunity for mutations resulting in somatic activation of oncogenes and tumour suppressor genes. The molecular abnormalities in ovarian cancer involve genes at each step in the complex pathway of cell regulation, which are summarized in Figure 32.1. These include growth factors (M-CSF, TGF-β), growth factor receptors (*fms*, EGFR, HER-2/*neu*), genes involved in signal transduction (*ras*), genes involved in transcriptional regulation (*myc*, *p53*) and loss of heterozygosity at various loci, which occurs in a proportion of epithelial ovarian cancers.

Oncogenes in sporadic ovarian cancer

Growth factors. There is good evidence that the response of ovarian cancer cells to growth factors is altered compared to normal ovarian epithelial cells. The proliferative response of ovarian cancer cells in culture to EGF (epidermal growth factor) and TGF-α (transforming growth factor α) is variable but usually less than in normal ovarian epithelium (Berchuck et al 1990), whereas the inhibitory effect of TGF-β (transforming growth factor β) is less marked in ovarian cancer cell lines than in normal ovarian epithelium (Berchuck et al 1992). TGF-β appears to function as an autocrine inhibitory factor in normal ovarian epithelial growth, and the loss of this regulatory loop may represent a step in the process of ovarian carcinogenesis. The macrophage colony-stimulating factor (M-CSF) is a ligand for a cell surface receptor encoded by the c-*fms* proto-oncogene. Normal ovarian epithelium does not express *fms*, whereas the majority of ovarian cancer cells do express the receptor (Kacinski et al 1990). M-CSF is a potent attractant for macrophages and can stimulate the invasiveness of cancer cell lines that express *fms*. It is possible that M-CSF regulates ovarian cancer cells via an autocrine pathway in cells expressing *fms*, as well as by a paracrine pathway through attraction of macrophages and consequent release of cytokines such as IL-1, IL-6 and TNF.

Growth factor receptors. The growth factor receptors are a family of cell membrane tyrosine kinases which act as receptors for the growth factors discussed above and are involved in signal transduction via autophosphorylation and phosphorylation of intracellular proteins. The EGF receptor (EGFR also referred to as *erb*B) and HER-2/*neu* (also referred to as *erb*B2) are structurally similar and both are overexpressed in human cancers. EGFR is expressed by most advanced-stage ovarian cancers and there is some evidence that EGFR-positive tumours have a worse prognosis than those not expressing the receptor (Berchuck et al 1991). HER-2/*neu* is overexpressed in approximately a third of ovarian cancers (Slamon et al 1989), and overexpression is associated with gene amplification.

Oncogenes involved in signal transduction. Although mutations of the *ras* oncogene occur in ovarian cancer they are relatively less frequent than in some other epithelial cancers. *Ki-ras* mutations in ovarian tumours almost exclusively involve codon 12, and are more frequent in borderline and invasive tumours of mucinous type than in serous tumours.

Nuclear oncogenes. Little is known about the role of most nuclear oncogenes in ovarian cancer. Amplification of c-*myc* and increased expression of the protein product has been described in approximately a third of ovarian cancers. Tashiro et al (1992) found an overall rate of overexpression of c-*myc* of 38% in a series of ovarian tumours.

Tumour suppressor genes in sporadic ovarian cancer

p53. Mutations of the *p53* gene are the most frequent genetic alteration in cancer, and occur most frequently in regions of the gene which show the greatest degree of conservation between *p53* proteins of different species. Immunohistochemical studies have revealed overexpression of the *p53* protein in 50% of advanced-stage ovarian cancers (Marks et al 1991). In most of these cases there are point mutations in conserved regions of the gene and the second copy of the gene has been deleted. Mutation of *p53* is less common in stage I disease than advanced-stage disease, and clonal analysis suggests that the *p53* mutation occurs just before metastasis (Jacobs et al 1992). No clear relationship between *p53* mutation and histological grade or prognosis has been established. The codons most frequently involved in *p53* mutations are the same as those described in other cancers. The pattern of mutations suggests that most have arisen through endogenous mutagenic processes, rather than exposure to a carcinogen.

Loss of heterozygosity. As tumour suppressor genes inhibit cell proliferation, both copies of the gene must be inactivated for neoplastic effect (i.e. they act recessively at a cellular level). The first hit is frequently a point mutation, whereas the second hit, inactivating the remaining wild-type copy of the gene, is often a larger event involving loss of a portion or the whole of a chromosome. The relatively large losses associated with the second hit are easier to identify than point mutations, and have been exploited as a method of mapping the location of tumour suppressor genes by loss of heterozygosity analysis. Studies of loss of heterozygosity (LOH) in ovarian cancer have revealed a number of regions with high frequencies of loss (Fig. 32.6).

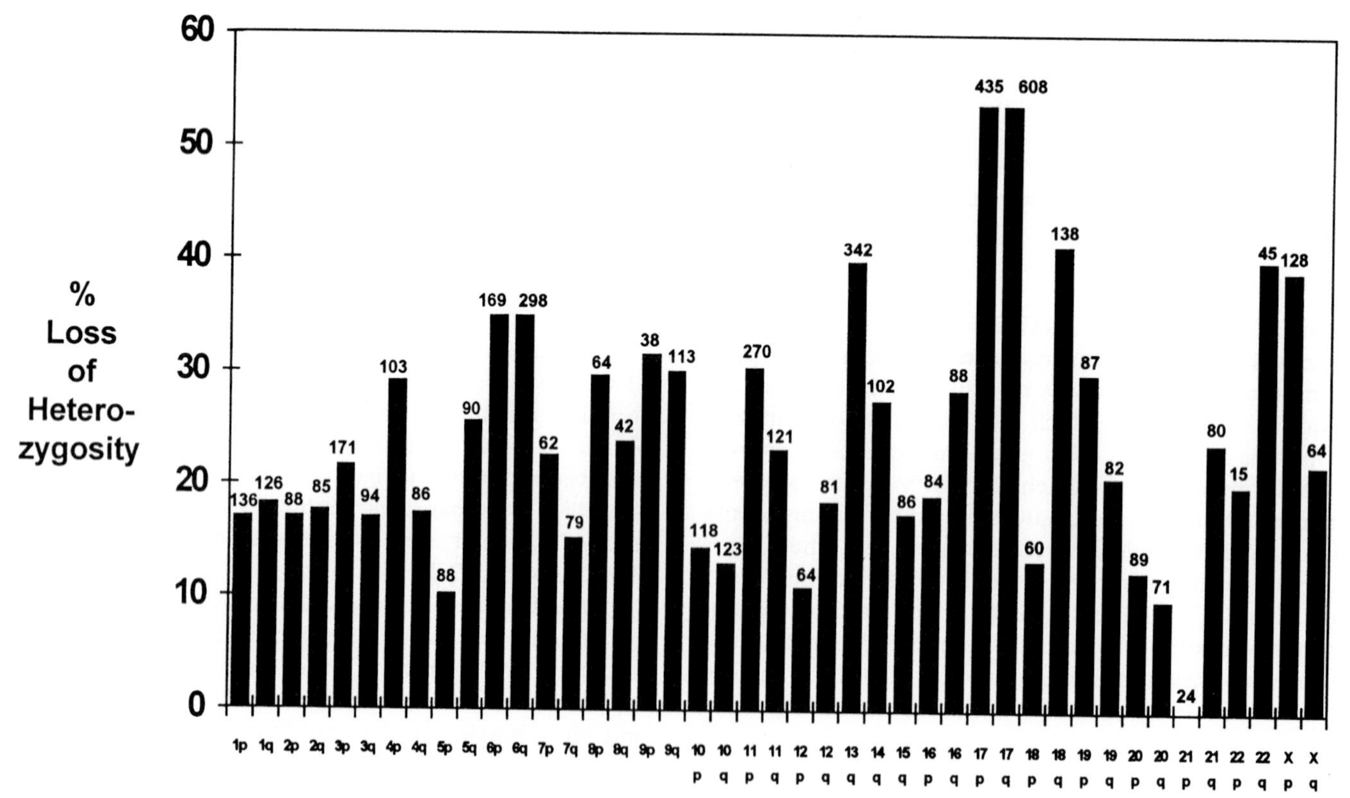

Fig. 32.6 Summary of report of the frequency of loss of heterozygosity at each chromosome arm in ovarian cancer. The data represent the number of tumours with LOH for the chromosome arm/the number of informative tumours for each chromosome arm. The number of tumours studied at each chromosome arm is shown at the top of each bar.

Losses have been observed on almost all chromosome arms and the background random rate of loss in ovarian cancer is high (15–25%). A high frequency of allelic deletion (>33%) based upon more than 50 tumours in at least three separate studies has been documented for seven chromosome arms: 6p, 6q, 13q, 17p (possibly associated with *p53*), 17q, 18q and Xp. A number of other chromosome arms have frequencies of loss in the range 25–33%, which may be above background rates: 4p, 8p, 9p, 9q, 11p, 14q, 16q, 19p and 21q. Further localization of putative tumour suppressor genes in regions with a high rate of LOH requires detailed analysis with a panel of polymorphic markers for the relevant chromosome arm. Available data suggest that a number of unidentified tumour suppressor genes are involved in ovarian carcinogenesis, and recent reports have defined deletion units on chromosome arms with the highest rates of LOH, including 6p, 6q, 11p, 13q, 17q and Xp.

BRCA1. The high rate of loss of heterozygosity on chromosome 17q in sporadic ovarian cancers was reported at the time that the *BRCA1* gene was mapped to 17q, and raised the exciting possibility that the same gene may be of importance in sporadic as well as familial ovarian cancer.

When the cloning of the *BRCA1* gene was reported, considerable effort was invested in searching for somatic *BRCA1* mutations in sporadic breast and ovarian cancers. Alongside the report of the cloning of *BRCA1*, Futreal et al (1994) described mutational analysis of a series of apparently sporadic breast and ovarian cancers from individuals without a known family history of ovarian cancer but with loss of heterozygosity on 17q. None of the cancers had somatic *BRCA1* mutations, although some had germline mutations. However, more recently two groups have described five somatic mutations in 64 cancers (Hosking et al 1995, Merajver et al 1995). This suggests that *BRCA1* mutations do occur in sporadic disease but are relatively uncommon. It is still possible that the spectrum of *BRCA1* mutations is different in sporadic tumours from that in familial cancer, and that the full story will be rather more subtle than is now apparent. The pattern of LOH on chromosome 17 suggests that, in addition to *BRCA1*, several unidentified tumour suppressor genes on the long arm of 17q are involved in ovarian carcinogenesis.

Endometrial cancer

A small proportion of endometrial cancers occur as part of the Lynch II syndrome, and it is possible that site-specific hereditary endometrial cancer exists as a distinct entity (Sandles et al 1992). The majority of cases of endometrial cancers are, however, sporadic. Although it is known that unopposed oestrogens are important in the aetiology of sporadic endometrial cancer, there is limited information about the molecular basis of this disease. Oestrogen and progesterone receptors are frequently expressed by endometrial cancers, and loss of expression is correlated with poor prognosis. In contrast to ovarian cancer only 25% of endometrial cancers are aneuploid, and this feature is associated with aggressive disease and poor prognosis. A number of recent studies have identified mutations of known oncogenes and tumour suppressor genes in endometrial cancer, but no genetic alterations specific to this cancer have been documented.

p53

Kohler et al (1992) reported immunohistochemical evidence of *p53* mutations in 21% of a series of 107 endometrial cancers. The results suggested that *p53* mutations were more frequent in advanced-stage than early stage disease, and were associated with non-endometrioid histology, positive peritoneal cytology and metastatic disease. These findings are consistent with other studies of *p53* in endometrial cancer. Mutations are usually in conserved regions of the gene with a similar distribution to *p53* mutations in ovarian cancer. Kohler et al (1993) also studied a series of 117 endometrial hyperplasias, none of which were found to have *p53* mutations, suggesting that this is a relatively late event in endometrial carcinogenesis.

Other oncogenes and growth factor receptors

A number of studies of *ras* mutations in endometrial cancer have been reported. *Ki-ras* mutations have been documented in approximately 20% of endometrial cancers analysed. Most of the mutations reported are in codon 12 and the remainder in codon 13. The relationship of prognostic factors to *Ki-ras* mutation is not yet clear. In contrast to *p53* mutation, *Ki-ras* mutation appears to be a relatively early event in endometrial carcinogenesis. The frequency of *Ki-ras* mutation in endometrial hyperplasia is similar to that in invasive disease (Enomoto et al 1993, Sasaki et al 1993). When *Ki-ras* mutations are present in areas of invasive endometrial cancer they are also in adjacent areas of atypical hyperplasia, but not simple or complex hyperplasia without atypia. Thus *Ki-ras* mutation appears to be involved in progression to atypical hyperplasia. Both overexpression and amplification of the *Erb*B2 oncogene have been reported in endometrial cancer. Small studies also suggest that endometrial cancer may be associated with amplification of c-*myc* and alterations of the retinoblastoma gene.

CLINICAL ASPECTS OF THE GENETICS OF GYNAECOLOGICAL CANCER

Clinical risk assessment

The first step in risk assessment is to obtain a detailed

family history, extending if possible to at least the second degree relatives of the individual seeking advice, and with confirmation of the diagnosis of cancers in the relatives. The assessment of risk is based largely on the recognition of certain patterns of cancer in the family. The association of breast with ovarian cancer strongly suggests the breast/ovarian syndrome caused by mutations in *BRCA1* or *BRCA2*, whereas the association of breast with cervical cancer does not fit a known pattern and is more likely to be coincidental. Confirmation of the precise site of cancers in relatives is therefore important.

Even with a complete family history it may not be possible to say with certainty that a particular family has an inherited predisposition and another does not. Ovarian cancer in a mother and daughter, for example, probably reflects inherited predisposition in about two-thirds of cases, but coincidence in the other one-third. Factors which are weighed in assessing the significance of the history are the number of cancers in the same genetic line of descent; the types of cancer and whether they fit a known pattern; and the ages at which they occurred, in general a younger onset favouring an inherited component. As more of the predisposing genes are identified and mutation testing is introduced in the next few years, precise confirmation of inheritance will become possible.

Assessment of the family history and individual risks may not be straightforward, and referral of families to a clinical geneticist or gynaecological oncologist with a special interest is recommended. In general, risk assessment has three stages:

1. an estimate of the probability that the family history reflects the presence of a predisposing gene;
2. an estimate of the probability that a given individual has inherited the genes, supposing it is present;
3. an estimate of the risks of ovarian cancer and other cancers (e.g. breast cancer) conferred by the gene at a given age (gene penetrance).

Although it is difficult to define precisely the minimum family history necessary to satisfy the description of a familial cancer syndrome, some broad guidelines can be given. Families in which two first-degree relatives have ovarian cancer, or two first-degree relatives have breast cancer and a third relative ovarian cancer, can be classified as breast/ovarian cancer families. The pattern of cancer in approximately 66% of such families is due to autosomal dominant inheritance of a gene such as *BRCA1* or *BRCA2* with high penetrance. Families in which one relative has ovarian or endometrial cancer and two or more first-degree relatives cancer of the colon can be classified as Lynch II syndrome families.

The daughter of an affected woman has a 50:50 chance of inheriting the predisposing gene from her mother. In such a family the risks of either breast or ovarian cancer in someone who has the gene is about 80% by age 70, averaged over the 40-year period from age 30. So a 35-year-old woman who has a 50:50 chance of having inherited the gene because her mother was affected, has a roughly 10% chance of developing breast or ovarian cancer by age 45, and a roughly 40% chance by age 70.

Risk assessment by gene analysis

Although the *BRCA1* gene and DNA repair genes have now been identified, analysis of these genes for mutations is not yet feasible in the clinical setting. The genes are large and the mutations are not localized to specific regions. Using currently available techniques, mutation detection is a lengthy, time-consuming and expensive process which can only be undertaken in the context of a research programme. This situation is likely to change in the foreseeable future, as new methods of screening for mutations are developed. Such progress will inevitably have major ethical implications which will require careful discussion with the family members concerned. Many of the women who are candidates for mutational analysis will already have been identified as being at high risk by virtue of their family history. The information will therefore be of most value to women without mutation, as they could be reassured that they were probably not at increased risk. On the other hand, there may be major psychological implications for women who are found to be gene carriers, and discrimination in obtaining employment, insurance and financial agreements is possible. In addition, it is far from clear that any improvement in life expectancy would follow the identification of genetic predisposition.

Prevention of familial cancer: clinical approaches

In principle, use of the oral contraceptive pill might be recommended for Lynch II and breast/ovary family members, since case control studies indicate a protective effect against sporadic ovarian and endometrial cancer. However, the effect of oral contraceptives on familial ovarian and endometrial cancer risk is uncertain. If the mechanisms of carcinogenesis in familial and sporadic disease are different, oral contraceptives may not provide the same degree of protection as for sporadic disease. Moreover, any benefits may be offset by an increased risk of breast cancer for women in breast/ovarian cancer families.

Prophylactic oophorectomy as a primary procedure is justifiable in women from breast/ovarian and Lynch II families, after completion of their family and after thorough counselling. Some cases of familial ovarian cancer may be part of a field change involving the peritoneal mesothelium as well as the ovarian epithelium, which share a common embryological origin. For this reason there is some doubt about the efficacy of oophorectomy as a preventive strategy. Although this is an interesting issue, its importance should not be exaggerated. Recent data suggest that intra-abdominal carcinomatosis following oophorectomy in women with a strong family history of ovarian cancer is uncommon. Some cases of intra-abdominal carcinomatosis following oophorectomy have been reported in which subsequent review of the oophorectomy specimen revealed a small focus of ovarian cancer (Chen et al 1985). Oophorectomy should therefore be accompanied by careful inspection of the abdomen and pelvis and thorough histological examination of the ovary.

In women from Lynch II families prophylactic oophorectomy should be accompanied by hysterectomy to prevent endometrial cancer. In women from breast/ovarian cancer families the main argument for hysterectomy is evidence that the risk of breast cancer is greater following cyclical combined HRT than continuous low-dose unopposed oestrogen replacement.

Screening women at risk of familial ovarian or breast cancer

The efficacy of ovarian cancer screening is unproven. However, in view of the size of the risk of ovarian cancer in this population it is reasonable to commence screening with either vaginal ultrasonography and serum CA125 measurement on an annual basis from the mid 20s, or 5 years prior to the earliest age of onset of ovarian cancer in the family.

Both CA125 and ultrasound are associated with a substantial risk of false positive results, which lead to unnecessary surgery, and it is essential to warn women clearly about this risk (Campbell et al 1993, Jacobs et al 1993). The false positive rate for both CA125 and ultrasonography is approximately 2–3% in postmenopausal women, and more in premenopausal women. It is therefore likely that a 30-year-old woman undergoing annual screening for up to 30 years will have a false positive result at some stage, with all the consequent anxiety and the risk of unnecessary surgery.

To minimize the risk of a false positive result, it is reasonable to advise that only one and not both of the tests should be used. Because the current, but scanty, evidence appears to suggest that ultrasound is the more sensitive test for preclinical disease, it must be regarded as the test of choice in this group of women at present. This situation may change with the development of new antibodies complementary to CA125.

Women in breast/ovarian cancer families may be advised to commence screening with mammography from the mid 30s, or 5 years prior to the earliest case of breast cancer in their family, although the value of mammography in premenopausal women is controversial. Women in Lynch II families should be advised to undergo regular colonoscopy and mammography in addition to ovarian cancer screening. Screening for endometrial cancer is not of proven efficacy but can be justified because of the particularly high risk in this group of women. Ultrasound measurement of endometrial thickness can be performed at the time of screening for ovarian size and morphology, and it is reasonable to add an outpatient form of endometrial sampling, such as Pipelle aspiration. These screening strategies are currently recommended on a pragmatic basis in view of the high risk of cancer, rather than on the basis of clear evidence of their efficacy.

Women with a family history not consistent with a familial syndrome

Most of the women who seek advice about a family history of gynaecological cancer have only one affected first-degree relative and do not fall into the group with a familial syndrome. Requests for advice from this group of women have increased dramatically following recent media publicity about screening for ovarian cancer and the identification of the *BRCA1* gene. Although women with one first-degree relative with ovarian cancer are at increased risk compared to the general population, the absolute risk remains small. They should be reassured that, although their risk of ovarian cancer may be increased severalfold, it remains low (lifetime risk of 2–5% vs. 1% in the general population).

Screening with either CA125 or ultrasound should not be offered routinely to these women, for two reasons. First, an improvement in prognosis for ovarian cancer through detection by screening has not been demonstrated. Secondly, because the incidence of ovarian cancer in this population is relatively low, the risk of a false positive result resulting in surgical investigation is likely to be more than 10 times that of a true positive result (i.e. the positive predictive value of screening is <10%). The value of screening women in this group and those without a family history awaits evaluation in large, well designed randomized controlled trials. Oophorectomy should not be recommended as a primary procedure but may be considered as a secondary procedure at the time of surgery for benign disease (e.g. hysterectomy).

Cancer prevention: molecular approaches

Genetic approaches may help in the identification of premalignant conditions amenable to conservative therapy. For example, there is no well documented precursor lesion for ovarian carcinoma. However, ovarian epithelial atypia, inclusion cysts and benign or borderline ovarian tumours may represent steps in the pathway of ovarian carcinogenesis (Puls et al 1992). Genetic studies may establish the relationship between these abnormalities and ovarian cancer, and consequently provide new opportunities for prevention.

Where known abnormalities confer a high risk of cancer

it may be possible to design strategies to correct the abnormality. In familial cancer syndromes it may ultimately be possible to transfer normal copies of the abnormal gene (e.g. *p53*, *BRCA1*) to the tissue at risk using tissue-specific viral vectors. In cervical cancer, work is in progress to develop a vaccine directed against the HPV types associated with the disease (Crawford 1993). It may be possible to generate an immune response to viral coat particles (L1 and L2) or to viral transforming proteins (E6 and E7) using either a protein vaccine or a presentation of these antigens in a viral or bacterial vector.

Although cervical cytology is the established method of screening for preinvasive change in the cervix, the sensitivity of a single test is no greater than 50%. Recent evidence suggests that greater sensitivity may be achieved by using a sensitive PCR (polymerase chain reaction)-based assay to detect HPV in cervical smears.

Future prospects for early detection of cancer

Knowledge of specific genetic alterations associated with cancer and the high sensitivity of molecular techniques such as PCR may provide new methods for detecting cancer. Because of the inaccessibility of the ovaries, any screening test for ovarian cancer would need to be based on the identification of a gene product in peripheral blood. The protein product of the *M-CSF* gene is detectable at elevated levels in the serum of ovarian cancer patients. It is possible that the products of other genes coding for secreted and cell surface proteins produced in abnormal forms or increased amounts in cancer will be markers for early-stage disease.

The opportunities may be even greater for cancers arising from accessible tissues such as the endometrium. Techniques such as PCR or ligase chain reaction can identify a small proportion of mutated copies of a gene in a background of many thousand-fold excess normal copies of the gene. Since it is a relatively simple outpatient procedure to obtain an endometrial sample, it may be possible to detect mutation of a gene associated with endometrial cancer at a very early stage of the disease. This approach has been used to detect mutations of *p53* and *K-ras* in urine, sputum and stool specimens in cancers of the bladder, lung and colon (Sidransky et al 1991). Such techniques may be used to identify early-stage disease, minimal residual disease and the early stages of recurrent disease.

Prognostic indicators

The behaviour of a malignancy is a consequence of the complex interaction of all of the genetic alterations which have accumulated during the process of carcinogenesis. Since different genetic alterations have different effects, and the set of genetic changes leading to a particular malignancy is not fixed, it is reasonable to infer that genetic analysis will provide important prognostic information. Evidence for this is emerging from studies of ovarian cancer. Although *p53* mutation does not appear to correlate with prognosis, there is evidence that *erb*B2 amplification is associated with decreased survival.

Several authors have investigated the relationship between loss of heterozygosity and tumour characteristics. Correlations with frequency of LOH in ovarian cancer have been reported for (i) histological type, LOH on chromosomes 6q, 13q, 17q and 19q being more frequent in serous than other histological types; (ii) FIGO stage of disease, with LOH on 17q more frequent in advanced-stage disease; and (iii) tumour grade. Zheng et al (1991) found a correlation between tumour grade and frequency of LOH at all loci analysed on nine chromosomes. They hypothesised that LOH on chromosomes 3 or 11 results in high-grade malignancy, whereas LOH on chromosome 6 is consistent with a well differentiated phenotype. Dodson et al (1993) found the average fractional allelic loss in high-grade tumours to be greater than that in low-grade tumours (39.5% vs. 16%). Chromosome arms 6p, 17p, 17q and 22q were frequently lost in both low- and high-grade tumours, whereas LOH on 13q and 15q was more common in high-grade tumours and LOH on 3p more common in low-grade tumours. These data raise the possibility that the pattern of LOH might be an independent prognostic indicator for ovarian cancer.

STRATEGIES FOR GENE THERAPY

The increase in understanding of carcinogenesis at a molecular level has raised the possibility that cancer can be treated by selectively targeting cells which have specific genetic abnormalities. A broad range of different methods for gene therapy have been suggested and numerous clinical trials are in progress.

Ex-vivo approaches to gene therapy

Ex-vivo techniques involve the removal of cells from the individual, manipulation of the cells in vitro and reinjection of altered cells. One approach is to remove tumour cells from a patient, insert genes in vitro which increase their immunogenicity, and reinject them into the patient in order to stimulate a systemic immune response that will recognize and destroy tumour cells. Suitable genes for this approach include cytokines which activate the immune system, such as the interleukins, and genes for MHC class I antigens. An alternative approach is to transfer a gene that activates a prodrug to become cytotoxic. For example, transfer of the thymidine kinase gene of the herpes simplex virus results in phosphorylation of the antiherpes drug ganciclovir and cell death due to inhibition of DNA polymerase. The potential of this approach is enhanced by the observation that adjacent cells which do not have the gene are also affected, presumably owing to diffusion of the phosphorylated drug (Culver et al 1992). A trial of intraperitoneal therapy using this strategy in stage III ovarian cancer is under way (Freeman et al 1993).

In-situ approaches to gene therapy

An exciting possibility is the correction of specific molecular genetic abnormalities responsible for carcinogenesis by inserting into cancer cells a normal copy of a tumour suppressor gene such as *p53*, or suppressing expression of an oncogene product such as *K-ras*. There is evidence that insertion of wild-type *p53* and antisense *K-ras* into tumour cells with abnormalities of these genes suppresses tumorigenicity (Harris & Hollstein 1993, Zhang et al 1993). It may also be possible to target genes involved in metastasis. Decreased expression of the *nm23* gene is associated with increased metastatic potential in some cancers, and transfection of *nm23* into melanoma cells decreases metastatic potential (Leone et al 1991).

The technical limitations of corrective gene therapy are currently twofold. First, in order to control a cancer in vivo the gene must be transferred to all tumour cells. The most hopeful method of gene transfer is the use of a recombinant virus, since viral replication and spread may overcome the difficulty of targeting tumour cells with a poor vascular supply, which limits other therapeutic approaches such as the use of monoclonal antibodies. Secondly, the vector used for gene transfer must be targeted to tumour but not normal cells. It may be possible to construct viral vectors which will bind to cell surface proteins expressed preferentially on tumour cells, or which require a transcription factor expressed in tumour cells but not normal cells. Ultimately a highly sophisticated therapeutic approach may involve a viral vector modified to contain a therapeutic gene, to recognize tumour cell surface antigens and require tumour-specific factors for transcription.

KEY POINTS

1. Oncogenes result in a gain in function which will take effect even in the presence of the remaining normal copy of the gene; tumour suppressor genes involve a loss of function that requires inactivation or deletion of both copies of the gene before cellular regulation is affected.
2. Several mutations (4–7) are required to cause cancer.
3. The genetic changes required for cancer usually occur in the somatic cells and are random events. However, some individuals develop oncogenic mutations in their germ cells which can then be passed on to their progeny.
4. Among gynaecological cancers inherited malignancies occur only in the ovary, endometrium and breast. These are rare, accounting for less than 5% of ovarian or endometrial cancers.
5. Two genes, termed *BRCA1* and *BRCA2*, have been identified. *BRCA1* is found in almost all families with both breast and ovarian cancer and in 40% of families with breast cancer alone.
6. These genes have high penetrance, with 80% of affected individuals developing a malignancy between 30 and 70 years of age.
7. Genetic advice to women who may have inherited a cancer gene should only be given by clinical geneticists or gynaecological oncologists with a special knowledge of these conditions.
8. The efficacy of screening such women is unproven. There is a substantial risk of false positive results.
9. Oophorectomy and hysterectomy should be considered if the risk of inheritance seems high.
10. Identifying the genetic basis for cancer opens the possibility of therapy targeted at the underlying abnormality.

Addendum

Since this chapter was completed the *BRCA2* gene has been cloned. Mutations of the *BRCA1* gene account for the majority of breast/ovarian cancer families and approximately one third of breast cancer families. Mutations of the *BRCA2* gene on chromosome 13q account for a further one third of breast cancer families and a small proportion of breast/ovarian cancer families. Both of these genes are large and their function is still unclear although they do have some similarities. At present mutation screening is largely confined to research laboratories due to the size of the genes, the cost of the analysis and the ethical/psychosocial implications of screening. However, the situation is changing rapidly and as the technology for mutation detection improves during the next few years mutation screening as a clinical service will become available. The complex financial, ethical and psychological implications of mutation detection will then need to be addressed.

REFERENCES

Aaltonen L A et al 1993 Clues to the pathogenesis of familial colorectal cancer. Science 260: 812–816
Alberts B, Bray D, Lewis J, Raff M, Robets K, Watson J D 1989 Molecular biology of the cell, 2nd edn. New York, Garland Publishing
Ames B N, Durston W E, Yamasaki E, Lee F D 1973 Carcinogens are mutagens: a simple test system combining liver homogenates for activation and bacteria for detection. Proceedings of the National Academy of Science USA 70: 2281–2285
Armitage P, Doll R 1954 The age distribution of cancer and a multi-stage theory of carcinogenesis. British Journal of Cancer 8: 1–12
Baker S J, Fearon E R, Nigro J M et al 1989 Chromosome 17 deletions and p53 gene mutations in colorectal carcinomas. Science 244: 217–221
Berchuck A, Rodriguez G, Kamel A, Soper J T, Clarke-Pearson D L, Bast R Jr 1990 Expression of epidermal growth factor receptor and HER-2/neu in normal and neoplastic cervix, vulva, and vagina. Obstetrics and Gynecology 76: 381
Berchuck A, Rodriguez G C, Kamel A et al 1991 Epidermal growth factor receptor expression in normal ovarian epithelium and ovarian cancer. I. Correlation of receptor expression with prognostic factors in patients with ovarian cancer. American Journal of Obstetrics and Gynecology 164: 669
Berchuck A, Rodriguez G, Olt G et al 1992 Regulation of growth of normal ovarian epithelial cells and ovarian cancer cell lines by transforming growth factor-beta. American Journal of Obstetrics and Gynecology 166: 676
Cairns J 1975 Mutation selection, and the natural history of cancer. Nature 255: 197–200
Campbell S, Bourne T, Bradley E 1993 Screening for ovarian cancer by transvaginal sonography and colour Doppler. European Journal of Obstetrics, Gynecology and Reproductive Biology 49: 33
Cavenee W K, Dryja T P, Phillips R A et al 1983 Expression of recessive alleles by chromosomal mechanisms in retinoblastoma. Nature 305: 779–784
Chen K T, Schooley J L, Flam M S 1985 Peritoneal carcinomatosis after prophylactic oophorectomy in familial ovarian cancer syndrome. Obstetrics and Gynecology 66: 93
Crawford L 1993 Prospects for cervical cancer vaccines. In: Lemoine N R, Wright N A (eds) The molecular pathology of cancer. Cold Spring Harbor Laboratory Press, pp 215–229
Crook T, Wrede D, Tidy J A, Mason W P, Evans D J, Vousden K H 1992 Clonal p53 mutation in primary cervical cancer: association with human papillomavirus-negative tumours. Lancet 339: 1070–1073
Culver K W et al 1992 In vivo gene transfer with retroviral vector-producer cells for treatment of experimental brain tumors. Science 256(5063): 1550–1552
DeKlein A, van Kessel A G, Grosveld G et al 1982 A cellular oncogene is translocated to the Philadelphia chromosome in chronic myelocytic leukemia. Nature 300: 765–767
Dodson M K, Hartmann L C, Cliby W A et al 1993 Comparison of loss of heterozygosity patterns in invasive low-grade and high-grade epithelial ovarian carcinomas. Cancer Research 53: 4456–4460
Durst M, Kleinheinz A, Hotz M 1985 The physical state of human papillomavirus type 16 DNA in benign and malignant genital tumours. Journal of General Virology 66: 1515–1522
Easton D F, Bishop D T, Ford D, Crockford G P 1993 Genetic linkage analysis in familial breast and ovarian cancer: results from 214 families. The Breast Cancer Linkage Consortium. American Journal of Human Genetics 52: 678
Easton D F, Ford D, Bishop D T et al 1995 Breast and ovarian cancer incidence in BRCA1 mutation carriers. American Journal of Human Genetics 56: 265–271
Enomoto T, Fujita M, Inoue M et al 1993 Alterations of the p53 tumor suppressor gene and its association with activation of the c-K-ras-2 protooncogene in premalignant and malignant lesions of the human uterine endometrium. Cancer Research 53: 1883
Fearon E R, Cho K R, Nigro J M et al 1990 Identification of a chromosome 18q gene that is altered in colorectal cancers. Science 247: 49–56
Fialkow P J 1976 Clonal origin of human tumours. Biochimica et Biophysica Acta 458: 283–321
Fishel R, Lascoe M K, Rao M R S et al 1993 The human mutator gene homolog MSH2 and its association with hereditary nonpolyposis colon cancer. Cell 75: 1027–1038
Ford D, Easton D F, Bishop D T et al 1994 Risks of cancer in BRCA1 mutation carriers. Lancet 343: 692–695
Freeman S M et al 1993 The ' bystander effect': tumor regression when a fraction of the tumor mass is genetically modified. Cancer Research 53: 5274–5283
Futreal P A, Liu Q, Shattuck-Eidens D et al 1994 BRCA1 mutations in primary breast and ovarian carcinomas. Science 266: 120–122
Hall J M, Lee M K, Newman B et al 1990 Linkage of early-onset familial breast cancer to chromosome 17q21. Science 250: 1684–1689
Harris C C, Hollstein M 1993 Clinical implications of the p53 tumor-suppressor gene. New England Journal of Medicine 329: 1318–1327
Harris H, Miller O J, Klein G, Worst P, Tachibana T 1969 Suppression of malignancy by cell fusion. Nature 223: 363–368
Hosking L et al 1995 A somatic BRCA1 mutation in an ovarian tumour. Nature Genetics 9(4): 343–344
Hudson J B, Bedell M A, McCance D J, Laimins L A 1990 Immortalisation and altered differentiation of human keratinocytes in vitro by the E6 and E7 open reading frames of human papillomavirus type 18. Journal of Virology 64: 519–526
Ionov Y, Peinado M A, Miakhosyan S, Shibata D, Penucho M 1993 Ubiquitous somatic mutations in simple repeated sequences reveal a new mechanism for colonic carcinogenesis. Nature 363: 558–561
Jacobs I, Davies A P, Bridges J et al 1993 Prevalence screening for ovarian cancer in postmenopausal women by CA 125 measurement and ultrasonography [see comments]. British Medical Journal 306: 1030
Jacobs I J, Kohler M F, Wiseman R W et al 1992 Clonal origin of epithelial ovarian carcinoma: analysis by loss of heterozygosity, p53 mutation, and X-chromosome inactivation. Journal of the National Cancer Institute 84: 1793
Kacinski B M, Carter D, Mittal K et al 1990 Ovarian adenocarcinomas express fms-complementary transcripts and fms antigen, often with coexpression of CSF-1. American Journal of Pathology 137: 135
Kinzler K W, Nilbert M C, Su L-K et al 1991 Identification of FAP locus genes from chromosome 5q21. Science 253: 661–665
Knudson A G 1971 Mutation and cancer: statistical study of retinoblastoma. Proceedings of the National Academy of Science USA 68: 820–823
Kohler M F, Berchuck A, Davidoff A M et al 1992 Overexpression and mutation of p53 in endometrial carcinoma. Cancer Research 52: 1622
Kohler M F, Nishii H, Humphrey P A et al 1993 Mutation of the p53 tumor-suppressor gene is not a feature of endometrial hyperplasias. American Journal of Obstetrics and Gynecology 169: 690
Krontiris T G, Cooper G M 1981 Transforming activity of human tumour DNAs. Proceedings of the National Academy of Science USA 78: 1811–1884
Land H, Parada L F, Weiberg R A 1983 Tumorigenic conversion of primary embryo fibroblasts requires at least two cooperating oncogenes. Nature 304: 596–602
Leach F S, Nicolaides N C, Papadopoulos N et al 1993 Mutations of a mutS homolog in hereditary nonpolyposis colorectal cancer. Cell 75: 1215–1225
Leone A, Flatow U, King C R et al 1991 Reduced tumor incidence, metastatic potential and cytokine responsiveness of *nm*23-transfected melanoma cells. Cell 65: 25–35
Lynch H T et al 1985 Hereditary nonpolyposis colorectal cancer (Lynch syndromes I and II). I. Clinical description of resource. Cancer 56(4): 934–938
Marks J R, Davidoff A M, Kerns B J et al 1991 Overexpression and mutation of p53 in epithelial ovarian cancer. Cancer Research 51: 2979
Merajver S D, Pham T M, Caduff R L et al 1995 Somatic mutations in the BRCA1 gene in sporadic ovarian tumours. Nature Genetics 9: 439–443
Miki Y, Swensen J, Shattuck-Eidens D et al 1994 Isolation of BRCA1, the 17q linked breast and ovarian cancer susceptibility gene. Science 266: 66–71

Peltomäki P et al 1993 Genetic mapping of a locus predisposing to human colorectal cancer. Science 260: 810–812

Puls L E, Powell D E, DePriest P D et al 1992 Transition from benign to malignant epithelium in mucinous and serous ovarian cystadenocarcinoma. Gynecologic Oncology 47: 53

Rous P 1911 A sarcoma of the fowl transmissible by an agent separable from the tumour cells. Journal of Experimental Medicine 13: 396–411

Sandles L G, Shulman L P, Elias S et al 1992 Endometrial adenocarcinoma: genetic analysis suggesting heritable site-specific uterine cancer. Gynecologic Oncology 47: 167

Santos E, Tronick S R, Aaronson S A, Pulciani S, Barbacid M 1982 T24 human bladder carcinoma oncogene is an activated form of the normal human homologue of BALB- and Harvey-MSV transforming genes. Nature 298: 343–347

Sasaki H, Nishii H, Takahashi H et al 1993 Mutation of the Ki-ras protooncogene in human endometrial hyperplasia and carcinoma. Cancer Research 53: 1906

Shirashawa J, Tomita Y, Sekiya S, Takamizawa H, Simizu B 1987 Integration and transcription of human papillomavirus type 16 and 18 sequences in cell lines derived from cervical carcinomas. Journal of General Virology 68: 583–591

Sidransky D, Von Eschenbach A, Tsai Y et al 1991 Identification of p53 mutations in bladder cancers and urine samples. Science 252: 706–709

Slamon D J, Godolphin W, Jones L A et al 1989 Studies of the HER-2/neu proto-oncogene in human breast and ovarian cancer. Science 244: 707

Smith S A, Easton D F, Evans D G, Ponder B A 1992 Allele losses in the region 17q12–21 in familial breast and ovarian cancer involve the wild-type chromosome. Nature Genetics 2: 128

Stehelin D, Varmus H E, Bishop J M, Vogt P K 1976 DNA related to the transforming gene(s) of avian sarcoma viruses is present in normal avian DNA. Nature 260: 170–173

Tashiro H, Miyazaki K, Okamura H, Iwai A, Fukumoto M 1992 c-myc over-expression in human primary ovarian tumours: its relevance to tumour progression. International Journal of Cancer 50: 828

Thibodeau S N, Bren G, Schaid D 1993 Microsatellite instability in cancer of the proximal colon. Science 260: 816–819

Vogelstein B, Kinzler W 1993 The multistep nature of cancer. Trends in Genetics 9(4):138–141

Vousden K H 1989 Human papillomaviruses and cervical cancer. Cancer Cells 1: 43–49

Vousden K H 1991 Human papillomavirus transforming genes. Seminars in Virology 2: 307–317

Zhang Y et al 1993 Retroviral vector-mediated transduction of K-ras antisense RNA into human lung cancer cells inhibits expression of the malignant phenotype. Human Gene Therapy 4: 451–460

Zheng J P, Robinson W R, Ehlen T, Yu M C, Dubeau L 1991 Distinction of low grade from high grade human ovarian carcinomas on the basis of losses of heterozygosity on chromosomes 3, 6, and 11 and HER-2/neu gene amplification. Cancer Research 51: 4045

33

The principles of radiotherapy and chemotherapy

H. E. Lambert C. C. Vernon

RADIOTHERAPY

Radiotherapy is the therapeutic use of ionizing radiation. It is used primarily for treating malignant tumours, including gynaecological cancers and in particular carcinoma of the cervix.

RADIATION PHYSICS

When living matter absorbs radiation energy, ionization of biological molecules occurs. Ionization is the result of radiation energy ejecting one or more electrons from an atom. Ionizing radiation as used for treatment is either electromagnetic or particulate.

Electromagnetic radiation

X-rays and γ-rays are identical types of electromagnetic radiation. X-rays for treatment purposes are produced by a machine called a linear accelerator, which accelerates electrons to high kinetic energy and then stops them abruptly on a target, which is usually made of tungsten or gold. Part of the kinetic energy of the electrons is converted to X-rays. γ-rays are emitted naturally by radioactive isotopes such as ^{60}cobalt as they decay to reach a stable form.

γ-rays and X-rays are characterized by a short wavelength and high frequency. They consist of a stream of photons (packets of energy) which are absorbed in tissue and which at high acceleration have sufficient power to break chemical bonds. This leads to biological change and can result in the death of a cell, hence their use in the treatment of cancer.

Particulate radiation

This consists of atomic subparticles, i.e. electrons (negative charges), protons (positive charges), neutrons (no charge) and negative iT mesons. At present only electrons are commonly used in radiotherapy, having been accelerated to high energy in a linear accelerator from which the tungsten target has been removed so that X-rays are not produced.

The gray

Radiation energy absorbed in tissue is measured in grays (Gy). One gray is the equivalent of 1 J/kg. Previously radiation energy was measured in rads, 1 Gy being equivalent to 100 rad. Particulate radiation causes ionization directly and X-rays and γ-rays indirectly by giving up their energy to eject fast-moving electrons from atoms.

RADIOBIOLOGY

The study of the effects of ionizing radiation on living matter is called radiobiology. The principal critical target in a cell is DNA. When this is damaged, cell metabolism and reproduction are affected. Ionizing radiation will act on both normal and cancer cells, and the problem for radiotherapy is to eliminate cancer cells without permanently damaging vital tissues. Recovery of normal tissue is usually better than that of malignant tissue, as long as the overall dose is not too large and it is given over a period of time. It is therefore the practice to fractionate the dose of radiation over several days or weeks.

SCHEDULING AND DOSE OF RADIOTHERAPY

Dose fractionation

Fractionated external beam therapy is usually given once daily 4–5 times a week. To attempt to improve cure rates, particularly in rapidly growing tumours, treatment can be accelerated by giving larger doses per fraction over a shorter time. This will increase the cell kill per fraction but will also interfere with normal cellular repair. Acceleration may also be carried out using normal-sized fractions twice daily, separated by at least 6 hours. Hyperfractionation, in which three or more small fractions are given each day, is also being examined in clinical trials. The theoretical reason for increasing the number of daily fractions is to allow sufficient time for normal tissue to regenerate but insufficient for tumour cells.

Dose prescription

The radiation dose prescribed includes the total dose to be given, the total number of fractions, the total time and the dose per fraction, for example 50 Gy in 25 fractions given five times weekly in 5 weeks at 2 Gy per fraction. For radical curative treatment, the greater the tumour volume the higher the radiation dose necessary to eliminate the cancer. For example, 50 Gy in 5 weeks is sufficient for microscopic foci in 90% of patients, but 6570 Gy in 6.5–7 weeks is needed to destroy a 2 cm mass. When there is no likelihood of cure but the patient is symptomatic, palliative radiotherapy has a valuable role to relieve pain. Doses are smaller and treatment time is reduced. If radiation fails, repeat treatment is of no value and will cause severe injury to normal tissues.

RADIOTHERAPY TECHNIQUES

Several techniques are used in the management of gynaecological cancer.

1. Teletherapy is external irradiation where the tumour is a 'long' distance – usually 100 cm – from the source of ionizing radiation.
2. Brachytherapy is either intracavitary or interstitial (inserted directly into tissues) irradiation where there is a 'short' distance between source and tumour (e.g. in the vagina and cervical canal).
3. Instillation of radioactive fluids into the pleural and peritoneal cavity or, more rarely, by intra-arterial infusion to the tumour site.

Teletherapy – external irradiation

Teletherapy is used to treat large volumes, such as in carcinoma of the cervix where the volume includes the tumour itself, the parametria and the regional lymph nodes. The size of the treatment volume and the overall dose will be influenced by the age and general condition of the patient. For example, arteriosclerosis or bowel disease such as diverticulitis both reduce bowel tolerance. The small bowel tolerates only relatively low doses of radiation but its mobility enables it to move in and out of the treatment area, thus reducing the dose it receives. Damage to the small bowel can result from surgical adhesions which immobilize the small bowel. Care must also be taken with the rectum and pelvic colon, which will be partly in the treatment volume.

Treatment planning

The aim of planning is to deliver a homogeneous dose to the tumour volume while giving only a low dose to surrounding normal tissues. The volume is measured in three dimensions: superior–inferior, anterior–posterior and right to left laterally. The dose of radiation which will be tolerated by normal tissues within the tumour volume must be known. Particular attention must be given to critical organs, such as the kidney or spinal cord, which tolerate only low doses of radiation. Accurate tumour localization is essential and is assessed by both clinical and surgical findings, with additional information from X-rays, ultrasound and computerized tomography (CT) scanning, and magnetic resonance imaging (MRI) when appropriate.

Planning procedure

The patient is placed on a mobile couch beneath a simulator – a diagnostic X-ray machine connected to a television screen which emulates a treatment machine (Fig. 33.1). The simulator defines the limits of the treatment volume, using a beam of light in place of the X-rays of the treatment machine. It will also take X-ray films for a permanent record.

The patient is positioned carefully with the help of a laser beam to ensure accurate replication at each treatment session. Cross-wires mounted in the light beam from the simulator define the size of the area to be treated (Fig. 33.2). This is marked on the patient with a semi-permanent dye, usually gentian violet, which will not wash off easily during the treatment period. The body contour at the volume centre is measured using pliable wire, or more accurately with CT. On to this contour the tumour volume will be drawn, either on paper or by using a CT planning computer.

For the tumour to receive an adequate dose without overdosing the skin or other tissues, several fields arranged at different entry points to the body are used (Fig. 33.3). A planning computer (Fig. 33.4) calculates field sizes, the dose from each field and the angles of the treatment machine to give a homogeneous distribution to the tumour. The computerized plan of the final radiation dose delivered to the pelvis for carcinoma of the cervix by a three-field arrangement is shown in Figure 33.5.

The most usual field arrangement is two to four fields, but a rotational or moving field and conformal techniques may also be used. In the former the radiation source rotates around the tumour centre to provide an even dose throughout the tumour volume, while reducing the total dose given to the normal tissues. This is time-consuming and is less used today with the advent of high-energy machines. In the latter technique the field is shaped around the tumour volume, again with the aim of reducing the dose to normal tissues. This is particularly useful where large radiation fields are needed, as in the combined irradiation of the pelvis and para-aortic nodes.

Lead compensators may be placed in the path of the radiation beam to absorb unnecessary radiation. The most frequently used compensators are wedge-shaped (Fig. 33.6). The wedges are made with angles from 15 to 60° to vary the amount of radiation absorbed. Sometimes compensators need to be designed specially for individual patients.

Choice of machine

The intensity of a beam of radiation decreases with depth in tissue, but high-energy machines spare skin by delivering more radiation below the skin surface at the same time

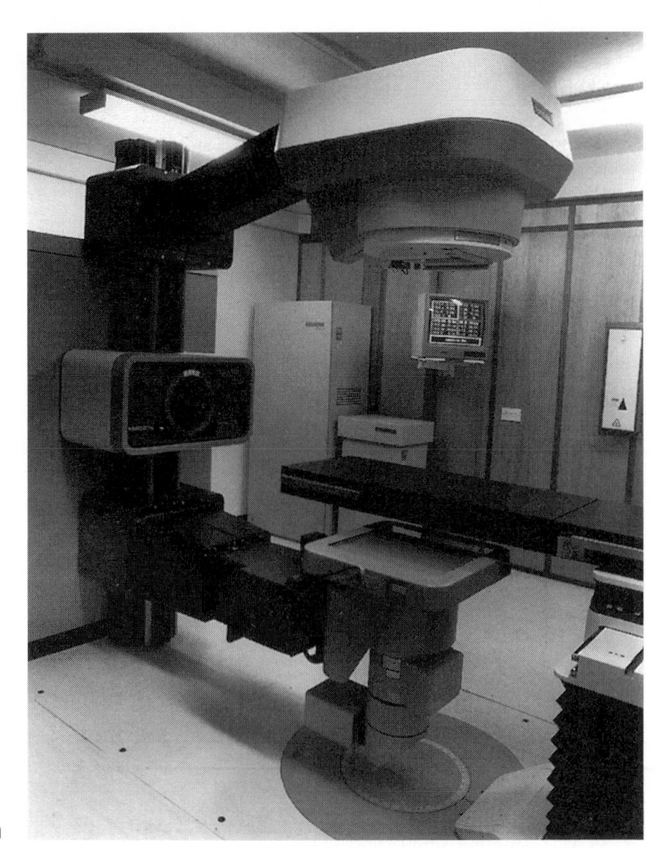
a

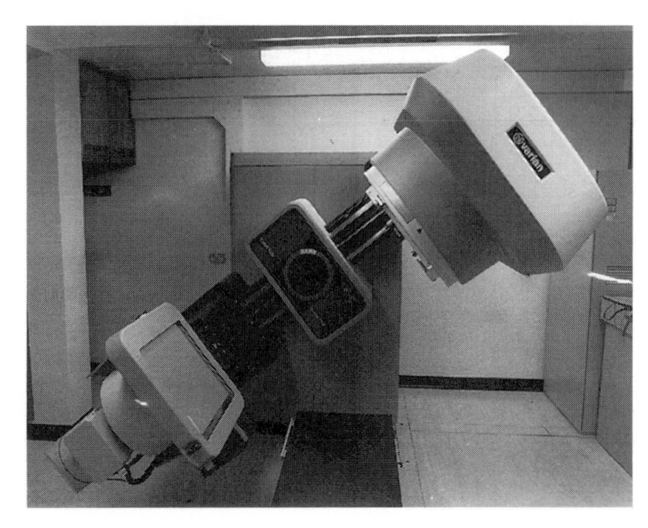

b

Fig. 33.1 **(a)** A Ximatron simulator with couch (manufactured by Varian TEM). **(b)** The gantry rotated.

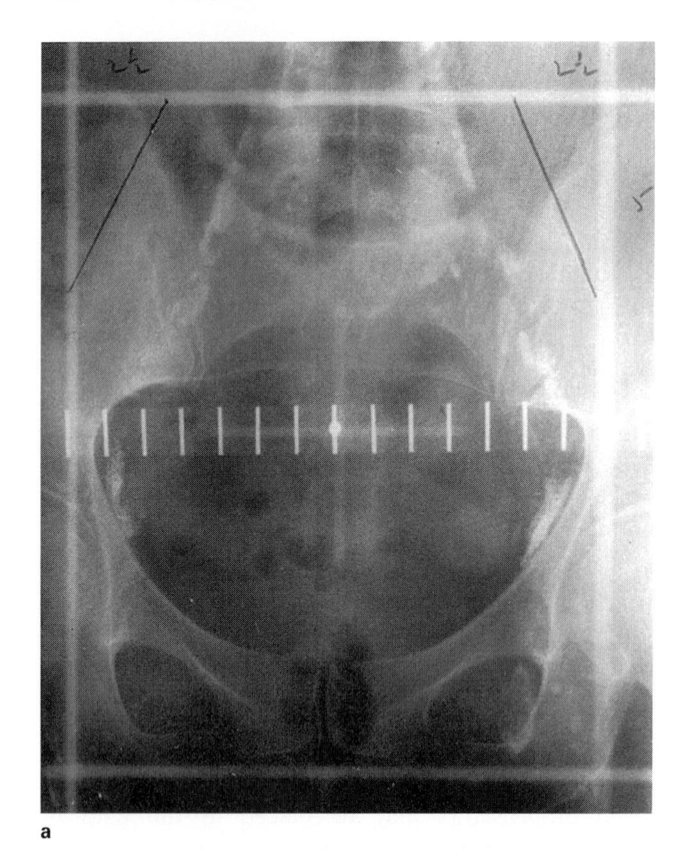

a

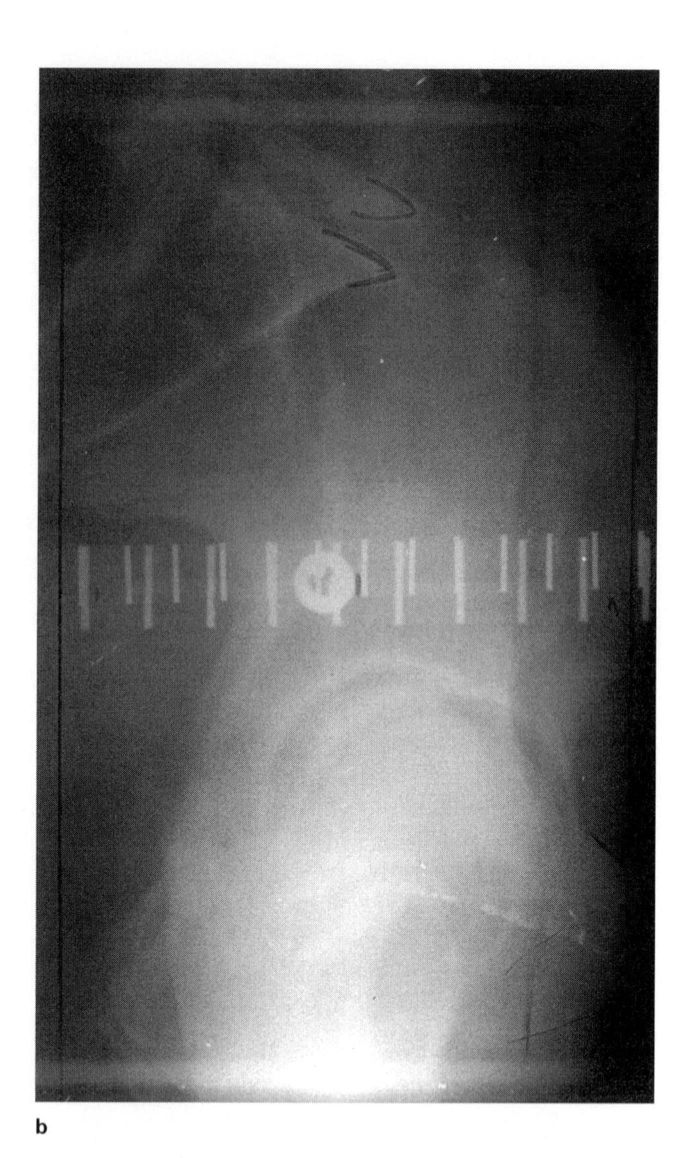

b

Fig. 33.2 **(a)** Anteroposterior X-ray of the treatment area (the pelvis) showing the superior, inferior and lateral margins. The triangular areas are protected from the beam. The patient has had a lymphangiogram. **(b)** Lateral X-ray of the treatment area.

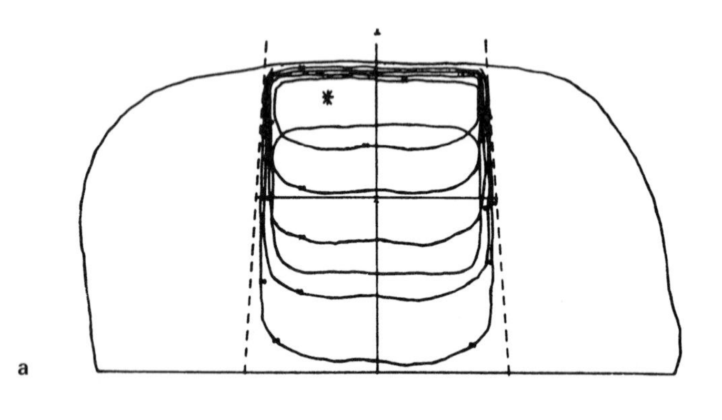

a

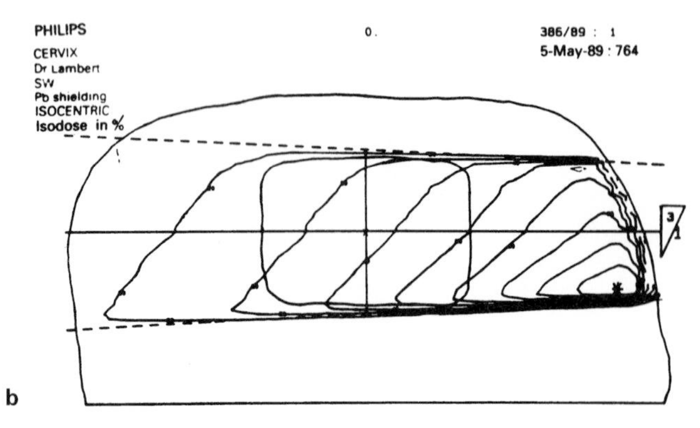

b

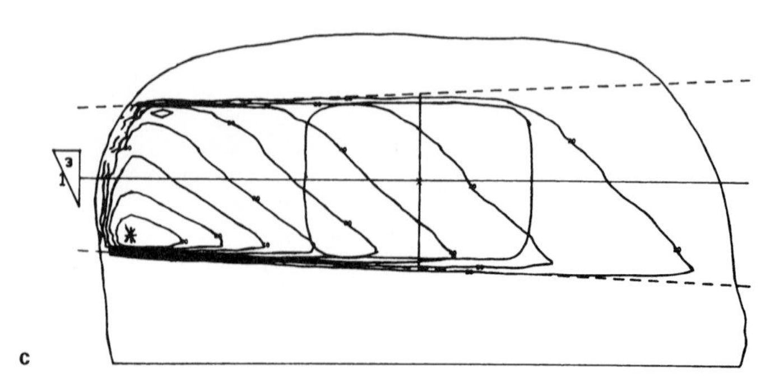

c

Fig. 33.3 Computer simulations of the isodose pattern of (**a**) the anterior field; (**b**) the left lateral field; (**c**) the right lateral field.

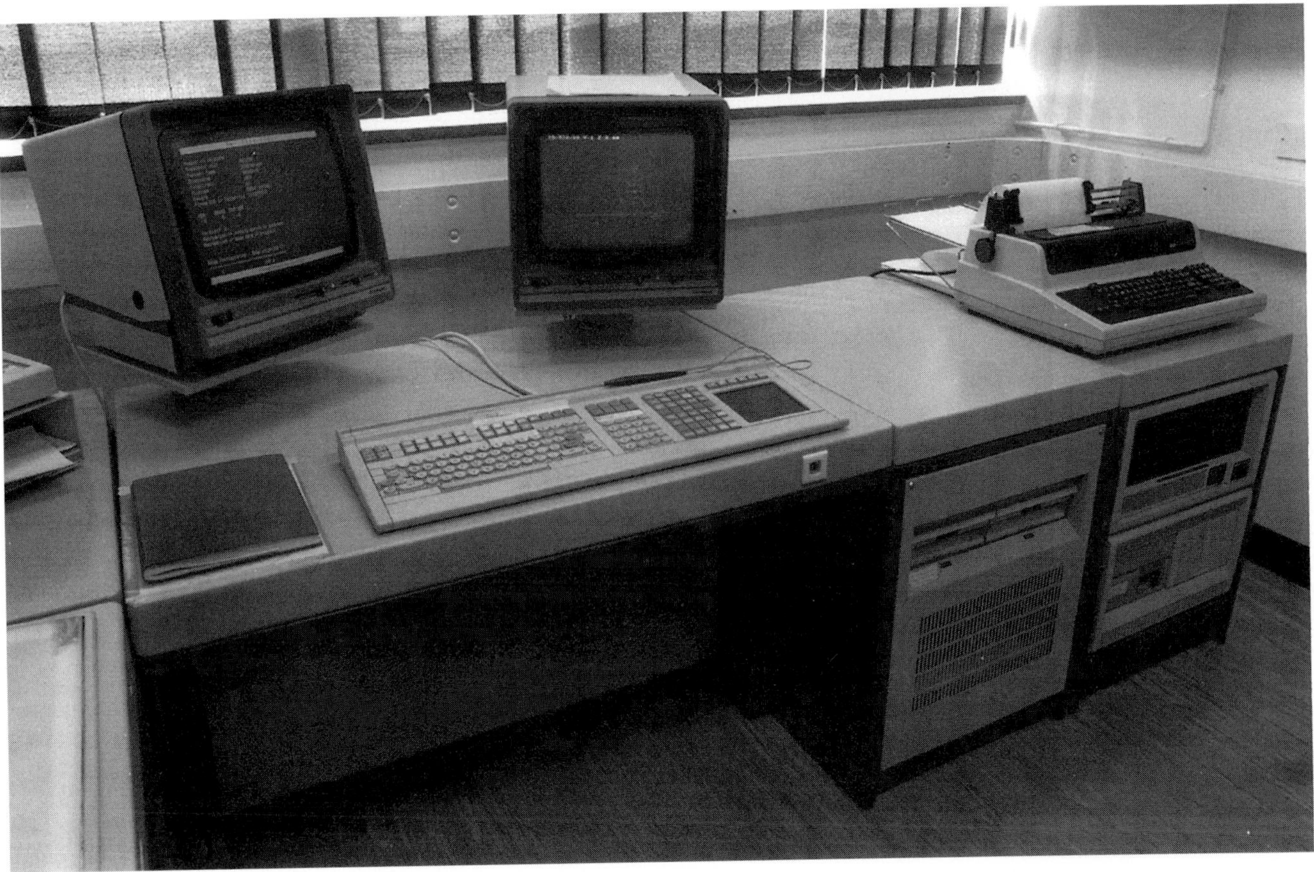

Fig. 33.4 The planning computer. A plan of the volume being prepared is shown on one screen and instructions are shown on the second. A permanent record is produced as in Figures 33.3 and 33.5.

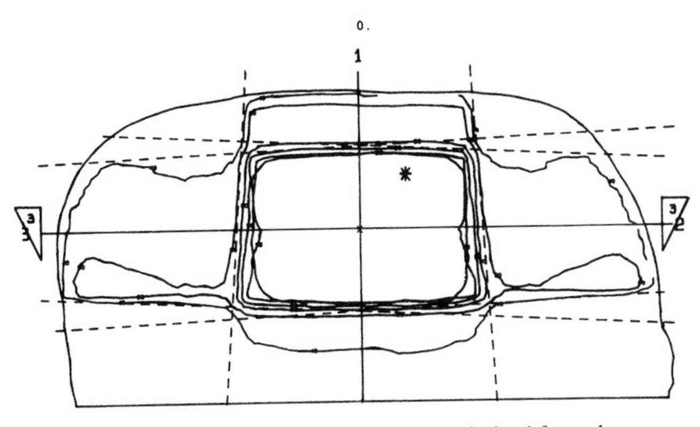

Fig. 33.5 The final tumour volume is shown derived from the summation of the isodoses from all three fields.

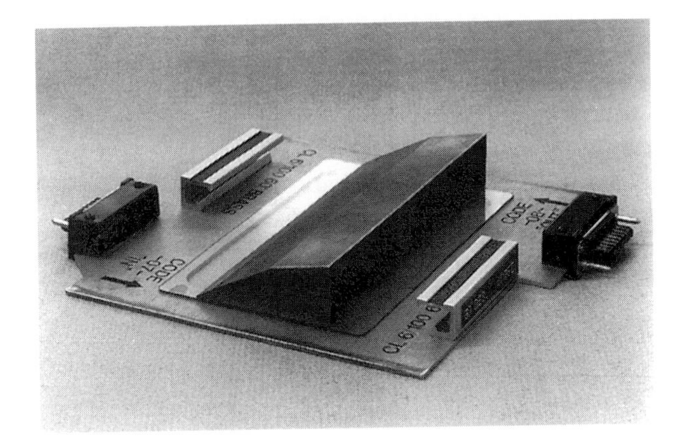

Fig. 33.6 A 60° wedge compensator.

as reaching deeply situated tumours. Such machines have included those with a ^{60}Co source releasing γ-rays of 1.3 meV energy, but it is more usual today to use linear accelerators which deliver X-rays of 4–8 meV.

Implementation of the plan

Treatment is carried out in a specially protected room with thick concrete walls, preventing radiation of personnel outside. The patient lies on the treatment couch in the same position as established with the simulator (Fig. 33.7). The machine angle, size of field and the use of wedges are carefully prepared for each treatment field. Radiographers, who set up and treat patients, use a control console outside the treatment room to start and stop the radiation and to set the dose and the time. Treatment time for each field is short, usually less than 1 minute. As the patient has to be alone during this time she is

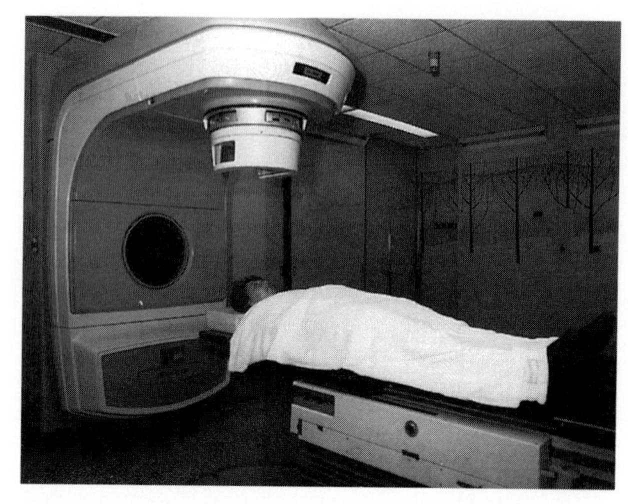

Fig. 33.7 Patient lying on the couch of a 6 meV Varian linear accelerator.

supervised using a television camera. A microphone enables patients to talk to staff and if they are distressed the treatment is stopped immediately, so the radiographers can re-enter the room. There are many safety precautions to prevent accidental overdosage and treatment machines are checked frequently.

Brachytherapy

Brachytherapy gives a very high dose of radiation from a source close to the tumour. Because radiation dose decreases with the square of the distance travelled, there is a very rapid fall-off of radiation around the source and less damage to normal tissues. For the same reason, this method is suitable only for treating small tumour volumes. In the past, the energy source used was radium-226, but because of its long half-life – approximately 1600 years – and because it produces a radioactive gas, radon, it has been replaced by other radioactive isotopes such as caesium-137 (^{137}Cs), which has a half-life of 33 years and produces no toxic gases.

Brachytherapy methods

Direct insertion. The commonest method of giving intracavitary radiation for gynaecological tumours is the Manchester system, in which a single uterine tube containing ^{137}Cs is passed through the cervix into the uterine cavity so that the inferior margin is flush with the external cervical os and smaller tubes, containing ^{137}Cs in plastic vaginal ovoids, are inserted into the lateral vaginal fornices. The tumour volume treated by these three radioactive sources is shown in Figure 33.8. This is a low dose rate treatment lasting for several days.

Afterloading. Most radiotherapy centres have replaced the direct insertion of radioactive sources into a patient with an afterloading system. This system allows

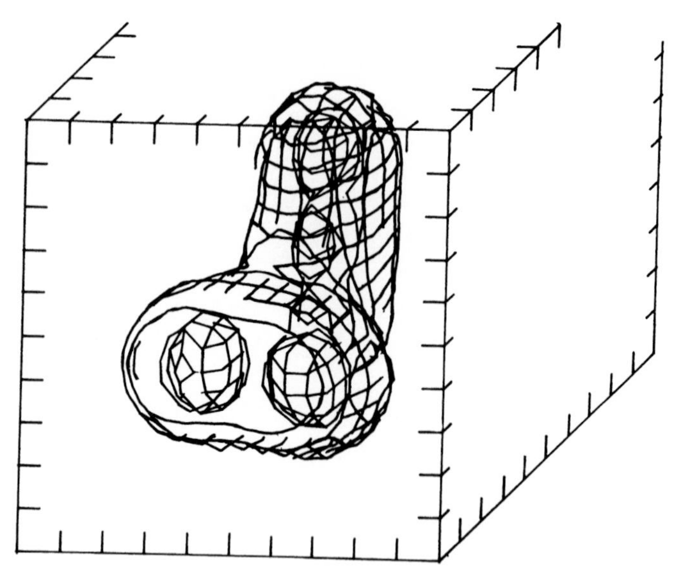

Fig. 33.8 The volume from the summation of three brachytherapy sources, an intrauterine tube and two vaginal ovoids. This shows the limits of the treatment volume and the rapid fall-off of the dose.

time to be taken over the positioning of source trains without hazard to the operator. Only after the accuracy of their placement has been verified with X-ray films are the radioactive sources inserted. In manual afterloading systems (Fig. 33.9), the active sources are inserted after the patient has returned to the ward, so eliminating radiation risk to theatre staff.

Remote afterloading systems are preferred as they allow complete staff protection. The patient is treated in a protected room for approximately 20 hours in the case of the Selectron, which uses ^{137}Cs, or for a few minutes with high dose-rate systems such as the High Dose Selectron, which uses ^{60}Co (Figs 33.10, 33.11). With high dose-rates severe damage to normal tissues is avoided by reducing and fractionating the total dose. All the techniques described are equally effective.

Intracavitary brachytherapy

The procedure is carried out under general anaesthetic. A pelvic examination, including cystoscopy and proctoscopy, is performed. For cervical cancer the bladder is catheterized, the cervix is dilated and the uterine length measured with a sound to ascertain the length of the uterine tube required. The width of the vaginal vault is assessed to decide on the size of applicator or applicators to be inserted. The uterine tube is inserted first and then the vaginal applicators. A gauze pack keeps the sources in place and away from the rectum to reduce the rectal dose, which can be checked with a dosimeter. A computer using information from X-rays is a better way of measuring the doses given to both the treatment volume and to normal tissues (see Fig. 33.8).

For carcinoma of the cervix the dose to be given can be

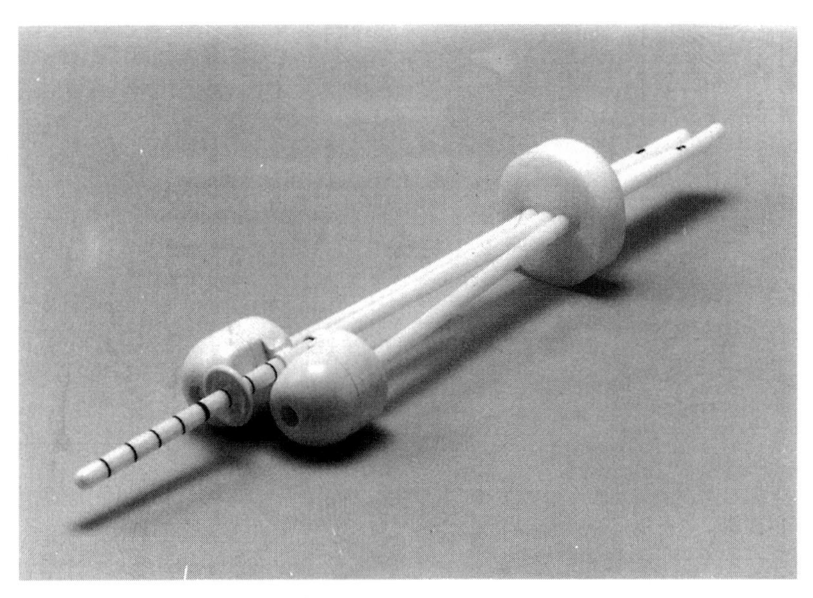

Fig. 33.9 The Amersham manual afterloading system for treating carcinoma of the cervix. There are three trains, a central one for the uterine tube and two lateral trains for the vaginal ovoids.

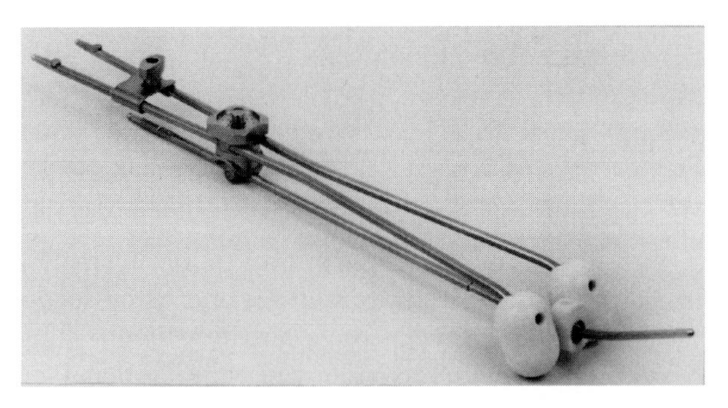

Fig. 33.10 Source train for Microselectron high dose-rate afterloading therapy. This shows a central uterine tube and two lateral vaginal ovoids.

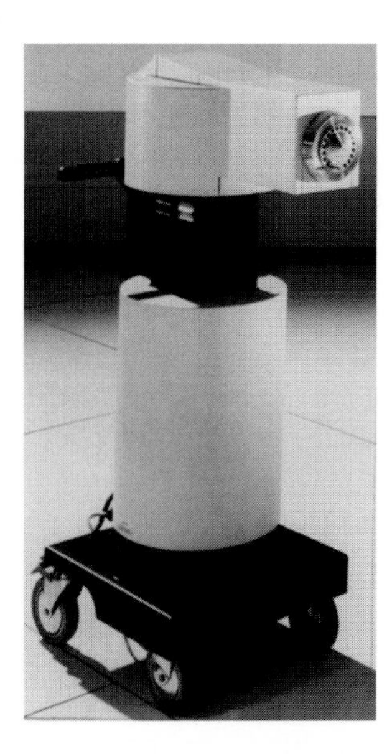

Fig. 33.11 The safe containing the radiation sources for the Microselectron.

calculated at reference point A, which in theory estimates the normal tissue dose where the ureter crosses the uterine artery. It is 2 cm lateral to the cervical canal and 2 cm superior to the lateral fornix. In practice this point is measured from the X-rays as 2 cm lateral to the centre of the uterine radioactive source and 2 cm superior to its inferior margin. A newer method of describing the given dose recommended by the ICRU (International Commission on Radiation Units and Measurements) measures the size of the tumour volume receiving full radiation dose. If the sole method of treatment is by low dose-rate intracavitary radiation, 80 Gy are given in two fractions. After external irradiation only one fraction of 20–30 Gy is required.

Interstitial brachytherapy

In some areas, treatment of small tumours with sparing of normal tissues can best be carried out by the insertion directly into the tumour of radioactive sources as needles, wires or seeds. An example is the insertion of radioactive needles for early cases of vaginal carcinoma. One such technique is to use a template (Fig. 33.12), which allows the insertion of guide tubes which can be afterloaded with active sources once X-rays have confirmed the correct position of the guides. Templates increase the accuracy of implants by ensuring that the sources are distributed in a regular fashion, giving a uniform dose to the treatment volume without 'hot' or 'cold' spots. The isotopes commonly used for this procedure are ^{192}Ir, ^{137}Cs and ^{125}I. For a radical course of treatment doses such as 60 Gy are given in 6 days.

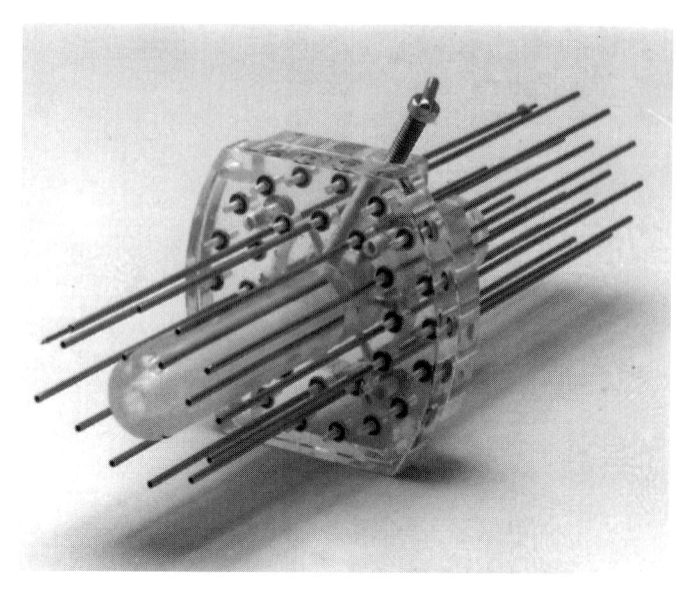

Fig. 33.12 A template (the 'Hammersmith hedgehog') for the interstitial treatment of carcinoma of the vagina.

Instillation of radioisotopes in solution

Radiotherapy for small-volume disease in the peritoneal, pleural or pericardial spaces can be given as a solution of radioisotopes. Early ovarian cancers have been treated using radioactive isotopes of either gold or phosphorus linked to carrier colloids. This gives a high dose of radiation but only to a depth of 4–6 mm, limiting therapy to small deposits on the pleural or peritoneal surfaces. Radioactive labelled monoclonal antibodies have been used in the same way in the hope that the antibody will target the radiotherapy to the tumour site.

RADIATION DAMAGE

The dose of radiation is limited by the tolerance of normal tissue. Large single fractions of radiation cause more damage than multiple small fractions for the same total dose. Normal tissue reactions occur both early and late. Early reactions take place during or immediately after a course of radiotherapy, but recovery is usually rapid. Late reactions occur from 1 year onwards, are permanent and usually slowly progressive. Skin, bowel and bone marrow proliferate rapidly and so are particularly susceptible to acute reactions during treatment. Tissues which divide slowly, such as kidney, show late reactions because the damage to DNA only becomes apparent when cells divide.

Early reactions

Skin

Except when the vulval or anal region is included, radiation damage to skin is largely avoided when treating pelvic tumours because megavoltage machines deliver their maximum dose below the skin surface and the use of multiple treatment fields reduces the dose to any particular area of skin. Epidermal cells turn over in 2–3 weeks, so any damage becomes apparent after that time. Erythema may be followed by dry desquamation or, with more severe damage, by moist desquamation. The basal cells are usually spared, allowing the skin to regrow.

Bowel

Cells in the intestinal mucosa are replaced every 3–6 days, leading to diarrhoea when bowel is included in the treatment volume. Most patients also complain of nausea and anorexia.

Bone marrow

The bone marrow is very sensitive to radiation and frequent blood counts are essential when large volumes of marrow are included in the treatment fields, as for example in whole abdominal radiotherapy for ovarian carcinoma. The white blood count and platelet count are affected early, but anaemia occurs later because of the longer life span of red blood cells.

Late complications

Bowel

Late but uncommon complications to both small and large bowel include bleeding, stenosis and malabsorption. These may require special diets and nutritional support with vitamin supplements. Exceptionally, surgical intervention such as excision of damaged bowel with or without a stoma is necessary. The poor blood supply after radiation damage makes surgery difficult and the security of bowel anastamoses uncertain.

Bladder and ureter

Bladder changes, including telangiectasiae, are common and occasionally cause haemorrhagic cystitis. Ureteric damage and vesicovaginal fistulae are rare.

Other organs

Late damage to liver and kidneys owing to damage to the vascular supply may cause cirrhosis or loss of renal function. The ovaries are particularly sensitive to radiation and even small doses can cause ovarian failure.

It is important to note that the endometrium is very resistant to radiotherapy and may well persist after radiotherapy for cervical cancer (Habeshaw & Pinion 1992). Hormone replacement therapy given in such cases should include progestogens to avoid the risk of inducing endometrial carcinoma.

CONCLUSION

Ionizing radiation is a sophisticated technique used for the treatment of cancer. It requires both highly technical machinery and expertise from specially trained personnel – engineers, physicists, doctors and radiographers. Side effects are usually slight, but complications can occur even after ideal treatment.

CHEMOTHERAPY

Cytotoxic chemotherapy developed from the realization that the effects on bone marrow cells of mustard gas used in World War I could be extended to the treatment of cancer. In the 1940s methotrexate and other antimetabolite drugs were discovered, and since that time many drugs have been found that are of potential use in cancer therapy. Of these, approximately 40 are now in general use.

DRUG EVALUATION

Before cytotoxic drugs can be used to treat cancer in humans they must first be tested for both their efficiency and their toxicity in animals. A promising drug is then studied in patients with advanced cancer to obtain pharmacological information (Phase 1). Sensitive tumours are identified in Phase 2, before a large number of patients with responsive tumours are treated to further define the drug's role (Phase 3).

PHARMACOLOGY

When considering the pharmacology of a drug, the following aspects must be investigated: absorption, distribution, metabolism and excretion. Drugs can only be taken orally if they are well absorbed from the alimentary tract. Parenteral administration – intravenous, intramuscular or intra-arterial – is the optimal route for most cytotoxic drugs. Of these, intravenous is by far the most common. Occasionally, in superficial tumours, cytotoxic drugs are given topically (5-fluorouracil) or by injection directly into the tumour (bleomycin).

The metabolism of drugs within the body is often unknown but several, including 5-fluorouracil, are metabolized in the liver. Most drugs are excreted in urine but a few are excreted in the alimentary tract via the bile duct. Only a very few drugs, such as the nitrosoureas and etoposide, cross the blood–brain barrier. This barrier can be overcome by intrathecal administration, and methotrexate is given this way in the treatment of lymphatic leukaemia (Table 33.1).

CLASSIFICATION

The most common classification of cytotoxic drugs is one based on their biochemistry. Drugs are divided into alkylating agents, antimetabolites, vinca alkaloids, antibiotics and miscellaneous.

CYTOTOXIC DRUGS COMMONLY USED IN GYNAECOLOGY

Alkylating agents

These drugs cross-link DNA strands by forming covalent bonds between highly reactive alkylating groups and nitrogen groups on the DNA helix. This either prevents division of the helix at mitosis or results in an imperfect division and cell death.

The most frequently used alkylating agents are cyclophosphamide, chlorambucil and melphalan. Newer agents include treosulfan and ifosfamide. Many alkylating agents may be taken orally. Cyclophosphamide is inactive until it is converted into its active metabolite in the liver (Table 33.1).

The toxic effects of alkylating agents are listed in Table 33.2. In particular they can cause vomiting if given in large doses, but this is seldom intractable. Most cause significant myelotoxicity, which can be cumulative. Alopecia is most marked with cyclophosphamide and ifosfamide. Both these last drugs are excreted in the urine in the form of active metabolites, which can cause a severe chemical cystitis when given in high doses unless mesna (sodium 2-mercaptoethanesulphonate) is administered at the same time to protect the bladder mucosa. In addition, ifosfamide may cause a fatal encephalopathy and must be given only after reference to a treatment nomogram.

Platinum agents

Cisplatin and carboplatin both contain platinum. They act in a similar way to alkylating agents. Both are given intravenously but, because of its severe nephrotoxicity, cisplatin requires a forced diuresis.

Cisplatin causes severe nausea and vomiting which require potent antiemetic therapy. Peripheral neuropathy can be disabling and is usually dose related. Cisplatin has little myelotoxicity except for anaemia, which frequently has to be corrected with blood transfusion.

Carboplatin has very little nephrotoxicity or neurotoxicity and also causes less vomiting. It may be given to outpatients, as it only requires a half-hour infusion unless vomiting is severe. Carboplatin is myelotoxic, a particular problem being thrombocytopenia. Impaired renal function increases thrombocytopenia, and so the drug is now usually given in a dose related to renal function, 'area under the curve' (AUC, Table 33.1), rather than surface area.

Antimetabolites

These compounds closely resemble metabolites essential

Table 33.1 Cytotoxic drugs: dosage, routes of administration and excretion

Drug	Route of administration	Dose (as a single agent)	Excretion
Alkylating agents			
Chlorambucil	Oral	10 mg/day or 10–14 days per month	Urine
Cyclophosphamide	Oral or i.v.	Oral 100–200 mg/day i.v. 500–1000 mg/week High dose 20–40 mg/kg	Bile Urine
Ifosfamide	i.v.	8–10 g/m^2 × 5 days 2–4-weekly	Urine
Melphalan	Oral	0.2 mg/kg/day × 5 days 4-weekly	Urine
Treosulphan	i.v. or oral	i.v. 5 g/m^2 3-weekly	Urine
Platinum compounds			
Cisplatin	i.v.	50–120 mg/m^2 weekly to 4-weekly	Urine
Carboplatin	i.v.	400 mg/m^2 or 5 × (EDTA clearance +25) mg 3–4-weekly	Urine
Antimetabolites			
Methotrexate	Oral, i.m. or i.v.	e.g. 100–1000 mg/m^2 with folinic acid rescue or 2.5–5 mg/day orally	Urine Bile
5-Fluorouracil	Oral or i.v.	Loading dose 12 mg/kg/day × 3 Maintenance 3–15 mg/kg/week	Urine
Vinca alkaloids			
Vincristine	i.v.	1–2 mg weekly	Bile
Vinblastine	i.v.	0.1–0.2 mg/kg weekly	Bile
Vindesine	i.v.	3–4 mg/m^2 weekly	Bile
Anthracyclines			
Doxorubicin (Adriamycin)	i.v.	60–75 mg/m^2 3-weekly Total dose <450 mg/m^2	Bile
Epirubicin	i.v.	75–90 mg/m^2 3-weekly	Bile
Mitozantrone	i.v.	14 mg/m^2 3-weekly	Bile
Other antibiotics			
Actinomycin D	i.v.	0.5 mg/day × 5 4-weekly	Bile
Mitomycin	i.v.	4–10 mg 6-weekly	Urine
Bleomycin	i.m., i.v., i.p. Malignant effusions	10–60 mg weekly 60 mg i.p. Maximum total dose 300 mg	Urine
Miscellaneous			
Dacarbazine (DTIC)	i.v.	250 mg/m^2/day × 5 3-weekly	Urine
Etoposide (VP 16)	Oral or i.v.	60–120 mg/m^2/day × 5 4-weekly	Urine
Lomustine (CCNU)	Oral	120 mg/m^2 6–8-weekly	Urine
Paclitaxel (Taxol)	i.v.	175 mg/m^2 over 3 h after premedication 3–4 weekly	Bile
Docetaxel (Taxotere)	i.v.	75–100 mg/m^2	Bile?

The doses shown are for general information only. The appropriate dose will vary in different circumstances and specific protocols should be consulted for detailed guidance.

for the synthesis of nucleic acids and proteins. They are incorporated into natural metabolic pathways and enzyme systems and disrupt the cellular mechanism. Each antimetabolite acts at different sites in the pathway of nucleic acid synthesis.

Methotrexate

Methotrexate is a folic acid antagonist. It inhibits the enzyme dihydrofolate reductase, which reduces dihydrofolate to tetrahydrofolate, the precursor of coenzymes essential for the formation of purines and pyrimidines, the nitrogen bases of DNA. These effects are bypassed by giving folinic acid. Folinic acid rescue is given from about 12 hours after the methotrexate dose to all patients receiving 100 mg or more. The commonest complication with methotrexate is oral ulceration. Because it is excreted in urine, the dose must be reduced in women with renal impairment or with large fluid collections such as ascites which delay excretion (Tables 33.1 and 33.2).

Table 33.2 The major toxic effects of some commonly used cytotoxic agents

Agent	Nausea & vomiting	Myelosuppression	Urological toxicity	Neuropathy	Others
Alkylating agents					
Chlorambucil	–	Moderate	–	–	Stomatitis, pulmonary fibrosis, hepatitis – all rare
Cyclophosphamide	Moderate	Moderate	Haemorrhagic cystitis	–	Alopecia; rare cardiomyopathy; very rare pulmonary fibrosis
Ifosfamide	Severe	Mild	Haemorrhagic cystitis	Confusion, tonic–clonic spasm, coma (rare)	Alopecia
Melphalan	Mild–moderate	Moderate	–	–	Rare pulmonary fibrosis
Treosulphan	Oral–moderate i.v. nil	Moderate	–	–	Very rare pulmonary fibrosis
Platinum agents					
Cisplatin	Very severe	Mild	Severe nephropathy	Moderate	Ototoxicity; hypomagnesaemia
Carboplatin	Moderate	Moderate–severe	Mild	Rare	Mild ototoxicity
Antimetabolites					
Methotrexate	Mild	Mild–moderate	Severe with high doses	–	Stomatitis; hepatitis with high doses
5-Fluorouracil	Mild	Moderate	–	–	Mucositis; dermatitis; alopecia with high doses
Vinca alkaloids					
Vincristine	–	–	Rare bladder atony	Severe: constipation, paralytic ileus, rare convulsions	Alopecia
Vinblastine	Mild	Moderate	–	Mild	Alopecia
Vindesine	Mild	Mild	–	Moderate: constipation, rare convulsions	Alopecia; stomatitis
Anthracyclines					
Doxorubicin	Severe	Moderate	–	–	Severe alopecia; severe cardiomyopathy if dose >450 mg/m^2
Epirubicin	Moderate	Moderate	–	–	Alopecia; mucositis; moderate cardiomyopathy
Mitozantrone	Mild	Moderate	Mild	–	Mild cardiomyopathy
Other antibiotics					
Actinomycin D	Moderate	Moderate–severe	–	–	Alopecia; mucositis; diarrhoea; fever; myalgia
Bleomycin	–	–	–	–	Fever; skin changes; pulmonary fibrosis and interstitial pneumonia
Mitomycin	–	Severe delayed	–	–	Stomatitis
Miscellaneous					
Dacarbazine (DTIC)	Severe	Severe	–	–	Photosensitivity; rare fever; alopecia; hepatitis
Etoposide (VP 16)	Moderate	Severe	–	–	Alopecia
Lomustine (CCNU)	Moderate	Severe delayed	Rare	–	–
Paclitaxel (Taxol)	Mild	Mild–moderate	–	Only at higher doses	Alopecia; hypersensitivity
Docetaxel (Taxotere)	Mild	Moderate–severe	–	Mild	Alopecia; hypersensitivity; skin rash; oedema

5-Fluorouracil

5-Fluorouracil is a pyrimidine analogue which blocks thymidine synthesis and inhibits the incorporation of uracil into DNA. Myelosuppression and mucositis are the most common toxic effects, but unless very high doses are given they are not usually severe (Table 33.2).

Vinca alkaloids

Vincristine, vinblastine and vindesine are derived from the periwinkle plant *Vinca rosea*. They act during the metaphase of mitosis, probably through toxicity to the microtubules of the mitotic spindle.

Peripheral and autonomic neuropathy are particular problems with vinca alkaloids, particularly vincristine. In addition, they are very irritant and are best injected into a fast-flowing drip. Vincristine is one of the very few chemotherapeutic drugs that is not myelotoxic.

Etoposide

Etoposide is a semisynthetic derivative of podophyllotoxin

that acts on cells in G2 in the cell cycle. Toxicity is shown in Table 33.2.

Antibiotics

Many antibiotics inhibit tumour cell division. Actinomycin D and doxorubicin (Adriamycin) form irreversible complexes with DNA. Bleomycin breaks up DNA chains, thus interfering with DNA replication.

Doxorubicin (Adriamycin)

Doxorubicin is a widely used anthracycline but causes marked alopecia and is myelosuppressive. It should always be given as a fast-running infusion as it is very irritant and will cause a necrotic ulcer if injected subcutaneously. Cardiomyopathy results from high cumulative doses unless the total dose is limited to 450 mg/m^2. As it is excreted in bile, an elevated bilirubin is an indication to reduce the dose. Newer anthracycline drugs epirubicin and mitozantrone appear to be as effective as doxorubicin but are much less cardiotoxic (Tables 33.1 and 33.2).

Bleomycin

Bleomycin is commonly included in multidrug regimens. It is not myelotoxic but sometimes causes a febrile reaction. Increased pigmentation of flexures is common. The most important toxic effect is a pulmonary fibrosis, which is dose related and not often seen at a cumulative dose less than 300 mg/m^2.

Taxols

Paclitaxel (Taxol) is the first of the taxanes to be identified and tested. It was first derived from the bark of the Pacific Yew tree, so production was very expensive, but new methods of synthesis from a precursor found in the needles of several species of yew have improved the supply and cost of the drug. It has a unique cytotoxic action, preventing depolymerization of microtubules. It is active in ovarian and breast cancer and in many other tumours (Spencer & Faulds 1994). Hypersensitivity reactions were common until a premedication cocktail of antihistamines, H_2 antagonists and steroids was devised. All patients develop total alopecia. Otherwise nausea and vomiting are mild and peripheral neuropathy is uncommon. On the whole it is very well tolerated. It is now usually given as a 3-hour infusion in a glass bottle through low absorbancy giving sets and filters supplied by Bristol-Myers Squibb, rather than a plastic bag and giving set. When combined with a platinum agent, taxol should be administered first to reduce toxicity and increase synergism. The reverse is the case for combination with Adriamycin.

Docetaxel (Taxotere) is a synthetic molecule with a structure similar to paclitaxel. There is less information about this drug, but at a dose of 100 mg/m^2 it does cause marked skin toxicity and oedema. Neutropenia seems to be more common at this dose than with paclitaxel at 175 mg/m^2, and some patients experience a sensory neuropathy and fatigue. A Japanese study using a dose of 75 mg/m^2 did not report these problems. There is little information on response rates.

Hormones

Progestins such as medroxyprogesterone acetate are used in endometrial cancer. There is little evidence that doses higher than 200 mg twice daily are more effective. Although widely regarded as free of side effects and toxicity, many patients do complain of fluid retention and there is some concern that prolonged use may increase the risk of cardiovascular disease. Tamoxifen, an antioestrogen widely used in breast cancer, may have a role in endometrial cancer (see Ch. 38). Glucocorticoids are often useful as antiemetics and in terminal care.

BIOLOGICAL AGENTS

Biological therapy includes methods of altering the host response to cancer and treatment with natural substances normally produced by the body but synthesized in the laboratory. Such treatment includes the use of vaccines, antibodies, activated lymphocytes or cytokines such as interleukin, interferon or tumour necrosis factor.

Interferons consist of a large family of molecules with similar but diverse and complex actions on the immune system, but with marked side effects which are dose limiting. Different members of the family have been used with varying success in leukaemias and renal cell carcinomas. They have been used in genital warts and cervical intraepithelial neoplasia with limited success. Low response rates have been reported in ovarian cancer. A place has yet to be defined for any of these agents in gynaecological cancer.

ROUTE OF ADMINISTRATION

Most cytotoxic drugs are given orally or intravenously. The intramuscular and intra-arterial routes are sometimes used and drugs are also instilled into the peritoneal or pleural cavities.

Oral chemotherapy

The alkylating agents are among the few drugs well absorbed by the oral route. Administration may be continuous on a daily basis, but is usually intermittent. For example, chlorambucil is often given 10 mg daily for 14 days every 28 days, to allow normal cells to recover.

Systemic chemotherapy

With intravenous and intramuscular administration drugs are normally given at intervals of 1–4 weeks. This pulsed treatment allows the bone marrow to recover and, although some cancer cells will also recover, there is a net loss of cancer cells in every cycle.

Intrapleural and intraperitoneal chemotherapy

Chemotherapy can be given into both the pleural and peritoneal cavities. Bleomycin has been used in this way for recurrent ascites or pleural effusions, but it acts mainly by stimulating an inflammatory reaction and forming adhesions. Tetracycline is equally effective. Cytotoxic drugs given systemically are far more effective at dealing with ascites and do not cause 'pocketing' from adhesions.

Use of the intraperitoneal route has been explored as a way of giving high concentrations of drugs into the peritoneal cavity, which acts as a reservoir, releasing the drugs slowly into the systemic circulation. This results in very high and prolonged local concentrations of drug. However, absorption of cytotoxic drugs directly into tumour nodules is limited as penetration will be only 3–6 cells deep. Some agents are unsuitable because they cause a severe local chemical peritonitis. Cisplatin can be given by this route, but if the dose is too high systemic complications ensue. This technique has yet to establish a place in routine therapy.

SINGLE-AGENT AND COMBINATION CHEMOTHERAPY

Drugs can be used alone or in combination. Combination chemotherapy in conditions such as Hodgkin's disease or germ cell ovarian tumours can be curative and is much more effective than single-agent regimens. However, combination regimens have yet to show clear-cut advantages in epithelial cancers.

The theoretical advantages of combination chemotherapy are:

1. Drugs acting at different cell sites can be combined to give a synergistic effect.
2. The ability of tumour cells to develop resistance to cytotoxic therapy is reduced.
3. Drugs with different toxicities can be combined to avoid the cumulative toxic effects of each individual drug.

SEQUENTIAL THERAPY

An alternative mechanism for preventing the development of drug resistance is to give different drugs in turn. This also allows for a shorter treatment time, as severely myelotoxic drugs can be alternated with those which have no effect on the bone marrow. This approach has been effective in treating germ cell tumours and trophoblastic disease (see Ch. 39) but not epithelial tumours.

DURATION OF THERAPY

The optimum duration of chemotherapy is unknown. A palpable tumour will contain 10^9–10^{12} cells, but even a clinically undetectable mass will still have 10^8 cells, so further chemotherapy is still needed. However, prolonged chemotherapy will cause toxicity. The bone marrow can become hypoplastic and the risk of developing leukaemia or other second cancers is increased. In practice, chemotherapy is usually given for 6–12 months, and there is substantial evidence that five courses of chemotherapy are as effective as eight in advanced ovarian carcinoma.

Rarely, where tumours release a specific tumour marker such as β-human chorionic gonadotrophin in trophoblastic disease marker measurements allow the treatment period to be more accurately defined for each patient. Sufficiently sensitive and specific tumour markers are not yet developed for the common gynaecological tumours.

CALCULATION OF DOSE

To give equivalent dosages to patients the dose of cytotoxic drugs is based on an estimate of the patient's surface area (m^2), calculated from height and weight. When myelotoxicity is encountered the dose is modified to prevent severe leukopenia or thrombocytopenia in subsequent courses. With renal or hepatic impairment doses of drugs excreted by the kidneys or metabolized by the liver are reduced. Carboplatin dosage is often based upon a measurement of renal function (see below).

TOXIC EFFECTS

The tissues affected by toxic effects include bone marrow; injection site; skin, hair and mucosa; gastrointestinal tract; reproductive system; heart; lungs; liver; renal system; and nervous system. A knowledge of these toxic effects is essential for the safe management of cytotoxic chemotherapy. The most common toxicities for each of the commonly used drugs are shown in Table 33.2. Patients in poor general condition will not tolerate intensive chemotherapy and, unless there are very exceptional circumstances, chemotherapy is not given in the presence of infection.

Myelosuppression

Myelosuppression occurs with almost all drugs because of their action on bone marrow stem cells, the exceptions being vincristine and bleomycin. The blood count must be checked regularly and before each course of treatment. Granulocytes have a life span of 4–5 days, leukopenia can appear soon after treatment has been given and, if severe (less than 0.5×10^9/l), can result in infections not only from infective organisms such as *Staphylococcus aureus* but also from opportunistic organisms which normally cause no problems in healthy individuals. Fungal infections also occur. Infections need to be treated aggressively as they can be life-threatening. Additional treatment is sometimes required, including bowel sterilization and granulocyte transfusions. Granulocyte colony-stimulating factors increase the tolerance of bone marrow to chemotherapy, reducing the incidence of secondary infections. The platelet count too can fall soon after treatment. Platelet transfusion may be required if spontaneous bleeding occurs. This is seldom a problem unless the platelet count falls below 25×10^9/l. Anaemia usually occurs only after several courses of chemotherapy because of the long half-life of red blood cells. Blood transfusion may be required.

Prolonged chemotherapy, particularly with alkylating agents such as chlorambucil, is associated with an increased incidence of myelogenous leukaemia. This is dose related.

Alimentary tract toxicity

Nausea and vomiting are common with chemotherapy. Doxorubicin causes moderate vomiting but it is particularly severe with cisplatin. This is principally due to a central nervous system effect. Antiemetic therapy includes steroids, the 5-hydroxytryptamine antagonists, high-dose metoclopramide and other drugs such as the phenothiazines.

Mouth ulcers are particularly common with the antimetabolites methotrexate and 5-fluorouracil. This ulceration can also affect small bowel mucosa, and in extreme cases results in infection leading to septicaemia.

Injection site

Some drugs given intravenously can give rise to phlebitis or thrombosis (e.g. vincristine and doxorubicin). This can be avoided by giving bolus injections into a free-running infusion. If such drugs leak out of the vein they can result in marked morbidity, including large painful ulcers and loss of function.

Skin and hair

Alopecia is a common problem with cyclophosphamide and the antibiotic cytotoxic drugs, in particular doxorubicin. The hair will regrow after chemotherapy is stopped, but a wig is required in the intervening period.

Hyperpigmentation of the skin can occur with treosulfan or bleomycin. At a dose of 100 mg/m^2 docetaxel has a high incidence of skin rashes.

Reproductive system

Chemotherapy may cause infertility, but many young women successfully treated for germ cell tumours have had normal pregnancies. Depending on the drugs given, fertility may return after some years but recovery is rare after procarbazine (used in Hodgkin's disease) and cyclophosphamide. Menstruation may cease permanently in women approaching the menopause, but there is usually only temporary cessation in young women.

Cytotoxic drugs during pregnancy, particularly in the first trimester, can result in abortion or congenital abnormalities. In theory, genetic damage to the fetus or to ova could cause abnormalities in later generations.

Heart

Doxorubicin can cause cardiomyopathy. This results initially in electrocardiogram changes or tachycardia, but can lead to heart failure. The risk is dose related. By keeping the total dose below 450 mg/m^2 and not using it in cases of impaired cardiac function, cardiotoxicity is rarely seen. The newer anthracycline drugs epirubicin and mitozantrone are less cardiotoxic. Cyclophosphamide is cardiotoxic when given in high doses after radiotherapy to the thorax.

Lungs

Bleomycin can cause pulmonary fibrosis and severe respiratory distress. Therefore, chest X-rays and respiratory function tests are essential before treatment. Anaesthesia after bleomycin also carries an increased risk, and anaesthetists need to be aware that the drug has been given in the past.

Liver

Toxic effects to the liver are not common. Methotrexate can cause hepatocellular damage resulting in abnormal liver function tests and very rarely jaundice, so caution must be exercised in patients with impaired hepatic function. Care must also be taken with drugs such as cyclophosphamide which are activated in the liver, or those excreted in the bile, such as doxorubicin.

Renal system

Nephrotoxicity is a serious complication of cisplatin and resulted in fatalities until forced diuresis was found to reduce renal damage. The toxicity is dose related. To avoid serious renal damage the serum creatinine should be measured before every course. If it increases by more than 25% over the pretreatment value, a creatinine or ethylenediaminetetraacetic acid (EDTA) clearance should be performed. If the clearance is less than 60 ml/min the dose should be reduced by 50%. If the clearance is less than 40 ml/min cisplatin should be discontinued. Carboplatin, an analogue of cisplatin, has virtually no renal toxicity.

The effect of metabolites from cyclophosphamide and ifosfamide on bladder mucosa has been mentioned previously.

Nervous system

Neurotoxicity is a common toxic effect with vincristine but is less common with other vinca alkaloids. It causes peripheral neuropathy, which gives tingling initially but loss of sensation and difficulty with walking can occur later. Vincristine can also affect the autonomic nervous system, causing severe constipation. This has been mistaken for a surgical emergency. Cisplatin also causes a dose-dependent peripheral neuropathy and high-tone deafness.

ROLE OF CHEMOTHERAPY

Chemotherapy can be given with either curative or palliative intent. It is the definitive mode of treatment in trophoblastic and germ cell tumours of the ovary, and has a major role in the palliation of recurrent and advanced gynaecological malignancies, particularly of the ovary and cervix.

Adjuvant chemotherapy, given in addition to surgery or radiotherapy, is used in carcinoma of the ovary where disease is known or suspected to be present after surgery, with the intent of prolonging disease-free survival. Neoadjuvant chemotherapy is given prior to definitive surgical or radiation therapy to reduce tumour bulk.

CONCLUSION

The role of chemotherapy in gynaecological cancer is limited. Only the rare trophoblastic and germ cell tumours are cured by drugs. Its use in solid tumours is adjunctive to surgery and radiotherapy, and will remain so unless new drugs with greater activity and tolerable toxicity become available. The drugs in use at present show considerable toxicity and can be life-threatening. They should only be given under specialist supervision.

Probably the most important contribution from chemotherapy is improved quality and duration of survival. This is particularly noticeable in patients with advanced ovarian carcinoma, in whom the median survival has been substantially extended although the 5-year survival figures have improved very little.

KEY POINTS

1. Most radiotherapy is given in the form of electromagnetic radiation, as either X-rays from a linear accelerator or as γ-rays from a radioactive isotope such as cobalt-60, or caesium-117 or iridium-192.
2. Tumour tissue recovers more slowly from radiation damage than does normal tissue, so radiotherapy is usually given in many fractions over weeks to exploit this difference.
3. Teletherapy is used to treat large volumes, and several fields are used with different entry points to the body to reduce the dose to skin and other normal tissues.
4. Intracavitary brachytherapy is used to treat small volumes, as there is a very rapid reduction in the dose of radiotherapy with increasing distance from the source.
5. Brachytherapy may be given at a low dose rate, lasting for several days, or at intermediate or high dose rates lasting for hours or minutes.
6. The main radiation complications following treatment of gynaecological cancers are to the gastrointestinal tract, the bladder and the bone marrow.
7. There are several different alkylating agents, each with a different toxicity spectrum but with similar antitumour activity.
8. Cisplatin has little myelotoxicity but causes severe nausea and vomiting, and can cause nephrotoxicity and peripheral neuropathy. Carboplatin has almost no nephrotoxicity or neurotoxicity but is myelotoxic and particularly prone to causing thrombocytopenia.
9. Although combination chemotherapy is much more effective than single-agent regimens in conditions such as Hodgkin's disease or germ cell ovarian tumours, a clear-cut advantage is not yet apparent in epithelial ovarian cancers.
10. Every cytotoxic agent has a characteristic pattern of toxicity which must be taken into account in its use, particularly in combinations.
11. Cytotoxic drugs should only be prescribed by those with specialized knowledge of their use, as toxicity can be fatal.
12. Chemotherapy can be curative in trophoblastic disease and ovarian germ cell tumours, but may only extend survival in other gynaecological malignancies, such as ovarian carcinoma, where cure rates are disappointing.

REFERENCES AND FURTHER READING

Balkwill F, Kelly S A, Malik S T A 1995 Cytokines. In: Peckham M, Pinedo H, Veronesi U (eds) Oxford textbook of oncology. Oxford, Oxford University Press, pp 103–117

Habeshaw T, Pinion S B 1992 The incidence of persistent functioning endometrial tissue following successful radiotherapy for cervical carcinoma. International Journal of Gynecological Cancer 2: 332–335

Rankin E M, Kaye S B 1990 Principles of chemotherapy. In: Sikora K, Halnan K E (eds) Treatment of cancer, 2nd edn. Chapman & Hall, London, pp 127–146

Spencer C M, Faulds D 1994 Paclitaxel: a review of its pharmacodynamic and pharmacokinetic properties and therapeutic potential in the treatment of cancer. Drugs 48: 794–847

Stewart S, Kam K C 1990 Radiotherapy techniques, planning and equipment. In: Sikora K, Halnan K E (eds) Treatment of cancer, 2nd edn. Chapman & Hall, London, pp 827–852

34

Premalignant disease of the lower genital tract

Pat Soutter

THE CERVIX

Terminology of cervical premalignancy

The terminology used to classify squamous cell lesions on the cervix has changed over the years in an attempt to reflect changing views of their nature (Table 34.1). Scheme 1 represents the original terms in use until Richart (1967) suggested scheme 2, incorporating the term 'cervical intraepithelial neoplasm' (CIN) to indicate the concept of cervical premalignancy as a continuum of change. Later, milder lesions thought to be due to human papilloma virus (HPV) infection were identified. The Bethesda terminology attempts simplification by grouping CIN I with HPV as a lesion with low potential for malignant change. The Bethesda terminology does not have wide support in the UK.

Table 34.1 Different terminologies for squamous cell cervical lesions

Scheme 1	Scheme 2	Bethesda scheme
	HPV changes	Low-grade lesions
Mild dysplasia	CIN I	Low-grade lesions
Moderate dysplasia	CIN II	High-grade lesions
Severe dysplasia	CIN III	High-grade lesions
Carcinoma-in-situ	CIN III	High-grade lesions

HPV = Human papilloma virus; CIN = cervical intraepithelial neoplasia

Adenocarcinoma-in-situ is recognized more frequently than before. It has become relatively more important where screening has reduced the numbers of squamous cancers without affecting the incidence of adenocarcinoma.

Pathology of cervical premalignancy

Cervical intraepithelial neoplasia

The diagnosis of CIN is based upon the architectural and cytological appearances of the cervical epithelium. Architectural features include differentiation, stratification and maturation, terms which are closely related but not synonymous. The proportion of the thickness of the epithelium showing differentiation is a useful feature to be taken into account when deciding the severity of a CIN. It is not the most important criterion, despite the fact that it is one of the easiest to assess. In CIN I (Fig. 34.1) at least the upper half of the epithelium usually shows good differentiation and stratification, whereas in CIN III differentiation may be very slight or even absent (Fig. 34.2).

Nuclear abnormalities are the most important combination of features to be taken into account when assessing CIN. The nuclei are examined using similar criteria to those employed by the cytologist in assessing a cervical smear: nuclear cytoplasmic ratio, hyperchromasia, nuclear pleomorphism and variation in size of nuclei. Both the overall number of mitotic figures and their height in the epithelium are assessed. The more superficially the mitot-

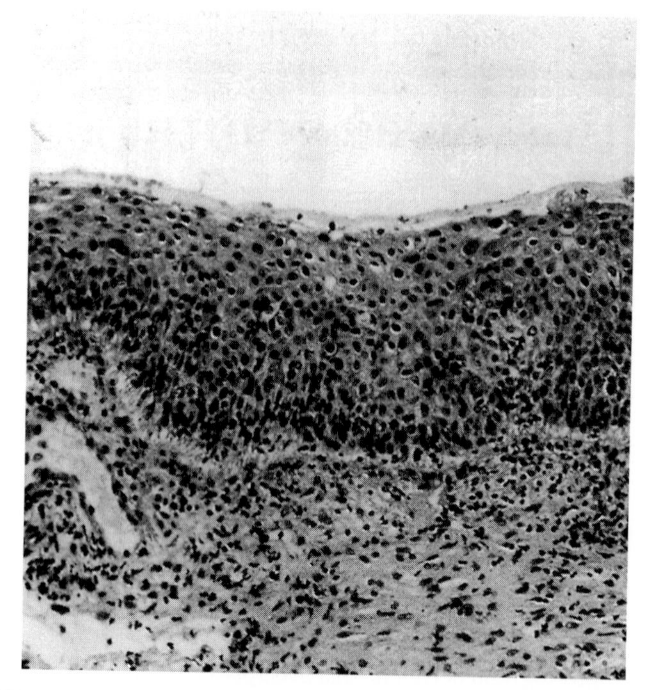

Fig. 34.1 CIN I. Haematoxylin and eosin × 170 (by kind permission of Dr M. C. Anderson).

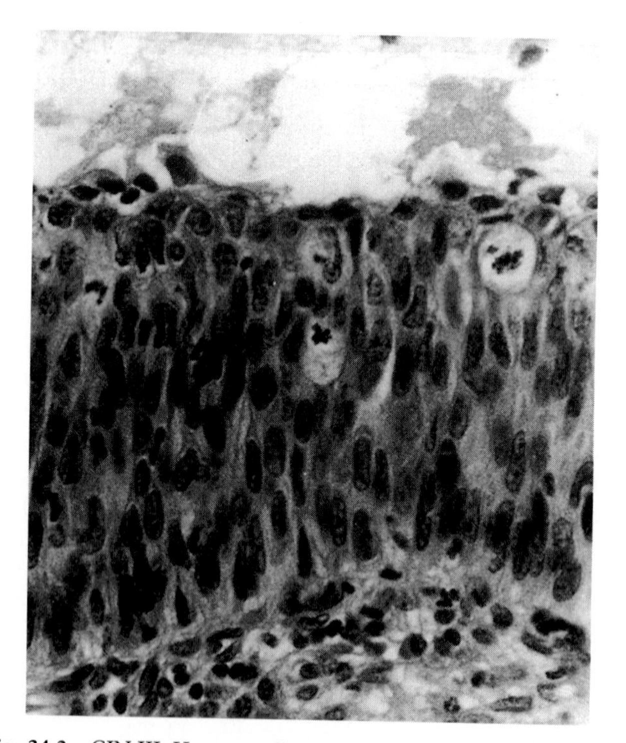

Fig. 34.2 CIN III. Haematoxylin and eosin × 170 (by kind permission of Dr M. C. Anderson).

ic figures are found, the more severe the CIN is likely to be. Abnormal configurations (three-group metaphases and multipolar mitotic figures) are more likely to be found in severe forms of CIN.

CIN may affect the gland crypts as well as the surface epithelium (Fig. 34.3). Anderson and Hartley (1980) showed that the mean depth of crypt involvement in women with CIN III was 1.25 mm and that the mean plus three standard deviations (taking in 99.7% of the population) was 3.8 mm. These figures suggested that treatment to a depth of 5 mm into the stroma would be sufficient to eradicate most CIN; however, practical experience has shown that treatment to 10 mm gives much better results without increasing morbidity (Soutter et al 1986a).

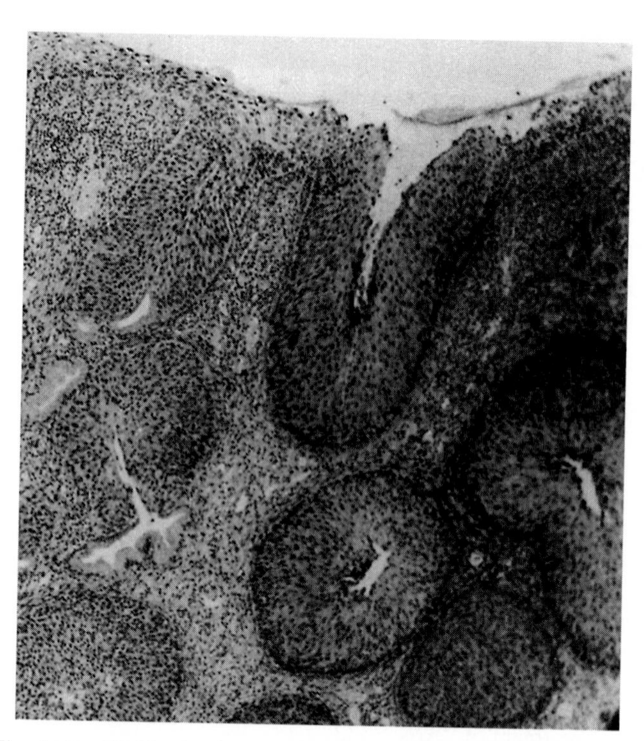

Fig. 34.3 CIN in gland crypts. The morphology of the abnormal epithelium in the involved crypts is similar to that on the surface. Normal columnar epithelium is recognizable in some crypts. Haematoxylin and eosin × 90 (by kind permission of Dr M. C. Anderson).

Adenocarcinoma-in-situ (AIS)

This underdiagnosed lesion is characterized by columnar cells with large hyperchromatic nuclei and prominent nucleoli (Fig. 34.4). The nuclei may be stratified and show abnormal mitotic figures. There is often gland budding and a 'back-to-back' arrangement. In some cases the whole of a gland may be involved, but often the lesion occurs as a sharply demarcated area in the deep portions of the glands. It may be multifocal. Early invasion is said to have occurred when these lesions are seen lying more deeply in the stroma than the normal glands.

The vast majority of women with AIS are detected by abnormal cytology, although in only half of these is an abnormality of the glandular cells recognized. In the remainder, the smear contains a squamous abnormality (Andersen & Arffmann 1989). In two-thirds of cases there is associated CIN or invasive squamous cancer, and it is usually only the squamous lesion which is recognized.

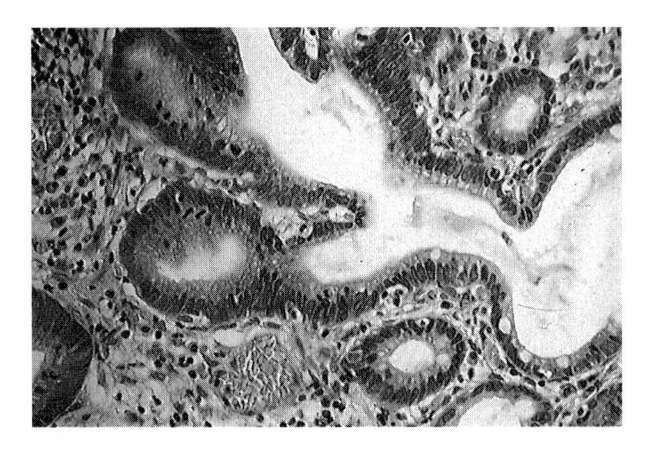

Fig. 34.4 A focal area of AIS showing gland budding, large hyperchromatic nuclei and nuclear stratification (by kind permission of Dr J. Pryse Davies).

There are no specific colposcopic features which identify AIS. It is often not detected until a cone biopsy or hysterectomy is performed.

In the great majority of cases the lesion lies in the transformation zone, close to the squamocolumnar junction (SCJ). Isolated AIS high in the endocervical canal some distance from the SCJ is rare. It follows that a cone biopsy with a good margin of excision in the endocervical canal will be adequate treatment for most cases of AIS.

Diagnostic precision

The histological diagnosis of these lesions is based largely upon subjective criteria. It is not surprising to find substantial inter- and intraobserver variation in the grading of CIN and the identification of AIS (Robertson et al 1989). Although the variation is greatest at the mild end of the spectrum, there is still a considerable amount of disagreement over severe lesions.

The scope for disagreement is inevitably increased when comparing two samples from the same lesion. In a study performed at Hammersmith Hospital, London, there were substantial differences between the colposcopically directed punch biopsy diagnosis and that based on a laser cone biopsy (Skehan et al 1990). This relative imprecision of histological grading of CIN makes it virtually impossible invariably to distinguish by punch biopsy a woman with CIN I from one with CIN III. This should be borne in mind when considering any discussion of the natural history of different grades of CIN and different treatment policies.

Malignant potential of CIN

Progression from CIN III to invasion

The malignant potential of CIN III is amply demonstrated by McIndoe et al (1984) in a crucial paper. A group of 131 patients who had been treated for CIN III and who continued to produce abnormal cytology for more than 2 years after the initial treatment were followed for 4–24 years. After 20 years' follow-up, 36% of these women had developed invasive disease. There was no evidence that the rate of conversion to invasive disease was slowing towards the end of this period.

Progression from CIN I to CIN III or invasion

Studies of progression from CIN I to CIN III are blighted by the difficulty in accurately determining the grade of the initial lesion. Those reports that relied upon cytology only to determine the initial diagnosis and to document progression or regression are invalidated by the poor correlation between the grade of cytologic abnormality and that of the histology (Soutter et al 1986b). Basing the diagnosis of CIN I upon a colposcopic assessment without punch biopsy, progression to CIN III was observed in 26% of women within 2 years (Campion et al 1986).

Which lesions to treat?

Given the clear malignant potential of untreated CIN III, the difficulty in identifying CIN I accurately and the high progression rate in women whose CIN I was not treated, it seems to be prudent to treat all women with CIN regardless of the grade of abnormality. There is no justification for treating subclinical HPV lesions.

Screening for cervical premalignancy

The objective of cervical screening is to reduce the incidence and the mortality from cervical cancer. When the screening programme detects early invasive disease it can be said to have been only partly successful, since the treatment of these early lesions carries a substantial morbidity, is not universally successful and is expensive. The objectives of cervical screening can only be achieved by detecting cervical premalignancy.

Cervical cytology

Cervical cytology is the only well established screening method. When a properly organized programme is implemented, substantial reductions in both incidence and mortality from cervical cancer are achieved (Anderson et al 1988). The vital elements of a successful programme are obtaining wide cover of the population at risk and taking effective action when a cytological abnormality is discovered.

To achieve wide cover, the confidence of the target population must be won. They must know about the programme, what it aims to achieve and how, and they must be convinced that the programme will be successful. If the quality of a cytology service is high, 3-yearly smears are virtually as effective as annual smears (IARC Working

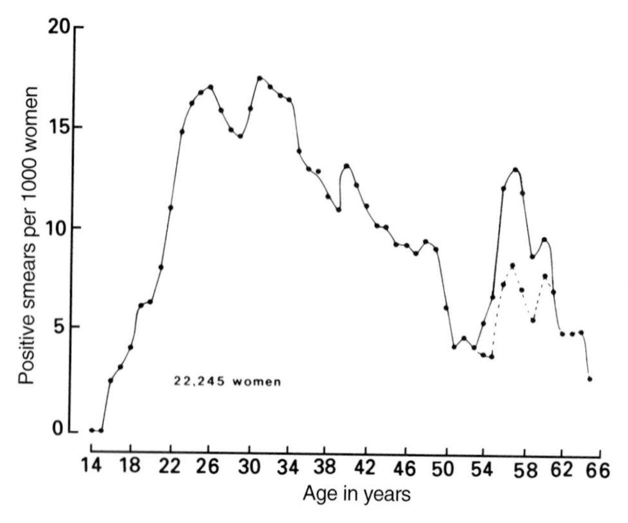

Fig. 34.5 Positive smears per 1000 women examined compared with age, plotted as a 3-year moving average, Queen Elizabeth Hospital, Gateshead, 1983. The second peak among the older women is due to smears being taken from women with symptoms and signs of malignancy. The dashed line corrects for this. (From Soutter et al 1984, with permission.)

Group 1986). In the UK the proportion of a screened population with positive smears (moderate–severe dyskaryosis) is highest in women aged 25–35 years (Fig. 34.5). A rational programme would therefore recommend 3-yearly smears for all at-risk women between 20 and 60 years of age. Indeed, the falling rate of positive smears in women over 50 years and data from Dundee (Wijngaarden & Duncan 1993) and Aberdeen suggest that screening might be stopped safely at 50 years of age in well-screened women.

In spite of the success achieved by cervical cytology, it is not without its shortcomings. A satisfactory sample must include cells from the relevant part of the cervix. The cytologist must scan the whole slide carefully to detect one of what may be a small number of abnormal cells. The assessment and definition of cytologic abnormality are subjective, with considerable interobserver variation. The process is laborious and tiring, and there is considerable scope for operator error, especially when the workload is high. Furthermore, cytology screening has little effect on the incidence of adenocarcinoma of the cervix (Nieminen et al 1995).

The imprecision of cervical cytology is evident from the many studies that report CIN II–III or invasive disease in about 50% of women with smears showing only mild dyskaryosis (Soutter et al 1986b, Flannelly et al 1994). The high risk associated with a mildly dyskaryotic smear is further illustrated by an annual incidence of invasive cancer of 208 per 100 000 women in patients with mild dyskaryosis followed up cytologically (Soutter & Fletcher 1994). This should be compared with the annual incidence of cervical cancer of 9 per 100 000 in UK women of a similar age.

There have been few satisfactory investigations of the accuracy of cervical cytology. Although false negative rates from 2.4 to 26% have been estimated by a variety of different types of study, there have been few in which a large asymptomatic population has been screened by cytology and the results corroborated by an alternative test such as colposcopy. In a study of this sort which enrolled over 400 women, the sensitivity of cytology was low (0.52) but the specificity high (0.94) (Kesic et al 1993). There is clearly scope for a more accurate and less labour-intensive screening method.

Cervicography

Cervicography is a method of detecting cervical pathology which uses the same principles as colposcopy. The cervix is visualized, 5% acetic acid is applied and, after allowing 1 minute for the effect of the acetic acid to become apparent, two photographs are taken of the cervix using a specially designed camera (Fig. 34.6). The film is developed as 35 mm slides and these are projected and interpreted by an experienced reviewer. Slides from between 30 and 50 patients can be reported on in an hour. The sensitivity of this method is high (89%) (Kesic et al 1993) but initial reports suggested low specificity. With increased experience and minor modifications to the reporting technique the specificity is now more satisfactory (92%) (Kesic et al 1993). This promising technique might be taken up first in countries which have no established cervical cytology service, or where it can be added to an established cytology screening programme either as an additional primary method or as a secondary screen of women with equivocal cytology.

Other new methods

HPV testing has been utilized as an adjunct to cytology screening but 5–15% of women, depending on their age,

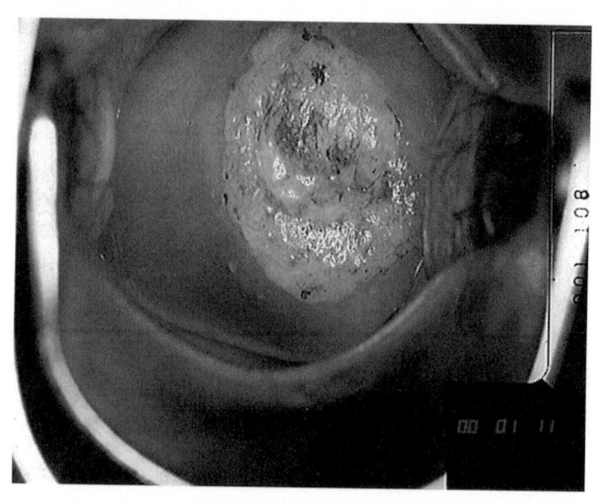

Fig. 34.6 Cervigram showing CIN III. A strongly staining acetowhite lesion with well demarcated, regular edges is seen.

have evidence of HPV infection using sensitive techniques. An alternative is to use a semiquantitative method which excludes those women with low copy numbers of HPV. A study of this technique in primary screening of a family planning clinic population showed a doubling in the sensitivity of the test for CIN II–III to 89–96% at the cost of a 5% false positive rate (Cuzick et al 1995). The false positive rate in the first round of screening may fall in subsequent rounds, and the very high sensitivity may mean that screening could safely be performed less frequently.

A number of innovative methods of identifying abnormal cells by computer image analysis are under investigation. One of these, the Papnet, was applied in screening 35 876 randomly chosen samples while the remaining 41 134 samples were screened by hand (Boon et al 1995). A histological diagnosis was obtained from all women with abnormal tests. CIN III was detected in 111 (0.31%) and 101 (0.24%) cases (NS) and invasive carcinoma in 24 (0.067%) and 13 (0.031%) ($P < 0.05$) women by Papnet and conventional screening respectively. The curiously termed 'accuracy rates' were also said to be superior for the Papnet system. No data were presented for the more difficult area of mild abnormalities, so it is possible that the marginal improvement in detection rates was obtained at the cost of higher referral rates. Depite showing promise, the results of using this system require much fuller analysis.

Colposcopy of the cervix

The basis of colposcopy

Eversion of the cervix. At puberty, during pregnancy or when the combined oral contraceptive pill is taken, the cervix enlarges. As it does so there is a tendency to eversion and to the exposure of columnar epithelium on the ectocervix (Fig. 34.7). The thin columnar epithelium appears red and the result is what is so often erroneously referred to as a 'cervical erosion'.

Squamous metaplasia. The columnar epithelium on the ectocervix is gradually replaced by a process of squamous metaplasia, spreading from the SCJ towards the cervical canal. The normal end result of this transformation is the replacement of the ectopic columnar epithelium with mature squamous epithelium (Fig. 34.7c). If squamous epithelium now covers the entrance to a cervical crypt and the columnar cells continue to secrete mucus in the crypt, a nabothian follicle results. This is the only clinical evidence of the prior existence of columnar epithelium in that area. When the cervix shrinks in the months and years following pregnancy and after the menopause, it gradually inverts, drawing the new SCJ up the endocervical canal (Fig. 34.7d).

The transformation zone. The region of the cervix in which this process of metaplasia occurs is called the transformation zone. In some women, the transformation zone may extend on to the vaginal walls. A common source of confusion in colposcopy is the loose use of the term 'transformation zone' when referring to that part of the true transformation zone where metaplastic or dysplastic epithelium can be seen colposcopically.

The genesis of squamous cervical neoplasia. Squamous neoplasia results from a disruption of the normal metaplastic process. Thus, CIN develops as a confluent lesion confined to an area of the cervix contiguous with the SCJ. It is this characteristic localization which enables the colposcope to be used in the assessment of CIN.

Referral for colposcopy

Prior to the advent of colposcopy cytologists recommended referral to a gynaecologist only after two successive severely dyskaryotic smears were obtained. The reason for this delaying policy was because a knife cone biopsy would

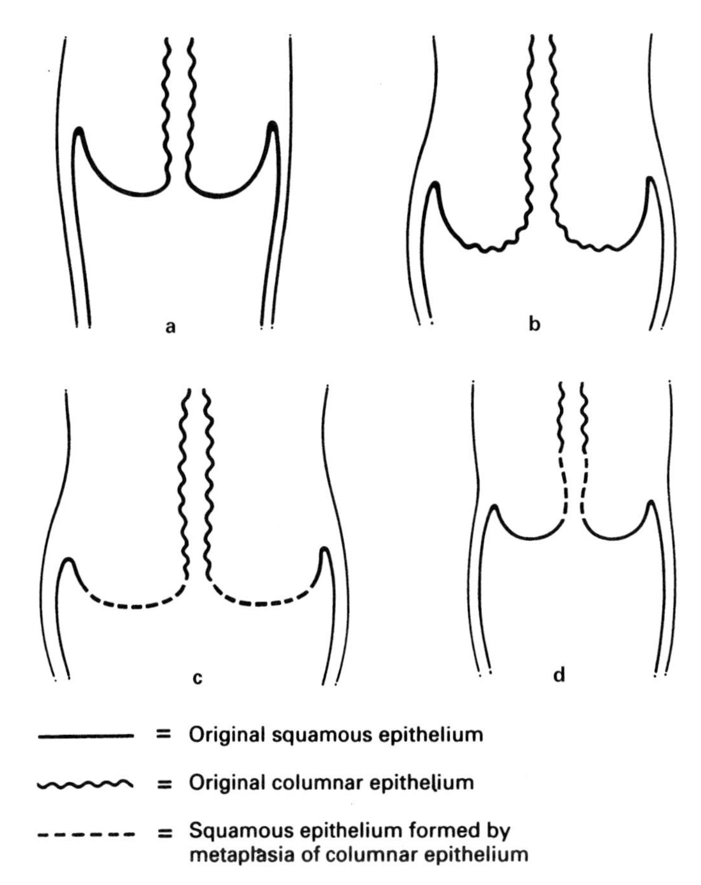

Fig. 34.7 The different stages in the development and involution of the cervix. (**a**) Before puberty the ectocervix is covered with squamous epithelium and columnar epithelium is usually confined to the endocervical canal. (**b**) The cervix enlarges and everts when oestrogen levels rise. This exposes columnar epithelium on the ectocervix. (**c**) The columnar epithelium on the ectocervix is replaced with squamous epithelium by a process of metaplasia. (**d**) Following the climacteric, when oestrogen levels fall, the cervix shrinks, drawing the squamocolumnar junction up the canal.

Table 34.2 Management of abnormal cervical cytology. This differs from the guidelines issued by the National Coordinating Network in 1993, in which a repeat smear was recommended for women with mild dyskaryosis. That was a controversial decision at the time and the results of subsequent studies have all supported immediate colposcopy.

Papanicolaou class		Histology	Action
I	Normal	0.1% CIN II–III	Repeat 3 years (unless clinical suspicion)
II	Inflammatory	6% CIN II–III	Repeat in 6 months (colposcopy after 3 abnormal)
	Borderline nuclear changes	20–37% CIN II–III	Repeat in 6 months (colposcopy after 2 abnormal)
III	Mild dyskaryosis	50% CIN II–III	Colposcopy
	Moderate dyskaryosis	50–75% CIN II–III	Colposcopy
IV	Severe dyskaryosis 'Positive' 'Malignant cells'	80–90% CIN II–III 5% Invasion	Colposcopy
V	Invasion suspected	50% Invasion	Urgent colposcopy
Abnormal glandular cells		? Adenocarcinoma of the cervix or endometrium	Urgent colpocospy

be required to determine whether or not there was a premalignant lesion on the cervix, and this operation had potentially serious consequences for the future obstetric prospects of the young women in whom these abnormalities were most often found.

That conservative policy is no longer justifiable. With colposcopy, the women who require treatment can be identified and those who do not can be reassured. In addition, the treatment can be carefully tailored to remove only the minimum of cervical tissue. Most women with CIN can be treated in the outpatient clinic with methods that do not prejudice their future fecundity. With the recognition that mild cytological abnormalities are associated with a high prevalence of significant histological abnormalities, it is apparent that the indications for referral need to be revised (Table 34.2). Nowadays, no woman with abnormal cytology should be treated without prior colposcopy.

Although the majority of women sent for colposcopy have abnormal smears, a suspicious-looking cervix is sufficient reason for referral even if the smear is negative. Such women sometimes have invasive cancer. Similarly, worrying symptoms such as postcoital bleeding should always be investigated by colposcopy, even if the smear is normal. Cervical cancer is found very occasionally in women with postmenopausal bleeding.

The colposcopic method

A detailed description of the author's personal method may be found elsewhere (Soutter 1993). Space permits only an outline description here.

Bimanual examination and the smear. A bimanual examination is essential to aid detection of frank invasive disease of the cervix, a uterine or an ovarian mass. A bivalve speculum is then introduced and a smear is taken. Deferring the smear until after the colposcopic inspection may reduce the risk of removing the epithelium one wishes to study (see below), but unfortunately it provides a less satisfactory sample for the cytologist (Griffiths et al 1989). Only if the os is narrowed or the SCJ out of sight up the canal is an endocervical brush used.

Preacetic acid examination. If the view of the cervix is obscured by a discharge this should be removed gently with saline. The preliminary inspection should include both the cervix and the upper vagina. At this stage of the examination there are three objectives: to identify leukoplakia; to exclude obvious evidence of invasive disease; and to identify viral condylomata.

Leukoplakia must be identified prior to the application of acetic acid, after which it may be impossible to differentiate from acetowhite epithelium. Because the hyperkeratinization of leukoplakia may conceal invasive disease, biopsy is mandatory.

Invasion is often obvious from the bizarre appearances of the surface of the cervix, which may appear grossly irregular, either raised or ulcerated (Fig. 34.8). This disorganization of the surface is usually recognizable even when atypical vessels cannot be identified or the area subsequently fails to turn white after the application of acetic acid. The atypical vessels seen on invasive lesions run a bizarre course and are often corkscrew- or comma-shaped (Fig. 34.9). They are large in diameter, abruptly appearing on and disappearing from the surface. They do not branch dichotomously like normal vessels.

Condylomata are usually obvious from their regular frond-like surface (Fig. 34.10), but biopsies should be taken, especially when they are located within the active part of the transformation zone where it is more difficult to be sure of their benign nature.

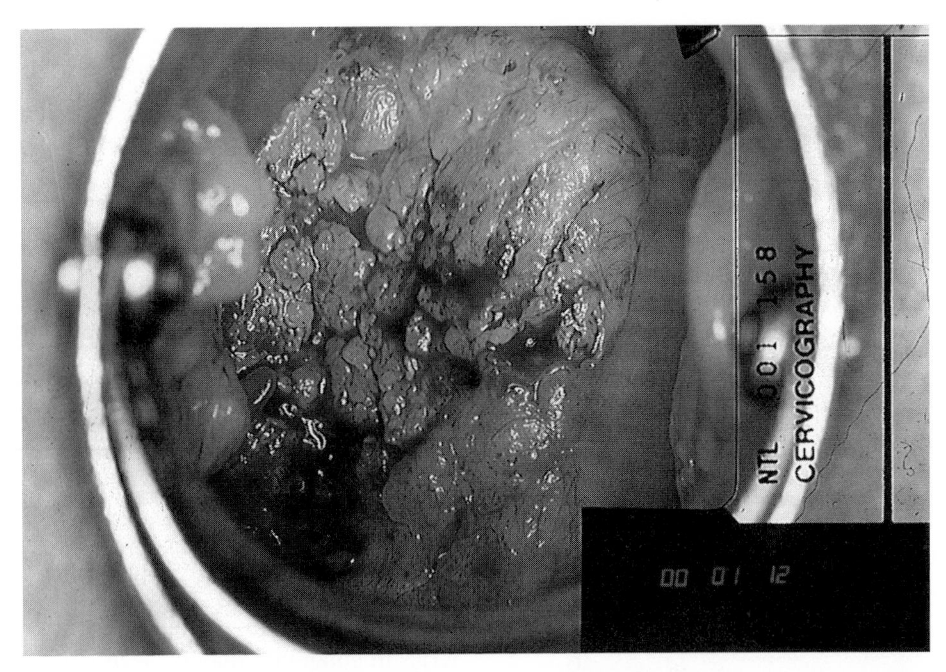

Fig. 34.8 A cervigram of a stage Ib cervical cancer showing the irregular surface.

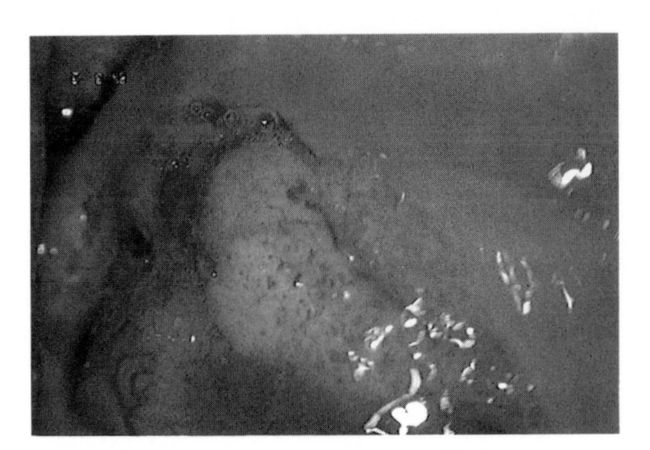

Fig. 34.9 This high-power view of a cervical tumour shows some short atypical vessels in the lower centre of the picture and longer stretches of atypical vessels above this area. Note also the irregular surface.

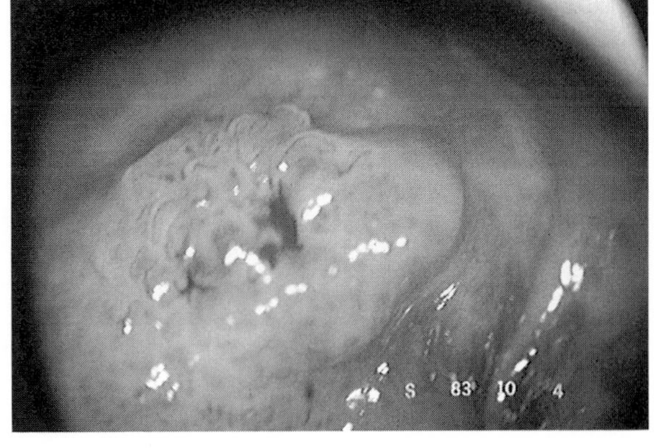

Fig. 34.10 A high-power view of a large cervical condyloma prior to the application of acetic acid. Note the regular form and the microvilli with looped capillaries on the top of the condyloma.

Acetic acid examination

A low-power inspection. Having completed the first inspection of the cervix, 5% acetic acid should be applied liberally and gently. This turns abnormal epithelium white, producing the so-called 'acetowhite' changes of CIN. It is important to allow sufficient time to elapse for faintly staining areas to show up. While waiting for any colour changes to occur, the cervix and vaginal fornices are inspected under low power in order to have the widest field of view possible, so that areas of faint acetowhite may be observed against the contrasting background of normal epithelium. After about 30 seconds it is usually possible to proceed. If a lesion has become visible, its outer limits should be determined first.

Identifying the SCJ. Next, the position of the SCJ must be ascertained to define the upper limits of the abnormality. Failure to identify the SCJ correctly is one of the main pitfalls in colposcopy. It is important to note that the SCJ is marked by the lower limit of normal columnar epithelium, not the upper limit of squamous, as these do not always lie at the same level. The higher the SCJ appears to lie in the canal the more difficult it becomes to assess the lesion accurately and, except when the cervix is very patulous, 5 mm represents the limit above which colposcopic evaluation becomes unsafe.

Determining the nature of the lesion. It is necessary only to decide whether or not a lesion with malignant potential is indeed present, and whether invasion may have already occurred. It is preferable to adopt a very conservative approach to the latter objective and to regard

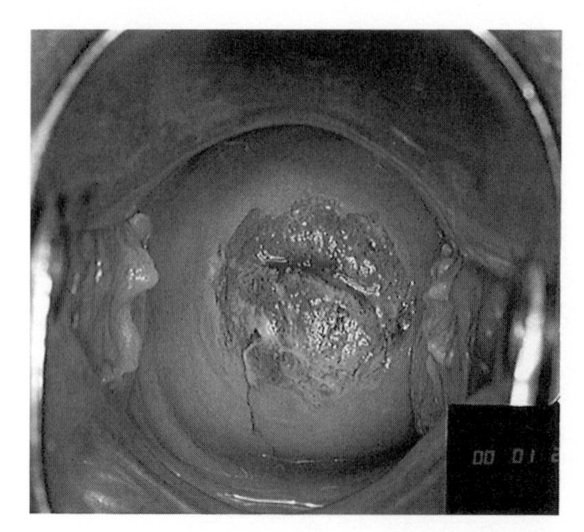

Fig. 34.11 A cervigram of a normal cervix with a large ectropion. The central portion of the cervix around the os is covered with normal columnar epithelium.

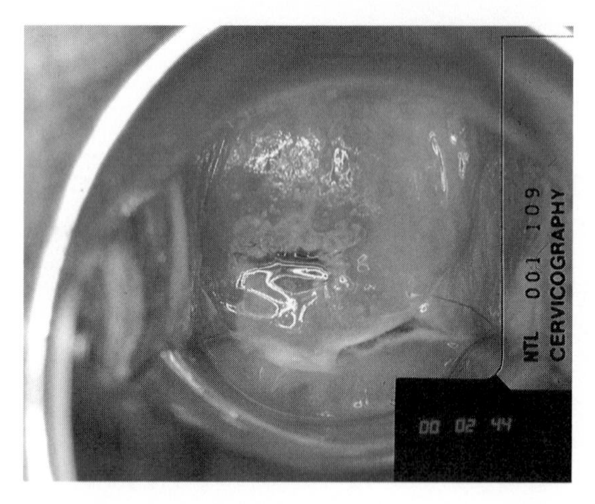

Fig. 34.12 This cervigram shows an area of faintly acetowhite epithelium around the cervical os; however, it is seen most clearly on the anterior lip in this photograph.

cases of severe CIN III as being potentially invasive. When determining the significance of a lesion the colposcopist assesses the colour, the margins and the vascular markings.

Non-malignant epithelium that becomes acetowhite. Not all areas of acetowhite change are abnormal. Columnar epithelium will blanch briefly after exposure to acetic acid. It may be identified by its villous or furrowed surface (Fig. 34.11). Squamous metaplasia has a glassy white appearance but can be hard to distinguish from CIN I (Fig. 34.12). After any form of treatment the cervix may develop areas of acetowhite, subepithelial fibrosis. This can be recognized by the radial arrangement of lines of fine punctation.

Wart virus lesions. Considering the difficulties the histopathologist has in differentiating CIN from wart virus lesions it is no surprise that flat viral lesions are difficult to identify with certainty colposcopically. In general they have faint, very irregular margins and isolated satellite

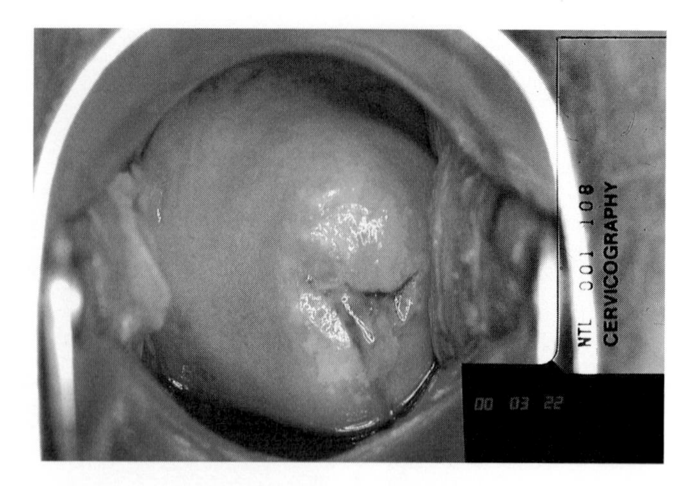

Fig. 34.13 A large, faintly acetowhite lesion with an irregular edge is visible on both lips of the cervix. Two satellite lesions are visible on the posterior lip at 6 o'clock below the main lesion.

lesions (Fig. 34.13). In early condylomata, looped capillaries in small villi may be seen (Fig. 34.10). The delicate fronds of fully formed condylomata are usually easy to identify, but all raised lesions on the active transformation zone must be biopsied lest they be invasive cancer.

Features of CIN. CIN are usually distinct acetowhite lesions with clear margins (see Fig. 34.6). They often show a mosaic vascular pattern, with patches of acetowhite separated by vessels like red weeds between white flagstones. Where the vessels run perpendicular to the surface, punctation is seen as the vessels are viewed end-on. This appears as red spots on a white background. In general, the more quickly and strongly the acetowhite changes develop, the clearer and more regular the margins of the lesion, and the more pronounced the mosaic or punctation, the more severe is the lesion likely to be. However, not all features will be equally marked and many CIN III lesions show only a strong matt-white colour.

Features of invasion. Frank early invasion is often obvious before acetic acid is applied (see above), but microinvasion may not become apparent until after the application of the acid. Although atypical vessels may be seen, the only indication of invasion is often a very marked mosaic pattern or coarse punctation – large-diameter, widely separated red spots (Fig. 34.14).

Because even expert colposcopists will fail to identify correctly every case of early invasion (Bekassy et al 1983), excisional treatment which removes the whole lesion for histological assessment merits wide use to avoid the risk of undertreating invasive disease.

Pitfalls in colposcopy

The first pitfall – the false SCJ caused by an abrasion. The SCJ should be identified by observing the lower limit of normal columnar epithelium, not the upper limit

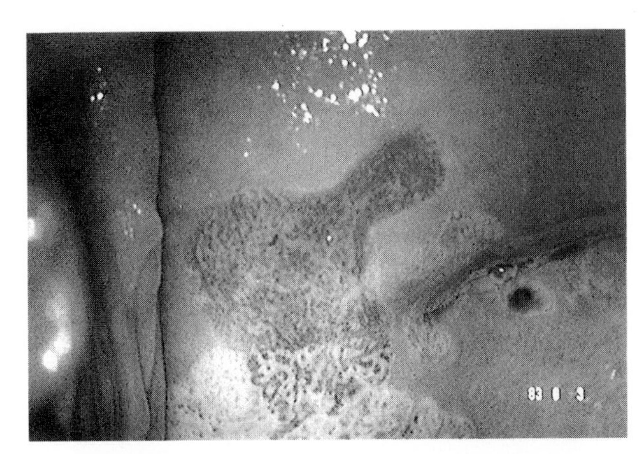

Fig. 34.14 This microinvasive lesion is a good example of coarse punctation.

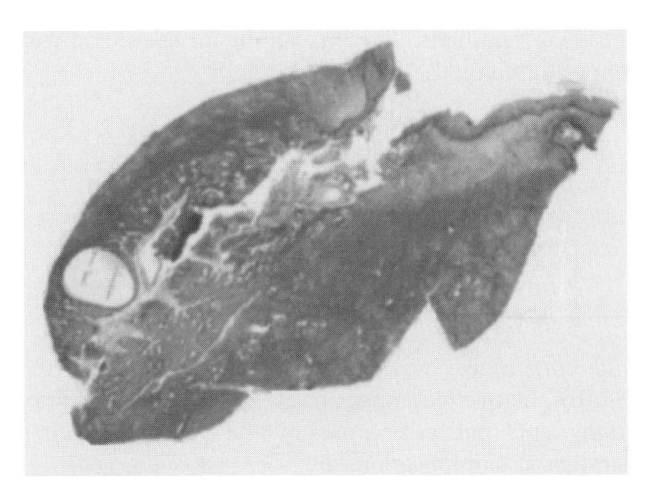

Fig. 34.15 An iatrogenic skip lesion can be seen in this cone biopsy performed in spite of a normal, satisfactory colposcopy because of severe dyskaryosis in a woman who had previously been treated with cervical electrodiathermy. The ectocervical end of this cone biopsy, to the top and right, is covered with normal squamous epithelium. The SCJ is near the external os and the lower canal is lined by columnar epithelium, but halfway up the canal, near the nabothian cyst on the left, is an isolated area of CIN III. In deeper sections this was shown to be an invasive tumour.

of squamous. The reason for this is the ease with which CIN and metaplastic epithelium can be detached from the underlying stroma, particularly at the SCJ, where the unwary may mistakenly regard the upper limit of acetowhite change as being synonymous with the SCJ. Careful inspection of the red epithelium at this junction will reveal a flat surface covered by spidery and often whorled blood vessels characteristic of exposed stroma. This can be distinguished from columnar epithelium, which has a soft, velvety-looking surface and blanches briefly when exposed to acetic acid.

The second pitfall – the SCJ in the canal. When the SCJ lies within the endocervical canal, if the upper part of the lesion is inspected from too acute an angle the assessment of both the length of the endocervical canal involved with CIN and the severity of the lesion becomes unreliable.

The third pitfall – the previously treated cervix. When a cervix has been treated previously for any reason, the topography of the transformation zone will have been altered. Areas of metaplasia, CIN or invasive disease in the canal or in cervical glands may have escaped destruction and may persist as isolated iatrogenic skip lesions surrounded by columnar epithelium, or covered by new squamous epithelium (Fig. 34.15). Such patients should always be treated by an excisional method.

The fourth pitfall – glandular lesions. It cannot be assumed that the rules of colposcopy apply to women with adenocarcinoma or AIS. AIS cannot be identified colposcopically, so a cone biopsy is an essential investigation in the management of a patient with abnormal glandular cells in her smear. Many of these patients also have CIN, which requires treatment in its own right. A cone biopsy which completely excises AIS is probably adequate therapy.

Treatment of CIN and AIS

Detailed descriptions of the techniques discussed may be found elsewhere (Soutter 1993). CIN was originally treated by radical hysterectomy, but it soon became evident that this was unnecessary and simple hysterectomy became the method of choice. In time, it was realized that cone biopsy was just as effective and now hysterectomy is reserved for those with difficult-to-treat recurrent disease or who have additional indications for hysterectomy. The introduction of colposcopy and a better appreciation of the limited location of CIN led to the introduction of more conservative methods of treatment.

Ablative methods

A large number of ablative methods are available (Table 34.3). The chief advantage of these (with the exception of radical electrodiathermy) is that general anaesthesia is not required. Cryotherapy is the one method most often associated with unsatisfactory results, but this has usually been due to inappropriate case selection. A disadvantage common to all these techniques is that they depend heavily upon the exclusion of invasion by colposcopy and directed biopsy. In addition, they are not applicable to all patients – some will always require an

Table 34.3 Methods of ablative treatment of CIN: in chronological order, with the longest established methods first

Method	Anaesthesia	Restrictions
Radical electrodiathermy	GA	Vaginal extension of CIN?
Cryotherapy	None	CIN III; large lesions
Laser vaporization	LA	None
'Cold' coagulation	None	Vaginal extension of CIN

GA = general anaesthesia; LA = local anaesthesia

excisional treatment. The indications for excisional treatment of CIN are:

1. any suspicion of invasive disease;
2. any suspicion of a glandular abnormality;
3. SCJ not clearly visible;
4. history of any previous cervical surgery;
5. elective method of treating any case of CIN?

Excisional methods

Knife cone biopsy was supplanted as the standard treatment by ablative techniques partly because of the complications and partly because of the need for general anaesthesia. Complications are:

1. intraoperative haemorrhage;
2. secondary haemorrhage;
3. pelvic infection;
4. cervical stenosis;
5. cervical incompetence.

The complications of laser cone biopsy are fewer than those of knife cone biopsy, the technique is far more precise (Larsson et al 1983) and the distortion of the cervix that results is much less, suggesting that there will be fewer problems in any subsequent pregnancies. In addition, laser cone biopsy can very often be performed under local anaesthesia (Partington et al 1987).

The ability to perform laser cone biopsy under local anaesthesia, the observation that the complications were no greater than in laser vaporization (Partington et al 1989) and anxieties about invasive cancer being missed led to a widening of the indications for excisional therapy and to the suggestion that laser excision should replace vaporization for most patients. The advent of large loop electrodiathermy excision of the transformation zone (LLETZ) made excisional treatment quicker and reduced the capital cost of the equipment required (Prendiville et al 1989). This technique employs a blended diathermy current and a loop of very thin stainless-steel wire (Figs 34.16 and 34.17). It has become the most widely used treatment for CIN in the UK, but the recurrent costs are much higher than for the laser.

Choice of technique

None of the different methods of treating CIN is more effective than any of the others when used appropriately by a well trained and experienced operator. Each has particular advantages of cost, ease of use, speed or precision. The particular method chosen will depend upon local circumstances. It seems sensible to the author to choose a method which will allow abnormalities to be excised under local anaesthesia. In spite of its greater capital cost, the laser does have the advantage that it may be used both to excise and to vaporize lesions when it is appropriate to do so. An example of the latter are large lesions which extend on to the sides of the cervix or beyond the cervix into the fornices.

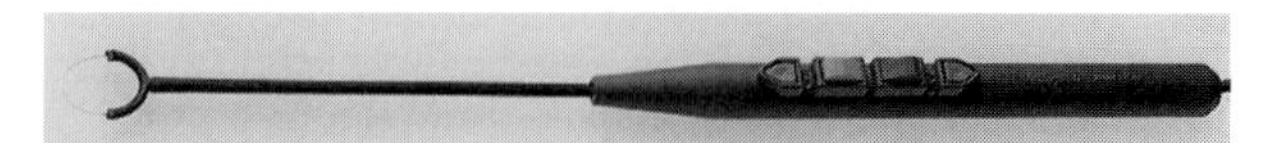

Fig. 34.16 One of the varieties of large wire loops used for LLETZ. (Figure supplied by Valleylab UK.)

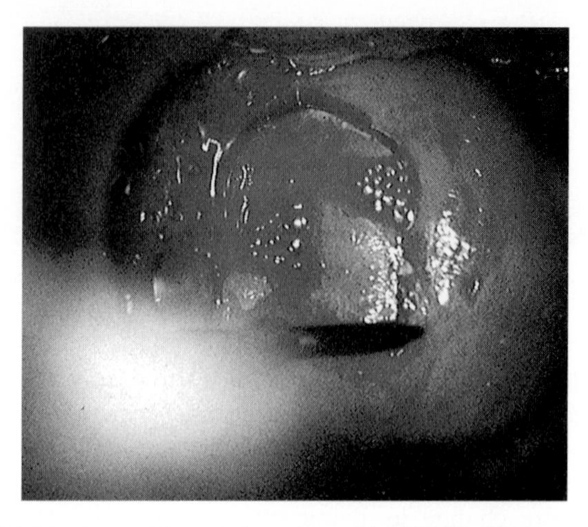

Fig. 34.17 A cone biopsy being taken with LLETZ. (Figure supplied by Valleylab UK.)

Treatment of adenocarcinoma-in-situ (AIS)

For most women with adenocarcinoma-in-situ (AIS), a cone biopsy with free margins is adequate treatment (Cullimore et al 1992). However, LLETZ is associated with a very much higher recurrence rate than knife cone biopsy and should probably not be used knowingly in a case of AIS (Widrich et al 1996). These problems with LLETZ in the treatment of AIS are probably due to removing too little of the endocervical canal. This problem does not occur with laser.

See and treat

'See and treat' means different things to different people. To some it means offering treatment at the first visit to women who meet certain criteria, including the colposcopy findings at that visit. To others it means treating all women referred to the clinic with certain cytological abnormalities, regardless of the colposcopy findings.

There are advantages to the hospital and to the women themselves in that an abnormality can be dealt with in one visit. The disadvantage is the extent of overtreatment that will result, depending on the criteria that are used to select women for immediate treatment (Brady et al 1994). Because the referral population differs greatly between clinics, it is not possible to define a set of rules that would be suitable for all clinics. Each centre must audit its own data and adjust its criteria accordingly. Unfortunately, cytology, colposcopy and histopathology are all subjective and prone to observer error, so that not even a pretreatment punch biopsy can be relied upon to identify accurately those who do not require treatment (Skehan et al 1990).

My own practice remains one of selective treatment, based upon the referral cytology, my colposcopic impression, a selective punch biopsy from lesions I am unsure about, and the result of the smear which I have taken in the clinic. To these factors I add the patient's age, being less conservative in older women, and the patient's own viewpoint: is she particularly anxious to be treated or would she prefer a more conservative approach if it is warranted? Provided I can see the SCJ clearly and the cytological abnormality is not glandular, I would rarely treat in the absence of a colposcopic abnormality. The only common exception would be a woman with a persistent moderate or severe dyskaryosis, especially if she had been treated before (Soutter 1993).

Results of treatment

Treated adequately, some 5% of patients treated for CIN will have recurrent disease within 2 years (Soutter et al 1986a, Paraskevaidis et al 1991). Thereafter, the number of recurrences is small. However, long-term follow-up is necessary as these women remain at a higher risk of CIN or invasive cervical cancer than the general population (Burghardt & Holzer 1980). In that study, the prevalence of invasive cancer in 1219 women treated by cone biopsy after colposcopic assessment was 574 per 100 000 during a follow-up of 4–20 years. All of the cancers were detected within 11 years. A further 2.21% were found to have recurrent CIN, but the authors did not specify how long after the initial treatment these were discovered. In addition, recurrent vaginal intraepithelial neoplasia (VAIN) was found in 3.8% of the 183 women in the 11 years after hysterectomy following incomplete excision by cone biopsy. All but one of these was treated with radiotherapy. A study combining the experience of four UK centres provided data on 36 435 woman-years of follow-up, with 896 women still under observation in the eighth year (Soutter et al unpublished). The cumulative rate of invasion after 8 years was 0.76% and the annual incidence of invasive cancer during this period was 85 per 100 000 women. The rates for women treated for CIN III were 1.31% and 142 per 100 000 women, respectively. Although most of the cancers were diagnosed in the first 5 years following treatment, because fewer women had been followed for longer than that, the risk of developing a cancer remained broadly similar throughout the 8 years. In the light of the results of this and other similar studies, annual cytological follow-up of patients treated for CIN by any method would seem to be prudent for at least 10 years.

THE VAGINA

Terminology and pathology of VAIN

The terminology and pathology of vaginal intraepithelial neoplasia (VAIN) is analogous to that of CIN (VAIN I–III). The main difference is that vaginal epithelium does not normally have crypts, so the epithelial abnormality remains superficial until invasion occurs. The common exception to this is found following surgery – usually hysterectomy – when abnormal epithelium can be buried below the suture line or in suture tracks.

Natural history of VAIN

VAIN is seldom seen as an isolated vaginal lesion. It is more usual for it to be a vaginal extension of CIN. In most cases it is diagnosed colposcopically prior to any treatment during the investigation of an abnormal smear. However, it may not be recognized until after a hysterectomy has been performed. When this happens, abnormal epithelium is likely to be buried behind the sutures used to close the vault. Consequently, a portion of the lesion will remain invisible and unevaluable (Fig. 34.18). In the series reported by Ireland and Monaghan (1988), 28% of those treated surgically proved to have unexpected invasive disease. Untreated or inadequately treated VAIN may progress to frank invasive cancer (Woodman et al 1984). Very rarely, VAIN may be seen many years after radiotherapy for cervical carcinoma, when it is probably a new lesion. Care must be taken in these women to ensure that postradiotherapy changes are not being misinterpreted as VAIN.

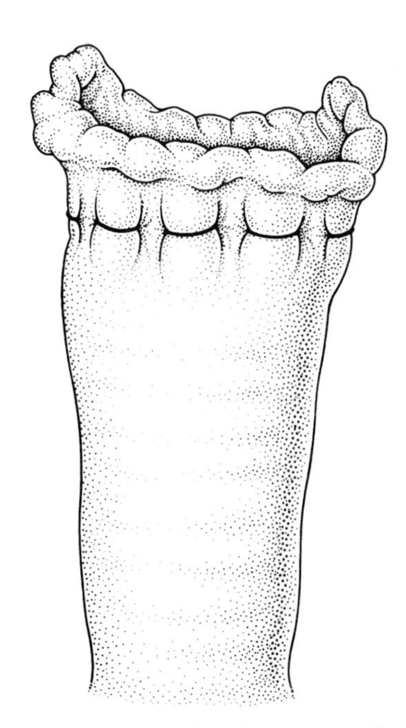

Fig. 34.18 Sutures in the vaginal vault isolate a cuff of the vagina above the suture line.

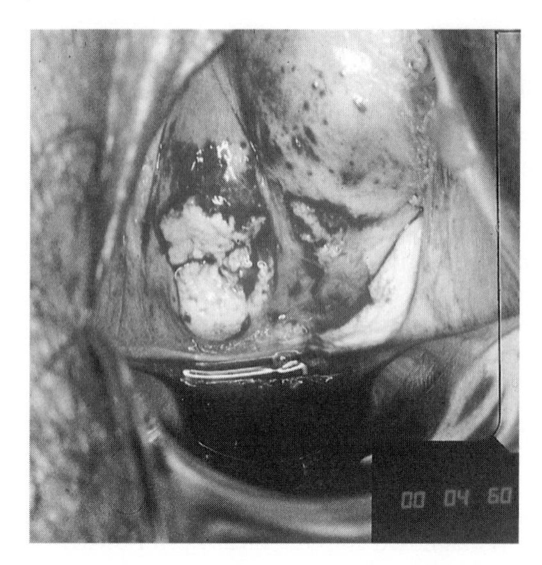

Fig. 34.19 VAIN after a hysterectomy. A patch of dense acetowhite epithelium is easily visible in the centre of the figure in the left vaginal angle. A second area of VAIN can be seen just above the speculum, spreading out of the right-angle.

Colposcopy of the vagina

Colposcopy of the vagina is more difficult than of the cervix, partly because of the greater area of epithelium to be examined, partly because the surface of the vaginal epithelium is very irregular, and partly because it is very difficult to view the vaginal walls at right-angles. If the patient has had a hysterectomy it is very difficult to see into the angles of the vagina and impossible to visualize epithelium that lies above the suture line or vaginal adhesions. The colposcopic features of VAIN are very similar to those of CIN, except that mosaic is seen less often (Fig. 34.19).

Treatment of VAIN

Carbon dioxide laser

Provided invasive disease has been excluded, laser vaporization is a satisfactory way of treating VAIN in women who have not undergone previous surgery. However, the report of invasive disease developing in two out of 14 posthysterectomy patients treated with the laser illustrated the dangers of overlooking disease buried above the suture line (Woodman et al 1984). Thus, although the laser may be useful in reducing the size of a lesion or in treating women who have not had a hysterectomy, it should not be used as the sole method of treatment in VAIN of the vaginal vault following hysterectomy. The same applies to the use of topical 5-fluorouracil.

Partial or total vaginectomy

Surgical excision of VAIN gives far more satisfactory results (Ireland & Monaghan 1988) and is the only effective option available to patients previously treated with

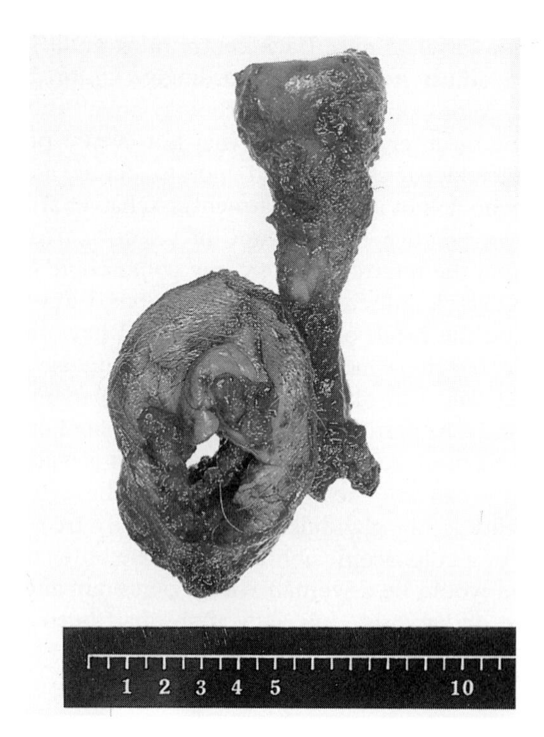

Fig. 34.20 A total vaginectomy, hysterectomy and vulvectomy performed by the vaginal route in an elderly woman with severe irritation from extensive VAIN and VIN 20 years after radiotherapy for cervical cancer (units in cm).

radiotherapy. The patients in Ireland and Monaghan's series were treated by an abdominal operation or by a combined abdominal and vaginal approach. This necessitates extensive pelvic dissection, which can be avoided by a vaginal approach (Fig. 34.20). Although the latter procedure is often very straightforward, it can prove to be extremely taxing in patients with a narrow introitus and no laxity of the vaginal vault.

Where the lesion involves a large area of the vagina there may be a place for laser vaporization to reduce the size of the lesion. The entire lesion is vaporized under general anaesthesia and, some months later when the effect of the laser treatment can be assessed, the vault of the vagina is excised. When this approach is unsuccessful, and in older patients, total vaginectomy or radiotherapy is required.

Radiotherapy

There can be no doubt that intracavitary radiotherapy is a highly effective treatment for VAIN (Hernandez-Linares et al 1980, Woodman et al 1988). The two major concerns about this form of therapy are the possibility of radiation-induced cancer and the effects it may have upon coital function. Radiation-induced second cancer in the vaginal vault may occur, but it is probably an extraordinarily rare event (Choo & Anderson 1982, Boice et al 1985). Brachytherapy to the vault of the vagina is unlikely to cause major coital problems if the patient and her spouse are encouraged to resume normal sexual relations as soon as possible (Woodman et al 1988). Where the area of disease is more extensive, no method of therapy is likely to be free of the risk of inducing sexual dysfunction.

Conclusions

The management of VAIN after hysterectomy in a young woman is likely to be surgical. If the lesion is extensive, prior laser therapy may be helpful in reducing the extent of disease. In older patients, especially when access is difficult, surgery offers few additional benefits but carries a potential for greater morbidity. Radiotherapy is therefore likely to be the treatment of choice. Whatever the circumstances it would be sensible for such patients to be evaluated and treated by those with experience of this unusual but troublesome condition.

THE VULVA

Vulval intraepithelial neoplasia (VIN) are seen more commonly than was the case 10–20 years ago. It is not certain whether this represents a real increase or is simply the result of a greater awareness of the problem. Bowen's disease, Bowenoid papulosis and erythroplasia of Queyrat are all terms for different clinical manifestations of VIN.

Pathology of premalignant disease of the vulva

Both squamous VIN and adenocarcinoma-in-situ (Paget's disease) occur on the vulva. The latter is very rare. The histological features and terminology of VIN are analogous to those of CIN and VAIN. In the same way, the histological appearance of Paget's disease is similar to the lesion seen in the breast. In a third of cases of Paget's disease there is an adenocarcinoma in underlying apocrine glands, and these carry an especially poor prognosis (Creasman et al 1975).

Natural history of VIN

Forty percent of women with VIN are younger than 41 years (Buscema et al 1980). Although histologically very similar to CIN and often occurring in association with it, VIN is said not to have the same malignant potential (Buscema et al 1980, Kaufman & Gordon 1986b). However, this opinion is based largely on studies of women who have been treated by excision biopsy or vulvectomy. This may not be true of untreated or inadequately treated patients: seven of eight such women progressed to invasive cancer within 8 years (Jones & Rowan 1994). Three of these were under 40 years of age.

Diagnosis and assessment of VIN

Intraepithelial disease of the vulva often presents as pruritus vulvae, but 20–45% are asymptomatic and are frequently found after treatment of preinvasive or invasive disease at other sites in the lower genital tract, particularly the cervix (Jones & McLean 1986, Kaufman & Gordon 1986a).

These lesions are often raised above the surrounding skin and have a rough surface. The colour is variable: white, due to hyperkeratinization; red, due to thinness of the epithelium; or dark brown, due to increased melanin deposition in the epithelial cells (Figs 34.21 and 34.22). They are very often multifocal.

However, the full extent of the abnormality is often not apparent until 5% acetic acid is applied (Fig. 34.23). After 2 minutes, VIN turns white and mosaic or punctation may

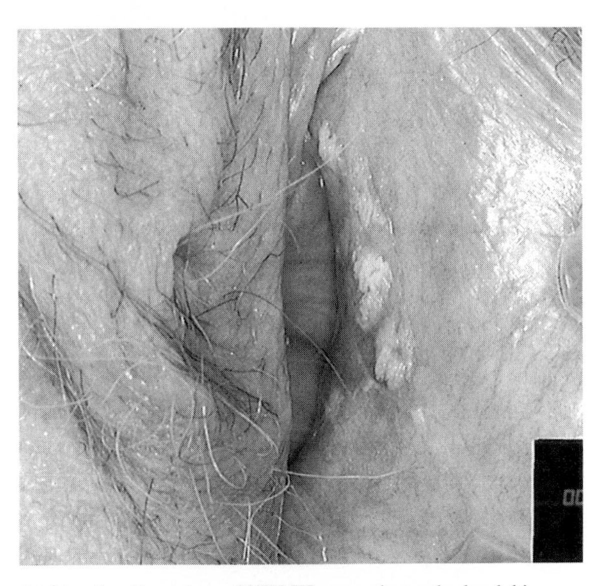

Fig. 34.21 Small patches of VIN III appearing as leukoplakia.

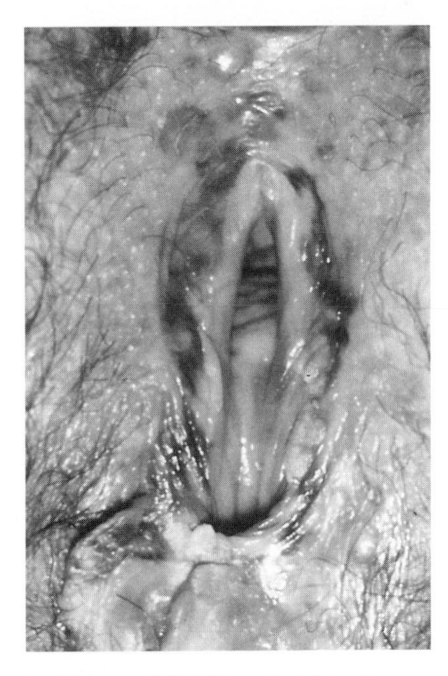

Fig. 34.22 A wide area of VIN III on the labia minora and the perineum seen as slightly raised, red lesions anteriorly, whitish lesions posteriorly and extensive dark brown lesions.

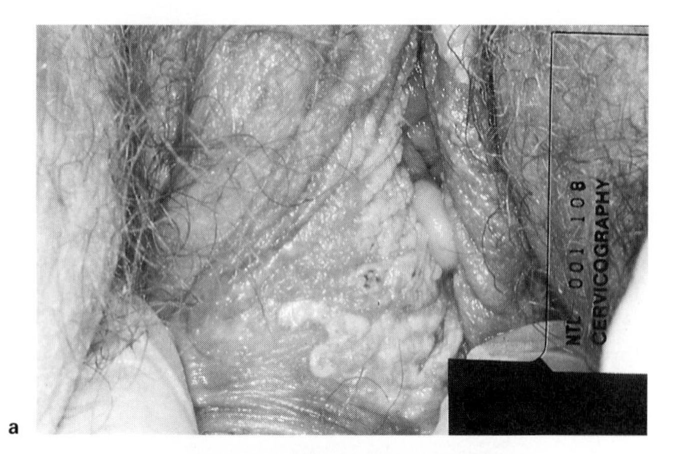

a

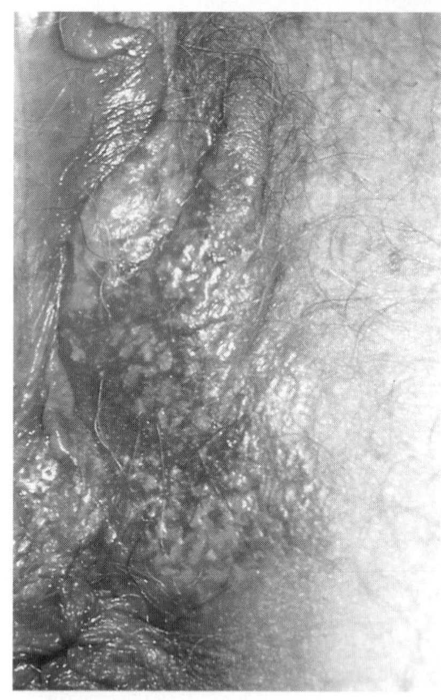

b

Fig. 34.23 **a** A patch of VIN III on the labium minorum after the application of acetic acid. **b** Paget's disease of the vulva. Note the red, crusted surface and clear margin.

be visible. Although these changes may be seen with the naked eye in a good light, it is much easier to use a hand lens or a colposcope. Toluidine blue is also used as a nuclear stain, but areas of ulceration give false positive results and hyperkeratinization gives false negatives.

Adequate biopsies must be taken from abnormal areas to rule out invasive disease. This can usually be done under local anaesthesia in the outpatient clinic, using a disposable 4 mm Stiefel biopsy punch or a Keyes punch.

Treatment of VIN

The treatment of VIN is difficult. Uncertainty about the malignant potential, the multifocal nature of the disorder and the discomfort and mutilation resulting from therapy suggest that recommendations should be cautious and conservative in order to avoid making the treatment worse than the disease. The youth of many of these patients is a further important consideration. Spontaneous regression of VIN III in women with the variant known as Bowenoid papulosis is well known (Friedrich 1972). These women are young, often present in pregnancy, have dark skin and the lesions are usually multifocal, papular and pigmented. However, progression to invasion does occur in young women (Planner et al 1987).

The documented progression of untreated cases of VIN III to invasive cancer underlines the potential importance of these lesions (Jones & Rowan 1994). If the patient has presented with symptoms, therapy is required. Asymptomatic patients, particularly under the age of 50, may be observed closely with biopsies repeated if there are any suspicious changes.

Medical therapy

The main role for medical treatment is in relieving symptoms in women for whom surgery may be avoided.

Provided invasion has been excluded as far as possible, topical steroids provide symptomatic relief for many women. A strong, fluorodinated steroid is usually required. This may be applied twice daily for not more than 6 months, because of the thinning of the skin which can result. Frequent review is necessary initially.

Topical 5-fluorouracil is painful and ineffective. Topical α-interferon produced promising results in one small series (Spirtos et al 1990).

Surgery

If the lesion is small an excision biopsy may be both diagnostic and therapeutic. If the disease is multifocal or covers a wide area, a skin graft may improve the cosmetic result of a skinning vulvectomy (Caglar et al 1986). However, the donor site is often very painful and a satisfactory result can be obtained in most patients without grafting.

Carbon dioxide laser

An alternative approach is to vaporize the abnormal epithelium with the carbon dioxide laser. Careful control of the depth of destruction is essential for good cosmetic results (Reid 1985). Given the very irregular surface of the vulva, it is very difficult to achieve a uniform depth of destruction. Moreover, the depth of treatment required for VIN is still unclear (Dorsey 1986). In some cases hair follicles may be involved for several millimetres below the surface (Mene & Buckley 1985), but it may not always be necessary to destroy the whole depth of involved appendages (Dorsey 1986). In any case, treatment of the whole vulva to such a depth would result in a third-degree burn which would need skin grafting. In practice, laser vaporization has proved to be disappointing in UK practice and is now seldom used (Shafi et al 1989).

Results

Assessment of the results of treatment should include a consideration of the length of follow-up. Surgical excision is associated with crude recurrence rates of 15–43% (Jones & McLean 1986, Shafi et al 1989). Short-term results from patients treated by laser were very promising (Leuchter et al 1984), but longer follow-up showed a re-currence rate similar to surgery (Shafi et al 1989). Close observation and rebiopsy are essential to detect invasive disease among those who relapse. Early invasion was detected in three (14%) of 21 patients with persisting signs of disease (Shafi et al 1989). Repeated treatments are commonly required.

VIN: conclusions

VIN is becoming more common, especially in young women. The treatment must be carefully tailored to the individual to avoid mutilating therapy whenever possible.

In view of the mutilating nature of treatment, the high recurrence rate and the uncertainty about the risk of invasion, there is a place for careful observation, especially of young women without severe symptoms. However, some of these untreated patients will develop vulvar cancer, so the importance of close follow-up must be emphasized to the patient and her general practitioner.

Paget's disease

This is an uncommon condition, similar to that found in the breast. Pruritus is the presenting complaint. The lesion is indistinguishable clinically from squamous intraepithelial neoplasia and the diagnosis must be made by biopsy (Fig. 34.23b).

Associated malignancies

In approximately one-third of patients there is an adenocarcinoma in the apocrine glands (Boehm & Morris 1971, Creasman et al 1975). This has a poor prognosis if the groin lymph nodes are involved, with no women surviving 5 years (Boehm & Morris 1971). Excluding underlying adnexal carcinomas, concomitant genital malignancies are found in 15–25% of women with Paget's disease of the vulva (Degefu et al 1986). These are most commonly vulval or cervical, but transitional cell carcinoma of the bladder (or kidney), and ovarian, endometrial, vaginal and urethral carcinomas have all been reported (Degefu et al 1986).

Treatment

The treatment of Paget's disease is very wide local excision, usually involving total vulvectomy because of the propensity of this condition to involve apparently normal skin (Creasman et al 1975). The specimen must be examined histologically with great care to exclude an apocrine adenocarcinoma.

ENDOMETRIUM

Premalignant disease of the endometrium is less well characterized than the equivalent lesions in the squamous epithelium of the cervix, vagina and vulva. This is partly because these lesions cannot be identified clinically and their detection is largely dependent on blind biopsy, which until recently required general anaesthesia.

Pathology of endometrial hyperplasia

Endometrial hyperplasia may be subdivided into cystic (simple) hyperplasia, adenomatous (complex) hyperplasia and atypical hyperplasia.

Simple hyperplasia is characterized by increased numbers of glands, which are often dilated or have an irregular outline. Some degree of crowding and reduction in the amount of endometrial stroma may be apparent but there is no cytological atypia (Figs 34.24 and 34.25). This is the most common hyperplasia (Table 34.4).

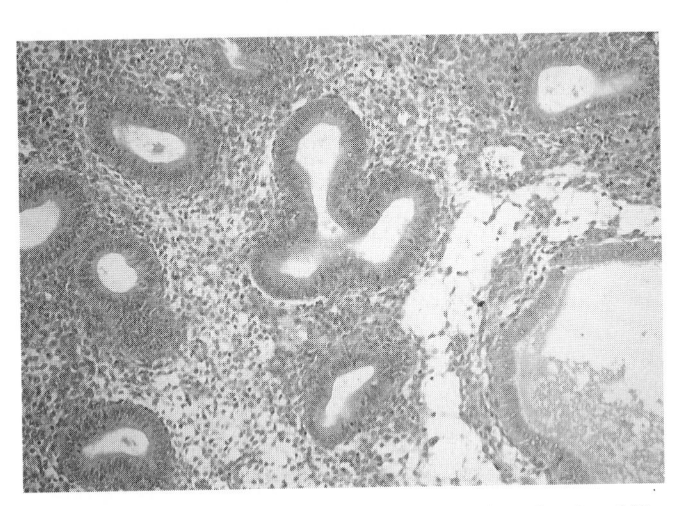

Fig. 34.24 Simple cystic hyperplasia. Haematoxylin and eosin × 100 (with kind permission of Dr Thomas Krausz).

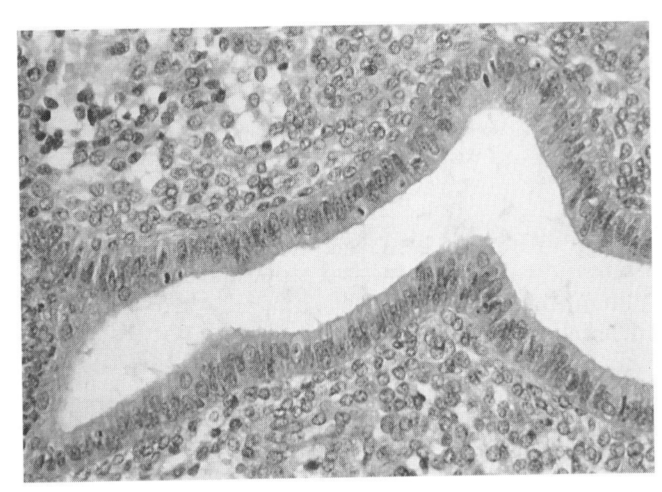

Fig. 34.25 Simple cystic hyperplasia. Haematoxylin and eosin × 250 (with kind permission of Dr Thomas Krausz).

Table 34.4 Frequency of endometrial hyperplasia and endometrial carcinoma in curettage specimens not associated with pregnancy (After Wentz 1974, Sherman 1978)

Histology	Detection rate (%)
Cystic hyperplasia	5.1
Adenomatous hyperplasia	2.6
Atypical hyperplasia	1.3
Carcinoma	2.6

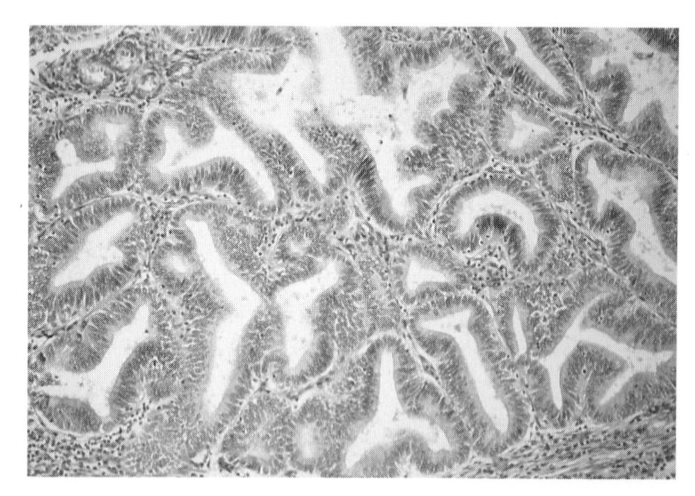

Fig. 34.26 Adenomatous hyperplasia without significant cytological atypia. Haematoxylin and eosin × 100 (with kind permission of Dr Thomas Krausz).

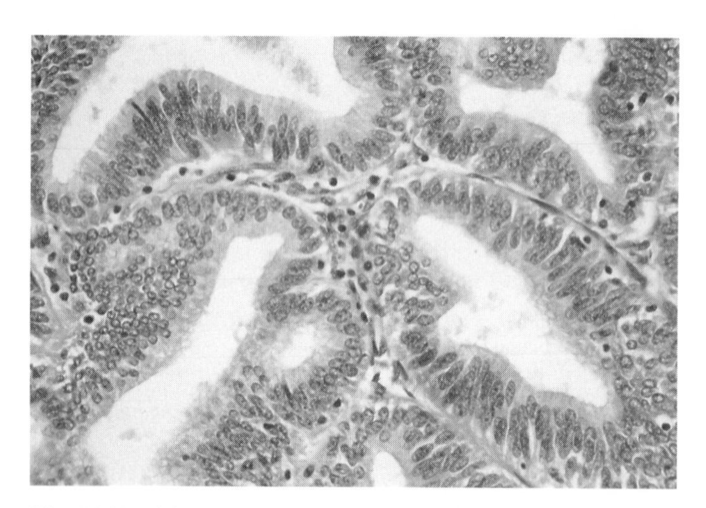

Fig. 34.27 Adenomatous hyperplasia without significant cytological atypia. Haematoxylin and eosin × 250 (with kind permission of Dr Thomas Krausz).

In adenomatous hyperplasia the glands have very irregular outlines showing marked structural complexity. In addition, the glands show 'back-to-back' crowding, with little intervening stroma (Figs 34.26 and 34.27).

Atypical hyperplasia is defined by the presence of glands showing nuclear atypia (Figs 34.28 and 34.29). Abnormal mitotic figures are often seen. These appearances may be accompanied by structural complexity. In severe cases, it may be impossible to differentiate from carcinoma (Figs 34.30 and 34.31).

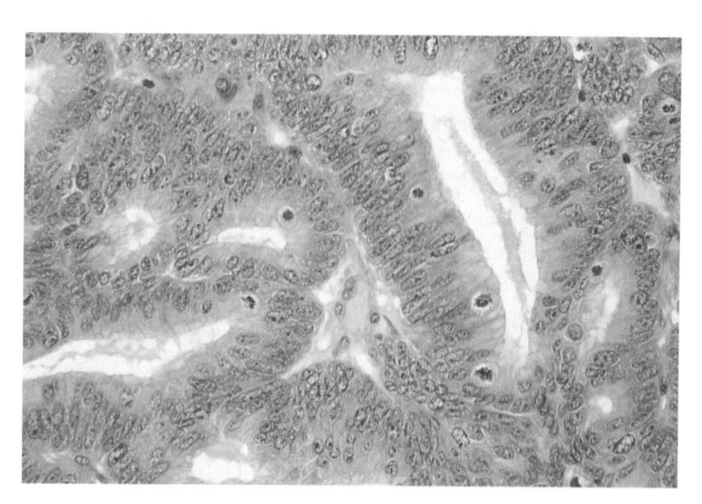

Fig. 34.28 Moderate atypical hyperplasia. Haematoxylin and eosin × 250 (with kind permission of Dr Thomas Krausz).

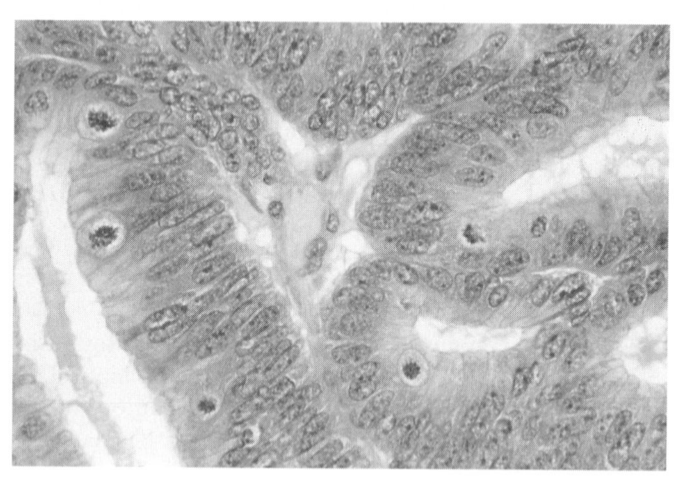

Fig. 34.29 Moderate atypical hyperplasia. Note the pseudostratification of the cells and the mitotic figures. The nuclei are plump, with some irregularity of the nuclear membrane and prominent nucleoli. Haematoxylin and eosin × 400 (with kind permission of Dr Thomas Krausz).

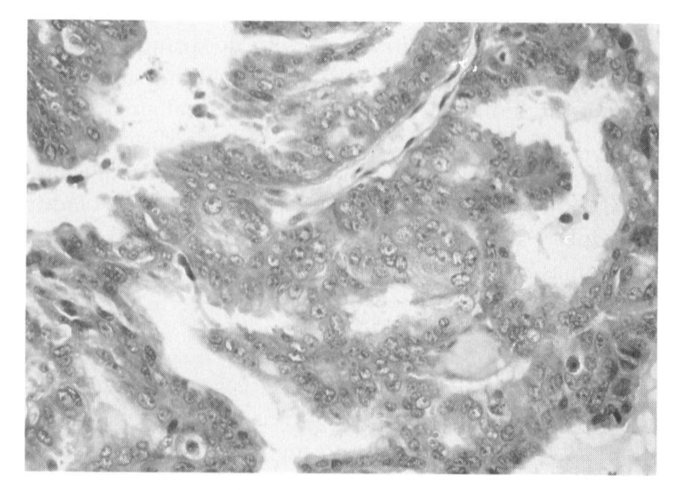

Fig. 34.30 Severe atypical hyperplasia. It is impossible to exclude invasive carcinoma from this material. Haematoxylin and eosin × 250 (with kind permission of Dr Thomas Krausz).

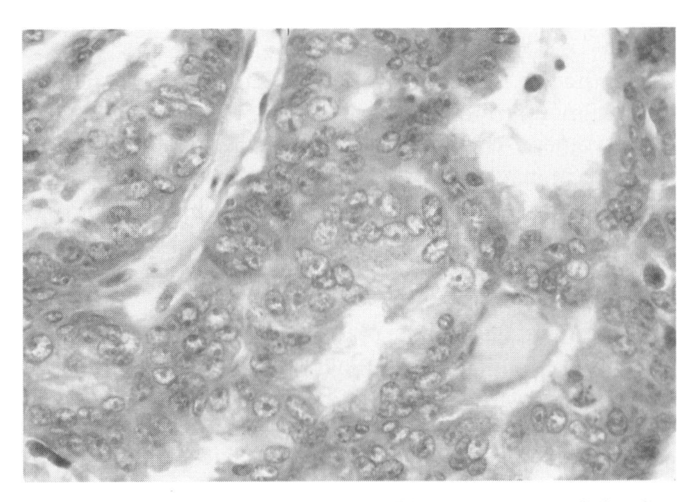

Fig. 34.31 Severe atypical hyperplasia. The nuclei are rounded and vesicular, with prominent nucleoli. Haematoxylin and eosin × 400 (with kind permission of Dr Thomas Krausz).

Aetiology of endometrial hyperplasia

1. Idiopathic
2. Anovulation
3. Exogenous oestrogens
4. Tamoxifen
5. Oestrogen-secreting tumour.

The majority of endometrial hyperplasias occur without any obvious predisposing cause. The most commonly recognized causes result in excessive oestrogen stimulation, unopposed by progesterone. This may arise from an endogenous source such as anovulatory cycles or an oestrogen-secreting tumour but exogenous, unopposed oestrogen administration and the oestrogenic effects of tamoxifen are more common causes.

Natural history of endometrial hyperplasia

The important practical considerations in the natural history of endometrial hyperplasias are:

1. coexisting endometrial carcinomas
2. coexisting ovarian carcinomas
3. risk of progression to endometrial carcinoma.

Cystic hyperplasia

Cystic hyperplasia is a common finding in postmenopausal women and anovulatory teenagers. It is not often seen in association with endometrial carcinoma or other pathology, and the risk of progression to endometrial carcinoma is 0.4–1.1% (McBride 1959, Kurman et al 1985, Lindahl & Willen 1994a,b).

Adenomatous hyperplasia

Adenomatous hyperplasia is not always identified separately in studies of endometrial hyperplasias, and mixed patterns with atypical changes are common. Thus there is little agreement in the literature about the rates of coexistent carcinoma or progression to invasion.

Table 34.5 Frequency of progression to carcinoma after diagnosis of hyperplasia

Reference	Cystic (%)	Adenomatous (%)	Atypical (%)
McBride 1959	0.4		
Gusberg & Kaplan 1963		10.4	
Wentz 1974		26.7	88.9
Sherman 1978		19.8	57.1
Kjorstad et al 1978			31.0*
Colgan et al 1983			33.3*
Kurman et al 1985	1.1	3.4	22.9
Lindahl & Willen 1994a	0.8	0	31.4
Baak et al 1994			22.6

*Some of these patients were treated with progestins

Estimates of the rate of progression to carcinoma in five studies range from none to 26.7% (Table 34.5). The highest rate comes from a study of women with persistent abnormalities, after two curettages more than 8 weeks apart. The low estimates in more recent studies in which the lesions were more clearly defined on the basis of the cytological features are more likely to reflect the level of risk for these lesions as currently defined.

Atypical hyperplasia

Coexistent carcinoma rates range from 25 to 50% (Tavassoli & Krausz 1978, Widra et al 1995). Clearly, this rate will depend upon the definition of the lesions included: no cancers were found in women without nuclear atypia (Widra et al 1995). It will also depend upon the readiness with which invasion is diagnosed in early cases without myometrial invasion. Only one of the 12 cases in one series invaded the myometrium and that was very superficial (Tavassoli & Krausz 1978); however, 17 of the 19 cases of cancer in another study did invade the myometrium (Janicek & Rosenshein 1994). Some women will have a concurrent endometrioid ovarian cancer.

The estimates of the risk of progression to endometrial carcinoma range from 22.6 to 88.9% (Table 34.5). Again, the highest rate comes from a study of women with persistent untreated atypical hyperplasia.

Morphometry may help to some extent in predicting the behaviour of these lesions (Colgan et al 1983, Baak et al 1994) but DNA ploidy is not useful.

Presentation of endometrial hyperplasia

The main presentations are abnormal uterine bleeding, infertility and postmenopausal bleeding. Premenopausal women will usually present with abnormal bleeding. Simple hyperplasia is most often found in women with infrequent, heavy periods, but complex and atypical hyperplasia do not give a characteristic pattern of bleeding. Some of these lesions are discovered in the course of infertility investigations. The largest group are women with postmenopausal or perimenopausal bleeding.

Investigation of endometrial hyperplasia

The main objectives of investigation of a woman found to have endometrial hyperplasia are to exclude invasive endometrial cancer or ovarian cancer, and to rule out an endogenous aberrant source of oestrogen secretion.

If endometrial hyperplasia has been diagnosed using an outpatient biopsy instrument, a formal examination under anaesthesia, hysteroscopy and curettage are required to palpate the adnexae and explore the endometrial and endocervical cavities. An ultrasound examination of the ovaries would be a sensible precaution, as would serum CA125 and oestradiol estimations.

Management of endometrial hyperplasia

The management will depend upon the severity of the abnormality and the patient's wishes for further children. The first step would be to discontinue oestrogen therapy or remove an oestrogen-secreting ovarian tumour.

Cystic hyperplasia

Cystic hyperplasia does not require special follow-up and may be managed on the basis of subsequent symptoms. Recurrent postmenopausal bleeding would require further investigation.

Adenomatous hyperplasia

Given the low risk of progression to carcinoma, there is no indication for hysterectomy or for progestin therapy in these women. As with women with cystic hyperplasia, subsequent management can probably be decided on the basis of further symptoms.

Atypical hyperplasia

Most women with atypical hyperplasia should have a hysterectomy and bilateral salpingo-oophorectomy because of the high risk of coexistent carcinoma. However, younger women who wish to preserve their fertility may be managed with medical therapy and repeated curettage. The data on medical treatment are few. Although both danazol and tamoxifen have been used in 52 women, only four had atypical hyperplasia. Similarly, a study of the use of a progesterone-containing IUCD included only four women with atypical hyperplasia.

Most data relate to the use of various progestins given for short-term courses or as continuous therapy for many years (Table 34.6). Most of the studies include only carefully selected cases, and the results of the different studies are not really comparable because of the selection criteria applied. The best results were obtained with moderately high doses of progestins – at least 20 mg/day of megestrol. If an adequate dose has been given it is probably safe to stop after 8–12 weeks, but Gal's (1986) experience of recurrence in both his patients who stopped indicates that there is not enough information to be sure of the optimum duration of therapy. One thing is clear: long-term follow-up is essential because recurrences may not appear for many years (Gal 1986, Ferenczy and Gelfand 1989).

Table 34.6 Studies of treatment of atypical hyperplasia with progestins

Reference	Lesion & no. of cases	Drug & dose	Short/long term	Persistence (%)	Recurrence (%)	Cancer (%)	Length of follow-up
Eichner & Abellera 1971	Adenomatous & atypical 16 cases	Megestrol 20 mg qid MPA 80 mg/day	Short term (6–9 weeks)	6	38	0	up to 4 yrs
Kjorstad et al 1978	Atypical 29 cases	Hydroxyprogesterone caproate 500 mg i.m. weekly	Short term (12 weeks)	24	31	31	3–10 yrs
Wentz 1985	Atypical 50 cases	Megestrol 20–40 mg qid	Short term (6–8 weeks)	0	0	0	1–5 yrs Most >4 yrs
Gal 1986	Atypical 32 cases	Megestrol 20–40 mg daily continuous	Long term	6	6*	0	2.5–12 yrs mean 5 yrs
Ferenczy & Gelfand 1989	Atypical 20 cases	MPA 20 mg/day continuous	Long term	50	25	25 mean 5.5 yrs	2–12 yrs mean 7 yrs
Lindahl & Willen 1994b	Atypical 10 cases	Medroxyprogesterone acetate 500 mg i.m. twice weekly	Short term (3 months)	0	10	0	5 yrs

* Both women who stopped megestrol recurred 10–18 months later

KEY POINTS

1. Both squamous (CIN) and glandular (AIS) premalignant lesions are seen on the cervix.
2. The diagnostic precision of small biopsies is not good. Invasive disease is not always detected and CIN II–III may be substantially underdiagnosed.
3. After 20 years about one-third of women with CIN III will develop invasive disease if untreated.
4. Progression of CIN I to CIN III or worse may occur in 26% of women within 2 years.
5. A well organized cervical cytology screening programme which reaches a large proportion of the population at risk, and which includes effective action when abnormal smears are detected, will reduce the incidence and mortality of cervical cancer.
6. The four pitfalls in colposcopy are the false SCJ caused by an abrasion; the SCJ in the canal; the previously treated cervix; and glandular lesions.
7. The majority of women with CIN can be treated in the outpatient department.
8. Excisional methods provide the whole lesion for histology without increasing the discomfort or complications for the patient.
9. Most cases of VAIN are seen after hysterectomy.
10. VAIN hidden above the vaginal suture line cannot be evaluated and early invasive cancer is common.
11. Surgical excision (preferably by the vaginal route) or intracavitary radiotherapy are the most effective treatments.
12. The malignant potential of VIN is uncertain but untreated cases can progress to invasion.
13. Treatment of VIN is mutilating and should be limited for the most part to symptomatic patients.
14. Atypical hyperplasia is the only form of endometrial hyperplasia with a significant risk of progression to malignancy, and the only one which merits surgical treatment.

REFERENCES

Andersen E S, Arffmann E 1989 Adenocarcinoma in situ of the uterine cervix: a clinico-pathologic study of 36 cases. Gynecologic Oncology 35: 1–7

Anderson G H, Boyes D A, Benedet J L et al 1988 Organisation and results of the cervical cytology screening programme in British Columbia, 1955–85. British Medical Journal 296: 975–978

Anderson M C, Hartley R B 1980 Cervical crypt involvement by intraepithelial neoplasia. Obstetrics and Gynecology 55: 546–550

Baak J P A, Kuik D J, Bezemer P D 1994 The additional prognostic value of morphometric nuclear arrangement and DNA-ploidy to other morphometric and stereological features in endometrial hyperplasias. International Journal of Gynecological Cancer 4: 289–297

Bekassy Z, Alm P, Grundsell H, Larsson G, Astedt B 1983 Laser miniconisation in mild and moderate dysplasia of the uterine cervix. Gynecologic Oncology 15: 357–362

Boehm F, Morris J M 1971 Paget's disease and apocrine gland carcinoma of the vulva. Obstetrics and Gynecology 38: 185–192

Boice J D, Day N E, Andersen A et al 1985 Second cancers following treatment for cervical cancer. An international collaboration among cancer registries. Journal of the National Cancer Institute 74: 955–975

Boon M E, Kok L P, Beck S 1995 Histologic validation of neural network-assisted cervical screening: comparison with the conventional procedure. Cell Vision 1: 23–27

Brady J L, Fish A N J, Woolas R P, Brown C L, Oram D H 1994 Large loop diathermy of the transformation zone: is 'see and treat' an acceptable option for the management of women with abnormal cervical smears? Journal of Obstetrics and Gynecology 14: 44–49

Burghardt E, Holzer E 1980 Treatment of carcinoma-in-situ: evaluation of 1609 cases. Obstetrics and Gynecology 55: 539–545

Buscema J, Stern J, Woodruff J D 1980 The significance of histologic alterations adjacent to invasive vulvar carcinoma. American Journal of Obstetrics and Gynecology 137: 902–909

Caglar H, Delgado G, Hreshchyshyn M M 1986 Partial and total skinning vulvectomy in treatment of carcinoma in situ of the vulva. Obstetrics and Gynecology 68: 504–507

Campion M J, McCance D J, Cuzick J, Singer A 1986 The progressive potential of mild cervical atypia: a prospective cytological, colposcopic and virological study. Lancet ii: 237–240

Campion M J, di Paola F M, Vellios F 1990 The value of cervicography in population screening. Journal of Experimental and Clinical Cancer Research 9 (Suppl): FC/107

Choo Y C, Anderson D G 1982 Neoplasms of the vagina following cervical carcinoma. Gynecologic Oncology 14: 125–132

Colgan T J, Norris H J, Foster W, Kurman R J, Fox C H 1983 Predicting the outcome of endometrial hyperplasia by quantitative analysis of nuclear features using a linear discriminant function. International Journal of Gynecological Pathology 1: 347–352

Creasman W T, Gallacher H S, Rutledge F 1975 Paget's disease of the vulva. Gynecological Oncology 3: 133–148

Cullimore J E, Luesley D M, Rollason T P et al 1992 A prospective study of conisation of the cervix in the management of cervical intraepithelial glandular neoplasia (CIGN) – a preliminary report. British Journal of Obstetrics and Gynaecology 99: 314–318

Cuzick J, Szarewski A, Terry G et al 1995 Human papillomavirus testing in primary cervical screening. Lancet 345: 1533–1536

Degefu S, O'Quinn A G, Dhurandhar H N 1986 Paget's disease of the vulva and urogenital malignancies: a case report and review of the literature. Gynecological Oncology 25: 347–354

Dorsey J H 1986 Skin appendage involvement and vulval intraepithelial neoplasia. In: Sharp F, Jordan J A (eds) Gynaecological laser surgery. Perinatology Press, New York, pp 193–195

Eichner E, Abellera M 1971 Endometrial hyperplasia treated by progestins. Obstetrics and Gynecology 38: 739–742

Ferenczy A, Gelfand M 1989 The biologic significance of cytologic atypia in progestogen-treated endometrial hyperplasia. American Journal of Obstetrics and Gynecology 160: 126–131

Flannelly G, Anderson D, Kitchener H C et al 1994 Management of women with mild and moderate cervical dyskaryosis. British Medical Journal 308: 1399–1403

Friedrich E G 1972 Reversible vulvar atypia. Obstetrics and Gynecology 39: 173–181

Gal D 1986 Hormonal therapy for lesions of the endometrium. Seminars in Oncology 13: Suppl 4: 33–36

Griffiths M, Turner M J, Partington C K, Soutter W P 1989 Should smears in a colposcopy clinic be taken after the application of acetic acid? Acta Cytologica 33: 324–326

Gusberg S B, Kaplan A L 1963 Precursors of corpus cancer. American Journal of Obstetrics and Gynecology 87: 662–678

Hernandez-Linares W, Puthawala A, Nolan J F, Jernstrom P H, Morrow C P 1980 Carcinoma in situ of the vagina: past and present management. Obstetrics and Gynecology 56: 356–360

IARC Working Group on Evaluation of Cervical Cancer Screening Programmes 1986 Screening for cervical squamous cancer: duration of low risk after negative results of cervical cytology and its implication for screening policies. British Medical Journal 293: 659–664

Ireland D, Monaghan J M 1988 The management of the patient with

abnormal vaginal cytology following hysterectomy. British Journal of Obstetrics and Gynaecology 95: 973–975
Janicek M, Rosenshein N B 1994 Invasive endometrial cancer in uteri resected for atypical endometrial hyperplasia. Gynecologic Oncology 52: 373–378
Jones R W, McLean M R 1986 Carcinoma in situ of the vulva: a review of 31 treated and five untreated cases. Obstetrics and Gynecology 68: 499–503
Jones R W, Rowan D M 1994 Vulval intraepithelial neoplasia III: a clinical study of the outcome in 113 cases with relation to the later development of invasive vulvar carcinoma. Obstetrics and Gynecology 84: 741–745
Kaufman R, Gordon A 1986a Squamous cell carcinoma in situ of the vulva. Part I. British Journal of Sexual Medicine 13: 24–27
Kaufman R, Gordon A 1986b Squamous cell carcinoma in situ of the vulva. Part II. British Journal of Sexual Medicine 13: 55–58
Larsson G, Gullberg B, Grundsell H 1983 A comparison of complications of laser and cold knife conisation. Obstetrics and Gynecology 62: 213–217
Kesic V I, Soutter W P, Sulovic V, Juznic N, Aleksic M, Ljubic A 1993 A comparison of cytology and cervicography in cervical screening. International Journal of Gynaecological Oncology 3: 395–398
Kjorstad K E, Welander C, Halvorsen T, Grude T, Onsrud M 1978 In: Brush M G, King R J B, Taylor R W (eds) Endometrial cancer. Baillière Tindall, London, pp 188–191
Kurman R J, Kaminski P F, Norris H J 1985 The behaviour of endometrial hyperplasia: a long-term study of 'untreated' hyperplasia in 170 patients. Cancer 56: 403–412
Leuchter R S, Townsend D E, Hacker N F, Pretorius R G, Lagasse L D, Wade M E 1984 Treatment of vulvar carcinoma in situ with the CO_2 laser. Gynecologic Oncology 19: 314–322
Lindahl B, Willen R 1994a Spontaneous endometrial hyperplasia. A prospective, 5 year follow up of 246 patients after abrasion only, including 380 patients followed up for 2 years. Anticancer Research 14: 2141–2146
Lindahl B, Willen R 1994b Spontaneous endometrial hyperplasia. A 5 year follow up of 82 patients after high dose gestagen treatment. Anticancer Research 14: 2831–2834
McBride J M 1959 Premenopausal cystic hyperplasia and endometrial carcinoma. Journal of Obstetrics and Gynaecology of the British Empire 66: 288–296
McIndoe W A, McLean M R, Jones R W, Mullins P R 1984 The invasive potential of carcinoma in situ of the cervix. Obstetrics and Gynecology 64: 451–458
Mene A, Buckley C H 1985 Involvement of the vulval skin appendages by intraepithelial neoplasia. British Journal of Obstetrics and Gynaecology 92: 634–638
Nieminen P, Kallio M, Hakama M 1995 The effect of mass screening on incidence and mortality of squamous and adenocarcinoma of cervix uteri. Obstetrics and Gynecology 85: 1017–1021
Paraskevaidis E, Jandial L, Mann E M F, Fisher P M C, Kitchener H C 1991 Pattern of treatment failure following laser for cervical intraepithelial neoplasia: implications for follow-up protocol. Obstetrics and Gynecology 78: 80–83
Partington C K, Soutter W P, Turner M J, Hill A S, Krausz T 1987 Laser excisional biopsy under local anaesthesia — an outpatient technique? Journal of Obstetrics and Gynaecology 9: 48–52
Partington C K, Turner M J, Soutter W P, Griffiths M, Krausz T 1989 Laser vaporisation versus laser excision conisation in the treatment of cervical intraepithelial neoplasia. Obstetrics and Gynecology 73: 775–779
Planner R S, Andersen H E, Hobbs J B, Williams R A, Fogarty L F, Hudson P J 1987 Multifocal invasive carcinoma of the vulva in a 25 year old with Bowenoid papulosis. Australian and New Zealand Journal of Obstetrics and Gynaecology 27: 291–295
Prendiville W, Cullimore J, Norman S 1989 Large loop excision of the transformation zone (LLETZ). A new method of management for women with cervical intraepithelial neoplasia. British Journal of Obstetrics and Gynaecology 96: 1054–1060
Reid R 1985 Superficial laser vulvectomy II. The anatomic and biophysical principles permitting accurate control over the depth of dermal destruction with the carbon dioxide laser. American Journal of Obstetrics and Gynecology 152: 261–271
Richart R M 1967 Natural history of cervical intraepithelial neoplasia. Clinics in Obstetrics and Gynecology 10: 748–784
Robertson A J, Anderson J M, Swanson Beck J et al 1989 Observer variability in histopathological reporting of cervical biopsy specimens. Journal of Clinical Pathology 42: 231–238
Robertson J H, Woodend B E, Crozier E H, Hutchinson J 1988 Risk of cervical cancer associated with mild dyskaryosis. British Medical Journal 297: 18–21
Shafi M I, Luesley D M, Byrne P et al 1989 Vulval intraepithelial neoplasia – management and outcome. British Journal of Obstetrics and Gynaecology 96: 1339–1344
Sherman A I 1978 Precursors of endometrial cancer. Israel Journal of Medical Science 14: 370–378
Sincock A M, Evans-Jones J, Partington C K, Steel S J 1987 Quantitative assessment of cervical neoplasia by hydrolysed DNA assay. Lancet ii: 942–943
Skehan M, Soutter W P, Lim K, Krause T, Pryse-Davies J 1990 Reliability of colposcopy and directed punch biopsy. British Journal of Obstetrics and Gynaecology 97: 811–816
Soutter W P 1993 A practical guide to colposcopy. Oxford, Oxford University Press
Soutter W P, Brough A K, Monaghan J M 1984 Cervical screening for younger women. Lancet ii: 745
Soutter W P, Wisdom S, Brough A K, Monaghan J M 1986a Should patients with mild atypia in a cervical smear be referred for colposcopy? British Journal of Obstetrics and Gynaecology 93: 70–74
Soutter W P, Abernethy F M, Brown V A, Hill A S 1986b Success, complications and subsequent pregnancy outcome relative to the depth of laser treatment of cervical intraepithelial neoplasia. Colposcopy and Gynecologic Laser Surgery 2: 35–42
Soutter W P, Fletcher A 1994 Invasive cancer of the cervix in women with mild dyskaryosis followed cytologically. British Medical Journal 308: 1421–1423
Soutter W P, Lopes AdB, Fletcher A, Monaghan J M, Duncan I D, Paraskevaidis E, Kitchener H C (unpublished) Invasive cervical cancer after conservative therapy for cervical intraepithelial neoplasia
Spirtos N M, Smith L H, Teng N N H 1990 Prospective randomised trial of topical α-interferon (α-interferon gels) for the treatment of vulval intraepithelial neoplasia III. Gynecologic Oncology 37: 34–38
Tavasolli F, Krausz F T 1978 Endometrial lesions in uteri resected for atypical endometrial hyperplasia. American Journal of Clinical Pathology 70: 770–779
Wentz W B 1974 Progestin therapy in endometrial hyperplasia. Gynecologic Oncology 2: 362–367
Wentz W B 1985 Progestin therapy in lesions of the endometrium. Seminars in Oncology 12: Suppl 1: 23–27
Widra E A, Dunton C J, McHugh M, Palazzo J P 1995 Endometrial hyperplasia and the risk of carcinoma. International Journal of Gynecological Cancer 5: 233–235
Widrich T, Kennedy A W, Myers T M, Hart W R, Wirth S 1996 Adenocarcinoma in situ of the uterine cervix: management and outcome. Gynecologic Oncology 61: 304–308
Wijngaarden van W J, Duncan I D 1993 Rationale for stopping cervical screening in women over 50. British Medical Journal 306: 967–971
Woodman C B J, Jordan J A, Wade-Evans T 1984 The management of vaginal intraepithelial neoplasia after hysterectomy. British Journal of Obstetrics and Gynaecology 91: 707–711
Woodman C B J, Mould J J, Jordan J A 1988 Radiotherapy in the management of vaginal intraepithelial neoplasia after hysterectomy. British Journal of Obstetrics and Gynaecology 95: 976–979

35

Malignant disease of the cervix

M. C. Anderson C. A. E. Coulter W. P. Mason W. P. Soutter

EPIDEMIOLOGY

Incidence

Invasive carcinoma of the cervix constitutes 4% of female malignancies in England and Wales. In 1989, 4147 cases of carcinoma of the cervix were registered (Office of Population Censuses and Surveys 1994). This is a slight increase from the 3879 cases registered in 1983 (Office of Population Censuses and Surveys 1987).

The incidence of invasive carcinoma in 1989 was 16 per 100 000 women in England and Wales. Throughout the world, the incidence of invasive disease varies widely: the cumulative risk of developing carcinoma of the cervix is 5.5% in Colombia by the age of 74, compared with 1.5% in England and Wales and 0.5% in Spain and Israel. Worldwide, cervical cancer is the second commonest cancer in women and is very nearly as common as breast cancer.

Age at presentation

In England and Wales the incidence of invasive cervical cancer has risen in the 25–34-year-old age group from approximately 6 per 100 000 in 1968 to about 16 per 100 000 in 1989 (OPCS 1994). The age-related distribution now shows two distinct peaks due to this rising rate in younger cohorts (Fig. 35.1), and in 1989 36% of cases were in women under 45 years old. In 1989 it was the commonest cancer in women aged 20–35, in whom it accounted for 25% of all cancers.

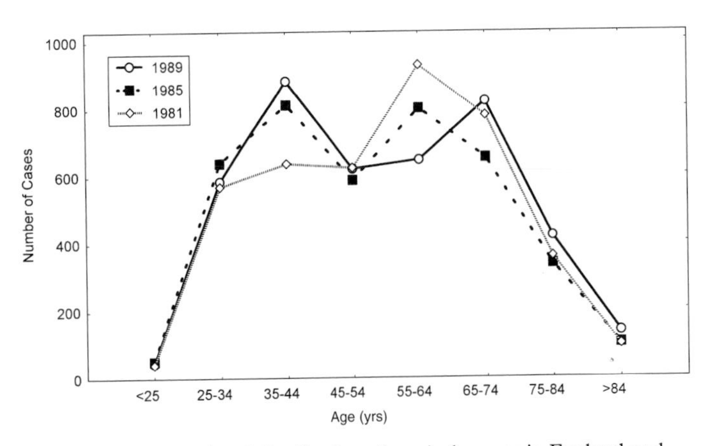

Fig. 35.1 Age-related distribution of cervical cancer in England and Wales in 1981, 1985 and 1989, showing the sharp increase in the younger cohorts of women (OPCS 1985, 1990, 1994). About 36% of cases in 1989 were in women less than 45 years of age. The shift of the 1981 peak in the 55–64-year-olds to a peak in 65–74-year-olds in 1989 is a cohort effect, as those born in the 1920s have had high rates throughout their lives.

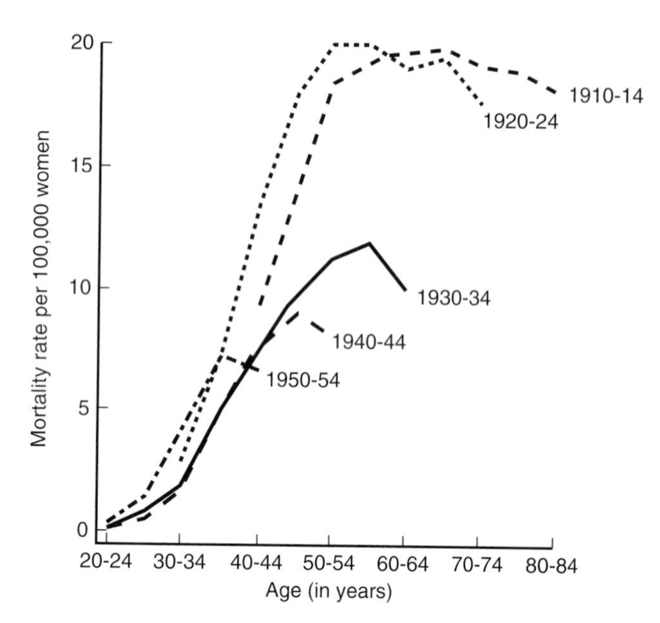

Fig. 35.2 Age-specific mortality rates by birth cohort, England and Wales, 1950–1994. (Reproduced from Sasieni et al 1995, with kind permission of *The Lancet*.)

It has been said that younger women have more aggressive disease but there is no evidence of this in women treated before 1981 (Meanwell et al 1988). There remains an anxiety that a poorer prognosis is apparent only in patients treated more recently (Dattoli et al 1989). The worse prognosis applied equally to women treated with surgery or with radiotherapy.

Mortality rates

In spite of the relatively static number of cervical cancers registered each year in England and Wales, the number of women dying from this disease has fallen dramatically since 1988 (Sasieni et al 1995). In the 1970s over 2000 women died of cervical cancer every year. The toll fell to 1781 in 1990, 1485 in 1993 and around 1370 in 1994. Between 1960 and 1988 the age-standardized mortality rate fell by 1–2% per year. Then the fall in mortality accelerated rapidly and was around 7% per year by 1994. The recent downturn in mortality rates in every birth cohort (Fig. 35.2) is probably due to the increased screening coverage of the population between 1988 and 1992.

ANATOMY

Origin of cervical neoplasia

The stratified squamous epithelium of the vagina and ectocervix meets the columnar epithelium of the uterine cavity at the squamocolumnar junction. In premenopausal women this squamocolumnar junction is usually situated just inside the external cervical os and can be readily visualized using a colposcope. The position of the squamocolumnar junction tends to lie inside the canal after the menopause. This is the site of origin of most preinvasive and invasive cervical neoplasia.

Gross anatomy

The cervix lies partly in the upper vagina and partly in the retroperitoneal space behind the bladder and in front of the rectum. It is related on each side to the terminal portion of the ureters as they swing anteriorly and medially below the uterine arteries into the bladder. The cardinal ligaments laterally and the uterosacral ligaments posterolaterally are inserted into the cervix and provide the main supports of the uterus.

Lymphatic drainage

The regional lymph drainage of the female genital organs follows a relatively well defined pattern. Cervical tumours spread via the parametrial lymphatics to the internal (hypogastric) and external iliac nodes, which surround the corresponding iliac vessels on the pelvic side wall. The lymph vessels ascend towards the network of nodes around the common iliac vessels on each side and amalgamate in a plexus surrounding the aorta and vena cava. The inferior margin of the aortic nodes is at the lower border of the fourth lumbar vertebra. The common iliac vessels commence to the right of the midline at the upper border of the same vertebra and pass in front of the sacroiliac joint on each side before bifurcating into external and internal branches.

AETIOLOGY

An association between sexual behaviour and the subsequent development of cervical carcinoma has been suggested for many years. This has generated considerable interest in the possibility that a sexually transmissible agent may be involved in the process.

Sexual history

The oft-quoted statement that nuns and virgins are immune from cervical cancer has been challenged in recent years. More critical examination of the evidence suggests that this contention is unlikely to be true (Griffiths 1991).

Two factors related to sexual behaviour – age at first intercourse and number of sexual partners – have been examined extensively. Rotkin (1973) reported a 50% excess of cases of cervical neoplasia in women who started sexual intercourse before their 20th birthday, supporting the proposal that the adolescent cervix may be more vulnerable to potential oncogenic agents. Several other studies have found a history of multiple sexual partners to be more significant than early age of first intercourse. Harris et al (1980) recorded a 14.2-fold increased risk of developing severe dysplasia with a past history of six or more partners, and this finding has been confirmed by others. There appears to be little correlation between the number of sexual acts and cervical neoplasia among women with two or less lifetime partners (Harris et al 1980).

Smoking

A strong epidemiological link between smoking and cervical neoplasia has been shown in studies which have controlled adequately for sexual behaviour (but see Ch. 31). A 12.7-fold greater risk of developing carcinoma-in-situ has been found after 12 years of smoking. The products of smoking, cotinine and nicotine, are found in higher concentrations in cervical mucus than in serum from women with cervical intraepithelial neoplasia (CIN). However, little is known about the direct effects of these agents on human epithelia. There are few data on the role of nitrosamines, the chemical carcinogens linked with the development of other smoking-related cancers, in the cervix.

Smoking reduces the number of Langerhans' cells present in the cervical epithelium in a dose-dependent manner. These cells, originally derived from macrophages, play a role in local immune surveillance within epithelia. Because their role is not fully understood, it is difficult to speculate upon the ways in which the reduction of Langerhans' cells may contribute to cervical neoplasia.

Contraception

No definite association between oral contraception and cervical neoplasia has been clearly demonstrated. Studies which have shown an increased risk in oral contraceptive pill users have often failed to control adequately for the sexual history of the women involved (Beral et al 1988). A lower incidence of cervical neoplasia has been demonstrated in women using a diaphragm, suggesting that a transmissible agent may be involved.

Male factor

In view of the association between sexual behaviour and cervical neoplasia it would be expected that factors relating to the male partner may influence the outcome. Kessler (1984) described a 2.7-fold increased risk of developing cervical neoplasia for a woman whose husband had previously been married to a woman with cervical carcinoma. Recent evidence seems firmly to refute the proposal of an association between penile and cervical cancer. The sexual history of the male partner may also influence the risk of a woman developing cervical neoplasia: a history of 15 or more partners is associated with a 7.8-fold increased risk of the current female partner developing cervical neoplasia (Buckley et al 1981). Several potent immunosuppressive agents are present in human seminal plasma. These may influence the development of cervical neoplasia by reducing the local immune response to viral infections or to cells transformed by other agents.

Infective agents

Agents that are known to infect the lower female genital tract have been studied in an attempt to find a link with cervical neoplasia. Of the non-viral agents, *Trichomonas vaginalis* and *Chlamydia trachomatis* have been studied recently. A twofold increased incidence of antibodies against *Chlamydia trachomatis* was found in women with CIN when compared with controls.

However, most research interest has concentrated upon viral agents. Both Epstein–Barr virus and cytomegalovirus are thought to infect the cervix, but neither has been linked to the development of cervical neoplasia. Early work on herpes simplex virus type 2 (HSV-2) did demonstrate a possible link with cervical neoplasia. In the laboratory HSV-2 has been shown to be a very weak oncogenic virus; however, analysis of many cervical tumours has failed to show any evidence of HSV-2 DNA. Despite early case-controlled studies linking previous infection with HSV-2 to cervical neoplasia, large population studies have shown that the presence of HSV-2 antibodies is related to sexual activity rather than cervical neoplasia.

Human papilloma viruses

Recent research has concentrated on the possible link between certain types of human papilloma virus (HPV) and cervical neoplasia. These are small DNA viruses which have no outer lipid-containing viral membrane. They cannot be grown in cell culture and so the development of adequate type-specific antibodies has been difficult. The distinction between different HPV types is based upon differences in DNA sequence (Howley & Schlegel 1988).

Over 50 different HPV types have now been described, of which at least nine infect the lower female genital tract. The sexual transmission of these viruses from male to female and from female to male has been shown to occur. The HPV types which infect the lower reproductive tract can be divided into two groups. One group, which includes types 6, 11, 31, 35, 42 and 50, is found in condylomata acuminata, low-grade CIN and only rarely in invasive tumours. The second group includes types 16, 18 and 33, and is associated with high-grade CIN and invasive tumours.

HPV types 16 and 18 have the ability to transform in vitro cells which can then cause tumours in immunocompromised animals. The transforming ability seems to depend upon two proteins produced by HPVs 16 and 18, the E6 and E7 proteins. The E7 protein has structural and functional homologies with two well-known viral transforming proteins, SV40 large T and EIA of adenovirus, and all three proteins bind the product of the retinoblastoma gene, a putative antioncogene. This may be the mechanism by which these proteins bring about cellular transformation. The E6 protein binds to the tumour suppressor *p53*, partly impairing its activity.

Integration of HPV DNA into the host genome may be an important early event in the neoplastic process. The majority of cervical carcinomas examined have integrated HPV sequences, whereas integration is uncommon in normal tissue and CIN. When integration occurs the circular HPV DNA is usually opened in the region which encodes for the E1 and E2 proteins. This will prevent any transcription of genes downstream from the break (e.g. E2), but will allow transcription of the upstream E6 and E7 proteins. The loss of E2 transcription may lead to the autonomous expression of E6 and E7, since it is E2 that controls early gene expression. This uncontrolled expression of the transforming proteins may be important in cellular transformation brought about by HPVs 16 and 18.

The prevalence of HPV infection in the normal population varies in different age groups and from country to country. In a study of women in Spain and Colombia, whose mean age was around 50 years, 4.6% and 13.3% had cervical HPV16 infection as judged by PCR assay (Muñoz et al 1992). Four studies of younger women found 20–40% infection rates (Bauer et al 1991, Ley et al 1991, Melkert et al 1993, Schiffman et al 1993). In one of very few longitudinal studies, 66% of a small group of normal German women tested positive to HPV16 on at least one occasion during a year (Schneider et al 1992). This and a larger, cross-sectional, study showing a 29.7% rate of infection, suggested that HPV16 infection may often be very transient (Fairley et al 1994). A study using a quantitative assay that detected all the HPV types thought to be oncogenic and excluded low copy numbers, found a 7.4% infection rate in women attending a family planning clinic in central London (Cuzick et al 1995). The rate fell from 10.2% in women under 30 years old to around 2% in the over 40s. There is also increasing evidence that HPV16 infection may be acquired commonly by non-sexual means, and is very common (20%) in children and teenagers (Muller et al 1995).

It is increasingly clear that HPV infection alone is not sufficient to induce cervical cancer. Possibly as many as four other genes may have to be modified to produce a potentially invasive phenotype (zur Hausen 1994). In addition, the affected cells must acquire the ability to escape recognition by the host's immune system.

Conclusions

There is much epidemiological evidence to suggest that part of the risk of developing cervical neoplasia is associated with sexual behaviour, and that a sexually transmissible agent may be involved in the process. It seems likely that HPV does play a role in the aetiology of cervical cancer, but there are other important factors at work.

PATHOLOGY

Malignant tumours of the cervix may be of squamous or glandular type; squamous cell carcinomas account for about 90% of invasive carcinomas and most of the remainder are adenocarcinomas. Preinvasive lesions are discussed in Chapter 34.

Squamous cell carcinoma

Early stromal invasion

This term has been dropped from the FIGO definitions of staging. It described the earliest recognizable stages of invasion, arising from CIN as minute prongs of malignant cells pushing through the basement membrane into the cervical stroma.

Microinvasive carcinoma (FIGO Stage Ia)

This has been modified yet again to describe a lesion which when measured in two dimensions has a maximum depth of invasion of not more than 5 mm from the nearest basement membrane and a maximum width of not more than 7 mm (Fig. 35.3). Stage Ia1 includes lesions which invade no more than 3 mm from the nearest basement

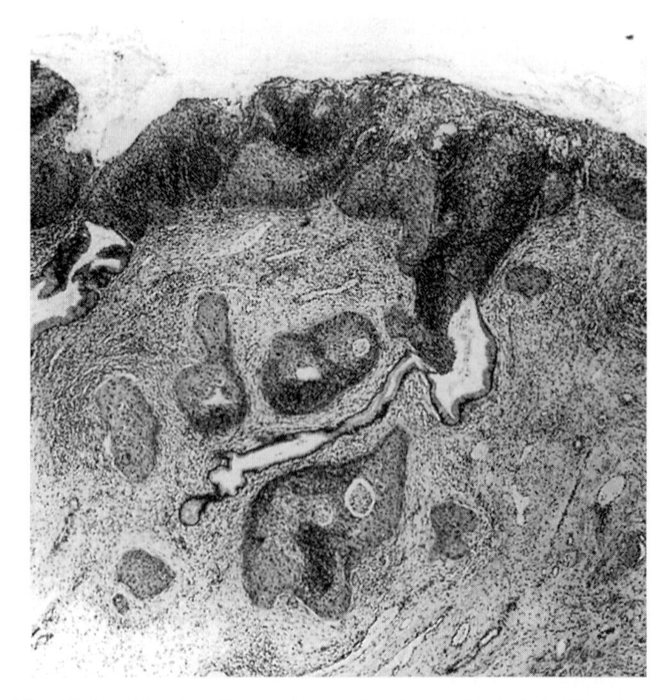

Fig. 35.3 Microinvasive carcinoma showing multiple foci of invasion arising from a gland crypt. The invasive islands are irregular in outline and partly show better differentiation than the overlying CIN. Haematoxylin and eosin × 42.

membrane, and Stage Ia2 encompasses the remaining lesions, which invade to between 3 and 5 mm.

For practical purposes it is advised that conservative treatment should only be contemplated where invasion is not greater than 3 mm from the nearest basement membrane and lymphatic channel involvement is not seen. Lesions larger than this, particularly when lymphatic channel involvement is seen, are probably best treated by radical hysterectomy.

Invasive squamous cell carcinoma

By the time they become clinically apparent most squamous cell carcinomas involve the external os and are visible on speculum examination. Some, however, remain entirely within the canal. These endocervical carcinomas can be very difficult to detect clinically. A squamous cell carcinoma may be either predominantly exophytic, growing out from the surface often as a papillary or polypoid excrescence, or mainly endophytic, infiltrating the surrounding structures. Ulceration and excavation are frequently seen.

The simplest and most widely used histological classification of squamous cell carcinoma subdivides the tumours into three groups: large-cell keratinizing; large-cell non-keratinizing; and small-cell non-keratinizing. These categories have been adopted by the World Health Organization. This classification depends on the histological cell type of the tumour, whereas from a clinical point of view, the grade (degree of differentiation) may be more important. Some so-called small-cell non-keratinizing carcinomas contain argyrophil cells and are akin to the small-cell anaplastic (oat cell) carcinoma of the bronchus with a correspondingly poor prognosis.

Invasive squamous cell carcinoma of the cervix infiltrates the tissue as irregular islands and cords of cells (Fig. 35.4). The intervening stroma often shows a dense chronic inflammatory reaction, representing an immune response by the host against the tumour.

Verrucous carcinoma is a rare variant of keratinizing squamous carcinoma. Progressive local invasion occurs but it rarely metastasizes to the lymphatic system. The relatively low mitotic rate in these tumours renders them rather resistant to radiotherapy. Surgery is therefore the treatment of choice.

Adenocarcinoma

Malignant tumours of glandular origin comprise 10–15% of cervical tumours. This figure is increasing, representing both an absolute increase in the number of cases of adenocarcinoma and an increase in the proportion of glandular tumours (Gallup & Abell 1977, Shingleton et al 1981).

Adenocarcinoma-in-situ was reported over 30 years ago and is being seen with increasing frequency. Microscopically, adenocarcinoma-in-situ generally retains the architectural pattern of the normal endocervical crypts, replacing the normal epithelium with an atypical epithelium showing loss of polarity, increased nuclear size, nuclear pleomorphism and anisokaryosis, mitotic activity, reduction in cytoplasmic mucin and, frequently, stratification (Fig. 35.5). The glandular abnormalities of the cervix appear to form a continuous spectrum of disease in exactly the same way as the squamous abnormalities. The less severe forms are referred to as glandular atypias, often divided into mild and severe.

A number of different histological patterns are found in invasive adenocarcinoma of the cervix. The endocervical type accounts for up to 90%. It is composed of crowded glands of variable size and shape, with budding and branching of the epithelium (Fig. 35.6), somewhat resem-

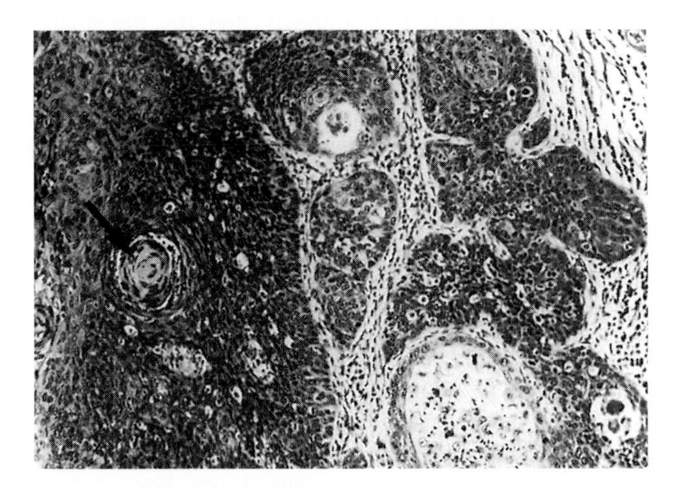

Fig. 35.4 Invasive squamous cell carcinoma. The invasive islands are composed of poorly differentiated cells, but an attempt at formation of a keratin pearl is marked by an arrow. Haematoxylin and eosin × 160.

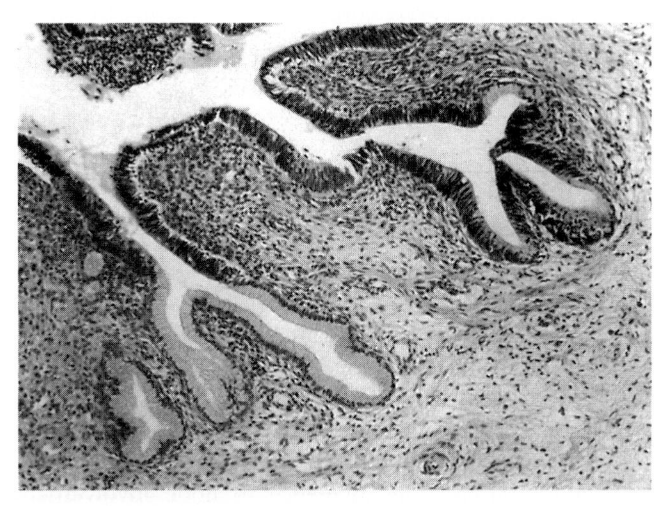

Fig. 35.5 Adenocarcinoma-in-situ. The abnormal epithelium follows the architectural outline of the normal crypts but the epithelium shows marked nuclear crowding, with loss of polarity and reduced mucin production. Haematoxylin and eosin × 160.

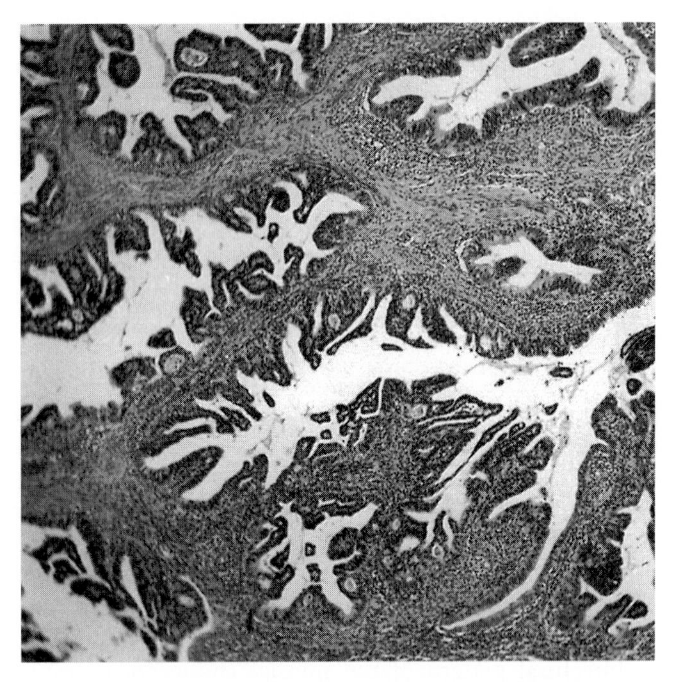

Fig. 35.6 Invasive adenocarcinoma of the cervix. Although the architectural pattern bears a superficial resemblance to normal cervical crypts, the pattern is excessively complex and papillary, with associated cellular abnormalities. Haematoxylin and eosin × 100.

bling that of normal endocervical epithelium. The terms 'adenoma malignum' and 'minimal deviation adenocarcinoma' have been used to describe a carcinoma in which the glandular pattern is particularly well differentiated and there is virtually no atypia of the epithelial cells. Tumours of endometrioid, clear cell, mucinous and papillary patterns are also seen.

NATURAL HISTORY

Carcinoma of the cervix spreads predominantly by either direct invasion or lymphatic permeation. The tumour may invade into the vaginal mucosa or into the myometrium of the lower uterine segment. Whereas spread into the parametrial tissues may occur as a continuous wave of infiltrating tumour, it is more common for there to be scattered foci of tumour in the parametrium, which only gradually become palpable as they coalesce.

Only 5% of small primary lesions which involve less than 20% of the cervix have histological evidence of parametrial disease, usually in parametrial nodes. In contrast, 48% of tumours invading more than 80% of the cervix are associated with parametrial extension, which is confluent in 23% (Burghardt et al 1988). If lymphatic spaces within the tumour are invaded, spread to the pelvic nodes may occur more often. The incidence of node involvement increases with the stage, grade and volume of the tumour (Table 35.1).

Survival following surgical treatment is closely related to the proportion of cervix involved. For example, 70% of patients with positive nodes survive for 5 years if the tumour invades less than 20% of the cervix, but only 54% survive if it involves more than 60% (Pickel et al 1988).

Table 35.1 Increased incidence of nodal metastases with increasing FIGO stage

	% Positive nodes	
FIGO stage	Pelvic	Para-aortic
Ib	16	7
II	30	16
III	44	35
IV	55	40

Forty percent of patients with carcinoma of the cervix die with uncontrolled pelvic disease leading to ureteric obstruction. Direct involvement of bone within the pelvis is common. Bloodstream metastases also occur, usually with poorly differentiated tumours and the higher stages of disease. The most common sites are the lungs, bones and liver.

STAGING

The FIGO classification is the most widely used (Table 35.2; FIGO 1995). It is recommended that bimanual examination under anaesthesia should be performed by more than one examiner. The intravenous urogram findings should be included, as should cystoscopy, but neither special imaging techniques nor subsequent operative findings alter the staging.

Surgical staging has been advocated, particularly to assess involvement of the para-aortic nodes. However, this delays the commencement of radiotherapy. The transperitoneal approach to the nodes, combined with radiotherapy, increases the incidence of bowel damage and is not recommended. The postoperative risk is less with a retroperitoneal approach, but it is unlikely that the information gained will lead to changes in management which will improve the prognosis. If para-aortic nodes are enlarged on imaging, fine-needle aspiration cytology may be performed under computerized tomography (CT) or ultrasound control without the need for surgery.

DIAGNOSIS AND INVESTIGATION

Presenting symptoms

The most common presenting features are postcoital or intermenstrual bleeding. A foul-smelling vaginal discharge may be the initial symptom. Anaemia may result from heavy vaginal bleeding. Pelvic and leg pain is uncommon in early tumours, but often occurs during later stages of the disease owing to spread to the pelvic side wall or invasion of the lumbosacral plexus.

Table 35.2 The FIGO staging classification for cervical cancer (FIGO 1995, Shepherd 1995)

Stage	Description
0	Preinvasive carcinoma (carcinoma-in-situ, CIN)
I	Carcinoma confined to the cervix (corpus extension should be disregarded)
Ia	Invasive cancer identified only microscopically. All gross lesions, even with superficial invasion, are Stage Ib cancers. Measured stromal depth should not be greater than 5 mm and no wider than 7 mm*
Ia1	Measured invasion no greater than 3 mm in depth and no wider than 7 mm
Ia2	Measured depth of invasion greater than 3 mm and no greater than 5 mm, and no wider than 7 mm
Ib	Clinical lesions confined to the cervix or preclinical lesions greater than Ia
Ib1	Clinical lesions no greater than 4 cm in size
Ib2	Clinical lesions greater than 4 cm in size
II	Carcinoma extending beyond the cervix and involving the vagina (but not the lower third) and/or infiltrating the parametrium (but not reaching the pelvic side wall)
IIa	Carcinoma has involved the vagina
IIb	Carcinoma has infiltrated the parametrium
III	Carcinoma involving the lower third of the vagina and/or extending to the pelvic side wall (there is no free space between the tumour and the pelvic side wall)
IIIa	Carcinoma involving the lower third of the vagina
IIIb	Carcinoma extending to the pelvic wall and/or hydronephrosis or non-functioning kidney due to ureterostenosis caused by tumour
IVa	Carcinoma involving the mucosa of the bladder or rectum and/or extending beyond the true pelvis
IVb	Spread to distant organs

*The depth of invasion should not be more than 5 mm from the base of the epithelium, either surface or glandular, from which it originates. Vascular space involvement, either venous or lymphatic, should not alter the staging

Tumours which spread into the bladder may cause haematuria or frequency of micturition. Spread of tumour into the rectum may cause tenesmus or rectal bleeding. Fistula formation may occur into either organ.

Clinical examination and initial investigations

The physical examination should include careful examination of the supraclavicular and inguinal nodes, and palpation of the abdomen for enlarged liver or kidneys. A preliminary speculum examination of the cervix should be performed prior to gentle digital examination. A smear may be taken from the cervix for cytology and a punch biopsy performed if there is an obvious lesion present. However, it should not be forgotten that the smear may be negative in the presence of invasive disease, and that a superficial biopsy may not confirm the diagnosis.

Bimanual examination may reveal a hard, friable, irregular, enlarged cervix which becomes fixed as the tumour spreads into the parametria. Rectovaginal examination is the best way of assessing parametrial and posterior spread. Mandatory investigations are a full blood count, urea and electrolytes, liver function tests, intravenous urogram and chest X-ray.

Examination under anaesthesia

Ideally, examination under anaesthesia should be performed by the gynaecologist and radiotherapist jointly. Rectovaginal examination is repeated in order to stage the tumour clinically. If there is any suspicion of rectal spread, proctoscopy and sigmoidoscopy are performed. Cystoscopy is not essential in patients who have early-stage disease, but must be performed if the disease appears locally advanced. Histological confirmation of the diagnosis is essential. Often parts of an exophytic tumour will detach easily from the cervix but if an adequate sample cannot be obtained in this way a wedge or cone biopsy should be obtained with a scalpel rather than using a small punch biopsy. The length of the uterine cavity is measured and curettings are taken from the endocervix and from the endometrial cavity.

Additional investigations

Other investigations may be performed but do not alter the FIGO staging of disease. Lymphangiography is not a routine test for staging. When assessed by surgical lymphadenectomy, lymphangiography correctly identified only 61% of women with positive nodes and 78% of those without nodal metastases (Lagasse et al 1979). Nodal disease was detected following lymphadenectomy in 21% of the women with negative lymphangiograms. Lymphangiography helps the planning of radiation fields and may be used to monitor the completeness of lymphadenectomy, but does not appear to be sufficiently accurate to be considered a routine diagnostic test.

CT scanning and abdominopelvic ultrasound may be used to estimate the size and extent of the primary tumour and to detect nodal disease. Neither is sufficiently accurate to merit routine use. The best imaging method is magnetic resonance imaging (MRI), especially when an endovaginal receiver coil is used (see Ch. 6). Although it gives reliable information about the primary tumour, MRI is unable to identify small metastatic deposits in lymph nodes.

TREATMENT

Microinvasive disease

No further treatment is required in young women if a colposcopically directed cone biopsy completely excises the lesion, if the depth of invasion is less than 3 mm, and if there is no marked lymph space involvement (Creasman et al 1985). However, in women who have completed their family a total hysterectomy is often performed. If marked lymphatic space involvement is present, or if invasion extends beyond 3 mm, there is a possibility of metastatic spread and more radical treatment should be considered.

In a report of the results of treatment of 200 cases of microinvasive disease as defined by FIGO in 1988, the recurrence rate was 3.5%, all being central recurrences (Oster & Rome 1994). Of these, 109 were cases of early stromal invasion of which two (1.8%) recurred, by comparison to five (5.5%) of the remainder, 23 of which had stromal invasion more than 3 mm. One (4.3%) of the 23 cases which would now be called Stage Ia2 recurred. There was one death from recurrent disease. However, only 23 of these 200 women were treated solely by cone biopsy; 101 underwent simple hysterectomy and the remainder were treated with radical hysterectomy or simple hysterectomy and lymphadenectomy, or some form of hysterectomy followed by radiotherapy.

Invasive cervical cancer

The definitive treatment for carcinoma of the cervix may involve either surgery or radiotherapy or a combination of both. Each patient should be staged and discussed jointly, although certain principles of management will develop in every unit. In many centres surgery is performed on the younger patient with lower-volume Stage Ib disease. This allows conservation of the ovaries, the preservation of a more normal vagina and avoidance of the long-term bowel and bladder sequelae sometimes seen after radiotherapy. Radiotherapy is used for older and less fit patients, regardless of the size of the tumour; for women with bulky Stage Ib and IIa tumours, or for more advanced disease.

Surgery

It is of great importance that the surgical procedure is carried out in a unit in which the Wertheim hysterectomy is regularly performed, as in less experienced hands this operation may be associated with mortality and considerable morbidity.

Preoperative care

It is not usually necessary to prepare the bowel rigorously, but a mild aperient and a small enema do ensure that the pelvis is not filled with distended loops of bowel and help to make the patient's first few postoperative days more comfortable. Cross-matching four units of blood is a sensible precaution as occasionally blood may be needed rapidly. A single dose of a broad-spectrum antibiotic given prophylactically with the premedication does reduce the risk of infective complications. Subcutaneous heparin must be started 8–24 hours prior to surgery and given in the dosage recommended for high-risk patients, 5000 IU tid.

Some patients may benefit especially from preoperative physiotherapy. This applies particularly to smokers. The anaesthetist should be consulted and warned about any potential difficulties. Epidural analgesia is a very valuable adjunct to the general anaesthetic, reducing blood loss and causing some constriction of the bowel, which thus occupies less space in the operative field. It may also be used to give postoperative analgesia.

The surgical procedure

Radical hysterectomy and pelvic lymphadenectomy. Either a high transverse or a midline incision may be used. In the former additional exposure is obtained by dividing the rectus muscles or their attachment to the pubic bone (Gleeson 1995).

The procedure commences with the lymphadenectomy. The role of lymphadenectomy is controversial. Whereas some believe it can be therapeutic, others regard it only as a means of refining the prognosis. The former group attempt a radical lymphadenectomy, but the latter are content to do no more than sample the nodes. Of those women treated surgically whose lymph nodes are positive at least 50% survive. Given that postoperative radiotherapy in this situation does not improve the prognosis (Morrow et al 1980, Fuller et al 1982), their survival can be attributed only to the complete surgical resection of metastatic disease. Because a sampling procedure is likely to miss at least 50% of positive nodes, radical resection of the pelvic lymph nodes is essential to maximize the removal of disease in the lymph nodes. The 5-year survival rate of patients with positive lymph nodes treated in the Hammersmith and the Samaritan hospitals is currently 72%.

The common iliac nodes are resected first and the dissection continues caudally until all of the iliac nodal groups have been resected (Figs 35.7 and 35.8). During the lymphadenectomy both ureters are reflected medially, attached to the parietal peritoneum. Any fixed and enlarged nodes are examined by frozen section. If they are positive the procedure is abandoned and the patient treated by irradiation. Resection of enlarged, mobile nodes should not preclude continuation of the procedure.

Following the lymphadenectomy the bladder is reflected inferiorly, the ureteric tunnels are defined and the uterine vessels divided (Fig. 35.9). The ureters are mobilized and reflected laterally by division of the small vessels running forwards to the bladder. The rectovaginal space is opened up and the rectum displaced posteriorly to define the uterosacral ligaments on each side of the rectum. These are divided as far posteriorly as possible. The cardinal ligaments and parametrial and paravaginal tissues are clamped and divided close to the pelvic side wall, taking care not to damage the internal iliac vein. In this way the uterus, cervix and upper third of the vagina are resected

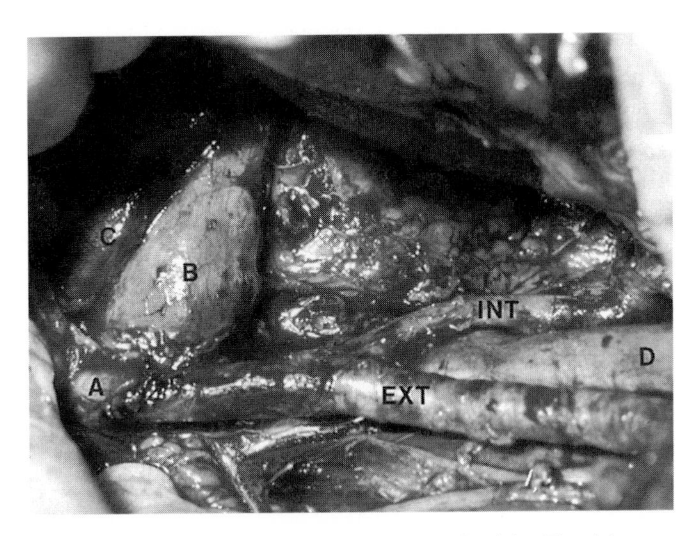

Fig. 35.7 The pelvis is viewed obliquely from the right. The right common iliac artery (A) is seen crossing over the left common iliac vein (B) as it runs behind the left common iliac artery (C). The right external iliac vein (D) can be seen first medial to the artery below the inguinal ligament. It then runs behind the common iliac artery and (not shown) joins the vena cava lateral to the artery. EXT, right external iliac artery; INT, right internal iliac artery.

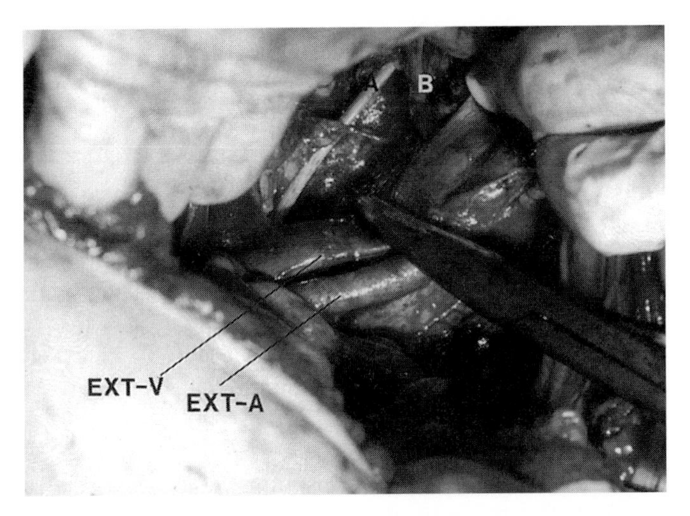

Fig. 35.8 The obturator nerve (A) and an abnormal obturator vein (B) are visible. EXT-A, right external iliac artery; EXT-V, right external iliac vein.

together with the related parametrial and uterosacral tissues. The more radical the resection of the parametria, the more common are postoperative voiding problems. This is why less radical procedures are sometimes adopted in patients with small lesions. Suction drains are inserted into the pelvis.

Radical trachylectomy. This new procedure removes the cervix and paracervical tissues but conserves the uterus. The objective is to give these women some chance of having children. A meticulous retroperitoneal lymph node dissection is performed as a separate, preliminary procedure and trachylectomy is undertaken at a later date

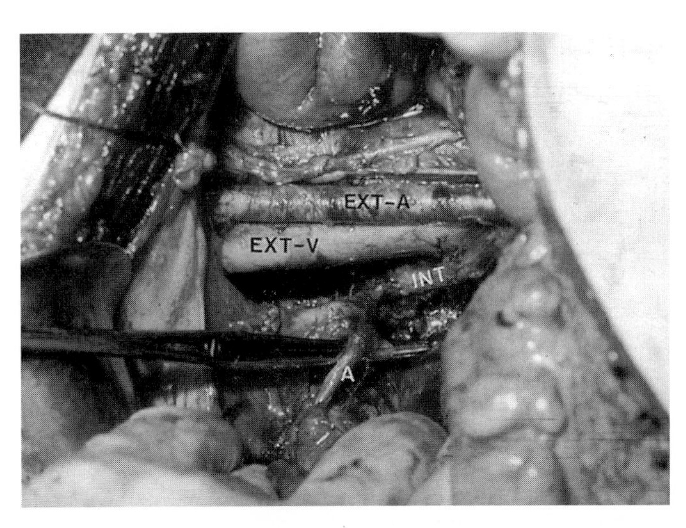

Fig. 35.9 Pelvis viewed from the left. The right uterine artery (A) is displayed by the forceps close to its origin from the internal iliac artery (INT). EXT-A, right external iliac artery; EXT-V, right external iliac vein.

only if careful examination of the lymph nodes confirms the absence of metastatic disease.

This procedure is suitable only for women with very early disease confined to the ectocervix, who are unlikely to have parametrial or lymph node metastases. The originator of this operation used laparoscopic retroperitoneal lymphadenectomy, but removed an average of only 13.4 nodes (D'Argent et al 1994). Of the 28 cases, 12 had microinvasive disease. After an average of 33 months follow-up one patient had died with para-aortic nodal disease and pulmonary metastases. Only 10 of the 28 women did not resume contraception and 11 pregnancies occurred in eight of the remaining patients, with five live births by caesarean section. There were two mid-trimester abortions and two premature deliveries. These results show that pregnancies are possible after radical trachylectomy, but more data are required on the mortality rate in what must be a very carefully selected group of low-risk women. This should still be regarded as an experimental technique.

Exenteration. Exenterative surgery – removing the bladder or rectum or both, together with the uterus – is usually reserved for women with a small central recurrence, usually following radiotherapy. The sooner the recurrence becomes evident after the initial therapy, the worse the prognosis and the less the likelihood of benefit from exenteration. Selective exenteration, conserving either bladder or rectum, is sometimes possible. With proper patient selection the results of exenterative surgery can be very worthwhile.

Postoperative care

The pulse and blood pressure must be monitored with

great care. The urinary output should exceed 30 ml/h and the intravenous fluids should be carefully adjusted to achieve this. Frusemide is rarely required. Any diminution in the urine output should be regarded as a possible sign of hypovolaemia due to occult blood loss, and the vital signs and peripheral circulation should be examined closely.

The drains should be kept in place until the loss is minimal. The urinary catheter is best left in situ until the patient is mobile. Thereafter, the residual urine volume should be checked by catheterizing the patient after she has 'emptied' her bladder herself. If the residual volume exceeds 100 ml, the bladder should be catheterized intermittently and the patient taught to do this herself so that if the problem does not resolve rapidly she may be discharged to continue self-catheterization at home. Alternatively, a suprapubic catheter may be used for postoperative bladder drainage. This is clamped when the patient is ready to begin attempting micturition, and the residual urine volumes may be measured via the suprapubic catheter.

The patient should be encouraged to mobilize as soon as possible, by both nursing staff and physiotherapist. As her general condition improves, opportunities should be created to allow her to discuss her feelings and her fears for the future. The effect of her illness and the operation upon her life, both at home and at work, and upon her self-image and sexuality, is a topic she may well wish to talk about. Experienced, caring nursing staff have a particularly important role in this aspect of her recovery.

Complications of surgery

The immediate complications of surgery include haemorrhage and damage to the urinary or intestinal tracts. Lacerations of the main pelvic veins or the vena cava will require careful repair with fine prolene or vicryl sutures. Vascular clamps may be invaluable. Ligation of one or both internal iliac arteries may be required, but the results of this procedure are often disappointing. Pressure with a hot pack for 2 minutes controls the bleeding in most cases, and allows preparation to be made for a further attempt to deal with the problem. Often, the field is cleared and the loss reduced by this manoeuvre sufficiently to expose the lacerated vessel. Prompt replacement of blood loss is essential, and fresh frozen plasma should be given if more than four units of blood are required. If postoperative bleeding occurs the site should be identified with arteriography as bleeding from pelvic vessels can be arrested by selective arterial embolization. Damage to ureter, bladder or bowel seldom gives rise to problems, provided it is recognized and repaired at the time.

The most feared postoperative complication is pulmonary embolism. There may be no evidence of a deep venous thrombosis in the legs, the clot having arisen in the pelvic veins. If there is any doubt about the diagnosis a ventilation perfusion (VQ) scan should be performed as an emergency, but heparin therapy should be started whenever there is strong clinical suspicion. In the absence of a pulmonary embolism it is probably wise to obtain confirmatory evidence before starting therapy for a suspected deep venous thrombosis.

Ureteric and bladder fistulae follow 1–2% of Wertheim hysterectomies. A trial of conservative management is sometimes worthwhile, but the patients usually prefer to opt for early surgical repair. Far more common than ureteric fistulae is the atonic bladder, with loss of bladder sensation. This almost invariably rectifies itself in time, but some women do need to undertake intermittent self-catheterization for several months.

Results of surgery

The overall 5-year survival rate after surgery for Stage Ib cervical carcinoma is around 82% (Monaghan et al 1990, FIGO 1995). For node-negative patients it is 87–91% and for node-positive women 51–67%.

Combinations of surgery and radiotherapy

If multiple lymph nodes are found to be involved histologically, or if the resection margins were narrow, postoperative radiotherapy should be considered. There is little evidence that radiotherapy increases survival in this situation but it may reduce the incidence of pelvic failure. Morrow reported that 84% of the recurrences in non-irradiated cases were found in the pelvis, compared with 50% in irradiated cases (Morrow et al 1980).

In spite of radical surgery radiotherapy can be given safely, but the dose is usually limited to 4500 cGy in 24 fractions over 5 weeks.

Preoperative intracavitary therapy is sometimes given but there is no evidence that this improves survival. Doses of 3500 cGy to point A are given in one or two low-dose rate insertions and surgery is performed 3–4 weeks later.

Radiotherapy

Radiotherapy for carcinoma of the cervix is given by intracavitary and external beam irradiation. The rapid fall-off in dose from intracavitary therapy gives effective treatment to the cervix and surrounding tissues, but the small bowel, rectum and bladder receive a relatively low dose.

External beam treatment is used to control spread within the pelvis, particularly to lymph nodes, and contributes to primary tumour control. As the disease becomes more advanced the balance between intracavitary and external beam treatment alters. Although it is possible to manage early-stage disease by intracavitary treatment alone, more advanced disease requires the combination of both techniques.

Intracavitary therapy

More details of intracavitary therapy are given in Chapter 33. Hollow radio-opaque intrauterine and intravaginal tubes, which act as carriers of the radioactive material, are placed in the uterine cavity and the vaginal fornices under general anaesthesia (Fig. 35.10). These afterloading systems allow the applicators to be positioned accurately before the radioactive sources are inserted, and avoid exposing theatre staff to unnecessary radiation. The sources may then be inserted either manually or remotely using a semi- or fully automated device, so that staff exposure is minimal or zero. High- or low-energy sources may be used (see Ch. 33) .

The dose is expressed at representative points in the pelvis. Point A is defined as the point 2 cm lateral to the central uterine canal and 2 cm above the external cervical os. This point is considered to lie in the paracervical region close to the uterine artery and the ureter. Point B is 5 cm lateral to the central uterine canal and 2 cm above the cervical os. The dose to point B is usually about one-third of the dose given to point A, owing to the rapid fall-off in dosage with intracavitary insertions.

In the Manchester system, 6600–7600 cGy were prescribed to point A in two treatments each lasting 70 hours 4–7 days apart. The currently used Amersham system is a modification of this technique. Various improvements have been implemented which allow for better staff protection and better geometrical arrangements of the radioactive sources.

If intracavitary irradiation is to be the only modality of treatment, a dose of 8000 cGy is given to point A in three insertions, with an interval of 1 week between each insertion. Following external beam therapy a dose of 2000–2500 cGy is given to point A in a single insertion.

Patients with small-volume Stage I tumours are treated by intracavitary treatment alone, but more advanced disease requires a combination of an intracavitary dose and external beam therapy. The rationale for the different techniques is that the risk of lymph node involvement increases with the size of the tumour and the proportion of cervix involved.

External beam therapy

External beam therapy is normally given first because it

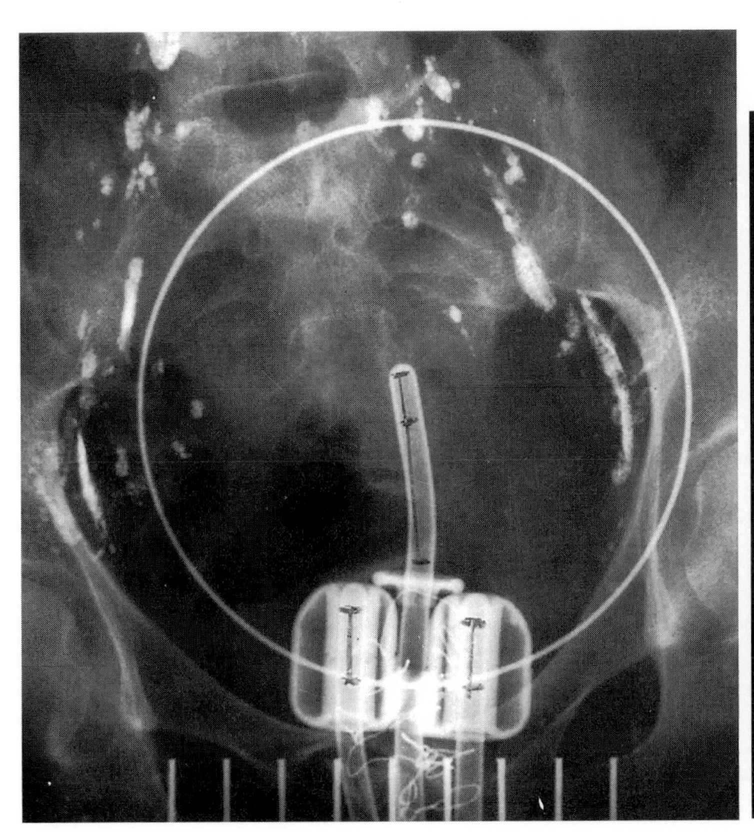

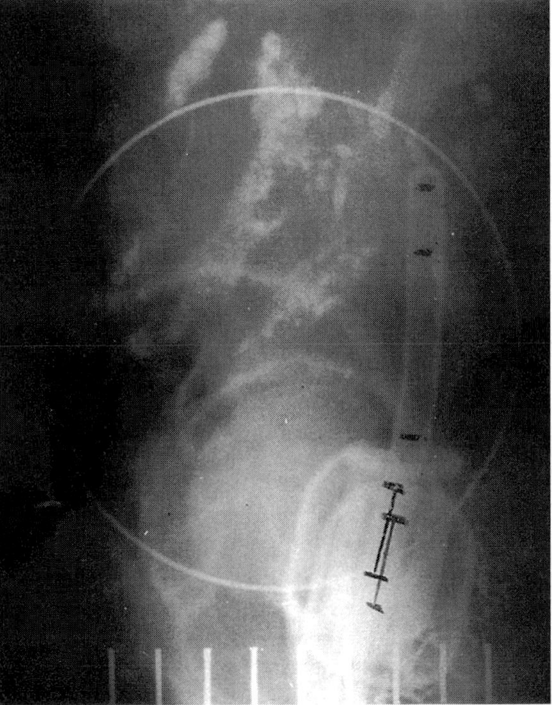

Fig. 35.10 These X-rays show an Amersham tube and ovoids in position. Contrast material from a previous lymphangiography can be seen in the lymph nodes.

shrinks the tumour mass, thus allowing a more satisfactory dose distribution from the intracavitary sources. A homogeneous dose of radiation is given to the pelvis through either three or four fields. The treatment volume extends from the junction between L4 and L5 to cover the common iliac nodes, to the lower border of the obturator foramen radiologically or the lower margin of the pubic symphysis by palpation. If the disease extends down the vagina the lower border must be taken to the introitus, which must be defined with a marker placed at a vaginal examination with the patient in the treatment position. The lateral margins of the field should lie 1 cm outside the bony margins of the pelvis.

The radiotherapy apparatus used is most commonly a linear accelerator working at an energy of 4 million electronvolts (MeV) or greater. A cobalt unit may be used, but gives a less satisfactory dose at depth and less well defined field margins. The dose to the rectum must not exceed 6000 cGy. The dose given to the pelvis varies depending upon the stage of the disease. Stage IIb–IVa cases receive 5000 cGy to the whole pelvis in 25 fractions in 5 weeks. If bulky disease is present in one parametrium a further 500 cGy may be given in 3–5 fractions to this area. Following this a caesium insertion is performed and a further 2000 cGy given to point A. If an insertion is not possible, the central dose may be taken to 5500–6000 cGy using external beam therapy alone.

About 35% of stage III patients have involved para-aortic nodes. However, it is difficult to assess the nodes accurately and to treat involved nodes effectively. Piver and Barlow (1977) treated biopsy-positive para-aortic nodes with more than 5500 cGy; 20% of patients died of the complications of treatment, usually small bowel stenosis. If para-aortic node treatment is contemplated lymphography or CT scanning should be performed, with directed fine-needle aspiration of suspicious nodes. In patients with disease outside the pelvis (Stage IVb), the treatment should be directed to relieving symptoms. If pelvic symptoms such as bleeding or offensive discharge are predominant, palliative treatment may be given to a small volume using opposed fields and giving a 3000 cGy midline dose in six treatments over 3 weeks. If pain is due to para-aortic node spread into the underlying vertebrae, palliative radiotherapy can be given but a high dose (5000 cGy midline dose in 5 weeks) is needed for control. If there is bone pain due to bloodborne metastases, a 1-week course of palliative radiotherapy may be given to a dose of 2500–3000 cGy in five treatments.

Results of radiotherapy

Tumour bulk and clinical stage are major predictors of the response to treatment, but squamous carcinomas and adenocarcinomas have a similar prognosis (Table 35.3). Substantial tumour regression during external beam therapy predicts a high chance of local tumour control and survival. If at the time of intracavitary treatment substantial tumour is still present, surgery or chemotherapy should be considered.

Table 35.3 Results of treatment by radiotherapy (Davidson et al 1989)

FIGO stage	5-year survival (%) Squamous carcinoma	Adenocarcinoma
I	79.9	81.8
II	61.9	65.9
III	39.9	29.8
IV	14.3	21.0
All stages	54.6	54.0

Radiotherapy complications

During radiotherapy most patients will suffer from diarrhoea. A low-residue diet is suggested and antidiarrhoeals such as Lomotil, codeine phosphate or loperamide are prescribed. The radiation reaction usually settles down within 2–3 weeks of completion of all therapy, but a minority of patients will continue to need antidiarrhoeal drugs.

If diarrhoea is associated with colicky pain or nausea, the possibility of small bowel damage must be considered and the treatment suspended. Treatment may be restarted at a lower daily dose, but if the problem persists radiotherapy may have to be abandoned.

Acute urinary symptoms are less common. If they are a problem, infection must be excluded. Occasionally anticholinergic agents may be helpful.

Late complications are related to dose and to pre-existing problems. Some 5–10% of patients develop long-term problems, which are usually related to the small or large bowel but may involve the urinary tract. These include subacute obstruction, diarrhoea due to radiation colitis, and haematuria due to radiation cystitis. The symptoms are often quite mild. Patients at high risk of developing radiation complications are those with poor nutritional status and recent weight loss, previous pelvic or abdominal surgery, severe vascular disease or pelvic inflammatory disease.

Complications may develop at any time after treatment, but symptoms of bowel damage occur on average after about 10 months and bladder symptoms after 22 months. Bowel and bladder symptoms should always be investigated, and it must not be assumed that they are due to recurrent malignant disease.

Management of complications must be individualized and early detection is of the greatest importance. Small bowel obstruction following radiotherapy should be managed conservatively only in its initial stages. If prolonged or repeated episodes occur, surgical intervention is imperative. Rectosigmoid constriction can normally be diagnosed from the clinical history and readily confirmed by barium studies. It can be managed without the need for a permanent colostomy in the majority of patients.

Vesicovaginal fistulae will occasionally occur in patients who have been treated entirely appropriately. Repair of such fistulae involves the provision of an alternative blood supply to the area, by either omental or myocutaneous grafting.

Chemotherapy

Radiotherapy and surgery are the only modalities that can cure cervical cancer, but chemotherapy can cause tumour regression. Single agents that have significant response rates include cisplatin, bleomycin and methotrexate. Combination regimens have been developed using these drugs and, as with ovarian cancer, cisplatin combinations appear to have the highest response rates.

The combination of 'neoadjuvant' chemotherapy and radiotherapy has not resulted in improved survival, as a good response to chemotherapy seems to occur only in women who also respond well to radiotherapy (Vermorken 1993). Combination of chemotherapy with surgery has given some very encouraging results but no randomized trials have reported yet.

SPECIAL TREATMENT PROBLEMS

Carcinoma of the cervical stump

Subtotal hysterectomy is not performed often, but this problem may occur in older patients. External beam radiotherapy to the usual dose should be given if bowel tolerance allows. To obtain a satisfactory dose, a medium caesium tube should be inserted together with ovoids. If this is not possible the external beam dose must be increased. The results are comparable with those in patients with an intact uterus.

Carcinoma after simple hysterectomy

Invasive carcinoma may be found after a hysterectomy for presumed preinvasive disease, or when cervical pathology was not suspected. The management and prognosis depend on the true stage of disease before the operation. If the patient was carefully evaluated before surgery and the invasive lesion was a small Ib tumour, the prognosis is good (Heller et al 1986). In studies where the outcome is poor, it is likely that the original lesion extended outside the cervix (Kinney et al 1992, Bissett et al 1994).

A 5-year survival of 82% may be achieved with radical parametrectomy, upper vaginectomy and pelvic lymphadenectomy (Kinney et al 1992). Alternatively, pelvic irradiation may be given to a dose of 4500 cGy in 5 weeks, followed by vault irradiation. Provided the lesion was originally Stage Ib, this offers a 5-year survival of 78%, similar to that for patients treated with an intact uterus (Heller et al 1986).

Table 35.4 The management of cervical cancer during pregnancy

Trimester	Stage I	Stages II–IV
First	Wertheim's hysterectomy	Vaginal termination & radiation
Second	Termination of pregnancy by hysterotomy & Wertheim's hysterectomy	Prostaglandin termination & radiotherapy
Third	Caesarean at 34/52 & Wertheim's hysterectomy	Caesarean at 34/52; start radiotherapy after 10 days

Carcinoma of the cervix during pregnancy

Management will depend on the stage at diagnosis, the gestational age and the wishes and beliefs of the patient and her partner (Table 35.4). When fetal survival is desired, delivery should be delayed until the fetus is mature rather than just potentially viable. The prognosis does not seem to be affected adversely by the pregnancy in women with early-stage disease (Van der Vange et al 1995).

Haemorrhage

If a patient presents with massive bleeding, bed rest and vaginal packing may arrest the haemorrhage. If this is not successful, treatment should begin with an intracavitary application giving 2000 cGy to point A. The haemoglobin in such a patient, and in any other, should always be restored to above 12 g/dl, as patients with a haemoglobin of less than that have a poorer survival.

Recurrence after radiotherapy

The patient should be assessed jointly with a gynaecological oncologist to ensure that the possibility of surgical salvage is not overlooked. The prognosis for those few women with central pelvic recurrence alone is relatively good with exenterative procedures, and such women should be carefully assessed and considered for such procedures in recognized gynaecological oncology units.

FOLLOW-UP

The continuing follow-up of these patients is of great importance to evaluate results, provide reassurance and to give symptomatic relief to those whose treatment has failed. It is recommended that there should be 3-monthly follow-up for 3 years, 6-monthly follow-up for 2 years and annual visits thereafter.

Counselling should be provided to support the patient throughout her treatment and help her to cope with all aspects of readjustment, including prevention of the sexual problems that tend to develop in these women and their partners. Premenopausal patients will have suffered functional ovarian ablation and may be treated with hormone replacement therapy if they are troubled by menopausal symptoms. Younger patients with a good prognosis should be encouraged to take hormone replacement therapy to reduce the risk of osteoporosis and cardiovascular disease. Hormone therapy should always include progestins if the patient has been treated by radiotherapy and retains her uterus. The endometrium is very resistant to radiotherapy (Habeshaw & Pinion 1992), and endometrial carcinoma may develop if unopposed oestrogens are given.

Radiotherapy will cause the vagina to contract, and it is important to remind patients who were sexually active to try and resume activity, often with the help of lubricants, within a couple of months of the completion of treatment. Dilators can be used to maintain vaginal patency. Patients need to be reassured that coitus will not cause the tumour to become active and that the cancer cannot be communicated to their partner.

KEY POINTS

1. In England and Wales the incidence of cervical cancer has been rising in the younger age groups. In 1989 36% of cases were in women aged less than 45 years.
2. The cause remains unknown, but is related in some way to sexual intercourse. HPV is thought to be implicated, but other factors are also required.
3. Conservative treatment of microinvasive lesions should only be considered where invasion is not greater than 3 mm from the nearest basement membrane and lymphatic channel involvement is not seen.
4. Squamous cell carcinoma is the most common type and has a similar prognosis to adenocarcinoma. Undifferentiated tumours have a poor prognosis.
5. Metastatic spread is mainly lymphatic, and involvement of the parametria is initially focal rather than confluent.
6. The size of the primary tumour and the proportion of the cervix it occupies are the most important indications of prognosis after the status of the lymph nodes.
7. Overall, 42% of women with cervical cancer die within 5 years.
8. Examination under anaesthesia is an essential step in determining the extent of disease, and in deciding on the optimum method of therapy.
9. Magnetic resonance imaging gives the best estimate of the size of the tumour but is not reliable in identifying nodal disease.
10. Surgery is most often performed on the younger patient with lower-volume Stage Ib disease.
11. Radiotherapy is used for older and less fit patients, regardless of the size of the tumour, for women with bulky Stage Ib and IIa tumours, or for more advanced disease.

REFERENCES

Bauer H M, Ting T, Chambero J C, Toschiro C T, Chimaro J et al 1991 Genital human papillomavirus infection in general university students as determined by PCR-based method. Journal of the American Medical Association 265: 472–477

Beral V, Hannaford P, Kay C 1988 Oral contraceptive use and malignancies of the genital tract: results from the Royal College of General Practitioners' oral contraception study. Lancet ii: 1331–1335

Bissett D, Lamont D W, Nwabineli N J, Brodie M M, Symonds R P 1994 The treatment of stage I carcinoma of the cervix in the west of Scotland 1980–1987. British Journal of Obstetrics and Gynaecology 101: 615–620

Buckley J D, Harris R W C, Doll R, Vessey M P, Willlams P T 1981 Case-control study of the husbands of women with dysplasia or carcinoma of the cervix uteri. Lancet ii: 1010–1014

Burghardt E, Haas J, Girardi F 1988 The significance of the parametrium in the operative treatment of cervical cancer. In: Burghardt E, Monaghan J M (eds) Operative treatment of cervical cancer. Clinical Obstetrics and Gynaecology, vol 2. Baillière Tindall, London, pp 879–888

Creasman W T, Fetter B F, Clarke-Pearson D L, Kaufmann L, Parker R T 1985 Management of stage Ia carcinoma of the cervix. American Journal of Obstetrics and Gynecology 153: 164–172

Cuzick J, Szarewski A, Terry G et al 1995 Human papillomavirus testing in primary cervical screening. Lancet 345: 1533–1536

D'Argent D, Brun J L, Roy M, Mathevet P, Remy I 1994 La trachélectomie élargie (TE): une alternative à l'hystérectomie radicale dans le traitment des cancers infiltrants développés sur la face externe du col utérin. Journal Obstetrique et Gynaecologique 2: 285–292

Dattoli M J, Gretz H F, Beller U et al 1989 Analysis of multiple prognostic factors in patients with stage Ib cervical cancer: age as a major determinant. International Journal of Radiation Oncology Biology and Physics 17: 41–47

Davidson S E, Symonds R P, Lamont D, Watson E R 1989 Does adenocarcinoma of uterine cervix have a worse prognosis than squamous carcinoma when treated by radiotherapy? Gynecologic Oncology 33: 23–26

Fairley C K, Chen S, Ugoni A, Tabrizi S N, Forbes A, Garland S M 1994 Human papillomavirus infection and its relationship to recent and distant sexual partners. Obstetrics and Gynecology 84: 755–759

FIGO 1995 Annual report on the results of treatment in gynaecological cancer, vol 22. International Federation of Gynaecology and Obstetrics, Stockholm

Fuller A F, Elliott N E, Kosloff C, Lewis J L 1982 Lymph node metastases from carcinoma of the cervix, Stages Ib and IIa:

implications for prognosis and treatment. Gynecological Oncology 13: 165–174
Gallup D G, Abell M R 1977 Invasive adenocarcinoma of the uterine cervix. Obstetrics and Gynecology 49: 596–603
Gleeson N C 1995 A modification of the Cherney incision in gynaecological oncology surgery. British Journal of Obstetrics and Gynaecology 102: 925–926
Griffiths M 1991 Nuns, virgins and spinsters. Rigoni–Stern and cervical cancer revisited. British Journal of Obstetrics and Gynaecology 98: 797–802
Habeshaw T, Pinion S B 1992 The incidence of persistent functioning endometrial tissue following successful radiotherapy for cervical carcinoma. International Journal of Gynecological Cancer 2: 332–335
Harris R W C, Briton L A, Cowdell R H et al 1980 Characteristics of women with dysplasia or carcinoma in situ of the cervix. British Journal of Cancer 42: 359–369
Heller P B, Barnhill D R, Mayer A R, Fontaine T P, Hoskins W J, Park R C 1986 Cervical carcinoma found incidentally in a uterus removed for benign indications. Obstetrics and Gynecology 67: 187–190
Howley P M, Schlegel R 1988 The human papillomaviruses. American Journal of Medicine 85: 155–158
Kessler I 1984 Natural history and epidemiology of cervical cancer with special reference to the role of herpes genitalis. In: McBrien D C H, Slater T F (eds) Cancer of the uterine cervix. Academic Press, London, pp 31–37
Kinney W K, Egorshin E V, Ballard D L, Podratz K C 1992 Long-term survival and sequelae after surgical management of invasive cervical carcinoma diagnosed at the time of simple hysterectomy. Gynecologic Oncology 44: 24–27
Lagasse L D, Ballon S C, Berman M L, Watring W G 1979 Pretreatment lymphangiography and operative evaluation in carcinoma of the cervix. American Journal of Obstetrics and Gynecology 134: 219–224
Ley C, Bauer H M, Reingold A et al 1991 Determinants of genital human papillomavirus infection in young women. Journal of the National Cancer Institution 83: 997–1003
Meanwell C A, Kelly K A, Wilson S et al 1988 Young age as a prognostic factor in cervical cancer: analysis of population based data from 10 022 cases. British Medical Journal 296: 386–391
Melkert P W, Hopman E, van den Brule A N et al 1993 Prevalence of HPV in cytomorphologically normal cervical smears, as determined by the polymerase chain reaction, is age dependent. International Journal of Cancer 53: 919–923
Monaghan J M, Ireland D, Mor-Yosef S, Pearson S E, Lopes A, Sinha D P 1990 Role of centralisation of surgery in Stage Ib carcinoma of the cervix: a review of 498 cases. Gynecological Oncology 37: 206–209
Morrow C P, Shingleton H M, Austin M J et al 1980 Is pelvic radiation beneficial in the postoperative management of stage Ib squamous cell carcinoma of the cervix with pelvic node metastases treated by radical hysterectomy and pelvic lymphadenectomy. Gynecologic Oncology 10: 105–110
Muller M, Viscidi R P, Ulken V et al 1995 Antibodies to the E4, E6, and E7 proteins of the human papillomavirus type 16 in patients with HPV associated diseases and in the normal population. Journal of Investigative Dermatology 104: 138–141
Muñoz N, Bosch F X, de Sanjosé S et al 1992 The causal link between human papillomavirus and invasive cervical cancer: a population-based case-control study in Colombia and Spain. International Journal of Cancer 52: 743–749
Office of Population Censuses and Surveys 1985 Cancer statistics: registrations in England and Wales 1981. MBI no. 13. HMSO, London
Office of Population Censuses and Surveys 1987 Cancer statistics: registrations in England and Wales 1983. MBI no. 15. HMSO, London
Office of Population Censuses and Surveys 1990 Cancer statistics: registrations in England and Wales 1985. MB1 no. 18. HMSO, London
Office of Population Censuses and Surveys 1994 Cancer statistics: registrations in England and Wales 1989. MBI no. 22. HMSO, London
Oster A G, Rome R M 1994 Microinvasive squamous cell carcinoma of the cervix: a clinico-pathological study of 200 cases with long-term follow-up. International Journal of Gynecological Cancer 4: 257–264
Pickel H, Haas J, Lahousen M 1988 Prognostic factors in cervical cancer on the basis of morphometric evaluation. In: Burghardt E, Monaghan J M (eds) Operative treatment of cervical cancer. Clinical Obstetrics and Gynaecology, vol 2. Baillière Tindall, London, pp 805–816
Piver M S, Barlow J Jr 1977 High dose irradiation to biopsy confirmed aortic node metastases from carcinoma of the uterine cervix. Gynecologic Oncology 3: 168–175
Rotkin I D 1973 A comparison review of key epidemiological studies in cervical cancer related to current searches for transmissible agents. Cancer Research 33: 1353–1367
Sasieni P, Cuzick J, Farmery E 1995 Accelerated decline in cervical cancer mortality in England and Wales. Lancet 346: 1566–1567
Schiffman M H, Bauer H M, Hoover R N et al 1993 Epidemiological evidence showing that human papillomavirus infection causes most cervical intraepithelial neoplasia. Journal of the National Cancer Institute 85: 958–964
Schneider A, Kirchhoff T, Meinhardt G, Gissmann L 1992 Repeated evaluation of human papillomavirus 16 status in cervical swabs of young women with a history of normal Papanicolaou smears. Obstetrics and Gynecology 79: 683–688
Shepherd J H 1995 Staging announcement – FIGO staging of gynaecological cancers; cervical and vulval. International Journal of Gynecological Cancer 5: 319
Shingleton H M, Gore H, Bradley D H, Soong S J 1981 Adenocarcinoma of the cervix. 1. Clinical evaluation and pathologic features. American Journal of Obstetrics and Gynecology 139: 799–814
Van der Vange N, Weverling G J, Ketting B W, Ankum W M, Samlal R, Lammes F B 1995 The prognosis of cervical cancer associated with pregnancy: a matched cohort study. Obstetrics and Gynecology 85: 1022–1026
Vermorken J B 1993 The role of chemotherapy in squamous cell carcinoma of the uterine cervix: a review. International Journal of Gynecological Cancer 3: 129–142
zur Hausen H 1994 Disrupted dichotomous intracellular control of human papillomavirus infection in cancer of the cervix. Lancet 343: 955–957

36

Benign disease of the vulva and vagina

W. P. Soutter

VULVA

INTRODUCTION

This chapter will be confined to a discussion of benign conditions and mention of malignant or premalignant disease will be made only in relation to differential diagnosis or management. Premalignant disease is discussed in Chapter 34 and invasive disease in Chapter 37. Similarly, only passing mention is made of sexually transmitted diseases, which are described in Chapter 56. Space does not permit an exhaustive description of all of the many conditions which may affect the vulva. Instead, the emphasis is on common or important conditions (not always the same thing), with the intention of providing the reader with a sound framework upon which to build. More information may be obtained from the excellent books by Dr Marjorie Ridley (1988) and by the late Dr Eduard Friedrich (1983).

Patients with vulval symptoms are frequently met in gynaecological practice. The complaint is often long-standing and distressing, and frequently induces a feeling of despair in both patient and doctor. A careful, sympathetic approach and a readiness to consult colleagues in other disciplines are essential. Even when it seems that no specific therapy can be offered, many patients are helped by the knowledge that there is no serious underlying pathology and by a supportive attitude.

ANATOMY AND HISTOLOGY

The vulva includes the mons pubis, the labia majora and minora, the clitoris, the vestibule of the vagina, the bulb of the vestibule and the greater vestibular glands (Bartholin's).

The mons pubis is a pad of fat anterior to the pubic symphysis and covered by hair-bearing skin. The labia majora extend posteriorly from the mons on either side of the pudendal cleft into which the urethra and vagina open. They merge with one another and the perineal skin anterior to the anus. They consist largely of areolar tissue and fat. The skin on their lateral aspects is pigmented and covered with crisp hairs. On the medial side the skin is smooth and has many sebaceous glands. The labia minora are small folds of skin which lie between the labia majora and which divide anteriorly to envelop the clitoris. The medial surfaces contain many sebaceous glands. The clitoris is an erectile structure analogous to the glans penis. Partly hidden by the anterior folds of the labia minora, the clitoris consists of a body of two corpora cavernosa lying side by side and connected to the pubic and ischial rami, and a glans of sensitive, spongy erectile tissue. The vestibule is that area between the labia minora into which the urethra and vagina open. The bulbs of the vestibule lie on either side of the vaginal opening and are elongated masses of erectile tissue. The greater vestibular glands lie posterior to the bulbs of the vestibule and are connected to the surface by short ducts.

HISTORY

The duration of the complaint, details of the onset and any precipitating factors must be elicited. Information about the treatments used so far is important, as many of these women will have already begun to use a variety of local preparations, some of which may be potentially harmful. The use of deodorants, bath gels, biological washing powders or shampoos may cause an allergic or irritation eczema. Wearing tight clothing, particularly nylon materials, may exacerbate the problem. Depression may be a result of the vulval condition rather than the cause, but it will still require treatment. A history of other illnesses or drug treatment may be relevant. The patient should be asked about other skin complaints. Sometimes a further line of enquiry is suggested by the findings on examination.

EXAMINATION

An examination for evidence of systemic disease or of a generalized skin condition is advisable. Pelvic and vaginal examination should be performed unless the patient is too uncomfortable to allow it. Cervical cytology and colposcopic examination of the cervix and vagina may be useful, and are mandatory if the vulval condition is thought to be premalignant. The vulva should be examined in a good light, preferably under low magnification. The colposcope is not ideal for this because of the narrow field of view, but it is often the best available option. Gentle pressure with a cotton-tipped applicator should be applied to erythematous areas to detect increased tenderness.

It is important to take biopsies liberally. These can readily be performed under local anaesthesia (Fig. 36.1) using a disposable 4 mm Stiefel biopsy punch or a Keyes punch. Silver nitrate or Monsel's solution will control the small amount of bleeding which results.

PRURITUS VULVAE

The term 'pruritus vulvae' properly refers to vulval irritation for which no cause can be found. In practice, many

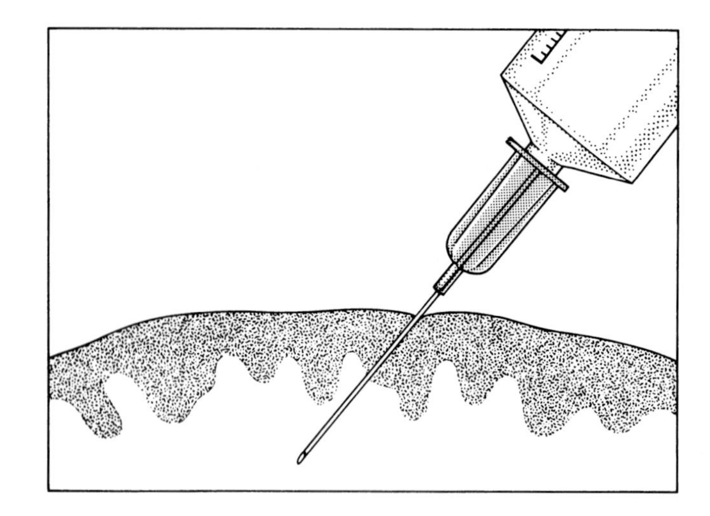

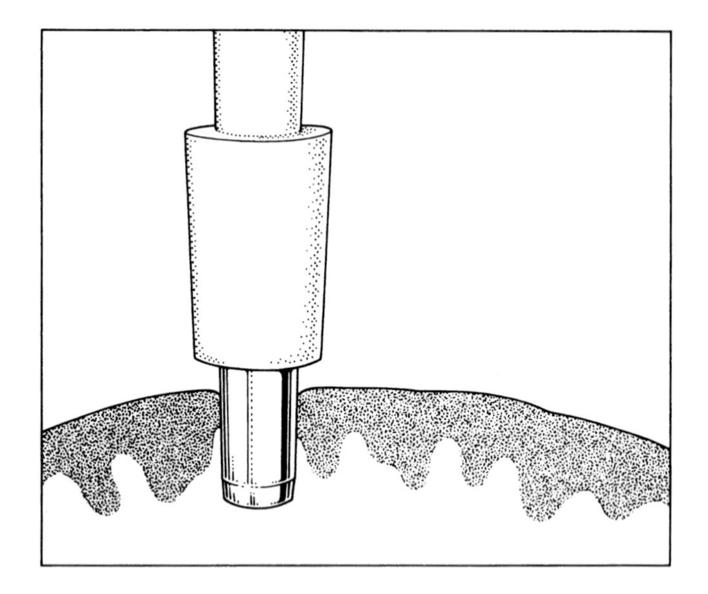

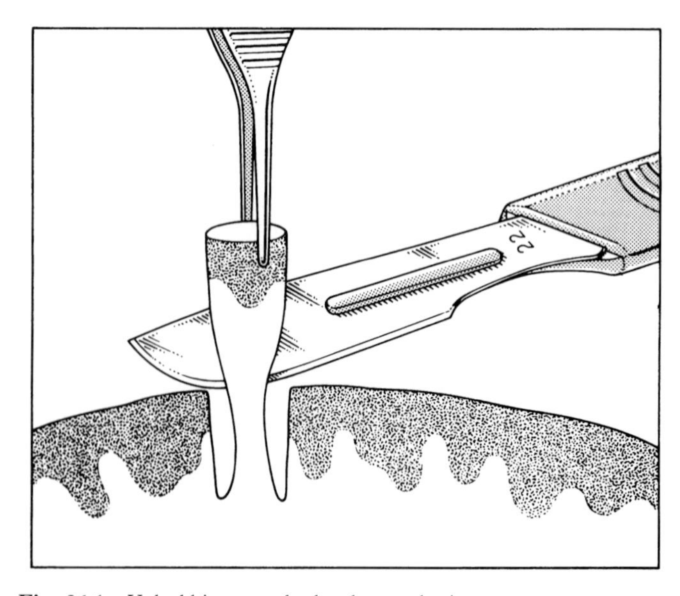

Fig. 36.1 Vulval biopsy under local anaesthesia.

gynaecologists use the term to describe this upsetting symptom regardless of whether or not a cause is evident. It should be distinguished from the burning sensation described by some women and discussed later.

Pruritus vulvae is commoner in older women and is most frequently encountered after the age of 40. The most common causes are lichen sclerosus and eczema due to an allergy or exposure to an irritant substance. Evidence of the latter is often obscured by the secondary effects of scratching – a thickening and whitening of the skin. The scratching initiates a vicious cycle, exacerbating the irritation and stimulating more scratching.

A vaginal discharge may give rise to vulval irritation. The discharge may be due to infection but some women seem to experience a profuse physiological discharge. Cautery of the cervix often gives disappointing results in such cases. A bland barrier ointment such as zinc and castor oil is sometimes useful in this situation. Threadworm infestation is very common in children and will cause pruritus ani and vulval irritation. Atrophic vaginitis responds to hormone replacement.

Occasionally a systemic illness may cause pruritus vulvae. Diabetes, uraemia and liver failure and low ferritin levels are all possible causes to consider.

If no specific cause is found, steps must be taken to remove any possible source of irritation or allergy. Vulval deodorants and perfumed additions to the bath water must be avoided. Simple, unperfumed soap should be used for vulval hygiene and for washing underwear. After washing, the vulva must be dried carefully and gently – if necessary a hair drier set at a low heat can be used. Loose-fitting cotton clothing should be worn to allow the evaporation of sweat. The patient would be well advised not to wear nylon tights.

Potent topical steroids, such as 0.1% diflucortolone valerate or 2.5% hydrocortisone, may be used two to three times per day for a few weeks. Thereafter, 1% hydrocortisone will usually suffice to maintain the improvement and to treat relapses. A sedative at night, such as hydroxyzine hydrochloride, can be useful to break the cycle of nocturnal itching and scratching. An antihistamine, terfenadine, taken during the day may help to relieve the itch without causing sedation.

It is important to treat depression appropriately. Even if the patient is not pathologically depressed she can benefit greatly from sympathetic support and understanding, and time must be set aside for this when necessary.

VULVAL PAIN

Vulval vestibulitis

This condition of unknown aetiology occurs in young women. The true incidence is unknown. The hallmarks are severe introital dyspareunia, tenderness to pressure in the vestibule, and erythema, particularly around the ducts of Bartholin and the minor vestibular glands. There is no completely satisfactory mode of treatment, but local steroid ointments are probably the first choice. Local injections of interferon have given variable success (Marinoff et al 1993). Vestibulectomy gives mixed results.

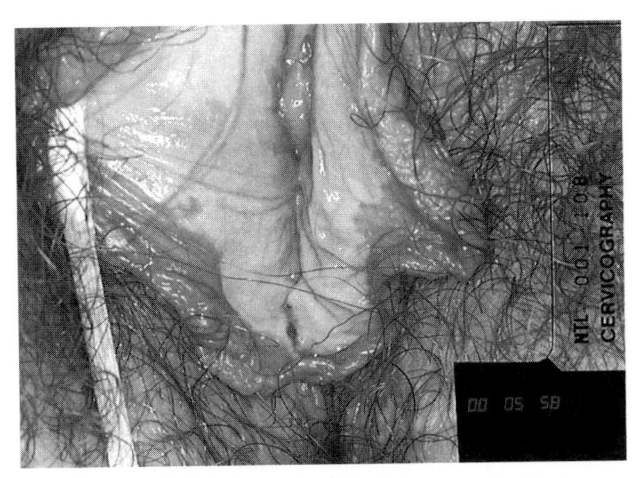

Fig. 36.2 Extensive area of acetowhite change.

Burning vulva syndrome

Vulvodynia is a term applied to a feeling of vulval burning (McKay 1989). These patients do not complain of pain when the vestibular ducts are touched, and they do not complain of dyspareunia. This condition is commonest in younger women. In most cases there is little or nothing to be seen on the vulva. Minor changes may be visible through the colposcope. Low-grade acetowhite changes (Fig. 36.2) and microvilli on the medial aspect of the labia minora have been attributed, perhaps wrongly, to infection with human papilloma virus, but the evidence that these changes contribute to the symptoms is scant (Dennerstein et al 1994). Vulvodynia may be caused by vulvovaginal infections, vulval dermatitis or any of the other dermatoses. Improvements have sometimes been obtained after laser vaporization of the minor vestibular glands when local inflammation has been evident. Amitriptyline in a dose of 20–60 mg per day may help.

Vulval or perineal neuralgia

Some women complain of vulval or perineal pain, but it is not clear whether they should be regarded as a separate group. These are often older patients, but both vulvodynia and vulval pain have many different causes, so considering them as separate entities is not particularly useful.

Neurological causes include spinal cord injury, meningeal cysts, diabetes and postherpetic neuralgia. Pudendal neuralgia is a syndrome described in men not unlike the vulval pain syndrome of women. No cause is known, but it seems

Table 36.1 Terminology of disorders of vulval skin and mucosa

Non-neoplastic disorders
Lichen sclerosus
Squamous cell hyperplasia (formerly hyperplastic dystrophy)
Other dermatoses
Vulval intraepithelial neoplasia (VIN)
Squamous VIN
VIN I Mild dysplasia
VIN II Moderate dysplasia
VIN III Severe dysplasia or carcinoma-in-situ, non-squamous VIN
Paget's disease

Note 1 Mixed epithelial disorders may occur. In such cases it is recommended that both conditions be reported. For example, lichen sclerosus with associated squamous cell hyperplasia (formerly classified as mixed dystrophy) should be reported as lichen sclerosus and squamous cell hyperplasia. Squamous cell hyperplasia with associated vulval intraepithelial neoplasia (formerly hyperplastic dystrophy with atypia) should be diagnosed as vulval intraepithelial neoplasia.

Note 2 Squamous cell hyperplasia is used for those instances in which the hyperplasia is not attributable to another cause. Specific lesions or dermatoses involving the vulva (e.g. psoriasis, lichen planus, lichen simplex chronicus, *Candida* infection, condyloma acuminatum) may include squamous cell hyperplasia, but should be diagnosed specifically and excluded from this category.

From International Society for the Study of Vulvar Disease (1989)

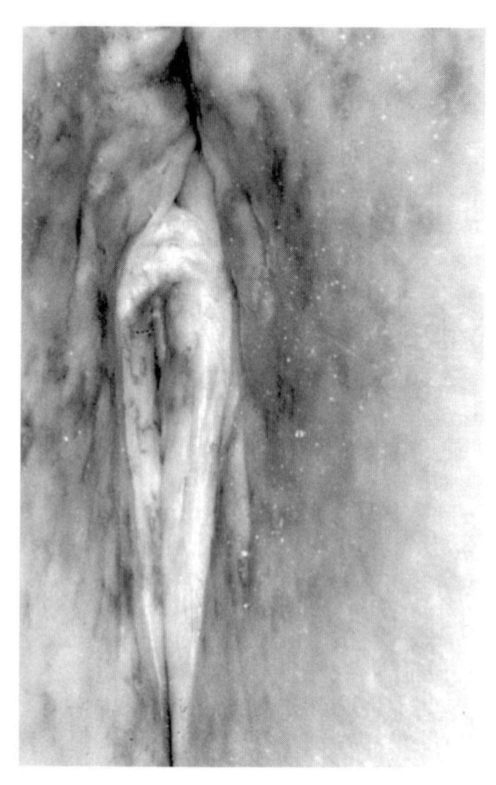

Fig. 36.3 Lichen sclerosus.

likely that some cases of both syndromes may be related to conditions such as trigeminal neuralgia and the dystonias.

Some of these women are clinically depressed and can be helped by appropriate therapy. When no abnormality is visible psychiatric advice should be sought, if only to rule out a psychosis. Once again sympathetic support is essential.

NON-NEOPLASTIC DISORDERS OF THE VULVA

In few areas has there been as much confusion over the terminology used as in that of vulvar 'dystrophies'. The latest recommended scheme is shown in Table 36.1. The non-neoplastic disorders have been separated from the potentially premalignant intraepithelial neoplasia, and only the non-neoplastic disorders will be discussed here.

Lichen sclerosus

This is the commonest condition found in elderly women complaining of vulvar itch, but may also be seen in children and, less commonly, in younger women. The cause is not known but the condition is associated with autoimmune disorders.

Although it most commonly affects the vulva and perianal skin, lesions do appear elsewhere. The lesion is white and the skin looks thin, with a crinkled surface (Fig. 36.3). The contours of the vulva slowly disappear and labial adhesions form. If the patient has been rubbing the area the skin will become thickened (lichenified). The diagnosis can usually be made clinically, but a biopsy should be performed whenever possible. Occasionally, even in a typical case, the histology is not characteristic.

There is much uncertainty about the risk to patients with lichen sclerosus of developing vulval cancer. Vulval intraepithelial neoplasia (VIN) and lichen sclerosus can coexist in the same patient, and many patients with invasive carcinoma also have lichen sclerosus in the surrounding skin. About 4% of women with lichen sclerosus develop invasive cancer (Meyrick Thomas et al 1988).

Although there is a 9% prevalence of thyroid disease, pernicious anaemia or diabetes in these patients, screening for these conditions may not be of value as in most cases the diagnosis has already been made by the time the patient presents with her vulval complaint (Meyrick Thomas et al 1988).

If the patient is asymptomatic no treatment is required. Mild itching may be helped by aqueous cream or 1% hydrocortisone ointment applied three times daily. More potent steroids may be required for short periods. If use of an ointment results in maceration, a cream base may be used. Some have suggested long-term use of potent steroid creams such as clobetasol propionate (Dalziel & Wojnarowska 1993). Some women benefit from 2% testosterone ointment, which should be applied twice or three times per day for 6 weeks. Thereafter the frequency can be reduced to once or twice a week. Excessive dosage will result in clitoral hypertrophy and increased facial hair (Friedrich 1983). There is virtually no place for vulvectomy for this condition, as the morbidity is not justified in the face of a high recurrence rate. The same may be said of laser vaporization.

Squamous cell hyperplasia

Squamous cell hyperplasia is a term applied in cases of histological evidence of hyperplasia with no clinical evidence of the cause (Fig. 36.4). Chronic rubbing of otherwise normal skin (lichen simplex), psoriasis, condylomata acuminata and infection with *Candida albicans* are among the diagnoses that must be excluded before this term may be applied. This stipulation is likely to reduce to near zero the number of cases assigned to this category on clinical grounds.

Other dermatoses

These problems are usually seen by dermatologists rather than by gynaecologists, but a knowledge of this area will help to identify those patients who should be referred. Space permits only a brief discussion of some of the more common lesions.

Allergic or irritant dermatitis

The patient will usually present with vulval itching. The skin is red and swollen and may later become thickened from constant scratching (lichenified). Secondary infection may occur. The list of potential irritants is endless, but includes detergents, perfume, synthetic materials, condom lubricants, chlorine in swimming pools, podophyllin, topical antihistamines, anaesthetics or antibiotics. After eliminating exposure to any potential irritant a 1% hydrocortisone ointment will prove helpful in most cases, but sometimes a stronger preparation is needed in the acute phase. Secondary infection may require treatment with local or systemic antibiotics. Aqueous cream should replace soap for washing the vulva.

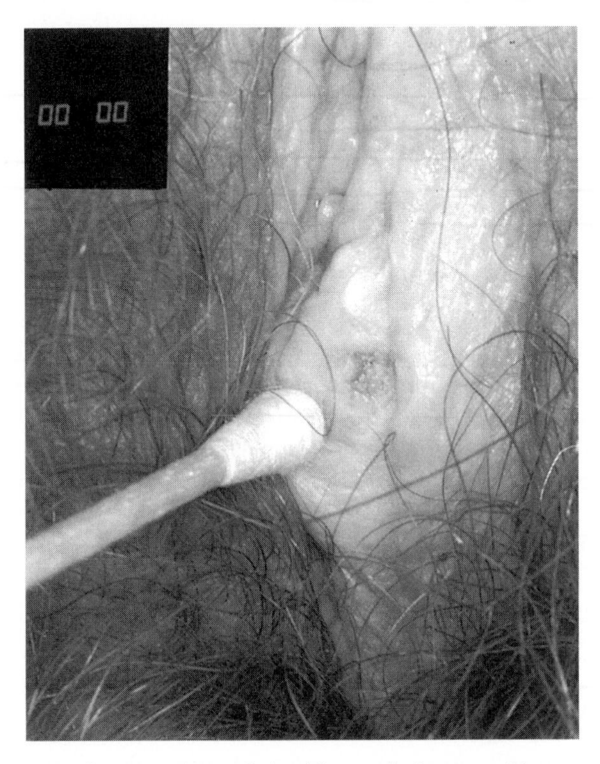

Fig. 36.4 Squamous hyperplasia with a small ulcer caused by scratching.

Psoriasis

It is unusual for a patient to present with isolated psoriasis of the vulva never having had the abnormality elsewhere. The lesion is red and sharply defined and often has a silvery scaling surface. This last may be absent in moist areas. The mucosal surfaces are rarely involved. Coal tar preparations should not be used on the vulva and treatment is usually begun with a strong steroid ointment (Ridley 1988).

Intertrigo

Any site where the skin remains moist is susceptible to inflammation and secondary infection. The lesions are red, moist and ill defined. Infection with *Candida* is particularly common, especially in obese diabetics. Occasionally psoriasis occurring in a flexure, or seborrhoeic dermatitis, may present in a similar fashion but both tend to occur at other sites at the same time. Topical antibiotic therapy may be required in combination with a mild steroid. General measures to keep the area dry and the skin surfaces separated are very helpful.

Lichen planus

This condition may occur on any part of the body and is often found in the mouth. In the skin it is usually a self-limiting and often asymptomatic condition. The lesions on the vulva are purple-white papules with a shiny surface and regular outline. The histology is diagnostic. If treatment is required, topical steroids are effective.

Erosive lichen planus

This uncommon variant of lichen planus occurs on the mucosal aspects of the labia minora and the vagina. This may cause pain and itching and, if the vagina is involved, may cause bleeding and dyspareunia due to vaginal adhesions. Unfortunately, it is often difficult to establish the diagnosis histologically. Systemic steroids can be helpful, but the prognosis is poor as the condition tends to persist. Gentle dilation with Sims dilators lubricated with clobetasol propionate cream may help to reverse the narrowing of the introitus that can occur. There may be a risk of malignancy.

Vulval ulcers

The causes of benign vulval ulcers are:

aphthous ulcers;
herpes genitalis;
primary syphilis;
Crohn's disease;
Behçet's disease;
Lipschutz ulcers;
Zoon's vulvitis;
lymphogranuloma venereum;
chancroid;
Donovanosis;
tuberculosis.

Aphthous ulcers

Simple aphthous ulcers, analogous to those seen in the mouth, may be found on the vulva. They are small and painful, with a yellow base, and are seen mainly on the labia majora. There is no associated constitutional upset and the ulcers are seldom as painful as those found in primary herpes.

Herpetic ulcers

The primary attack of herpes genitalis usually presents as an extremely painful vulval ulceration, together with general malaise, fever and often inguinal lymphadenopathy. Some intact vesicles may still be visible. There is often an associated herpetic pharyngitis. Severe headache should suggest the possibility of viral meningitis. Herpes genitalis is described more fully in Chapter 56.

Syphilitic ulcers

The chancre of primary syphilis is an indurated painless ulcer. There may be several chancres. If secondary infection occurs the ulcer may become tender. The majority occur on the vulva but the cervix may be involved.

Crohn's disease

Crohn's disease may affect the vulva or perineum in 25–30% of cases, and this often precedes the appearance of intestinal symptoms by many years. The ulcers look like knife cuts in the skin. Later, when bowel disease is evident, oedema, discharging sinuses and irregular ulcers are more common.

Behçet's disease

Behçet's disease is a chronic condition characterized by oral, genital and ocular ulceration. It may be many years before all of these features are evident. The oral ulcers are often not severe but the vulval lesions can be very erosive. They can last for several months and leave extensive scarring. It can be difficult to distinguish from Crohn's disease and there are no diagnostic histological features. There is no specific treatment. Oestrogen-dominant oral contraceptives are said to have a beneficial effect in some cases, and topical and systemic steroids are also used.

Lipschutz ulcers

Lipschutz ulcers affect mainly the labia minora and introitus. They can be acute in onset, with an associated fever and lymphadenopathy. Often no cause can be found, but they may be due to Epstein–Barr virus.

Zoon's vulvitis

This is a rare and ill-defined condition originally described on the penis. It is less common in women, in whom it presents as red, erosive plaques on the vulva. The diagnosis depends upon the histological findings. There is an intense dermal infiltrate of plasma cells with haemosiderin deposits. It responds to potent topical steroids.

'Tropical' infections causing vulval ulceration

Lymphogranuloma venereum, a tropical infection due to certain subtypes of *Chlamydia trachomatis*, causes a painless vulval ulcer which heals after 3–4 weeks. Inguinal lymphadenopathy develops a few weeks later. Chancroid, infection with *Haemophilus ducreyi*, is a very common cause of genital ulceration in tropical parts of the world, but outbreaks have occurred in western countries. Donovanosis can cause chronic, spreading ulcers and is most common in southeast Asia and India. Tuberculosis is a rare but important cause of vulval ulceration and inguinal lymphadenopathy.

Disorders of pigmentation

Melanosis vulvae (lentigo) is the commonest pigmented lesion on the vulva, producing asymptomatic light-brown macules which are frequently multiple and can appear anywhere on the vulva. Because they can be difficult to differentiate conclusively from melanoma or VIN, excision biopsy is recommended. Benign naevi may also be difficult to identify with certainty. Biopsy should be the rule for pigmented lesions.

Vitiligo is an area of depigmentation. It does not cause symptoms but may be mistaken for lichenification or lichen sclerosus.

VULVAL NEOPLASIA

VIN are discussed in Chapter 34 and vulval cancer in Chapter 37.

BENIGN TUMOURS

Ectopic tissues

Occasionally, breast tissue may be found on the vulva. It commonly presents during pregnancy as a firm, mobile vulval mass. Endometriosis may also be found on the vulva, often after implantation in a surgical wound such as an episiotomy. This does not always exhibit cyclic changes.

Cystic lesions

Epidermoid and sebaceous cysts can be difficult to differentiate, but the distinction is academic as the management of both is excision. Mucinous cysts may arise from the minor vestibular glands (Fig. 36.5), whereas mesonephric cysts are found on the labia majora. Cysts on the anterior part of the vulva may have arisen from peritoneum carried into the vulva by the round ligament (cysts of the canal of Nuck). Cysts may arise around the urethra in Skene's ducts or in suburethral glands.

Bartholin's cyst

These cysts arise from the duct of Bartholin's gland, which lies in the subcutaneous tissue below the lower third of the labium majorum. When the duct becomes blocked a tense retention cyst forms. The patient usually presents only after infection has supervened and a painful abscess has formed. Incision and marsupialization of the abscess and antibiotic therapy give excellent results. The pus from the abscess should be sent for culture in media suitable for the detection of gonococcal infection.

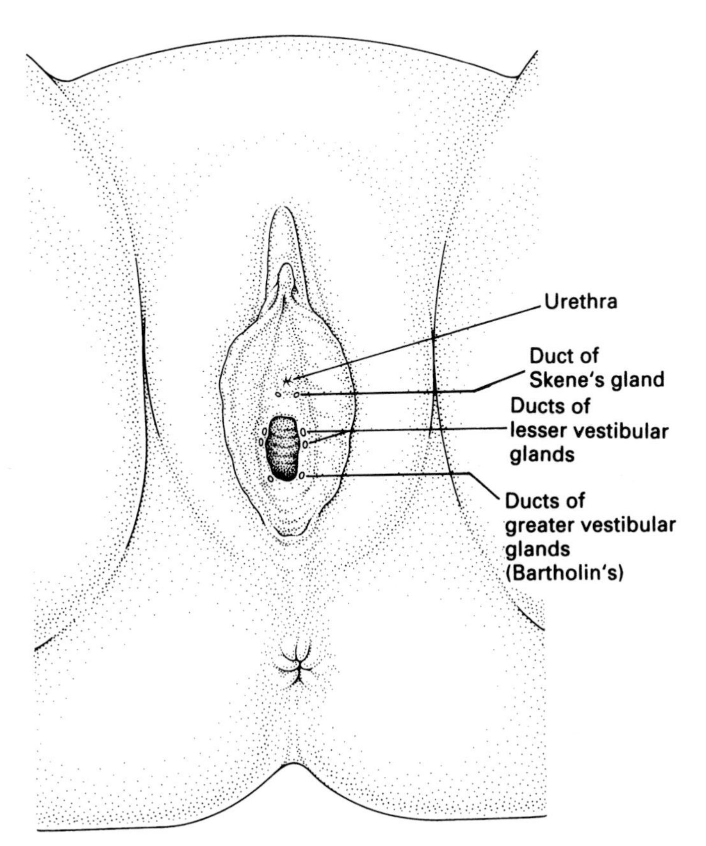

Fig. 36.5 The vulval glands.

Non-epithelial tumours

Lipomas and fibromas are the commonest benign tumours of the vulva which arise from other than the epithelial tissues. The benign angiokeratoma may be difficult to distinguish from a melanoma, especially if the initial red colour has given way to the later brown or black hue and the lesion has begun to bleed due to trauma. Many other benign tumours may be found on the vulva (Fox & Buckley 1988) but the diagnosis is nearly always made on histological rather than clinical grounds.

Epithelial tumours

Squamous papillomata and 'skin tags' are common, benign and similar in appearance. Folliculitis – infection of hair follicles – may be caused by shaving or depilatory creams. Infestation with lice may present in this way. Any precipitating cause should be dealt with. Topical antiseptics or even systemic antibiotics may be required.

Secondary syphilis may present as a maculopapular rash which can affect the vulva. Condyloma lata are sessile papules seen on the vulva and perianal skin. These may ulcerate and are highly infectious. A generalized lymphadenopathy is common at this stage.

Condyloma acuminata are small papules which are sometimes sessile and often polypoid (Fig. 36.6). They are caused by infection with human papilloma virus, usually type 6/11. Acetowhite changes and 'microwarts', seen best under low-power magnification, have been attributed to human papilloma virus infection but this may not be correct. Microwarts may be no more than a variation of normal warts. The majority of condylomata acuminata can be treated satisfactorily in the outpatient department by the sparing application of 80% trichloroacetic acid, a very corrosive liquid. Care must be taken not to injure the adjacent normal skin. Podophyllin is less effective and more toxic. If the lesions are large and widespread, removal under general anaesthesia will probably be required using electrodiathermy or carbon dioxide laser. The advantage of the latter is that its greater precision permits removal of the lesion without subsequent scarring, and with more rapid healing. Laser treatment of the vulva is discussed more fully in Chapter 34.

The rare keratoacanthoma might well be mistaken for invasive squamous cancer because of its rapid growth over a matter of weeks. Spontaneous involution usually begins after about 6 months. The centre of this well demarcated, regular dome contains a plug of keratin, which may sug-

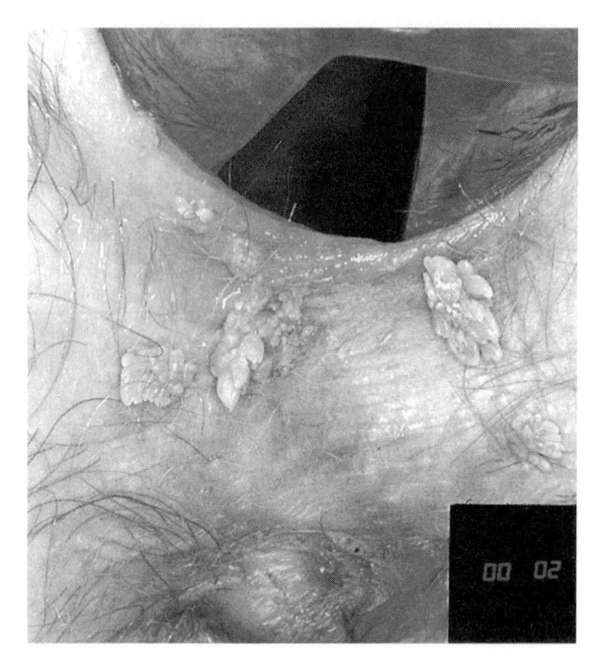

Fig. 36.6 Small genital warts at the fourchette.

gest the diagnosis, but complete excision of the lesion is required for histological confirmation.

TRAUMA TO VULVA OR VAGINA

A torn hymen following a first attempt at intercourse may result in profuse, frightening haemorrhage and transfusion may be indicated. Suture of the bleeding vessel under general anaesthesia should be accompanied by one or more radial incisions in the hymen to prevent a recurrence.

Trauma is usually the result of falling astride a sharp object such as a fence. It may result from sexual abuse, sometimes self-inflicted. It may also occur following normal sexual intercourse, particularly in a postmenopausal woman who has not had intercourse for some time. In these cases the laceration is usually at the vault of the vagina in the posterior fornix.

An indwelling catheter may be necessary and ice packs will give some comfort. Damage to the vagina, rectum, urethra, bladder or ureter may also occur. Pain relief with opiates and replacement of blood loss may be needed urgently. Examination under anaesthesia is often required to determine the extent of the damage. A closed haematoma is best managed conservatively but bleeding lacerations will require suture. Devitalized tissues will need to be excised and tears in the bowel or bladder must be repaired in layers. Occasionally a hysterectomy must be performed.

CONGENITAL ABNORMALITIES

Congenital abnormalities of the vulva and vagina are discussed in Chapters 1, 11 and 13.

MISCELLANEOUS CONDITIONS

Occasionally prolapse of the urethral mucosa will occur, usually in children or elderly women. This can become infarcted. An everted, inflamed portion of the urethral mucosa is called a caruncle. It may be asymptomatic, but it can be painful and cause dysuria and dyspareunia. In elderly women swelling and erythema of the urethral meatus may just be the result of atrophy, which will be improved by oestrogen therapy. Excision or cautery are required for caruncle and urethral prolapse.

VAGINA

INTRODUCTION

Many of the disorders that affect the vagina are discussed in depth elsewhere in this book: congenital abnormalities will be found in Chapters 1, 11 and 13; infections in Chapter 56: psychosexual problems in Chapter 27; atrophic changes in Chapter 25; prolapse in Chapter 51; intraepithelial disease in Chapter 34; and cancer in Chapter 37. The purpose of this short section is to discuss briefly some of these problems as symptom complexes, and to refer the reader to those parts of this book where more detailed information may be found.

ANATOMY AND HISTOLOGY

The upper two-thirds of the vagina are derived from the mullerian duct and the lower third from the ectoderm of the cloaca. The vagina is related anteriorly to the bladder above and the urethra below. Posteriorly, the vault of the vagina is covered with the peritoneum of the pouch of Douglas. It thus becomes closely related to loops of small or large bowel. Below this, it is closely related to the anterior wall of the rectum until the perineal body separates it from the anal canal. The ureters run close to the cervix over each side of the vaginal vault to the bladder. Laterally, the vagina is supported by the lower portion of the cardinal ligaments until it reaches the pelvic floor, where it is invested by the medial part of the levator ani muscles (pubococcygeus). Lateral to the vagina most of the tissue is areolar, except at the level of the perineal body.

The vagina is lined by stratified squamous epithelium. When the transformation zone of the cervix has extended on to the vagina, clefts or glands partly lined by columnar epithelium will be seen deep to the squamous epithelium.

VAGINAL DISCHARGE

Because there is almost always some escape of vaginal or cervical secretions it can be difficult sometimes to assess the significance of a vaginal discharge, and often the patient is just seeking reassurance. The best guide is to ask whether the amount or character of the discharge has altered from the patient's usual pattern.

Physiological discharge

A physiological discharge is usually clear or whitish in colour. Part of this secretion comes from the cervix and, unless the patient is taking an oral contraceptive, the normal cyclical fluctuation may be evident with an increase in flow just before ovulation. Physiological secretion is increased following a pregnancy and women using oral contraception often note an additional loss. Irritation may result from a copious physiological secretion and does not always indicate infection. Similarly, some women find the smell of normal secretion offensive. A marked recent increase in the volume of discharge, accompanied by irritation, suggests the presence of infection. A bloodstained discharge should always arouse suspicion.

Speculum examination will show a healthy-looking vagina with a small amount of mucoid discharge. An area of ectopy (an erosion) may be visible on the cervix, but this is a normal finding in premenopausal women and is seldom responsible for symptoms. Because it is not possible to exclude infection from the clinical appearance, a swab sent for microscopy and culture is required.

Cytolytic vaginosis

This is due to excess lactobacilli in the vagina causing a thick white cheesy discharge. It is frequently misdiagnosed as *Candida*. The patient may complain of pruritus and dyspareunia, with a cyclical increase in symptoms in the luteal phase. A Gram-stained film or wet preparation should be examined. Treatment consists of weak sodium bicarbonate douches three times a week.

Bacterial vaginosis

Bacterial vaginosis is a common syndrome often overlooked by gynaecologists. It appears to be caused not by one but by several different organisms (see Ch. 56). *Gardnerella vaginalis* is one of these but is often found in asymptomatic women. It would seem either that simultaneous infection with multiple organisms is required or that some hitherto undetected pathogen is the cause. The characteristic features are a vaginal pH over 5.0 and a fishy odour, made more obvious by adding a drop of 10% potassium peroxide to a drop of the discharge on a slide. Microscopy of the discharge will show 'clue cells': epithelial cells covered by bacteria. Sophisticated gas chromatographic analysis of the discharge adds little to the diagnostic armamentarium save expense. Investigations for other sexually transmitted disease should be instituted (Ch. 56).

Metronidazole is the treatment of choice as a single 2 g dose. This may be repeated in 24 hours. In resistant cases 400 mg bd is prescribed for 7 days. The patient must not drink alcohol while taking metronidazole to avoid the risk of an antebuse reaction. Metronidazole often causes nausea and should be taken after food. An alternative treatment is vaginal clindamycin cream.

Monilial vaginitis

Candida spp. are frequently found in the vagina of asymptomatic women. Symptoms result when the numbers of organisms increase, for reasons which are often not apparent. Diabetic patients, women using oral contraception or taking broad-spectrum antibiotics, pregnant patients and the immunosuppressed are all particularly prone to *Candida* infection. Such patients will complain of vaginal irritation, dysuria, dyspareunia and a vaginal discharge. The discharge may be recognizable in severe cases, when it is thick and white, like cottage cheese. The vulva may be reddened and sore looking, and the vagina and cervix inflamed and covered with adherent lumps of the discharge. Microscopy will show the characteristic hyphae or spores (Fig. 36.7). In cases of doubt, a high vaginal swab should be sent for culture.

A convenient treatment is a single 500 mg pessary of clotrimazole with 1% clotrimazole cream for any external lesions. In recurrent cases it may be worth asking the sexual partner to apply clotrimazole to his penis, but there is doubt about the value of this approach.

If the infection persists or recurs frequently, culture of the *Candida* species and determination of the sensitivity to antifungal agents is advisable. Provided the organism is sensitive, single doses of the oral agents fluconazole 150 mg or itraconazole 200 mg may be prescribed on the first day of the period for 6 months, provided the patient is not pregnant and has no evidence of liver or renal impairment. These may be combined with oral nystatin 500 000 IU qid and nystatin pessaries bd for 3–4 months.

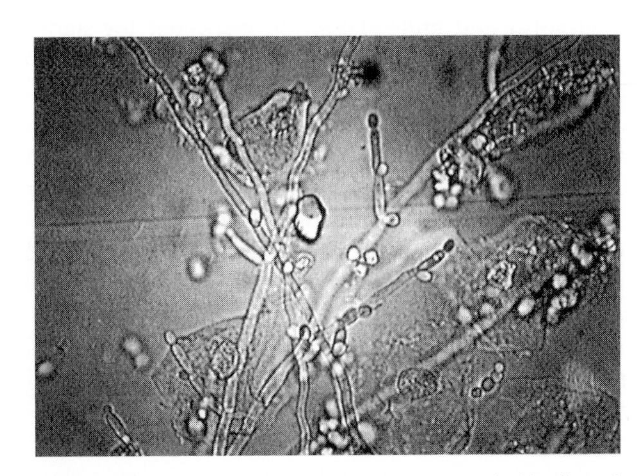

Fig. 36.7 Microscopy of vaginal discharge shows typical hyphae of *Candida*.

Women with recurrent vulvovaginal candidiasis may have subtle deficiencies in their cell-mediated immunity.

Trichomonal vaginitis

This condition is caused by a motile protozoon. It is sexually transmitted but may be asymptomatic for long periods. It usually causes a foul-smelling, mucopurulent discharge. The patient may complain of dysuria, dyspareunia and vulvovaginal irritation. The vulva and vagina may be very inflamed. The vagina and cervix are often covered by petechial haemorrhage, giving the so-called 'strawberry cervix'.

A wet film will demonstrate the motile organisms, but the diagnosis may be confirmed by culture. As with bacterial vaginosis, it may be prudent to screen the patient for other sexually transmitted diseases (Ch. 56).

Treatment is with metronidazole 200 mg tid for 7 days, or as a single dose of 2 g.

Miscellaneous causes of vaginal discharge

A number of other problems may present as a vaginal discharge. A foreign body (e.g. a tampon) will cause a purulent, bloodstained discharge whose cause will be all too obvious on speculum examination. A bloody discharge may result from tumours of the vagina, cervix or uterus. Atrophic vaginitis may cause a vaginal discharge, but endometrial pathology must be ruled out before commencing oestrogen therapy.

Vaginal discharge in children

A vaginal discharge in a young child is often due to infection secondary to atrophic vaginitis. A foreign body is sometimes found, or occasionally threadworms are involved. In the older child evidence of sexual abuse must be sought (see Ch. 56). Only very rarely is a vaginal tumour responsible.

The vulva and anus should be inspected for signs of trauma. Atrophic changes should be noted. If possible, swabs should be taken from the vagina for culture and, if indicated, from the rectum and urethra. It is usually possible to perform a gentle rectal examination using the little finger to detect a foreign body in the vagina. In cases of doubt, a general anaesthetic is necessary to allow an adequate inspection of the vagina without frightening the child. A paediatric laryngoscope is particularly useful for this.

Any foreign body should be removed and the vagina gently cleansed under general anaesthesia. Appropriate oral antibiotics should be given for any infection. If atrophic vaginitis has contributed, the sparing application of topical oestrogen to the vulva for 2 weeks should suffice.

DYSPAREUNIA

Dyspareunia may result from one of many causes, most of which have little to do with the vagina itself. Primary dyspareunia often has a psychological background and may require expert counselling (see Ch. 27). Secondary dyspareunia is more often due to organic disease, especially when the pain is felt only after full insertion has occurred. Pelvic inflammatory disease, endometriosis and pelvic or vaginal tumours are not infrequent causes. Introital, secondary dyspareunia may result from vaginal infection, atrophic changes, or after surgery to the perineum, most commonly an episiotomy. Dyspareunia may result from vulval disease. Radiotherapy to the pelvis or vagina will often cause fibrosis of the pelvic floor and contracture of the vagina. Great care must be taken in the management of these patients to prevent this complication (Chs 33 and 35).

Examination may reveal spasm of the levator muscles in women with a psychological cause for their symptom, but may also be seen in women with a physical cause. Tact and gentleness are essential – it may not be prudent to pursue an attempt at vaginal examination at this stage. Women who complain of dyspareunia due to vulvodynia appear to have no obvious abnormality. Their problem has been discussed earlier in this chapter. A tender perineal scar may be evident in a woman complaining of dyspareunia following childbirth, but some of these women also have a psychological overlay which requires help. Occasionally, a tender adhesion may be detected in the vagina. Atrophic changes or vaginal infection may sometimes prove to be the cause.

Retroversion of the uterus is seldom an explanation in itself for dyspareunia. More usually, associated endometriosis or pelvic inflammatory disease is the culprit. An ovarian tumour or a fibroid uterus may present with dyspareunia.

If no cause is evident, laparoscopy is very useful. Quite marked endometriosis or pelvic inflammatory disease may be undetected by bimanual examination. If no pathology is found after a careful inspection of the pelvic organs, the patient may be reassured that no serious disease exists. Specialized investigations may be indicated (see Ch. 27) and referral for sexual therapy may be appropriate.

Treatment will depend upon the cause. General advice about coital technique may be helpful, particularly in employing sufficient foreplay to ensure adequate arousal and in adopting coital positions which allow the woman to control insertion and the depth of penetration (see Ch. 27).

ATROPHIC VAGINITIS

Symptoms of vaginal atrophy occur in many women after

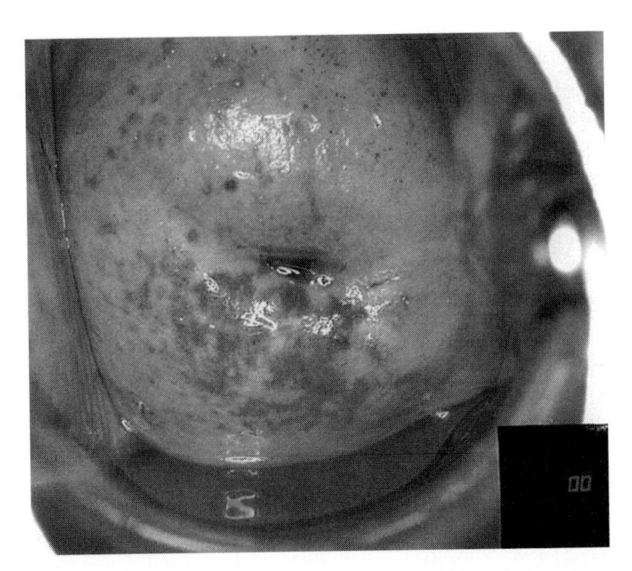

Fig. 36.8 Atrophic changes on the cervix. The epithelium is thin and easily traumatized. On the anterior lip there are small petechial haemorrhages which have coalesced on the posterior lip.

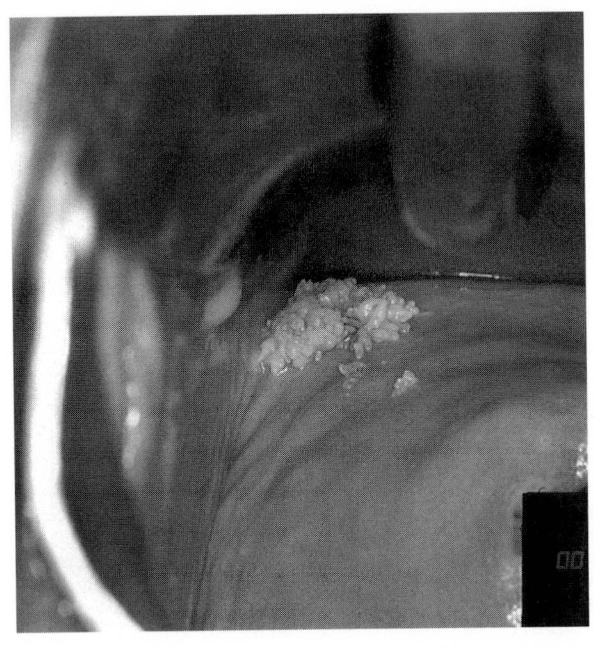

Fig. 36.9 These vaginal condylomata have turned bright white after the application of 5% acetic acid.

the menopause. Vaginal dryness, dyspareunia, superimposed infection and bleeding are common problems. These are often associated with symptoms due to atrophy of the lower urinary tract: dysuria, frequency and urgency.

Examination will show pale, thinned vaginal epithelium, often with petechial haemorrhage (Fig. 36.8). In extreme cases the vulva becomes atrophied, the labia shrink and the introitus contracts.

When bleeding has occurred, a cervical smear and endometrial biopsy are mandatory to exclude malignancy. Vaginal ultrasound examination of the endometrial thickness is a very useful adjunct to these (see Ch. 6).

Appropriate hormone replacement therapy will reverse all these symptoms of end-organ failure. There is little logic in prescribing an oestrogen cream for local application. It is more expensive, more inconvenient and, dose for dose, has systemic effects that are similar to oral or parenteral therapy.

Prepubertal children may develop a vaginal discharge, sometimes bloodstained, as a result of secondary infection following atrophic vaginitis (see above).

BENIGN TUMOURS

Tumours in the vagina are uncommon. Condyloma acuminata are by far the most common seen (Fig. 36.9). The frondlike surface is usually characteristic, but it is wise to await the result of a biopsy before instituting treatment.

Endometriotic deposits may be seen in the vagina. They are most common in an episiotomy wound and may lie deep to the epithelium.

Simple mesonephric (Gartner's) or paramesonephric cysts may be seen, especially high up near the fornices. If asymptomatic, they are best not treated. If treatment is required, marsupialization is effective and safer than excision.

Adenosis – multiple mucus-containing vaginal cysts – is a rare condition which even more rarely gives rise to symptoms. A variety of abnormalities are reported in the daughters of women who took diethylstilboestrol during their pregnancy. Most of these are of no significance (see Ch. 37).

VAGINAL NEOPLASIA

VIN are discussed in Chapter 34 and vaginal cancer in Chapter 37.

KEY POINTS

1. Vulval lesions should be biopsied liberally under local anaesthetic.
2. If no specific cause is found for pruritus vulvae, general advice, sympathetic handling, a steroid ointment and a sedative at night are often helpful.
3. Some patients benefit from antidepressant therapy.
4. There is no place for vulvectomy in the management of lichen sclerosus.
5. Vulval disease may be a manifestation of a systemic disorder.
6. Infection should be excluded in any woman complaining of a vaginal discharge.
7. A vaginal discharge is frequently due to increased physiological secretions.

REFERENCES

Dalziel K L, Wojnarowska F 1993 Long term control of vulval lichen sclerosus after treatment with long term clobetasol propionate, a potent topical steroid cream. Journal of Reproductive Medicine 38: 25–72

Dennerstein G J, Scurry J P, Garland S M et al 1994 Human papilloma virus vulvitis: a new disease or an unfortunate mistake? British Journal of Obstetrics and Gynaecology 101: 992–998

Friedrich E G 1983 Vulvar disease, 2nd edn. Saunders, Philadelphia

Fox H, Buckley C H 1988 Non-epithelial and mixed tumours of the vulva. In: Ridley C M (ed) The vulva. Churchill Livingstone, Edinburgh, pp 235–262

International Society for the Study of Vulvar Disease 1989 New nomenclature for vulvar disease. Report of the Committee on Terminology. American Journal of Obstetrics and Gynecology 73: 769

McKay M 1989 Vulvodynia – a multifactorial clinical problem. Archives of Dermatology 125: 256–262

Marinoff S C, Turner M L, Hirsch R P, Richard G 1993 Intralesional α interferon: cost effective therapy for vulvar vestibulitis syndrome. Journal of Reproductive Medicine 38: 19–24

Meyrick Thomas R H, Ridley C M, McGibbon D H, Black M M 1988 Lichen sclerosus and autoimmunity: a study of 350 women. British Journal of Dermatology 118: 41–46

Ridley C M 1988 The vulva. Churchill Livingstone, Edinburgh

37

Malignant disease of the vulva and vagina

W. P. Soutter   H. E. Lambert

CANCER OF THE VULVA

INTRODUCTION

Invasive vulvar cancer is an uncommon and unpleasant but potentially curable disease even in elderly, unfit women if referred early and managed correctly from the outset. If mismanaged, the patient with vulvar cancer is condemned to a miserable, degrading death. The surgical treatment appears deceptively simple, but few gynaecologists and their nursing colleagues acquire sufficient experience of this disease to offer the highest quality of care for these women. All too often, an inadequate initial attempt at surgery is made and the patient referred for specialist care only after recurrent disease is evident.

There were about 852 new cases of carcinoma of the vulva in 1989 in England and Wales, and the annual incidence is approximately 3.1/100 000, making it about five times less common than cervical cancer (Office of Population Censuses and Surveys (OPCS) 1994). The majority of these women are elderly (Fig. 37.1; OPCS 1994). With increased life expectancy this cancer will be seen more frequently.

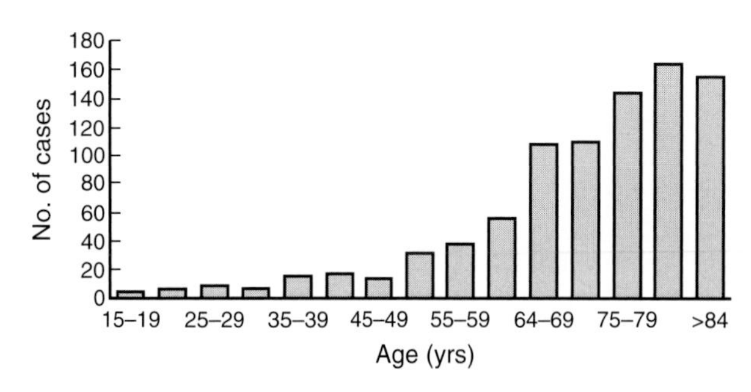

Fig. 37.1 The age-specific distribution of vulval carcinoma (OPCS 1994).

AETIOLOGY

Little is known of the aetiology of vulvar cancer. A viral factor has been suggested by the detection of antigens

Table 37.1 Groin recurrences in women who did not undergo any form of groin node surgery. None had clinically suspicious lesions in the groin, all were regarded as 'low-risk cases'. In many, groin node surgery was omitted because of associated medical problems

Reference	Depth of lesion (mm)	Diameter of lesion (cm)	Number evaluable	Groin recurrence	DoD with groin disease
Magrina et al 1979	≤ 5	≤ 2	35	4	3
Hacker et al 1984a	> 1	≤ 2	23	2	2
Bryson et al 1991	NK	≤ 2	27	6	NK
Sutton et al 1991	≤ 1	≤ 2	10	0	0
Kelly et al 1992	≤ 1	≤ 2	13	0	0
Lingard et al 1992	NK	NK	20	7	7
			128	19 (14%)	

DoD, died of disease; NK, not known

induced by herpes simplex virus type 2 (HSV2) and of DNA from type 16/18 human papilloma virus (HPV) in vulval intraepithelial neoplasia (VIN), and also by the association of a history of genital warts with vulval cancer (Brinton et al 1990). The significance of this viral association remains uncertain. The majority of genital condylomata contain HPV 6/11, not now considered to have any oncogenic potential, and very few contain HPV 16, the type found in invasive lesions (Bergeron et al 1987).

Table 37.2 Tumour thickness and positive groin nodes (Modified from Sedlis et al 1987)

Tumour thickness (mm)	Number of cases	% with positive nodes
< 1	32	3.1
1–2	56	8.9
2–3	59	18.6
3–4	68	30.9
4–5	57	33.3

ANATOMY

The gross anatomy is discussed in Chapters 2 and 36.

Lymphatic drainage

The lymph drains from the vulva to the inguinal and femoral glands in the groin and then to the external iliac glands. Drainage to both groins occurs from midline structures – the perineum and the clitoris – but some contralateral spread may take place from other parts of the vulva (Iversen & Aas 1983). Direct spread to the pelvic nodes along the internal pudendal vessels occurs only very rarely, and no direct pathway from the clitoris to pelvic nodes has been demonstrated consistently.

PATHOLOGY

Most invasive cancers (85%) are squamous. Some 5% are melanomas and the remainder are made up of carcinomas of Bartholin's gland, other adenocarcinomas, basal cell carcinomas, and the very rare verrucous carcinomas, rhabdomyosarcomas and leiomyosarcomas.

In a third of cases of Paget's disease there is an adenocarcinoma in underlying apocrine glands; these carry an especially poor prognosis (Boehm & Morris 1971, Creasman et al 1975).

NATURAL HISTORY

Microinvasive disease

The definition of microinvasion of the vulva has proved extremely problematical. The purpose is to identify a group of women with invasive carcinoma who could safely be treated without inguinofemoral lymphadenectomy. The potential for disaster if lymphadenectomy is wrongly omitted is all too clear (Table 37.1).

Although it was initially suggested that up to 5 mm invasion into the stroma might be acceptable (Rutledge et al 1970, Wharton et al 1974), subsequent reports have suggested lower limits. Some have suggested 2 mm (Friedrich & Wilkinson 1982), others preferred 1 mm (Iversen et al 1981), and further reports emphasize the importance of lymphatic or vascular invasion and the degree of differentiation (Parker et al 1975) or confluence (Hoffman et al 1983). However, all these have been retrospective studies and most of the subjects were women in whom invasive disease was not suspected initially but found in a specimen removed in the treatment of vulval intraepithelial disease.

The Gynaecological Oncology Group undertook a prospective study of women with vulval cancer treated with radical vulvectomy and groin node dissection between November 1977 and February 1984. Superficial vulval cancer was identified in 272 of 558 women (Sedlis et al 1987). The Group chose tumour thickness rather than depth of stromal invasion, which they found impracticable in their material. They found positive nodes even in women with tumours less than 1 mm thick (Table 37.2). They concluded that the risk of nodal disease was best assessed by a combination of factors. A later study of the whole group of 558 patients concurred that several factors were independent predictors of positive groin nodes (Homesley et al 1993). It was not possible to define a group free of risk. Finally, it is important to remember that prognostic factors worked out on one population must be tested against a second population to confirm their general applicability. This has never been done in this disease. It seems that the safest course is to perform groin node dissection in all cases of clinical carcinoma, regardless of the depth of invasion or the thickness of the tumour.

Frank invasion

Invasive disease involves the labia majora in about two-thirds of cases and the clitoris, labia minora or posterior fourchette and perineum in the remainder (Cavanagh et al 1985). The tumour usually spreads slowly, infiltrating local tissue before metastasizing to the groin nodes. Spread to the contralateral groin occurs in about 25% of those cases with positive groin nodes, so bilateral groin node dissection is required in all cases with metastatic disease in the groin lymph nodes (Monaghan 1985a). Pelvic node involvement is not common (1.4–16.1%; Cavanagh et al 1985) and haematogenous spread to bone or lung is rare. Death is a long, unpleasant process, and is often due to sepsis and inanition or haemorrhage. Uraemia from bilateral ureteric obstruction may supervene first. Such is the abject misery of this demise that all patients with resectable vulvar lesions should be offered surgery regardless of their age and general condition.

CLINICAL STAGING

The FIGO classification is shown in Table 37.3. In spite of the apparent limitations of this classification, it does give a reasonable guide to the prognosis. The main drawback was reliance on clinical palpation of the groin nodes, which is notoriously inaccurate (Monaghan 1985a). Now that the surgical findings are incorporated in the staging evaluation, the prognostic value of staging is greatly improved.

Table 37.3 The FIGO staging of vulvar cancer (1995)

Stage	Definition
Stage Ia	Confined to vulva and/or perineum, 2 cm or less maximum diameter. Groin nodes not palpable. Stromal invasion no greater than 1 mm
Stage Ib	As for Ia but stromal invasion greater than 1 mm
Stage II	Confined to vulva and/or perineum, more than 2 cm maximum diameter. Groin nodes not palpable
Stage III	Extends beyond the vulva, vagina, lower urethra or anus; or unilateral regional lymph node metastasis
Stage IVa	Involves the mucosa of rectum or bladder; upper urethra; or pelvic bone; and/or bilateral regional lymph node metastases
Stage IVb	Any distant metastasis, including pelvic lymph node

DIAGNOSIS AND ASSESSMENT

Most patients with invasive disease (71%) complain of irritation or pruritus and 57% note a vulvar mass or ulcer (Monaghan 1985a). It is usually not until the mass appears that medical advice is sought. Bleeding (28%) and discharge (23%) are less common presentations. One of the major problems in invasive vulvar cancer is the delay between the first appearance of symptoms and referral for a gynaecological opinion. This is only partly due to the patient's reluctance to attend. In many cases the doctor fails to recognize the gravity of the lesion and prescribes topical therapy, sometimes without examining the woman. Delays of over 12 months are common, occurring in 33% of a large series collected in Florida (Cavanagh et al 1985).

Because of the multicentric nature of female lower genital tract cancer (Hammond & Monaghan 1983), the investigation of a patient with vulvar cancer should include inspection of the cervix and cervical cytology. The groin nodes must be palpated carefully and any suspicious nodes sampled by fine-needle aspiration. A chest X-ray is always required and an intravenous pyelography or lymphangiography may sometimes be helpful. Thorough examination under anaesthesia and a full-thickness generous biopsy are the most important investigations. The examination should note particularly the size and distribution of the primary lesion, especially the involvement of the urethra or anus, and secondary lesions in the vulval or perineal skin must be sought. The groins should be re-examined under general anaesthesia when the diagnostic biopsies are taken, as previously undetected nodes may be palpated at that time.

TREATMENT

Surgery

Surgery is the mainstay of treatment. The introduction of radical vulvectomy reduced the mortality from 80% to 40% (Taussig 1940, Way 1960). However, to control lymphatic spread these techniques removed large areas of normal skin from the groins and primary wound closure was rarely achieved. Modifications of this en bloc excision were devised to allow primary closure and to reduce the considerable morbidity (Fig. 37.2; Monaghan 1986, Cavanagh et al 1990). Although these variations did reduce the rate of wound breakdown without any apparent loss of efficacy, the morbidity remained high and impaired psychosexual function was common (Andersen & Hacker 1983). Much work in the past decade has aimed at reducing the morbidity still further without compromising the efficacy of the treatment.

Separate groin incisions

In pursuit of an effective treatment with lower morbidity,

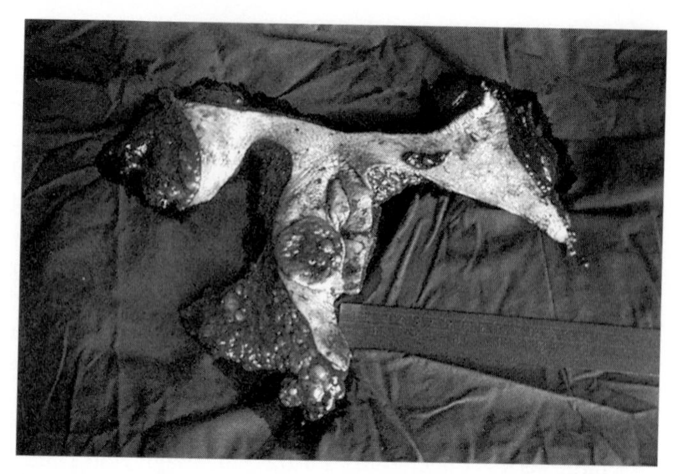

Fig. 37.2 A specimen from a radical vulvectomy and groin node dissection en bloc using a modified incision removing a minimum of skin from the groins. This operation would now only be used in women with clinical involvement of the groin nodes. Note the large amount of subcutaneous tissue removed from the vulva seen on the right.

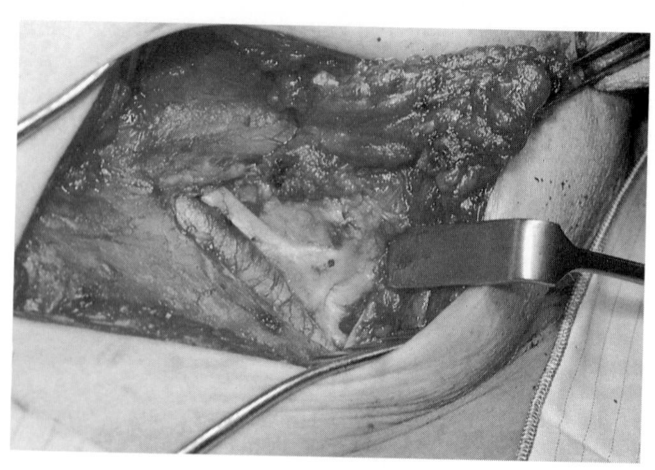

Fig. 37.4 The fascia lata overlying the femoral nerve, lateral to the femoral artery, has been preserved, but the femoral artery and the triangle medial to it have been meticulously dissected down to the surface of the adductor longus muscle posteriorly.

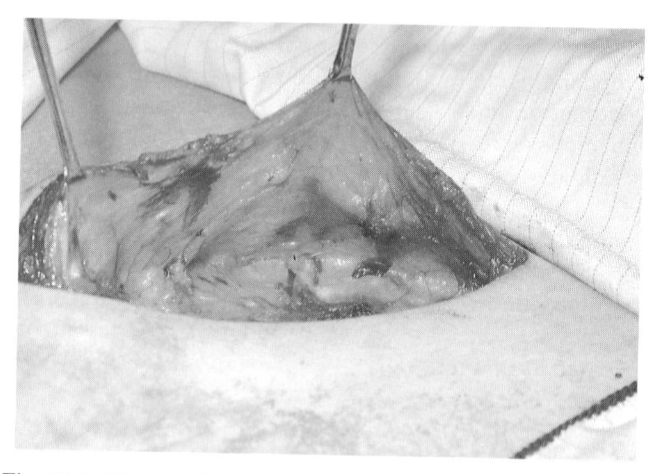

Fig. 37.3 The superficial plane deep to Camper's fascia is defined carefully, thus preserving sufficient subcutaneous fat to provide an adequate blood supply to the skin flap.

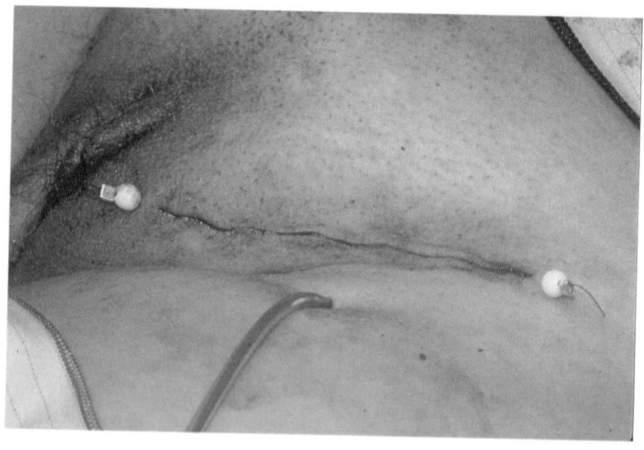

Fig. 37.5 The linear incision heals by first intention in the majority of cases, with greatly reduced morbidity.

the en bloc dissection of the groin nodes in continuity with the vulva was replaced by an operation using three separate incisions. This technique was originally suggested by Taussig (1940). This depended on the principle that lymphatic metastases developed initially by embolization. Therefore, in the early stages of spread there would be no residual tumour in the lymphatic channels between the tumour and the local lymph nodes in the groin. Many studies have since attested to the reduced morbidity of this method without loss of efficacy (Byron et al 1962, Ballon & Lamb 1975, Hacker et al 1981, Cavanagh et al 1990, Helm et al 1992, Grimshaw et al 1993). However, care needs to be taken in undercutting the skin edges so as to leave sufficient subcutaneous fat to provide a blood supply for the skin without, on the other hand, leaving superficial nodes in situ (Fig. 37.3). The deep femoral nodes are removed by excising the cribriform fascia over the femoral vessels and removing the fat and nodes anterior to the vessels and from the femoral triangle medial to the vessels (Fig. 37.4). The linear incision closes without tension and usually heals well (Fig. 37.5). Recurrent tumour in the bridge of skin between the groin and the vulva has occasionally been reported (Hacker et al 1981, Schulz & Penalver 1989, Sutton et al 1991, Grimshaw et al 1993). This is most likely to occur when the lymph nodes are extensively involved, and such women are better treated with an en bloc technique.

Ipsilateral lymphadenectomy

Spread to the contralateral groin from a lesion placed on one side of the vulva is very unusual without the ipsilateral nodes being involved (Homesley et al 1991, Grimshaw et al 1993; Table 37.4). This has led to the suggestion that, in the absence of clinical suspicion of groin node involvement, ipsilateral lymphadenectomy is sufficient to detect lymph node disease *provided the lesion is not centrally placed or bilateral.* If nodal disease is found in one groin, the opposite groin must also be explored.

Superficial inguinal lymphadenectomy

A further modification of groin node lymphadenectomy, applicable to women without clinical evidence of nodal disease, was the limitation of the dissection to the superficial nodes lying anterior to the cribriform fascia (DiSaia et al 1979). The rationale for this suggested change was the belief that lymphatic drainage from the vulva passes first to the superficial inguinal nodes before subsequently going to the femoral nodes deep to the cribriform fascia (Way 1948, Parry-Jones 1960, Borgno et al 1990). The superficial nodes were sent for frozen section. Deep femoral lymphadenectomy was performed only if the pathologist identified lymphatic metastases. This placed a great responsibility upon the pathologist, who would have to identify and examine rapidly an average of 18 nodes from each groin (Helm et al 1992). Inevitably mistakes will occur, with tragic consequences (Berman et al 1989). It is unlikely that postoperative radiotherapy will prove an adequate substitute for complete surgical clearance of the groin in this situation (see below).

Table 37.4 Inguinal node metastases in women with carcinoma of the vulva (Modified from Homesley et al 1991)

Nodal status	Midline lesions (n = 301)	Unilateral lesions (n = 287)	Total (n = 588)
Negative	61%	70%	65%
Bilateral	15%	6%	11%
Unilateral	24%	24%	24%
Ipsilateral		21%	
Contralateral		3%	
All positive	39%	30%	35%

Superficial lymphadenectomy does reduce still further the risk of troublesome lymphoedema and wound breakdown (DiSaia et al 1979, Helm et al 1992). However, because few women survive after recurrence in the groin, it is essential to ensure that this modified lymphadenectomy is as effective as standard inguinofemoral lymphadenectomy (Podratz et al 1982, Lingard et al 1992, Tilmans et al 1992, Piura et al 1993). Most of the experience with this technique has been obtained in women with a low risk of nodal disease, but several authors have commented upon an apparent increase in nodal recurrences (Table 37.5).

Hacker and his colleagues (1984a) noted that three of 26 patients who had a modified lymphadenectomy (1) or no lymphadenectomy (2) developed a groin recurrence. All three died, as did one other woman treated with radical local excision, giving a mortality rate of 15.4% for the conservative treatment of superficially invasive tumours. No groin recurrence was seen in 58 patients who were treated with inguinofemoral lymphadenectomy because of more advanced disease, and only one of these women died (mortality rate 1.7%). They commented that 'patients with greater than 1 mm of stromal invasion require at least ipsilateral inguinal–femoral lymphadenectomy'.

Berman and his group (1989) reported one nodal recurrence in 50 superficially invasive Stage I vulval cancers. The patient died. The M. D. Anderson group described the results of radical wide excision and selective inguinal node dissection in 32 women with tumours invading more than 1 mm into the stroma (Burke et al 1990). They excluded all patients with invasion less than 1 mm because most of those patients 'had no clinically identifiable tumour and were undergoing resection for suspected carcinoma in situ'. Only two patients were found to have groin node disease and the dissection was extended to include the deep femoral glands. Both received postoperative radiotherapy to the groins and whole pelvis, and were alive with no evidence of disease at 32 and 56 months. Helm and his associates described a similar experience in their matched, retrospective comparison of traditional radical vulvectomy with a triple-incision technique incor-

Table 37.5 Groin recurrence after superficial inguinal lymphadenectomy. None had clinically suspicious groin nodes

Reference	Depth of lesion (mm)	Diameter of lesion (cm)	Other criteria	Vulval surgery	Number evaluable	Groin recurrence	DoD with groin disease
DiSaia et al 1979	≤5	≤1	Non-clitoral, nodes negative	WLE	16	0	0
Hacker et al 1984a	≤5	≤2	No suspicious nodes	WLE	3	1	1
Berman et al 1989	<5	≤2	No suspicious or positive nodes	WLE	50	1	1
Burke et al 1990	>1	0.5–6.5	No suspicious nodes	WLE	32	1	0
Sutton et al 1991	1–5	≤2	No suspicious nodes	MRV	36	1	1
Kelly et al 1992	<1	≤2	No suspicious nodes	Various	11	1	0
Stehman et al 1992a	≤5	≤2	No suspicious or positive nodes	WLE	121	9	5
Helm et al 1992			All Stages	Various	32	3	1
					301	17 (5.7%)	9 (3.0%)

DoD, died of disease; WLE, wide local excision; MRV, modified radical vulvectomy

porating superficial lymphadenectomy in most cases (Helm et al 1992). The outcome in the 32 women in each group was similar, but they expressed concern that the four women with positive nodes in the conservative group seemed to have done rather badly.

At Indiana University, modified radical hemivulvectomy and superficial inguinal lymphadenectomy was performed on 36 women with lesions 2 cm in diameter or less, invading less than 5 mm into the stroma and without clinically suspicious nodes (Sutton et al 1991). One tumour recurred in the groin and the vulva less than 3 months after surgery, and this woman died a few months later in spite of further surgery and radiotherapy. The authors expressed concern at a possible increase in recurrent disease.

The M. D. Anderson Centre reported their experience with 24 cases of minimally invasive carcinoma, defined as lesions invading less than 1 mm (Kelly et al 1992). Most of these were women without a clinical tumour who were thought to have only VIN III. However, four patients (17%) developed recurrent VIN and four more developed an invasive recurrence (17%)! One of the invasive recurrences was in the groin of a woman whose superficial node dissection had been negative. She was treated with surgery and radiotherapy and was disease-free at 27 months. Two other cases of groin node recurrence in women with lesions invading less than 1 mm have been reported, one following wide local excision only (Atamdede & Hoogerland 1989) and one after a superficial lymphadenectomy (Van der Velden et al 1992). The authors of this chapter have themselves seen a third woman with a tiny, minimally invading lesion on the vulva who presented with groin node disease. Two of these women died of their disease and the third almost certainly did so, as she had multiple groin and pelvic nodes involved, but no follow-up was reported.

The only prospective study of conservative surgery has been performed by the Gynecological Oncology Group (Stehman et al 1992a). This examined the role of ipsilateral superficial inguinal lymphadenectomy and modified radical hemivulvectomy in 121 women with primary carcinoma of the vulva, 2 cm or less in maximum diameter, 5 mm or less in thickness, without vascular space invasion and with no suspicious groin nodes. Patients found to have positive lymph nodes at primary surgery were withdrawn. Although this was a highly selected, low-risk group of patients, invasive disease recurred in 19 women (15.6%). There were nine (7.3%) groin and ten (8.3%) vulval recurrences. Six of the groin recurrences occurred on the same side as the lymphadenectomy. At the time of the report, five of the nine women with recurrence in the groin had died, as had two of the ten with vulval recurrences. These results were compared with a historical group of 96 similar patients who had been treated with radical vulvectomy and bilateral inguinofemoral lymphadenopathy. Six (6.3%) of these developed a vulval recurrence, one (1.0%) developed a pelvic recurrence, but none recurred in the groin. The recurrence-free survival was significantly better in the historical controls ($P = 0.0028$). The authors expressed concern at the high rate of recurrent disease and noted especially the groin recurrences. They speculated very reasonably that this might be due to undetected disease in the femoral nodes.

This combined experience of superficial lymphadenectomy is not very reassuring. Even when applied to a low-risk population it seems to be associated with an unacceptably high risk of recurrent disease in the groin, which is ultimately fatal in most cases.

Deep femoral lymphadenectomy with preservation of the cribriform fascia

A study in Turin has suggested that the deep femoral nodes may be excised without removing the fascia lata or the cribriform fascia (Micheletti et al 1990). An earlier study of 50 female cadavers confirmed that these nodes lie medial to the femoral vein and can be seen through the fossa ovalis (Borgno et al 1990). The altered technique suggested by this anatomical information was used in 42 women with vulval cancer. An average of nine nodes were removed from each groin, a number similar to cadaver studies. The 5-year survival rates of 91.4% and 86.7% in 14 and 18 women with Stages I and II respectively are comparable to those reported in the literature. However, the wound complication rate remained high owing to retention of the ‘butterfly’ incision in the first 25 patients. This technique may allow the radical removal of superficial and deep groin lymph nodes with reduced morbidity, and is worthy of further investigation.

Pelvic lymphadenectomy

There is little value in performing a pelvic node dissection, as this probably has no therapeutic value (Shimm et al 1986) and as radiation therapy to the groins and pelvis gives superior results when the groin nodes are involved (Homesley et al 1986).

Modified radical vulvectomy

The major cause of psychosexual morbidity and of damage to body image comes from vulvectomy, particularly the removal of the clitoris and mons pubis. This has led some surgeons to devise more limited operations on the primary tumour when this has been small and unifocal (DiSaia et al 1971, Hacker et al 1984a). In all of these, the objective has been to obtain a margin of apparently healthy tissue of 2–3 cm all round the lesion. This is often impossible with lesions adjacent to the urethra or anus, but every effort must be made to maximize the margins even if this means sacrificing the lower 1–2 cm of the urethra or parts of the anus. The latter will sometimes make a colostomy necessary.

The risk of local recurrence is related to the size of the tumour-free margin (Heaps et al 1990). These authors recommended aiming for a tumour-free margin of only 1 cm, but the lesion may extend much further than is obvious to naked-eye inspection, so obtaining a wider zone of healthy tissue would be prudent. Not only are wide lateral margins required, but the dissection must be taken down to the deep fascia in exactly the same way as a traditional radical vulvectomy. These 'wide local excisions', 'hemivulvectomies' or 'modified radical vulvectomies' are very radical operations indeed, but in suitable cases do permit preservation of the clitoris and part of the vulva. The effect on psychosexual function has not been studied in depth, but it does seem likely that these procedures are less damaging (DiSaia et al 1979).

The reported vulval recurrences following radical local excision are shown in Table 37.6. The recurrence rate of 6.3% is a little disappointing for what are generally small, low-risk tumours. However, very few of these women subsequently died of their disease because vulval recurrences are fairly readily treated (Tilmans et al 1992, Piura et al 1993). A retrospective comparison of radical vulvectomy with modified radical vulvectomy found no difference in recurrence rates or cancer deaths in a small study with 45 patients in each group (Hoffman et al 1991). However, there were differences between the groups, not least in the length of follow-up, which was much shorter in the modified vulvectomy patients. More importantly, it was impossible to say why the women had been assigned to a particular form of treatment. There must be a substantial risk of an undetected bias in any study of this sort.

A similar, but much larger, study was undertaken at the M. D. Anderson Centre (Rutledge et al 1991). This consisted of an analysis of the records of 365 women with carcinoma of the vulva treated between 1944 and 1990. A Cox proportional hazards model was used to identify factors which predicted recurrence and death. This technique allows the effect of all known variables to be evaluated individually and together. An analysis of the 176 Stage I–II lesions treated with curative intent showed no difference in the disease-free survival or the survival corrected for death from intercurrent disease between women treated with radical vulvectomy and those who underwent radical local excision. Although this is reassuring, it should be noted that only 27 women were treated with radical local excision and few of these had been followed for more than 2 years (Mitchell, personal communication).

Complications

The complication rate depends on the surgical method, but all share common problems. The most common complication is wound breakdown and infection. With the triple-incision technique this is seldom more than a minor problem. Conservative therapy with liquid honey packs is all that is required for the occasional de-hiscence. Osteitis pubis is a rare but very serious compli-cation that requires intensive and prolonged antibiotic therapy. Thromboembolic disease is always a greatly feared complication of surgery for malignant disease, but the combination of perioperative epidural analgesia to ensure good venous return with subcutaneous heparin begun 12–24 hours before the operation seems to reduce this risk. Secondary haemorrhage occurs from time to time. Chronic leg oedema may be expected in 14–21% of women (Hacker et al 1981, Grimshaw et al 1993). Numbness and paraesthesia over the anterior thigh is common owing to the division of small cutaneous branches of the femoral nerve. Loss of body image and impaired sexual function undoubtedly occur but the patients' responses to surgery are enormously

Table 37.6 Vulval recurrences and deaths following conservative vulval surgery

Reference	Depth of lesion (mm)	Diameter of lesion (cm)	Other criteria	Vulval surgery	Groin surgery	Number evaluable	Vulval recurrence	DoD with vulval disease
DiSaia et al 1979	≤5	≤1	Non-clitoral, nodes negative	WLE	SIL	16	0	0
Hacker et al 1984a	9/10 < 1	≤2	No suspicious nodes	WLE	None	11	1	1
Hacker et al 1984a	≤5	≤2	No suspicious nodes	WLE	SIL	3	0	0
Hacker et al 1984a	≤5	≤2	No suspicious nodes	WLE/MRV	IFL	14	0	0
Burrell et al 1988	>1	0.7–4.5	Included suspicious nodes	MRV	IFL	28	0	0
Berman et al 1989	<5	≤2	No suspicious or positive nodes	WLE	SIL	50	4	0
Burke et al 1990	>1	0.5–6.5	No suspicious nodes	WLE	SIL	32	2	0
Hoffman et al 1991	>1	≤6	Included suspicious nodes	MRV	Various	45	1	0
Sutton et al 1991	≤1	≤2	No suspicious nodes	WLE	None	10	0	0
Sutton et al 1991	1–5	≤2	No suspicious nodes	MRV	SIL	36	3	0
Kelly et al 1992	>1	≤2	No suspicious nodes	WLE	Various	18	3	0
Stehman et al 1992a	≤5	≤2	No suspicious or positive nodes	WLE	SIL	121	10	2
						384	24 (6.3%)	3 (0.8%)

DoD, died of disease; WLE, wide local excision; MRV, modified radical vulvectomy; SIL, superficial inguinal lymphadenectomy; IFL, inguinofemoral lymphadenectomy

variable and probably depend on the woman's age, upbringing and attitude to life.

Conclusions

The emphasis of current research in the surgical treatment of vulval carcinoma is in reducing morbidity, especially for the young women in whom the disease appears to be becoming more common. However, reduced morbidity must not be gained at the cost of increased recurrence and mortality. There is little solid evidence on which to base a decision as to the best practice. Whereas most agree that an en bloc dissection of the inguinofemoral nodes and the vulva remains the optimum treatment for women with clinically suspicious nodes, there is no general agreement as to the best management for early invasive disease.

Groin node dissection. Given the available evidence, the lack of consistent results and the very high mortality associated with groin recurrences, it seems that the safest course is to perform a groin node dissection in all cases with more than 1 mm stromal invasion and to remove both superficial and deep nodes en bloc (Hacker et al 1984a, Monaghan 1985a). A possible exception might be women with what appears to be VIN III in whom a small, superficial focus of invasion is found histologically. These might not require lymphadenectomy. It certainly does not make sense to omit groin node dissection in elderly women, because they have a higher incidence of nodal disease (Homesley et al 1993). Individual women with selected Stage I–II lesions may prefer to take the risk of unilateral lymphadenectomy, but very careful pathological and clinical assessment would be necessary to advise on the degree of risk. Separate incisions in the groin are recommended in cases without clinically suspicious nodes, but en bloc excision with the vulva is probably required in other cases. The technique of deep femoral lymphadenectomy which preserves the cribriform fascia is worth investigation.

Vulval dissection. Because recurrent disease on the vulva does not carry such a high risk of mortality, and because it is the vulval surgery which has the greatest impact upon a woman's body image and sexuality, there is more to be gained and less to lose from conservative vulval surgery. Although the evidence supporting radical local excision is far from conclusive it would seem to offer a reasonable approach, provided the principles of wide lateral and deep margins are observed. The benefits will be far less in anterior and clitoral lesions. Large or multicentric lesions will still require radical vulvectomy to achieve adequate local control. Such tumours may benefit from preoperative irradiation (see below).

The role of radiotherapy

For many years radiotherapy to the vulva was avoided because severe late morbidity was common with the machines available and the techniques used. Severe acute reactions in the vulval epithelium and severe late radiation reactions, such as vulvar fibrosis, atrophy or even necrosis, made radiotherapy to this organ difficult. Modified techniques now permit radiation to the vulva without undue morbidity.

Technique

At Hammersmith Hospital, radiotherapy is given in two fractions per day at least 6 hours apart. This approach enables a large percentage of the total dose to be given over a short period of time, and avoids delays in treatment caused by acute local reactions. Preoperative treatment consists of 1.5 Gy per fraction given to a total dose of 45 Gy in 30 fractions, 5 days per week for 3 weeks. Surgery can be carried out 2–3 weeks later, when healing is usually complete. Those rare women who are unsuitable for surgery receive 45 Gy in 3 weeks to the vulva, followed by a 2-week break before continuing with the same fractionation regimen to a total dose of 65 Gy. Whereas photons are used for opposed radiation fields to the whole of the vulva, smaller vulval lesions are treated with electrons on direct perineal fields because of their limited depth of penetration, thus reducing the radiation effect on organs close to the vulva. This regimen is well tolerated and the reduced treatment time allows the prescribed dose to be given without interruption.

Interstitial radiotherapy has a place in the non-surgical management of cancer of the vulva as an alternative to electrons, particularly if the lower vagina is involved. It is carried out by the insertion of needles afterloaded with iridium-192. A plastic template, such as the Hammersmith Hedgehog, ensures an even distribution. The procedure is carried out under general anaesthesia. For small lesions when interstitial therapy is used alone, the total dose should be no higher than 65 Gy given over 6–7 days to prevent serious morbidity. Sometimes external and interstitial radiotherapy are given sequentially, the interstitial treatment being given 2 weeks after the end of external beam therapy. The total dose remains 65 Gy. The importance of the size of the total dose was shown in a report of interstitial radiotherapy, combined in most cases with external radiation, in which six of 10 patients developed radionecrosis when doses of 70–90 Gy were given (Hoffman et al 1990).

Primary radical radiotherapy

Radiotherapy is considered as primary radical treatment only for patients who are unfit for surgery. With modern anaesthesia and current surgical techniques, such cases are very few.

Preoperative radiotherapy to the vulva

Patients with large tumours which extend very close to or involve the urethra, vagina or anus may benefit from preoperative radiotherapy alone or with chemotherapy to facilitate subsequent surgery and reduce morbidity. Preoperative radiotherapy can be given to the vulva without serious complications, and substantially reduces the size of the lesions (Acosta et al 1978, Hacker et al 1984b, Boronow et al 1987, Rotmensch et al 1990).

Postoperative radiotherapy to the vulva

Heaps et al (1990) concluded that a surgical disease-free margin of less than 8 mm was associated with a 50% chance of recurrence. If further surgery is not going to be possible, postoperative radiotherapy to the vulva should be considered. The radiotherapy field may not always need to cover the whole vulva but can be confined to the site of disease in early lateral lesions (Thomas et al 1991).

Radiotherapy for groin node disease

Some 20% of women with positive groin nodes will have metastatic disease in the pelvic lymph nodes. Radiotherapy to the groin and pelvic nodes is more effective than pelvic lymphadenectomy in the management of women with positive groin nodes if given after a complete inguinofemoral lymphadenectomy (Homesley et al 1986) and is now given to all women with more than microscopic disease of one groin node. A total dose of 45–50 Gy in 1.8–2.0 Gy fractions is administered to the midplane of the pelvis in opposed anterior and posterior fields, using a midline block to protect the vulva. In addition, 45–50 Gy, measured 2–3 cm from the anterior surface, is given to the centre of the inguinal and femoral nodes. Using this technique, both the time to recurrence and the survival are improved.

Preoperative radiotherapy to the groins and pelvis may be of value in women with clinically detectable disease in the nodes (Boronow et al 1987). Only one of seven had residual disease at surgery following radiotherapy, compared with seven of nine to whom radiotherapy was not given. Some authors have even suggested radiotherapy as an alternative to inguinofemoral lymphadenectomy (Perez et al 1993). However, this opinion was based upon a retrospective review of a highly selected group of 37 women treated over a period of 22 years. In contrast, the Gynecological Oncology Group prematurely terminated a prospective randomized controlled trial comparing radiotherapy with inguinofemoral lymphadenectomy in a group of women with clinically non-involved nodes because of the higher recurrence rate ($P = 0.033$) and mortality ($P = 0.035$) in the radiation group (Stehman et al 1992b). The 20% of those who were found to have positive nodes at surgery received postoperative radiotherapy to the groin and pelvis. Five (18.5%) groin relapses occurred in the radiation-only group, compared to none in the groin dissection regimen. Although radiation is a useful supplement to inguinofemoral lymphadenectomy, it is not an effective substitute.

Concurrent chemoradiotherapy

Concurrent radiotherapy and chemotherapy has been used for vulval carcinoma in a small number of cases and remains an experimental procedure.

Conclusion

Surgery remains the mainstay of treatment, but radiotherapy has a proven role in the treatment of groin node disease after inguinofemoral lymphadenectomy. It may also prevent local recurrence in the vulva when there is an insufficient tumour-free margin. Radiotherapy may be used for the preoperative treatment of advanced disease. Chemotherapy may add to the efficacy of radiotherapy when used concurrently, but this has not yet been demonstrated by randomized studies.

Recurrent disease

Although most women with recurrence in the groin die in spite of treatment, surgical excision of a vulval recurrence can be effective, especially if the recurrence is delayed for more than 2 years (Shimm et al 1986, Grimshaw et al 1993). However, in the majority of patients only palliative treatment is possible and this is usually radiotherapy, either external or interstitial.

Chemotherapy may be given with the radiotherapy or alone. As well as regimens using 5-fluorouracil, other cytotoxic combinations have been assessed. The EORTC used a continuous low-dose regimen designed for elderly women consisting of bleomycin, methotrexate and CCNU given as a 6-week cycle repeated three times, depending on response and toxicity (Durrant et al 1990). Although 60% of 28 women with inoperable or recurrent tumours showed a response, toxicity was unacceptably high, particularly stomatitis and infection secondary to myelosuppression. Single-agent chemotherapy using bleomycin or cisplatin can give a few partial responses, but is usually ineffective (Deppe et al 1979, Thigpen et al 1986).

Results of treatment

Corrected survival rates from two recent publications are shown in Table 37.7 (Homesley et al 1993, Grimshaw et al 1993). These use the 1988 FIGO staging which includes the surgical findings, so Stages I and II do not have groin lymph node involvement. However, Stages III and

Table 37.7 Survival by FIGO Stage (1988) (Homesley et al 1993, Grimshaw et al 1993)

FIGO Stage	Corrected 5-year survival (%)	
	Grimshaw et al (1993)	Homesley et al (1993)
I	97	98
II	85	85
III	46	74
IV	50	31

IV are more heterogeneous. The overall 5-year corrected survival in the British study was 74.6% (Grimshaw et al 1993).

UNCOMMON TUMOURS OF THE VULVA

Melanoma

Approximately 5% of melanomas in women occur on the vulva, and this is the second most common carcinoma of the vulva (Monaghan & Hammond 1984, Morrow & DiSaia 1976). Melanin production is variable, and the lesions range from black to completely amelanotic. The most usual presenting complaint is of a lump or an enlarging mole. Pruritus and bleeding are less common.

The prognosis is strongly related to the depth of invasion (Clark et al 1969, Breslow 1970, Podratz et al 1983). Because of the absence of a well defined papillary dermis in much of the vulvar skin, levels of invasion as defined by Clark and co-workers (1969) are unsuitable for use on vulvar skin (Chung et al 1975), and measurement of the thickness of the lesion as suggested by Breslow (1970) may be more reproducible. No patient from the Sloan-Kettering series died with a lesion with less than 1 mm penetration but thereafter the outlook was bleak (Chung et al 1975).

Local invasion occurs in an outward direction as well as downward, so excision margins must be very wide, 3–5 cm being suggested for all but the most superficial lesions (White & Polk 1986). Approximately one-third of patients have inguinal lymph node metastases at presentation and 2.6% have distant spread (Morrow & DiSaia 1976). When the nodes are negative, the 5-year survival is approximately 56%, falling to 14% when the nodes are positive (Morrow & DiSaia 1976). Involvement of urethra or vagina, or the presence of satellite lesions, all worsen the prognosis.

It is probable that the minimum therapy should be wide local excision (this usually requires a radical vulvectomy) without lymphadenectomy unless there is clinical evidence of groin disease (White & Polk 1986, Davidson et al 1987). If the groin nodes are removed, the operation should be performed en bloc rather than through separate incisions because of the melanoma's propensity to spread unseen by lateral intradermal infiltration (Karlen et al 1975). Radiation therapy is ineffective (White & Polk 1986) and adjuvant chemotherapy and immunotherapy have no proven value. Chemotherapy has not proved effective in the treatment of recurrent disease (Seeger et al 1986).

Verrucous carcinoma

This slowly growing neoplasm is seen rarely on the vulva (Gallousis 1972, Isaacs 1976). Both macroscopically and histologically it resembles condyloma acuminata and the diagnosis can be difficult. Generous biopsies are required to provide sufficient material for the pathologist. The treatment is surgery, usually a radical vulvectomy but very occasionally wide local excision. The place of lymphadenectomy is debatable, as lymph node metastases are uncommon. Radiotherapy is ineffective and may result in anaplastic transformation (Krausz & Perez-Mesa 1966).

Basal cell carcinoma

This tumour is rarely found on the vulva. Wide local excision gives excellent results in most cases.

Bartholin's gland carcinoma

Usually an adenocarcinoma, this tumour may be squamous, transitional cell type, or even mixed squamous and adenocarcinoma (Cavanagh et al 1985). It has often spread widely to pelvic and groin nodes before the diagnosis is made. It must be distinguished from adenoid cystic carcinoma, which is similar to the tumour found in salivary glands and which seldom gives rise to metastatic disease (Webb et al 1984, Cavanagh et al 1985). The treatment is surgery but because of its deep origin, part of the vagina, levatores ani and the ischiorectal fat must be removed.

Sarcoma

This is a particularly rare tumour. Leiomyosarcomas may be difficult to distinguish from their benign counterpart histologically, but the presence of more than 10 mitoses per high-power field serves to differentiate the two. These tumours tend to grow slowly and metastasize late. In contrast, rhabdomyosarcomas are rapidly growing, aggressive tumours. A radical vulvectomy and groin node dissection is the usual treatment, but local recurrence is common and haematogenous spread is unaffected by this treatment (DiSaia et al 1971, Cavanagh et al 1985).

CONCLUSIONS

The main problems with carcinoma of the vulva are delay in presentation and diagnosis, and inadequate initial therapy. Surgery remains the cornerstone of treatment but, in carefully selected cases, this can be made less extensive than in the past. Even when radical surgery is necessary, new techniques have reduced the morbidity enormously. Radiotherapy has an important role to play in the treatment of patients with metastatic groin node disease.

CANCER OF THE VAGINA

INTRODUCTION

Invasive vaginal cancer is rare. With 184 cases in England and Wales in 1981, the incidence was 0.7/100 000 women (OPCS 1985). However, like the cervix, the vagina has a range of premalignant lesions, many of which may be previously unrecognized extensions of cervical abnormalities. Coincident with the rise in prevalence of cervical intraepithelial neoplasia (CIN) is an increase in the frequency with which vaginal intraepithelial neoplasia (VAIN) is seen.

AETIOLOGY

Irritation, immunosuppression, infection

There is little firm evidence of aetiological agents. The irritation caused by procidentia and vaginal pessaries has been suggested but this is an infrequent association (Al-Kurdi & Monaghan 1981, Benedet et al 1983). A field effect in the lower genital tract has been suggested by the observation of multicentric neoplasia involving cervix, vagina and vulva (Hernandez-Linares et al 1980, Weed et al 1983), and both immunosuppression and infection with HPV have been suggested (Weed et al 1983, Carson et al 1986).

Radiation-induced vaginal cancer

The aetiological role of radiotherapy is hard to determine, but is no longer simply a theoretical question in view of the proposal that preinvasive disease of the vaginal vault after hysterectomy should be treated by radiotherapy (Woodman et al 1988).

Evidence for radiation-induced vaginal cancer

Three studies have raised a concern that women less than 40 years old, treated with radiotherapy for cervical cancer, may be at a high risk of subsequently developing vaginal cancer 10–40 years later. A high proportion of those women who developed a primary vaginal cancer after radiotherapy for cervical cancer were less than 40 years of age when treated for their first cancer (Barrie & Brunschwig 1970, Choo & Anderson 1982). Futoran and Nolan (1976) reported the appearance of a primary vaginal cancer in eight of 42 women treated with radiotherapy for Stage I cervical cancer when less than 40 years of age, and followed for 10 years or more.

Evidence for the defence

However, only 50 (1.54%) of 3239 patients treated for cervical cancer, most with radiotherapy, subsequently developed a primary vaginal neoplasm, and only 29 of these had invasive lesions (Choo & Anderson 1982). Furthermore, an international collaborative study of cancer registers recorded only 48 cancers of the vagina or vulva (ICD7–176) in 25 995 women treated with radiotherapy for cervical cancer and followed for 10 or more years (Boice et al 1985). The proportion of women treated with surgery and followed for 10 or more years and who were recorded as developing a vaginal or vulval cancer was similar (seven of 5125) to that seen following radiotherapy. These data suggest that if vaginal cancer is induced by radiotherapy it is a very rare event.

Diethylstilboestrol

For some time the prevalence of clear cell adenocarcinoma of the vagina was thought to be increased by intrauterine exposure to diethylstilboestrol (Herbst et al 1971). With the accrual of more information the risks now seem to be very low and lie between 0.1 and 1.0 per 1000 (Coppleson 1984, Herbst 1984). Whereas vaginal adenosis and minor anatomical abnormalities of no significance (e.g. cervical cockscomb) are common following intrauterine diethylstilboestrol exposure, the only lesion of any significance that is seen more commonly is CIN (Robboy et al 1984). Uterine malformations may be more common and may result in impaired fecundity in a small minority of cases.

ANATOMY

The anatomy of the vagina is described in Chapters 2 and 36.

PATHOLOGY

The great majority (92%) of primary vaginal cancers are squamous. Clear cell adenocarcinomas, malignant melanomas, embryonal rhabdomyosarcomas and endodermal sinus tumours are the commonest of the small number of other tumours seen very rarely in the vagina. These are discussed separately.

NATURAL HISTORY

Although the upper vagina is the commonest site for invasive disease, about 25–30% is confined to the lower vagina, usually the anterior wall (Pride et al 1979, Monaghan 1985b, Gallup et al 1987). Squamous vaginal cancer spreads by local invasion initially. Lymphatic spread occurs by tumour embolization to the pelvic nodes from

Table 37.8 FIGO staging for vaginal cancer (Pettersson 1995)

Stage	Definition
Stage 0	Intraepithelial neoplasia
Stage I	Invasive carcinoma confined to vaginal mucosa
Stage II	Subvaginal infiltration not extending to pelvic wall
Stage III	Extends to pelvic wall
Stage IVa	Involves mucosa of bladder or rectum
Stage IVb	Spread beyond the pelvis

the upper vagina and to both pelvic and inguinal nodes from the lower vagina (Monaghan 1985b). Haematogenous spread is unusual.

CLINICAL STAGING

The FIGO clinical staging is shown in Table 37.8.

DIAGNOSIS AND ASSESSMENT

Before making a diagnosis of primary vaginal cancer, the following criteria must be satisfied: the primary site of growth must be in the vagina; the uterine cervix must not be involved; and there must be no clinical evidence that the vaginal tumour is metastatic disease (Pettersson 1995). To this list, Murad and colleagues (1975) would add that the patient should not have had any antecedent genital cancer. Choo and Anderson (1982) dissent from this view, which they regard as too restrictive. In their series, 11 of the 14 invasive vaginal cancers following radiation therapy for cervical cancer occurred after an interval of more than 10 years, and three were of a different histological type.

The most common presenting symptom is vaginal bleeding (53–65%), with vaginal discharge (11–16%) and pelvic pain (4–11%) being less common (Pride et al 1979, Gallup et al 1987). The rate of detection of asymptomatic cancer with vaginal cytology varies greatly (10–42%) depending on the patient population studied, and most of the disease thus detected is at an early stage (Pride et al 1979, Choo & Anderson 1982, Gallup et al 1987).

The most important part of the pretreatment assessment of invasive cancer of the vagina is a careful examination under anaesthesia. Colposcopy will identify coexisting VAIN and help to define the location of the lesion. A combined vaginal and rectal examination will help to detect extravaginal spread. Cystoscopy and proctosigmoidoscopy are indicated if anterior or posterior spread is suspected. A generous, full-thickness biopsy is essential for adequate histological evaluation. A chest X-ray and an intravenous pyelogram are the only radiological investigations required routinely, but lymphangiography can help occasionally in Stage II cases to determine the need for teletherapy. Transrectal ultrasound and magnetic resonance imaging can be used to define the size and extent of the lesion.

TREATMENT AND COMPLICATIONS

Radiotherapy

Invasive vaginal cancer is usually treated with radiotherapy. Early cases, Stage I–IIa, may be treated entirely with interstitial therapy with iridium-192. In the Hammersmith Hospital this is afterloaded into three concentric rings of stainless-steel guide needles located by a specially designed template (Branson et al 1985). The two outer rings of needles are located in the paravaginal space by being inserted through the perineum under general anaesthesia. The inner ring is located in grooves on a vaginal obturator. The objective is to achieve a tumour dose of 70–80 Gy in two fractions, each over 72 hours, 2 weeks apart. Cases with parametrial involvement receive teletherapy to the pelvis as for carcinoma of the cervix, with a tumour dose of 45 Gy followed by interstitial or intracavitary therapy to a total dose of 70–75 Gy. The field may be extended to include the groins if the tumour involves the lower half of the vagina.

Complications of radiotherapy

Vaginal stenosis may occur and is more likely when advanced tumours are treated (Puthawala et al 1983). The overall prevalence of vaginal stenosis is 25–32% (Pride et al 1979, Puthawala et al 1983, Gallup et al 1987) and is an undoubted problem for sexually active patients. Mucosal ulceration, either immediate or delayed, can be a distressing complication but conservative therapy, sometimes aided by grafts, is usually effective. Approximately 10% of patients develop a fistula or other serious complication (Pride et al 1979, Puthawala et al 1983, Gallup et al 1987) and these are almost invariably associated with teletherapy for advanced disease (Pride et al 1979). Vesicovaginal and rectovaginal fistulae and small bowel complications are especially frequent if previously irradiated patients are treated with radiotherapy (Choo & Anderson 1982).

Surgery

A Stage I lesion in the upper vagina can be adequately treated by radical hysterectomy (if the uterus is still present), radical vaginectomy and pelvic lymphadenectomy (Ball & Berman 1982, Johnston et al 1983) (Fig. 37.6). Exenteration is required for more advanced lesions and carries the problems of stomata. However, surgery may be the treatment of choice for women who have had prior pelvic radiotherapy (Choo & Anderson 1982).

RESULTS

Probably as a result of the small numbers of cases in the reported series, the 5-year survival figures described for Stage I range widely from 64 to 90%, and for Stage II

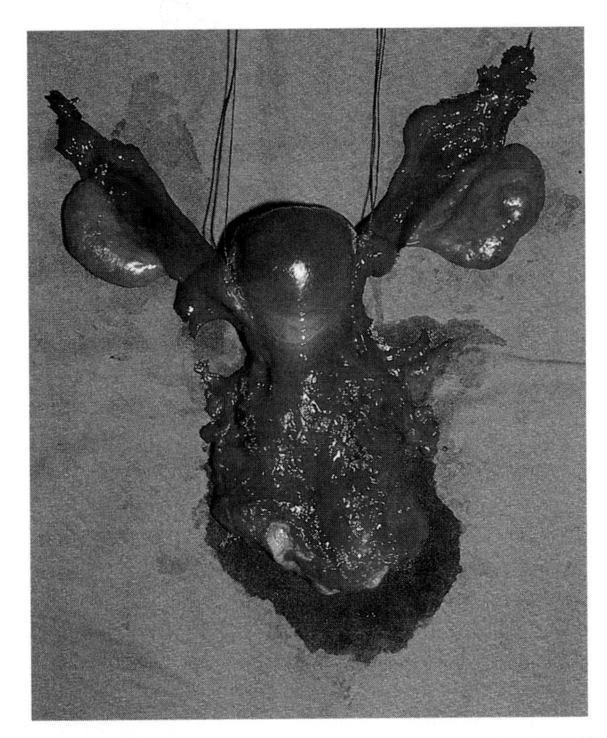

Fig. 37.6 Radical hysterectomy and total vaginectomy for Stage I carcinoma extending into the middle third of the vagina.

Table 37.9 Five-year survival rates for vaginal cancer

	Perez & Camel (1982)		Kucera et al (1985)	
Stage	No. of cases	% Alive	No. of cases	% Alive
0	15	90		
I	39	90	67	75
IIa	39	58		
IIb	21	32		
II			120	46
III	12	40	191	29
IV	8	0	83	19

from 29 to 66% (Monaghan 1985b). The results of therapy in more advanced disease are less satisfactory, with 5-year figures for Stage III of 17–49% (Monaghan 1985b). Some of the best results in a reasonably sized series are quoted by Perez and Camel (1982) and the largest series reported is by Kucera and colleagues (1985) (Table 37.9).

CONCLUSIONS

Invasive vaginal cancer is a rare tumour more often seen in association with an antecedent cervical malignancy. Radiotherapy is the main treatment method. Interstitial therapy offers good cure rates in Stages I–IIa, with only a small risk of seriously impairing vaginal function. Teletherapy is added for more advanced cases. Previous pelvic radiotherapy greatly increases the risk of serious complications and individualization of treatment regimens is essential for the best results.

UNCOMMON VAGINAL TUMOURS

Clear cell adenocarcinoma

The relation of this rare tumour to intrauterine exposure to diethylstilboestrol is discussed under Aetiology. The histology is characterized by vacuolated or clear areas in the cytoplasm and a hobnail appearance of the nuclei of cells lining the lumen of glands. Radical surgery or radical radiotherapy is required for invasive lesions. As most are situated in the upper vagina they may be treated as cervical lesions. Lymph node metastases and 5-year survival figures are equivalent to those for cervical cancer (Herbst & Scully 1983).

Malignant melanoma

Vaginal melanoma has a 5-year survival rate of only 7% (Lee et al 1984). Vaginal bleeding and discharge are the commonest presenting symptoms. The prognosis depends upon the depth of epithelial invasion. Radical surgery and radiotherapy are of little value if the lesion is deeply invasive because of its propensity to metastasize early via the bloodstream. There is at present no effective chemotherapy.

Rhabdomyosarcoma (sarcoma botryoides)

Some 90% of these rare tumours occur in children less than 5 years old. They present with vaginal bleeding and a grape-like mass in the vagina. The appearance of cross-striations in the rhabdomyoblasts is characteristic of this tumour. The results of radical surgery are poor (Huffman 1968), but chemotherapy alone with VAC (vincristine, actinomycin D and cyclophosphamide) now gives 'cure' in 82% of cases (Raney et al 1983). Indeed, Dewhurst (1985) reported seven alive and well out of a small personal series of nine children followed for 4–19 years.

Endodermal sinus tumour

These very rare tumours may resemble rhabdomyosarcomas but histology shows a primitive adenocarcinoma. Most occur in infants under the age of 2. Although surgery used to be the mainstay of treatment, with an occasional long-term survivor (Dewhurst & Ferreira 1981), chemotherapy with regimens used for this tumour in other sites may offer a hope for more long-term cures (Wiltshaw 1985).

KEY POINTS

1. The prognosis for vulval cancer is good if the lesion is treated adequately at an early stage.
2. Even elderly and relatively unfit women should be treated surgically.
3. There is no place for superficial inguinal lymphadenectomy in the treatment of vulval carcinoma.
4. Inguinofemoral lymphadenectomy should be carried out in all but a small minority of cases, which usually present as VIN rather than clinical invasion.
5. Cases suitable for local radical excision must be chosen with great care – many will need radical vulvectomy.
6. Radiotherapy should be used to treat the pelvis and groins of women with positive groin nodes.
7. Radiotherapy may have a role in treating large tumours prior to surgery, but this remains an experimental approach.
8. Radiotherapy rarely, if ever, causes a vaginal carcinoma.
9. The risks of vaginal cancer in diethylstilboestrol-exposed women now appear to be very low indeed.
10. Early vaginal cancer may be treated with surgery or interstitial brachytherapy, but more advanced cases are better treated with radiotherapy.

REFERENCES

Acosta A A, Given F T, Frazier A B, Cordoba R B, Luminari A 1978 Preoperative radiation therapy in the management of squamous cell carcinoma of the vulva: preliminary report. American Journal of Obstetrics and Gynecology 132: 198–206

Al-Kurdi M, Monaghan J M 1981 Thirty-two years experience in management of primary tumours of the vagina. British Journal of Obstetrics and Gynaecology 88: 1145–1150

Andersen B L, Hacker N F 1983 Psychosexual adjustment after vulvar surgery. Obstetrics and Gynecology 62: 457–462

Atamdede F, Hoogerland D 1989 Regional lymph node recurrence following local excision for microinvasive vulvar carcinoma. Gynecologic Oncology 34: 125–128

Ball H G, Berman M L 1982 Management of primary vaginal carcinoma. Gynecologic Oncology 14: 154–163

Ballon S C, Lamb E J 1975 Separate incisions in the treatment of carcinoma of the vulva. Surgery, Gynecology and Obstetrics 140: 81–84

Barrie J R, Brunschwig A 1970 Late second cancers of the cervix after apparent successful initial radiation therapy. American Journal of Roentgenology and Therapeutic Nuclear Medicine 109: 109–112

Benedet J L, Murphy K J, Fairey R N, Boyes D A 1983 Primary invasive carcinoma of the vagina. Obstetrics and Gynecology 62: 715–719

Bergeron C, Ferenczy A, Shah K, Naghashfar Z 1987 Multicentric human papillomavirus infections of the female genital tract: correlation of viral types with abnormal mitotic figures, colposcopic presentation and location. Obstetrics and Gynecology 69: 736–742

Berman M L, Soper J T, Creasman W T, Olt G T, DiSaia P J 1989 Conservative surgical management of superficially invasive Stage I vulvar carcinoma. Gynecologic Oncology 35: 352–357

Boehm F, Morris J M 1971 Paget's disease and apocrine gland carcinoma of the vulva. Obstetrics and Gynecology 38: 185–192

Boice J D, Day N E, Andersen A et al 1985 Second cancers following treatment for cervical cancer. An international collaboration among cancer registries. Journal of the National Cancer Institute 74: 955–975

Borgno G, Micheletti L, Barbero M et al 1990 Topographic distribution of groin lymph nodes. Journal of Reproductive Medicine 35: 1127–1129

Boronow R C, Hickman B T, Reagan M T et al 1987 Combined therapy as an alternative to exenteration for locally advanced vulvovaginal cancer. American Journal of Clinical Oncology 10: 171–181

Branson A N, Dunn P, Kam K C, Lambert H E 1985 A device for interstitial therapy of low pelvic tumours – the Hammersmith Perineal Hedgehog. British Journal of Radiology 58: 537–542

Breslow A 1970 Thickness, cross-sectional areas and depth of invasion in the prognosis of cutaneous melanoma. Annals of Surgery 172: 902–908

Brinton L A, Nasca P C, Mallin K, Baptiste M S, Willbanks G D, Richart R M 1990 Case control study of cancer of the vulva. Obstetrics and Gynecology 75: 859–866

Bryson S C, Dembo A J, Colgan T J, Thomas G M, DeBoer G, Lickrish G M 1991 Invasive squamous cell carcinoma of the vulva: defining low and high risk groups for recurrence. International Journal of Gynecological Cancer 1: 25–31

Burke T W, Stringer C A, Gershenson D M, Edwards C L, Morris M, Wharton J T 1990 Radical wide excision and selective inguinal node dissection for squamous cell carcinoma of the vulva. Gynecologic Oncology 38: 328–332

Burrell M O, Franklin E W, Campion M J, Crozier M A, Stacy P W 1988 The modified radical vulvectomy with groin dissection: an eight year experience. American Journal of Obstetrics and Gynecology 159: 715–722

Byron R L, Lamb E J, Yonemoto R H, Kase S 1962 Radical inguinal node dissection in the treatment of cancer. Surgery, Gynecology and Obstetrics 114: 401–408

Carson L F, Twiggs L B, Fukushima M, Ostrow R S, Faras A J, Okagaki T 1986 Human genital papilloma infections: an evaluation of immunologic competence in the genital neoplasia–papilloma syndrome. American Journal of Obstetrics and Gynecology 155: 784–789

Cavanagh D, Ruffolo E H, Marsden D E 1985 Cancer of the vulva. In: Cavanagh D, Ruffolo E H, Marsden D E (eds) Gynecologic cancer – a clinicopathological approach. Appleton-Century-Crofts, Connecticut, pp 1–40

Cavanagh D, Fiorica J V, Hoffman M S et al 1990 Invasive carcinoma of the vulva – changing trends in surgical management. American Journal of Obstetrics and Gynecology 163: 1007–1015

Choo Y C, Anderson D G 1982 Neoplasms of the vagina following cervical carcinoma. Gynecologic Oncology 14: 125–132

Chung A F, Woodruff J M, Lewis J L 1975 Malignant melanoma of the vulva: a report of 44 cases. Obstetrics and Gynecology 45: 638–646

Clark W H, From L, Bernadino E A, Mihm M C 1969 The histogenesis and biologic behaviour of primary human malignant melanomas of the skin. Cancer Research 29: 705–726

Coppleson M 1984 The DES story. Medical Journal of Australia 141: 487–489

Creasman W T, Gallacher H S, Rutledge F 1975 Paget's disease of the vulva. Gynecologic Oncology 3: 133–148

Davidson T, Kissin M, Westbury G 1987 Vulvo-vaginal melanoma: should radical surgery be abandoned? British Journal of Obstetrics and Gynaecology 94: 473–476

Deppe G, Cohen C J, Bruckner H W 1979 Chemotherapy of squamous cell carcinoma of the vulva: a review. Gynecologic Oncology 7: 345–348

Dewhurst J 1985 Malignant disease of the genital organs in childhood. In: Shepherd J H, Monaghan J M (eds) Clinical gynaecological oncology. Blackwell, London, pp 270–285

Dewhurst J, Ferreira H P 1981 An endodermal sinus tumour of the

vagina in an infant with 7-year survival. British Journal of Obstetrics and Gynaecology 88: 859–862
DiSaia P J, Rutledge F, Smith J P 1971 Sarcoma of the vulva. Obstetrics and Gynecology 38: 180–184
DiSaia P J, Creasman W T, Rich W M 1979 An alternative approach to early cancer of the vulva. American Journal of Obstetrics and Gynecology 133: 825–832
Durrant K R, Mangioni C, Lacave A J et al 1990 Bleomycin, methotrexate, and CCNU in advanced inoperable squamous cell carcinoma of the vulva: a phase II study of the EORTC Gynaecological Cancer Cooperative Group (GCCG). Gynecologic Oncology 37: 359–362
Friedrich E G, Wilkinson E J 1982 The vulva. In: Blaustein A (ed) Pathology of the female genital tract, 2nd edn. Springer-Verlag, New York, pp 13–58
Futoran R J, Nolan J F 1976 Stage I carcinoma of the uterine cervix in patients under 40 years of age. American Journal of Obstetrics and Gynecology 125: 790–797
Gallousis S 1972 Verrucous carcinoma – report of three vulvar cases and review of the literature. Obstetrics and Gynecology 40: 502–507
Gallup D G, Talledo O E, Shah K J, Hayes C 1987 Invasive squamous cell carcinoma of the vagina: a 14-year study. Obstetrics and Gynecology 69: 782–785
Grimshaw R N, Murdoch J B, Monaghan J M 1993 Radical vulvectomy and bilateral inguinal–femoral lymphadenectomy through separate incisions – experience with 100 cases. International Journal of Gynecological Cancer 3: 18–23
Hacker N F, Leuchter R S, Berek J S, Castaldo T W, Lagasse L D 1981 Radical vulvectomy and bilateral inguinal lymphadenectomy through separate groin incisions. Obstetrics and Gynecology 59: 574–579
Hacker N F, Berek J S, Lagasse L D, Neiberg R K, Leuchter R S 1984a Individualisation of treatment for Stage I squamous cell vulvar carcinoma. Obstetrics and Gynecology 63: 155–162
Hacker N F, Berek J S, Juillard G J F, Lagasse L D 1984b Preoperative radiation therapy for locally advanced vulvar cancer. Cancer 54: 2056–2061
Hammond I G, Monaghan J M 1983 Multicentric carcinoma of the female genital tract. British Journal of Obstetrics and Gynaecology 90: 557–561
Heaps J M, Fu Y S, Montz F J, Hacker N F, Berek J S 1990 Surgical–pathological variables predictive of local recurrence in squamous cell carcinoma of the vulva. Gynecologic Oncology 38: 309–314
Helm C W, Hatch K, Austin J M et al 1992 A matched comparison of single and triple incision techniques for the surgical treatment of carcinoma of the vulva. Gynecologic Oncology 46: 150–156
Herbst A L 1984 Diethylstilboestrol exposure – 1984. New England Journal of Medicine 22: 1433–1435
Herbst A L, Scully R E 1983 Newsletter – Registry for research on hormonal transplacental carcinogenesis.
Herbst A L, Ulfelder H, Poskanzer D C 1971 Adenocarcinoma of the vagina; association of maternal stilbestrol therapy with tumour appearance in young women. New England Journal of Medicine 284: 878–881
Hernandez-Linares W, Puthawala A, Nolan J F, Jernstrom P H, Morrow C P 1980 Carcinoma in situ of the vagina: past and present management. Obstetrics and Gynecology 56: 356–360
Hoffman J S, Kumar N B, Morley G W 1983 Microinvasive squamous carcinoma of the vulva: search for a definition. Obstetrics and Gynecology 61: 615–618
Hoffman M, Greenberg S, Greenberg H et al 1990 Interstitial radiotherapy for the treatment of advanced or recurrent vulvar and distal vaginal malignancy. American Journal of Obstetrics and Gynecology 162: 1278–1282
Hoffman M S, Roberts W S, Finan M A et al 1991 A comparative study of radical vulvectomy and modified radical vulvectomy for the treatment of invasive squamous cell carcinoma of the vulva. Gynecologic Oncology 45: 192–197
Homesley H D, Bundy B N, Sedlis A, Adcock L 1986 Radiation therapy versus pelvic node resection for carcinoma of the vulva with positive groin nodes. Obstetrics and Gynecology 68: 733–740
Homesley H D, Bundy B N, Sedlis A, Yorand E, Berek J S, Jahshan A, Mortel R 1991 Assessment of current International Federation of Gynaecology and Obstetrics staging of vulvar carcinoma relative to prognostic factors for survival (a Gynecological Oncology Group Study). American Journal of Obstetrics and Gynecology 164: 997–1004
Homesley H D, Bundy B N, Sedlis A et al 1993 Prognostic factors for groin node metastasis in squamous cell carcinoma of the vulva (a Gynecologic Oncology Group Study). Gynecologic Oncology 49: 279–283
Huffman J W 1968 The gynecology of childhood and adolescence. W B Saunders, Philadelphia
Isaacs J H 1976 Verrucous carcinoma of the female genital tract. Gynecologic Oncology 4: 259–269
Iversen T, Aas M 1983 Lymph drainage from the vulva. Gynecologic Oncology 16: 179–189
Iversen T, Abeler V, Aalders J 1981 Individualised treatment of Stage I carcinoma of the vulva. Obstetrics and Gynecology 57: 85–89
Johnston G A, Klotz J, Boutselis J G 1983 Primary invasive carcinoma of the vagina. Surgery, Gynecology and Obstetrics 156: 34–40
Karlen J R, Piver M S, Barlow J J 1975 Melanoma of the vulva. Obstetrics and Gynecology 45: 181–185
Kelly J L III, Burke T W, Tornos C, Morris M, Gershenson D M, Silva E G, Wharton J T 1992 Minimally invasive vulvar carcinoma: an indication for conservative surgical therapy. Gynecologic Oncology 44: 240–244
Kraus F T, Perez-Mesa C 1966 Verrucous carcinoma: clinical and pathological study of 105 cases involving oral cavity larynx and genitalia. Cancer 19: 26–38
Kucera H, Langer M, Smekal G, Weghaupt K 1985 Radiotherapy of primary carcinoma of the vagina: management and results of different therapy schemes. Gynecologic Oncology 21: 87–93
Lee R B, Buttoni L, Dhru K, Tamimi I I 1984 Malignant melanoma of the vagina: a case report of progression from preexisting melanosis. Gynecologic Oncology 19: 238–245
Lingard D, Free K, Wright R G, Battistutta D 1992 Invasive squamous cell carcinoma of the vulva: behaviour and results in the light of changing management regimens. Australian and New Zealand Journal of Obstetrics and Gynaecology 32: 137–145
Magrina J F, Webb M J, Gaffey T A, Symmonds R E 1979 Stage I squamous cell cancer of the vulva. American Journal of Obstetrics and Gynecology 134: 453–459
Micheletti L, Borgno G, Barbero M et al 1990 Deep femoral lymphadenectomy with preservation of the fascia lata – preliminary report on 42 invasive vulvar carcinomas. Journal of Reproductive Medicine 35: 1130–1133
Monaghan J M 1985a Management of vulvar carcinoma. In: Shepherd J H, Monaghan J M (eds) Clinical gynaecological oncology. Blackwell, London, pp 133–153
Monaghan J M 1985b Management of vaginal carcinoma. In: Shepherd J H, Monaghan J M (eds) Clinical gynaecological oncology. Blackwell, London, pp 154–166
Monaghan J M 1986 Bonney's gynaecological surgery, 9th edn. Baillière Tindall, Eastbourne, pp 121–128
Monaghan J M, Hammond I G 1984 Pelvic node dissection in the treatment of vulvar carcinoma – is it necessary? British Journal of Obstetrics and Gynaecology 91: 270–274
Morrow C P, DiSaia P J 1976 Malignant melanoma of the female genitalia: a clinical analysis. Obstetrical and Gynecologic Survey 31: 233–271
Murad T M, Durant J R, Maddox W A et al 1975 The pathologic behaviour of primary vaginal carcinoma and its relationship to cervical cancer. Cancer 35: 787–794
Office of Population Censuses and Surveys 1985 Cancer statistics – registrations 1981. HMSO, London, pp 27, 39
Office of Population Censuses and Surveys 1994 Cancer statistics registrations in 1989. HMSO, London, MB1 No 22
Parker R T, Duncan I, Rampone J, Creasman W 1975 Operative management of early invasive epidermoid carcinoma of the vulva. American Journal of Obstetrics and Gynecology 123: 349–355
Parry-Jones E 1960 Lymphatics of the vulva. Journal of Obstetrics and Gynaecology of the British Commonwealth 67: 919–928
Perez C A, Camel H M 1982 Long term follow-up in radiation therapy of carcinoma of the vagina. Cancer 49: 1308–1315

Perez C A, Arneson A N, Galakatos A, Samanth H K 1973 Malignant tumours of the vagina. Cancer 31: 36–44
Perez C A, Grigsby P W, Galakatos A et al 1993 Radiation therapy in management of carcinoma of the vulva with emphasis on conservative therapy. Cancer 71: 3707–3716
Pettersson F 1995 Annual report on the results of treatment in gynecological cancer. International Federation of Gynecology and Obstetrics (FIGO) Volume 22
Piura B, Masotina A, Murdoch J, Lopes A, Morgan P, Monaghan J 1993 Recurrent squamous cell carcinoma of the vulva: a study of 73 cases. Gynecologic Oncology 48: 189–195
Podratz K C, Symmonds R E, Taylor W F 1982 Carcinoma of the vulva: analysis of treatment failures. American Journal of Obstetrics and Gynecology 143: 340–351
Podratz K C, Gaffey T A, Symmonds R E, Johansen K L, O'Brien P C 1983 Melanoma of the vulva: an update. Gynecological Oncology 16: 153–168
Pride G L, Schultz A E, Chuprevich T W, Buchler D A 1979 Primary invasive squamous carcinoma of the vagina. Obstetrics and Gynecology 53: 218–225
Puthawala A, Syed A M N, Nalick R, McNamara C, DiSaia P J 1983 Integrated external and interstitial radiation therapy for primary carcinoma of the vagina. Obstetrics and Gynecology 62: 367–372
Raney R B, Crist W M, Maurer H M, Foulkes M A 1983 Prognosis of children with soft tissue sarcoma who relapse after achieving a complete response. Cancer 52: 44–50
Robboy S J, Noller K L, O'Brien P et al 1984 Increased incidence of cervical and vaginal dysplasia in 3980 diethylstilbestrol-exposed young women. Journal of the American Medical Association 252: 2979–2983
Rotmensch J, Rubin S J, Sutton H G et al 1990 Preoperative radiotherapy followed by radical vulvectomy with inguinal lymphadenectomy for advanced vulvar carcinomas. Gynecologic Oncology 36: 181–184
Rutledge F N, Smith J P, Franklin E W 1970 Carcinoma of the vulva. American Journal of Obstetrics and Gynecology 106: 1117–1130
Rutledge F N, Mitchell M F, Munsell M F et al 1991 Prognostic indicators for invasive carcinoma of the vulva. Gynecologic Oncology 42: 239–244
Schulz M J, Penalver M 1989 Recurrent vulvar carcinoma in the intervening tissue bridge in early invasive stage disease treated by radical vulvectomy and bilateral groin node dissection through separate incisions. Gynecologic Oncology 35: 383–386
Sedlis A, Homesley H, Bundy B N et al 1987 Positive groin nodes in superficial squamous cell vulvar cancer. American Journal of Obstetrics and Gynecology 156: 1159–1164
Seeger J, Richman S P, Allegra J C 1986 Systemic therapy of malignant melanoma. Medical Clinics of North America 70: 89–94
Shimm D S, Fuller A F, Orlow E L, Dosorctz D E, Aristizabal S A 1986 Prognostic variables in the treatment of squamous cell carcinoma of the vulva. Gynecologic Oncology 24: 343–358
Stehman F B, Bundy B N, Dvoretsky P M, Creasman W T 1992a Early Stage I carcinoma of the vulva treated with ipsilateral superficial inguinal lymphadenectomy and modified radical hemivulvectomy: a prospective study of the Gynecologic Oncology Group. Obstetrics and Gynecology 79: 490–497
Stehman F B, Bundy B N, Thomas G et al 1992b Groin dissection versus radiation in carcinoma of the vulva: a Gynaecological Oncology Group Study. International Journal of Radiation Oncology, Biology and Physics 24: 389–396
Sutton G P, Miser M R, Stehman F B, Look K Y, Ehrlich C E 1991 Trends in the operative management of invasive squamous carcinoma of the vulva at Indiana University, 1974 to 1988. American Journal of Obstetrics and Gynecology 164: 1472–1481
Taussig F J 1940 Cancer of the vulva – an analysis of 155 cases (1911–1940). American Journal of Obstetrics and Gynecology 40: 764–779
Thigpen J T, Blessing J A, Homesley H D, Lewis G C 1986 Phase II trials of cisplatin and piperazinedione in advanced or recurrent squamous cell carcinoma of the vulva: a Gynecologic Oncology group study. Gynecologic Oncology 23: 358–363
Thomas G, Dembo A J, Bryson S C P et al 1991 Changing concepts in the management of vulvar cancer. Gynecologic Oncology 42: 9–21
Tilmans A S, Sutton G P, Look K Y, Stehman F B, Ehrlich C E, Hornback N B 1992 Recurrent squamous carcinoma of the vulva. American Journal of Obstetrics and Gynecology 167: 1383–1389
Van der Velden J, Kooyman C D, Van Lindert A C M, Heintz A P M 1992 A Stage Ia vulvar carcinoma with an inguinal lymph node recurrence after local excision. A case report and literature review. International Journal of Gynecological Cancer 2: 157–159
Way S 1948 The anatomy of the lymphatic drainage of the vulva and its influence on the radical operation for carcinoma. Annals of the Royal College of Surgeons of England 3: 187–209
Way S 1960 Carcinoma of the vulva. American Journal of Obstetrics and Gynecology 79: 692–698
Webb J B, Isoti M, O'Sullivan J C, Azzopardi J G 1984 Combined adenoid cystic and squamous carcinoma of Bartholin's gland. British Journal of Obstetrics and Gynaecology 91: 291–295
Weed J C, Lozier C, Daniel S J 1983 Human papilloma virus in multifocal, invasive female genital tract malignancy. Obstetrics and Gynecology 62: 83S–87S
Wharton J T, Gallagher S, Rutledge F N 1974 Microinvasive carcinoma of the vulva. American Journal of Obstetrics and Gynecology 118: 159–162
White M J, Polk H C 1986 Therapy of primary cutaneous melanoma. Medical Clinics of North America 70: 71–87
Wiltshaw E 1985 Chemotherapy of ovarian carcinoma and other gynaecological malignancies. In: Shepherd J H, Monaghan J M (eds) Clinical gynaecological oncology. Blackwell, London, pp 215–238
Woodman C B J, Mould J J, Jordan J A 1988 Radiotherapy in the management of vaginal intraepithelial neoplasia after hysterectomy. British Journal of Obstetrics and Gynaecology 95: 976–979

38

Malignant disease of the uterus

M. A. Quinn   M. C. Anderson   C. A. E. Coulter   W. P. Soutter

INTRODUCTION

Carcinoma of the endometrium has been the poor relation of gynaecological malignancies, with the majority of cases being treated outside major oncology centres. Such an approach has stemmed from a belief that this cancer carries a uniformly good prognosis. However, despite the preponderance of early-stage disease, the overall survival in the UK is only 60% and the survival corrected for death from other causes is a mere 68% (Office of Population Censuses and Surveys 1988, Black et al 1993). It is a sad fact that the best therapy for this disease has yet to be defined, and that treatment protocols still rely heavily on historical data rather than being based on prospective randomized trials. Confusion and controversy relate to a number of basic areas in the management of patients with corpus cancer, including the place of radiation therapy, radical surgery and adjuvant treatment with hormones. This chapter aims to give an overview of existing information relating to the natural history of the disease, and thereby to provide a rational approach to the care of women with this cancer.

EPIDEMIOLOGY

The median age of patients with endometrial cancer is 61 years, with 75–80% of women being postmenopausal and 3–5% being less than 40 years old (Fig. 38.1). Note the steep rise in incidence in the years immediately before the menopause and the plateau thereafter (Fig. 38.2). It is curious that a tumour thought to be oestrogen dependent should become commoner when endogenous levels of oestrogen are falling.

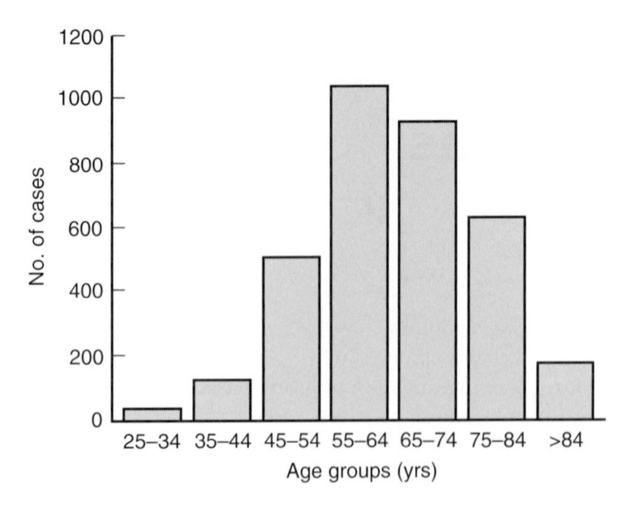

Fig. 38.1 The numbers of cases of endometrial cancer by age.

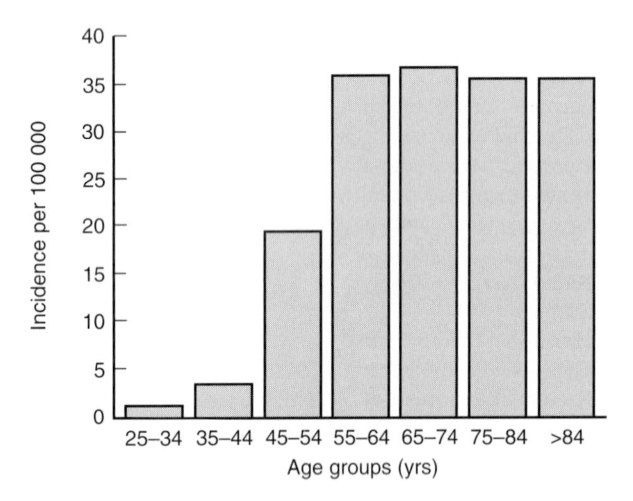

Fig. 38.2 The incidence of endometrial cancer by age.

Geographical and racial variation in incidence

The incidence of corpus cancer varies markedly, not only from country to country, but between different racial groups in one geographical area. The highest incidence is in white North Americans who have a rate approximately seven times higher than the Chinese. Asian women who migrate to the USA very quickly develop incidence rates similar to the local population.

AETIOLOGY

The aetiology of endometrial cancer is unknown but several factors are known to increase or decrease the likelihood of developing endometrial cancer (Table 38.1). Most of these risk factors relate to postmenopausal women, but women under 40 who develop endometrial cancer have a high incidence of anovulation, especially due to polycystic ovarian syndrome. They are often obese – 45% of women in one series weighed more than 80 kg.

Table 38.1 Factors known to alter the risk of developing endometrial cancer

Increase	Decrease
Obesity, especially upper body	Oral contraceptives
Carbohydrate intolerance	Progestogens
Nulliparity	? Smoking cigarettes
Late menopause	
Polycystic ovarian syndrome	
Unopposed oestrogen therapy	
Functioning ovarian tumours	
Personal history of breast or colon carcinoma	
Family history of breast, colon or endometrial carcinoma	
Tamoxifen therapy	

However, premenopausal women over 40 do not seem to share the same risk factors as younger women, having in particular a low incidence of nulliparity (Quinn et al 1985a).

Body weight, diet and carbohydrate metabolism

Most of the known risk factors for the development of this cancer appear to share a common basis – excessive unopposed oestrogen stimulation of the endometrium. The major circulating oestrogen in postmenopausal women is oestrone, derived from aromatization of peripheral androgens, mainly Δ_4-androstenedione. This conversion takes place in a wide variety of body sites, particularly in fat and muscle. A doubling in body weight results in a doubling of peripheral conversion, and continuous exposure allows nuclear uptake and resultant protein synthesis and cell growth to occur. In addition, there is an association between obesity and reduced levels of sex hormone-binding globulin, which leads to an increase in free oestrogen being available to target organs. A number of case-control studies have identified an increased risk with high fat intake (Shu et al 1993), especially fried foods (Potischman et al 1993). Upper body obesity (waist–thigh circumference ratio) seems to be a risk factor independent of weight.

Carbohydrate metabolism

The mechanism by which disturbed carbohydrate metabolism influences the risk of development of endometrial cancer is unclear. Postmenopausal women with diabetes mellitus have increased oestrogen and reduced gonadotrophin levels independent of body weight (Quinn et al 1981). Whether women with endometrial carcinoma have an altered oestrogen metabolism independent of the effect of weight remains controversial.

Oestrogen production by ovarian tumours

The ovarian tumours classically associated with oestrogen production are the granulosa–theca cell tumours, with approximately 10% of cases (reported range 2.5–23%) being associated with endometrial cancer and 50% (reported range 22–72%) with endometrial hyperplasia. Ovarian epithelial cancers may also be responsible for steroid production, probably by a process of stromal luteinization. In one series, seven of nine mucinous carcinomas, five of six endometrioid carcinomas and all eight Krukenberg tumours showed an increase in oestrogen secretion (Rome et al 1981). The ovarian stroma from postmenopausal women with endometrial cancer has been shown to produce more androgens than that of women without endometrial cancer, and luteinizing hormone and insulin may be important in this regard (Nagamani et al 1992).

Exogenous oestrogens

The association between exogenous oestrogens and endometrial cancer is discussed in Chapter 31. The administration of unopposed oestrogens leads to a risk of developing endometrial cancer from seven to 10 times that of the general population. Indeed, a recent prospective study showed that 10% of women developed adenomatous hyperplasia every year (PEPI 1995).

The addition of a progestogen to oestrogen therapy for 12–14 days each month reduces the risk, possibly to less than that of the general population. There is some evidence that progestins given as infrequently as every 6 months can prevent the induction of hyperplasia (Kemp et al 1989).

Personal or family history of cancer

Women with a personal history of breast or colon cancer are at increased risk of developing endometrial cancer. The gene responsible for the Lynch II syndrome, a familial predisposition to non-polyposis colon cancer, endometrial cancer and ovarian cancer, has recently been located on chromosome 2p 22-21. Called MSH2, it encodes a protein important in the DNA mismatch repair pathway (Fishel et al 1994).

Tamoxifen therapy

Women who take tamoxifen are exposed to a risk of oestrogenic-type effects on the uterus. This includes polyps, fibroids, glandular hyperplasia and, less commonly, cancers including perhaps sarcomas. Cancers associated with tamoxifen may be of poorer prognostic type (Magriples et al 1993). The risk of neoplasia increases with duration of use; the effect of dose is controversial. Women with breast cancer undoubtedly benefit from adjuvant tamoxifen with a better survival than controls in all studies: the uncertainty about its value affects only women at high risk of breast cancer enrolled in studies of the use of tamoxifen as a prophylactic (Neven et al 1994). Women with breast cancer have approximately a twofold higher incidence of endometrial cancer (Adami et al 1987), so comparisons of tamoxifen-treated women must be with other breast cancer patients. Such a comparison has shown an increase in the annual incidence of endometrial cancer from 0.2/1000 women to 1.6/1000 women (Fisher et al 1994). Although the relative risk is large, the absolute risk of endometrial cancer is still very small in tamoxifen-treated women. In a study of 75 000 women with breast cancer, 990 were known to have died for some reason other than breast cancer – only two died from endometrial cancer (Early Breast Cancer Trialists' Collaborative Group 1992).

Oral contraception

Women who have ever used combined oral contraceptives have a substantially reduced risk (perhaps 50% or less) of developing corpus cancer, especially after 10 or more years of use. Protection is present even 20 years after discontinuation (Stanford et al 1993).

The identification of risk factors is of value only if such factors can be manipulated to change the incidence of the disease (e.g. altered diet) or alternatively, if screening programmes can be introduced, especially in high-risk populations. Few data exist on how many women with endometrial cancer have a risk factor that can be manipulated, but screening is attracting increasing interest from researchers.

PATHOLOGY

Malignancy may develop in either the glands or the stroma of the endometrium. Endometrial adenocarcinoma, derived from the endometrial glandular cells, is overwhelmingly the most common malignant tumour arising in the body of the uterus; the stroma is the origin of the much rarer endometrial stromal sarcoma. The even more uncommon malignant mixed mullerian tumour is composed of both glandular and stromal elements. The sarcomas are discussed separately.

Endometrial carcinoma is usually seen as a raised, rough, perhaps papillary area occupying at least half the endometrium. Endometrial carcinomas often arise in the fundal region of the uterus; the internal os is rarely involved early in the disease. Myometrial invasion may be obvious to the naked eye. There seems to be no correlation between the degree of exophytic growth of the tumour within the uterine cavity and the presence of myometrial invasion.

Endometrial carcinoma is not a single tumour; it is a group of distinct subtypes (Poulsen et al 1975):

1. Adenocarcinoma not otherwise specified (endometrioid).
2. Adenocarcinoma with benign squamous change (adenoacanthoma).
3. Adenosquamous (mixed) carcinoma.
4. Papillary serous adenocarcinoma.
5. Clear cell carcinoma.
6. Squamous cell carcinoma.

Endometrioid adenocarcinoma

The commonest endometrial carcinoma is referred to as endometrioid adenocarcinoma, the glandular pattern of which generally resembles that of normal proliferative-phase endometrium, although sometimes showing extreme complexity of the glands and cribriform pattern (Fig. 38.3). Multilayering of the epithelial cells is nearly always seen.

Endometrial adenocarcinoma with squamous metaplasia (adenoacanthoma)

Up to 25% of endometrioid-pattern endometrial adenocarcinomas contain areas of squamous metaplasia. Those tumours in which the squamous component is morphologically benign are commonly termed 'adenoacanthoma' (Christopherson et al 1983). The squamous change is seen as islands of typical squamous epithelium, very often situated within the gland lumina or as surface or diffuse squamous metaplasia (Fig. 38.4).

Adenosquamous carcinoma

An adenosquamous carcinoma is a carcinoma of the endometrium composed of malignant glands with a morphologically malignant squamous element. Histologically the glandular element always predominates, making up at least 70% of the tumour.

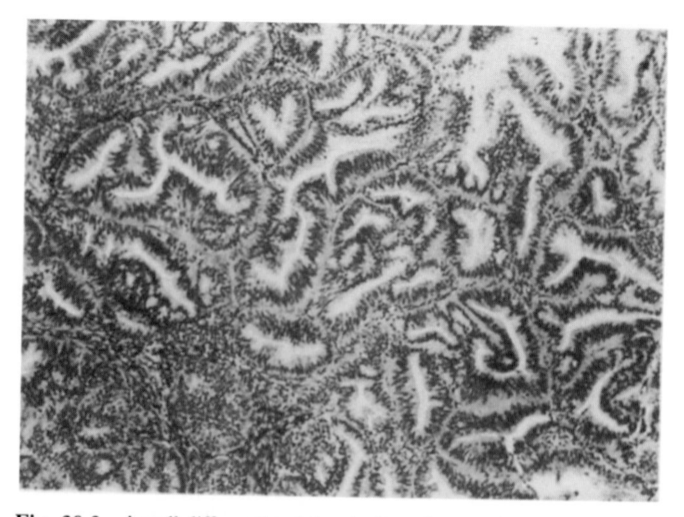

Fig. 38.3 A well differentiated (grade 1) endometrial carcinoma of endometrioid pattern. Haematoxylin and eosin × 170.

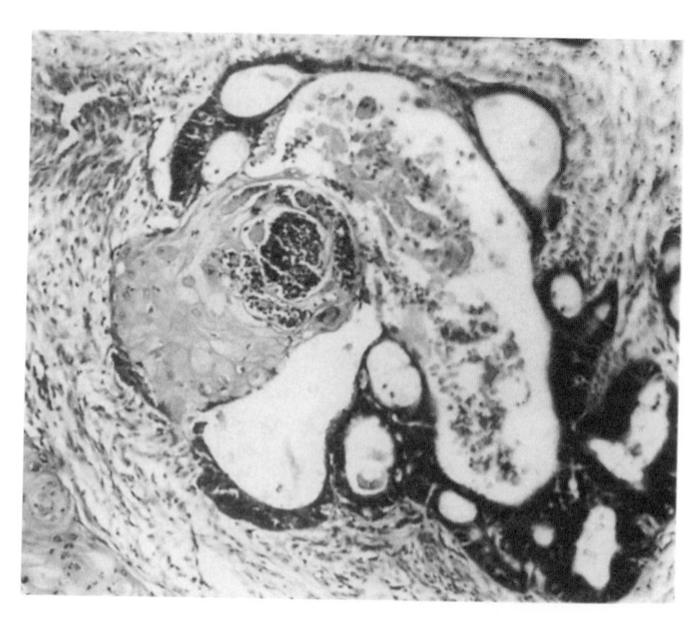

Fig. 38.4 Adenocarcinoma with benign squamous metaplasia (adenoacanthoma). Haematoxylin and eosin × 195.

Papillary serous and clear cell carcinomas

Less common variants of endometrial adenocarcinoma are the papillary serous and clear cell carcinoma. These are both associated with a poor prognosis.

NATURAL HISTORY

Endometrial hyperplasia

Simple glandular hyperplasia is no longer considered to be a premalignant condition but complex hyperplasia, especially with atypical cells, is an ominous finding. Approximately 10–20% of all cases with atypia will have an underlying carcinoma present, and invasive cancer will develop later in up to 50% of cases. Whether morphometric features will provide a better clue to neoplastic risk is still debatable (Baak et al 1992).

All women with hyperplasia without cytological atypia may be treated with cyclical or continuous progestogens for 6 months and then undergo rebiopsy. Women with lesions showing cytological atypia who have finished childbearing should be offered a hysterectomy. The management of younger women with atypical hyperplasia is more difficult. Hyperplasia is discussed further in Chapter 34.

Spread of disease

Endometrial carcinoma spreads by invading the myometrium. In some cases it extends over the endometrial surface before penetrating the muscle layer. The more deeply it invades, the greater is the likelihood of lymphatic or, less commonly, vascular involvement. Unlike cervical carcinoma, in which lymphatic spread usually occurs to

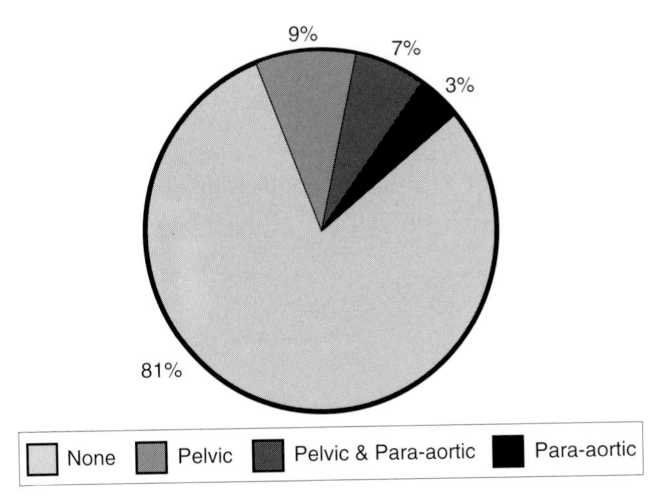

Fig. 38.5 Lymph node involvement in clinical Stage I endometrial carcinoma (after Ayhan et al 1994).

Table 38.2 Incidence of nodal involvement when disease is clinically confined to corpus (modified from Creasman et al 1987)

Grade	No. of cases	Depth of myometrial invasion				
		None ($n = 86$)	Inner 1/3 ($n = 281$)	Mid 1/3 ($n = 115$)	Outer 1/3 ($n = 139$)	All cases ($n = 621$)
		Positive pelvic nodes (%)				
Grade 1	180	0%	3%	0%	11%	2.8%
Grade 2	288	3%	5%	9%	19%	8.7%
Grade 3	153	0%	9%	4%	34%	18.3%
All cases	621	1.2%	5.3%	6.1%	25.2%	9.3%
		Positive para-aortic nodes (%)				
Grade 1	180	0%	1%	5%	6%	1.7%
Grade 2	288	3%	4%	0%	14%	4.9%
Grade 3	153	0%	4%	0%	24%	11.1%
All cases	621	1.2%	2.8%	0.9%	17.3%	5.5%

the pelvic nodes before the para-aortic nodes become involved, direct spread to the para-aortic nodes is common. The result is that 50% of nodal disease in women with apparently early endometrial cancers is found in the para-aortic region (Fig. 38.5). Lymphatic spread may rarely include the supraclavicular or the inguinal nodes. Spread to the cervix may occur by extension along the surface, but infiltration of the lymphatics or cervical stroma is more common. This is difficult to assess clinically (see below). Direct infiltration into the parametria is uncommon except when the cervix is involved.

In those with metastatic disease, spread to the ovaries is common. Sometimes a second, primary tumour will be found in the ovaries. Transperitoneal spread occurs either when myometrial invasion reaches the serosal surface or via the fallopian tubes. This will involve the peritoneal surfaces and omentum in the same way as ovarian carcinoma. Clear cell and papillary serous carcinomas have a propensity to spread in this way, often without deep myometrial invasion.

Prognostic factors

Many prognostic factors have been studied in this disease but only a few are incorporated in the FIGO staging system. Most are closely interrelated, so that multivariate analysis is required to determine which are of critical importance. The objective of refined prognostic schemes is to identify a low-risk group of women who do not need adjuvant therapy. When effective adjuvant treatment becomes available it will also be valuable to be able to define a high-risk group who require additional therapy.

Factors which are significant only in univariate analysis:

1. Lymph node involvement.
2. Capillary-like space involvement.
3. Histological subtype.
4. Peritoneal cytology.
5. Body morphology.
6. Steroid receptor status.
7. CA125 level.

It may seem surprising that lymph node involvement is not as important as other factors. This may be partly due to incomplete sampling failing to detect involved nodes, especially para-aortic nodes, and partly to the effects of spread by other routes. Depth of myometrial penetration is a more important guide to the likelihood of nodal metastases than tumour grade (Table 38.2; Creasman et al 1987). Serous papillary and clear cell cancers had the highest risk of spread to para-aortic nodes. Only 10% of cases subsequently proven to have nodal spread had clinically enlarged nodes. Palpation of nodes is a very unreliable way of identifying disease!

Patients with clear cell cancers have an overall survival of less than 50%. Serous papillary carcinoma of the endometrium, histologically similar to serous papillary cancer of the ovary, has a very poor prognosis and a pattern of spread akin to ovarian malignancy.

Positive peritoneal washings are present in approximately 12–15% of all cases of endometrial cancer, with half of these having no histological evidence of extrauterine spread. The prognostic value of positive cytology remains uncertain in the absence of other evidence of extrauterine spread (Yazigi et al 1983, Kadar et al 1992).

An elevated serum CA125 value at diagnosis suggests a high risk of subsequent recurrence (Rose et al 1994) but is less effective at predicting myometrial invasion than ultrasound (Lehtovirta et al 1994).

Factors which remain significant after multivariate analysis:

1. Stage of disease.
2. Myometrial invasion.
3. Degree of differentiation.

Table 38.3 FIGO surgical staging of endometrial carcinoma

Stage		Description
Stage	Ia G123	Tumour limited to endometrium
	Ib G123	Invasion < half myometrium
	Ic G123	Invasion > half myometrium
Stage	IIa G123	Endocervical glandular involvement only
	IIb G123	Cervical stromal invasion
Stage	IIIa G123	Tumour invades serosa and/or adnexae and/or positive peritoneal cytology
	IIIb G123	Vaginal metastases
	IIIc G123	Metastases to pelvic and/or para-aortic lymph nodes
Stage	IVa	Tumour invades bladder and/or bowel mucosa
	IVb	Distant metastases including intra-abdominal and/or inguinal lymph nodes

G123 refers to the grade of the tumour. For example, a grade 2 tumour invading to the serosal surface of the uterus with no metastatic disease would be stage IIIa G2

4. Ploidy status.
5. Tumour size.
6. Age.
7. Morphometric assessment.

The current FIGO (International Federation of Gynaecology and Obstetrics) staging criteria are shown in Table 38.3. The stage distribution and 5-year survival in a study of the Norwegian population, using the new FIGO system, are shown in Table 38.4 alongside the survival figures for the old, clinical system. It should be noted that the analysis of the surgically staged patients was restricted to those women who underwent a total abdominal hysterectomy and bilateral salpingo-oophorectomy and for whom full staging details were available. This excluded a group of women whose prognosis was much worse. As a result, these Norwegian survival figures are better than those of the whole population from the Norwegian series, whose overall crude 5-year survival rate was 73.1%. These figures are also better than those recorded in the United Kingdom, where the crude overall 5-year survival is only around 60% (Office of Population Censuses and Surveys 1988, Black et al 1993).

Few large studies have examined all of the factors mentioned above. In those that have looked at the commonly available clinical and histological factors, the most important, in descending order, have been myometrial invasion, age and stage of disease (Abeler et al 1992). Histological grade often appears in this list too. Most clinicians use stage, myometrial invasion, tumour grade and age as their main indicators of prognosis, but will also consider the size of the tumour and any evidence of lymph node metastases.

Endometrial Carcinoma Prognostic Index for Stage I (ECPI-1 Score)

The depth of myometrial invasion, DNA ploidy and the morphometric parameter, mean shortest nuclear axis, have been combined together to provide an Endometrial Carcinoma Prognostic Index for Stage I (ECPI-1). The score was developed in a prospective study of a population of women with Stage I endometrial carcinoma who had been followed for 5 years but its value has been confirmed in a second study of a different population of women. This showed only a 3% mortality in women with a favourable score and an 84.6% mortality in those with an unfavourable score (Baak et al 1995). This method uses fixed material for all the measurements, so these techniques could be applied widely by sending samples to specialized laboratories.

SCREENING

The methods available to screen asymptomatic women for endometrial neoplasia are as follows:

1. Endometrial biopsy.
2. Aspiration curettage.
3. Endometrial lavage.
4. Endometrial brush sponge.
5. Endometrial aspiration.
6. Papanicolaou smear of cervix.
7. Vaginal pool smear.
8. Progestogen challenge test.
9. Vaginal ultrasound.

Given the number of available devices and tests, it can be surmised that no one method is perfect and that no data currently available support the value of these tests in reducing the morbidity and mortality of the disease.

Endometrial sampling

Endometrial sampling techniques involve the use of various ingenious devices to obtain a sample of endometrial tissue for histological or cytological examination. The former is easier for the pathologist to interpret. Most studies have been performed in patients about to undergo diagnostic curettage, and the value of these instruments as a tool for screening the asymptomatic population is not yet clear. Koss et al (1982) obtained a sensitivity of 80% in a study of just over 2000 asymptomatic women, 80% of whom were postmenopausal. However, adequate samples for assessment were obtained in only 80% of women screened, with a fall-off in successful sampling with advancing age.

Vaginal or cervical cytology

Although cervical smears may occasionally detect endometrial cancer there is no evidence that cervical cancer screening programmes have a major impact on the morbidity and mortality from endometrial cancer (Mitchell et al 1993).

Table 38.4 Surgical FIGO stage distribution and 5-year survival. Note that these data were obtained only from women who were able to undergo full surgical staging and treatment. The crude 5-year survival for the whole population was 73.1%

	Surgically staged[1]		Clinically staged[2]
Stage	% of cases	% 5-year survival	% 5-year survival
I	81.3	82.9	86
II	11.2	70.8	66
III	5.9	39.2	44
IV	1.7	27.3	16
All stages		78.1	73

[1]Abeler et al (1992); [2]Pettersson (1995)

Progestogen challenge test

The progestogen challenge test is based on the hypothesis that endometrial cancer is oestrogen dependent and that a withdrawal bleed following postmenopausal progestogen administration is indicative of the presence of oestrogen-stimulated endometrium. The role of this test in a population setting is yet to be defined, although preliminary studies are promising (Macia et al 1993).

Vaginal ultrasound

Vaginal ultrasound has been used to detect endometrial carcinoma by measuring the thickness of the endometrium (Osmers et al 1990). In this study of 103 women with postmenopausal bleeding and 283 asymptomatic postmenopausal women, a cut-off value of 4 mm was used. All of the symptomatic group underwent curettage and all 23 women with complex or atypical hyperplasia or carcinoma had an endometrial thickness greater than 4 mm. Surprisingly, 3.5% of the asymptomatic group had endometrial cancers detected by ultrasound. This high prevalence suggests a selection bias for high-risk characteristics, or overdiagnosis of endometrial carcinoma.

Conclusions

It remains to be shown whether any benefits would accrue to individual women or to society from screening for endometrial cancer. Although a combination of vaginal ultrasound and outpatient endometrial biopsy may have the sensitivity and, possibly, the specificity necessary the women detected would still need to undergo a hysterectomy and bilateral salpingo-oophorectomy. Given that most women with endometrial carcinoma present at an early stage of disease, the advantage of screening may be quite small. Not knowing how quickly these tumours grow, it is impossible to calculate how frequently screening would be needed. This would apply particularly to poorly differentiated tumours which are the poor prognosis tumours one would most want to detect early but which are most likely to progress rapidly between screening examinations.

DIAGNOSIS AND INVESTIGATION

Presenting symptoms

The vast majority of women diagnosed as having endometrial cancer present with abnormal bleeding. The remainder have a discharge or pain, or are referred because of an abnormal screening test.

Postmenopausal bleeding

Postmenopausal bleeding is the most common presenting symptom as 75–80% of women with the disease are in this age group. The most common mistake made which delays the diagnosis is to assume that vaginal spotting is due to atrophic vaginitis. A woman not taking hormone replacement therapy who bleeds after the menopause has a 10% risk of having a genital cancer, and a further 10% risk of significant pathology (Gredmark et al 1995; Table 38.5). This large study of 475 women has the advantage of being population based. A cervical smear and endometrial biopsy should be performed in all cases of postmenopausal or perimenopausal bleeding, no matter what the clinical diagnosis may be. The same is required for a woman on hormone replacement therapy with irregular bleeding.

Postmenopausal discharge

Diagnostic curettage in the patient with postmenopausal discharge due to a pyometra will reveal a carcinoma in about 50% of cases, and it is usually in these women that the rare, pure squamous carcinoma is found.

Pelvic pain

The presence of pain usually indicates metastatic disease. It is often due to nerve compression on the pelvic side wall. Pyometra may present with a constant dull pain or cramping pain.

Table 38.5 Prevalence of pathology in 475 women complaining of postmenopausal bleeding. (After Gredmark et al 1995)

Pathology	Number	Percentage
Adenocarcinoma	37	8.1
Squamous cervical carcinoma	6	1.3
Ovarian or tubal carcinoma	3	0.7
Secondary carcinoma	1	0.2
All carcinomas	47	10.3
Benign or borderline ovarian tumours	6	1.3
Adenomatous endometrial hyperplasia	25	5.5
Atypical endometrial hyperplasia	8	1.8
Cervical dysplasia (CIN)	9	2.0
All 'benign tumours' requiring surgery	48	10.5
Cervical polyps	42	9.2
Cystic hyperplasia	12	2.6
All 'simple' conditions	54	11.8

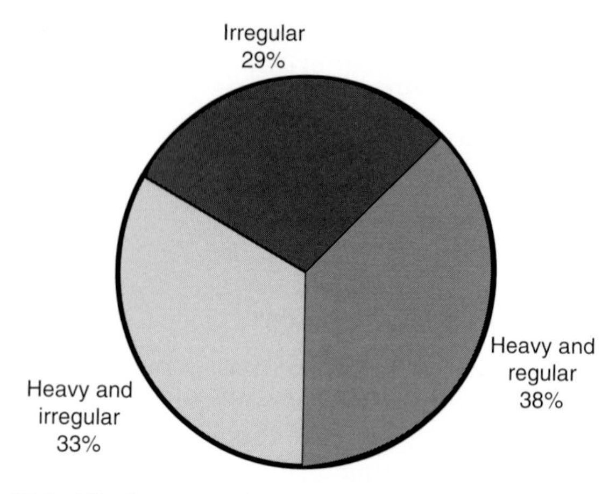

Fig. 38.6 Bleeding pattern in 106 premenopausal women with endometrial carcinoma (Quinn et al 1985a).

Symptoms in premenopausal women

Premenopausal women with endometrial carcinoma usually present with irregular bleeding, but over one-third complain of heavy but regular periods (Fig. 38.6).

Clinical examination

Physical examination will seldom suggest the diagnosis of endometrial carcinoma, but there are several signs worth looking out for in women with postmenopausal or perimenopausal bleeding. Enlarged lymph nodes in the groin or supraclavicular fossa may be found. A metastatic focus in the vagina may lie behind the blades of the speculum, commonly on the anterior wall, and be missed by the unwary. The uterus may be enlarged – an unusual finding in a postmenopausal woman – or spread to the adnexae or parametrium may be felt. The breasts should be palpated because breast cancer can sometimes present with the symptoms caused by uterine or ovarian spread.

Outpatient investigation of postmenopausal or perimenopausal bleeding

Until very recently, dilatation and curettage under general anaesthesia was mandatory for women with these symptoms. This was justified by the 10% prevalence of malignancy and the further 10% with significant pathology, but this policy results in 'unnecessary' investigation for the remaining 80% of women. Recognition of this problem has led many investigators to design devices to permit sampling of the endometrium in the outpatient department without general anaesthesia.

Outpatient endometrial biopsy

Using the Sharman curette in a dedicated clinic, Kitchener's group in Aberdeen (Shaker et al 1991) were able to avoid admission for 81% of their patients with postmenopausal bleeding. As the only gynaecological unit serving a stable population, they can be confident in the accuracy of their claim not to have missed any cases of endometrial carcinoma.

Others have used a narrower plastic cannula (Pipelle®, Z-sampler®) which is easier to insert in the uterus and has a tightly fitting plunger that provides adequate suction to obtain excellent samples of endometrium and is very acceptable to patients (Eddowes 1990). Most studies have shown that this instrument detects endometrial carcinoma and atypia with acceptable reliability (Stovall et al 1991, Reid et al 1993, Batool et al 1994). The main reason for discrepancy appears to be hyperplasia on an endometrial polyp (Reid et al 1993). However, it is important to remember that not even curettage under general anaesthesia is 100% reliable (Word et al 1958, MacKenzie & Bibby 1978).

If the biopsy is benign, or if no tissue is obtained after an apparently satisfactory insertion of the Pipelle into the cavity, it is reasonable to reassure the woman that intrauterine malignancy is very unlikely. She should be asked to return to the clinic if the bleeding recurs. In that event, hysteroscopy and curettage under general anaesthesia are required.

Ultrasound

It is not always possible to insert the endometrial biopsy instrument into the uterus in the clinic. A failure rate of around 20% may be expected (Shaker et al 1991, Batool et al 1994). In this situation, vaginal ultrasound can help to 'rule out' endometrial carcinoma in those postmenopausal women whose endometrium is less than 4 mm thick (Osmers et al 1990). In the remainder, curettage under general anaesthesia is necessary. The combination of vaginal ultrasound followed by Pipelle endometrial biopsy would seem to offer a high sensitivity for significant endometrial pathology (Van den Bosch et al 1995).

Ultrasound will also help to detect ovarian pathology. However, it is important to remember that some ovarian tumours will not be seen with vaginal ultrasound because of their size or position high in the pelvis. If the ovaries are not seen clearly with a vaginal transducer, an abdominal scan may be needed.

Outpatient hysteroscopy

With modern instruments it is possible to perform hysteroscopy in the outpatient department (Hill et al 1992). However, this requires experience and skill if it is to be used safely and effectively. As hysteroscopes are substantially thicker than the Pipelle, local anaesthesia and cervical dilatation are required in 29% of cases, and it is likely that insertion will fail more frequently. Even in experienced hands it can be very difficult to diagnose endometrial carcinoma through the hysteroscope, and a biopsy is always needed to settle the issue one way or the other. Unfortunately, only very tiny biopsies can be taken under direct vision through the hysteroscope: the instrument must be removed to allow adequate samples to be obtained. For these reasons, it may prove to add little to the Pipelle in the outpatient setting.

Other investigations

The need to perform a cervical smear should never be forgotten. With a 1.3% prevalence of invasive cervical cancer, colposcopy may be a useful additional investigation that could be incorporated easily into the examination.

Inpatient investigations

If carefully controlled and well organized facilities for the outpatient management of these women are not available, all patients with abnormal bleeding and a normal cervix should be investigated under general anaesthesia. Even if outpatient facilities are available, the same would apply to any woman with suspicious clinical or ultrasound findings, recurrent bleeding, or a histological sample suggestive of hyperplasia or endometrial carcinoma.

The bimanual examination should be repeated under general anaesthesia. The surgeon should look especially for cervical, vaginal, parametrial or adnexal disease. Hysteroscopy is valuable in assessing the status of the endocervix and uterine cavity. Should the endocervix be seen to be involved, a fractional curettage should be performed for confirmation. The presence of stromal invasion of the cervix, or carcinomatous tissue contiguous with endocervical glands, are the criteria required to diagnose cervical involvement by a primary endometrial tumour. However, clinical determination of cervical involvement is not very accurate (see discussion below).

Additional investigations to assess possible metastatic disease

If the diagnosis of endometrial carcinoma is confirmed, a chest X-ray is essential and some recommend an intravenous urogram. A full blood count, urea, creatinine and electrolyte estimations are required, as is urinalysis for sugar and protein.

Magnetic resonance imaging is the investigation of choice if extrauterine spread in the pelvis is suspected, but ultrasound can give very useful information provided the limitations of its accuracy are kept in mind. The positive and negative predictive values for deep myometrial invasion are 71.4% and 98% (Lehtovirta et al 1994). Estimation of serum CA125 levels may be of some value.

MANAGEMENT

The number of women who are medically unfit and unable to undergo surgery is shrinking. This, together with the inaccuracy of clinical staging and the importance of prognostic factors which can be identified surgically, led FIGO to introduce a surgicopathological staging scheme (see Table 38.3).

Stage I

Surgical treatment

The treatment of choice in patients with endometrial cancer is total abdominal hysterectomy and bilateral salpingo-oophorectomy, especially since clinical staging is so inaccurate (Cowles et al 1985). The adnexae are removed because of the risk that they will be involved with tumour, rather than to eliminate any hormonal influence they may have.

Role of lymphadenectomy. One purpose of lymphadenectomy is to spare the many women without nodal disease the side effects of radiotherapy. The overall rate of severe complications is in the region of 5%, but the complication rate of radiotherapy is higher in older women (11% vs. 2%), who are least able to undergo lymphadenectomy (Corn et al 1994). Thus those who would benefit most from lymphadenectomy are least likely to be fit enough for the procedure. Moreover, lymph node sampling increased the risk of severe radiotherapy complications from 1 to 7% in one retrospective study which included women treated over a 30-year period (Corn et al 1994). However, no increase in severe complications was noted following external beam radiotherapy given to women with positive pelvic lymph nodes after a complete pelvic lymphadenectomy in a prospective, international study, which began recruitment in 1982 and used modern radiotherapy techniques (COSA-NZ-UK 1996). A policy of lymphadenectomy will spare some women radiotherapy, but those found to have nodal disease might have a higher complication rate because of the additional surgery. The net result of this balance in the COSA-NZ-UK study was in fact a reduction in the rate of severe radiotherapy complications from 4.4 to 1.6% in women who underwent a complete pelvic lymphadenectomy. However, this was not a randomized selection and the women selected for lymphadenectomy were younger and lighter than the other patients in the trial.

The effect of lymphadenectomy on survival is controversial, as there has been no prospective trial addressing this question. One retrospective study of 425 cases of endometrial cancer concluded that selective pelvic lymphadenectomy was useful for prognostic purposes but did not confer a therapeutic benefit (Candiani et al 1990). The prospective COSA-NZ-UK study came to the same conclusion (COSA-NZ-UK 1996). In complete contrast, a retrospective American study of 649 women treated over a 21-year period suggested that multiple-site node sampling did improve 5-year survival from around 70% to around 90% (Kilgore et al 1995).

An approach used by some is to identify patients at high risk of node involvement and to perform a complete bilateral pelvic lymphadenectomy only in suitable patients. Obesity is the major surgical determinant. If pelvic nodes are obviously involved, then a para-aortic dissection is performed. Otherwise, the para-aortic nodes are not removed unless enlarged. This approach obviates the need for adjuvant irradiation in most 'high-risk' patients. Given that all women with positive para-aortic nodes die, pelvic lymphadenectomy alone may suffice (Belinson et al 1992).

Operative approach. A midline subumbilical incision, which can be extended above the umbilicus if required, is used if para-aortic lymphadenectomy is contemplated. Alternatively, a transverse incision will allow adequate exposure of the pelvis. In the obese patient it is best not to straighten out the abdominal wall by pulling up the panniculus of fat over the pubic symphysis: retraction of this excess fat is often tiring, exposure can be suboptimal and the incidence of wound infection in the skin fold is very high. Immediately the abdominal cavity is entered, 100 ml of sterile saline should be instilled into the pelvis to bathe the uterus, bladder and pouch of Douglas, and then aspirated. The specimen should be mixed with 1000 units of heparin to prevent a clot forming which could trap malignant cells.

Once the peritoneal washings have been taken, a thorough laparotomy should be performed with particular attention being paid to the liver, omentum, uterine adnexae and retroperitoneal node-bearing areas. A simple total hysterectomy and bilateral salpingo-oophorectomy should then be completed. Removal of a vaginal cuff, once thought to be mandatory, does not reduce the recurrence rate or improve survival, and nor does radical hysterectomy. Likewise, manoeuvres to occlude the cervix and fallopian tubes to prevent intraoperative spill of tumour are unnecessary.

The uterus may now be opened off the operating table and the depth of myometrial invasion assessed if lymphadenectomy is to be considered. The specimen may then be placed on ice and sent immediately to the pathology laboratory for histology, ploidy and receptor analysis. Alternatively, a piece of the carcinoma can be snap-frozen in liquid nitrogen and stored for analysis at a later date. At this point a decision as to lymph node removal is made. This may be considered in patients with poorly differentiated disease, clear cell or serous papillary tumours, lesions which invade half or more of the myometrium, and those which are seen to involve the cervix or adnexae.

Vaginal hysterectomy and bilateral salpingo-oophorectomy. The morbidity of vaginal hysterectomy is less than with abdominal hysterectomy, a factor that becomes more important in the older and often unfit population with endometrial cancer. The experience of endometrial carcinoma in two Italian centres is that operative mortality after abdominal hysterectomy is 2.4–2.7%, compared to no deaths after the vaginal approach (Candiani et al 1978, Scarselli et al 1992). Severe complications were also much less common after the vaginal approach. The 5-year survival figures were indistinguishable. It should be noted that the ovaries were removed vaginally in virtually all of these cases. Indeed, failure to remove the ovaries resulted in poorer 5-year survival figures (Candiani et al 1978). The vaginal approach should probably be used more often, possibly in conjunction with laparoscopic removal of the adnexae if vaginal adnexectomy is unsuccessful.

Radiotherapy

Radiotherapy is usually given after surgery to those who have adverse prognostic features. A comparison of preoperative radiotherapy for all patients, with selective postoperative therapy given to only 30% of women, showed identical 5-year survival figures (Bean et al 1978). By waiting until after surgery, 70% of these patients avoided unnecessary irradiation.

Radiotherapy for carcinoma of the endometrium may consist of brachytherapy to the vaginal vault, external beam therapy (teletherapy) to the whole pelvis, or both combined. Postoperative vault irradiation reduces the incidence of vault recurrence (Graham 1971, Piver et al 1979) and is given to all patients. However, some centres do omit brachytherapy in women with superficial well differentiated tumours (Fig. 38.7). In others, brachytherapy is not given to women who will receive teletherapy.

The dose of brachytherapy given depends on whether or not teletherapy is to be given. If no teletherapy is required, a dose in the region of 60 Gy is administered to the surface of the vagina. This is reduced to 30 Gy if teletherapy has

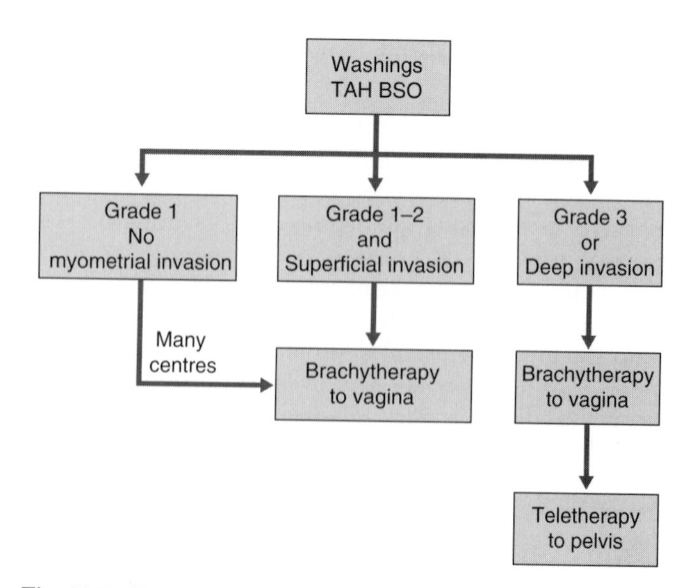

Fig. 38.7 Treatment plan for Stage I endometrial carcinoma.

been given. In many centres high dose-rate machines are used. In these the total dose is reduced by some 30–40% and is given in 3–6 fractions of 6 Gy.

External beam therapy is reserved for women with poor prognostic factors such as invasion more than halfway through the myometrium, high-grade tumours, and large tumours. The technique is similar to that used for cervical cancer, delivering a total dose of 40–45 Gy in fractions no greater than 1.8 Gy over 4–5 weeks. Although this is standard treatment, the only prospective randomized controlled study of teletherapy in Stage I disease showed no improvement in survival for women given radiotherapy (Aalders et al 1980). Pelvic recurrence was more common in women who did not receive teletherapy, but distant metastases were more common in those who did. There was a suggestion of survival benefit in women with high-grade tumours and deep myometrial invasion.

Radiation is more effective combined with surgery than when given alone (Bickenback 1967). However, if the patient is not fit for surgery two caesium insertions delivering 60 Gy to point A may be used for well differentiated tumours. If the curettings were poorly differentiated, 45 Gy may be given in 5 weeks to the whole pelvis, followed by a single insertion delivering 20–25 Gy to point A.

Adjuvant progestogen therapy

Because of the known response of advanced and recurrent endometrial cancers to progestational agents, the use of such therapy in the absence of residual disease has seemed an attractive proposition, especially as adjuvant hormonal treatment seems to reduce the recurrence risk in patients with postmenopausal breast cancer. A number of trials have been undertaken in patients with Stage I and Stage II disease using a variety of progestogens, a variety of routes of administration and a variety of time periods, during which the hormone has been prescribed. Few randomized trials have shown a survival benefit, but all published studies suffer from the inclusion of patients with low-risk tumours, thereby decreasing the likelihood of detecting a therapeutic benefit in the treated group (Kneale 1986).

Stage II

Clinical assessment of cervical involvement with fractional curettage is very unreliable. Only 52.4–56.3% are confirmed as Stage II after the hysterectomy (Onsrud et al 1982, Berman et al 1982, Abeler et al 1992). In contrast, understaging is much less common. In prospective studies, 5.5–8.7% of clinical Stage I cancers are found to have cervical involvement only after the hysterectomy has been performed (Mangioni et al 1993, Ayhan et al 1994). About half of all FIGO Stage II cancers by the new surgical system will be diagnosed in this way.

Overall, patients with Stage II tumours have a survival rate about 20% less than those with tumour confined to the corpus. However, women with only microscopic evidence of spread to the cervix have a prognosis similar to those with Stage I disease (Berman et al 1982, Zablow et al 1994). In a large prospective study of women who were thought to have Stage I tumours, the 91 in whom involvement of the cervix was found after histological examination of the uterus had an 86% relapse-free survival rate at 7 years, compared to 92% in the 723 women with Stage Ib–Ic disease (Mangioni et al 1993). The increased risk in Stage II thus appears to be confined largely to those with clinical involvement of the cervix.

Similarly, the depth of invasion into the cervix correlates with mortality (Berman et al 1982), but cervical invasion is also closely related to the degree of myometrial invasion and the grade of tumour and may not be an independent risk factor (Morrow et al 1991). In a study of Stage I–II endometrial cancer, depth of myometrial invasion was strongly associated with prognosis but involvement of the cervix was not (Lindahl et al 1994), further suggesting that subclinical involvement of the cervix need not be included as an additional risk factor to be considered when deciding whether postoperative radiotherapy is required.

From the above it will be apparent that the management of patients with endometrial cancer involving the cervix depends on whether spread is microscopic or macroscopic. In those patients in whom spread to the cervix is occult, the diagnosis being made on endocervical curettage or in the operative specimen, management may be identical to those patients with Stage I disease. The need for radiotherapy may be decided on the basis of depth of myometrial invasion and grade of tumour. The prognosis for such women is very similar to Stage I cases (Onsrud et al 1982, Zablow et al 1994) and does not seem to be improved by postoperative teletherapy, which does increase the risk of serious complications (Onsrud et al 1982).

On the other hand, when the cervix is obviously involved with tumour the prognosis is much worse, falling to between 30 and 59% (Berman et al 1982, Onsrud et al 1982, Zablow et al 1994). If surgically fit, such patients may be treated with radical hysterectomy, bilateral pelvic lymphadenectomy and para-aortic node sampling. Alternatively, and much more commonly in Britain, radiation is chosen, using a regimen similar to that used for cervical cancer. Teletherapy to a dose of 50 Gy is given to the whole pelvis in 5.5 weeks, followed by brachytherapy to deliver 20 Gy to point A.

Stage III

The rare patient with parametrial extension of disease or vaginal involvement should have a computed tomography (CT) scan of the pelvis and upper abdomen performed. Should the spread of disease be confined to the pelvis, then radiation therapy is the treatment of choice, given in a manner similar to Stage II.

On the other hand, when there is clinical spread to the adnexae, a laparotomy should still be undertaken to define accurately the extent of the disease and to remove as much tumour as possible. Following removal of the pelvic disease, omentectomy should be performed in the same way as for patients with primary ovarian malignancies. The prognosis for women who are in Stage III solely because of ovarian involvement is better than one might expect. Patients with metastases to the tubes or ovaries found incidentally at surgery have a 5-year survival of approximately 80%, about five times higher than when other pelvic structures or the vagina are involved.

Stage IV

The lungs are the most common site of metastases in patients presenting with extrapelvic disease, followed by peripheral lymph nodes and bladder. Over 20% of patients will have disease at multiple sites. Management needs to be individualized, with the primary aim being control of symptoms and local control of tumour growth. Radiation therapy, cytotoxic drugs and hormonal therapy may all be required. One study has stressed that cytoreduction may improve outcome when extrapelvic disease is found at laparotomy (Goff et al 1994).

The use of whole-abdominal irradiation with a pelvic boost for patients with intra-abdominal spread which has been optimally debulked has been reported to be very successful, with a 5-year survival of over 70% (Greer & Hamberger 1983).

MANAGEMENT AFTER INITIAL SURGERY

Follow-up after treatment for endometrial cancer has three broad objectives:

1. To detect recurrent disease that can be treated effectively.
2. To detect and treat complications of treatment.
3. To manage other problems related to the diagnosis.

Detecting recurrence

Unfortunately, most recurrences are ultimately fatal and most present with symptoms, but isolated vaginal disease can be treated successfully. Careful inspection and palpation of the whole length of the vagina should be performed at every visit, remembering that the recurrence may be located in the lower vagina. Vaginal cytology is not likely to be very helpful.

Regular ultrasound examinations of the pelvis or chest X-rays are of little value in the absence of symptoms, as metastatic disease in the pelvis or chest seldom responds to treatment.

Complications of therapy

Most surgical complications become apparent soon after the operation, but radiotherapy complications may not become evident for several years. These include haematuria from radiation cystitis; diarrhoea, melaena or rectal spasm from radiation colitis; small bowel obstruction from radiation ileitis; vaginal stenosis; or lymphoedema of the legs. Fortunately, these are all uncommon.

Hormone replacement therapy

The association of endometrial cancer with oestrogens has long been regarded as evidence to proscribe the use of oestrogen replacement therapy in these women. However, five papers describe the apparently safe use of oestrogens in women treated for Stage I–II disease (reviewed by Wren 1994). If all the disease has been removed by surgery or destroyed by radiotherapy, subsequent hormonal treatment can have no deleterious effects on the tumour. It is probably safe to prescribe oestrogens in this setting if the woman has menopausal symptoms or if she is at high risk of osteoporosis. This would be especially true for younger women. Women with poor-prognosis disease might obtain adequate relief from menopausal symptoms with medroxyprogesterone acetate.

Breast cancer

Women with endometrial cancer have a higher risk of developing breast cancer. They should be offered mammography and taught self-palpation.

RECURRENT DISEASE

Approximately 70% of all recurrences following primary treatment present within the first 2–3 years. Early recurrences carry a grave prognosis, presumably because of the inherent aggressiveness of the tumour. The common sites of treatment failure are the pelvis and vagina, the peritoneal cavity, lungs, liver, bone and inguinal or supraclavicular nodes (Fig. 38.8).

Radiotherapy

Vault recurrence is more common in the non-irradiated patient (Lotocki et al 1983). If there is no other, more distant spread, radiation may cure 33–60% of cases with isolated vaginal recurrence (Phillips et al 1982, Morgan et al 1993).

Radiotherapy is also of great value for palliation of symptoms, particularly relief of pain and discomfort due to bony and nodal metastases.

Surgery

Very few of these patients are fit enough to be considered for exenterative surgery.

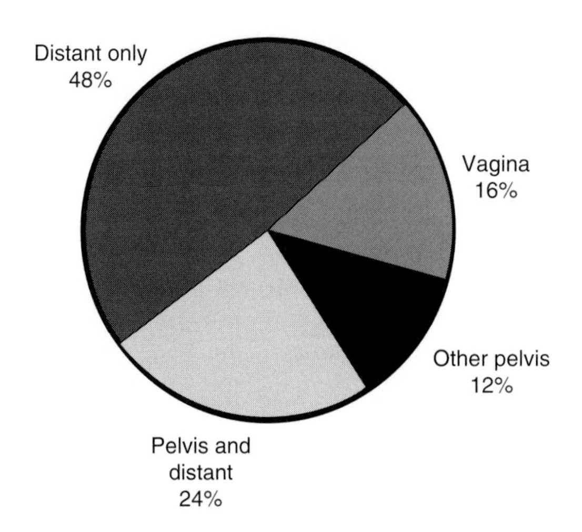

Fig. 38.8 Location of recurrent disease (after Burke et al 1990).

Hormonal therapy

Progestogen therapy has for many years been used in patients with recurrent endometrial carcinoma. The response rate is probably around 15–20%. A 52% response rate may be expected in patients with grade 1 adenocarcinoma, as opposed to a 15% response rate in patients with grade 3 cancers (Kohorn 1976). Tumours which recur more than 3 years after primary treatment are more responsive to progestogens, but recurrences which are widespread, are intra-abdominal or have been previously irradiated show lower response rates. The factors associated with tumour response to progestogens are:

1. Tumour differentiation.
2. Disease-free interval.
3. Site of recurrence.
4. Number of metastases.
5. Prior irradiation.
6. Steroid receptor status.

Approximately 80% of progestogen receptor-positive and 70% of oestrogen receptor-positive tumours respond to progestogen treatment, whereas only 11% of progestogen receptor-negative and 5% of oestrogen receptor-negative tumours respond. Unfortunately, recurrent tumour is often inaccessible for biopsy and only data on the primary tumour are available. None the less, this gives an excellent guide to response (Quinn et al 1985b). The most commonly used progestin is medroxyprogesterone acetate at an oral dose of 200 mg twice or three times a day. Higher doses are probably no more effective.

Tamoxifen has the ability to increase intracellular progestogen receptor content and may be of value in advanced disease; response rates to tamoxifen alone vary from 0 to 60% (Quinn & Campbell 1989). These probably depend on previous treatment, with higher response rates seen in patients previously responding to progestogens. The use of combination therapy has been studied by Rendina et al (1984), who added tamoxifen to medroxyprogesterone acetate in patients who relapsed or initially failed to respond to the progestogen. Patients who relapsed after an initial response to medroxyprogesterone acetate had a 62% response to the combination, whereas 48% of patients who initially had no response to medroxyprogesterone acetate responded to the combination. Whether tamoxifen and progestogens should be given simultaneously or sequentially awaits further clarification. Aminoglutethimide, an aromatase inhibitor which causes adrenal blockade, has also been used successfully in advanced endometrial cancer (Quinn 1989).

Cytotoxic chemotherapy

The use of cytotoxic therapy in patients with advanced endometrial cancer is a less attractive option than hormonal therapy, since many of these women are elderly and medically unfit. None the less, cytotoxic agents do have a small role following the failure of hormonal therapy. Single agents known to have activity include Adriamycin (response rate 19–38%), cisplatin (response rate 4–42%), cyclophosphamide (response rate 21%) and hexamethylmelamine (response rate 30%). Combination therapy has so far not proved superior to single-agent therapy (Thigpen et al 1987). The efficacy of paclitaxel in this situation is under investigation.

Results of treatment of recurrent disease

About 80% die within 2 years (Abeler et al 1992). Only 6% survive for 5 years after recurrence and only 0.6% are alive after 10 years. With these very poor results it is important not to make the treatment worse than the disease.

RESULTS OF TREATMENT

The crude overall 5-year survival rate in the United Kingdom is in the region of 60% and the corrected survival rate is around 68% (Office of Population Censuses and Surveys 1988, Black et al 1993). This is substantially worse than the crude rate of 73.1% reported from Norway (Abeler et al 1992). Although it is possible that these better results are due to differences in ascertainment of cases, this is unlikely. Careful review of the Norwegian cases resulted in 4% being excluded because the true diagnosis was a benign condition. Only 1.1% were excluded because of another condition with a potentially worse prognosis. An alternative explanation for the better survival rate may be that 75% of the women were treated in the Norwegian Radium Hospital by a specialist team.

The impression that this is a 'benign cancer' is mistaken. Fortunately, the prognosis is better in younger women than in the elderly, and most women present at Stage I. However, with an ageing population this cancer is likely to become still more common. It is important that these women should be given treatment which maximizes their prognosis with the minimum morbidity.

The surgical treatment has generally become less radical over the years, with the abandonment of modified radical hysterectomy and the removal of a cuff of vagina by most surgeons. The role of lymphadenectomy remains controversial. It is seldom performed in UK practice but is advocated by many in the USA. Vaginal hysterectomy and bilateral salpingo-oophorectomy may have been underutilized because of the technical difficulties in removing the adnexae vaginally. The advent of laparoscopic adnexectomy has both offered an alternative and reawakened interest in the vaginal approach (Richardson et al 1995).

The role of radiation therapy is somewhat ambiguous. Although there are some data to support the use of brachytherapy, the small amount of information available on teletherapy suggests that it is of only limited value. In spite of this paucity of information, few clinical oncologists would be willing to give up their use of teletherapy for high-risk disease. A large international trial to explore this important issue is overdue. The main problem remains the control of metastatic disease. In the absence of effective and tolerable chemotherapy or novel alternative therapies, the limitations of current treatment options must be acknowledged.

UTERINE SARCOMA

Sarcomas of the uterus are often highly malignant but rare tumours with an incidence of approximately 2/100 000 women over the age of 20. They account for 3–5% of all uterine cancers. These tumours are more common in black women and in women who have undergone previous pelvic irradiation. The literature relating to these tumours is beset by differences in histological classification. This situation is further complicated by difficulties in determining the malignant status of some of the smooth muscle tumours. No staging system for these tumours has been proposed by FIGO, but a clinical staging scheme similar to that used for endometrial carcinoma is often used (Table 38.6). This scheme allows a comparison of results from different centres and a rational approach to therapy.

Table 38.6 Staging system for uterine sarcomas

Stage I	Sarcomas confined to the uterus
Stage II	Sarcomas involving the corpus and cervix
Stage III	Sarcomas spreading beyond the uterus, but not outside the pelvis
Stage IV	Sarcomas spreading outside the pelvis or into the bladder or rectum

Endometrial stromal sarcomas

These tumours derive from the stromal cells of the endometrium rather than the glandular cells from which the common adenocarcinoma develops.

Endometrial stromal nodule

This is a rare, benign tumour composed of endometrial stroma in the myometrium. Clinically it looks like a fibroid. Its main importance is the need to differentiate this benign lesion from a malignant endometrial stromal sarcoma.

Low-grade endometrial stromal sarcoma

The low-grade endometrial stromal sarcoma has previously been known as endolymphatic stromal myosis, endolymphatic stromatosis or stromal endometriosis. This neoplasm arises from endometrial stroma, from adenomyosis and occasionally from pelvic endometriosis (Hendrickson & Kempson 1987).

The tumour may be polypoid and protrude into the uterine cavity, but an infiltrating growth pattern is more characteristic, resulting in an area of thickening of the uterine wall. Microscopically (Fig. 38.9) the tumour cells resemble those of normal endometrial stroma; nuclear atypia is usually slight. The most striking feature of the low-grade endometrial stromal sarcoma, and the origin of the alternative name of endolymphatic stromal myosis, is the nature of the infiltrating margin of the tumour. Broad, rounded bands and sharp finger-like processes of stromal cells infiltrate extensively into the myometrium between the muscle fibres and into the lymphatic spaces. Mitotic figures are generally fewer than 10 per 10 high-power fields.

Prior to surgery this lesion is usually thought to be a fibroid. Abnormal vaginal bleeding and pain are the most common symptoms. Extrauterine spread into the broad

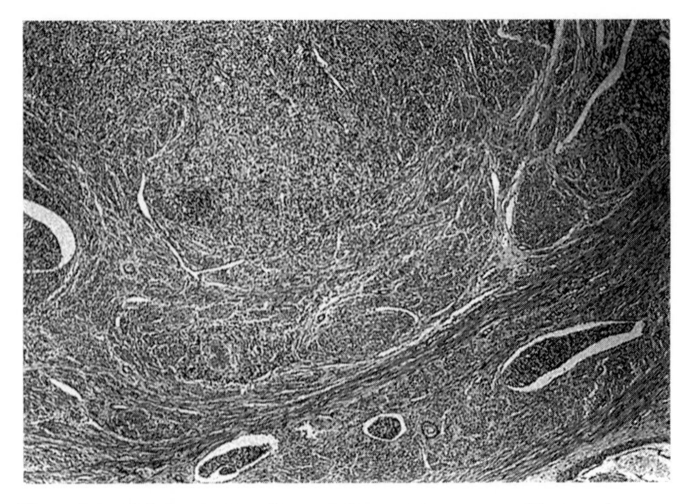

Fig. 38.9 A low-grade endometrial stromal sarcoma with prominent lymphatic channel involvement. Haematoxylin and eosin × 64.

or cardinal ligaments, the adnexae or to other intra-abdominal organs is detected at operation in 20–30% of cases. The most appropriate management is probably a total abdominal hysterectomy and bilateral salpingo-oophorectomy, with wide excision of the parametria, but most cases are not diagnosed until after the hysterectomy. The surgical removal of all visible extrauterine disease is very worthwhile, but pelvic lymphadenectomy is of doubtful value. The ovaries should be removed, partly because of the risk of occult metastatic disease and partly because of possible stimulation by oestrogens.

This is a slowly growing neoplasm which tends to recur late. The recurrence rate in early-stage disease has been reported to be as high as 50% in some series (Piver et al 1984), but further treatment is often effective. This may include surgery, progestogen therapy or irradiation. CA125 may be a good marker for recurrence.

Recurrence is commoner when the tumours are more than 5 cm in diameter or there is venous or parametrial extension. In such cases there may well be a case for adjuvant progestin therapy or pelvic radiotherapy post-operatively.

High-grade endometrial stromal sarcoma

The uterus harbouring a high-grade stromal sarcoma is usually enlarged, and the tumour appears as a polypoid mass extending into the uterine cavity from the endometrium. The mass is characteristically round with a smooth surface, a feature that often distinguishes this tumour from the rather unusual polypoid variant of endometrial carcinoma, which has a rough or papillary surface. Necrosis of the tumour is often a prominent naked-eye feature.

Microscopically, the resemblance to endometrial stromal cells is less obvious than is seen in the low-grade endometrial stromal sarcoma (Fig. 38.10). The cells are oval or spindle-shaped and may show considerable pleomorphism. Mitotic figures are numerous, always exceeding 10 per 10 high-power fields and often amounting to as many as 40 or 50 per 10 high-power fields. The tumour is richly vascular, but blood vessel and lymphatic channel involvement is much less frequently seen than in the low-grade variant. Areas of necrosis are frequently present.

High-grade endometrial stromal sarcoma is an aggressive tumour which occurs most commonly after the menopause. It usually presents as postmenopausal bleeding or irregular vaginal bleeding or discharge. Many complain of pelvic pain.

The treatment of choice is total abdominal hysterectomy and bilateral salpingo-oophorectomy. The overall survival of patients with this rare sarcoma is considerably less than 50%. Adjuvant pelvic irradiation is used in the hope of improving local control. Adriamycin or progestogens (Katn et al 1987) may be used in recurrent disease.

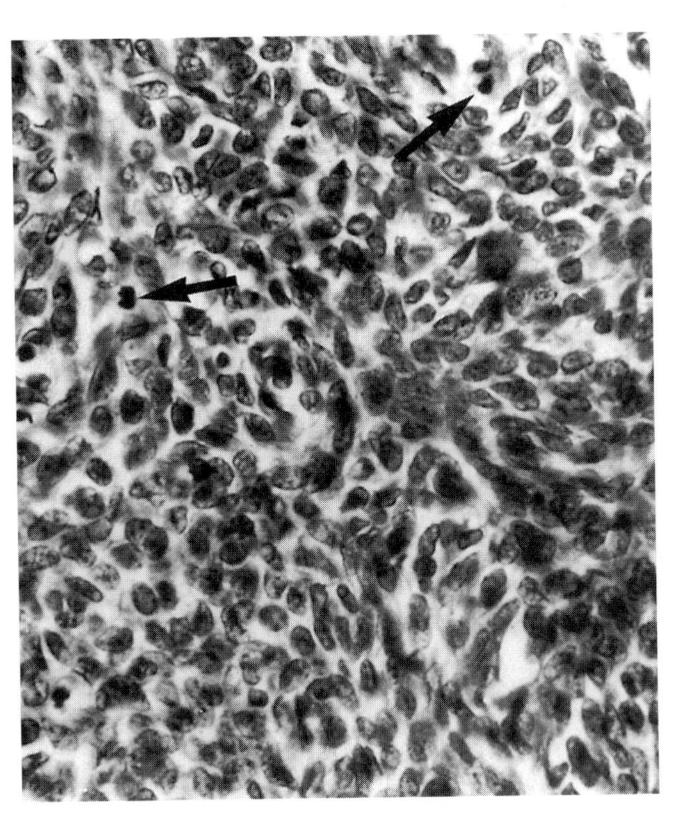

Fig. 38.10 A high-grade endometrial stromal sarcoma. Nuclear crowding and pleomorphism are apparent and, although mitotic figures (arrowed) are not conspicuous, this tumour contains more than 10 mitotic figures per 10 high-power fields. Haematoxylin and eosin × 650.

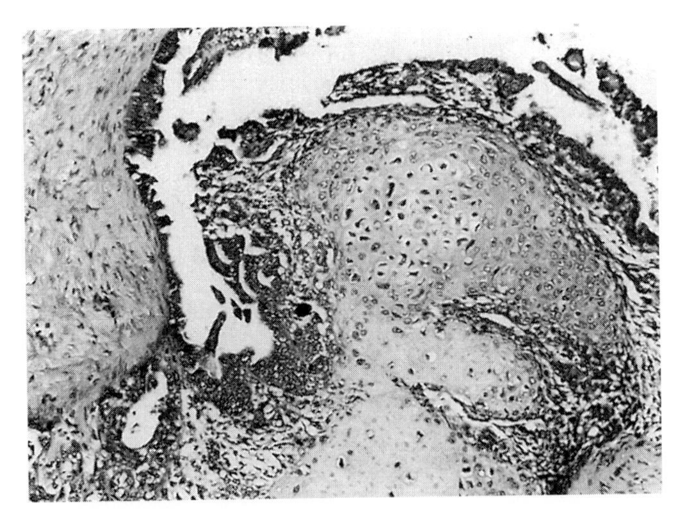

Fig. 38.11 Malignant mixed mullerian tumour. Malignant papillary epithelium and malignant cartilage are both present in this illustration. Haematoxylin and eosin × 195.

Malignant mixed mullerian tumour

The malignant mixed mullerian tumour is composed of malignant glands in malignant stroma (Fortune & Ostor 1987). In the past, different terms have been used to describe it; those that contain homologous mesenchymal elements have been called 'carcinosarcoma' and those with heterologous elements have been known as 'mixed mesodermal tumours'.

The neoplasm characteristically distends the uterine cavity and occasionally protrudes through the external cervical os. Areas of haemorrhage and necrosis are often prominent and myometrial invasion may be very obvious, as many of these tumours present at a fairly advanced stage. Multicentric tumour masses may be found.

The microscopic features of the malignant mixed mullerian tumour are striking and characteristic (Fig. 38.11). Both the epithelial and mesenchymal elements are malignant. Most frequently the carcinomatous element is of an endometrioid pattern, although often poorly differentiated. On occasion, squamous cell carcinoma is the sole epithelial component. The stromal element may be homologous or heterologous. The homologous malignant mixed mullerian tumour contains a mesenchymal element composed of cell types that are normally found in the uterus, such as leiomyosarcoma, endometrial stromal sarcoma, fibrosarcoma and the often-encountered undifferentiated sarcoma. The heterologous elements are rhabdomyosarcoma, osteosarcoma and chondrosarcoma.

The average age of patients with these aggressive cancers is 60 years, and presentation is usually with abnormal bleeding, pain or a mass. These tumours have a similar pattern of spread and prognosis to poorly differentiated adenocarcinomas, with spread to the cervix and regional nodes being common (Gallup et al 1989). They should be managed in a similar fashion to endometrial cancer. Postoperative pelvic irradiation may improve local pelvic control. Cisplatin and Adriamycin may be used for patients with recurrent or advanced disease.

Myometrial tumours

Leiomyosarcoma

This tumour is the malignant counterpart of the leiomyoma and is the most common pure sarcoma of the uterus (Hendrickson & Kempson 1987). Its incidence is commonly quoted as 0.67/100 000 women. Although the true figure is unknown, it might be reasonable to suggest that perhaps two or three women per 1000 with smooth muscle tumours of the uterus have a leiomyosarcoma.

The gross appearance of a leiomyosarcoma may not differ significantly from that of a leiomyoma. Leiomyosarcomas have been described as having a cut surface that appears paler, perhaps more yellow, than a leiomyoma, with areas of haemorrhage and necrosis. Adhesions and evidence of gross invasion into the surrounding myometrium may be present, but this is seldom of diagnostic value. Leiomyosarcomas are frequently found in uteri that contain leiomyomas, but they can also occur singly, and are more likely to be solitary than a leiomyoma. The peak age incidence of leiomyosarcoma is about 10 years later than leiomyoma.

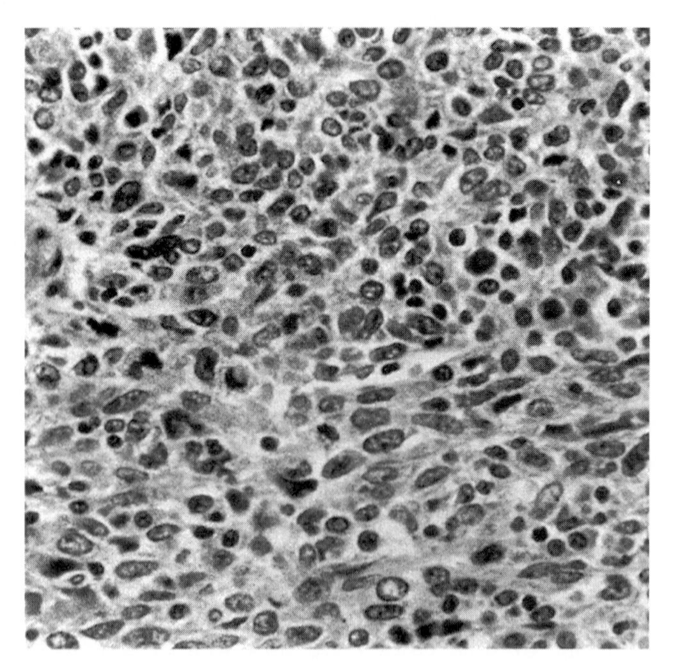

Fig. 38.12 Leiomyosarcoma. Although a few cells are spindled, most are poorly differentiated and show marked nuclear pleomorphism. Haematoxylin and eosin × 720.

Microscopically, well differentiated leiomyosarcomas are composed of elongated cells with regular nuclei that are little different from those of leiomyoma (Fig. 38.12). At the other end of the spectrum, a poorly differentiated leiomyosarcoma is composed of rounded and pleomorphic cells that have virtually no resemblance to normal smooth muscle cells. Areas of necrosis and haemorrhage, sometimes obvious to the naked eye, are also seen microscopically.

The 5–10% of leiomyosarcomas that arise from a fibroid have a better prognosis than those that originate in normal myometrium. This is especially true if the surrounding muscle is not involved. Some 20% of patients are nulliparous. A history of pelvic irradiation is uncommon (5%) and the majority of patients present with menometrorrhagia or postmenopausal bleeding. Other presenting symptoms include vaginal discharge, pelvic pain or pressure and weight loss. Rarely, a sarcoma is detected when fibroids enlarge rapidly. In over 80% of cases the diagnosis is not made until hysterectomy is performed, with the remainder being detected on curettage.

In those patients in whom a preoperative diagnosis is made, the treatment of choice is total abdominal hysterectomy and bilateral salpingo-oophorectomy. Washings from the pelvis should be taken. Given the propensity for leiomyosarcomas to spread within the abdomen and to lymph nodes, a full staging procedure similar to that for patients with ovarian cancer is performed on fit patients.

The role of adjuvant treatment, either radiotherapy or chemotherapy, has not been accurately defined in patients with early-stage disease. Recurrences are more common with tumours with more than 10 mitoses per 10 high-power fields and in patients with positive washings or lymph node involvement. Although cytotoxic agents such as vincristine, actinomycin and cyclophosphamide in combination, as well as Adriamycin and DTIC either alone or in combination, have proven activity in advanced or recurrent cases, their use in an adjuvant setting has not been shown to improve survival in any randomized trials. Cisplatin is also active in these tumours.

Other myometrial tumours

Atypical smooth muscle tumours include leiomyoblastoma, clear cell leiomyoma and epithelioid leiomyoma. The majority of patients are premenopausal and present with irregular bleeding, pain and abdominal distension. The diagnosis is usually made following hysterectomy. Recurrences occur in approximately 10% of cases and are more likely when the mitotic count is more than one per 10 high-power fields.

Intravenous leiomyomatosis is the rare situation in which there are fibrous growths into the uterine veins and beyond. Again, most women are premenopausal and these growths may be oestrogen dependent. Occasionally the major veins are involved, and a direct surgical approach offers the best chance of cure.

Benign metastasizing leiomyoma is similar but venous infiltration is absent and nodules are usually found in the pulmonary circulation. Progression is more common in the younger patient and respiratory failure may ensue. Again, oestrogen dependence has been suggested.

Leiomyomatosis peritonealis disseminata occurs in premenopausal women, often with a history of oral contraceptive use, and in up to 50% cases associated with pregnancy. The condition is marked by the presence of small nodules arising from the visceral and parietal peritoneal surfaces, and treatment is usually by surgical excision. Surgical castration may help regression. The prognosis is usually good.

KEY POINTS

1. The overall 5-year survival for cancer of the uterus in the United Kingdom is only 60% (corrected survival 68%).
2. The incidence of corpus cancer varies markedly, not only from country to country, but between different racial groups in the one geographical area.
3. Oral contraceptive use substantially protects against the later development of endometrial cancer.
4. Most of the known risk factors for the development of this cancer share a common basis: excessive or unopposed oestrogen stimulation of the endometrium.
5. Postmenopausal bleeding is the most common presenting symptom, as 75–80% of women with the disease are in this age group.
6. Over one-third of premenopausal patients present with heavy but regular periods.
7. Patients with endometrial tumour involving the cervix have a survival rate about 25% less than those with tumour confined to the corpus, but this risk is confined largely to those with gross extension to the cervix.
8. Clear cell tumours, papillary serous carcinomas and grade 3 tumours all have a poor prognosis.
9. The depth of myometrial invasion and tumour grade are the most important clinical prognostic indicators.
10. Total abdominal hysterectomy and bilateral salpingo-oophorectomy is the treatment of choice for Stage I disease.
11. Vault irradiation reduces the incidence of vault recurrence and might be omitted only in superficial, well differentiated tumours.
12. Stage II disease should be treated with radiotherapy or radical hysterectomy if the cervix is macroscopically involved.
13. Isolated vaginal recurrence in the non-irradiated patient has a good prognosis if treated with radiotherapy.
14. The value of adjuvant progestin therapy is not established.
15. Progestins given for recurrent disease produce a response in 15–20% of cases.

REFERENCES

Aalders J, Abeler V, Kolstad P, Onsrud V 1980 Postoperative external irradiation and prognostic parameters in Stage I endometrial carcinoma. A clinical and histopathological study of 540 patients. Obstetrics and Gynecology 56: 419–427

Abeler V M, Kjørstad K E, Berle E 1992 Carcinoma of the endometrium in Norway: a histopathological and prognostic survey of a total population. International Journal of Gynecological Cancer 2: 9–22

Adami H-O, Krusemo U B, Bergkvist L, Persson I, Pettersson B 1987 On the age-dependent association between cancer of the breast and of the endometrium. A nationwide cohort study. British Journal of Cancer 55: 77–80

Ayhan A, Tuncer R, Tuncer Z S, Yüce K, Küçükali T 1994 Correlation between clinical and histopathological risk factors and lymph node metastases in early endometrial cancer (a multivariate analysis of 183 cases). International Journal of Gynecological Cancer 4: 306–309

Baak J P A, Wisse-Brekelmans E C, Fleege J C, Van der Putten H W, Bezemer P D 1992 Assessment of the risk of endometrial cancer in hyperplasia, by means of morphological and morphometric features. Pathology Research Practice 188: 856–859

Baak J P A, Snijders W P, van Diest P J, Armee-Horvath E, Kenemans P 1995 Confirmation of the prognostic value of the ECPI-1 score in FIGO Stage I endometrial cancer patients with

long follow up. International Journal of Gynecological Cancer 5: 112–116
Batool T, Reginald P W, Hughes J H 1994 Outpatient pipelle endometrial biopsy in the investigation of postmenopausal bleeding. British Journal of Obstetrics and Gynaecology 101: 545–546
Bean H A, Bryant A J, Carmichael J A, Mallik A 1978 Carcinoma of the endometrium in Saskatchewan 1966–1971. Gynecologic Oncology 6: 503–514
Belinson J L, Lee K R, Badger G J, Pretorius R G, Jarrell M A 1992 Clinical Stage I adenocarcinoma of the endometrium – analysis of recurrences and the potential benefit of staging lymphadenectomy. Gynecologic Oncology 44: 17–23
Berman M L, Afridi M A, Kanbour A I, Ball H G 1982 Risk factors and prognosis in Stage II endometrial cancer. Gynecologic Oncology 14: 49–61
Bickenback W 1967 Factor analysis of endometrial cancer in relation to treatment. Obstetrics and Gynecology 29: 632–637
Black R J, Sharp L, Kendrick S W 1993 Trends in cancer survival in Scotland. Edinburgh, Information and Statistics Division, Directorate of Information Services, National Health Service in Scotland
Burke T W, Heller P B, Woodward J E, Davidson S A, Hoskins W J, Park R C 1990 Treatment failure in endometrial carcinoma. Obstetrics and Gynecology 75: 96–101
Candiani G B, Mangioni C, Marzi M M 1978 Surgery in endometrial cancer: age, route and operability rate in 854 Stage I and II fresh consecutive cases: 1955–76. Gynecologic Oncology 6: 363–372
Candiani G B, Belloni C, Maggi R, Colombo G, Frigoli A, Carinelli S G 1990 Evaluation of different surgical approaches in the treatment of endometrial cancer at FIGO Stage I. Gynecologic Oncology 37: 6–8
Christopherson W M, Connelly P J, Alberhasky R C 1983 Carcinoma of the endometrium. V. An analysis of prognosticators in patients with favourable subtypes and stage I disease. Cancer 51: 1705–1709
Corn B W, Lanciano R M, Greven K M et al 1994 Impact of improved irradiation technique, age and lymph node sampling on the severe complication rate of surgically staged endometrial cancer patients: a multivariate analysis. Journal of Clinical Oncology 12: 510–515
COSA-NZ-UK Endometrial Cancer Study Groups 1996 Pelvic lymphadenectomy in high risk endometrial cancer. International Journal of Gynecological Cancer 6: 102–107
Cowles T A, Magrina J F, Masterson B J, Capen C V 1985 Comparison of clinical and surgical staging in patients with endometrial carcinoma. Obstetrics and Gynecology 66: 413–416
Creasman W T, Morrow P, Bundy B W, Homesley H D, Graham J E, Heller P B 1987 Surgical pathological spread patterns of endometrial cancer. A Gynaecologic Oncology Group study. Cancer 60: 2035–2041
Early Breast Cancer Trialists' Collaborative Group 1992 Systemic treatment of early breast cancer by hormonal, cytotoxic, or immune therapy. Part 1. Lancet 339: 1–15
Eddowes H A 1990 A more acceptable technique for out-patient endometrial biopsy. British Journal of Obstetrics and Gynaecology 97: 961–962
Fishel R, Lescoe M K, Rao M R S et al 1994 The human mutator gene homolog MSH2 and its association with hereditary nonpolyposis colon cancer. Cell 77: 167–172
Fisher B, Costantino J P, Redmond C K et al 1994 Endometrial cancer in tamoxifen treated breast cancer patients: findings from the National Surgical Adjuvant Breast and Bowel Project (NSABP) B-14. Journal of the National Cancer Institute 86: 527–537
Fortune D W, Ostor A G 1987 Mixed mullerian tumours of the uterus. In: Fox H (ed) Haines and Taylor: Obstetrical and gynaecological pathology, 3rd edn. Churchill Livingstone, Edinburgh, pp 457–478
Gallup D G, Gable D S, Talledo O E, Otken L B 1989 A clinical-pathologic study of mixed mullerian tumours of the uterus over a 16 year period: the Medical College of Georgia experience. American Journal of Obstetrics and Gynecology 161: 533–539
Goff B A, Goodman A, Munty H G, Fuller A F Jr, Nikrui N, Rice L W 1994 Surgical Stage IV endometrial cancer: a study of 47 cases. Gynecologic Oncology 52: 237–240
Graham J 1971 The value of preoperative or postoperative treatment by radium for carcinoma of the uterine body. Surgery, Gynecology and Obstetrics 132: 855–860
Gredmark T, Kvint S, Havel G, Mattsson L-A 1995 Histopathological findings in women with postmenopausal bleeding. British Journal of Obstetrics and Gynaecology 102: 133–136
Greer B E, Hamberger A D 1983 Treatment of intraperitoneal metastatic adenocarcinoma of the endometrium by the whole-abdomen moving-strip technique and pelvic boost irradiation. Gynecologic Oncology 16: 365–373
Hendrickson M R, Kempson R L 1987 Pure mesenchymal neoplasms of the uterine corpus. In: Fox H (ed) Haines and Taylor: Obstetrical and gynaecological pathology, 3rd edn. Churchill Livingstone, Edinburgh, pp 411–456
Hill N C W, Broadbent J A M, Magos A L, Baumann R, Lockwood G M 1992 Local anaesthesia and cervical dilatation for outpatient diagnostic hysteroscopy. Journal of Obstetrics and Gynaecology 12: 33–37
Kadar N, Homesley H D, Malfetano J H 1992 Positive peritoneal cytology is an adverse factor in endometrial carcinoma only if there is other evidence of extrauterine disease. Gynecologic Oncology 46: 145–149
Katn L, Merino M J, Sakamoto H, Schwartz P E 1987 Endometrial stromal sarcoma: a clinicopathological study of 11 cases with determination of estrogen and progestin receptor levels in three tumours. Gynecologic Oncology 26: 87–97
Kemp J F, Fryer J A, Baber R J 1989 An alternative regimen of hormone replacement therapy to improve patient compliance. Australian and New Zealand Journal of Obstetrics and Gynaecology 29: 66–69
Kilgore L C, Partridge E E, Alvarez R D et al 1995 Adenocarcinoma of the endometrium: survival comparisons of patients with and without pelvic node sampling. Gynecologic Oncology 56: 29–33
Kneale B L G 1986 Adjunctive and therapeutic progestins in endometrial cancer. Clinics in Obstetrics and Gynaecology 13: 789–809
Kohorn E I 1976 Gestagens and endometrial carcinoma. Gynecologic Oncology 4: 398–411
Koss L G, Schreiber K, Moussouris H, Oberlander S G 1982 Endometrial cancer and its precursors: detection and screening. Clinics in Obstetrics and Gynecology 25: 419–461
Lehtovirta P, Cacciatore B, Ylöstalo 1994 Serum CA 125 levels and sonography in the preoperative assessment of myometrial invasion of endometrial cancer. British Journal of Obstetrics and Gynaecology 101: 532–535
Lindahl B, Ranstam J, Willén R 1994 Five year survival rate in endometrial carcinoma stages I-II: influence of degree of tumour differentiation, age, myometrial invasion and DNA content. British Journal of Obstetrics and Gynaecology 101: 621–625
Lotocki R J, Copeland L J, DePetrillo A D, Muirhead W 1983 Stage I endometrial adenocarcinoma: treatment results in 835 patients. American Journal of Obstetrics and Gynecology 146: 141–145
Macia M, Novo A, Ces J, Gonzalez M, Quintana S, Codesido J 1993 Progesterone challenge test for the assessment of endometrial pathology in asymptomatic postmenopausal women. International Journal of Gynecology and Obstetrics 40: 145–149
MacKenzie I Z, Bibby J G 1978 Critical assessment of dilatation and curettage in 1029 women. Lancet ii: 566–568
Magriples V, Naftolm F, Schwartz P E, Carcangiv M L 1993 High-grade endometrial carcinoma in tamoxifen-treated breast cancer patients. Journal of Clinical Oncology 11: 485–490
Mangioni C, De Palo G, Marubini E, Del Vecchio M 1993 Surgical pathological staging in apparent Stage I endometrial carcinoma. International Journal of Gynecological Cancer 3: 373–384
Meanwell C A, Kelly K A, Wilson S et al 1988 Young age as a prognostic factor in cervical cancer: analysis of population based data from 10,022 cases. British Medical Journal 296: 386–391
Mitchell H, Giles G, Medley G 1993 Accuracy and survival benefit of cytological prediction of endometrial carcinoma on routine cervical smears. International Journal of Gynaecological Pathology 12: 34–40
Morgan J D, Reddy S, Sarin P, Yordan E, De Geest K, Hendrickson F R 1993 Isolated vaginal recurrences of endometrial carcinoma. Radiology 189: 609–613
Morrow C P, Bundy B N, Kurman R J et al 1991 Relationship between

surgical–pathological risk factors and outcome in clinical stage I and II carcinoma of the endometrium: a Gynecologic Oncology Group study. Gynecologic Oncology 40: 55–65
Nagamani M, Stuart C A, Doherty M G 1992 Increased steroid production by the ovarian stromal tissue of postmenopausal women with endometrial cancer. Journal of Clinical Endocrinology and Metabolism 74: 172–176
Neven P, Muylder X de, Van Belle Y, Campo R, Vanderick G 1994 Tamoxifen and the uterus. British Medical Journal 309: 1313–1314
Office of Population Censuses and Surveys 1988 Cancer survival 1981 registrations. HMSO, London, MB1 88/1
Onsrud M, Aalders J, Abeler V, Taylor P 1982 Endometrial carcinoma with cervical involvement (Stage II): prognostic factors and value of combined radiological–surgical treatment. Gynecologic Oncology 13: 76–86
Osmers R, Völksen M, Schauer A 1990 Vaginosonography for early detection of endometrial carcinoma? Lancet 335: 1569–1571
PEPI – Writing Group for PEPI Trial 1995 Effects of oestrogen or oestrogen/progestin regimens on heart disease risk factors in postmenopausal women. Journal of the American Medical Association 273: 199–208
Pettersson F 1995 Annual report on the results of treatment in gynaecological cancer, vol 22. International Federation of Gynaecology and Obstetrics, Stockholm
Phillips G L, Prem K A, Adcock L L, Twiggs L B 1982 Vaginal recurrence of adenocarcinoma of the endometrium. Gynecologic Oncology 13: 323–328
Piver M S, Yazigi R, Blumenson L, Tsukada Y 1979 A prospective trial comparing hysterectomy, hysterectomy plus vaginal radium, and uterine radium plus hysterectomy in Stage I endometrial carcinoma. Obstetrics and Gynecology 54: 85–89
Piver M S, Rutledge F N, Copeland L, Walster K, Blumenson L, Suh O 1984 Uterine endolymphatic stromal myosis: a collaborative study. Obstetrics and Gynecology 64: 173–178
Potischman N, Swanson C A, Brinton L A et al 1993 Dietary associations in a case-control study of endometrial cancer. Cancer Causes Control 4: 239–250
Poulsen H E, Taylor C W, Sobin L H 1975 In: Histological typing of female genital tract tumours. International histological classification of tumours no 13. World Health Organization, Geneva, p 64
Quinn M A 1989 Endocrine aspects of human uterine sarcoma. American Journal of Obstetrics and Gynecology 159: 88
Quinn M A, Campbell J J 1989 Tamoxifen therapy in advanced or recurrent endometrial carcinoma. Gynecologic Oncology 32: 1–3
Quinn M A, Ruffe H, Brown J B, Ennis G 1981 Circulating gonadotrophins and urinary oestrogens in postmenopausal diabetic women. Australian and New Zealand Journal of Obstetrics and Gynaecology 21: 234–236
Quinn M A, Kneale B J, Fortune D W 1985a Endometrial carcinoma in premenopausal women: a clinicopathological study. Gynecologic Oncology 20: 298–306
Quinn M A, Cauchi M, Fortune D 1985b Endometrial carcinoma: steroid receptors and response to medroxyprogesterone acetate. Gynecologic Oncology 21: 314–319
Reid P C, Brown V A, Fothergill D J 1993 Outpatient investigation of postmenopausal bleeding. British Journal of Obstetrics and Gynaecology 100: 498
Rendina G M, Donadio C, Fabri M, Mazzoni P, Nazzicone P 1984 Tamoxifen and medroxyprogesterone therapy for advanced endometrial carcinoma. European Journal of Obstetrics, Gynaecology and Reproduction 17: 285–291
Richardson R E, Bournas N, Magos A L 1995 Is laparoscopic hysterectomy a waste of time? Lancet 345: 36–41
Rome R, Fortune D W, Quinn M A, Brown J B 1981 Functioning ovarian tumours in postmenopausal women. Obstetrics and Gynecology 57: 705–710
Rose P G, Sommers R M, Reale F R, Hunter R E, Fournier L, Nelson B E 1994 Serial serum CA 125 measurements for evaluation of recurrence in patients with endometrial carcinoma. Obstetrics and Gynecology 84: 12–16
Scarselli G, Savino L, Ceccherini R, Barciulli F, Massi G B 1992 Role of vaginal surgery in the 1st stage of endometrial cancer. European Journal on Gynaecological Oncology 13: Suppl 1: 15–19
Shaker A G, Anderson M, Kitchener H C 1991 An outpatient approach to the management of post-menopausal bleeding. British Journal of Obstetrics and Gynaecology 98: 488–490
Shu X O, Zheng W, Potischman N et al 1993 A population-based case-control study of dietary factors and endometrial cancer in Shanghai, People's Republic of China. American Journal of Epidemiology 137: 155–165
Stanford J L, Brinton L A, Berman M L et al 1993 Oral contraceptives and endometrial cancer: do other risk factors modify the association? International Journal of Cancer 54: 243–248
Stovall T G, Photopulos G Y, Poston W M, Ling F W, Sandles L G 1991 Pipelle endometrial sampling in patients with known endometrial carcinoma. Obstetrics and Gynecology 77: 954–956
Thigpen T, Vance R, Lambeth B et al 1987 Chemotherapy for advanced or recurrent gynaecological cancer. Cancer 60: 2104–2116
Van den Bosch T, Vandendael A, Schoubroeck v D, Wranz P A B, Lombard C J 1995 Combined vaginal ultrasonography and office endometrial sampling in the diagnosis of endometrial disease in postmenopausal women. Obstetrics and Gynecology 85: 349–352
Word B, Gravlee C, Wideman G L 1958 The fallacy of simple uterine curettage. Obstetrics and Gynecology 12: 642–648
Wren B G 1994 Hormonal therapy following female genital tract cancer. International Journal of Gynecological Cancer 4: 217–224
Yazigi R, Piver S, Blumenson L 1983 Malignant peritoneal cytology as a prognostic indicator in Stage I endometrial cancer. Obstetrics and Gynecology 62: 359–362
Zablow A, Adams M, Gregori C, Breen J L, Sanfilippo L J 1994 Stage II adenocarcinoma of the endometrium treated by two standard regimens of combined preoperative irradiation and surgery. International Journal of Gynecological Cancer 4: 265–271

39

Trophoblastic diseases

G. J. S. Rustin

INTRODUCTION

The spectrum of trophoblastic diseases extends from benign hydatidiform moles, which usually resolve spontaneously, to life-threatening choriocarcinoma. Virtually all patients are now potentially curable, provided they are correctly diagnosed and the appropriate therapy is administered early enough in the course of disease. Only doctors in specialist centres gain adequate experience in treating these rare tumours. However, with the incidence of hydatidiform mole ranging from 0.5 to 2.5/1000 pregnancies, most obstetric units will see at least one case per year. A woman who has had a hydatidiform mole has approximately a 1000-fold greater chance of developing choriocarcinoma than one who has had a live birth. Continued awareness and education are required, not just about the optimal management and follow-up of molar pregnancy, but also so that choriocarcinoma developing after non-molar pregnancy is detected as early as possible.

PATHOLOGY OF GESTATIONAL TROPHOBLASTIC DISEASE

A World Health Organization scientific group (1983) clarified the clinical and pathological definitions of the various conditions that make up gestational trophoblastic disease. This term includes the diseases detailed below, as well as two conditions which are not followed by malignant sequelae. These are hydropic degeneration – an aborted conceptus containing excessive fluid, or liquefaction of placental villous stroma without undue trophoblastic hyperplasia – and placental site reaction – the presence of trophoblastic cells and leukocytes in a placental bed.

Complete hydatidiform mole

This term is derived from the Greek word *hydatis* meaning a drop of water, and the Latin word *mola* meaning a mass. It is defined as an abnormal conceptus without an embryo, with gross hydropic swelling of the placental villi and usually pronounced trophoblastic hyperplasia, having both cytotrophoblastic and syncytial elements. The villous swelling leads to central cistern formation, with a concomitant compression of the maturing connective tissue that has lost its vascularity. A classic mole resembles a bunch of grapes.

Partial hydatidiform mole

This is an abnormal conceptus with an embryo or fetus that tends to die early, with a placenta subject to focal and villous swelling leading to cistern formation and focal trophoblastic hyperplasia, usually involving the syncytiotrophoblast only. The unaffected villi appear normal and vascularity of the villi disappears following fetal death. Unequivocal choriocarcinoma has never been recorded after partial hydatidiform mole, but chemotherapy has been given to some women because of metastases or elevated human chorionic gonadotrophin (hCG) levels. Most studies suggest that complete is more common than partial hydatidiform mole.

Invasive mole

This is a tumour invading the myometrium and is characterized by trophoblastic hyperplasia and persistence of placental villous structures. It commonly results from complete hydatidiform mole, and may do so from partial hydatidiform mole. It does not often progress to choriocarcinoma. It may metastasize, but does not progress like a true cancer and may regress spontaneously.

Gestational choriocarcinoma

This is a carcinoma arising from the trophoblastic epithelium that shows both cytotrophoblastic and syncytiotrophoblastic elements. It may arise from conceptions that give rise to a live birth, a stillbirth, an abortion at any stage, an ectopic pregnancy or a hydatidiform mole. The lack of villous structures distinguishes choriocarcinoma morphologically from invasive mole. Over 50% of cases of choriocarcinoma are preceded by hydatidiform mole in most series.

Placental site trophoblastic tumour

This tumour arises from the trophoblast of the placental bed and is composed mainly of cytotrophoblastic cells. This accounts for the relatively low level of hCG associated with this condition. About one case of this tumour is seen for every 100 cases of invasive mole and choriocarcinoma. Pathologists may initially consider it as atypical choriocarcinoma. It was earlier called trophoblast pseudotumour of the uterus, but the term 'placental site trophoblastic tumour' is now preferred because of the malignant behaviour reported in some cases. Complete surgical excision is the preferred treatment, as these tumours are not as chemosensitive as choriocarcinoma (Lathrop et al 1988).

Gestational trophoblastic tumours

This term is used to denote those conditions that require more active intervention, usually chemotherapy, and includes invasive mole, choriocarcinoma and placental site tumours. The reliance on persistently elevated hCG levels for diagnosis and the frequent absence of tissue for histology make it often impossible to differentiate between invasive mole and choriocarcinoma, so the term 'gestational trophoblastic tumour' covers both diseases.

EPIDEMIOLOGY

The very high incidence of hydatidiform mole in Asia, parts of Africa and South and Central America may have been exaggerated by many hospital-based studies due to selection bias (Bracken 1987). Japanese population studies report an average incidence of about 2.5/1000 pregnancies, compared to a nationwide Chinese incidence of 0.78/1000 pregnancies. Studies in the USA report incidence rates from 0.5 to 1.08/1000 pregnancies, whereas a recent study from England and Wales showed an incidence of 1.54/1000 live births. Large differences in incidence in different racial groups have not been confirmed.

Studies from many countries show that the risk of hydatidiform mole increases progressively in women aged over 40, reaching almost one in three live births in those aged over 50. The risk is also slightly higher in pregnancies of those aged less than 15 years. Increasing gravidity does not appear to increase the risk of hydatidiform mole. However, a woman who has had a hydatidiform mole has a greater than 20-fold increased chance of having a further one; the rate for a second hydatidiform mole is 0.8–2.9% and for a third 15–28% (Bagshawe et al 1986).

A recent case-control study has suggested that low oestrogen levels may be associated with a disruption of normal ovulation, and predispose to choriocarcinoma. Other reported weak associations include prior miscarriages, artificial insemination by donor, longer duration of smoking and reduced carotene intake. Oral contraception appears to be unrelated.

Genetics

Complete hydatidiform mole appears to result from fertilization of an egg from which the nucleus has been lost or inactivated. The chromosomal complement arises by androgenesis and there are no maternal chromosomes, although the mitochondrial DNA is of maternal origin (Lawler & Fisher 1987). In most cases the paternal contribution stems from a duplication of a haploid sperm or from two different sperm. The 10% of hydatidiform mole that are heterozygous do not appear to have a higher chance of progressing to choriocarcinoma than the homozygous ones. Although both homozygous and heterozygous cases of choriocarcinoma have been reported, one would expect all cases of gestational choriocarcinoma to be androgenetic, whereas non-gestational tumours showing trophoblast differentiation would contain just maternal chromosomes.

Genetic studies show partial hydatidiform mole to be triploid, with one maternal and two paternal chromosome sets. It is thought to arise via dispermy. This genetic distinction is important, as choriocarcinoma has never been shown to develop from a partial mole. Flow cytometry on nuclei prepared from fresh or formalin-fixed paraffin-embedded tissue is very useful in confirming the triploid nature of partial hydatidiform mole. Twin pregnancies with a hydatidiform mole and normal fetus occasionally occur, and some of these pregnancies result in a live birth.

PRESENTATION

Hydatidiform mole

The great majority of hydatidiform moles are detected between 8 and 24 weeks of gestation, with a peak around 14 weeks. Vaginal bleeding is the most common presenting symptom. Many women pass molar tissue mixed with blood clot per vaginam. A fluid like prune juice, consisting of old blood, may be seen. This blood loss can lead to severe anaemia, especially in malnourished women. Acute life-threatening haemorrhage can occasionally occur. The uterus is large for dates in approximately half the patients at presentation. Theca lutein cysts are also common. These cysts may cause abdominal pain due to torsion or rupture, and commonly take up to 4 months to regress following evacuation. Pre-eclampsia and hyperemesis gravidarum are seen in about a quarter of these patients.

Clinical hyperthyroidism is uncommon, although increased thyroid function may be detected biochemically. This is probably due to the high levels of hCG, which is thyrotropic in bioassays. There is a correlation between hCG levels and endogenous thyroid function, but only those with hCG levels over 100 000 IU/l are overtly thyrotoxic. The possibility of thyrotoxicosis must be mentioned to an anaesthetist prior to evacuation because of the danger of precipitating a thyroid crisis. Symptoms due to uterine perforation, pelvic sepsis and disseminated intravascular coagulopathy can occur. Severe symptoms due to trophoblastic pulmonary embolization sometimes develop after evacuation, but these usually resolve with supportive care. The major long-term risk after molar pregnancy is the development of either invasive mole or choriocarcinoma. In the prechemotherapy era the risk of choriocarcinoma after hydatidiform mole was estimated to be less than 3%. The risk of developing invasive mole depends upon the criteria used for its identification, but probably 90% of hydatidiform moles resolve spontaneously.

There are several factors which have been shown to be associated with an increased risk of gestational trophoblastic tumour (Table 39.1). There is little relationship between histological grading of hydatidiform mole and subsequent clinical course.

Table 39.1 Factors increasing the risk of chemotherapy after hydatidiform mole

Pre-evacuation hCG level>100 000 IU/l*
Uterine size>gestational age*
Large (>6 cm) theca lutein cysts*
Maternal age >40 years*
Medical induction hysterectomy or hysterotomy†
Oral contraceptive before hCG falls to undetectable level†

Factors* plus previous molar pregnancy, hyperthyroidism, toxaemia, trophoblastic emboli and disseminated intravascular coagulation were considered high-risk by Goldstein et al (1981); † considered increased risk by Stone and Bagshawe (1979)

Invasive mole and choriocarcinoma

Invasive mole is seen in the early months following the evacuation of hydatidiform mole, and is only rarely recognized in the absence of such a history. Some centres diagnose invasive mole if the hCG level is still elevated at 8–10 weeks, giving an incidence of about 25%. Using high levels at 6 months gives an incidence of about 7%. A few cases of metastatic invasive mole with characteristic villi on histology have been seen in deposits in the lungs, cervix, vagina, vulva and even the brain. Apart from problems associated with these metastases, the symptoms of invasive mole are due to the invasive trophoblast. These include vaginal bleeding, amenorrhoea, infertility, abdominal pain and symptoms resulting from uterine perforation (Table 39.2). Histology is the only way of differentiating invasive mole from choriocarcinoma. The symptoms may be identical, but whereas all invasive moles are preceded by a hydatidiform mole, only about 50% of choriocarcinomas have a history of prior molar pregnancy. The remainder follow a live birth, stillbirth, abortion or ectopic pregnancy, which may have occurred up to several years previously. Choriocarcinoma occasionally presents in postmenopausal women.

Invasive mole can metastasize to virtually any part of the body. The commonest site is the lungs, where it is usually asymptomatic (Fig. 39.1). Pleuritic pain and haemoptysis can occur, owing to tumour invasion or following pulmonary infarction. Dyspnoea is seen with more extensive metastases. Dyspnoea and signs of pulmonary hypertension can also result from the rare growth of choriocarcinoma in the pulmonary arterial bed.

The vagina is the next commonest site of metastases. Their great vascularity makes them appear densely reddened. They bleed easily and may be missed without careful visual inspection. Cerebral metastases may present

Table 39.2 Differential diagnosis and distinguishing features

Diagnosis	Investigation
Molar pregnancy	
Pregnancy	Ultrasound
Abortion	Ultrasound
Partial hydatidiform mole	Histology, genetics
Toxaemia of pregnancy	Ultrasound
Hyperemesis gravidarum	Ultrasound
Ovarian cysts	Ultrasound, hCG
Invasive mole, choriocarcinoma	
Abortion	Ultrasound
Menorrhagia	hCG
Amenorrhoea, infertility	hCG
Metastases from any tumour	hCG Colour if superficial; histology (if safe); distribution: vagina and lung, common; bone and lymph nodes, rare
Pulmonary hypertension	hCG

hCG, human chorionic gonadotrophin

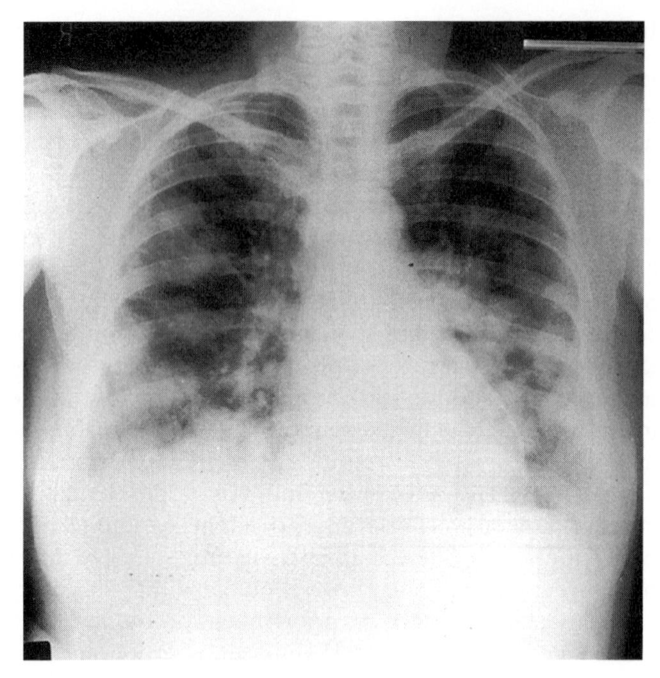

Fig. 39.1 Classic cannonball metastases in a woman with choriocarcinoma. Serum hCG should always be measured in a woman of reproductive age with such an X-ray.

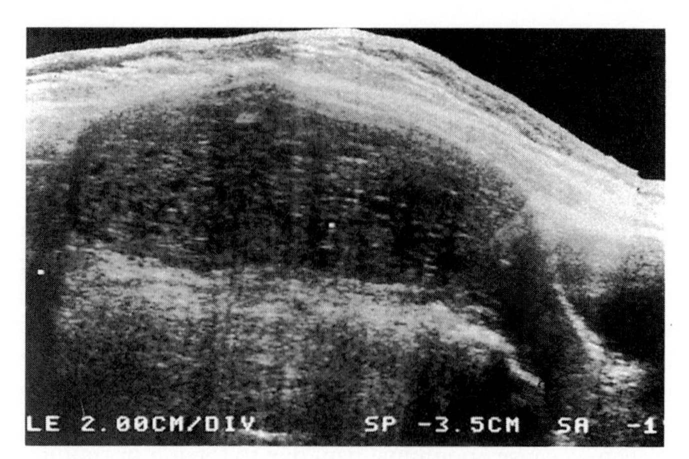

Fig. 39.2 Pelvic ultrasound of a woman with a hydatidiform mole, showing the characteristic snowstorm pattern.

suddenly as a cerebrovascular accident. Symptoms may be non-specific, such as headache, fits or loss of consciousness, or related to the site of neurological damage. Liver metastases are usually now discovered incidentally on scans. Purple skin deposits are sometimes seen. Lymph node and bone deposits are so rare that histological review is advisable.

INVESTIGATIONS

hCG estimation

In trophoblastic tumours hCG comes close to being the ideal tumour marker. It is a placental hormone that is secreted by the syncytiotrophoblast, and serves to maintain corpus luteum function and preserve progesterone secretion during the early stages of gestation. In a normal pregnancy it can be detected about 5 days after conception, and reaches its peak at 8–10 weeks of pregnancy. Although syncytiotrophoblast is the physiological source of hCG, an hCG-like substance has been detected in a wide variety of normal human tissues and low levels can be measured in normal human plasma.

The α subunit of hCG is nearly identical to the α units of thyroid-stimulating hormone, follicle-stimulating hormone and luteinizing hormone. The β subunit shares many similarities with the β subunits of other glycoprotein hormones, but the carboxyl terminal end contains unique amino acid sequences giving distinct antigenic characteristics. Immunoassays that utilize the intact hCG molecule as immunogen may be influenced by luteinizing hormone levels. A good assay detects down to 2 IU/l in serum.

Assays on urine are useful in the long-term follow-up of patients, although the background noise on urine assays tends to be higher than in serum, so that values up to the equivalent of 30 IU/l may not be significant. Urine estimations should be based on timed collections or be related to creatinine concentration. The preferred preservative for immunoassay is merthiolate (Thiomersal 100 mg per 24-h collection). Pregnancy tests will be positive in most patients with trophoblastic diseases, but may miss some cases due to the lower sensitivity.

In an attempt to distinguish between normal placenta and trophoblastic tumours many placental proteins have been investigated, including pregnancy-specific B_1 glycoprotein, human placental lactogen and inhibin. Their clinical value remains unclear.

Diagnosis and determining prognosis

Hydatidiform mole

In a woman thought to be pregnant, ultrasound scanning of the pelvis is the investigation most likely to confirm the presence of hydatidiform mole (Table 39.2). Hydatidiform mole produces a characteristic pattern of echoes that appear like a snowstorm (Fig 39.2). The presence of a live fetus must be excluded on ultrasound by carefully searching for a gestational sac and fetal heart. Large ovarian cysts are commonly visualized on the ultrasound and should be observed. It is advisable to demonstrate an elevated hCG level prior to evacuation. A chest X-ray should be performed to exclude trophoblastic emboli or metastases of invasive mole or choriocarcinoma. The products obtained at evacuation are usually the only tissue available for histology. Biopsy of vaginal metastases should not be performed, as this frequently leads to profuse bleeding which may be difficult to control. A full blood count is required to check for anaemia and two units of blood should be cross-matched prior to evacuation. T_3 and T_4 should be measured prior to surgery if there is any suspicion of thyrotoxicosis.

Invasive mole and choriocarcinoma

Choriocarcinoma may be excluded by a normal serum hCG level (<2 IU/l). An elevated level could be due to pregnancy, residual placental elements, ovarian germ cell tumour, placental site tumour, trophoblast differentiation in a carcinoma (most frequently gastric), or ectopic production from a variety of different tumours. Non-trophoblastic tumours are rarely associated with hCG levels >1000 IU/l.

Histological confirmation of the diagnosis is not required if there is a history of a recent molar pregnancy, the hCG level is grossly elevated and the distribution of disease is typical of choriocarcinoma. Provided pregnancy has been excluded in patients with grossly elevated levels of hCG, even without a history of a mole, it is safer to treat them as choriocarcinoma than to risk biopsying a metastasis. Needle biopsies of the liver or other sites have resulted in fatal haemorrhage; delay in starting therapy while the patient is recovering from surgical biopsies allows the tumour to grow. Clinical examination should include inspection of the vagina for metastases. The only routine staging investigations required are posteroanterior and lateral chest X-rays and pelvic ultrasound. Cerebrospinal fluid hCG should be measured if the patient fits into the high-risk prognostic group (see later), or has lung metastases and is in the middle-risk group. Cerebrospinal fluid levels of hCG that are more than 1/60 of the serum level indicate the presence of brain metastases, though a normal ratio does not exclude them.

A computed tomography (CT) scan of the brain is only required if there is clinical suspicion of brain metastases or the hCG ratio is abnormal. Magnetic resonance imaging (MRI) should be performed if, despite suspicions of a cerebral metastasis, the CT scan is normal. MRI sometimes detects lesions missed on CT scan, especially in the posterior fossa. MRI is the investigation of choice if spinal metastases are suspected. CT scans of the chest will detect metastases missed on chest X-ray, but in our experience have not led to a change in management and are not performed routinely. Scans of the abdomen are only performed if there is clinical suspicion of disease there. Pelvic arteriograms are rarely performed now except in patients who have severe vaginal haemorrhage after eradication of the mole. Radioimmunolocalization using radiolabelled antibody against hCG can locate drug-resistant deposits of tumour, which may then be resected. This method of imaging can sometimes detect deposits missed on CT or ultrasound scans, and may differentiate between viable and necrotic deposits (Begent et al 1987).

Prior to starting therapy a full blood count is required and renal and hepatic function must be assessed. Thyroid function should be measured. The blood group of the patient and her partner responsible for the most recent or molar pregnancy is required for the prognostic score (see later).

Staging

A staging system has been considered by the International Federation of Gynaecology and Obstetrics. This groups patients with a molar pregnancy as stage 0; lesions confined to the uterus without any metastases as stage I; lesions extending outside the uterus but confined to genital organs as stage II; lung metastases as stage III; and other metastatic sites as stage IV. This staging system is not used by most major trophoblastic disease centres as it does not help in treatment planning.

Follow-up after treatment

Postmolar pregnancy

Following the diagnosis of a molar pregnancy, follow-up is essential to detect those women who require chemotherapy for invasive mole or choriocarcinoma. Follow-up relies upon measurement of hCG in serum or urine. The serum half-life of hCG is approximately 24–36 hours. After a full-term normal delivery, serum and urine hCG become undetectable (<2 IU/l) within 10–20 days, but a small proportion of women have detectable hCG for longer periods. After a non-molar abortion hCG takes a few days longer to become undetectable, partly because the level is higher early in pregnancy and possibly due to retained products of conception. Following evacuation of a hydatidiform mole in a series of patients who did not require chemotherapy, hCG levels were still detectable in 3% of women until 20–22 weeks following evacuation (Bagshawe et al 1986). However, an early normalization of hCG suggests a shorter follow-up as, among 5124 patients, none of the 42% in whom the hCG level was undetectable by 7 weeks postevacuation required chemotherapy. Regular hCG estimations will detect a plateau or rise in hCGlevel, which would indicate persistence or growth of trophoblast.

A national follow-up service for hydatidiform mole patients has been in operation in the UK since 1972. Patients are registered centrally and then automatically sent boxes with prepaid returnable postage, containing tubes and a letter requesting that urine or serum samples be returned to one of three assay centres. It is recommended that hCG measurements be performed every 2 weeks until the limit of detection is reached, monthly during the first year after evacuation and 3-monthly during the second year. Measurements should continue for at least 6 months after the hCG has been undetectable because of the occasional late recrudescence. It is advisable to confirm that the hCG is undetectable for 6 months before starting another pregnancy. hCG must be monitored after all further pregnancies because of the 2% chance of a second hydatidiform mole and the slightly increased risk of choriocarcinoma arising either from a subsequent mole or normal pregnancy. Follow-up is not necessary after hydropic degeneration because of the low risk of malignant sequelae, but when the diagnosis is in doubt it is necessary to ensure that hCG remains undetectable in 3-monthly measurements.

Post chemotherapy

The author's policy is to continue hCG follow-up for life, because of the potential of choriocarcinoma to recur after several years.

Investigations for monitoring therapy

The close linear relationship between the number of choriocarcinoma cells present and the serum concentration of hCG allows for a more accurate assessment of response than for any other tumour. It is estimated that only 10^4–10^5 cells are required to produce a serum concentration of 1 IU/l. hCG levels can sometimes rise during the early days of drug therapy, even though the tumour is chemo-sensitive. This is thought to be related to tumour lysis. Serum hCG levels should be monitored at least weekly during therapy.

A plateau above the normal range may be due to cross-reaction of the assay with luteinizing hormone if the patient has become menopausal. However, a plateau or rising levels usually indicate drug resistance. Owing to the accuracy of hCG monitoring, repeat X-rays and scans are required only to confirm resolution of metastases or uterine or ovarian abnormalities at the end of treatment, or to detect surgically resectable masses in patients with drug-resistant disease. Radiological abnormalities may persist for some time after the hCG has become normal, before finally resolving.

TREATMENT

Evacuation of hydatidiform mole

Patients with clinical and ultrasound features suggestive of hydatidiform mole should have any significant blood loss replaced and the uterus evacuated by suction. Even a large hydatidiform mole can be evacuated with little blood loss. The need for chemotherapy after evacuation of hydatidiform mole is two- to threefold greater in patients who have undergone a medical induction, hysterectomy or hysterotomy than in those in whom the mole has been evacuated by vacuum or surgical curettage, or who have aborted spontaneously. If bleeding is severe after uterine evacuation, use of ergometrine is sometimes unavoidable. The single contraction produced by this agent appears to be less likely to produce embolization of trophoblast than the repeated contractions induced by oxytocin or prostaglandin. Many gynaecologists perform a second dilatation and curettage routinely 2 weeks later or, if there is persistent bleeding, following the initial evacuation. Because curettage cannot remove invasive mole from the myometrium, further dilatation and curettages are of no value. Hysterectomy should be avoided because of the intense vascularity and high risk of uncontrollable bleeding.

We advise patients not to take oral contraceptives until hCG has been normal for 3 months after molar evacuation, because of the increased chance of requiring chemotherapy found by us but not by some other investigators.

Prophylactic chemotherapy

Prophylactic chemotherapy following hydatidiform mole has been abandoned by certain centres because of unacceptable toxicity in women who had a high chance of never requiring chemotherapy. There is a suggestion from non-randomized studies that those patients who received prophylaxis had less chance of requiring subsequent chemotherapy than those not given prophylactic chemotherapy. Actinomycin D 12 μg/kg for 5 days following evacuation is advocated by the New England Trophoblastic Disease Center for women who fit into their high-risk group following evacuation of hydatidiform mole (Table 39.1). The arguments for prophylactic chemotherapy are less persuasive in those centres which treat a considerably smaller percentage of their patients following a molar pregnancy. The major attraction of prophylactic chemotherapy is for those patients in whom follow-up is likely to be difficult.

Selection of cases for chemotherapy

Chemotherapy may be given because of persistence or complications of invasive mole; because choriocarcinoma has been diagnosed; or, in some centres, as prophylaxis with the aim of preventing malignant sequelae. Criteria for treatment vary between different centres and it is often difficult to compare results between reported series. The World Health Organization Scientific Group (1983) agreed that treatment should be started if any of the following applies after a hydatidiform mole:

1. A high level of hCG more than 4 weeks after evacuation (serum level >20 000 IU/l; urine levels >30 000 IU/l).
2. Progressively increasing hCG values at any time after evacuation.
3. Histological identification of choriocarcinoma at any site, or evidence of central nervous system, renal, hepatic or gastrointestinal metastases, or pulmonary metastases >2 cm in diameter or >3 in number.

Persistent uterine haemorrhage with an elevated hCG is an indication for therapy in most centres. The major risk in delaying treatment in the patient with very high levels of hCG is uterine perforation. There is considerable disagreement about management of patients with persisting hCG levels. Some centres give chemotherapy to patients in whom hCG is detectable at a defined time, such as 8–10 weeks after evacuation. Others treat all patients who have a stationary hCG level for 2, 3 or more consecutive weeks. This results in approximately 27% of molar patients receiving chemotherapy. The policy at the Charing Cross Hospital since 1973 has been to allow the hCG to remain detectable for up to 4–6 months after evacuation, as spontaneous disappearance of hCG can take that long. This results in less than 8% of molar patients requiring chemotherapy.

Surgery

Apart from evacuation as discussed above, surgery has only a limited role. Uterine perforation is best managed by local resection of tumour and uterine repair. Hysterectomy may be required for persistent heavy bleeding, but this usually settles on chemotherapy. Angiographic embolization may be used to control bleeding if uterine preservation is desired. Surgical removal of drug-resistant disease has a curative role in the rare patient in whom the disease is limited to resectable sites. Elective hysterectomy has been used in the hope of reducing the need for or the duration of chemotherapy in patients not wishing to retain their reproductive potential. However, many such patients still require a full course of chemotherapy.

Prognostic scoring factors

The spectrum of gestational trophoblastic disease extends from persistence of a small focus of trophoblast in the uterus to widespread metastases. Obviously they do not all require the same intensity of treatment. Retrospective analysis has shown that various factors are related to survival (Table 39.3). To stratify treatment according to prognostic factors, Bagshawe, in 1976, devised a scoring system in which a weighting was applied for each factor. Each was assumed to act as an independent variable and their effects were assumed to be additive. This system, which defined low-, medium- and high-risk groups, was used successfully in several centres. Over the years it has been simplified and Table 39.3 shows the system adopted by the World Health Organization. Between 1958 and 1982, of the 860 patients treated for gestational trophoblastic tumours at the Charing Cross Hospital, 223 were in the high-risk group and 47% died; 232 fitted into the middle-risk group, of whom 1.3% died; and 405 fell into the low-risk group, of whom one died from an intercurrent tumour.

Chemotherapy

Patients for whom chemotherapy is considered necessary require the care of a doctor well versed in the use of cytotoxic drugs, a subject which is beyond the scope of this chapter (see Ch. 33). The three drugs with the greatest activity against gestational trophoblastic tumours are methotrexate, actinomycin D and etoposide. 6-Mercaptopurine, vincristine, cyclophosphamide, cisplatin and hydroxyurea also have proven activity. 5-Fluorouracil has been used successfully in China but not elsewhere (Song et al 1979). Primary drug resistance has been seen only rarely after methotrexate and actinomycin D, but not yet after etoposide. Drug resistance developing during treatment is a problem, especially in patients with a high prognostic score (see above). The prognostic group must be

Table 39.3 Scoring system based on prognostic factors

Prognostic factors	Score			
	0	1	2	4
Age (years)	<39	>39		
Antecedent pregnancy	Hydatidiform mole	Abortion	Term	
Interval*	4	4–6	7–12	12
hCG (IU/l)	$<10^3$	10^3–10^4	10^4–10^5	$>10^5$
ABO groups (female × male)		0 × A A × 0	B AB	
Largest tumour, including uterine tumour		3–5 cm	>5 cm	
Site of metastases		Spleen, kidney	Gastrointestinal tract, liver	Brain
Number of metastases identified		1–4	4–8	>8
Prior chemotherapy			Single drug	2 or more

The total score for a patient is obtained by adding the individual scores for each prognostic factor.
Total score: <4=low risk; 5–7 = middle risk; >8=high risk.
*Interval time (in months) between end of antecedent pregnancy and start of chemotherapy.

determined so that patients at higher risk of developing drug resistance are given combination chemotherapy from the start.

Low-risk patients

There is general agreement that methotrexate followed by folinic acid is the preferred treatment for the low-risk group, provided renal and hepatic function are normal. The most proven regimen is given over 8 days (Table 39.4). To prevent relapse, treatment should be repeated every 14 days and continued until the hCG level has been undetectable (<2 IU/l) for about 6 weeks (Fig. 39.3). Provided patients drink at least 2 litres of fluid a day they are unlikely to develop mucositis. Apart from occasional cases of chemical pleurisy, other side effects are very uncommon. Of 347 low-risk patients treated at the Charing Cross Hospital between 1974 and 1986, all entered complete remission and only one died, from intercurrent lymphoma (Bagshawe et al 1989). However, 69 (20%) had to change treatment because of drug resistance and 23 (6%) needed to change treatment because of drug-induced toxicity.

Short infusions of higher doses of methotrexate are used in some centres, but owing to differences in patient selection it is impossible to compare results. Actinomycin D 1.25 mg/m² has been recommended, but nausea, vomiting, alopecia, skin rashes and myelosuppression become problems with repeated courses. Etoposide cannot be recommended in this patient group as it invariably causes alopecia and its long-term carcinogenic properties are unknown.

Table 39.4 Low-risk regimen

Day	Treatment
1	Methotrexate (MTX) 50 mg i.m. at noon
2	Folinic acid (FA) 6 mg i.m. at 6.00 p.m. (30 h later)
3	MTX 50 mg i.m. at noon
4	FA 6 mg i.m. at 6.00 p.m.
5	MTX 50 mg i.m. at noon
6	FA 6 mg i.m. at 6.00 p.m.
7	MTX 50 mg i.m. at noon
8	FA 6 mg i.m. at 6.00 p.m.

Note: Courses are repeated after an interval of 6 days. Start each course on the same day of the week.

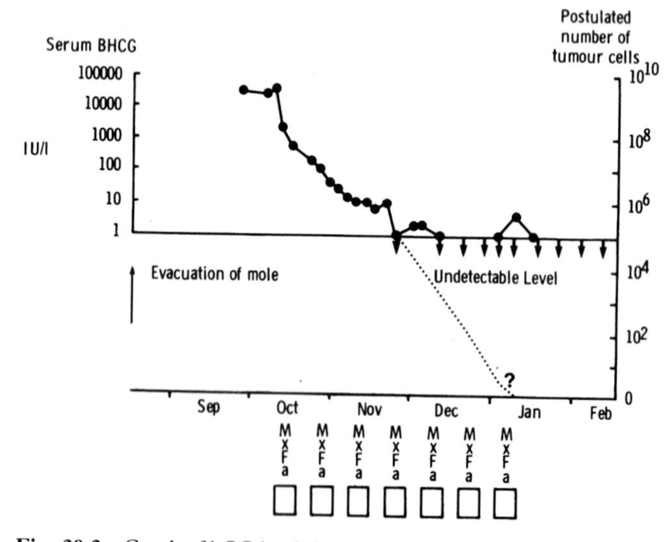

Fig. 39.3 Graph of hCG levels in a woman who required low-risk chemotherapy with methotrexate (Mx) and folinic acid (Fa) because of high levels of hCG following evacuation of hydatidiform mole. If chemotherapy had been stopped when the serum hCG became undetectable, approximately 10^5 tumour cells were postulated to have been still present. Cell numbers associated with the hCG level are shown on the right-hand vertical axis.

Medium-risk patients

This group was designed so that a range of drugs could be introduced sequentially, reserving the more toxic high-risk regimens for patients with a higher score of adverse prognostic factors. Many centres divide their patients into only low- and high-risk groups, and since the high-risk regimens have become less toxic this approach appears sensible. The middle-risk regimen is maintained at the Charing Cross Hospital because it allows for the introduction as a single agent of new drugs shown to be active in resistant patients. The medium-risk regimen, which is continued for 8–10 weeks after hCG has become undetectable, is shown in Table 39.5. At the Charing Cross Hospital 103 patients were treated in this group between 1973 and 1980. There have been three deaths, all due to drug resistance.

Table 39.5 Medium-risk patients: cycling regimen

Day	Drug	Dosage
Regimen A		
1 and 3	Etoposide	250 mg/m² in 500 ml 150 mmol NaCl i.v.
Regimen B		
1	Hydroxyurea	500 mg p.o. 12-hourly for 2 doses
2	Methotrexate (MTX)	50 mg i.m. at noon
3	Folinic acid (FA)	6 mg i.m. at 6.00 p.m.
	6-Mercaptopurine (6MP)	75 mg p.o.
4	MTX	50 mg i.m. at noon
5	FA	6 mg i.m. at 6.00 p.m.
	6MP	75 mg p.o.
6	MTX	50 mg i.m. at noon
7	FA	6 mg i.m. at 6.00 p.m.
	6MP	75 mg p.o.
8	MTX	50 mg i.m. at noon
9	FA	6 mg i.m. at 6.00 p.m.
	6MP	75 mg p.o.
Regimen C		
1–5	Actinomycin D	0.5 mg for 5 days

Note: Courses are given in the sequence ABACA, with intervals usually of 6 drug-free days between courses.

High-risk patients

Only 31% of patients in this group survived if given single-agent methotrexate (Bagshawe et al 1989). Several intensive multidrug regimens have been developed. These include CHAMOCA, developed at the Charing Cross Hospital, and MAC III used in Boston (Goldstein & Berkowitz 1982). Since 1979, patients in the high-risk group at the Charing Cross Hospital have received a weekly alternating regimen called EMA/CO (Table 39.6, Fig. 39.4). This regimen is given on the same day each week unless the total white cell count falls below 1.5×10^9/l or platelets below 75×10^9/l or mucosal ulceration develops. Of 27 patients who received EMA/CO as initial therapy, 93% survived and one patient relapsed; of 20 who received EMA/CO after prior therapy, 74% survived and five patients relapsed (Newlands et al 1986). In patients who develop drug resistance, cisplatin 75 mg/m^2 and etoposide 100 mg/m^2 can lead to a durable remission when substituted for the CO of EMA/CO.

In patients with extensive pulmonary metastases deaths may occur due to respiratory failure, which can be exacerbated by too-aggressive initial therapy. Ventilation or high-dose steroids have not been shown to be of any value in this situation, so extracorporeal membrane oxygenation is now being assessed.

Table 39.6 EMA/CO regimen for high-risk patients

Course 1 EMA	
Day 1	Actinomycin D 0.5 mg i.v. stat Etoposide 100 mg/m^2 in 200 ml N/S over 30 min Methotrexate 300 mg/m^2 i.v. 12-h infusion
Day 2	Actinomycin D 0.5 mg stat Etoposide 100 mg/m^2 i.v. in 200 ml N/S over 30 min Folinic acid 15 mg p.o. or i.m. bd for 4 doses starting 24 h after the start of methotrexate 5-day drug-free interval to course 2
Course 2 CO	
Day 1	Vincristine 1.0 mg/m^2 i.v. stat (maximum 2.0 mg) Cyclophosphamide 600 mg/m^2 i.v. infusion over 20 min 6-day drug-free interval

If there is no mucositis, patients normally start each course on the same day of the week.
Note: Intervals between courses should not be increased unless white blood count $<1.5 \times 10^9$/l or platelets $<75 \times 10^9$/l or mucositis develops. If mucositis develops, delay next course until it has healed. Continue alternating courses 1 and 2 until the patient is in complete remission or there is evidence of drug resistance.
N/S = 150 mmol NaCl.

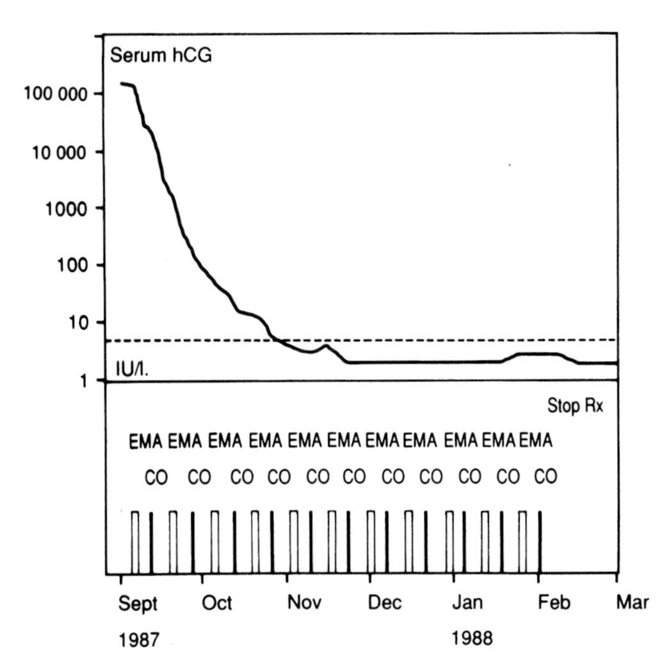

Fig. 39.4 Graph of hCG levels of a woman who required chemotherapy with EMA/CO for high-risk choriocarcinoma.

Central nervous system metastases

In countries without adequate hydatidiform mole follow-up, and in patients presenting with choriocarcinoma following an abortion or term delivery, there is an incidence of central nervous system metastases of 3–15%. Since 1980 we have used the EMA/CO regimen for these patients, with the dose of methotrexate increased to 1 g/m^2 and 12.5 mg of methotrexate is given intrathecally with each course of CO. Of 18 patients who presented with central nervous system metastases 13 (72%) are surviving disease-free (Rustin et al 1989). Because of the vascular nature of these tumours and the 22% incidence of early deaths we now attempt early surgical excision to prevent intracerebral haemorrhage. Although radiotherapy has been used in other centres their reported results do not approach the 72% survival we have obtained without radiotherapy.

LONG-TERM SIDE EFFECTS OF THERAPY

Patients are advised against pregnancy for a year after chemotherapy, to avoid confusing a further pregnancy with relapse and to reduce the risk of delayed teratogenicity. A study of 445 long-term survivors following chemotherapy showed that 86% of patients wishing to have a further pregnancy succeeded in having at least one live birth (Rustin et al 1984). The incidence of congenital abnormalities was no greater than expected.

The incidence of second tumours has also been investigated. One case of myeloid leukaemia and one case of breast cancer were found in 457 long-term survivors followed for a mean period of 7.8 years (Rustin et al 1983). The expected number for this group of women would have been 3.5 second tumours.

KEY POINTS

1. Virtually all patients with trophoblastic disease are curable.
2. Referral to specialist centres is essential.
3. The incidence is 1–2:1000 live births and is increased with increasing maternal age.
4. Hydatidiform mole usually presents with vaginal bleeding and amenorrhoea, and the uterus is often large for dates.
5. Choriocarcinoma may present in a similar way but is notorious for its protean manifestations. Symptoms related to cerebral metastases may be the first sign of disease.
6. The diagnosis of gestational trophoblastic tumours is usually made by finding elevated hCG levels. Provided pregnancy is excluded, a histological diagnosis is not required.
7. Ultrasound is useful in the diagnosis of hydatidiform mole. A chest X-ray should be performed.
8. Cerebrospinal fluid hCG levels should be measured in high-risk cases and in medium-risk cases with lung metastases.
9. hCG levels should be monitored after every molar pregnancy for at least 6 months after they have become undetectable, and again after every subsequent pregnancy.
10. Hydatidiform mole should be evacuated by suction and chemotherapy given if the hCG levels remain >20 000 IU/l more than 4 weeks after evacuation, or if the hCG increases progressively.
11. Apart from evacuation of hydatidiform mole, surgery has only a limited role.
12. When chemotherapy is required the regimen should be chosen according to the prognostic score.
13. Patients should avoid pregnancy for 1 year after chemotherapy. A large majority who wish to conceive again will be successful.

ACKNOWLEDGEMENTS

The author wishes to thank Professor K. D. Bagshawe, Dr E. S. Newlands and Dr R. H. J. Begent and his other colleagues at Charing Cross Hospital, without whom this review would not have been possible. He is also indebted to the gynaecologists who have referred patients.

REFERENCES

Bagshawe K D 1976 Risk and prognostic factors in trophoblastic neoplasia. Cancer 38: 1373–1385

Bagshawe K D, Dent J, Webb J 1986 Hydatidiform mole in England and Wales 1973–83. Lancet ii: 673–677

Bagshawe K D, Dent J, Newlands E S, Begent R H J, Rustin G J S 1989 The role of low-dose methotrexate and folinic acid in gestational trophoblastic tumours (GTT). British Journal of Obstetrics and Gynaecology 96: 795–802

Begent R H J, Bagshawe K D, Green A J, Searle F 1987 The clinical value of imaging with antibody to human chorionic gonadotrophin in the detection of residual choriocarcinoma. British Journal of Cancer 55: 657–660

Bracken M B 1987 Incidence and aetiology of hydatidiform mole: an epidemiological review. British Journal of Obstetrics and Gynaecology 94: 1123–1135

Goldstein D P, Berkowitz R S 1982 Gestational trophoblastic neoplasms. W B Saunders, Philadelphia, p 143

Goldstein D P, Berkowitz R S, Bernstein M R 1981 Management of molar pregnancy. Journal of Reproductive Medicine 26: 208–212

Lathrop J C, Lauchlan S, Nayak R, Ambler M 1988 Clinical characteristics of placental site trophoblastic tumor. Gynecologic Oncology 31: 32–42

Lawler S D, Fisher A 1987 Genetic studies in hydatidiform mole with clinical correlations. Placenta 8: 77–88

Newlands E S, Bagshawe K D, Begent R H J, Rustin G J S, Holden L, Dent J 1986 Developments in chemotherapy for medium- and high risk patients with gestational trophoblastic tumours (1979–1984). British Journal of Obstetrics and Gynaecology 93: 63–69

Rustin G J S, Rustin F, Dent J, Booth M A, Salt S, Bagshawe K D 1983 No increase in second tumours after cytotoxic chemotherapy for gestational trophoblastic tumours. New England Journal of Medicine 308: 473–477

Rustin G J S, Booth M, Dent J, Salt S, Rustin F, Bagshawe K D 1984 Pregnancy after cytotoxic chemotherapy for gestational trophoblastic tumours. British Medical Journal 288: 103–106

Rustin G J S, Newlands E S, Begent H J, Dent J, Bagshawe K D 1989 Weekly alternating chemotherapy (EMA/CO) for treatment of central nervous system metastases of choriocarcinoma. Journal of Clinical Oncology 7: 900–903

Song H, Xia Z, Wu B, Wang Y 1979 20 years' experience in chemotherapy of choriocarcinoma and malignant mole. Chinese Medical Journal 92: 677–687

Stone M, Bagshawe K D 1979 An analysis of the influences of maternal age, gestational age, contraceptive method, and the mode of primary treatment of patients with hydatidiform moles on the incidence of subsequent chemotherapy. British Journal of Obstetrics and Gynaecology 86: 782–792

World Health Organization Scientific Group 1983 Gestational trophoblastic diseases. Technical Report Series 692. WHO, Geneva

FURTHER READING

Berkowitz R S, Goldstein D P, Bernstein M R 1984 Modified triple chemotherapy in the management of high-risk metastatic gestational trophoblastic tumours. Gynecologic Oncology 19: 173–181

Buckley J D, Henderson B E, Morrow C P, Hammond C B, Kohorn E I, Austin D F 1988 Case-control study of gestational choriocarcinoma. Cancer Research 48: 1004–1010

Rustin G J S, Bagshawe K D 1984 Gestational trophoblastic tumours. Critical Review in Oncology/Haematology, CRC Press Inc. 3: 103–142

40

Benign tumours of the ovary

J. C. Girling W. P. Soutter

INTRODUCTION

Benign ovarian cysts are common, frequently asymptomatic and often resolve spontaneously. They are the fourth most prevalent gynaecological cause of hospital admission. By the age of 65 years, 4% of all women in England and Wales will have been admitted to hospital for this reason.

Ninety percent of all ovarian tumours are benign, although this varies with age. Among surgically managed cases the frequency of malignant tumours is 13% in premenopausal women and 45% in postmenopausal women. Thus the major concerns are to exclude malignancy and to avoid cyst accidents, without causing undue morbidity or impairing future fertility in younger women.

Ovarian tumours may be physiological or pathological, and may arise from any tissue in the ovary. Most benign ovarian tumours are cystic, and the finding of solid elements makes malignancy more likely. However, fibromata, thecomata, dermoids and Brenner tumours usually have solid elements.

PATHOLOGY (Table 40.1)

Physiological cysts

Physiological cysts are simply large versions of the cysts that form in the ovary during the normal ovarian cycle.

Table 40.1 Pathology of benign ovarian tumours

Physiological cysts
Follicular cysts
Luteal cysts
Benign germ cell tumours
Dermoid cyst
Mature teratoma
Benign epithelial tumours
Serous cystadenoma
Mucinous cystadenoma
Endometrioid cystadenoma
Brenner
Benign sex cord stromal tumours
Theca cell tumour
Fibroma
Sertoli–Leydig cell tumour

Most are asymptomatic, being found incidentally as a result of pelvic examination or ultrasound scanning. Although they may occur in any premenopausal woman, they are most common in young women. They are an occasional complication of ovulation induction, when they are commonly multiple. They may also occur in premature female infants and in women with trophoblastic disease.

Follicular cyst

Lined by granulosa cells, this is the commonest benign ovarian tumour and is most often found incidentally. It results from the non-rupture of a dominant follicle, or the failure of normal atresia in a non-dominant follicle. A follicular cyst can persist for several menstrual cycles and may achieve a diameter of up to 10 cm. Smaller cysts are more likely to resolve, but may require intervention if symptoms develop or if they do not resolve after 8–12 weeks. Occasionally oestrogen production may persist, causing menstrual disturbances and endometrial hyperplasia.

Luteal cyst

Less common than follicular cysts, these are more likely to present as a result of intraperitoneal bleeding, and this is more commonly on the right side, possibly as a result of increased intraluminal pressure secondary to ovarian vein anatomy. They may also rupture, characteristically on day 20–26 of the cycle. Corpora lutea are not considered to be luteal cysts unless they are greater than 3 cm in diameter.

Benign germ cell tumours

Germ cell tumours are among the commonest ovarian tumours seen in women less than 30 years of age. Overall, only 2–3% are malignant but in the under-20s this proportion may rise to a third. Malignant tumours are usually solid, although benign forms also commonly have a solid element. Thus the traditional classification into solid or cystic germ cell tumours, signifying malignant or benign, respectively, may be misleading. As the name suggests, they arise from totipotential germ cells and may therefore contain elements of all three germ layers (embryonic differentiation). Differentiation into extraembryonic tissues results in ovarian choriocarcinoma or endodermal sinus tumour. When neither embryonic nor extra-embryonic differentiation occurs, a dysgerminoma results.

Dermoid cyst (mature cystic teratoma)

The benign dermoid cyst is the only benign germ cell tumour which is common. It results from differentiation into embryonic tissues and accounts for around 40% of all ovarian neoplasms. It is most common in young women with a median age of presentation of 30 years (Comerci et al 1994). It is bilateral in about 11% of cases. However, if the contralateral ovary is macroscopically normal, the chance of a concealed second dermoid is very low (1–2%), particularly if preoperative ultrasound has failed to demonstrate typical features (see Ch. 6).

These are usually unilocular cysts less than 15 cm in diameter, in which ectodermal structures are predominant. Thus they are often lined with epithelium like the epidermis, and contain skin appendages, teeth, sebaceous material, hair and nervous tissue. Endodermal derivatives include thyroid, bronchus and intestine, and the mesoderm may be represented by bone and smooth muscle.

Occasionally only a single tissue may be present, in which case the term monodermal teratoma is used. The classic examples are carcinoid, and struma ovarii, which contains hormonally active thyroid tissue. Primary carcinoid tumours of the ovary rarely metastasize but 30% may give rise to typical carcinoid symptoms (Saunders & Hertzman 1960). Thyroid tissue is found in 5–20% of cystic teratomas. The term 'struma ovarii' should be reserved for tumours composed predominantly of thyroid tissue, and as such comprise only 1.4% of cystic teratomas. Only 5–6% of struma ovarii produce sufficient thyroid hormone to cause hyperthyroidism. Some 5–10% develop carcinoma.

The majority (60%) of dermoid cysts are asymptomatic. However, 3.5–10% may undergo torsion. Less commonly (1–4%) they may rupture spontaneously: either suddenly, causing an acute abdomen and a chemical peritonitis, or slowly, causing chronic granulomatous peritonitis. As the latter may also arise following intraoperative spillage great care should be taken to avoid this event, and thorough peritoneal lavage must be performed if it does occur. During pregnancy rupture is more common owing to external pressure from the expanding gravid uterus, or to trauma during delivery.

About 2% are said to contain a malignant component, usually a squamous carcinoma in women over 40 years old. Poor prognosis is indicated by non-squamous histology and capsular rupture. Among women aged under 20 years, up to 80% of ovarian malignancies are due to germ cell tumours (see Ch. 41).

Mature solid teratoma

These rare tumours contain mature tissues just like the dermoid cyst, but there are few cystic areas. They must be differentiated from immature teratomas, which are malignant (see Ch. 41).

Benign epithelial tumours

The majority of ovarian neoplasia, both benign and malignant, arise from the ovarian surface epithelium. They are therefore essentially mesothelial in nature, deriving from the coelomic epithelium overlying the embryonic gonadal ridge, from which develop Mullerian and Wolffian structures. Therefore, this may result in development along endocervical (mucinous cystadenomata), endometrial (endometrioid) or tubal (serous) pathways, or uroepithelial (Brenner) lines, respectively. Although benign epithelial tumours tend to occur at a slightly younger age than their malignant counterparts, they are most common in women over 40.

Serous cystadenoma

This is the most common benign epithelial tumour and is

bilateral in about 10% of cases. It is usually a unilocular cyst with papilliferous processes on the inner surface, and occasionally on the outer surface. The epithelium on the inner surface is cuboidal or columnar and may be ciliated. Psammoma bodies are concentric calcified bodies which occur occasionally in these cysts, but more frequently in their malignant counterparts. The cyst fluid is thin and serous. They are seldom as large as mucinous tumours.

Mucinous cystadenoma

These constitute 15–25% of all ovarian tumours and are the second most common epithelial tumour. They are typically large, unilateral, multilocular cysts with a smooth inner surface. A recent specimen at Hammersmith Hospital weighed over 14 kg! The lining epithelium consists of columnar mucus-secreting cells. The cyst fluid is generally thick and glutinous.

A rare complication is pseudomyxoma peritonei, which is more often present before the cyst is removed rather than following intraoperative rupture. Pseudomyxoma peritonei is most commonly associated with mucinous tumours of the ovary or appendix. Synchronous tumours of the ovary and appendix are common. These are usually well differentiated carcinomas or borderline tumours (Wertheim et al 1994). It results in seedling growths which continue to secrete mucin, causing matting together and consequent obstruction of bowel loops. The 5-year survival rate is approximately 50%, but by 10 years as few as 18% are still alive.

Endometrioid cystadenoma

Most of these tumours are malignant, as benign endometrioid cysts are difficult to differentiate from endometriosis.

Brenner

These account for only 1–2% of all ovarian tumours, and are bilateral in 10–15% of cases. They probably arise from Wolffian metaplasia of the surface epithelium. The tumour consists of islands of transitional epithelium (Walthard nests) in a dense fibrotic stroma, giving a largely solid appearance. The vast majority are benign, but borderline or malignant specimens have been reported. Almost three-quarters occur in women over the age of 40 and about half are incidental findings, being recognized only by the pathologist. Although some can be large the majority are less than 2 cm in diameter. Some secrete oestrogens, and abnormal vaginal bleeding is a common presentation.

Clear cell (mesonephroid) tumours

These arise from serosal cells showing little differentiation, and are only rarely benign. The typical histological appearance is of clear or 'hobnail' cells arranged in mixed patterns.

Benign sex cord stromal tumours

Sex cord stromal tumours represent only 4% of benign ovarian tumours. They occur at any age, from prepubertal children to elderly postmenopausal women. Many of these tumours secrete hormones and present with the results of inappropriate hormone effects.

Granulosa cell tumours

These are all **malignant** tumours but are mentioned here because they are generally confined to the ovary when they present, and so have a good prognosis. However, they do grow very slowly and recurrences are often seen 10–20 years later. They are largely solid in most cases. Call–Exner bodies are pathognomonic but are seen in less than half of granulosa cell tumours. Some produce oestrogens and most appear to secrete inhibin.

Theca cell tumours

Almost all are benign, solid and unilateral, typically presenting in the sixth decade. Many produce oestrogens in sufficient quantity to have systemic effects, such as precocious puberty, postmenopausal bleeding, endometrial hyperplasia and endometrial cancer. They rarely cause ascites or Meig's syndrome.

Fibroma

These unusual tumours are most frequent around 50 years of age. Most are derived from stromal cells and are similar to thecomas. They are hard, mobile and lobulated, with a glistening white surface. Less than 10% are bilateral. Whereas ascites occurs with many of the larger fibromas, Meig's syndrome – ascites and pleural effusion in association with a fibroma of the ovary – is seen in only 1% of cases.

Sertoli–Leydig cell tumours

These are usually of low-grade malignancy. Most are found around 30 years of age. They are rare, being less than 0.2% of ovarian tumours. They are often difficult to distinguish from other ovarian tumours because of the variety of cells and architecture seen. Many produce androgens and signs of virilization are seen in three-quarters of patients. Some secrete oestrogens. They are usually small and unilateral.

Table 40.2 Histological distribution of benign ovarian neoplasms treated surgically by age (as %) and percentage of all neoplasms which are benign (n = 650) (Modified from Koonings et al 1989)

Histology	Age in years							All ages	
	⩽19	20–29	30–39	40–49	50–59	60–69	⩾70	% of all benign tumours in each group	% of each histology group which is benign
Epithelial	30	27	30	51	63	73	88	38	57
Germ cell	70	72	66	46	21	16	0	58	97
Sex cord	0	1	4	3	17	11	12	4	66
% benign	92	94	81	59	50	47	71	100	75

AGE DISTRIBUTION OF OVARIAN TUMOURS

In younger women the most common benign ovarian neoplasm is the germ cell tumour, and among older women the epithelial cell tumour. The percentage of ovarian neoplasms which are benign also changes with the age of the woman (Table 40.2).

PRESENTATION

Benign ovarian tumours can be asymptomatic or present with pain, abdominal swelling, pressure effects, menstrual disturbances, hormonal effects or an abnormal cervical smear.

Asymptomatic

Many benign ovarian tumours are found incidentally in the course of investigating another unrelated problem, or during a routine examination while performing a cervical smear or at an antenatal clinic. As pelvic ultrasound, and particularly transvaginal scanning, is now used more frequently, physiological cysts are detected more often. Where ultrasound was used in trials of screening for ovarian cancer, the majority of tumours detected were benign. Many simple cysts will resolve spontaneously if observed over a period of 2–3 months. Use of gonadotrophin suppression by an oral contraceptive pill will further encourage the resolution of physiological cysts. Unfortunately, it is not possible with ultrasound to differentiate reliably between benign and malignant ovarian disease, especially when the tumour is small (Campbell et al 1989). Colour-flow Doppler imaging may help in this regard (Bourne et al 1993).

Pain

Acute pain from an ovarian tumour may result from torsion, rupture, haemorrhage or infection. Torsion usually gives rise to a sharp, constant pain caused by ischaemia of the cyst. Areas may become infarcted. Haemorrhage may occur into the cyst and cause pain as the capsule is stretched. If the cyst is large the bleeding may be sufficient to give rise to a haemolytic jaundice, so leading the unwary to wrongly diagnose malignancy. Intraperitoneal bleeding mimicking ectopic pregnancy may result from rupture of the tumour. This happens most frequently with a luteal cyst. Chronic lower abdominal pain sometimes results from the pressure of a benign ovarian tumour, but is more common if endometriosis or infection is present.

Abdominal swelling

Patients seldom note abdominal swelling until the tumour is very large. A benign mucinous cyst may occasionally fill the entire abdominal cavity. The bloating of which women so often complain is rarely due to an ovarian tumour.

Miscellaneous

Gastrointestinal or urinary symptoms may result from pressure effects. In extreme cases oedema of the legs, varicose veins and haemorrhoids may result. Sometimes uterine prolapse is the presenting complaint in a woman with an ovarian cyst.

Occasionally the patient will complain of menstrual disturbances, but this may be coincidence rather than due to the tumour. Rarely, sex cord stromal tumours present with oestrogen effects such as precocious puberty, menorrhagia and glandular hyperplasia, breast enlargement and postmenopausal bleeding. Secretion of androgens may cause hirsutism and acne initially, progressing to frank virilism with deepening of the voice or clitoral hypertrophy. Very rarely indeed thyrotoxicosis may occur.

Infrequently, a patient with an abnormal cervical smear will be found to have an ovarian tumour and removal is followed by resolution of the cytological abnormality. Surprisingly, these tumours are often benign.

DIFFERENTIAL DIAGNOSIS

The differential diagnosis of benign ovarian tumours is broad, reflecting the wide range of presenting symptoms:

Pain
Ectopic pregnancy
Spontaneous abortion
Pelvic inflammatory disease
Appendicitis
Meckel's diverticulum
Diverticulitis

Abdominal swelling
Pregnant uterus
Fibroid uterus
Full bladder
Distended bowel
Ovarian malignancy
Colorectal carcinoma

Pressure effects
Urinary tract infection
Constipation

Hormonal effects
All other causes of menstrual irregularities, precocious puberty and postmenopausal bleeding.

A full bladder should be considered in the differential diagnosis of any pelvic mass. In premenopausal women a gravid uterus must always be considered. Fibroids can be impossible to distinguish from ovarian tumours. Rarely, a fimbrial cyst may grow sufficiently to cause anxiety.

Ectopic pregnancy may present as a pelvic mass and lower abdominal pain, especially if there has been chronic intraperitoneal bleeding. Often a ruptured, bleeding corpus luteum will be mistaken for an ectopic gestation. It may be difficult to differentiate between appendicitis and an ovarian cyst. Cooperation between gynaecologist and surgeon is essential to avoid unnecessary surgery on simple ovarian cysts in young women, and the effects this may have upon subsequent fertility. Pelvic inflammatory disease may give rise to a mass of adherent bowel, a hydrosalpinx or pyosalpinx.

If the tumour is ovarian, malignancy must be excluded. In the vast majority of cases this can only be done by a laparotomy. Even then, careful histological examination may be necessary to exclude invasion. Frozen section will only rarely be of value. A pelvic mass may also be caused by a rectal tumour or diverticulitis. Hodgkin's disease may present as a pelvic mass with enlarged pelvic lymph nodes.

INVESTIGATION

The investigations required will depend upon the circumstances of the presentation. The patient presenting with acute symptoms will usually require emergency surgery, whereas the asymptomatic patient or the woman with chronic problems may benefit from more detailed preliminary assessment.

Gynaecological history

Details of the presenting symptoms and a full gynaecological history should be obtained, with particular reference to the date of the last menstrual period, the regularity of the menstrual cycle, any previous pregnancies, contraception, medication and family history (particularly of ovarian cancer).

General history and examination

Indigestion or dysphagia might indicate a primary gastric cancer metastasizing to the pelvis. Similarly, a history of altered bowel habit or rectal bleeding should be sought as evidence of diverticulitis or rectal carcinoma. However, ovarian carcinoma may also present with these features.

If the patient has presented as an acute emergency, evidence of hypovolaemia should be sought. Hypotension is a relatively late sign of blood loss, as the blood pressure will be maintained for some time by peripheral and central venous vasoconstriction. When decompensation of this mechanism occurs it often does so very rapidly. It is vital to recognize the early signs: tachycardia and cold peripheries.

The breasts should be palpated and evidence of lymphadenopathy sought in the neck, the axillae and the groins. The chest should be examined for signs of a pleural effusion. Some patients may have ankle oedema. Very occasionally foot drop may be noted as a result of compression of pelvic nerve roots. This would not occur with a benign tumour but suggests a malignancy with lymphatic involvement.

Abdominal examination

The abdomen should be inspected for signs of distension by fluid or by the tumour itself. Dilated veins may be seen on the lower abdomen. Gentle palpation will reveal areas of tenderness, and peritonism may be elicited by asking the patient to cough or alternately suck in and blow out her abdominal wall. Male hair distribution may suggest a rare androgen-producing tumour.

The best way of detecting a mass that arises from the pelvis is to palpate gently with the radial border of the left hand, starting in the upper abdomen and working caudally. This is the reverse of the process taught to every medical student for feeling the liver edge. Use of the right hand alone is the commonest reason for failing to detect pelviabdominal masses.

Shifting dullness is probably the easiest way of demonstrating ascites but it remains a very insensitive technique.

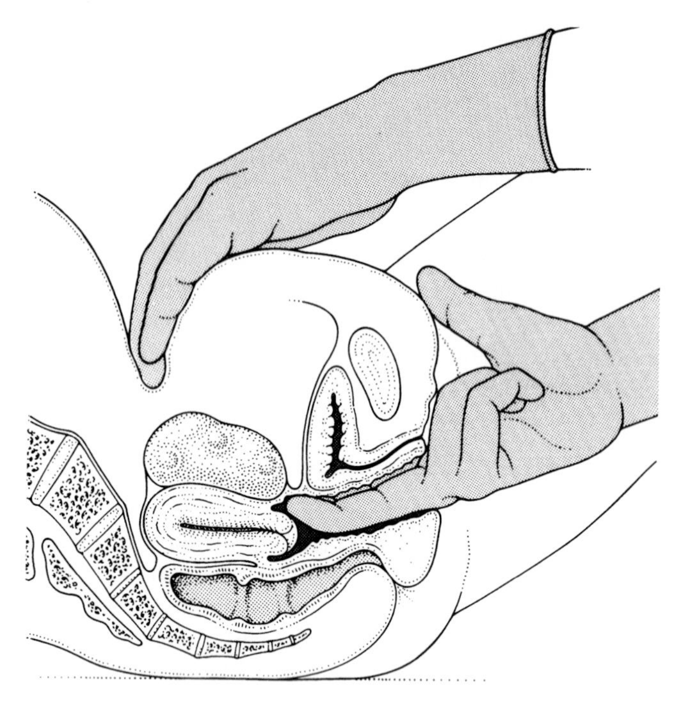

Fig. 40.1 Bimanual examination involves palpating the pelvic organs between both hands.

It is always worth listening for bowel sounds in any patient with an acute abdomen. Their complete absence in the presence of peritonism is an ominous sign.

Bimanual examination

This is an essential component of the assessment because, even in expert hands, ultrasound examination is not infallible. By palpating the mass between both the vaginal and abdominal hands, its mobility, texture and consistency, the presence of nodules in the pouch of Douglas and the degree of tenderness can all be determined (Fig. 40.1). Although it is impossible to make a firm diagnosis with bimanual examination, a hard irregular fixed mass is likely to be invasive.

Ultrasound

The techniques of transabdominal and transvaginal ultrasound are discussed in detail in Chapter 6. It can demonstrate the presence of an ovarian mass with reasonable sensitivity and fair specificity and, although it cannot distinguish reliably between benign and malignant tumours, solid ovarian masses are more likely to be malignant than their cystic counterparts. The use of colour-flow Doppler may increase the reliability of ultrasound in this area (Bourne et al 1993). Neither CT scanning nor MRI has significant advantages over ultrasound in this situation, and both are more expensive.

Ultrasound-guided diagnostic ovarian cyst aspiration

This investigation has been introduced gradually into gynaecological practice from the subspecialty of assisted reproduction, where ultrasound-guided egg collection is now commonplace. This has happened without the benefit of appropriate trials to indicate its potential efficacy.

Unfortunately, this technique has up to a 71% false negative rate and a 2% false positive rate for the cytological diagnosis of malignancy (Diernaes et al 1987). The degree of risk of dissemination of malignant cells along the needle track or into the peritoneal cavity is not established.

The second potential role of a diagnostic cyst aspiration is to distinguish between functional and benign cysts, and in the latter case to determine the type. This is not reliably achieved, even when apparently simple cysts are selected. The inability to inspect the ovarian capsular surface and the peritoneal cavity, and the lack of knowledge concerning the long-term behaviour of cysts following aspiration, are also important limitations. Overall, ultrasound-guided aspiration of ovarian cysts cannot be recommended as a first-line diagnostic tool.

Radiological investigations

A chest X-ray is essential to detect metastatic disease in the lungs or a pleural effusion which may be too small to detect on auscultation. Occasionally an abdominal X-ray may show calcification, suggesting the possibility of a benign teratoma. An intravenous urogram is often performed, but is seldom useful. A barium enema is indicated only if the mass is irregular or fixed, or if there are bowel symptoms. A CT scan is seldom indicated.

Blood test and serum markers

It is always sensible to measure the haemoglobin, and an elevated white cell count would suggest infection. Platelet count and clotting screen may be useful in the rare case of a large intra-abdominal bleed. Blood may be cross-matched if necessary.

Serum markers have yet to establish a role in the routine management of most ovarian tumours (see Ch. 41). However, a raised serum CA125 is strongly suggestive of ovarian carcinoma, especially in postmenopausal women. Women with extensive endometriosis may also have elevated levels, but the concentration is usually not as high as is seen with malignant disease. The β-human chorionic gonadotrophin concentration might be measured to exclude an ectopic pregnancy, but trophoblastic tumours and some germ cell tumours secrete this marker. Oestradiol levels may be elevated in some physiological follicular cysts and sex cord stromal tumours. Androgen concentrations may be increased in Sertoli–Leydig tumours. Raised α-fetoprotein levels suggest a yolk sac tumour.

MANAGEMENT

The management will depend upon the severity of the symptoms, the age of the patient and therefore the risk of malignancy, and her desire for further children.

The asymptomatic patient (Fig. 40.2)

The older woman

Women over 50 are far more likely to have a malignancy (Fig. 40.3 and Table 40.2) and have less to gain from the conservative management of a pelvic mass more than 5 cm in diameter (Rulin & Preston 1987). Physiological cysts are, by definition, unlikely. However, the capacity of the postmenopausal ovary to generate benign cysts is greater than previously thought, occurring in up to 17% of asymptomatic women (Levine et al 1992). Over 50% of small, simple cysts will resolve spontaneously and almost 30% will remain static (Levine et al 1992). Even in this age group, only 29–50% of all ovarian cysts will be malignant (Table 40.2). Therefore, efforts have been made to safely avoid unnecessary surgery in this older age group. Evaluation of the cyst with tumour markers, ultrasound and colour-flow Doppler studies and careful follow-up suggests that simple unilateral cysts less than 3 cm (or maybe even 5 cm) with CA125 less than 35 U/ml and normal vascular resistance patterns are likely to be benign and may safely be managed conservatively (Goldstein 1993).

The role of laparoscopic surgery in the assessment and treatment of apparently benign cysts in this age group is controversial (Parker 1995, Fowler & Carter 1995). Whereas the small cysts described above may be managed without surgery, there may be a small role for the laparoscopic assessment and treatment of larger (perhaps up to 10 cm) but otherwise apparently benign cysts. None the less, this should only be in the hands of those who are both laparoscopically experienced and prepared to perform definitive surgery for an unexpected ovarian carcinoma under the same anaesthetic. Complete and intact removal of the cyst should be achieved. For the more general gynaecologist the open approach is still recommended.

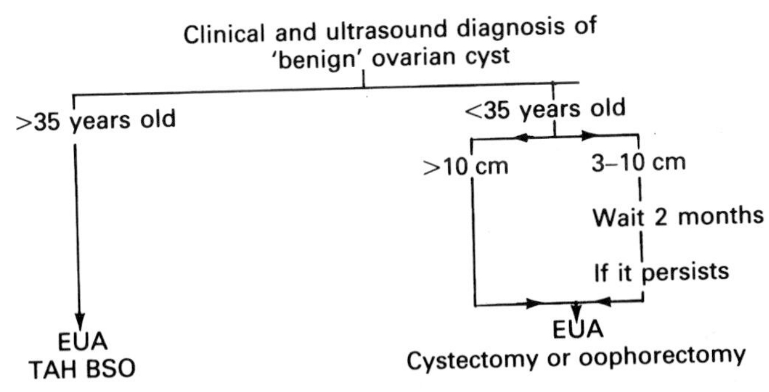

Fig. 40.2 Management of what appears on clinical and ultrasound grounds to be a benign ovarian cyst in an asymptomatic patient. EUA, examination under anaesthesia; TAH BSO, total abdominal hysterectomy and bilateral salpingo-oophorectomy.

Premenopausal women

Women under 35 are both more likely to wish to have the option of further children and less likely to have a malignant epithelial tumour. However, ovarian cysts more than 10 cm in diameter are unlikely to be physiological or to resolve spontaneously. A normal follicular cyst up to 3 cm in diameter requires no further investigation. A clear unilocular cyst of 4–10 cm identified by ultrasound should be re-examined 8 weeks later for evidence of diminution in size. The use of a combined oral contraceptive is unlikely to accelerate the resolution of a functional cyst (Steinkampf & Hammond 1990), and hormonal treat-

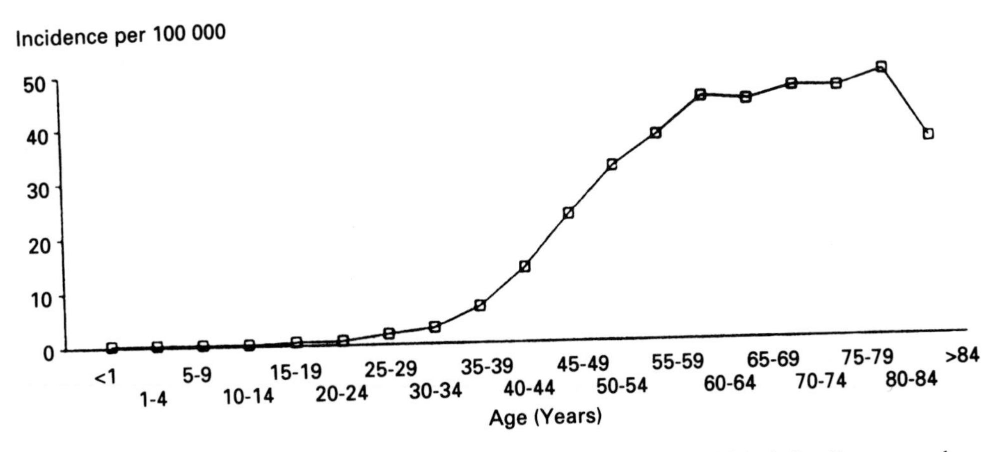

Fig. 40.3 The incidence of ovarian cancer in England and Wales (Office of Population Censuses and Surveys 1985). Note how uncommon ovarian cancer is before the age of 35.

ment of endometriosis does not usually benefit an endometrioma. If the cyst does not get smaller, laparoscopy or laparotomy will be indicated.

The criteria for observation of an asymptomatic ovarian tumour are: a premenopausal woman; age less than 35; a unilateral tumour; unilocular cyst without solid elements; tumour 3–10 cm in diameter; and no free fluid or masses suggesting omental cake or matted bowel loops.

The patient with symptoms

If the patient presents with severe acute pain or signs of intraperitoneal bleeding an emergency laparoscopy or laparotomy will be required. More chronic symptoms of pain or pressure may justify pelvic ultrasound if no mass can be felt, but ultrasound is unlikely to contribute to the investigation of a woman in whom both ovaries can be clearly felt to be of a normal size.

The pregnant patient

An ovarian cyst in a pregnant woman may undergo torsion or bleed. There is said to be an increased incidence of these complications in pregnancy, although the evidence for this is poor. Very occasionally it can prevent the presenting fetal part from engaging. A dermoid cyst may rupture or leak slowly, causing peritonitis. However, an ovarian cyst is usually discovered incidentally at the antenatal clinic or on ultrasound, and occasionally at caesarean section.

The pregnant woman with an ovarian cyst is a special case because of the dangers of surgery to the fetus. These have probably been exaggerated in the past and no urgent operation should be postponed solely because of a pregnancy. Thus, if the patient presents with acute pain due to torsion or haemorrhage into an ovarian tumour, or if appendicitis is a possibility, the correct course is to undertake a laparotomy regardless of the stage of the pregnancy. The likelihood of labour ensuing is small. However, the operation should be covered by tocolytic drugs and performed in a centre with intensive neonatal care facilities when possible.

If an asymptomatic cyst is discovered it is prudent to wait until after 14 weeks' gestation before removing it. This avoids the risk of removing a corpus luteal cyst upon which the pregnancy might still be dependent. In the second and third trimesters the management of an asymptomatic ovarian cyst may be either conservative or surgical. The risks to the mother and fetus of an elective procedure need to be balanced against the chances of a cyst accident, an unexpected malignancy and spontaneous resolution. Cysts less than 10 cm in diameter which have a simple appearance on ultrasound are unlikely to be malignant or to result in a cyst accident, and may therefore be followed ultrasonographically: many will resolve spontaneously (Thornton & Wells 1987). If the cyst is unresolved 6 weeks postpartum, surgery may be undertaken then. The role for cyst aspiration in pregnancy, either diagnostically or therapeutically, is small.

Ovarian cancer is uncommon in pregnancy, occurring in less than 3% of cysts. However, a cyst with features suggestive of malignancy on ultrasound, or one that is growing, should be removed surgically. The tumour marker CA125 is not useful in the pregnant woman, since elevated levels occur frequently as an apparently physiological change. Management may need to include a caesarean hysterectomy, bilateral salpingo-oophorectomy and omentectomy.

The female fetus

Fetal ovarian androgen synthesis commences at 12 weeks' and oestradiol and progesterone at 20 weeks' gestation. Thus small follicular cysts up to 7 mm in diameter may occur in up to a third of newborn girls. However, larger cysts are rare and are usually isolated findings. Most are follicular, although luteal cysts, cystic teratomata and granulosa cell tumours also occur. They may undergo torsion or haemorrhage, and occasionally necrosis of the pedicle may result in the 'disappearance' of the ovary. Rarely, small bowel compression may cause polyhydramnios, but diaphragmatic splinting and consequent pulmonary hypoplasia does not seem to occur. Most resolve spontaneously, either antenatally or, more commonly, postnatally. Consideration may need to be given to the antenatal aspiration of a very large cyst if it is felt that it may obstruct labour or be ruptured during vaginal delivery, although this is reported rarely. Therefore, delivery by caesarean section is not indicated. Cysts which have not resolved by 6 months of age should be explored surgically.

The prepubertal girl

Ovarian cysts are uncommon and often benign. Teratomata and follicular cysts are the most common. Theca and granulosa cell tumours may secrete hormones. Presentation may be with abdominal pain or distension, or precocious puberty, either isosexual or heterosexual. Management depends upon relief of symptoms, exclusion of malignancy and conservation of maximum ovarian tissue without jeopardizing fertility.

TREATMENT

Treatment is mostly surgical, although there may be a few women in whom cyst aspiration is indicated.

Therapeutic ultrasound-guided cyst aspiration

The theoretical advantages of this technique are that

surgery is avoided and cyst accidents are reduced. However, it assumes that the cyst fluid is unable to re-accumulate, and that both physiological (likely to resolve spontaneously) and malignant cysts can be reliably excluded beforehand. Cytological assessment of the aspirated fluid is routinely performed but cannot be relied upon to confirm a benign diagnosis (see above).

The role of this technique therefore remains controversial. The best candidate is a young woman with a unilateral, unilocular, anechoic, thin-walled cyst less than 10 cm in diameter. The recurrence rate is 27% if the fluid is clear and 68% if it is bloodstained (De Crespigny et al 1989). A tumour in a young woman that appears to be largely solid on ultrasound is likely to be a germ cell tumour, and requires removal. An acutely painful ovary may be due to torsion, and surgery is essential.

There may be a small place for cyst aspiration in women in whom surgery is considered to be high risk, either because of coexisting medical problems or because dense pelvic adhesions envelop the ovaries.

Examination under anaesthesia

Prior to any laparoscopy or laparotomy for a suspected ovarian tumour, it is prudent to perform a bimanual examination under anaesthesia to confirm the presence of the mass.

Laparoscopic procedures

The indications for laparoscopy are uncertainty about the nature of the mass, or a tumour suitable for laparoscopic surgery, i.e.:

age less than 35 years;
ultrasound shows no solid component;
simple ovarian cyst;
benign cystic teratoma;
endometrioma.

Laparoscopy may be of value if there is uncertainty about the nature of the pelvic mass. Thus it may be possible to avoid a laparotomy when there is no pathology. However, it can be difficult to exclude ovarian disease in the presence of marked pelvic inflammatory disease.

The second indication for laparoscopy is if the patient has a cyst suitable for laparoscopic surgery (Nezhat et al 1989). This decision should be made after a full history and careful bimanual examination, ultrasound assessment and a thorough laparoscopic appraisal of the whole abdominal cavity, particularly the contralateral ovary. The patient should be aware of the possibility of and give consent for a laparotomy, in case malignancy is found or unexpected laparoscopic complications are encountered.

The advantages are those of laparoscopic surgery in general: less postoperative pain, shorter hospital stay and quicker return to normal activities. It may also result in less adhesion formation than an open procedure, although the evidence is not convincing. It is probable that approximation of the ovarian capsule edges after cystectomy is important in this respect, although some experts believe that non-closure does not result in adhesion formation or reduced fertility. However, the consequences of spillage of cyst contents, incomplete excision of the cyst wall and an unexpected histological diagnosis of malignancy are considerable disadvantages. Up to 83% of malignant ovarian tumours found by chance at a laparoscopic operation for a 'cyst' are treated inadequately (Maiman et al 1991).

Laparoscopic surgery is best reserved for women under 35 in whom the likelihood of malignant disease is small and in whom conservation of ovarian tissue is more important. These operations require considerable expertise in laparoscopic manipulation and should not be attempted without appropriate training.

The following laparoscopic procedures have been used in the management of ovarian cysts:

aspiration and fenestration;
cystectomy – intraperitoneal, with or without cyst puncture;
cystectomy – extra-abdominal;
oophorectomy or salpingo-oophorectomy.

Aspiration and fenestration (removal of a window of the cyst wall, for histological analysis) has several disadvantages and cannot be recommended. Recurrence, spillage of cyst contents and failure to diagnose a malignant tumour are all possible, even if the inner surface of the cyst is carefully inspected (ovarian cystoscopy), the fluid sent for cytological assessment and careful peritoneal lavage performed. Frozen section is also unreliable and cannot be recommended routinely. It has been suggested that aspiration is reserved for physiological cysts, but in general their benign course means that they should not be subjected to surgery unless they fail to resolve spontaneously. Aspiration may be combined with cystectomy.

Cystectomy may be performed using two or three 5 mm puncture trocars, one inserted suprapubically in the midline and the others lateral to the inferior epigastric vessels. The ovarian capsule is incised with either scissors, diathermy or CO_2 laser, and either blunt or hydrodissection used to separate the cyst. The CO_2 laser may be particularly useful to vaporize the inner wall of endometriomas. The cyst is then removed, either through a large portal or in a laparoscopic bag without dissemination of the contents.

Alternatively, following laparoscopic assessment of the cyst a minimal suprapubic transverse skin incision allows the ovary to be grasped under laparoscopic view and pulled on to the skin. The parietal peritoneum under the skin incision is only incised once the ovary has been grasped. This extra-abdominal approach is particularly appropriate for the management of larger cysts, and seems to combine the best aspects of laparoscopic and 'traditional' surgery.

Prior to oophorectomy, the course of the ureter must be established. The broad ligament and round ligament are coagulated and cut. Endoloops, extracorporeal knots or the Endo-GIA stapler may be used to ligate the infundibulo-pelvic ligament and ovarian vessels.

Laparotomy

A clinical diagnosis may not be possible without a laparotomy, and even then histological examination is essential for a confident conclusion. Frozen section is seldom of value in this situation as thorough examination of a tumour is required to exclude invasive disease.

If there is any possibility of invasive disease a longitudinal skin incision should be used, to allow adequate exposure in the upper abdomen. If wider exposure is required after making a transverse incision, the ends of the wound can be extended cranially to fashion a flap from the upper edge of the wound (Fig. 40.4). A sample of ascitic fluid or peritoneal washings should be sent for cytological examination at the beginning of the operation. It is essential to explore the whole abdomen thoroughly and to inspect *both* ovaries.

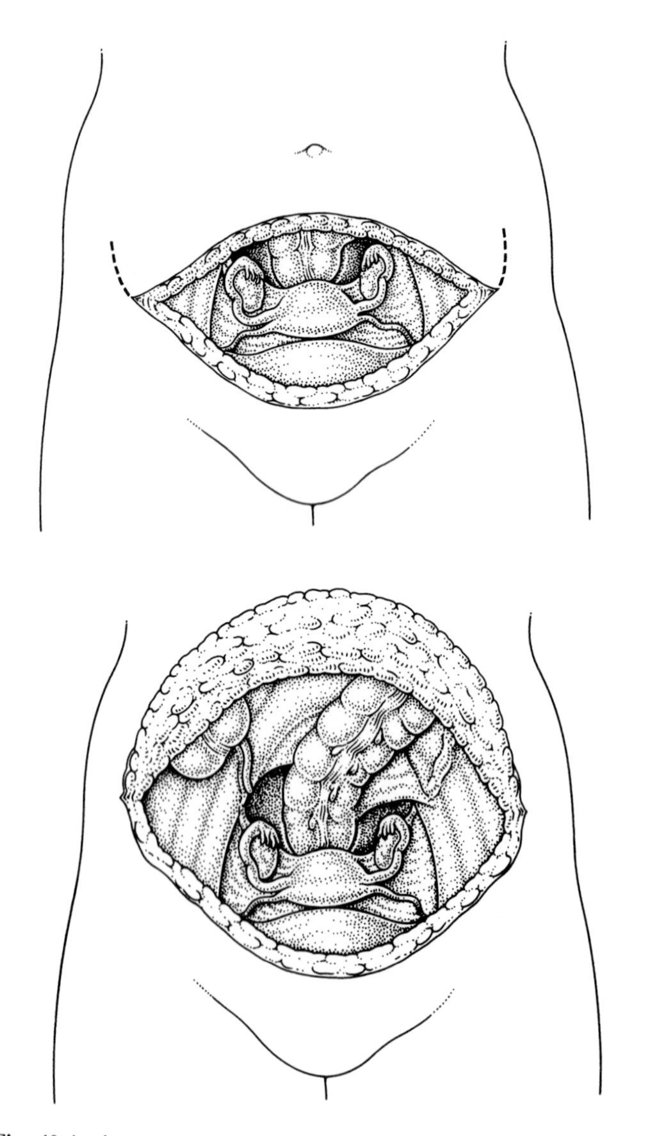

Fig. 40.4 A transverse wound may be enlarged by extending the ends cranially to create a flap from the upper edge.

Table 40.3 Distribution of malignant ovarian tumours treated surgically, by cell type at different ages, as percentages (n = 180) (Modified from Koonings et al 1989)

	Age in years							
Histology	≤19	20–29	30–39	40–49	50–59	60–69	≥70	All ages
Epithelial	0	33	69	94	96	100	100	86
Germ cell	80	33	8	2	2	0	0	7
Sex cord	20	33	21	4	2	0	0	7

In a woman less than 35 years of age an ovarian tumour is very unlikely to be malignant. Even if the mass is a primary ovarian malignancy, it is likely to be a germ cell tumour which is responsive to chemotherapy (Tables 40.2 and 40.3). Thus, ovarian cystectomy or unilateral oophorectomy are sensible and safe treatments for unilateral ovarian masses in this age group (Bianchi et al 1989). It is often said that the contralateral ovary should be bisected and a sample sent for histology in case the tumour is malignant. In practice, most gynaecologists would be unwilling to biopsy an apparently healthy ovary lest this result in infertility from periovarian adhesions. This would be especially true if the tumour was thin-walled and cystic, but even apparently solid tumours may be benign. Bilateral dysgerminomas are not common, even allowing for microscopic disease in an apparently normal ovary. Even when the lesion is bilateral, every effort should be made to conserve ovarian tissue. This policy is made possible by the effectiveness of modern chemotherapy for germ cell tumours and is discussed further in Chapter 41.

Since epithelial cancer is so much more likely in a woman over the age of 44 with a unilateral ovarian mass, she is probably best advised to have a total abdominal hysterectomy, bilateral salpingo-oophorectomy and infracolic omentectomy. However, there is evidence to suggest that unilateral oophorectomy in selected cases of epithelial carcinoma confined to one ovary may give results as good as the traditional radical approach (Mangioni et al 1989). It would seem reasonable to individualize the treatment of women 35–44 years of age, where there are greater benefits to the patient from a conservative approach and where the risks may well be less. If conservative surgery is planned, preliminary hysteroscopy and curettage of the uterus are essential to exclude a concomitant endometrial tumour, a thorough laparotomy is especially important and an appropriate plan of action must be decided in advance with the patient should more widespread disease be found.

KEY POINTS

1. Asymptomatic, benign ovarian cysts in young women often resolve spontaneously.
2. Ultrasound cannot reliably exclude malignancy.
3. Ovarian cysts are very rarely malignant before the age of 35, especially when less than 10 cm in diameter.
4. Solid ovarian tumours are often malignant – in young women these are usually germ cell or sex cord stromal tumours.
5. There is only a limited place for aspiration of cysts.
6. Conservative management is appropriate for most young women:
   observation of cystic lesions <10 cm;
   laparoscopic treatment should be considered;
   unilateral oophorectomy, even for solid lesions.
7. Women over 45 with a unilocular ovarian cyst greater than 5 cm or with any other type of ovarian tumour should usually be advised to have a total abdominal hysterectomy and bilateral salpingo-oophorectomy.
8. A bimanual examination under anaesthesia should be performed prior to any surgery for ovarian tumours to confirm that a mass is still palpable.

REFERENCES

Bianchi U A, Favalli G, Sartori E et al 1989 Limited surgery in non-epithelial ovarian cancer. In: Conte P F, Ragni N, Rosso R, Vermorken J B (eds) Multimodal treatment of ovarian cancer. Raven Press, New York, pp 119–126

Bourne T H, Campbell S, Reynolds K M 1993 Screening for early familial ovarian cancer with transvaginal ultrasonography and colour flow imaging. British Medical Journal 306: 1025–1029

Campbell S, Bhan V, Royston P, Whitehead M I, Collins W P 1989 Transabdominal ultrasound screening for early ovarian cancer. British Medical Journal 299: 1363–1367

Comerci J T, Licciardi F, Bergh P A, Gregori C, Breen J L 1994 Mature cystic teratoma: a clinicopathological evaluation of 517 cases and review of the literature. Obstetrics and Gynecology 84: 22–28

De Crespigny L C, Robinson H P, Davoren R A, Fortune D 1989 The 'simple' ovarian cyst: aspirate or operate? British Journal of Obstetrics and Gynaecology 96: 1035–1039

Diernaes E, Rasmussen J, Soersen T, Hasche E 1987 Ovarian cysts: management by puncture? Lancet i: 1084

Fowler J M, Carter J R 1995 Laparoscopic management of the adnexal mass in postmenopausal women. Journal of Gynecologic Techniques 1: 7–10

Goldstein S R 1993 Conservative management of small postmenopausal cystic masses. Clinical Obstetrics and Gynecology 36 (2): 395–401

Koonings P P, Campbell K, Mishell D R, Grimes D A 1989 Relative frequency of primary ovarian neoplasms: a 10 year review. Obstetrics and Gynecology 74: 921–926

Levine D, Gosink B, Wolf S I, Feldesman M R, Pretorius D H 1992 Simple adnexal cysts: the natural history in postmenopausal women. Radiology 184: 653–659

Maiman M, Seltzer V, Boyce J 1991 Laparoscopic excision of ovarian neoplasms subsequently found to be malignant. Obstetrics and Gynecology 77: 563–565

Mangioni C, Chiari S, Colombo N et al 1989 Limited surgery in epithelial ovarian cancer. In: Conte P F, Ragni N, Rosso R, Vermorken J B (eds) Multimodal treatment of ovarian cancer. Raven Press, New York, pp 127–132

Nezhat C, Winer W K, Nezhat F 1989 Laparoscopic removal of dermoid cysts. Obstetrics and Gynecology 73: 278–281

Office of Population Censuses and Surveys 1985 Cancer statistics registration 1981. HMSO, London

Parker W H 1995 Laparoscopic management of the adnexal mass in postmenopausal women. J Gynecol Tech 1: 3–6

Rulin M C, Preston A L 1987 Adnexal masses in postmenopausal women. Obstetrics and Gynecology 70: 579–581

Saunders A M, Hertzman V O 1960 Malignant carcinoid teratoma of the ovary. Canadian Medical Association Journal 83: 602–605

Steinkampf M P, Hammond K R 1990. Hormonal treatment of functional ovarian cysts: a randomised, prospective study. Fertility and Sterility 54: 775–777

Thornton J G, Wells M 1987 Ovarian cysts in pregnancy: does ultrasound make traditional management inappropriate? Obstetrics and Gynecology 69: 717–720

Wertheim I, Fleischhacker D, McLachlin C M, Rice L W, Berkowitz R S, Goff B A 1994 Pseudomyxoma peritonei: a review of 23 cases. Obstetrics and Gynecology 84: 17–21

41

Carcinoma of the ovary and fallopian tube

M. C. Anderson   H. E. Lambert   G. J. S. Rustin   W. P. Soutter

CARCINOMA OF THE OVARY

EPIDEMIOLOGY

Carcinoma of the ovary is commoner in developed areas, such as Europe and the United States of America, than in underdeveloped areas. In the United Kingdom there were approximately 5800 cases in 1989. The lifetime risk of developing ovarian cancer (1.4%) is higher than that for either cancer of the cervix (1.25%) or the endometrium (1.1%) but lower than that for cancer of the breast (7.1%). Deaths from ovarian cancer outnumber those from carcinoma of the cervix and body of the uterus combined.

Most ovarian tumours are of epithelial origin. These are rare before the age of 35 years, but the incidence increases with age to a peak in the 50–70-year-old age group. Just under half occur in women aged 45–65 years (Fig. 41.1).

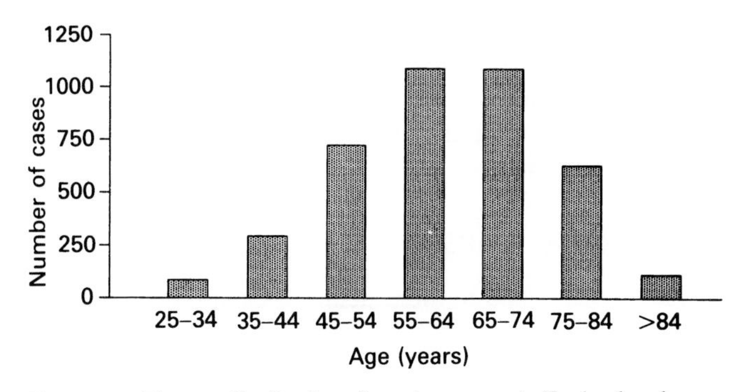

Fig. 41.1 The age distribution of ovarian cancer in England and Wales in 1981 (Office of Population Censuses and Surveys 1988).

Most epithelial tumours are advanced at diagnosis, so less than 25% of women with ovarian cancer are alive at 5 years. Eventually 80–85% of women with ovarian cancer will die from their disease. Only 3% of ovarian cancers are seen in women younger than 35 years and the vast majority of these are non-epithelial cancers such as germ cell tumours.

AETIOLOGY

'Incessant ovulation' theory

The factors which lead to the development of ovarian carcinoma are not known. Epithelial tumours are most frequently associated with nulliparity, an early menarche, a late age at menopause and a long estimated number of years of ovulation (Hildreth et al 1981). The infrequent occurrence of carcinoma of the ovary in women of high parity is thought to be due to the suppression of continuous ovulation, and there is now good evidence that oral contraceptives play a protective role (Vessey et al 1987). However, a very large case-control study which confirmed the protective effect of parity also showed that the risk fell with increasing age at first birth in a population in which use of oral contraceptives was very limited (Adami et al 1994). This and other anomalies cast doubt upon the 'incessant ovulation' theory.

Infertility treatment

There is an association between infertility and both ovarian and endometrial cancer. This link appears to be strongest in women with unexplained infertility (Venn et al 1995). However, a pooled analysis of several case-control studies showed a small increased risk for ovarian cancer in infertile women treated with 'fertility drugs' (odds ratio 2.8, 95% CI 1.3–6.1) (Whittemore et al 1992) and 12 cases of granulosa cell tumours were reported after ovarian stimulation (Willemsen et al 1993). A later paper showed that use of clomiphene for more than a year was associated with an increased risk of borderline or invasive ovarian tumours (relative risk 11.1, 95% CI 1.5–82.3) (Rossing et al 1994). Subsequently, a large study of women who underwent IVF (in-vitro fertilization) showed no increased risk in up to 15 years after ovarian stimulation (Venn et al 1995). However, these women would not have been treated more than five or six times at most. Overall, these various studies do suggest the possibility of a link between ovulation induction, but only after prolonged treatment.

GENETIC FACTORS

These are described in more detail in Chapter 32.

Familial cancer

Inheritance plays a significant role in about 5% of epithelial ovarian cancers. These tumours are usually serous adenocarcinomas.The lifetime risk for a woman with one affected close relative is 2.5%, twice the risk in the general population. If there are two affected close relatives, the lifetime risk increases to 30–40% (Ponder et al 1992). A particular feature of familial cancers is the relatively early age at which they occur. It is unusual to find families with multiple cases of only ovarian cancer. More commonly, there are cases of breast or colorectal cancer in the family. The Lynch syndrome consists of families with colorectal cancer, endometrial cancer and ovarian cancer (Watson & Lynch 1992).

One of the two genes responsible for about two-thirds of familial breast cancer has been identified (Miki et al 1994). This gene, *BRCA1*, located on chromosome 17q, is probably associated with one-third of families with multiple breast cancer and 80% of families with both breast and ovarian cancer (Ponder 1994). A woman who has inherited the *BRCA1* gene in a well documented family has a 60% risk of breast cancer by 50 years of age, and a 90% lifetime risk. However, the risk of ovarian cancer is much more variable, being equally high in some families but much lower in others. This suggests allelic heterogeneity, or two closely linked genes.

The coding sequence mutations and allelic loss seen in affected kindreds suggest that *BRCA1* is a tumour-suppressor gene. Because loss of heterozygosity in 17q had been noted in 60% of sporadic ovarian carcinomas, it was thought that spontaneous somatic mutations in *BRCA1* might be involved in the development of non-familial cancers (Eng et al 1994). Unexpectedly, no purely somatic *BRCA1* mutations were found in 32 breast and 12 ovarian cancers (Futreal et al 1994). Four of these women had germ cell mutations. However, five somatic mutations were subsequently found in 64 cancers, suggesting that *BRCA1* mutations do occur in sporadic disease but are relatively uncommon (Hosking et al 1995, Merajver et al 1995).

Management of women with a family history of ovarian cancer

Genetic testing for *BRCA1* will become a possibility in the near future. However, there are many difficulties in the provision of such a service, even in thoroughly documented families with multiple cancers that can clearly be shown to be due to *BRCA1* (King et al 1993). The problems in interpreting the results in women with only one or two affected relatives will be very much greater. There may be a spectrum of mutations, with very different levels of risk. Even a negative test result may not provide the expected reassurance.

Once identified, women with a high risk of ovarian cancer are difficult to manage. None of the available screening tests are particularly effective. Annual ovarian ultrasonography with colour-flow Doppler studies are recommended, but it is very uncertain how much protection this offers. Prophylactic bilateral oophorectomy, usually combined with hysterectomy, is also recommended for clearly defined high-risk women after completion of their family. This does not remove the risk entirely, as cases of carcinoma of the peritoneum have occurred after this procedure.

MOLECULAR BIOLOGY

Much effort has been invested in studying the biology of ovarian cancer in the hope that improved understanding would lead to better treatment or prevention. In recent years, the search has focused on the overexpression of potential oncogenes and on the role of cytokines. HER-2/*neu* (c-*erbB*-2) is an oncogene that codes for an epidermal growth factor (EGF) receptor-like molecule. It is overexpressed in about 30% of ovarian carcinomas and may indicate a poor prognosis (Berchuck et al 1990). Inactivating antibodies to the extracellular portion of the HER-2/*neu* gene product can inhibit the growth of cells that overexpress the gene (Bast et al 1992).

Mutations in the tumour-suppressor gene *p53* are observed in up to half of women with advanced disease (Marks et al 1991). The lower incidence of mutations in early-stage disease may suggest that *p53* mutations are a late event in the development of ovarian cancer. Alternatively, such mutations may result in rapid progression of disease.

Most ovarian and endometrial tumours overexpress CSF-1 (M-CSF: macrophage colony-stimulating factor) and its receptor encoded by the proto-oncogene c-*fms*. CSF-1 can stimulate the growth of tumour cell lines and transfection of the cells with a dominant negative mutant c-*fms* gene inhibits cell growth. This suggests that CSF-1 and c-*fms* can cause an autocrine stimulation of tumour growth. There is also evidence of persistent autocrine stimulation by transforming growth factor-α (TGFα) and epidermal growth factor (EGF), both acting through the EGF receptor (EGFR) (Rodriguez et al 1991). Paracrine stimulation by cytokines produced by macrophages may also influence both the growth and invasiveness of tumour cells. Tumour necrosis factor-α (TNFα) appears to be particularly potent in this regard (Naylor et al 1995).

CLASSIFICATION OF OVARIAN TUMOURS

Ovarian tumours can be solid or cystic. They may be benign or malignant, and in addition there are those which, despite having some of the features of malignancy, lack any evidence of stromal invasion. These are called borderline tumours.

The most commonly used classifications of ovarian tumours was defined by the World Health Organization (Serov et al 1973). This is a morphological classification that attempts to relate the cell types and patterns of the tumour to tissues normally present in the ovary. The primary tumours are thus divided into those that are of epithelial type (implying an origin from surface epithelium), those that are of sex cord gonadal type (also known as sex cord stromal type, or sex cord mesenchymal type, and originating from sex cord mesenchymal elements), and those that are of germ cell type (originating from germ cells). A simplified version of the WHO classification is given in Table 41.1.

Table 41.1 Histological classification of ovarian tumours

I	Common epithelial tumours (benign, borderline or malignant)
	A Serous tumour
	B Mucinous tumour
	C Endometrioid tumour
	D Clear cell (mesonephroid) tumour
	E Brenner tumour
	F Mixed epithelial tumour
	G Undifferentiated carcinomas
	H Unclassified tumour
II	Sex cord stromal tumours
	A Granulosa stroma cell tumour
	B Androblastoma: Sertoli–Leydig cell tumour
	C Gynandroblastoma
	D Unclassified tumour
III	Lipid cell tumours
IV	Germ cell tumours
	A Dysgerminoma
	B Endodermal sinus tumour (yolk sac tumour)
	C Embryonal cell tumour
	D Polyembryoma
	E Choriocarcinoma
	F Teratoma
	G Mixed tumours
V	Gonadoblastoma
VI	Soft tissue tumours not specific to ovary
VII	Unclassified tumours
VIII	Metastatic tumours

PATHOLOGY OF EPITHELIAL TUMOURS

Well-differentiated epithelial carcinomas tend to be more often associated with early-stage disease, but the degree of differentiation does correlate with survival, except in the most advanced stages. Diploid tumours tend to be associated with earlier-stage disease and a better prognosis. Histological cell type is not of itself prognostically significant. Comparing patients stage for stage and grade for grade, there is no difference in survival in different epithelial types. However, mucinous and endometrioid lesions are likely to be associated with earlier stage and lower grade than serous cystadenocarcinomas.

Serous carcinoma

Gross features

The majority of serous carcinomas show a mixture of solid

and cystic elements, although a significant minority are predominantly cystic. Serous carcinomas have a propensity to bilaterality, ranging from 50 to 90%.

Microscopical features

The better-differentiated tumours have an obviously papillary pattern with unequivocal stromal invasion, and psammoma bodies (calcospherules) are often present (Fig. 41.2). None of these features is diagnostic of serous tumours alone. Endometrioid and clear cell carcinomas and, to a lesser extent, mucinous carcinomas, may all form papillary structures. The term 'papillary carcinoma of the ovary' should therefore not be used as a diagnosis.

At the other end of the spectrum is the anaplastic tumour composed of sheets of undifferentiated neoplastic cells in masses within a fibrous stroma. Occasional glandular structures may be present to enable a diagnosis of adenocarcinoma to be made. All gradations between these two are seen, sometimes in the same tumour.

Mucinous carcinoma

Gross features

Malignant mucinous tumours comprise about 10% of malignant tumours of the ovary. They are typically multilocular, thin-walled cysts with a smooth external surface, containing mucinous fluid. The locules vary in size, and often the tumour may be composed of one major cavity with many smaller daughter cysts apparently within its wall. Mucinous tumours are among the largest tumours of the ovary and may reach enormous dimensions: a cyst diameter of 25 cm is quite commonplace.

A mucinous cystadenocarcinoma may look the same as a benign tumour. Some malignant tumours may exhibit obvious solid areas, perhaps with necrosis and haemorrhage. The more advanced carcinomas will show the stigmata of ovarian malignancy, with adhesions to adjacent viscera and malignant ascites.

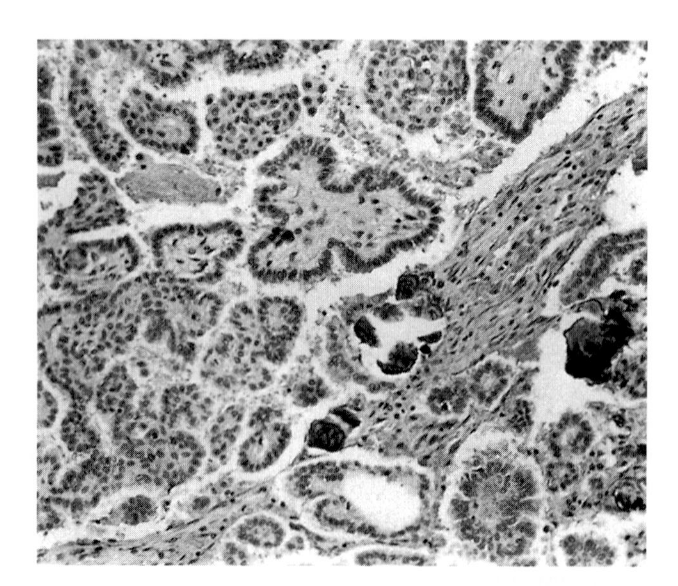

Fig. 41.2 Serous papillary cystadenocarcinoma. A well-differentiated (grade 1) serous carcinoma. The papillary pattern is obvious and a group of psammoma bodies is present at the lower right. Haematoxylin and eosin × 180.

Microscopic features

Mucinous adenocarcinomas present a variety of histological appearances (Fig. 41.3). The better-differentiated examples are composed of cells that retain a resemblance to the tall, picket-fence cells of the benign tumour, although stromal invasion is present. As differentiation is lost, the cells become less easily recognizable as being of mucinous type and their mucin content diminishes.

Endometrioid carcinoma

These are ovarian tumours that resemble the malignant neoplasia of epithelial, stromal and mixed origin that are found in the endometrium (Czernobilsky et al 1970).

Gross features

There is little to characterize an ovarian tumour as being of endometrioid type by naked-eye examination. Most are cystic, often unilocular, and contain turbid brown fluid. The internal surface of the cyst is usually rough with rounded, polypoid projections and solid areas, the appearances of which are usually distinct from those of the papillary excrescences seen in serous tumours.

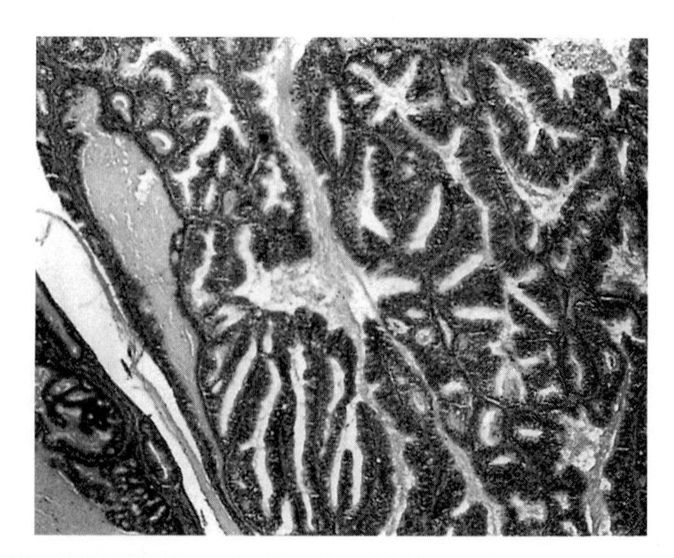

Fig. 41.3 Mucinous adenocarcinoma of the ovary. Haematoxylin and eosin × 180.

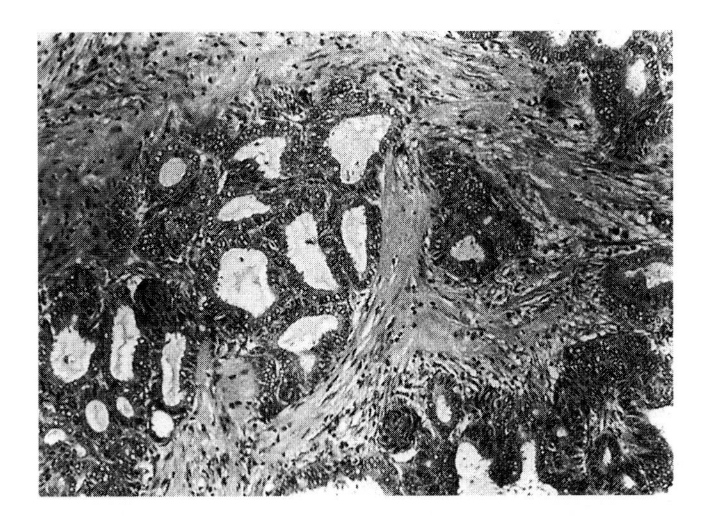

Fig. 41.4 Endometrioid carcinoma of the ovary. Haematoxylin and eosin × 180.

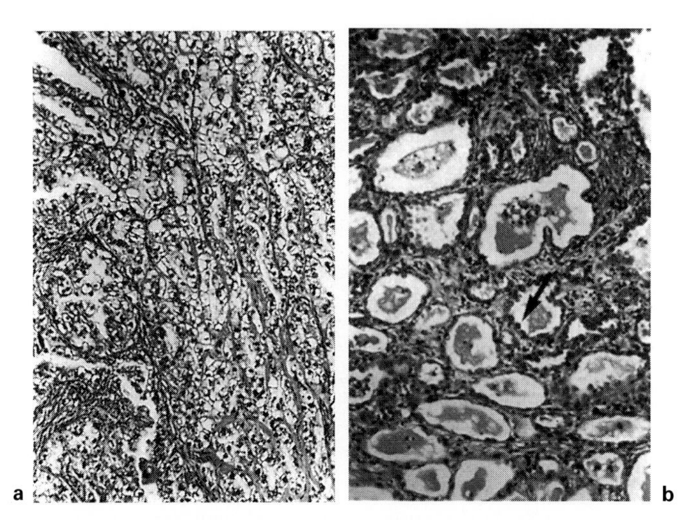

Fig. 41.5 Clear cell carcinoma of the ovary. **(a)** A moderately differentiated glandular pattern composed entirely of clear cells. Haematoxylin and eosin × 170. **(b)** A tubulocystic area showing prominent 'hobnail' cells (arrow). Haematoxylin and eosin × 230.

Microscopical features

Endometrioid carcinomas resemble the endometrioid carcinomas of the endometrium (Fig. 41.4). The pattern is predominantly tubular and may resemble proliferative endometrium. The epithelium is tall and columnar, with a high nuclear cytoplasmic ratio. Endometrioid carcinomas of the ovary are more likely to be papillary than are primary endometrial carcinomas. Five to 10% of cases are seen in continuity with recognizable endometriosis. Ovarian adenoacanthoma, with benign-appearing squamous elements, accounts for almost 50% in some series of endometrioid tumours.

Associated endometrial carcinoma

It is important to note that 15% of endometrioid carcinomas of the ovary are associated with endometrial carcinoma in the body of the uterus. Although this is sometimes due to a primary in one site and a secondary at the other, in most cases these are two separate primary tumours.

Clear cell carcinoma (mesonephroid)

These are the least common of the malignant epithelial tumours of the ovary, accounting for 5–10% of ovarian carcinomas (Anderson & Langley 1970).

Gross features

There is nothing characteristic about the gross appearances of the clear cell tumour to distinguish it from the other cystadenocarcinomas of the ovary. Most are thick-walled, unilocular cysts containing turbid brown or blood-stained fluid, with solid, polypoid projections arising from the internal surface. About 10% are bilateral.

Microscopical features

Clear cell carcinomas of the ovary are characterized by the variety of their architectural patterns, which may be found alone or in combination in any individual tumour (Fig. 41.5). The appearance from which the tumours derive their name is the clear cell pattern but, in addition, some areas show a tubulo-cystic pattern with the characteristic 'hobnail' appearance of the lining epithelium. The third major pattern is papillary.

Association with endometriosis and endometrioid tumours

Because there is a very strong association between clear cell tumours of the ovary and ovarian endometriosis, and because clear cell and endometrioid tumours frequently coexist, it has been suggested that the clear cell tumour may be a variant of endometrioid tumour.

Borderline epithelial tumours

Ten per cent of all epithelial tumours of the ovary are of borderline malignancy (Ovarian Tumour Panel of RCOG 1983). These show varying degrees of nuclear atypia and an increase in mitotic activity, multilayering of neoplastic cells and formation of cellular buds, but no invasion of the stroma. Most borderline tumours remain confined to the ovaries, and this may account for their much better prognosis. Peritoneal lesions are present in some cases, and although a few are true metastases many remain stationary and even regress after removal of the primary. The histological diagnosis of borderline malignancy can be difficult, particularly in mucinous tumours (Fig. 41.6).

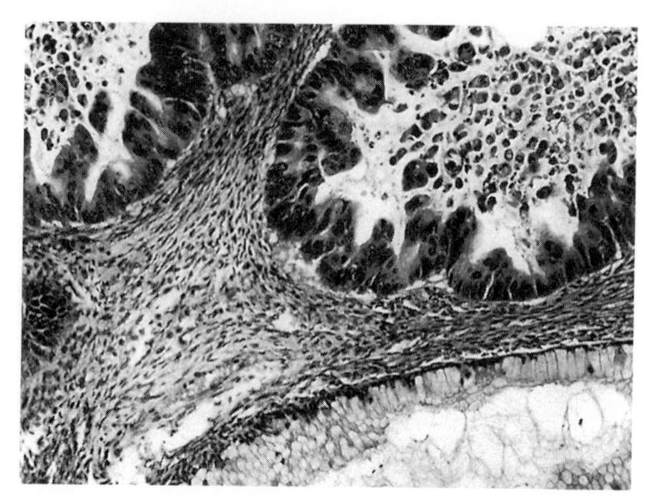

Fig. 41.6 A borderline mucinous tumour with multilayering of the epithelium but no evidence of stromal invasion.

Most borderline tumours are serous or mucinous in type. Other borderline tumours are rare.

NATURAL HISTORY

Approximately two-thirds of patients present with disease spread beyond the pelvis. This is probably due to the insidious nature of the signs and symptoms of carcinoma of the ovary, but may sometimes be due to a rapidly growing tumour. Because of the non-specific nature of most of these symptoms, a diagnosis of ovarian cancer is seldom considered until the disease is in an advanced stage.

Metastatic spread

The pelvic peritoneum and other pelvic organs become involved by direct spread. The peritoneal fluid, flowing to lymphatic channels on the undersurface of the diaphragm, carries malignant cells to the omentum, to the peritoneal surfaces of the small and large bowel and liver and to the parietal peritoneal surface throughout the abdominal cavity and on the surface of the diaphragm. Metastases on the undersurface of the diaphragm may be found in up to 44% of what otherwise seems to be Stage I–II disease. Intraperitoneal metastases are superficial and seldom involve the substance of the organ beneath. Even when the surface of the bowel is extensively involved, the muscularis layer is seldom infiltrated.

Lymphatic spread is generally thought to be mainly along the lymphatics that run with the ovarian vessels to the para-aortic region at the level of the renal vessels. These nodes may be involved in 19% of Stages I–II and in 65% of Stages III–IV. However, pelvic lymph node involvement occurs more often than previously reported (Table 41.2; Burghardt et al 1991). Spread may also occur to nodes in the neck or inguinal region.

Table 41.2 Pelvic and para-aortic node metastases (Burghardt et al 1991)

	Nodes involved (%)	
	Pelvic	Para-aortic
Stage I–II	30	19
Stage III–IV	67	65

Table 41.3 FIGO staging for primary ovarian carcinoma

Stage	FIGO definition
I	Growth limited to ovaries
	Ia Growth limited to one ovary no ascites; no tumour on external surface; capsule intact
	Ib Growth limited to both ovaries no ascites; no tumour on external surfaces; capsule intact
	Ic Tumour either Stage Ia or Ib but tumour on surface of one or both ovaries; or with capsule ruptured; or with ascites present containing malignant cells; or with positive peritoneal washings
II	Growth involving one or both ovaries with pelvic extension
	IIa Extension and/or metastases to the uterus or tubes
	IIb Extension to other pelvic tissues
	IIc Tumour either Stage IIa or IIb but tumour on surface of one or both ovaries; or with capsule ruptured; or with ascites present containing malignant cells; or with positive peritoneal washings
III	Growth involving one or both ovaries with peritoneal implants outside the pelvis or positive retroperitoneal or inguinal nodes. Superficial liver metastases equals Stage III
	IIIa Tumour grossly limited to the true pelvis with negative nodes but with histologically confirmed microscopic seeding of abdominal peritoneal surfaces
	IIIb Tumour with histologically confirmed implants on abdominal peritoneal surfaces none exceeding 2 cm in diameter. Nodes are negative
	IIIc Abdominal implants greater than 2 cm in diameter or positive retroperitoneal or inguinal nodes
IV	Growth involving one or both ovaries with distant metastases. If pleural effusion is present there must be positive cytology to allot a case to Stage IV. Parenchymal liver metastasis equals Stage IV

Haematogenous spread usually occurs late in the course of the disease. The main areas involved are the liver and the lung, although metastases to bone and brain are sometimes seen.

CLINICAL STAGING

The staging of ovarian cancer as defined by FIGO is shown in Table 41.3. Peritoneal deposits on the surface of the liver do not make the patient Stage IV: the parenchyma must be involved. Similarly, the presence of a pleural effusion is insufficient to put the patient in Stage IV unless malignant cells are found on cytological examination of the pleural fluid.

DIAGNOSIS

Abdominal pain or discomfort are the commonest presenting complaints, and distension or feeling a lump the next most frequent. Patients may complain of indigestion, urinary frequency, weight loss or, rarely, abnormal menses or postmenopausal bleeding. A hard abdominal mass arising from the pelvis is highly suggestive, especially in the presence of ascites. A fixed, hard, irregular pelvic mass is usually best felt by combined vaginal and rectal examination (Fig. 41.7). The neck and groin should also be examined for enlarged nodes.

Haematological investigations include a full blood count, urea, electrolytes and liver function tests. A chest X-ray is essential. It is sometimes advisable to carry out a barium enema to differentiate between an ovarian and a colonic tumour and to assess bowel involvement from the ovarian tumour itself. An intravenous pyelogram is sometimes useful.

Imaging techniques

Ultrasonography may help to confirm the presence of a pelvic mass and detect ascites before it is clinically apparent. It is also a relatively reliable tool for examining the liver parenchyma and may detect enlarged pelvic or para-aortic lymph nodes.

Computed tomography of the abdomen and pelvis is used as an alternative to ultrasonography, but is more expensive and less accurate in the pelvis. Magnetic resonance imaging (MRI) is being assessed in a few centres as it is particularly useful for examining the pelvis (Johnson et al 1984). Radioimmunoscintigraphy is still a research tool but it has some value in detecting spread of ovarian tumour within the abdomen. None of these techniques will detect small peritoneal metastases.

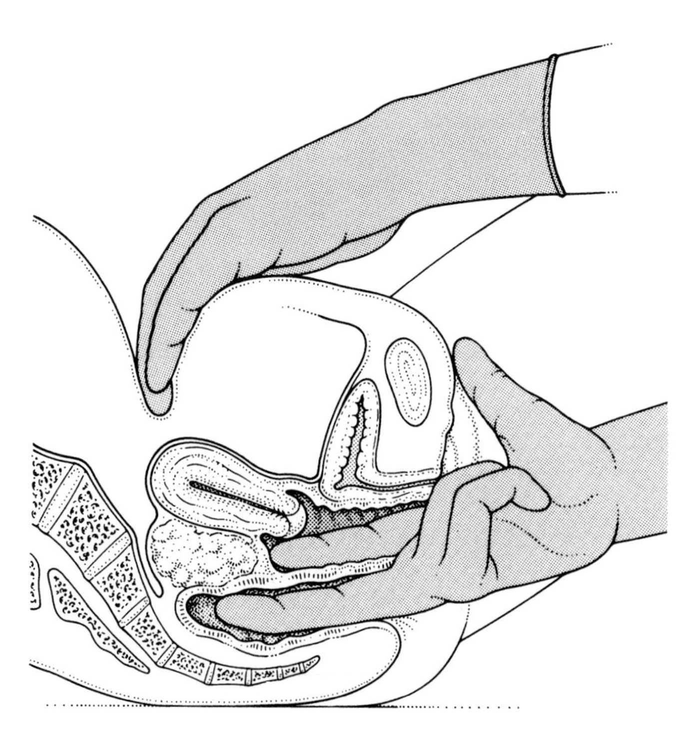

Fig. 41.7 A combined vaginal and rectal examination allows more accurate assessment of the pouch of Douglas.

The most accurate method for assessing lymph node involvement is biopsy at the time of surgery. Lymphangiography is accurate only to a degree, as it cannot detect micrometastases and false positive results are frequent.

Cytology

In patients with pleural effusion or ascites, specimens of fluid may be examined cytologically for the presence of malignant cells. It is seldom justifiable to perform a paracentesis for cytology. That can be deferred until the laparotomy. Fine-needle aspiration of clinically suspicious lymph nodes in the groin or neck can be very valuable.

Markers for epithelial tumours

None of the markers currently available is sufficiently accurate or truly specific to detect ovarian cancer at an early stage. The most useful marker, CA125, derived from a human cancer line, is usually raised in advanced ovarian cancer but it can also be raised in benign conditions such as endometriosis. Using CA125 estimations to monitor women receiving chemotherapy is a useful method for assessing response, and can reduce the need for scans. A persistent rise in CA125 may precede clinical evidence of recurrent disease by several months in some cases. However, the values can be normal in the presence of small tumour deposits.

Carcinoembryonic antigen (CEA) is abnormal most often in mucinous cystadenocarcinoma. Concentrations in excess of 20 ng/ml are suggestive of ovarian tumour. The tumour-associated antigens OCCA and OCA are raised in both serous and mucinous cystadenocarcinoma (Van Nagell 1983).

Sensitivity may be increased by using a panel of tumour markers. For example, combining assays for CA125, HMFG1 and HMFG2 (human milk factor globulin), and H17E2 (an epitope of placental alkaline phosphatase), increased the detection rate to 95% in 85 patients with advanced disease (Dhokia et al 1987). Similar work using CA125, HMFG2 and placental alkaline phosphate (PLAP) found elevated levels of at least one marker in all patients with advanced disease and in seven of 11 with Stage I or II ovarian cancer (Ward et al 1987).

Screening

Because carcinoma of the ovary tends to be asymptomatic

in the early stages and most patients present with advanced disease, efforts have been made to define a tumour marker which could be used for screening purposes. So far, none has become available which is truly specific and which is suitable for the early detection of epithelial carcinoma (Lambert 1987, Oram & Jeyarajah 1994).

Tumour markers

The only marker assessed in a prospective trial of screening is CA125 (Jacobs et al 1993). Ultrasound was used for all women with abnormal values. In this study of 22 000 women, 11 cancers were detected but seven of these were Stage III or IV. Seven women with normal CA125 values subsequently presented with ovarian cancer, two within a year. Thus only four curable cancers were detected, seven incurable tumours were found and seven other cancers were missed.

New markers with promise for the future include macrophage colony-stimulating factor (MCSF) (Suzuki et al 1993); inhibin, a marker for mucinous cancers (Burger 1993) and granulosa cell tumours; and OVX1 (Xu et al 1993). A combination of CA125, MCSF and OVX1 gave 98% sensitivity in patients with Stage I disease but 11% false positive results (Woolas et al 1993).

Ultrasound for screening

After very disappointing results with conventional ultrasound methods, colour flow transvaginal ultrasound was assessed in 1601 women with a family history of ovarian cancer (Bourne et al 1993). A laparotomy or laparoscopy was performed in 61 of these women as a result of an abnormal scan. Six of these had ovarian cancer, five were Stage Ia and three of these were borderline tumours.

Conclusion

In our present state of knowledge, and with the available technology, screening the general population is neither useful nor safe. High-risk patients may take part in trials to assess new screening techniques but should not be led to believe that these have proven value. This subject is well reviewed by Oram and Jeyarajah (1994).

SURGERY

The exploration

Surgery is the mainstay of both the diagnosis and the treatment of ovarian cancer. A vertical incision is required for an adequate exploration of the upper abdomen. A sample of ascitic fluid or peritoneal washings with normal saline, which must be taken for cytology, should be obtained before any manipulation of the tumour to avoid contamination.

The pelvis and upper abdomen are explored carefully, including the omentum, subdiaphragmatic areas, the paracolic gutters, large and small bowel and small bowel mesentery. Such an exploration is not possible with a low transverse incision. In the absence of gross upper abdominal disease, suspicious areas should be biopsied. A sample for cytology may be taken from the diaphragm with an Ayre's spatula (Griffiths 1987).

Therapeutic objective

The therapeutic objective of surgery for ovarian cancer is the removal of all tumour. Whereas this is achieved in the majority of Stage I cases and in some Stage II, it is probably impossible in more advanced disease. Because of the diffuse spread of tumour throughout the peritoneal cavity and the retroperitoneal nodes, microscopic deposits will persist in almost all cases even when all macroscopic tumour appears to have been excised. Thus, although surgery alone may be curative in many Stage I cases, additional therapy is essential for most of the remainder.

Conservative surgery in Stage I disease

The resection of all visible tumour usually requires a total hysterectomy and bilateral salpingo-oophorectomy, but in a young nulliparous woman with a unilateral tumour and no ascites, unilateral salpingo-oophorectomy may be justifiable after careful exploration to exclude metastatic disease. Curettage of the uterine cavity should be performed to exclude a synchronous endometrial tumour. Some recommend that the normal-looking ovary be biopsied, but the risk of occult spread to that ovary is small and biopsy may impair fertility, negating the purpose of the conservative operation. If the tumour is subsequently found to be poorly differentiated, or if the washings are positive, a second operation to clear the pelvis will be necessary.

Maximal cytoreductive surgery in advanced disease

Maximal cytoreductive surgery aims to remove all macroscopic tumour and to remove tissue such as the omentum, to which microscopic spread is common. The minimum operation consists of a total abdominal hysterectomy and bilateral salpingo-oophorectomy and infracolic omentectomy. Some surgeons also include pelvic and para-aortic lymphadenectomy, either as a sampling procedure or as a radical removal of retroperitoneal nodes.

Even if no disease is apparent in the upper abdomen, infracolic omentectomy is advisable because microscopic spread can be present when the omentum looks normal. Even when the omentum is extensively infiltrated it is usually possible to free it from adherent loops of small bowel and to separate it from the transverse colon and stomach. If a limited area of the small bowel or its mesentery is involved it can be resected. However, multiple or extensive resections of small bowel are limited by the need to preserve a functional length of intestine, and such patients will still have a poor prognosis.

If the pelvic tumour is large or densely adherent to the pelvic side wall and the colon, it is usually easier to enter the retroperitoneal space at the pelvic brim in order to ligate the ovarian vessels, dissect the ureter from the pelvic peritoneum and mobilize the tumour. The mass can often be freed from the bladder and rectum by peeling the tumour-bearing visceral peritoneum off the underlying organ. The uterine vessels may be ligated at the pelvic side wall and a hysterectomy performed. Sometimes resection of part of the bladder or removal of the sigmoid colon and rectum is necessary. Primary reanastomosis is often possible. Resection of the pelvic colon is indicated if obstruction is imminent, but in most other circumstances the prognosis is unlikely to be greatly improved.

Observing a high incidence of pelvic and para-aortic node metastases in their patients, Burghardt and colleagues (1991) attempted a complete clearance initially of only the pelvic nodes, and more recently of pelvic and para-aortic nodes, to the level of the renal vessels. It remains to be seen whether radical lymphadenectomy will make a major impact upon the survival of women with this dreadful disease.

Feasibility and morbidity of cytoreductive surgery

The proportion of patients optimally cytoreduced depends on the attitudes and experience of the surgical team. Gynaecological oncologists who are fully trained in this type of surgery, with experienced anaesthetists and nurses, will successfully cytoreduce patients with advanced disease more often than those with less experience or enthusiasm. Approximately 75% of women with advanced ovarian cancer are amenable to optimal surgery. The post-operative morbidity is surprisingly low for a poor-risk group, and seems to relate more to the experience of the team looking after the patient than to the amount of surgery performed.

The value of maximal cytoreductive surgery in advanced disease

For the past 10–15 years gynaecological oncologists have been advocating maximal cytoreductive surgery in advanced ovarian cancer, in the belief that this would improve the prospects for survival and make tumours more amenable to chemotherapy. This view is undergoing revision in the light of more recent data.

Many studies show that women with minimal or no residual disease after surgery have a better prognosis than those in whom more disease remained after surgery. However, it is likely that the latter group includes the more aggressive tumours with an intrinsically worse prognosis. Griffiths and co-workers (1979) showed that women with no or minimal residual disease (<1.5 cm) after primary surgery survived longer than those with larger residual masses, and that patients with residual masses <1.5 cm following surgery did as well as those whose metastases were small from the outset. These data suggested that surgical intervention could indeed influence the prognosis. Unfortunately, an analysis of more modern data has failed to confirm these findings (Hoskins et al 1992).

It has become clear that the prognosis is adversely affected by the volume of metastatic disease at the outset, even when maximum cytoreduction has been successfully performed (Hacker et al 1983). Similarly, women who have undergone bowel surgery as part of successful cytoreduction have a worse prognosis than those without bowel surgery, even if cytoreduction was unsuccessful (Potter et al 1991).

No prospective controlled trials of primary cytoreductive surgery have been reported. However, a study of two different chemotherapy regimens showed no survival advantage for those women operated upon in units with higher rates of successful cytoreduction (Bertelsen 1990). A subsequent meta-analysis of over 6000 cases was based on the principle that groups of women with higher rates of successful cytoreduction should have better survival rates if the surgery was contributing to the outcome (Hunter et al 1992). In this study, maximal cytoreductive surgery had no significant effect on median survival once the effects of chemotherapy had been taken into account.

Although it seems likely that primary cytoreductive surgery can improve the quality of life for women with advanced ovarian cancer (Blyth & Wahl 1982) and increase their ability to tolerate chemotherapy, any effect on survival will probably be small. Removal of the majority of the tumour volume should always be attempted, and is likely to be successful in some 75% of cases. However, resection of bowel should not be performed except when obstruction is imminent. The meticulous removal of all tiny tumour nodules is unlikely to be helpful. Similarly, radical lymphadenectomy cannot be recommended.

Intervention debulking surgery

An alternative approach when initial surgery has left bulky disease is a planned second laparotomy after two to four courses of cytoreductive chemotherapy in those women who respond. The chemotherapy is then resumed as soon as possible after the second operation. A relatively small British study did not show any benefit from this approach (Redman et al 1994). The results of a larger EORTC study are more encouraging (Van der Berg et al 1995). These suggest that the median survival in this poor prognosis group may be increased by 6 months and that the survival at 3 years may be improved from 10 to 20%. This interesting area requires further study.

Second-look surgery

Second-look surgery is defined as a planned laparotomy at the end of chemotherapy. The objectives are first to determine the response to previous therapy in order to document accurately its efficacy and to plan subsequent management, and secondly to excise any residual disease. Although there is no doubt that second-look surgery gives the most accurate indication of the disease status, laparotomy being more accurate in this respect than laparoscopy, the balance of evidence suggests that neither the surgical resection of residual tumour nor the opportunity to change the treatment has any effect whatever on the patient's survival. Second-look procedures therefore have no place outside clinical trials at the present time.

SELECTING PATIENTS FOR POSTOPERATIVE TREATMENT

In Stage I carcinoma of the ovary where the tumour is confined to the ovaries there is a need to define those cases where adjuvant therapy is indicated to prevent recurrent disease. While FIGO Stage Ic includes cases with capsular penetration by tumour, rupture of the capsule, and ascites or positive peritoneal washings, there is little evidence that each of these has the same prognostic value.

Dembo (1992) considered that dense adherence of a malignant ovarian cyst should be considered as Stage II disease. Thereafter, only differentiation of the tumour, a large volume of ascites and positive peritoneal washings were of prognostic significance in Stage I disease. Vergote et al (1993) found that grade of tumour was the most important prognostic indicator for disease-free survival in 290 patients with Stage I disease. This was followed by DNA ploidy and substage. Poor differentiation of the tumour and aneuploidy indicated a poor prognosis. Dense adhesions, ascites, extracapsular growth and rupture during surgery were no longer prognostic once these factors had been accounted for. Rupture of the tumour capsule during surgery has no effect on survival, but the prognosis is much worse when rupture has occurred before the operation (Sjovall et al 1994). A randomized trial by the Gynecological Oncology Group (GOG) found that the survival at 5 years was over 90% in patients with low- to intermediate-grade tumours confined to the ovaries, whether they received adjuvant therapy or not (Young et al 1990).

These data suggest that women with Stage Ia or Ib disease and well or moderately differentiated tumours may not require further treatment. The benefit of adjuvant therapy for an intermediate group, Stage Ic, with low- to intermediate-grade tumours but with a surgically ruptured cyst, dense adhesions, extracapsular growth or ascites, is uncertain.

All other patients with invasive ovarian carcinoma require adjuvant therapy. There is no evidence that adjuvant therapy affects the outcome in women with borderline tumours.

RADIOTHERAPY

Indications for radiotherapy

Radiotherapy has only a very small role to play in the management of ovarian carcinoma. Even in early-stage disease, where Dembo et al (1979) found that adjuvant whole-abdominal radiotherapy led to improved survival, it has been superseded by the platinum drugs. This work remains of historical importance, as it emphasized that the whole abdominal cavity is at risk of occult metastases.

In more advanced cases radiotherapy is ineffective, as the radiation doses that can be given to the upper abdomen fail to sterilize macroscopic deposits. It can, however, be useful as a palliative treatment for painful recurrences in the pelvis, or for metastases in bone or brain.

External radiotherapy to the whole abdomen has also been used as a consolidation therapy, following adjuvant chemotherapy, in patients found to have little or no residual disease at second-look surgery. In a randomized study of over 200 patients treated with carboplatin chemotherapy, no advantage was found in those receiving consolidation radiotherapy compared to those who received consolidation chemotherapy with carboplatin (Lambert et al 1993). Although there was no significant morbidity in this study, this has not always been the case in other non-randomized studies using consolidation radiotherapy. The conclusion is that there is no role for consolidation therapy using whole-abdominal radiotherapy.

Radioactive isotopes

Radioactive isotopes of either gold (^{198}Au) or phosphorus (^{32}P) linked to carrier colloids have been used intraperitoneally for many years in early carcinoma of the ovary. They have been used alone and in combination with external radiotherapy. These isotopes are both β emitters and have short half-lives of 2.69 and 14.2 days, respectively. Radioactive phosphorus has replaced gold as it is safer because it has no additional γ radiation (see Ch. 33).

When given intraperitoneally, radioactive substances are absorbed directly on to the peritoneal surface and are taken up by macrophages lining the peritoneal cavity or floating free. This gives a high dose of radiation but to an effective depth of only 4–6 mm, thereby limiting therapy to the peritoneal surface and to small microscopic deposits on its surface. Colloid-linked isotopes enter the lymphatic circulation by the diaphragmatic lymphatics to reach the mediastinal lymphatics and then the general circulation. They are poorly absorbed by the retroperitoneal nodes (Currie et al 1981).

Although cure rates of approximately 90% for Stage I disease have been reported after treatment with intraperitoneal radioactive isotopes, it is only recently that randomized studies have been carried out. Vergote et al (1992a) randomized 347 patients with epithelial ovarian cancer without residual tumour after primary laparotomy to either six courses of 50 mg/m^2 cisplatin given 3-weekly, or to intraperitoneal ^{32}P instilled on the first postoperative day. Patients with extensive intraperitoneal adhesions had whole-abdominal irradiation instead of ^{32}P. Both overall survival and disease-free survival were similar in the two groups, but there was a high incidence of late bowel complications in the radioactive phosphorus group. A similar study in patients with early-stage ovarian cancer with poor prognostic features is being carried out by the GOG, comparing intraperitoneal ^{32}P with three courses of intravenous cisplatin and cyclophosphamide. There are no reported studies comparing intraperitoneal ^{32}P with no treatment in early-stage ovarian cancer (Cannistra 1993). The combination of intraperitoneal and external radiotherapy has been shown to be too toxic to merit further study (Klaassen et al 1985).

The overall conclusion is that there is no evidence to show that the use of intraperitoneal ^{32}P prolongs survival in early ovarian cancer, but there is evidence of an increased incidence of bowel complications.

Monoclonal antibodies such as HMFG1, HMFG2, AUA1 and H17E2 react with antigens produced by ovarian carcinomas. A pilot study using radioactive monoclonal antibody as adjuvant therapy in patients with no or minimal macroscopic disease at second-look surgery following chemotherapy for ovarian cancer showed greatly improved survival, but only for those patients who had no evidence of disease at second-look surgery (Hird et al 1993). This included patients with Stage III disease at diagnosis compared retrospectively with similar patients in a study by the North Thames Ovary Group. In order to determine whether this form of maintenance therapy is truly effective, a prospective study is now under way comparing no further therapy with intraperitoneal radioactive monoclonal antibody therapy in patients with no residual disease at second-look surgery following chemotherapy.

Radiotherapy – conclusions

Postoperative abdominopelvic radiotherapy for early ovarian carcinoma no longer has a role in the management of ovarian cancer. Chemotherapy has replaced radiotherapy in the management of early ovarian cancer and has always been used for advanced disease for which radiotherapy is ineffective. Intraperitoneal colloid-bound radioactive phosphorus has not been proved to have any advantage over chemotherapy for early-stage disease, and can cause serious late bowel problems. Intraperitoneal radioactive antibody therapy is still a research tool.

CHEMOTHERAPY

Chemotherapy plays a major role in treating ovarian carcinoma of epithelial origin except for the very earliest stages when surgery alone is sufficient. Chemotherapy is given postoperatively to prolong both clinical remission and survival, and for palliation in advanced and recurrent disease. Chemotherapy is commenced as soon as possible after surgery, and it is recommended that the treatment delay should never be more than 6 weeks. Chemotherapy is usually given for five or six cycles at 3–4-weekly intervals. Randomized trials by Hakes et al (1992) and the North Thames Ovary Group (1995) comparing five cycles of chemotherapy with 10 and eight cycles respectively in Stages III and IV ovarian cancer showed no clinical benefit to support prolonging treatment beyond five cycles.

Single agents

Alkylating agents, antimetabolites and antitumour antibiotics

The most commonly used chemotherapeutic agents in carcinoma of the ovary have been the alkylating agents. They have been in use for several decades, with reported response rates of 35–65%, and with 5–15% still responding after 2 years. The most commonly used alkylating agents are chlorambucil, melphalan, cyclophosphamide, ifosfamide and treosulfan. Chlorambucil and melphalan can be given orally and are still used, particularly in elderly patients, as they are well tolerated, usually causing no more than mild nausea. They are toxic to the bone marrow and should be given in intermittent courses. Altretamine (hexamethylmelamine), derived from melamine, is thought to act by alkylation. It is given orally and has activity even when tumours have become resistant to more classic alkylating agents (Manetta et al 1990). Other drugs showing some activity include the antimetabolites 5-fluorouracil and methotrexate, and the antitumour antibiotics such as doxorubicin, epirubicin and mitoxantrone. Etoposide (VP16) also shows some activity in ovarian cancer.

Platinum drugs

The platinum drugs, cisplatin and its analogue carboplatin, are heavy metal compounds which cause cross-linkage of DNA strands in a similar fashion to alkylating agents. These are considered to be the most effective drugs in general use in the management of ovarian carcinoma, and are the most widely used cytotoxic drugs, either alone or in combination. A prospective randomized study (Lambert & Berry 1985) compared cisplatin with cyclophosphamide in advanced ovarian cancer and showed better response and survival rates with cisplatin. The dose of cisplatin as a single agent is usually 75 mg/m^2.

Cisplatin is a very toxic drug. Until the advent of the 5HT antagonists (ganesetron and ondansetron) severe nausea and vomiting, sometimes lasting several days, was a serious problem. Permanent renal damage will occur unless cisplatin is given with adequate hydration with intravenous fluids. Peripheral neuropathy and hearing loss are reported with increasing cumulative doses. Electrolyte disturbances, such as hypomagnesaemia, are seen occasionally. Unlike with most chemotherapeutic agents marrow toxicity is not usually a problem, with the exception of anaemia.

Carboplatin is as effective as cisplatin in the treatment of ovarian cancer (Wiltshaw 1985, Advanced Ovarian Cancer Trialists Group 1991). The advantage of carboplatin over cisplatin is that it causes less nausea and vomiting and has no significant renal toxicity. Neurotoxicity is rare and hearing loss is subclinical. The lack of renal toxicity means that there is no need to give carboplatin with intravenous hydration. The dose is calculated in relation to the glomerular filtration rate, using the area under the curve (AUC) formula (Calvert et al 1989). This method allows a higher dose of carboplatin to be given when renal function is normal. Leucopenia and thrombocytopenia, the dose-limiting toxicities of carboplatin, can be severe in the presence of renal impairment.

New drugs

Paclitaxel (Taxol), the first drug containing the taxane ring structure to be used, is one of three new drugs that have recently been found to have significant activity in ovarian cancer. The other two which appear to be promising are docetaxol (Taxotere), which also has the taxane ring, and gemcitabine.

Paclitaxel is derived from the bark of the Pacific yew tree (*Taxus brevifolia*) and has a mechanism of action which is unique among cytotoxic drugs. It acts by promoting polymerization of microtubules, making them excessively stable. This leads to blocking of cell division and tumour growth. In initial studies paclitaxel was found to be the most active drug ever tested in patients with cisplatin-resistant ovarian cancer, with a response rate of 22% in a study of 1000 heavily pretreated patients (Trimble et al 1993). A recent report using single-agent paclitaxel in Stage IV patients showed an overall response rate of 32% (Gore et al 1995).

A prospective randomized Canadian–European trial showed that a 3-hour infusion of 175 mg/m^2 was the best of the options tested (Swenerton et al 1993). This has been adopted in the UK but a lower dose of 135 mg/m^2 is used in the USA.

Sensory neuropathy and neutropenia are more common with the higher dose and infusions for 24 hours resulted in a higher incidence of grade 4 neutropenia. Other forms of toxicity, such as myalgia and arthralgia, were dose dependent but were never severe.

Hypersensitivity reactions, such as angioedema, respiratory distress, hypotension or generalized urticaria, were a serious problem with paclitaxel when it was first assessed but these are now very rare since the introduction of a premedication regimen of dexamethasone 20 mg, diphenhydramine 50 mg and ranitidine or cimetidine given prior to paclitaxel. Nausea and vomiting is very mild with paclitaxel. Body hair loss is usually total, irrespective of dose and schedule, as are asymptomatic cardiovascular symptoms such as bradycardia and hypotension.

Docetaxol (Taxotere) is a semisynthetic taxoid derived from the needles of the European yew tree (*Taxus baccata*). This means that, unlike paclitaxel, this drug can be manufactured from an easily renewable source. However, semisynthetic production of the latter is now being developed. Early studies indicate that docetaxol has similar activity to paclitaxel, but it has an unusual skin toxicity and can produce marked oedema. Gemcitabine, which is also showing some activity in cisplatin-resistant ovarian cancer, differs from the taxoid-based drugs in being a pyrimidine antimetabolite.

Combination chemotherapy

Combination chemotherapy has the theoretical advantage that it allows ovarian cancer to be treated by several drugs, all of which have shown some activity when used singly. Drugs which act in different ways on the cell cycle and which have different toxicities can be combined, reducing the chance of resistance occurring. Despite many relatively small studies over the years and evidence of an increased response rate, there has been very little evidence of longer survival compared to single-agent therapy. A meta-analysis which looked at over 3000 patients in 16 randomized trials comparing a single alkylating agent with a non-cisplatin combination found no survival advantage for the combination (Advanced Ovarian Trialists Group 1991).

Trials which compared a single alkylating agent with drug combinations that included cisplatin consistently showed a significantly better clinical response for the combination but no significant improvement in survival. The same was true of those studies where a non-platinum combination regimen was compared to the same combination with cisplatin added. It was thought that this lack of survival benefit might be due to platinum treatment of the failures in the non-platinum arm.

The overview also used data from six randomized studies to compare cisplatin alone with cisplatin in a combination regimen. Despite not reaching statistical significance, there was a long-term survival advantage for the combination. However, in these retrospective trials the dose of cisplatin in the single-agent arm was suboptimal, and the survival difference may have been due to this factor rather than to any advantage in a combination regimen.

To discover whether platinum-based combination therapy would improve survival over platinum alone requires a large number of patients to detect the modest survival differences that would be expected with current chemotherapy. The International Collaborative Ovarian Neoplasm Group are comparing single-agent carboplatin with the combination CAP (cyclophosphamide, doxorubicin, cisplatin) (ICON2). The study was commenced in 1992 and interim results reported in 1995 show no good evidence of a survival difference between CAP and carboplatin.

However, a combination of paclitaxel with cisplatin has shown better survival rates than conventional combination therapy in patients with advanced ovarian cancer (McGuire et al 1996). On the basis of this study, the GOG now consider a paclitaxel and cisplatin combination to be the standard chemotherapy for ovarian cancer, but these results await confirmation by a similar, ongoing EORTC trial. In 1995 the MRC began a randomized trial of paclitaxel with carboplatin compared to carboplatin alone or CAP. This should show whether taxol combinations are superior to platinum drugs used alone. Unfortunately, with current therapy the most powerful determinant of prognosis remains the biological behaviour of the tumour itself.

Experimental chemotherapy

Despite improved results in the treatment of advanced ovarian cancer with platinum-based chemotherapy, which have led to useful prolongation of survival, the continued fall in survival curves after 5 years with current therapies is not dramatically changing the long-term survival rates. Only 20–30% will survive 5 years, and approximately 15–20% are curable with the therapeutic approaches used at present. This is an improvement compared to the 5–10% cure rate obtained with single alkylating agents, but shows that the outlook for patients with advanced ovarian cancer remains very poor (Ozols & Young 1991). As well as looking at new drugs such as paclitaxel, other approaches being examined include dose intensification with platinum compounds, intraperitoneal chemotherapy and reversal of drug resistance.

Dose intensification

There are no data at present to show that dose intensification of platinum drugs beyond the upper limits of standard therapy improve survival, and there may well be a plateau in the dose–response curve. Toxicity will ultimately limit the dose of chemotherapy that can be tolerated. Although colony-stimulating factors can alleviate marrow toxicity to some extent, repeated high doses of carboplatin can cause cumulative toxicity which is resistant to treatment, particularly thrombocytopenia. New methods of dealing with marrow toxicity with high-dose carboplatin have been the use of autologous bone marrow transplantation or peripheral blood progenitor cell infusion. With dose intensification, non-haematological toxicity becomes the dose-limiting problem, particularly nephrotoxicity and neurotoxicity with high-dose cisplatin. Protective agents, such as amifostine and glutathionine, are under investigation. In contrast to cisplatin, if bone marrow toxicity is circumvented carboplatin can be escalated to 2000 mg/m^2 before renal and hepatotoxicity become dose-limiting.

Intraperitoneal chemotherapy

The intraperitoneal use of cytotoxic drugs is of particular interest in ovarian cancer, which tends to recur or persist within the peritoneal cavity even at a late stage of the disease. With intraperitoneal therapy much higher concentrations of drugs can be achieved with less toxicity.

Cisplatin is considered to be the best drug currently available, because it is both effective with a peritoneal/plasma AUC ratio of between 30:1 and 50:1, and lacks intraperitoneal toxicity even at high doses. However, systemic toxicity with high doses remains a problem. Various trials of intraperitoneal cisplatin, either alone or combined with other drugs such as etoposide, have demonstrated that complete remission rates of approximately 30% are obtainable in patients who have had an initial response to the platinum analogues and who have small-volume peritoneal disease (<1–2 cm) at relapse or persisting after conventional systemic chemotherapy. The impact on long-term survival is unknown. Paclitaxel may replace cisplatin for intraperitoneal therapy as the latter has been found to have a high volume of distribution within the peritoneal cavity, extremely low plasma levels and a peritoneal/plasma AUC of approximately 1000:1.

The role for intraperitoneal chemotherapy is probably small, as the depth of drug penetration is only a few millimetres, restricting benefit for this procedure to those with either minimal or microscopic residual disease. It is uncertain whether intraperitoneal chemotherapy is superior to systemic treatment, and randomized trials are therefore being carried out in previously untreated patients with Stage III disease with small-volume residuum after surgery, comparing intravenous cisplatin and cyclophosphamide with intraperitoneal cisplatin and intravenous cyclophosphamide. In addition, an EORTC study is comparing intraperitoneal cisplatin as consolidation therapy with observation alone in patients with advanced ovarian cancer with a pathological complete remission. For the present, intraperitoneal chemotherapy must be considered to be a research tool only.

OTHER TREATMENTS

Hormonal therapy

Cytoplasmic oestrogen and progesterone receptors have been detected in malignant ovarian tumours (Soutter & Leake 1987) but the use of progestogens in recurrent disease, except for giving a feeling of wellbeing, has been disappointing. Other hormones have also been of little value, but there is the occasional partial remission and disease is stabilized in approximately 14% of cases. Hormones which have been used include progestins such as megestrol, and other drugs such as tamoxifen, cyproterone acetate and the GnRH analogues goserelin and leuprorelin.

Hormone replacement therapy (HRT) is used increasingly in premenopausal women treated for ovarian cancer. A retrospective study which assessed 373 patients given HRT showed no detrimental effect on the prognosis (Eeles et al 1991).

Immunotherapy

The role of immunotherapy in ovarian carcinoma has been evaluated over many years but must be considered of unproven benefit at the present time. Early investigations were concerned with non-specific immunotherapy, using BCG (Bacille Calmette–Guérin) or *Corynebacterium parvum*. These, together with chemotherapy, appeared to lead to prolongation of response. A combination of α-interferon and low-dose doxorubicin gave encouraging results in patients with relapsing ovarian cancers (Welander 1987). α-interferon is currently being assessed in a prospective study by the Yorkshire Ovarian Group, to evaluate its role in prolonging disease-free and overall survival following chemotherapy in advanced ovarian carcinoma.

Intraperitoneal immunotherapy has been used over the last decade in a similar fashion to intraperitoneal chemotherapy, that is, for minimal residual disease, particularly after initial chemotherapy. Drugs used for this approach include *C. parvum* (Bast et al 1983b) and intraperitoneal recombinant α-interferon, (Berwick et al 1986). Complications were common with all these approaches, including severe peritoneal fibrosis. In a similar group of patients alternating recombinant α_2-interferon with cisplatin, pathological complete remissions were obtained in seven of 14 patients (Nardi et al 1990). The use of intraperitoneal immunotoxins, such as pseudomonas exotoxin and recombinant ricin A chain, attached to monoclonal antibodies is also being investigated. The use of monoclonal antibodies against the transferrin receptor or against tumour-associated antigens is under investigation (Bookman & Bast 1991, Bookman 1992).

TREATMENT OF PERSISTENT OR RECURRENT DISEASE

Most patients with advanced epithelial ovarian carcinoma will either not respond to initial treatment or will recur. In either case, cure is not a realistic goal and treatment can only be palliative, with quality of life being the first consideration. The longer the interval between the end of postoperative chemotherapy and the recurrence of the neoplasm, the greater the likelihood of the patient responding to second-line chemotherapy. The first sign of recurrence may be a persistent rise in the level of the tumour marker CA125. At present, treatment is usually delayed until the patient is symptomatic because cure is not possible at this stage. In 1995 the MRC launched a randomized trial to determine whether immediate therapy before the onset of symptoms is more beneficial than delaying therapy until recurrence is clinically apparent.

When cisplatin- or carboplatin-based chemotherapy was the initial therapy, repeating treatment with a platinum analogue is effective if there has been an interval of 6 months or longer between the end of platinum treatment and recurrence. However, when there is progression of disease on treatment, or within 6 months of platinum chemotherapy, other drugs or new experimental treatments should be considered if the patient's condition warrants it. Paclitaxel has been shown to be the most active drug at present available for platinum-resistant patients, giving response rates of approximately 30% (Vergote et al 1992b), but unfortunately remissions are usually short, with a median duration of 4 months. Oral altretamine (hexamethylmelamine) has also shown activity in platinum-resistant ovarian cancer, but with only a 14% objective response rate. High-dose iphosphamide with mesna has been found useful as salvage treatment in patients resistant to cisplatin or carboplatin (Markman et al 1992b), and oral etoposide has some efficacy as salvage treatment. The hormones detailed earlier, in particular the GnHR analogues, are sometimes useful in stabilizing disease.

RESULTS – EPITHELIAL TUMOURS

Borderline epithelial tumours

Borderline ovarian epithelial tumours have a good 5-year prognosis but the death rate continues to rise slowly thereafter. DNA ploidy appears to be the most important prognostic factor. Patients with diploid Stage I tumours have a very good prognosis but those with aneuploid tumours have a 19-fold increased risk of dying (Kaern et al 1993). Patients with aneuploid tumours are more likely to be older and to have mucinous tumours or severe atypia. The 5-year survival for serous borderline epithelial tumours is 90–95% and at 15 years is 72–86%. For mucinous tumours the survival rates are 81–91% at 5 years and 60–85% at 15 years. Stage is also a prognostic indicator for survival, being nearly 100% at 5 years for Stage I but dropping to 65–87% for Stage III.

Invasive epithelial ovarian cancer

Survival for epithelial ovarian cancer is dependent on several prognostic factors. These include stage, grade, size of residual tumour at the end of initial surgery, DNA ploidy, overexpression of some oncogenes, age over 50 years, performance status and the histological diagnosis of clear cell carcinoma.

The importance of stage can be seen from the 5-year survival figures, which range from 60 to 70% in Stage I disease to 10% in Stage III–IV. Since the majority of patients present with advanced disease, the overall 5-year survival in the UK is only 23% (Office of Population Censuses and Surveys 1988).

Whereas Stage I tumours with grade 1 or 2 histology have a 5-year survival rate of over 90% (Young et al 1990), some other Stage I cases have a worse prognosis, which may be identified by study of some of the factors mentioned above. The most important is poor differentiation of the tumour. Ploidy is also important in both early and advanced disease, with diploid tumours surviving significantly longer than those with aneuploid tumours.

In more advanced tumours stage is more important than grade for even well-differentiated tumours. Size of residual tumour at the end of initial surgery has been shown to be highly significant in terms of prognosis, although the effect of cytoreductive surgery is disputed. Age is a less important prognostic factor than residual disease, stage or grade, but older women do have a worse prognosis.

Recent work assessed the value of oncogenes as prognostic indices in ovarian carcinoma. Five oncogenes were studied by multiparameter flow cytometry in 80 patients. The oncogenes were epidermal growth factor receptor (EGFR), insulin-like growth factor 1 receptor, c-*erbB*-2, c-*ras* and c-*myc*. Overexpression of at least one oncogene was evident in up to one-third of patients, and EGFR, c-*ras* and c-*myc* indicated a worse prognosis. EGFR was the most sensitive predictor (Van Dam et al 1993).

The survival figures for cancer of the ovary have changed little over the last 20 years and remain poor for women with advanced disease, despite more radical surgery and improvements in chemotherapy. Most studies do show some improvement in median survival in patients with minimal residual disease following surgery, and who respond to postsurgical treatment. However, this benefit has not been sufficiently long-lasting to affect 5-year survival rates. There is no doubt that even if long-term survival has not been improved, modern cytotoxic therapy has improved the quality of life for many patients with advanced ovarian cancer in spite of the side effects.

NON-EPITHELIAL TUMOURS

Non-epithelial tumours constitute approximately 10% of all ovarian cancers. Because of their rarity and their sensitivity to intensive chemotherapy, it is especially appropriate to refer these patients for specialist care.

Sex cord stromal tumours

Granulosa and theca cell tumours

The most common sex cord stromal tumours are the granulosa and theca cell tumours. These often produce steroid hormones, in particular oestrogens, which can cause postmenopausal bleeding in older women and sexual precocity in prepubertal girls. The hormones may cause cystic glandular hyperplasia, or occasionally carcinoma of the endometrium (Fox & Langley 1976). Theca cell tumours are usually benign. The majority of those that are malignant contain both granulosa and theca cells, the malignant element originating in the granulosa cell. Granulosa cell tumours occur at all ages, but are found predominantly in postmenopausal women. The staging system for these tumours is the same as for epithelial tumours. Most present as Stage I. Bilateral tumours are present in only 5% of cases.

Pathology. Granulosa cell tumours are normally solid although, when they become large, cystic spaces may develop and some tumours are predominantly cystic. As with most tumours of the sex cord-stromal group, the cut surface is often yellow, reflecting the presence of neutral lipid which is related to sex steroid hormone production. Areas of haemorrhage are also common.

A variety of histological appearances are seen in granulosa cell tumours: follicular, insular, trabecular, moiré-silk and diffuse (sarcomatoid). These may occur separately but are more usually found in combination. The most characteristic pattern is the microfollicular, in which the tumour cells are arranged in large groups in which are numerous Call–Exner bodies, small rounded cavities that often contain dense eosinophilic material of basement membrane type or nuclear debris (Fig. 41.8).

Treatment. The surgical treatment is the same as for epithelial tumours. Unilateral oophorectomy is indicated only in young women with Stage Ia disease. The effect of adjunctive therapy is difficult to assess, as granulosa cell tumours can recur up to 20 years after the initial diagnosis (Lamont & Ashton 1975). For advanced and recurrent disease, radiotherapy used to be the treatment of choice as these tumours are thought to be moderately radiosensitive but this has been largely replaced by chemotherapy as for epithelial tumours.

Because of the rarity of this tumour the efficacy of chemotherapy is unknown, but regimens similar to those for epithelial ovarian cancer are used in advanced and recurrent disease. In cases of late recurrence, further surgery should be considered before any other therapy is given. The 5-year survival is around 80% overall, but recurrence is associated with a high mortality (Evans et al 1980).

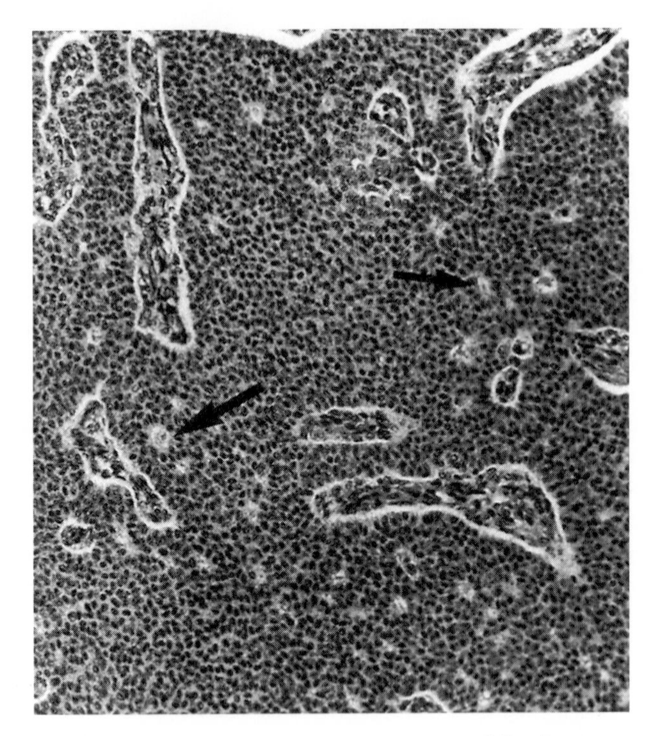

Fig. 41.8 A granulosa cell tumour showing a microfollicular pattern. Call–Exner bodies are shown with the arrows. Haematoxylin and eosin × 170.

Sertoli–Leydig cell tumours

Half of these rare neoplasia produce male hormones, which can cause virilization. Rarely oestrogens are secreted. The prognosis for the majority who have localized disease is good, and surgery as for granulosa cell tumours is the treatment of choice. Chemotherapy may be used for metastatic or recurrent disease.

Germ cell tumours

Dysgerminomas

Dysgerminomas are uncommon ovarian tumours accounting for 2–5% of all primary malignant ovarian tumours. Originating in the germ cells, 90% occur in young women less than 30 years old. They behave in a similar way to seminoma in men, spreading mainly by lymphatics to para-aortic, mediastinal and supraclavicular glands. All cases need to be investigated by chest X-ray, CT scanning and lymphangiogram. Serum AFP and βhCG must be assayed to exclude the ominous presence of elements of choriocarcinoma, endodermal sinus tumour or teratoma. Occasionally some cases of pure dysgerminoma have raised levels of βhCG and, in metastatic disease, placental alkaline phosphatase and lactate dehydrogenase are usually elevated. Pure dysgerminomas have a good prognosis as they are normally Stage I tumours (75%), most being Stage Ia (Scully 1982).

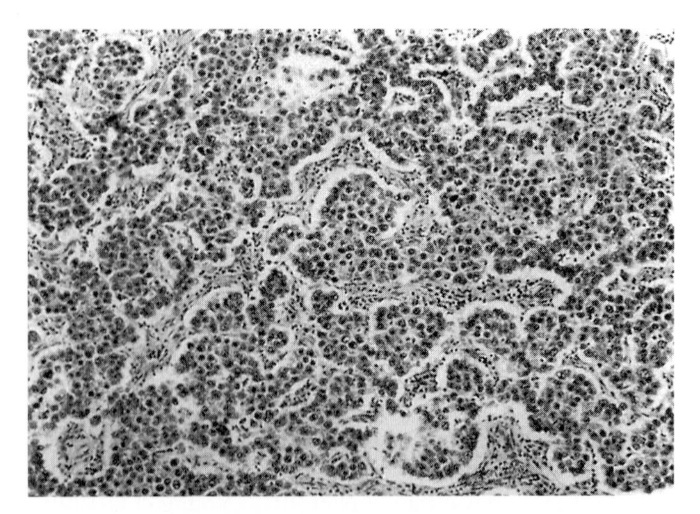

Fig. 41.9 A dysgerminoma with the typical large, pale round cells separated by fibrous septae in which a lymphocytic infiltrate is prominent. Haematoxylin and eosin × 200.

Pathology (Gordon et al 1981). Dysgerminomas are solid tumours which have a smooth or nodular bosselated external surface. They are soft or rubbery in consistency, depending upon the proportion of fibrous tissue contained in them. They may reach a considerable size: the mean diameter is 15 cm. Approximately 10% are bilateral; they are alone among malignant germ cell tumours in having a significant incidence of bilaterality.

Dysgerminoma is composed of groups of large, round tumour cells separated by fibrous tissue septae infiltrated by lymphocytes (Fig. 41.9). The tumour cells possess abundant pale, slightly eosinophilic cytoplasm which contains glycogen, lipid and alkaline phosphatase, the last being situated predominantly in the periphery of the cell. A minimal lymphocytic response, a high mitotic count, capsular penetration, and intraovarian lymphatic or vascular invasion are all associated with a decreased survival.

Immature teratoma, yolk sac tumour or choriocarcinoma are found in 6.7–13.8% of dysgerminomas. Very thorough sampling of all dysgerminomas must be undertaken by the histopathologist to exclude the presence of these more malignant germ cell elements, as this indicates a worse prognosis.

Treatment. A germ cell tumour should be suspected prior to surgery if a young woman has what appears to be a predominantly solid tumour on ultrasound examination. Such patients should be referred to a gynaecological oncologist.

Early disease is treated by surgery. In young women with Stage Ia disease, unilateral oophorectomy may suffice but in older patients hysterectomy and bilateral salpingo-oophorectomy is recommended. Women are suitable for conservative surgery if they have a unilateral encapsulated tumour, no ascites, no evidence of abnormal lymph nodes at surgery and a negative CT scan of the para-aortic nodes.

In the past radiotherapy was used for metastatic or recurrent disease, and good results were obtained in cases of pure dysgerminoma with whole-abdominal radiotherapy. As this is a very radiosensitive tumour, doses as low as 2000–2500 cGy in 2–3 weeks to the pelvis and para-aortic nodes were recommended, unless the nodes were grossly involved, when 3000–4000 cGy were needed. The mediastinal and supraclavicular nodes were also treated if there was evidence of para-aortic node involvement.

However, chemotherapy has replaced radiotherapy in the treatment of metastatic and recurrent dysgerminoma, particularly in the young age groups in which this tumour is most common, as fertility is likely to be preserved. Chemotherapy may be given prior to surgery if the diagnosis has been made histologically by Tru-cut biopsy. Chemotherapy is the treatment of choice for mixed tumours with other malignant elements, as these are not radiosensitive. The regimens used are discussed below.

Other germ cell tumours

Germ cell tumours other than dysgerminoma also occur in young women under 30. Their very poor prognosis has been greatly improved by combination chemotherapy. Their derivation from germ cells is shown in Figure 41.10 (Teilum 1965). Mature teratomas are benign, the most common being the cystic teratoma or dermoid cyst found at all ages, but particularly in the third and fourth decades.

Tumour markers are of value in diagnosis, in monitoring therapy and in early detection of recurrence. The two main markers are α-fetoprotein (AFP), produced by yolk sac cells, and βhCG from the syncytiotrophoblast.

Pathology of yolk sac (endodermal sinus) tumours (Kurman & Norris 1976). Yolk sac tumour is the second most common malignant germ cell tumour of the ovary, making up 10–15% overall and reaching a higher proportion in children. It may present as an acute abdomen owing to rupture of the tumour following necrosis and haemorrhage.

The tumour is usually well encapsulated and solid. Areas of necrosis and haemorrhage are often seen, as are small cystic spaces. Its consistency varies from soft to firm and rubbery, and its cut surface is slippery and mucoid.

The yolk sac tumour is characterized by the presence of a variety of patterns. The background of the tumour is a loose vacuolated network of microcysts lined by flat cells of mesothelial appearance. The most characteristic feature is the endodermal sinus (Schiller–Duval body). A constant finding is periodic acid–Schiff (PAS)-positive hyaline globules containing AFP and other metabolic products of the normal yolk sac.

Pathology of immature teratomas. These tumours are solid and often malignant. It should be noted that solid teratomas are not all of immature type. Immature teratomas are composed of a wide variety of tissues and comprise about 1% of all ovarian teratomas.

The tumours are unilateral in almost all cases, and appear as solid masses with smooth and bosselated surfaces. The cut surface shows mainly solid tissue, although small cystic spaces are visible. The tumour is very heterogeneous and areas of bone and cartilage may be apparent and hair may be seen. The most conspicuous feature is usually the soft, pale pink to cream-coloured immature neural tissue. Both the gross appearance and the histology may resemble a benign teratoma owing to the presence of these mature elements. The amount of embryonal tissue and its degree of atypia and mitotic activity correlate with the prognosis. Rosettes of tightly packed neuroectodermal cells with dark nuclei are usually the most conspicuous feature (Fig. 41.11).

A careful search must be made for elements of yolk sac tumour and choriocarcinoma; the presence of these may have a bearing on prognosis and treatment, particularly if the teratoma is of low grade. Blood levels of βhCG and AFP should be estimated to exclude their presence, even when the tumour appears to be a straightforward immature teratoma.

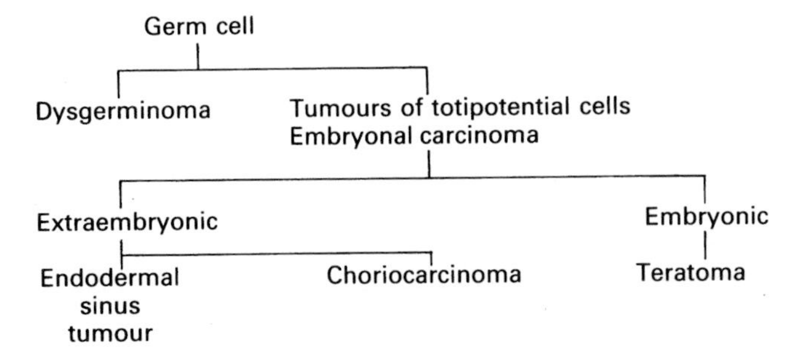

Fig. 41.10 The derivation of germ cell tumours.

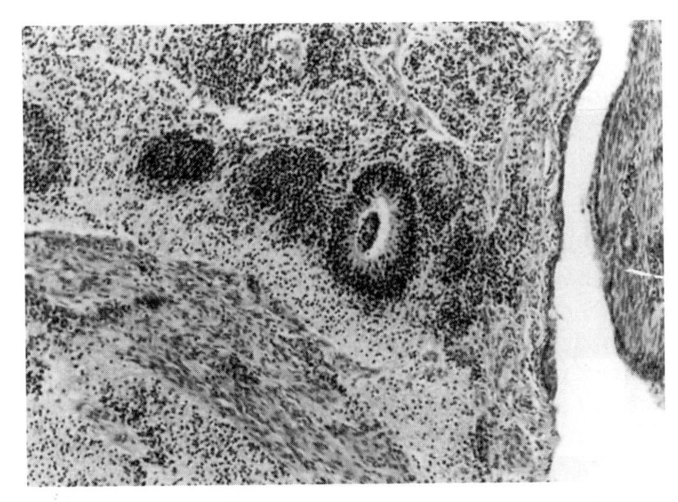

Fig. 41.11 An immature teratoma with prominent neuroectodermal tissue and a well-formed rosette. Haematoxylin and eosin × 170.

Chemotherapy for non-epithelial tumours

Following conservative surgery to establish the diagnosis, remove the primary lesion and stage the disease, the main treatment is combination chemotherapy, except for Stage I malignant teratomas, which may be followed up closely.

Many combinations have been used, the most common being VAC (vincristine, actinomycin D and cyclophosphamide) (Cangir et al 1978). These regimens, which were given for periods of up to 2 years, have now been superseded by much shorter courses of cisplatin chemotherapy given in combination with bleomycin and etoposide (BEP), which is curative in the 90% of patients with testicular teratoma without adverse features such as very high tumour markers, very bulky disease or involvement of the liver or central nervous system.

More intensive regimens are being evaluated for patients with adverse features. A short but intensive course of chemotherapy, the POMB/ACE regimen, is given at the Charing Cross Hospital. This regimen alternates cisplatin, vincristine, methotrexate and bleomycin with actinomycin D, cyclophosphamide and etoposide. Cycles are repeated every 2 weeks for three to five courses. This regimen does not interfere with fertility, and children born to mothers who have received this chemotherapy develop normally with no evidence of endocrine dysfunction (Newlands & Bagshawe 1987).

OVARIAN CARCINOMA – CONCLUSIONS

Epithelial ovarian carcinoma is still a difficult tumour to treat, partly because of its late presentation and partly because no truly effective therapy has yet been developed. Surgery remains an important part of the management. Prolonged survival is only possible when the tumour can be virtually completely excised. Chemotherapy has had a major impact on the rare, germ cell tumours. Although less effective in the common epithelial malignancies, chemotherapy does substantially extend the life expectancy of many patients.

CANCER OF THE FALLOPIAN TUBE

Cancers of the fallopian tube can be either primary or secondary. Most tumours involving the fallopian tube are metastatic from ovarian cancer, but secondary spread from the breast and gastrointestinal tract also occur. Primary carcinoma is usually unilateral. It is thought to be extremely rare, comprising only 0.3% of gynaecological malignancies. However, only early fallopian tube carcinomas can be distinguished with certainty from ovarian disease. A study of the use of CA125 in screening for ovarian carcinoma detected three cases of early fallopian tube carcinoma and 19 ovarian tumours (Woolas et al 1994). This prevalence of fallopian tube lesions is 25-fold greater than expected. This may be due to a greater sensitivity of CA125 for these tumours or, more probably, they are more common than is realized.

Most present after the menopause, the mean age being 56 years. Many of the patients are nulliparous (45%) and infertility is reported in up to 71% of these women. Tumour spread is identical to that of ovarian cancer, and metastases to pelvic and para-aortic nodes are common.

PATHOLOGY

Because of the histological similarity between serous ovarian carcinoma and primary tubal carcinoma, strict criteria must be applied before the diagnosis of tubal carcinoma can be made. Carcinoma of the fallopian tube usually distends the lumen with tumour. The tumour may protrude through the fimbrial end and the tube may be retort-shaped, resembling a hydrosalpinx. It is typically very similar to the serous adenocarcinoma of the ovary histologically (Fig. 41.12). The predominant pattern is papillary, with a gradation through alveolar to solid as the degree of differentiation decreases.

STAGING

The FIGO clinical staging is similar to that used for ovarian cancer (Table 41.4). Probably because of the difficulty in distinguishing between advanced ovarian and advanced fallopian tube carcinoma, 74% of fallopian tube carcinomas are diagnosed at Stage I–IIa; the remaining 26% are Stage IIb–IV (Hellström et al 1994).

CLINICAL PRESENTATION AND MANAGEMENT

Most cases of cancer of the fallopian tube are diagnosed at laparotomy: the diagnosis is seldom considered preoperatively. The usual presenting symptom is postmenopausal

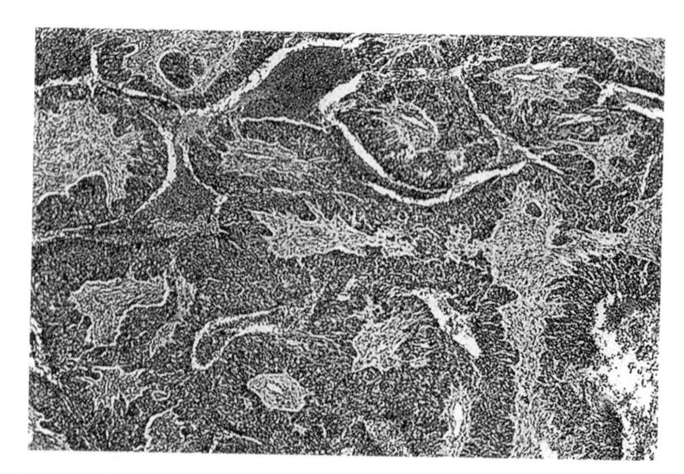

Fig. 41.12 A rather poorly differentiated serous adenocarcinoma of the fallopian tube in which the papillary pattern is still recognizable. Haematoxylin and eosin × 100.

Table 41.4 FIGO staging for fallopian tube carcinoma

Stage	FIGO definition
0	Carcinoma in situ – limited to the tubal mucosa
I	Growth limited to the fallopian tubes
	Ia One tube involved with extension into the submucosa or muscularis. Not penetrating the serosal surface. No ascites
	Ib Both tubes involved but otherwise as for Ia
	Ic One or both tubes with extension through or onto the tubal serosa; or ascites with malignant cells; or positive peritoneal washings
II	Growth involving one or both fallopian tubes with pelvic extension
	IIa Extension or metastases to the uterus or ovaries
	IIb Extension to other pelvic organs
	IIc Stage IIa or IIb plus ascites with malignant cells; or positive peritoneal washings
III	Tumour involves one or both fallopian tubes with peritoneal implants outside the pelvis or positive retroperitoneal or inguinal nodes. Superficial liver metastases equals Stage III. Tumour appears limited to the true pelvis but with histologically proven malignant extension to the small bowel or omentum
	IIIa Tumour is grossly limited to the true pelvis with negative lymph nodes but with histologically confirmed microscopic seeding of abdominal peritoneal surfaces
	IIIb Tumour involving one or both tubes with histologically confirmed implants of abdominal peritoneal surfaces, none exceeding 2 cm in diameter. Lymph nodes are negative
	IIIc Abdominal implants greater than 2 cm in diameter or positive retroperitoneal or inguinal nodes
IV	Growth involving one or both fallopian tubes with distant metastases. If pleural effusion is present there must be positive cytology. Parenchymal liver metastases equals Stage IV

Note: Staging for fallopian tube cancer is by the surgical pathological system. Operative findings designating stage are determined prior to tumour debulking.

bleeding and the diagnosis should be considered particularly if the patient also complains of a watery discharge and lower abdominal pain. Unexplained postmenopausal bleeding or abnormal cervical cytology without obvious cause demands a careful bimanual examination and pelvic ultrasound. Laparoscopy may be required in doubtful cases.

The management of cancer of the fallopian tube is as for cancer of the ovary, with surgery to remove gross tumour. This will almost always involve a total abdominal hysterectomy and bilateral salpingo-oophorectomy. Postoperative chemotherapy will be required with platinum analogues for all but the earliest cases. The treatment of carcinoma metastatic to the fallopian tube is determined by the management of the primary tumour.

RESULTS

The overall 5-year survival rate is around 35%. The prognosis is improved if the tumour is detected early. The 5-year survival for Stage I is in the region of 70%. The 5-year survival for Stage Ia cases is in the region of 70%, but in Stages Ib–IIIc survival falls to 25–30% (Hellström et al 1994). Chemotherapy with platinum agents improves the survival.

KEY POINTS

1. Epithelial ovarian cancer most often occurs between the ages of 45 and 65 years. The disease is usually advanced at presentation, and except when confined to the ovaries and well or moderately well differentiated, it has a poor prognosis.
2. Oral contraceptive use protects against the development of ovarian cancer.
3. Inheritance plays a significant role in approximately 5% of epithelial ovarian cancers. The *BRCA1* gene is associated with 80% of families with both breast and ovarian cancer, but the risk of ovarian cancer alone is variable. *BRCA1* does not appear to be responsible for many sporadic cases of ovarian cancers.
4. Population screening for ovarian cancer is not yet justified with the techniques evaluated so far.
5. Standard treatment at the present time is surgery followed by a platinum-based chemotherapy regimen. This approach allows many women to lead a relatively symptom-free life for periods of up to 2–3 years.
6. Chemotherapy of epithelial ovarian tumours with platinum agents, either alone or in combination, will prolong the patient's life but is unlikely to result in an improved long-term survival. New chemotherapeutic drugs such as paclitaxel have not been assessed for long enough to establish whether they will lead to an improvement in this situation, but early studies with paclitaxel are promising, particularly in combination with the platinum analogues.
7. At present the biological factors inherent in each tumour, rather than treatment, determine survival.
8. Germ cell tumours occur in young women. They have a much better prognosis than the epithelial tumours. Chemotherapy for germ cell tumours is effective even in advanced and recurrent cases, and fertility can be preserved. A young woman with a solid ovarian tumour should be referred to a gynaecological oncologist. If the diagnosis is made postoperatively she should always be referred to a specialist team.
9. Primary carcinoma of the fallopian tube is treated like ovarian carcinoma.

REFERENCES

Acheson E D, Gardner M J, Pippard E C, Grime L P 1982 Mortality of groups of women who manufactured gas masks from chrysotile and crocidolite asbestos: a 40 year follow-up. British Journal of Industrial Medicine 39: 344–348

Adami H-O, Hsieh C-C, Lambe M et al 1994 Parity, age at first childbirth, and risk of ovarian cancer. Lancet 344: 1250–1254

Advanced Ovarian Cancer Trialists Group 1991 Chemotherapy in advanced ovarian cancer: an overview of randomised clinical trials. British Medical Journal 303: 884–893

Anderson M C 1987 Histopathology – a guide to prognosis and treatment. In: Sharp F, Soutter W P (eds) Ovarian cancer – the way ahead. The Seventeenth Study Group of the Royal College of Obstetricians and Gynaecologists. Royal College of Obstetricians and Gynaecologists, London, pp 55–68

Anderson M C, Langley F A 1970 Mesonephroid tumours of the ovary. Journal of Clinical Pathology 23: 210–218

Barker G H, Orledge J, Wiltshaw E 1981 Involvement of the central nervous system in patients with ovarian carcinoma. British Journal of Obstetrics and Gynaecology 88: 690–699

Bast R C, Klug T I, St John E et al 1983a A radio-immunoassay using a monoclonal antibody to monitor the course of epithelial ovarian cancer. New England Journal of Medicine 309: 883–887

Bast R C, Berek J S, Obrist R et al 1983b Intraperitoneal immunotherapy of human ovarian carcinoma with corynebacterium parvum. Cancer Research 43: 1395–1401

Bast R C, Xu F J, Rodriguez G C et al 1992 Inhibition of breast and ovarian tumour cell growth by antibodies and immunotoxins reactive with distinct epitopes on the extracellular domain of HER-2/*neu* (c-*erbB2*). In: Sharp F, Mason W P, Creasman W (eds) Ovarian cancer 2: Biology, diagnosis and management. Chapman & Hall, London, pp 67–71

Benedet J L, White G W, Fairey R N, Boyes D A 1977 Adenocarcinoma of the fallopian tube: experience with 41 patients. Obstetrics and Gynecology 50: 654–657

Berchuck A, Kamel A, Whitaker R et al 1990 Overexpression of HER-2/*neu* is associated with poor survival in advanced ovarian cancer. Cancer Research 50: 4087–4091

Bertelsen K 1990 Tumour reduction surgery and long term survival in advanced ovarian cancer: a DACOVA study. Gynecologic Oncology 38: 203–209

Berwick J S, Hacker N F, Lichtenstein A et al 1986 Intraperitoneal recombinant α-interferon for 'salvage' immunotherapy in Stage III epithelial ovarian carcinoma: Gynecologic Group Study. Seminars in Oncology 13: 61–71

Blyth J G, Wahl T P 1982 Debulking surgery: does it increase the quality of survival? Gynecologic Oncology 14: 396-406

Bookman M A 1992 Immunotoxin therapy in ovarian cancer. In: Sharp F, Mason W P, Creasman W (eds) Ovarian cancer 2: Biology, diagnosis and management. Chapman & Hall, London pp 153–160

Bookman M A, Bast R C 1991 The immunobiology and immunotherapy of ovarian cancer. Seminars in Oncology 18: 270–291

Bourne T H, Campbell S, Reynolds K M et al 1993 Screening for early familial ovarian cancer with transvaginal ultrasonography and colour blood flow imaging. British Medical Journal 306: 1025–1029

Burger H G 1993 Clinical utility of inhibin measurements. Journal of Clinical and Endocrinological Metabolism 76: 1391–1396

Burghardt E, Girardi F, Lahousen M, Tamussino K, Stettner H 1991 Patterns of pelvic and paraaortic lymph node involvement in ovarian cancer. Gynecologic Oncology 40: 103–106

Calvert A H, Newell D R, Gumbrell S et al 1989 Carboplatin dosage: prospective evaluation of a simple formula based on renal function. Journal of Clinical Oncology 7: 1748–1757

Cancer and Steroid Hormone Study of the Centre for Disease Control and the National Institute of Child Health and Human Development 1987 The reduction in risk of ovarian cancer associated with oral contraceptive use. New England Journal of Medicine 316: 650–655

Cangir A, Smith J , van Eys J 1978 Improved prognosis in children with ovarian cancers following modified VAC (vincristin sulfate, dactinomycin and cyclophosphamide) chemotherapy. Cancer 42: 1234–1238

Canney P S, Moore M, Wilkinson P M, Jones R D 1984 Ovarian cancer antigen CA125: a prospective clinical assessment of its role as a tumour marker. British Journal of Cancer 50: 765–769

Cannistra S A 1993 Cancer of the ovary. New England Journal of Medicine 329: 1550–1559

Chen S S, Brochner R 1985 Assessment of morbidity and mortality in primary cytoreductive surgery for advanced ovarian cancer. Gynecologic Oncology 20: 109–195

Cramer D W, Welch W R, Scully R E, Wojciechowski C A 1982 Ovarian cancer and talc: a case controlled study. Cancer 50: 371–376

Creasman W T, Clarke-Pearson D L 1984 Ovarian cancer: post-operative management. In: Forastiere A A (ed) Gynecologic cancer – contemporary issues in clinical oncology. Churchill Livingstone, Edinburgh, pp 139–255

Currie J L, Bagne F, Harris C et al 1981 Radioactive chromic phosphate suspension: studies on distribution, dose absorption and effective therapeutic radiation in phantoms, dogs and patients. Gynecologic Oncology 12: 193–218

Czernobilsky B, Silverman B B, Mikuta J J 1970 Endometrioid carcinoma of the ovary. A clinicopathologic study of 75 cases. Cancer 26: 1141–1152

Dembo A J 1987 Epithelial ovarian cancer: radiotherapy for minimal disease. In: Sharp F, Soutter W P (eds) Ovarian cancer – the way ahead. The Seventeenth Study Group of the Royal College of Obstetricians and Gynaecologists. Royal College of Obstetricians and Gynaecologists, London, pp 409–425

Dembo A J 1992 Epithelial ovarian cancer: the role of radiotherapy. International Journal of Radiation Oncology Biology and Physics 22: 835–845

Dembo A J, Bush R S, Beale F A et al 1979 The Princess Margaret Hospital Study of ovarian cancer: Staged I, II and asymptomatic III presentations. Cancer Treatment Reports 63: 249–254

Dembo A J, Davy M, Stenwig A E et al 1990 Prognostic factors in patients with Stage I epithelial ovarian cancer. Obstetrics and Gynecology 75: 263–273

Denham J W, MacLennan K A 1984 The management of primary carcinoma of the fallopian tube: experience of 40 cases. Cancer 53: 166–172

Dhokia B, Canney P, Pectasides D et al 1987 A new immunoassay using monoclonal antibodies HMFG1 and HMFG2 together with an existing marker CA125 for the serological detection and management of epithelial ovarian cancer. British Journal of Cancer 54: 891–895

Eeles R A, Tan S, Wiltshaw E et al 1991 Hormone replacement therapy and survival after surgery for ovarian cancer. British Medical Journal 302: 259–262

Eng C, Stratton M, Ponder B et al 1994 Familial cancer syndromes. Lancet 343: 709–713

Epenetos A A, Britton K E, Mather S et al 1982 Targeting of iodine-123-labelled tumour-associated monoclonal antibodies to ovarian, breast and gastro-intestinal tumours. Lancet ii: 999–1004

Evans A T, Gaffey T A, Malkasian G D, Annegers J F 1980 Clinicpathologic review of 118 granulosa and 82 theca cell tumours. Obstetrics and Gynecology 55: 231–238

Fox H 1985 Pathology of surface epithelial tumours. In: Hudson C N (ed) Ovarian cancer. Oxford University Press, Oxford, pp 72–93

Fox H 1987 Prognostic indices in ovarian tumours of borderline malignancy with particular reference to morphometric analysis. In: Sharp F, Soutter W P (eds) Ovarian cancer – the way ahead. The Seventeenth Study Group of the Royal College of Obstetricians and Gynaecologists. Royal College of Obstetricians and Gynaecologists, London, pp 69–78

Fox H 1992 Novel approaches to the management of gynecological malignancies: Proceedings of a satellite symposium held in Cairns, Australia, on 22 September 1991. International Journal of Gynecological Cancer 2 (Suppl 1)

Fox H, Langley F A 1976 Tumours of the ovary. Heinemann, London, pp 119–137

Friedlander M L, Hedley D W, Taylor I W et al 1984 Influence of cellular DNA content on survival in advanced ovarian cancer. Cancer Research 44: 397–400
Futreal P A, Liu Q, Shattuck-Eidens D et al 1994 BRCA1 mutations in primary breast and ovarian carcinomas. Science 266: 120–122
Gordon A, Lipton D, Woodruff J D 1981 Dysgerminoma; a review of 158 cases from the Emil Novak ovarian tumor registry. Obstetrics and Gynecology 58: 497–504
Gore M E, Rustin G, Slevin M et al 1995 Single agent paclitaxel in previously untreated patients with Stage IV epithelial ovarian cancer [abstract]. Proceeding of the American Society for Clinical Oncology 14: 269
Griffiths C T 1987 Carcinoma of the ovary: surgical objectives. In: Sharp F, Soutter W P (eds) Ovarian cancer – the way ahead. The Seventeenth Study Group of the Royal College of Obstetricians and Gynaecologists. Royal College of Obstetricians and Gynaecologists, London, pp 235–244
Griffiths C T, Parker L M, Fuller A F J 1979 Role of cytoreductive surgical treatment in the management of advanced ovarian cancer. Cancer Treatment Reports 63: 235–240
Gruppo Interregional Cooperativo Oncologico Ginecologia 1987 Randomised comparison of cisplatin with cyclophosphamide/cisplatin and with cyclophosphamide/doxorubicin/cisplatin in advanced ovarian cancer. Lancet ii: 353–359
Hacker N F, Berek J S, Lagasse L D et al 1983 Primary cytoreductive surgery for epithelial ovarian cancer. Obstetrics and Gynecology 61: 413–420
Hakes T B, Chalas E, Hoskins W J et al 1992 Randomised prospective trial of 5 versus 10 cycles of cyclophosphamide, doxorubicin and cisplatin in advanced ovarian carcinoma. Gynecologic Oncology 45: 284–289
Hamilton T, O'Dwyer P, Young R et al 1990 Phase I trial of buthionine sulfoximine (BSO) plus melphalan (L-PAM) in patients with advanced cancer. Proceedings of the American Society for Clinical Oncology 9: 73
Hammersmith Oncology Group and the Imperial Cancer Research Fund 1984 Antibody-guided irradiation of malignant lesions: three cases illustrating a new method of treatment. Lancet i: 1441–1443
Heintz A P M, Hacker N F, Berek J S et al 1986 Cytoreductive surgery in ovarian carcinoma: feasibility and morbidity. Obstetrics and Gynecology 67: 783–788
Hellström A-C, Silfverswärd C, Nilsson B, Pettersson F 1994 Carcinoma of the fallopian tube. A clinical and histopathological review. The Radiumhemmet series. International Journal of Gynecologic Cancer 4: 395–400
Hildreth N G, Kelsey J L, LiVolsi V A et al 1981 An epidemiological study of epithelial carcinoma of the ovary. American Journal of Epidemiology 114: 389–405
Hird V, Maraveyas A, Snook D et al 1993 Adjuvant therapy of ovarian cancer with radioactive monoclonal antibody. British Journal of Cancer 68: 403–406
Hosking L, Trowsdale J, Nicolai H et al 1995 A somatic BRCA1 mutation in an ovarian tumour. Nature Genetics 9: 343–344
Hoskins W J, Bundy B N, Thigpen J T, Omura G A 1992 The influence of cytoreductive surgery on recurrence-free interval and survival in small-volume stage III epithelial ovarian cancer: a Gynecologic Oncology Group study. Gynecologic Oncology 47: 159–166
Hunter R W, Alexander N D E, Soutter W P 1992 Meta-analysis of surgery in advanced ovarian carcinoma: is maximum cytoreductive surgery an independent determinant of prognosis? American Journal of Obstetrics and Gynecology 166: 504–511
Jacobs I, Bridges J, Reynolds C et al 1988 Multimodal approach to screening for ovarian cancer. Lancet i: 268–271
Jacobs I, Davies A P, Bridges J et al 1993 Prevalence screening for ovarian cancer in postmenopausal women by CA125 measurement and ultrasonography. British Medical Journal 306: 1030–1034
Johnson I R, Symonds E M, Kean D M, Worthington B S 1984 Imaging ovarian tumours by nuclear magnetic resonance. British Journal of Obstetrics and Gynaecology 91: 260–264
Kaern J, Tropé C G, Kristensen V M et al 1993 DNA ploidy: the most important prognostic factor in patients with borderline tumors of the ovary. International Journal of Gynecologic Cancer 3: 349–358
Kaye S B, Lewis C R, Paul J et al 1992 Randomised study of two doses of cisplatin with cyclophosphamide in epithelial ovarian cancer. Lancet 340: 329–333
King M C, Rowell S, Love S M 1993 Inherited breast and ovarian cancer. What are the risks? What are the choices? Journal of the American Medical Association 269: 1975–1980
Klaassen D, Starravald A, Shelly W et al 1985 External beam pelvic radiotherapy plus intraperitoneal radioactive chromic phosphate in early stage ovarian cancer: a toxic combination. A National Cancer Institute of Canada Clinical Trials Group Report. International Journal of Radiation Oncology Biology and Physics 11: 1801–1804
Krebs H B, Goplerud D R, Kilpatrick S J et al 1986 Role of CA125 as a tumour marker in ovarian carcinoma. Obstetrics and Gynecology, 67: 473–477
Kurman R J, Norris H J 1976 Endodermal sinus tumour of the ovary; a clinical and pathological analysis of 71 cases. Cancer 38: 2404–2419
Lambert H E 1987 The value of CA125 serum assay in the management of ovarian cancer. British Journal of Obstetrics and Gynaecology 94: 193–195
Lambert H E, Berry R J 1985 High dose cis-platinum compared with high dose cyclophosphamide in the management of advanced epithelial ovarian cancer Stage III and IV: a report from the North Thames Co-operative Group. British Medical Journal 290: 889–893
Lambert H E, Rustin G, Gregory W, Nelstrop A 1993 A randomised trial comparing single agent carboplatin with carboplatin followed by radiotherapy for advanced ovarian cancer: A North Thames Ovary Study group. Journal of Clinical Oncology 11: 440–448
Lambert H E, Rustin G J S, Gregory W et al 1995 A randomised trial of 5 versus 8 courses of cisplatin or carboplatin in advanced ovarian pregnancy [abstract]. Brtish Journal of Cancer 72, Suppl XXV: 7
Lamont C A R, Ashton P W 1975 Observations on granulosa cell tumours. In: Watteville H D E (ed) Diagnosis and treatment of ovarian neoplastic alterations. Exerpta Medica, Amsterdam, pp 241–248
Lawton F, Chan K K, Hilton C et al 1987 Intervention debulking surgery. In: Sharp F, Soutter W P (eds) Ovarian cancer – the way ahead. The Seventeenth Study Group of the Royal College of Obstetricians and Gynaecologists. Royal College of Obstetricians and Gynaecologists, London, pp 285–296
Longo D L, Young R C 1979 Cosmetic talc and ovarian cancer. Lancet ii: 349–351
Luesley D M, Lawton F G, Chan K K et al 1987 Second look laparotomy. In: Sharp F, Soutter W P (eds) Ovarian cancer – the way ahead. The Seventeenth Study Group of the Royal College of Obstetricians and Gynaecologists. Royal College of Obstetricians and Gynaecologists, London, pp 297–312
McGuire W P, Rowinsky E K 1991 Old drugs revisited, new drugs, and experimental approaches in ovarian cancer therapy. Seminars in Oncology 18: 255–269
McGuire W P, Hoskins W J, Brady M F et al 1996 Comparison of combination therapy with paclitaxel and cisplatin versus cyclophosphamide and cisplatin in patients with suboptimal stage III ovarian cancer. International Journal of Gynecologic Cancer 6, Suppl 1: 2–8
Malkasian G D, Decker D G, Webb M J 1975 Histology of epithelial tumours of the ovary. Clinical usefulness and prognostic significance of the histological classification and grading. Seminars in Oncology 2: 191–202
Manetta A, MacNeill C, Lyter J A et al 1990 Hexamethylmelamine as a single second-line agent in ovarian cancer. Gynecologic Oncology 36: 93–96
Markman M, Berek J S, Blessing J A et al 1992a Characteristics of patients with small-volume residual ovarian cancer unresponsive to cisplatin-based IP chemotherapy: lessons learned from a Gynaecology Oncology Group phase II trial of IP cisplatin and recombinant alpha-interferon. Gynecologic Oncology 45: 3–8
Markman M L, Hakes T, Reichman B et al 1992b Ifosfamide and mesna in previously treated advanced epithelial ovarian cancer. Activity in platinum resistant disease. Journal of Clinical Oncology 10: 243–248
Marks J R, Davidoff A M, Kerns B J M et al 1991 Overexpression and

mutation of p53 in epithelial ovarian cancer. Cancer Research 51: 2979–2984
Merajver S D, Pham T M, Caduff R L et al 1995 Somatic mutations in the BRCA1 gene in sporadic ovarian tumours. Nature Genetics 9: 439–443
Miki Y, Swensen J, Shattuck-Eidens D et al 1994 A strong candidate for the breast and ovarian cancer susceptibility gene BRCA1. Science 266: 66–71
Musemeci R, De Palo G, Korda K et al 1980 Retroperitoneal metastases from ovarian carcinoma: reassessment of 365 patients studied with lymphography. American Journal of Roentgenology 134: 449–452
Nardi M, Cognetti F, Pollera C F et al 1990 Intraperitoneal recombinant alpha-22-interferon alternating with cisplatin as salvage therapy for minimal residual-disease ovarian cancer: a phase II study. Journal of Clinical Oncology 8: 1036–1041
Naylor M S, Burke F, Balkwill F R 1995 Cytokines and ovarian cancer. In: Sharp F, Mason P, Blackett T, Berek J (eds) Ovarian cancer 3. London, Chapman & Hall, pp 89–97
Newlands E S, Bagshawe K D 1987 Advances in the treatment of germ cell tumours of the ovary. In: Bonnar J (ed) Recent advances in obstetrics and gynaecology. Churchill Livingstone, Edinburgh, pp 143–156
Office of Population Censuses and Surveys 1988 Monitor MB1 88/1 Cancer Survival 1981 registrations, HMSO, London
Oram D H, Jeyarajah A R 1994 The role of ultrasound and tumour markers in the early detection of ovarian cancer. British Journal of Obstetrics and Gynaecology 101: 939–945
Order S E, Rosenheim N, Klein J L et al 1981 The integration of new therapies and radiation in the management of ovarian cancer. Cancer 48: 590–596
Ovarian Tumour Panel of the Royal College of Obstetricians and Gynaecologists 1983 Ovarian epithelial tumours of borderline malignancy: pathological features and current status. British Journal of Obstetrics and Gynaecology 90: 743–750
Ozols R F, Young R C 1991 Ovarian cancer: where to next? Seminars in Oncology 18: 307–310
Piver M S, Baker T 1986 The potential optimal cytoreductive surgery in advanced ovarian cancer at a tertiary medical centre: a prospective study. Gynecologic Oncology 24: 1–8
Ponder B 1994 Breast cancer genes – searches begin and end. Nature 371: 279
Ponder B A J, Peto J, Easton D F 1992 Familial ovarian cancer. In: Sharp F, Mason W P, Creasman W (eds) Ovarian cancer 2: Biology, diagnosis and management. London, Chapman & Hall, pp 3–7
Potter M E, Partridge E E, Hatch K D, Soong S-J, Austin J M, Shingleton H M 1991 Primary surgical therapy of ovarian cancer: how much and when? Gynecologic Oncology 40: 195–200
Redman C W E, Warwick J, Luesley D M, Varma R, Lawton F G, Blackledge G P R 1994 Intervention debulking surgery in advanced epithelial ovarian cancer. British Journal of Obstetrics and Gynaecology 101: 142–146
Rodriguez G C, Berchuck A, Whitaker R S et al 1991 Epidermal growth factor expression in normal ovarian epithelium and ovarian cancer. II. Relationship between receptor expression and response to epidermal growth factor. American Journal of Obstetrics and Gynecology 164: 745–750
Rosenoff S H, Devita V T, Hubbard S, Young R C 1975 Peritoneoscopy in the staging and follow-up of ovarian cancer. Seminars in Oncology 2: 223–228
Rossing M A, Daling J R, Weiss N S, Moore D E, Self S G 1994 Ovarian tumours in a cohort of infertile women. New England Journal of Medicine 331: 771–776
Scrapart G, Smith J P, Routledge F, Eclosse L 1978 The treatment for dysgerminoma of the ovary. Cancer 41: 986–990
Scully R E 1982 Special ovarian tumours and their management. International Journal of Radiation Biology and Physics 8: 1419–1421
Serov S F, Scully R E, Sobin L H 1973 International classification of tumours no 9. Histological typing of ovarian tumours. World Health Organization, Geneva
Sjovall K, Nilsson B, Einhorn N 1994 Different types of rupture of the tumour capsule and the impact on survival in early ovarian carcinoma. International Journal of Gynecologic Cancer 4: 333–336
Sorbe B, Frankendal B, Verres B 1982 Importance of histological grading in the prognosis of epithelial ovarian cancer. Obstetrics and Gynecology 59: 576–582
Soutter W P, Leake R E 1987 Steroid hormone receptors in gynaecological cancers. In: Bonnar J (ed) Recent advances in obstetrics and gynaecology. Churchill Livingstone, Edinburgh, pp 175–194
Suzuki M, Ohwada M, Aida I et al 1993 Macrophage colony-stimulating factor as a tumour marker for epithelial ovarian cancer. Obstetrics and Gynecology 82: 946–950
Swenerton K, Eisenhauer E, Huinink WtB et al 1993 Taxol in relapsed ovarian cancer. High vs low dose and short vs long infusion: a European–Canadian study coordinated by the NCI Canada Clinical Trials Group. Proceedings of the American Society for Clinical Oncology 12: 810
Teilum G 1965 Classification of endodermal sinus tumours (mesoblastoma vitellinum) and so called 'embryonal carcinoma' of the ovary. Acta Pathologica Microbiologica 64: 407
Thigpen J T, Vance R B, Khansur T 1993 Second-line chemotherapy for recurrent carcinoma of the ovary. Cancer 71: 559–564
Trimble E L, Adams J D, Vena D et al 1993 Paclitaxel for platinum-refractory ovarian cancer: Results from the first 1,000 patients registered to National Cancer Institute Treatment Referral Centre 9103. Journal of Clinical Oncology 11: 2405–2410
Van Dam P A, Vergote I B, Lowe D G et al 1993 Epidermal growth factor receptor expression is an independent prognostic factor in ovarian cancer. International Journal of Gynecologic Cancer 3, (Suppl 1): 51
Van der Berg M E, van Lent M, Buyse M et al 1995 The effect of debulking surgery after induction chemotherapy on the prognosis in advanced epithelial ovarian cancer. New England Journal of Medicine 332: 629–634
Van Nagell J R 1983 Tumour markers in gynaecologic malignancies. In: Griffiths C T, Fuller A F (eds) Gynecologic Oncology, Martinus Nijhoff, Boston, pp 63–79
Venn A, Watson L, Lumley J, Giles G, King C, Healy D 1995 Breast and ovarian cancer incidence after infertility and in vitro fertilisation. Lancet 336: 995–1000
Vergote I B, De Vos L N, Abeler V M et al 1992a Randomized trial comparing cisplatin with radioactive phosphorus or whole abdominal irradiation as adjuvant treatment of ovarian cancer. Cancer 69: 741–749
Vergote I B, Himmelmann A, Frankendal B et al 1992b Hexamethylmelamine as a second line therapy in platinum resistant ovarian cancer. Gynecologic Oncology 47: 282–286
Vergote I B, Trope C G, Kaern J et al 1993 Identification of high-risk Stage I ovarian carcinoma. Importance of DNA ploidy. International Journal of Gynecologic Cancer 3 (Suppl 1): 51
Vessey M, Metcalfe A, Wells C, McPherson K, Westhoff C, Yeates D 1987 Ovarian neoplasms, functonal cysts and oral contraceptives. British Medical Journal 294: 1518–1520
Ward B G, Cruikshank D J, Tucker D R, Love S 1987 Independent expression in serum of three tumour associated antigens, CA125, placental alkaline phosphatase and HMFG 2 antigen in ovarian carcinoma. British Journal of Obstetrics and Gynaecology 94: 696–698
Watson P, Lynch H T 1992 Hereditary ovarian cancer. In: Sharp F, Mason W P, Creaman W (eds) Ovarian cancer 2: Biology, diagnosis and management. London, Chapman & Hall, pp 9–15
Welander C E 1987 Use of interferon in the treatment of ovarian cancer as a single agent and in combination with cytotoxic drugs. Cancer 59: 617–619
Wharton J T, Edwards C I, Rutledge F N 1984 Long term survival after chemotherapy for advanced epithelial ovarian carcinoma. American Journal of Obstetrics and Gynecology 148: 997–1005
Whittemore A, Harris R, Intyre J, The Collaborative Ovarian Cancer Group 1992 Characteristics related to ovarian cancer risk: collaborative analysis of twelve US case-control studies. II. Invasive epithelial cancer in white women. American Journal of Epidemiology 136: 1184–1203
Willemsen W, Kruitwagen R, Bastiaans B, Hanselaar T, Rolland R

1993 Ovarian stimulation and granulosa-cell tumour. Lancet 341: 986–988
Wiltshaw E 1985 Ovarian trials at the Royal Marsden. Cancer Treatment Reports 12: 67–71
Wiltshaw E, Kroner T 1976 Phase II study of cis-cishlorodiammine platinum (II) (RSC-119875) in advanced adenocarcinoma of the ovary. Cancer Treatment Reports 60: 55–60
Wiltshaw E, Raju K S, Dawson I 1985 The role of cytoreductive surgery in advanced carcinoma of the ovary: an analysis of primary and secondary surgery. British Journal of Obstetrics and Gynaecology 92: 522–527
Woolas R P, Xu F J, Jacobs I J et al 1993 Elevation of multiple serum markers in patients with Stage I ovarian cancer. Journal of the National Cancer Institutes 85: 1748–1751
Woolas R, Jacobs I, Prys Davies A et al 1994 What is the true incidence of primary fallopian tube carcinoma? International Journal of Gynecologic Cancer 4: 384–388
Xu F J, Yu Y H, Daly L et al 1993 The OVX1 radioimmunoassay complements CA125 for predicting the presence of residual ovarian carcinoma at second look surgical surveillance procedures. Journal of Clinical Oncology 11: 1506–1510
Young R C, Chabner B A, Hubbard S P et al 1978 Advanced ovarian adenocarcinoma: a prospective clinical trial of melphalan (L-PAM) versus combination chemotherapy. New England Journal of Medicine 299: 1261–1266
Young R C, Walton L A, Ellenberg S S et al 1990 Adjuvant therapy in stage I and stage II epithelial ovarian cancer: results of two prospective randomized trials. New England Journal of Medicine 322: 1021–1027

42

Benign disease of the breast

J. McCue W. Svensson J. Lynn

INTRODUCTION

Breast cancer is such an emotive disease that on discovering a breast-related symptom many women fear the worst. In fact, around 90% of these women will have benign pathology. The easiest way to reassure them is with a prompt and accurate diagnosis which lays the foundation for treatment. This is most easily achieved in a 'one-stop' clinic where immediate radiological and cytological facilities are available, so that the majority of patients leave with a diagnosis at the end of their first appointment. Unfortunately, this option is expensive in resource allocation and is thus available in only a minority of institutions.

The approach to the patient on first presentation will be described initially. As with any clinical problem the process starts with the history and examination, followed by special investigations. After a discussion of the merits of the diagnostic modalities available, the conditions and their treatment will be described.

HISTORY

If the main symptom is of a lump it is important to discover how long it has been present, whether it has grown, if it is painful and whether it varies with the menstrual cycle.

The most commonly presenting breast symptom is mastalgia. It is necessary to determine whether the pain truly originates in the breast or whether it is referred from elsewhere, e.g. the oesophagus or the heart. It is important to know the site, severity and duration of pain, and whether it is bilateral. Relationship to the menstrual cycle often provides a key to diagnosis. If this relationship is uncertain, a daily pain chart kept over a period of 2–3 months may help to confirm a link.

Information to elicit about nipple discharge includes the colour of the discharge and whether it comes from one or both nipples.

It is important to know if the patient is on the oral contraceptive pill or taking any other hormonal agent. A history of current pregnancy or breastfeeding may be significant, and a family history of breast disease is essential.

EXAMINATION

The examination should take place in a warm and com-

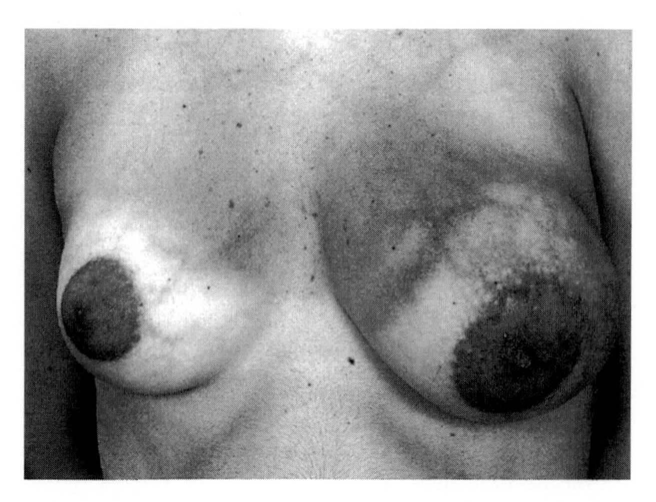

Fig. 42.1 The left breast is clearly larger, more dependent and has visible distended veins. The cause was a giant fibroadenoma.

fortable environment where the patient's privacy is maintained at all times. The patient should be in a semi-recumbent position on a couch. Adequate lighting is necessary to enable a thorough inspection of the breasts, with the arms at the side and above the head. This may reveal an asymmetry in breast contour as well as evidence of previous scarring (Fig. 42.1). If either nipple is inverted the patient should be asked how long this has been the case.

Palpation of the breasts is performed with the fingers flexing at the metacarpophalangeal joints. All four quadrants should be examined in turn plus the axillary tail. If the patient presents with a lump it is useful to ask her to localize it before starting palpation. Feeling the asymptomatic breast first will give you an idea of the normal breast consistency. If a lump is found, the following characteristics should be noted: position, consistency and fixity (both deep and superficial), and specifically whether the lump feels discrete or not. The patient who complains of a nipple discharge should be asked to express a small quantity for analysis for haemoglobin, cytology and culture. Examination of the axillary and supraclavicular glands completes the examination. Palpable lymphadenopathy increases suspicion of a breast carcinoma, but can also occur with an inflammatory process.

INVESTIGATIONS

The aim of imaging is first, to provide a probable diagnosis, and secondly, to help exclude the presence of cancer, thereby reducing the need for more invasive interventions. Ultrasound and mammography are the most frequently used methods of imaging (Table 42.1).

Palpable masses within the breast are best imaged with ultrasound in patients under the age of 35. Over the age of 35, mammography and/or ultrasound should be performed. If there has been recent mammography ultrasound may be the investigation of choice, particularly if there is a previous history of cysts or the palpable lump is thought to be a cyst. If clinically the lesion is suspicious of malignancy, a tissue diagnosis should also be obtained, unless the imaging is unequivocally benign.

Table 42.1 Indications for imaging and the advantages of the different techniques

Indications for mammography	Indications for breast ultrasound
Over 50 years old Breast screening **Over 35 years old** No recent mammogram and a palpable mass and clinical suspicion of carcinoma **Under 35 years old** Very strong clinical suspicion of malignancy and normal breast ultrasound and cytology	**Under 35 years old** Clinically benign mass and no significant risk factors for breast cancer **Over 35 years old** *Benign or equivocal solitary mass* Can be biopsied under direct vision if indicated *Cysts* Can be diagnosed reliably and needling avoided *Multiple masses* Solid lesions can be differentiated from cysts and suspicious areas can be biopsied or needled *Abscess cavities* Can be identified and drained by needle aspiration *Augmented breast* Not obscured by a prosthesis so silicone granuloma and leakage are more easily diagnosed than by mammography *Pregnant woman* Because mammography is contraindicated by slight radiation risk

Whenever possible imaging should precede fine-needle aspiration or core biopsy, as these can cause changes within the breast tissue which can be indistinguishable from the mammographic and ultrasound appearance of carcinoma. If fine-needle aspiration precedes imaging at least a fortnight should elapse before mammography, and up to 3 months before ultrasound, to allow the changes caused by haematoma and bruising to subside. Earlier imaging may be unhelpful because, if there is a suspicious abnormality, it may not be possible to determine whether or not it is due to the aspiration. Core biopsies may require a longer period before mammography. The changes may take up to 3 months to subside on both mammography and ultrasound.

Mammography

Mammography should be performed on a modern dedicated mammography unit by a radiographer who has had mammography training under the supervision of a recognized breast screening training centre. Interpretation should be performed by an experienced radiologist with suitable breast imaging training. Best results are obtained in units with a sufficiently high throughput to ensure that expertise is maintained.

In the absence of a palpable mass, mammography is not recommended in the under 35-year-old because it is a screening procedure. The risks of mammography causing breast cancer are greater in young or large breasts than in old or small breasts. Law (1993) has estimated, for the United Kingdom, that for women aged 30–34 one cancer is likely to be caused for every three detected, if two views are taken for each breast. At age 40–44 it is one for every 30 detected, whereas at 50–54 it decreases to one for every 90 detected. Because of the cumulative effect of radiation, mammographic screening is certainly not indicated below the age of 40, and between the ages of 40 and 50 the benefits are not yet clear. Over the age of 50 there is a clear benefit from breast screening.

Mammography is helpful in the staging and evaluation of a known carcinoma at any age, and over the age of 35 is of use for screening the contralateral breast for an occult second primary. Its main use in the evaluation of palpable lumps is for the demonstration of microcalcifications, and to evaluate the margins and extent of lesions.

Ultrasound

Ultrasound should be performed by an experienced radiologist or ultrasonographer using a high-resolution linear array probe (7–10 MHz) on an ultrasound machine with colour Doppler designed for high-resolution small parts soft-tissue imaging. Many benign lesions can now be diagnosed ultrasonographically with a high degree of certainty, reducing the need for open biopsy. If fine-needle aspiration cytology (FNAC) is not performed, serial ultrasound measurement with high-definition images can confirm the absence of change in ultrasonically benign lesions.

Under the age of 35 ultrasound is the imaging modality of choice for a palpable mass. Over 35 it may also be the most useful, though the indications for mammography are stronger.

Ultrasound is of less help in screening for impalpable cancers than is mammographic screening, and is rarely if ever helpful in identifying microcalcification demonstrated mammographically. Conversely, it is often very useful for identifying and localizing the impalpable mammographic mass for ultrasound diagnosis, or to allow ultrasound guided FNA, core biopsy or wire localization for open excision biopsy. Ultrasound-guided interventions are preferable to mammographic guidance, both for the experienced operator and the patient, as the patient lies in a comfortable supine position rather than sitting up for mammographic procedures. Ultrasound is real-time imaging and always allows optimum placement of needle tips under direct vision.

Ductography

Ductography is the demonstration of a duct by injection of X-ray contrast after cannulation of the duct. Indications are continuing discharge after previous surgery, and suspicion of a ductal abnormality despite a normal ultrasound examination. Most intraductal lesions of any size, such as intraductal papillomata, are demonstrated on ultrasound (Fig. 42.2).

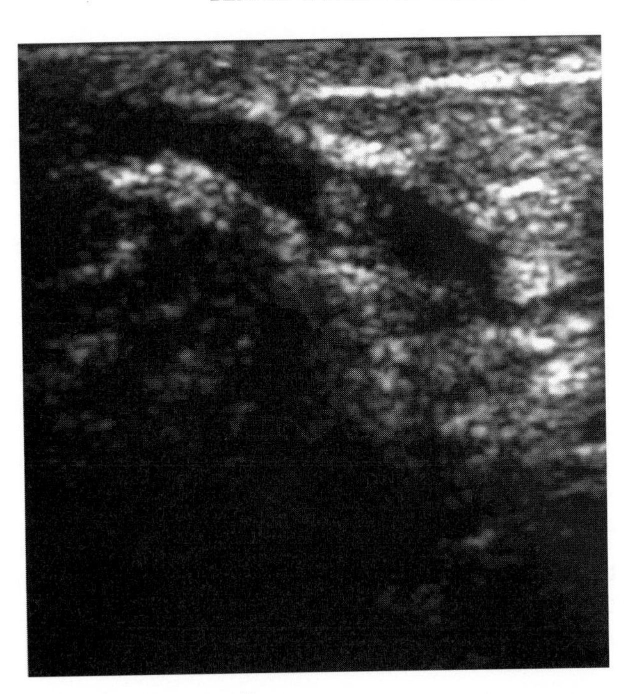

Fig. 42.2 Intraductal papilloma.

Thermography, like transillumination, does not have sufficient specificity or sensitivity to be recommended as a routine examination.

Magnetic resonance imaging

Magnetic resonance imaging (MRI), especially with dedicated coils and i.v. contrast agents, is showing great promise but still needs further evaluation to determine its place in the current imaging of breast problems. At present, cost and availability of equipment are also important additional considerations.

Fine needle aspiration cytology (FNAC)

The emergence of breast FNAC has produced a major change in the management of breast symptoms over the past decade, with a substantial reduction in the need for open biopsy. For optimal results FNAC requires a consistent sampling technique in conjunction with reporting by a skilled cytopathologist. Results can be generated within minutes; this allows planning of treatment and, for those with benign disorders, has the potential to allay patient fears.

FNAC should be performed with a 21 g needle. Local anaesthesia is rarely required, but for the particularly anxious patient EMLA cream can be used topically. The lump is 'fixed' between the thumb and index finger of the surgeon's non-dominant hand. Once the needle has entered the lump, suction is applied to the syringe and is maintained during several passes through the lump. The suction is then released and the needle withdrawn. The contents of the syringe are smeared over two slides; one is sealed with fixative and the other is air dried.

Increasingly, the trend is to allocate breast cytology reports a numerical score:

Grade	Meaning
5	Diagnostic for malignancy
4	Highly suspicious for malignancy
3	Atypical features seen
2	Benign cells only
1	Scanty aspirate
0	No epithelial cells seen

The majority of patients reported as grade 3 will have a benign diagnosis. In general, the aspirate from those with benign lumps is less cellular than from those with malignancy.

Histological biopsy

Tru-cut biopsy has fallen from favour as FNAC has emerged. It is more traumatic for the patient and necessitates local anaesthesia. Its place is now usually confined to those institutions where good cytology facilities are lacking, or when FNAC has been unhelpful.

Diagnosis is usually reached by a combination of clinical and radiological assessment with either FNAC or Tru-cut results. Open biopsy is now most commonly performed for reasons of diagnostic uncertainty. Specific indications for biopsy in cases of clinically benign breast disease include cytological or radiological suspicion, heightened patient anxiety and a breast cyst that either recurs or persists after two attempts at aspiration. Recommendations for open biopsy based on age are contentious, with arbitrary limits set at either 35 or 40 years.

SCREENING DETECTED IMPALPABLE LESIONS

This new category has been generated by the growth of breast screening programmes. As with palpable lesions, a diagnosis must be achieved by a combination of radiological, pathological and clinical means. Further mammographic or ultrasonographic views may clinch the diagnosis, along with ultrasound-guided or stereotactic aspiration. Where uncertainty still exists, open targeted biopsy should be performed. Guide-wire localization is the most commonly used technique, although other methods are available. The specimen should always be X-rayed to confirm that the relevant area has been excised.

ABNORMALITIES OF DEVELOPMENT AND INVOLUTION

In the past there have been a variety of names given to the condition of painful, often lumpy, breasts, including benign mammary dysplasia, fibroadenosis and chronic mastitis. Histological analysis of breast tissue from these women has often shown similar features to those with apparently normal asymptomatic breasts. To resolve this dilemma, the concept of abnormalities of development and involution (ANDI) has been established by the Cardiff Breast Clinic as a framework for benign breast disorders. This proposes that there is a gradation from normal, through mild abnormality (disorder) to more pronounced abnormality which presents as frank disease. The scheme encompasses not merely painful nodularity but also other conditions, such as fibroadenomas, adolescent hypertrophy and cystic disease.

PAIN AND/OR NODULARITY

The most common reason for a patient to seek medical attention with breast-related symptoms is pain. From the outset anxiety can be alleviated by the knowledge that pain is a most unusual presenting symptom for breast cancer.

To pinpoint the exact cause for the pain it is important to establish whether the pain originates in the breast itself, and whether it is cyclical or non-cyclical in nature. Cervical spondylosis, cardiac pain, pleurisy, oesophageal lesions and Tietze's disease may all mimic breast pain. This latter condition is a painful costochondritis deep to the breast. Non-steroidal analgesics are commonly of benefit.

Non-cyclical breast pain is most commonly seen in the perimenopausal age group. The most likely underlying causes such as duct ectasia, fat necrosis and sclerosing adenosis, are discussed later in the chapter.

CYCLICAL MASTALGIA

Many patients are relieved to hear that cyclical breast pain affects the majority of women to varying degrees at some point in their reproductive life. The condition is usually considered an aberration of the normal cyclical changes, quite possibly hormonal in origin. Major hormonal events, e.g. pregnancy and the menopause, frequently relieve cyclical mastalgia and spontaneous remission is common. Characteristically, pain occurs in the few days leading up to the onset of menstruation, when the breasts feel swollen and areas of nodularity may be evident. However, the relationship between nodularity and pain is not constant. In more severe cases the patient may only be pain-free for a few days after menstruation. Usually both breasts are affected, particularly in the upper outer quadrant. A pain chart kept by the patient over a 2–3-month period may help to demonstrate the cyclical nature of the pain (Fig. 42.3).

Investigation

Careful clinical examination coupled with a sympathetic

BREAST PAIN CHART

Patient name:

Month	1	2	3	4	5	6	7	8	9	10	11	12	13	14	15	16	17	18	19	20	21	22	23	24	25	26	27	28	29	30	31

Note the degree of breast pain you experience on each day by filling in the relevant square

■ severe pain

◩ mild pain

• no pain

Note when your period starts with the letter "P" for each day

Fig. 42.3 Breast pain chart.

explanation of the condition will satisfy around 85% of patients. The remainder require medical treatment. The majority of patients are relieved to learn they do not have cancer, or any problem likely to lead to breast cancer. Mammography often has a therapeutic effect, although in the absence of a dominant nodule this should be reserved for those over the age of 35.

Areas of focal nodularity are extremely common and should be investigated as any other lump in the breast. In patients over the age of 35 mammography is the first line of investigation whereas under 35 ultrasound is the investigation of choice. FNAC can be performed but may have a lower diagnostic yield than in other breast conditions. Open biopsy should resolve any element of suspicion, and be employed freely in patients over the age of 35. Features of normal breast involution, i.e. fibrosis, adenosis, apocrine change and microcyst formation, will be evident on histological examination.

Treatment

Randomized controlled trials have confirmed the efficacy of four drugs in the treatment of cyclical mastalgia.

γ-Linolenic acid

Empirical treatment with oil of evening primrose was noted to produce a reduction in breast pain. This oil is rich in γ-linolenic acid, an essential fatty acid. It was subsequently demonstrated that women with mastalgia have abnormal fatty acid profiles, which tend to correct after several months' treatment with γ-linolenic acid. Essential fatty acids are intimately related with lipid metabolism and consequently affect such diverse functions as cellular membrane flexibility, hormone receptor affinity and cholesterol transport. γ-Linolenic acid (GLA) is now the first-line drug for the treatment of cyclical mastalgia. It is almost free of side effects and is popular with patients. A pain response rate is seen in approximately 60% of patients. Unfortunately, on cessation of treatment, pain may recur after several months in up to 50% of responders.

Hormonal agents

Danazol. Danazol is a synthetic steroid which combines androgenic activity with antioestrogenic and antiprogestogenic activity. A prospective randomized double-blind trial using danazol in the dose 200 mg bd showed a significant improvement in breast pain, tenderness and nodularity. In cyclical mastalgia a response rate approaching 80% can be anticipated. Unfortunately, side effects, most notably virilization, reduce patient compliance. Use of this drug should therefore be reserved for those unresponsive to GLA.

Bromocriptine. This drug stimulates dopamine receptors and inhibits prolactin release. Mastalgia is relieved in approximately 60% of patients. Again, the side effects, especially nausea, vomiting and dizziness, preclude widespread use of the drug. A gradual increase in dose may reduce the frequency of complications.

Tamoxifen. Tamoxifen, an oestrogen receptor antagonist, has been shown to be of benefit in the treatment of cyclical mastalgia.

Many of the old theories, e.g. water retention or neurosis, have been discounted. Although widely used, the efficacy of pyridoxine is unproven.

EPITHELIAL HYPERPLASIA

A suspicious aspirate (grade 3 or 4) may indicate a diagnosis of epithelial hyperplasia. This results from exaggerated proliferation of the ductal epithelium. Severe hyperplasia doubles the risk of breast carcinoma, which is further increased in the presence of cellular atypia or a positive family history. Diagnosis is confirmed by open biopsy. Those with cellular atypia warrant close surveillance.

SCLEROSING ADENOSIS

Sclerosis may occur during the process of involution and may give rise to diagnostic confusion. Distortion of the terminal duct lobular unit is seen, perhaps provoked by an adjacent scar. Rarely, in complex lesions, epithelial hyperplasia is noted. Clinical presentation is either with a breast lump or an abnormality detected on screening mammography. FNAC may enable a diagnosis to be made, but any doubt warrants excision biopsy.

Unfortunately, benign lesions such as sclerosing adenosis and radial scars may often be indistinguishable in appearance from carcinomas, both mammographically and ultrasonically. This also applies to scars within the breast, when there is a question of the possibility of recurrence at the site of previous excision of a carcinoma. Radial scars can sometimes be differentiated from cancers mammographically by their radiolucent centre. On ultrasound a similar increased echo appearance within the centre of the lesion may give the suspicion that it contains fat rather than the low echogenic appearance which is associated with tumour. Colour Doppler can be used to determine the extent and number of vessels within suspicious lesions of this nature and, as a general rule, tumours are associated with an increased number of irregular vessels, whereas benign lesions such as scars and radial scars are frequently relatively avascular. Ultrasound can be used for frequent follow-up of such areas if excision biopsy for diagnosis is unlikely to alter the management of the case.

CYSTIC BREAST DISEASE

This is a condition which affects over 5% of women. It most commonly occurs in the decade before the menopause. In contrast with ANDI, in which cysts are also an integral component, in cystic breast disease the cysts are usually larger. Macroscopically the cysts may have a bluish appearance and are known eponymously as the 'blue-domed cyst of Bloodgood'.

Cysts probably arise as an aberration of senile involution associated with active secretion of apocrine epithelium. There may be an underlying hormonal imbalance. One theory suggests that altered central regulation of prolactin may be involved, and levels of essential fatty acids are lower than in the general population.

Characteristically, breast cysts are discrete, smooth, rounded lumps. The upper outer quadrant is most commonly affected. If tensely filled with fluid, the cyst may cause pain. Multiple cysts occur in 50% of affected women, with a small percentage reporting over 20 cysts (Fig. 42.4).

Investigation

Mammographically cysts may classically present with a localized opacity with a surrounding halo, but more frequently are ill defined and not clearly seen. Ultrasound gives a definitive diagnosis of cyst in most cases, and aspiration is not usually necessary unless the ultrasound appearances raise suspicions of a concomitant tumour.

Approximately 2% of patients with breast cysts may have a coexistent carcinoma, and so all women presenting over the age of 35 should undergo mammography. Radiographically cysts present a localized opacity with a surrounding halo.

If definitive ultrasound is not performed the cyst should be aspirated. The fluid varies in colour from pale yellow to green. Unless the fluid is bloodstained cytological analysis is unwarranted, as the risk of carcinoma is negligible. After aspiration one should check to ensure there is no residual lump and a further examination should take place 4 weeks later to confirm that the cyst has not reaccumulated. Excision biopsy is required for cytological uncertainty or if the cyst repeatedly refills.

There is an increased risk of breast carcinoma in patients with breast cysts, and the tendency is most marked in those with multiple cysts, who should undergo regular

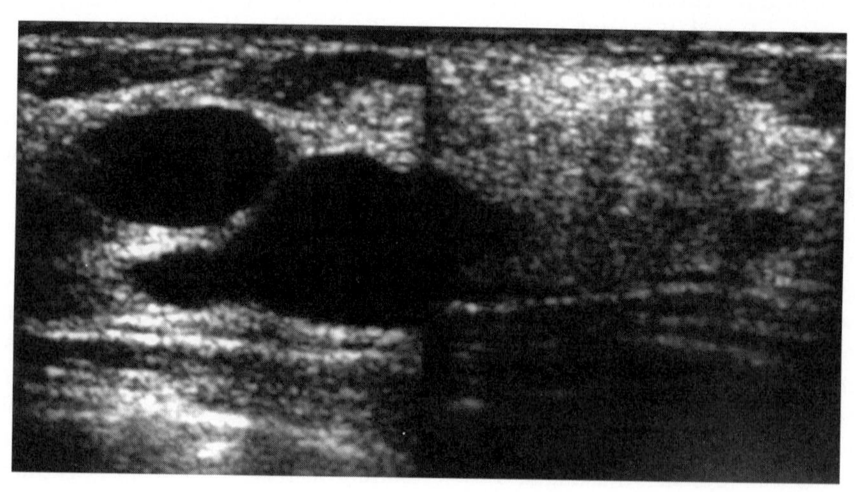

Fig. 42.4 Breast cyst.

mammography. Danazol may be effective at reducing the numbers of cysts and the associated discomfort.

FIBROADENOMA

The contemporary view is that these lesions are also aberrations of normal breast development. Clonal analysis has shown that both epithelial and stromal cells are polyclonal, confirming that fibroadenomas, which develop from a whole lobule, are hyperplastic. Furthermore, hyperplastic lobules, histologically indistinguishable from fibroadenomata, are commonly present in the breasts of normal young women. Fibroadenomas are most commonly found in early adult life, and are particularly prevalent in Negroid races. Up to the mid-30s fibroadenomas are a commoner cause of breast lumps than carcinoma. Juvenile fibroadenomas are occasionally seen in adolescent girls.

The usual presentation is with a discrete, firm breast lump, most commonly situated in the upper outer quadrant of the breast. Because of their mobility these lumps are popularly known as breast mice. Fibroadenomas may be multiple in up to 20% of cases. Most lumps are 1–2 cm in diameter at presentation; those over 5 cm are defined as giant fibroadenomas (Figs 42.5 and 42.6).

Investigation

Although the vast majority of clinically diagnosed fibroadenomas are benign, up to 5% will subsequently be shown to be carcinomas. Consequently these lesions warrant investigation even if a subsequent conservative policy is to be employed.

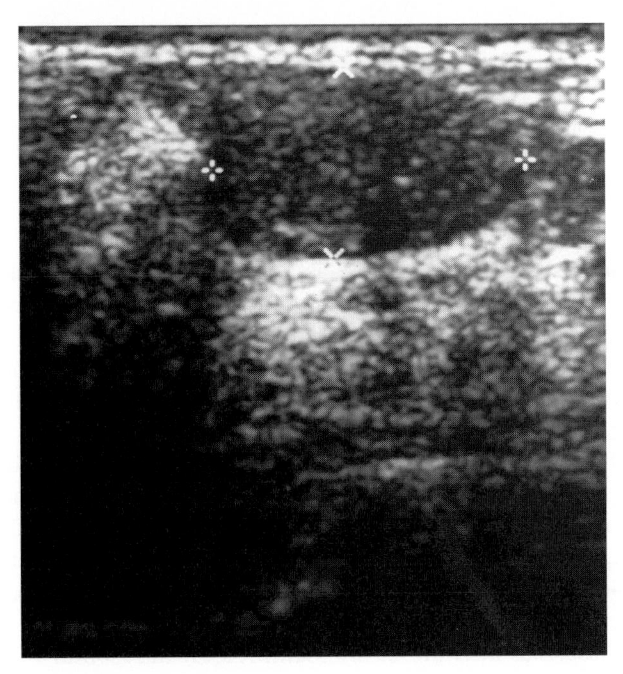

Fig. 42.5 Fibroadenoma.

Definitive and reliable diagnosis of fibroadenoma can be achieved by a combination of ultrasound investigation and FNAC. Ultrasound of the breast should be performed in those under 35. Characteristic features are of a mostly hypoechoic and homogeneous lesion, but up to 10% may show intratumoural calcification. Mammography is the investigation of choice for those over the age of 35, although ultrasound may be required if the breasts are dense. FNAC can now accurately distinguish benign from malignant disease, although false positive results have been reported.

Treatment

Fibroadenomas are hormonally dependent, and so may enlarge during pregnancy or use of the oral contraceptive pill but regress during the puerperium or on cessation of oral contraception. Evidence is accumulating that not all fibroadenomas continue to grow. Up to 30% disappear

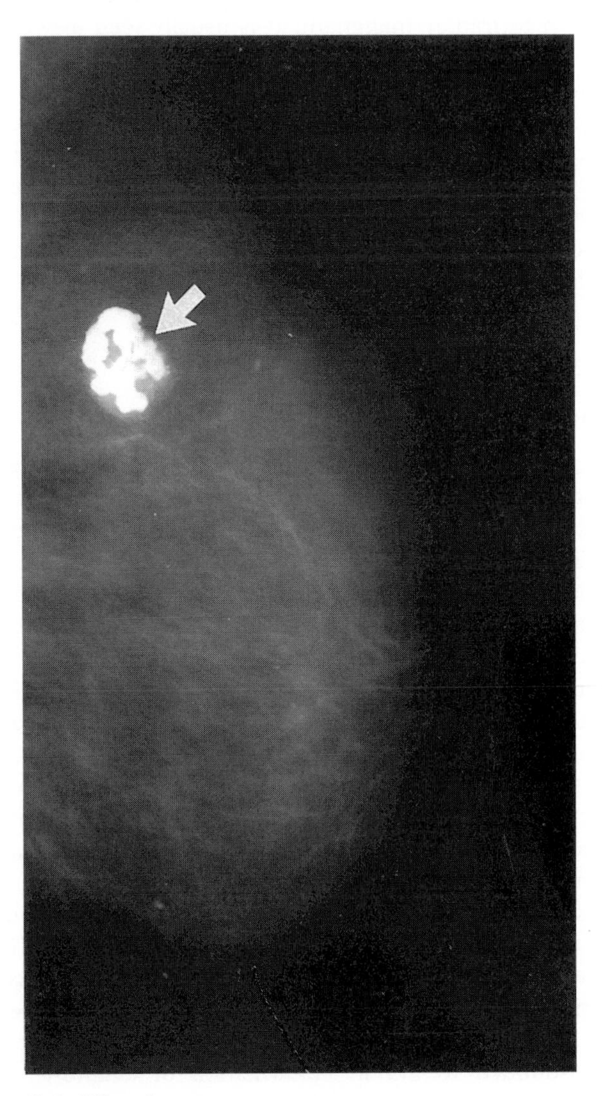

Fig. 42.6 Fibroadenoma.

spontaneously over a period of months, but a similar proportion will increase in size. Armed with this information the patient, in conjunction with her doctors, can decide whether the cytologically diagnosed fibroadenoma should be removed. The majority of women still elect for excision if offered the choice. A conservative policy should not be followed unless good cytological facilities are available. The fear of mistaking a carcinoma for a fibroadenoma is obviously greater in the older patient. Many units would routinely excise all presumed fibroadenomas in patients over 35 because of this worry. If surgical excision is performed the lump should be removed through a cosmetic incision, usually under general anaesthesia. Follow-up ultrasound should be arranged after approximately 4 months in those women who do not undergo surgery.

PHYLLOIDES TUMOURS

This is an unusual condition allied to fibroadenomas, although with a pattern of behaviour which can vary from benign to frankly malignant. It is usually seen in women over the age of 40. The lumps are bosselated and may grow in size rapidly to produce pressure necrosis and ulceration of the overlying breast skin. Macroscopically the lesions may be centrally necrotic and the more malignant variants show sarcomatous stroma. Local recurrence can be a problem; more rarely, metastasis occurs via the bloodstream. These tumours should be excised with a wide margin of surrounding tissue (Fig. 42.7).

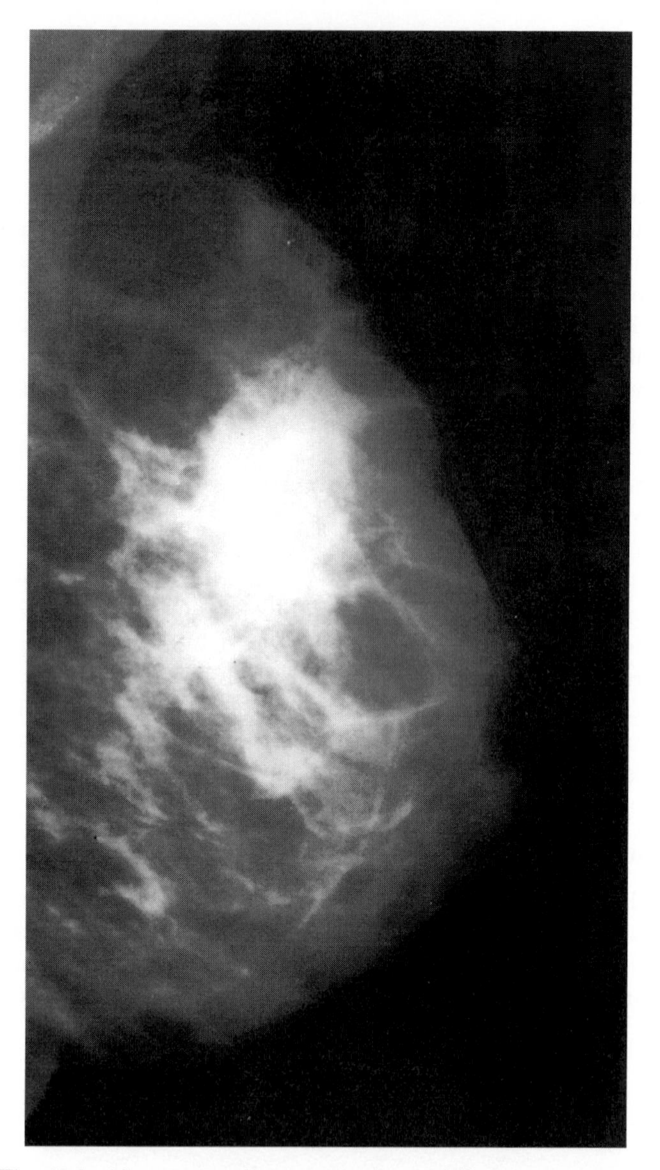

Fig. 42.7 Mammogram demonstrating large calcified cystosarcoma phylloides. This lesion recurred locally twice but remained histologically benign.

BENIGN TUMOURS OF THE BREAST

Duct papilloma

Characteristically these tumours produce a bloodstained nipple discharge. Unless there are multiple papillomas the discharge issues from a single duct. Occasionally, a lump is felt lying deep to the areola. Mammography and cytological examination of the aspirate has largely replaced mammary dochography in the diagnosis of this condition. Microdochectomy (excision of a single duct) is the treatment of choice. Dilated ducts are easily identified on ultrasound and the intraductal papillomas within are also easily identified, provided they do not completely occlude and fill the duct. Usually they are obvious, extending into the duct lumen with fluid around them or, if they are large, fluid can be seen tracking around them from the dilated portion of duct.

Lipomas can be diagnosed with certainty on ultrasound because they either have the same echogenicity as subcutaneous or breast fat, or have a slightly increased echogenicity with a similar echo pattern. Frequently, patients have lipomas elsewhere in the body which can also be ultrasounded to aid in confirmation of diagnosis. On mammography the lower density of lipomas makes their diagnosis easy if they are associated with dense breasts with a high proportion of parenchyma, but in fatty breasts they are indistinguishable from the surrounding fat.

Oil cysts can be identified mammographically if they have a calcified rim or lie within parenchyma. Within the fat they often cannot be identified because of the lack of difference of density. On ultrasound it may not be possible to differentiate oil cysts from ordinary cysts, because they may be echo free or contain echos and have similar appearances to fluid-filled cysts. If there is an oil/water mixture the fluid level is well identified on ultrasound as well as on mammography.

Sebaceous cysts are easily identified on ultrasound from their position, the fact that they are well defined and the internal echos are usually increased owing to the lipid content.

Lymph nodes may be isoechoic with the surrounding fat in a mainly fatty breast, but in a breast with a large proportion of parenchyma they usually have an oval shape, with a slightly more translucent cortex and a slightly increased echogenic medulla. The vessels entering the hilum of the cortex can frequently be demonstrated with the aid of colour Doppler. Reactive, hypertrophied lymph nodes retain their anatomical structure and appearance, whereas lymph nodes that have been invaded by tumour from a breast primary are usually masses of reduced echogenicity, often similar in echogenicity to the primary tumour. As in other parts of the body it is not always possible to exclude the presence of tumour from a node which appears to be hypertrophied with a normal architecture.

INFECTIVE LESIONS OF THE BREAST

Mastitis of infancy

Some breast enlargement is seen in over 50% of newborn babies of either sex. This is a reaction to maternal hormones and can result in production of a small amount of 'witch's milk'. Occasionally infection with subsequent abscess formation supervenes. Antibiotics (the infection is usually staphylococcal) are required for the treatment of mastitis. Systemic upset occurs in the baby with an abscess. Treatment is by open incision and drainage under general anaesthetic, administered by a paediatric anaesthetist, combined with antibiotics.

Infection in the lactating woman

The commonest breast infection, acute mastitis and its complications, has declined in frequency with an improvement in standards of hygiene. Prompt and appropriate treatment is necessary to minimize what can be a miserable condition when the patient is already under strain coping with the demands of a new baby.

Infection usually arises in conjunction with a cracked nipple. Bacteria colonize the broken skin and may enter the duct system via the nipple. Staphylococci, the commonest organism involved, are found in the nasopharynx of 50% of neonates by day 2. Stasis due to poor milk drainage facilitates infection.

The early days of breastfeeding are most prone to infection. Clinical features include breast pain, swelling and tenderness and constitutional upset may occur. Fluctuance is a late feature of abscess formation, as are skin changes which suggest the abscess may be about to discharge spontaneously.

Treatment

If treated early with antibiotics, mastitis may resolve. Flucloxacillin is the drug of choice, or erythromycin in those with penicillin allergy. The patient should be encouraged to continue breastfeeding.

Failure to respond to antibiotics should raise the suspicion of abscess formation. Continued treatment with antibiotics will result in an 'antibioma', a firm loculated mass. Ultrasound will reliably show such a collection. Application of topical skin anaesthetic (EMLA cream) permits diagnostic aspiration; any pus obtained should be sent for bacteriological analysis. Previously, incision and drainage under general anaesthetic followed by daily dressings was the gold standard in the management of breast abscesses. The incision was placed over Langer's lines and deepened to permit digital breakdown of the abscess septa. Recent evidence has emerged to suggest that repeated needle aspiration with oral antibiotics, or incision under topical anaesthetic combined with daily irrigation, are satisfactory alternatives.

Infection in the non-lactating woman

Acute peripheral abscesses

These occur mainly in immunosuppressed patients. They are much rarer than lactating abscesses but the clinical features and management are otherwise similar.

Duct ectasia

This is a disease of the ageing breast and can be considered an aberration of normal breast involution. It is the commonest cause of nipple discharge in older women. This discharge varies from creamy white to green or black, and usually emerges from more than one duct. Other clinical features include pain, nipple retraction and lumpiness.

The histological features of subareolar duct dilatation containing inspissated material and a mild surrounding inflammatory infiltrate have been observed in 25% of female postmortem specimens (Fig. 42.8).

Treatment

Surgery is indicated for troublesome symptoms or suspicion of malignancy. Single duct involvement can be treated by microdochectomy. Excision of the major duct complex (Hadfield's operation) is warranted when more than one duct is diseased. Unfortunately, almost 20% of patients report further sepsis after surgery.

Periareolar infection and mamillary fistula

Periareolar infection is characterized by inflammation, mostly with plasma cells, around non-dilated ducts. Smoking appears to be an important aetiological factor. A

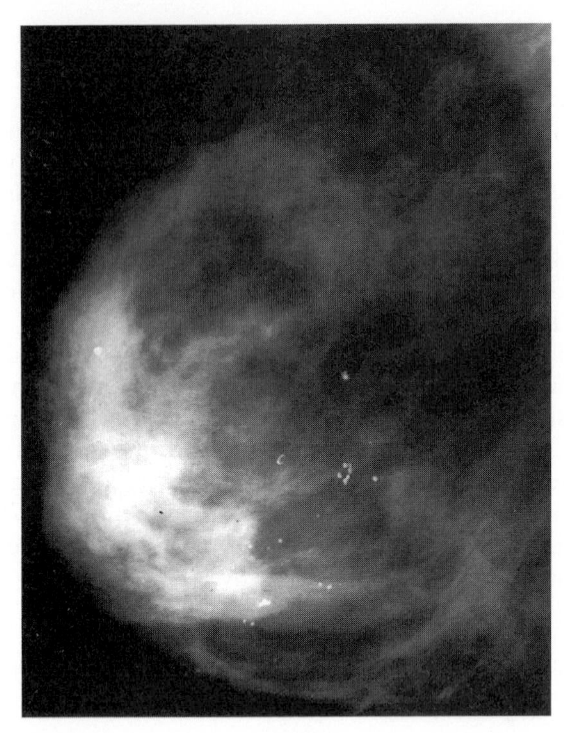

Fig. 42.8 Mammogram showing diffuse, coarse calcification typical of duct ectasia.

wide spectrum of bacteria, including anaerobes, is involved in its pathogenesis. Most patients present with periareolar pain and tenderness, often accompanied by a mass. About one-fifth of patients have nipple discharge and nipple retraction can develop.

Treatment

Initial treatment is with antibiotics active against anaerobic organisms, e.g. augmentin or metronidazole plus a cephalosporin. Suspected abscess formation can be confirmed on diagnostic aspiration. Evacuation of pus should be managed by incision and drainage or repeated aspiration plus antibiotic therapy.

Periductal mastitis often recurs owing to persisting inflammation from the diseased duct. Following incision and drainage of a periareolar abscess, nearly one-third of patients will develop a mamillary fistula. This abnormal communication between the skin at the areolar margin and the duct system results in a purulent discharge from the fistula and the nipple. Surgical management consists of laying open the fistula and allowing it to heal by granulation or excision, or primary closure of the fistula under antibiotic cover, which gives a better cosmetic result. Nipple eversion must be achieved or further infection will ensue.

Unusual infections

Tuberculosis is a major health threat in the third world and, although rare, is undergoing a slight resurgence in industrialized countries. Rarely the breast can be involved with either primary or, more commonly, secondary infection. Tuberculous breast infection can be an unusual presentation of the acquired immune deficiency syndrome.

The early feature is an ill-defined swelling, with later development of multiple chronic abscesses and sinus formation. Acute abscess formation can occur due to secondary infection of a tuberculous lesion with pyogenic bacteria.

Diagnosis is achieved by bacteriological analysis, with biopsy if required. Both antituberculous chemotherapy and surgery may be necessary for treatment.

Rare breast infections include syphilis, actinomycoses, mycotic, helminthic and viral infections.

CONGENITAL ABNORMALITIES AND COSMETIC CONSIDERATIONS

A number of developmental anomalies may be seen by the surgeon with a breast practice.

Accessory nipples and breasts

These are found anywhere in the milk line from axilla to groin, although they are rarely seen below the waist. Present in 1–2% of the population, they can be the site of all diseases affecting normally positioned breasts. During lactation these supernumerary breasts swell; if the duct system is developed lactation can occur; otherwise the tissue involutes. Excision is warranted on grounds of discomfort, cosmesis or disease development.

Absent or hypoplastic breasts

True absence of the breast and nipple complex can occur and in the majority of cases is associated with an abnormality of the underlying pectoral muscle. Breast hypoplasia is seen when the nipple is present but underlying breast tissue is absent. Rarely the nipple alone is deficient.

The breasts are normally asymmetrical, the left being slightly larger than the right. The patient's perception as well as the degree of asymmetry will dictate whether surgical intervention is appropriate. These women are often severely affected psychologically and can benefit enormously from plastic surgery. Disparity between the sides can be corrected by increasing the size of the smaller breast, reducing the larger or by a combination of these methods.

An absent areola can be constructed by 'borrowing' tissue from the other breast, labia minora grafts or skin tattooing. Prosthetic nipples are available but less realistic.

Reduction mammoplasty

Massive uncontrolled development of breast tissue may develop in adolescent girls. This condition, known as juvenile hypertrophy, is due to overgrowth of periductal connective tissue without lobule formation. These young women are embarrassed by their physique and are troubled by neck, back and shoulder pain, as well as excoriation beneath their breasts. Ideally, surgery should be deferred until at least the age of 17. The results are good in skilled hands and suspension mammoplasty is effective for women with sagging breasts.

Augmentation mammoplasty

Modern society projects an image of the desirable woman as possessing large breasts. It is not surprising, therefore, that some patients request augmentation. Careful screening is needed to ensure that unnecessary operations are avoided. There are, however, women who do benefit from an increase in breast size. Methods currently available include silicone implants, saline-filled prostheses and muscle flaps.

Recognized complications of prosthetic surgery include infection, prosthesis migration or implantation leakage (Figs 42.9, 42.10 and 42.11). Capsular contracture around silicone prostheses is reported in between 10 and 40% of patients, although prior tissue expansion may reduce this prevalence. There has been considerable speculation over the safety of silicone prostheses, in particular subsequent breast cancer risk or the development of autoimmune disease, and in 1992 the US Food and Drug Administration restricted their use to research and breast reconstruction.

However, a large epidemiological study of women who had previously received silicone prostheses showed that they have a lower risk of breast carcinoma than the general population. The situation regarding autoimmune disease is less clear-cut. Although a small retrospective study showed no significant difference in incidence of arthritis or

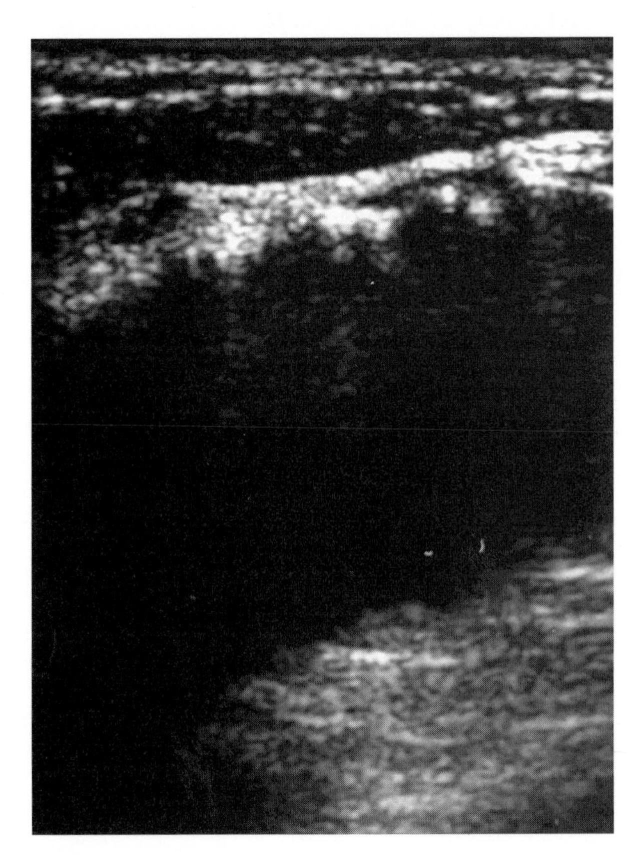

Fig. 42.9 Breast prosthesis with granulomata from silicone implant.

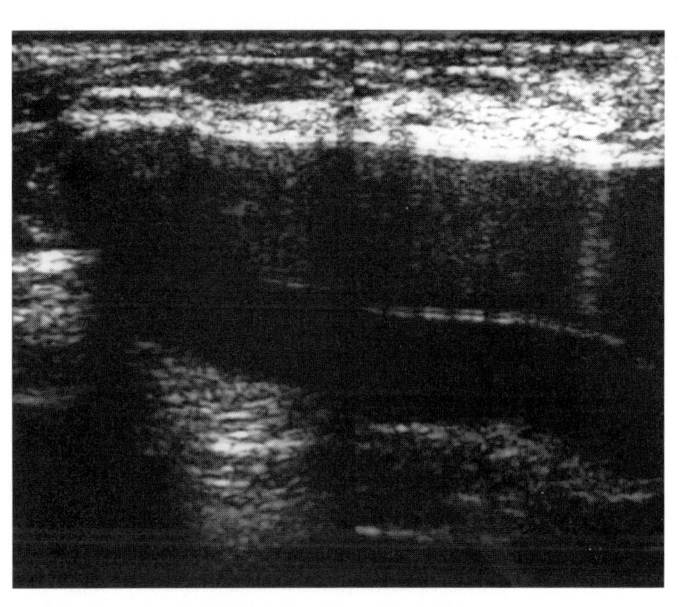

Fig. 42.10 Breast prosthesis: normal appearance with reverberation artefact in its centre.

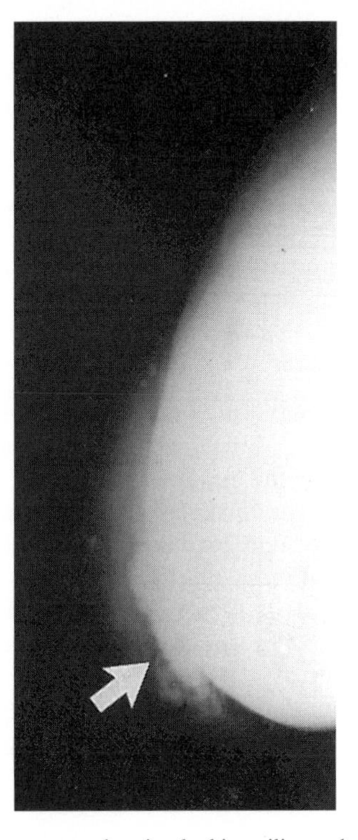

Fig. 42.11 Mammogram showing leaking silicone breast prosthesis (arrowed) which caused pain, lumpiness and local inflammation.

autoimmune disease between implant and control groups, reports of scleroderma appear to be overrepresented in the literature. Of course, the coexistence of silicone implants and autoimmune pathology does not prove causality, and no significant difference in autoantibody levels has been demonstrated between implant recipients and a control population. There is also concern that the children of women with implants may be affected by either transplacental or transmammary delivery of silicone. Until this controversy is resolved it is probably prudent to advise women with silicone prostheses against breastfeeding, because of the potential effect on their babies.

Silicone implants and the associated postoperative scarring due to cosmetic and reconstructive surgery can make subsequent mammographic interpretation difficult. Modified views may improve visualization of breast parenchyma. Ultrasound is much more helpful in the evaluation of palpable abnormalities. Even after removal of silicone prostheses, residual spiculated silicone granulomas may simulate carcinoma on mammography.

MISCELLANEOUS CONDITIONS

Fat necrosis

This condition is most prevalent in plump middle-aged women. A history of trauma, most commonly seat-belt injury, is reported in about 50% of affected patients. The major significance of fat necrosis is that it mimics many of the features of breast carcinoma, e.g. skin tethering or dimpling, with a poorly defined painless lump. Less commonly the patient may complain of non-cyclical mastalgia.

Investigation is by mammography in conjunction with FNAC. Calcification and fibrosis may be seen mammographically, again leading to confusion with carcinoma. Open biopsy is indicated if the results of these investigations are inconclusive.

Haematoma

These are clearly seen as fluid-filled low-echogenic areas within the breast. If the blood has clotted within the haematoma it is often seen as heterogenous echogenicity within the low-echogenic area. It is often possible to differentiate haematomas from abscesses using colour Doppler, as there is no significant increase in blood flow around haematomas, compared with the markedly increased blood flow around infected areas such as abscesses within the breast. Ultrasound allows localization of both haematomas and abscesses for aspiration with a broad needle under ultrasound control.

Galactocoele

This rare cystic lesion always dates from lactation. It presents in a subareolar position and contains milk, either liquid or inspissated. Treatment by aspiration is usually successful. Ultrasound diagnosis is usually definitive.

Mondor's disease

Thrombophlebitis of the superficial veins of the breast and anterior chest wall is known as Mondor's disease. The inflamed vein is palpable as a subcutaneous cord, and elevation of the arms throws the adjacent skin into a furrow. Mondor's disease is a self-limiting complaint but symptomatic relief may be required in the early stages when the area is painful.

Enlarged Montgomery's tubercles

Montgomery's tubercles are sebum-producing glands which open on to the areola. Blockage of the draining duct will produce an areolar lump, which can become secondarily infected. Excision may be necessary for troublesome symptoms.

KEY POINTS

1. If possible, imaging of the breast should precede fine-needle aspiration to avoid difficulties in interpretation due to the changes caused by the aspiration.
2. Ultrasound can now diagnose many benign lesions with a high degree of certainty, and is the imaging method of choice for women under 35.
3. X-ray mammography is not recommended for women less than 35 years old except if required to evaluate a known carcinoma.
4. Fine-needle aspiration performed with a consistent technique and reported by an experienced cytopathologist is rapid and has a high degree of accuracy.
5. Cyclical breast pain is very common and 85% of patients are satisfied with explanation alone. The remainder may be treated with γ-linolenic acid, danazol, tamoxifen or bromocriptine.
6. Women with multiple breast cysts have an increased risk of breast cancer.
7. About 5% of what are thought clinically to be fibroadenomas are in fact malignant. Investigation with ultrasound and fine-needle aspiration is required.
8. Breast abscesses can usually be treated with repeated needle aspiration.

SUGGESTED READING

Asch R H, Greenblatt R B 1977 The use of an impeded androgen – danazol – in the management of benign breast disorders. American Journal of Obstetrics and Gynecology 127: 130–134

Goldberg R P, Hall F M, Simon M 1983 Preoperative localization of non-palpable breast lesions using a wire marker and a perforated mammographic grid. Radiology 146: 833–835

Klein D L, Sickles E A 1982 Effects of needle aspiration on the mammographic appearance of the breast: a guide to the proper timing of the mammography examination. Radiology 145: 44

Law J 1993 Variations in individual radiation dose in a breast screening programme and consequences for the balance between associated risk and the benefit. British Journal of Radiology 66: 394–397

Mansel R E 1983 Classification of mastalgia – the Cardiff system. In: Benign breast disease. Royal Society of Medicine, London, pp 33–41

Mansel R E, Wisbey J R, Hughes L E 1982 Controlled trial of the anti gonadotrophin danazol in painful nodular benign breast disease. Lancet i: 928–930

Moskowitz M, Russell P, Fidler J, Sutorius D J, Law E J, Holle J 1975 Breast cancer screening. Preliminary report of 207 biopsies performed in 4128 volunteer screenees. Cancer 36: 2245–2250

Preece P E, Hughes L E, Mansel R E, Baum M, Bolton P M, Gravelle I H 1976 Clinical syndromes of mastalgia. Lancet ii: 670–673

Sackier J M, Wood C B 1988 The treatment of fibroadenoma and phylloides tumours. In: Ioannidou-Mouzaka L, Philippakis M, Angelakis P (eds) Mastology. Elsevier, Amsterdam, pp 151–156

Snyder R E 1980 Specimen radiography and pre-operative localization of non-palpable breast cancer. Cancer 46: 950–956

Svensson W E, Tohno E, Cosgrove D O, Powles T J, Al Murrani B, Jones A 1992 Effects of fine needle aspiration on the ultrasound appearance of the breast. Radiology 185: 709–711

Tokunaga M, Land C E, Yamamoto T 1984 Breast cancer among atomic bomb survivors. In: Boice J D Jr, Fraumani J F (eds) Radiation carcinogenesis: epidemiology and biological significance. Raven Press, New York, p 45

43

Malignant disease of the breast

J. Marsden M. Baum

EPIDEMIOLOGY

Breast cancer is the most common malignancy affecting women in North America and in most of Europe. The UK has the highest mortality rate in the world. It is the commonest single cause of all deaths in women aged 35–55 years, but is most commonly seen in women between 55 and 85 (Fig. 43.1). In the UK, 1 in 12 women will develop breast cancer. Incidence rates of breast cancer are approximately six to seven times higher in the western world than in underdeveloped countries.

Within any particular country, an increase in socio-economic status is accompanied by an increase in incidence; this may account for the recent rise in the incidence of breast cancer in low-risk countries. Racial characteristics appear to be less important than environmental factors: immigrants gradually assume the incidence rates of their adopted country.

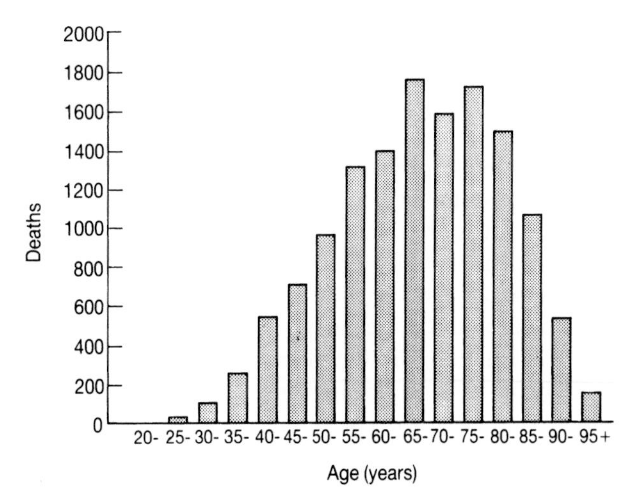

Fig. 43.1 The age-related death rate from breast cancer in England and Wales in 1988 (Office of Population Censuses and Surveys).

AETIOLOGY AND RISK FACTORS

There is no single identifiable factor or group of factors which can identify the majority of women who will develop breast cancer (Hulka & Stark 1995). A small percentage of women are at higher risk, i.e. those with a family history of breast cancer or women who have a diagnosis of atypical ductal or lobular hyperplasia as a chance finding on a breast biopsy.

The role of oestrogens

Evidence for the oestrogen dependency of breast cancer has been derived from in-vitro and animal models and epidemiological studies that have demonstrated an increased incidence of breast cancer in women who have undergone prolonged exposure to endogenous oestrogens. Thus an early menarche, late menopause, nulliparity, an older age at first conception and obesity have all been shown to be associated with an increased risk. Women are also 100 times more likely to develop the disease than men. Despite this, no clinical studies in humans have definitively demonstrated that the administration of exogenous oestrogens promotes the growth or dissemination of breast cancer cells.

The contraceptive pill

Breast cancer may be present for years before it becomes clinically apparent. Hence, women may have been prescribed an oral contraceptive when the disease was occult. Breast cancer patients with a history of contraceptive pill use present at an earlier stage than those who have never received the pill, but this has been attributed to surveillance bias (Vessey et al 1983). No detrimental effect on prognosis has been observed in pill users. Some studies have shown that the longer the duration of contraceptive pill use, the greater the incidence of breast cancer in premenopausal women. However, this appears to be associated with starting the contraceptive pill at a younger age (Rookus & van Leeuwen 1994).

Hormone replacement therapy

A meta-analysis of the use of hormone replacement therapy (HRT) in postmenopausal women indicated a relative risk of subsequently developing breast cancer of 1.07 (Dupont & Page 1991). More recent data from the American nurses' health study estimates that oestrogen alone, and combined oestrogen and progesterone preparations taken for more than 5 years, increase both the incidence and death rate by almost 50% (Colditz et al 1995). These increased risks have to be set against the reduced risk of fractures and of ischaemic heart disease (McPherson 1995). Calculation of the ultimate risk/benefit ratio is dependent upon a number of unknown factors, not least of which is whether the risk of breast cancer falls to background levels soon after stopping hormone replacement therapy or remains elevated for a prolonged period. Current risk analysis suggests that replacement therapy is beneficial when taken for up to 5 years at least.

Dietary factors

Fat consumption has been shown to stimulate breast cancer cells in experimental animal models. Case-controlled and cohort studies have not shown consistent conclusions about the importance of dietary saturated or unsaturated fats, nor the age at which dietary restriction would be important if the incidence of breast cancer were to be reduced. Abdominal-type obesity is associated with an increased risk of breast carcinoma in postmenopausal women. This may be because it provides an endocrine environment favouring the promotion of breast cancer growth in genetically susceptible women (Stoll 1994).

Radiation

The breasts are particulary susceptible to the carcinogenic effects of ionizing radiation. The effect is dose dependent and sensitivity appears to be greatest in childhood, but persists at a slowly reducing rate until the end of the fourth decade at least. The dose of radiation with mammography is less than 1.5 mGy and carries a negligible risk.

Familial breast cancer

A two- to threefold increase in incidence occurs in first-degree relatives of women who develop breast cancer under 50 years of age. However, familial aggregation of cases does not necessarily imply an inherited predisposition.

Inherited breast cancers account for about 5% of all cases, and the genetic inheritance is complex. They are characterized by an early age at presentation (i.e. < 50 years), occurrence of bilateral disease, involvement of several relatives and sometimes a history of related cancers of the colon, ovary or endometrium. Two genes, *BRCA-1* (chromosome 17q) and *BRCA-2* (chromosome 13q), probably account for about two-thirds of familial breast cancers; inherited mutations in the *p53* gene on chromosome 17p are implicated in a small number of cases.

Inherited mutations in the *BRCA-1* gene have been estimated to account for about 80% of families with early onset of multiple breast and ovarian epithelial cancers. Women in *BRCA-1* families with breast cancer are at high risk of developing a second primary breast cancer and ovarian cancer (Easton et al 1994). No male breast cancers have been seen in *BRCA-1* families, whereas several cases are present in the *BRCA-2* set.

The *BRCA-1* gene has been identified and testing should become possible (Ponder 1994). The implications for a patient shown to be at high risk emphasize the importance of counselling before testing.

Prevention of breast cancer

As no clear causative factors have emerged for breast cancer, studies can only be carried out in women who are at moderately high risk of disease. Any preventative agent must have a low risk profile.

Family history clinics. These provide the opportunity for identifying patients who are at high risk and evaluating strategies which may further improve their identification and management. Women at high risk often undergo annual breast examination, although this is of unproven value and the role of mammography in women from the age of 35 years is controversial. Data from screening the general population below the age of 50 have not demonstrated a reduction in mortality, and there are no data available on mammography in these younger, high-risk women.

Prevention trials. There are currently three different types of prevention trials under way. The tamoxifen prevention trials are under way in the UK, USA, Europe and Australasia. A trial of reduction of fat intake in high-risk women is in progress in Canada. This study will need 12 000 women in the dietary restriction intervention arm to remain compliant with the diet for 5–10 years. A chemoprevention study of contralateral breast cancer using the synthetic retinoid fenretinide is being carried out in Italy.

Surgery for prevention. Prophylactic mastectomy is the standard treatment in many centres for women with in-situ carcinoma because of the risk of subsequent invasive disease. Women at very high risk for genetic reasons may be offered bilateral prophylactic mastectomies. The psychological effects of this have yet to be fully evaluated, but it should be reserved for women in those families with an undoubted genetic predisposition who have a 50:50 chance of inheriting the gene. The mutilation of this approach may be reduced by reconstructive surgery (see below).

PATHOLOGY

There are two common forms of invasive breast cancer: ductal carcinoma and lobular carcinoma. There are in addition several 'special' forms of invasive breast cancer, as well as carcinoma-in-situ.

Invasive lobular carcinoma

These constitute 5% of invasive cancers. The microscopic appearance is characterized by a fibrous matrix through which run loose strands of small tumour cells in a linear arrangement known as Indian filing. The tumour cells also tend to grow circumferentially around ducts and lobules (targetoid growth).

Synchronous or metachronous bilateral carcinomas are not uncommon. Rarely are calcifications seen on mammography. The prognosis is similar to invasive ductal carcinoma, but lobular disease can exhibit an unusual spread of metastases, for example, meningeal infiltration in the central nervous system and diffuse retroperitoneal or serosal spread in the abdomen. The presence of signet ring cells in the latter can cause diagnostic difficulty.

Invasive ductal carcinoma

Approximately 70–80% of breast cancers are of this type. Histologically three grades of malignancy are described, according to the amount of tubular differentiation, degree of nuclear pleomorphism and number of mitotic figures. This grading system is related to prognosis. Vascular and nerve invasion indicates a worse prognosis.

Special types

These are rare, except from screening programmes, and all tend to have a favourable prognosis.

Tubular carcinoma

Pure tubular carcinoma is well differentiated and over 75% of the neoplastic elements resemble normal breast ductules. It is rare in its pure form but is commoner in screen-detected cases.

Medullary carcinoma

Often found in younger patients, these are solid, well circumscribed tumours with a marked lymphocytic infiltrate. The prognosis is relatively good.

Mucinous (colloid or gelatinous) carcinoma

Here strands or clusters of tumour cells are surrounded by abundant extracellular mucus. This tumour is thought to have a good prognosis.

Papillary carcinoma

This is usually found in elderly patients and classically presents with a nipple discharge. The tumour is well circumscribed and growth is characterized by papillary structures, often with foci of intraductal papillary growth.

In-situ carcinoma

There are two types of in-situ breast disease: ductal (DCIS) and lobular (LCIS). Lobular in-situ disease can be considered to arise from the epithelium of breast lobules, whereas ductal disease arises from the epithelium of terminal ductules.

LCIS. Lobular carcinoma-in-situ is found primarily in premenopausal women, where it is usually an incidental finding in a breast biopsy carried out for other reasons. This diagnosis does not mean that the patient will invariably develop invasive disease. Over the subsequent 20 years, about 30% will develop an invasive carcinoma, which may be either ductal or lobular and is just as likely to be in the opposite breast. There is still debate as to whether these women should be managed by observation alone or by prophylactic bilateral mastectomy.

DCIS. This may present as a nipple discharge, a palpable lump, an incidental finding at biopsy or as a screening abnormality on mammography (associated with calcification). The risk of developing invasive disease after biopsy alone is 20–30% but, in contrast to LCIS, the subsequent invasion occurs at the site of the original lesion. It is subdivided into two broad categories: (a) large cell or comedo and (b) small cell or papillary or cribriform type. The former has the greater potential to progress to invasive disease. It is not known how best to treat DCIS. There is controversy as to whether it always progresses to invasive disease or not. A national UK trial is currently evaluating the use of postbiopsy radiotherapy and tamoxifen treatment for screen-detected DCIS.

BREAST SCREENING

The NHS breast screening programme was instituted in 1988 following guidelines recommended by the Forrest Report in 1987, the aim being to reduce mortality from breast cancer by 25%. Women between the ages of 50 and 65 are invited for mammography every 3 years. Successful implementation requires a high participation of the eligible population.

Randomized controlled trials of women over 50 years of age offered screening compared with unscreened controls demonstrate that cause-specific mortality is decreased overall by 29% (Nyström et al 1993). Mortality does not appear to be reduced in women under 50.

Interval cancers, defined as those arising between screenings, has fuelled debate over the optimum period between screening mammograms. However, these cancers are usually high grade and more aggressive than screen-detected ones, and so decreasing the screening interval may not significantly influence their incidence.

A cancer screening procedure should result in the early detection and treatment of precancerous lesions with minimal upset, both constitutionally and psychologically, to the patient. Debate exists over several aspects of breast screening:

1. Lead time bias – cancers are detected at an earlier stage without any effect on overall survival, the patient has to live with the knowledge of their disease for a longer period of time.
2. Length time bias – mammography detects slower-growing, less aggressive tumours.
3. Selection bias – trials generally recruited from volunteers who are usually more health conscious and have a lower all-cause mortality.
4. 20–25% of detected lesions are DCIS – the natural history and optimum management are unknown.
5. False positive results – can generate unnecessary investigations and biopsy. Women should be aware of these facts before consenting to screening.

PRESENTATION

Breast lump

This is the commonest presentation of breast cancer. It is usually painless and discovered by chance or incidentally as part of a routine examination. The majority occur in the upper outer quadrant and axillary tail of the breast. Simultaneous bilateral carcinomas are rare (0.1–2%).

Axillary lymph node enlargement

Clinical assessment of axillary nodes is often inaccurate. Up to 40% of patients with breast cancer who have clinically normal axillary nodes actually have metastatic axillary disease. Rarely, axillary lymphadenopathy may be the only sign of an occult carcinoma.

Nipple discharge

This is an infrequent presenting symptom, being found in less than 2% of cases. A palpable lump is usually also present. Single duct discharge indicates a local cause, such as intraduct papilloma or carcinoma. Multiduct or bilateral discharge is usually due to a physiological disorder, such as duct ectasia.

Skin changes

The stroma surrounding a cancer can become fibrosed, shorten Cooper's ligaments and cause dimpling of the overlying skin or inversion of the nipple (Fig. 43.2). Oedema (peau d'orange) occurs when dermal lymphatics are infiltrated by tumour.

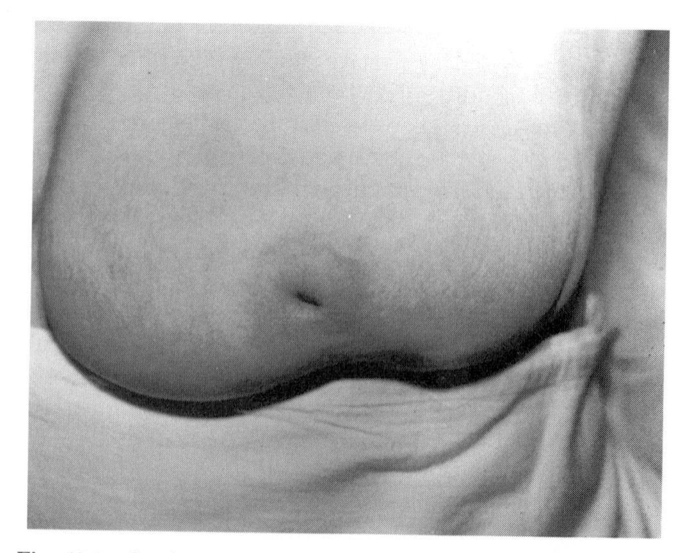

Fig. 43.2 Carcinoma of the left breast causing skin and nipple retraction.

Paget's disease

The characteristic changes of nipple discharge, ulceration and inflammation appear as a slowly growing red, raw or dry scaly patch which replaces the nipple and areola. This usually occurs in association with an underlying intraduct or infiltrating ductal carcinoma which has spread from the proximal ducts. This is palpable in only 40% of cases, but can be seen on a mammogram.

Inflammatory carcinoma

Clinically this mimics acute inflammation with erythema, swelling and tenderness. It accounts for up to 4% of all cancers and is often rapidly progressive.

Breast cancer in pregnancy

Only 0.4–5% of all cancers are diagnosed during pregnancy. Unfortunately, they often present at a late stage, as a lump may be mistaken for an adaptive change of lactation. Breast engorgement can also mask abnormalities. The prognosis is similar to the non-pregnant population when matched for age and stage.

Advanced disease

Breast cancer can be locally advanced with fixation or ulceration at presentation, or the patient may present because of symptoms from widespread metastases in the liver, skeleton or brain, without palpable evidence of a breast primary.

DIFFERENTIAL DIAGNOSIS

The differential diagnosis of breast cancer includes a number of benign, neoplastic and inflammatory conditions that can mimic malignancy. Most benign breast tumours are well defined clinically, radiographically and ultrasonographically, but confusion may arise particularly in middle and older age groups.

Although occasionally associated with underlying intraduct carcinoma, nipple discharge is more commonly seen with inflammatory lesions (e.g. duct ectasia), intraduct papillomata, endocrine disease (e.g. hyperprolactinaemia) or drug therapy (e.g. psychotrophics). Plasma cell mastitis and breast abscess produce changes similar to inflammatory carcinoma, whereas the periductal fibrosis associated with duct ectasia mimics malignancy by inversion of the nipple.

Dermatitis or eczema of the areola may suggest Paget's disease, but in the former the nipple is usually spared. Lastly, traumatic fat necrosis can produce marked fibrosis which may simulate carcinoma on both clinical and mammographic examination.

INVESTIGATION

The most important investigations in patients with breast problems are clinical examination, mammography, aspiration cytology and ultrasound scanning. The positive predictive value of these combined is high, with a low false positive rate. The aim of investigations is to determine the nature of the breast abnormality. Confirmation of a cancer will enable the patient to be fully counselled before definitive treatment.

Mammography

This involves compression of the breast between two plates – usually two views are obtained, craniocaudal and oblique. Most significant lesions present as densities (these may be irregular or spiculated), architectural distortions, oedema or calcifications within the breast (Fig. 43.3). Up to 10% of cancers will not be visible on mammography. Calcifications may be benign, malignant or indeterminate in nature. Malignant calcifications vary in size, density, alignment and may be clustered, linear

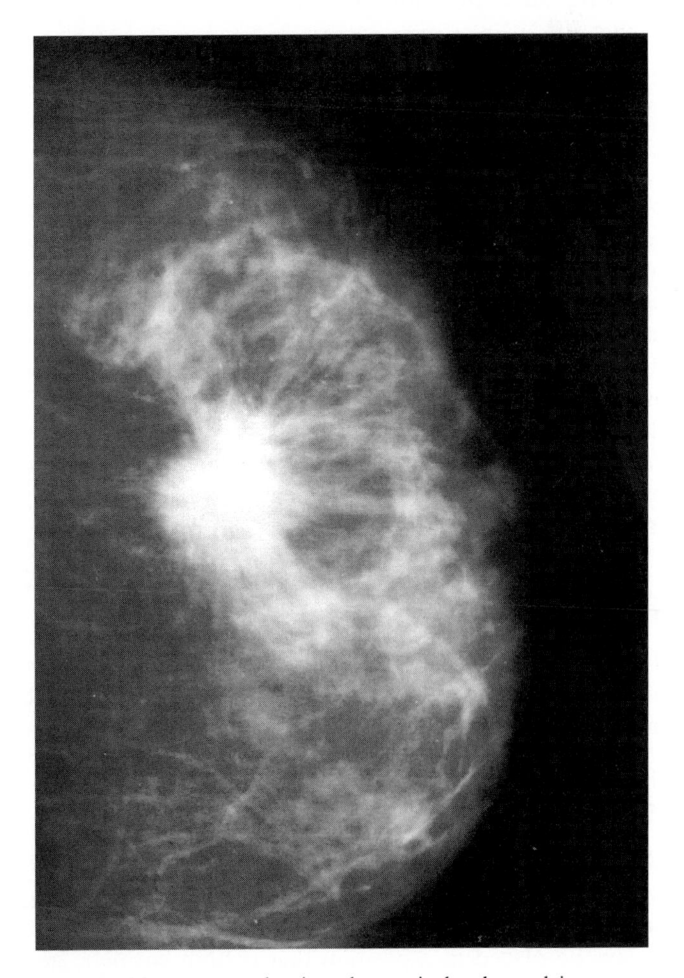

Fig. 43.3 Mammogram showing a large spiculated mass lying centrally. This was a carcinoma.

or branching. They are usually indicative of DCIS and, to a lesser extent, invasive disease. Benign calcifications, in contrast, are commonly uniform in size and density.

In addition to its use in screening, mammography can be used to detect the presence of multifocal or contralateral disease and recurrent cancer. Impalpable but mammographically suspicious lesions may be localized prior to surgical excision by placing a percutaneous hook needle alongside the lesion under mammographic guidance. Limited excision based on palpation of the needle tip is then carried out and excision of the lesion can be confirmed by specimen radiology.

Ultrasound scan

This can be used to evaluate breast lumps and as an adjunct to mammography, especially in the differentiation between solid and cystic masses. Malignant lesions are usually irregular, of mixed echogenicity and highly vascular on colour Doppler scanning (see Ch. 6).

Fine-needle aspiration cytology

Aspiration cytology is a safe and reliable outpatient procedure. It has a high sensitivity, specificity and positive predictive value. Good results are dependent on the expertise of both the clinician and the cytologist. The results are reported as follows (Trott 1991): C0 – no cells; C1 – blood and debris; C2 – benign epithelial cells; C3 – atypical cells; C4 – cells suspicious of carcinoma; C5 – carcinoma. This investigation can be used in clinically palpable lumps or in the evaluation of impalpable mammographic lesions. In the latter case, a C5 cytology cannot be used to differentiate between in-situ and invasive disease. The aspirate may also be used for hormone receptor analysis, flow cytometry and tumour markers. The commonest complication is haematoma formation. Infection and pneumothorax have been documented, but are extremely rare.

Trucut biopsy

This can be used to confirm the nature of a suspicious lump and also to provide material for grading and research purposes.

Excision biopsy

Despite the above investigations, there are a small proportion of breast lumps whose nature cannot be determined and excision biopsy is required. The breast incision should always be placed in a position that is both cosmetic and could be incorporated in a further resection if it proved to be a carcinoma.

Table 43.1 The UICC TNM staging system for breast cancer

T Tumour size	
T0	Impalpable
T1a/b	2 cm
T2a/b	2–5 cm
T3a/b	>5 cm
T4a	Direct chest extension
T4b	Skin infiltration or oedema or peau d'orange or satellite nodules in same breast
T4c	T4a + T4b
	(a = no deep fixation; b = with deep fixation)
N Nodal status	
N0	No palpable nodes
N1a	Palpable homolateral axillary nodes Clinically non-malignant
N1b	Palpable homolateral axillary nodes Clinically malignant
N2	Palpable fixed malignant nodes
N3	Clinically malignant homolateral clavicular nodes or oedema of arm
M Metastases	
M0	No clinically apparent distant metastases
M1	Distant metastases apparent

Staging investigations

Preoperative laboratory and radioimaging investigations have a low yield and high false positive rate and are not routinely necessary in the assessment of a patient known to have a primary breast cancer (Ciatto et al 1988).

STAGING

Breast cancer is staged by the TNM system based on UICC criteria (Table 43.1). This has been promoted to enhance the comparison of results of trials worldwide and provide information that can be used to choose treatment regimens. It is, however, observer biased, dependent on the extent of axillary surgery, the completeness of excision and the staging investigations that are carried out. It will soon be overtaken by more sophisticated systems (Barr & Baum 1992).

TREATMENT

Breast cancer should be regarded as a systemic disease from the outset, where long-term survival is determined by the control of micrometastases. The aims of treatment are to achieve the best cosmesis without compromising local control and to provide optimum survival with minimal adverse toxicity and psychological morbidity. Treatment of patients within randomized prospective trials greatly facilitates the evaluation of different therapies. The care of a patient with breast cancer is best catered for by a multidisciplinary approach between surgeon, medical oncologist and radiotherapist. Specially trained nurse counsellors provide invaluable support for the patient.

Surgery

In patients with operable cancer, breast conserving surgery with radiotherapy can provide similar disease control and equivalent survival to mastectomy, with a superior cosmetic result (Fisher et al 1989). Conservative surgery should only be undertaken when a good cosmetic result can be achieved without compromising local control. It would be inappropriate for a large tumour in a small breast, multifocal disease, when the risk of recurrence in the conserved breast is high (e.g. tumour extending to the margins of excision, the presence of extensive intraduct disease) or if the patient herself chooses mastectomy. The psychological outcome has been shown to be similar in patients undergoing conservative or more radical surgery, indicating that it is the diagnosis itself which affects mental wellbeing (Fallowfield et al 1986).

All patients undergoing radical surgery should be offered reconstruction. There is no evidence that immediate reconstructive surgery influences the course of the disease or delays the detection of recurrence. The aim of reconstruction is to match the projection and ptosis of the unaffected breast. There are many techniques, including subpectoral insertion of a silicone implant, tissue expanders and myocutaneous latissimus dorsi or rectus abdominis flaps (Watson et al 1995, and see below).

Treatment of the axilla

The degree of axillary lymph node involvement after initial surgery is the most powerful predictor of outcome. It must be emphasized that treating the axilla does not affect survival but it will provide local control of disease. In addition, it will identify premenopausal patients with positive nodes who might benefit from adjuvant treatment. Limited node biopsy or sampling may provide this prognostic information, but at the cost of inadequate local control – recurrence in a previously treated axilla is more difficult to manage. Formal axillary surgery avoids this problem. A level III dissection is associated with a less than 2% local recurrence rate. However, there are complications of lymphoedema (<5%), neurovascular damage and restricted shoulder movement.

Radical axillary radiotherapy achieves equivalent local control rates but prognostic information is lost. Avoiding combined surgery and radiotherapy has dramatically reduced the incidence of severe lymphoedema. New methods of staging in the axilla are being evaluated, such as antigen targeting but, at present, surgery provides the most accurate means of risk assessment.

Risk evaluation and prognosis

The risk of distant metastases is high when axillary lymph nodes are affected. A proportion of patients without involved nodes will have a poor prognosis, but at present there is no accurate method of identifying these women. Other prognostic factors, such as tumour size, grade, indices of tumour proliferative activity measured by flow cytometry, and expression of the c-*erb*B-2 oncogene, can be used to decide which of these patients should receive adjuvant therapy.

Adjuvant systemic treatment

The aim is to eradicate micrometastatic disease. Adjuvant systemic therapy can reduce the relative risk of recurrence or death by 30% at 10 years (Early Breast Cancer Trialist's Collaborative Group 1992). The results from this meta-analysis of 133 randomized trials involving 75 000 women have more clearly defined the benefits of different adjuvant treatments in pre- and postmenopausal women.

Combination chemotherapy

This has the greatest effect in patients under 50, reducing the annual rate of death by 16% and recurrence by 28%. More than 6 months' treatment does not confer added benefit.

Preoperative chemotherapy is currently being evaluated for its ability to downstage tumours and so allow conservative surgery. Its effects on disease-free and overall survival are also being examined (Bonnadonna et al 1990).

Ovarian ablation

Whether performed by surgery, radiotherapy or drugs, ovarian ablation confers a similar reduction in death and recurrence rates to chemotherapy in premenopausal women. Current trials are investigating the role of GnRH (gonadotrophin-releasing hormone) agonists as an alternative to ovarian ablation, either in direct comparison with chemotherapy or as an addition to conventional cytotoxic adjuvant therapy.

Tamoxifen

Tamoxifen reduces the annual rate of death by 17% and the recurrence rate by 25%, but survival benefits are greater in women older than 50. Significant responses are seen in both oestrogen receptor-positive and -negative patients. The optimum duration of treatment has yet to be defined. It decreases the risk of developing a contralateral breast cancer by 39% in the same age group, and a reduction in mortality associated with cardiovascular deaths has been observed.

More recently, long-term tamoxifen usage has been shown to be associated with thickening of the endometrium and possibly endometrial hyperplasia or carcinoma. This seems to apply particularly to a dose of 40 mg/day. Prior to the introduction of tamoxifen, women with breast cancer had a twofold increased risk of developing endometrial cancer within 5 years of the diagnosis of breast cancer (Adami et al 1987). The relative risk increased with age from 1.24 in women under 50 to 2.73 over 69 years of age.

The true relative risk of tamoxifen still has to be fully evaluated (Fisher et al 1994). The worst-case scenario suggests a relative risk of 3.0 for use of tamoxifen for more than 2 years. This would represent an increase in incidence from 3 per 10 000/year to 9 per 10 000/year. Monitoring the endometrium of women on adjuvant tamoxifen has produced an additional burden on already overstretched gynaecological services in the UK.

Table 43.2 Treatment of the complications of advanced breast cancer

Complication	Treatment
Vertebral collapse	Radiotherapy plus decompression
Long bone fracture	Internal fixation plus radiotherapy
Hypercalcaemia	Rehydration, calcium-lowing agents
Pleural effusions	Drainage plus pleural cytotoxics plus pleurodesis
Liver pain, cachexia	Oral corticosteroids
Cerebral secondaries	Dexamethasone Radiotherapy
Rampant local disease	Chemotherapy Radiotherapy

Treatment of the elderly

Elderly patients with breast cancer should receive treatment that effectively controls their disease long term. If they are fit, with operable disease, a wide local excision plus radiotherapy, or modified mastectomy if more appropriate, with adjuvant tamoxifen should be offered. If unfit they should receive tamoxifen and have a wide local excision under local anaesthetic, with or without radiotherapy (Dixon 1992).

Treatment in pregnancy

Any women presenting with a breast lump during pregnancy must be investigated with aspiration cytology. Mammography is safe if the fetus is shielded. Treatment decisions should be the same as for any women with breast cancer, but the use of adjuvant therapy has to be weighed against the risks of damage to the fetus. Termination may be advised during the first trimester if chemotherapy is planned, but at present there is no evidence of adverse effects on the fetus in the later stages of the pregnancy if teratogenic drugs are avoided. Radiotherapy is usually avoided until after delivery or following termination. Tamoxifen is contraindicated as the effects on the embryo are unknown. When matched for stage, survival does not appear to be affected adversely by pregnancy.

Follow-up after primary treatment

The aim is to detect and treat recurrence at an early stage. Routine restaging investigations do not appear to confer any survival advantage over a regular history, examination, mammography and additional tests as dictated by patient symptoms (Tomiak & Piccart 1993). Psychological problems are common. Some 30% of patients have significant depression and anxiety 1 year after diagnosis. The identification of these patients needs to be improved.

Treatment of metastatic disease

Metastatic disease is incurable: the prognosis for patients with advanced disease has not altered over the last 30 years, and once metastatic disease is detected the average duration of survival is 2 years. Palliation of disease while maintaining a good quality of life is the management goal.

Endocrine treatment is usually the first-line therapy. Chemotherapy is indicated in endocrine-resistant disease, rapidly progressive or life-threatening disease, and in younger patients.

The response to first-line endocrine therapy is usually around 25–30%, but may be as high as 60% in oestrogen receptor-positive tumours. Tamoxifen is the drug of choice in postmenopausal women; goserelin can be used in premenopausal patients. Second-line hormonal treatment is indicated if there is no response, or relapse at multiple sites. The main classes of drugs in this instance are progestogens or aromatase inhibitors. Approximately 30% of patients will respond.

Response rates to chemotherapy are of the order of 60%, and the average duration of response is 6 months. Combinations containing doxorubicin appear to be most effective (A'Hern et al 1993).

Secondaries may arise at any site and should be treated appropriately by the relevant specialist. The treatment of problems commonly encountered in advanced disease is summarized in Table 43.2. Close liaison between hospital staff, the palliative care team and the general practitioner is essential, not only in managing the changes in therapy that are often necessary but also to provide emotional support for the patients and their relatives.

BREAST RECONSTRUCTION

Júlio Edi Chaves,
Sirlei dos Santos Costa

Very few diseases have undergone such a revolution in treatment in the last 20 years as breast cancer. After almost a century of mutilating surgery, 'Halstedian' prin-

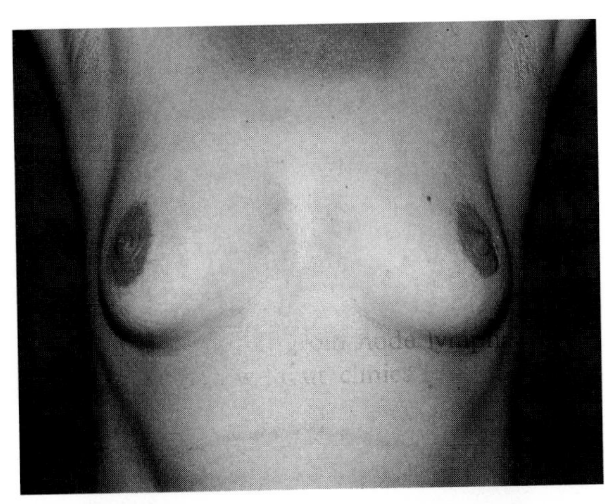

Fig. 43.4 A 34-year-old woman with a central tumour in her left breast. A biopsy was taken prior to referral.

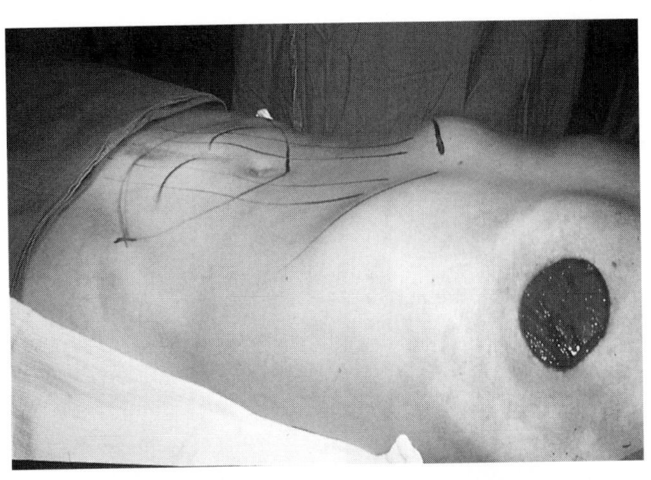

Fig. 43.5 The same patient after a periareolar mastectomy and axillary lymphadenectomy to level III. The preoperative marking of the TRAM flap is shown. A previous longitudinal incision did not interfere with the flap.

ciples were abandoned and an era of conservative surgery began. Initially, conservative surgery was intended to treat small tumours, less than 2 cm in diameter, with no evidence of axillary spread. Quandrantectomy aimed to achieve surgical resection margins of 2–4 cm (Fisher et al 1989). Since then lumpectomy or tumorectomy have been employed where lesser margins were accepted. Quadrantectomy and lumpectomy produce similar survival rates but the latter has a 2.6-fold higher local recurrence rate despite better cosmetic results (Veronesi et al 1994). Conservative surgery is now applied more often than in the past, but without reconstructive surgery a good cosmetic result often can only be achieved at the cost of inadequate margins. Reconstructive surgery aims to provide an excellent cosmetic result without sacrificing radicality of local excision (Slavin & Goldwyn 1988).

Breast reconstruction is best done at the time of primary surgery. This ensures that radicality is not sacrificed and avoids the need for a second operation, admission to hospital and period of convalescence. It is likely that the psychological trauma due to loss of body image is reduced (Rowlan et al 1995). Initially, breast reconstruction aimed only to restore an acceptable appearance when the woman was fully clothed. Now, the aim is to construct a breast which appears normal even when naked.

Our preferred procedure combines radical local excision, axillary dissection through the incision on the breast and reconstruction with a myocutaneous flap using the rectus muscle. The radical excision and careful axillary dissection obviates the need for postoperative radiotherapy in most cases, thus conserving the cosmetic advantages of the reconstruction (Dixon 1995).

The operation lasts from 4 to 5 hours and is performed simultaneously by the breast surgeon and the plastic surgeon in separate operative fields. The reconstruction of the nipple and areola is usually performed under local anaesthesia a few weeks later in the outpatient clinic

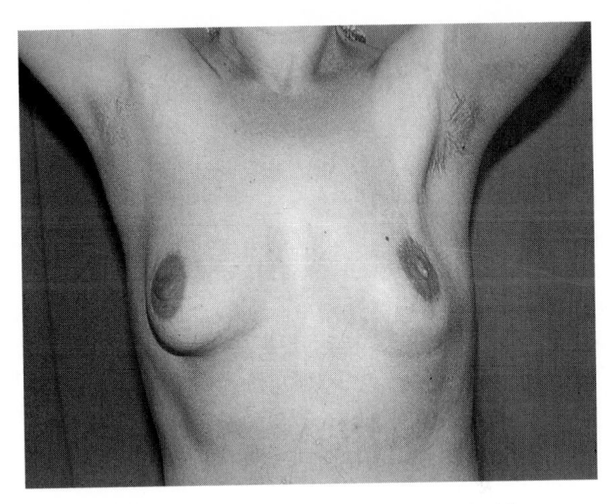

Fig. 43.6 The patient 4 months after the operation, with a reconstructed nipple and areola. The mastectomy scar is on the periareolar line.

(Figs 43.4–43.6). It is unusual to need to perform mammoplasty on the opposite breast to achieve symmetry.

A modified radical mastectomy is performed through a circumareolar incision, removing the tumour and the entire breast with wide tumour-free surgical margins. The axillary dissection is performed through the same incision to level III, in most cases dividing the tendon of the pectoralis minor. Avoiding an incision near the axilla reduces postoperative pain, causes fewer problems with the shoulder and improves the speed of postoperative recovery. A pocket on the chest wall is created to receive the flap. It is desirable to preserve the inframammary crease.

Myocutaneous flaps are created from both rectus muscles with an incision extending from 2 cm above the umbilicus to 2–3 cm above the pubic arch. Both muscles are used to reduce the risk of fat necrosis. The flap is

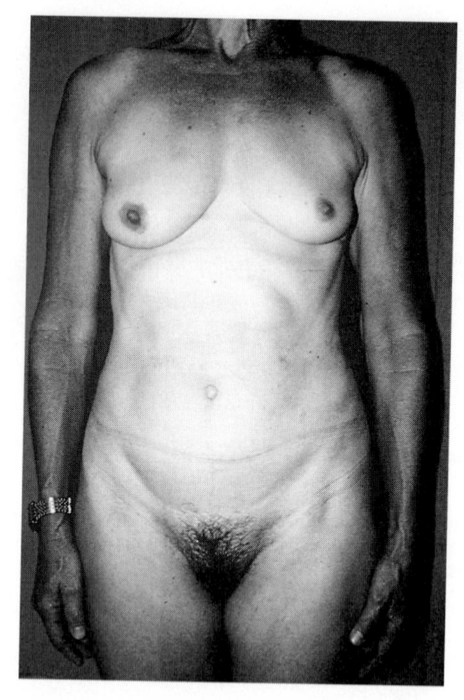

Fig. 43.7 A 42-year-old woman with a large central tumour in her right breast.

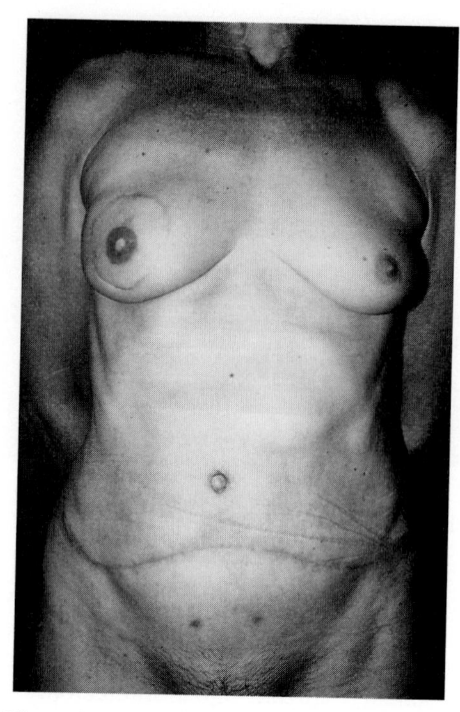

Fig. 43.8 The patient after TRAM and nipple–areola reconstruction. Note the scar on the donor area of the abdomen.

somewhat extended laterally in the region of the anterior superior iliac spine. After making the skin incision, the abdominal wall is dissected up to the chest and the vascular pedicle containing the superior epigastric vessels is carefully identified and mobilized. The myocutaneous flap is elevated, the rectus fascia is incised and the lower ends of the rectus muscle and inferior epigastric vessels are divided.

The flaps are rotated gently and delivered through a previously created subcutaneous tunnel into the chest pocket. They are anchored gently to the anterior chest wall without tension and the abdominal wound is closed (Figs 43.7 and 43.8). The chest wound is closed and the flap is fashioned to the shape and size of the contralateral breast. The tailoring of the flap to create a natural-looking breast is probably the most demanding part of the procedure. A few weeks later the nipple and areola are reconstructed under local anaesthesia, using skin from the inguinal area. A tattoo is not required. Complications include infections, wound breakdown and necrosis of the flap. These occur in less than 9% of cases, when minor complications are included.

A more recently developed method which we use increasingly often is a free myocutaneous flap created from the rectus muscle. The inferior epigastric artery, the dominant blood vessel to the rectus muscle (Moon & Taylor 1988), is carefully conserved and reanastamozed to the local blood supply, most commonly the thoracodorsal pedicle (Grotting et al 1989). The advantages of this technique are a reduced disruption of the abdominal wall because only a small part of one rectus muscle is required; reduced dissection of the chest wall; greater versatility in positioning the breast mound; and better preservation of the inframammary crease.

The team looking after women with breast cancer has a range of different options available. The best results are obtained when the options chosen are most appropriate for the individual woman. Reconstructive surgery plays an important part in this armamentarium, allowing radical local surgery to be used without sacrificing cosmesis.

KEY POINTS

1. Breast cancer is the most common cause of death in women under 55 years of age in the developed world. Environmental factors appear to play an important role in determining the incidence.
2. Early age at menarche and a late menopause are independent risk factors.
3. A family history of breast cancer in a first-degree relative increases the risk of developing breast cancer.
4. Familial breast cancers account for 5% of all breast cancers. Mutations in the *BRCA-1* and *BRCA-2* genes account for more than 80% of families with a high risk of early-onset breast cancer.

5. Benign breast disease probably does not predispose towards breast cancer.
6. The modern low-dose pill probably does not increase the incidence of breast cancer. Prognosis from breast cancer does not appear to be affected in either previous or current users of the contraceptive pill.
7. The evidence for the effect of hormone replacement therapy on breast cancer incidence is conflicting, but tends to suggest no increase in risk.
8. Mammographic screening appears to reduce the mortality in women over 50 years of age. Some 20–25% of screen detected lesions are DCIS, the natural history of which is unknown.
9. Most patients present with a lump in the breast, but skin changes or inversion of the nipple may be the first sign.
10. Breast cancer usually presents at a more advanced stage in pregnancy, but the prognosis remains the same, stage for stage.
11. Premenopausal patients with a palpable tumour should have axillary surgery and those with positive nodes be offered adjuvant chemotherapy.
12. Postmenopausal patients should receive adjuvant tamoxifen therapy, irrespective of nodal and oestrogen receptor status.

REFERENCES

Adami H-O, Krusemo U B, Bergkvist L, Persson I, Pettersson B 1987 On the age-dependent association between cancer of the breast and of the endometrium. A nationwide cohort study. British Journal of Cancer 55: 77–80

A'Hern R P, Smith I E, Ebbs S R 1993 Chemotherapy and survival in advanced breast cancer: the inclusion of doxorubicin in Cooper type regimens. British Journal of Cancer 67: 801–805

Barr L C, Baum M 1992 Time to abandon TMN staging of breast cancer? Lancet 339: 915–917

Bonnadonna G, Veronesi U, Brambilla C et al 1990 Primary chemotherapy to avoid mastectomy in tumours with diameters of 3 cm or more. Journal of the National Cancer Institute 82: 1539–1545

Ciatto S, Pacini P, Azzini V et al 1988 Preoperative breast cancer investigations: a multicentre study. Cancer 61: 1038–1040

Colditz G A, Hankinson S E, Hunter D J et al 1995 The use of oestrogens and progestins and the risk of breast cancer in postmenopausal women. New England Journal of Medicine 332: 1589–1593

Dixon J M 1992 Treatment of elderly patients with breast cancer. British Medical Journal 304: 996–997

Dixon J M 1995 Surgery and radiotherapy for early breast cancer. British Medical Journal 311: 1515–1516

Dupont W D, Page D L 1991 Menopausal estrogen replacement therapy and breast cancer. Archives of Internal Medicine 151: 67–72

Early Breast Cancer Trialist's Collaborative Group 1992 Systemic treatment of early breast cancer by hormonal, cytotoxic or immune therapy I. Lancet 339: 1–15

Early Breast Cancer Trialist's Collaborative Group 1992 Systemic treatment of early breast cancer by hormonal, cytotoxic or immune therapy II. Lancet 339:71–85

Easton D F, Narod S, Ford D, Steel M on behalf of the Breast Cancer Linkage Consortium 1994 The genetic epidemiology of BRCA1. Lancet 344: 761

Fallowfield L J, Baum M, Maguire G P 1986 Effects of breast conservation on psychological morbidity associated with diagnosis and treatment of primary breast cancer. British Medical Journal 293: 1331–1334

Fisher B, Redmond C, Poisson R et al 1989 Eight year results of a randomized trial comparing total mastectomy and lumpectomy with or without radiotherapy in the treatment of breast cancer. New England Journal of Medicine 320: 822–828

Fisher B, Constantino J P, Redmond C et al 1994 Endometrial cancer in tamoxifen-treated breast cancer patients: findings from the National Surgical Adjuvant Breast and Bowel Project (NSABP) B-14. Journal of the National Cancer Institute 86: 527–537

Grotting J C, Urist M D, Maddox W A, Vasconez L O 1989 Conventional TRAM flap versus free microsurgical TRAM flap for immediate breast reconstruction. Plastic and Reconstructive Surgery 83: 828–841

Hulka B S, Stark A T 1995 Breast cancer: cause and prevention. Lancet 346: 883–887

McPherson K 1995 Breast cancer and hormonal supplements in postmenopausal women. British Medical Journal 311: 699–700

Moon H K, Taylor G I 1988 The vascular anatomy of the rectus musculocutaneous flaps based on the deep superior epigastric system. Plastic and Reconstructive Surgery 82: 815–832

Nyström L, Rutqvist L E, Wall S et al 1993 Breast cancer screening with mammography: overview of Swedish randomised trials. Lancet 341: 973–978

Ponder B 1994 Searches begin and end. Nature 371: 279

Rookus M A, van Leeuwen F E 1994 Oral contraceptives and risk of breast cancer in women aged 20–54 years. Lancet 344: 844–851

Rowlan J H, Dioso J, Holland J C, Chaglassian T, Kinne D 1995 Breast reconstruction after mastectomy: who seeks it, who refuses? Plastic and Reconstructive Surgery 95: 812–822

Slavin S A, Goldwyn R M 1988 The midabdominal rectus abdominis myocutaneous flap: review of 236 flaps. Plastic and Reconstructive Surgery 81: 189–197

Stoll B A 1994 Breast cancer: the obesity connection. British Journal of Cancer 69: 799–801

Tomiak E, Piccart M 1993 Routine follow-up of patients after primary therapy for early breast cancer: changing concepts and challenges for the future. Annals of Oncology 4: 144–204

Trott P A 1991 Aspiration cytodiagnosis of the breast. Diagnostic Oncology 1: 79–87

Veronesi S et al 1994 Breast cancer: conservative approaches. World Journal of Surgery 18: 72–74

Vessey M, Baron J, Doll R, McPherson K, Yates D 1983 Oral contraceptives and breast cancer: final report of an epidemiological study. British Journal of Cancer 47: 455–462

Watson J D, Sainsbury J R C, Dixon J M 1995 Breast reconstruction after surgery. British Medical Journal 310: 117–121

44

Supportive care for gynaecological cancer patients: psychosocial and emotional aspects

Lawrence Goldie Jennifer Peebles Stephen Kirkham Pat Soutter

A woman suffering from cancer needs more than treatment for her disease if she is to avoid becoming a cancer cripple – a person whose life and personality are circumscribed by her disease. This applies equally to those who survive and to those whose lives are shortened. Those who care for her must be prepared to stand by her in the mental and physical turmoil to come, helping her to tap those hidden resources that lie within us all. Such a prospect is bound to be painful for the carers but the rewards are great. This chapter aims to provide an overview of the psychological and physical needs of women with cancer and their families, and the ways in which additional psychological and physical support may be provided.

BEING TRUTHFUL

It is in the nature of gynaecological malignancies that the possibility of cancer is uppermost in the mind of the patient even before the investigations that confirm their worst fears. This is unlike cancer in other parts of the body, where the patient can be unaware of the nature of her condition until told.

Whether or not to be truthful in these circumstances is no longer an issue (Goldie 1982). The problem is how best to help the woman to cope with the knowledge of her disease and its implications. This should not be seen as a task that can be disposed of in one interview, nor should it be seen as the sole responsibility of one individual. Support will be required for an extended period of time, in a variety of different forms and from a number of different individuals, but the prime responsibility lies with the physician who is caring for her.

In order to deal effectively with this situation, doctors must understand their own feelings and be aware of the natural devices they may use to avoid what is always a difficult duty, and one for which they have received no training.

Until relatively recently it was common for patients not to be told that they had cancer. The diagnosis and prognosis were imparted to the nearest relative who was left with the unenviable responsibility of telling some, all, or none of the truth to the patient and the rest of the family. This reluctance to inform the patient of the diagnosis may have stemmed from a genuine belief that she did not wish to be confronted with the truth. Although that is the case for some, there are more who do want information about their illness (Hinton 1979). Indeed, it is almost impossible to administer cytotoxic chemotherapy or radiotherapy without the patient realizing the diagnosis. Not to talk openly with the woman about her illness denies her the opportunity of talking about her fears, many of which will be inappropriate anxieties about possible effects of the cancer or the treatment.

More often the decision not to tell the truth (or to totally obscure it by euphemism) is a subconscious defence mechanism generated by the doctor. First, he has no wish to provoke the emotional anguish that such grave news will bring, and he fears the outpouring of emotion that may follow. The doctor may feel in danger of being overcome if exposed to this emotional maelstrom. As a result, he tries to be 'emotionally detached'. A carapace of cold professionalism prevents a doctor from responding to the patient's distress. Intellectual detachment may still be necessary, but it is not appropriate to stand aside emotionally. Now the doctor has to earn respect, not as a physician but as a human being. In this situation he or she is very vulnerable, and may well wish to avoid an emotional encounter.

One mechanism for self-protection is to impart the bad news just before going to theatre, or when late for a busy clinic. This provides an apparently valid excuse for not facing the inevitable emotional turmoil that ensues. These avoidance techniques may be entirely subconscious or simply due to thoughtlessness.

This behaviour is understandable. Young doctors in particular may have little personal experience of tragedy. Moreover, in the earliest years of their training student doctors are exhorted to know all the answers. Although they may be thoroughly trained in the various organic disease processes, little emphasis is given to the psychological and emotional dimensions of disease. When an operation or treatment has failed they may feel that they have failed personally. Some of the attitudes that are learnt as a student may now need to be discarded. Although doctors dealing with these tragic situations can improve their ability to cope effectively and sensitively, expert help from fully trained individuals is essential.

BREAKING THE NEWS TO THE PATIENT

When a diagnosis of cancer is made, one of the doctor's first responsibilities is breaking the news to the patient. The manner in which this responsibility is undertaken determines the subsequent relationship between the patient and the doctor. Trust and respect established at this time will ease future care for both.

Organizing the interview

Uninterrupted time without a bleep or telephone is difficult to find, but time spent now will save many hours later. A fabric of half-truths and evasion is exhausting and time-consuming to maintain. It is important to allow sufficient time for these consultations. They should never be undertaken in a hurry, or in the open ward or corridor, but be allotted time and quiet. Although it is often difficult within the constraints of a busy clinic, arrangements should be made to prevent interruptions by bleeps, telephone calls or other people. When time has been allocated, the doctor will tend to indicate by his body language that he has time to listen. No conversation of worth can be initiated by a doctor showing signs of impatience. Should it be impossible to provide a reasonable length of time (at least 20 minutes) then it is perhaps better to make a specific arrangement to see the patient again at the end of the clinic. The difficulty in finding time must never be used as an excuse to avoid a difficult and painful situation. This may also be an opportunity to introduce another member of the team who will be providing psychosocial help. This may be a specially trained counsellor, nurse, doctor or psychotherapist. Joint interviews can be helpful for the patient when the two staff members work in concert, and they are also useful for the staff to learn from one another.

Patients' frequent dissatisfaction with the explanations given to them may not be due solely to a failure of communication or lack of time. They may not retain the information or may even repress it when the content of the conversation is emotionally distressing. Hogbin and Fallowfield (1989) have suggested that tape recording 'bad news' consultations and giving the tapes to the patients to take away with them may help them understand the problem, overcome failures of recall and explain the diagnosis to their relatives. The fact that the consultation was recorded also had the effect that the doctor would often attach more importance to the consultation than hitherto. However, this approach may prevent the interview from achieving the degree of privacy and intimacy which is necessary for a real interaction.

BACUP, the British Association of Cancer United Patients, provides a series of leaflets which explain simply the nature of different cancers and their modes of treatment. These are often very helpful for patients. Main addresses are as follows: 3 Bath Place, Rivington Street, London EC2A 3JR, local information service 0171 613 2121, counselling service 696 9000, Freefone information 0800 18 11 99, 10.00 am–7.00 pm Monday–Thursday, 10.00–5.30 Friday. Glasgow office: 30 Bell Street, Glasgow

G1 1LG, 0141 553 1553, office hours. Many areas also have local support groups to which patients can be referred.

Give the patient opportunities to ask

Simple questions such as 'Have I made myself clear?' or 'Is there anything I have not explained?' will give the patient a cue to speak. Clinicians should be conscious of their body language, avoid interposing large desks between them and the patient, and try to sit at the same level and maintain eye contact. If an authoritarian posture is avoided, patients will be more likely to express their fears and feelings.

Reply honestly to questions

The clinician should always be realistic and avoid giving false reassurance. At the same time, it is important not to deny the patient all hope. Encouraging a positive but realistic attitude will help. The importance of this stage cannot be emphasized too strongly. If the doctor forms an open and honest relationship when there is hope for cure, his help will be far easier for the patient to accept if disease recurs or her condition becomes terminal.

Allow the expression of feelings

To do this effectively the doctor should empty his mind of any preconceptions about what may occur. This is difficult, because a doctor is trained to deduce what will happen in a certain set of circumstances. A doctor may think that he or she knows what it feels like to be the patient and respond accordingly. This is possibly the biggest obstacle to sensitivity. He may be seeing only a reflection of himself and may mistakenly attribute his own preconceptions and reactions to the patient. When doctors become ill themselves they often realize how wrong they have been in their assumptions about how patients feel and their responses to treatment.

Pain, grief and anger can be forcefully expressed physically, or in tears or a 'breakdown'. These emotions are natural and normal. Ideally their expression should be seen as beneficial and acceptable to both patient and doctor. If the doctor is uncomfortable in the presence of these emotions, an immediate barrier is erected. Time spent in examining this discomfort and endeavouring to understand it is intensely rewarding. Mindless reassurance benefits only those who reassure. Far better to look at one's own fears and fantasies, 'examine them, become acquainted with them, accept them and then bury them with full military honours'! By trying to protect ourselves from the possibility of failure or of saying the wrong thing, we doctors fail to discover our full potential in such circumstances and do not grow as people.

Some women will wish to cope with this news by denial. They should not be assaulted with the truth but allowed to come to terms with the situation in their own time. No response is needed other than gentle reiteration of the truth when requested. Denial may, in part, be responsible for a woman's apparent lack of understanding after the initial interview. In this case it should be carefully noted for use in further meetings.

BREAKING THE NEWS TO THE FAMILY

The conspiracy of silence

Relatives often ask that the patient should not be told the diagnosis. This wish can sometimes be very strongly stated, occasionally amounting to an absolute veto. It is worth discovering whether this is because their own fears are too great to face, or whether they wish to protect the patient. It is frequently the former, but if it is the latter it is useful to look at the relationship that already exists. If this is good the family normally wish to cope together, and know that with their help the patient will cope as well. It is when the patient's ability to cope has been thought inadequate in the past that the fear is the greatest. If the opportunity is given to discuss the woman's illness, with care and support for the whole family to cope as never before, a very positive outcome can result. The alternative is that the strain of pretence will undermine patient and family alike, with both sides usually being aware of the game being played, even if this is not admitted (Twycross & Lack 1983).

Modern cancer treatment, involving radical surgery, chemotherapy and radiotherapy, can hardly be carried out without the patient realizing that she has cancer. Even if the medical and nursing staff collude with relatives to conceal the diagnosis, day-to-day discussion and comparison of treatments with other patients will usually result in her guessing the truth. If an open approach is not adopted it imposes an almost intolerable burden on the person who is fully informed. There is a tragic irony in the situation where the nearest relative has been told the diagnosis but tries to preserve a façade, while the patient who has guessed the truth attempts to maintain a brave face for the benefit of her relatives. She then has to face alone the prospect of death, and the relatives live separated from her by this conspiracy of silence. How much better to be able to discuss their fears with each other and to provide the close emotional support that they have shared in their relationship thus far.

Telling the children

Children also need to be given information about their mother's condition to a degree dependent on their maturity. If she is frequently absent or not well enough to care for and play with them as she did prior to her illness, they may become excessively demanding, disobedient or show other signs of disturbance because they feel inexplicably rejected. Without reassurance, a child may feel responsible for his mother's illness and subsequent death. Many adults still bear feelings of guilt over how they treated their mother before her death. Frequently they were not told of the prognosis and now regret and resent the lost opportunities for giving her their time and love before her demise. Such unresolved guilt feelings not infrequently give rise to significant problems in personality and emotional adjustment in adolescents and adults. A child's understanding of illness and death, although not the same as an adult's, is often underestimated. Children can often accept the inevitable more easily than their elders.

PROBLEMS SPECIFIC TO WOMEN WITH GYNAECOLOGICAL CANCER

The gynaecologist must appreciate feminine attitudes to the menarche, menopause, menstruation and fertility. These attitudes will vary with age, social class and ethnic grouping. In younger women, gynaecological cancer may require treatment which produces sterility. Whereas an infertile woman may receive sympathy for her inability to conceive, a young woman who has had radical surgery or radiotherapy often receives no such consideration because survival from the malignant condition is considered paramount, and her infertility may be disregarded by others as relatively unimportant. Her sterility may affect her prospects of marriage or a current relationship. Women who have had children may not be unduly concerned about their reproductive abilities, but still exhibit marked anxiety over their perceived loss of femininity and sexual function. The treatment of gynaecological cancer often produces a premature menopause, and oestrogen replacement is sometimes mistakenly withheld.

The genital region is psychologically very special, being both exquisitely sensitive and primal in sexual arousal. A malignancy – literally something 'bad' – in this area is especially disturbing and significantly different in its emotional effects from cancers in other parts of the body. Surgical and radiological treatments invade and expose these private parts. Reactions will vary according to the fantasies and feelings of the individual woman about her genitalia prior to developing cancer. The over-publicized and greatly exaggerated association of cervical cancer with sexual promiscuity is a particularly potent source of unjustified and unnecessary guilt in some women.

PROBLEMS DURING AND AFTER TREATMENT

Simple questions such as 'What particularly worries you about the treatment?' provide an opportunity for the patient to express her fears. The exploration of these anxieties may be undertaken in a formal setting, or informally when the time seems opportune; on a one-to-one basis or in group therapy. There is some evidence that support of this sort may prolong the survival of cancer patients (Spiegel et al 1989).

The patient's view of time

People who are ill and receiving treatment are abstracted from the world of arranged time. For a patient waiting for results of histological examination, a week may seem an eternity. It is important to keep the patient informed at each stage of investigation and treatment, and to explain the often mundane reasons for any delay. She will frequently assume that a delay in the results of a blood test, for example, means a serious turn for the worse rather than the more prosaic reason that the sample has been mislaid or not collected from the ward.

Fears about treatment and side effects

Almost invariably a patient's fears about treatment and possible side effects are worse than the reality. Surgery is often more easily understood, but fears about anaesthesia are extremely common and often overlooked. Specific reassurance about premedication, the induction of anaesthesia and the management of postoperative pain should be given by the surgeon.

Chemotherapy and radiotherapy are potent sources of anxiety because, in the public consciousness, the frequency and severity of side effects are usually exaggerated. For example, most women expect complete hair loss after chemotherapy and should be reassured when this will not occur. If alopecia is anticipated a suitable wig should be chosen at the start of treatment, so that it can be matched to the woman's natural colour if necessary and so that it will be available when needed. Nausea and vomiting are a common problem but, with the use of prophylactic antiemetics, the treatment becomes more tolerable.

Sexual activity after treatment

When a sexually active woman undergoes radical gynaecological surgery or radiotherapy she will be concerned about her future ability to enjoy sexual activity and whether it will be as pleasurable for her partner as before her illness. However, she may be too embarrassed to ask about such matters and some may regard it as 'tasteless' or 'inappropriate' to discuss because of the gravity of her illness.

The quality of a woman's life has to be considered in relation to what it was before she became ill. An unsatisfactory relationship prior to the illness may be improved by a couple having to cope with cancer. Alternatively, a poor relationship may just simply continue to be poor, devoid of intimacy and affection. A counsel of perfection is that the doctor should be experienced in dealing with sexual problems in both the male and the female, but this is seldom the case. However, simple enquiries and a willingness to listen may be all that is required. Occasionally a patient will not have resumed sexual intercourse because she was not told that a shortened vagina can stretch with coital activity. Atrophic vaginitis is another potential cause of coital difficulty.

Loss of libido is more difficult to treat. It may arise from an altered body image – 'I am not a real woman any more' – or there may be unresolved guilt about sexual activity because of the fear of an association between sexual intercourse and cancer. Frequently all that is required is a sympathetic hearing, a full discussion and the removal of misconceptions. Occasionally, testosterone implants may be of value in the stimulation of libido. Whether this is a placebo effect or not remains undetermined.

The effect of the diagnosis on the male partner is often overlooked and close enquiry may be required to elicit an admission of difficulties. Almost invariably, when the patient admits to sexual difficulties she will also quickly add that her partner is 'very understanding', whether he is or not. Some men become impotent. This may be due to fear on his part that he may damage his partner in some way; others may feel that they can 'catch' cancer themselves. A cessation of normal sexual activity can make the patient feel unloved and make her fear that her partner is being unfaithful. Indeed, it is not uncommon for an affected male partner to regain his potency with another woman whom he regards as 'intact'. To complicate matters further these motivations may be entirely subconscious.

It cannot be emphasized too strongly that preparation is better than avoidance and silence. While the patient is in hospital undergoing treatment simple explanations and reassurance, preferably to both the woman and her partner, can prevent problems arising. Sexual function should be enquired into at the early follow-up visits, so that if any problems have occurred they can be recognized and dealt with before they become entrenched behaviour patterns. Sometimes this will require skilled psychotherapeutic help.

Returning to normal life

Prior to leaving hospital the patient should be warned that some of her relatives and friends may show some degree of embarrassment, appear ill at ease, or even avoid her. They simply do not know what to say, or how to behave. This situation may be eased if she herself brings up the subject of her illness, in order to give her relatives and friends an opportunity to voice their fears and concerns about her health, both present and future.

The woman may have been the central supporting figure in a household of some complexity and may have provided the main economic support. The very act of returning to work is often a significant milestone in recovery. Although attitudes are changing rapidly, the diagnosis of cancer may mean the end of her previous employment. Apart from the obvious anxieties about her prognosis and family relationships, financial worries can be an immense source of stress for the patient. The follow-up appointment is a suitable occasion to explore this area, with such questions as 'Are you back at work yet?' or 'The finances must be difficult with you not working'. Some employers and companies may discriminate against employees who have had cancer but are to all intents and purposes cured. Often a letter from the doctor can help, or he may be able to facilitate the intervention of social services where the patient is unaware of financial assistance that may be available.

Review appointments provide an excellent opportunity for reassurance and the reduction of unnecessary anxiety. A patient who is in the seventh year of follow-up following a Wertheim hysterectomy may not be aware that the chances of recurrence are very small because she has not been told that simple fact. At each visit the patient should be told the outcome of any investigations or examinations, and these should be presented in as optimistic and positive fashion as honesty and the clinical situation permit. Women often put on weight because of comfort eating and lack of exercise. They should be encouraged to avoid this and to take a pride in their appearance – to return to normal life.

RECURRENCE OF DISEASE AND CESSATION OF ACTIVE THERAPY

For the woman who hopes to be cured, the discovery of recurrence of cancer is a time of great despair, rage and fear. This is often worse than the time of initial diagnosis. The three causes of anguish and anger described most commonly by patients are: delay in diagnosis; not being told the diagnosis until they were too ill to complete unfinished business; and return of the cancer when they felt they had been assured of cure. The resentment at having been cheated is great. For some it is simply having the cancer; for some the word 'cure' has probably been 'heard' rather than said; but all feel that false hope has been given. The balance between false hope and no hope is difficult to achieve but important. The anger may spill over, not only to medical staff but to the family, God and the world, and is often accompanied by spiritual pain. If this anger is accepted and understood the path to acceptance is cleared. If it is not understood, and especially if it is met by a defensive attitude, it increases as unresolved or unexpressed anger and may lead to depression. Permanent, intermittent or transitory denial of the prognosis represents a necessary defence against a massive assault on the mind and emotions, and should be treated as such and the patient allowed to accept her situation at her own pace.

Hope

Cessation of active therapy means that the woman may

now be facing a terminal illness. For her family and friends this knowledge is accompanied by new fears: the course of the disease, disfigurement, dependency, loss of self-respect and dignity, dying and the manner of dying. Open discussion and acknowledgement of these anxieties with all concerned will help towards emotional security. Stopping treatment need not remove all hope. The nature of hope is to be flexible: hope for cure can be replaced with hope for a time of reasonable life; for an opportunity to complete unfinished business; or for the time to witness a particular family or personal milestone.

Loneliness and a feeling of being apart are not only hard to bear in themselves but also heighten other symptoms. This isolation is sometimes imposed by the woman herself when the thought of parting becomes intolerable. Sometimes it is imposed by medical staff, family and friends. The doctor, who can be the first person to prevent isolation, is often in a dilemma himself. With the cessation of active treatment, the identity of a doctor as the provider of physical cure disappears. To step into the role of providing emotional support is difficult. This may be why contact with the oncologist or gynaecologist is sometimes severed. This breach ends an important relationship and the patient feels unsupported and abandoned. It is impossible to overestimate the benefit of an offer of palliative care and occasional follow-up appointments, even if little physical help can be provided.

It is important at this stage to reassure the patient that she will not be abandoned. Her treatment will now be focused on her symptoms rather than on her tumour. It is vital to watch and listen with care, and to respond to what is seen and heard. It is always possible to deal honestly with her without moving into stark truth (Saunders & Baines 1989). Now the patient has to face the more immediate prospect of death. The immediate reaction may be disbelief or denial. She may react with anger, either immediately or at a later stage. Depression is common. These different emotions may occur at any time and daily alternation between one and another is possible.

Although most patients welcome the truth it will take some time and much discussion on several occasions for her to face her situation fully. She needs to feel that she can survive as an integrated caring person, whatever length of time she has and whatever the disease or treatment does to her until such time as she loses consciousness. She will require a considered, truthful answer to each of her questions. The doctor has to decide exactly what is meant by each question. 'Am I going to be all right, doctor?' could mean: 'Is there any hope of a cure?' or 'Will my death be painful?' or 'Will you abandon me?'. It may be more appropriate, when faced with an ambiguous question, to reply with 'Tell me what you mean'. This provides the patient with a cue to express her fears and ask the questions she feels need answers. Bland reassurance rarely provides more than transient comfort. It is only by giving the patient an opportunity to voice her hidden fears that her mental anguish can be relieved. She will find it difficult to talk about her impending death and will need gentle encouragement. The situation is obviously made easier if there has been an open, truthful relationship at an earlier stage of the disease.

During this time many patients ruminate over their past lives and ponder their mistakes and omissions. Essentially, the process is one of trying to find some order and meaning in their life and impending death. At this stage many personal and family quarrels can be resolved and reconciliations with estranged siblings and children may be achieved. The personal growth which can occur at this stage is substantial, and personalities can be transformed as mental peace and acceptance of the inevitable are achieved.

Fear of symptoms

Fear of symptoms now causes anxiety, not only for themselves but for the significance they bear. If this is discussed fully with patients and relatives, the anxiety is diminished and the future can be faced with greater confidence that problems will be taken seriously. This is particularly true when dealing with pain. The comment is often made that the pain is bearable now but 'supposing it becomes worse?'. Even mild pain should be taken seriously, so that confidence is established that pain can and will be treated effectively. The underlying constant fear of the patient and her carers is that they will be asked to cope with more than they are able. When further investigations and X-rays are necessary, waiting for results can be truly torture and delay seems interminable, so speed of reply is important.

Support from family, friends and professional carers

Family and friends who do not offer support may simply not know what to do or say, and it may be sufficient to show them that simple, truthful exchange is not damaging. Apparently callous demands that a wife or mother continues to fulfil her domestic duties, particularly those of providing food, can cover extreme anguish. The thought of loss is unbearable and best countered by assuming normality. This may be painful for the woman and anger others unless its cause is understood.

Help from a palliative care centre is best sought early, so that home care nurses and hospice staff are trusted friends by the time death approaches. A woman who feels alone or needs to escape from domestic responsibility often responds well to day care at a unit where she can be herself and find companionship with other cancer sufferers. The atmosphere in a good day centre is not false jollity but tranquillity, care and true happiness. Occasion may arise when symptom control can be better achieved by a short admission. Not only does the patient feel better, but the hospice is no longer perceived by the patient or her family as just a place to die. This is especially useful when young children are involved, as they have a chance to trust the staff and not to associate them only with grief and fear.

A dedicated hospice may not be available, but it would be wrong to think that anything else is inadequate. The tranquillity of a hospice is difficult to achieve elsewhere, but there is nothing sacrosanct or special about much of the expertise and care. When there is true commitment it does not take an inordinate time or effort to become familiar with the ethos of hospice care, or to acquire the expertise to provide palliative medicine.

The partner of a terminally ill woman may also feel isolated, emotionally and physically impotent, fearful of not being adequate, and unable to bear the thought of death and loss. Close involvement in emotional support and physical care will ease the burden if sufficient confidence and help can be given.

Physical needs

When physical love has been important it is now more so; when it has not been important its need is now felt. Loving touch may be avoided for fear that it may lead to more sexual intimacy. This can be overcome if both partners discuss these anxieties. The woman may not show love for fear of sex, and the man may be just as fearful of coitus causing hurt or damage. If there is libido on both sides and coitus is not possible, methods of mutual masturbation can be explained provided patient, partner and doctor or nurse are comfortable.

For a woman to be sexually complete she must feel secure. For a woman to face the future when she is terminally ill she must also feel secure. Respect, trust and love are needed to establish security. Fear, distrust and anger need to be dispelled. Respect includes self-respect, and this may have been absent even before the occurrence of cancer. Altered body image can only make it worse. To acknowledge the hurt of emaciation, hair loss, discharges, colostomy or urostomy is difficult, and sharing this difficulty helps. Love of the person rather than the body must be constantly reinforced. This can be something that has never been believed by the woman and it is hard work. There is an opportunity to engender new self-respect by true love and respect in the nursing, in discussing openly and equally, in courteous and caring examination. It is all too easy when busy and anxious and when dealing with a profoundly ill patient to forget even the common courtesies afforded to the bodily fit: to talk standing over the bed; to talk over a woman's head; not to knock on her door; to speak to a nurse when the woman is being washed or on a commode; or to refer to 'the cervix in bed 19'. To discover that caring is positive rather than just 'not negative' is rewarding for medical staff and patients alike.

SPIRITUAL AND PHYSICAL PAIN

The depression which may follow the patient's realization of the severity of her illness should not be confused with an endogenous depression. When an individual is faced with the imminent prospect of death, depression and grief are appropriate, not pathological reactions. Moreover, the patient's mental state will profoundly affect her symptomatology.

The symptom most feared by patients and their families is pain. It was Cicely Saunders who first discussed the concept of 'total pain', which includes psychological, physical, social, spiritual components as well as physical pain. Mental pain may present as a physical pain which is only poorly controlled by large doses of parenteral analgesics. When a better psychological adjustment is achieved, the quantity of analgesia required may be markedly reduced. Saunders and Baines (1989) have stressed the role of symptom control, but also point out that this requires time and close contact with the patient to give her the confidence to impart her deeper feelings, whether they be of anger, depression, guilt or regret. When a physician learns to accept mental pain as inevitable, he is freed from feelings of inadequacy and futility which inhibit intimate discussion of the patient's hopes and fears.

'Factors that lower the pain threshold include fear, anger, sadness and boredom. Sympathy, understanding, companionship, diversional activity and elevation of mood raise the pain threshold' (Twycross & Lack 1983). 'Good communication which allows expression of fears and anxiety and that conveys understanding and support can be a powerful means of alleviating pain. In some instances the relief of persistent pain may require no more than providing the honest communication that has previously been denied to the patient' (Lichter 1987).

It is a feature of all aspects of modern life that inadequate attention is given to spiritual problems. The effect of this neglect on both the dying and those caring for them is spiritual pain. Religion is a component of spirituality but is not always the total. 'Man is not destroyed by suffering, he is destroyed by meaningless suffering' (Frankl 1987). Thus the pain suffered can incorporate guilt: at having led an insufficiently caring life, at not having been strong enough to fight the cancer, at having failed God or of having deserved the cancer; anger with God for having failed; anger at being chosen to suffer; grief for the family, the world and things undone. All need to be expressed and understood even if answers cannot be offered.

PAIN CONTROL

This is managed best by following some simple general rules (Regnard & Mannix 1989).

Determine the cause of the pain

It is futile to try to manage pain in the patient with advanced cancer without first making at least a tentative diagnosis of the mechanism of production of the pain. Not all pains are due to the cancer itself: previous treatment and incidental causes are also important. Because of this a clear clinical assessment must be made, with a history of the site, areas of radiation, duration, aggravating and relieving factors, as well as a relevant clinical examination. A few investigations may be appropriate, although as a general rule very ill patients should only be subjected to even simple investigations if it is clear that different results will lead to differences in management.

Treatment goals

Treatment goals must be realistic. The aim is to free the patient from the limitations imposed upon her life by pain or by the analgesics required. The pain must be attacked both with analgesics and with measures designed to improve her ability to endure the pain by restoring her sense of personal worth and by providing her with opportunities for creative and meaningful activity.

It is almost always possible to achieve a full night's sleep free from pain. The next step is to try to ensure that the patient is sufficiently comfortable to be able to continue to engage in social intercourse and to make arrangements for her life.

Route and frequency of drug administration

Whenever possible analgesics should be given by mouth. Adequate analgesia is obtained only by the regular administration of an adequate dose of an appropriate drug at time intervals which take into account the compound's pharmacokinetics. This prevents breakthrough pain. Pethidine is not a useful drug for long-term pain control because of its short duration of action.

Choosing the correct analgesic

The mainstay of pain control remains the opioid analgesics, and the WHO have put forward a three-stage ladder for the management of pain, involving non-opioid analgesics, mild opioids and strong opioids, each stage also involving the appropriate use of other drugs which may help in pains of varying cause. Some authorities believe that even this three-stage ladder is more complicated than it need be, suggesting that large doses of weak opioids such as codeine have no advantage over small doses of strong opioids, and indeed may have disadvantages, such as an even greater tendency to cause constipation.

Generally speaking it is better to be familiar with a small number of drugs and use them well, rather than changing between a larger variety. In the UK, the drug of first choice has long been oral morphine, originally as an aqueous solution, and more recently as controlled-release tablets. Where oral administration is impossible, subcutaneous diamorphine is the usual drug of choice. The only practical difference between morphine and diamorphine lies in their solubility, diamorphine being more highly soluble than any salt of morphine. Both need be given regularly every 4 hours, in individually titrated doses increased every 2–3 days until effective control of the pain has been achieved. This may require anything from 2.5 to 200 mg per dose. The controlled-release tablets can be given every 12 hours.

In the early stages of treatment, nausea and vomiting are common and can be relieved by low doses of haloperidol, 1.5–3 mg at night (Regnard & Mannix 1989). Constipation is an almost invariable consequence of narcotic analgesia and prophylactic laxatives should be given routinely. A combination of a stool softener with a mild stimulant such as codanthramer (poloxamer plus danthron) is essential.

It has recently been recognized that both morphine and diamorphine need to be used with caution in renal failure, because of the accumulation of active metabolites. Phenazocine (Narphen) is an alternative which may be safer, although it is only available as tablets; 5 mg of phenazocine is approximately equivalent to 25 mg oral morphine. For patients who are stable transdermal fentanyl may be an option, but it is not possible to titrate analgesics against pain using a preparation which involves a new dose only every 3 days.

Presumably all pains are ultimately controllable by morphine, if enough is given to render the patient comatose, but this is hardly helpful to the patient. There is undoubtedly variation in how readily different pains respond to the strong opioids, but perhaps the best practical approach is to say that an opioid-responsive pain is one which can be completely controlled with opioids alone without significant drowsiness.

If this cannot be achieved, alternative measures need to be considered. A short course of palliative radiotherapy can be very helpful for bony metastases. NSAIDs are also useful for bone pain and for pain which is aggravated by movement. Corticosteroids relieve nerve entrapment pain by reducing local oedema. Tricyclic antidepressives such as dothiepin or amitriptyline may help soft tissue pelvic pains, and an antimuscarinic such as propantheline or hyoscine (hydrobromide sublingually or butylbromide parenterally) alleviates colic. Nerve-blocking procedures such as epidurals or intrathecal injections of neurolytics may be useful in a limited number of sites if there is resistant pain, but there may be a price to pay in terms of weakness or diminished continence.

CONTROL OF ALIMENTARY SYMPTOMS

Oral symptoms

Oral candidosis is probably the commonest cause of an uncomfortable mouth in patients with advanced malignant disease. It may show the classic signs of thrush, but can also present as angular stomatitis or atrophic glossitis. Cultures may be unhelpful because of the frequency of subclinical infection and false negatives. All forms of oral candidosis should respond to a week's course of nystatin suspension, if the patient is given adequate instruction in its use, based on the knowledge that it is a local rather than systemic antifungal. Fluconazole is a simpler, equally effective but more expensive alternative. A dry mouth is often related to treatment with antimuscarinic drugs, and the drug chart should be reviewed regularly to ensure that all medications are indeed still necessary.

Dysphagia is uncommon in women with gynaecological malignancy. It can be broadly classified into mechanical or neuromuscular dysphagia. The first is predominantly for solids and may improve with corticosteroids or endo-oesophageal stenting. The latter affects mainly liquids and occasionally responds to corticosteroids, but may need percutaneous endoscopic gastrostomy placement.

Anorexia, nausea and vomiting

Anorexia is a common accompaniment of any advanced cancer, and in severe cases can present as refractory nausea. Both glucocorticosteroids and progestogens, particularly megestrol acetate, have been reported to be helpful in anorexia. However, the use of corticosteroids is limited by long-term side effects and it is unwise to use dexamethasone in a dose larger than 2 mg daily (prednisolone 15 mg daily) for more than 2 months or so. It is advisable to check the urine occasionally for glycosuria.

Nausea and vomiting are common problems and, just as with pain, it is important to characterize what the patient is experiencing as precisely as possible before prescribing rational drug treatment based on a knowledge of the mechanism of action of the antiemetics. Although the first dose or two may need to be given parenterally, regular oral administration is the best way of keeping these symptoms at bay.

It is occasionally necessary to distinguish between regurgitation and true vomiting, because patients frequently refer to regurgitation as 'being sick', although antiemetics will clearly have no effect. A positive response to the simple if distasteful question 'Does it taste the same on the way up as it did on the way down?' virtually excludes true vomiting.

Stimulation of the chemoreceptor trigger zone (CTZ) by drugs, hypercalcaemia and tumour metabolites usually causes predominant nausea with intermittent vomiting. This usually responds to those antiemetics that block the CTZ by their antidopaminergic action, such as the phenothiazines (prochlorperazine 10 mg tds) and haloperidol (1.5–3 mg nocte). Metoclopramide and domperidone also have an antidopaminergic action, but may be less effective. As indicated above, anorexia may be so severe as to manifest as nausea. Sometimes sickness that is refractory to other treatments will respond to a moderate dose of corticosteroids.

Vomiting associated with dizziness or precipitated by movement normally responds to a vestibular tranquillizer such as sublingual hyoscine hydrobromide, cyclizine or cinnarizine. Vomiting with little or no preceding nausea usually indicates raised intracranial pressure or intestinal obstruction. If the vomits are only occasional, but of large volume, there may be gastric stasis, in which case a prokinetic such as metoclopramide, domperidone or cisapride may be helpful.

Intestinal obstruction

Intestinal obstruction is not uncommon in gynaecological malignancies, particularly where the primary site is the ovary or cervix. Although cancers may present with acute intestinal obstruction at a single site, it is much more common for advanced disease to cause intermittent subacute obstruction at several points, which in turn produces narrowed segments and reduces peristalsis. Because of this, colic is not normally a prominent feature of obstruction in this group, and indeed troublesome colic sometimes reflects a more limited number of blockages which may be amenable to surgical intervention.

It is difficult to lay down rules for drug regimens in obstruction, but certain principles may be listed:

1. There is rarely any need for intravenous rehydration or nasogastric drainage unless surgical correction is a feasible option. Indeed, a certain degree of dehydration may reduce swelling in distended loops of bowel, and therefore help symptoms to settle.
2. Parenteral steroids in high doses, such as dexamethasone 8 mg daily or more, may help to enlarge narrowed segments and relieve obstruction.
3. Patients should be prescribed a pure faecal softener such as docusate sodium, in doses up to 200 mg tds, to help to coax faecal matter past the intestinal narrowings. Peristaltic stimulants should generally be avoided as they increase the likelihood of colic.
4. Colic frequently responds to antimuscarinics such as hyoscine butylbromide or propantheline.
5. Cyclizine is probably the antiemetic of choice in this situation. It may not be possible completely to control vomiting but the vast majority of patients are able to cope at home if vomiting is reduced to about once each day. If more severe vomiting continues to be a problem the most effective antiemetic is

methotrimeprazine, a sedating phenothiazine which has blocking effects at many different sites. The drawback of methotrimeprazine is that the full antiemetic effect is not achieved until there is significant drowsiness.

6. There is a vicious cycle in intestinal obstruction, in which obstruction leads to distension, which causes intestinal hypersecretion, giving rise to further distension. This cycle can often be broken using parenteral octreotide, a synthetic analogue of somatostatin, in doses of 300–600 μg daily.

Constipation and diarrhoea

Constipation is a very much more common problem than diarrhoea, and often requires large doses of combinations of faecal softeners and peristaltic stimulants. Wherever possible, constipation should be controlled by oral laxatives rather than relying on local rectal measures, because the delayed transit time affects the whole length of the gut. The most useful single preparation is probably codanthramer, which in the UK is marketed in two strengths of suspension as well as two strengths of capsule. The stronger formulations are generally preferable, not only because patients then do not need to take so much, but also because the proportions of constituents are different, so that it is less likely to cause colic.

Diarrhoea is unusual, and spurious diarrhoea due to constipation and infective causes must be excluded. It is important also to take a history to exclude malabsorption. Formal tests of malabsorption are cumbersome, but in this patient group with a very limited prognosis a history suggestive of malabsorption, frequent passing of offensive stools that are pale and are difficult to flush away, warrants a trial of pancreatic replacement therapy.

CONTROL OF RESPIRATORY SYMPTOMS

Dyspnoea

Dyspnoea is probably one of the most difficult symptoms to manage. This is partly because a low pO_2 is not the direct cause of the breathlessness, so that giving extra oxygen is often of only marginal benefit. Instead, the breathlessness is caused by a perceived imbalance between the work done in breathing and the gas levels which are achieved. Of course reversible causes must be corrected, but often dyspnoea is due to pulmonary infiltration which makes the lungs stiff and increases the work associated with breathing, rather than impairing gas exchange. In these cases, reassurance that suffocation will not occur can be the single most helpful action. Other possibilities include the use of a variety of drugs, especially small doses of opioids, to try to reduce the brain's ability to compare respiratory effort with gas exchange. These are all sedative and there may be some price to pay in terms of drowsiness. Steroids can help to reduce the stiffness of the lungs.

Cough

In the assessment of cough it is important to distinguish dry from moist cough, since the former may respond well to antitussives, of which the most effective is probably linctus methadone 5–10 ml up to three times daily. Simple antitussives are unlikely to provide the answer in a productive cough, where antibiotics, antimuscarinics and steroids are more likely to be of benefit.

PSYCHOLOGICAL SYMPTOMS

There is an important distinction to be made between sadness which is normal and not treatable, and depression which is normal and eminently treatable. Depression can present with atypical emotions such as anger and guilt, and can be difficult to diagnose because so many of the somatic features are common in the patient with advanced cancer. However, early morning waking should be treated as being highly indicative of at least a mild depressive state. Even in the absence of depression, a tricyclic antidepressive is more likely to help this kind of sleep disturbance than a benzodiazepine hypnotic, which will generally only help problems with the onset of sleep.

Problems of confusion are more commonly due to delirium than dementia, and standard medical texts provide lists of possible causes. Drug toxicity is by far the most important because it is both frequent and treatable. The most common culprits are antidepressives, antimuscarinics and opioids, although any sedative drug can be implicated.

COMBATING LONELINESS AND LOSS OF SELF-RESPECT

Towards the end of the illness, the patient can no longer live a normal life and is relatively immobile. She remains mentally alert but is bored and may feel herself to be a burden. At such a time it is possible for occupational therapists and physiotherapists to find ways of encouraging the patient's creativity and making the best of her physical capacity. This allows her to use the time in a creative and fulfilling way. Feelings of loneliness and isolation are particularly difficult to endure, and are not helped by mere physical proximity of other people. These women need to be helped to retain a sense of their own personal worth. They need to feel that others want to share time with them: a joke, a chat or a moment of reflection; and that their opinions are still sought and valued.

FAMILY REACTIONS

The family and friends will often exhibit similar reactions of grief, anger or denial. They need time to express their feelings. Children need to be included. Any attempts to protect them are usually unhelpful. They need explanations of the disease and its treatment, and occasionally they will need reassurance that the disease is not contagious or hereditary and that it is not their fault. There is no emotional or psychological advantage in shielding them from the situation, because they will have to face the inevitable traumatic reality of bereavement in the foreseeable future. Financial and social problems also have to be considered. Relatives may wish to protect the patient from these worries, but avoiding discussion of these matters increases the patient's feelings of isolation.

ALTERNATIVE CARE SPECIALISTS

In the past these have been regarded sceptically by the medical establishment, with just cause in some cases. The desperation of those unfortunate individuals with terminal malignant disease leads them to grasp at any hope of treatment, however unlikely its provenance. Naturopathy and homoeopathy have their advocates and reported successes but, unlike some conventional medical therapy, they have not been subjected to scientific evaluation. Recent studies have attempted to evaluate 'alternative' therapies as adjuncts to conventional treatment, with apparently discouraging results (Bagenal et al 1990).

The burgeoning interest in alternative medicine is probably an expression of the desire of patients to be treated as individuals rather than have their care focused solely on the disease process. The organic model of disease which is implicit in modern scientific treatment excludes consideration of the mental or psychological dimension of illness.

The success of the organic model hitherto has probably reinforced the neglect of psychological aspects, which are not so amenable to study by scientific methods. That the mind has profound effects on bodily function and vice versa is demonstrated both in common parlance ('she lost the will to live') and by profound effects of hysterical disturbance on the motor and sensory nervous systems, as described by Breure and Freud at the turn of the century. The Cartesian dichotomy between mind and body has permeated western thought for centuries and, possibly because of this, the mental process has been regarded as qualitatively a different form of existential activity from physical function. This assumption has perhaps militated against efforts to search for a mechanism linking the two. That the two are interdependent is becoming more firmly established. Intensive counselling and supportive therapy have significantly improved the mean survival time of women with breast cancer (Spiegel et al 1989). It is not unreasonable to surmise that there may be some mechanism whereby the immune system is activated or depressed by the mental state and that this may influence tumour growth.

DYING

Dying has taken on a negative connotation because it is no longer accepted as a natural event of life. Rather, death is viewed as something contrary to nature. It is in part for the medical profession to place death in the context of life. Birth is accompanied by physical inconveniences but the beginning of life is still celebrated as glorious. Death is equally significant, and its lasting effects on the dying person's loved ones are as important. We should strive not just for death with dignity but for death with style.

For the medical profession this asks two things: first, that death should not be seen as a failure of medicine; and secondly, that each doctor becomes acquainted with death and comfortable in its presence. The latter means being at the bedside, even for a short while, and participating in death.

Kubler-Ross (1970) defined the stages of dying as denial, anger, bargaining, depression and acceptance. This helps understanding but is confusing if taken too literally: the intensity of each stage may vary widely and may last for moments only or many months. Nor is it entirely a one-way street. Ideally, by the time a woman is dying denial and anger will have been dealt with as discussed above. Depression may be deep sadness rather than clinical depression. It is natural to mourn for life and family. Intense grief is hard for carers too, and medical staff may be driven to inappropriate reactions. Excessive sedation may lead to a distraught patient unable to express her grief. 'Jollying along is to be avoided because it conveys a clear message that only cheerful positive feelings are acceptable' (Lichter 1987). This does not mean that laughter or everyday chat are inappropriate: they can help to defeat solitude and make the woman feel that, even dying, she is still a normal person.

Despite the sadness, hope and love can lead to serenity. Hope now will be that death can be dignified and that the family will be close. Many women are helped by the feeling that they can still be useful in helping their families to grieve, and welcome the chance to make their own death a less frightening and dreadful event for those for whom they care.

The needs of the family must also be attended to: as death comes closer the patient's emotional pain tends to lessen but that of the relatives does not (Hinton 1994a). This is particularly true immediately prior to death, when the patient tends to withdraw. 'The person who is frightened and insecure has a greater need of close physical contact than the person who is strong and independent' (Parkes 1978). This is true of relatives, patients and staff.

Tender nursing care gives great comfort and anxieties

which seem too trivial to show to others are shared. Nurses often have great insight into the woman's needs, and time to share this insight is important.

Even in a hospital setting it can be mutually helpful for relatives and friends to help with the physical care. It is painful to see children with a dying mother, and the instinctive desire is to protect them from terminal illness and death. However, there is ample evidence that they cope remarkably well and like to be involved with the caring. Children who are shut away from the illness and the surrounding grief find their own grieving more difficult. The fear that they have been the reason for this death is lessened if they are able to love and be loved. The aim is to allow a woman to die as the person she has always been, and mothers even of adult children tend to protect until the end unless they are helped to see the needs of the child. If the emotional and physical needs of patient and family are met, they can achieve acceptance and true serenity and feel a pride in having done so.

Physical needs of the dying

When asked early in the course of the disease, almost all women wish to die at home. As the disease progresses this number decreases (Hinton 1994a). The most common symptoms in the terminal phase of the disease are pain, weakness, nausea, vomiting and dyspnoea (Hinton 1994b). The severity of these problems occasionally necessitates admission. However, some can be overcome, pain in particular. Many of the problems of unrelieved pain arise from the actions and the mistaken beliefs of the patient or family. All these difficulties are due to poor communication with the patient and can be avoided by giving full explanations about drug use, anticipating the common responses, anxieties and misunderstandings and dispelling the unrealistic fears about drug tolerance and addiction (Twycross 1981).

Paradoxically, hospice patients more frequently die at home, largely because of the confidence given by the promise of a bed if things become too difficult. The family do not feel that admission for the last few days is a failure on their part. This is important in the period of mourning (Hinton 1994a).

If admission becomes necessary then the local palliative care unit tends to be preferred. However, this is not always possible and is relatively expensive. Hospital admission is the obvious alternative but providing care for a dying person in a busy unit is difficult and, although most relatives are happy with the care of their dying relatives, hospitals do receive more criticism than hospice or home.

General areas of dissatisfaction

Inadequate symptom control is a problem in hospices and hospitals alike. The undesirable nature of dying on busy acute wards, difficulties in obtaining information and lack of adequate community services and out of hours support are other common problems (Hinton 1994a) The noise, lack of privacy and the difficulty of providing adequate nursing care in a busy acute unit are problems that are hard to overcome. Privacy in side wards or hospice beds within a hospital setting still needs extra nursing time, which is expensive. However, some areas can be addressed, in particular the provision of information. The question most frequently asked is, when will death occur. During the pre-dying stage of the disease an accurate answer cannot be given and an attempt to do so should be avoided because it causes distress, whether the predicted time is too short or longer than was expected. It is helpful to acknowledge how hard it must be to accept that the doctor cannot really predict when death will occur. When death is imminent then it is important that the carers are kept adequately informed all the time. They wish to know not just how long it is going to be but also need help in understanding how the woman probably feels, and what is required of them. Unless reassured they may feel that sitting doing nothing is not sufficient, and need to be told that simply holding a hand or being quietly present is quite sufficient.

COMMUNITY CARE

The general practitioner

Good communication with the general practitioner is important from the outset. He should have detailed information about the initial problem and prognosis. His knowledge of the family setting may be extremely helpful where there are problems with the patient's adjustment to the diagnosis, family pressures, or her return to work. He can play a central role in mobilizing help for the patient and family from local services and organizations at all stages of the disease.

Social services

The diagnosis of malignant disease may have social effects far beyond loss and bereavement. The economic effects of loss of income may have disastrous consequences for family finances. More importantly, the patient may be a single parent, or the prime carer of an elderly, infirm parent or a disabled husband. The patient, who has to face the prospect of death, may be even more distressed by concern over her family's welfare. The social worker should be involved, not only to enlist what help social services can offer but also to contact other members of the family and close friends to try to solve what the patient may regard as insurmountable problems.

Domiciliary nursing services and hospice care

Domiciliary terminal care teams have been an important

development of the hospice movement. These may be community based, hospice based or located in a general hospital. The Douglas MacMillan and Marie Curie Foundation nurses have had special training in terminal care and bereavement counselling. Selection ensures that these nurses do not have family commitments which would prevent them from being available 24 hours a day and 7 days a week. This availability and support is greatly appreciated by families, and makes a home death possible where it would not otherwise be feasible. Only a small percentage of patients die in a hospice. Hospices will continue as centres for research, for the training of staff to work in home care teams, and for those patients with problems considered too intractable for home care.

Support organizations

There are often local branches of BACUP, CancerLink or other local organizations which run support groups. These offer a range of services, from group therapy to leaflets and advice phone lines. These can often be very helpful, not only to the patient but also to the family both during her illness and afterwards during the period of bereavement. Cancerlink central office is as follows: 11–21 Northdown Street, London N1 9BN; Freefone helpline 0800 132 905 and Asian Cancer Information helpline 0800 590 415.

BEREAVEMENT

Family and friends

Bereavement is the complex of emotions felt by those close to the patient who has died. This painful condition takes many months or years to heal. Numbness, shock and disbelief are common. The best preparation for bereavement is sympathetic handling of the patient's and family's problems throughout her illness.

There may be displaced anger, which may be directed towards the staff but is subconsciously felt towards the deceased because they have 'left' the bereaved. Anger may be directed inappropriately at the staff, especially if there appear to have been delays in diagnosis or problems with treatment. Feelings of guilt may be because of unresolved family disputes or failure to be present at the time of death, or because they did not feel able to look after the patient at home. Time and opportunities should be allowed for the family to express their feelings. If anger is displayed, a confrontational or authoritarian approach should be avoided. Questions should be answered honestly and often the real cause of the anger will then become apparent.

Immediate expressions of grief may vary. Certain ethnic groups have a cultural necessity to express their grief in a noisy and demonstrative fashion, and every effort should be made to allow this without disturbing other patients. An apparent absence of emotion commonly indicates that an abnormal grief reaction will develop. Abnormal grief reactions should be noted so that early intervention by the medical team, GP or bereavement counsellors can avert significant psychological disturbance. CRUSE Bereavement Care is an organization which specialises in the care of widows and widowers: 126 Sheen Road, Richmond, Surrey TW9 1UR, 0181 940 4818; helpline Monday–Friday 9.30 am–5.00 pm, 0181 332 7227.

Attempts to obliterate grief reactions by the use of psychotropic drugs are usually unhelpful and occasionally bring about dependence in the vulnerable personality. If an abnormal grief reaction is established, the help of a skilled psychotherapist should be sought sooner rather than later.

The staff

Saunders and Baines (1989) use the concept of 'staff pain'. They emphasize that the staff also need to grieve the loss of the patient and emphasize the importance of group support for staff to allow opportunities to express these feelings. In the context of the general gynaecological ward group meetings are probably not appropriate, but all members of staff in close contact with dying patients should offer each other support, if only in an informal way. Needs will vary. It may be a junior nurse who does not understand the need for, and hence disapproves of, a radical and possibly mutilating operation, or chemotherapy, or she may feel that she acted ineptly or inadequately at the time of death (Goldie 1990). The gynaecological surgeon or oncologist may become imperceptibly more depressed with every treatment failure, or may seek refuge by adopting a cold, impersonal attitude, avoiding non-professional contact with patients and family. He may try to deal with these feelings of loss and sadness by denial or repression. Exhaustion, frustration and despair can overtake the doctor or nurse. Recognition of these feelings and acceptance of help in coming to terms with them is the only way to retain the resilience and humanity required for the task.

KEY POINTS

1. Most patients prefer to be told the truth about their condition.
2. Supportive care is not the sole responsibility of one person but the onus lies with her doctor.
3. Staff need to be aware of their own feelings and attitudes to illness and death.
4. Staff must watch and listen carefully and respond to what they observe, rather than have any preconceived ideas about the woman's feelings and needs.
5. Time with the patient must be protected from interruption and adequate time allocated.

6. Accepting the inevitability of mental pain in the patient frees the physician from feelings of inadequacy.
7. There must be no conspiracy of silence in the family, and children need to be included.
8. Many sexual problems can be avoided by simple discussion and encouragement.
9. Analgesia should usually be given orally in regular doses.
10. Intravenous fluids should be avoided in obstruction unless it is clear that surgical correction is a feasible option.
11. Cyclizine and haloperidol are very useful for controlling nausea in obstruction.
12. The general practitioner can play a central role in mobilizing local help.
13. Bereavement affects both family and staff. Both need to mourn.

REFERENCES

Bagenal F S, Easton D F, Harris E, Chilvers C E D, McElwain T J 1990 Survival of patients with breast cancer attending Bristol Cancer Help Centre. Lancet 336: 606–610

Frankl V E 1987 Man's search for meaning, 5th edn. Hodder and Stoughton, London

Goldie L 1982 Ethics of telling the patient. Journal of Medical Ethics 8: 128–133

Goldie L 1983 Doctors in training and the dying patient. Journal of the Royal Society of Medicine 76: 995

Goldie L 1984 Psychoanalysis in the NHS general hospital. Psychoanalytic Psychotherapy 1: 23–24

Goldie L 1988 The interdisciplinary treatment of cancer: cooperation or competition. In Psychiatric Oncology – Proceedings of the 2nd and 3rd Meetings of the British Psychosocial Oncology Group 1985 and 1986

Goldie L 1990 Ethical dilemmas for nurses and their emotional implications. Psychoanalytic Psychotherapy 5: 125–138

Hinton J 1979 Comparison of places and policies for terminal care. Lancet i: 29–32

Hinton J 1994a Can home care maintain an acceptable quality of life for patients with terminal cancer and their relatives? Journal of Palliative Medicine 8: 183–196

Hinton J 1994b Which patients with terminal cancer are admitted from home care? Journal of Palliative Medicine 8: 197–210

Hogbin B, Fallowfield L 1989 Getting it taped: the 'bad news' consultation with cancer patients. British Journal of Hospital Medicine 41: 330–333

Kubler-Ross E 1970 On death and dying. Tavistock, London

Lichter I 1987 Communication in cancer care. Churchill Livingstone, Edinburgh

Parkes C M 1978 Psychological aspects in the management of terminal diseases. Edward Arnold, London

Regnard C, Mannix K 1989 Pain relief in advanced cancer. Haigh and Hochland, Manchester

Spiegel D, Bloom J R, Kraemer H C, Gottheh E 1989 Effect of psychosocial treatment on survival of patients with metastatic breast cancer. Lancet ii: 888–891

Saunders C, Baines M 1989 Living with dying. Oxford Medial Publications, Oxford

Twycross R G 1981 Rehabilitation in terminal cancer patients. International Rehabilitation Medicine 3: 135–144

Twycross R G, Lack S A 1983 Symptom control in far advanced cancer: pain relief. Pitman Medical, Tunbridge Wells

SECTION 4

Urogynaecology

45

Classification of urogynaecological disorders

S. L. Stanton

INTRODUCTION

If the body were sometimes divided into specialties by physiological rather than anatomical boundaries, there would be no need for an explanation of urogynaecology. As it is, this specialty represents an interface between gynaecologist and urologist. Physiological events or disease affecting gynaecological organs invariably affect the urinary tract, as they will also sometimes affect the adjacent alimentary system.

It is increasingly recognized that colorectal surgeons have an important role in the management of pelvic floor disorders. The studies of Snooks et al (1984) and Sultan et al (1993) show the traumatic effects of vaginal delivery on the pelvic floor and anal sphincters. Wall and De Lancey (1991) have succinctly summarized the need for a holistic approach involving gynaecologists, urologists and colorectal surgeons in the management of pelvic floor disorders.

Following the introduction of subspecialization by the American College of Obstetricians and Gynecologists, the Royal College of Obstetricians and Gynaecologists considered and then recommended subspecialization in 1982. Four subspecialties were created, among them urogynaecology. This comprised the following disorders: congenital anomalies, incontinence, voiding difficulties, urinary fistulae, bladder neuropathy, genital prolapse, urgency and frequency and urinary tract infection. By common consent, all 'supravesical' conditions and neoplasia arising anywhere in the urinary tract belong to the realm of urology. To these might now be added functional disturbances of the lower bowel, comprising faecal and flatal incontinence, disordered motility, descending perineum and rectal prolapse (in collaboration with colorectal colleagues).

TERMINOLOGY

As in any developing branch of medicine and science, old terms and definitions have become inadequate. To provide a common language for both clinician and researcher, the International Continence Society (ICS) formed a standardization committee in 1973 to draw up and revise standards of terminology of lower urinary tract function.

Five reports have appeared; the latest supersedes the others (Abrams et al 1988). Since then a further four reports have been produced: bladder training (1990), intestinal reservoirs (1996), pelvic organ prolapse and pelvic floor dysfunction (1996), and pressure–flow studies of voiding, urethral resistance and urethral obstruction (1996).

The term 'stress incontinence' was coined by Sir Eardley Holland in 1928, and meant the loss of urine during physical effort. It came to be used not only as a symptom and sign, but also as a diagnostic term. As the pathophysiology of urinary incontinence became more clearly understood, it was apparent that the term 'stress incontinence' was ambiguous as it could be applied to a symptom, a sign and a diagnosis – indeed, the symptom and sign of stress incontinence can be found in most types of incontinence.

Nowadays the term 'stress incontinence' is retained for the symptom of involuntary loss of urine on physical exertion and the sign of urine loss from the urethra immediately on increase in abdominal pressure. The term 'genuine stress incontinence' was proposed by the ICS in 1976 (Bates et al 1976) to mean the condition of involuntary loss of urine when the intravesical pressure exceeds the maximum urethral pressure in the absence of a detrusor contraction. This condition has a number of synonyms: urethral sphincter incompetence, stress urinary incontinence, anatomical stress incontinence and pressure equalization incontinence. I prefer the term 'urethral sphincter incompetence' because this accurately describes the pathophysiology of this condition.

In a similar way, the term 'dyssynergic detrusor dysfunction' was introduced by Hodgkinson et al in 1963 and other synonyms followed: urge incontinence, uninhibited bladder, bladder instability/unstable bladder. In 1979, the ICS defined an unstable bladder as one 'shown objectively to contract, spontaneously or on provocation during the filling phase, while the patient is attempting to inhibit micturition. Unstable contractions may be asymptomatic and do not necessarily imply a neurological disorder'. The contractions are phasic. Another term, 'low compliance', is used to mean a gradual increase in detrusor pressure without a subsequent decrease during bladder filling. The term 'detrusor hyperreflexia' is used for phasic uninhibited contractions when there is objective evidence of a relevant neurological disorder. Terms to be avoided include 'hypertonic', 'spastic' and 'automatic'.

CLASSIFICATION

Congenital anomalies (see Ch. 1)

The subject of congenital anomalies reaffirms the principle that a lesion affects multiple systems. Often these present to the urologist as a primary urological problem (e.g. bladder exstrophy, horseshoe kidney). The gynaecologist's expertise lies in the area of diagnosis and management of dubious sexuality or later, when reconstructive surgery may be required for epispadias or haematocolpos.

Incontinence

Urinary incontinence forms the major proportion of urogynaecology. It is defined by the ICS as 'an involuntary loss of urine which is objectively demonstrable and a social or hygienic problem'.

Incontinence is considered to be involuntary; for two categories of patients further explanation is needed. In a child under 3 years of age control of continence has not yet developed; however, careful observation shows that the normal child is dry between involuntary voids, whereas the incontinent child is wet the whole time. On the other hand, the mentally frail patient may be incontinent because she has lost her social consciousness and appreciation of the need to be dry.

The social isolation caused by incontinence is demonstrated by 25% of patients delaying for more than 5 years before seeking advice, owing to embarrassment (Norton et al 1988). Ostracism and rejection by relatives may lead to an elderly patient being institutionalized solely because of incontinence; paradoxically, some allegedly 'caring' institutions will not accept an elderly patient if she is incontinent.

There is a growing awareness that incontinence should be objectively demonstrable using urodynamic studies which will define the cause and detect other conditions such as voiding disorders.

The hygienic aspect of incontinence occupies some 25% of nursing time in hospitals, and unless managed, urinary odour is offensive to both patient and relatives alike.

Incontinence may be divided into urethral and extraurethral conditions (Fig. 45.1).

Urethral conditions

1. The commonest form is urethral sphincter incompe-

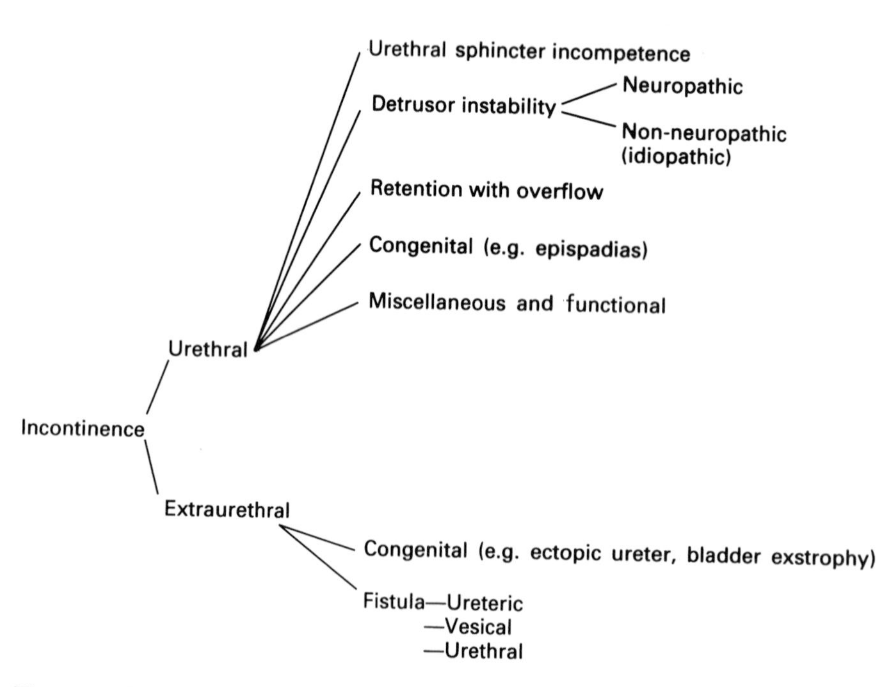

Fig. 45.1 Classification of incontinence.

tence (genuine stress incontinence), which can present from childhood (see Ch. 48). This condition has several causes and is treatable by pelvic floor exercises or surgery.

2. *Detrusor instability* (see Ch. 49): Depending on its cause, this may be subdivided into neuropathic (hyperreflexia) or non-neuropathic (idiopathic). Some patients with instability and a competent sphincter mechanism may remain dry. If, however, there is any coexistent sphincteric incompetence, the patient may complain of stress incontinence or urge incontinence.

3. *Urinary retention and overflow* (see Ch. 50): This may be acute or chronic; the former is usually sudden in onset and painful. There may be an obvious cause, such as an impacted pelvic mass. Chronic retention, on the other hand, is often painless and insidious and frequently undetected, so errors in diagnosis are often made. It occurs more commonly in the elderly as a result of neuropathy, e.g. peripheral diabetic neuropathy or stenosis of the lumbar spinal canal.

4. *Congenital disorders*: Epispadias is usually detected during childhood, but occasionally it is not diagnosed until adult life.

5. *Miscellaneous*: These causes include urethral diverticulum, urinary tract infection (temporary and commonest in the elderly), faecal impaction, drugs (such as α-adrenergic blocking agents) and functional disorders. These are rare, and the patient should be fully investigated and all the above causes excluded before this diagnosis is made. The loss of social awareness of the need to be continent is usually associated with dementia or a space-occupying lesion of the frontal cortex.

Extraurethral conditions

These are distinguished from urethral conditions by the symptom of continuous incontinence. The congenital disorders include ectopic ureter and bladder exstrophy. Urinary fistulae in the western world are largely iatrogenic, the majority occurring after abdominal hysterectomy for benign conditions (see Ch. 53). Other causes include pelvic carcinoma and its attendant surgery or radiotherapy. In the developing world, obstetrical causes such as obstructed labour with an impacted vertex are commoner. If the fistula is small, skill and patience are required to detect it.

Voiding difficulties (see Ch. 50)

These are uncommon in the female and are frequently undiagnosed. If untreated they can lead to recurrent urinary tract infection or retention following otherwise successful bladder-neck surgery for incontinence.

Urinary fistulae

These have already been referred to and are dealt with at length in Chapter 53.

Bladder neuropathy

This is rightfully dealt with by the urologist, but it is important for the gynaecologist to be aware of and recognize these disorders.

Genital prolapse

Prolapse should not be considered in isolation as it is sometimes associated with genuine stress incontinence or with perineal descent and faecal incontinence (see Ch. 51). The latter conditions represent an important interface with the colorectal surgeon.

Urgency and frequency

These symptoms can of course be part of a urinary disease process, such as urinary tract infection or detrusor instability, but can often present as single or combined symptoms in the absence of an obvious pathology (see Ch. 52).

Urinary tract infection (see Ch. 54)

This is of common interest to the obstetrician/gynaecologist, urologist and nephrologist, and the experience of all three may be required for difficult cases. However, the majority of patients are treated by the general practitioner without referral to hospital, although urinary tract infection is frequently unproven. Inadequate treatment during pregnancy can lead to acute pyelonephritis and abortion and, if neglected in later life, can lead to chronic pyelonephritis, hypertension and later renal failure.

CONCLUSION

This classification is an introduction to urogynaecology and the ensuing chapters will cover more depth. For more specialized reading a list of selected books is given after the references.

KEY POINTS

1. As trauma or denervation commonly affects the whole of the pelvic floor the concept of urogynaecology needs to be broadened to include certain functional lower bowel disorders.
2. It is important to recognize and use the internationally agreed terminology as agreed by the International Continence Society.
3. Incontinence has a variety of causes which may need urodynamic studies to diagnose them.
4. Stress incontinence means a symptom and a sign, and not a diagnosis.

REFERENCES

Abrams P, Blaivas J, Stanton S L, Andersen J 1988 Standardization of terminology of lower urinary tract function. International Continence Society. Scandinavian Journal of Urology and Nephrology (suppl) 114: 5–19

Bates P, Bradley W, Glen E et al 1976 First report on standardization of terminology of lower urinary tract function. International Continence Society. British Journal of Urology 48: 39–42

Bump R, Bo K, Brubaker L, De Lancey J, Klarskov P et al 1996 Standardization of female pelvic organ prolapse and pelvic floor dysfunction. ICS Committee on Standardization of Terminology.

Griffiths D, Hofner K, van Mastrigt R, Rollema H, Spangberg A et al 1996 Standardization of terminology of lower urinary tract function: pressure flow studies of voiding, urethral resistance and urethral obstruction.

Hodgkinson C P, Ayers M, Drukker B 1963 Dyssynergic detrusor dysfunction in the apparently normal female. American Journal of Obstetrics and Gynecology 87: 717–730

Norton P, MacDonald L, Sedgwick P, Stanton S L 1988 Distress and delay associated with urinary incontinence, frequency and urgency in women. British Medical Journal 297: 1187–1189

Snooks S, Barnes P, Swash M 1984 Damage to innervation of the voluntary anal and periurethral sphincter musculature in incontinence: an electrophysiological study. Journal of Neurology, Neurosurgery and Psychiatry 47: 1269–1273

Snooks S, Swash M, Henry M, Setchell M 1984 Injury to innervation of pelvic floor sphincter musculature in childbirth. Lancet ii: 546–550

Sultan A, Kamm M, Hudson C, Thomas J, Bartram C 1993 Anal sphincter disruption during vaginal delivery. New England Journal of Medicine 329: 1905–1911

Thuroff J, Hedlund H, Hinman F Jnr, Hohenfeller M, Mansson W et al 1996 ICS standardization of assessment and terminology of functional characteristics of intestinal urinary reservoirs.

Wall L L, De Lancey J 1991 The politics of prolapse: a revisionist approach to disorders of the pelvic floor in women. Perspectives in Biology and Medicine 34: 486–496

SUGGESTED READING

Mundy A, Stephenson T, Wein A 1994 Urodynamics; principles, practice and application, 2nd edn. Churchill Livingstone, Edinburgh

Ostergard D, Bent A 1996 Urogynecology and urodynamics: theory and practice, 4th edn. Williams & Wilkins, Baltimore

Sand P, Ostergard D 1995 Urodynamics and evaluation of female incontinence. Springer-Verlag, London

Stanton S L 1997 Clinical urogynaecology, 2nd edn. Churchill Livingstone, London (in press)

Stanton S L, Tanagho E 1986 Surgery of female incontinence, 2nd edn. Springer-Verlag, Heidelberg

Wall L, Norton P, De Lancey J 1993 Practical urogynaecology. Williams & Wilkins, Baltimore

Zacharin R F 1988 Obstetric fistula. Springer-Verlag, Vienna

46

The mechanism of continence

P. Hilton

INTRODUCTION

Urinary incontinence may be defined as a condition in which involuntary loss of urine is a social or hygienic problem, and is objectively demonstrable. Continence, then, is the ability to retain urine within the bladder between voluntary acts of micturition. In order to comprehend fully the pathological processes which lead to the development of urinary incontinence, a clear understanding of the normal mechanisms for the maintenance of continence is of course fundamental; this in turn must be based on a knowledge of the morphology and physiology of the bladder and urethra, and their supporting structures.

ANATOMY OF THE LOWER URINARY TRACT

The bladder

Detrusor

The bladder muscle or detrusor is often described as consisting of three distinct smooth muscle layers, the outer being oriented longitudinally, the middle circularly and the inner longitudinally. There is, however, frequent interchange of fibres between bundles, and separate layers are not easily defined. Moreover, from a functional point of view the detrusor appears to be constructed so as to contract as a single syncytial mass. With the exception of the muscle fibres of the superficial trigone, all areas of the detrusor show similar histological and histochemical characteristics. In distinction from other smooth muscle cells within the urinary tract, those of the detrusor are shown to contain significant amounts of acetylcholinesterase, in keeping with their abundant cholinergic parasympathetic nerve supply.

Trigone

The smooth muscle of the trigone, in contrast to that of the rest of the bladder, is easily visualized as two distinct layers (Fig. 46.1a). The deep trigonal muscle is in all respects similar to the detrusor; the superficial muscle in this region, however, has several distinguishing features. It is relatively thin, and consists of small muscle bundles; the cells themselves are devoid of acetylcholinesterase and have a more sparse cholinergic nerve supply. It may be

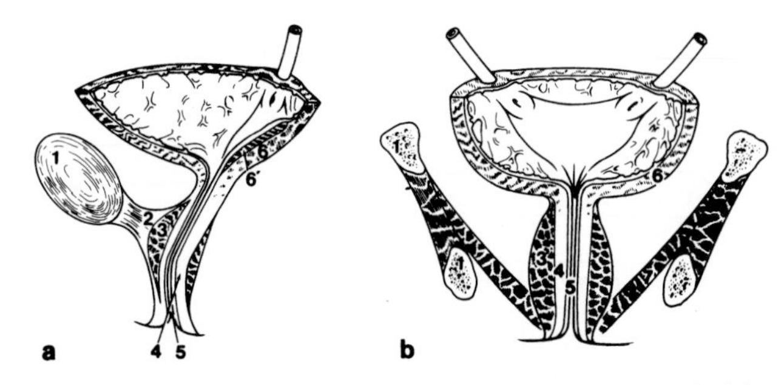

Fig. 46.1 Schematic diagrams of female bladder and urethra in (**a**) sagittal and (**b**) coronal sections. 1, pubic symphysis/rami; 2, posterior pubourethral ligaments; 3, intrinsic striated muscle (rhabdosphincter urethrae); 4, intrinsic smooth muscle; 5, mucosa and submucosal vascular tissues; 6, smooth muscle of detrusor/deep trigone; 6^1, smooth muscle of superficial trigone; 7, extrinsic striated muscle/levator ani. (From Hilton 1986, with permission)

traced distally where it fades out in the proximal urethra, forming a low crest on the posterior wall, and proximally, where it is continuous with the ureteric smooth muscle. Indeed, it has been suggested that although the bulk of this muscle is too small for it to be of any relevance to bladder-neck or urethral function, it may have significance in the control of the ureterovesical junction during voiding, thereby preventing ureteric reflux.

Bladder neck

The smooth muscle of the bladder neck is also distinct from that of the detrusor. In the male a well-defined preprostatic smooth muscle sphincter is present, consisting of small-diameter muscle bundles. In the female, however, although the smooth muscle is similarly distinct from the detrusor in terms of muscle bundle size, the orientation of bundles is largely oblique or longitudinal, and they appear to have little or no sphincter action.

Urothelium

The mucosal lining of the bladder is consistent in appearance in all regions in the distended state, and is made up of two or three layers of transitional cells. When empty, however, except over the trigone, the bladder lining is thrown up into extensive rugae and the urothelium may be up to six cells thick.

The urethra

The normal female urethra is between 30 and 50 mm in length from internal to external meatus. Its structure, in particular that of the smooth and striated muscle components, has been the subject of considerable debate.

Urethral smooth muscle

It was previously held by many workers that the smooth muscle of the bladder and that of the urethra were in direct continuity, the inner longitudinal and outer oblique layers of urethral muscle being continuous with the inner and outer longitudinal layers of the detrusor. Yet, whereas morphologically they may appear continuous, histochemically they are different in that the urethral smooth muscle cells are devoid of the acetylcholinesterase which is found in profusion within the cells of the detrusor.

Urethral and periurethral striated muscle

Controversy has also surrounded the striated muscle components of the urethra. It was previously considered that the external striated urethral sphincter and the periurethral striated muscle of the levator ani were in continuity. There is now increasing evidence that they are distinct. The intrinsic striated portion of the urethral sphincter mechanism (the external sphincter, or rhabdosphincter urethrae) consists of bundles of circularly arranged fibres, maximum in bulk at the midurethral level anteriorly, thinning laterally and being almost totally deficient posteriorly (Fig. 46.1). The extrinsic periurethral muscle of the levator ani has no direct contiguity with the urethra, being separated from it by a distinct connective tissue septum. Its muscle bundles lie in general terms lateral to the urethra, the most medial fibres being inserted into the anterolateral vaginal walls, and their bulk is maximal at the junction of the middle and lower thirds of the urethra, i.e. at a somewhat lower level than the intrinsic striated muscle. It has also been demonstrated that these muscles are histochemically distinct, and of different functional specialization. The intrinsic striated muscle is made up of small-diameter muscle fibres, rich in acid-stable myosin adenosine triphosphatase and possessing numerous mitochondria; they are therefore classified as slow twitch fibres, and are thought to be responsible for the striated muscle contribution to urethral closure at rest. By contrast, the extrinsic periurethral striated muscles are made up of a heterogeneous population of fibres, some of which show the above characteristics of slow twitch muscle whereas others are rich in alkaline-stable adenosine triphosphatase, characteristic of fast twitch muscle. The latter fibres are suspected to contribute an additional reflex component to aid urethral closure on stress.

Mucosa and submucosa

The epithelial lining of the urethra is of two types. Proximally it is continuous with that of the bladder and consists of pseudostratified transitional cells; distally it is continuous with introital skin, and consists of non-keratinized stratified squamous cells. The junction between the two varies with age and oestrogen status, and may be of significance with regard to the prevention of ascending infection.

Within the submucosa of the female urethra two prominent venous plexuses have been identified: a distal one whose structure varies little with age, and a proximal one beneath the bladder neck, where marked age-related changes are seen. In women of reproductive age the vessels are highly folded, thin-walled and with numerous arteriovenous anastomoses, giving a cavernous appearance to the submucosa not seen in postmenopausal women. These findings have been interpreted as indicating that the urethral vascular system plays a major role in the closure of the urethra in young women. The role of mucosal softness in the effective occlusion of the urethral lumen has been emphasized (see below), and it is perhaps in this context that the vascularity of the urethra has its significance.

The pubourethral ligaments

The endopelvic fascia, and more specifically the pubourethral ligaments, have been considered to form the most important suspensory mechanism for the female urethra. Zacharin (1963) described these structures as consisting of a single anterior and paired posterior ligaments, the latter being of much greater functional significance. Three anatomical expansions of the posterior ligaments have been described: posteriorly to the paraurethral tissues, laterally to the levator fascia, and recurrently, beneath the subpubic arch towards the anterior ligament, forming the so-called intermediate ligament. These 'ligaments' contain large numbers of smooth muscle bundles, which extend upwards towards the lower fibres of the bladder, and indeed have been shown to be histologically identical with the detrusor, possessing an abundant presumptive cholinergic nerve supply.

DeLancey (1988) has described a different view of the anatomy of the urethral supports, based on a series of dissections and histological sections of cadaveric pelves. He found two arches of striated muscle in relation to the distal urethra – the *compressor urethrae* and the *urethrae vaginal sphincter* – contraction of which compresses the urethra distally. In the region of the proximal urethra he found the anterior vaginal wall to have both muscular (to the pelvic diaphragm) and fascial (to the arcus tendineus fasciae pelvis) attachments. Contraction of the pelvic diaphragm therefore tends to pull the vagina against the proximal urethra, and the latter against the posterior surface of the pubic symphysis.

Although morphologically very different, these two descriptions have similar functional implications, indicating that the urethral supports may have both active and passive roles in the maintenance of the normal spatial relationships of urethra, bladder and pelvis.

NEUROLOGICAL CONTROL OF MICTURITION

The main function of the bladder is to convert the continuous excretory process of the kidneys into a more convenient intermittent process of evacuation. In order to achieve this the bladder must serve first as an efficient – i.e. continent – low-pressure reservoir whose function interferes minimally with the individual's other activities, and secondly it must allow the intermittent voluntary relinquishment of its reservoir function, within socially acceptable limits with respect to time and place, to allow voiding. These two requirements call for an extraordinarily complex neural control to coordinate sensory input from and motor output to bladder and urethra in reciprocal fashion (Fig. 46.2).

Innervation of the detrusor

Parasympathetic supply

The bladder muscle is diffusely and richly supplied with cholinergic nerve fibres, to the extent that each individual muscle cell may be supplied by one or more cholinergic nerves. The cell bodies of these fibres lie either within the pelvic plexus or within the bladder wall itself. These postganglionic fibres are supplied by preganglionic fibres with cell bodies in the intermediolateral grey columns of the sacral segments S2–S4.

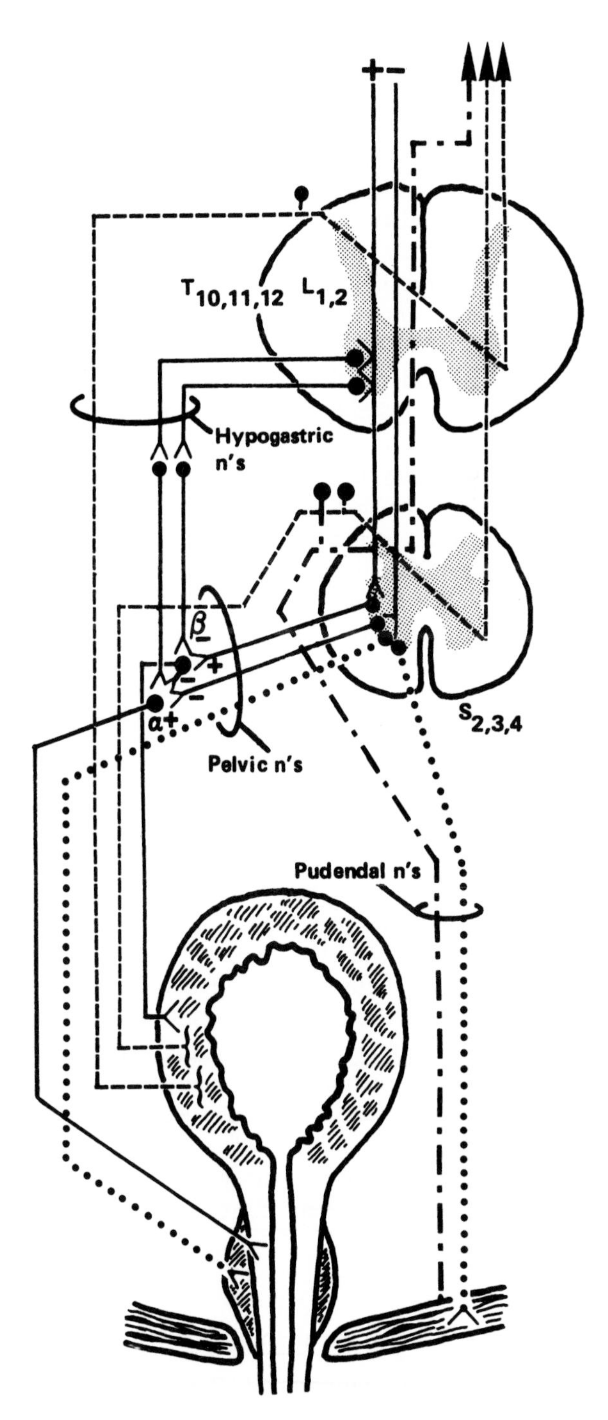

Fig. 46.2 Peripheral nerve supply to the lower urinary tract: ——, visceral efferents (parasympathetic and sympathetic); - - - -, visceral afferents; ••••, somatic efferents; – • – • – •, somatic afferents.

Sympathetic supply

Several authors have reported noradrenergic terminals to be present throughout the bladder in small numbers, and in greater concentration in the bladder neck. Others, however, found such terminals to be surprisingly sparse, and have suggested that those fibres that are present in the bladder wall are associated with blood vessels. The preganglionic fibres terminating on these postganglionic noradrenergic fibres have their cell bodies in the intermediolateral grey areas of the thoracic and lumbar segments T10–L2. They travel in the sympathetic chain and then via the lumbar splanchnic nerves to the superior hypogastric plexus. From there the right and left hypogastric nerves ramify within the pelvic plexus. It is suggested that sympathetically mediated inhibition of the bladder depends not on direct effects from noradrenergic fibres on the detrusor but indirectly, by inhibition of the excitatory parasympathetic supply within the ganglia of the pelvic plexus.

There is clear evidence that acetylcholine, acting as transmitter from the parasympathetic efferents, is responsible for the detrusor contraction during micturition. Noradrenaline, however, may be either excitatory or inhibitory, depending on the predominant receptor type. In several mammalian species α receptor sites, producing contraction in response to noradrenaline binding, have been shown to predominate in the bladder base, whereas β receptors, producing relaxation, are predominant in the dome.

Visceral afferent supply

Visceral afferent fibres may be identified travelling with both sacral and thoracolumbar visceral efferent nerves. Sacral afferents have been shown to be evenly distributed between muscle and submucosa throughout the bladder; they appear to convey the sensations of touch, pain and bladder distension, and are essential to complete normal micturition. Afferents in the thoracolumbar nerves become activated only during marked bladder distension, and their transection seems to have little effect on voiding.

All the above findings conform to the hypothesis that the sympathetic innervation of the bladder, along with the associated thoracolumbar visceral afferent supply, is concerned mainly with the filling and storage phases of the micturition cycle, whereas the parasympathetic supply and accompanying sacral afferent fibres are important for normal voiding.

Innervation of the urethral smooth muscle

Sympathetic and parasympathetic efferent and associated visceral afferent fibres from the vesical plexus also innervate the urethra. Parasympathetic efferents terminate in the urethral smooth muscle, and cholinergic stimulation produces contraction. The functional significance of this muscle, however, remains in some doubt. The orientation of its fibres suggests little sphincteric action, and its parasympathetic innervation suggests importance with respect to voiding function; contraction produces shortening and widening of the urethra along with detrusor contraction during micturition.

Sympathetic efferents also innervate the intrinsic smooth muscle, which possesses predominantly α-adrenoreceptor sites. Although there are no sex differences in adrenergic innervation of the bladder body, the sympathetic innervation of the bladder neck and urethra in the female is much less dense than in the male, where it has been suggested to have a genital rather than urinary function, preventing reflux ejaculation of semen.

Innervation of striated muscle

Intrinsic urethral striated muscle

It was long held that the rhabdosphincter urethrae was supplied by somatic efferent fibres via the pudendal nerves, but it has now been shown that this muscle is supplied via the pelvic splanchnic nerves travelling with the parasympathetic fibres to the intrinsic smooth muscle of the urethra. This is analogous to the puborectalis muscle, the other pelvicaudal component of the pelvic floor muscle.

Extrinsic periurethral striated muscle

In contrast to the intrinsic striated muscle sphincter, the extrinsic periurethral muscle of the levator ani is innervated by motor fibres from the perineal branch of the pudendal nerve. This is in common with the other sphincter cloacae component, the external anal sphincter. The above findings have clinical significance in that first, pudendal blockade would not be expected to reduce urethral resistance to a major extent, since the intrinsic striated sphincter will be unaffected, and secondly, electromyogram activity recorded from the external anal sphincter or pelvic floor does not necessarily correlate with activity of the external urethral sphincter.

Associated somatic afferent fibres also travel with the pudendal nerves; they ascend via the dorsal columns to convey proprioception from the pelvic floor.

Central nervous connections

The connections of the lower urinary tract within the central nervous system are extraordinarily complex, and many discrete centres with influences on micturition have been identified: within the cerebral cortex, in the superior frontal and anterior cingulate gyri of the frontal lobe, and the paracentral lobule; within the cerebellum, in the anterior vermis and fastigial nucleus; and within subcortical areas, including the thalamus, the basal ganglia, the limbic system, the hypothalamus, and discrete areas of the mesencephalic pontine medullary reticular formation. The full function and interactions of these various areas are incompletely understood, although the effects of ablation and tumour growth in humans and stimulation studies in animals have given some insights.

The centres within the cerebral cortex are important in the perception of sensation from the lower urinary tract and the inhibition and subsequent initiation of voiding. Lesions of the superior frontal or anterior cingulate gyri impair conscious and subconscious inhibition of the micturition reflex, and are therefore associated with symptoms of urgency and incontinence. The paracentral lobule appears to be more concerned with sphincteric function, and lesions are likely to result in urinary retention resulting from impaired sensation and spasticity of the pelvic floor.

The thalamus is the principal relay centre for pathways projecting to the cerebral cortex, and ascending pathways activated by bladder and urethral receptors synapse on neurons in specific thalamic nuclei which have reciprocal connections with the cortex. Electrical stimulation of the basal ganglia in animals leads to suppression of the detrusor reflex, whereas ablation has resulted in detrusor hyperreflexia; patients with Parkinsonism commonly are shown to have detrusor instability on cystometric examination.

Within the pontine reticular formation are two closely related areas with inhibitory and excitatory effects on the sacral micturition centre in the conus medullaris. Lesions of the cord below this always lead to incoordinate voiding, with failure of urethral relaxation during detrusor contraction; lesions above this level may be associated with normal, though involuntary, micturition.

PHYSIOLOGY OF THE LOWER URINARY TRACT

From the definitions given above it is self-evident that continence is dependent on 'the powers of urethral resistance exceeding the forces of urinary expulsion', that is, continence is maintained when the maximum urethral pressure exceeds the bladder pressure, or when the urethral closure pressure is positive. Normal micturition may be said to result from the controlled reversal of this equilibrium, and incontinence from its uncontrolled reversal. The important aspects of the control of continence, therefore, are first, those factors which maintain low intravesical pressure, and secondly, those which ensure that the urethral pressure remains high – or at least higher than intravesical pressure – at all times during the filling and storage phases of the micturition cycle.

Behaviour of the bladder

The intravesical pressure is dependent upon a number of factors (Fig. 46.3), including the following:

1. *Hydrostatic pressure at the bladder neck.* Liquid in the bladder, when in hydrostatic equilibrium, has a vertical gravitational pressure gradient and the measured pressure must therefore be referred to a standard level. For clinical practice the intravesical pressure is defined as the pressure in the bladder with respect to atmospheric pressure, measured at the level of the upper border of the symphysis pubis. In terms of the maintenance of continence, the critical pressure is that acting at the bladder neck, which tends to work against the closure forces of the urethra; this has a hydrostatic element dependent on the head of fluid above it; this, of course, increases with increasing bladder volume, although it rarely amounts to more than 10 cmH_2O.
2. *Transmission of intra-abdominal pressure.* The bladder is normally an intra-abdominal organ, and is therefore subject to pressures transmitted from adjacent viscera and elsewhere within the abdominal cavity. This is not of great importance in the resting situation, since pressures transmitted to the bladder are low and are generally transmitted equally to bladder neck and proximal urethra; this effect may, however, be critical in the maintenance of continence in the face of stress (see below).
3. *Tension in the bladder wall.* This is in part a passive phenomenon related to the distensibility or viscoelastic properties of the bladder wall itself, and in part an active

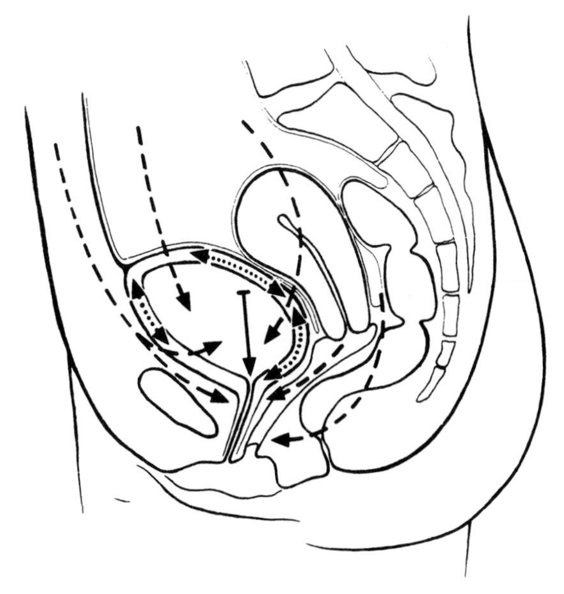

Fig. 46.3 Factors determining the intravesical pressure, and which are therefore of relevance to the maintenance of urethral closure pressure: ——, hydrostatic pressure at the bladder neck; – – – –, transmission of intra-abdominal pressure; ••••, passive and active tension in the bladder wall. (From Hilton 1992, with permission)

phenomenon due to the contractility of the detrusor muscle and its neurological control.

Viscoelasticity of the bladder

During rapid stepwise filling of the bladder the detrusor pressure rises rapidly and afterwards decays exponentially with time (Fig. 46.4a); this time dependence is similar to that expected of a passive viscoelastic solid. However, under the near-static conditions of physiological filling, the detrusor's behaviour is more accurately described as elastic. That is, the detrusor pressure rises little as the bladder volume increases from zero to functional capacity (Fig. 46.4b).

Contractility of the bladder and its neural control

The neurological control of detrusor contractility is dependent upon a sacral spinal reflex under the control of several higher centres, as considered earlier. This basic reflex arc is best considered as a loop (Fig. 46.5) extending from sensory receptors within the bladder wall, through the pelvic plexus and via visceral afferent fibres travelling with the pelvic splanchnic nerves, to enter the spinal cord in the S2–S4 level, via internuncial neurons within the cord synapsing with cell bodies in the intermediolateral grey area of the same sacral levels, and thence via parasympathetic fibres in the pelvic splanchnic nerves through the pelvic plexus to the smooth muscle cells of the detrusor. The stretch receptors or proprioceptors within the bladder wall are in effect connected in series with muscle cells, and are therefore stimulated by both passive stretch and by active contraction of the detrusor. Once a critical level of stretch is achieved impulses pass in the afferent limb of the reflex arc, and the resultant efferent discharge leads to a detrusor contraction.

The higher control over the basic visceral reflex arc is mediated through descending pathways from the pontine reticular formation. Although both excitatory and inhibitory centres have been located in this region, their net effect is primarily an inhibitory one and their normal influence is therefore to prevent contraction of the detrusor, and thus to encourage the maintenance of a low intravesical pressure during the filling phase of the micturition cycle.

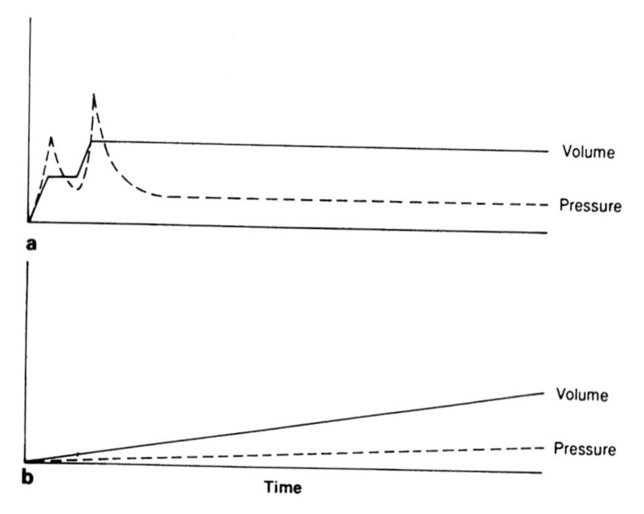

Fig. 46.4 The behaviour of the bladder in terms of pressure and volume changes with time during (**a**) rapid stepwise filling and (**b**) slow continuous (physiological) filling. (From Hilton 1992, with permission)

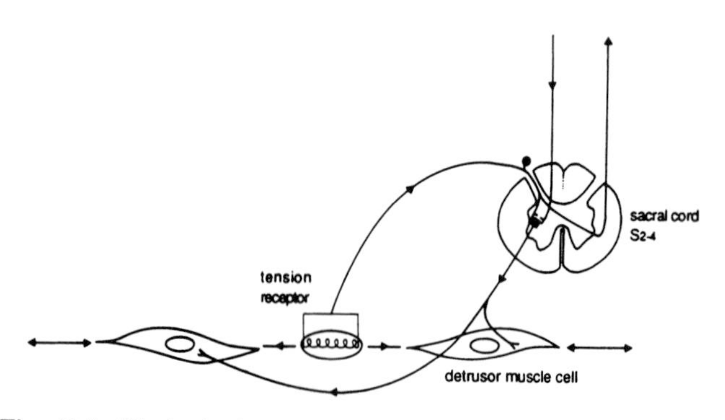

Fig. 46.5 The basic visceral reflex arc concerned in detrusor contractility.

Urethra

In order to maintain continence it is vital not only that the intravesical pressure should remain low during the storage phase of the micturition cycle, but also that the urethral lumen should seal completely. Three components of urethral function are necessary to achieve this hermetic property: urethral inner wall softness, inner urethral compression and outer wall tension. Whereas the closure of any elastic tube can be obtained if sufficient compression is applied to it, the efficiency of closure is dramatically increased if its lining possesses the property of plasticity, or the ability to mould into a watertight seal.

There has been much debate over the morphological components that contribute to the functional characteristics of softness, compression and tension in the urethra. Several authors have commented on the vascularity of the urethra and pointed out that the submucosal vascular plexuses far exceed the requirements of a blood supply for the organ. Some have suggested a significant vascular contribution to urethral closure, although others have found no specific features to suggest an important occlusive role for the urethral vascular supply. Nevertheless, whatever the contribution of the urethral blood supply to the measured intraluminal pressure, it is likely to be of significance as regards the plasticity of the urothelium and submucosa.

The structures leading to inner wall compression by virtue of their contribution to outer wall tension can be and have been quantified in terms of the urethral pressure profile (Fig. 46.6). These structures may include the intramural elastic fibres, the intrinsic smooth and striated muscle, and the extrinsic or periurethral striated muscle.

From urethral pressure studies undertaken at various stages during radical pelvic surgery, Rud and colleagues (1980) showed that approximately one-third of the resting urethral pressure is due to striated muscle effects, one-third to smooth muscle effects and one-third to its vascular supply.

Whatever the relative importance of the above factors to active wall tension, it should be remembered that these same structures also contribute a passive or elastic tension, together with the supporting elements of collagen and elastin.

The usual level of continence in the female is not, as one might expect, in the midurethra at the level of maximum resting pressure, but at the bladder neck. This region in the female has no sphincteric circular smooth muscle and is virtually devoid of striated muscle; it would therefore seem that the passive elastic tension is the most important factor leading to closure at the bladder neck and proximal urethra (Fig. 46.6). It is recognized, however, that 20–50% of women have incompetence at the bladder-neck level, and depend on distal mechanisms for continence.

In midurethra the most prominent structural feature is the intrinsic striated muscle, or rhabdosphincter. Electron microscopic and histochemical evidence suggests that this may be responsible for the bulk of active urethral tone at rest. Electromyographic studies, histochemical evidence and urethral pressure measurements all suggest that the periurethral striated muscles have their maximum effect at a level slightly distal to that of the resting urethral pressure profile (Fig. 46.6) and do not contribute greatly to the maintenance of continence at rest. It is likely, however, that these muscles play a significant role in the maintenance of urethral closure in the face of increased intra-abdominal pressure (see below).

Resting urethral closure pressure profile

Intravesical pressure

Atmospheric pressure

Stress urethral closure pressure profile

Fig. 46.6 Schematic drawing of the female bladder and urethra in coronal section. Below are shown urethral closure pressure profiles at rest (middle) and on stress (bottom) to demonstrate the morphological and functional correlation. (From Hilton 1990, with permission)

THE NORMAL MICTURITION CYCLE

From the background information contained in previous sections it is now possible to discuss the mechanisms whereby urine is retained within the bladder during the filling and storage phases, and evacuated during the voiding phase of the normal micturition cycle (Fig. 46.7).

Filling and storage phase

The bladder normally fills with urine by a series of peristaltic contractions at a rate of between 0.5 and 5 ml/min;

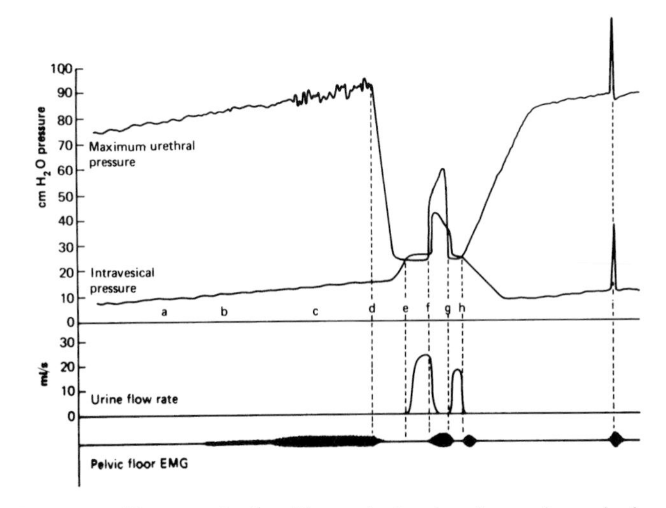

Fig. 46.7 The normal micturition cycle showing changes in urethral and intravesical pressure, urine flow rate and pelvic floor electromyogram (EMG). **a** Phase of subconscious inhibition; **b** phase of conscious (suppressible) inhibition; **c** phase of reinforced (unsuppressible) inhibition; **d** initiation or transition; **e** voiding; **f** interruption of micturition by pelvic floor contraction; **g** resumption of micturition; **h** end of void; **i** increase in intra-abdominal pressure due to a cough. (From Hilton 1986, with permission)

under these conditions the bladder pressure increases only minimally. Even during the course of cystometry at rapid filling rates, in normal individuals the pressure rises by no more than 15 cmH_2O from empty to cystometric capacity. Urethral closure, meanwhile, is maintained by the combined passive and active effects of its smooth and striated muscle components, its elastic content and its blood supply. The hermetic efficiency is accentuated by the softness of its mucosa.

During the early stages of bladder filling, proprioceptive afferent impulses from stretch receptors within the bladder wall pass via the pelvic nerves to sacral dorsal roots S2–S4. These impulses ascend in the cord via the lateral spinothalamic tracts and a detrusor motor response is subconsciously inhibited by descending impulses from the subcortical micturition centres (Fig. 46.7a).

As the bladder volume increases further afferent impulses ascend to the cerebral cortex, and the sensation of bladder filling associated with the desire to micturate is first consciously appreciated usually at between 200 and 300 ml, or half the functional bladder capacity. The inhibition of detrusor contraction is now cortically mediated, although the desire to void may be further suppressed to subconscious levels again, given sufficient distracting afferent stimuli. Although descending impulses inhibit preganglionic parasympathetic cell bodies in the sacral cord, there may also be excitatory effects on the sympathetic neurons in the thoracolumbar region, causing increased efferent discharge to the β-adrenoreceptors within the bladder (and/or further inhibition within the pelvic plexus of parasympathetic fibres to the bladder), leading to its relaxation, and to α-adrenoreceptors in the proximal urethra (and/or further excitation within the pelvic plexus of postganglionic parasympathetic fibres to the urethra), leading to a slight increase in urethral pressure (Fig. 46.7b).

With further filling, impulses within the visceral afferent fibres accompanying the sympathetic efferents to thoracolumbar roots T10–L2 ascend to the cerebral cortex, and a further desire to void is appreciated; reinforced conscious inhibition of micturition then occurs while a suitable site and posture for micturition are sought. During this time, in addition to the cortical suppression of detrusor activity, there may also be a voluntary pelvic floor contraction in an attempt to maintain urethral closure; this may be evidenced by a further increase in urethral closure pressure and by marked fluctuations in urethral pressure as the sensation of urgency becomes increasingly severe (Fig. 46.7c).

Initiation phase

When a suitable time, site and posture for micturition have been selected the process of voiding commences. This may be considered in two phases – the initiation, or transition from the non-voiding state, and micturition itself. Several theories have been propounded to explain the transition phase, although the process is perhaps best viewed as combining features of several of these.

Relaxation of the pelvic floor may be shown to occur early in the process, both radiologically and electromyographically; it is likely that simultaneous relaxation of the intrinsic striated muscle also occurs, since a marked fall in intraurethral pressure is seen before the intravesical pressure rises, during both voluntary and provoked voiding, and the same has been shown in response to sacral nerve stimulation (Fig. 46.7d).

A few seconds later the descending inhibitory influences from the cerebral cortex acting on the sacral micturition centre are suppressed, allowing a rapid discharge of efferent parasympathetic impulses via the pelvic nerves, to cause contraction of the detrusor, and probably also to pull open the bladder neck and shorten the urethra; simultaneous inhibition of the efferent sympathetic discharges via the thoracolumbar outflow to the pelvic plexus probably also occurs, encouraging detrusor contraction and urethral relaxation. Depending on the relationship between the force of detrusor contraction and the residual urethral resistance, the intravesical pressure may rise to a variable extent (usually less than 60 cmH_2O). When the falling urethral and increasing intravesical pressures equate, urine flow will commence (Fig. 46.7e).

Voiding phase

The application of physical laws to explain the mechanism of continence is often considered inappropriate and misleading. In considering the bladder during micturition, however, the law of Laplace may be useful. It states that the pressure (P) in a vessel varies directly with the mural tension (T), and inversely with the radius (R). Since the bladder at the initiation of micturition takes on a nearly spherical shape, and has walls which are thin in comparison to its radius, its behaviour may be usefully expressed by the basic formula of the law as applied to a sphere: $P = 2T/R$. As the mural tension rises in the absence of voiding the intravesical pressure also rises. When a critical opening pressure is achieved, urine will start to flow and the bladder radius will fall. The pressure, however, usually remains constant during voiding, and the mural tension must therefore fall. Once initiated, therefore, the process of micturition requires little to sustain it. Although active tension is required throughout, the effectiveness of detrusor contraction increases as the muscle fibres shorten, and therefore decreasing forces are required as micturition proceeds.

If micturition is voluntarily interrupted midstream, this is usually achieved by a contraction of the periurethral striated muscle of the pelvic floor. In association with this contraction the urethral pressure rises rapidly to exceed the intravesical pressure, and therefore urine flow stops.

The detrusor, being a smooth muscle, is much slower to relax, and therefore goes on contracting against the closed sphincter. That is, an isometric contraction occurs, and again applying the law of Laplace, the intravesical pressure rises (Fig. 46.7f). If micturition is resumed by relaxation of the pelvic floor, both urethral and intravesical pressures will return to their previous voiding state (Fig. 46.7g).

At the end of micturition the intravesical pressure gradually falls as urinary flow diminishes (Fig. 46.7h). The pelvic floor and intrinsic striated muscle are contracted and flow is interrupted in midurethra; the few drops of urine left in the proximal urethra are milked back into the bladder by the intrinsic mechanisms discussed above which contribute to the hermetic closure of the urethra and bladder neck competence. Simultaneously the subconscious inhibition of the sacral micturition centre is reapplied as the filling phase of the cycle recurs.

Mechanism of stress continence

The above discussion of the normal micturition cycle relates to the events occurring in a patient essentially at rest, and assumes that intravesical pressure is unaffected by extravesical influences. Acute intra-abdominal pressure rises due to coughing, or more sustained pressure variations due to straining or movement, would easily exceed the normal resting maximum urethral closure pressure and result in incontinence unless additional influences were brought to bear on the mechanism of continence.

The factors that maintain the positive urethral pressure at rest (i.e. which ensure that the urethral pressure exceeds the bladder pressure) have been considered above. This positive closure pressure is also maintained in symptom-free women in the face of intra-abdominal pressure rises (Fig. 46.7i) by at least two mechanisms.

First, there is a passive or direct mechanical transmission of the intra-abdominal increase to the proximal urethra (Fig. 46.8). This effect is dependent upon the normal spatial relationships between the bladder and urethra, and on their fixation in a retropubic position by the posterior pubourethral ligaments. The extent of this transmission of intra-abdominal pressure to the urethra may be quantified by means of urethral pressure profiles recorded during stress (see Fig. 46.6). The pressure transmission ratio is defined as the increment in urethral pressure as a percentage of the simultaneously recorded increment in intra-abdominal pressure; this parameter may be recorded at several points along the urethra, and a pressure transmission profile can be constructed which details the transmission of intra-abdominal pressure rises from bladder neck to external urethral meatus. Using this technique it has been shown that in normal women transmission of intra-abdominal pressure rises is effective throughout the proximal three-quarters of the urethral length, i.e. throughout that portion of the urethra lying above the urogenital diaphragm (Fig. 46.9).

Secondly, an active or neuromuscular effect on transmission may be important in stress continence. It may also be shown by simultaneous bladder and urethral pressure measurements that in a region around the third quarter of the functional urethral length, pressure transmission ratios often exceed 100% (Figs 46.6 and 46.9). It has been suggested that this may reflect a reflex pelvic floor contraction in response to stress, augmenting urethral closure (Fig. 46.8). Certainly the observed pressure changes do fit closely with the current concepts of the anatomy of the region, and an active neuromuscular element in the maintenance of normal stress continence is accepted by many authors.

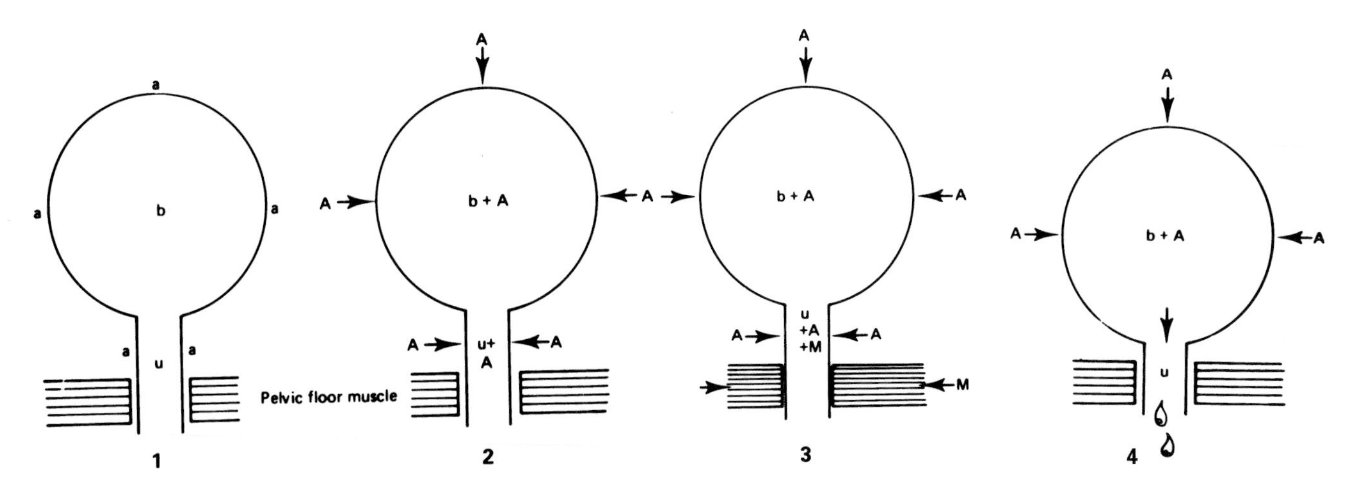

Fig. 46.8 Diagram to show the relationship between bladder, urethra and pelvic floor in (1) the resting state and on stress, to illustrate the passive (2) and active (3) components of pressure transmission to the proximal urethra aiding stress continence. When these components are ineffective (4) stress incontinence results. a, resting intra-abdominal pressure; A, intra-abdominal pressure when straining; b, intravesical pressure; u, intraurethral pressure; M, pressure exerted by the pelvic floor muscles. (From Hilton 1987, with permisssion)

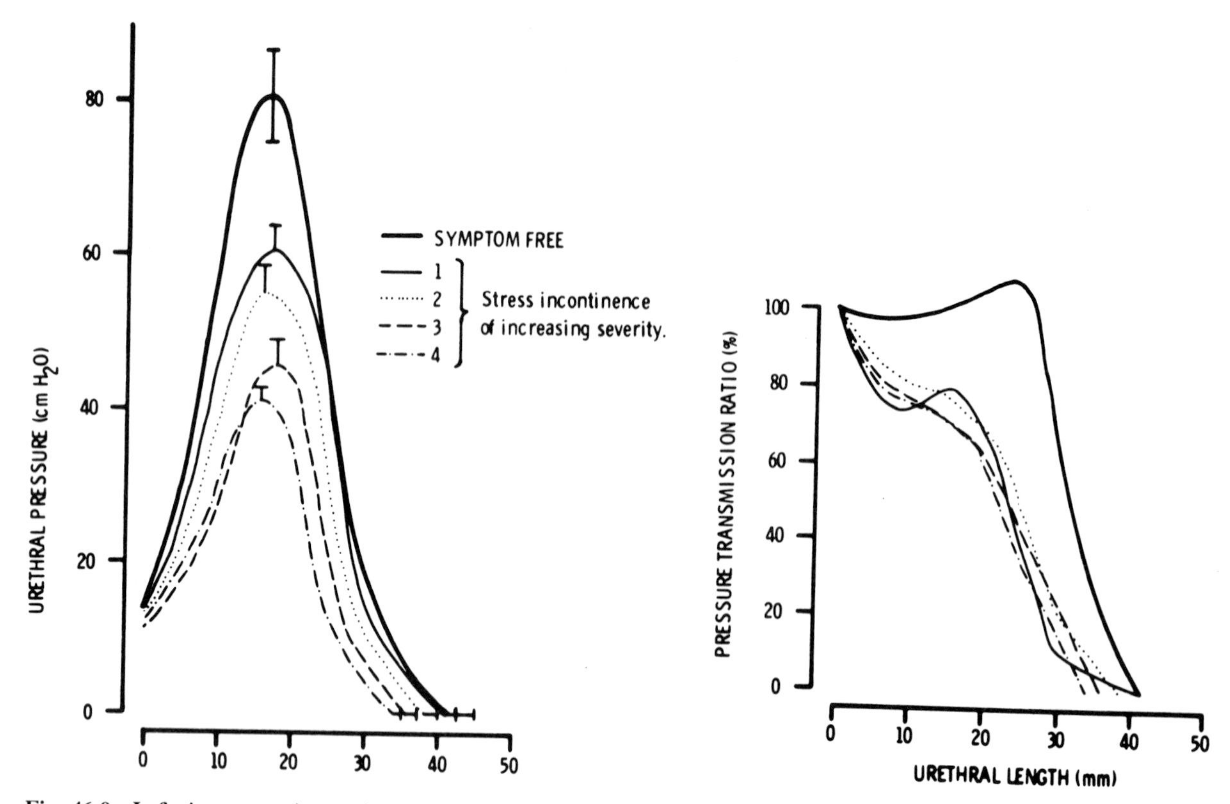

Fig. 46.9 **Left**: Average resting urethral pressure profiles and **right**: pressure transmission profiles in a group of symptom-free women and four groups with stress incontinence of varying severity. (From Hilton & Stanton 1983a, with permission)

PATHOPHYSIOLOGY OF URINARY INCONTINENCE

General considerations

The pathophysiology of several causes of incontinence is considered in greater detail in this volume in chapters relating to individual conditions; here, general comments are made in so far as the pathophysiology relates to abnormalities of the micturition cycle as described above.

Assuming an intact lower urinary tract, urine flow occurs only when the intravesical pressure exceeds the maximum urethral pressure, or when the maximum urethral closure pressure becomes zero or negative. In general terms this may occur as a result of:

1. A fall in urethral pressure associated with an increase in intravesical pressure (Fig. 46.10a) – as in normal voiding or in many cases of detrusor instability, primarily those of idiopathic or psychosomatic origin, or those resulting from neurological lesions above the level of the pontine micturition centre.
2. An increase in intravesical pressure associated with an increase in urethral pressure, the latter being insufficient to maintain a positive closure pressure (Fig. 46.10b) – as in detrusor instability with associated detrusor–sphincter dyssynergia, resulting from neurological lesions above the sacral but below the pontine micturition centre.
3. An abnormally steep rise in detrusor pressure during bladder filling (Fig. 46.10c) – a situation considered by some workers to be analogous to detrusor instability, but perhaps better considered as impaired bladder compliance. This may be seen in chronic inflammatory conditions such as tuberculosis or interstitial cystitis and also following pelvic irradiation. A similar situation also accounts for the incontinence often seen in chronic urinary retention, where the bladder pressure rises acutely at the end of filling.
4. A loss of urethral pressure alone, without any coincident change in intravesical pressure (Fig. 46.10d) – as in urethral instability.
5. Where on stress the intravesical pressure rises to a greater extent than the intraurethral pressure (Fig. 46.10e) – as in stress incontinence. This effect may arise from inherent weakness of the urethra itself (intrinsic sphincter incompetence) or, more commonly, from impairment of urethral support (genuine stress incontinence). There is increasing evidence that this defect may result at least in part from a degree of denervation of the pelvic floor, as a normal accompaniment of ageing and as a consequence of childbirth. Alterations in the biochemistry or mechanical properties of pelvic connective tissues are also known to occur progressively with increasing age; the endocrine effects of pregnancy may also accelerate this process.

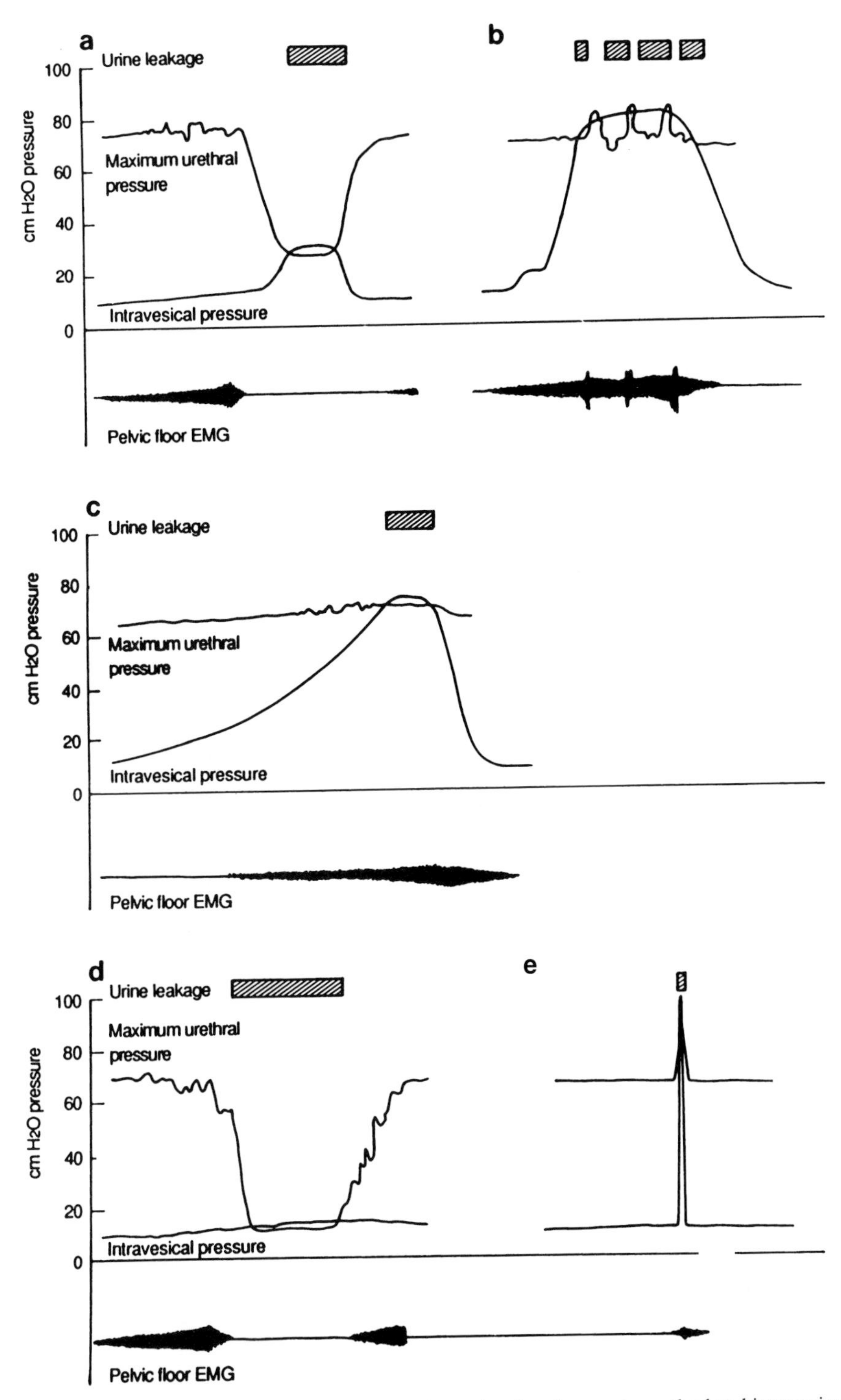

Fig. 46.10 Mechanisms of urinary incontinence showing changes in urethral and intravesical pressure and pelvic floor electromyogram (EMG) at various stages of bladder filling, in different types of incontinence. **a** Normal voiding or detrusor instability; **b** detrusor instability with detrusor–sphincter dyssynergia; **c** impaired bladder compliance; **d** urethral instability; **e** genuine stress incontinence.

EFFECTS OF CONTINENCE SURGERY ON MECHANISMS OF CONTINENCE

Well over 100 different operations have been described for the treatment of genuine stress incontinence, reflecting not merely the inadequacy of any single procedure to deal satisfactorily with all cases, but also uncertainties about the nature of the problem, and the mechanism of its cure.

The aims of incontinence surgery have been variously

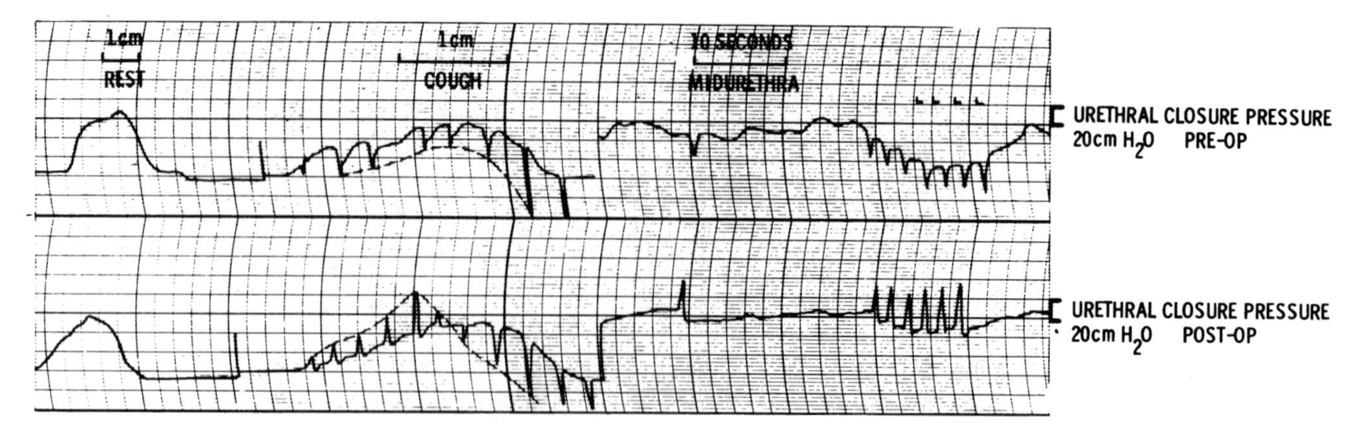

Fig. 46.11 Example of pre- and postoperative urethral closure pressure recordings in a patient undergoing successful Burch colposuspension. L, demonstrated urinary leakage during preoperative trace. (From Hilton & Stanton 1983b, with permission)

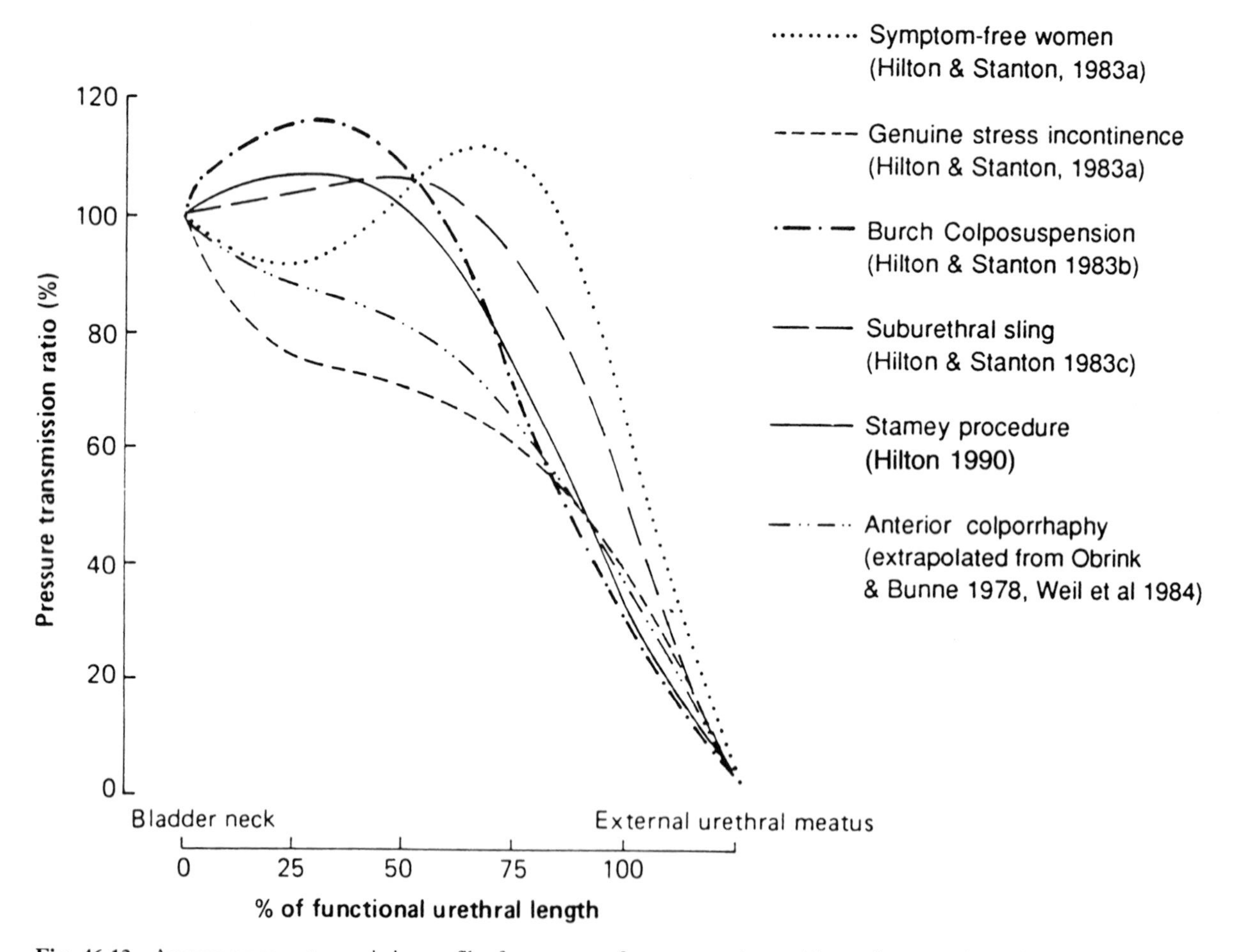

Fig. 46.12 Average pressure transmission profiles for symptom-free women, those with genuine stress incontinence, and patients undergoing successful treatment for stress incontinence using a variety of surgical procedures.

defined as tightening of the pubocervical fascia, elevation of the bladder neck, restoration of the posterior urethrovesical angle, increasing urethral pressure, increasing functional urethral length, and increasing urethral resistance. There is, however, little information as to the extent to which these aims are achieved by the various surgical techniques. Cure rates between 40 and 97% have been reported, but which aspects of the procedures, or of urethral function, determine success or failure is still poorly understood.

Urethral pressure profiles have been recorded at rest and on stress, before and after a variety of incontinence operations, including the anterior colporrhaphy, Burch colposuspension, Marshall–Marchetti–Krantz, suburethral sling and Stamey endoscopic bladder-neck suspension procedures. Although marked changes are noted in the resting urethral profile peroperatively, these are short-lived and could not account for the success of surgery. In stress profiles, however, improvements in pressure transmission in midurethra are consistently found following successful surgical treatment (Figs 46.11 and 46.12). Although results of these various studies are qualitatively similar, there are considerable quantitative differences: improvements in transmission vary from only a few percent with the anterior repair to well over 100% with the colposuspension.

The nature of the improvement in urethral pressure transmission following surgery is uncertain. It has previously been suggested that it is simply due to elevation of the bladder neck and proximal urethra into the abdominal pressure zone, thereby allowing improved passive transmission to the region. This would explain transmission ratios approaching 100%, but it clearly could not explain ratios over 100%, as noted above. It is possible that the elevation of the bladder neck not only allows improved passive transmission, but also promotes greater efficiency of the pelvic floor reflex, with accentuation of urethral closure by active means. The distribution of pressure transmission along the urethra following successful suprapubic surgery is quite different from that seen in healthy women (Fig. 46.12), and the delay between intravesical and urethral pressure rises on coughing – around 10 ms – is too short to involve a neuromuscular reflex.

It would seem more likely, therefore, that the improved transmission has a mechanical rather than a neuromuscular basis. The most obvious anatomical change following successful suprapubic incontinence surgery is the relocation of the urethra in a high retropubic position, and it is possible that downward pressure from abdominal viscera on coughing compresses the urethra against the posterior surface of the symphysis, accentuating urethral closure.

It appears that those operations which give the best results in terms of cure of stress incontinence are those which produce maximum urethral and bladder-neck elevation – and at the same time the greatest enhancements in pressure transmission – but are also those with the greatest risk of increasing urethral resistance; operations which produce lesser degrees of elevation may cause fewer postoperative voiding difficulties, but are also less likely to cure stress incontinence. This principle has been proven for the colposuspension in particular, and seems likely to apply to incontinence surgery in general.

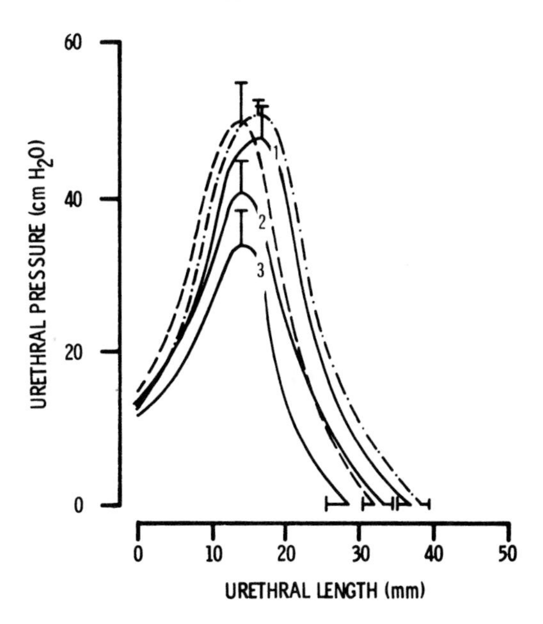

Fig. 46.13 Average resting urethral pressure profiles for stress incontinent patients according to previous surgical history. – • –, No pelvic surgery (n = 58); —, one (n = 25), two (n = 14) and three or more (n = 7) previous unsuccessful incontinence operations; — — —, previous pelvic surgery other than for incontinence (n = 16). (From Hilton & Stanton 1983a, with permission)

Little research has been done into the effects of unsuccessful incontinence surgery on bladder and urethral function. It has, however, been shown that the improvements in pressure transmission noted following successful surgery are not found following unsuccessful surgery. It has also been shown that following some failed procedures a reduction in resting urethral closure pressure may ensue, and that the more unsuccessful procedures a patient has undergone, the less efficient her urethral closure is likely to be (Fig. 46.13).

CONCLUSIONS

If dysfunction of the urinary tract is to be effectively managed, the choice of treatment must be optimal. This choice must be based on a firm knowledge of the normal mechanisms of continence, and of the mechanisms whereby this normal control may break down. Only in the light of this knowledge can the meaningful investigation of the individual incontinent patient be carried out. The results of this investigation, taken in conjunction with a knowledge of the effects of various treatment modalities, should allow the selection of a rational and specific therapy for each patient.

KEY POINTS

1. The urethral sphincter mechanism contains both slow and fast twitch muscle fibre, to produce continuous closure at rest and additional closure on effort, respectively. The former predominate in the intrinsic rhabdosphincter urethrae; the latter are found in the extrinsic periurethral muscle of the levator ani.
2. The epithelial lining of the mucosa and submucosal venous plexuses of the urethra are probably also important in its hermetic closure, and the passive elastic properties of the tissues at the bladder neck are of considerable importance in the majority of women.
3. The bladder and urethra have complex parasympathetic and sympathetic innervation, coordinated by multiple centres within the CNS, whose predominant influence is inhibition of the sacral micturition reflex.
4. Continence is maintained by direct mechanical transmission of intra-abdominal pressure to the proximal urethra and by reflex pelvic floor contraction in the face of increased intra-abdominal pressure.
5. Successful continence surgery is related to elevation of the bladder neck and to improvement in abdominal pressure transmission to the proximal urethra. In some patients excessive bladder-neck elevation may lead to voiding difficulty.

SUGGESTED READING

Definitions and terminology

Abrams P, Blaivas J, Stanton S L, Andersen J 1990 The standardisation of terminology of lower urinary tract function. British Journal of Obstetrics and Gynaecology 97: (Suppl 6)

Anatomy of the lower urinary tract

DeLancey J O 1988 Structural aspects of the extrinsic continence mechanism. American Journal of Obstetrics and Gynecology 72: 296–301

Gosling J A, Dixon J, Critchley H O D, Thompson S A 1981 A comparative study of human external sphincter and periurethral levator ani muscle. British Journal of Urology 53: 35–41

Gosling J A, Dixon J, Humpherson J R 1983 Functional anatomy of the urinary tract. Churchill Livingstone, Edinburgh

Huisman A B 1983 Aspects of the anatomy of the female urethra with special relation to urinary continence. In: Ulmsten U (ed) Contributions to gynaecology and obstetrics, vol 10: Female stress incontinence. Karger, Basel, pp 1–31

Zacharin R F 1963 The suspension mechanism of the female urethra. Journal of Anatomy 97: 423–427

Neurological control of micturition

Bradley W E, Timm T W, Scott F B 1974 Innervation of the detrusor muscle and urethra. Urological Clinics of North America 1: 3–27

Fletcher T F, Bradley W E 1978 Neuroanatomy of the bladder–urethra. Journal of Urology 119: 153–160

Torrens M 1984 Neurophysiology. In: Stanton S L (ed) Clinical gynaecological urology. C V Mosby, St Louis, pp 13–21

Physiology of the lower urinary tract

Asmussen M, Ulmsten U 1983 On the physiology of continence and pathophysiology of stress incontinence in the female. In: Ulmsten U (ed) Contributions to gynaecology and obstetrics, vol 10: Female stress incontinence. Karger, Basel, pp 32–50

Constantinou C E 1985 Resting and stress urethral pressures as a clinical guide to the mechanism of continence. Clinics in Obstetrics and Gynaecology 12: 343–356

Rud T 1980 The urethral pressure profile in continent women from childhood to old age. Acta Obstetrica et Gynaecologica Scandinavica 59: 331–335

Rud T, Andersson K-E, Asmussen M, Hunting A, Ulmsten U 1980 Factors maintaining the intraurethral pressure in women. Investigative Urology 17: 343–347

Wein A 1986 Physiology of micturition. Clinics in Geriatric Medicine 2(4): 689–699

The mechanics and hydrodynamics of bladder and urethra

Coolsaet B L R A 1984 Cystometry. In: Stanton S L (ed) Clinical gynecological urology. C V Mosby, St Louis, pp 59–81

Griffiths D J 1980 Urodynamics. Adam Hilger, Bristol

Hilton P 1981 Urethral pressure measurement by microtransducer: observations on the methodology, the pathophysiology of genuine stress incontinence and the effects of its treatment in the female. MD Thesis, University of Newcastle-upon-Tyne

Hilton P 1990 Urethral pressure profilometry in the female. In: George N, O'Reilly P, Weiss R (eds) Diagnostic techniques in urology. W B Saunders, Philadelphia, pp 309–335

Zinner N R, Ritter R C, Sterling A M 1976 The mechanism of micturition. In: Williams D I, Chisholm G D (eds) Scientific foundations of urology. Heinemann, London, pp 39–51

Pathophysiology of urinary incontinence

Anderson R S 1984 A neurogenic element to urinary genuine stress incontinence. British Journal of Obstetrics and Gynaecology 91: 41–46

Enhorning G E 1961 Simultaneous recording of the intravesical and intraurethral pressure. Acta Chirurgica Scandinavica: 276 (suppl): 1–68

Hilton P 1988 Clinical algorithms. Urinary incontinence in women. British Medical Journal 295: 426–432

Hilton P, Stanton S L 1983a Urethral pressure by microtransducer: the results in symptom-free women and in those with genuine stress incontinence. British Journal of Obstetrics and Gynaecology 90: 919–933

Lose G, Colstrup H 1991 Pathophysiologic subdivision of genuine stress incontinence. Neurourology and Urodynamics 10: 247–256

Snooks S J, Badenoch D F, Tiptaft R C, Swash M 1985 Perineal nerve damage in genuine stress urinary incontinence. British Journal of Urology 57: 422–426

Smith A R B, Hosker G L, Warrell D W 1989 The role of partial denervation of the pelvic floor in the aetiology of genitourinary prolapse and stress incontinence of urine. A neurophysiological study. British Journal of Obstetrics and Gynaecology 96: 24–28

Smith A R B, Hosker G L, Warrell D W 1989 The role of pudendal nerve damage in the aetiology of genuine stress incontinence in women. British Journal of Obstetrics and Gynaecology 96: 29–32

Versi E 1991 The significance of an open bladder neck in women. British Journal of Urology 68: 42–43

The effects of incontinence surgery on continence mechanisms

Hertogs K, Stanton S L 1985 Mechanism of urinary continence after colposuspension: barrier studies. British Journal of Obstetrics and Gynaecology 92: 1184–1188

Hilton P 1986 The mechanism of continence. In: Stanton S L, Tanagho E A (eds) Surgery of female incontinence, 2nd edn. Springer-Verlag, Berlin, pp 1–21

Hilton P 1987 Surgery for urinary stress incontinence. In: Monaghan J M (ed) Rob and Smith's operative surgery: Gynaecology and obstetrics, 4th edn. Butterworths, London, pp 105–126

Hilton P 1989 A clinical and urodynamic comparison of the abdomino-vaginal sub-urethral sling and Stamey endoscopic bladder neck suspension in the treatment of genuine stress incontinence. British Journal of Obstetrics and Gynaecology 96: 213–220

Hilton P, Stanton S L 1983b A clinical and urodynamic assessment of the Burch colposuspension for genuine stress incontinence. British Journal of Obstetrics and Gynaecology 90: 934–939

Obrink A, Bunne G 1978 The margin to incontinence after three types of operation for stress incontinence. Scandinavian Journal of Urology and Nephrology 12: 209–214

Weil A, Reyes H, Bischof P, Rottenberg R D, Krauer F 1984 Modifications of the urethral resting and stress profiles after different types of surgery for urinary stress incontinence. British Journal of Obstetrics and Gynaecology 91: 46–55

47

Urodynamic investigations

S. M. Creighton

INTRODUCTION

Lower urinary tract symptoms are common and objective assessment is important. An accurate and detailed history and examination provide a framework for the diagnosis, but there is often a discrepancy between the patient's symptoms and the urodynamic findings. Jarvis et al (1980) found the clinical diagnosis to be accurate in only 65% of cases. Cardozo and Stanton (1980) reviewed 200 patients and found that 35% of those with detrusor instability on cystometry actually complained of both stress and urge incontinence. As the results of surgery are jeopardized by pre-existing detrusor instability, urodynamic studies on patients with symptoms of both urge and stress incontinence would seem, from these studies, to be necessary.

When stress incontinence is the sole symptom, Farrar et al (1975) found that the clinical and cystometric diagnoses agreed in 96% of cases, and concluded that urodynamic investigations were superfluous in these patients. The poor predictive value of symptoms in those patients with a mixed clinical picture was again confirmed.

In patients with neurological disorders the symptoms may be even less likely to correlate with the urodynamic findings. Blaivas et al (1979) showed a 27% improvement in patients with multiple sclerosis treated empirically, but an 81% improvement when the treatment was based on the urodynamic findings.

Urodynamic studies are also important to exclude voiding disorders (which can be asymptomatic) and in the evaluation of the success or failure of surgical or conservative treatment. Bates et al (1973) studied patients with recurrent incontinence following bladder-neck surgery and found that 50% of those complaining of stress incontinence postoperatively had urodynamic diagnosis of detrusor instability.

BASIC TESTS

Midstream urine specimen

A midstream urine specimen must be taken from all patients presenting with urinary symptoms. A urine infection may be responsible for some or all of their symptoms and, if present, must be treated before invasive urodynamic studies are performed. A significant bacteriuria is considered to be 100 000 organisms per millilitre of urine, and is usually associated with pyuria. The presence of epithelial cells, erythrocytes and casts is also noted.

Invasive urodynamic studies, if performed competently and cleanly, have a less than 2% risk of urinary tract infection (Walter & Vejlsgaard 1978).

Urinary diary

A urinary diary is a simple record of the patient's fluid intake and output (Fig. 47.1). It should be completed by all patients for 1 week. It also records episodes of leakage, and whether or not these were precipitated by urgency or activity. These diaries aid diagnosis and are more accurate than attempted recall by the patient. An idea of the functional capacity of the bladder is obtained, and overdrinking as a cause of incontinence can be excluded. The diary can also be used as a baseline for bladder retraining (Fig. 47.1).

DAY: monday.

TIME	INTAKE (ml)	OUTPUT (ml)	LEAKAGE: ACTIVITY	Amount	Urge	Wet Bed
07.00		350	Getting out of bed	Soaked Pad.	Yes	
08.00	200	75			Yes	
08.30	200	50			Yes	
08.50		100			Yes	
09.30	240	75			Yes	
10.00		50			Yes	
11.30	120	100			Yes	
12.30		100			Yes	
1.15	240	75			Yes	
1.50	240	50			Yes	
2.30		50			Yes	
3.50	240	120	Getting to toilet.	Few Drops	Yes	
4.40		100			Yes	
5.15	240	50			Yes	
6.00		50			Yes	
7.10	100	100	washing up	Soaked Pad.	Yes	
8.20	120	100			Yes	
9.30		75			Yes	
10.15		50			Yes	
11.00	240	75			Yes	
2.00		100				
4.30	100	150				
TOTAL	2280	2045				

Fig. 47.1 Urinary diary showing the input and output for each day. The patient records the timing and amount of leakage and precipitating events.

Pad test

Two types of pad test are in common use. A simple pad test can be performed on all patients presenting with incontinence, and also as an easy follow-up measure for incontinence surgery. The patient, with a comfortably full bladder, wears a sanitary towel and performs some simple exercises, including coughing, sitting and standing, bending to pick objects from the floor and hand-washing for 5–10 minutes. The test is positive if the pad becomes damp.

The extended pad test is a more lengthy and objective measurement of leakage, and can be used to confirm or refute leakage in those patients complaining of stress incontinence which has not been demonstrated on cystometry. The International Continence Society pad test takes 1 hour. The patient wears a preweighed sanitary towel, drinks 500 ml of water and rests for 15 minutes. She then performs half an hour of gentle exercise, such as walking and climbing stairs. She then performs 15 minutes of more provocative exercise, including bending, standing and sitting, coughing, hand-washing, and running if possible. The sanitary towel is then removed and reweighed. An increase in weight of greater than 1 g is considered a significant loss.

UROFLOWMETRY

Uroflowmetry is a simple non-invasive investigation and can be easily performed in an outpatient department. Flowmeters are relatively inexpensive and give a permanent graphic record.

Indications

Measurement of the flow rate is indicated in women with complaints of hesitancy or difficulty in voiding, with neuropathy or with a past history of urinary retention. It can also be used to evaluate patients before incontinence surgery to exclude voiding difficulties which may be aggravated by bladder-neck surgery.

Measurements

The flow rate is defined as the volume of urine (in ml) expelled from the bladder each second (Fig. 47.2). The flow time is the total duration of micturition and includes interruptions in a non-continuous flow. The maximum flow rate is the maximum measured rate of flow, and the average flow is the volume voided divided by the flow time. The total volume voided is therefore the area under the curve. The two most useful parameters are the maximum flow rate and the voided volume. In patients with intermittent flow the same parameters can be used, but time intervals between flow episodes must be discounted.

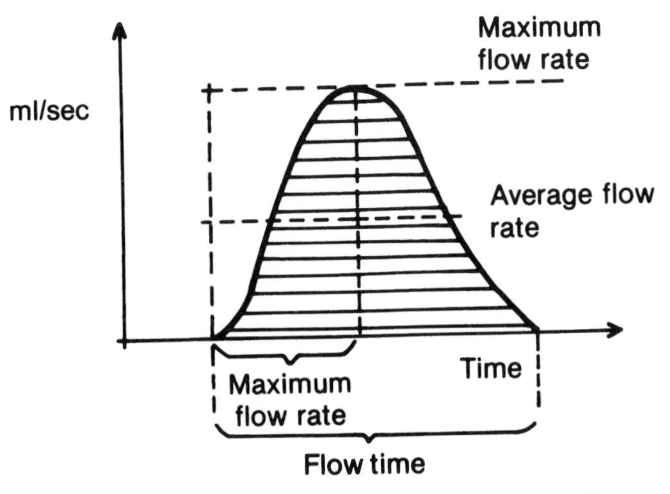

Fig. 47.2 Diagrammatic representation of a urinary flow rate. The shaded area represents voided volume.

Equipment

There are three main types of flowmeter. The earliest models used a strain-weighing transducer which measured the rate of change of the weight of urine voided, which was converted into a flow rate.

The rotating disc flowmeter has a disc which is spun at a constant speed. As the patient voids on to the disc the inertia of the urine reduces its speed. The flow rate can be calculated from the amount of power needed to maintain the disc spinning at a constant speed. This is a simple and relatively inexpensive system, but is more fragile and more liable to mechanical failure.

The capacitance flowmeter has a metal strip capacitor attached to a plastic dipstick inserted vertically into the jug containing the voided urine (Fig. 47.3). The rate and volume changes are measured by a change in electrical conductance across the capacitor. This is the most expensive type of flowmeter, but is robust and very reliable.

Abnormal flow rates

Nomograms for peak and average urine flow rates in

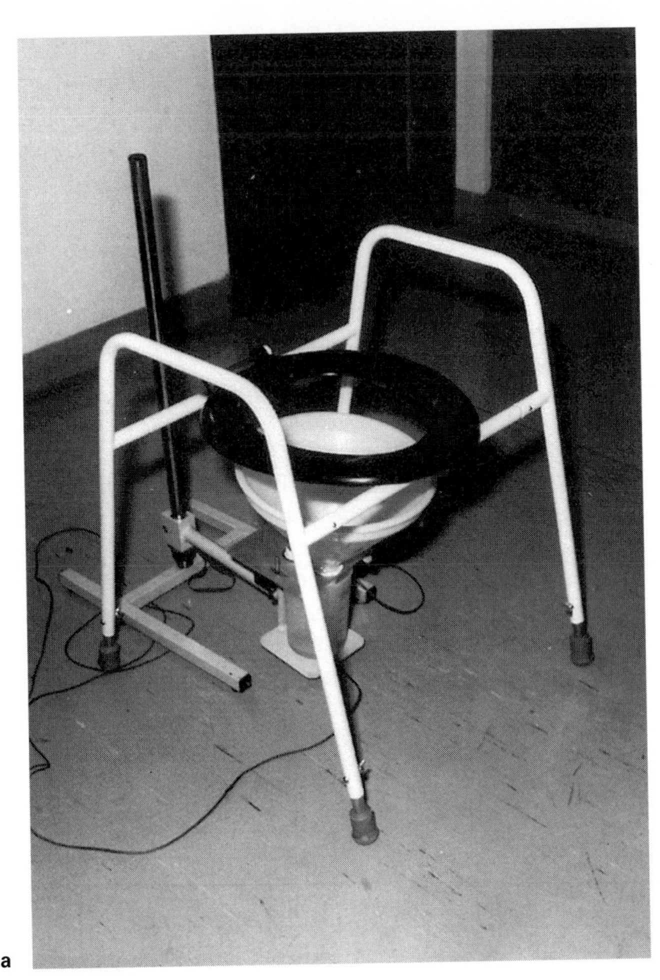
a

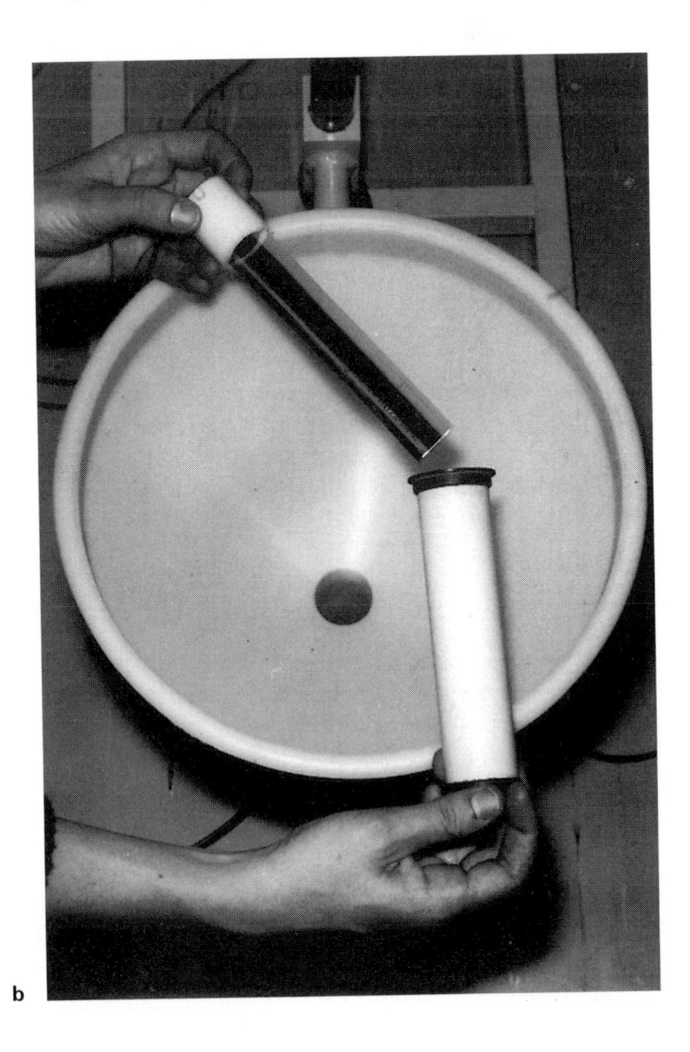
b

Fig. 47.3 (**a**) Capacitance urinary flowmeter; (**b**) the capacitance strip.

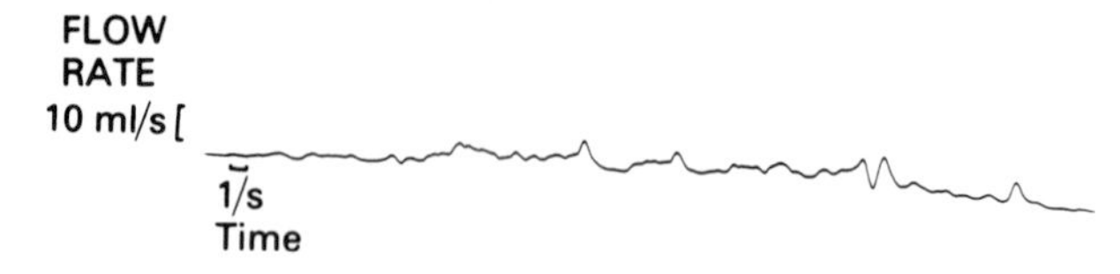

Fig. 47.4 Urinary flow rate showing a prolonged flow with a low maximum peak flow rate suggestive of a voiding disorder.

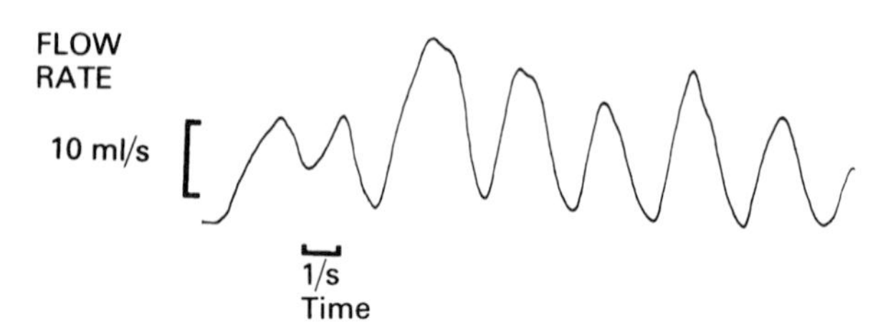

Fig. 47.5 A straining flow rate also suggestive of a voiding disorder.

women have been constructed from flow rates of 249 normal women (Haylen et al 1988). These allow comparison of a single value with a standard flow rate. A flow rate below 15 ml/s on more than one occasion is taken as abnormal in female patients. The voided volume should be above 150 ml, as flow rates on smaller volumes than this are not reliable.

A low peak flow rate and a prolonged voiding time suggest a voiding disorder (Fig. 47.4). Straining can give abnormal flow patterns with interrupted flow (Fig. 47.5). More useful detailed information is obtained by the addition of simultaneous voiding pressure measurements.

CYSTOMETRY

Cystometry involves the measurement of the pressure/volume relationship of the bladder during filling and voiding, and is the most useful test of bladder function. It is a simple and accurate investigation and is easy to perform, taking between 15 and 20 minutes per patient.

Indications

Cystometry is indicated in the investigation of the following bladder disorders:

1. Multiple symptoms, i.e. urge incontinence, stress incontinence and frequency.
2. Voiding disorder.
3. Prior to any bladder-neck surgery.
4. Previous unsuccessful incontinence surgery.
5. Neuropathic bladder disorders.

Ideally, urodynamic studies should be performed on every patient. However, when access to investigations is limited it is reasonable to manage patients with clear-cut symptoms conservatively. When conservative treatments fail or surgery is contemplated, urodynamics should be performed.

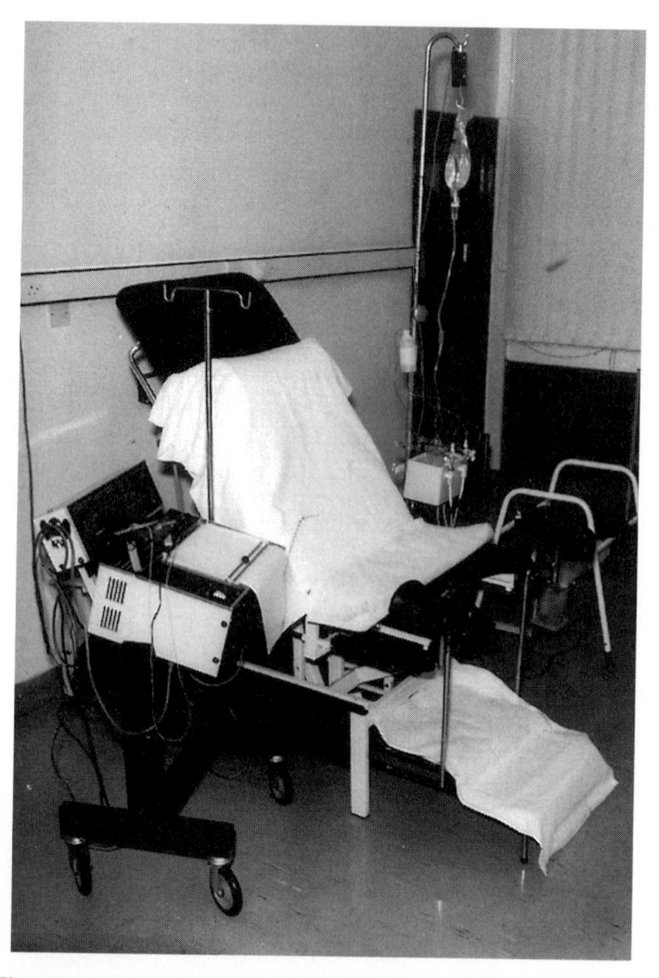

Fig. 47.6 Urodynamic equipment. From left to right: a twin-channel cystometry unit, patient couch, patient unit with transducer and uroflowmeter.

Equipment

Modern twin-channel cystometry requires a transducer, a recorder and an amplifying unit (Fig. 47.6). Bladder pressure is measured using a fluid-filled line or a solid microtip pressure catheter. For the former, a 1 mm fluid-filled catheter (such as an epidural cannula) is inserted into the bladder with a filling line and connected to an external pressure transducer. To measure abdominal pressure a rectal catheter is required; a fluid-filled 2 mm diameter catheter covered with a rubber finger cot to prevent blockage with faeces is inserted into the rectum (Fig. 47.7). The microtip transducer catheter has a transducer mounted on the tip of a solid catheter and has a diameter of about 7 French gauge. It is inserted into the bladder and the level of the bladder neck is taken as being approximately level with the upper edge of the pubic symphysis: this is the zero reference for all measurements, which are made in centimetres of water (cmH_2O).

The external transducer is cheaper and less fragile, but the microtip transducer is more accurate as it eliminates

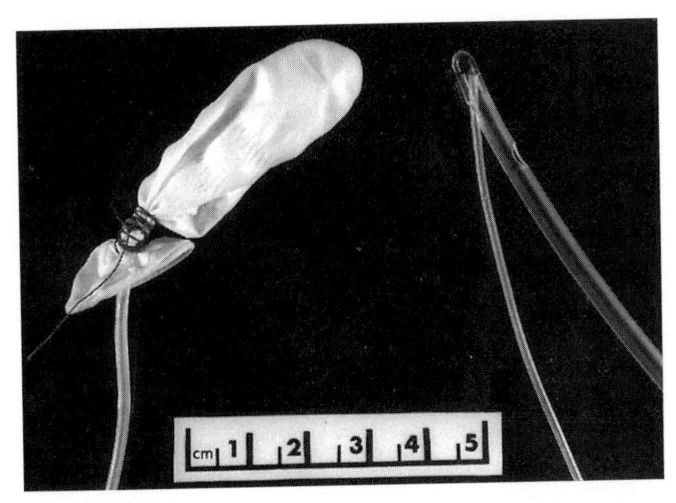

Fig. 47.7 Pressure lines for cystometry. From left to right: bladder and rectal filling lines.

error, owing to the column of water in the connecting catheter; it is more expensive and more easily damaged.

The bladder is filled using a 12 FG catheter with a continuous infusion of normal saline at room temperature. The standard filling rate is between 10 and 100 ml/min and is provocative for detrusor instability. Slow-fill cystometry at a rate below 10 ml/min is indicated in patients with neuropathic bladders. Rapid filling at over 100 ml/min is rarely used, but can be a further provocative test for detrusor instability.

Measurements

The parameters measured are the intravesical pressure (P_{ves}; measured with the bladder transducer) and the intra-abdominal pressure (P_{abd}) measured with the rectal line. The detrusor pressure (P_{det}) is obtained by subtracting the abdominal pressure from the intravesical pressure, and if twin-channel cystometry is used this subtracted value is displayed concomitantly. The filling and voided volumes are also displayed.

Method

Prior to performing the cystometry, the patient voids on the flowmeter. Any residual urine on subsequent catheterization of the patient is noted. During filling the patient is asked to indicate her first desire to void and the maximal desire to void, and these volumes are noted. The presence of systolic detrusor contractions is observed, and whether it is associated with urgency. Any precipitating factors, such as coughing or running water, are also noted. Any detrusor pressure rise during filling and on standing is again recorded.

At the end of filling, the filling line is removed and the patient stands. She is asked to cough and leakage is noted. Provocative tests for detrusor instability, such as listening to running water and hand-washing, are performed at this stage. The patient then transfers to the commode and voids with the pressure transducer still in place. Once urinary flow is established she is asked to interrupt the flow if possible.

Normal cystometry

The following are parameters of normal bladder function:

1. Residual urine of less than 50 ml.
2. First desire to void between 150 and 200 ml.
3. Capacity (taken as strong desire to void) of greater than 400 ml.
4. Detrusor pressure rise on filling which does not return to the baseline when filling stops.
5. Absence of systolic detrusor contractions.
6. No leakage on coughing.
7. A detrusor pressure rise on voiding (maximum voiding pressure) of less than 70 cmH_2O, with a peak flow rate of greater than 15 ml/s for a volume over 150 ml.
8. The patient should be able to interrupt her urine flow on command; failure to do so is not necessarily abnormal.

Abnormal cystometry

If leakage on coughing occurs in the absence of a rise in detrusor pressure, genuine stress incontinence is diagnosed (Fig. 47.8). It is therefore a diagnosis of exclusion, as cystometry by itself cannot indicate bladder-neck or urethral function; radiographic imaging or the addition of urethral function tests is required. Detrusor instability is diagnosed if, during the filling phase, spontaneous or provoked detrusor contractions occur which the patient cannot suppress (Fig. 47.9). Systolic detrusor instability is shown by phasic contractions, whereas low compliant detrusor instability is diagnosed when the pressure rise on filling is greater than 15 cmH_2O and does not settle after filling is stopped.

AMBULATORY MONITORING

Criticism has recently been expressed about the accuracy of simple cystometry. The test period is short and the rate of filling is not physiological. The test also renders the patient immobile and bladder abnormalities produced by movement may be missed. Some abnormalities of bladder function may escape detection during standard cystometry, giving a false negative result. This has led to the introduction of ambulatory monitoring using portable data storage units attached to the patients for periods of several hours (Griffiths et al 1989, Webb et al 1991).

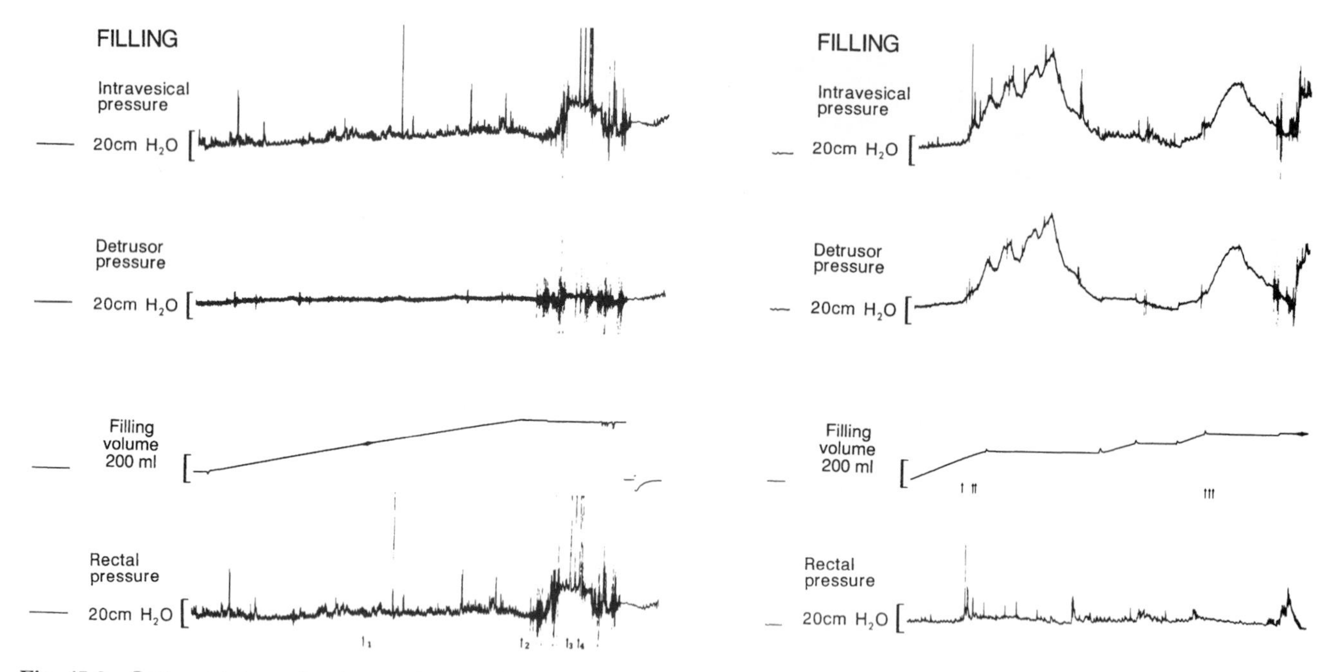

Fig. 47.8 Cystometric trace showing genuine stress incontinence. The detrusor line remains flat. Each arrow (1–4) indicates a cough, when leakage occurred.

Fig. 47.9 Cystometric trace showing detrusor instability. The arrows indicate where the patient complained of urgency and leakage occurred.

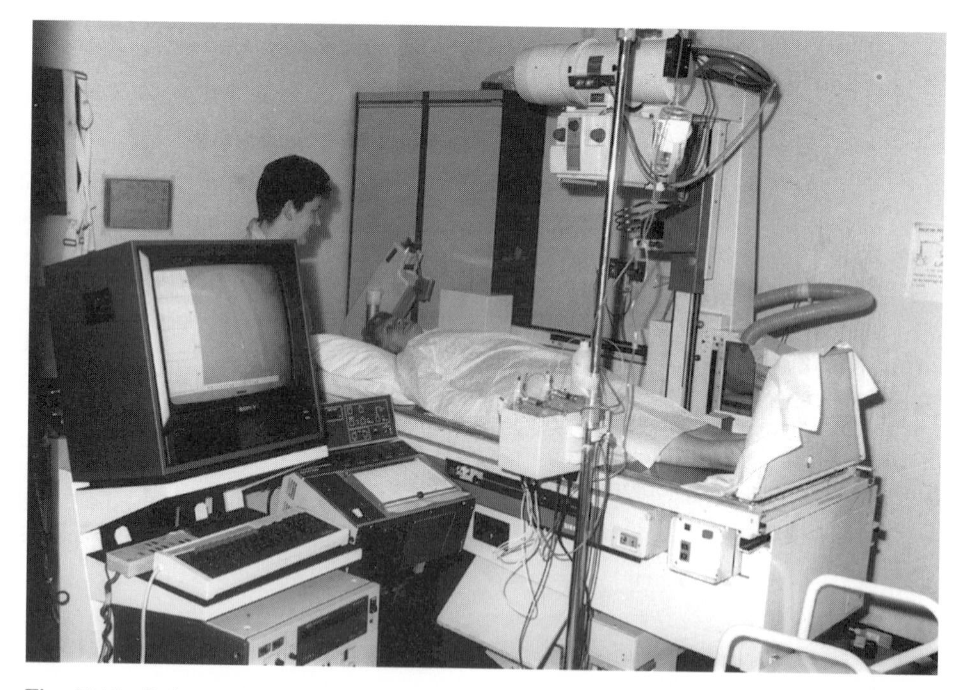

Fig. 47.10 Patient undergoing a videocystourethrogram. The patient lies on an X-ray table which is then tilted vertically for the voiding phase.

Technique

The portable data storage unit is light (about 0.75–1 kg) and the patient can wear it attached to a shoulder strap or belt. Most units collect data at a rate of 1 Hz while rectal and detrusor pressures are recorded independently by transducers mounted on small-gauge catheters. The test period lasts up to 24 hours and the patient is allowed home during this time. They are encouraged to mobilize and continue normal daily activities, including gentle exercise. Fluids are not restricted and antibiotic cover is usually given with a broad-spectrum antibiotic.

Results

Although this is a new technique, results are encouraging. Several studies have shown it to be more accurate than standard cystometry (Van Waalwijk et al 1991). Robertson et al (1994) found significant differences between conventional cystometry and ambulatory monitoring, including pressure rise on filling, voided volumes and maximum detrusor pressure on voiding. Detrusor instability was found in 38% of a group of 17 patients with ambulatory monitoring, compared to none when the same patients were measured with conventional fast-flow (100 ml/min) cystometry. There is some evidence that detrusor instability developing after colposuspension may actually have been present before and was not detected by routine cystometry (Khullar et al 1994a).

The technique does still have some disadvantages. Ambulatory monitoring is time-consuming and sometimes technically difficult. The equipment is expensive (currently about £9400 plus VAT) and fragile, which is important when patients are being discharged home with equipment in situ. Discomfort is a problem but is usually mild and more common in male than female patients. At present ambulatory monitoring is not widely available, and tends to be reserved for patients where routine cystometry gives conflicting or unexpectedly negative results.

RADIOLOGY

General radiology

A plain abdominal X-ray is useful when symptoms suggest bladder calculi. Osteitis pubis is a rare complication of the Marshall–Marchetti–Krantz procedure, presenting with suprapubic pain, and is diagnosed on an anteroposterior pelvic X-ray. Sacral and lumbar spine X-rays are indicated if a congenital abnormality is suspected, e.g. spina bifida and meningomyelocele, which are important causes of neuropathic bladder disorders in children. Spinal cord trauma and tumours can also cause disturbances of micturition. Disc prolapse is common and is demonstrated on a myelogram.

Intravenous urography

Intravenous urography is not indicated in most women with lower urinary tract symptoms. It is, however, indicated in patients with neuropathic bladders, suspected ureterovaginal fistulae or haematuria.

Videocystourethrography

Videocystourethrography (VCU) is radiological screening of the bladder synchronized with pressure studies of the bladder recorded with a sound commentary on video (Fig. 47.10). This study is regarded in some centres as a fundamental investigation, but Stanton et al (1988) reviewed 200 cases of urinary incontinence following failed surgery and concluded that VCU was shown to have an advantage over a cystometrogram in only a few selected groups of patients. VCU is indicated in patients complaining of postmicturition dribble, which may be due to diverticula (Fig. 47.11), where incontinence occurs on standing up, where ureteric reflux may be a cause of urinary symptoms associated with pain, or in the investigation of a neuropathic bladder. It is not necessary in the routine evaluation of female incontinence.

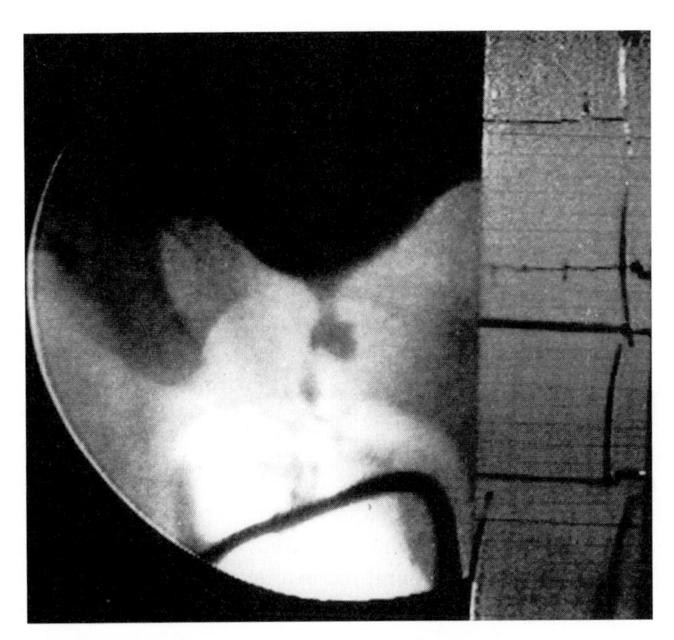

Fig. 47.11 VCU showing a urethral diverticulum.

Technique

On arrival the patient voids into a flowmeter and then lies on a tilting X-ray table. Routine filling cystometry is performed using a contrast medium such as Urografin 35% to fill the bladder. At the maximum desire to void, the filling line is removed and the patient tilted upright and positioned in the erect lateral oblique position. She is asked to cough and strain. Leakage, bladder-neck opening and bladder-base descent are all noted. Any ureteric reflux and detrusor contractions are also noted. The patient then commences voiding and, once the flow is established, she is asked to interrupt it. The ability to milk back urine from the urethra is noted.

All data are recorded on a twin-channel recorder and displayed at the same time as the bladder image. A sound commentary can also be recorded.

Micturating cystogram

This investigation also involves radiological screening of the bladder but without pressure or flow measurements, and is therefore less useful in the investigation of incontinence. Its main value is to demonstrate vesicoureteric reflux, abnormalities of bladder and urethral anatomy, e.g. diverticula, and bladder and urethral fistulae. It is not useful in incontinence.

Lateral chain X-rays

A lateral pelvic X-ray with a metallic bead chain can be used to outline the urethra and bladder neck. Downward and backward displacement of the bladder neck during coughing and straining can be demonstrated (Hodgkinson et al 1958). Lateral chain X-rays have been advocated in the assessment of patients with failed incontinence surgery. This is based on the premise that if the bladder neck has not been moved upwards and forwards compared with the preoperative position, the operation is a technical failure (Stamey 1983). Radiographic evaluation of the posterior urethral angle has, however, proved neither reliable nor consistent in clinical practice. Wall et al (1991) examined lateral chain X-rays on 98 women undergoing one of four different bladder procedures, and confirmed that no useful information was obtained regarding the dynamics of incontinence or its surgical cure. This technique has since been discontinued in some units.

INVESTIGATIONS OF URETHRAL FUNCTION

Urethral pressure measurement

To maintain continence the urethral pressure must remain higher than the intravesical pressure, and various methods of measuring urethral pressure have been devised. It is usually measured with a catheter-tip dual-sensor microtransducer, although in the past resistance to fluid or gas and intraluminal balloons have all been used. The two transducers are 12 mm long and 1.6–2.3 mm in diameter, mounted on a 7 FG catheter at the tip and 6 cm along the catheter (Fig. 47.12). The microtip transducer is easy to use but fragile and expensive.

Technique

The bladder is filled with 250 ml of physiological saline and the catheter passed so that both sensors are within the bladder. The catheter is then connected to a catheter withdrawal mechanism set at a standard speed of 5 cm/min, and also to a chart recorder. The static urethral pressure is the urethral intraluminal pressure along its length with the bladder at rest. The dynamic urethral pressure (the urethral closure pressure) is the difference between the maximal urethral pressure and the intravesical pressure while the patient gives a series of coughs. Women with stress incontinence have a lower urethral closure pressure than continent women, and this is directly proportional to the severity of their incontinence (Hilton 1984).

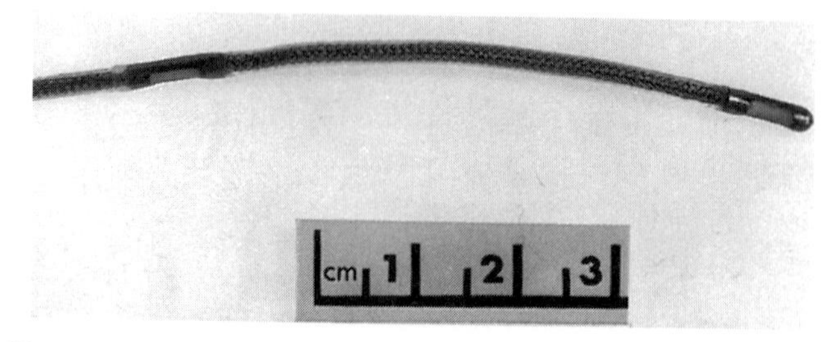

Fig. 47.12 Gaeltec urethral pressure catheter.

Clinical value

Urethral pressure measurements are useful in defining the physical properties; however, their value in clinical practice is not certain. The static urethral pressure profile is of no clinical value. The dynamic urethral pressure profile more closely approximates to the clinical problem, but there is a large overlap for both the functional urethral length and the urethral closure pressure between normal and stress-incontinent women, and it may not be possible to separate the two groups on urethral pressure profile alone. The urethral pressure profile also may not be reproducible when repeated in the same patient. Richardson (1980) studied 144 patients and found a 92% specificity but only a 41% sensitivity in the evaluation of stress-incontinent women. Versi et al (1986) compared the urethral pressure profile with VCU as the 'gold standard' investigation and found that accurate diagnosis was not possible with the urethral pressure profile alone.

A low urethral closure pressure has been implicated as a risk factor for surgical failure. This appears to be restricted to women under 50 years, and some clinicians have suggested these women may be less suitable for colposuspension (Sand et al 1987) and should have a sling-type procedure. Other authors have disagreed with this and show good cure rates with colposuspension despite low urethral closure pressures (Richardson et al 1991). Currently low urethral closure pressure is an interesting research finding but does not prohibit the patient from successful colposuspension.

Valsalva leak-point pressure

Valsalva leak-point pressure (VLPP) is the bladder pressure at which leakage occurs during a slow Valsalva manoeuvre. It is a new term and has been proposed as a measure of the resistance of the urethral sphincter to increased intra-abdominal pressure (Badlani et al 1993). It is highly reproducible but no correlation has been demonstrated with maximum urethral closure pressure. VLPP has been shown to have a high specificity (100%) but poor sensitivity (69.2%) in the diagnosis of genuine stress incontinence (Alcalay et al 1994), and its clinical usefulness is at present not clear.

Urethral electrical conductance

This is a relatively new technique using changes in electrical conductance to detect movement of urine along the urethra (Plevnik et al 1985). Two gold-plated electrodes are mounted on a 7 FG catheter. A non-stimulatory voltage of 20 mV is applied and the electrode connected to a meter calibrated in mA. The current measured between the two electrodes is proportional to whatever substance is between them. The conductance of urine is much higher than that of urothelium, and causes a deflection on the meter. Therefore, entry of urine into the urethra can be sensitively detected. The catheter is either short and positioned in the distal urethra (distal urethral electrical conductance, DUEC; Fig. 47.13) or long and lies at the bladder neck (bladder-neck electrical conductance, BNEC). Urethral electrical conductance profiles can be measured by withdrawing the BNEC catheter at a fixed speed from the bladder to the external meatus (Fig. 47.14). DUEC measurement is used during cystometry following removal of the filling line, to detect stress incontinence more accurately than just by observation. Three different patterns of DUEC have been shown. Types 1 and 2 patterns (deflections of greater than 8 mA, with a quick return to the baseline; Fig. 47.15a) are associated with a cystometric diagnosis of stress incontinence, and type 3 (deflections of greater than 8 mA lasting longer than 3 s; Fig. 47.15b) is associated with a cystometric diagnosis of detrusor instability (Peattie et al 1988a). Any reduction in urethral pressure is invariably associated with an increase in urethral electrical conductance if the two parameters are measured simultaneously in women with genuine stress incontinence (Hilton & Mayne 1988). DUEC has been suggested as an alternative screening test to cystometry for the detection of incontinence (Creighton et al 1991).

BNEC is performed in the investigation and treatment of patients with detrusor instability and sensory urgency. Both of these conditions can demonstrate bladder-neck opening associated with urgency and, if this occurs, it can be used for biofeedback (Peattie et al 1988b).

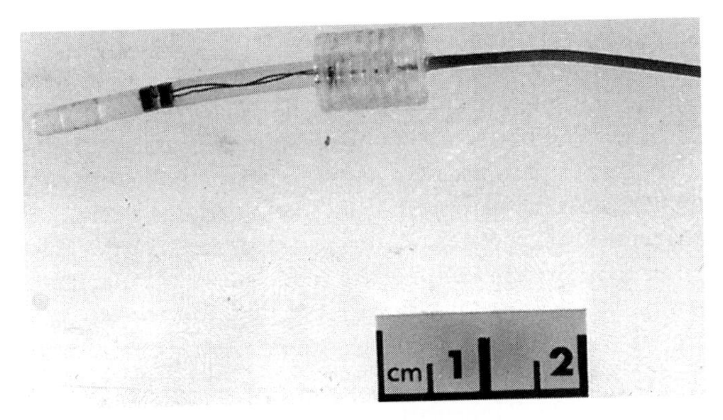

Fig. 47.13 DUEC catheter. The two gold-plated brass electrodes can be seen mounted towards the tip of the catheter.

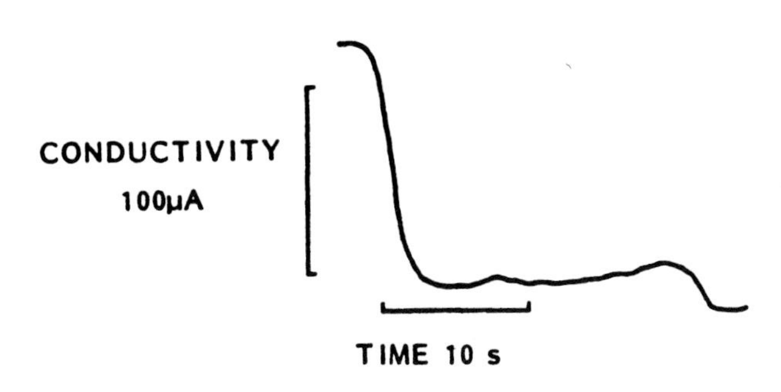

Fig. 47.14 Urethral electrical conductance profile.

Urethral sensitivity

Urethral sensitivity thresholds have been measured in women with both detrusor instability and sensory urgency to determine whether altered urethral sensitivity is an aetiological factor. Initial studies were done by applying a stimulatory electrical current through two electrodes mounted on a Foley urethral catheter (Powell & Fenely 1980). Attempts at making this technique more accurate and assessing different sections of the urethra were made by applying the stimulus via much smaller urethral electric

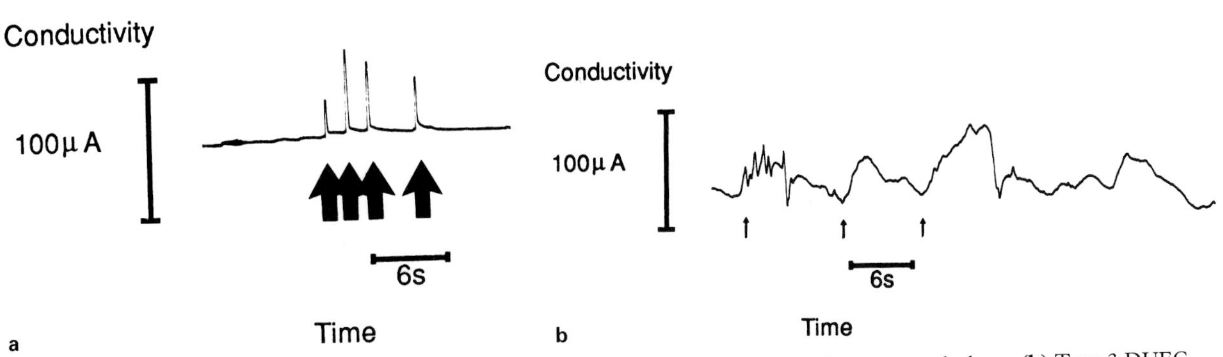

Fig. 47.15 (**a**) Type 1 DUEC pattern. At each cough a spike of increase in conductance demonstrates leakage. (**b**) Type 3 DUEC pattern. In this pattern the coughs provoke a more sustained rise in urethral electrical conductance.

conductance catheters (Creighton et al 1994a). Results are as yet conflicting and this investigation is currently not used in routine clinical practice.

CYSTOURETHROSCOPY

Cystoscopy establishes the presence of disease in the bladder or urethra. It is indicated in a small group of women with incontinence but is not a part of the routine investigation of incontinence as it gives little information about the function of the bladder neck.

Cystoscopy is indicated where there is:

1. A reduced bladder capacity at cystometry.
2. Recent (<2 years) history of urinary symptoms, e.g. frequency and urgency.
3. A suspected urethrovaginal or vesicovaginal fistula.
4. Suspicion of interstitial cystitis.
5. Haematuria not related to urinary tract infection.
6. A need to exclude neoplasm in the presence of persistent urinary infection.

Cystoscopy also comprises part of the operative technique in needle suspension operations for incontinence, such as the Stamey and Raz procedures, to ensure that no sutures have passed through the bladder or urethra and that the sutures are correctly placed at the bladder neck.

Technique

Cystoscopy is a sterile technique and can be performed under general or local anaesthetic. If it is used to assess reduced bladder capacity during urodynamic studies, it must be performed under a general anaesthetic. The urethra is difficult to examine in women and is best done by withdrawing the cystoscope and using a urethroscope sheath. Residual urine should be noted, although it is not always accurate if the patient has not recently voided.

Bladder capacity is the volume at which filling usually stops, using a litre bag under gravity feed. The mucosa should be inspected for abnormalities, such as signs of infection, and tumour. A note is made on the state of the bladder and urethral mucosa and the presence of normally situated ureteric orifices. Interstitial cystitis may be suspected by the presence of linear splits which bleed on decompression, and a reduced capacity. If diverticula are present an attempt must be made to see inside to exclude carcinoma and calculi. Bladder calculi may be present, particularly in patients with neuropathic bladder and/or indwelling catheters. Abnormal areas must be biopsied.

Most makes of cystoscope are similar and, as they are often not interchangeable, it is preferable to stick to one kind. A standard set should include a cystoscope, urethroscope sheath, 0°, 30° and 70° telescopes, a catheterizing bridge and a fibreoptic light. A biopsy forceps is essential, as is a method for dilating the urethra, such as an Otis urethrotome or a set of Hegar dilators. Flexible cystoscopes are available and can be more suitable for cystoscopy under local anaesthetic, but have the disadvantage that instrumentation such as biopsy is not feasible.

ULTRASOUND

Ultrasound is becoming more widely used in gynaecological urology. Its most simple use is in the estimation of postmicturition residual urine volume, and to assess the bladder neck and surrounding area.

Postmicturition urine estimation

This useful technique obviates the need for urethral catheterization with its risk of infection. It is indicated in the investigation of patients with voiding difficulties, either idiopathic or preoperative, and also occasionally following postoperative catheter removal. The bladder is scanned in two planes and three diameters are measured. As the bladder only approaches a spherical shape when it is full, a correction factor has to be applied. Several different formulae have been devised: the most common is to multiply the product of three diameters (height × width × depth) by a figure of 0.625 (Hakenberg et al 1983). This has an error rate of 21%, which is acceptable.

Bladder neck

Ultrasound scanning of the bladder neck is used as an alternative to radiological screening (with its radiation hazard) but is undergoing evaluation. It obviates the need for contrast and catheterization, avoids irradiation and provides good visualization of structures around the bladder neck.

Ultrasound of the bladder neck has been performed using the transabdominal approach (White et al 1980); recently rectal, vaginal and perineal probes have also been used. Transabdominal scanning is more difficult in the obese patient and does not utilize a fixed reference point when assessing bladder-neck descent. This means that any movement of the patient or the transducer will introduce artefact into the measurements. Intraurethral ultrasonography of the urethral sphincter has recently been described (Kirschner-Hermas et al 1994). Preliminary reports look interesting but findings have not yet been related to clinical symptoms or their treatments.

Vaginal, rectal and perineal probes use the pubic symphysis as a fixed reference. The rectal probe is less acceptable to patients and difficulties arise with rotation of the probe, causing loss of the image.

Transvaginal ultrasound

The vaginal probe has been used successfully to investigate the bladder neck. Descent of the bladder base, together with bladder neck opening, has been demonstrated in a majority of patients with stress incontinence but not in controls (Quinn et al 1988). However, bladder-neck opening also occurs with detrusor instability, and this may be difficult to distinguish from stress incontinence unless there is concomitant bladder pressure recording. The potential for distortion of the bladder neck by the probe has not been fully assessed. Transvaginal ultrasonography has recently been used to measure bladder wall thickness (Khullar et al 1994b) (Fig. 47.16). Women with urodynamically diagnosed detrusor instability were found to have significantly thicker bladder walls than those with genuine stress incontinence, and this has been proposed as a screening and diagnostic test.

Perineal ultrasound

Perineal scanning is the most readily available and least expensive technique, as standard equipment which is already available can be used. It is less likely to cause pelvic distortion, is more acceptable to the patient and is feasible in the obese patient (Fig. 47.17). It has been shown to be as accurate as lateral chain urethrocystography in the assessment of patients with failed incontinence surgery, and has the advantages (listed above) of carrying no radiation risk. The equipment is accurate, portable and available in most gynaecology departments (Gordon et al 1989). It may be of use in the determination of causes of failed incontinence surgery (Creighton et al 1994b).

Urethral ultrasound

Urethral cysts and diverticula can be examined using ultrasound. The disadvantage of this method is that unless

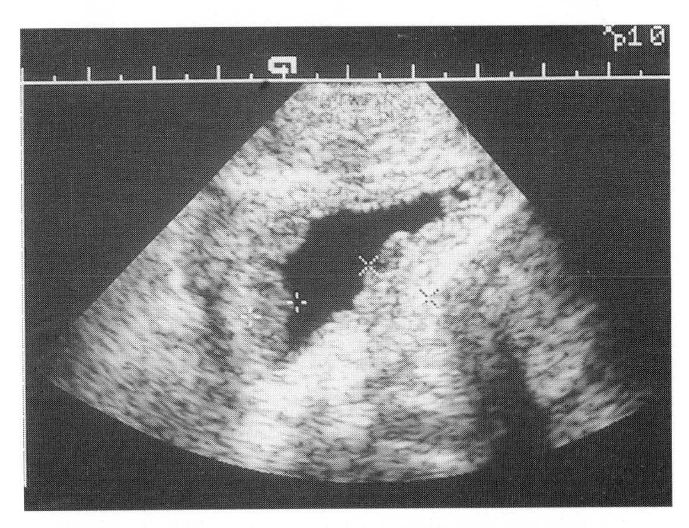

Fig. 47.16 Transvaginal ultrasound picture showing measurement of bladder wall thickness. (With kind permission of V. Khullar)

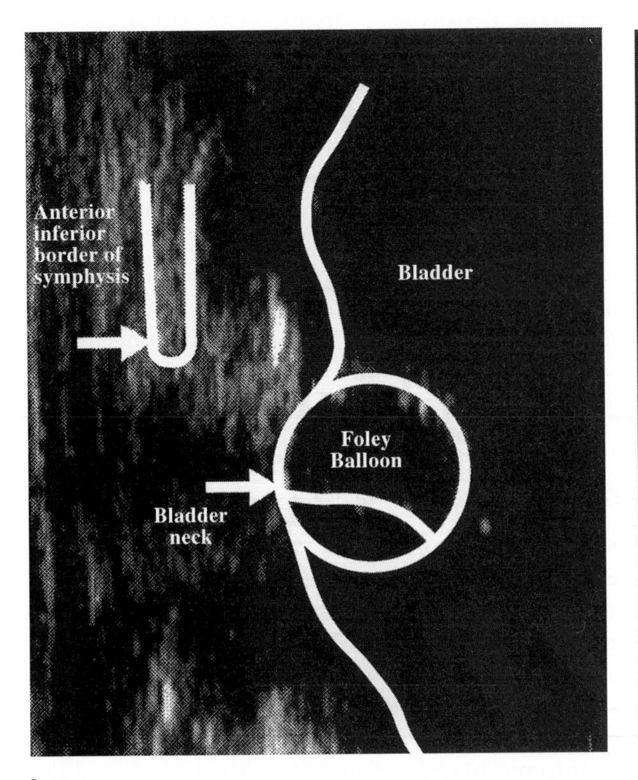

a

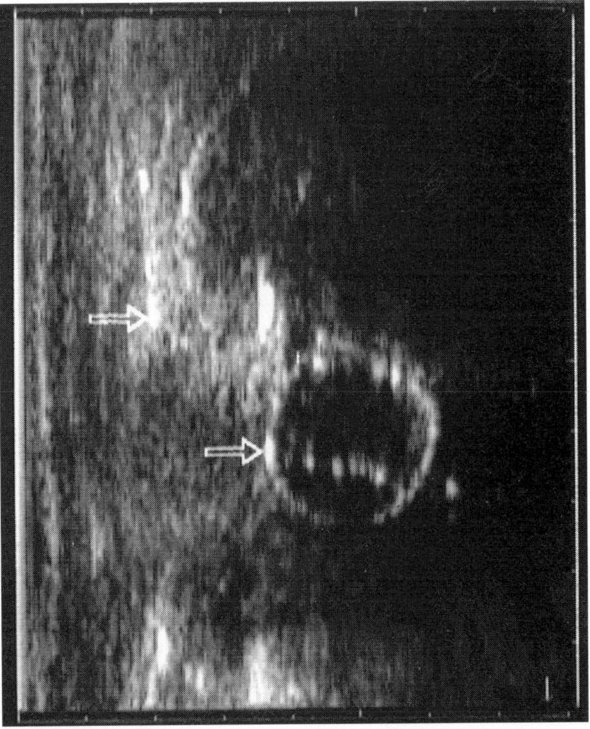

b

Fig. 47.17 Perineal ultrasound of the bladder neck. **(a)** Bladder at rest. Arrows mark the inferior border of the pubic symphysis and the bladder neck, which is demarcated by a Foley catheter. **(b)** Diagrammatic representation of the scan.

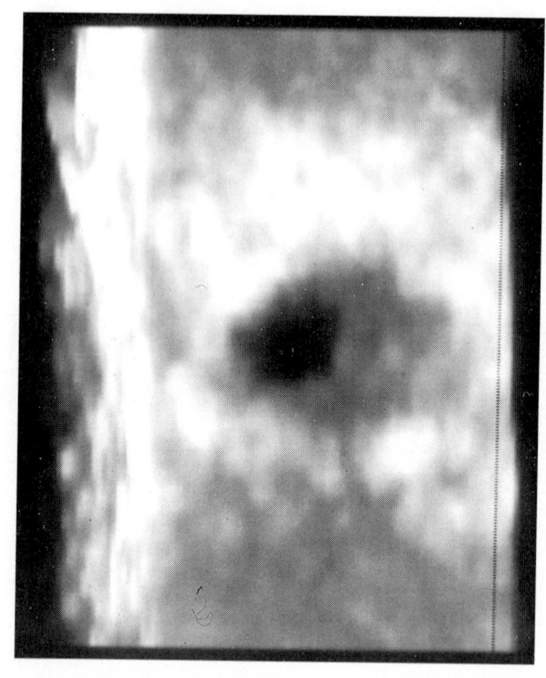

Fig. 47.18 Three-dimensional ultrasound of urethra. (With kind permission of V. Khullar)

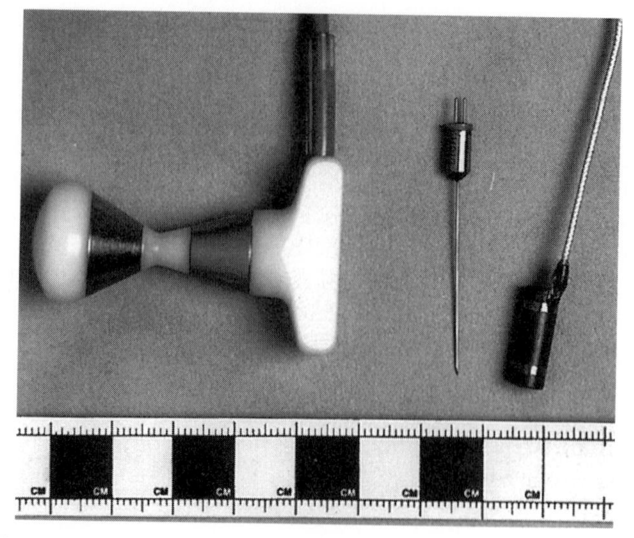

Fig. 47.19 Electrodes for electromyography. From left to right: anal plug electrode, concentric needle electrode and urethral ring electrode.

the opening of the diverticulum is seen directly, the two cannot be differentiated.

Three-dimensional ultrasound of the urethra and urethral sphincter has recently been described (Khullar et al 1994c). This uses a perineal probe which records 150 ultrasound 'slices' as the probe scans 90° on its axis. A three-dimensional image is reconstructed, giving views of the urethra and rhabdosphincter (Fig. 47.18). Evidence of damage to the rhabdosphincter is present in some women with severe genuine stress incontinence.

ELECTROPHYSIOLOGICAL TESTS

Electromyography

Electromyography is the study of bioelectrical potentials generated by smooth and striated muscles, and can be used to evaluate pelvic floor damage in women with urinary or faecal incontinence and prolapse. A motor unit comprises a motor nerve and the fibres it innervates. The potential it generates during contraction is called the motor nerve unit potential, and this can be measured using electromyography. If denervation occurs the remaining nerves sprout collaterals to reinnervate the muscle fibres, thus increasing the dispersion of the motor unit so that more fibres of a particular unit will fire together at one time. This is seen on electromyography as an increase in the amplitude, duration and number of phases of the action potential. If reinnervation is present, polyphasic potentials are seen.

Partial denervation has been proposed as the mechanism by which childbirth contributes to the aetiology of stress incontinence. Allen and Warrell (1987) performed transvaginal electromyography on primiparous women before and after delivery, and detected a highly significant increase in mean motor unit potential duration which was positively associated with birthweight and length of second stage of labour. Smith and Warrell (1984) studied anal sphincter density in patients with stress incontinence and/or prolapse, and found an increased fibre density in all groups compared to normal controls.

Electromyography can be performed using surface electrodes such as anal or vaginal plugs and ring electrodes mounted on a urethral catheter, or it can be performed using needle electrodes inserted into the external anal sphincter or periurethral muscles (Fig. 47.19). Single-fibre needles give a more selective recording and allow measurement of motor unit fibre density. A single-fibre reading is more difficult to obtain than concentric needle signals: 55% of patients were successfully sampled in the former compared to 85% in the latter (Krieger 1990).

Sacral reflexes

Sacral reflexes indicate the integrity of the sacral reflex arc by measuring the conduction time between a stimulus and an evoked muscle contraction. Electrical stimuli can be applied to the skin over the clitoris while recording from the pelvic floor muscle using an electromyography needle, a ring electrode on a Foley catheter or an anal plug electrode. This technique has been used in the investigation of neurogenic bladder disorders, although its usefulness in the detection of 'lower motor neuron' bladder disorders is not clear.

Pudendal terminal motor latencies

Terminal motor latency in the pudendal nerve has been used extensively to investigate neurogenic disorders of the pelvic floor. Motor latency, however, reflects only the conduction velocity of the fastest-conducting muscle fibres, whereas terminal motor latency will be prolonged if there is demyelination of the nerve between the site of stimulation and the muscle. The pudendal nerve is difficult to access and must be stimulated using a fingerstall-mounted electrode applied to the ischial spine via rectal examination.

Weak responses with an increased latency have been observed in women with urethral sphincter incompetence. Snooks et al (1984) found an increased pudendal nerve latency to the anal sphincter in women following a vaginal delivery, compared to women following caesarean section. Smith et al (1989) found that terminal motor latency to the urethral sphincter (perineal terminal latency) was prolonged in women with stress incontinence.

These techniques have been invaluable in the study of pelvic floor damage sustained during childbirth and its contribution to the later development of incontinence.

KEY POINTS

1. Clinical history is often not a good predictor of urodynamic findings.
2. Urinary infection must be excluded before any urodynamic investigation takes place.
3. Peak urinary flow rate measurement is indicated in all women with voiding difficulty, particularly prior to continence surgery, which may aggravate this.
4. Stress incontinence diagnosed on cystometry is a diagnosis of exclusion; it is assessed by leakage in the absence of detrusor contractions.
5. Cough-induced detrusor instability may clinically mimic genuine stress incontinence.
6. All patients undergoing repeat continence surgery must have urodynamic studies performed.
7. Intravenous urography is not indicated in the routine investigation of incontinent women.
8. Cystoscopy must be performed in the case of recurrent urinary tract infections to exclude malignancy.
9. Ultrasound is becoming more widely used in the assessment of the incontinent patient, with the advantage that radiological screening can be avoided.
10. Partial denervation of the pelvic floor following childbirth contributes to the development of both incontinence and prolapse.

REFERENCES

Alcalay M, Griffiths C, Stanton S L 1994 Comparison of Valsalva leak point pressure and stress urethral profilometry in the evaluation of genuine stress incontinence. Abstracts of 24th Annual Meeting, International Continence Society, Prague: 39–40

Allen R E, Warrell D W 1987 The role of pregnancy and childbirth in partial denervation of the pelvic floor. Neurourology and Urodynamics 6: 183–184

Badlani G H, Ravalli R, Moscovitz M O 1993 A tool for the objective assessment of passive urinary incontinence. Contemporary Urology July: 29–35

Bates C P, Loose H, Stanton S L 1973 Objective study of incontinence after repair operations. Surgery, Gynecology and Obstetrics 136: 17–22

Blaivas J G, Bhimani G, Labib K B 1979 Vesicourethral dysfunction in multiple sclerosis. Journal of Urology 122: 342–345

Cardozo L D, Stanton S L 1980 Genuine stress incontinence and detrusor instability: a review of 200 patients. British Journal of Obstetrics and Gynaecology 87: 184–190

Creighton S M, Plevnik S, Stanton S L 1991 Distal urethral electric conductance (DUEC) – a preliminary assessment of its role as a quick screening test for incontinent women. British Journal of Obstetrics and Gynaecology 98: 160–172

Creighton S M, Plevnik S, Stanton S L 1994a Urethral sensitivity in the aetiology of sensory urgency. British Journal of Urology 73: 190–195

Creighton S M, Clark A, Pearce J M, Stanton S L 1994b Perineal bladder neck ultrasound: appearances before and after continence surgery. Ultrasound Obstetrics and Gynecology 4: 428–433

Farrar D J, Whiteside C G, Osbourne J L, Turner-Warwick R T 1975 A urodynamic analysis of micturition symptoms in the female. Surgery, Gynecology and Obstetrics 141: 875–881

Gordon D, Pearce J M, Norton P, Stanton S L 1989 Comparison of ultrasound and lateral chain urethrocystography in the determination of bladder neck descent. American Journal of Obstetrics and Gynecology 160: 182–185

Griffiths C J, Assi M S, Styles R A, Ramsden D D, Neal D R 1989 Ambulatory monitoring of bladder and etrusor pressure during natural filling. Journal of Urology 142: 780–784

Hakenberg O W, Ryall R L, Langlois S L, Marshall V R 1983 The estimation of bladder volume by sonocystography. Journal of Urology 130: 249–251

Haylen B T, Ashby D, Frazer M I, Sutherst J R, West C 1988 Peak and average urine flow rates in a normal female population: the Liverpool nomograms. Neurourology and Urodynamics 7: 176–178

Hilton P 1984 Urethral pressure measurement. In: Stanton S L (ed) Clinical gynecologic urology. C V Mosby, St Louis, pp 110–126

Hilton P, Mayne C J 1988 Urethral pressure variations; the correlation between pressure measurement and electrical conductance in genuine stress incontinence. Neurourology and Urodynamics 7: 175–176

Hodgkinson C P, Doub H, Keely W 1958 Urethrocystograms: metallic bead technique. Clinics in Obstetrics and Gynecology 1: 668–677

Jarvis G J, Hall S, Stamp S, Millar D R, Johnson A 1980 An assessment of urodynamic examination in the incontinent woman. British Journal of Obstetrics and Gynaecology 87: 893–896

Khullar V, Salvatore S, Cardozo L D, Abbot D, Hill S, Kelleher C 1994a Ambulatory urodynamics: a predictor of de novo detrusor instability after colposuspension? Neurourology and Urodynamics 13(4): 443–444

Khullar V, Salvatore S, Cardozo D, Bourne T H, Abbott D, Kelleher C 1994b A novel technique for measuring bladder wall thickness in

women using transvaginal ultrasound. Ultrasound Obstetrics and Gynecology 4: 220–223
Khullar V, Salvatore S, Cardozo L D, Hill S, Kelleher C J 1994c Three dimensional ultrasound of the urethra and urethral sphincter – a new diagnostic technique. Neurourology and Urodynamics 13(4): 352–353
Kirschner-Hermas R, Keln H M, Muller V, Schafer W, Kokse G 1994 Intraurethral ultrasonography in women with stress incontinence. British Journal of Urology 74: 315–318
Krieger M S 1990 MD Thesis: The electrophysiological investigation of genuine stress incontinence and voiding difficulty in women. Sydney University, Australia
Peattie A B, Plevnik S, Stanton S L 1988a Distal urethral electric conductance (DUEC) test: a screening test for female urinary incontinence? Neurourology and Urodynamics 7: 173–174
Peattie A B, Plevnik S, Stanton S L 1988b The use of bladder neck electrical conductance (BNEC) in the investigation and management of sensory urge incontinence in the female. Journal of the Royal Society of Medicine 81: 442–444
Plevnik S, Holmes D M, Janez J, Mundy A R, Vrtacnik P 1985 Urethral electrical conductance (UEC) – a new parameter for the evaluation of urethral and bladder function: methodology of the assessment of its clinical potential. Proceedings of the 15th International Continence Society Meeting, London
Powell P H, Feneley R C L 1980 The role of urethral sensation in clinical urology. British Journal of Urology 52: 539–541
Quinn M J, Beynon J, Mortenson N J, McSmith P J B 1988 Transvaginal endosonography: a new method to study the anatomy of the lower urinary tract in urinary stress incontinence. British Journal of Urology 62: 414–418
Richardson D A 1980 Value of the cough pressure profile in the evaluation of patients with stress incontinence. American Journal of Obstetrics and Gynecology 155: 808–811
Richardson D A, Ramahi A, Chalas E 1991 Surgical management of stress incontinence in patients with low urethral pressure. Gynecologic and Obstetric Investigation 31: 106–109
Robertson A S, Griffiths C J, Ramsden P D, Neal D E 1994 Bladder function in healthy volunteers: ambulatory monitoring and conventional urodynamic studies. British Journal of Urology 73: 242–249
Sand P K, Boweb L W, Panganiban R, Ostergard D R 1987 The low pressure urethra as a factor in failed retropubic urethropexy. Obstetrics and Gynecology 69: 399–402
Smith A R B, Warrell D W 1984 A neurogenic aetiology of stress urinary incontinence and uterovaginal prolapse. Proceedings of the 14th International Continence Society Meeting, Innsbruck, pp 485–487
Smith A R B, Hosker G L, Warrell D W 1989 The role of pudendal nerve damage in the aetiology of genuine stress incontinence in women. British Journal of Obstetrics and Gynaecology 96: 29–32
Snooks S J, Setchell M, Swash M, Henry M M 1984 Injury to innervation of pelvic floor sphincter musculature in childbirth. Lancet ii 2: 546–550
Stamey T A 1983 Endoscopic suspension of the vesical neck. In: Raz S (ed) Female urology. W B Saunders, Philadelphia, pp 267–268
Stanton S L, Krieger M S, Ziv E 1988 Videocystourethrography: its role in the assessment of incontinence in the female. Neurourology and Urodynamics 7: 172–173
van Waalwijk van Doorn E S C, Remmers A, Jankneft R A 1991 Extramural ambulatory urodynamic monitoring during natural filling and normal daily activities: evaluation of 100 patients. Journal of Urology 146: 124–131
Versi E, Cardozo L D, Studd J, Cooper D 1986 Evaluation of urethral pressure profilometry for the diagnosis of genuine stress incontinence. World Journal of Urology 4: 6–9
Wall L L, Helms M, Peattie A, Pearce M, Stanton S L 1991 Bladder neck mobility and the outcome of surgery for genuine stress urinary incontinence. Journal of Reproductive Medicine 39: 429–435
Walter G J, Vejlsgaard R 1978 Diagnostic catheterization and bacteriuria in women with urinary incontinence. British Journal of Urology 50: 106–108
Webb R J, Ramsden P D, Neal D E 1991 Ambulatory monitoring and electronic measurement of urinary leakage in the diagnosis of detrusor instability and incontinence. British Journal of Urology 68: 148–152
White R D, McQuown D, McCarthy T A, Ostergard D R 1980 Real time ultrasonography in the evaluation of urinary stress incontinence. American Journal of Obstetrics and Gynecology 138: 235–237

48

Urethral sphincter incompetence

S. L. Stanton

DEFINITIONS

When a woman coughs and loses urine the condition used to be called stress incontinence, a term coined by Sir Eardley Holland in 1928. Today, investigations have shown that many conditions can cause stress incontinence and therefore it is preferable to use the term to refer only to symptoms and signs. In 1976, the International Continence Society (ICS) adopted the term 'genuine stress incontinence', which was defined as involuntary urethral loss of urine when the intravesical pressure exceeds the maximum urethral pressure in the absence of detrusor activity (Abrams et al 1988). I prefer the term 'urethral sphincter incompetence', which conveys the pathophysiology more precisely. In the USA the term 'stress urinary incontinence' or 'anatomic stress incontinence' is still commonly used.

We retain the symptom to indicate the patient's statement of involuntary urine loss on physical effort and the sign to denote observation of urine loss from the urethra synchronous with physical exertion.

AETIOLOGY

The mechanism of continence is dealt with in Chapter 46.

Urethral sphincter incompetence is due to two causes: descent of the bladder neck and proximal urethra, so that there is failure of equal transmission of intra-abdominal pressure to the proximal urethra, leading to reversal of the normal pressure gradient between the bladder and urethra and resulting in a negative urethral closure pressure. Alternatively, the intraurethral pressure at rest is below the intravesical pressure. The factors responsible for this are:

1. Congenital weakness of the bladder neck, e.g. epispadias (see Fig. 48.1). The urethra and bladder neck are imperfectly formed owing to faulty migration and midline fusion of mesoderm, resulting in a widened bladder neck, a short urethra and defective smooth and striated musculature. The symphysis and clitoris are split.

Less obvious congenital weakness presents in the early teens, when healthy nulliparous girls exercise and find that they are incontinent. Nemir and Middleton (1954) and Thomas et al (1980) have shown that 5–10% of young girls have regular troublesome stress incontinence. In the evolutionary change from the horizontal to the vertical position, women have come to rely on a poorly constructed pelvic floor to support the bladder neck; it may fail to do so adequately during times of physical effort (Fig. 48.2). This is aggravated by genetic variation in collagen and other connective tissue. Keane et al (1992) have shown a reduction in total collagen and a decrease in type I in nulliparous premenopausal women with urethral sphincter incompetence.

Weakness and malformation of the bladder neck found in epispadias produce incontinence resistant to conventional bladder-neck elevating procedures, and are corrected by increasing the urethral resistance, i.e. using an artificial urinary sphincter.

2. Childbirth, leading to denervation of smooth and striated components of the sphincter mechanism and pelvic floor and pubocervical fascia (Snooks et al 1984, Sayer et al 1989).

3. Menopause: oestrogen deficiency may lead to further weakness of bladder-neck supports and loss of hermetic sealing of the urothelium.

4. Trauma: fracture of the pelvic ring and symphysial diastasis with avulsion diastasis with avulsion of the

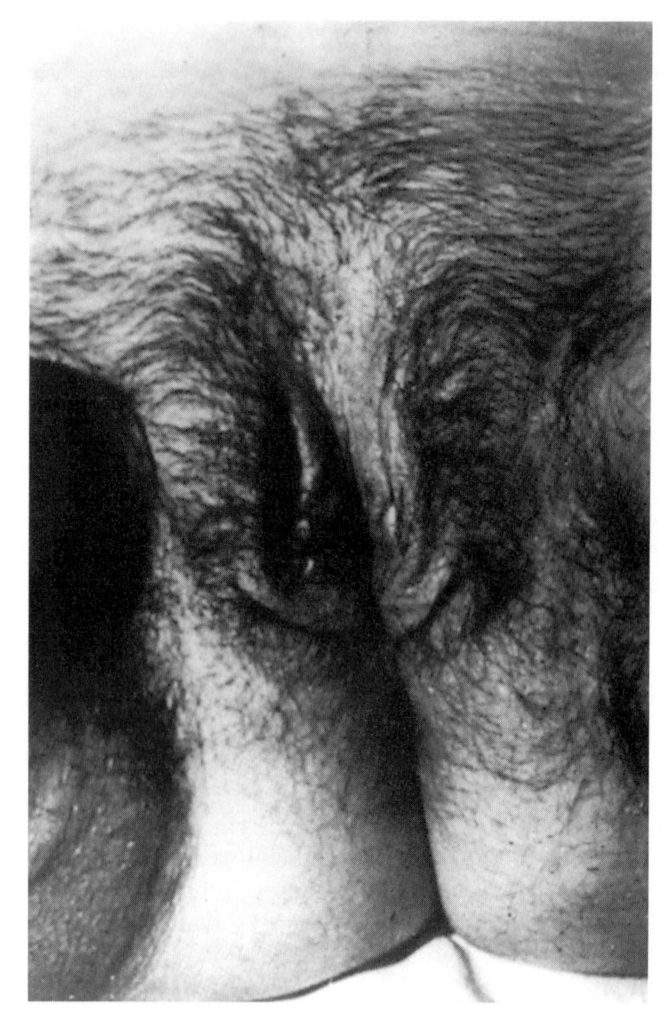

Fig. 48.1a Female epispadias showing separation of clitoris.

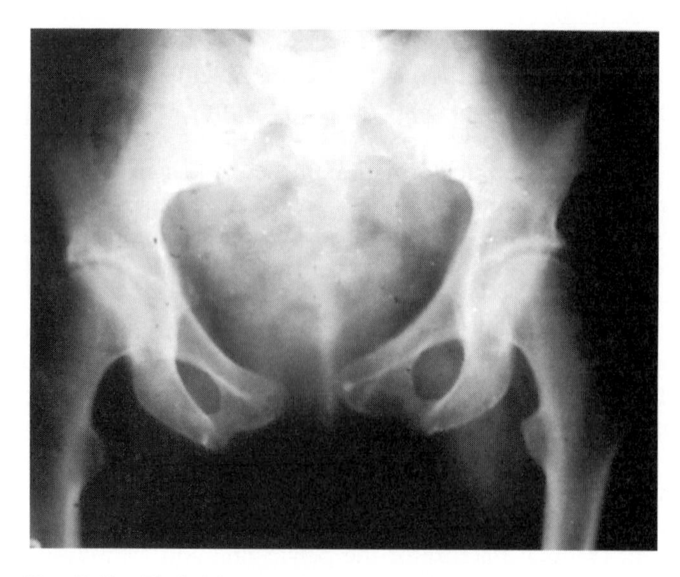

Fig. 48.1b Underlying symphyseal separation.

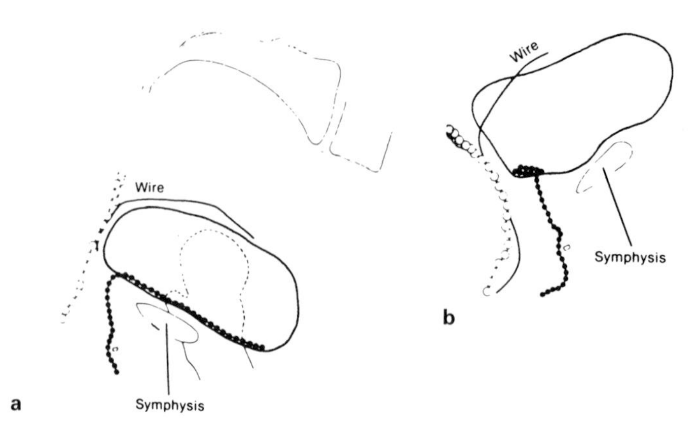

Fig. 48.2 **a** Chain cystourethrogram with patient in the non-straining lateral position on all fours showing urethra exiting from a high position in the bladder and supported by the symphysis. **b** Patient erect, showing bladder neck junction at lowest level of bladder and without symphysial support. (From Hodgkinson 1970, with permission)

bladder neck from its attachment to the back of the symphysis by the pubourethral ligaments (Stanton et al 1981).

5. Fibrosis of the urethra and urethral musculature secondary to bladder-neck surgery, for either continence or prolapse.

PRESENTATION

Symptoms

The classic symptom of urethral sphincter incompetence is stress incontinence; however, frequency, urge incontinence and incontinence on standing are also complained of by many patients (Cardozo & Stanton 1980; Fig. 48.3). Usually stress incontinence is worse in the week preceding the menstrual period. Interruption of the urinary stream can be confirmed objectively in about 83% of patients with sphincter incompetence and in 87% of patients with detrusor instability, so the symptom is of no use in differentiating between the two.

The patients are usually multiparous and symptoms commonly occur in pregnancy and deteriorate in the postnatal period and in successive pregnancies (Francis 1960, Stanton et al 1980).

Signs

There are no special general or neurological features on clinical examination.

Epispadias will be readily recognized. Anterior vaginal wall descent (cystourethrocoele) will be present in about 50% of women with sphincter incompetence.

It is helpful to assess whether other genital prolapse is present and to detect pathology such as uterine or ovarian enlargement, so that surgery for that can be carried out at the same time as continent surgery.

The vaginal capacity and mobility (indicators of vaginal

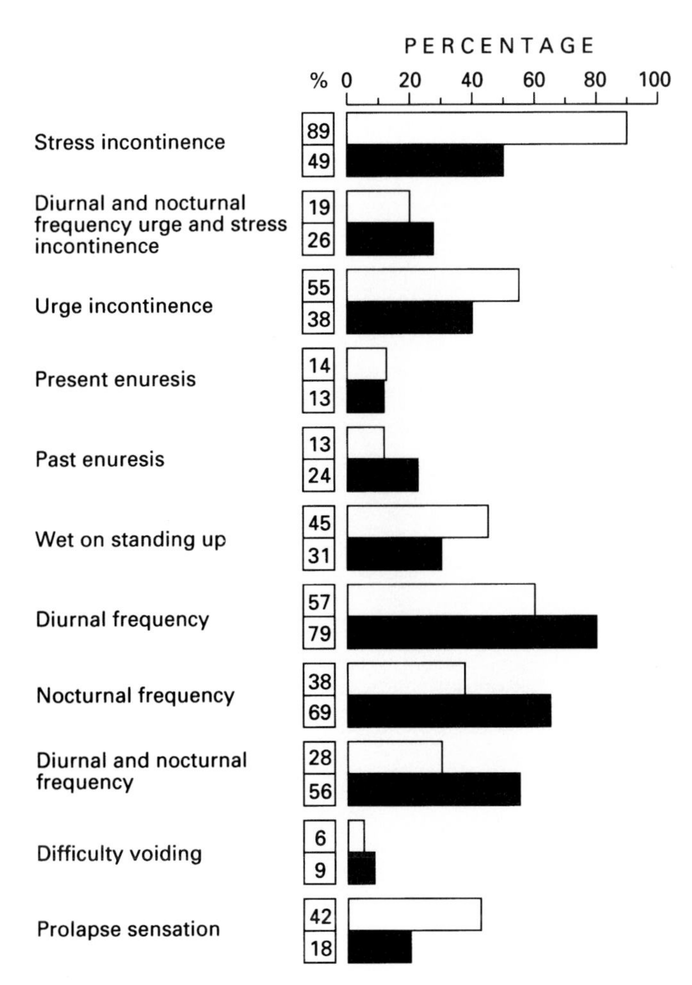

Fig. 48.3 Prevalence of symptoms associated with urethral sphincter incompetence and detrusor instability. (From Cardozo & Stanton 1980, with permission). □ = Genuine stress incontinence; ■ = detrusor instability. Stress incontinence is dominant; other symptoms include urgency, diurnal and nocturnal frequency.

scarring) need to be assessed, as these may be relevant in determining the choice of any continence surgery.

INVESTIGATIONS

The bladder is not a reliable witness. Many clinicians have demonstrated the discrepancy between clinical findings and urodynamic studies (Haylen & Frazer 1987, Ng & Murray 1989). The difficulty lies in the complexity of the history. Stress incontinence alone is likely to indicate sphincter incompetence and a combination of stress incontinence, urge incontinence and frequency is more likely to suggest detrusor instability. In a consecutive group of 800 women attending the urodynamic clinic, approximately 50% were diagnosed by urodynamic studies as having urethral sphincter incompetence. Of these only 3% had the symptom and sign of stress incontinence and 1.5% (6) had the sole symptom of stress incontinence (Haylen & Frazer 1987). Of the total group, 85% had urgency, urge incontinence and stress incontinence but only 25% had detrusor instability on testing. It was similar with voiding disorders: 53% had two symptoms suggestive of voiding disorder, which was confirmed in only 10% on testing. The aims of urodynamic studies are:

1. To confirm the symptoms (e.g. incontinence or voiding difficulty).
2. To make a diagnosis.
3. To detect other abnormalities, e.g. detrusor instability.
4. To refine the course of treatment.
5. To confirm the cure.

A full description of urodynamic studies is given in Chapter 47; the following tests are useful to investigate a diagnosis of sphincter incompetence.

A negative midstream urine specimen should precede all urodynamic studies to avoid risk of invasive procedures aggravating urinary tract infection and because the subsequent results will be unreliable.

Pad test

A pad test is a simple, inexpensive and non-invasive method of demonstrating urinary loss when this is unproven on a clinical examination or cystometry or videocystourethrography. Of the many varieties, a 1-hour test as recommended by the ICS (Abrams et al 1988) is probably the most reliable (Mayne & Hilton 1988). However, the pad test does not confirm the cause of leakage.

Urethral electric conductance

Measurement of change in distal urethral electric conductance will confirm urinary leakage and may indicate whether this is due to sphincter incompetence, urethral or detrusor instability (Peattie et al 1989).

Cystometry and videocystourethrography

The cystometric diagnosis of urinary leakage will indicate the presence of detrusor instability or voiding difficulty; only if detrusor instability is absent is the diagnosis of urethral sphincter incompetence made by exclusion.

The combination of cystometry and radiological screening with recording on video tape, together with a sound commentary, allows other diagnoses to be made, including the cause of incontinence on assuming the upright position, the presence of a urethral diverticulum (see Fig. 47.11) and occasionally the presence of a urinary fistula (Fig. 48.4). It otherwise adds little to the assessment of straightforward urethral sphincter incompetence (Stanton et al 1988).

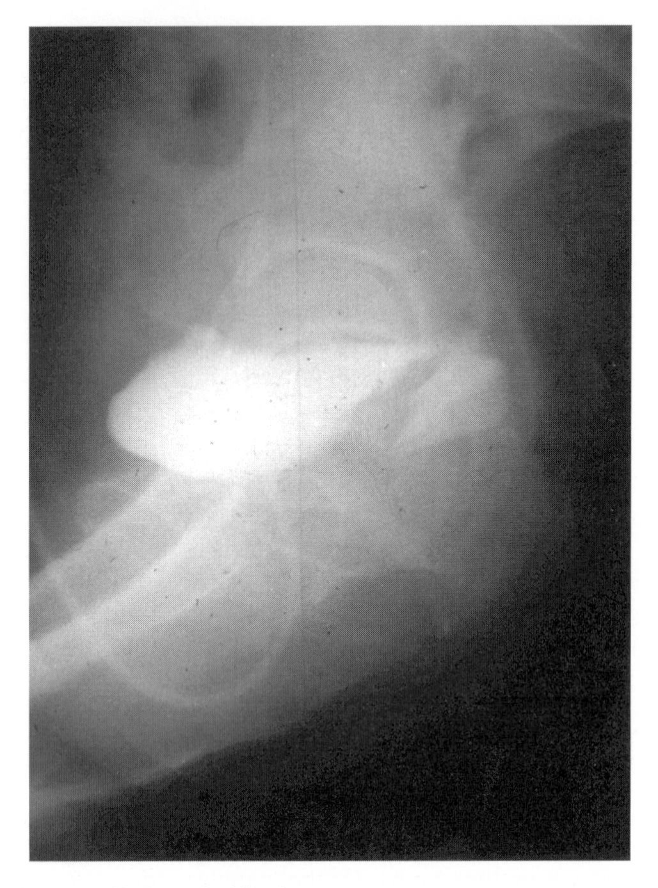

Fig. 48.4 Vesicovaginal fistula.

Radiology

A plain anteroposterior pelvic radiograph will detect symphysial diastasis when associated with a pelvic fracture (Fig. 48.5) or a full bladder associated with chronic retention and overflow (Fig. 48.6), although the latter can be detected without irradiation using ultrasonography.

Intravenous urography would demonstrate an ectopic ureter; it is necessary when incontinence is present from birth, or when continuous incontinence follows pelvic surgery, in order to exclude a ureteric fistula.

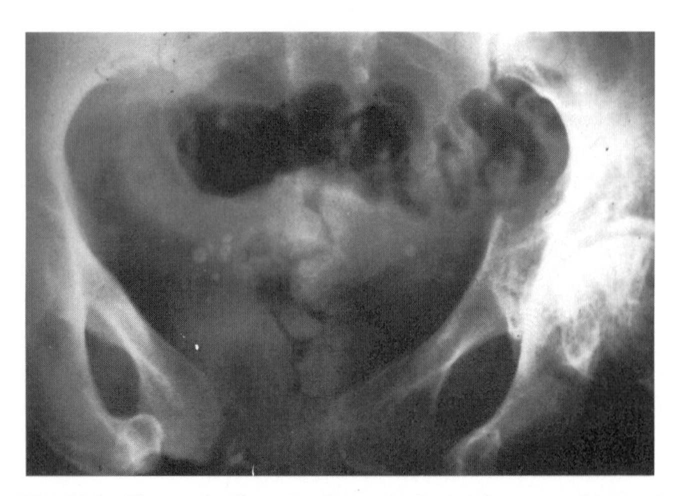

Fig. 48.5 Traumatic diastasis of symphysis and fractures of internal ring.

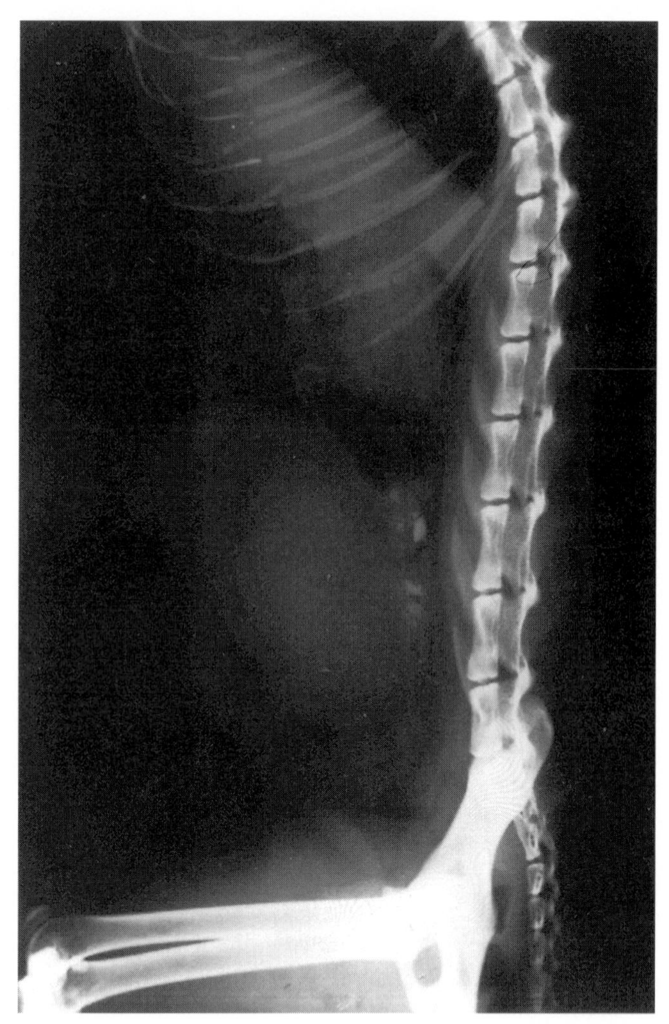

Fig. 48.6 Lateral radiograph showing full bladder associated with chronic retention and overflow. (Courtesy of Victor E. Travis)

Uroflowmetry

The measurement of urine flow is simple and non-invasive and although it is not directly necessary for the diagnosis of sphincter incompetence, it will detect unsuspected voiding difficulty (which may compromise any intended bladder-neck surgery). On its own it serves only as a screening test and gives more information when combined with intravesical pressure measurement.

Urethral pressure profilometry

The role of urethral pressure profilometry in the diagnosis of urethral sphincter incompetence remains controversial and undecided. Versi et al (1986) declared that 'the overlap between normal and GSI [USI] was so great as to make accurate diagnosis impossible'. Sand and colleagues

(1987) measured the urethral closure pressure and took a cut-off of 20 cmH_2O to detect the problem of the low-pressure urethra, which they said was a significant feature of failed continent surgery. Hilton (1988) reviewed the concept of the unstable urethra as a cause of sphincter incompetence, and found that a relative change of 30% of maximum urethral closure pressure was the best discriminant to detect this.

The main disadvantages of the urethral pressure are the relative inflexibility of the catheter, leading to artefact, and the marked overlap in results between continent and incontinent patients.

Ultrasonography

Ultrasound will detect incomplete bladder emptying, which may be responsible for stress incontinence. It will also allow estimation of the position and excursion of the bladder neck, which is relevant to the diagnosis of urethral sphincter incompetence and may help in the analysis of failure of conventional surgery and in the definitive choice of surgery (Creighton et al 1991). Examples of bladder neck position and excursion are shown in Figure 47.17.

Electrophysiological studies

Snooks et al (1984) demonstrated denervation of the sphincter mechanism and pelvic floor after childbirth. In complex cases of sphincter incompetence, especially where multiple bladder-neck surgeries are being performed and further surgery is contemplated, it may be worthwhile measuring the electromyographic activity of these structures using a single-fibre electrode (Krieger et al 1988) and terminal motor latencies in the perineal branch of the pudendal nerve.

TREATMENT

Conservative and surgical treatments are used depending on the patient's condition and urodynamic diagnosis. Conservative therapy is indicated when:

1. The patient refuses or is undecided about surgery.
2. The patient is mentally or physically unfit.
3. Childbearing continues.
4. There is uncontrolled detrusor instability or voiding difficulty.

Conservative treatment

1. The continuous indwelling catheter remains a simple method of managing urinary incontinence. However, it predisposes to urinary tract infection and may be uncomfortable to wear. For long-term use suprapubic insertion is preferable and the 'add-a cath' method of insertion (Bard) using a Foley silastic catheter (either 12 or 16 French gauge) is recommended (Lawrence et al 1989; Fig. 48.7). If there is urethral leakage, urethral closure may be performed.

2. For mild sphincter incompetence, wearing a tampon or a reusable foam pessary may temporarily cure incontinence by elevating the bladder neck (Fig. 48.8). This is recommended for patients who are incontinent at known times.

3. Absorbent pads are useful when incontinence is mild. The latest are made of a gel substance which absorbs many times its volume of water. The pads have a water-repellent backing and absorb urine without it leaking back to the patient's skin (to make damp) or forward, so making

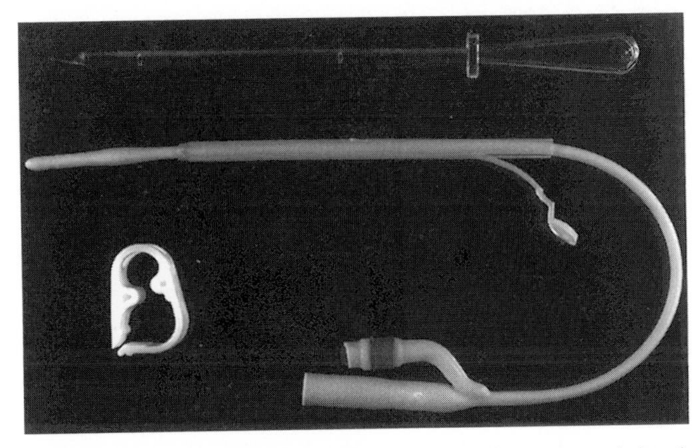

Fig. 48.7 'Add-a' suprapubic catheter showing the trocar and sheath containing Foley catheter (Bard).

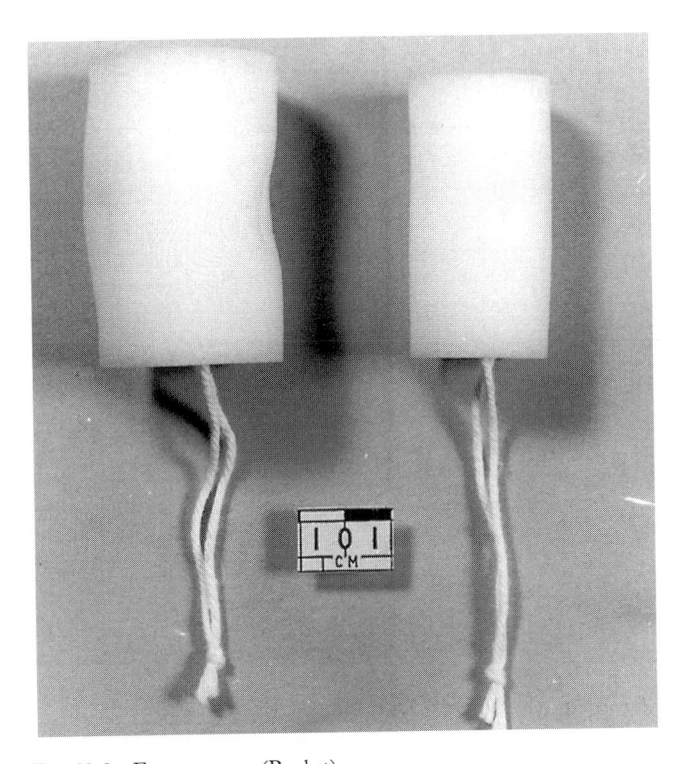

Fig. 48.8 Foam pessary (Rocket).

the patient's clothing wet. Good examples are the pads manufactured by Conveen.

4. The use of electronic vaginal devices to cure sphincter incompetence has had a variable popularity over the past 20 years. The technique of using short-term electrical stimulation via vaginal or anal electrodes with daily treatments of 20 minutes over a period of 30 days has been found effective (Plevnik et al 1986). The current used was up to 90 mA with a frequency of 20 Hz and pulse duration 0.75 ms.

5. There are a variety of exercises to enhance pelvic floor tone and control incontinence. However, the exercise regimens are rarely objectively tested and often carried out for inadequate periods of time, so improvement in incontinence is unsatisfactory. Tapp et al (1989) found that about 50% of women awaiting surgery for urethral sphincter incompetence were improved with 6 months of physiotherapy alone. Marginally more were improved when faradism was added.

At least 1 hour of exercise a day for 3 months is required to show any improvement, which lasts only while the exercises are being carried out. The easiest one to teach is to interrupt the urinary stream and then to practise this at other times.

Interferential therapy can also be used to improve pelvic floor tone (Bridges et al 1988).

6. Vaginal cones were designed by Plevnik (1985), an engineer from the former Yugoslavia, as a method of actively and passively exercising the pelvic floor (Figs 48.9 and 48.10). Since the patient knows the weight of the cone she is able to retain with her pelvic floor muscles, she can monitor her progress. More than 70% of patients are cured or improved, and 90% find it an acceptable method of treatment (Bridges et al 1988, Peattie et al 1988).

7. There are several new mechanical devices which are commercially available: they either occlude the urethra or support the bladder neck. Of the former, Reliance (UroMed) is placed inside the urethra and replaced after each void and FemAssist (Insight Medical UK Ltd) is

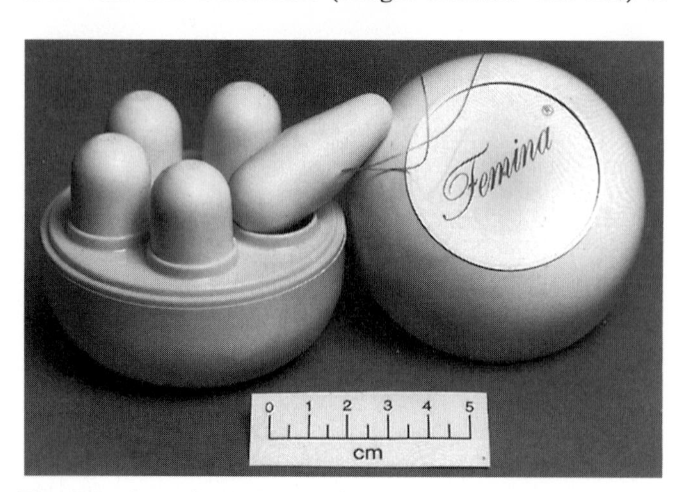

Fig. 48.9 A set of vaginal cones (Colgate Medical).

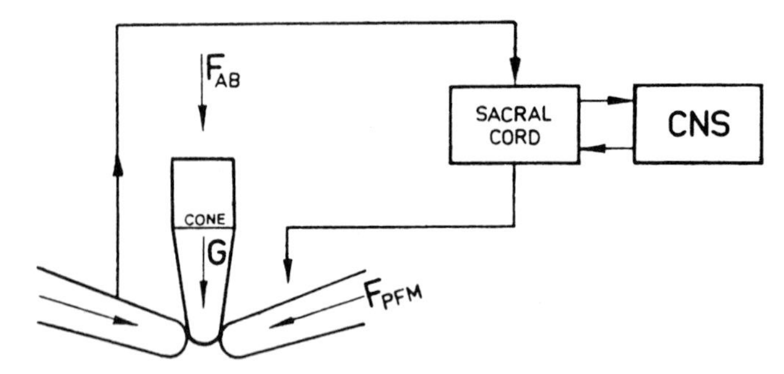

Fig. 48.10 Diagrammatic representation of forces on the cones when in situ. G = weight of cone; F_{AB} = force due to abdominal pressure; F_{PFM} = force developed by pelvic floor muscle; CNS = central nervous system.

positioned on the external urethral meatus and remains there by light suction. It is re-usable and replaced weekly. A multi-centre trial of the Reliance device (Staskin et al 1995) has shown a 31% incidence of urinary tract infection (40% were asymptomatic), a 27% patient withdrawal due to discomfort and medical reasons and 78% of the remainder were dry at 1 year follow-up. Supportive devices include the Conveen continence guard (Coloplast) and Introl (Johnson & Johnson). Thyssen & Lose (1996) found that the continence guard cured 41% without any urinary tract infection and with only 15% of withdrawals for discomfort.

Surgical treatment

Continence surgery is indicated when conservative measures have failed or the patient wants definitive treatment now. If detrusor instability and voiding difficulty are present, the patient should be warned that surgery may make either condition worse. If the patient has not completed her family bladder-neck surgery can be performed, but if she subsequently conceives and is dry, a caesarean section should be performed to avoid further pelvic floor trauma. The patient should be counselled that it is wise to avoid heavy lifting after any urethrovesical suspension operation, certainly for at least 2 months.

Choice of operation

The choice of operation is influenced by the clinical features and urodynamic data. An elderly or frail patient is less likely to make energetic demands on the site of operation and will benefit from a shorter operation of 20–30 minutes, with a relatively pain-free postoperative period to aid mobilization. A younger and fitter patient will require more extensive surgery as she is more likely to be more physically active and will cope better with the pain of a major operation. In general, vaginal operations and endoscopic bladder-neck suspensions are quicker and less painful, but may not be as durable as the urethrovesical suspension operations.

Table 48.1 Clinical and urodynamic features

Access	Operation	Mechanism	Clinical indications	Urodynamic effects/ complications
Vaginal	Anterior colporrhaphy	Elevates bladder neck from below	Elderly; physically frail	Minimal recurrence of stress incontinence
	Periurethral injection (e.g. GAX collagen)	Prevents premature bladder-neck opening	Mild urethral sphincter incompetence – primary and failed surgery; physically frail	Transient urinary retention
Vaginal and suprapubic	Endoscopic bladder neck suspension (Raz and Stamey)	Elevates from above; enhances pressure transmission in proximal urethra	Elderly; physically frail	Suture can pull through causing recurrence
Suprapubic	Marshall–Marchetti–Krantz	Elevates bladder neck from above	Urethral sphincter incompetence without cystocoele	Osteitis pubis
	Colposuspension	Elevates bladder neck	Primary or secondary urethral sphincter incompetence with or without cystocoele	Voiding difficulty; detrusor instability
	Sling	Elevates bladder neck from above; supports proximal urethra	Proximal urethra needs support; contracted vagina	Voiding difficulty and urinary tract infection; sling erosion; detrusor instability
	Artificial urinary sphincter	Increases urethral resistance	Neurogenic reconstructive surgery; failed conventional bladder neck surgery	Erosion, mechanical failure

GAX collagen, glutaraldehyde cross-linked bovine collagen

Urodynamic studies will indicate whether surgery is required to correct bladder-neck descent and support the bladder neck, or whether urethral resistance has to be enhanced, or whether both are necessary. The flow rate and maximum voiding pressure will suggest whether there is need for caution with an operation likely to produce obstruction.

To choose the operation, the clinical and urodynamic features of the patient and characteristics of each operation have to be matched (Table 48.1).

Jarvis (1994) carried out a meta-analysis of the overall results of surgery for urethral sphincter incompetence. The analysis has the disadvantage that the initial indications and outcome measures differ from study to study, so a limited interpretation must be placed on the findings. He does, however, support the contention that there is no single operation that could be offered to all women.

Continence operations

Anterior colporrhaphy. A number of clinicians have now demonstrated that the anterior colporrhaphy has a lower success rate for cure of urethral sphincter incompetence than suprapubic operations (Bergman et al 1989). In our own study on 26 patients, at the end of 2 years six no longer complained of stress incontinence but only 14 (54%) were objectively cured (Stanton et al 1991). The advantage of an anterior colporrhaphy is that it will correct coexistent anterior vaginal wall prolapse and is unlikely to cause either voiding difficulty or detrusor instability. Apart from a low cure rate of urethral sphincter incompetence, the operation may produce narrowing and scarring of the vaginal tissues, which may render further bladder-neck surgery more difficult.

In comparing results for anterior colporrhaphy, it is obvious that different surgical techniques exist. Some surgeons claim that the pubocervical fascia is found on the vaginal aspect of the bladder and plicate that, whereas others take the pubocervical fascia as being adherent to the undersurface of the anterior vaginal wall flap, and use that for plication.

Periurethral injection. Periurethral injections are simple procedures for restoring continence. GAX collagen (glutaraldehyde cross-linked bovine collagen: Bard Contigen) is a day-case local anaesthetic procedure which restores continence by preventing premature bladder-neck opening. In a 2-year follow-up it achieved a 68% subjective and 48% objective cure (Monga et al 1995; Fig. 48.11).

Endoscopic bladder neck suspension operation. The Stamey (1973) operation consists of needle insertion of a suture either side of the bladder neck, anchored by a buffer below the pubocervical fascia and tied above on top of the rectus sheath at a tension sufficient to close the bladder neck. Raz (1981) modified this to include a wider blunt dissection to free the endopelvic fascia from the back of the pubis, and inserted helical sutures into the deep endopelvic fascia, including part of the vaginal wall (Fig. 48.12).

I prefer the Raz technique and use it for the elderly woman. I use a no. 2 proline suture on a small 4 trocar pointed Mayo needle and a 15° angle Stamey needle to retrieve the suture. I tighten sufficiently to elevate the bladder neck and support it. A small vertical vaginal incision is used on either side of the bladder neck to insert the suture and a small suprapubic incision is placed in each iliac fossa, to retrieve and tie the suture on to the rectus sheath.

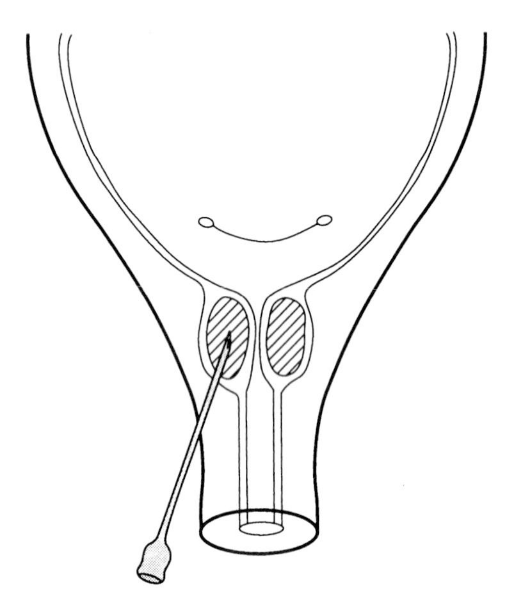

Fig. 48.11 Periurethral injection of material under the submucosa.

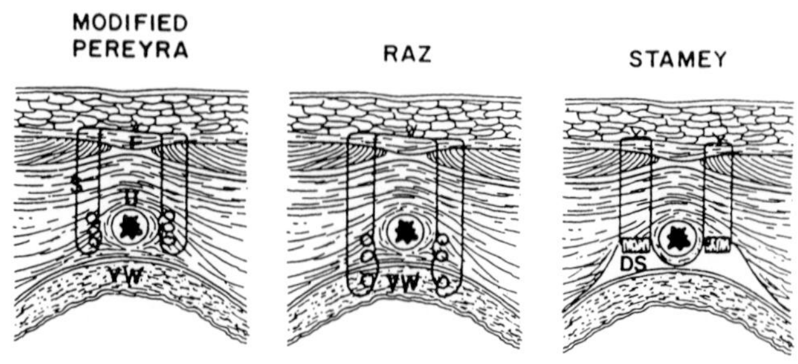

Fig. 48.12 Comparison of modified Pereyra, Raz and Stamey operations: coronal section of bladder neck and surrounding tissues. VW = Vaginal wall; U = urethra; S = suture; DS = dacron support; F = fascia.

Whichever technique is used, cystoscopy is essential after all needle passes have been completed to ensure that no suture has passed through the bladder and that the sutures are at the level of the bladder neck.

Marshall–Marchetti–Krantz (MMK) operation. The MMK is probably the most widely used suprapubic procedure. The sutures are inserted between paraurethral tissues along the proximal half of the urethra and the periosteum or perichondrium of the symphysis pubis. Krantz (1986) prefers one suture of 2.0 braided Mersilene and uses a double bite and anchors this to the perichondrium. The main complications are osteitis pubis (0.5–5% of cases) and sometimes difficulty in finding tissue behind the symphysis in which to anchor the suture. The procedure will not correct a cystocoele.

Colposuspension. The original description by Burch in 1961 has changed little, apart from a more specific direction as to where to place the supporting sutures (Stanton 1986).

Before commencing, it is important to ensure that the vagina has adequate capacity and mobility so that the lateral fornices can be elevated towards each ipsilateral iliopectineal ligament. If not, the operation is unlikely to be technically feasible and an alternative procedure should be considered. If an enterocoele or rectocoele is present, they are likely to be made worse by this operation and ought to be corrected at the same time.

The abdomen and perineum are prepared in a sterile fashion and a urological drape (3 M-1071) is used to allow the operator to dissect with one finger in the vagina. A Foley catheter is inserted and a low Pfannenstiel incision or a combination of Pfannenstiel and Cherney incision is used, if a previous lower abdominal incision is present; this avoids a tedious dissection and sometimes inadvertent opening of the peritoneum. After having dissected the base of the bladder medially, two to three Ethibond no. 1 sutures (polybutylate-coated polyethylene; Ethicon) are inserted, 1 cm apart and starting as cephalad as possible, between endopelvic fascia (incorporating the whole thickness of the anterior vaginal wall if the fascia is thin) and the ipsilateral iliopectineal ligament (Fig. 48.13). To avoid the suture sliding through the fascia when later tied to the iliopectineal ligament, and to aid haemostasis, the suture is tied on the endopelvic fascia. I try and avoid placing sutures distal to the bladder neck because of their tendency to produce voiding disorders. To do this, I gently pull on the Foley catheter and determine by feel whether there is room for a further suture more distally. The procedure is repeated on the other side. After completing haemostasis the sutures are tied, a vacuum drain is left in the retropubic space and a suprapubic catheter inserted. A long-term follow-up has shown that for primary surgery

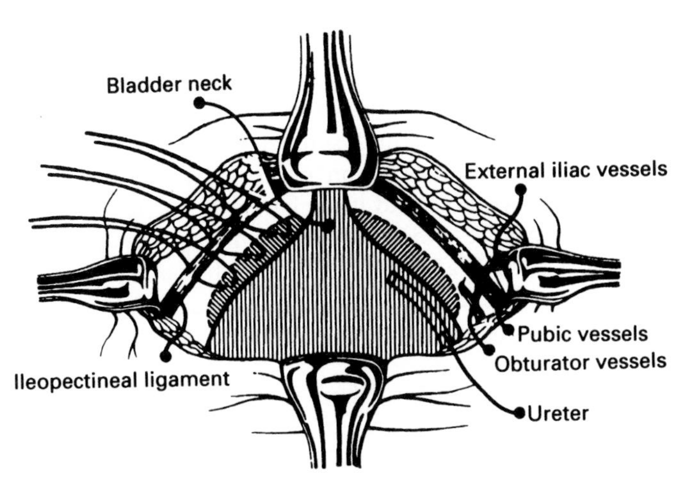

Fig. 48.13 Schema of colposuspension as exposed by a Pfannenstiel incision.

the colposuspension has an objective cure rate of 85% at 5 years, which falls to 69% at 10 years. The success rate for secondary surgery is 67% and 62% respectively (Alcalay et al 1995).

I would suggest the following order for additional procedures. If an enterocoele repair is required, the uterosacral ligaments should be coapted at the beginning of the operation. If a hysterectomy is necessary this should be carried out as an abdominal procedure, with careful attention to vault haemostasis and support. The colposuspension is then performed and finally, if a posterior repair is required, this is carried out as the last procedure.

Laparoscopic colposuspensions have been reported by many authors. However, the high complication rate (1–10% bladder or ureteric injury) and lower success rate compared to conventional colposuspension throw some doubt on its role until the technique can be improved.

Sling procedures. There are many varieties, depending on routes of access, type of material used and sling tension.

Most gynaecologists prefer a synchronous vaginal and suprapubic approach. This has the advantage of seeing exactly where the sling is placed and anchoring it at the bladder neck if required. It may be more effective in producing haemostasis and in avoiding sling erosions than the suprapubic approach alone. The disadvantage is the potential of the vaginal incision for infection, which is relevant when inorganic tissue is used. I prefer the single abdominal incision and use a 'blind tunnel' technique to insert the sling under the bladder neck, and then anchor it to each iliopectineal ligament.

Sling materials are either organic or inorganic. The former is either autogenous (from rectus fascia or, if unavailable, fascia lata) or from animal tissues, e.g. porcine dermis. Inorganic materials are stronger, more consistent and readily available. However, if infection occurs the sling may have to be removed. Meshes such as Marlex

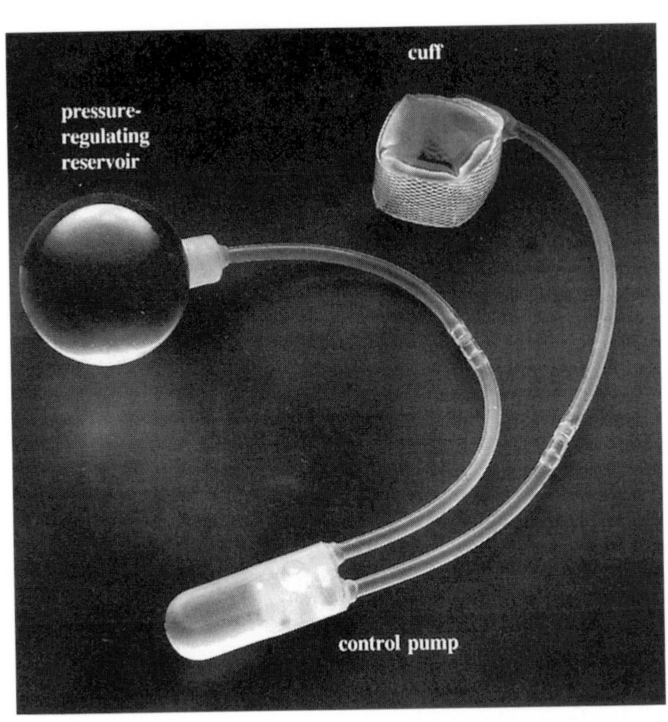

Fig. 48.14 Artificial urinary sphincter 800 showing cuff, reservoir and pump.

(polypropylene) allow fibroblasts to grow into them and become inextricably bound with body tissues, and are difficult to remove subsequently.

I prefer silastic bonded to Dacron, which is strong and does not bond to body tissues, but causes a fibrous sheath to form around the sling (Stanton et al 1985). The silastic sling must be sutured using a non-absorbable suture, and to avoid obstruction I place the sling under minimal tension, just sufficient to support the bladder neck and produce some elevation.

The cure rates for stress incontinence vary between 75% and 95%, depending on whether it is a primary or secondary procedure and whether subjective or objective evaluation is used. Our results (Chin & Stanton 1995) show an objective success rate of 71% at 5 years. Complications include urinary retention, voiding difficulty and sling erosion. The intention is to provide proximal support to the bladder neck and sometimes bladder-neck elevation. The sling is used as a primary and secondary procedure, particularly where vaginal capacity and mobility are decreased.

Artificial urinary sphincter (Fig. 48.14). The artificial urinary sphincter has been in use since 1973. It is indicated in the female for resistant urethral sphincter incompetence where conventional surgery has failed and the options of continued incontinence, catheter drainage or a diversion are not acceptable. The indications therefore are persistent incontinence in a patient who is mentally alert and manually dexterous. There should be no urinary infection, a bladder capacity greater than 250 ml, controlled detrusor instability and no voiding difficulty or upper urinary tract dilatation.

I have now implanted 30 sphincters and have an objective overall cure or improvement rate of 66%.

Postoperative catheter regimen

I usually use a suprapubic catheter (e.g. Bonanno) as this allows the patient to void spontaneously without removing the catheter. It is clamped on the second day and removed once the patient is able to void in excess of 150–200 ml and the evening and early morning residual urines are less than 150–200 ml respectively.

MANAGEMENT OF RECURRENT INCONTINENCE

The management will depend on the cause, which is likely to be one of the following:

1. Persistent urethral sphincter incompetence because the procedure was either incorrectly chosen or inadequately performed.
2. Occurrence of detrusor instability.
3. Overflow retention.
4. A fistula – ureteric, vesical or urethral.

Clinical and urodynamic assessments will differentiate between these. If urethral sphincter incompetence persists, either further elevation or an increase in urethral resistance is required and if the latter, an artificial urinary sphincter may be chosen. The alternative is a continent diversion, such as a Mitrofanoff (Woodhouse et al 1989).

CONCLUSION

The precise mechanism of urethral sphincter incompetence has not yet been fully explained. Improved investigation, particularly of urethral function, is required. The balance between invasiveness and information must be carefully assessed. Conservative methods are usually without long-term side effects and should be tried first, unless the patient wishes immediate surgical correction. The many operations again demonstrate that none is supreme. The operation to be used is chosen by considering both clinical and urodynamic features. Recurrent incontinence is managed according to its cause and urodynamic assessment is essential.

KEY POINTS

1. Urethral sphincter incompetence is due to either descent of the bladder neck or a decrease in urethral resistance or pressure.
2. Vaginal delivery is the commonest cause of urethral sphincter incompetence.
3. 50% of patients will have some cystourethrocoele present when urethral sphincter incompetence exists.
4. If stress incontinence is the sole symptom chosen to diagnose urethral sphincter incompetence, only 1.5% of patients attending with incontinence will present like this.
5. Most patients with sphincter incompetence will present with both stress incontinence and urge incontinence, and urodynamic studies are usually required to make an exact diagnosis.
6. Urodynamic studies are equally necessary to detect detrusor instability and voiding difficulty, as well as to diagnose the cause of incontinence.
7. A battery of tests, rather than one single test, may be required to diagnose urethral sphincter incompetence.
8. Conservative measures will cure or improve 50% of patients, but exercises have to be maintained.
9. The choice of surgery depends upon the patient's characteristics, and particularly the position of the bladder neck and urethral resistance. Each continence operation also has its own characteristics.
10. Elderly or frail patients need an operation with a brief operating time, low postoperative morbidity and a quick recovery.

REFERENCES

Abrams P, Blaivas G, Stanton S L, Andersen J 1988 Standardisation of terminology of lower urinary tract function. Scandinavian Journal of Urology and Nephrology (Suppl) 114: 5–19

Alcalay M, Monga A, Stanton S L 1995 Burch colposuspension – a 10–20-year follow-up. British Journal of Obstetrics and Gynaecology 102: 740–745

Bergman A, Ballard C, Cooning P 1989 Primary stress incontinence and pelvic relaxation: prospective randomised comparison of three different operations. 19th Annual Meeting of the International Continence Society, Ljubljana. Neurourology and Urodynamics 8: 334–335

Bridges N, Denning J, Ollah K, Farrar D 1988 A prospective trial comparing interferential therapy and treatment using cones in patients with symptoms of stress incontinence. Proceedings of the 18th Annual Meeting of the International Continence Society, Oslo. Neurourology Urodynamics 7: 267–268

Burch J 1961 Urethrovaginal fixation to Cooper's ligament for correction of stress incontinence, cystocele and prolapse. American Journal of Obstetrics and Gynecology 81: 281–290

Cardozo L, Stanton S L 1980 Genuine stress incontinence and detrusor instability: a review of 200 patients. British Journal of Obstetrics and Gynaecology 87: 184–190

Chin Y K, Stanton S L 1995 A follow-up of silastic sling for genuine stress incontinence. British Journal of Obstetrics and Gynaecology 102: 143–147

Creighton S M, Clark A, Pearce J M, Stanton S L 1991 Perineal bladder neck ultrasound: appearances before and after continence surgery. Submitted for publication

Francis W 1960 The onset of stress incontinence. Journal of Obstetrics and Gynaecology of the British Empire 67: 899–903
Haylen B T, Frazer M I 1987 Is the investigation of most stress incontinence really necessary? Proceedings of 17th Annual Meeting of ICS. Neurourology and Urodynamics 6: 188–189
Hilton P 1988 Unstable urethral pressure: towards a more relevant definition. Neurourology and Urodynamics 6: 411–418
Hodgkinson C P 1970 American Journal of Obstetrics and Gynecology 108: 1141–1168
Holland E 1928 Cited in Jeffcoate T N 1967 Principles of gynaecology, 3rd edn. Butterworths, London
Jarvis G 1994 Surgery for genuine stress incontinence. British Journal of Obstetrics and Gynaecology 101: 371–374
Keane D, Sims T, Bailey A, Abrams P 1992 Analysis of pelvic floor electromyography and collagen studies in pre-menopausal nulliparous females with genuine stress incontinence. Neurourology and Urodynamics 11: 308–309
Krantz K 1986 Marshall–Marchetti–Krantz. In: Stanton S L, Tanagho E (eds) Surgery: female incontinence, 2nd edn. Springer-Verlag, Heidelberg, pp 87–93
Krieger M, Gordon D, Stanton S L 1988 Single fibre EMG: a sensitive tool for evaluation of the urethral sphincter. Proceedings of the 18th Annual Meeting of the International Continence Society, Oslo. Neurourology and Urodynamics 7: 239–240
Lawrence W, McQuilkin P, Mann D 1989 Suprapubic catheterisation. British Journal of Urology 63: 443
Mayne C J, Hilton P 1988 The short pad test: standardization of method and comparison with the one hour test. Neurourology and Urodynamics 7: 443
Monga A, Robinson D, Stanton S L 1995 Periurethral collagen injection for genuine stress incontinence: a 2-year follow-up. British Journal of Urology 76: 156–160
Nemir A, Middleton R 1954 Stress incontinence in nulliparous women. American Journal of Obstetrics and Gynecology 68: 1166–1168
Ng R, Murray A 1989 Place of routine urodynamics in the management of female GSI. Neurourology and Urodynamics 8: 307–308
Peattie A, Plevnik S, Stanton S L 1988 Vaginal cones: a conservative method of treating genuine stress incontinence. British Journal of Obstetrics and Gynaecology 95: 1049–1053
Peattie A, Plevnik S, Stanton S L 1989 Is the bladder really an unreliable witness? Proceedings of the 19th Annual Meting of the International Continence Society, Ljubljana. Neurourology and Urodynamics 8: 303–304
Plevnik S 1985 New method for testing and strengthening of pelvic floor muscles. Proceedings of the 15th Annual Meeting of the International Continence Society, London: 267–268
Plevnik S, Janez J, Vrtacnik P, Trsinar B, Vodusek D 1986 Short term electrical stimulation: home treatment for urinary incontinence. World Journal of Urology 4: 24–26
Raz S 1981 Modified bladder neck suspension for female stress incontinence. Urology 17: 82–85
Sand P, Bower L, Panganibani R, Ostergard D 1987 The low pressure urethra as a factor in failed retropubic urethropexy. Obstetrics and Gynecology 69: 399–402
Sayer T, Dixon J, Hosker G, Warrell D 1989 Histological study of pubo-cervical fascia in women with stress incontinence of urine. International Urogynaecology Journal 1: 18
Snooks S, Swash M, Setchell M, Henry M 1984 Injury to innervation of the pelvic floor and sphincter musculature in childbirth. Lancet ii: 546–550
Stamey T 1973 Cystoscopic suspension of the vesical neck for urinary incontinence. Surgery, Gynecology and Obstetrics 136: 547–554
Stanton S L 1986 Colposuspension. In: Stanton S L, Tanagho E (eds) Surgery of female incontinence, 2nd edn. Springer-Verlag, Heidelberg, pp 95–103
Stanton S L, Kerr Wilson R, Harris V G 1980 Incidence of urological symptoms in normal pregnancy. British Journal of Obstetrics and Gynaecology 87: 897–900
Stanton S L, Cardozo L, Riddle P 1981 Urological complications of traumatic diastasis of the symphysis pubis. British Journal of Urology 53: 453–454
Stanton S L, Brindley G S, Holmes D 1985 Silastic sling for urethral sphincter incompetence in women. British Journal of Obstetrics and Gynaecology 92: 747–750
Stanton S L, Chamberlain G V P, Holmes D 1991 Comparison between anterior colporrhaphy and colposuspension in the correction of genuine stress incontinence. Submitted for publications
Stanton S L, Krieger M, Ziv E 1988 Videocystourethrography: its role in the assessment of incontinence in the female. Proceedings of the 18th Annual Meeting of the International Continence Society, Oslo. Neurourology and Urodynamics 7: 172–173
Staskin D, Sant G, Sand P et al 1995 Use of an expandable urethral insert for GSI. Long-term results of a multi-center trial. Neurourology and Urodynamics 5: 420–422
Tapp A, Hills B, Cardozo L 1989 Randomised study comparing pelvic floor physiotherapy with the Burch colposuspension. 19th Annual Meeting of the International Continence Society, Ljubljana. Neurourology and Urodynamics 8: 356–357
Thomas T M, Plymat K, Blannin J, Meade T 1980 Prevalence of urinary incontinence. British Medical Journal 281: 1243–1245
Thyssen H, Lose G 1996 New disposable vaginal device (continence guard) in the treatment of female stress incontinence. Acta Obstetrica Gynologica Scandinavica 75: 170–173
Versi E, Cardozo L, Studd J, Cooper D 1986 Evaluation of urethral pressure profilometry for diagnosis of genuine stress incontinence. World Journal of Urology 4: 6–9
Woodhouse C R J, Malone P, Curry J, Reilly T 1989 The Mitrofanoff principle for continent urinary diversions. British Journal of Urology 63: 53–57

49

Detrusor instability

L. Cardozo

INTRODUCTION

The normal adult human bladder is stable and does not contract except during micturition, which is under voluntary control. Conversely, an unstable bladder is one which contracts involuntarily or can be provoked to do so. Raised bladder pressure was first reported in certain neurological conditions over 60 years ago (Rose 1931, Langworthy et al 1936) but its clinical significance was not appreciated until 1963, when Hodgkinson et al demonstrated urinary incontinence as a result of detrusor contractions in 64 neurologically normal women. They called this condition 'dyssynergic detrusor dysfunction'. Various other names have been used, including uninhibited detrusor, detrusor reflex instability, overactive bladder, and detrusor hyperreflexia – the latter is now reserved for abnormal detrusor activity secondary to a neuropathy. The term 'detrusor instability' was coined by Bates et al (1970) to describe 'the objectively measured loss of ability to inhibit detrusor contraction even when it is provoked to contract by filling, change of posture, coughing, etc.' More recently the International Continence Society (Bates et al 1981) has defined an unstable bladder as one that is shown objectively to contract, spontaneously or on provocation, during the filling phase while the patient is attempting to inhibit micturition.

INCIDENCE

Detrusor instability is a common condition and it has been suggested that it may be a variant of normal, occurring in about 10% of the population who have not learnt bladder control at the appropriate age. We have shown that 10% of postmenopausal women complaining of climacteric symptoms, but without urological complaints, have unstable bladders (Versi & Cardozo 1988). In the adult female population detrusor instability is the second commonest cause of urinary incontinence, after genuine stress incontinence, accounting for 30–50% of cases investigated (Moolgaoker et al 1972, Torrens & Griffiths 1974). Among the elderly detrusor instability is the commonest cause of urinary incontinence (Castleden & Duffin 1985), and has been shown to exist in as many as 80% of those presenting for urodynamic assessment because of urinary incontinence (Malone-Lee & Wahedeny 1993).

AETIOLOGY

No specific underlying cause for detrusor instability has been identified but some probabilities are idiopathic, psychosomatic, neuropathic (hyperreflexia), incontinence surgery and outflow obstruction (men).

During infancy, prior to potty training it is normal for the bladder to contract uninhibitedly at a critical volume and an unstable bladder may be the result of poorly learnt bladder control. Zoubek et al (1990) studied 46 toilet-trained children all of whom developed isolated urinary frequency. In 40% of cases a 'trigger' was identified prior to the onset of symptoms. This often involved problems at school. All cases were self-limiting or resolved following counselling or removal of the 'trigger'. There is a strong association between childhood nocturnal enuresis and detrusor instability presenting in adult life (Whiteside & Arnold 1975).

In the majority of women who suffer from detrusor instability no cause can be found, although some have neurotic personality traits (Freeman et al 1985), and they may respond well to psychotherapy. The psychoneurotic status of women with detrusor instability has been assessed by several authors, with conflicting results. Walters et al (1990) evaluated 63 women with incontinence and 27 continent controls using formal psychometric testing. They reported no difference in the test results between women with genuine stress incontinence and those with detrusor instability. Women with detrusor instability scored significantly higher than controls on the hypochondriasis, depression and hysteria scales. They concluded that these abnormalities may be related to incontinence in general and not to the specific diagnosis. Norton et al (1990) psychiatrically assessed 117 women attending the urodynamic clinic prior to urodynamic investigation. There was no increased psychiatric morbidity in women with detrusor instability compared to women with genuine stress incontinence. Interestingly, women in whom no urodynamic abnormality could be detected had the highest scores for anxiety and neuroticism.

These levels were comparable to those of psychiatric outpatients. Moore and Sutherst (1990) have evaluated the response to treatment of detrusor instability, using oxybutynin, in relation to psychoneurotic status. Poor responders had a higher mean psychoneurotic score than responders, although one-third of poor responders were normal. Patients who responded well to therapy had scores similar to normal urban females. Many women with detrusor instability therefore show little evidence of psychoneuroticism. Using validated generic and disease-specific quality of life questionnaires we have shown that detrusor instability more severely adversely affects the quality of life of sufferers than does genuine stress incontinence (Kelleher et al 1993).

Neurological lesions such as multiple sclerosis and spinal injuries may cause uninhibited bladder contractions, which play an aetiological role in only a small group of women with detrusor hyperreflexia. Following incontinence surgery there is an increased incidence of detrusor instability (Cardozo et al 1979, Steel et al 1985) for which no specific cause has been found, but it may be due to extensive dissection around the bladder neck as it is more commonly seen after multiple previous operations. Alternatively, the problem in some women may be failure to diagnose the abnormality prior to surgery, or due to relative outflow obstruction caused by the operation itself. Outflow obstruction is rare in women and does not seem to cause detrusor instability in the same way that prostatic hypertrophy does in men. The increased incidence of detrusor instability in the elderly may be due to the onset of occult neuropathy, e.g. senile atherosclerosis or dementia.

PATHOPHYSIOLOGY

The motor nerve supply to the bladder is via the parasympathetic nervous system (S2, 3, 4), specifically by the pelvic nerve. Its effects are mediated by acetylcholine acting on muscarinic receptors (Kinder & Mundy 1985). Sympathetic innervation is derived from the hypogastric nerve and acts predominantly on β receptors, causing relaxation of the detrusor. Other neurotransmitters, including adenosine triphosphate and vasoactive intestinal polypeptide, may also play a minor role (Burnstock et al 1972, Gu et al 1983). A detrusor contraction is initiated in the rostral pons. Efferent pathways emerge from the sacral spinal cord as the pelvic parasympathetic nerves and run forwards to the bladder. Acetylcholine is released at the neuromuscular junction and results in a coordinated contraction. Thus a balance between sympathetic and parasympathetic stimulation is required for normal detrusor function.

The pathophysiology of detrusor instability remains a mystery. In-vitro studies have shown that the detrusor muscle in cases of idiopathic detrusor instability contracts more than normal detrusor muscle. These detrusor contractions are not nerve mediated and can be inhibited by the neuropeptide vasoactive intestinal polypeptide (Kinder & Mundy 1987). Other studies have shown that increased α-adrenergic activity causes increased detrusor contractility (Eaton & Bates 1982). There is evidence to suggest that the pathophysiology of idiopathic and obstructive detrusor instability is different. From animal and human studies on obstructive instability it would seem that the detrusor develops postjunctional supersensitivity, with reduced sensitivity to electrical stimulation of its nerve supply but a greater sensitivity to stimulation with acetylcholine (Sibley 1985). If outflow obstruction is relieved the detrusor can return to normal behaviour and reinnervation may occur (Speakman et al 1987).

Relaxation of the urethra is known to precede contraction of the detrusor in a proportion of women with detrusor instability (Wise et al 1993a). This may represent primary pathology in the urethra which triggers a detrusor contraction, or may merely be part of a complex sequence of events which originate elsewhere. It has been postulated that incompetence of the bladder neck, allowing passage of urine into the proximal urethra, may result in an uninhibited contraction of the detrusor. However, Sutherst and Brown (1978) were unable to provoke a detrusor contraction in 50 women by rapidly infusing saline into the posterior urethra using modified urodynamic equipment.

Recently Brading and Turner (1994) have suggested that the common feature in all cases of detrusor instability is a change in the properties of the smooth muscle of the detrusor which predisposes it to unstable contractions. This change is caused by a long-term reduction in the functional innervation of the bladder wall. They dispute the concept of 'hyperreflexia', that is, increased motor activity to the detrusor, as the underlying mechanism in detrusor instability.

CLINICAL PRESENTATION

Detrusor instability usually presents with a multiplicity of symptoms. Those most commonly seen are:

Urgency
Frequency (>7 times per day)
Nocturia (>once per night)
Urge incontinence
Stress incontinence
Nocturnal enuresis
Coital incontinence.

The most common symptoms are urgency and frequency of micturition, which occur in about 80% of patients (Cardozo & Stanton 1980). However, there are numerous other causes of urgency and frequency (Table 49.1).

Some women void frequently because they drink numerous cups of tea or coffee each day, and this polyuria should be differentiated from small volumes voided frequently, by means of a frequency/volume chart. Most women who are incontinent develop voluntary frequency, initially in order to try to leak less. Nocturia is also a common symptom in detrusor instability, occurring in almost 70% of cases (Cardozo & Stanton 1980). However, being woken from sleep for some other reason and voiding because one is awake does not constitute nocturia. There is an increasing incidence of nocturia, with increasing age, and it is normal, over the age of 70 years, to void twice, and over the age of 80 years to void three times during the night.

Table 49.1 Common causes of frequency and urgency of micturition

Urological	Urinary tract infection Detrusor instability Small-capacity bladder Interstitial cystitis Chronic urinary retention/residual Bladder mucosal lesion, e.g. papilloma Bladder calculus Urethral syndrome Urethral diverticulum Urethral obstruction
Gynaecological	Pregnancy Genuine stress incontinence Cystocoele Pelvic mass, e.g. fibroids Previous pelvic surgery Radiation cystitis/fibrosis Postmenopausal urogenital atrophy
Sexual	Coitus Sexually transmitted disease Contraceptive diaphragm
Medical	Diuretic therapy Upper motor neuron lesion Impaired renal function Congestive cardiac failure (nocturia) Hypokalaemia
Endocrine	Diabetes mellitus Diabetes insipidus Hypothyroidism
Psychological	Excessive drinking Habit Anxiety

Urge incontinence is usually preceded by urgency (a strong and sudden desire to void) and is due to an involuntary detrusor contraction. However, some women are unaware of any sensation associated with their detrusor contractions and just notice that they are wet. There seems to be a strong correlation between nocturnal enuresis, either childhood or current, and idiopathic detrusor instability (Whiteside & Arnold 1975). Some women complain of incontinence during sexual intercourse and they can be broadly divided into two groups: those who leak during penetration and tend to have genuine stress incontinence, and those who wet themselves at orgasm. The most common pathology among the latter is detrusor instability (Hilton 1988).

The most noticeable feature of the symptomatology of detrusor instability is its infinite variability. Some patients may be severely incapacitated when at work but virtually asymptomatic when they go on holiday; others complain of severe urgency and frequency in the mornings but void normally during the rest of the day; and others say that they wet themselves when they do the washing up, or put the door key in the lock.

There are no specific clinical signs in women with detrusor instability but it is always worth looking for vulval excoriation and stress incontinence. Occasionally an underlying neurological lesion such as multiple sclerosis will be discovered by examining the cranial nerves and S2, 3 and 4 outflow.

INVESTIGATIONS

Urine culture

A midstream specimen of urine should be sent for microscopy, culture and sensitivity in all cases of incontinence. An infection may contribute to the symptomatology, and investigations, which are mainly invasive, may exacerbate this. Such investigations are certainly uncomfortable when an infection is present and the results may be inaccurate.

Frequency/volume chart

It is our practice to send all patients a frequency/volume chart with their appointment for urodynamic investigations, so that when they arrive we can evaluate their fluid

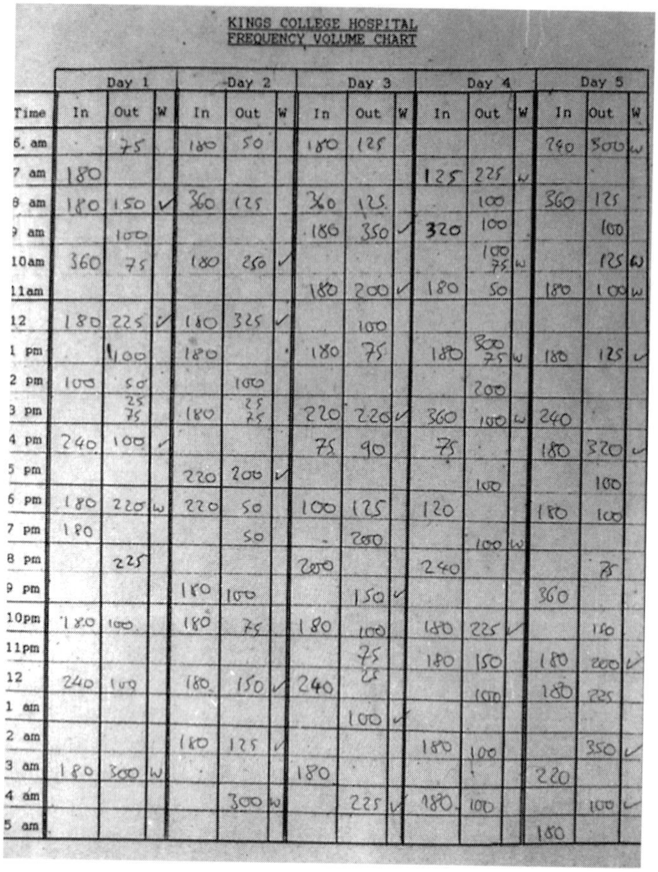

KINGS COLLEGE HOSPITAL
FREQUENCY VOLUME CHART

Time	Day 1 In	Day 1 Out	Day 1 W	Day 2 In	Day 2 Out	Day 2 W	Day 3 In	Day 3 Out	Day 3 W	Day 4 In	Day 4 Out	Day 4 W	Day 5 In	Day 5 Out	Day 5 W
6. am		75		180	50		180	125					240	500	w
7 am	180									125	225	w			
8 am	180	150	✓	360	125		360	125			100		360	125	
9 am		100					180	350	✓	320	100			100	
10am	360	75		180	250	✓					100 75	w		125	w
11am							180	200	✓	180	50		180	100	w
12	180	225	✓	180	325	✓		100							
1 pm		100		180			180	75		180	300 75	w	180	125	✓
2 pm	100	50			100						200				
3 pm		25 75		180	25 75		220	220	✓	360	100	w	240		
4 pm	240	100	✓				75	90		75			180	320	✓
5 pm				220	200	✓					100			100	
6 pm	180	220	w	220	50		100	125		120			180	100	
7 pm	180				50			200			100	w			
8 pm		225					200			240				75	
9 pm				180	100			150	✓				360		
10pm	180	100		180	75		180	100		180	225	✓		150	
11pm								75		180	150		180	200	✓
12	240	100		180	150	✓	240	25			100		180	225	
1 am								100	✓						
2 am				180	125	✓				180	100			350	✓
3 am	180	300	w				180						220		
4 am					300	w		225	✓	180	100			100	✓
5 am													180		

Fig. 49.1 Frequency volume chart from a woman with detrusor instability.

intake and voiding pattern. They are asked to complete the chart (Fig. 49.1) for 5 days, but are told that they need not measure their voided volumes when at work if this proves difficult. Some women find that this is a useful exercise, similar to home bladder drill.

Uroflowmetry

Although voiding difficulties are uncommon in women, a large chronic urinary residual may present with symptoms of urgency and frequency of micturition, so it is relevant to measure the urine flow rate prior to urodynamic assessment. Usually, in uncomplicated idiopathic detrusor instability the flow rate is high and the voiding time short, with only a small volume being passed each time.

Cystometry

The diagnosis of detrusor instability is made when detrusor contractions are seen on a cystometrogram. The recorded detrusor pressure rise may take different forms on the cystometrogram trace. Most commonly, uninhibited systolic contractions occur during bladder filling (Fig. 49.2). Not all cases of detrusor instability will be diagnosed on supine filling alone (Turner-Warwick 1975). Some show an abnormal detrusor pressure rise on the change of posture and may void precipitately on standing (Fig. 49.3), or there may be detrusor contractions provoked by coughing which manifest as stress incontinence (Fig. 49.4) Sometimes a steep detrusor pressure rise occurs during bladder filling (Fig. 49.5). This usually represents low compliance of the detrusor but may be due to involuntary detrusor activity in some cases. It can be difficult to differentiate between systolic (phasic) detrusor instability and low compliance, which may coexist. Both conditions usually produce the same symptoms.

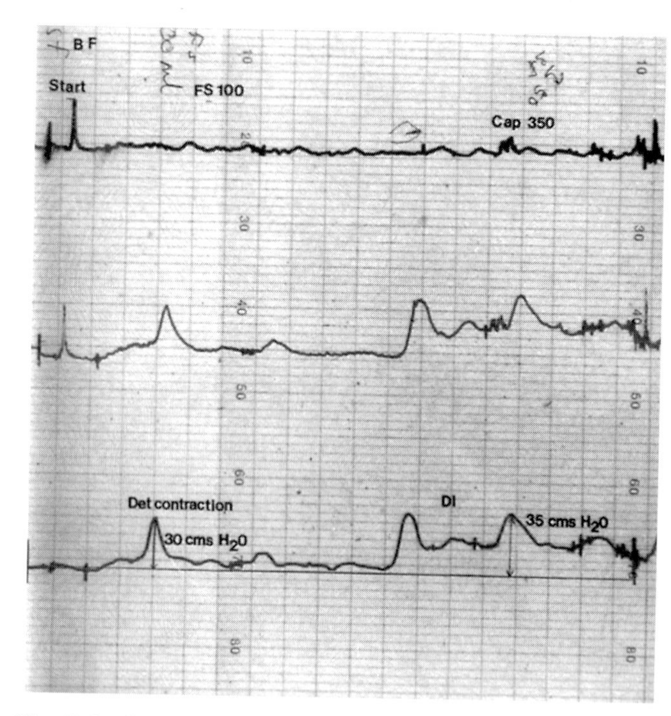

Fig. 49.2 Cystometrogram showing systolic detrusor contractions during bladder filling. FS100 = first sensation 100 ml; DI = detrusor instability.

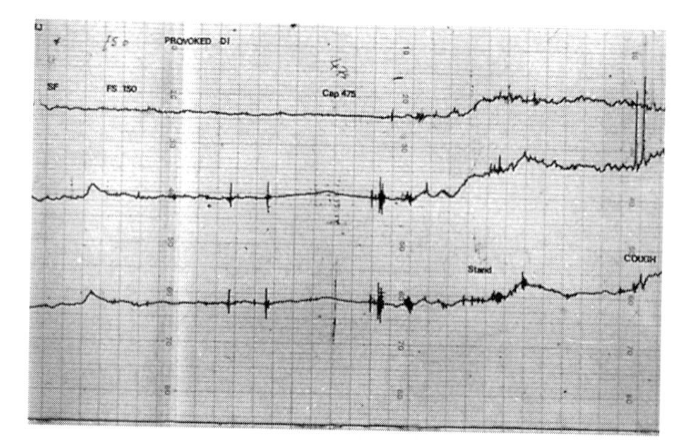

Fig. 49.3 Cystometrogram showing an uninhibited detrusor contraction on standing. SF = Start filling; FS150 = first sensation 150 ml; DI = detrusor instability.

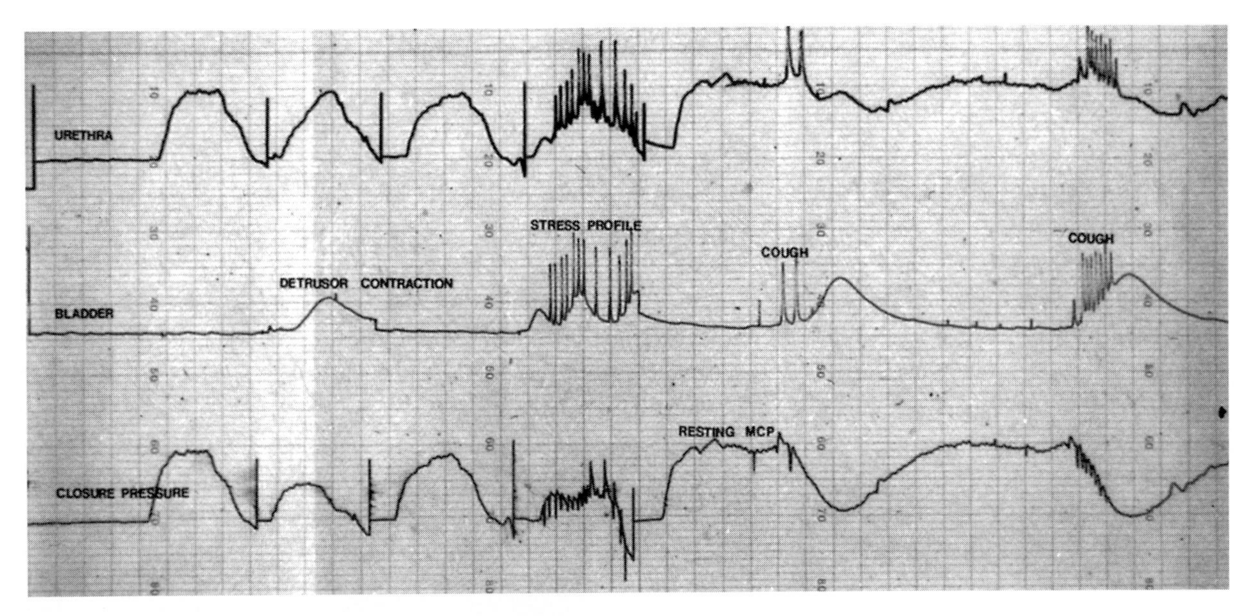

Fig. 49.4 Urethral pressure profile trace showing detrusor contractors in response to coughing. MCP = Maximum closure pressure.

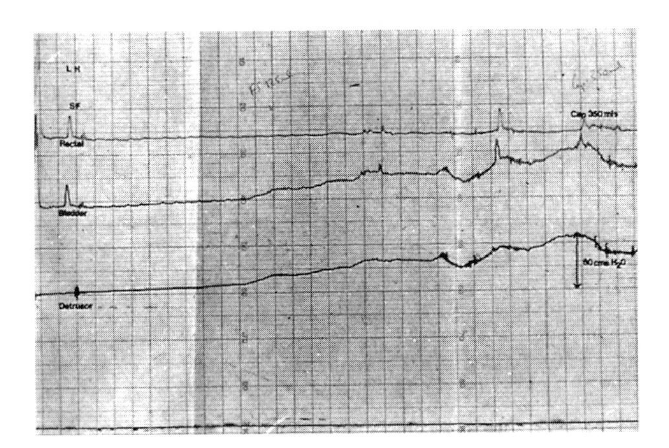

Fig. 49.5 Cystometrogram showing a low compliance bladder. SF = start filling.

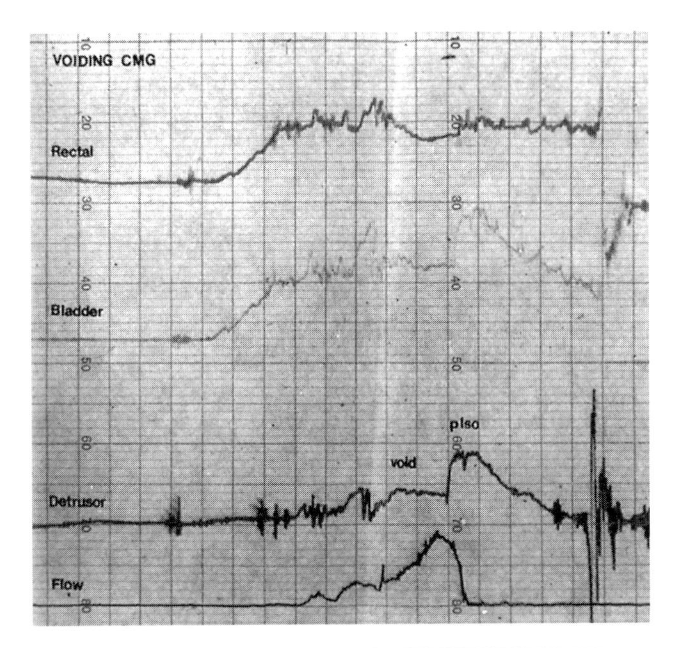

Fig. 49.6 Cystometrogram showing a large isometric detrusor contraction. PISO = Isometric contraction pressure.

During the cystometrogram it is important to ask the patient about her symptoms and relate them to the recorded changes. Most patients will complain of urgency when a detrusor contraction occurs, or urge incontinence if the detrusor pressure exceeds the urethral pressure. Thus, in order to diagnose or exclude detrusor instability subtracted provocative cystometry must be employed. Other common, although not universal, features of the cystometrogram in women with detrusor instability are early first sensation, small bladder capacity and inability or difficulty in interrupting the urinary stream. The latter may be associated with a high isometric detrusor contraction (Fig. 49.6) or, if videocystourethrography is performed, slow or absent milk-back of contrast medium from the proximal urethra into the bladder.

In the absence of subtracted cystometry single-channel cystometry provides a useful screening test with fairly high levels of sensitivity, although rather poor specificity (Sutherst & Brown 1984, Cutner et al 1992).

Ambulatory urodynamics

Ambulatory monitoring is becoming popular and is believed to be more physiological and therefore more accurate in the diagnosis of detrusor instability (Griffiths et al 1989) (Fig. 49.7). In a large study of women with

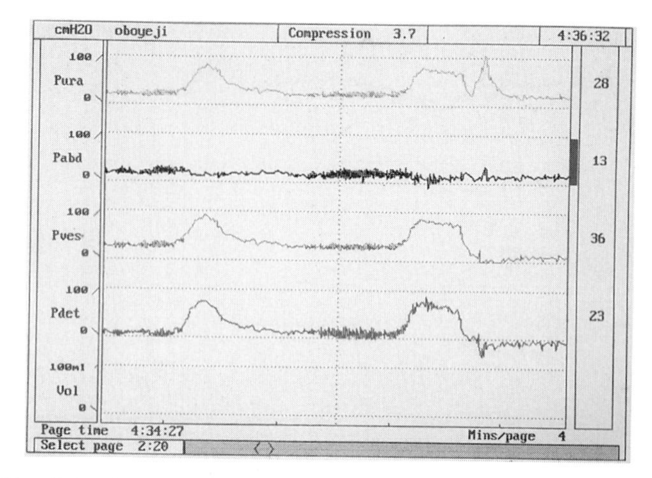

Fig. 49.7 Cystometrographic recording obtained during ambulatory monitoring – detrusor instability.

symptoms of urinary incontinence but normal laboratory urodynamic investigation, detrusor instability was detected in 65% of cases on ambulatory testing (Khullar & Cardozo unpublished data 1994). The presence of uninhibited detrusor contractions has also been detected in asymptomatic 'normal' controls during ambulatory monitoring (van Waalwijk van Doorn et al 1992), and therefore a consensus needs to be reached regarding the definition of 'normal'.

Ambulatory urodynamics has recently been used to evaluate the efficacy of oxybutynin in the treatment of detrusor instability (van Waalwijk van Doorn & Zwiers 1990). The frequency and amplitude of the uninhibited detrusor contractions was significantly reduced by the medication during the treatment period.

Cystourethroscopy

Endoscopy is not helpful in diagnosing detrusor instability but may be used to exclude other causes for the symptoms, such as a bladder tumour or calculus. Coarse trabeculation of the bladder may be noted in long-standing cases of detrusor instability. This can also be seen during videocystourethrography (Fig. 49.8).

Other urodynamic tests are of limited benefit in detrusor instability. Urethral pressure profilometry (Hilton & Stanton 1983) may reveal coexistent urethral instability but its clinical significance is uncertain. A positive bladder-neck electric conductance test (Holmes et al 1989) has been found to correlate well with the symptom of urgency, but this test has not gained widespread popularity and requires further evaluation.

Additional information may be acquired by undertaking videocystourethrography with pressure and flow studies, rather than subtracted cystometry, although this will not increase the diagnostic accuracy. However, when severe

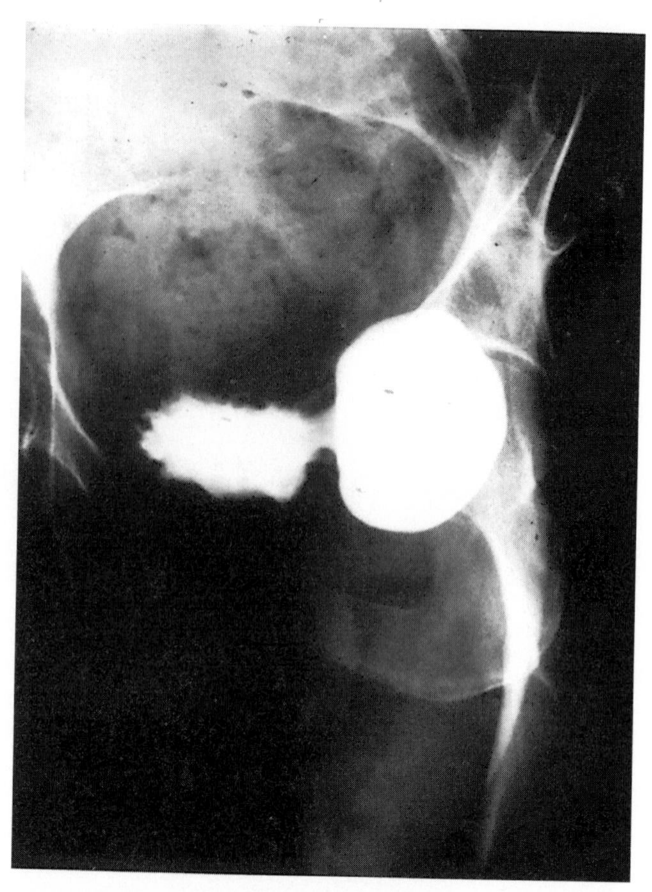

Fig. 49.8 Trabeculated bladder secondary to long-standing detrusor instability, with a large diverticulum on the left.

detrusor instability has caused upper urinary tract damage vesicoureteric reflux may be observed (Fig. 49.9).

TREATMENT

Not all women with detrusor instability require treatment. Once the problem has been explained to them some will be able to control their own symptoms by behaviour modification, such as drinking less and avoiding tea, coffee and alcohol (which are bladder stimulants). However, most women with detrusor instability request treatment, and although many different therapies have been tried none has proved universally satisfactory. The major therapeutic interventions which are currently in use attempt to either improve central control, as in behavioural intervention, or alter detrusor innervation using drugs or surgical denervation techniques. When these measures fail to adequately control the patient's symptoms over a long period of time augmentation cystoplasty may be undertaken. Conventional bladder-neck surgery (as is used to treat genuine stress incontinence) rarely cures women with detrusor instability and may make the symptoms of urgency and frequency worse.

Methods of treatment currently employed are drug

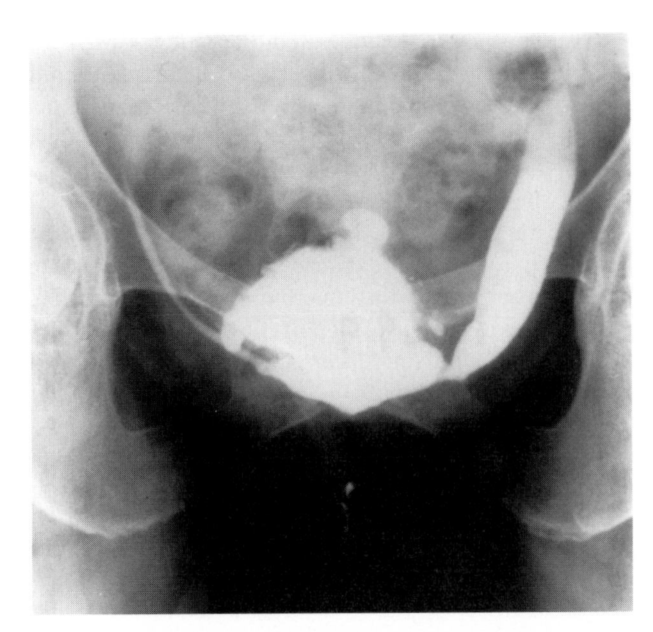

Fig. 49.9 Detrusor hyper-reflexia with a trabeculated bladder and vesicoureteric reflux with a hydro-ureter on the left.

therapy, behavioural intervention, maximal electrical stimulation, acupuncture, augmentation cystoplasty and urinary diversion. Other types of treatment which have been tried include vaginal denervation (Hodgkinson & Drukker 1977, Warrell 1977, Ingelman-Sundberg 1978), caecocystoplasty, selective sacral neurectomy (Torrens & Griffiths 1974), cystodistension (Ramsden et al 1976, Higson et al 1978, Pengelly et al 1978) and bladder transection (Mundy 1983). All give some short-term benefit in carefully selected cases but may produce significant morbidity, and none has stood the test of time.

General management

All incontinent women benefit from advice regarding simple measures which they can take to help alleviate their symptoms. Many women drink far too much, and they should be told to limit their fluid intake to between 1 and 1.5 litres per day and to avoid tea, coffee and alcohol if these exacerbate their problem. The use of drugs which affect bladder function, such as diuretics, should be reviewed and if possible stopped. If there is coexistent genuine stress incontinence then pelvic floor exercises with or without electrical treatment such as faradism may be helpful.

It is usually preferable in cases of mixed incontinence to treat detrusor instability prior to resorting to surgery for the urethral sphincter incompetence. Such treatment may obviate the need for surgery (Karram & Bhatia 1989). In addition there is aways the risk that the incontinence operation may exacerbate the symptoms of detrusor instability.

For younger women who leak only when exercising, a tampon in the vagina during sporting activities may be helpful. For a peri- or postmenopausal woman hormone replacement therapy is unlikely to cure the problem, but may increase the sensory threshold of the bladder and may also make urinary symptoms easier to cope with. The most degrading aspect of urinary incontinence for many patients is the odour and staining of their clothes, and this can be helped by good advice regarding incontinence pads and garments.

Drugs

Drugs which may be useful in the treatment of detrusor instability fall into three main categories:

1. Those that inhibit bladder contractility.
2. Those that increase outlet resistance.
3. Those that decrease urine production.

In practice only the first group are prescribed regularly. Neurotransmission in the detrusor is cholinergic, and so most of the agents used to treat detrusor instability have some anticholinergic properties. Unfortunately, it is very difficult to assess the clinical benefit of drugs prescribed for this condition because they may act at more than one site, have different effects in vitro and in vivo, and may have different short- and long-term effects. Many drugs have been tried but few are in regular clinical use (Wein 1986).

The following types of drugs inhibit bladder contractility (the efficacy of those in brackets is uncertain):

1. Anticholinergic agents
2. Musculotropic relaxants
3. Tricyclic antidepressants
4. (Calcium-channel blockers)
5. (β-adrenergic agonists)
6. (α-adrenergic antagonists)
7. (Prostaglandin inhibitors).

Anticholinergic agents

The detrusor is innervated by the parasympathetic nervous system (pelvic nerve), the sympathetic nervous system (hypogastric nerve) and by non-cholinergic, non-adrenergic neurons. The motor supply arises from S2, 3 and 4 and is conveyed by the pelvic nerve. The neurotransmitter at the neuromuscular junction is acetylcholine, which acts upon muscarinic receptors. Antimuscarinic drugs should therefore be of use in the treatment of detrusor instability. Atropine is the classic anticholinergic drug with antimuscarinic activity; however, its non-specific mode of action makes it unacceptable for clinical use because of the high incidence of side effects. All anticholinergic agents produce competitive blockade of acetylcholine receptors at postganglionic parasympathetic receptor sites. They all, to a lesser or greater extent, have the typical side effects of dry mouth, blurred vision, tachycardia, drowsiness and constipation. Unfortunately, virtually all the drugs which are truly beneficial in the management of detrusor instability produce these unwanted side effects.

Propantheline bromide is a related drug with fewer side effects. It is a quaternary ammonium analogue with both antimuscarinic and antinicotinic properties, which acts at both the ganglionic level and at the neuromuscular junction. Blaivas et al (1980) have shown that intramuscular injection of propantheline abolishes involuntary detrusor contractions in 79% of cases of detrusor instability. However, 50% of patients required short-term intermittent self-catheterization for resulting urinary retention. When given orally in a dose of 15 mg four times daily it is often ineffective. The dose may therefore be increased as high as 90 mg four times daily, but introduced slowly to minimize side effects. Gastrointestinal absorption is aided by taking the drug before meals (Gibaldi & Grundhofer 1975). Propantheline is cheap, with few side effects, and is particularly useful when frequency of micturition is a major problem. Unfortunately there have been no good recent clinical trials.

Emepronium bromide has anticholinergic activity at both peripheral and ganglionic levels and has to be taken in doses above 200 mg tds. Unfortunately, it is poorly absorbed from the gastrointestinal tract (Ritch et al 1977) and at high doses causes oesophageal ulceration. Emepronium carragenate, which is available in some parts of Europe, does not have this problem and has been shown to improve symptoms when administered in high doses (Massey & Abrams 1986).

Musculotropic relaxants

These drugs are mainly smooth muscle relaxants which act predominantly on the bladder. Their side effects are anticholinergic. Oxybutynin, a tertiary amine, is probably the most effective drug currently available for the treatment of detrusor instability. Given in the maximum recommended dose of 5 mg three times daily many women find the side effects less tolerable than the symptoms of detrusor instability. The worst problems seems to be a very dry mouth and throat, with a lingering bad taste. However, oxybutynin does cause significant improvement in the symptom of urgency, but this may be at the expense of an increased urinary residual volume (Cardozo et al 1987). In those patients who can tolerate this drug a 70% improvement rate can be expected.

In a large randomized double-blind multicentre study conducted by Thuroff et al (1991) the degree of symptomatic improvement and objective improvement in urodynamic parameters was significantly greater for those treated with oxybutynin than with either propantheline or placebo. However, the dose of propantheline was too low to be considered effective therapy for the majority of women with detrusor instability.

Oxybutynin is contraindicated in patients with glaucoma. It has a half-life of only 5 hours and is therefore rapidly effective following ingestion. A dose may be taken as prophylaxis to control symptoms for short periods, when the individual feels it is necessary (Burton 1994). Alternatively, the side effects may be reduced by lowering the dose to 3 mg three times daily (Moore et al 1990) without significantly reducing the efficacy. Intravesical administration of oxybutynin is an effective and useful alternative for patients with detrusor hyperreflexia who need to self-catheterize, or who suffer from 'bypassing' an indwelling catheter (Madersbacher & Jilg 1990).

Flavoxate is a tertiary amine with a papaverine-like effect on smooth muscle. It is still commonly prescribed in a dose of 200 mg three times daily, but is poorly absorbed from the gut and in clinical trials its effect has not been shown to be superior to that of placebo (Briggs et al 1980, Chapple et al 1990).

Tricyclic antidepressants

These drugs have a complex pharmacological action. Imipramine has anticholinergic, antihistamine and local anaesthetic properties. It may increase outlet resistance caused by peripheral blockage of noradrenaline uptake, and it also acts as a sedative. The side effects are anticholinergic, together with tremor and fatigue. Imipramine is particularly useful for the treatment of nocturia and nocturnal enuresis (Castleden et al 1981). Imipramine together with propantheline may be used to treat the combined symptoms of diurnal frequency and nocturia. A dose of up to 150 mg may be given safely, but the standard dosage is 50 mg twice daily. Other tricyclic antidepressants such as amitriptyline may be substituted for imipramine if specific side effects are a problem. A tricyclic given prophylactically before sexual intercourse may be a benefit to patients with coital incontinence at orgasm (Cardozo 1988).

Other drugs

Antidiuretic hormone analogues. Synthetic vasopressin (DDAVP) has been shown to reduce nocturnal urine production by up to 50%. It can be used for children or adults with nocturia or nocturnal enuresis, but must be avoided in patients with hypertension, ischaemic heart disease or congestive cardiac failure (Hilton & Stanton 1982). There is good evidence to show that it is safe to use in the long term (Rew & Rundle 1989, Knudsen et al 1989).

Oestrogen. Oestrogen deficiency following the menopause causes changes in all layers of the urethra, which has abundant oestrogen receptors (Tapp & Cardozo 1986), but the bladder itself possesses fewer receptors. There have been few placebo-controlled trials using objective as well as subjective outcome measures, but a meta-analysis of the worldwide literature would suggest that oestrogens may produce some symptomatic improvement in urinary symptoms, including urgency and frequency of micturition (Fantl et al 1994). In addition, sensory urgency, which may be due to generalized urogenital atrophy, does respond to oestrogen replacement therapy (Fantl et al 1988, Wise et al 1993b).

Capsaicin. The pungent ingredient found in red chillies is a neurotoxin of substance P containing (C) nerve fibres. Patients with detrusor hyperreflexia secondary to multiple sclerosis appear to have abnormal C fibre sensory innervation of the detrusor, which leads to premature activation of the holding reflex arc during bladder filling (Fowler et al 1992). Intravesical application of capsaicin dissolved in 30% alcohol solution appears to be effective for up to 6 months. The effects are variable (Chandiramani et al 1994) and the long-term safety of this treatment has not yet been evaluated.

Drugs may be used in combination in order to produce the greatest beneficial effect on symptoms with the least side effects. Similarly, drugs can be used in combination with other forms of treatment, such as bladder retraining. The choice of drug for each patient would depend on their predominant symptoms and their tolerance of side effects.

Behavioural therapy

As continence is normally learned during infancy it is logical to suppose that it can be relearned during adult life. Various different forms of bladder re-education have been tried, including bladder drill, biofeedback and hypnotherapy.

Bladder discipline was first described as a method of treating urgency incontinence by Jeffcoate and Francis (1966) in the belief that this type of incontinence was exacerbated or even caused by underlying psychological factors. Since then Frewen (1970) has shown that many women with detrusor instability are able to correlate the onset of their symptoms with some untoward event, which can be identified by taking a careful history. He showed that both inpatient and outpatient bladder drill can be effective forms of treatment for many such women.

The technique for performing inpatient bladder drill has been established by Jarvis (1989) and is shown below.

Technique for bladder drill

1. Exclude pathology and admit to hospital (if possible).
2. Explain rationale to patient.
3. Instruct the patient to void every one-and-a-half hours during the day (either she waits or is incontinent).
4. When one-and-a-half hours is achieved, increase by half an hour and continue with 2-hourly voiding, etc.
5. Allow a normal fluid intake (1500 ml/24 h).
6. The patient keeps a fluid balance chart.
7. She meets a successful patient.
8. She receives encouragement from patients, nurses and doctors.

Jarvis and Millar (1980) performed a controlled trial of bladder drill in 60 consecutive incontinent women with idiopathic detrusor instability. They showed that following inpatient treatment 90% of the bladder drill group were continent and 83.3% remained symptom-free after 6 months. In the control group 23.2% were continent and symptom-free due to the placebo effect. Despite the excellent early results it has been shown that up to 40% of patients relapse within 3 years (Holmes et al 1983).

Although home bladder drill is not as effective as hospital inpatient bladder drill it is obviously considerably cheaper and can be initiated by a general practitioner or continence adviser. It provides general awareness regarding appropriate voiding habits, and should therefore be advocated for all patients with detrusor instability.

Biofeedback

Biofeedback is a form of learning or re-education in which the patient is given information about a normally unconscious physiological process in the form of an auditory, visual or tactile signal. The objective effects of biofeedback in the treatment of detrusor instability can be recorded on a polygraph trace, but the subjective changes may be difficult to separate from the placebo effect. This technique was originally described by Cardozo et al (1978a). Thirty women aged between 16 and 65 years of age suffering from idiopathic detrusor instability which was resistant to conventional therapy were treated in two centres (Cardozo et al 1978b). Some 80% of the women were cured or significantly improved subjectively and 60% were cured or improved objectively. Long-term follow-up revealed a relatively high relapse rate (Cardozo & Stanton 1984) consistent with the long-term effects of bladder drill. Other reports suggest that bladder training with or without biofeedback can be effectively used to treat incontinence due to detrusor instability (Millard & Oldenberg 1983, Burgio et al 1986). However, this type of treatment is time-consuming and requires trained personnel, and currently biofeedback is used almost exclusively to treat children with maladaptive voiding problems.

Hypnotherapy

Hypnotherapy can be used in one of two ways: either symptom removal by suggestion alone, or by attempting to help the patient disclose hidden emotions or memories which may be pathogenic. Freeman and Baxby (1982) treated 61 women with idiopathic detrusor instability using 12 sessions of hypnosis over a period of 1 month. They achieved an overall improvement rate of over 80%, but unfortunately at 2-year follow-up only nine of the women remained symptom free (Freeman 1989). This type of treatment is not currently employed in the management of detrusor instability.

Acupuncture

Acupuncture is thought to act by increasing levels of endorphins and encephalins in the cerebrospinal fluid. Encephalins are known to inhibit detrusor contractility in vitro (Klarskov 1987). Naloxone, an opiate antagonist, conversely causes decreased bladder capacity and increased detrusor pressure (Murray & Feneley 1982). Several studies have shown symptomatic improvement (Philp et al 1988) or decreased frequency and urinary leakage (Pigne et al 1985) in patients with detrusor instability treated with acupuncture. Gibson et al (1990) utilized infrared low-power laser on acupuncture points successfully initially, but unfortunately there was a high relapse rate at 6 months. We have found that acupuncture is as effective as oxybutynin in the treatment of symptoms associated with idiopathic low compliance and that it is acceptable to patients but time-consuming for the operator (Kelleher et al 1993).

Maximal electrical stimulation

Electrical stimulation, applied either vaginally or anally, may inhibit spontaneous detrusor contractions and thus represents a therapeutic alternative for the management of detrusor instability (Plevnik et al 1986). The neurophysiological basis for the resulting prolonged bladder inhibition remains unclear. The technique is safe and inexpensive and can be performed by specialist nurses. A success rate (cure or significant improvement) of 77% on objective follow-up at 1 year after an average initial treatment regimen of seven sessions has been reported by Eriksen et al (1989).

We have compared maximal electrical stimulation with oxybutynin in women with detrusor instability (Wise et al 1992). Both treatments were associated with a significant reduction in symptoms. Although 20% of the women who received oxybutynin withdrew due to treatment side effects, maximal electrical stimulation was universally acceptable and should therefore be considered as an alternative to pharmacological agents.

All forms of bladder retraining in the treatment of detrusor instability are advantageous because there are few unpleasant side effects and no patient is ever made worse. Mild to moderate detrusor instability can be cured or significantly improved by re-educating the bladder. However, the relapse rate is very high, and although this type of treatment avoids the morbidity associated with surgery and the side effects of drug therapy, it requires skilled personnel and is time-consuming for both the patient and the operator.

Transvesical phenol

Originally described for the treatment of detrusor hyperreflexia (Ewing et al 1982), this treatment has since been used for women with idiopathic detrusor instability. Through a 30° cystoscope a 35 cm semirigid needle is inserted under the bladder epithelium midway between the ureteric orifice and the bladder neck and 10 ml of 6% aqueous phenol is injected on each side. In the largest published series, Blackford et al (1984) reported improvement for at least 1 year in 88 of 116 women treated. They found that the response to treatment was best in those women over the age of 55. A number of side effects and complications were recorded, of which transient postoperative haematuria was the most common. However, they said that there was no significant morbidity. Other workers in the field have been less enthusiastic about the long-term results of transvesical phenol and more concerned about the incidence of significant complications (Rosenbaum et al 1988). This form of treatment is now rarely employed.

Surgery

Various different surgical techniques have been described for the treatment of detrusor instability, but currently the most commonly performed operation is the 'clam' cystoplasty (Mundy & Stephenson 1985). The bladder is bisected almost completely and a patch of gut (usually ileum) equal in length to the circumference of the bisected bladder (about 25 cm) is sewn in place. This often cures the symptoms of detrusor instability (McRae et al 1987) but inefficient voiding may result. Patients have to learn to strain to void, or may have to resort to clean intermittent self-catheterization, sometimes permanently. In addition, mucus retention in the bladder may be a problem, but this can be partially overcome by ingestion of 200 ml of cranberry juice each day (Rosenbaum et al 1989). The chronic exposure of the ileal mucosa to urine may lead to malignant change. There is a 5% risk of adenocarcinoma arising in ureterosigmoidostomies, where colonic mucosa is exposed to N-nitrosamines found in both urine and faeces, and a similar risk may apply to enterocystoplasty. Biopsies of the ileal segment taken from patients with 'clam' cystoplasties show evidence of chronic inflammation of villous atrophy (Nurse & Mundy 1987).

A possible alternative surgical intervention is autoaugmentation (Cartwright & Snow 1989), which avoids bowel and electrolyte problems and, as it is extraperitoneal, may be preferable for patients who have undergone previous abdominal surgery. Kennelly et al (1994) report good results in five patients with small, poorly compliant bladders and vesicoureteric reflux.

As a last resort for those women with severe detrusor instability or hyperreflexia who cannot manage clean intermittent catheterization, it may be more appropriate to perform a urinary diversion. Usually this will utilize an ileal conduit. This is particularly useful in young disabled women, as it is often easier for them or their carers to empty a bag rather than change wet underclothing or incontinence pads.

CONCLUSION

Detrusor instability is a common condition affecting people of all ages. It is characterized by multiple symptoms which, although not life-threatening, may cause much embarrassment and a very restricted lifestyle. Our lack of understanding of the underlying pathology of detrusor instability is reflected in the many different methods of treatment which are currently employed, none of them wholly satisfactory. Conventional bladder-neck surgery is not useful in the treatment of detrusor instability unless there is concomitant urethral sphincter incompetence, and therefore it is important to make an accurate diagnosis before treatment is commenced.

Surgical procedures such as augmentation cystoplasty are reserved for women with severe symptoms in whom other forms of treatment have been tried and failed. Behavioural intervention seems to be the best type of treatment of idiopathic detrusor instability because it may produce a permanent cure without any significant morbidity or side effects. However, the majority of patients are still treated with drug therapy, which they may need to take indefinitely as symptoms usually return once the tablets are discontinued.

Fortunately, detrusor instability is a disease of spontaneous exacerbations and remissions and therefore short courses of drug therapy, when symptoms are at their worst, may be sufficient for the sufferer to maintain a normal lifestyle. Although it is rare to cure a patient completely with any form of treatment, most can have their symptoms significantly reduced. The elucidation of the patient's main complaints is therefore of great importance. As the pathophysiology of the condition becomes clearer we can expect significant advances in the management of detrusor instability.

KEY POINTS

1. Detrusor instability is a disease of spontaneous exacerbations and remissions.
2. Detrusor instability may occur in 10% of the normal population and be asymptomatic.
3. It is the second commonest cause of incontinence in young and middle-aged women but the commonest cause in the elderly.
4. The cause of idiopathic detrusor instability is unknown but many patients have a neurotic personality trait.
5. The diagnosis of detrusor instability can be suggested by symptoms but confirmed only on cystometry.
6. Bladder retraining and behaviour modification are important treatments which can be augmented by anticholinergic drug therapy.
7. Most anticholinergic drugs require to be given at dosage which will produce parasympathetic side effects.
8. Mild instability can be cured or improved by bladder retraining but the relapse rate is high.
9. Where instability and genuine stress incontinence coexist, it is preferable to treat the instability first.

REFERENCES

Bates C P, Whiteside C G, Turner-Warwick R T 1970 Synchronous cine-pressure–flow cystourethrography with special reference to stress and urge incontinence. British Journal of Urology 50: 714–723

Bates C P, Bradley W, Glen E et al 1981 International Continence Society: Fourth report of the standardisation of terminology of lower urinary tract function. British Journal of Urology 53: 333–335

Blackford W, Murray K, Stephenson T P, Mundy A R 1984 Results of transvesical infiltration of the pelvic plexus with phenol in 116 patients. British Journal of Urology 56: 647–649

Blaivas J G, Labib K B, Michalik S J, Zayed A A H 1980 Cystometric response to propantheline in detrusor hyperreflexia. Therapeutic implications. Journal of Urology 124: 259–262

Brading A F, Turner W H 1994 The unstable bladder: towards a common mechanism. British Journal of Urology 73: 3–8

Briggs R S, Castleden C M, Asher M J 1980 The effect of flavoxate on uninhibited detrusor contractions and urinary incontinence in the elderly. Journal of Urology 123: 665–666

Burgio K L, Robinson J C, Engel B T 1986 The role of biofeedback in Kegel exercise training for stress incontinence. American Journal of Obstetrics and Gynecology 154: 64–88

Burnstock G, Dumsday B, Smythe A 1972 Atropine resistant excitation of the urinary bladder: the possibility of transmission via nerve releasing a purine nucleotide. British Journal of Pharmacology 44: 51–61

Burton G 1994 A randomised cross over trial comparing oxybutynin taken three times a day or taken 'when needed'. Neurourology and Urodynamics 13: 351–352

Cardozo L D 1988 Sex and the bladder. British Medical Journal 296: 587–588

Cardozo L D, Stanton S L 1980 Genuine stress incontinence and detrusor instability: a review of 200 cases. British Journal of Obstetrics and Gynaecology 87: 184–190

Cardozo L D, Stanton S L 1984 Biofeedback: a five year review. British Journal of Urology 56: 220

Cardozo L D, Stanton S L, Allan V 1978a Biofeedback in the treatment of detrusor instability. British Journal of Urology 50: 250–254
Cardozo L D, Abrams P H, Stanton S L, Feneley R C L 1978b Idiopathic detrusor instability treated by biofeedback. British Journal of Urology 50: 521–523
Cardozo L D, Stanton S L, Williams J E 1979 Detrusor instability following surgery for genuine instability. British Journal of Urology 51: 204–207
Cardozo L D, Cooper D, Versi E 1987 Oxybutynin chloride in the management of idiopathic detrusor instability. Neurourology and Urodynamics 6: 256–257
Cartwright P C, Snow B W 1989 Bladder autoaugmentation: partial detrusor excision to augment the bladder without use of bowel. Journal of Urology 142: 1050
Castleden C M, Duffin H M 1985 Factors influencing outcome in elderly patients with urinary incontinence and detrusor instability. Aging 14: 303–307
Castleden C M, George C F, Renwick A G, Asher M J 1981 Imipramine – a possible alternative to current therapy for urinary incontinence in the elderly. Journal of Urology 125: 318–320
Chandiramani V A, Peterson T, Beck R O, Fowler C J 1994 Lessons learnt from 44 intravestial instillations of capsaicin. Neurourology and Urodynamics 13: 348–349
Chapple C R, Parkhouse H, Gardener C, Milroy E J G 1990 Double blind placebo-controlled cross over study of fluroxates in the treatment of idiopathic detrusor instability. British Journal of Urology 66: 491–494
Cutner A, Wise B S, Cardozo L D, Burton G, Abbott D, Kelleher C J 1992 Single channel cystometry as a screening test for abnormal detrusor activity. Neurourology and Urodynamics 11(4): 455–456
Eaton A C, Bates C P 1982 An *in vitro* physiological, study of normal and unstable human detrusor muscle. British Journal of Urology 54: 653–657
Eriksen B C, Bergmann S, Eik-Nes S H 1989 Maximal electro-stimulation of the pelvic floor in female idiopathic detrusor instability and urge incontinence. Neurourology and Urodynamics 8: 219–230
Ewing R, Bultitude M E, Shuttleworth K G D 1982 Subtrigonal phenol injection for urge incontinence secondary to detrusor instability in females. British Journal of Urology 54: 689–692
Fantl J A, Wyman J F, Anderson R L, Matt D W, Bump R C 1988 Postmenopausal urinary incontinence: a comparison between non-estrogen supplemented and estrogen supplemented women. Obstetrics and Gynecology 71: 823–828
Fantl J A, Cardozo L D, McLish D 1994 The Hormones and Urogenital Therapy Committee. Estrogen therapy in the management of urinary incontinence in postmenopausal women: a meta-analysis. Obstetrics and Gynecology 83: 12–18
Fowler C J, Jewkes D, McDonald W I, Lynn B, DeGroat W C 1992 Intravesical capsaicin for neurogenic bladder dysfunction. Lancet 339: 1239
Freeman R M 1989 Hypnosis and psychomedical treatment. In: Freeman R M, Malvern J (eds) The unstable bladder. Wright, Bristol, pp 73–80
Freeman R M, Baxby K 1982 Hypnotherapy for incontinence caused by the unstable detrusor. British Medical Journal 284: 1831–1834
Freeman R M, McPherson F M, Baxby K 1985 Psychological features of women with idiopathic detrusor instability. Urologia Internationalis 40: 247–259
Frewen W K 1970 Urge and stress incontinence: fact and fiction. Journal of Obstetrics and Gynaecology of the British Commonwealth 1977: 932–934
Frewen W K 1984 The significance of the psychosomatic factor in urge incontinence. British Journal of Urology 56: 330
Gibaldi M, Grundhofer S 1975 Biopharmaceutic influences on the anticholinergic effect of propantheline. Clinical Pharmacology and Therapeutics 18: 457–461
Gibson J S, Pardley J, Neville J 1990 Infra-red low power laser therapy on acupuncture points for treatment of the unstable bladder. Proceedings of the 20th Meeting of the International Continence Society, pp 146–147
Griffiths C J, Assi M, Styles R A, Ramsden P D, Neal D E 1989 Ambulatory monitoring of bladder and detrusor pressure during natural filling. Journal of Urology 142: 780–784
Gu J, Restorick J M, Blank M et al 1983 Vasoactive intestinal polypeptide in the normal and unstable bladder. British Journal of Urology 54: 252–255
Higson R H, Smith J C, Whelan P 1978 Bladder rupture: an acceptable complication of distension therapy? British Journal of Urology 50: 529–534
Hilton P 1988 Urinary incontinence during sexual intercourse: a common but rarely volunteered symptom. British Journal of Obstetrics and Gynaecology 95: 377–381
Hilton P, Stanton S L 1982 Use of desmopressin (DDAVP) in nocturnal urinary frequency in the female. British Journal of Urology 54: 252–255
Hilton P, Stanton S L 1983 Urethral pressure measurement by microtransducer: the results in symptom-free women and those with genuine stress incontinence. British Journal of Obstetrics and Gynaecology 90: 919–933
Hodgkinson C P, Drukker B H 1977 Infravesical nerve resection for detrusor dyssynergia (the Ingleman-Sundberg operation). Acta Obstetrica Gynecologica Scandinavica 56: 401–408
Hodgkinson C P, Ayers M A, Drukker B H 1963 Dyssynergic detrusor dysfunction in the apparently normal female. American Journal of Obstetrics and Gynecology 87: 717–730
Holmes D M, Stone A R, Barry P R, Richards C J, Stephenson T P 1983 Bladder training – 3 years on. British Journal of Urology 55: 660–664
Holmes D, Plevnik S, Stanton S L 1989 Bladder neck electric conductivity in female urinary urgency and urge incontinence. British Journal of Obstetrics and Gynaecology 96: 816–820
Ingleman-Sundberg A 1978 Partial bladder denervation for detrusor dyssynergia. Clinical Obstetrics and Gynaecology 21: 797–805
Jarvis G T 1989 Bladder drill. In: Freeman R, Malvern J (eds) The unstable bladder. Wright, Bristol, pp 55–60
Jarvis G T, Millar D R 1980 Controlled trial of bladder drill for detrusor instability. British Medical Journal 281: 1322–1323
Jeffcoate T N A, Francis W J A 1966. Urgency incontinence in the female. American Journal of Obstetrics and Gynecology 94: 604–618
Karram M M, Bhatia N W 1989 Management of coexistent stress and urge urinary incontinence. Obstetrics and Gynecology 73: 4–7
Kelleher C, Khullar V, Cardozo L D 1993 Psychoneuroticism and quality of life in healthy incontinent women. Neurourology and Urodynamics 12(4): 393–394
Kelleher C J, Filsche J, Burton G, Cardozo L D 1994 Acupuncture and the treatment of irritative bladder symptoms. Acupuncture in Medicine 12(1): 9–12
Kennelly M J, Gormley E A, McGuire E J 1994 Early clinical experience with adult bladder autoaugmentation. Journal of Urology 152: 303–306
Kinder R B, Mundy A R 1985 Atropine blockade of neuro-mediated stimulation of the human detrusor. British Journal of Urology 57: 418–421
Kinder R B, Mundy A R 1987 Pathophysiology of idiopathic detrusor instability and detrusor hyperreflexia – an *in vitro* study of human detrusor muscle. British Journal of Urology 60: 509–515
Klarskov P 1987 Gukephaline inhibits presynaptically the contractility of urinary tract smooth muscle. British Journal of Urology 59: 31–35
Knudsen U B, Rittig S, Pedersen J P, Norgaard J P, Djurhuus J C 1989 Long-term treatment of nocturnal enuresis with desmopressin – influence on urinary output and haematological parameters. Neurourology and Urodynamics 8: 348–349
Langworthy D R, Kolb L G, Dees J E 1936 Behaviour of the human bladder freed from cerebral control. Journal of Urology 36: 577–597
McRae P, Murray K H, Nurse D E, Stephenson J P, Mundy A R 1987 Clam entero-cystoplasty in the neuropathic bladder. British Journal of Urology 60: 523–525
Madersbacher H, Jilg S 1991 Control of detrusor hyperreflexia by the intravesical instillation of oxybutynin hydrochloride. Paraplegia 29: 84–90
Malone-Lee J, Wahedena I 1993 Characterisation of detrusor contractile function in relation to old age. British Journal of Urology 72: 873–880
Massey J A, Abrams P 1986 Dose titration in clinical trials: an example

using emepronium caragenate in detrusor instability. British Journal of Urology 58: 125–128
Millard R J, Oldenberg B F 1983 The symptomatic, urodynamic and psycho-dynamic results of bladder re-education programmes. Journal of Urology 130: 717–719
Moolgaoker A S, Ardran G M, Smith J C, Stallworthy J A 1972 The diagnosis and management of urinary incontinence in the female. British Journal of Obstetrics and Gynaecology 79: 481–497
Moore K H, Sutherst J R 1990 Response to treatment of detrusor instability in relation to psychoneurotic status. British Journal of Urology 66: 486–490
Moore K H, Hay D M, Irvine A E, Watson A, Goldstein M 1990 Oxybutynin hydrochloride (3 mg) in the treatment of women with idiopathic detrusor instability. British Journal of Urology 66: 479–485
Mundy A R 1983 The long-term results of bladder transection for urge incontinence. British Journal of Urology 55: 642–644
Mundy A R, Stephenson T P 1985 Clam ileocystoplasty for the treatment of refractory urge incontinence. British Journal of Urology 57: 647–651
Murray K H, Feneley R C L 1982 Endorphins – a role in lower urinary tract function? The effect of opioid blockade on the detrusor and urethral sphincter mechanism. British Journal of Urology 54: 638–640
Norton K R W, Bhat A V, Stanton S L 1990 Psychiatric aspects of urinary incontinence in women attending an outpatient clinic. British Medical Journal 31: 271–272
Nurse D E, Mundy A R 1987 Cystoplasty infection and cancer. Neurourology and Urodynamics 343–344
Pengelly A W, Stephenson T P, Milroy E J G, Whiteside C G, Turner-Warwick R 1978 Results of prolonged bladder distension as treatment for detrusor instability. British Journal of Urology 50: 243–245
Philp T, Shah P J R, Worth P H L 1988 Acupuncture in the treatment of bladder instability. British Journal of Urology 61: 490–493
Pigne A, Degansac C, Nyssen C, Barratt J 1985 Acupuncture and the unstable bladder. In Proceedings of the 15th International Continence Society Meeting, pp 186–187
Plevnik S, Janez J, Vrtacnik P, Trsinar B, Vodusek D B 1986 Short-term electrical stimulation: home treatment for urinary incontinence. World Journal of Urology 4: 24–26
Ramsden P D, Smith J C, Dunn M, Ardran G M 1976 Distension therapy for the unstable bladder: late results including an assessment of repeat distensions. Journal of Urology 48: 623–629
Rew D A, Rundle J S H 1989 Assessment of the safety of regular DDAVP therapy in primary nocturnal enuresis. British Journal of Urology 63: 352–353
Ritch A E S, George C F, Castleden C M, Hall M R P 1977 A second look at emepromium bromide in urinary incontinence. Lancet 1: 504–505
Rose D K 1931 Clinical application of bladder physiology. Journal of Urology 26: 91–105
Rosenbaum T P, Shah P J R, Worth P H L 1988 Transtrigonal phenol – the end of an era? Neurourology and Urodynamics 7: 294–295
Rosenbaum T P, Shah P J R, Rose G A, Lloyd-Davies R W 1989 Cranberry juice helps the problem of mucus production in enterouroplastics. Neurourology and Urodynamics 8: 344–345
Sibley G N A 1985 An experimental model of detrusor instability in the obstructed pig. British Journal of Urology 57: 292–298
Speakman M J, Brading A F, Gilpin C J, Dixon J S, Gilpin S A, Gosling J A 1987 Bladder outflow obstruction – cause of denervation supersensitivity. Journal of Urology 183: 1461–1466
Steel S A, Cox C, Stanton S L 1985 Long-term follow-up of detrusor instability following the colposuspension operation. British Journal of Urology 58: 138–142
Sutherst J R, Brown M 1978 The effect on the bladder pressure of sudden entry of fluid into the posterior urethra. British Journal of Urology 50: 406–409
Sutherst J R, Brown M 1984 Comparison of single and multichannel cystometry in diagnosing bladder instability. British Medical Journal 288: 1720–1722
Tapp A J S, Cardozo L D 1986 The postmenopausal bladder. British Journal of Hospital Medicine 35: 20–23
Thuroff J W, Burke B, Ebner A et al 1991 Randomised double-blind multicentre trial on treatment of frequency, urgency and incontinence related to detrusor hyper-activity: oxybutynin versus propantheline versus placebo. Journal of Urology 145: 813–817
Torrens M J, Griffiths H B 1974 The control of the uninhibited bladder by selective sacral neurectomy. British Journal of Urology 46: 639–644
Turner-Warwick R T 1975 Some clinical aspects of detrusor dysfunction. Journal of Urology 113: 539–544
van Waalwijk van Doorn E S C, Zwier W 1990 Ambulatory monitoring to assess the efficacy of oxybutynin in patients with mixed incontinence. European Urology 18: 49–51
van Waalwijk van Doorn E S C, Remmers A, Janknegt R A 1992 Conventional and extramural ambulatory urodynamic testing of the lower urinary tract in female volunteers. Journal of Urology 47: 1319–1326
Versi E, Cardozo L D 1988 Oestrogens and lower urinary tract function. In: Studd J W W, Whitehead M (eds) The menopause. Blackwell Scientific Publications, Oxford, pp 76–84
Walters M D, Taylor S, Schoenfeld L S 1990 Psychosexual study of women with detrusor instability. Obstetrics and Gynaecology 75: 22–26
Warrell D W 1977 Vaginal denervation of the bladder nerve supply. Urology International 32: 114–116
Wein A J 1986 Pharmacology of the bladder and urethra. In: Stanton S L, Tanagho E (eds) surgery of female incontinence, 2nd edn. Springer-Verlag, Heidelberg, pp 229–250
Whiteside C G, Arnold G P 1975 Persistent primary enuresis: a urodynamic assessment. British Medical Journal 1: 364–369
Wise B G, Cardozo L D, Cutner A, Kelleher C, Burton G 1992 Maximal electrical stimulation: an acceptable alternative to anticholinergic therapy. International Urogynecology Journal 3(3): 270
Wise B G, Cardozo L D, Cutner A, Benness C J, Burton G 1993a The prevalence and significance of urethral instability in women with detrusor instability. British Journal of Urology 72: 26–29
Wise B G, Benness C J, Cardozo L D, Cutner A 1993b Vaginal oestradiol for lower urinary tract symptoms in post-menopausal women. A double blind placebo-controlled study. In Proceedings of the 7th International Congress on the Menopause, Stockholm, p 15
Zoubek J, Bloom D, Sedman A B 1990 Extraordinary urinary frequency. Pediatrics 85: 1112–1114

50

Voiding difficulties

S. L. Stanton

INTRODUCTION

Voiding disorders in the female are important: they are frequently underdiagnosed and often badly managed. In the male, high bladder pressures lead to back-pressure effects on the kidney, with the development of hydronephrosis. Fortunately these rarely occur in the female; none the less, she may be left with disturbing symptoms of difficulty in bladder emptying, recurrent urinary tract infections and a chronically overdistended bladder.

There is a spectrum of disease. Voiding disorders can be asymptomatic or may commence with symptoms of poor stream, hesitancy, incomplete emptying and straining to void. This may lead to chronic retention, or chronic retention can develop de novo. Acute retention can also occur de novo, and may either resolve or lead to chronic retention.

DEFINITIONS

Voiding disorders in the female are rarely defined in textbooks of either urology or gynaecology, and have not yet been included in the standardization of terminology of lower urinary tract function, published by the International Continence Society (Appendix II). I would suggest the following working definitions:

1. *Acute retention* – the sudden onset of painful or painless inability to void over 12 hours, requiring catheterization with removal of a volume equal to or greater than normal bladder capacity. Acute retention is usually painful, but in the presence of a neurological lesion or following an epidural anaesthetic it may be painless. It seems reasonable to set a time limit and to state that it needs catheterization, as this should provide confirmation of retention. Finally, the volume should be at least equal to normal bladder capacity; sometimes the patient is catheterized unnecessarily and a volume very much less than bladder capacity is removed. That patient may be falsely labelled as having acute retention.

2. *Chronic retention* – insidious and painless failure of bladder emptying where catheterization yields a volume equal to at least 50% of normal bladder capacity. This can include the presence of residual urine after bladder-neck surgery. Otherwise the cause of chronic retention is often obscure.

PATHOPHYSIOLOGY

Voiding in the female can occur via one of three mechanisms. These are a detrusor contraction, an increase in abdominal pressure generated by abdominal wall muscles and diaphragm, or relaxation of the pelvic floor and urethral sphincter mechanism. Voiding disorders therefore result when these mechanisms fail, i.e. when the detrusor is unable to contract or maintain an effective contraction, when the urethral sphincter mechanism fails to relax, or when there is a combination of both. In suprasacral neurological lesions there is synchronous failure of detrusor contraction and urethral sphincter relaxation (detrusor–sphincter dyssynergia), resulting in a voiding disorder.

Acute and chronic retention can occur following a variety of causes. Acute retention may be recognized as a well defined entity, but chronic retention may be less readily recognized.

AETIOLOGY

Voiding disorders and urinary retention may be classified in the following way.

Neurological

Three main levels of neurological lesion are recognized: above the pons (suprapontine lesions), between the pons and parasympathetic outflow (cord lesions) and distal to the sacral parasympathetic outflow (peripheral lesions). All can produce voiding disorders. Suprapontine disorders (e.g. cerebrovascular accidents and Parkinson's disease) will cause voiding disorder but detrusor–sphincter dyssynergia does not occur. Cord lesions (e.g. spinal cord injury or multiple sclerosis) frequently cause voiding difficulties and retention is present in the early phases of spinal cord injury. About 25% of multiple sclerosis patients will present with acute retention. Detrusor–sphincter dyssynergia will occur in this group. Peripheral lesions (e.g. prolapsed intervertebral disc, diabetic autonomic neuropathy and other peripheral autonomic neuropathies) cause acontractile failure of the detrusor.

Painful conditions of the vulva and perineum (e.g. following posterior repair or with prolapsed haemorrhoids) will reflexly inhibit micturition.

Pharmacological

Epidural anaesthesia (especially in labour) and certain drugs, e.g. tricyclic antidepressants, anticholinergic agents, α-adrenergic stimulants and ganglion-blocking drugs, may all predispose to voiding disorder. The epidural in labour is the most commonly encountered pharmacological cause. Following delivery under epidural, nursing or medical staff fail to enquire about voiding and painless retention develops. In neglected cases, up to 4 litres of urine can be withdrawn. This produces a grossly overdistended bladder which may fail to function and leave the patient with retention for up to 3 months or more. Some patients will have permanent voiding disorders.

Inflammatory

Painful inflammatory lesions around the anogenital region, such as genital herpes, acute vulvovaginitis, urthritis or cystitis, can all precipitate acute retention of urine.

Obstructive

Postoperative urethral oedema (e.g. following anterior colporrhaphy) frequently causes voiding difficulties and up to 50% of patients fail to void spontaneously on the day following bladder-neck surgery, hence the conventional use of either a urethral or suprapubic catheter. As most operations for continence will produce some urethral obstruction, it is a sensible prophylaxis to catheterize patients at operation until they are able to void spontaneously.

Other causes of obstruction include an impacted pelvic mass (e.g. retroverted gravid uterus, uterine fibroids or an ovarian cyst), foreign bodies in the urethra, an ectopic ureterocoele, and a bladder polyp or a carcinoma occluding the internal urethral meatus. Rarely, urethral distortion associated with a cystocoele causes retention.

Bladder overdistension

Overdistension after failure to catheterize for retention develops insidiously, is much more common in the female than in the male and is difficult to treat effectively. Denervation, ischaemia of the detrusor muscle fibres and distraction of the detrusor syncytium are likely sequelae of overdistension, and are responsible for the continuation of voiding difficulty.

Psychogenic

This group should only be diagnosed after the above organic conditions can be excluded.

INCIDENCE

In a population attending a urodynamic clinic for a wide variety of gynaecological urology disorders, up to 2% may have asymptomatic voiding difficulty and up to 25% may have symptomatic proven voiding difficulty.

PRESENTATION

Voiding disorders are associated with symptoms of poor flow, intermittent stream, incomplete emptying, straining to void and hesitancy. Hilton and Laor (1989) reviewed these symptoms and compared them with urodynamic findings in a group of women attending a urodynamic clinic. Symptoms of poor or intermittent urinary stream correlated best with urodynamic evidence of voiding difficulty. When acute retention has developed, the patient has not voided and may be in pain. Chronic retention presents with frequency and then overflow incontinence. All of these may be associated with symptoms of a primary cause. Urine infection may occur with the residual urine, and these symptoms will be present as well.

Clinical examination will disclose a palpable bladder and there may be signs of the primary cause. A neurological examination should be carried out, including inspection of the back for stigmata of underlying neurological lesion, e.g. spina bifida occulta.

INVESTIGATION

Urine culture and sensitivity

A midstream sample of urine should be sent for analysis on all patients with voiding difficulty, as urinary infection may occasionally produce acute retention and infection is often a sequel to incomplete bladder emptying.

Urinary diary

An accurate record of fluid intake and output is important and a urinary diary can be easily maintained by the patient. When catheterization is carried out for acute retention it is essential to note the amount of urine removed. Not only does this confirm acute retention, but it may give some guide as to the severity of bladder distension and therefore a prognosis as to when spontaneous voiding may resume.

Uroflowmetry

Measurement of free urine flow rate is a good guide to voiding function. Flow rates consistently below 15 ml/s for a volume of >150 ml indicate impaired voiding, and this may be a precursor of retention. However, a flow rate of >15 ml/s may still be associated with voiding disorder if accompanied by a high maximum voiding pressure. The shape of the curve is also important. Compare the normal bell-shaped cone (Fig. 50.1) with the attenuated and intermittent flow rate of the patient with voiding difficulty (Fig. 50.2).

Cystometry

The combination of uroflowmetry and cystometry provides the best information about bladder function. Both the filling and voiding phases will help establish whether there is a neuropathic component. Suprapontine and cord lesions above S2, 3 and 4 may show systolic (phasic) detrusor contractions and a reduced bladder capacity (Fig. 50.3). Peripheral lesions of the cord will show residual urine, late desire to void and a large-capacity bladder with a normal pressure rise (Fig. 50.4). Both may show an inability to produce a voluntary and sustained detrusor contraction.

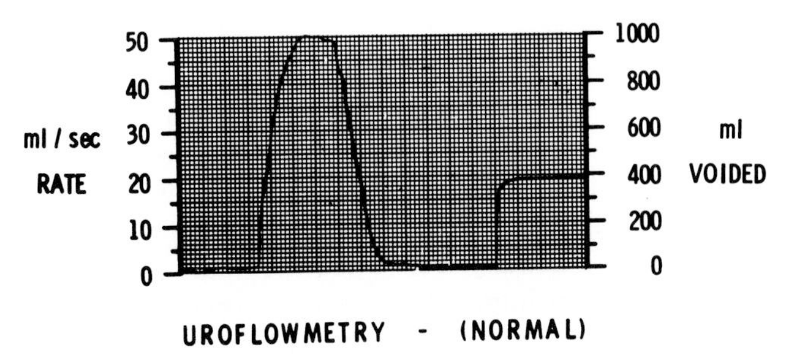

Fig. 50.1 Normal flow rate.

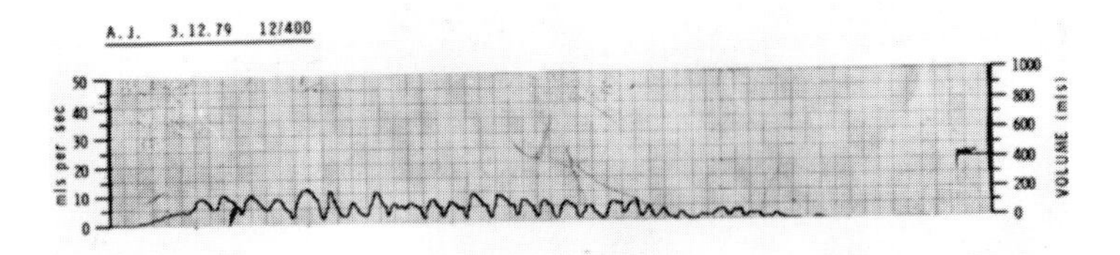

Fig. 50.2 Flow rate showing voiding difficulty with an attenuated flow, not exceeding 15 ml/s.

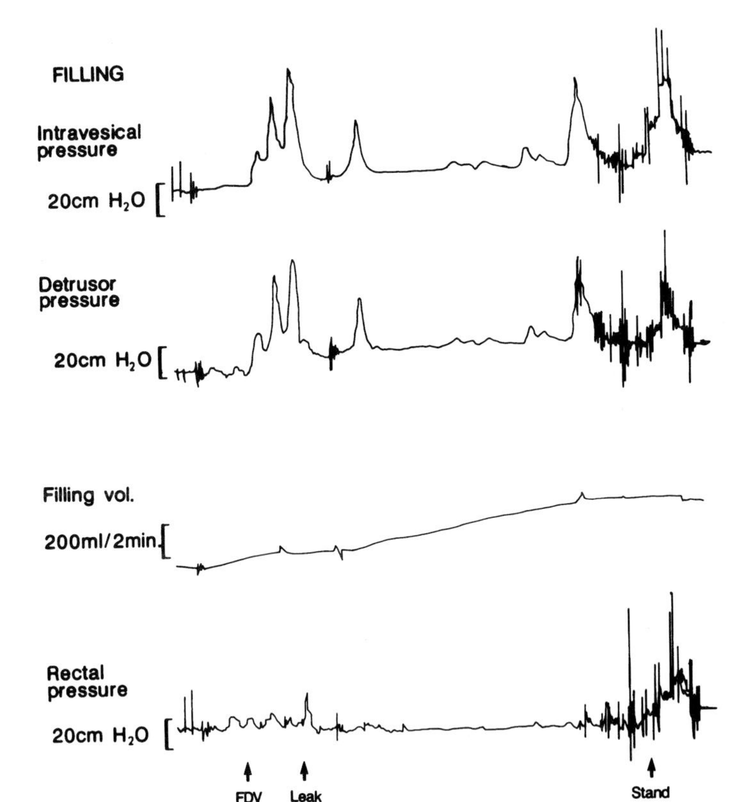

Fig. 50.3 Cystometry showing systolic detrusor contractions.

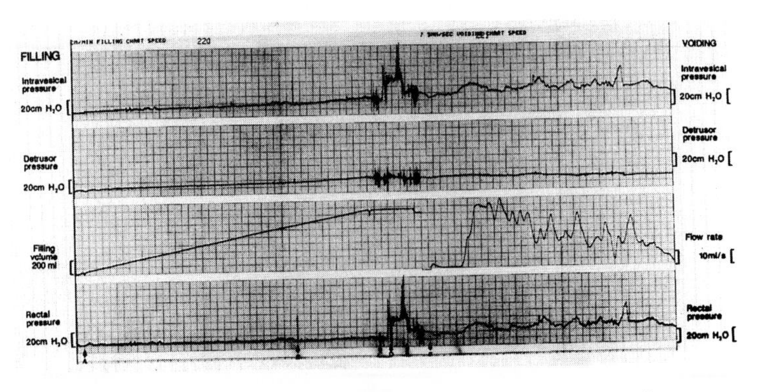

Fig. 50.4 Cystometry showing a peripheral (lower motor neuron) lesion with a residual urine, delayed desire to void and a large-capacity bladder. A, start; B, first desire to void; C, stop filling; D, stand; E, cough; F, start to void.

Radiology

A plain abdominal X-ray will disclose a large residual urine (Fig. 50.5). A lumbosacral spine X-ray is important to exclude congenital (e.g. sacral agenesis; Fig. 50.6) or acquired (prolapsed intervertebral disc) lesions. Both will produce a peripheral neurological disorder.

Intravenous urography is less useful than it was as ultrasound now produces comparable information on back-pressure effects on the ureter and kidney.

Videocystourethrography (the combination of cystometry, uroflowmetry and radiological screening during bladder filling and voiding, recorded with sound on a video tape) provides a comprehensive study of bladder function, but whether this is necessary in all cases of voiding difficulty is debatable. In addition to the information provided by cystometry, it will also show abnormal bladder morphology secondary to voiding difficulty, e.g. sacculation and diverticulum formation, and the presence of vesicoureteric reflux (Fig. 50.7).

Ultrasonography

Abdominal ultrasound scanning will provide an estimate of residual urine to within 20%, which is sufficiently accurate. Intravesical lesions such as an ectopic ureterocoele can be demonstrated.

Cystourethroscopy

Difficulty in instrumentation of the urethra will show if there is significant urethral narrowing (e.g. distal urethral stenosis). Cystoscopy demonstrates whether there is any intravesical pathology and whether or not trabeculation, sacculation and diverticulum formation have occurred. These indicate long-standing obstruction but not its cause.

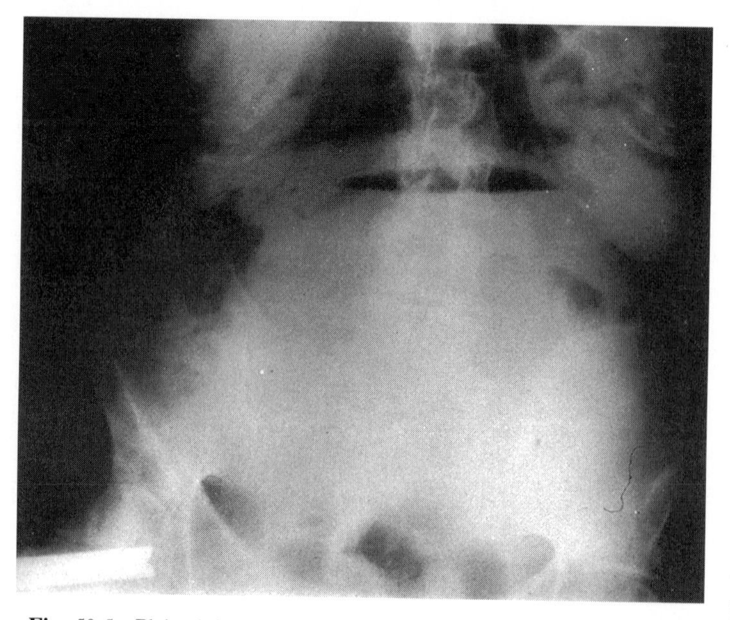

Fig. 50.5 Plain abdominal X-ray showing large residual urine.

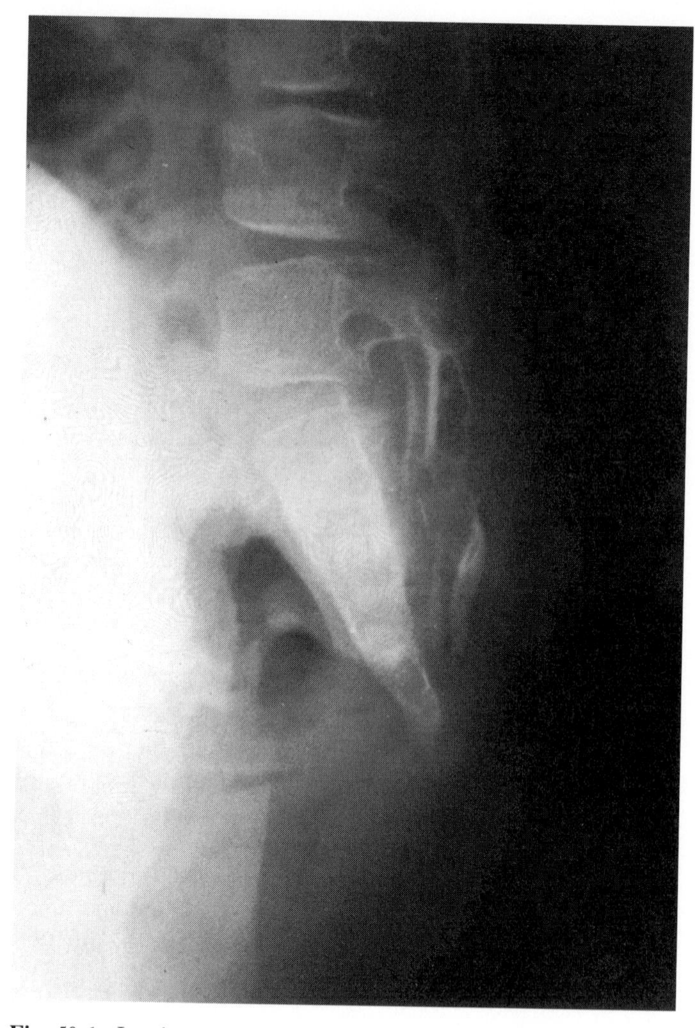

Fig. 50.6 Lumbosacral spine X-ray showing sacral agenesis.

Electrophysiological tests

Concentric or single-fibre electromyography of the pelvic floor and urethral sphincter mechanism with terminal motor latency studies of the perineal branch of the pudendal nerve will indicate whether denervation or nerve damage to these structures has occurred.

TREATMENT

Principles of therapy

Both the primary condition and its effects on the bladder may need treatment, and in the case of acute retention these may be simultaneous.

Catheterization is either urethral or suprapubic: urethral is quickest and simplest. The disadvantages are that this is an uncomfortable method of catheterization. If maintained for longer than 24 hours it is associated with a higher incidence of urinary tract infection than a suprapubic catheter, and it is impossible to see whether a patient can resume spontaneous voiding with a urethral catheter in place. However, it is ideal for short-term catheterization.

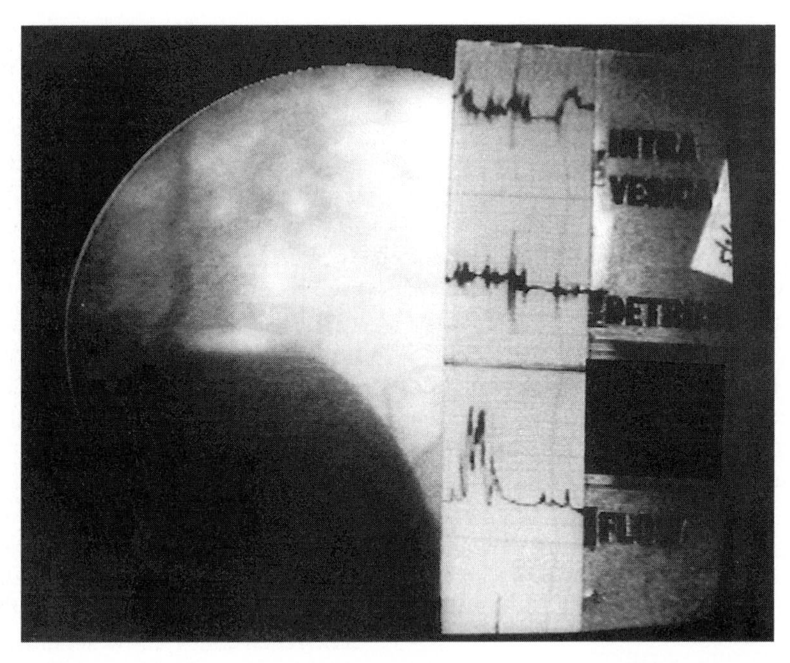

Fig. 50.7 Videocystourethrogram image showing vesicoureteric reflux.

Clean intermittent self-catheterization is a clean (and not sterile) technique to enable the patient (or her partner) to catheterize herself intermittently for the management of chronic urinary retention. The catheters are disposable and are changed once a week (Fig. 50.8). A suprapubic catheter is ideal if the catheter is required for more than 24–48 hours. Its main use is following pelvic and especially bladder-neck surgery. Its disadvantages include the requirement of a doctor for its insertion; caution must be taken during insertion to avoid bowel injury.

Drugs may be used either to treat symptoms of voiding difficulty or as an adjunct to catheterization; they are often ineffective. They may either relax the sphincter mechanism or stimulate the detrusor to contract.

α-Adrenergic blocking agents (phenoxybenzamine 10 mg bd) are non-selective α-blocking agents, with the unwanted side effects of tachycardia and fainting due to α_2 stimulation. Prazosin (0.5–3 mg daily in divided doses) and indoramin (50–200 mg daily in divided doses) are selective α_1-blocking agents. Baclofen (5 mg tds – 25 mg qds) is a striated muscle relaxant used to treat spasticity and diazepam (10–15 mg nocte) acts centrally as a muscle relaxant and has an anxiolytic effect; both may be used for sphincteric relaxation.

Muscarinic agents (e.g. bethanechol chloride 20–100 mg qds) should be used with caution in the elderly; in asthmatic patients and those with cardiovascular disease or parkinsonism. Anticholinesterase agents such as distigmine bromide (5 mg/day) have been tried but have little proven effect. The E_2 and $F_{2\alpha}$ prostaglandins will cause detrusor contractions in vitro, but have an inconsistent effect when administered intravesically to patients with retention.

Prophylaxis

It is a simple and wise precaution to measure the free urine flow rate in any patient who is to have continence surgery; most of these procedures are obstructive and any predisposition to a voiding difficulty will result in retention.

Asymptomatic voiding difficulty

These patients need supervision to avoid urinary tract infection. Upper tract dilatation rarely occurs in the female unless associated with a neuropathy.

Symptoms only

Patients with only symptoms of voiding difficulty may be treated with α-adrenergic blocking agents in the dosages detailed above. Lying and standing blood pressures and an

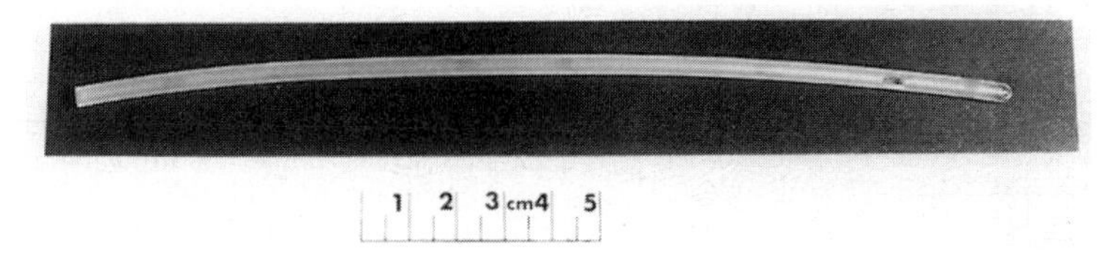

Fig. 50.8 Disposable female self-catheter.

electrocardiogram should be taken beforehand. The dosage will often be limited by the side effects of hypotension.

Retention

Acute retention

Where the cause is likely to recur, simply relieving retention and then removing the catheter is likely to lead to retention again. Equally, if the amount withdrawn is greater than 1 litre, the bladder is unlikely to recover immediately. In these situations it is sensible to use a suprapubic catheter and this will ensure that spontaneous voiding can be easily re-established.

When there is not an obvious cause and an amount of less than 1 litre is removed, a Foley catheter can be left in place for 24–48 hours.

Chronic retention

This includes conditions without an obvious cause as well as postoperative and postpartum retention.

Postoperative and postpartum retention are best managed by a suprapubic catheter or the use of clean intermittent self-catheterization. For the latter, the patient should be manually dexterous and able to carry out self-catheterization 3–4 times a day, depending on the amounts of urine removed. Most patients develop a subclinical urinary tract infection and antibiotics are only required if symptoms of urinary infection are present.

For some causes of chronic retention an Otis urethrotomy may be helpful.

A suprapubic catheter can remain in place for many months and is ideal for the patient who is not manually dexterous. Once the patient is voiding amounts of greater than 150–200 ml and the evening and early morning residual urines are less than 200 ml, the catheter can be removed.

Some conditions (e.g. distal urethral stenosis) will benefit from an Otis urethrotomy. The epithelium and submucosa of the urethra is cut in three longitudinal incisions at 4, 7 and 12 o'clock, and a large Foley catheter (26 French gauge) is left in place for 5–7 days.

For patients with chronic retention (due to inefficient or absent reflex micturition, usually after spinal cord injury) who have been resistant to conservative therapy, electrostimulation using a sacral anterior root stimulator of S2, 3 and 4 may be tried. If detrusor–sphincter dyssynergia is present, complete sacral rhizotomy of S2–S5 is offered as well. A three-channel stimulator for both sides of S2, 3 and 4 is implanted with cables led to three independent receivers to allow separate stimulation of S2, 3 and 4. It is activated by a battery-driven oscillator block placed over the three independent receivers (Brindley 1994).

CONCLUSION

Voiding difficulties form a spectrum of disorders ranging from symptoms only to established retention. Often these are poorly recognized and inadequately treated. Prevention, early diagnosis and treatment with catheterization where indicated, are key points.

KEY POINTS

1. Voiding disorders may be asymptomatic and occasionally lead to upper tract dilatation.
2. Normal voiding in the female occurs by detrusor contraction, pelvic floor relaxation or abdominal straining. Failure of incoordination of the first two may lead to voiding difficulty.
3. The epidural in labour is a potent cause of undiagnosed urinary retention and subsequent voiding difficulty.
4. Symptoms of poor or intermittent urinary stream are the best markers of voiding difficulty.
5. Uroflowmetry is the simplest screening test: when combined with cystometry this will be sufficient to diagnose most voiding disorders.
6. Treatment is directed towards bladder emptying and management of the primary cause.
7. Drug therapy has little proven clinical effect.

REFERENCES

Brindley G 1994 Electrical stimulation in vesicourethral dysfunction: practical devices. In: Mundy A, Stephenson T, Wein A (eds) Urodynamics: principles, practice and application, 2nd edn. Churchill Livingstone, London, pp 489–493

Hilton P, Laor D 1989 Voiding symptoms in the female: the correlation with urodynamic voiding characteristics. Neurourology and Urodynamics 8: 308–310

FURTHER READING

Hilton P 1990 Bladder drainage. In: Stanton S L (ed) Clinical urogynaecology, 2nd edn. Churchill Livingstone, London

Shaw P J R 1992 Voiding difficulties and retention. In: Stanton S L (ed) Clinical urogynaecology, 2nd edn. Churchill Livingstone, Edinburgh (in press)

Snooks S J, Swash M 1984 Abnormalities of the innervation of the urethral striated musculature in incontinence. British Journal of Urology 56: 401–405

Stanton S L, Ozsoy C, Hilton P 1983 Voiding difficulties in the female: prevalence, clinical and urodynamic review. Obstetrics and Gynecology 61: 144–147

Worth P 1986 Urethrotomy. In: Stanton S L, Tanagho E A (eds) Surgery of female incontinence, 2nd. edn. Springer-Verlag, Heidelberg

51

Vaginal prolapse

Stuart L. Stanton

CLASSIFICATION

A prolapse is the protrusion of an organ or structure beyond its normal anatomical confines. This is classified according to its anatomical location, and in the vagina it is convenient to start from the anterior and move to the posterior vaginal wall.

The pelvis may be divided into three compartments: anterior, middle and posterior. The anterior compartment contains the urethra (urethrocele) and bladder (cystocele). The middle compartment comprises uterine vault descent and enterocele, and the posterior compartment contains the rectum (rectocele) (Fig. 51.1). An enterocele may contain small bowel as well as omentum. Some amount of vaginal wall laxity is normal and prolapse is a matter of degree rather than being absolute. There are many grading classifications: none is perfect and some are very complex and impractical. Conventionally, any descent within the vagina is graded as first degree, descent to the introitus as second degree, and third degree is when the prolapse has descended outside the introitus. This is simple but lacks accuracy for scientific comparison.

A more complex system to overcome this has been devised by the International Continence Society Committee for Standardization of Terminology (ICS 1994). It uses the hymen as a fixed point of reference and measurements are taken from this on the anterior and posterior vaginal walls and to the vaginal apex. In addition, the genital hiatus, width of the perineal body and total vaginal length are measured (Fig. 51.2) and recorded on a grid form (Fig. 51.3). Once the measurements have been completed the prolapse can also be staged from 0 to IV, depending on the severity and extent of prolapse. For all of these measurements the conditions of the examination must be specified, i.e. straining down, traction and position of the subject.

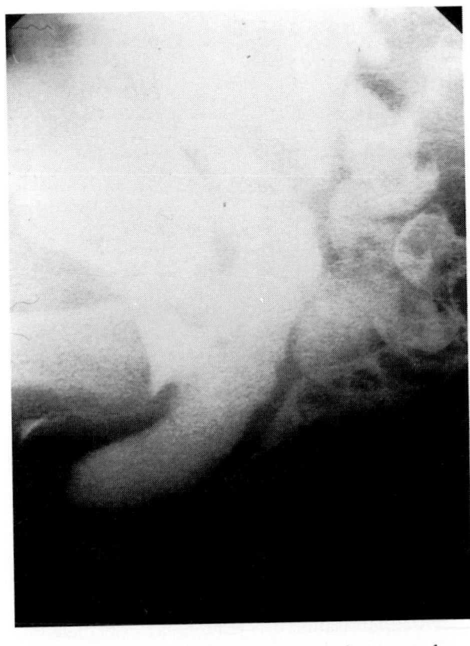

Fig. 51.1 **a** Cystourethrocele. **b** Rectocele and enterocele. **c** Pelvic fluoroscopy showing enterocele and rectum in process of emptying (by kind permission of Dr Margie Kahn).

Prolapse is common and may be associated with urinary symptoms. It is benign, but third-degree uterine prolapse with a cystocele may cause ureteric obstruction and is therefore potentially fatal (Fig. 51.4). The ureters are also at risk of being traumatized during vaginal hysterectomy.

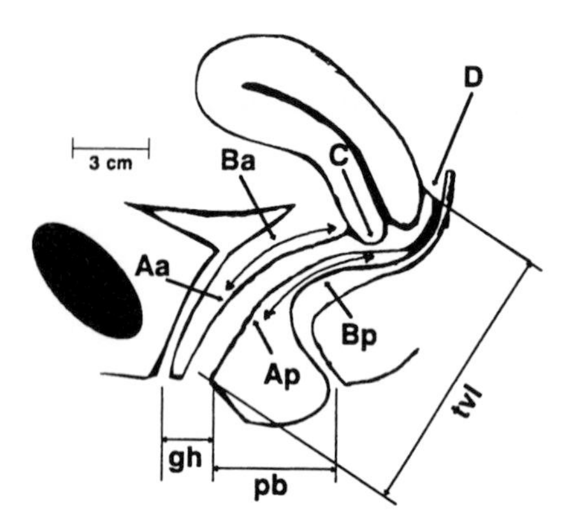

Fig. 51.2 Graphic representation of points used to quantify prolapse. gh = genital hiatus, pb = perineal body, tvl = total vaginal length. Point Aa is midline point of the anterior vaginal wall 3 cm proximal to the external urethral meatus. Ba is most distal/dependent position of the anterior vaginal wall from the vaginal vault or anterior fornix to Aa. C = most distal/dependent edge of cervix or vault. D = location of posterior fornix. Bp = most distal/dependent point on posterior vaginal wall from vault or posterior fornix to Ap. Ap = point on midline posterior vaginal wall 3 cm proximal to hymen. (ICS Standardisation of Terminology of Female Pelvic Organ Prolapse and Pelvic Floor Dysfunction 1994)

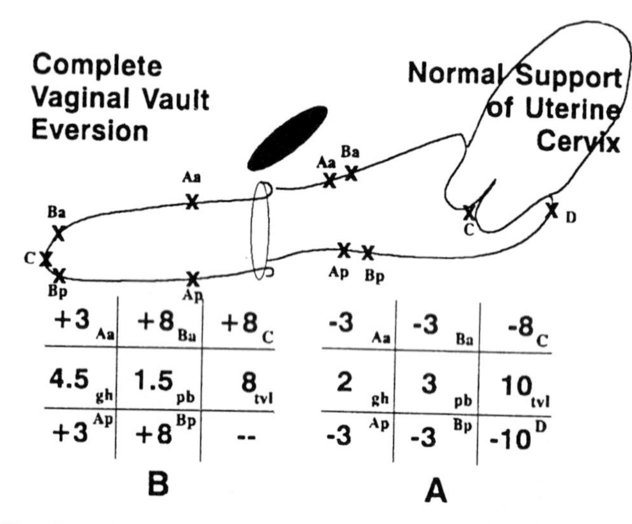

+3 Aa	+8 Ba	+8 C
4.5 gh	1.5 pb	8 tvl
+3 Ap	+8 Bp	--

-3 Aa	-3 Ba	-8 C
2 gh	3 pb	10 tvl
-3 Ap	-3 Bp	-10 D

Fig. 51.3 Line diagram to show contrasting measurement between normal support and post hysterectomy vaginal eversion. **a** (right) normal support of uterus and cervix. **b** (left) complete vaginal vault eversion. (ICS Standardisation of Terminology of Female Pelvic Organ Prolapse and Pelvic Floor Dysfunction 1994)

INCIDENCE

Cystourethrocele is the most common type of prolapse, followed by uterine descent and then rectocele. A urethrocele occurring on its own is rare. The enterocele is more common following abdominal or vaginal hysterectomy or colposuspension.

Approximately 20% of patients waiting for gynaecological surgery are due to have repair of a prolapse (Stallworthy 1971). The incidence rises in the elderly, constituting 59% of one series of patients who underwent major gynaecological surgery (Lewis 1968). With improved general health, better care in labour and shorter duration of first and second stages and a tendency towards smaller families, it is likely that prolapse may become less common.

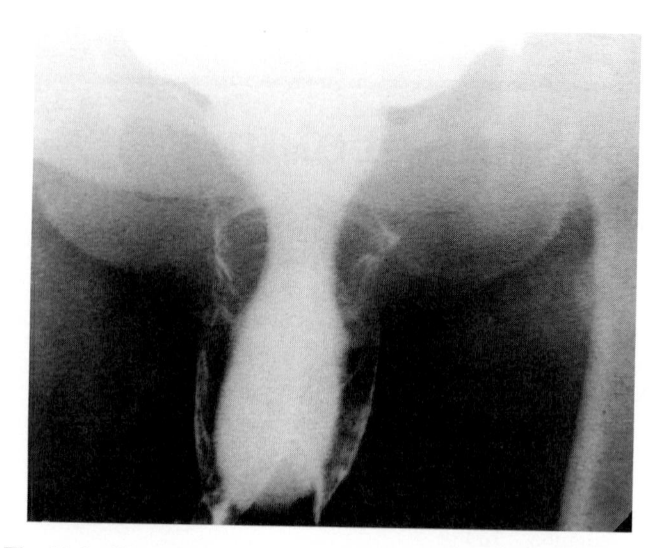

Fig. 51.4 X-ray showing marked cystocele with uretero-vesical junctions outside the vagina (by kind permission of Dr Margie Kahn).

PELVIC ANATOMY

The pelvic viscera are supported by the pelvic floor, which is composed of muscle, fascia and ligamentous supports.

Pelvic floor

The pelvic floor includes the levator ani, internal obturator and piriform muscles, and superficial and deep perineal muscles (Fig. 51.5). The levator ani (which is in two parts, pubococcygeal and iliococcygeal) is covered by pelvic fascia and arises from the pelvic surface of the pubic bone (lateral to the symphysis pubis) and posteriorly from the ischial spine. In between, it takes its origin from the internal obturator fascia (tendinous arch). The pubococcygeal muscle fans out and forms two parts, which are inserted differently. The anterior fibres decussate around the vagina and pass to the perineal body and anal canal. Although anteriorly the fibres of the pubococcygeal muscle are in close relation to the urethra, they are not structurally attached to it (Gosling 1981). Posterior fibres join the raphe formed by the iliococcygeal muscle. The deeper fibres of each side unite behind the anorectal junction to form the puborectal muscle, which slings the anorectal junction from the pubic bone. The fibres of the iliococcygeal muscle proceed downwards medially and backwards to be inserted into the last two pieces of the coccyx and into a median fibrous raphe that extends from the tip

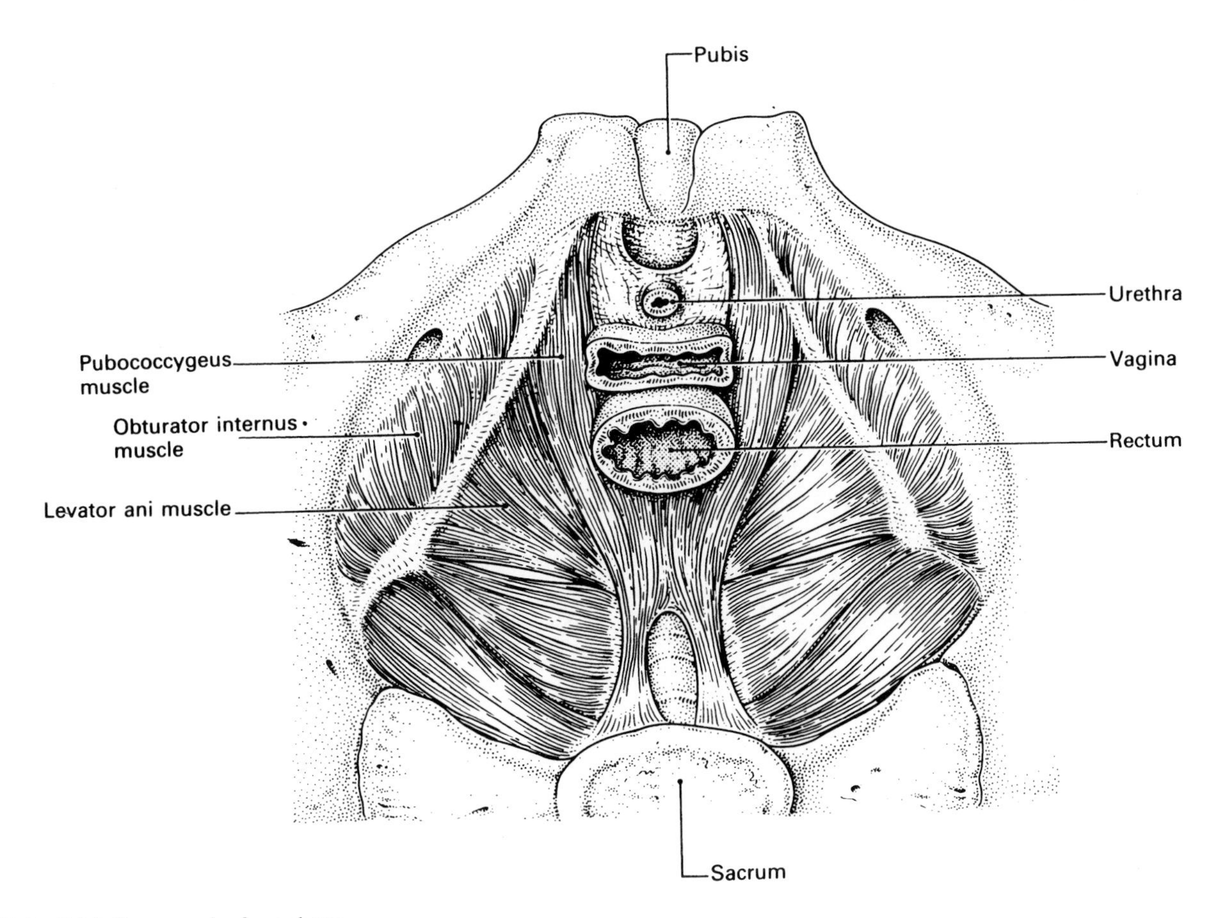

Fig. 51.5 Pelvic floor muscles from above.

of the coccyx to the anus. The muscle is supplied by the anterior primary rami of S3 and S4.

The coccygeal muscle is a flat, triangular muscle arising from the ischial spine and in the same place as the iliococcygeal muscle. It is inserted into the lateral margin of the lower two pieces of the sacrum and the upper two pieces of the coccyx. Its nerve supply is the anterior primary rami S3 and S4.

Both of these muscles act as support for the pelvic viscera and as sphincters for the rectum and vagina. Contraction of the pubococcygeal muscle will also arrest the urinary stream.

These muscles are aided by the muscles of the urogenital diaphragm – the superficial and deep perineal muscles that originate from the ischial rami and are inserted into the perineal body (Fig. 51.6). They are supplied by the perineal branch of the pudendal nerve (S2 and S4) and brace the perineum against the downward pressure from the pelvic floor. The muscles are covered superiorly by fascia continuous with that over the levator ani and internal obturator muscles, and inferiorly by fascia called the perineal membrane.

Pelvic ligaments

The pelvic ligaments are condensations of pelvic fascia that sling the cervix, uterus and upper part of the vagina from the walls of the pelvis. They include the following.

1. The pubocervical ligament (pubocervical fascia) extends from the anterior aspect of the cervix to the back of the body of the pubis.
2. The lateral cervical ligament (transverse cervical, Mackenrodt or cardinal ligaments) extends from the lateral aspect of the cervix and upper vagina to the pelvic side walls. It is the lower part of the broad ligament and nerves and vessels pass through from the pelvic side walls to the uterus. The ureter passes underneath it to the urethrovesical junction. The upper edge of the broad ligament contains the ovarian vessels.
3. The uterosacral ligament extends from the back of the uterus to the front of the sacrum.
4. The posterior pubourethral ligament extends from the posterior inferior aspect of the symphysis to the anterior aspect of the middle third of the urethra and on to the bladder (Fig. 51.7). It maintains elevation of the bladder neck and prevents excess posterior displacement of the urethra (Gosling 1981). It may facilitate micturition and is important in maintaining continence.
5. The round ligament, which is not ligamentous but is formed of smooth muscle, passes from the uterine cornu through the inguinal canal to the labia majus. It is believed

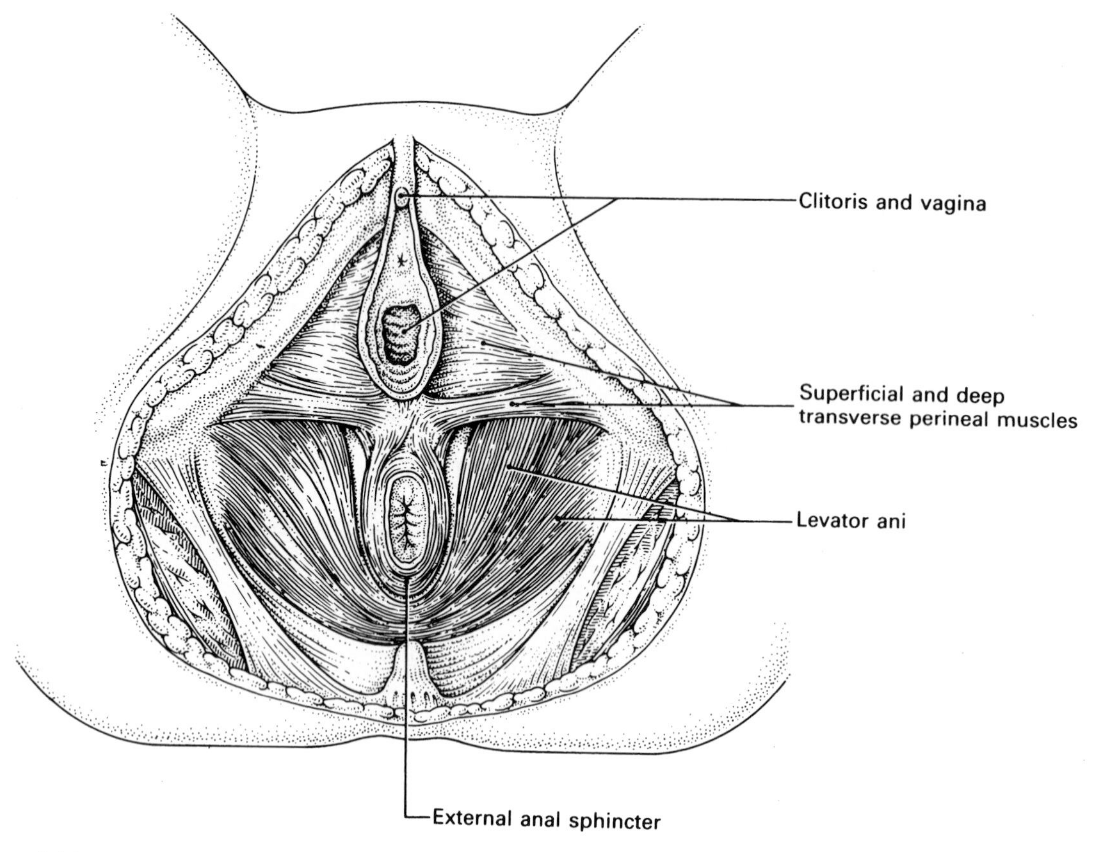

Fig. 51.6 Superficial and deep perineal muscles.

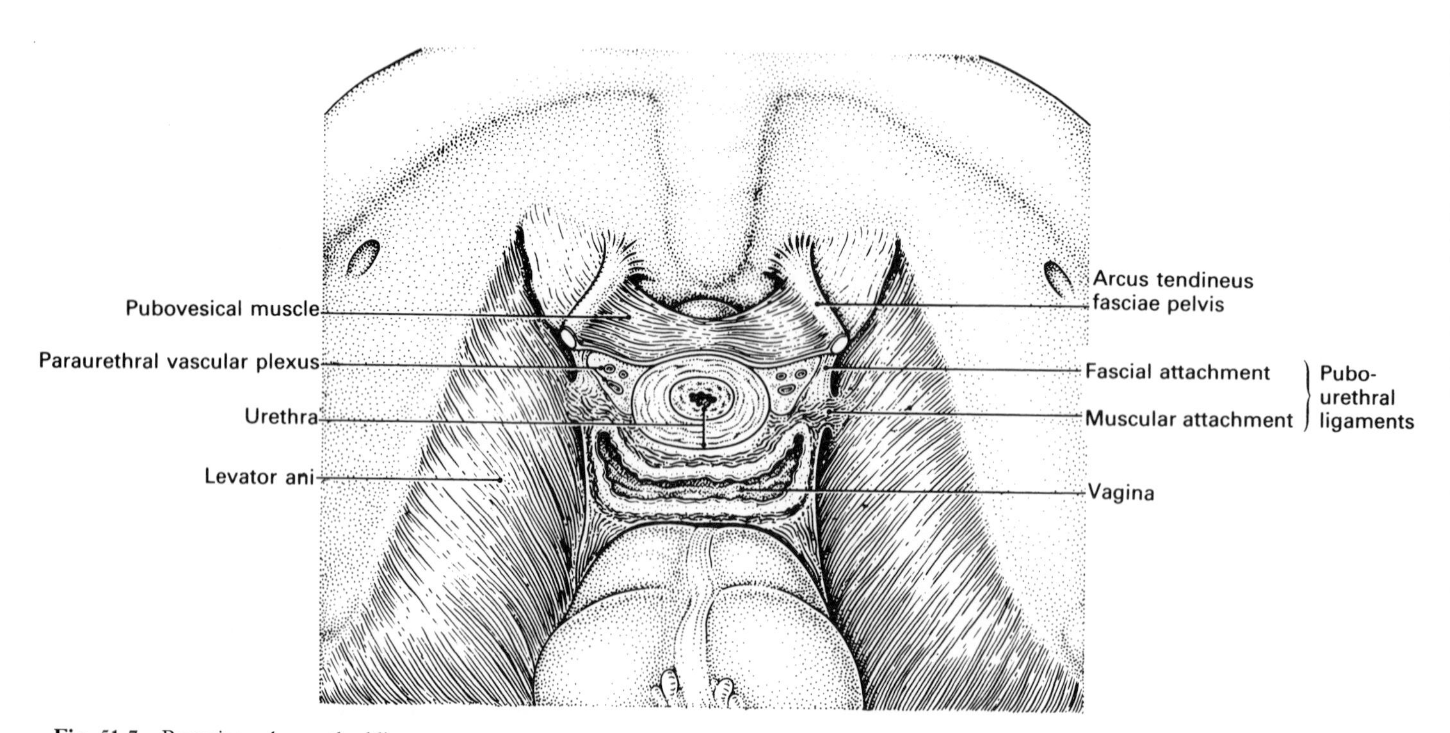

Fig. 51.7 Posterior pubo-urethral ligaments.

to keep the uterus anteflexed but probably plays little part in actually supporting it.

Structures involved in prolapse

A cystocele occurs because the bladder descends either centrally through the pubocervical fascia, or laterally where a break has developed between the attachment of pubocervical fascia from the white line (arcus tendineus) of the pelvic side wall. A large cystocele will carry both the ureterovesical junctions and the lower end of the ureters with it, so that these protrude outside the vagina. This can result in ureteric obstruction, and ureteric damage occurs when these structures are not recognized at surgery.

A urethrocele occurs because of loss of support by the pubocervical fascia and posterior pubourethral ligaments. The latter are probably the most important structures supporting the urethrovesical junction and maintaining continence.

Descent of the uterus and cervix occurs when the lateral cervical ligaments become weakened. Sometimes, particularly in prolapse associated with nulliparity, the cervix elongates and the uterus descends without any cystocele but with an enterocele; condensations of pelvic fascia are inadequately developed and lack their normal resilience.

Vault prolapse occurs following abdominal or vaginal hysterectomy, owing to failure to support the vault adequately using the lateral cervical ligaments or to inadequate strength of these ligaments, or to failure to correct an enterocele at the time of hysterectomy. It usually contains small bowel or omentum, and may accompany uterine descent or follow a colposuspension. It used to be a common sequel to vaginal hysterectomy until its prevention was noted and a prophylactic high fascial repair performed (Hawksworth & Roux 1958). Failure despite this may be caused by the presence of deep urethrovesical and uterorectal peritoneal pouches.

A rectocele represents increased hiatus between the left and right portions of the levator ani muscle, and may be accompanied by tears in the rectovaginal septum (Richardson 1993). However, care must be used in interpreting imaging of rectoceles as up to 77% of healthy women may show a rectocele on defecography (Shorvon et al 1989).

AETIOLOGY

Congenital weakness of pelvic floor ligaments and fascia may be found with spina bifida or bladder exstrophy, or when there is an underlying abnormality in connective tissue – principally collagen and elastin, e.g. type IV Ehlers–Danlos syndrome. Joint hypermobility, which is a clinical marker for connective tissue abnormalities, has been shown to be associated with a higher prevalence of genital prolapse than is normal joint mobility (Norton et al 1995). Congenital shortness of the vaginal and deep uterovesical or uterorectal peritoneal pouches may also be responsible (Jeffcoate 1967). Finally, Bump (1993) showed that in relation to parity, black women have less chance of developing a prolapse than do white women, presumably owing to a different structure of connective tissue and a greater tendency to form keloid.

Factors which may initiate prolapse include prolonged or difficult labour, bearing down before full dilatation, multiparity, a baby weighing more than 4 kg and forceful delivery of the placenta. Other causes include chronically raised intra-abdominal pressure due to pulmonary disease, heavy lifting, chronic straining during bowel movement, ageing and oestrogen deficiency, and vitamin C deprivation.

Electrophysiological studies have shown that there are denervation changes in the pelvic floor (and anal sphincter) following vaginal delivery, and that these may lead to prolapse and temporary and sometimes permanent urinary or faecal incontinence (Snooks et al 1984, Swash 1984, Allen et al 1990, Sayer et al 1990).

Where prolapse and stress incontinence coexist it is likely that the collagen is weaker and there is more denervation than in patients with prolapse only.

The role of positions other than squatting for delivery is believed by some clinicians to be instrumental in causing prolapse. Indeed, in countries where squatting is the normal position of delivery and where women return early to heavy physical work, the incidence of prolapse is lower.

PRESENTATION

Symptoms

Symptoms of prolapse depend not necessarily on the size but on the site and type of prolapse. The discomfort experienced is usually caused by abnormal tension on nerves in the tissues that are being stretched.

Cystocele and cystourethrocele

Prolapse of the bladder and urethra may lead to dragging discomfort, the sensation of a lump in the vagina and urinary symptoms, the most common of which is stress incontinence. This will be present if there is descent of the urethrovesical junction or if delivery and repeated operations have produced scarring around the urethra and bladder neck, leading to inadequate urethral closure. About 50% of patients with urethral sphincter incompetence and stress incontinence have a cystourethrocele; therefore prolapse is not the sole cause of this condition. Voiding difficulty can occur if a large cystocele is present and the bladder neck is anchored normally. This can lead to overflow incontinence. It can be corrected temporarily by replacing the prolapse manually. If sufficient urine is being voided but a chronic residual urine remains, the patient may complain of frequency and inadequate emptying, and a urinary tract infection may supervene.

Urgency and frequency are found in association with cystocele and its correction may relieve these symptoms, although not invariably. It is therefore unwise to perform a repair operation just for these symptoms, especially without excluding other causes of urgency and frequency (e.g. detrusor instability) beforehand. A patient with incontinence may develop frequency and urgency as a self-induced habit to keep the bladder empty. She voids at frequent intervals, believing that incontinence is better controlled if the bladder is kept as empty as possible. From time to time, while endeavouring unsuccessfully to find a toilet, she may experience urgency. If this pattern is repeated, urgency becomes an established symptom. Certainly these symptoms are often linked, and cure of one may lead to cure of both (Stanton et al 1976).

Uterine descent

Uterine descent may cause low backache, which is relieved by lying flat or temporarily using a ring pessary to support the prolapse. A patient with procidentia may complain of protrusion of the cervix and a bloodstained, sometimes purulent, vaginal discharge.

Enterocele or vault prolapse

An enterocele or vault prolapse may produce only vague symptoms of vaginal discomfort. Because an enterocele is often associated with other prolapse, it can be difficult to ascribe separate symptoms to it. Rarely, dehiscence of the vault may occur and the patient complains of acute pain; small bowel may be seen at the vulva (Fig. 51.8). This can strangulate and is an acute abdominal emergency.

Rectocele

This gives rise to symptoms of backache, a lump in the vagina and incomplete bowel emptying; the patient may have discovered that digital reduction of the rectocele allows completion of bowel action.

Signs

Certain predisposing conditions to prolapse, such as chronic cough and constipation, may be present. A patient complaining of prolapse should be examined in the lithotomy or left lateral position using a Sims' speculum. Stress incontinence is most likely to be demonstrated if the bladder is full. The patient is asked to cough or bear down, and any anterior wall prolapse or uterine descent will be demonstrated by retracting the posterior vaginal wall. Sometimes the patient may have to stand up to show prolapse or stress incontinence. Enterocele and rectocele can be demonstrated by using the speculum to retract the anterior vaginal wall. If the rectocele protrudes and obscures an enterocele, it can be reduced by the examining finger, and an enterocele will be either seen at the tip of the examining finger or felt as an impulse on coughing. Further differentiation can be made by asking the patient to cough while the rectum and vagina are simultaneously examined. If the cervix protrudes outside the vagina it may be ulcerated and hypertrophied, with thickening of the epithelium and keratinization. Carcinoma of the cervix is not a sequel to long-standing procidentia but may be a coincidental finding. A full pelvic examination should always be performed to exclude a pelvic mass that might cause prolapse.

Differential diagnosis

A variety of conditions can mimic prolapse of the anterior

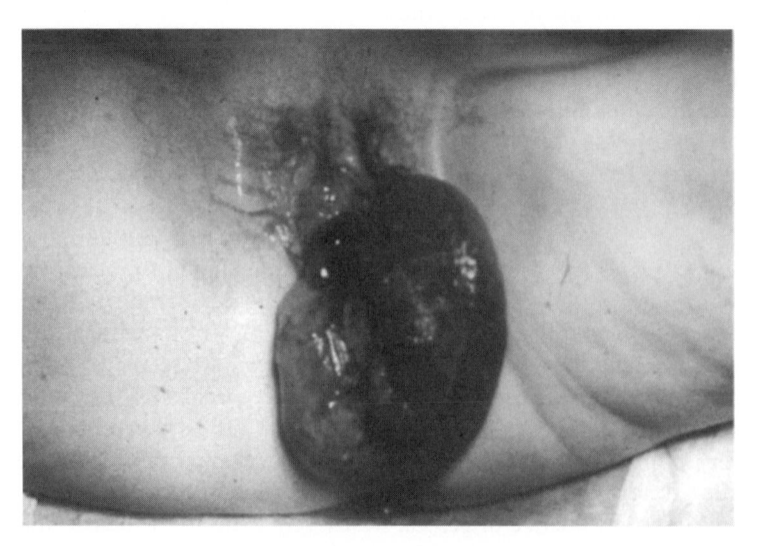

Fig. 51.8 Dehiscence of vault and presentation of small bowel at the vulva.

vaginal wall, such as congenital anterior vaginal wall cyst (e.g. a remnant of the mesonephric duct system or Gartner's duct), a urethral diverticulum, metastases from a uterine tumour (e.g. choriocarcinoma or adenocarcinoma) and an inclusion dermoid cyst following trauma or surgery. Procidentia can be confused with a large cervical or endometrial polyp or chronic uterine inversion.

INVESTIGATION

When urinary symptoms are present a midstream specimen of urine must be sent for culture and sensitivity testing before any investigations are undertaken. Urodynamic studies should be carried out, and include twin-channel cystometry and uroflowmetry. If there is frequency a urinary diary should be completed and an early morning urine sample sent for acid-fast bacilli culture. If there is doubt about bladder capacity, a cystoscopy should be performed under general anaesthetic. The anterior vaginal wall can be very adequately imaged using perineal ultrasound with simultaneous bladder pressure recordings (Creighton et al 1992). This avoids the disadvantage of X-ray irradiation. However, simultaneous imaging of the remainder of the pelvis is best obtained using radiological techniques. Pelvic fluoroscopy has been described by Altringer et al (1995) and entails the introduction of barium contrast into the bladder, small bowel, vagina and rectum. The patient sits on a commode and is encouraged first to contract her pelvic floor muscles, then to strain down, and then to evacuate bladder and rectum. Unfortunately, the technique reveals prolapse which may not be visible clinically and vice versa, and validation of this technique is still required.

Magnetic resonance imaging (MRI) has been attempted for all compartments (Yang et al 1991). However, the difficulty of effectively demonstrating prolapse in the supine position and without simultaneously being able to provide a reliable measure of intra-abdominal pressure and cost, limits the practical usefulness of this technique at present.

For posterior compartmental prolapse a defecating proctogram will show anatomical changes. For the functional and anatomical evaluation, scintigraphic defecography has been developed. Technetium 99m-labelled 'porridge' is introduced into the rectum and a γ-camera image records the descent of the pelvic floor and rectum, together with the mean evacuation times of the rectum and rectocele and the amount retained within the rectocele (Hutchinson et al 1993).

TREATMENT

It is important to ensure that the woman's symptoms are caused by prolapse and not by other pelvic or spinal conditions. The patient should be told that, provided there is no urinary tract obstruction or infection, prolapse carries no risk to life. It is preferable to have completed childbearing because a successful pelvic floor repair can be disrupted by a further vaginal delivery. Coital activity must be taken into account and narrowing of the vagina carefully avoided. Obese patients should be referred to a dietitian for dietary control, and chronic cough and constipation should be corrected as far as possible. Ulceration of the cervix (after first excluding any neoplastic lesion) may be managed by reducing the uterine prolapse and applying oestrogen cream, if not contraindicated. The ulcer will usually heal within 7 days.

Prevention

Shortening the first, and particularly the second, stage of delivery with increased operative intervention and a decline in parity are likely to decrease the incidence of prolapse. The role of episiotomy is uncertain and controversial. Postnatal exercises have little proven scientific evidence to support their benefit, but are traditionally advised. Hormone replacement therapy given at the time of the menopause may help prevent the development of postmenopausal prolapse, but is unlikely to alter established prolapse.

Medical

Before safe anaesthesia and surgery, prolapse was managed by a variety of ingenious pessaries of differing shapes and sizes. Today the role of the pessary is more restricted and is indicated as follows:

1. During and after pregnancy (awaiting involution of tissues);
2. As a therapeutic test to confirm that surgery might help;
3. When the patient has not completed her childbearing, or is medically unfit or refuses surgery and prefers conservative management;
4. For relief of symptoms while the patient is awaiting surgery.

In the past pessaries were made of vulcanized rubber and had to be changed every 3 months. Today they are made of inert plastic and can be left in place for up to a year, provided there are no adverse symptoms or signs. The most common pessary is ring-shaped and is available in a variety of sizes. Shelf pessaries may be helpful. The two main complications are vaginal ulceration (if the pessary is too large or there is loss of vaginal sensation) and incarceration leading to vaginal discharge and bleeding (when the pessary has been forgotten and not changed for several years).

When prolapse occurs during pregnancy, reposition of the prolapse and insertion of a ring pessary, with additional vaginal packing if necessary, and bed rest may be sufficient.

Physiotherapy and electrical stimulation of the pelvic floor muscles have a minor role in the management of established prolapse.

Surgical

The surgical repair of prolapse is one of the oldest gynaecological procedures. The majority of operations are performed through the vagina, and the abdominal route is reserved for recurrence or more complex prolapse. The aims of surgery are to correct the prolapse, to maintain continence and to preserve coital function.

Cystourethrocele

Traditionally an anterior colporrhaphy or anterior repair has been used to correct cystocele or cystourethrocele and stress incontinence. Nowadays it is less frequently used for stress incontinence, because it has a lower success rate than urethrovesical suspension procedures. The essential features are a vertical anterior vaginal wall incision and dissection to display the proximal two-thirds of the urethra, the urethrovesical junction and part of the bladder base. The urethrovesical junction is repositioned higher in the pelvis using one of two Kelly sutures (Fig. 51.9). The cystocele is then reduced by the insertion of several interrupted sutures in the overlying pubocervical fascia, which is found attached to the underside of the vaginal skin. Surplus vaginal skin is excised and the wound closed with an interrupted or continuous suture.

There are many variations on this procedure. Pacey (1949) emphasized the importance of locating the edge of the pubococcygeal muscle and coating this in the midline. Ingelman-Sundberg (1946) advocated cutting the pubococcygeal muscle behind the midpoint and uniting the anterior portion in the midline to form a further support for the bladder neck, while laterally fixing the posterior portion of the muscle.

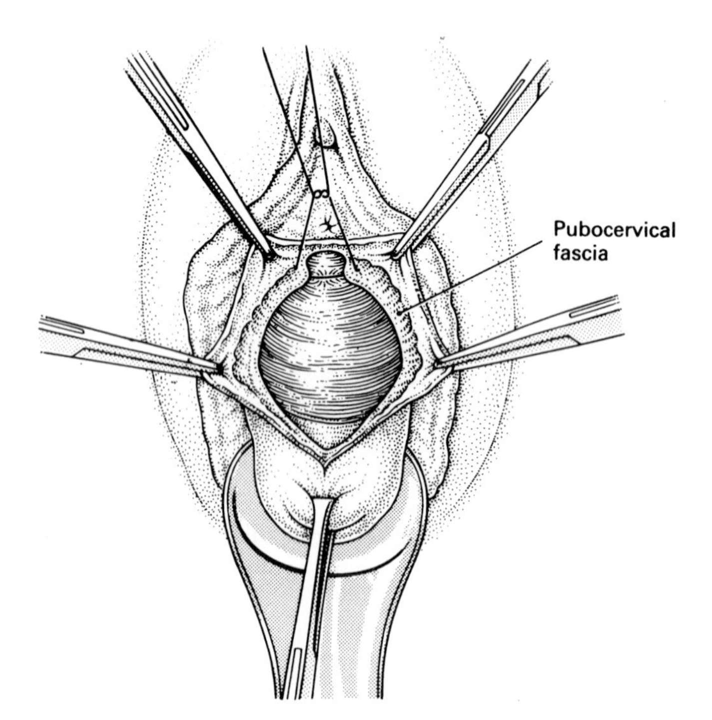

Fig. 51.9 Fascial repair in anterior colporrhaphy.

Approximately 50% of patients will suffer postoperative urinary retention following an anterior repair, which can be avoided by using a suprapubic catheter. This allows the patient to void spontaneously and is more comfortable and less prone to urinary infection than a urethral catheter. The catheter is clamped on the second postoperative day and is removed when the patient is voiding amounts greater than 200 ml, with a residual urine volume of less than 150 ml.

One of the most important complications that can occur following an anterior colporrhaphy is the development of incontinence in a patient who was hitherto dry. It is likely to be caused by interference with the sphincter mechanism during dissection, leading to inadequate support and elevation of that region.

If the cystocele coexists with a first- or second-degree uterine prolapse and a rectocele, a Manchester repair can be performed. This is an older procedure and less commonly used today. It consists of amputation of the cervix, and an anterior and posterior repair. Its disadvantages are:

1. The uterus is left behind, and this can prolapse further or may contain unsuspected disease, or be the future site for a carcinoma. Bonnar et al (1970) found unsuspected lesions in 26% of uteri removed at hysterectomy for prolapse.
2. It does not effectively allow an enterocele to be corrected.

The Burch colposuspension can very effectively correct a cystocele accompanied by stress incontinence caused by urethral sphincter incompetence (Burch 1961) (Fig. 51.10). The lateral fornices are approximated and sutured to the ipsilateral iliopectineal ligaments, producing elevation of the bladder neck and reduction of the cystourethrocele (Stanton et al 1976, Stanton & Cardozo 1979). Enteroceles and rectoceles are complications of this procedure.

An alternative to the anterior colporrhaphy is the paravaginal repair, which corrects breaks in the pubocervical fascia by reattaching it to the white line using permanent sutures. This can be performed abdominally (Richardson et al 1981, Youngblood 1993) or vaginally (Shull et al 1994).

Uterine prolapse

The vaginal hysterectomy is the preference today for correction of uterine prolapse.

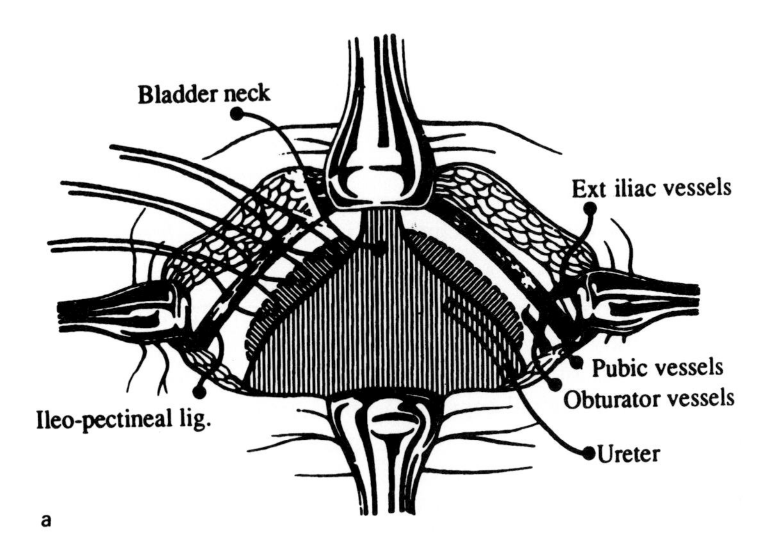

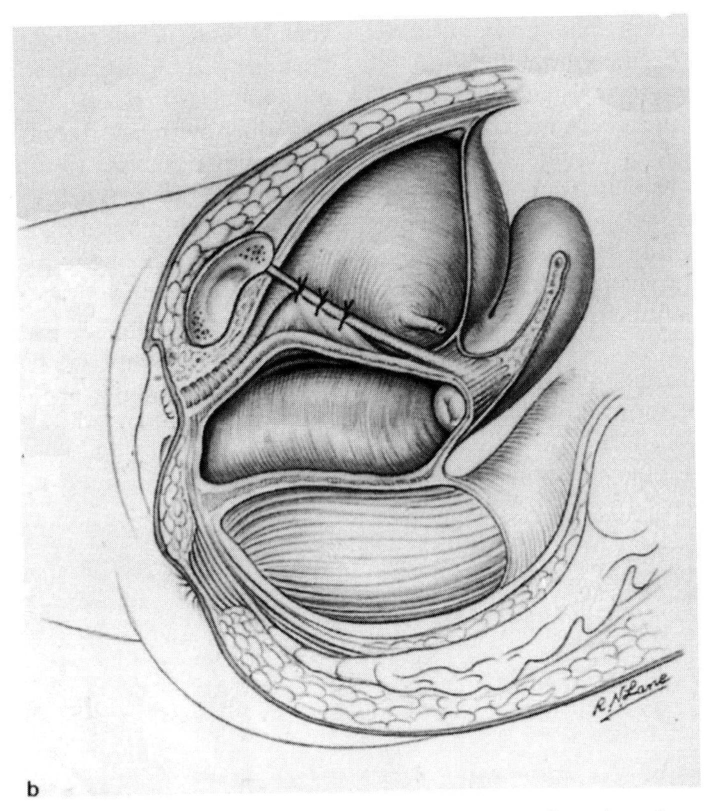

Fig. 51.10 Burch colposuspension. **a** plan view looking down through a Pfannenstiel incision. **b** sagittal view at end of colposuspension.

The vaginal hysterectomy can be combined with an anterior or posterior colporrhaphy and correction of an enterocele by coaptation of the uterosacral ligaments. Indeed, most surgeons carry out prophylactic coaptation of these ligaments at the time of hysterectomy, to avoid a future enterocele and vault prolapse.

A vaginal hysterectomy is indicated:

1. For uterine prolapse: a uterus up to 20 weeks in size (1100 g) may be removed by vaginal morcellation (Magos et al 1996);
2. For recurrent uterine prolapse following a Manchester repair;
3. When the patient is obese. Pitkin (1976) has shown that abdominal wound complications are seven times more common in women weighing more than 90 kg who have undergone abdominal hysterectomy. With a vaginal hysterectomy there is no difference in morbidity or length

of stay when comparing obese women and those of normal weight (Pitkin 1977);

4. Where a painful abdominal wound is undesirable and early ambulation is advantageous (e.g. in pulmonary disease or the elderly);

5. Where non-malignant uterine pathology (e.g. dysfunctional uterine bleedings) exists and where it is technically feasible to remove the uterus.

The assessment for vaginal hysterectomy is important. The subpubic arch should be sufficiently wide to accommodate two fingers, which will allow the operator access to the uterus. There should be sufficient vaginal capacity to allow surgery to be carried out, and clinical experience, with the help of an episiotomy, will determine this. Unless morcellation is intended the uterus should not be larger than 14 weeks in size. It is wise to avoid vaginal hysterectomy where there is the likelihood of bowel adhering to the fundus of the uterus, following previous pelvic surgery, or where ventrosuspension has been performed.

The principles of vaginal hysterectomy include careful upward displacement of the bladder and ureters, ligation of each main pedicle and repair of any enterocele. The ovaries are inspected, and if there is ovarian pathology or the woman is over 50 years of age, vaginal oophorectomy can easily be accomplished at the same time (Sheth 1991). The pedicles are then approximated to each other in pairs to reform the roof of the vault. The uterosacral ligaments are united and the vaginal skin closed, first securing the posterior fornix skin to the new vault. If a vaginal hysterectomy alone is performed, bladder drainage is unnecessary.

When the woman wishes to retain her uterus a sacrohysteropexy is performed. The junction of the cervix and uterus is attached to the anterior longitudinal ligament over the first sacral vertebra by an inorganic graft such as Teflon, which should then be peritonealized.

Enterocele or vault repair

Most enteroceles can be repaired at the time of abdominal surgery, by coaptation of the uterosacral ligaments. The more extensive procedure described by Moschowitz has the danger of inclusion of a ureter when inserting the pursestring sutures into the pouch of Douglas peritoneum, and as there is little inherent strength in this peritoneum it seems an unnecessary procedure.

The initial decision to use the vaginal suprapubic route of access depends on the patient's general state and whether or not she wishes to continue intercourse. The vaginal route is simpler and provides a relatively painfree postoperative recovery, but may preclude intercourse if an overenthusiastic repair is performed. In an older patient it is frequently impossible to find adequate or convincing uterosacral ligaments to bring together. The sacrospinous fixation operation (Nichols 1982) does not compromise vaginal size, but the surgery is carried out under limited visibility and damage to pudendal vessels and nerves is a recognized hazard. There is a significant risk of cystocele and stress incontinence following this procedure. If intercourse is not intended it is easier to obliterate the vagina, placing successive pursestring sutures to include the uterosacral ligaments and then the levator ani, and finally the superficial perineal muscles.

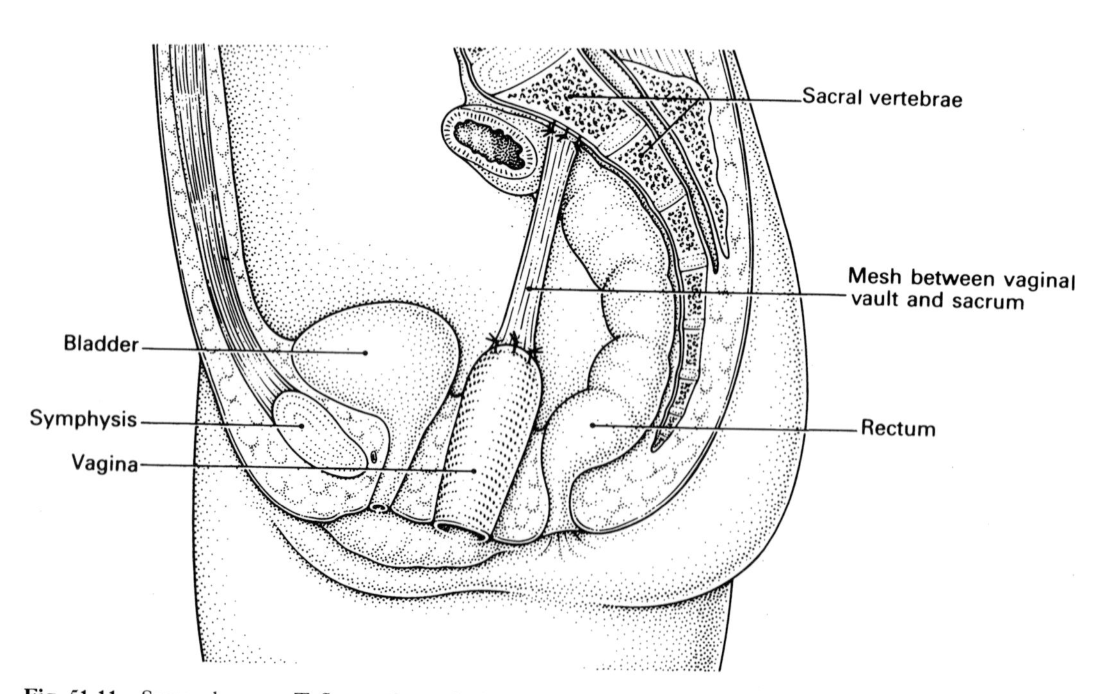

Fig. 51.11 Sacrocolpopexy. Teflon mesh attached to vault and to anterior longitudinal ligament over sacral 1 vertebra.

Where there is recurrent prolapse and intercourse is intended, most clinicians prefer the abdominal route. With the sacrocolpopexy (Birnbaum 1973; Fig. 51.11) the vault is attached by a non-absorbable mesh (Terylene or Teflon) to the anterior longitudinal ligament of the first sacral vertebra. Care has to be taken here because the venous plexus is in front of this ligament and the pelvic nerves are lateral. The mesh is peritonealized, to avoid bowel becoming trapped underneath it.

Results indicate that although this a very effective operation for support of the vault, stress incontinence may occur in 7–33% of patients according to series in the literature, presumably owing to excess tension on the anterior vaginal wall interfering with the urethral sphincter mechanism. Our own series of 41 cases had a cure rate of vault prolapse of 88%; one case developed stress incontinence de novo and four suffered deterioration in their stress incontinence (Valaitis & Stanton 1994).

Laparoscopic sacrocolpopexy has been undertaken in a number of centres with interesting results, but the technique has by no means been validated, nor are long-term results yet available.

Vault procedures have been critically reviewed by Wall and Stanton (1988).

Rectocele

Because of complications following posterior colporrhaphy, namely dyspareunia and bowel symptoms, this operation should not be carried out as a routine accompaniment to anterior colporrhaphy in the management of pelvic floor prolapse; instead, there should be sound indications for its use: a symptomatic rectocele producing a lump; incomplete rectal evacuation or needing digitation or splinting to aid evacuation; or slackness at intercourse. Any patient with coincident bowel dysfunction, such as faecal incontinence or constipation, may need anorectal investigation before undergoing surgery (Kahn & Stanton 1996).

The operations to correct rectocele are the conventional posterior colporrhaphy, endorectal or transrectal repair and placement of a mesh between the vagina and rectum to support the rectovaginal fascia. Laparoscopic repair of enterocele still requires validation and is of uncertain value.

The technique of posterior colporrhaphy involves dissection of the levator ani muscles and rectum via a vertical posterior vaginal wall incision. The levator muscles and then the superficial perineal muscles are sutured together; any excess vaginal skin is minimally excised and the wound closed with a continuous locking stitch to avoid vaginal wall shortening.

Bladder drainage may be required, especially in elderly patients because they may not immediately resume spontaneous micturition following pelvic surgery.

To minimize the risk of postoperative infection by anaerobic organisms, 1 g metronidazole is given rectally 2 hours prior to surgery.

CONCLUSION

Pelvic floor weakness resulting in prolapse with or without incontinence is a common gynaecological entity. Because of the involvement of bowel and bladder, a pelvic floor reconstruction team with colorectal, urological and gynaecological expertise is invaluable for dealing with complex prolapse.

KEY POINTS

1. Prolapse may be due to congenital disorders such as collagen and elastin weakness, as well as to denervation and muscle trauma following childbirth.
2. Additional aetiological factors include chronic straining on defecation and oestrogen deficiency at the menopause.
3. Only 50% of patients with a cystourethrocele have stress incontinence.
4. Prolapse is benign, except where third-degree uterine prolapse may be associated with ureteric obstruction.
5. A large enterocele may require prompt surgery, as vault dehiscence with extrusion of bowel can occur.
6. Surgery is the most usual form of treatment for prolapse, but should be deferred until childbearing and vaginal delivery have been completed or an elective caesarean section chosen.
7. The anterior repair is a reliable cure for a cystourethrocele but not for the correction of stress incontinence.
8. Ultrasound and radiological imaging may be helpful with the investigation of the more complex prolapse.
9. Dyspareunia can follow a rectocele and its choice should be carefully indicated.

REFERENCES

Allen R, Hosker G, Smith A, Warrell D 1990 Pelvic floor damage and childbirth: a neurophysiological study. British Journal of Obstetrics and Gynaecology 97: 770–779

Altringer W, Saclaraides T, Domingez J, Brubaker L C 1995 Four contrast defecography: pelvic 'floor-oscopy'. Diseases of the Colon and Rectum 38: 695–699

Birnbaum S J 1973 Rational therapy for the prolapsed vagina. American Journal of Obstetrics and Gynecology 115: 411–419
Bonnar J, Kraszewski A, Davis W 1970 Incidental pathology at vaginal hysterectomy for genital prolapse. British Journal of Obstetrics and Gynaecology 77: 1137–1139
Bump R 1993 Racial comparisons and contrasts in urinary incontinence and pelvic organ prolapse. Obstetrics and Gynecology 81: 421–425
Burch J C 1961 Urethro-vaginal fixation to Cooper's ligament for correction of stress incontinence. American Journal of Obstetrics and Gynecology 100: 768–774
Creighton S, Pearce J, Stanton S L 1992 Perineal video-ultrasonography in the assessment of vaginal prolapse – early observations. British Journal of Obstetrics and Gynaecology 99: 310–313
Gosling J 1981 Why are women continent? Proceedings of symposium on 'The incontinent woman'. Royal College of Obstetricians and Gynaecologists, London
Hawksworth W, Roux J 1958 Vaginal hysterectomy. British Journal of Obstetrics and Gynaecology 65: 214–228
Hutchinson R, Mostafa A, Grant et al 1993 Scintifigraphic defecography: quantitative and dynamic assessment of ano-rectal function. Diseases of the Colon and Rectum 36: 1132–1138
ICS 1994 Standardisation of terminology of female pelvic organ prolapse and pelvic floor dysfunction. International Continence Society Committee on Standardisation of Terminology
Ingelman-Sundberg A 1946 Operative technique in stress incontinence of urine in the female. Nordisk Medicine 32: 2297–2299
Jeffcoate T N A 1967 Principles of gynaecology, 3rd edn. Butterworths, London
Kahn M, Stanton S L 1996 Posterior colporrhaphy: its effect on bowel and sexual function. British Journal of Obstetrics and Gynaecology (in press)
Lewis A C 1968 Major gynaecological surgery in the elderly. Journal of the International Federation of Gynaecology and Obstetrics 6: 244–258
Magos A, Bournas N, Sinha R, Richardson R, O'Connor H 1996 Vaginal hysterectomy for the large uterus. British Journal of Obstetrics and Gynaecology 103: 246–251
Nichols D 1982 Sacrospinous fixation for massive eversion of the vagina. American Journal of Obstetrics and Gynecology 142: 901–904
Norton P, Baker J, Sharp H, Warenski J 1995 Genito-urinary prolapse and joint hypermobility. Obstetrics and Gynecology 85: 225–228
Pacey K 1949 Pathology and repair of genital prolapse. Journal of Obstetrics and Gynaecology of the British Empire 56: 1–15
Pitkin R M 1976 Abdominal hysterectomy in obese women. Surgery, Gynecology and Obstetrics 142: 532–536
Pitkin R M 1977 Vaginal hysterectomy in obese women. Obstetrics and Gynecology 49: 567–569
Richardson A C 1993 The recto-vaginal septum revisited: its relationship to rectocele and its importance in rectocele repair. Clinical Obstetrics and Gynecology 36: 976–983
Richardson A C, Edmonds P, Williams N 1981 Treatment of stress incontinence due to paravaginal and fascial defect. Obstetrics and Gynecology 57: 357–363
Sayer T, Dixon H, Hosker G, Warrell D 1990 A study of paraurethral connective tissue in women with stress incontinence of urine. Neurourology and Urodynamics 9: 319–320
Sheth S 1991 Place of oophorectomy at vaginal hysterectomy. British Journal of Obstetrics and Gynaecology 98: 662–666
Shorvon R, McHugh S, Diamant N et al 1989 Defaecography in normal volunteers: results and implications. Gut 30: 1737–1749
Shull B, Benn S, Kuehl T 1994 Surgical management of prolapse of the anterior vaginal segment: an analysis of support defects, operative morbidity and anatomic outcome. American Journal of Obstetrics and Gynecology 171: 1429–1439
Snooks S, Swash M, Henry M, Setchell M 1984 Injury to innervation of the pelvic floor musculature in childbirth. Lancet ii: 546–550
Stallworthy J A 1971 Prolapse. British Medical Journal 1: 499–500, 539–540
Stanton S L, Cardozo L D 1979 Results of colposuspension operation for incontinence and prolapse. British Journal of Obstetrics and Gynaecology 86: 693–697
Stanton S L, Williams J E, Ritchie D 1976 Colposuspension operation for urinary incontinence. British Journal of Obstetrics and Gynaecology 83: 890–895
Swash M 1984 Ano-rectal incontinence: electrophysiological tests. British Journal of Surgery (Suppl): S14–S22
Valaitis S, Stanton S L 1994 Sacrocolpopexy: a retrospective study of a clinician's experience. British Journal of Obstetrics and Gynaecology 101: 518–522
Wall L, Stanton S L 1988 Alternatives for repair of post hysterectomy vault prolapse and enterocele. Contemporary Obstetrics and Gynecology Sept: 32–48
Yang A, Mostwyn J, Rosenheim N, Zerhouni E 1991 Pelvic floor descent in women: dynamic evaluation with fast MRI and cinematic display. Radiology 179: 25–33
Youngblood J 1993 Paravaginal repair for cystourethrocele. Clinical Obstetrics and Gynecology 36: 960–966

52

Frequency, urgency and the painful bladder in the female

A. K. Monga   A. B. Peattie

INTRODUCTION

Frequency, urgency and pain are sensory symptoms affecting the lower urinary tract. They result in poorer quality of life scores than all other urinary symptoms, including incontinence (Kelleher et al 1994). Successful management requires careful patient evaluation and a knowledge of possible causes, including disease outside the urinary tract. Frequency is defined as the passage of urine more than seven times during the waking hours and/or being awakened from sleep twice or more to micturate, whereas urgency is a sudden strong desire to micturate which if not relieved may lead to urge incontinence (Fig. 52.1).

Prevalence

Epidemiological studies have produced varying estimates, with 7.2–20% of women complaining of frequency and 15% complaining of urgency (Bungay et al 1980, RCGP 1981–82). These figures increase to 23% in the elderly (Diokno et al 1986) and 32% in patients with neurological disease (McGrother et al 1987). There is a paucity of reported figures of the prevalence of painful micturition. Milne et al (1972) found that 3% of 200 women had pain on passing urine and a further 21% reported having pain in the past. It is probable that the prevalence of these symptoms is underestimated, as embarrassment prevents 25% of women seeking professional help, despite experiencing severe urinary symptoms for more than 5 years (Norton et al 1988).

Aetiology

Symptoms may be due to bladder or urethral disorder or dysfunction, but systemic disease may also produce urinary tract symptomatology (Fig. 52.1). The bladder may be physically or functionally small due to a number of causes. The urethral syndrome or a urethral diverticulum may give rise to these symptoms, as may diabetes mellitus, diabetes insipidus and hypercalcaemia.

CONDITIONS OUTSIDE THE BLADDER

Urinary frequency and urgency may be the presenting symptoms of a pelvic mass which reduces bladder capacity by external compression; treatment is to remove the mass. Compression symptoms are also common during late pregnancy, although frequency and urgency in early preg-

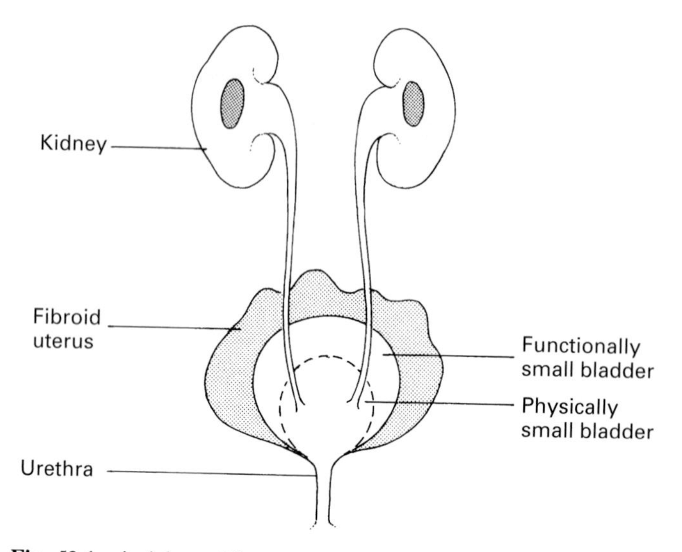

Fig. 52.1 Aetiology of frequency and urgency.

nancy are thought to be a response to increased plasma volume. In later life it is uncertain whether oestrogen deficiency results in frequency and urgency, although the lower urinary tract contains oestrogen-dependent tissues of endodermal origin; benefit from oestrogen replacement is debatable and progestogens exacerbate these symptoms (Benness et al 1991). It is increasingly apparent that urinary and bowel symptoms often coexist, and increased urinary frequency and urgency are reported in women with irritable bowel syndrome (Monga et al 1994). In addition, chronic constipation and faecal impaction are important causes of frequency and urgency in the elderly.

The amount of urine produced will affect the frequency of micturition. Diuretic therapy increases urinary output and is therefore best taken in the morning. Diabetes mellitus and insipidus will be associated with urinary frequency due to increased urinary output. Similarly, an excessive fluid intake will produce frequency: some patients drink large quantities by habit, or have a psychiatric disorder. The usual daily fluid intake is around 2 litres, which varies according to climate and social circumstances. A daily intake of greater than 3 litres will automatically lead to greater urinary production and frequency.

Renal disease

Polyuria is one of the symptoms of chronic renal failure; measurement of the blood urea and electrolyte concentrations and creatinine clearance will demonstrate the degree of renal dysfunction. A midstream urine specimen (MSU) may reveal bacterial infection and granular casts, and urine osmolality should be noted.

After surgery

Radical hysterectomy is known to cause bladder and urethral dysfunction, probably due to disruption of the pelvic nerve plexus which supplies the lower urinary tract. Reports of the incidence of bladder disturbance vary from 16 to 80%, but problems include genuine stress incontinence, frequency and urgency, detrusor instability, voiding disorders and disturbed urethral function (Scotti et al 1986). Symptoms are not transient and persist at 5-year follow-up (Dwyer & O'Callaghan 1993). Whether abdominal hysterectomy causes urinary symptoms remains contentious (Griffith-Jones et al 1991). Bladder-neck surgery for genuine stress incontinence may also result in urgency and frequency. When frequency and urgency are the main problems, infection, detrusor instability and urethral instability must all be considered.

BLADDER DISEASE

The physically small bladder

The conditions discussed in this section cause a reduction in bladder capacity as a consequence of chronic inflammation.

Tuberculosis, schistosomiasis and recurrent urinary tract infection due to conventional organisms

Bladder lesions are always secondary to renal tuberculosis, with infection starting around the ureteric orifices. There is inflammation with granulation and ulceration of the mucous membrane. Fibrous tissue forms in the bladder wall, leading to contraction of the bladder and a reduced capacity. An intravenous urogram is appropriate, as bladder changes are never present without changes in the radiological appearances of the pelvicalyceal system. By this stage conventional triple therapy will not reverse changes in the bladder.

Fibrosis and calcification of the entire lower urinary tract, including the bladder (with resultant urinary frequency), can occur following infection with *Schistosoma haematobium*. Diagnosis is made by identification of ova in urine specimens.

The vast majority of recurrent urinary tract infections are due to reinfection with Gram-negative aerobic bacteria of colonic origin. Recurrent infection causes chronic inflammation and fibrosis.

After radiation

Radiation cystitis can occur as a complication of radiotherapy for pelvic malignancy. Symptoms may occur immediately after completion of treatment or many years later, and are related to field and fraction size as well as total radiation dosage. They include frequency, urgency, suprapubic pain and occasionally haematuria. Acute symptoms usually respond to simple analgesia, but later fibrosis may ensue, causing a physically small bladder with decreased compliance. A 25% reduction in bladder capacity is reported (Parkin et al 1988). Symptoms of frequency and pain may be of sufficient severity to warrant bladder augmentation or a urinary diversion. Cystoscopy reveals a whitened bladder mucosa with characteristic telangiectasia. If the bladder capacity at cystoscopy is 300 ml or greater, then by adjustment of fluid load the patient should be able to achieve a frequency of micturition that is acceptable.

Interstitial cystitis

Interstitial cystitis is one of the most disabling chronic conditions and presents with severe frequency, urgency, lower abdominal pain, dysuria and haematuria in the absence of bacterial cystitis. Hunner (1914) examined a group of women with prolonged symptoms of cystitis: cystoscopy revealed ulcers with a granulomatous base and white urothelial scars, both surrounded by a hyperaemic area which bled when touched. The aetiology remains obscure but infection, allergy, psychosomatic dysfunction and neurogenic disorders have been considered and discredited. Histological findings include infiltration with lymphocytes, plasma cells and mast cells (Larsen et al 1982). These, in conjunction with an increased incidence of coexistent autoimmune disease and the presence of positive antinuclear antibody, have suggested an autoimmune basis but have subsequently been shown to be an immunological response to the disease (Anderson et al 1989). Current theories suggest that the aetiology is related to a dysfunctional epithelium allowing increased leakage of urea. There is an inability to repair the normal protective coat composed of glycosaminoglycans and proteoglycans (Stein & Parsons 1994).

Reported prevalence varies from 5% (Hand 1949) to 50% (Hanash & Pool 1970) in patients with recurrent cystitis. It is more common in caucasians, with a 9:1 female preponderance (Parsons 1994). The majority of patients are between 40 and 60 years of age. The lack of agreement in reported prevalence suggests that diagnostic criteria vary. In an attempt to standardize diagnosis, the National Institute of Arthritis, Diabetes, Digestive and Kidney Diseases published its consensus criteria (1988). The most salient points are listed in Table 52.1. Diagnosis is based on the typical symptom complex, cystoscopic findings of petechial submucosal haemorrhage, fissures, linear scars and Hunner's ulcer (the latter is present in 8% of patients). Bladder biopsies are not pathognomonic but will exclude malignancy.

Table 52.1 Consensus criteria for diagnosis of interstitial cystitis

Automatic exclusions	Automatic inclusions
<18 years age	Hunner's ulcer
Bladder tumour	
Urogenital malignancy	*Positive factors*
Radiation cystitis	
TB cystitis	Pain on bladder filling relieved by emptying
Cyclophosphamide cystitis	Glomerulations at cystoscopy
Bacterial cystitis	Low bladder compliance
Vaginitis	
Active herpes	
Urethral diverticulum	
Bladder calculus	
Daytime frequency <5 in 12 hours	
Nocturia <2	
Duration <12 months	
Capacity >400 ml	
Detrusor instability	
Symptom relief with antibiotics	

The functionally small bladder

Acute inflammation

Infectious cystitis. Common presenting symptoms include frequency, dysuria, suprapubic pain and hesitancy. In addition there may be a fever, loin pain and haematuria, but symptoms alone are not enough for a diagnosis of cystitis due to urinary tract infection. Bacteriological examination of the urine reveals pus cells indicative of inflammation and significant bacteriuria (>10^5 organisms/ml). Treatment comprises a high fluid intake (approx 3 l/day) and appropriate antibiotics. Once an MSU has been sent for culture and sensitivity it is appropriate to treat the symptomatic patient with trimethoprim, amoxycillin or nitrofurantoin. Symptomatic relief may be obtained by alkalinization with potassium citrate or sodium bicarbonate. For women with recurrent problems advice about perineal toilet and voiding before and after sexual intercourse are simple measures that may be helpful.

Chemical cystitis. The symptoms are identical to infection. A careful history, including use of irritant perfumed soap, bubble bath and perineal deodorants, may help to avoid the causative agent.

Detrusor instability

Detrusor instability or motor urge incontinence is characterized by involuntary detrusor contractions which the patient cannot suppress. The commonest presenting symptoms are frequency and urgency. The diagnosis is made by subtracted cystometry. This topic is discussed further in Chapter 49.

Sensory urgency

This condition is diagnosed by exclusion: the patient complains of urgency but on cystometric testing no abnormality is detected – more specifically, detrusor instability is absent. The incidence is difficult to determine as the condition is often managed and classed with motor urge incontinence or detrusor instability. Precise volumes for first sensation have been suggested but are not in routine use; however, heightened perception of bladder volume has been demonstrated (Creighton et al 1991). MacCaulay et al (1987) found equal anxiety scores in women with sensory urgency and detrusor instability, but those with sensory urgency scored higher on hysteria scales. Six percent of patients attending for urodynamics in our unit have sensory urgency, compared to 31% with detrusor instability. It is difficult to justify treating these patients similarly as it is recognized that anticholinergic medication for detrusor instability has troublesome side effects and poor results.

The aetiology of this condition is unclear; it is not known whether it represents a prodromal form of detrusor instability or whether it is a discrete clinical entity. Some cases of detrusor instability are missed during conventional subtracted cystometry, and it is possible that these are labelled as sensory urgency. Unfortunately, ambulatory monitoring detects detrusor contractions in asymptomatic controls as well as those with sensory urgency, and therefore its diagnostic role is uncertain (van Waalwijk van Doorn et al 1992, Robertson et al 1994).

Neither cystometry nor urethral pressure measurement provide helpful information about bladder-neck activity. Urethral electric conductance (UEC) has shown that bladder-neck opening correlates well with symptoms of urgency (Peattie et al 1988). UEC uses the principle that urothelium and urine have different electric impedances and a specially designed conductivity catheter can detect opening of the bladder neck. In patients with sensory urgency the recording obtained showed marked variation, associated with the sensation of urgency.

Poor habit

Although children are taught to control detrusor contractions and to void voluntarily at the appropriate time and place, this control can deteriorate. Voiding at first sensation or 'prophylactically' before leaving home may lead to a vicious cycle of frequency and urgency and a reduced functional capacity.

Voiding disorder

Urinary frequency and urgency may be associated with chronic retention and overflow incontinence (see Ch. 50).

Neuropathic bladder

Patients with suprasacral lesions who retain cortical control will have detrusor–sphincter dyssynergia, which may cause severe frequency, and urgency with incomplete bladder emptying.

Long-term catheterization

As a consequence of chronic catheterization the bladder can become fibrotic and contracted. If the catheter is removed severe urgency and frequency may be encountered.

URETHRAL CONDITIONS

Urethral syndrome

This term has been applied to a symptom complex comprising frequency, urgency, dysuria and voiding disorder, where no cause can be found and symptoms persist despite all attempts at treatment. The prevalence of the condition is unknown. At initial presentation the patient is often misdiagnosed as having a urinary tract infection. Treatment with antibiotics may give symptomatic relief, but the symptoms return and may become refractory to antibiotic therapy. The other common feature is suprapubic pain, often described as a feeling of pressure and relieved by micturition. Sometimes the pain is more localized to the vagina or the urethra, and relief of pain is thought to be associated with relaxation of the urethral sphincter. The spectrum of symptoms includes hesitancy, dribbling and intermittent stream, suggesting urethral sphincter dysfunction as a possible cause.

There are many proposed aetiologies, including infection with fastidious organisms not identified by standard culture techniques; urethral sphincter spasm; urethral obstruction; neuropathy; oestrogen deficiency; trauma; and psychological problems. Diagnosis is made by exclusion of infection, malignancy and detrusor instability. *Chlamydia* infection diagnosed from urethral swabs may be identified in one-third of patients presenting with the symptom complex (Stamm et al 1980).

Urodynamic investigation has revealed a high urethral pressure in some of these patients (Raz & Smith 1976, McGuire 1978), which may be associated with increased anal sphincter tone. On passage of a urethral catheter resistance will be noted and movement of the catheter may replicate the patient's symptoms. Palpation of the levatores ani may also produce symptoms, which the patient can learn to control by relaxing the levatores. Not all patients with urethral syndrome have urodynamic evidence of sphincter dysfunction. Other investigators have assessed the sensitivity of the urethral mucosa and demonstrated hypersensitivity in patients with frequency, dysuria and associated suprapubic discomfort (Powell et al 1981).

Urethral instability

About 6% of patients with lower urinary tract symptoms exhibit pressure variation of 15 cmH_2O or more at the point of maximum urethral pressure (Clarke 1992). The existence of urethral instability is debated, but it appears to cause frequency and urgency and its presence increases the risk of urinary incontinence. The diagnosis is often missed because urethral pressure profilometry is not performed.

Urethral diverticulum

A urethral diverticulum can cause frequency, urgency, dysuria and a postvoid dribble. It is believed to arise from inflammation in the paraurethral glands and is found mainly in parous patients. Urethral diverticula are usually found in the distal third of the vaginal side of the urethra, but complex structures which corkscrew around the entire urethra may be found. A tender mass may be palpated on vaginal examination and pus can sometimes be milked out of the urethra. Gonorrhoea must be excluded and appropriate antibiotic therapy should be started before surgical excision. Occasionally a calculus, or rarely a malignancy, may be encountered in the diverticulum.

HISTORY

Patients presenting with urinary frequency and urgency need to be questioned about associated incontinence, which may imply the presence of detrusor instability. Dysuria can be found with urinary tract infection, urethral syndrome or a urethral caruncle, and if haematuria is present then bladder carcinoma, calculus, urinary tract infection or interstitial cystitis must be excluded. There may be predisposing factors to urinary tract infection that can be elicited from the history, e.g. first intercourse ('honeymoon cystitis'), use of the contraceptive diaphragm and recurrent episodes of infection possibly associated with bladder calculus or renal disease. A voiding disorder due to bladder or pelvic floor dysfunction may be suspected with complaints of hesitancy, poor stream and incomplete bladder emptying, though a pelvic mass must also be ruled out. Frequency can be due to diuretic therapy and inappropriate timing may cause nocturia. The date of the last menstrual period must be ascertained, as pregnancy is a well recognized cause of urinary frequency. The past medical history will reveal any relevant pelvic surgery or radiotherapy.

EXAMINATION

Abdominal examination will identify a full bladder, pelvic mass or pregnancy, but a neurological assessment is essential to exclude an upper motor neuron lesion, with special attention to the S2–S4 dermatomes, which innervate the bladder.

Pelvic examination may reveal a urethral caruncle, whereas expression of pus through the external urethral meatus after examination may suggest a urethral diverticulum. Tenderness on bimanual palpation of the bladder may be found with interstitial cystitis; tenderness on palpation of the pelvic floor muscles has been found in the urethral syndrome. A large fibroid uterus, ovarian cyst or pregnancy may produce symptoms by pressure on the bladder.

INVESTIGATIONS

MSU

Urinary tract infection should always be excluded. Examination of urine is also necessary if tuberculosis or schistosomiasis are suspected.

Miscellaneous

Blood tests for renal function and urine osmolality may be appropriate, and if the patient has delivered an infant over 4.5 kg a blood glucose test may be indicated. If acute urethritis is suspected then a urethral swab will be needed.

Urinary diary

A urinary diary is a simple record of the patient's fluid intake and output, and episodes of urgency are recorded. Each patient should complete this for 1 week prior to investigation. These diaries are more accurate than patient recall and provide an assessment of frequency and functional bladder capacity (Fig. 52.2), and indicate where excessive intake is causing urinary frequency.

Subtracted cystometry

Having ruled out infection or the more obvious causes of symptoms, urodynamic tests are necessary. Twin-channel subtracted cystometry will diagnose detrusor instability or genuine stress incontinence.

Urethral electric conductance

This test may be performed at the same time as cystometry. In cases of sensory urgency or detrusor instability distinct fluid movements can be detected when the patient experiences urgency (Fig. 52.3). This may imply that these two conditions are part of the same disease process; however, not all cases of sensory urgency progress to detrusor instability.

Urethral pressure profilometry (UPP)

UPP measurement may identify urethral instability.

Cystoscopy

This is indicated in cases of haematuria, recurrent urinary

DAY: TUES 24 MARCH

TIME	INTAKE (ml)	OUTPUT (ml)	LEAKAGE			
			ACTIVITY	Amount	Urge	Wet Bed
7^{30}		350				
7^{40}	100					
8^{00}		100				
8^{00}	240					
8^{40}		250				
9^{00}	150		SNEEZING	1	NO	
10^{00}	180					
10^{15}		275				
10^{30}	180					
11^{00}	240					
11^{30}		250				
12^{00}	240					
12^{30}	80					
13^{15}		180				
14^{00}	150					
15^{00}	150		RUNNING	1	NO	
15^{15}		250				
16^{30}	80					
18^{00}	150					
19^{00}		300				
19^{30}	300					
20^{00}	300					
20^{15}		180				
20^{30}	300					
21^{00}	100					
21^{20}		400				
21^{40}	100					
22^{10}		200				
23^{00}		200				
03^{00}		250ml				
TOTAL	3040	3185				

Fig. 52.2 Urinary diary showing excess intake of fluid.

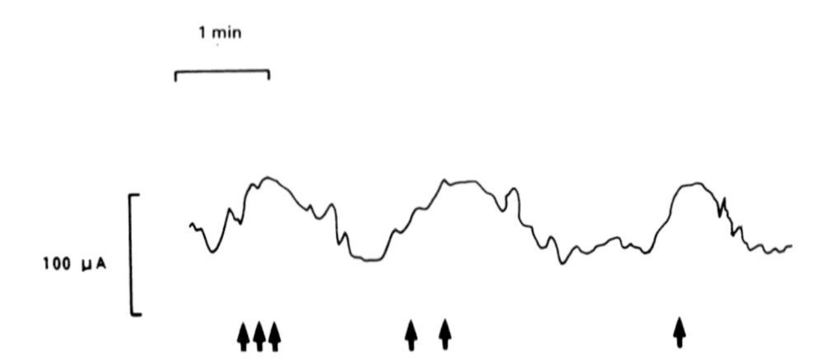

Fig. 52.3 Bladder-neck urethral electrical conductance, showing bladder-neck opening on experiencing urgency.

tract infection, suspected urethral syndrome, urethral diverticulum and interstitial cystitis.

TREATMENT

Treatment must be directed towards the cause with antibiotics for infection, restriction of fluid intake and medical referral in renal failure, adjustment of diuretic therapy and neurological referral as appropriate.

Bladder retraining

Bladder retraining has been successfully employed in the management of urinary urgency. The patient uses timed voiding to overcome her urgency, and by slowly increasing the voiding interval an acceptable daily frequency can be achieved. Jarvis (1982) reported that more than 50% of women with sensory urgency were symptom-free and objectively dry 6 months after treatment with bladder drill. Frewen (1980) felt that voluntary frequency may be a factor in the genesis of detrusor instability, and advocated bladder training in all cases of frequency and urgency, whether due to sensory urgency or to detrusor instability. More recently, functional electrical stimulation and acupuncture have been advocated for women with urge symptoms, with improvement cure rates of 83% (Eriksen et al 1989) and 76% (Philip et al 1988) respectively.

Biofeedback

Biofeedback is the process of providing visual or auditory evidence of the status of an autonomic function so that the patient may exert control over that function. It has been used for the management of detrusor instability (Cardozo et al 1978). Using bladder-neck measurement the rises in electrical conductivity associated with urgency have been noted to precede detrusor contraction by a few seconds. Voluntary closure of the bladder neck using conductivity recording as feedback abolished that sensation of urgency. After a course of biofeedback therapy 93% of patients were cured of symptoms (Peattie et al, unpublished work).

Drugs

Drug therapy for frequency and urgency is the same as that for detrusor instability. Oxybutynin hydrochloride, propantheline bromide and imipramine are used for their anticholinergic effect (see Ch. 49). If frequency is a solitary complaint then desmopressin may be utilized. Oestrogen replacement may provide symptom relief in some patients.

Interstitial cystitis

Many different treatments have been tried, but with little

success. Hunner (1930) tried surgical removal of the affected portion of the bladder, but recurrence was common and made surgery unacceptable. Instillations of silver nitrate or dimethylsulphoxide have given some relief, but again recurrence of symptoms is common. As pain is a feature denervation of the bladder or bilateral sacral neurectomy has been reported, but again with poor results. Cystodistension seemed to show promise, but again symptomatic relief was only transient (Badenoch 1971). Psychiatric therapy has been tried, as many patients were found to have high emotional or neurotic symptom scores, but the chronicity and severity of symptoms may account for this finding. Bladder retraining is a worthwhile treatment, with 88% reporting some improvement (Parsons & Koprowski 1991, Chaiken et al 1993). More recently laser treatment to affected areas has shown promise, but awaits further evaluation (Malloy & Shanberg 1994). This chronic condition is notoriously difficult to manage and patients usually become long-term attenders at clinics. In some patients bladder augmentation or urinary diversion procedures are necessary to alleviate symptoms.

Urethral syndrome

Treatment is tailored to symptoms: antibiotics, oestrogen replacement therapy, psychotherapy and biofeedback have limited success. Urethral dilatation is advocated for voiding difficulty but must be performed with caution, as scarring may cause symptom deterioration. The best results are reported in patients managed by observation alone, when spontaneous remission occurs in 85–100% of women (Carson et al 1980, Zufall 1978).

Reconstructive surgery

Where other treatments fail and symptom severity destroys a patient's quality of life, then reconstructive bladder surgery such as substitution cystoplasty should be considered and urological opinion sought. If all fails, or the patient is too frail for major surgery, then long-term catheterization may alleviate symptoms.

SUMMARY

The causes of urinary frequency and urgency in the female are numerous. A diligent history and examination will indicate the most likely cause and investigations can be tailored accordingly. Some conditions are readily amenable to treatment but others have a chronic course, where only symptomatic relief is available and patients require thorough explanation. In some patients the symptoms are so debilitating that major reconstructive surgery or long-term catheterization is necessary.

KEY POINTS

1. Frequency and urgency are common symptoms but embarrassment or a feeling that these symptoms are normal prevents many women seeking advice.
2. Frequency and urgency can be caused by many lesions outside the urinary tract.
3. The urinary diary is a simple and inexpensive investigation, and also serves as a basis for treatment.
4. Simple treatment measures such as antibiotics for urinary tract infection, fluid restriction and adjustment of diuretic therapy may be all that is required.
5. Bladder drill may achieve improvement in up to 80% of patients.
6. Surgery and chronic catheterization should only be considered when other methods have failed.

REFERENCES

Anderson J B, Parivar F, Lee G et al 1989 The enigma of interstitial cystitis — an autoimmune disease? British Journal of Urology 63: 58–63

Badenoch A W 1971 Chronic interstitial cystitis. British Journal of Urology 43: 718–720

Benness C, Gangar K, Cardozo L, Cutner A, Whitehead M 1991 Do progestogens exacerbate urinary incontinence in women on HRT? Neurourology and Urodynamics 10: 316–317

Bungay G T, Vessey M P, McPherson C K 1980 Study of symptoms in middle life with special reference to the menopause. British Medical Journal 281: 181–183

Cardozo L D, Stanton S L, Hafner J, Allan V 1978 Biofeedback in the treatment of detrusor instability. British Journal of Urology 50: 250–254

Carson C C, Segura J W, Osborne D M 1980 Evaluation and treatment of the female urethral syndrome. Journal of Urology 124: 609–610

Chaiken D C, Blaivas J G, Blaivas S T 1993 Behavioural therapy for the treatment of refractory interstitial cystitis. Journal of Urology 149: 1445–1448

Clarke B 1992 Urethral instability. Australian and New Zealand Journal of Obstetrics and Gynaecology 32: 270–275

Creighton S M, Pearce J M, Robson I, Wang K, Stanton S L 1991 Sensory urgency: how full is your bladder? British Journal of Obstetrics and Gynaecology 98: 1287–1289

Diokno A C, Brock B M, Brown M B, Herjog A R 1986 Prevalence of urinary incontinence and other urological symptoms in the non institutionalised elderly. Journal of Urology 136: 1022–1025

Dwyer P L, O'Callaghan D 1993 Urinary dysfunction following radical hysterectomy, is there spontaneous improvement with time? Neurourology and Urodynamics 12: 429–430

Eriksen B C, Bergmann S, Eik-Nes S H 1989 Maximal electrostimulation of the pelvic floor in female idiopathic detrusor instability and urge incontinence. Neurourology and Urodynamics 8: 219–230

Frewen R K 1980 The management of urgency and frequency of micturition. British Journal of Urology 52: 367–369
Griffith-Jones M D, Jarvis G J, McNamara H M 1991 Adverse urinary symptoms after total abdominal hysterectomy – fact or fiction? British Journal of Urology 67: 295–297
Hanash K A, Pool T L 1970 Interstitial and haemorrhagic cystitis: viral, bacterial and fungal studies. Journal of Urology 104: 705–706
Hand J R 1949 Interstitial cystitis: report of 223 cases. Journal of Urology 61: 291–292
Hunner G L 1914 A rare bladder ulcer in women. Transactions of the Southern Surgical and Gynecological Association 27: 247
Hunner G L 1930 Neurosis of the bladder. Journal of Urology 24: 567
Jarvis G J 1982 The management of urinary incontinence due to primary vesical sensory urgency by bladder drill. British Journal of Urology 54: 374–376
Kelleher C J, Cardozo L D, Khullar V, Salvatore S, Hill S 1994 Symptom scores and the subjective severity of urinary incontinence. Neurourology and Urodynamics 13: 373–374
Larsen S, Thompson S A, Hald T 1982 Mast cells in interstitial cystitis. British Journal of Urology 54: 283–286
MacCaulay A J, Stern R S, Holmes D M, Stanton S L 1987 Micturition and the mind: psychological factors in the aetiology and treatment of urinary symptoms in women. British Medical Journal 294: 540–543
McGrother C W, Castleden C M, Duffin J, Clarke M 1987 A profile of disordered micturition in the elderly at home. Age and Ageing 16: 105–110
McGuire E J 1978 Reflex urethral instability. British Journal of Urology 50: 200–204
Malloy T R, Shanberg A M 1994 Laser therapy for interstitial cystitis. Urologic Clinics of North America 21: 141–144
Milne J S, Williamson J, Maule M M, Wallace E T 1972 Urinary symptoms in older people. Modern Geriatrics 2: 198–212
Monga A K, Marrero J M, Maxwell J D, Stanton S L 1994 Is there an irritable bladder in the irritable bowel syndrome? Neurourology and Urodynamics 13: 450–451
National Institute of Arthritis, Diabetes, Digestive and Kidney Diseases 1988 Summary of the Workshop on Interstitial Cystitis 1988. National Institutes of Health, Bethesda, Maryland. Journal of Urology 140: 203–206
Norton P A, MacDonald L D, Sedgewick P M, Stanton S L 1988 Distress and delay associated with urinary incontinence, frequency and urgency in women. British Medical Journal 297: 1187–1189
Parkin D E, Davis J A, Symmonds R P 1988 Urodynamic findings following radiotherapy for cervical carcinoma. British Journal of Urology 61: 213
Parsons C L 1994 Interstitial cystitis. In: Kursh E D, McGuire E J (eds) Female urology. J B Lippincott, Philadelphia, pp 421–438
Parsons C L, Koprowski P F 1991 Interstitial cystitis: successful management by increasing urinary voiding intervals. Urology 37: 207–212
Peattie A B, Plevnik S, Stanton S L 1988 What is the current needed to close the gate? Journal of the Royal Society of Medicine 81: 442–444
Philip T, Shah P J R, Worth P H L 1988 Acupuncture in the treatment of bladder instability. British Journal of Urology 61: 490–493
Powell P H, George N J R, Smith P J B, Feneley R C L 1981 The hypersensitive female urethra – cause of recurrent frequency and dysuria. Proceedings of the International Continence Society 11th AGM, Lund, pp 81–82
Raz S, Smith R B 1976 External sphincter spasticity syndrome in females. Journal of Urology 115: 443–446
RCGP Office of Population Censuses and Surveys 1981–82. DHSS morbidity statistics from general practice third national study, studies on medical and population subjects, No. 36
Robertson A S, Griffiths C J, Ramsden P D, Neal D E 1994 Bladder function in healthy volunteers: ambulatory monitoring and conventional urodynamic studies. British Journal of Urology 73: 242–249
Scotti R J, Bergman A, Bhatia N N 1986 Urodynamic changes in urethrovesical function after radical hysterectomy. Obstetrics and Gynecology 68: 111–116
Stamm W E, Wagner K F, Amsel R et al 1980 Causes of the acute urethral syndrome in women. New England Journal of Medicine 303: 409–415
Stein P C, Parsons C L 1994 Proteoglycan core protein syndecan in bladder biopsies. World Journal of Urology 12: 15–20
van Waalwijk van Doorn E S C, Remmers A, Janknegt R A 1992 Conventional and extramural ambulatory urodynamic testing of the lower urinary tract in female volunteers. Journal of Urology 47: 1319–1326
Zufall R 1978 Ineffectiveness of treatment of urethral syndrome in women. Urology 12: 337–339

53

Fistulae

Paul Hilton

INTRODUCTION

A fistula may be defined as an abnormal communication between two or more epithelial surfaces. In the context of gynaecology we are concerned primarily with fistulae between the genital tract (vagina, cervix, uterus or perineum, in decreasing order of occurrence) and either the urinary tract (bladder, urethra or ureter) or the gastrointestinal tract (rectum, colon, anal canal or small bowel).

Multiple or complex fistulae are common, particularly after attempts at surgical repair. Dual involvement of the bowel and urinary tract is regularly seen, and concurrent involvement of, for example, ureter and bladder, or bladder and urethra, is often seen in strategically placed or large urinary fistulae. They may also involve an intervening cavity so that the fistulous nature of an inflammatory mass may not be immediately obvious.

Rarer forms may occur, for example a salpingocolic fistula in association with actinomycosis or tuberculosis. Although such pathologies are interesting and important as causes of diagnostic confusion and therapeutic difficulty, in view of their rarity they are not considered further in this chapter.

AETIOLOGY AND EPIDEMIOLOGY

The aetiology of urogenital fistulae is varied, and may be broadly categorized into congenital or acquired, the latter being divided into obstetric, surgical, radiation, malignant and miscellaneous causes. The same factors may be responsible for intestinogenital fistulae, although inflammatory bowel disease is an additional important aetiological factor here. In most third-world countries over 90% of fistulae are of obstetric aetiology, whereas in the UK over 70% follow pelvic surgery (Table 53.1).

Congenital fistulae are strictly outside the scope of this chapter, and readers are advised to refer to Chapters 1 and 45 for further information. Some cases of ectopic ureter may discharge into the vagina and are described simply because their presentation may be delayed into the teens or adult life, and may therefore lead to confusion with acquired fistulae or other causes of incontinence. This occurs particularly if the abnormal ureter is draining only a small or poorly functioning part of the renal tissue. Under these circumstances the abnormal tissue may be insufficient to show up as a soft tissue shadow on a plain X-ray, and so poorly functional that it is not easily seen on excretion urography. A high index of clinical suspicion is

Table 53.1 Aetiology of urogenital fistulae in two series, from the north of England (Hilton, unpublished) and from southeast Nigeria (Hilton & Ward 1995)

Aetiology	NE England (n = 85)		SE Nigeria (n = 2485)	
	%	%	%	%
Obstetric	11.8		93.3	
Obstructed labour		1.2		81.4
Caesarean section		3.5		6.8
Ruptured uterus		2.4		5.1
Forceps		2.4		
Breech extraction		1.2		
Abruption		1.2		
Surgical	75.3		2.5	
Abdominal hysterectomy		42.4		0.8
Radical hysterectomy		9.4		
Urethral diverticulectomy		8.2		
Colporrhaphy				0.8
Vaginal hysterectomy		2.4		0.6
TAH + colporrhaphy		1.2		
TAH + colposuspension		1.2		
LAVH		1.2		
Cystoplasty + colposuspension		1.2		
Colposuspension		1.2		
Sling		1.2		
Needle suspension		1.2		
Cervical stumpectomy		1.2		
Subtrigonal phenol injection		1.2		
Transurethral resection (tb)		1.2		
Lithoclast		1.2		
Suture to vaginal laceration				0.3
Radiation	10.5		0.0	
Malignancy	0.0		2.0	
Miscellaneous	2.4		2.2	
Catheter associated		1.2		
Trauma		1.2		0.6
Infection				0.6
Coital injury				1.1
Total	100.0		100.0	

required if the diagnosis is not to be overlooked (Fig. 53.1).

Obstetric

The underlying factors responsible for the development of obstetric fistulae may be considered in physical, biosocial, cultural and geographical or political terms. The basic physical factors responsible for obstetric fistula development include obstructed labour, accidental injury at the time of caesarean section, forceps delivery, craniotomy or symphysiotomy, traditional surgical practices including circumcision and gishiri, and complications of criminal abortion.

The overwhelming proportion are complications of neglected obstructed labour. During normal labour the bladder is displaced upwards and the anterior vaginal wall, bladder base and urethra are compressed between the fetal head and the posterior surface of the pubis. No harm results if this occurs for a short time, but in prolonged obstructed labour the intervening tissues are devitalized by ischaemia. Usually the anterior vaginal wall and underlying bladder neck are affected, although sometimes the area of necrosis is higher, in which case the anterior lip of the cervix and underlying trigone are involved. Compression of the soft tissues posteriorly between the sacral promontory and the presenting part may occur at the same time, with necrosis at the posterior vaginal wall and the underlying rectum. The devitalized area separates as a slough, usually between the third and 10th days of the puerperium, with the resulting incontinence (Fig. 53.2).

Accidental injury to the vaginal wall during a difficult operative delivery may involve damage to the underlying bladder wall, particularly if the tissues are devitalized by prolonged pressure. Forcible rotation of the head with Kielland's forceps is particularly liable to produce such an injury by shearing stresses. The bladder is particularly exposed to injury following symphysiotomy if the pubic bones are too widely separated by forced abduction of the thighs. In these circumstances the unsupported bladder neck is very likely to be damaged, especially if the head is rotated and extracted with forceps. The posterior wall of the bladder may be accidentally incised during lower segment caesarean section or repair of a ruptured uterus,

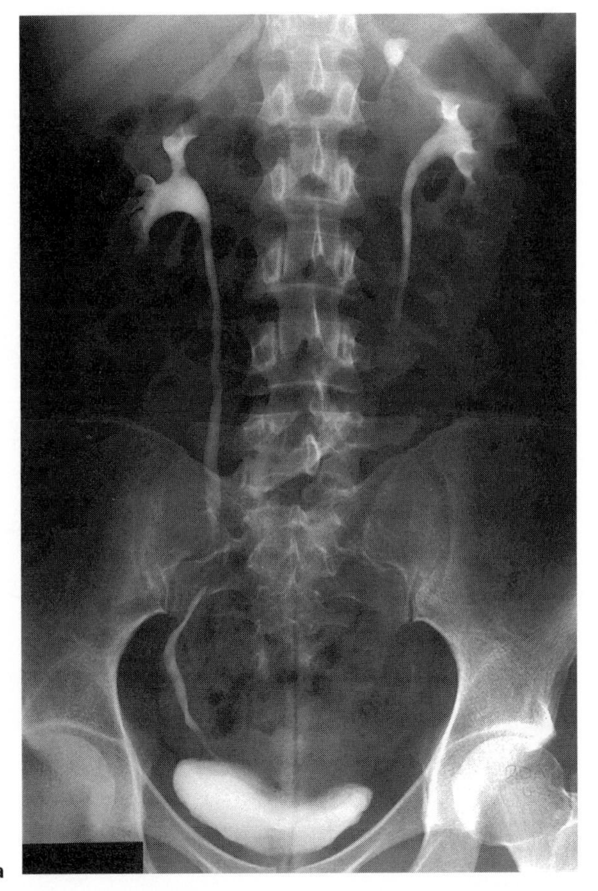

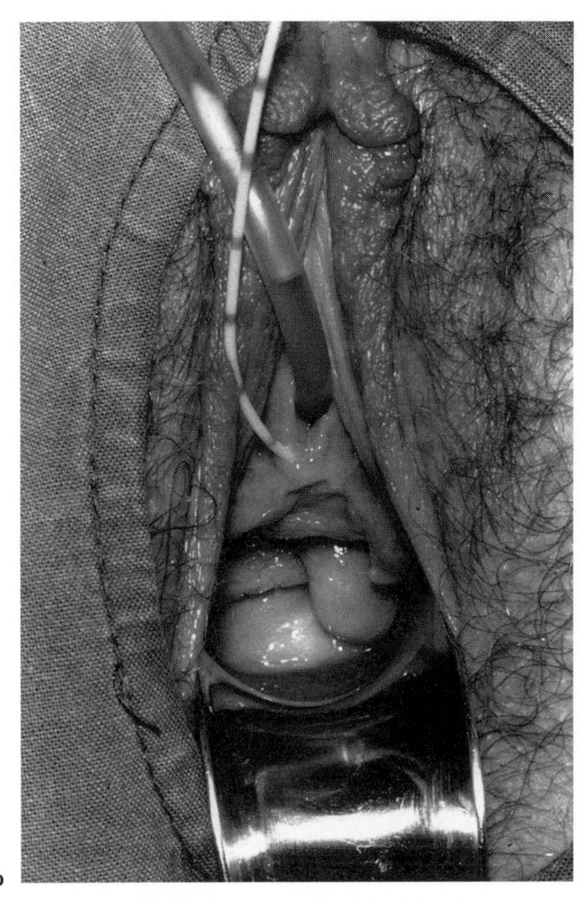

Fig. 53.1 **(a)** Intravenous urogram from patient presenting with continuous urinary incontinence; a small discrete left upper pole element is visible, although the upper pole ureter is not clearly seen. **(b)** Appearance of the vulva in the same patient, with urethral catheter in place and a ureteric catheter placed in the ectopic ureteric opening just below the external urethral meatus.

particularly if the bladder is not reflected sufficiently far downwards before the lower segment is opened. During the reflection itself the bladder may be torn, especially if a previous operation has made it densely adherent to the lower segment. If the bladder injury goes undetected at the time urinary leakage through the abdominal wound soon develops. This is usually followed by vaginal incontinence when urine finds its way through the uterine incision. The abdominal leakage then dries up as the bladder drains through the resulting vesicocervical fistula. Alternatively, sutures may be passed through the posterior bladder wall during repair of the uterine incision. The appearance of urinary incontinence in these cases is delayed until sloughing of the intervening bladder tissue caught up in the suture.

The perineum and posterior vaginal wall are of course at risk from even the most straightforward delivery, although primiparity, forceps delivery, birthweight over 4 kg and occipitoposterior position have been found to be significant risk factors associated with third-degree tears (Sultan et al 1994). Even when identified and repaired, this increases the risk of rectovaginal fistula.

Traditional surgical practices play a significant role in the aetiology of obstetric fistulae in several parts of Africa. Among the Hausa, Fulani and Kanuri tribes of northern Nigeria the practice of gishiri is commonly employed to treat a wide variety of conditions, including obstructed labour, infertility, dyspareunia, amenorrhoea, goitre, backache and dysuria. The traditional cut made with a razor blade or knife through the vaginal introitus is sometimes superficial, but may result in fistula formation (Fig. 53.3). Because the incisions are usually made linearly into healthy tissues, repair is often much easier than those resulting from pressure necrosis.

Circumcision has been practised in various forms in much of north Africa, and is still practised widely in Sudan and other Muslim cultures. The most extreme form, pharaonic circumcision, involves removal of the labia minora, most of the labia majora, the mons veneris, and often the clitoris (Fig. 53.4), the introitus being reduced to pinhole size. The effect in labour is to produce significant delay in the second stage. This will often necessitate wide episiotomy, often with an anterior incision to allow delivery, and contributes to the development of both

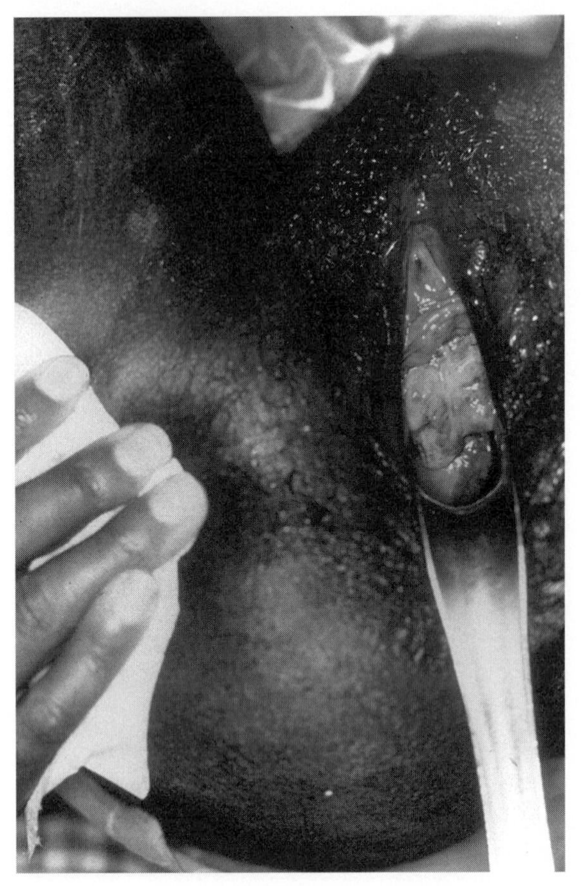

Fig. 53.2 Puerperal patient following prolonged obstructed labour. An area of devitalized tissue is seen on the anterior vaginal wall, about to slough, with resultant fistula formation.

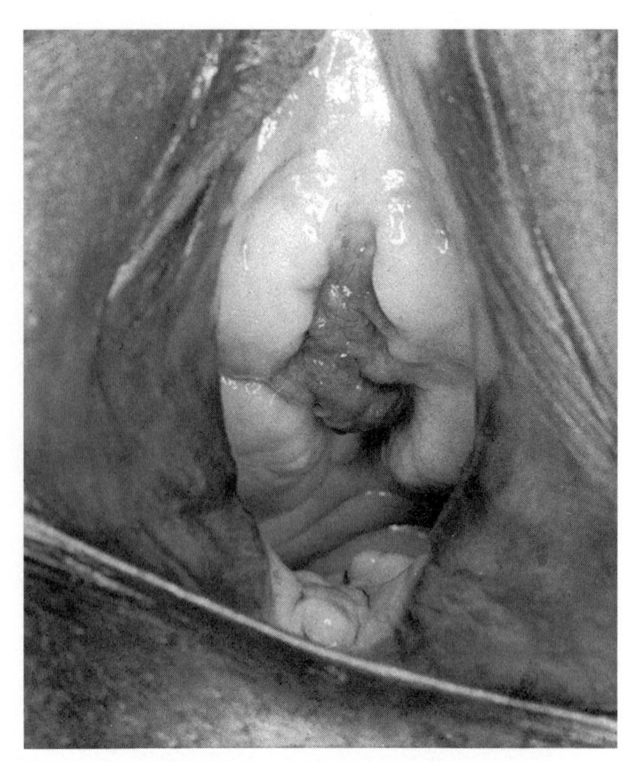

Fig. 53.3 Vesicovaginal fistula resulting from gishiri cut in a young Hausa girl.

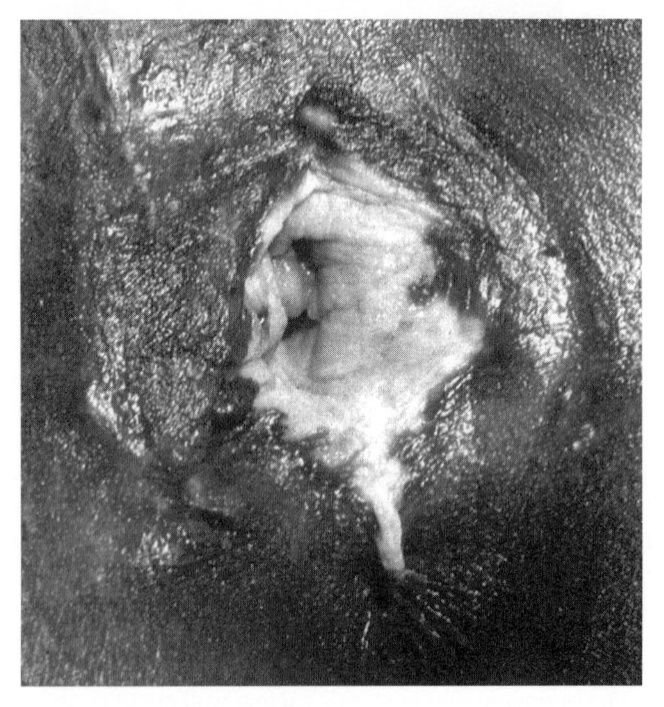

Fig. 53.4 Pharaonic circumcision.

vesicovaginal fistulae and rectovaginal fistulae or third-degree tears.

Tahzib (1983, 1985) reported on the epidemiological determinants of vesicovaginal fistulae in northern Nigeria. In 84% of cases obstructed labour was the major aetiological factor; 33% had undergone gishiri, and in 15% this was felt to be the main aetiological factor.

In considering obstetric fistulae, however, it is perhaps as much, if not more, relevant to consider not simply the direct physical injury to the lower urinary tract, but also the social, cultural and geographical influences. Obstructed labour is most often due to a contracted pelvis. This usually results from stunting of growth by malnutrition and untreated infections in childhood and adolescence. Where women retain a subservient role in society, and standards of education are limited, early marriage and the absence of family planning services results in an early start to childbearing; where first pregnancies occur soon after the menarche, before growth of the pelvis is complete, this also contributes to obstruction in labour.

The influence of these factors is illustrated in the epidemiological studies alluded to earlier. Tahzib (1983) reported that over 50% of the cases of vesicovaginal fistulae seen in northern Nigeria were aged under 20; over 50% were in their first pregnancy, and only 1 in 500 had received any formal education. Murphy (1981) reported

Table 53.2 Epidemiological aspects of obstetric fistula as illustrated in five studies from Nigeria, Ethiopia and Pakistan

	Northern Nigeria Murphy (1981) n = 100	Northern Nigeria Tahzib (1983) n = 1443	Ethiopia Kelly & Kwast (1993) n = 309	Southeast Nigeria Hilton & Ward (1995) n = 2485	Pakistan Ahmad (WHO 1989) n = 325
Mean age (yrs)	20	21	22	28	32
Mean parity	?	1.6	2.1	3.5	?
% in 1st pregnancy	65	52	63	31	15
Divorced/deserted (%)	54% divorced/sep'd	?	52% deserted	10% divorced/sep'd	?
Literacy (%)	8	0.2	?	29	?
Delivered at home (%)	?	64	58	27	?

from the same area that 88% of patients had married at 15 years of age or less, and 33% had delivered their first child before the age of 15. In different third-world societies, however, these factors do seem to have variable influence and, for example, in southeast Nigeria (Hilton & Ward 1995) and the northwest frontier of Pakistan (Ahmad, cited in WHO 1989), fistula patients seem to be somewhat older and of higher parity; they also appear to have a higher literacy rate, and to be more likely to remain in a married relationship after the development of their fistula (Hilton & Ward 1995). It is likely that the development of fistulae here reflects other biosocial variations (Table 53.2). It is clear that in these populations, even where skilled maternity care is available, uptake may be poor. Mistrust of hospital is commonplace, antenatal care poorly attended and delivery commonly conducted at home by elderly relatives or unskilled traditional birth attendants. Where labour is prolonged, transfer to hospital may only be used as a last resort.

Surgical

Genital fistula may occur following a wide range of surgical procedures within the pelvis (see Table 53.1 and Fig. 53.5). It is often supposed that this complication results from direct injury to the lower urinary tract at the time of operation. Certainly on occasions this may be the case; careless, hurried or rough surgical technique makes

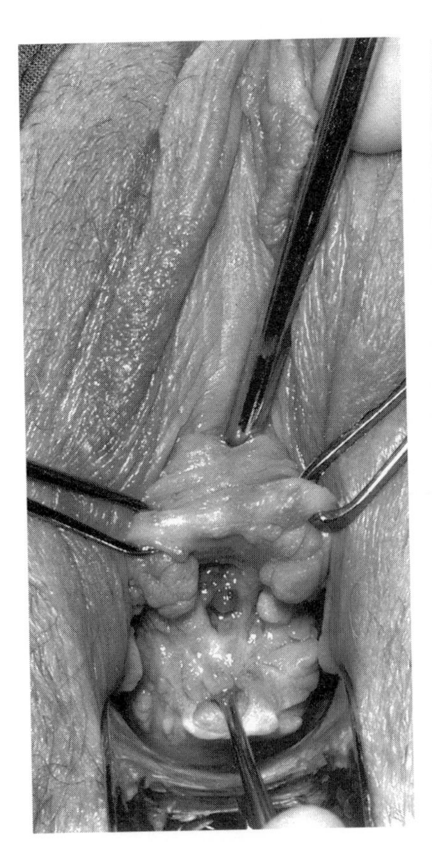
a

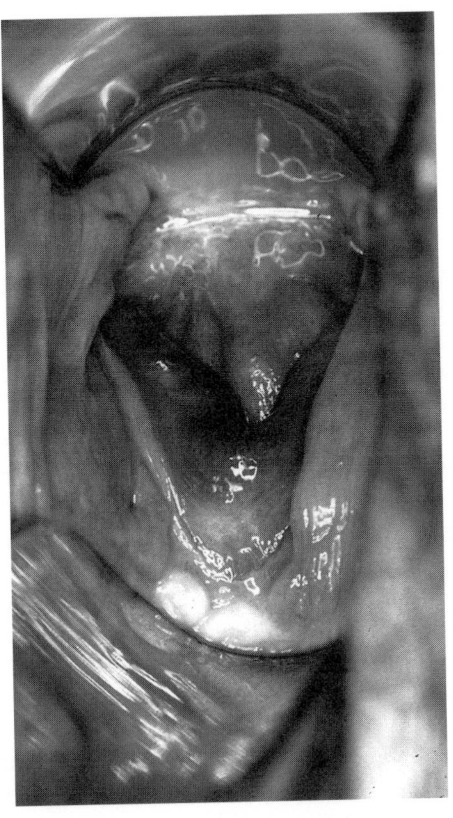
b

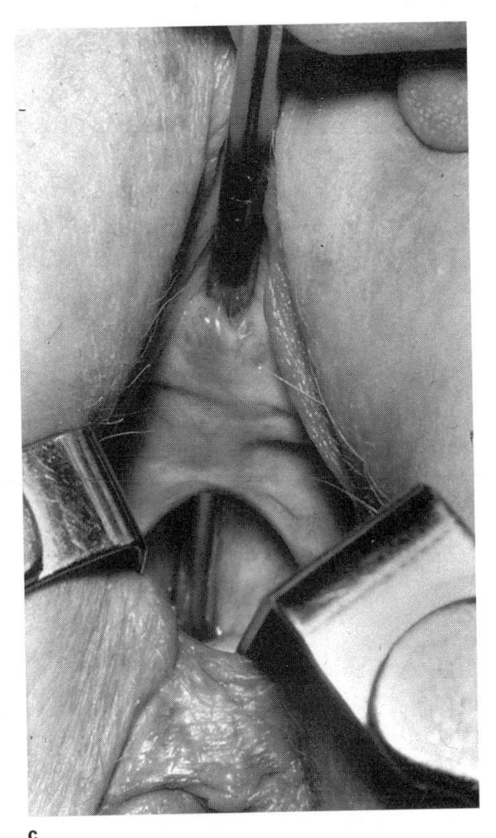
c

Fig. 53.5 Urogenital fistulae of varying aetiologies. **(a)** (left) Urethrovaginal fistula resulting from urethral diverticulectomy; **(b)** (centre) Large vesicovaginal fistula following radical hysterectomy; the right ureteric orifice is seen in the edge of the fistula; **(c)** (right) Postradiation fistula.

Table 53.3 Risk factors for postoperative fistulae

Risk factor	Pathology	Specific example
Anatomical distortion		Fibroids
		Ovarian mass
Abnormal tissue adhesion	Inflammation	Infection
		Endometriosis
	Previous surgery	Caesarean section
		Cone biopsy
		Colporrhaphy
	Malignancy	
Impaired vascularity	Ionizing radiation	Preoperative radiotherapy
	Metabolic abnormality	Diabetes mellitus
	Radical surgery	
Compromised healing		Anaemia
		Nutritional deficiency
Abnormality of bladder function		Voiding dysfunction

injury to the lower urinary tract much more likely. However, of 85 fistulae referred to the author in the UK over the last 8 years, 64 have been associated with pelvic surgery and 49 followed hysterectomy; of these, only four presented with leakage of urine on day 1. In other cases compromise to the blood supply may result in tissue necrosis and subsequent leakage; or, alternatively, a small pelvic haematoma may develop in association with the vaginal vault which subsequently becomes infected and discharges, with the characteristic puff of haematuria, 5–10 days later; incontinence follows shortly thereafter.

Although it is important to remember that the majority of surgical fistulae follow apparently straightforward hysterectomy in skilled hands, several risk factors may be identified that make direct injury more likely (Table 53.3). Obviously anatomical distortion within the pelvis by ovarian tumour or fibroid will increase the difficulty, and abnormal adhesions between bladder and uterus or cervix following previous surgery, or associated with previous sepsis, endometriosis or malignancy, may make fistula formation more likely. Preoperative or early radiotherapy may decrease vascularity and make the tissues in general less forgiving of poor technique.

Issues of training and surgical technique are, of course, also important. The ability to locate and if necessary dissect out the ureter must be part of routine gynaecological training, as should the first aid management of lower urinary tract injury when it arises. The use of gauze swabs to separate the bladder from the cervix at caesarean section or hysterectomy should be discouraged: sharp dissection with a knife or scissors does less harm, especially where the tissues are abnormally adherent.

It has recently been shown that there is a high incidence of abnormalities of lower urinary tract function in fistula patients (Hilton 1995b); whether these abnormalities antedate the surgery, or develop with or as a consequence of the fistula, cannot be answered from these data. It is the view of some, however, that patients with a habit of infrequent voiding (Turner-Warwick 1993, personal communication), or with inefficient detrusor contractility, may be at increased risk of postoperative urinary retention; if this is not recognized early and managed appropriately, the risk of fistula formation may be increased.

Radiation

As noted above, preoperative pelvic irradiation increases the risk of postoperative fistula development, but irradiation itself may be a cause of fistula (Fig. 53.5c). The obliterative endarteritis associated with ionizing radiation in therapeutic dosage proceeds over many years, and may be aetiological in fistula formation long after the primary malignancy has been treated. Of the nine radiation fistulae in the author's series, the fistula developed at intervals between 1 and 30 years following radiotherapy. Not only does this ischaemia produce the fistulae, it also causes significant damage in the adjacent tissues, so that ordinary surgical repair has a high likelihood of failure and modified surgical techniques are required.

Malignancy

The treatment of pelvic malignancy by either surgery or radiotherapy is associated with a risk of fistula development, but tissue loss associated with malignant disease itself may result in genital tract fistula. Carcinoma of the cervix, vagina and rectum are the most common malignancies to present in this way. It is relatively unusual for urothelial tumours to present with fistula formation, other than following surgery or radiotherapy. The development of a fistula may be a distressing part of the terminal phase of malignant disease; it nevertheless deserves not simply compassion, but full consideration of the therapeutic or palliative possibilities.

Inflammatory bowel disease

Inflammatory bowel disease is the most significant cause of intestinogenital fistulae in the UK, although these rarely present directly to the gynaecologist. Crohn's disease is by far the most important, and appears to be increasing in frequency in the western world. A total fistula rate approaching 40% has been reported, and in females the involvement of the genital tract may be up to 7%.

Ulcerative colitis has a small incidence of low rectovaginal fistulae. Diverticular disease can produce colovaginal fistulae and, rarely, colouterine fistulae, with surprisingly few symptoms attributable to the intestinal pathology. The possibility should not be overlooked if an elderly woman complains of faeculent discharge or becomes incontinent without concomitant urinary problems (Fig. 53.6).

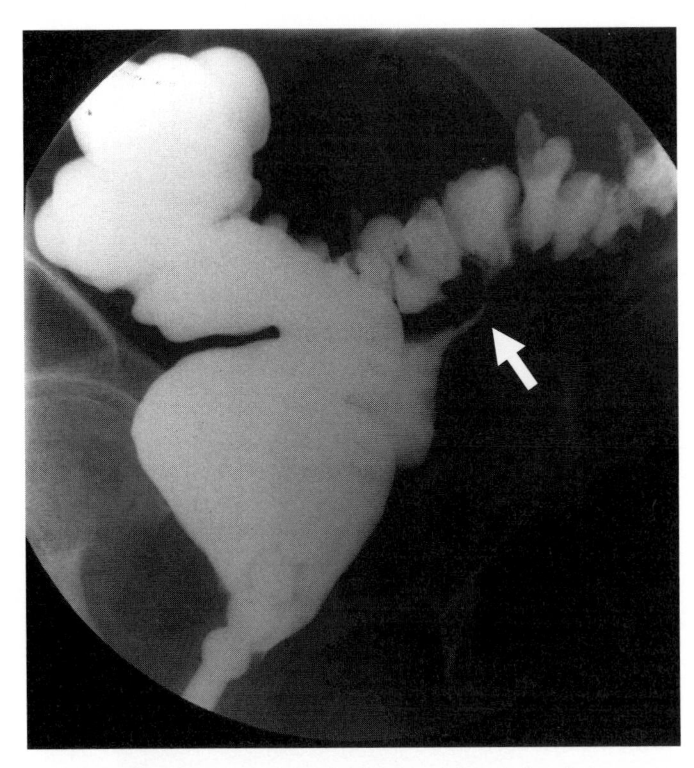

Fig. 53.6 Barium enema from patient complaining of vaginal discharge; demonstrates extensive diverticular disease and obvious colovaginal fistula (arrowed).

Miscellaneous

Among other miscellaneous causes of fistulae in the genital tract, the following should be considered:

- Infection
  - Lymphogranuloma venereum
  - Schistosomiasis
  - Tuberculosis
  - Actinomycosis
  - Measles
  - Noma vaginae
- Other
  - Penetrating trauma
  - Coital injury
  - Neglected pessary
  - Other foreign body
  - Catheter-related injury.

PREVALENCE

The prevalence of genital fistulae obviously varies from country to country and continent to continent as the main causative factors vary. Accurate figures are impossible to obtain, as those areas with the highest overall prevalence are also those with the poorest systems of health data collection. Recent data from the Regional Health Authority Information Units in England and Wales suggests an average of seven fistula repairs per health region per year over the last 5 years, and a national incidence of approximately 120 per year (95% confidence interval 80–160) (Hilton 1995a). Other estimates range between 135 (Lawson 1990, personal communication) and 350 (Kelly 1983) fistulae per year in the UK, with a posthysterectomy fistula rate of approximately 1 per 1300 operations (Lawson 1990, personal communication).

In the studies of Sultan et al (1994) third-degree tears followed 0.6% of vaginal deliveries, and in 6% of these (1 in 3000 deliveries overall) a rectovaginal fistula resulted.

In the developing world many fistula sufferers are unknown to the medical services, being separated from their husbands and ostracized from society. Although the true prevalence in the developing world is unknown, particularly high prevalence rates are reported in Nigeria, Ethiopia, Sudan and Chad. The estimated third-world prevalence is 1–2 per 1000 deliveries, with perhaps 50 000–100 000 new cases each year. Although several units exist in Nigeria, Ethiopia and Sudan, which deal with 100–700 cases per year, these nowhere nearly meet the demand and there are estimated to be perhaps 500 000 untreated cases worldwide (Waaldijk & Armiya'u 1993).

CLASSIFICATION

Many different fistula classifications have been described in the literature on the basis of anatomical site; these are often subclassified into simple cases (where the tissues are healthy and access good) (Fig. 53.7a) or complicated (where there is tissue loss, scarring, impaired access, involvement of the ureteric orifices, or the presence of coexistent rectovaginal fistula) (Fig. 53.8). Urogenital fistulae may be classified into urethral, bladder neck, subsymphysial (a complex form involving circumferential loss of the urethra, with fixity to bone), mid-vaginal, juxtacervical or vault fistulae, massive fistulae extending from bladder neck to vault, and vesicouterine or vesicocervical fistulae (Fig. 53.9). It is interesting to note that whereas over 60% of fistulae in the third world are mid-vaginal, juxtacervical or massive (reflecting their obstetric aetiology), such cases are relatively rare in western fistula practice; by contrast 50% of the fistulae managed in the UK are situated in the vaginal vault (reflecting their surgical aetiology) (Hilton 1995a).

PRESENTATION

Fistulae between the urinary tract and the female genital tract are characteristically said to present with continuous urinary incontinence, by both day and night. In patients with large fistulae the volume of leakage may be such that they rarely feel any sensation of bladder fullness, and normal voiding may be infrequent. Where there is extensive tissue loss, as in obstetric fistulae from obstructed labour,

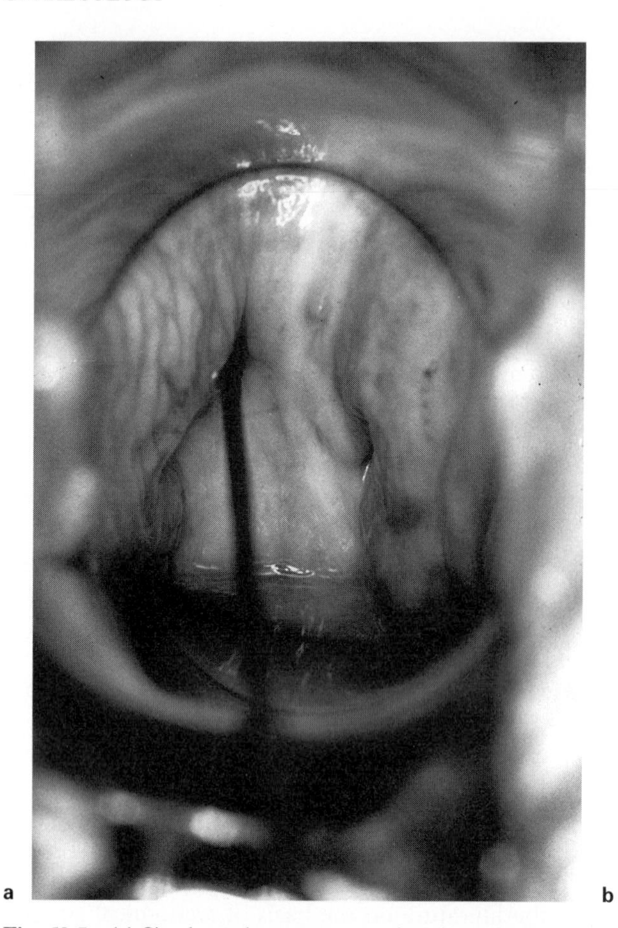

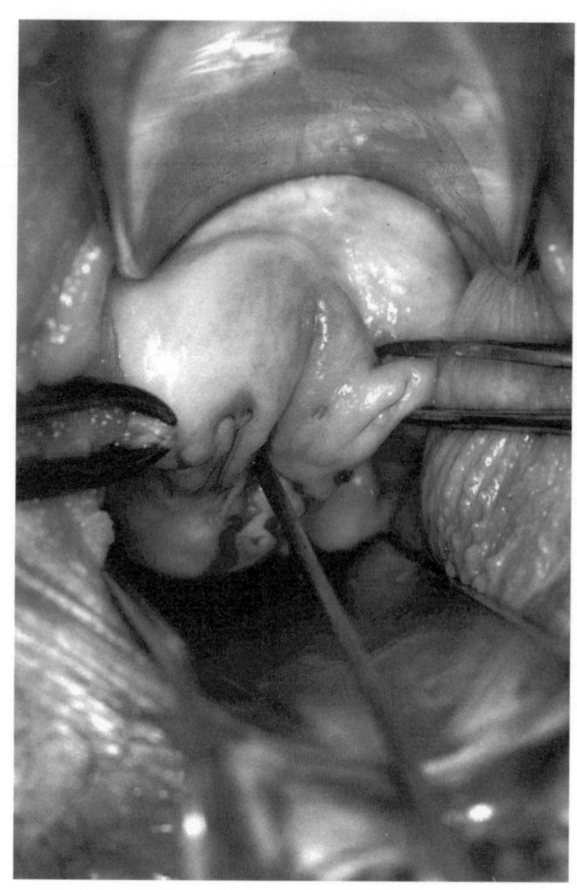

Fig. 53.7 **(a)** Simple posthysterectomy vault vesicovaginal fistula; **(b)** Same case illustrating tissue mobility and ease of access for repair per vaginam.

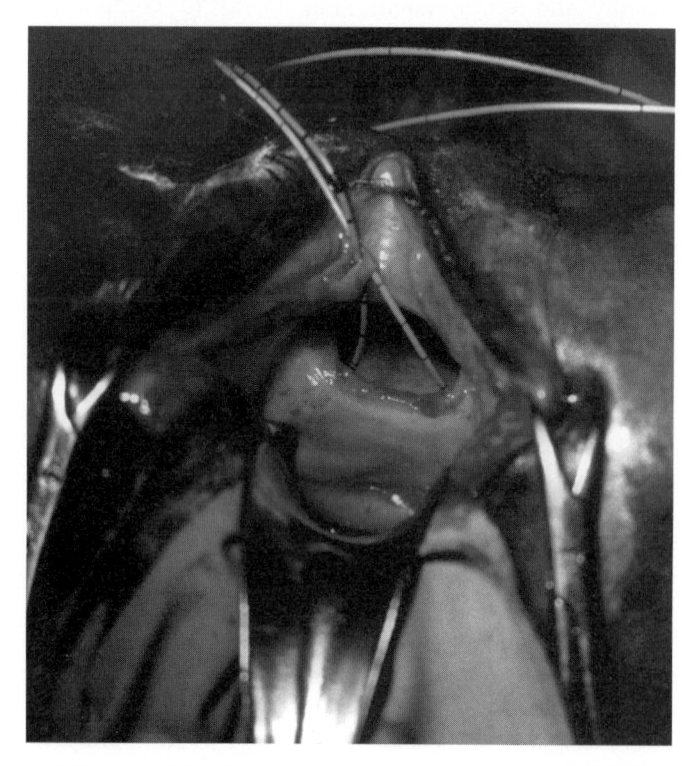

Fig. 53.8 Complex obstetric fistula; a massive vesicovaginal fistula with involvement of both ureteric orifices, and coexistent rectovaginal fistula.

or radiation fistulae, this typical history is usually present, the clinical findings gross and the diagnosis rarely in doubt. With postsurgical fistulae, for example, the history may be atypical and the orifice small, elusive or occasionally completely invisible. Under these circumstances the diagnosis can be much more difficult, and a high index of clinical suspicion must be maintained.

Occasionally a patient with an obvious fistula may deny incontinence, and this is presumed to reflect the ability of the levator ani muscles to occlude the vagina below the level of the fistula. Some patients with vesicocervical or vesicouterine fistula following caesarean section may maintain continence at the level of the uterine isthmus, and complain of cyclical haematuria at the time of menstruation, or menouria (Falk & Tancer 1956, Youssef 1957). In other cases patients may complain of little more than a watery vaginal discharge, or intermittent leakage which seems posturally related. Leakage may appear to occur specifically on standing or on lying supine, prone, or in the left or right lateral positions, presumably reflecting the degree of bladder distension and the position of the fistula within the bladder; such a pattern is most unlikely to be found with ureteric fistulae.

Although in the case of direct surgical injury leakage may occur from day 1, in most surgical and obstetric fistu-

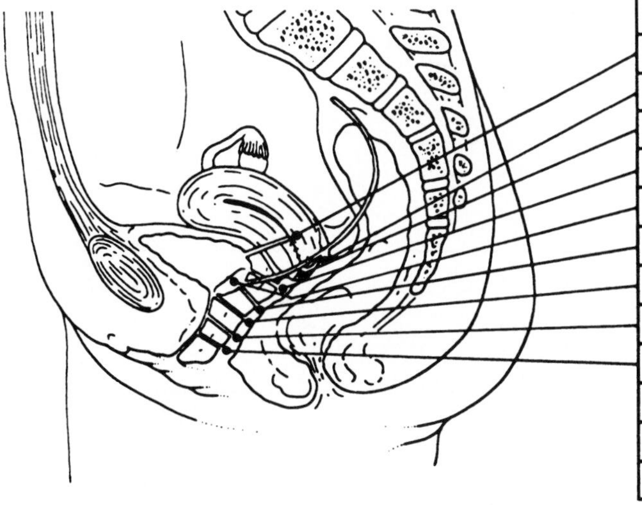

Site	NE England n=85 Hilton, unpublished	SE Nigeria n=2485 Hilton & Ward, 1995
Vesico-cervical/uterine	5.9	3.0
Uretero-vaginal	5.9	4.6
Vault	51.7	0.1
Juxta-cervical	0.0	29.4
Massive	1.2	18.2
Mid-vaginal	10.6	16.7
Bladder neck	10.6	5.3
Sub-symphysial	0.0	3.3
Urethro-vaginal	14.1	4.8
Multiple	0.0	3.7
Unspecified	0.0	10.9
Total	100.0	100.0

Fig. 53.9 Classification of urogenital fistulae by site. Table shows the distribution of types in the UK (Hilton, author's unpublished series) and Nigeria (Hilton & Ward 1995).

lae symptoms develop between 5 and 14 days after the causative injury; the time of presentation, however, may be quite variable. This will depend to some extent on the severity of symptoms, but as far as obstetric fistulae in the third world are concerned, is determined more by access to health care. In a recent review of cases from Nigeria the average time for presentation was over 5 years, and in some cases over 35 years, after the causative pregnancy (Hilton & Ward 1995).

Urethrovaginal fistulae distal to the sphincter mechanism will often be asymptomatic and require no specific treatment. Some may lead to obstruction, and are more likely to present with postmicturition dribbling than other types of incontinence; they can therefore be very difficult to recognize. More proximally situated urethral fistulae are perhaps most likely to present with stress incontinence, since bladder neck competence is frequently impaired.

Ureteric fistulae occur from similar aetiologies to bladder fistulae, and the causative mechanism may be one of direct injury by incision, division or excision, or of ischaemia from strangulation by suture, crushing by clamp or stripping by dissection (Yeates 1987). The presentation may therefore be similarly variable. With direct injury leakage is usually apparent from the first postoperative day. Urine output may be physiologically reduced for some hours following surgery, and if there is significant operative or postoperative hypotension oliguria may persist for longer. Once renal function is restored, however, leakage will usually be apparent promptly. With other mechanisms obstruction is likely to be present to a greater or lesser degree, and the initial symptoms may be of pyrexia or loin pain, with incontinence occurring only after sloughing of the ischaemic tissue, from around 5 days up to 6 weeks later.

With intestinal fistulae the history may be much more misleading. A small communication with the large bowel may cause only an offensive discharge. Even fistulae of obstetric origin may be rendered relatively asymptomatic by the cicatrization of the vagina which occurs following sloughing. A small high posterior horseshoe-shaped fistula may only become apparent during division of constricting bands for the repair of a vesicovaginal fistula. Most typically, however, patients will complain of incontinence of liquid stool, and flatus, and although they may often be unsure as to whether stool is from the vagina or the anus, the sensation of flatus from the vagina is rarely misinterpreted.

INVESTIGATIONS

If there is suspicion of a fistula, but its presence is not easily confirmed by clinical examination with a Sims' speculum, further investigation will be necessary to confirm or fully exclude the possibility. Even where the diagnosis is clinically obvious, additional investigation may be appropriate for full evaluation prior to deciding on treatment.

Microbiology

Urinary infection is surprisingly uncommon in fistula patients, although especially where there have been previous attempts at surgery urine culture should be undertaken and appropriate antibiotic therapy instituted. Urine culture is not easily obtained when a fistula produces severe incontinence, but a pipette may be used to obtain a small intravesical sample for investigation.

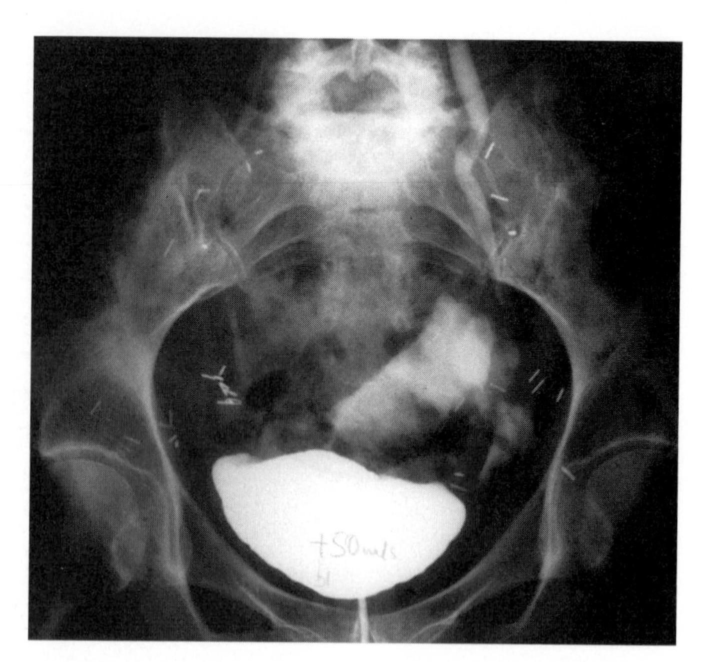

Fig. 53.10 Intravenous urogram (with simultaneous cystogram) demonstrating a complex surgical fistula occurring after radical hysterectomy. After further investigation including cystourethroscopy, sigmoidoscopy, barium enema and retrograde cannulation of the vaginal vault to perform fistulography, the lesion was defined as a ureterocolovesicovaginal fistula.

Dye studies

When the diagnosis is in doubt it is important first to confirm that the discharge is urinary, secondly that the leakage is extraurethral rather than urethral, and thirdly to establish the site of leakage. Although other imaging techniques undoubtedly have a role (see below) carefully conducted dye studies remain the investigation of first choice.

Excessive vaginal discharge, or the drainage of serum from a pelvic haematoma postoperatively, may simulate a urinary fistula. If the fluid is in sufficient quantity to be collected, biochemical analysis of its urea content compared to that of urine and serum will confirm its origin. Phenazopyridine may be used orally (200 mg tds), or indigo carmine intravenously, to stain the urine and hence confirm the presence of a fistula. The identification of the site of a fistula is best carried out by the instillation of coloured dye (methylene blue or indigo carmine) into the bladder via a catheter with the patient in the lithotomy position. The traditional 'three swab test' has its limitations and is not recommended; the examination is best carried out with direct inspection; multiple fistulae may be located in this way. It is important to be alert for leakage around the catheter which may spill back into the vagina, creating the impression of a fistula. It is also important to ensure that adequate distension of the bladder occurs, as some fistulae do not leak at small volumes; conversely, some fistulae with an oblique track through the bladder wall may leak at small volumes, but not at capacity. If leakage of clear fluid continues after dye instillation a ureteric fistula is likely, and this is most easily confirmed by a 'two dye test', using phenazopyridine to stain the renal urine and methylene blue to stain the bladder contents (Raghavaiah 1974).

Dye tests are less useful for intestinal fistulae, although a carmine marker taken orally may confirm their presence. Rectal distension with air via a sigmoidoscope may be of more value; if the patient is kept in a slight head-down position and the vagina filled with saline, the bubbling of any air leaked through a low fistula may be detected.

Imaging

Excretion urography

Although intravenous urography is a particularly insensitive investigation in the diagnosis of vesicovaginal fistula, knowledge of upper urinary tract status may have a significant influence on the treatment measures applied, and should therefore be looked on as an essential investigation for any suspected or confirmed urinary fistula. Compromise to ureteric function is a particularly common finding when a fistula occurs in relation to malignant disease or its treatment (by radiation or surgery).

Dilatation of the ureter is characteristic in ureteric fistula, and its finding in association with a known vesicovaginal fistula should raise suspicion of a complex ureterovesicovaginal lesion. Despite being essential for the diagnosis of ureteric fistula, intravenous urography is not completely sensitive, although the presence of a periureteric flare is highly suggestive of extravasation at this site (Fig. 53.10).

Retrograde pyelography

Retrograde pyelography is a more reliable way of identifying the exact site of a ureterovaginal fistula, and may be undertaken simultaneously with either retrograde or percutaneous catheterization for therapeutic stenting of the ureter (see below).

Cystography

Cystography is not particularly helpful in the basic diagnosis of vesicovaginal fistulae, and a dye test carried out under direct vision is likely to be more sensitive. It may, however, occasionally be useful in achieving a diagnosis in complex fistulae (Fig. 53.10) or vesicouterine fistulae, where a lateral view may show the cavity of the uterus filled with radio-opaque dye behind the bladder.

Fistulography

This is a special example of the X-ray technique commonly referred to as sinography. For small fistulae a ureteric catheter is suitable, although if the hole is large enough a small Foley catheter may be used to deliver the radio-opaque dye; this is particularly of value for fistulae for which there is an intervening abscess cavity. If a catheter will pass through a small vaginal aperture into an adjacent loop of bowel the nature of the fistula may become apparent from the radiological appearance of the lumen and haustrations, although further imaging studies are usually required to demonstrate the underlying pathology.

Colpography and hysterosalpingography

If a fistula opening cannot be directly identified colpography or hysterography may occasionally be helpful. If a large Foley catheter with a large balloon is distended in the lower vagina, injection of a non-viscous opaque medium under pressure may outline a fistulous track to an adjacent organ. However, failure to demonstrate a fistula by this means does not exclude its presence. If a patient with a vesicouterine fistula has no history of incontinence but complains of cyclical haematuria, contrast studies carried out through the uterus may be more rewarding than cystography. Again, a lateral view is necessary to detect the anterior leak.

Barium enema, barium meal and follow-through

Either or both of these may be required for the evaluation of the intestinal condition when an intestinal fistula is present above the anorectum. Apart from confirming the presence of a fistula, evidence of malignant or inflammatory disease may be identified.

Ultrasound, computed tomography and magnetic resonance imaging

These may occasionally be appropriate for the complete assessment of complex fistulae. Endoanal ultrasound and MRI are particularly useful in the investigation of anorectal and perineal fistulae.

Examination under anaesthesia

Careful examination, if necessary under anaesthetic, may be required to determine the presence of a fistula and is deemed by several authorities to be an essential preliminary to definitive surgical treatment (Chassar Moir 1967, Lawson 1978, Jonas & Petri 1984, Lawson & Hudson 1987). A malleable silver probe is invaluable for the exploration of the vaginal walls, and tissue forceps or plastic surgical skin hooks helpful to put tension on the tissues for the identification of small fistulae (see Fig. 53.7b). If the probe passes directly into the rectum it may be felt digitally or seen via the proctoscope; in the bladder or urethra it may be identified by a metallic click against a silver catheter, or seen by a cystoscope; in either case the diagnosis is then obvious.

It is also important at the time of examination to assess the available access for repair vaginally, and the mobility of the tissues (see Fig. 53.7a & b). The decision between the vaginal and abdominal approaches to surgery is thus made; when the vaginal route is chosen it may be appropriate to select between the more conventional supine lithotomy with a head-down tilt and the prone (reverse lithotomy) with head-up tilt (Fig. 53.11). This may be

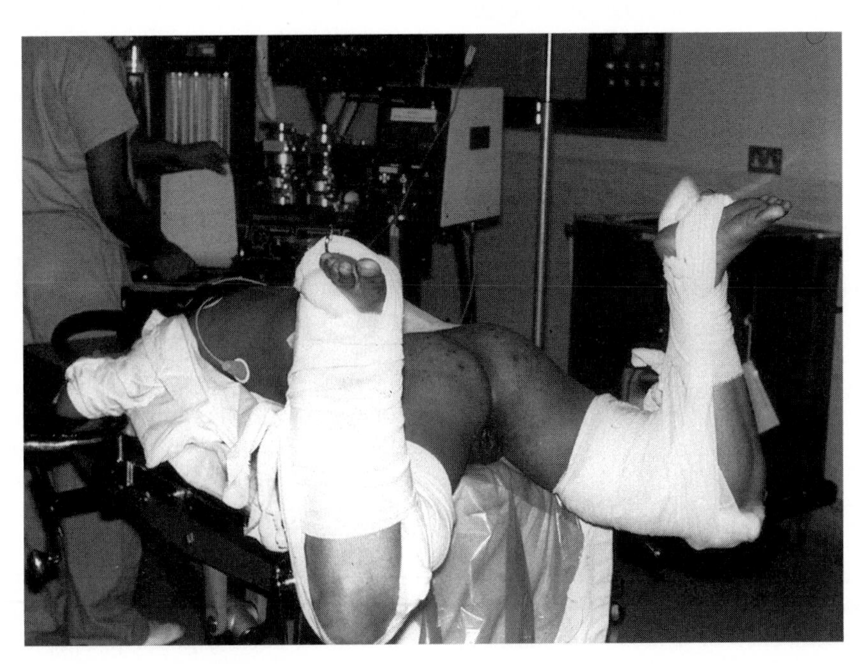

Fig. 53.11 Patient in the prone (reverse lithotomy) position with head-up tilt, in preparation for repair of a fixed subsymphysial fistula.

particularly useful in allowing the operator to look down on to bladder neck and subsymphysial fistulae, and is also of advantage in some massive fistulae in encouraging the reduction of the prolapsed bladder mucosa (Lawson 1967).

Endoscopy

Cystoscopy

Although some authorities suggest that endoscopy has little role in the evaluation of fistulae, it is the author's practice to perform cystourethroscopy in all but the largest defects. Although in some obstetric and radiation fistulae the size of the defect and the extent of tissue loss and scarring may make it difficult to distend the bladder, nevertheless much useful information is obtained. The exact level and position of the fistula should be determined, and its relationship to the ureteric orifices and bladder neck is particularly important. With urethral and bladder-neck fistulae failure to pass a cystoscope or sound may indicate that there has been circumferential loss of the proximal urethra, a circumstance which is or considerable importance in determining the appropriate surgical technique and the likelihood of subsequent urethral incompetence. Similar considerations may apply to investigation of the lower bowel following major obstetric injuries in which segmental circumferential loss of the upper rectum may have occurred.

The condition of the tissues must be carefully assessed. Persistence of slough means that surgery should be deferred, and this is particularly important in obstetric and postradiation cases. Biopsy from the edge of a fistula should be taken in radiation fistulae, if persistent or recurrent malignancy is suspected. Malignant change has been reported in a long-standing benign fistula, and so where there is any doubt at all about the nature of the tissues biopsy should be undertaken (Hudson 1968). In areas of endemicity evidence of schistosomiasis, tuberculosis and lymphogranuloma may become apparent in biopsy material, and again it is important that specific antimicrobial treatment is instituted prior to definitive surgery.

If calculi are identified in the bladder, vaginal vault or diverticula, either clinically, radiologically or endoscopically, their removal prior to any attempt at surgical correction is essential.

Sigmoidoscopy and proctoscopy

These examinations are important for the diagnosis of inflammatory bowel disease, which may not have been suspected before the occurrence of a fistula. Biopsies of the fistula edge or any unhealthy-looking area should always be obtained.

MANAGEMENT

Immediate management

Before epithelialization is complete an abnormal communication between viscera will tend to close spontaneously, provided that the natural outflow is unobstructed. Normal continence mechanisms, however, involve the intermittent physiological contraction of urethral and anal sphincters (see Ch. 46). As a result, although spontaneous closure of genital tract fistulae does occur, it is the exception rather than the rule. Bypassing the sphincter mechanisms, or diverting flow around the fistula, for example by urinary catheterization or defunctioning colostomy, may, however, encourage closure.

The early management is of critical importance and depends on the aetiology and site of the lesion. If surgical trauma is recognized within the first 24 hours postoperatively immediate repair may be appropriate, provided that extravasation of urine into the tissues has not been great.

The majority of surgical fistulae are, however, recognized between 5 and 14 days postoperatively, and these should be treated with continuous bladder drainage. It is worth persisting with this line of management in vesicovaginal or urethrovaginal fistulae for 6–8 weeks, since spontaneous closure may occur within this period (Davits & Miranda 1991).

Obstetric fistulae developing after obstructed labour should also be treated by continuous bladder drainage, combined with antibiotics to limit tissue damage from infection. Indeed, if a patient is known to have been in obstructed labour for any significant length of time, or is recognized to have areas of slough on the vaginal walls in the puerperium, prophylactic catheterization should be undertaken. If sloughing of the rectal wall has also occurred faecal discharge will adversely affect spontaneous healing, and temporary defunctioning colostomy should be performed.

The management of ureterovaginal fistulae is beyond the skill of most gynaecologists, and even those with specialist skills in urogynaecology are likely to liaise with urological and radiological colleagues in this situation. Whereas in the past ureteric reimplantation has been looked on as the preferred approach in most cases, the use of stents, inserted either endoscopically or percutaneously, is successful in the majority of cases (Chang et al 1987). Where stenting cannot be achieved, or does not result in closure of the fistula, definitive surgery should be undertaken at 4–6 weeks, unless progressive calyceal dilatation demands earlier intervention.

The immediate management of obstetric third-degree tears has traditionally been thought to provide a good outcome. Recent data suggest that about half of patients sustaining such injuries will have subsequent defecatory symptoms as a result of sphincter disruption rather than denervation, and 6% may end up with rectovaginal fistulae (Sultan et al 1994). Whether primary repair by a more experienced surgeon, or delayed repair, would improve outcome has not been investigated.

It is important to appreciate that some fistulae may be associated with few or slight symptoms, and even if persistent these do not require surgical treatment. Small distal urethrovaginal fistulae, uterovesical fistulae with menouria, and some low rectovaginal fistulae may fall into this category.

Palliation and skin care

During the waiting period from diagnosis to repair incontinence pads should be provided in generous quantities so that patients can continue to function socially to some extent. Fistula patients usually leak very much greater quantities of urine than those with urethral incontinence from whatever cause, and this needs to be recognized in terms of provision of supplies.

The vulval skin may be at considerable risk from ammoniacal dermatitis, and liberal use of silicone barrier cream should be encouraged. Steroid therapy has been advocated in the past as a means of reducing tissue oedema and fibrosis, although these benefits are refuted and there may be a risk of compromise to subsequent healing (Jonas & Petri 1984). Local oestrogen has been recommended by some authors (Kelly 1983, Jonas & Petri 1984), and although empirically one might expect benefit in postmenopausal women, or those obstetric fistula patients with prolonged amenorrhoea, the evidence for this is lacking.

Nutrition

Because of social ostracism and the effects of prolonged sepsis, patients with obstetric fistulae may also suffer from malnutrition and anaemia. To maximize the prospects for postoperative healing it is essential, therefore, that the general health of the patient should be optimized. Where there is severe inflammatory bowel disease the question of elemental diet, or even total parenteral nutrition, may need to be considered in consultation with the gastroenterologist involved.

Physiotherapy

Obstetric fistulae are commonly associated with lower limb weakness, foot drop and limb contracture. In a group of 479 patients studied prospectively 27% had signs of peroneal nerve weakness at presentation and a further 38%, despite having no current signs, gave a history of relevant symptoms (Waaldijk & Elkins 1994). Early involvement of the physiotherapist in the preoperative management and rehabilitation of such patients is essential.

Antimicrobial therapy

In tropical countries the treatment of malaria, typhoid, tuberculosis and parasitic infections should be rigorously undertaken before elective surgery. Opinions differ on the desirability of prophylactic antibiotic cover for surgery, some avoiding their use other than in the treatment of specific infection, and some advocating broad-spectrum treatment in all cases. The author's current practice is for single-dose prophylaxis in urinary fistulae, and 5 days' cover for intestinal fistulae, in each case using metronidazole and cefuroxime.

Bowel preparation

Although surgeons vary in the extent to which they prepare the bowel prior to rectovaginal fistula repair, it is the author's preference to carry out formal preparation in all cases of intestinogenital fistula, whatever the level of the lesion. A low-residue diet should be advised for a week prior to admission, followed by a fluid-only diet for 48 hours preoperatively. Polyethylene glycol 3350 (Kleneprep), four sachets in 4 litres of water over a 4-hour period, or alternatively sodium picosulphate (Picolax) 10 mg repeated after 6 hours, is given orally on the day before operation. Bowel washout should be carried out on the evening before surgery, and if bowel content is not completely clear this should be repeated on the morning of surgery.

Counselling

Surgical fistula patients are usually previously healthy individuals who entered hospital for what was expected to be a routine procedure, and they end up with symptoms infinitely worse than their initial complaint. Obstetric fistula patients in the developing world are social outcasts. In both situations, therefore, these women are invariably devastated by their situation. It is vital that they understand the nature of the problem, why it has arisen, and the plan for management at all stages. Confident but realistic counselling by the surgeon is essential, and the involvement of nursing staff or counsellors with experience of fistula patients is also highly desirable. The support given by previously treated sufferers can also be of immense value in maintaining patient morale, especially where a delay prior to definitive treatment is required.

General principles of surgical treatment

Details of individual operations are outside the scope of this chapter, and readers wishing for further information about this aspect of fistula management are referred to operative surgical texts or more specific texts on the subject, e.g. Chassar Moir (1967), Lawson & Hudson (1987), Zacharin (1988), Mundy (1993), Waaldijk (1994).

Timing of repair

The timing of surgical repair is perhaps the single most

contentious aspect of fistula management. Although shortening the waiting period is of both social and psychological benefit to what are always very distressed patients, one must not trade these issues for compromise to surgical success. The benefit of delay is to allow slough to separate and inflammatory change to resolve. In both obstetric and radiation fistulae there is considerable sloughing of tissues, and it is imperative that this should have settled before repair is undertaken. In radiation fistulae it may be necessary to wait 12 months or more. In obstetric cases most authorities suggest that a minimum of 3 months should be allowed to elapse, although Waaldijk (1994) has recently advocated surgery as soon as slough is separated.

With surgical fistulae the same principles should apply, and although the extent of sloughing is limited, extravasation of urine into the pelvic tissues inevitably sets up some inflammatory response. Although early repair is advocated by several authors, again most would agree that 10–12 weeks postoperatively is the earliest appropriate time for repair.

Pressure from patients to undertake repair at the earliest opportunity is always understandably great, but is never more so than in the case of previous surgical failure. Such pressure must, however, be resisted, and 8 weeks is the minimum time that should be allowed between attempts at closure.

Route of repair

Many urologists advocate an abdominal approach for all fistula repairs, claiming the possibility of earlier intervention and higher success rates in justification. Others suggest that all fistulae can be successfully closed by the vaginal route (Waaldijk 1994). Such arguments have little merit, and both approaches have their place. Surgeons involved in fistula management must be capable of both approaches, and have the versatility to modify their techniques to select the one most appropriate to the individual case. Where access is good and the vaginal tissues sufficiently mobile, the vaginal route is usually most appropriate. If access is poor and the fistula cannot be brought down, the abdominal approach should be used. Although such difficulties can sometimes be handled vaginally, where there is concurrent involvement of ureter or bowel in a surgical fistula, an abdominal procedure may be used to advantage.

Overall more surgical fistulae than obstetric fistulae are likely to require an abdominal repair, although in the author's series from the UK, and those reviewed from Nigeria, two-thirds of cases were satisfactorily treated by the vaginal route regardless of aetiology (Table 53.4).

Table 53.4 Route of primary repair (i.e. first repair at referral centre) of urogenital fistulae in two series, from the north of England (Hilton, unpublished) and from southeast Nigeria (Hilton & Ward 1995)

Route of repair (primary procedure)	NE England (n = 85)		SE Nigeria (n = 2485)	
	%	%	%	%
Abdominal	33 .8		17.0	
Transperitoneal		13.0		} 13.4
Transvesical		13.0		}
Ureteric reimplantation/ stenting		3.9		3.0
Ureterosigmoid transplantation		0.0		0.6
Ileal conduit		2.6		0.0
Vaginal lithotomy	63.6		80.0	
Layer dissection		39.0		
Layer dissection + Martius graft		18.2		
Colpocleisis		6.4		
Vaginal reverse lithotomy	2.6		3.0	
Total	100.0		100.0	

Instruments

All operators have their own favoured instruments, although those described by Chassar Moir (1967) and Lawson (1967) are eminently suitable for repair by any route (Fig. 53.12). The following are particularly useful:

- Series of fine scalpel blades on the no. 7 handle, especially the curved no. 12 bistoury blade;
- Chassar Moir 30° angled-on-flat and 90° curved-on-flat scissors;
- Cleft palate forceps;
- Judd–Allis, Stiles and Duval tissue forceps;
- Millin's retractor for use in transvesical procedures, and Currie's retractors for vaginal repairs;
- Skin hooks to put the tissues on tension during dissection;
- Turner-Warwick double-curved needle holder is particularly useful in areas of awkward access, and has the advantage of allowing needle placement without the operator's hand or the instrument obstructing the view.

Dissection

Great care must be taken over the initial dissection of the fistula, and one should probably take as long over this as over the repair itself. Preliminary infiltration with 1 in 200 000 solution of adrenaline may help separate planes and reduce oozing. The fistula should be circumcised in the most convenient orientation, depending on size and access. All things being equal, a longitudinal incision should be made around urethral or mid-vaginal fistulae, so that during repair sutures tend to close the bladder neck; conversely, vault fistulae are better handled by a transverse elliptical incision, so that during repair sutures do not tend to approximate the ureters (Fig. 53.13a)

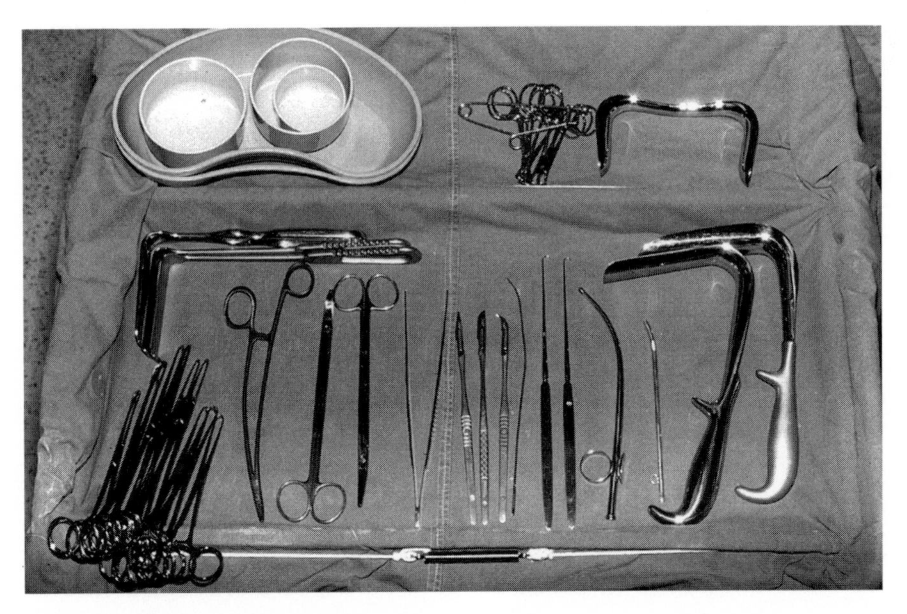

Fig. 53.12 Fistula repair instruments.

The tissue planes are often obliterated by scarring, and dissection close to a fistula should therefore be undertaken with a scalpel or scissors (Fig. 53.13b). Sharp dissection is easier with countertraction applied by skin hooks, tissue forceps or retraction sutures. Blunt dissection with small pledgets may be helpful once the planes are established, and provided one is away from the fistula edge. Wide mobilization should be performed, so that tension on the repair is minimized (Fig. 53.13c).

There are arguments over the benefits of excision of the fistula track itself. Excision of the bladder walls is probably unwise, as it enlarges the defect and may increase the amount of bleeding into the bladder. Limited excision of the scarred vaginal wall is, however, usually appropriate (Fig. 53.13d).

Bleeding is rarely troublesome with vaginal procedures, except occasionally with proximal urethrovaginal fistulae. Diathermy is best avoided, and pressure or underrunning sutures preferred.

Suture materials

Although a range of suture materials have been advocated over the years, and a range of opinion still exists, the author's view is that absorbable sutures should be used throughout all urinary fistula repair procedures. Polyglactin (Vicryl) 2/0 suture on a 25 mm heavy taper-cut needle is preferred for both the bladder and vagina, and polydioxanone (PDS) 4/0 on a 13 mm round-bodied needle is used for the ureter; 3/0 sutures on a 30 mm round-bodied needle are used for bowel surgery, polydioxanone (PDS) for the small bowel, and either polydioxanone (PDS) or braided polyamide (Nurolon) for large bowel reanastomosis.

Specific repair techniques

Vaginal procedures

Dissection and repair in layers. There are two main types of closure technique applied to the repair of urinary fistulae, the classic saucerization technique described by Sims (1852), and the much more commonly used dissection and repair in layers. Sutures must be placed with meticulous accuracy in the bladder wall, care being taken not to penetrate the mucosa, which should be inverted as far as possible. The repair should be started at either end, working towards the midline, so that the least accessible aspects are sutured first (Fig. 53.13e). Interrupted sutures are preferred and should be placed approximately 3 mm apart, taking as large a bite of tissue as feasible. Stitches that are too close together, or the use of continuous or purse-string sutures, tend to impair blood supply and interfere with healing. Knots must be secure with three hitches so that they can be cut short, leaving the minimum amount of material within the body of the repair.

With dissection and repair in layers the first layer of sutures in the bladder should invert the edges (Fig. 53.13e); the second adds bulk to the repair by taking a wide bite of bladder wall, but also closes off dead space by catching the back of the vaginal flaps (Fig. 53.13f). After testing the repair (Fig. 53.13g) (see below) a third layer of interrupted mattress sutures is used to evert and close the vaginal wall, consolidating the repair by picking up the underlying bladder wall (Fig. 53.13h).

Saucerization. The saucerization technique involves converting the track into a shallow crater, which is closed without dissection of bladder from vagina using a single row of interrupted sutures. The method is only applicable to small fistulae, and perhaps residual fistulae after closure

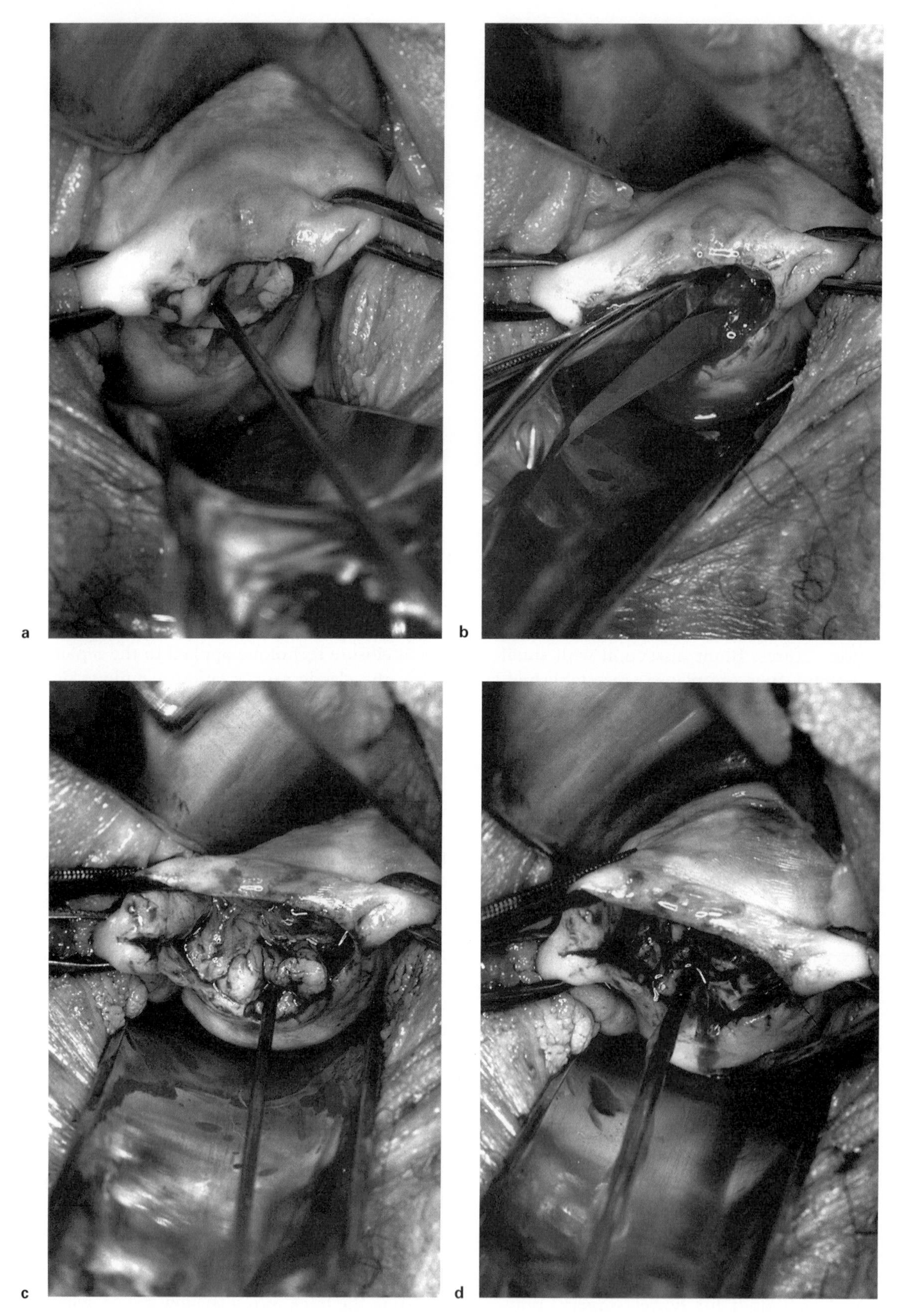

Fig. 53.13 Series of operative photographs demonstrating steps of repair of typical posthysterectomy vault fistula. **(a)** Fistula circumcised using no. 12 scalpel; **(b)** Sharp dissection around fistula edge; **(c)** Fistula fully mobilized; **(d)** Vaginal scar edge trimmed.

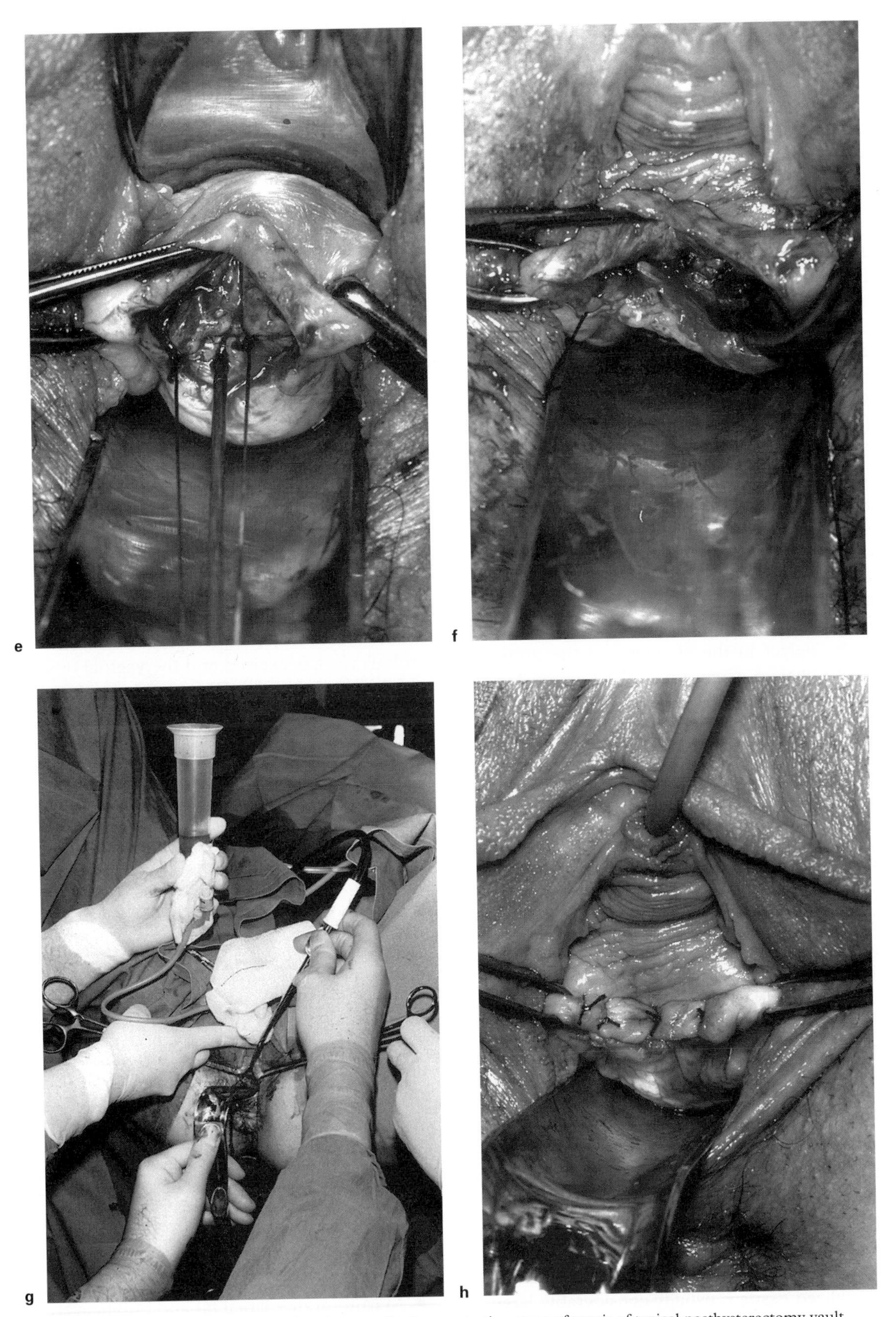

Fig. 53.13, cont'd. Series of operative photographs demonstrating steps of repair of typical posthysterectomy vault fistula. **(e)** First two sutures of first layer of repair in place lateral to the angles of the repair; **(f)** Second layer completed, sutures catching back of vaginal flaps to close off dead space; **(g)** Testing the repair with methylene blue dye instillation; **(h)** Final layer of mattress sutures in the vaginal wall.

of a larger defect; in other situations the technique does not allow secure closure without tension.

Vaginal repair procedures in specific circumstances. The conventional dissection and repair in layers as described above is entirely appropriate for the majority of mid-vaginal fistulae, although modifications may be necessary in specific circumstances. In juxtacervical fistulae in the anterior fornix vaginal repair may be feasible if the cervix can be drawn down to provide access. Dissection should include mobilization of the bladder from the cervix. The repair must be undertaken transversely to reconstruct the underlying trigone and prevent distortion of the ureteric orifices.

Vault fistulae, particularly those following hysterectomy, can again usually be managed vaginally. The vault is incised transversely and mobilization of the fistula is often aided by deliberate opening of the pouch of Douglas (Lawson 1972). The peritoneal opening does not require to be closed separately, but is incorporated into the vaginal closure.

With subsymphysial fistulae involving the bladder neck and proximal urethra as a consequence of obstructed labour, tissue loss may be extensive and fixity to underlying bone a common problem. The lateral aspects of the fistula require careful mobilization to overcome disproportion between the defect in the bladder and the urethral stump. A racquet-shaped extension of the incision facilitates exposure of the proximal urethra. Although transverse repair is often necessary, longitudinal closure gives better prospects for urethral competence.

Where there is substantial urethral loss reconstruction may be undertaken using the method described by Chassar Moir (1967) or Hamlin and Nicholson (1969). A strip of anterior vaginal wall is constructed into a tube over a catheter. Plication behind the bladder neck is probably important if continence is to be achieved. The interposition of a labial fat or muscle graft not only fills up the potential dead space, but provides additional bladder-neck support and improves continence by reducing scarring between bladder neck and vagina.

With very large fistulae extending from bladder neck to vault, the extensive dissection required may produce considerable bleeding. The main surgical difficulty is to avoid the ureters. They are usually situated close to the superolateral angles of the fistula, and if they can be identified they should be catheterized (see Fig. 53.8). Straight ureteric catheters passed transurethrally, or double pigtail catheters, may both be useful in directing the intramural portion of the ureters internally; nevertheless, great care must be taken during dissection.

Radiation fistulae present particular problems in that the area of devitalized tissue is usually considerably larger than the fistula itself. Mobilization is often impossible, and if repair in layers is attempted the flaps are likely to slough; closure by colpocleisis is therefore required. Some have advocated total closure of the vagina, although it is preferable to avoid dissection in the devitalized tissue entirely, and to perform a lower partial colpocleisis converting the upper vagina into a diverticulum of the bladder. It is usually necessary to fill the dead space below this with an interposition graft (see below).

Abdominal procedures

Transvesical repair. Repair by the abdominal route is indicated when high fistulae are fixed in the vault and are therefore inaccessible per vaginam. Transvesical repair has the advantage of being entirely extraperitoneal. It is often helpful to elevate the fistula site by a vaginal pack, and the ureters should be catheterized under direct vision. The technique of closure is similar to that of the transvaginal flap-splitting repair, except that for haemostasis the bladder mucosa is closed with a continuous suture.

Transperitoneal repair. It is often said that there is little place for a simple transperitoneal repair, although a combined transperitoneal and transvesical procedure is favoured by urologists and is particularly useful for vesicouterine fistulae following caesarean section. A midline split is made in the vault of the bladder; this is extended downwards in a racquet shape around the fistula. The fistulous track is excised and the vaginal or cervical defect closed in a single layer. The bladder is then closed in two layers.

For ureteric fistulae not manageable by stenting reimplantation is considered preferable to reanastomosis of the ureter itself, which carries a greater risk of stricture. Several techniques are described for ureteroneocystostomy, and the most appropriate will depend on the level of the fistula and the nature of the antecedent pathology. The most widely used techniques are direct reimplantation using a psoas hitch, or the creation of a flap of bladder wall, the Boari–Ockerblad technique. There are few lesions which are too high for this approach, although where there is significant deficiency it may be necessary to perform an end-to-side anastomosis between the injured ureter and the good contralateral ureter, i.e. ureteroureterostomy, or to interpose of a loop of small bowel.

Interposition grafting

Several techniques have been described to support fistula repair in different sites. In each case the interposed tissue serves to create an additional layer in the repair, to fill dead space, and to bring in new blood supply to the area. The tissues used include:

- Martius graft – labial fat and bulbocavernosus muscle passed subcutaneously to cover a vaginal repair; this is particularly appropriate to provide additional bulk in a colpocleisis, and in urethral and bladder-neck fistulae may help to maintain competence of closure mechanisms by reducing scarring.

- Gracilis muscle passed either via the obturator foramen or subcutaneously (Hamlin & Nicholson 1969) is used as above.
- Omental pedicle grafts (Kiricuta & Goldstein 1972, Turner-Warwick 1976) may be dissected from the greater curve of the stomach and rotated down into the pelvis on the right gastroepiploic artery; this may be used in any transperitoneal procedure, but has its greatest advantage in postradiation fistulae.
- Peritoneal flap graft (Jonas & Petri 1984) is an easier way of providing an additional layer in transperitoneal repair procedures, by taking a flap of peritoneum from any available surface, most usually the paravesical area.

Testing the repair

The closure must be watertight and so should be tested at the end of vaginal repairs by the instillation of dye into the bladder under minimal pressure; a previously unsuspected second fistula is occasionally identified this way. Testing after abdominal procedures is impractical.

Postoperative management

Fluid balance

The nursing care of patients who have undergone fistula repair is of critical importance, and obsessional postoperative management may do much to secure success. As a corollary, however, poor nursing may easily undermine what has been achieved by the surgeon. A strict fluid balance must be kept and a daily fluid intake of at least 3 litres, and output of 100 ml/h, should be maintained until the urine is clear of blood. Haematuria is more persistent following abdominal than vaginal procedures, and intravenous fluid is therefore likely to be required for longer in this situation.

Bladder drainage

Continuous bladder drainage in the postoperative period is crucial to success, and where failure occurs after a straightforward repair it is almost always possible to identify a period during which free drainage was interrupted. Nursing staff should check catheters hourly throughout each day, to confirm free drainage and check output. Catheters should of course drain into a sterile closed drainage system with a non-return valve (Hilton 1987). In circumstances where supplies of sterile disposables are limited, or where standards of nursing are poor, as in many developing countries, open drainage has been advocated, with good success and low infection rates (Ward 1989, personal communication). Bladder irrigation and suction drainage are no longer recommended.

Views differ as to the ideal type of catheter. The calibre must be sufficient to prevent blockage, although whether the suprapubic or urethral route is used is to a large extent a matter of individual preference. A urethral Foley catheter should probably be avoided following bladder-neck fistulae, and either a suprapubic catheter or a non-balloon urethral catheter sutured in place would be preferable. The bladder should not be distended to insert a suprapubic catheter after a vaginal repair, although it could be inserted preoperatively by the technique of cutting on to a sound. The author's usual practice is to use a 'belt and braces' approach of both urethral and suprapubic drainage initially, so that if one becomes blocked free drainage is still maintained. The urethral catheter is removed first, and the suprapubic retained and used to assess residual volume until the patient is voiding normally (Hilton 1987).

Where there are problems with free drainage, or leakage becomes apparent during the postoperative period, the following steps should be taken:

- Ensure that the catheter is secured, and not kinked.
- Check that fluid intake has been adequate.
- Try to establish whether any leakage is vaginal or urethral, i.e. bypassing the catheter.
- Gently flush the catheter – only a small volume of saline should be used, with minimal pressure on the syringe.
- If the problem is one of bypassing, but flushing the catheter does not solve it, it may be worth trying an anticholinergic drug, e.g. probanthine or oxybutynin, to reduce any unstable detrusor activity.
- If a urethral catheter is in place it may rarely be appropriate to replace this, depending on the fistula type; this should only be after consultation with the surgeon.

The duration of free drainage depends on the fistula type. Following repair of surgical fistulae, 12 days is adequate. With obstetric fistulae up to 21 days' drainage may be appropriate, and following repair of radiation fistulae 21–42 days is required. In any of these situations it is wise to carry out dye testing (see below) prior to catheter removal if there is any doubt about the integrity of the repair. Where a persistent leak is identified free drainage should be maintained for 6 weeks.

Mobility and thromboprophylaxis

The biggest problem in ensuring free catheter drainage lies in preventing kinking or drag on the catheter. Restricting patient mobility in the postoperative period helps with this, and some advocate continuous bed rest during the period of catheter drainage. If this approach is chosen patients should be looked on as being at moderate to high risk for thromboembolism, and prophylaxis must be employed (THRIFT 1992); the author's practice is to use both graduated compression stockings and low-dose subcutaneous heparin, starting preoperatively and continued until the patient is fully mobile postoperatively.

Antibiotics

Antibiotic cover is advised for all intestinovaginal fistula repairs. If prophylactic antibiotics are not used at urogenital fistula repair, catheter urine specimens should be collected for culture and sensitivity every 48 hours; only symptomatic infection need be treated in the catheterized patient.

Bowel management

If patients are restricted to bed following urogenital fistula repair, a laxative should be administered to prevent excessive straining at stool. Following abdominal repair of intestinovaginal fistulae patients should either have a nasogastric tube inserted or be kept nil by mouth until they are passing flatus; the majority prefer the latter approach. Once oral intake is allowed, or following vaginal repair of rectovaginal fistulae, a low-residue diet should be administered until at least the fifth postoperative day. Enemas and suppositories should be avoided, although a mild aperient such as dioctyl sodium (Docusate) is advised to ease initial bowel movements.

Subsequent management

On removal of the catheter most patients will feel the desire to void frequently, since the bladder capacity will be functionally reduced having been relatively empty for so long. In any case it is important that they do not become overdistended, and hourly voiding should be encouraged and fluid intake limited. It may also be necessary to wake them once or twice through the night for the same reason. After discharge from hospital patients should be advised to gradually increase the period between voiding, aiming to be back to a normal pattern by 4 weeks postoperatively.

Tampons, pessaries, douching and penetrative sex should be avoided until 3 months postoperatively.

PROGNOSIS

Results

It is difficult to compare the results of treatment in different series, since the lesions involved and the techniques of repair vary so greatly. Cure rates should be considered in terms of closure at first operation, and vary from 60 to 98% (Turner-Warwick et al 1967, Hamlin & Nicholson 1969, Chassar Moir 1973, Hudson et al 1975, Kelly 1979, Godwin & Scardino 1980, Patil et al 1980, O'Connor 1980, Wein et al 1980, Elkins et al 1988, Lee et al 1988, Ahmad (cited by WHO 1989), Hilton 1995a, Hilton & Ward 1995). On average one might anticipate 80% cures with 10% failures and, in the case of obstetric fistulae at least, 10% suffering from postfistula stress incontinence (see below).

Of the 85 patients in the author's series managed in the UK, three (3.5%) healed without operation, three declined surgery, one (with coexistent detrusor instability) was asymptomatic on medical treatment, two (2.4%) underwent primary urinary diversion, and one patient with a radiotherapy fistula died from recurrent disease during the course of assessment. Of the remaining 75 who have undergone repair surgery, 70 (93%) were cured by the first

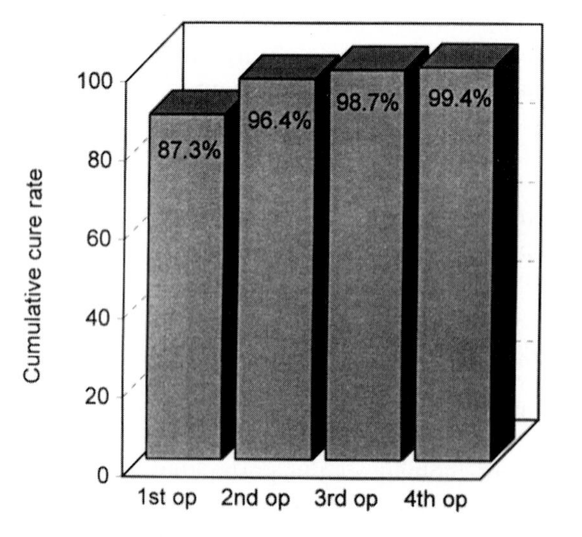

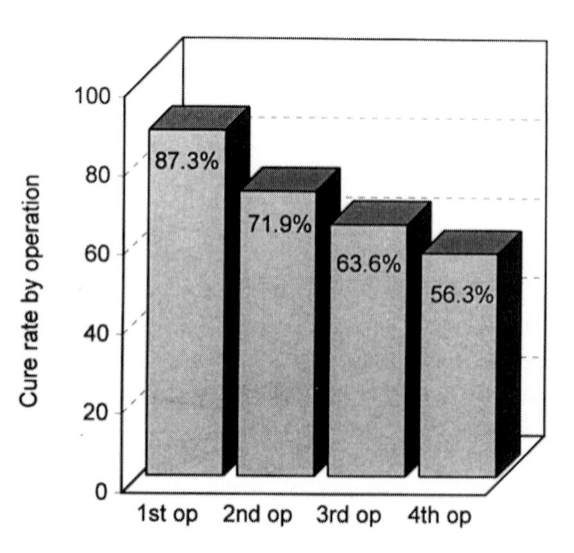

Fig. 53.14 (left) Cumulative success rate of obstetric fistula surgery, after a first, second, third and fourth operation (n = 2485); (right) Success rates for first and subsequent operations (Hilton & Ward 1995).

operation; of the 41 fistulae following simple hysterectomy all were cured at their first operation.

Of the largely obstetric fistulae reviewed from Nigeria (Hilton & Ward 1995), 87.3% were cured by a first operation and 99.4% eventually successfully anatomically repaired, with only 0.6% undergoing urinary diversion.

A law of diminishing returns has previously been reported (Lawson 1978). Although repeat operations are certainly justified, the success rate decreases progressively with increasing numbers of previous unsuccessful procedures (Hilton & Ward 1995) (Fig. 53.14). It cannot be overemphasized that the best prospect for cure is at the first operation, and there is no place for the well-intentioned occasional fistula surgeon, be they gynaecologist or urologist.

Post-fistula stress incontinence

Stress incontinence has long been recognized as a complication of vesicovaginal fistulae (Lawson 1967). It is most likely to occur in obstetric fistula patients when the injury involves the sphincter mechanism, particularly if there is tissue loss (Waaldijk 1994), although it has also been reported in a large proportion of surgical fistulae involving the urethra or bladder neck (Hilton 1995b). It affects at least 10% of all fistula patients.

The extent of scarring in the area means that conventional approaches to bladder-neck elevation may be technically difficult and of limited success. The use of a labial musculofat graft in the initial repair may reduce the likelihood of the complication (Waaldijk 1994) and a number of other techniques have been attempted (Hudson et al 1975, Waaldijk 1994). The implantation of an artificial urinary sphincter, or neourethral reconstruction, might from a theoretical point of view be appropriate (Hilton 1990), but the former would be prohibitively expensive, and both excessively morbid for use in the developing world. Periurethral injections hold promise as a minimally invasive technique particularly appropriate in the situation of urethral insufficiency with a relatively fixed immobile urethra, and have recently been reported with initial success in postfistula stress incontinent patients (Hilton et al 1995).

Subsequent pregnancy

Although many patients with obstetric vesicovaginal fistula will experience amenorrhoea for 2 years or more after the causative pregnancy (Hilton & Ward 1995), where tissue loss is not great hypothalamic function often returns to normal immediately after successful repair, and fertility may be relatively normal. Most authorities emphasize need for caesarean section in any subsequent pregnancy (Lawson 1978). Kelly (1979), however, reported on 33 patients who became pregnant within 1 year of fistula repair, 12 of whom were delivered vaginally without damage to the repair. The criteria he used for attempting vaginal delivery were: that the fistula arose from a non-recurring cause (i.e. malpresentation as opposed to pelvic contraction); that an interposition graft had been utilised in the repair; and that the labour be conducted under skilled supervision in hospital.

The management of delivery in women who have had a previous third-degree tear has not been prospectively studied, although it has been suggested that there may be benefit in assessing the sphincter by endoanal ultrasound; prior to delivery where minor defects are present potentially traumatic vaginal delivery should be avoided, and where more major defects are identified caesarean section might be offered (Sultan et al 1994).

PREVENTION

It is estimated by the World Health Organization (WHO) that there are approximately 500 000 maternal deaths per year worldwide, and it is clear that the prevalence of obstetric fistulae and maternal mortality rates are closely related. Indeed, one might look on the vesicovaginal fistula patient as being the 'near miss' maternal death. In recognition of this fact, WHO, through their 'Safe Motherhood Initiative', established a technical working group to investigate the problems of prevention and management of obstetric fistulae. The recommendations from that working group included the extension of antenatal and intrapartum care; the transfer of women in prolonged labour for delivery by skilled personnel; the identification of areas where fistulae are still prevalent, so that resources could be mobilized to deal with fistulae more effectively; and the creation of specialized centres for management, training and research, with a specific aim of treating existing cases within 5 years (WHO 1989). One thousand years ago Avicenna recognized the problems of early childbearing, saying: 'in cases where women are married too young the physician should instruct the patient in the ways of preventing pregnancy. In these patients the bulk of the fetus may cause a tear in the bladder which results in incontinence of urine which is incurable and remains until death' (Hilton 1995a). Clearly, the achievement of the WHO's aims and recommendations is critically dependent on major social change in areas of endemicity. Without improvement in the status of women, an extension of primary education, deferment of marriage and childbearing, improved nutritional status and contraceptive services, and skilled attendants in childbirth throughout the world, the problem of obstetric fistulae will remain with us well into the next millennium.

In the developed world our concern must lie with the prevention and management of fistulae following gynaecological surgery. Primarily we need to be aware of those factors increasing the likelihood of lower urinary tract injury during surgery, and must recognize the limits of our own, and perhaps more importantly our trainees', surgical skills. We should not expect staff in training to undertake surgery in cases where risk factors are known to be present without adequate supervision and support. We should be equally aware of the signs of injury in the postoperative period, and should have standard regimens for the management of patients with voiding difficulty in the postoperative period if bladder overdistension and the risk of late damage is to be avoided. One might perhaps anticipate that with advances in minimally invasive surgery and techniques of endometrial ablation, the need for hysterectomy, and the risk of surgical vesicovaginal fistula, might reduce considerably. Hysterectomy will, however, always be necessary for fibroids, endometriosis, sepsis and malignancy, and these carry the greatest risk of lower urinary tract injury. If these are the only cases on which our trainees can train, then there is a danger that surgical skills in general may decline, in the same way that skills in vaginal breech delivery and rotational forceps delivery have declined with the increasing use of caesarean section.

KEY POINTS

1. In developing countries over 90% of fistulae are of obstetric origin, and are due to pressure necrosis from prolonged obstructed labour.
2. In the UK approximately 75% of fistulae follow pelvic surgery, and half of these cases are associated with simple abdominal hysterectomy.
3. The characteristic presentation, with continuous urinary leakage and reduced frequency and bladder sensation, is not always present in patients with small fistulae, and a high index of suspicion must be maintained if the diagnosis is not to be missed. With intestinal fistulae the history may be similarly misleading.
4. The best estimate is that vesicovaginal fistula complicates 1 in 1300 hysterectomies; this is rarely due to direct injury, and most often results from tissue ischaemia or subclinical haematoma or infection. Although poor surgical technique increases the risk, the mere development of a fistula following hysterectomy does not imply negligence.
5. Where bladder damage is suspected, or fistula confirmed following surgery or childbirth, catheterization should be undertaken and continuous drainage maintained; spontaneous healing may occur up to 8 weeks after the initiating event.
6. The possibility of inflammatory bowel disease should always be considered in patients with intestinogenital fistulae even in the absence of specific bowel symptoms. Of the inflammatory causes Crohn's disease is the most important, and surgical treatment should ideally only be undertaken when the bowel pathology is quiescent.
7. Biopsy of the fistula edge or any unhealthy looking local tissue should be undertaken before embarking on repair of radiation, inflammatory or potentially infective fistulae.
8. Malnutrition, anaemia and infection should be treated before attempting surgical closure; this applies most particularly in patients with obstetric fistulae in the developing world.
9. Surgery for urogenital or intestinogenital fistulae should only be undertaken by surgeons with the appropriate training and experience, and with the versatility to undertake the most appropriate operation by the most appropriate route.
10. Layered closure with avoidance of tension on the suture lines, good haemostasis and obliteration of dead space are important technical points for successful closure.
11. Interposition grafting with pedicled fat or muscle may be a useful adjunct in fistula surgery, by providing an additional layer to the repair, filling dead space, bringing new blood supply and encouraging tissue mobility.
12. Successful anatomical closure of a urinary or intestinal fistula is not necessarily associated with restoration of complete functional normality. Incompetence of sphincter mechanisms may occur, with residual stress urinary incontinence, faecal soiling or incontinence of flatus.
13. Diversion of urinary or faecal stream should rarely be required as definitive measures for the management of fistula patients.

REFERENCES

Chang R, Marshall F F, Mitchell S 1987 Percutaneous management of benign ureteral strictures and fistulas. Journal of Urology 137: 1126–1131

Chassar Moir J 1967 The vesico-vaginal fistula, 2nd edn. Baillière, London

Chassar Moir J 1973 Vesico-vaginal fistulae as seen in Britain. Journal of Obstetrics and Gynaecology of the British Commonwealth 80: 598–602

Davits R J A M, Miranda S I 1991 Conservative treatment of vesico-vaginal fistulas by bladder drainage alone. British Journal of Urology 68: 155–156

Elkins T E, Drescheer C, Martey J O, Fort D 1988 Vesicovaginal fistula revisited. Obstetrics and Gynecology 72: 307–312

Falk F C, Tancer M L 1956 Management of vesical fistulas after Caesarean section. American Journal of Obstetrics and Gynecology 71: 97–106

Godwin W E, Scardino P T 1980 Vesico-vaginal and uretero-vaginal fistulas: a summary of 25 years of experience. Journal of Urology 123: 370–374

Hamlin R H J, Nicholson E C 1969 Reconstruction of urethra totally destroyed in labour. British Medical Journal 2: 147–150

Hilton P 1987 Catheters and drains. In: Stanton S L (ed) Principles of gynaecological surgery. Springer-Verlag, London, pp 257–283

Hilton P 1990 Surgery for genuine stress incontinence: which operation for which patient. In: Drife J O, Hilton P, Stanton S L (eds) Micturition – Proceedings of the 21st RCOG Study Group.

Springer-Verlag, London, pp 225–246
Hilton P 1995a Sims to SMIS – an historical perspective on vesico-vaginal fistulae. In: Studd J W W (ed) The Yearbook of the RCOG, 1994. RCOG, London, pp 7–16
Hilton P 1995b Urodynamic findings in patients with urogenital fistula. International Urogynecology Journal 6(4): 243 (abstract)
Hilton P, Ward A 1995 Epidemiological and surgical aspects of urogenital fistulae: a review of 25 years' experience in Nigeria. International Urogynecology Journal 6(4): 243 (abstract)
Hilton P, Ward A, Molloy M, Umana O 1995 Periurethral injection of autologous fat for stress incontinence after fistula repair: a preliminary report. International Urogynecological Journal 6(4): 243 (abstract)
Hudson C N 1968 Malignant change in an obstetric vesico-vaginal fistula. Proceedings of the Royal Society of Medicine 61: 121–124
Hudson C N, Hendrickse J P de V, Ward A 1975 An operation for restoration of urinary continence following total loss of the urethra. British Journal of Obstetrics and Gynaecology 82: 501–504
Jonas U, Petri E 1984 Genitourinary fistulae. In: Stanton S L (ed) Clinical gynecologic urology. C V Mosby, St Louis, pp 238–255
Kelly J 1979 Vesico-vaginal fistulae. British Journal of Urology 51: 208–210
Kelly J 1983 Vesico-vaginal fistulae In: Studd J W W (ed) Progress in obstetrics and gynaecology, 3rd edn. Churchill Livingstone, Edinburgh, pp 324–333
Kelly J, Kwast B E 1993 Epidemiologic study of vesicovaginal fistulas in Ethiopia. International Urogynecology Journal 4: 278–281
Kiricuta I, Goldstein A M B 1972 The repair of extensive vesicovaginal fistulas with pedicled omentum: a review of 27 cases. Journal of Urology 108: 724–727
Lawson J B 1967 Injuries to the urinary tract. In: Lawson J B, Stewart D B (eds) Obstetrics and gynaecology in the tropics and developing countries. Edward Arnold, London, pp 481–522
Lawson J B 1972 Vesical fistulae into the vaginal vault. British Journal of Urology 44: 623–631
Lawson J B 1978 The management of genito-urinary fistulae. Clinics in Obstetrics and Gynaecology 5: 209–236
Lawson J B, Hudson C N 1987 The management of vesico-vaginal and urethral fistulae. In: Stanton S L, Tanagho E A (eds) Surgery for female urinary incontinence, 2nd edn. Springer-Verlag, Berlin, pp 193–209
Lee R A, Symmonds R E, Williams T J 1988 Current status of genitourinary fistula. Obstetrics and Gynecology 72: 313–319
Mundy A R 1993 Urodynamic and reconstructive surgery of the lower urinary tract. Churchill Livingstone, Edinburgh
Murphy M 1981 Social consequences of vesico-vaginal fistula in northern Nigeria. Journal of Biosocial Sciences 13: 139–150
O'Connor V J 1980 Review of experience with vesico-vaginal fistula repair. Journal of Urology 123: 367–369
Patil U, Waterhouse K, Laungani G 1980 Management of 18 difficult vesico-vaginal and urethro-vaginal fistulas with modified Ingleman-Sundberg and Martius operations. Journal of Urology 123: 653–656
Raghavaiah N V 1974 Double-dye test to diagnose various types of vaginal fistulas. Journal of Urology 112: 811–812
Sims J M 1852 On the treatment of vesico-vaginal fistula. American Journal of the Medical Sciences XXIII: 59–82
Sultan A H, Kamm M A, Hudson C N, Bartram C I 1994 Third degree obstetric anal sphincter tears: risk factors and outcome of primary repair. British Medical Journal 308: 887–891
Tahzib F 1983 Epidemiological determinants of vesico-vaginal fistulas. British Journal of Obstetrics and Gynaecology 90: 387–391
Tahzib F 1985 Vesico-vaginal fistula in Nigerian children. Lancet ii: 1291–1293
Thromboembolic Risk Factors (THRIFT) Consensus Group 1992 Risk of and prophylaxis for venous thromboembolism in hospital patients. British Medical Journal 305: 567–574
Turner-Warwick R 1976 The use of the omental pedicle graft in urinary tract reconstruction. Journal of Urology 116: 341–347
Turner-Warwick R T, Wynne E J C, Handley-Ashken M 1967 The use of the omental pedicle graft in repair and reconstruction of the urinary tract. British Journal of Surgery 54: 849–853
Waaldijk K 1994 Step-by-step surgery of vesico-vaginal fistulas. Campion, Edinburgh
Waaldijk K, Armiya'u Y D 1993 The obstetric fistula: a major public health problem still unresolved. International Urogynecology Journal 4: 126–128
Waaldijk K, Elkins T E 1994 The obstetric fistula and peroneal nerve injury: an analysis of 947 consecutive patients. International Urogynecology Journal 5: 12–14
Wein A J, Malloy T R, Carpiniello V L, Greenberg S H, Murphy J J 1980 Repair of vesico-vaginal fistula by a suprapubic transvesical approach. Surgery Gynecology and Obstetrics 150: 57–60
World Health Organization 1989 The prevention and treatment of obstetric fistulae: a report of a Technical Working Group. WHO, Geneva
Yeates W K 1987 Uretero-vaginal fistulae. In: Stanton S L, Tanagho E A (eds) Surgery for female urinary incontinence, 2nd edn. Springer-Verlag, Berlin, pp 211–227
Youssef A F 1957 'Menouria' following lower segment caesarean section: a syndrome. American Journal of Obstetrics and Gynecology 73: 759–767
Zacharin R F 1988 Obstetric fistula. Springer-Verlag, Vienna

SECTION 5

Genitourinary infections

54

Urinary tract infection

A. J. France

INTRODUCTION

Urinary tract infections (UTIs) are important because 20% of women aged 20–65 years suffer one attack per year, approximately 50% of women develop a UTI during their lives and there is a prevalence rate of 5% per year of asymptomatic or covert bacteriuria in non-pregnant women between the ages of 21 and 65. UTI is a common reason for visiting a general practitioner, accounting for between 1 and 6% of consultations. Among working women, days lost from work as a result of UTIs account for about one-tenth of those due to respiratory infections. Depending upon the survey, between 12 and 25% of cases of chronic renal failure are attributed to chronic pyelonephritis. Before the antibiotic era febrile UTIs, especially in children, were life-threatening with a mortality of 20% and a morbidity of 20%, mostly from hypertension and renal failure. Although 60% healed spontaneously, the patient was often seriously ill for 6–8 weeks.

TERMINOLOGY

UTIs are defined by the presence of viable microorganisms within the urinary tract, although it may be difficult to distinguish between contamination, colonization or infection. The term 'bacteriuria' is used to define the presence of living bacteria in freshly voided urine or urine obtained via suprapubic aspiration. In 1956 Kass proposed that the isolation of more than 100 000 colony-forming units (cfu) or organisms per millilitre of midstream-voided urine should be used to differentiate probable contamination from covert infection or asymptomatic bacteriuria (ASB).

Cystitis indicates inflammation of the bladder but is often used by patients to indicate any UTI. Another term, 'the urethral syndrome', has a variety of meanings depending upon the author. It is sometimes interchangeable with 'frequency dysuria syndrome' (FDS) with or without bacteriuria.

Acute bacterial pyelonephritis indicates acute infection of the kidneys. More confusion occurs over the term 'chronic pyelonephritis'. This consists of chronic inflammation of renal and tubular tissue, with scarring and shrinkage secondary to interstitial fibrosis. There is accompanying reduction in the glomerular filtration rate, tubular function and ability to concentrate urine.

BACTERIOLOGY

UTIs are usually caused by Gram-negative aerobic organisms originating from the gut flora. In 80–90% of first infections, *Escherichia coli* is isolated. The outer genital and periurethral bacterial flora usually reflect the gut flora, e.g. *Pseudomonas, Klebsiella.* With subsequent infections *E. coli* are seen in around 70% of cases, although more unusual organisms occur after antibiotic therapy, surgery, or the presence of obstruction or stones. *Proteus* species are often associated with renal calculi.

Many bacteriology laboratories merely report the presence of coliform bacteria in the culture. In doing so, they adopt the pragmatic view that antibiotic sensitivities are a more important part of the result than precise species identification. In the author's experience *E. coli* is the most commonly isolated organism. *Klebsiella*, *Proteus* and enterococci are less commonly encountered. It is my experience that staphylococcal UTI is very rare. I believe the high isolation rate in other studies may reflect contamination with staphylococci which normally reside on the skin.

AETIOLOGY

Virulence factors

The ability to adhere to epithelial surfaces and resistance to phagocytosis are the main features of virulent organisms.

Host factors

The maintenance of an infection-free urinary tract relies first, on regular and complete flushing of the system with a steady flow of urine from the kidneys, and secondly, the presence of friendly flora in the vagina and vulva. Anatomical abnormalities and neurological diseases may interfere with the flushing. The friendly flora are disrupted by sexual activity, particularly when spermicides are used. Hooton et al (1991) found that *E. coli* bacteriuria was considerably increased in diaphragm-spermicide users as well as spermicidal foam–condom users. Colonization of the vagina with *E. coli* was transient in oral contraceptive pill users, but longer lasting for spermicide users. Fihn et al (1985) reported 26.6 episodes of UTI per 1000 patient-months in diaphragm users, compared to 8.9 for oral contraceptive users.

Vaginal intercourse was examined in Strom et al's (1987) case control study for UTI. The authors found that sexual intercourse in the previous 48 hours had an odds ratio for UTI of 58.1 and was the most important single factor in the development of UTIs.

Although the symptoms of acute UTI resolve within a few days of starting antibiotics, the epithelium may take weeks to recover fully. During this recovery period its resistance to further infection is impaired and recurrent infection is more likely.

NATURAL HISTORY

The prevalence of UTIs varies with age and sex. There is a 10-fold increase in incidence for adolescent girls compared to boys, and this continues through adult life until around 55 years, when the incidence of UTIs in men and women is equal, mostly as a consequence of prostatic problems in men.

It is difficult to attribute primary mortality to UTIs, although they often complicate other illnesses and conditions. Approximately 12% of cases of chronic renal failure are now attributed to chronic pyelonephritis.

On average, 5% of women at their first antenatal clinic have ASB and, unlike the non-pregnant state, only 3% of these individuals lose their bacteriuria over the course of the pregnancy. The prevalence of ASB increases with parity, and in women with prior ASB 40% had infection documented during pregnancy. Several studies have shown that ASB does have an effect on maternal health. Between 10 and 30% of women with ASB developed acute pyelonephritis during the pregnancy; they have lower haemoglobins, which improves with eradication of the ASB, and hypertension is commoner, especially in association with renal scars. There is no significant effect on renal function but a significant number of patients with ASB have chronic renal disease. Some studies suggest a greater risk of prematurity, an increase in perinatal mortality and a higher incidence of mental retardation. However, most studies have not been large enough to investigate these problems effectively.

Whereas UTIs in adult life have little influence on renal function this cannot be said for the elderly, where bacteriuric individuals have a mean glomerular filtration rate 20% less than non-bacteriuric controls. In addition, over a 2-year follow-up period the glomerular filtration rate declined four to six times as much in the bacteriuric individuals. It would thus appear that the nephrosclerotic changes associated with ageing are accelerated by UTIs.

PRESENTATION

Symptoms

In adult women the archetypal attack of acute cystitis is heralded by the abrupt onset of one or more of the following symptoms: urinary frequency, dysuria, nocturia, urgency, haematuria, malodorous urine, suprapubic pain, and nausea. In some cases the patient recognizes that sexual intercourse may be the precipitating factor. In acute pyelonephritis, loin pain and fever are more common, although the symptoms of cystitis may coexist. In children the symptoms of urinary tract infection may be non-specific abdominal pain, or simply failure to thrive. In elderly patients the classic symptoms are usually absent. UTI is a common cause of confusion or loss of mobility in a previously fit elderly woman. Thus the clinician should have no difficulty recognizing UTI in young and middle-aged adults, but must be aware of the paucity of classic symptoms at the two extremes of life. It must be remembered that urethral strictures can occur in women and that the symptoms of poor flow rate may not be apparent to the patient.

The complete history should include an enquiry about previous UTIs, particularly during childhood and pregnancy. Contraceptive practice may influence advice regarding treatment and prevention (see below). A family history of tuberculosis should alert the clinician to this chronic but treatable condition.

Not all patients are good witnesses. In some patients with recurrent urinary symptoms it is often enlightening to have the patient keep a record of the time of day and the volume every time she passes urine. This introduces an objective measurement, which is useful when assessing the severity of her symptoms and monitoring the response to treatment.

Predisposing factors

These are discussed in detail above. In summary, the clinician should enquire about:

1. Diabetes mellitus, which may cause glycosuria – an enriched culture medium.
2. The presence of foreign bodies such as stones or catheters.
3. Recent instrumentation of the urinary tract.
4. Neurological disorders or anticholinergic drugs, which may cause incomplete bladder emptying.
5. Coexisting pelvic disease, including tumours and inflammatory bowel disease which may directly invade the bladder or alter its mechanical properties.
6. Contraceptive practice and sexual activity.

Physical signs

In acute cystitis/urethritis suprapubic tenderness is often present; alternatively, palpation in this region will provoke a desire to pass urine. The patient may be restless. Fever is unusual. In acute pyelonephritis the patient looks ill. She is usually pyrexial (temperature >38°C) and has a tachycardia. Loin tenderness is a common finding and is bilateral if both kidneys are infected. Septicaemia must be suspected when hypotension accompanies the tachycardia. In young adults with septicaemia the supine blood pressure may be normal but postural hypotension is invariable.

In children and the elderly the physical signs may be misleading by their atypical nature. The absence of the common physical findings does not exclude significant UTI in these age groups.

If a neuropathic bladder is suspected then the skin over the buttocks must be examined for sensory loss. Spinal cord lesions and damage to the sacral nerve roots may be detected in this manner.

INVESTIGATIONS

Inspection

Infected urine may look cloudy. Commercial 'stick tests' are useful to detect glycosuria proteinuria and haematuria. Some sticks will also reveal the presence of nitrites in the urine, which indicates bacterial infection.

Urine microscopy and culture

This is desirable in all cases of suspected UTI. Microscopy of a fresh specimen of urine from a patient with a UTI will detect bacteria and pus cells in abundance. The presence of casts indicates renal disease. The presence of pus cells and subsequent failure to isolate a pathogen is called sterile pyuria, and alerts the clinician to the possibility of tuberculosis. The presence of haematuria in the absence of pus cells or bacteria suggests pathologies other than infection.

The urine is cultured on selective media such as MacConkey or CLED. This helps to restrict the growth of contaminants but allows recognition of most pathogens after 24-hour culture. Identification and antibiotic sensitivity testing complete the microbiological report. If tuberculosis is suspected, at least three early-morning urine samples must be collected and cultured for mycobacteria. The patient is asked to collect the whole of her early-morning urine sample. The laboratory will concentrate the sample by centrifugation, thus improving the detection rate. Radiometric culture methods, e.g. Bactec, have considerably shortened the culture time before mycobacteria are detected and their sensitivities determined.

If there is a significant delay between collecting a sample of urine and plating it on culture medium the final culture result may be misleading, because it will not be a true reflection of urinary tract flora. The inevitable contamination of the sample with skin flora during collection can lead to an overgrowth of these organisms on the culture medium. In an attempt to overcome this problem, some clinicians use a dipslide system. Briefly, a slide coated with solid culture medium is dipped into the urine specimen and then transported to the laboratory in a sealed container. The resulting colonies remain fixed in one place and do not mix, as happens in liquid media. This system has a number of disadvantages: first, there is no microscopy, and so red cells, white cells, casts and crystals will not be detected. Secondly, the technique has a false positive rate of up to 10% and a false negative of up to 3%. Thus a negative dipslide result does not mean the urinary tract is healthy.

If a sexually transmitted disease is suspected the reader is referred to Chapter 56 for further details.

Imaging

Ultrasound examination

Ultrasound examination is a well tolerated investigation with no recognized hazards. It is used to measure the dimensions of the kidneys and to detect obstruction of their drainage. It will also reveal residual urine following incomplete bladder emptying.

Plain abdominal radiograph

This investigation will detect the presence of most stones and foreign bodies. It may also show the calcification which can accompany some chronic infections such as tuberculosis and bilharzia.

Isotope renogram

This investigation gives three important pieces of information:

1. The relative contribution made by each kidney to total renal function.
2. The presence of obstructed drainage of each kidney.
3. Vesicoureteric reflux (VUR) while voiding urine. Merrick et al (1977) showed that isotope techniques were at least as good as conventional micturating cystourethrography at detecting VUR in children with UTI. They pointed out that the isotope method was cheaper, did not require catheterization and involved a lower dose of radiation.

Renal scintigraphy

Renal scintigraphy detects functioning proximal tubular cells. Its application in patients with UTI is the demonstration of renal scars. Monsour et al (1987) showed that renal scintigraphy was superior to ultrasound or intravenous urography when searching for early renal scars in children under the age of 5 years. Over this age the three examinations were equally sensitive. A further application of DMSA scintigraphy is the sequential measurement of renal function in patients without severe renal impairment.

Intravenous urography

Intravenous urography now has limited application in the investigation of the urinary tract. Ultrasound and isotope studies are superior to or equally as sensitive as intravenous urography. A further disadvantage is the relatively high dose of radiation of intravenous urograms. The one area where it is superior is in the demonstration of precise anatomical relations of the ureter. This may be helpful when planning surgical operations involving the ureters.

Logical approach to imaging

The combination of a plain abdominal radiograph and ultrasound has been compared with traditional intravenous urography (Lewis-Jones et al 1989, Spencer et al 1990) in the investigation of patients with UTI. Both have similar sensitivities and concur in 96% of cases. Intravenous urography involves a greater dose of radiation, more radiographer's time and more expensive consumables: £25 vs. £3 per investigation. It seems wise to commence with a plain abdominal radiograph and ultrasound. In most cases of UTI in adults this will be normal and no further imaging is warranted. However, if an abnormality is detected the clinician may wish to proceed with further imaging studies, as described above.

Blood tests

Plasma creatinine and urea concentrations are important measurements of renal function and should be performed in all cases other than solitary episodes of cystitis in adult women. The fasting plasma glucose concentration and oral glucose tolerance test are superior to tests for glycosuria when considering diabetes mellitus.

MANAGEMENT

General principles

The management and prevention of UTIs are closely related. Often the patient's management should include advice as to how further infections can be avoided.

Many women and girls can be saved from the needless prescription of antibacterial agents if they are given – and abide by – some simple instructions. These can be either verbal or written in the form of a handout (ideally both). They should include basic information about the source of the bacteria that invade the urinary tract from the patient's own bowel, and how important it is to wipe the perineum from front to back to avoid faecal contamination of the urethra, especially during an episode of diarrhoea. Potentially irritant vaginal deodorants and bubble baths should be avoided and a high standard of perineal hygiene maintained.

The adult patient with recurrent UTI should drink a minimum of 2 litres of fluid daily – more if exercising strenuously or staying in a warm climate. This should be increased to 3 litres or more daily if symptoms of UTI are suspected, irrespective of the degree of urgency and frequency of micturition or painful dysuria. Keeping a bladder chart may be the best way of reinforcing this advice. Regular and complete bladder emptying must be taught and the concept of double micturition emphasized to those with residual bladder urine after voiding. Women working on assembly lines and girls who abhor unhygienic school lavatories are very prone to acquire overstretched bladders and a tendency to VUR if they are unable to void regularly.

The complaint of postcoital UTI symptoms provides the ideal opportunity to review contraceptive methods, perhaps advising the oral contraceptive rather than the condom if there is much irritation with the latter, and asking the patient to be sure to void as soon as is decently possible after intercourse. Likewise, the use of spermicidal gels is undesirable in women with recurrent UTIs.

Sometimes, however, antibacterial drugs must be given. Their use where appropriate will be discussed in the following sections.

Asymptomatic bacteriuria

Most women with ASB do not require antibacterial treatment. There are, however, certain well defined groups of female patients who do need treatment for ASB. These include pregnant women and women with renal scars from previous infection acquired in childhood.

Symptomatic lower urinary tract infections

The ideal duration of antibiotic therapy for uncomplicated UTI is often debated. Single-dose therapies carry a risk of failure, whereas regimens lasting longer than the duration of symptoms are unlikely to be completed as prescribed. Most practitioners and their patients will find a 3-day course acceptable (Brumfitt & Hamilton-Miller 1994).

The choice of antibiotic will be determined by information on local sensitivity patterns. Trimethoprim, augmentin and ciprofloxacin are effective in most cases. Cephalosporins have an unacceptably high risk of precipitating vaginal candidiasis and should be avoided in this setting.

Acute pyelonephritis

Acute pyelonephritis is a medical emergency, especially in pregnancy, as Gram-negative bacteraemia, endotoxin shock and disseminated intravascular coagulation can occur. Antibiotics must be given intravenously as soon as the blood culture has been collected. Do not delay the antibiotics while waiting for a urine sample.

Gentamicin, third-generation cephalosporins, augmentin and ciprofloxacin are suitable best-guess antibiotics while waiting for the result of cultures. Persistent high concentrations of gentamicin can be nephrotoxic and ototoxic. Unfortunately, fear of these toxicities and failure to grasp the importance of a loading dose usually leads to inadequate doses being given. Thus underdosing is more common than overdosing (Parker & Davey 1993). The traditional approach to using aminoglycosides three times daily has been challenged. Prins et al (1993) have shown that once-daily dosing with gentamicin is at least as effective and is less nephrotoxic than divided doses. Whichever regimen is used, the clinician will need the support of a microbiologist and/or infectious diseases physician.

Careful monitoring and support of the cardiovascular system is an important part of the management of this acute infection. The place of intravenous corticosteroids in Gram-negative septicaemia has recently been challenged, and there is clear evidence that they offer no benefit.

A 'clotting screen' to measure the concentrations of platelets, prothrombin, fibrinogen and fibrin split products will assist in deciding whether disseminated intravascular coagulation has occurred. Expert haematological help is advised if this is diagnosed to decide whether heparin should be given to all but the pregnant patient.

Chronic pyelonephritis

When bacteriuria is diagnosed in a patient with chronic pyelonephritis, antibacterial therapy should be given irrespective of whether the patient is asymptomatic or symptomatic. Failure to do so may lead to worsening of renal scarring. This applies particularly to infants and small children, who have a greater tendency to VUR and consequently more easily convert a lower into an upper urinary tract infection. A 10-day course of oral antibacterial treatment is needed.

If it is decided to use long-term suppressive therapy it is very important to avoid drugs such as nitrofurantoin, as this can cause peripheral neuropathy, eosinophilic lung infiltrates or irreversible pulmonary fibrosis when given to a patient with only marginal renal decompensation.

Long-term suppressive therapy

All pregnant women with a history of recurrent UTI should receive suppressive therapy for the duration of the pregnancy. Women with more than two episodes of UTI per annum should be considered for long-term suppressive therapy and reviewed after 2 years of antibiotics. Patients with neuropathic bladders, indwelling catheters, a reduced bladder volume from radiotherapy or interstitial cystitis, or those with ileal conduits, should not receive long-term suppressive chemotherapy but be treated only when they have symptoms highly suggestive of urinary infection together with proven bacteriuria.

The suppressive dose usually employed is one-quarter or one-third of that given for the management of an acute episode. Thus the patient whose acute infection might be treated with 250 mg amoxycillin every 8 hours should receive a long-term dose of 250 mg amoxycillin daily. The drug is best given in the late evening before retiring, so that, in the patient without nocturia at least, a high antibacterial concentration remains in the urine for a prolonged period.

Individual antibacterial agents

Only a selection of the many possible drugs can be given

Table 54.1 Antibacterial agents for intravenous use in acute pyelonephritis (doses for adults with normal renal function)

Drug	Dose	Dose interval (h)
Gentamicin[1]	1–1.7 mg/kg	8
Cefotaxime	1–2 g	8–12
Ceftazidime	1–2 g	8
Augmentin	1–2 g	68
Ciprofloxacin[2]	200–400 mg	12

[1] Remember the loading dose for gentamicin.
[2] Oral ciprofloxacin has a high bioavailability and a 250 mg tablet achieves superior serum concentrations than a 100 mg intravenous dose at much lower cost.

Table 54.2 Oral antibacterial agents for acute lower urinary tract infection and chronic pyelonephritis. The doses are for adults with normal renal function. For long-term suppressive therapy the stated dose is given once only at night

Drug	Treatment course		Suppressive dose (mg nocte)
	Dose (mg)	Frequency (times daily)	
Amoxycillin	500	3	250
Augmentin	375	3	375
Trimethoprim	200	2	200
Ciprofloxacin	250–500	2	250

(Tables 54.1 and 54.2). Which one to choose depends on individual circumstances. In women of childbearing potential it is better to use drugs known to be safe in pregnancy. In women taking a low-dose oestrogen contraceptive the interaction with drugs such as rifampicin must be remembered, and also in a few there may be a possible reduction in the contraceptive effect of the pill with high doses of ampicillin.

URINARY TRACT TUBERCULOSIS

There may occasionally be an underlying tuberculous infection of the urinary tract in patients who also show significant bacteriuria with expected urinary tract pathogens such as *E. coli*, *Proteus* spp. or enterococci. Diagnostic suspicion should be high in immigrant families who have come from a country where there is still much tuberculosis, any patient with a suspect chest X-ray, so-called sterile pyuria or frank haematuria, or a strongly positive tuberculin test outside the context of a recent BCG immunization.

In addition to an abnormal chest X-ray there is usually a characteristic appearance on ultrasound and intravenous urography, often showing hydronephrosis and/or a small bladder with a straight or stretched-looking ureter in between. An autonephrectomy may already have taken place, with loss of function on one side. Calcium often lies over the renal shadow. Six early-morning urine cultures should be taken for acid-fast bacilli and a tuberculin test performed. A practical point in the collection of specimens for culture is that augmentin (co-amoxiclav) and quinolones (e.g. ciprofloxacin) have excellent antimycobacterial activity. These antibiotics should be avoided when investigating for possible tuberculosis.

Apart from possible surgical relief of obstruction, or the insertion of a stent in the lower ureter to prevent obliteration by fibrosis, antituberculous chemotherapy should start as soon as the diagnosis is reasonably certain. A 3-week course of prednisolone 20 mg daily at the start of antituberculous chemotherapy helps to keep the lower ureter patent.

Four-drug treatment is usually recommended, with modification to two-drug treatment in 2 months when the results of the sensitivity of the tubercle bacilli are known. A total of 9 months' chemotherapy is given, provided that one of the drugs used is rifampicin. Depending on the patient's weight, standard once-daily doses of isoniazid, rifampicin, ethambutol and pyrazinamide should be given initially. Because of the teratogenic potential of antituberculous drugs, expert advice should be sought in the choice of chemotherapy for a pregnant patient with urinary tract tuberculosis. Isoniazid and ethambutol are probably the least likely to upset the fetus. A radiographic check of the patency of the urinary collecting system should be made after a few weeks of treatment to ensure free drainage. Surgical intervention will be necessary if obstruction occurs.

Tuberculosis is a notifiable infectious disease in the UK. Although renal tuberculosis is rarely infectious to the patient's contacts it is important to notify the community medicine specialist so that other members of the family can be screened for occult infection.

URINARY TRACT SCHISTOSOMIASIS (BILHARZIA)

As with urinary tract tuberculosis, routine coliform pathogens may also be found in the urine of a patient with underlying schistosomiasis. This helminthic infestation is contracted from washing or bathing in fresh water harbouring the cercarial stage of the lifecycle of *Schistosoma haematobium*. The cercariae penetrate the skin and migrate to the liver, where the sexual forms copulate, and the gravid female then moves to the venous plexuses around the bladder or rectum. There she lays her eggs, whose tiny spines erode through the bladder wall and enter the urine to be shed during micturition. The lifecycle of the worm is completed by the rupture of the ova in fresh water, releasing a ciliated miracidium which finds its way into a freshwater snail. There it undergoes asexual reproduction and emerges as a free-swimming cercaria ready to invade another human being.

This disease cannot spread in the UK. It is usually acquired in the near east, east Africa and South America. Early symptoms which may be ignored by the patient are 'swimmer's itch' at the site of entry of the cercaria.

Months or years later terminal haematuria may be noted, especially by the male. Damage with chronic inflammation, calcification and fibrosis can take place throughout the urinary tract, leading to obstructive uropathy, a tiny non-distensible bladder and renal failure. At the same time the worm load in the liver may cause chronic cirrhosis with portal hypertension.

Diagnosis is made by finding schistosomal ova in terminal specimens of urine or in a biopsy taken at proctoscopy from what may appear to be a healthy rectal mucosa. A characteristic heaped-up appearance may be seen on the inflamed bladder lining at cystoscopy, and again biopsy may reveal ova. There is usually, but not invariably, an eosinophilia. A schistosomal enzyme-linked immunosorbent assay test should be positive within a few months of contracting the infestation.

If treatment is given promptly and the worm load is not huge, cure can be effected with a single oral dose of praziquantel. Assuming that the individual is not re-exposed to the infestation, a second dose of praziquantel is rarely needed.

KEY POINTS

1. Urinary infections are a significant cause of morbidity in women aged 20–65 years.
2. Infections can present with only 10^2 or 10^3 organisms per ml of urine, and even in the presence of sterile urine.
3. Up to 80% of recurrent infections are reinfection.
4. Between 10 and 30% of women with asymptomatic bacteriuria develop acute pyelonephritis during pregnancy.
5. Predisposing factors include diabetes mellitus, foreign body, instrumentation of the urinary tract and incomplete bladder emptying.
6. Prevention entails a high standard of perineal hygiene, avoidance of vaginal deodorants and bubble baths.
7. Management includes drinking at least 2 litres of fluid a day, regular and complete bladder emptying and voiding after intercourse.
8. Asymptomatic bacteriuria may not require treatment unless there is vesico ureteric reflux, renal scarring or failure to thrive in an infant.
9. Symptomatic lower urinary infection requires at least a 3-day course of antibiotics and follow-up within 2–3 weeks.
10. Urinary tract infection in a patient with a neuropathic bladder, indwelling catheter or ileal conduit should only be treated when it is symptomatic or there is proven bacteriuria.
11. Note that certain antibiotics may reduce the effectiveness of the oral contraceptive pill.

REFERENCES AND FURTHER READING

Asscher A W, Brumfitt W (eds) 1986 Microbial diseases in nephrology. John Wiley, Chichester
Brumfitt W, Hamilton-Miller J M T 1994 Consensus viewpoint on management of urinary infections. Journal of Antimicrobial Chemotherapy 33 (suppl A): 147–153
Fihn S D, Latham R H, Roberts P, Running K, Stamm W E 1985 Association between diaphragm use and urinary tract infection. Journal of the American Medical Association 254: 240–245
Hooton T M, Hillier S, Johnson C, Roberts P L, Stamm W E 1991 *Escherichia coli* bacteriuria and contraceptive method. Journal of the American Medical Association 265: 64–69
Kass E H 1956 Asymptomatic infections of the urinary tract. Transactions of the Association of American Physicians 69: 56–64
Lewis-Jones H G, Lamb G H R, Hughes P L 1989 Can ultrasound replace the intravenous urogram in the preliminary investigation of urinary tract disease? British Journal of Radiology 62: 977–980
Maskell R 1988 Urinary tract infection in clinical and laboratory practice. Edward Arnold, London
Merrick M V, Uttley W S, Wild R 1979 A comparison of two techniques of detecting vesico-ureteric reflux. British Journal of Radiology 52(622): 792–795
Monsour M, Azmy A F, MacKenzie J R 1987 Renal scarring secondary to vesicoureteric reflux. Critical assessment and new grading. British Journal of Urology 70: 320–324
Nimmo M J, Merrick M V, Allan P L 1987 Measurement of relative renal function. A comparison of methods and assessment of reproducibility. British Journal of Radiology 60: 861–864
Parker S E, Davey P G 1993 Once daily aminoglycoside dosing. Lancet 341: 346–347
Prins J M, Buller H R, Kuijper E J, Tange R A, Speelman P 1993 Once versus thrice daily gentamicin in patients with serious infections. Lancet 341: 335–339
Smith C C, Morris L, Wallace E T, Gray J A 1973 Comparison of two commercially available dipinocula with standard bacteriological assessment of bacteriuria. British Journal of Urology 45: 323–326
Spencer J, Lindsell D, Mastorakou I 1990 Ultrasonography compared with intravenous urography in the investigation of urinary tract infection in adults. British Medical Journal 301: 221–224
Strom B L, Collins M, West S L, Kreisberg J, Weller S 1987 Sexual activity, contraceptive use and other risk factors for symptomatic and asymptomatic bacteriuria. Annals of Internal Medicine 107: 816–823

55

Pelvic inflammatory disease

A. Moors   C. D. Bevan   E. J. Thomas

INTRODUCTION

Pelvic inflammatory disease (PID) is defined as 'the acute clinical syndrome associated with ascending spread of microorganisms (unrelated to pregnancy or surgery) from the vagina or cervix to the endometrium, fallopian tubes, and/or contiguous structures' (Weström & Wølner-Hanssen 1993).

The public health significance of PID is indisputable, with up to one in nine American women of reproductive age reporting that they have received treatment for pelvic infection (Aral et al 1991). An estimated one million women seek treatment for PID in the United States at an annual cost of $4.2 billion (Washington & Katz 1991). The situation in the non-industrialized world is undoubtedly worse, although a lack of accurate epidemiological data makes it difficult to quantify. Certainly, in sub-Saharan Africa bilateral fallopian tube occlusion secondary to salpingitis is the predominant cause of infertility.

Although it is apparent that PID poses a major threat to the reproductive health of young women and is a significant drain on health care resources, it also represents an often neglected area of modern medical practice. However, significant inroads into the control of this disease have been achieved. Intense educational campaigns and attention to improving contact tracing and treatment have been effective in substantially reducing the incidence and prevalence of acute salpingitis in Sweden over the last two decades (Fig. 55.1; Weström 1988). Investment in such proven strategies will pay dividends in the long term.

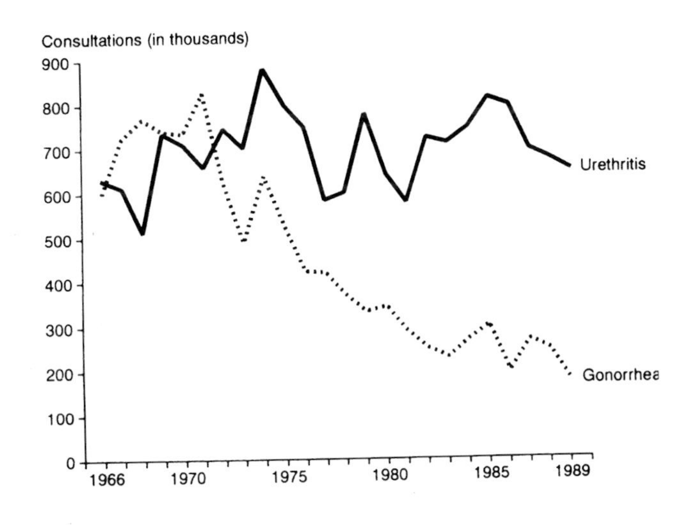

Fig. 55.1 Mean incidence (per 1000 women aged 15–39 in Lund) of first or repeat episodes of acute salpingitis in 5-year periods from 1960.

EPIDEMIOLOGY

The epidemiological study of PID is flawed by diagnostic and reporting uncertainty. Unfortunately, PID is a term that lacks precise clinical definition and there are no diagnostic tests available which are simple, safe and specific. To compound the problem, many cases are either asymptomatic or run a very benign clinical course. Thus, most studies will tend to underreport its true incidence and prevalence. Most of the information available is variably derived from national surveys of self-reported PID, hospital discharge data, returns from genitourinary medicine clinics and outpatient visiting data.

The incidence of PID is strongly correlated with the prevalence of sexually transmitted diseases, and has increased in most countries, reflecting the worldwide epidemic of STDs. A small proportion of infections might be of endogenous origin, but those arising from a focus outside the genital tract cannot strictly be defined as PID.

Of the estimated 10–15% of women of reproductive age in the United States who have had at least one episode of PID, the highest annual incidence is among sexually active women in their teenage years. Of those hospitalized with acute PID in 1988, it was notable that 43% were younger than 25 years of age and 34% underwent major surgery as a direct result of the infection (National Institutes of Health 1991). However, a downward trend in the cumulative incidence of self-reported PID has been identified in the United States between 1982 and 1988 (Aral et al 1991). Although this is encouraging, an increase in the proportion of asymptomatic PID might account for it.

Chlamydia trachomatis and *Neisseria gonorrhoeae* are probably the most prevalent sexually transmitted bacteria in the western world, and one or both of these microorganisms have been implicated in at least 60% of cases of PID in young women. The relative importance of individual species of microorganism as aetiological agents in PID depends on the population studied and the prevalence of the agent within that population. In the United Kingdom, uncomplicated gonococcal infections in women have halved in frequency during the last decade, while at the same time the rate of chlamydial infections has continued to rise (Catchpole 1992), such that *C. trachomatis* is probably now the major aetiological pathogen in PID. A similar pattern in the United States is illustrated by Fig. 55.2, which uses the syndrome of non-specific urethritis in men as a proxy for chlamydial infections.

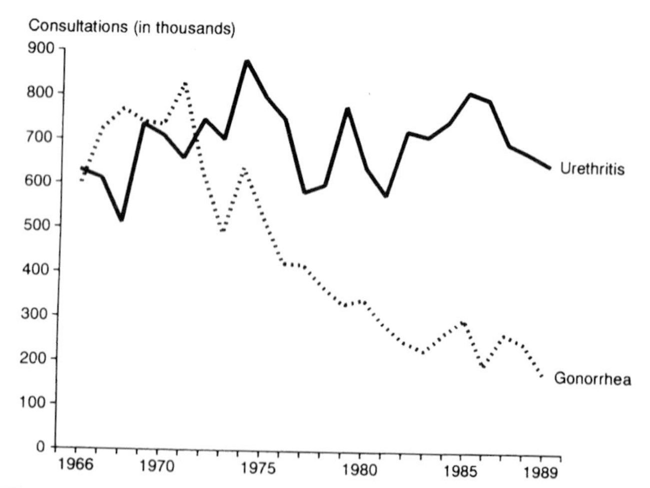

Fig. 55.2 Total consultations for non-specific urethritis and gonorrhoea among men in the United States from 1966 to 1989.

The most accurate data on PID in Europe, and probably worldwide, come from the city of Lund and its surrounding rural districts in southern Sweden. This is the only department for inpatient treatment of gynaecological disorders in the area, and patients are routinely laparoscoped to detect PID. Thus, few symptomatic cases are missed. However, since there is no screening for asymptomatic PID, their figures must be considered an underestimate of the true incidence.

From 1960 to 1984 the proportion of patients with gonorrhoea-associated PID decreased from 49 to 8%. This decline mirrors that observed in much of the industrialized world. The yearly incidence of genital chlamydial infections also decreased from 49 to 27 per 1000 women between 1970 and 1981. The most important factor influencing this decrease in gonorrhoea and chlamydial infection seemed to be a more conservative attitude to sex and changes of partners in young people during the last decade, allied to the public health care measures mentioned above (Weström et al 1992).

The incidence of PID in the developing world is more difficult to assess, available data often being based on point prevalence studies of the different STDs. Gonococcal infection rates of up to 15% have been reported in pregnant women in many African countries, and as high as 20% in Kenya and Zaire (Miotti et al 1992). Surveys of Ugandan women have found the prevalence of PID to range from 6% up to 19% (Arya et al 1980).

The high STD prevalence in many African countries can be attributed to the high proportion of teenagers and young adults within the total population, early sexual debut, multiple sexual partners, the abundance of migrant labour and a delay in the treatment of STDs. In addition, ritual practices such as female circumcision are strongly associated with PID.

Unless effective contraception programmes are linked to STD control programmes, changes in the epidemiology of gonococcal and chlamydial infection are predicted to result in accelerated population growth in the developing world.

The evidence for a role for ulcerating STDs, especially chancroid, as cofactors in HIV transmission, is strong (Piot & Laga 1989). Studies involving non-ulcerative STDs are less conclusive, but if found to be associated with an increased risk of HIV transmission the overall risk in the developing world would be large, since they are highly prevalent.

MICROBIOLOGY AND PATHOGENESIS

The majority of cases of acute PID are believed to occur as a result of ascending canalicular spread of microorganisms from the lower to the upper genital tract. This is evidenced by their simultaneous isolation in the endocervix, endometrium, fallopian tube and peritoneal cavity, in association with a continuum of histopathological changes, i.e. cervicitis, endometritis and salpingitis. Pathogens that gain access to the peritoneal cavity can then spread to the surfaces of the abdominal viscera and cause periappendicitis, perisplenitis and perihepatitis. Although parametrial spread of *Mycoplasma hominis* has been demonstrated in animal models, there is no good evidence to support this mechanism in the pathogenesis of PID in humans.

PID is predominantly a disease of young sexually active women, with at least 75% of cases occurring in women under the age of 25. In general, the pathogens identified in the upper genital tract of women with PID will be either sexually transmitted microorganisms or facultative and anaerobic microorganisms, which would normally be considered to be part of the flora of the lower genital tract. *N. gonorrhoeae* was the first microorganism to be recognized as an aetiological agent in PID, and traditionally the disease had been described as either of gonococcal or non-gonococcal origin. It is now recognized that a large proportion of non-gonococcal disease is in fact caused by *C. trachomatis*.

C. trachomatis and *N. gonorrhoeae* are described as 'primary' pathogens in PID, as it is believed they damage the protective mechanisms within the endocervix and the tubal mucosa by causing an acute inflammatory response. This subsequently allows endogenous bacteria from the vagina and cervix to ascend into the upper genital tract, where they act as 'secondary invaders'. Identification of microorganisms from fallopian tube samples by culture appears to be directly related to the severity of disease. STDs are usually only isolated in women who present early and have relatively mild disease, whereas the isolation of 'endogenous' microorganisms occurs more frequently in women with advanced disease.

The presence of a mixed 'polymicrobial' infection leads to tissue destruction, which favours the formation of tubo-ovarian abscesses where strictly anaerobic microorganisms predominate and STDs are rarely isolated.

Neisseria gonorrhoeae

Gonococci selectively adhere to and invade non-ciliated secretory cells in the mucosa of the fallopian tube, where they are protected from the host's immune defence mechanisms. After crossing the epithelium, gonococci are released from the basal surface by exocytosis and then invade the subepithelial space (Fig. 55.3). Whereas only the secretory cells are infected, it is the ciliated cells of the tubal mucosa that are damaged in gonococcal PID. Either they slough off, or ciliary stasis occurs, probably as a result of gonococcal toxin production. Gonococcal antigen also activates the complement cascade, producing an acute polymorphonuclear response that in turn switches on the 'common inflammatory pathways'. Cell death and tissue destruction ensue, providing the ideal situation for invasion by endogenous anaerobic microorganisms.

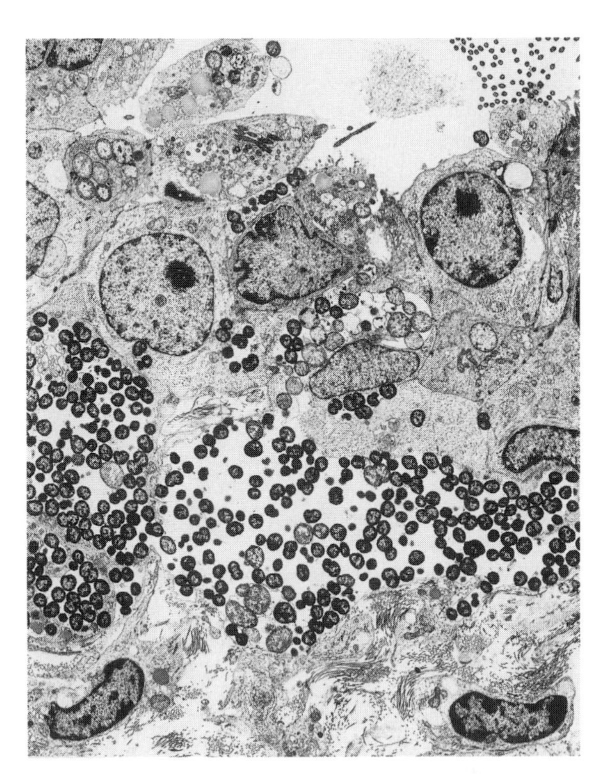

Fig. 55.3 Human oviduct in organ culture 42 hours after infection with gonococci. Gonococci have penetrated the tissue both within and between cells to set up an expanding focus of infection at junction of the basal epithelium with connective tissue. Magnification × 960. (Courtesy of Professor M. E. Ward, Molecular Microbiology, Southampton General Hospital)

Chlamydia trachomatis

Chlamydiae are small bacteria that are obligate intracellular parasites.

C. trachomatis adheres to the columnar epithelial cells of the endocervix and the epithelial surfaces of the endometrium and fallopian tubes. Endocytosis results in the metabolically inert but infectious elementary body (EB) being taken into the cytoplasm of the cell. Within the endosomal vacuole, which is apparently protected from immune surveillance, the EB changes into the larger vegetative reticulate body (RB) over a period of 24 hours. The RB multiplies by binary fission, producing intracellular inclusions that contain thousands of RBs (Fig. 55.4). The RBs subsequently condense again within the inclusion into EBs and, in 48–72 hours, cell lysis occurs, releasing the infectious forms into the extracellular fluid, where they can then attach to new cells and repeat the cycle.

It is unlikely that the upper genital tract damage seen in chlamydial PID is caused by the local effects of chlamydial replication alone. More probably the host's humoral

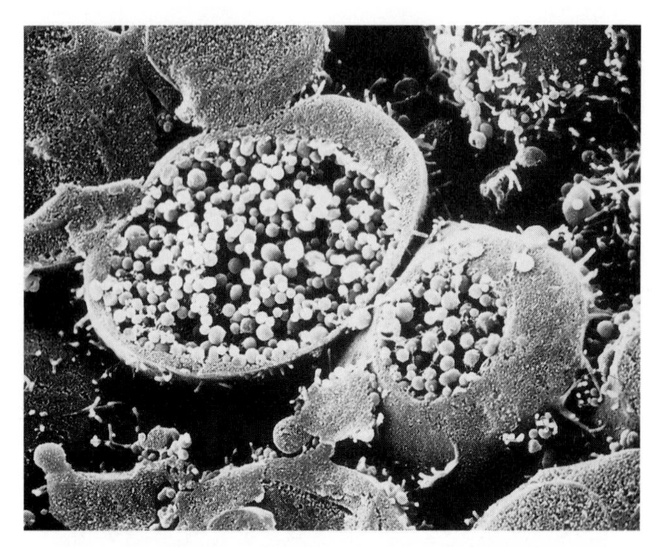

Fig. 55.4 Field emission scanning electron micrograph of freeze-fractured chlamydia-infected tissue culture cells. Note how the chlamydial elementary bodies occupy virtually the whole of the cytoplasm. Magnification × 8500. (Courtesy of Professor M. E. Ward, Molecular Microbiology, Southampton General Hospital)

and cell-mediated immune response to *C. trachomatis* determines the extent of tubal damage. Chlamydiae appear to be capable of influencing the immune response in ways that are beneficial to their survival, such that persistent – i.e. viable but non-replicating – forms remain in the cells of the human upper genital tract, serving as subclinical pockets of antigenic stimulation. Primary chlamydial infection in monkeys is self-limiting, but repeat inoculation produces extensive tubal scarring (Patton et al 1989). This may well be a delayed hypersensitivity-type response, either to the presence of persistent chlamydial antigen in the genital tract or perhaps provoked by ubiquitous heat shock proteins (HSP). Similar mechanisms may be responsible for much of the morphological damage seen in women following chlamydial PID, as there does appear to be a strong correlation between the finding of antibodies to HSP and PID, tubal factor infertility and ectopic pregnancy (Paavonen & Lehtinen 1994).

Mycoplasma

The role that mycoplasma may play in the aetiology of PID is uncertain, as they are part of the normal vaginal flora in the genital tract of more than 50% of healthy sexually active women. Mycoplasma are rarely isolated from fallopian tube specimens of women with PID and, although acute antibody responses do occur in a minority of women, this may simply reflect exposure of the immune system to the microorganism as a result of epithelial damage in the genital tract.

Bacterial vaginosis

There is much speculation as to the part that bacterial vaginosis (BV) may play in the pathogenesis of PID. In BV there is a profound disturbance of the vaginal flora, such that anaerobes prevail. These microorganisms are frequently isolated in the fallopian tubes of women with advanced disease. However, it is not clear whether BV has an important aetiological role in PID or is just a cofactor. The chronological relationship between BV and the development of acute PID has not yet been determined, and the reported association of BV and PID may just reflect changes in the vaginal ecosystem that occur as a result of infection by a 'primary pathogen'.

PATHOLOGY

The pathological changes that occur in the genital tract during the acute phase of PID and the resultant morphological damage that follows may be overt or occult. In women with mild PID the pelvic organs are not much affected. The serosal surface of the fallopian tubes appears reddened (hyperaemic) and the tubes are oedematous but freely mobile, with patent abdominal ostia. There may be a sticky purulent exudate on the serosal surface of the pelvic organs and exuding from the fimbrial ends of the tube. If no pus is present, it should be possible to express some from the fallopian tube by manipulation of the distal end.

Moderately severe disease is associated with marked changes. The inflammation and oedema of the fallopian tubes is more pronounced and, as a result, tubal mobility may be limited. Patchy fibrin deposits are seen on the serosal surfaces and loose adhesions may form between the pelvic and abdominal viscera. These subsequently become organized with collagen as a result of fibroblastic activity. In the majority of cases these are permanent, although there is evidence that they may resolve spontaneously in some women (Wølner-Hanssen & Weström 1983). The distal end of the fallopian tube often appears phimotic and the tubes may not be patent. In severe disease, occlusion of the tubal ostia as a result of the fimbria sticking together results in the formation of a pyosalpinx, often with marked distortion of the normal pelvic anatomy. The pelvic peritoneum is intensely congested and the pelvic organs become adherent, resulting in the formation of a complex inflammatory mass. If the infectious process has not been sealed off in the fallopian tube, then a tubo-ovarian abscess (TOA), the most severe manifestation of PID, may develop. The pathogenesis of TOA is not well understood and up to 50% of women who present with TOA give no reliable history of a preceding episode of PID (Walker & Landers 1991). Nevertheless, it is likely that development of a TOA is the natural progression when PID is not arrested either by medical intervention or by the host's natural defence mechanisms.

The extent of tubal damage after an episode of PID varies and the adnexae are not always affected to the same degree. At best, in mild disease there will be complete restitution of tubal morphology with no effect on function. At worst, distal tubal occlusion with hydrosalpinx formation, intramural fibrosis and damage to the tubal mucosa occur, impairing function, often irreversibly.

Histological examination of the fallopian tubes of women with tubal factor infertility often shows marked dilation of the tubal lumen. The plicae are flattened and covered by a single layer of flattened columnar cells, with an associated plasma cell infiltrate in the submucosa. The secretory cells either lose their microvilli or become thickened, with clubbed appendages, and extensive areas of the mucosa have no ciliated epithelial cells. Electron microscopic studies reveal extensive vacuole formation within the cytoplasm of the secretory cell and a reduction in intracellular organelles and secretory granules (Patton et al 1989). The ciliated epithelial cells have few cilia and the beat frequency is significantly reduced (Fig. 55.5).

The chronic sequelae of PID, i.e. tubal factor infertility, ectopic pregnancy and chronic pelvic pain, are largely the result of these changes in tubal morphology. Pelvic adhesions distort normal anatomical and functional relationships. Ovum pick-up mechanisms may be affected, leading to lower conception rates. Intraluminal adhesions between plicae and deciliation or ciliary dyskinesia may also inhibit progression of the ovum or blastocyst through the fallopian tube, increasing the likelihood of an ectopic pregnancy.

CLINICAL MANIFESTATIONS AND DIAGNOSIS

Early diagnosis is of paramount importance in the management of women with acute upper genital tract infection, as delay will result in late treatment, with an attendant increased risk of complications. Classically, women with PID are described as presenting with subacute lower abdominal pain that is dull in nature and usually bilateral. Less than 10% of laparoscopically confirmed salpingitis is unilateral (Jacobson & Weström 1969). They also have a fever, purulent vaginal discharge, bilateral adnexal tenderness with cervical excitation, and an elevated erythrocyte sedimentation rate (ESR). However, it is now recognized that there is a wide spectrum of disease presentation, which extends from the woman with mild disease, who may have little evidence of systemic upset, to the seriously ill woman with life-threatening pelvic sepsis. A number of other gynaecological and surgical conditions where lower abdominal pain is the principal presenting complaint also mimic the clinical picture of acute PID, causing diagnostic uncertainty. Furthermore, there is increasing evidence that there may be a substantial number of women with acute upper genital tract infection whose

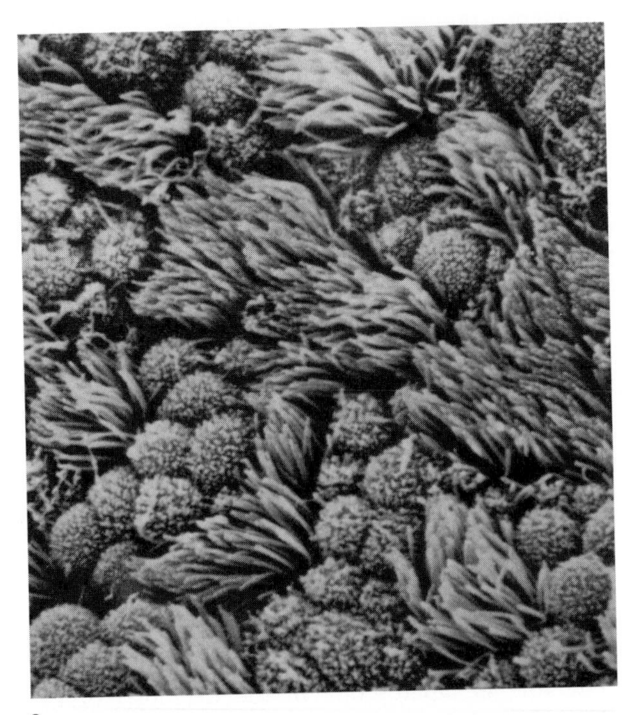

a

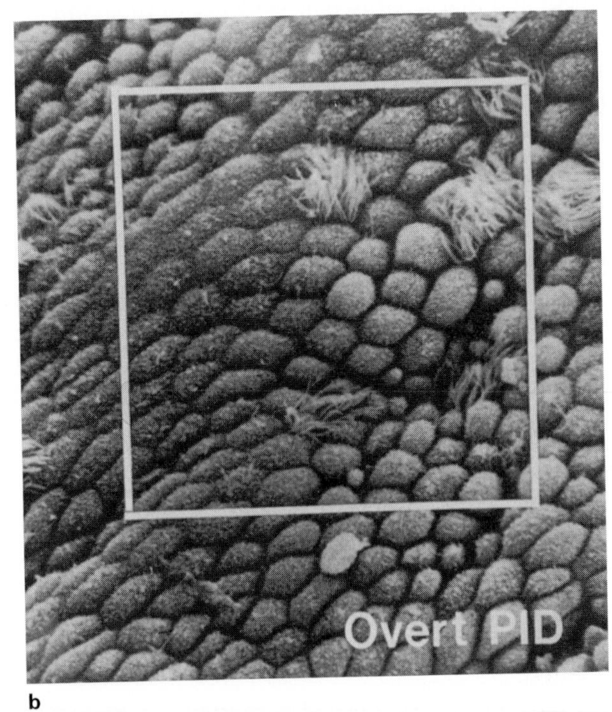

b

Fig. 55.5 (**a**) Scanning electron micrograph of lumen of normal fallopian tube ampulla. The non-ciliated secretory cells are rounded in shape and are covered by microvilli. The long slender cilia project above the secretory epithelial cells (× 2400). (**b**) After overt PID the secretory epithelial cells appear smooth and flattened. Few microvillous projections are present on their surfaces. Widespread deciliation of the mucosal surface is observed (× 1200).

condition goes unnoticed because it is atypical or asymptomatic (Moore et al 1982), and yet the extent of tubal damage in these women is the same as in symptomatic disease (Patton et al 1989). The diagnosis is made retrospectively when they present with complications or sequelae such as infertility.

Table 55.1 Minimum criteria for clinical diagnosis of PID

Lower abdominal tenderness
Bilateral adnexal tenderness
Cervical motion tenderness
No evidence of a competing diagnosis

Microbial aetiology and clinical presentation

It is not possible to determine the microbial aetiology of a given case of PID on clinical grounds, but there are a number of reported differences between women whose PID is due to an STD and those with non-STD associated disease, that may suggest likely aetiology and guide antibiotic therapy.

The onset of symptoms in women with STD-associated PID occurs more frequently in the early follicular phase of the menstrual cycle than in women who have non-STD disease. Women with gonococcal PID invariably present a florid clinical picture, but evidence of systemic disturbance is often not marked. The onset of symptoms is acute, with the complaint of abdominal pain usually of less than 3 days' standing. Pyrexia >38°C and a palpable adnexal mass are common findings. In contrast, the clinical course of chlamydial PID is generally of a more indolent nature. Women present later, with little systemic upset and apparently milder disease (Svensson et al 1980). Pyrexia >38°C is unusual but the ESR is often raised >30 mm/h. A study comparing gonococcal and chlamydial PID suggested that laparoscopic evidence of tubal inflammation in women with chlamydial disease is more pronounced than might be expected from the clinical picture (Svensson et al 1980), but this finding has not been supported by more recent investigations which have shown that *C. trachomatis* causes the same degree of tubal damage as *N. gonorrhoeae* (Wølner-Hanssen et al 1991, Bevan et al 1994).

Women with non-STD-associated disease are usually older than 35 and often have had one or more previous episodes of upper genital tract infection. The disease runs a much more severe course, often with a palpable adnexal mass and a major degree of systemic upset.

Diagnosis

PID is a complex condition for which there is no ideal algorithm to aid diagnosis. Many observational studies have confirmed that the specificity of clinical diagnosis is low, with an overall clinical misdiagnosis of PID occurring in about 35% of all cases when laparoscopy is used for confirmation.

There have been a number of suggested combinations of 'clinical criteria' that should be fulfilled for a diagnosis of PID, but they have never been evaluated objectively (Hager et al 1983, Method 1988). When selecting diagnostic criteria for PID it is clearly important to choose those which have a low diagnostic threshold for women with mild or atypical disease, but at the same time are accurate (sensitive and specific) for severe disease.

It is now evident that historical, clinical and laboratory findings are not consistently useful in the diagnosis of PID, either individually or in combination (Kahn et al 1991). Therefore, their inclusion as diagnostic indicators in any chosen set of criteria will reduce the sensitivity of diagnosis. As a result, women with mild, atypical or asymptomatic upper genital tract infection may be missed and not receive appropriate early treatment for their disease. It has therefore been proposed that the criteria shown in Table 55.1 should be all that is required to trigger early antibiotic treatment for probable PID in women with milder presentations (Rolfs 1991).

This suggestion is in an important departure from the laboratory and laparoscopy-based investigation of PID which has been previously advocated. Although it is accepted that some unnecessary antibiotic therapy will be administered as a result of taking this approach, this would be set against the potential benefit of earlier intervention in a larger number of cases of PID.

In women with a more severe presentation hospitalization is mandatory and further investigation required. The most important competing diagnoses to rule out are ectopic pregnancy and appendicitis, as failure to do so could have disastrous consequences. It is often extremely difficult to distinguish between mild PID and an early ectopic pregnancy on clinical grounds, and so until a pregnancy has been excluded by the use of a sensitive pregnancy test it is not safe to make a diagnosis of PID (see Ch. 55). Generally, women with appendicitis have been symptomatic for a shorter period of time and have more pronounced gastrointestinal symptoms. They are clinically more unwell, with signs localizing to the right iliac fossa. Laparoscopy should be employed more frequently in the diagnosis and management of the acute abdomen in young women suspected of having acute appendicitis (Patterson-Brown et al 1986).

Laparoscopy

The role of laparoscopy in the diagnosis of PID was firmly established in the large cohort study from Lund University, Sweden (Jacobson & Weström 1969). This work described the classic appearances of the pelvic organs, considered essential for visual confirmation of PID (see

Pathology). Moreover, it demonstrated convincingly that without the aid of laparoscopy it is often not possible to differentiate on clinical grounds alone between women with acute PID and those with other important pathological conditions. Only 65% of women with classic symptoms and signs of PID had laparoscopic evidence of the disease, whereas 23% had no abnormality detected and the remaining 12% had other pathological conditions, including ectopic pregnancy, endometriosis and ovarian accidents.

With wider use it has become increasingly clear that the interpretation of laparoscopic findings in some cases of suspected PID may not always be straightforward. Changes in the appearance of the fallopian tubes during the menstrual cycle and the effects of carbonic anhydrase in the peritoneal cavity can produce a false impression of serosal hyperaemia. Operator expectation bias may mean that hyperaemia and oedema in the absence of a purulent exudate is overinterpreted, with a resultant false positive diagnosis. On the other hand, if laparoscopy is performed too early in an evolving upper genital tract infection, before overt signs of tubal involvement are present, a false negative diagnosis may be made. Hager et al (1983) further refined Jacobson and Weström's criteria in order to standardize and improve the sensitivity of laparoscopic diagnosis of PID (Table 55.2). More recently, *C. trachomatis* has been identified in the fallopian tubes of women with a clinical diagnosis of acute PID but with apparently normal tubes at laparoscopy (Stacey et al 1992). This emphasizes the inconsistency of visual diagnosis for detecting upper genital tract infection, as it is likely that these cases represent an acute endosalpingitis, the antecedent of acute salpingitis.

Despite the recognized shortfalls of laparoscopy, it has always been accepted as the 'gold standard' for diagnosis in PID; nevertheless, this role has recently been challenged. In a study comparing visual diagnosis with histopathological diagnosis of endometrial and fimbrial biopsies, Sellors et al (1991) found laparoscopy to be only 50% sensitive and 80% specific for diagnosing acute PID. It is therefore probably best to err on the side of caution and administer empirical antibiotic therapy to women with equivocal findings at laparoscopy, while waiting for histological confirmation of PID.

Because of the expense and the potential morbidity associated with laparoscopy, some groups believe it should only be used when the diagnosis is uncertain or when a woman is severely ill. Diagnostic models utilizing multivariate logistic analysis suggest that perhaps only one-third of women hospitalized with suspected PID need undergo laparoscopy (Hagdu et al 1986). Unfortunately, by focusing solely on its role in diagnosis, this approach means that the other advantages that laparoscopy offers in the management of women with PID are lost. Laparoscopic grading of disease severity (Table 55.2) gives guidance as to appropriate antibiotic regimens and length of treatment required, as this cannot be judged on the basis of clinical findings alone (Svensson et al 1980, Patton et al 1989, Bevan et al 1995). In addition, there is increasing evidence that other therapeutic laparoscopic measures carried out at the time of diagnosis may also improve long-term outcome in women with PID (Reich & McGlynn 1987).

Table 55.2 Hager's criteria for laparoscopic diagnosis and grading of disease severity

Mild	Erythema, oedema and a purulent exudate present on manipulation of mobile fallopian tubes
Moderate	Gross purulent material present, with greater erythema and oedema. The fallopian tubes may not be freely mobile nor patent
Severe	Pyosalpinx or inflammatory complex Abscess

Tubal factor infertility is five times more likely after a single episode of severe PID than after an episode of mild PID (Weström 1994), but without laparoscopic assessment of the extent of tuboperitoneal damage the prognosis for future fertility cannot be objectively determined at the time of diagnosis.

There appears to be no economic disadvantage in laparoscoping all women who are admitted to hospital with suspected PID, as opposed to treating them empirically with antibiotics and adopting a 'wait and see' policy (Method et al 1987). Given that at least a third of women admitted with suspected PID who are managed expectantly do not have the disease, and in view of the advantages that accrue from early visual confirmation of PID, laparoscopy should be considered in all hospitalized cases.

SEQUELAE

Most women recover completely following an episode of PID, although extrapolation from infertility data (Hull 1985) and the reported levels of symptomatic sequelae following hospitalization for PID, indicate that the long-term outcome for some women has considerable implications for the provision of gynaecological services (Buchan et al 1993).

The likelihood of developing tubal factor infertility following PID is determined by the severity and number of episodes of disease. Follow-up of the Lund cohort indicates that 8% of women attempting to conceive after one episode of PID have tubal factor infertility, whereas after two episodes 19.5% are affected and after three or more episodes the figure rises to 40%. Only 0.6% of women experience tubal factor infertility after a single episode of mild disease, but this figure rises to 21.4% after an episode of severe disease.

Damage to the fallopian tubes after PID is a well-documented risk factor for ectopic pregnancy, and in this same series the ectopic pregnancy rate was 9.1% compared to a rate of 1.4% in the control group (Weström et al 1992).

Although attention has focused on tubal infertility and ectopic pregnancy following PID, other serious sequelae are common. Chronic abdominal pain occurs frequently and contributes to the high rates of hospitalization and the 10-fold increase in hysterectomy rate seen in women following PID (Buchan et al 1993).

RISK ASSESSMENT

Determination of risk factors for PID, especially those that are modifiable, is an essential step towards successful disease prevention. Demographic and social indicators of risk such as race, socioeconomic status, age and marital status are markers of disease risk but are not modifiable. The behavioural risk factors discussed below can be modified and should be targeted in campaigns for prevention of PID.

Sexual history

Young age at sexual debut, a high frequency of sexual intercourse and multiple sexual partners have all been associated with increased risk of PID (Washington et al 1991). Young age at first intercourse is correlated with sexual promiscuity and an increased susceptibility to PID because of the presence of cervical ectopy, which provides target cells for chlamydial and gonococcal infections. The role of sperm as vectors carrying organisms to the upper genital tract, allied to myometrial activity during coitus, may explain the increased risk of PID with frequency of sexual intercourse (Grodstein & Rothman 1994).

Barrier contraception

Barrier methods of contraception include the condom, diaphragm and cervical cap. When diligently used, the condom is highly effective in reducing the risk of transmission of the sexually transmitted infections causing PID. Diaphragm use, especially in conjunction with spermicides, also appears to decrease a woman's risk for PID.

Oral contraception

The relationship between oral contraceptives and risk of PID is not so clear cut. In vitro studies suggest that natural resistance to genital chlamydial infection may vary during the menstrual cycle and may be modified by hormonal contraceptives (Mahmoud et al 1994). Epidemiological studies demonstrate a two- to threefold increase in the prevalence of cervical chlamydial infection in oral contraceptive users, compared to women using another method or no contraception (Washington et al 1991). The explanation for these findings may be that oral contraceptive use alters the susceptibility of mucosal cells to chlamydia infection, possibly by facilitating the development of cervical ectopy. Immune function may also be modified by pill use.

In the upper reproductive tract oral contraceptive use appears to provide some protection against symptomatic infection. In addition, PID in women using oral contraceptives seems to be clinically and laparoscopically less severe. These observations are supported by Weström's cohort study which also identified lower rates of tubal infertility among oral contraceptive users (Weström et al 1992). The presence of thicker cervical mucus, an atrophic endometrium and decreased menstrual blood loss may inhibit bacterial invasion and proliferation, explaining these findings among the pill users.

Intrauterine contraception

Controversy surrounds the relationship between the use of an intrauterine contraceptive device (IUCD) and development of PID. Vessey, in a large cohort study, calculated a relative risk of 10.5 for acute PID amongst IUCD users (Vessey et al 1981). However, the control group consisted largely of women using an oral contraceptive or diaphragm, and there is good evidence that these methods of birth control may reduce the risk of PID. Such methodological inconsistencies are common and, in the most objective studies, the increase is in the range of 1.5–2.6 (Washington et al 1991). A recent WHO study showed that the highest risk of PID occurred during the first 20 days after insertion, but then dropped to a much lower rate thereafter (Farley et al 1992). The introduction of organisms into the endometrial cavity during IUCD insertion is probably the critical factor, and those women at low risk for STDs may similarly be at low risk of developing PID with IUCD use. To minimize this risk, IUCD insertion should be carried out under strict aseptic conditions, with appropriate antibiotic prophylaxis following cervical screening, and IUCDs should not be changed more regularly than their recommended life span.

Other risk factors

Of the other risk variables vaginal douching has been associated with PID, although this may be a marker of infection rather than a true risk factor. Cigarette smoking has been postulated as increasing the risk of PID, but this may only be indicative of risk-taking behaviour. If the suspected relationship between bacterial vaginosis and PID is confirmed, it will increase the importance of surveillance and treatment of those women affected (Hay & Taylor-Robinson 1992).

TREATMENT

Because of the polymicrobial nature of PID, broad-spectrum treatment is recommended and is usually initiated before the microbial aetiology is established. It is therefore usually empirical in nature. *C. trachomatis* and *N. gonorrhoeae* are the two most commonly encountered aetio- logical agents and provide the focus for most treatment regimens. In addition, a variety of endogenous anaerobic and aerobic bacteria have been isolated from women with PID, but the importance of anaerobic antibacterial cover in the absence of pelvic abscess has been questioned. The antibiotic chemotherapy of bacterial STDs and PID has recently been comprehensively reviewed by Corcoran and Ridgway (1994).

Tetracyclines have formed the mainstay of treatment of acute chlamydial infections, with macrolides used as an alternative in pregnancy. However, lengthy courses of treatment are required, leading to problems with compliance. The quinolones, in particular ofloxacin and ciprofloxacin, have been assessed for potential use against chlamydial infections. Regardless of their efficacy, however, they are more expensive, their use involves a 7-day course and they are contraindicated in pregnancy. Azithromycin, one of the newer macrolides, seems to offer the best prospect for short-course PID therapy. A single 1 g dose taken orally is as effective as a 7-day course of doxycycline in lower genital tract chlamydial infection, and is also promising in treating uncomplicated gonorrhoea.

Where penicillinase-producing *N. gonorrhoeae* is not a major problem, penicillin is the mainstay of genital gonococcal treatment, usually in the form of a single oral dose of amoxycillin with probenicid. Combining clavulanic acid with penicillin improves its spectrum to include activity against otherwise resistant *N. gonorrhoeae*. Cephalosporins are widely used to treat gonorrhoea in the United States, a single intramuscular dose of ceftriaxone being most commonly used, although cefuroxime and cefoxitin are effective in equivalent dosages.

Ciprofloxacin is active against both Gram-positive and Gram-negative bacteria, and a single intramuscular dose is effective in acute uncomplicated gonorrhoea. Concerns have been expressed, however, about the emergence of quinolone resistance. Spectinomycin is in widespread use for the treatment of gonorrhoea caused by penicillin-resistant organisms, or in a penicillin-allergic patient, although resistance has been described.

Many antibacterial regimens have been assessed for the treatment of PID, but invariably focus only on short-term objectives rather than their efficacy in preventing long-term sequelae. The choice of regimen tends to be governed by local prescribing guidelines, patterns of antibacterial resistance, predicted patient compliance and accurate microbiological diagnosis. Whichever regimen is chosen, evaluation and treatment of symptomatic PID should be prompt (Table 55.3). Delay of care for 3 or more days in gonorrhoea- or chlamydia-associated PID leads to a threefold increased risk of ectopic pregnancy or tubal infertility (Hillis et al 1993).

Table 55.3 Guidelines for management of PID in the UK (Ridgway G L 1994, personal communication)

Second- or third-generation cephalosporin +/– probenecid in antigonococcal dose (intramuscular or intravenous)
Tetracycline 500 mg 12-hourly (intravenous) or doxycycline 100 mg twice daily (orally, continued for 10–14 days)
Consider metronidazole (intravenous or oral) for up to 14 days

If patients resume sexual intercourse with an untreated, infected partner, the chances of reinfection are high. More than 50% of the sexual partners of women with PID will have evidence of a genital tract infection. They should be treated either empirically with regimens effective against *C. trachomatis* and *N. gonorrhoeae*, or following accurate microbiological diagnosis. This crucial aspect of treatment is often neglected by gynaecologists, and if efficient contact tracing and treatment cannot be effected, women with PID should be referred to a genitourinary physician.

Although radical surgery is rarely necessary in the management of acute PID, aggressive laparoscopic surgery should be considered. Laparoscopic surgical techniques can be utilized to drain purulent fluid, lyse bowel adhesions and excise acute and necrotic tubo-ovarian adhesions. There is some evidence that early laparoscopic treatment of tubo-ovarian abscess leads to more rapid short-term recovery and preservation of normal anatomy (Reich & McGlynn 1987).

As an adjunct to the antibacterial and surgical management of acute PID, the role of non-steroidal anti-inflammatory agents in the prevention of long-term sequelae has been considered, but as yet remains unclear. The development of new, highly specific anti-inflammatory agents may offer better prospects.

PREVENTION

Because PID and its sequelae cause widespread suffering and drain limited health care resources, investments in prevention are likely to pay dividends. The successful strategies employed in Sweden to control genital chlamydia and gonorrhoea have significantly reduced the occurrence of symptomatic PID, and should be implemented elsewhere.

Primary prevention of PID is dominated by preventing both exposure to and acquisition of chlamydial and gonococcal infection. Intense, culturally sensitive educational campaigns should aim to raise professional and public awareness of healthy sexual behaviour. These should employ both the mass media and a community-based approach. Young people can be targeted in schools from as early as 12 years of age, and the message continually reinforced later. Health care providers should be encouraged to update their knowledge about the prevention, recognition and proper treatment of PID and associated STDs.

Clinicians must routinely enquire about high-risk sexual behaviour, and encourage screening tests for those at risk. Finally, the search for bacterial STD vaccines is being pursued with renewed vigour and offers hope for future primary prevention of PID.

Once a lower genital tract infection is acquired, secondary prevention is aimed at reducing the incidence of upper genital tract infection and preventing further transmission within the community. Increasing public awareness of the signs and symptoms of lower genital tract infection, and encouraging prompt health care evaluation, should allow earlier therapeutic intervention. The development of simple inexpensive rapid tests for the detection of chlamydial and gonococcal cervicitis will further expedite this process. The increasing availability of effective single-dose antibacterial therapy should improve patient compliance and allow for easier treatment of sexual contacts.

Because substantial tubal damage has already occurred in most women presenting with symptoms of acute PID, interventions have been largely disappointing. This observation reinforces the importance of primary and secondary preventive measures.

KEY POINTS

1. PID poses a major threat to female reproductive health.
2. *C. trachomatis* is now the major aetiological pathogen in PID seen in the industrialized world.
3. Many cases of PID are either asymptomatic or run a very benign clinical course.
4. The incidence of PID is strongly correlated with the prevalence of sexually transmitted diseases.
5. PID is clinically misdiagnosed in about 35% of cases when laparoscopy is used for confirmation.
6. Laparoscopy should be considered in all hospitalized cases of PID, as it provides valuable diagnostic and prognostic information as well as an acute therapeutic option.
7. Despite apparent clinical and microbiological cure in PID, current therapeutic regimens do not guarantee preservation of normal reproductive function.
8. Delay of treatment for 3 or more days in gonorrhoea- or chlamydia-associated PID leads to a threefold increased risk of ectopic pregnancy or tubal infertility.
9. The likelihood of developing tubal factor infertility following PID is determined by the severity and number of episodes of disease.
10. Effective treatment of PID must include contact tracing and treatment of sexual partners.

REFERENCES

Aral S O, Mosher W D, Cates W 1991 Self-reported pelvic inflammatory disease in the United States, 1988. Journal of the American Medical Association 266: 2570–2573

Arya O P, Taber S R, Nsanze H 1980 Gonorrhoea and female infertility in rural Uganda. American Journal of Obstetrics and Gynecology 138: 929–932

Bevan C D, Johal B J, Mumtaz G, Ridgway G L, Siddle N C 1995 Clinical, laparoscopic and microbiological findings in acute salpingitis: report on a United Kingdom cohort. British Journal of Obstetrics and Gynaecology 102: 407–414

Buchan H, Vessey M, Goldacre M, Fairweather J 1993 Morbidity following PID. British Journal of Obstetrics and Gynaecology 100: 558–562

Catchpole M 1992 Sexually transmitted diseases in England and Wales: 1981–1990. Communicable Disease Report Review 2: R1–R7

Corcoran G D, Ridgway G L 1994 Antibiotic chemotherapy of bacterial sexually transmitted diseases in adults: a review. International Journal of STD and AIDS 5: 165–171

Farley T M M, Rosenberg M J, Rowe P J, Chen J H, Meirik O 1992 Intrauterine devices and pelvic inflammatory disease: an international perspective. Lancet 339: 785–788

Grodstein F, Rothman K J 1994 Epidemiology of pelvic inflammatory disease. Epidemiology 5: 234–242

Hagdu A, Weström L, Brooks C A, Reynolds G H, Thompson S E 1986 Predicting acute pelvic inflammatory disease: a multivariate analysis. American Journal of Obstetrics and Gynecology 155: 954–960

Hager W D, Eschenbach D A, Spence M R, Sweet R I 1983 Criteria for diagnosis and grading of salpingitis. Obstetrics and Gynecology 61: 113–114

Hay P E, Taylor-Robinson D 1992 Diagnosis of bacterial vaginosis in a gynaecology clinic. British Journal of Obstetrics and Gynaecology 99: 63–66

Hillis S D, Joesoef R, Marchbanks P-A, Wasserheit J N, Cates W, Weström L 1993 Delayed care of pelvic inflammatory disease as a risk factor for impaired fertility. American Journal of Obstetrics and Gynecology 168: 1503–1509

Hull M G 1985 Population study of causes, treatment, and outcome of infertility. British Medical Journal 291: 1693–1697

Jacobson L, Weström L 1969 Objectivised diagnosis of acute pelvic inflammatory disease. American Journal of Obstetrics and Gynecology 105: 1088–1098

Kahn J G, Walker C K, Washington A E, Landers D V, Sweet R L 1991 Diagnosing pelvic inflammatory disease. A comprehensive analysis and considerations for developing a new model. Journal of the American Medical Association 266: 2594–2604

Mahmoud E A, Hamad E E, Olsson S-E, Mardh P-A 1994 Antichlamydial activity of cervical secretion in different phases of the menstrual cycle and influence of hormonal contraceptives. Contraception 49: 265–274

Method M W 1988 Laparoscopy in the diagnosis of pelvic inflammatory disease. Journal of Reproductive Medicine 33: 901–906

Method M W, Urnes P D, Neahring R 1987 Economic considerations in the use of laparoscopy for diagnosing pelvic inflammatory disease. Journal of Reproductive Medicine 32: 759–764

Miotti P G, Chiphangwi J D, Dallabetta G A 1992 The situation in Africa. Baillière's Clinical Obstetrics and Gynaecology 6: 165–186

Moore D E, Foy H M, Daling J R et al 1982 Increased frequency of serum antibodies to *Chlamydia trachomatis* in infertility due to distal tubal disease. Lancet ii 8298: 574–577

National Institutes of Health, Expert Committee on Pelvic

Inflammatory Disease 1991 Pelvic inflammatory disease. Sexually Transmitted Diseases 18: 46–64
Paavonen J, Lehtinen M 1994 Immunopathogenesis of chlamydial pelvic inflammatory disease: the role of heat-shock proteins. Infectious Diseases in Obstetrics and Gynaecology 1–6
Patterson-Brown S, Eckersley J R, Sims A J, Dudley H A 1986 Laparoscopy as an adjunct to decision making in the 'acute abdomen'. British Journal of Surgery 73: 1022–1044
Patton D L, Moore D E, Spadoni L R, Soules M R, Halbert S A, Wang S 1989 A comparison of the fallopian tube's response to overt and silent salpingitis. Obstetrics and Gynecology 73: 622–630
Piot P, Laga M 1989 Genital ulcers, other sexually transmitted diseases, and the sexual transmission of HIV. British Medical Journal 298: 623–624
Reich H, McGlynn F 1987 Laparoscopic treatment of tubo-ovarian and pelvic abscess. Journal of Reproductive Medicine 32: 747–752
Rolfs R T 1991 'Think PID'. New directions in prevention and management of pelvic inflammatory disease. Sexually Transmitted Diseases 18 (2): 131–132
Sellors J, Mahony J, Goldsmith C et al 1991 The accuracy of clinical findings and laparoscopy in pelvic inflammatory disease. American Journal of Obstetrics and Gynecology 164: 113–120
Stacey C, Munday P, Thomas B, Gilchrist C, Taylor-Robinson D, Beard R 1992 *Chlamydia trachomatis* in the fallopian tubes of women without laparoscopic evidence of salpingitis. Lancet 336: 960–963
Svensson L, Weström L, Ripa K T, Mårdh P-A 1980 Differences in some clinical and laboratory parameters in acute salpingitis related to culture and serological findings. American Journal of Obstetrics and Gynecology 138: 1017–1021
Vessey M P, Yeates D, Flavel R, McPherson K 1981 Pelvic inflammatory disease and the intrauterine device: findings in a large cohort study. British Medical Journal 282: 855–857
Walker C K, Landers D V 1991 Pelvic abscesses: new trends in management. Obstetrical and Gynecological Survey 46: 615–624
Washington A E, Katz P 1991 Cost of and payment source for pelvic inflammatory disease: trends and projections, 1983 through 2000. Journal of the American Medical Association 266: 2565–2569
Washington A E, Aral S O, Wølner-Hanssen P, Grimes D A, Holmes K K 1991 Assessing risk for pelvic inflammatory disease and its sequelae. Journal of the American Medical Association 266: 2581–2586
Weström L 1988 Decrease in incidence of women treated in hospital for acute salpingitis in Sweden. Genitourinary Medicine 64: 59–63
Weström L 1994 Sexually transmitted diseases and infertility. Sexually Transmitted Diseases 21 (2) suppl: S32–S37
Weström L, Wølner-Hanssen P 1993 Pathogenesis of pelvic inflammatory disease. Genitourinary Medicine 69: 9–17
Weström L, Joesoef R, Reynolds G, Hagdu A, Thompson S E 1992 Pelvic inflammatory disease and fertility. Sexually Transmitted Diseases 19: 185–192
Wølner-Hanssen P, Weström L 1983 Second-look laparoscopy after acute salpingitis. Obstetrics and Gynecology 61: 702–704
Wølner-Hanssen P, Mårdh P-A, Svensson L, Weström L 1983 Laparoscopy in women with chlamydial infection and pelvic pain: a comparison of patients with and without salpingitis. Obstetrics and Gynecology 61: 299–303
Wølner-Hanssen P, Eschenbach D A, Paavonen J, Thorpe E, Pettinger M, Holmes K K 1991 Acute salpingitis: relationship of manifestations to infection with *Chlamydia trachomatis* or *Neisseria gonorrhoeae*. In: Bowie R B et al (eds) Chlamydial infections: Proceedings of the Seventh International Symposium on Human Chlamydial Infections. Cambridge University Press, Cambridge, pp 311–314

56

Sexually transmitted diseases

G. R. Kinghorn   C. J. F. Priestley

INTRODUCTION

In the UK, the hospital service for treating sexually transmitted diseases (STDs) was first established by statute in 1917. The clinics provided open patient access without the need for general practitioner referral, confidentiality regarding attendance and diagnosis, and free treatment. This service has now evolved into the specialty of genitourinary medicine (GUM), whose major functions are the diagnosis and treatment of patients suffering from STDs and the control of STDs within the community.

The *Health of the Nation* White Paper, published in July 1992, identified HIV/AIDS and sexual health as key areas for improvement. The general objectives are listed in Table 56.1. Specific targets were set for reducing the incidence of gonorrhoea and the rate of conceptions among the under-16s. It must be remembered that both STDs and pregnancy may be unwanted results of unprotected sexual intercourse. Close liaison between GUM and other disciplines, such as gynaecology, family planning and health education and promotion services, is essential to develop strategies to achieve these objectives.

Table 56.1 General objectives in the key areas of HIV/AIDS and sexual health (*The Health of The Nation – Strategy for Health in England*)

To reduce the incidence of HIV infection
To reduce the incidence of other sexually transmitted diseases
To develop further and strengthen monitoring and surveillance
To provide effective services for diagnosis and treatment of HIV and other STDs
To reduce the number of unwanted pregnancies
To ensure the provision of effective family planning services for those people who want them

GUM clinics provide rapid diagnosis and effective contact tracing, which are important for the control of STDs. They need to be accessible and acceptable to patients; their siting within hospital outpatient departments and close links with allied disciplines have aided other efforts to destigmatize attendance. Early treatment of STDs can prevent complications and reduce transmission; patient education is also regarded as an essential part of management.

EPIDEMIOLOGICAL ASPECTS

Increasing incidence

There has been a dramatic increase in the reported incidence of STDs during the past 25 years. The sexual revolution of the 1960s, facilitated by the wider availability of reliable contraception and changing sexual mores, was followed by a rising incidence of all STDs. This trend was augmented by earlier sexual maturity in girls and earlier age of onset of sexual activity in both sexes. The change in sexual behaviour among young women is manifest as a falling ratio of male:female patients for most STDs, which now approaches 1. In the UK the importance of prostitutes as vectors of STD transmission has declined, although they remain of major importance in disease transmission in developing countries. Prostitution is often linked to drug use: the exchange of sex for drugs is particularly risky.

Other sociological changes which contribute to the increased incidence of STD include urbanization, increased mobility among the young, and the greater ease of worldwide travel. Sexual tourism is increasingly common. This last factor has also promoted the importation of unusual tropical STDs and antibiotic-resistant infections. It is a strange paradox that, despite the availability of effective treatment during the past 40 years, STDs have become more common in many countries.

Changing pattern

In the UK during the past decade the traditional bacterial venereal diseases have become less common, whereas those infections caused by *Chlamydia*, viruses and other non-specific genital conditions have become more widespread. The reasons for this changing pattern are not fully understood, but may partially reflect the effectiveness of control methods for bacterial infections contrasting with the difficulties encountered with diseases due to other microorganisms. The changing pattern of STD is mirrored by the changed aetiology of STD complications, such as pelvic inflammatory disease and neonatal ophthalmia, where chlamydial infections now far outnumber gonococcal infections.

IMPACT OF HIV/AIDS

The advent of the acquired immune deficiency syndrome (AIDS) has focused attention upon sexual behaviour and emphasized the importance of STD control. On a worldwide basis, the commonest method of human immunodeficiency virus (HIV) transmission is by heterosexual intercourse. In sub-Saharan Africa and southeast Asia there is widespread infection among young women, and consequent vertical transmission in pregnancy.

In 1990 a programme was started by the Communicable Disease Surveillance Centre (CDSC) to monitor the prevalence of HIV infection in England and Wales. It used unlinked anonymous testing of blood specimens collected from antenatal and GUM clinics. This has confirmed that, in the UK, HIV infection is still relatively confined to well defined risk groups: homosexual or bisexual men; injecting drug users; and haemophiliacs. Infection in women is increasing, particularly in London, but remains mostly restricted to consorts of men in the above groups; injecting drug users; and women who were probably infected abroad, particularly in sub-Saharan Africa. There remains considerable uncertainty as to the rate at which it will spread to a wider heterosexual population.

Attempts to understand and modify risky sexual behaviour are crucial in curbing the spread of HIV. In addition, it is well recognized that STDs, particularly those causing genital ulceration, are important cofactors in HIV transmission. This knowledge must lead to redoubled efforts to control STDs as an essential, attainable objective in AIDS prevention.

Table 56.2 Markers for women at risk of STD

Age	15–34 years (maximal incidence 20–24)
Marital status	Single, separated or divorced
	Married before the age of 20
Occupation	Patient or consort with mobile job
Medical history	Previous STD
	Previous termination of pregnancy
	Multiple pregnancies before age 20
	Previous parasuicide or drug abuse
	Previous abnormal cervical cytology
Social history	Newly living away from home
	Disturbed family background
	Previously in care of local authority
	History of prostitution
	Late booking for antenatal care
	Self-applied tattoos

At-risk groups

The major risk groups show considerable overlap with those of other medical conditions, e.g. women requesting termination of pregnancy or with increased obstetric hazards (Table 56.2).

Changed sexual behaviour as a consequence of the HIV threat dramatically reduced the incidence of all STDs among gay men, although a recent increase in the incidence of gonorrhoea in this group suggests that a new generation needs to be educated about safe sex. However, there has been far less of a change among heterosexuals. A high rate of sexual partner change, which is the single most important factor in determining risk for STD, remains common in many groups of young people. It is not necessarily related to social class, to educational attainment or to standards of personal hygiene.

STDs not infrequently occur in apparently stable relationships, where neither partner admits infidelity. It is important to recognize that many STDs have long latent phases and that there are asymptomatic carriers in both sexes.

ROUTINE ASSESSMENT OF FEMALE PATIENTS

The history and examination are identical to the routine assessment of the gynaecological patient. A good history will contain details of the presenting symptoms, associated local or constitutional features, menstruation and contraceptive practice. Parity, and previous obstetric, medical and surgical history are noted; current drug therapy, including self-medication, and drug allergies are also recorded. A sexual history which includes detailed information about recent partner change, partner symptoms and their geographical origin is essential, and enquiries about risk factors for HIV infection should be routine.

One of the commonest complaints is of vaginal discharge, which may be due to a wide variety of physiological and pathological causes. It may also be the presenting complaint in women who suspect they may have been exposed to an STD. In these the true reason for seeking medical advice may only become apparent when a detailed sexual history is taken.

Routine examination will include inspection of the external anogenital area in a good light, most easily performed in the lithotomy position; palpation of the inguinal lymph glands and any vulval swelling; speculum examination of the vagina and cervix; and bimanual pelvic examination. Where indicated by the history or other findings a full physical examination may be required.

Precise details of routine microbiological investigations will vary between clinics, but will usually include microscopy of a wet film preparation of vaginal secretions and Gram-stained smears from the urethra, cervix and vagina. Urethral and cervical swabs are usually taken for gonococcal culture and *Chlamydia trachomatis* culture or antigen detection, and a high vaginal swab may be cultured. If reliable results are to be obtained specimens must be taken from the appropriate site, inserted into appropriate transport media, and be suitably stored and transported to the laboratory. Serological tests for syphilis (STS) are performed routinely in all new patients. Anonymous testing for HIV is performed in many GUM and antenatal clinics. If the patient requests a named HIV test, this can be performed on the same sample as the STS; pretest counselling is mandatory.

PRINCIPLES OF MANAGEMENT

Although the effective drug treatment of STD is often simple, there are also psychological and social consequences for each affected individual which require additional management. The principles of management are listed below:

1. Establish a firm diagnosis before treatment.
2. Investigate for multiple infections.
3. Use simple dosage regimens, preferably single-dose.
4. Confirm cure clinically and microbiologically.
5. Trace sexual contacts.
6. Educate patients and counsel them in a non-judgemental way.

STDs occur together, so that in patients presenting with genital warts, for example, screening for other infections should be mandatory. This principle is more easily forgotten with other sexually transmitted conditions, such as unwanted pregnancy in young girls, in whom surgical intervention may inadvertently result in ascending complications of unsuspected accompanying cervical or vaginal infection. However, many centres are now screening women prior to coil insertion or termination of pregnancy.

Control of STD demands that a precise diagnosis is reached before treatment is commenced, that follow-up is completed to ensure that both clinical and microbiological cure is achieved, and that contact tracing is routinely carried out. The last is most easily achieved by non-judgemental presentation of the facts in order to seek patient cooperation. In only a small proportion of cases will home visits by a health adviser be necessary.

BACTERIAL DISEASES

Syphilis

Syphilis is one of four human treponemal diseases whose causative organisms are morphologically indistinguishable and which cannot be differentiated by the results of serological tests. In developed countries infectious syphilis has decreased markedly in incidence during the past decade, and is now more common in homosexual men than in heterosexuals. However, in the USA there has been a resurgence of syphilis associated with HIV, particularly among 'crack' cocaine users and prostitutes. The non-venereal treponematoses – yaws, pinta and endemic syphilis – may cause concern in immigrant populations, when detected by routine antenatal screening tests for syphilis. In the developing countries syphilis remains a significant cause of morbidity and mortality among women and neonates.

Clinical features

Syphilis is a chronic systemic disorder caused by infection with *Treponema pallidum*, in which periods of florid clinical manifestations are interspersed by periods of latency when the disease is detectable only by serological tests. Both sexually acquired and congenital syphilis are subdivided into early and late disease. With the possible exception of the pregnant woman, who may potentially transmit infection to the fetus at any stage of the disease, those with late disease of longer than 2 years' duration are not infectious to others. Early syphilis includes the primary, secondary and early latent stages.

The primary chancre, a raised round indurated and usually painless ulcer, appears about 3 weeks after infection (Fig. 56.1). The incubation period can vary between 9 and 90 days. The chancre is usually single, sited on the external genitalia, and accompanied by bilateral non-tender rubbery inguinal lymphadenopathy. The untreated lesion will resolve spontaneously within 3–8 weeks. Presentation with secondary syphilis is more common in women when the primary lesion has been hidden in the vagina or on the cervix. Constitutional symptoms of fever, headache, bone and joint pains are accompanied by signs of a generalized non-irritant rash, most prominent on flexor surfaces and present on the palms and soles. Initially the rash is macular, but later becomes papular

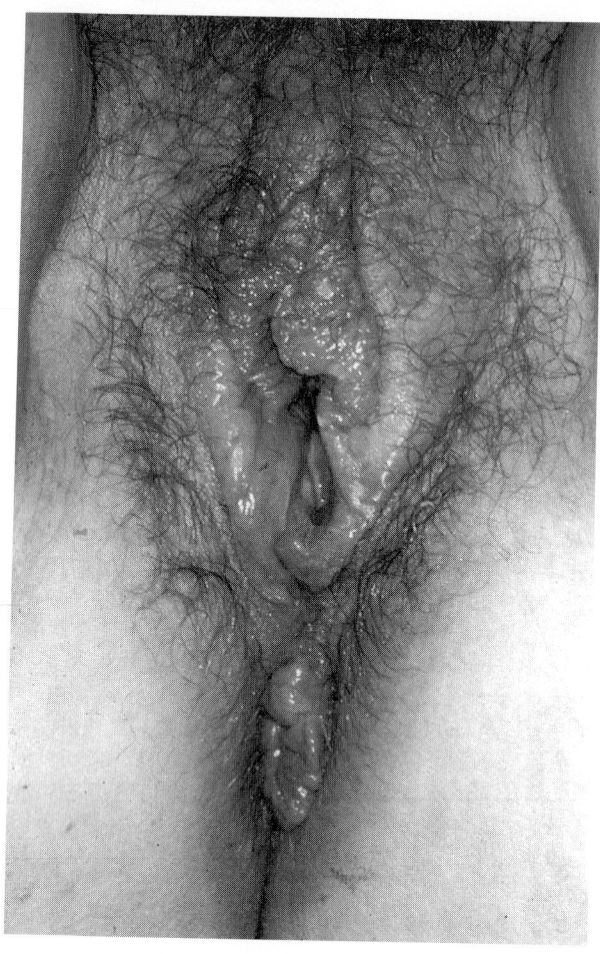

Fig. 56.1 Primary syphilis: this pregnant patient has a chancre at the fourchette with local oedema in the labia. She also has a trichomonal discharge.

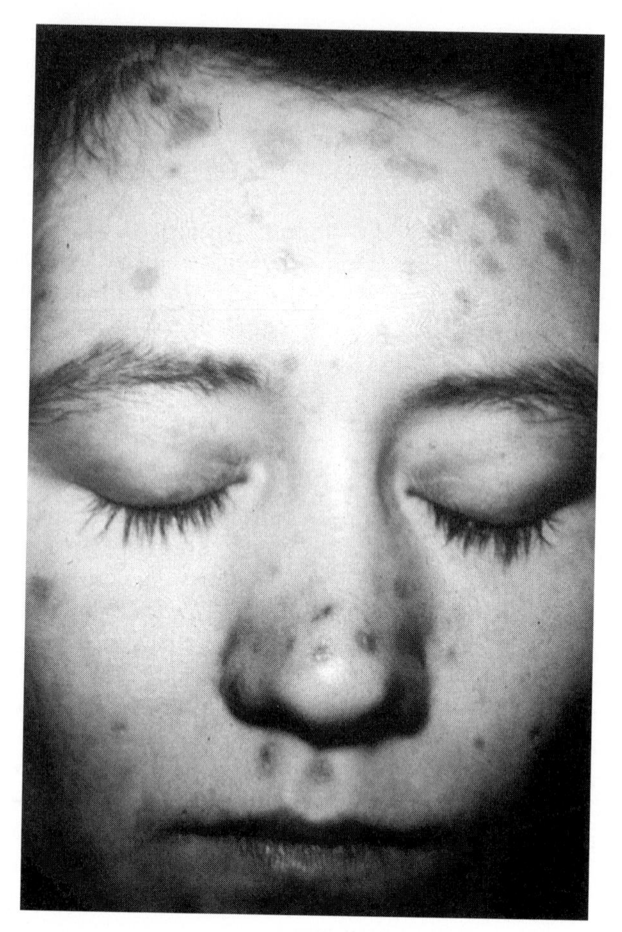

Fig. 56.2 Secondary syphilis: the maculopapular rash.

then nodular (Fig. 56.2). In moist areas – the genitals, the anus and beneath the breasts – condylomata lata appear. These, like the erosive lesions on mucous membranes, are highly infectious. Generalized painless lymphadenopathy is common; there may also be iritis, hepatitis or neurological manifestations.

Even without treatment all lesions will resolve and the patient will pass into the latent stage. The untreated patient may have persistent latent infection or may progress after several years to develop either tertiary gummatous syphilis, characterized by chronic inflammation of skin, bones, mucous membranes and, occasionally, viscera, or quaternary syphilis, typified by neurological and cardiovascular disease.

Congenital syphilis

Maternal syphilis often has an adverse effect on the pregnancy. *T. pallidum* can infect the fetus transplacentally at any time, typically leading to intrauterine death and midtrimester abortion. In surviving fetuses intrauterine growth retardation and prematurity are likely.

Congenital infection may be readily apparent at birth (Fig. 56.3). In less severely infected infants clinical manifestations can be delayed for weeks, months or years. There is no primary stage, as the bloodborne infection is systemic from the outset. Many of the early features are similar to those of acquired secondary syphilis, but skin rashes are often bullous, hepatosplenomegaly is common, and nasopharyngitis with a highly infectious nasal discharge (the 'snuffles') occurs (Fig. 56.4a–c). With delayed presentation, bone involvement causing pseudoparesis appears during the first months after birth (Fig. 56.4d). Hutchinson's triad of interstitial keratitis leading to corneal scarring, nerve deafness and notched permanent incisor teeth may result when the diagnosis is not made until childhood.

Diagnosis

In primary and secondary syphilis the diagnosis is rapidly confirmed with dark-ground microscopy by demonstrating *T. pallidum* in serum from abraded lesions. Serological tests become positive in late primary disease, reach maximal titres in the secondary stage and decline slowly during the latent phase. Table 56.3 shows common patterns of

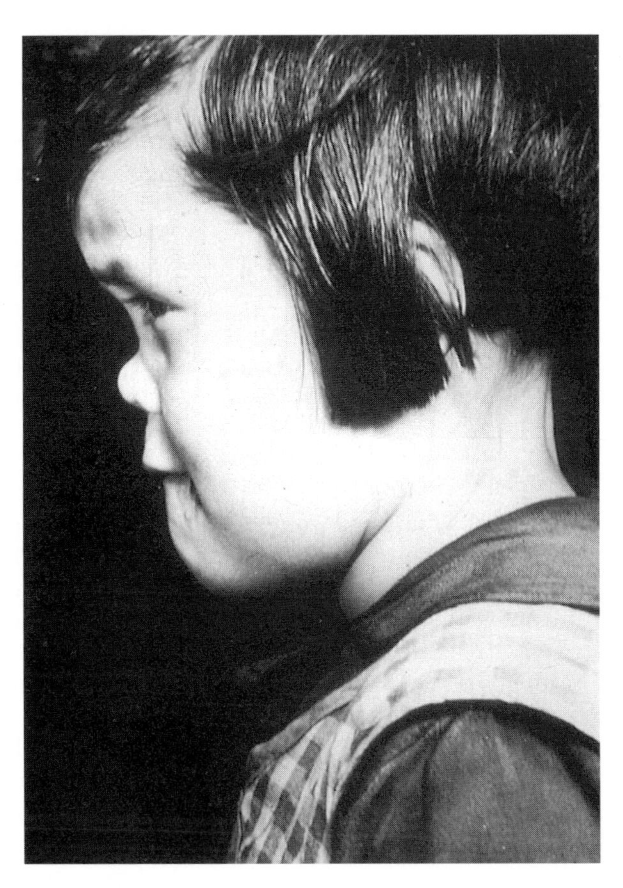

Fig. 56.3 Congenital syphilis: the typical facies has a depressed nasal bridge, frontal bossing and a prominent lower jaw.

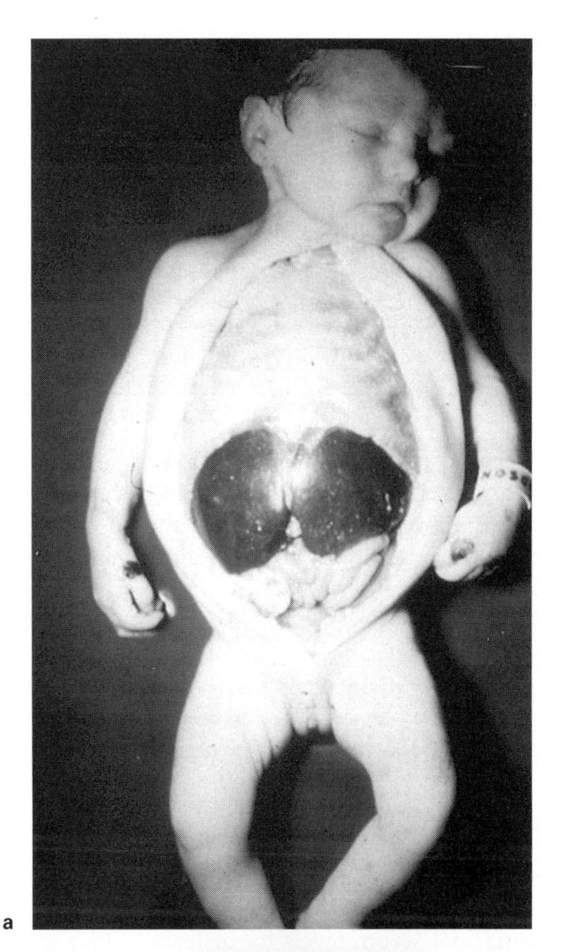

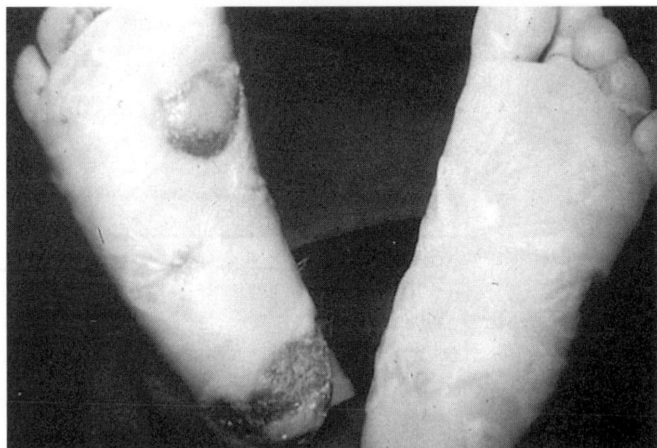

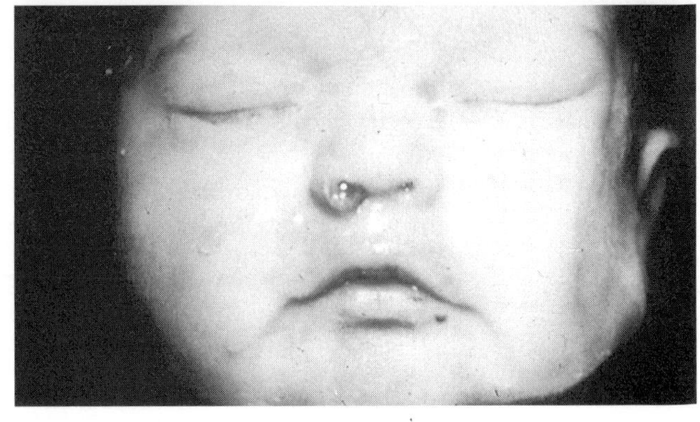

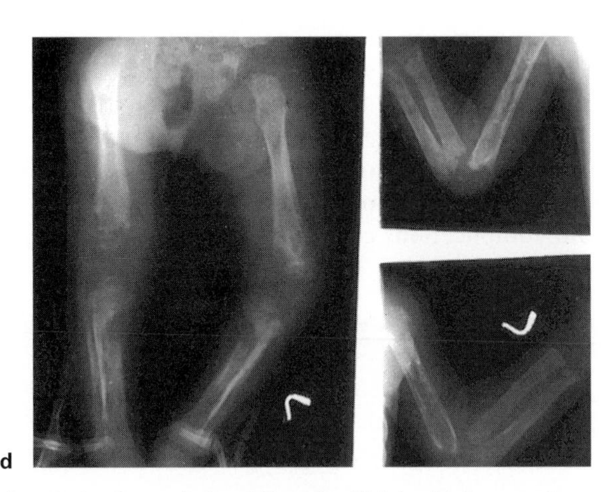

Fig. 56.4 Congenital syphilis: **(a)** stillbirth with hepatosplenomegaly; **(b)** bullous rash seen here on the feet; (**c**) serous nasal discharge; (**d**) lytic bone lesions.

syphilis serology. Although the reagin tests, such as those of the Venereal Disease Research Laboratories (VDRL), may revert to negative spontaneously, it is unusual for the highly sensitive, specific treponemal antibody tests such as the TPHA and fluorescent treponemal antibody

Table 56.3 Common patterns of syphilis serology

VDRL	TPHA	FTA	Likely diagnosis
+	–	–	False positive – repeat to exclude primary syphilis
+	+/–	+	Primary syphilis – dark-ground may be positive
+	+	+	Untreated or recently treated syphilis – probably beyond primary stage
–	+	+	Treated or partially treated syphilis – any stage Untreated latent or late syphilis
–	+	–	Treated syphilis
–	–	+	Very early primary syphilis

(FTA-absorbed) to become completely negative, even after treatment. Biological false positive reagin tests are occasionally seen during pregnancy; the specific treponemal tests will generally be negative, although false positive FTA-absorbed tests have been reported. The serological tests should always be repeated to exclude early syphilis.

Recently developed enzyme immunoassay (EIA) tests to detect antitreponemal IgM and IgG appear to be both sensitive and specific. Because they can be automated, they are likely to be used increasingly for screening purposes.

Treatment

These organisms remain sensitive to penicillin, which is still the treatment of choice. Preparations which maintain treponemacidal serum levels for at least 7 days are used: for example, Bicillin 3 ml (containing procaine penicillin 900 000 IU) i.m. daily for 10–14 days. In late disease treatment is given for longer and repeated courses may be required. In neurosyphilis and cardiovascular syphilis, intravenous penicillin is often given for at least 14 days, requiring hospital admission. In penicillin-allergic patients either tetracycline or erythromycin 2 g daily for 15 days is used, but treatment success is less assured.

Congenitally infected babies are treated with procaine penicillin 500 mg/kg i.v. daily for 10 days. Babies born to mothers treated with penicillin at any stage of pregnancy do not need additional therapy.

Prevention

A further fall in the incidence of acquired syphilis will depend upon adoption of safer sexual practices. Congenital syphilis is totally preventable and antenatal testing remains cost-effective despite the low prevalence of syphilis in developed countries. Some clinicians recommend additional insurance courses of penicillin treatment in all subsequent pregnancies.

Gonorrhoea

This infection, caused by *Neisseria gonorrhoeae*, reached a peak incidence in the UK during the mid 1970s and has since declined. In 1992 a total of 14 283 cases were reported from STD clinics. Gonorrhoea remains a common cause of morbidity in women and neonates worldwide, and antibiotic resistance is increasingly encountered in developing countries.

The organism is highly infectious and is transmissible prior to the onset of symptoms. Gonorrhoea has a short incubation period, usually 2–5 days. Asymptomatic infections are common in women, especially during pregnancy, and also occur in men. This results in late presentation with complications, and facilitates disease transmission.

Clinical features

At least half of all infected women have no symptoms and present as the result of contact-tracing procedures. When present, symptoms are similar to those of other lower genital tract infections, consisting of excessive vaginal discharge and dysuria.

Examination may reveal no abnormality but there may be signs of cervicitis, with a mucopurulent cervical discharge (Fig. 56.5). It is unusual to observe a urethral discharge in women. Rectal and pharyngeal infections are asymptomatic in the majority of cases and are more difficult to eradicate.

Complications

Complications may be local, ascending or distant. Acute local complications include skenitis, resulting in pain and swelling at the urinary meatus, and bartholinitis, causing painful unilateral vulval swelling which is fluctuant if an abscess has formed. The major ascending complication is pelvic inflammatory disease, which occurs in about 15% of infected women. Gonococcal pelvic inflammatory disease often starts at the time of menstruation.

Distant complications consist of perihepatitis and septi-

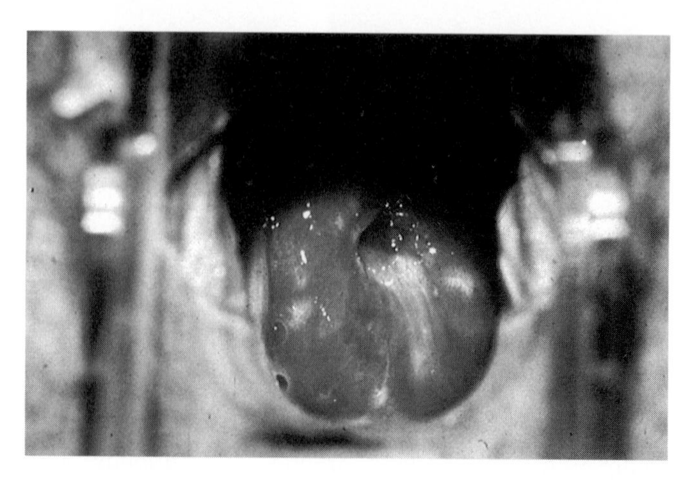

Fig. 56.5 Gonococcal cervicitis: the purulent endocervical discharge.

caemia. Gonococcal perihepatitis results from spread of infection to the liver capsule, which may then form adhesions to the abdominal wall. Patients complain of pain in the right upper abdomen which is worse on coughing, deep breathing and on flexing the trunk. The pain may be referred to the right shoulder and may be accompanied by nausea and vomiting. Pyrexia, abdominal tenderness and signs of lower genital tract infection are usually present, and pelvic inflammatory disease may coexist.

Septicaemia is most often due to gonococci with particular growth requirements; these organisms are usually very sensitive to penicillin. Pregnancy appears to be a predisposing factor. In the non-pregnant woman menstruation may precede bacteraemia. This is usually a relatively benign illness, characterized by low-grade fever; asymmetrical arthralgia, tenosynovitis and arthritis affecting wrists, elbows, knees and small joints of the hand; a skin rash, occurring in crops which have a typical evolution through papular and pustular stages to leave a haemorrhagic lesion showing central necrosis sited over joints and the peripheral aspects of limbs (Fig. 56.6).

In pregnancy, gonorrhoea may be associated with early abortion, intrauterine growth retardation, prematurity and postpartum sepsis. Gonococcal ophthalmia neonatorum usually begins 2–7 days after birth, with severe bilateral conjunctivitis (Fig. 56.7). This can lead to keratitis and blindness unless promptly treated. Gonococcal ophthalmia is a notifiable disease.

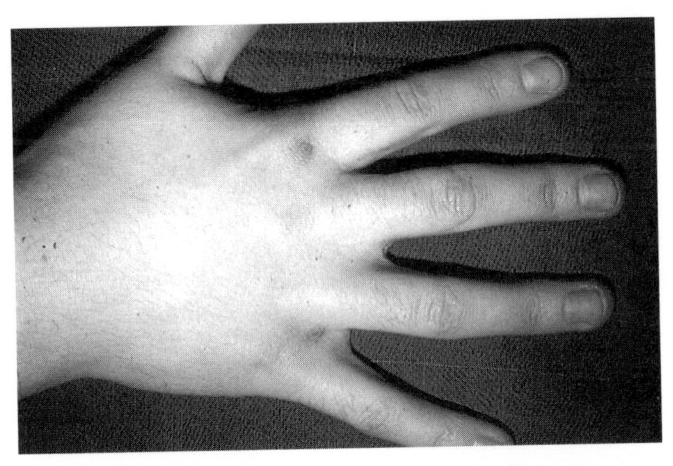

Fig. 56.6 Skin lesions caused by systemic gonococcal infection.

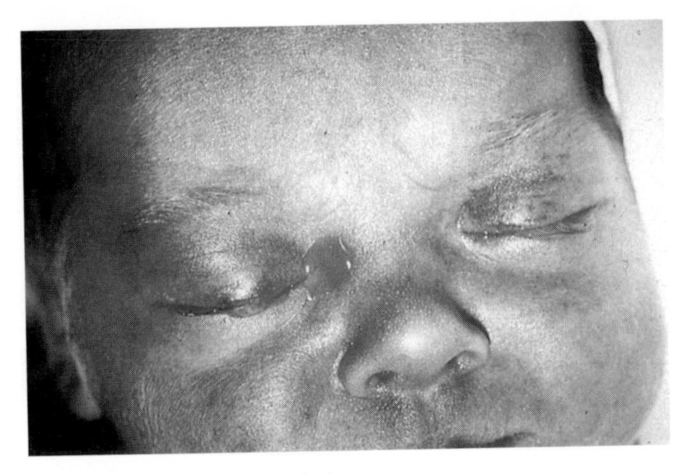

Fig. 56.7 Gonococcal ophthalmia neonatorum.

Although most men with gonorrhoea will develop an overt urethritis with dysuria and a urethral discharge, the male consorts of women with complicated gonorrhoea are often asymptomatic carriers of *N. gonorrhoeae.*

Diagnosis

Typically the organism infects columnar epithelium. In women the appropriate sites to test for infection are the endocervix, the urethra, the rectum and the pharynx. If bacteraemia is suspected, blood cultures are also necessary. Microscopic identification of Gram-negative intracellular diplococci allows a presumptive diagnosis to be made and the treatment to be begun. Cultures are more sensitive, permit antibiotic sensitivity testing and are always desirable for confirmation.

Treatment

Gonorrhoea can usually be cured with a single dose of a suitable antibiotic. In the UK penicillin remains effective; it is usually given as amoxycillin and probenecid. Elsewhere in the world, due to either plasmid-borne β-lactamase production or chromosomally mediated factors, penicillin resistance is the rule, rendering the drug useless. This is often accompanied by resistance to aminoglycosides, tetracyclines, sulphonamides and other antibiotics. Suitable single-dose regimens are shown in Table 56.4.

In complicated infections continuous therapy is given. In gonococcal pelvic inflammatory disease it is important to remember that concurrent infection with *Chlamydia*, mycoplasmas, anaerobes and other facultative pathogens is common. Thus, initial antibiotic regimens usually include metronidazole, and will change from penicillin-based to tetracycline-based after the first 2–3 days.

Gonococcal ophthalmia is preventable and prophylaxis should continue in developing countries where infection rates remain high and antenatal maternal screening is not possible. Erythromycin (1%) or 1% tetracycline eye

Table 56.4 Single-dose regimens for gonorrhoea

Medication	Dosage
Spectinomycin	2–4 g i.m.
Amoxycillin	3 g by mouth
with probenecid 1 g by mouth	
Cefuroxime	1 g by mouth
Ciprofloxacin	250 mg by mouth
Doxycycline	300 mg by mouth
Minocycline	300 mg by mouth

ointments can be used. Established neonatal disease is treated with a β-lactam stable antibiotic such as cefotaxime 100 mg/kg/day i.v. in three divided doses. It is probably unnecessary to use additional topical antibiotics, although regular saline irrigation to remove inflammatory exudate from the eyes is required.

It is essential that contact tracing is performed in all gonococcal infections, and both parents of infected babies should be examined as a matter of urgency.

Chlamydial infections

Chlamydia trachomatis is probably the commonest sexually transmitted bacterial pathogen in developed countries. This unusual Gram-negative bacterium behaves like a virus in that it replicates intracellularly. It is responsible for at least half of all cases of non-specific genital infection, which includes non-specific urethritis in the male and related conditions in the female. In 1992 there were a total of 107 916 cases of non-specific genital infection reported from STD clinics in the UK.

Clinical features

In women, early chlamydial infections are often silent and may remain so for months and possibly years. Most women are diagnosed as a result of routine screening, if complications occur, or if their partner presents with non-gonococcal urethritis (NGU). Symptomatic chlamydial infection may present with a wide variety of manifestations. Urethral involvement may lead to dysuria and frequency; *Chlamydia* is a cause of the urethral syndrome in young women. Cervical infection may be associated with an excessive discharge and postcoital or intermenstrual bleeding. Examination may show congested, oedematous cervical ectopy with small follicles, or there may be unexpected contact bleeding from the endocervical canal (Fig. 56.8). Often there are no abnormal signs.

Complications of local infection include skenitis and bartholinitis. Ascending infection may cause endometritis, which may manifest as painful and excessive menstrual loss. The most important complication of *Chlamydia* infection is pelvic inflammatory disease (PID), which may be acute, subacute or 'silent'. *Chlamydia* is now recognized to be associated with at least 50% of cases of acute PID in developed countries. It is also a more common cause of perihepatitis than is the gonococcus (Fig. 56.9). Periappendicitis, in which inflammation begins in the serosal layer and adhesions form between the appendix and adjacent structures, is recognized as another chlamydial complication presenting as right iliac fossa pain in young sexually active women.

Late sequelae of PID are chronic pelvic pain and tubal damage, the latter potentially resulting in infertility or ectopic pregnancy. The risk of tubal damage increases with delayed treatment or multiple episodes of PID. Early treatment can result in complete functional resolution, but serological evidence of previous *Chlamydia* infection has been found in a high proportion of women with tubal infertility.

In those who are genetically predisposed, chlamydial infection is a common precipitating cause of Reiter's syndrome in men. This syndrome is more common in women than was previously thought, and should be considered as part of the differential diagnosis of arthropathy in young persons, especially if associated with dermatological, mucosal, conjunctival and genital symptoms.

In pregnancy, chlamydial infection may be asymptomatic or may present as vaginal discharge, bleeding or the urethral syndrome as in non-pregnant women. However, it has also been associated with chorioamnionitis, spontaneous abortion, intrauterine growth retardation, premature rupture of membranes, preterm birth, perinatal death, and puerperal sepsis. It has been suggested that acute infection during pregnancy, as evidenced by a specific IgM response, is more damaging than pre-existing infection.

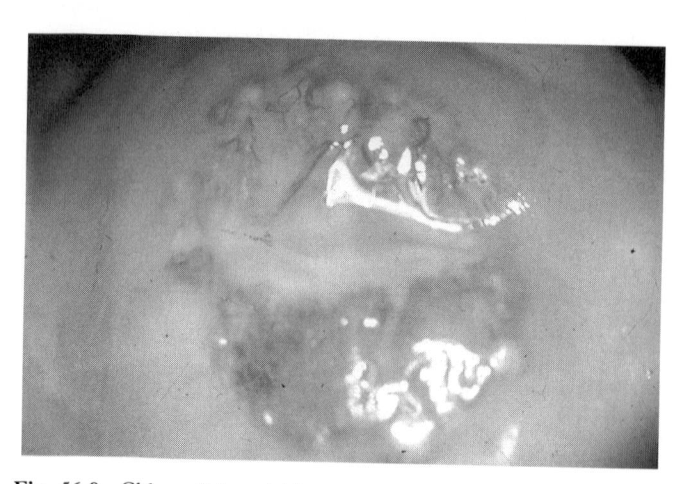

Fig. 56.8 Chlamydial cervicitis: a purulent discharge and inflamed follicles are seen.

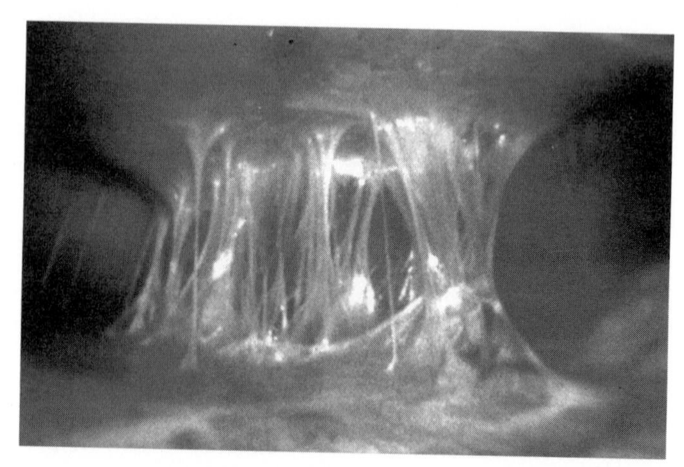

Fig. 56.9 Chlamydial perihepatitis: 'violin-string' adhesions are visible.

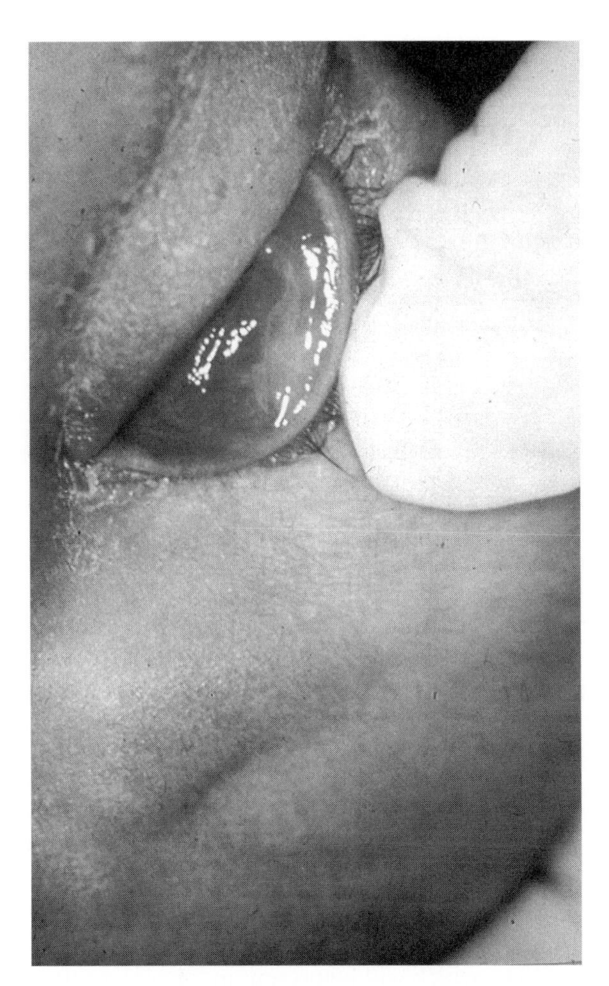

Fig. 56.10 Chlamydial ophthalmitis: the conjunctiva is swollen and inflamed.

The incidence of *Chlamydia* infection in women attending for termination of pregnancy (TOP) is 5–15%; untreated, these women are at least three times more likely to develop post-TOP sepsis than untreated women. Tragically, some of these may later present with infertility.

Chlamydia is also a common cause of neonatal disease. There is a 50–70% risk of transmission from an infected mother to the neonate during delivery. The associated conjunctival infection presents later than that due to the gonococcus – between 4 and 14 days, often after discharge from hospital (Fig. 56.10). An accompanying nasopharyngeal infection may later progress to afebrile pneumonitis and otitis media.

Diagnosis

Whatever method is used for diagnosis, it is essential that specimens are correctly obtained, transported, and stored. Swabs with cotton tips and metal or plastic shafts appear to be best for taking samples, which should contain columnar epithelial cells rather than exudate. Endocervical swabs should be taken after mopping the cervix to remove excess exudate. Taking urethral swabs in addition may increase the sensitivity of diagnostic methods. In salpingitis, tubal specimens in addition are desirable.

Chlamydia can be demonstrated in cell culture, for which a special transport medium and prompt delivery to the laboratory are necessary. Detection of *Chlamydia* antigen can be as or more reliable than culture, as living organisms are not required. Direct fluorescent antibody (DFA) tests are highly sensitive and specific, and should probably be regarded as the reference standard; however, there is a limit to the numbers that can be processed in the laboratory. Antigen detection using enzyme linked immunosorbent assay (ELISA) techniques is more suitable for large-batch testing, but is probably less reliable. Detection of chlamydial DNA using nucleic acid hybridization and amplification by polymerase chain reaction (PCR) is very sensitive but is at present unsuitable for routine diagnosis. *Chlamydia* serology to detect micro-immunofluorescent antibody has no place in the diagnosis of lower genital tract infections, but can be useful in the diagnosis of ascending infection and distant complications.

Treatment

Because available tests for the detection of *C. trachomatis* infections are not 100% sensitive, if only those sexual partners who were *Chlamydia* positive were treated it is likely that a significant number of infections would be missed, increasing the risks of reinfection and complications. Therefore in GUM clinics contact tracing is vigorously pursued and the index patient's sexual partner(s) will be treated whether or not *Chlamydia* is detected in them.

Uncomplicated *Chlamydia* infections are usually treated with systemic tetracycline or erythromycin 1–2 g daily for 7–14 days. The failure rate of 2.5% can mostly be attributed to a failure to treat both partners concurrently, or poor compliance with treatment, including taking tetracyclines with milk products. The 4-quinolone ofloxacin 400 mg daily appears effective in the treatment of *C. trachomatis* infections, as does azithromycin. The latter, although expensive, can be given as a single dose of 1 g orally, which may prove useful where compliance is a problem.

Complicated *Chlamydia* infection is often treated with a 21-day course of doxycycline, and the addition of metronidazole is recommended in PID as concomitant anaerobic infection is common.

Women who are pregnant, lactating or not using adequate contraception should be given erythromycin stearate. This may be poorly tolerated. Clindamycin appears to be effective but is not yet licensed in the UK for use in pregnancy.

Chlamydial disease of the neonate requires prolonged systemic therapy with oral erythromycin ethyl succinate suspension 50 mg/kg/day in four divided doses before feeds for 3 weeks. Tetracycline eye ointment can be added in the treatment of conjunctivitis and may speed up healing. Both parents should be investigated.

VIRAL DISEASES

Genital warts

Genital warts (condylomata acuminata) are the commonest viral STD in the UK. The annual incidence has increased more than threefold in the past decade, to 84 600 cases in 1992. They are caused by human papilloma viruses (HPV): these are small, non-enveloped icosahedral DNA viruses which have a particular tropism for epithelial cells. At least 60 different types have been recognized. Genital warts are almost always associated with infection caused by HPV types 6 or 11, and occasionally 16, 18 or 31. Subclinical HPV infection is very common. Patients with clinical warts are merely a subgroup of the total population affected. The factors governing the appearance of warts are not known. The main method of acquisition is by sexual transmission. Vertical transmission may also occur; infection from common warts is considered to be rare. The incubation period varies from a few weeks to 9 months, perhaps longer in some cases.

Clinical features

Warts vary in appearance according to their site and causative viral type. In women they can occur anywhere in the anogenital region, but most commonly appear on the vulva at sites of maximal trauma during intercourse (Fig. 56.11). In warm moist areas they are filiform but tend to be flatter upon keratinized skin. Although some women complain of an associated itch, this is usually the result of concomitant infections.

The growth of warts is favoured by warmth and moisture. They often proliferate in pregnant women, rarely posing obstetric problems, and regress spontaneously in the puerperium. Cervical warts are seen in less than 1 in 10 affected women, although a third will have evidence of warty change on cervical cytology or colposcopy (Fig. 56.12). Warts in men may be equally difficult to visualize, and show a wide variety of appearances and sites.

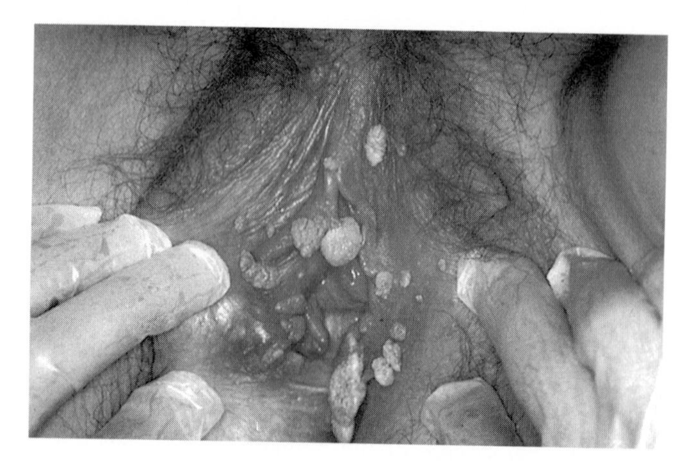

Fig. 56.11 Vulval warts.

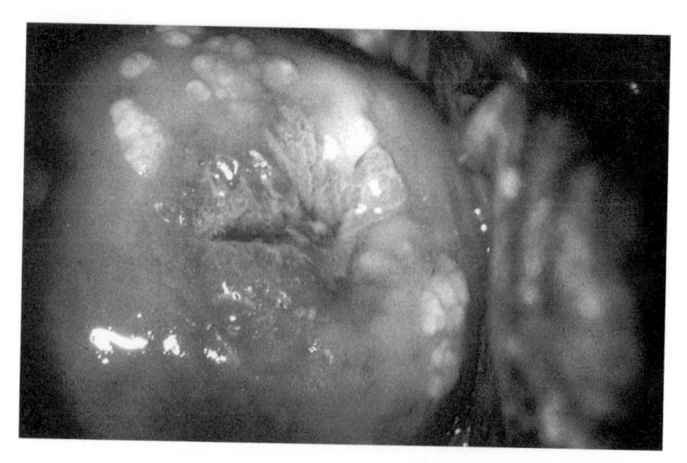

Fig. 56.12 Cervical warts.

Although warts are distinctive in appearance, biopsy is necessary if there is any suspicion about the nature of the lesion. This is especially true on the cervix. Warts characteristically show papillomatosis, acanthosis and koilocytotic changes.

Patients presenting with warts should be screened for other STDs, which will be present in 25%. A further 25% will have other genital infections such as candidiasis. Cervical cytology should be performed routinely. Colposcopic examination of the cervix and vagina is recommended if warts are present on the cervix. Patients with moderate or severe dyskaryosis on cervical cytology should undergo immediate colposcopy. Present recommendations are that those with lesser abnormalities should have a repeat smear after 6 months, and colposcopy performed if the abnormality persists; however, there is much debate as to whether mild dyskaryosis warrants immediate colposcopy or cytological surveillance.

Complications

It is generally accepted that genital HPV infection plays an important role in the development of malignant epithelial transformation of the cervix, vagina, vulva and anus, although other cofactors are necessary. Subclinical and latent infections with HPV types 16 or 18 appear to have the highest risk. In men, HPV 6 and 11 infections can rarely develop into a giant Buschke–Lowenstein tumour, which is a locally aggressive non-metastasizing verrucous carcinoma prone to secondary bacterial infection.

Vertical transmission may uncommonly cause anogenital warts to appear within the first year of life. Very rarely, juvenile laryngeal papillomatosis may develop. The appearance of anogenital warts in older infants must raise the possibility of sexual abuse.

Treatment

There are several local chemical and destructive treatment methods, each with its own practical limitations. Recurrence after apparent treatment success is common.

Podophyllin. A plant extract prepared in ethanolic solution or in tincture of benzoin, podophyllin is applied to warts as a paint, left to dry, and then washed off 4 hours later to prevent chemotrauma to healthy adjacent epithelium. It is best applied by medical or nursing staff. Podophyllin should not be used in pregnancy. It is potentially teratogenic and systemic absorption has resulted in serious maternal toxicity, affecting the liver, heart, kidneys and nervous system.

Podophyllotoxin. This is the main active ingredient of podophyllin. Liquid and cream preparations are now available, which, although expensive, allow self-treatment. Although this is usually reserved for men, studies have shown that self-treatment of external warts in women appears safe and effective.

Trichloroacetic acid. In 90–100% saturated solution this is a caustic agent which is useful to treat isolated, keratinized flat warts which respond poorly to podophyllin. Injudicious application can result in scarring.

Destructive methods. These include cryotherapy, which can be administered either by closed systems containing nitrous oxide or carbon dioxide with variable-sized probes, or by liquid nitrogen applied directly to the wart on swabs. Curettage, diathermy and laser therapy may also be used; these methods may require anaesthesia and inpatient admission.

Other chemical treatments. These include 5-fluorouracil, which has been used successfully to treat intraurethral warts. The α- and β-interferons given by subcutaneous or intramuscular injection have been studied intensively, with disappointing results. This is the only form of treatment with a potential action on the causative virus rather than merely on the resultant warts. Future treatment regimens may include topically applied interferon inducers as an adjunct to existing chemical and destructive therapies in an attempt to reduce relapse rates.

The partners of individuals with warts should always be examined, if necessary using a colposcope.

Genital herpes

The human herpes viruses are characterized by lifelong persistence of infection and the potential for reactivation, resulting in repeated disease episodes.

Genital herpes is caused by the herpes simplex virus (HSV) types 1 and 2, which are large complex DNA viruses. In the UK during the past decade there has been a large increase in the reported cases of genital herpes. This is partially a reflection of increased awareness and better diagnostic methods, but is principally a true increase in incidence matching those of other STDs.

Transmission occurs by contact with a person who is shedding virus, with or without symptomatic lesions. The incubation period is 2–14 days. Apparently longer incubation periods are usually due to 'non-primary first episodes'. It is becoming apparent from seroprevalence studies employing type-specific antibody tests that asymptomatic acquisition of HSV-2 infection may be the rule rather than the exception. In some parts of the UK HSV-1 causes 50% of first episodes. This may reflect changes in sexual practices. HSV-1 may be transmitted in monogamous relationships from orolabial lesions to the genitals of the partner, especially if they have pre-existing candida infection or vulval skin disease.

Clinical features

First episodes are often severe in women. They are less severe in those previously infected with orolabial herpes. Symptoms are both local and constitutional. Pain, dysuria and discharge are commonly associated with flu-like symptoms.

The lesions begin as erythematous plaques, which vesiculate and then form extremely tender superficial ulcers which possess an erythematous halo and a yellow or grey base. These are often accompanied by bilateral inguinal lymphadenopathy. Lesions are widespread in women and affect the introitus, labia majora, perineum, vagina and cervix (Figs 56.13 and 56.14). Untreated, a primary episode lasts for 3–4 weeks.

Complications of first episodes are common. There may be secondary bacterial infection of lesions. Autoinoculation to distant sites occurs, especially to the fingers and eyes. Local neurological complications include a sacral radiculomyelopathy causing self-limiting hyperaesthesia in the buttocks, thighs or perineum, decrease in sensation over the sacral dermatomes and difficulty in bladder and bowel emptying. Acute urinary retention can occur as a result of this neuropathy, or simply due to severe pain (Fig. 56.15). A self-limiting meningitis is sometimes seen. Severe, potentially fatal encephalitis is an extremely rare complication more typical in immunosuppressed individuals. Fulminating disseminated HSV infection is a very rare complication of primary infection in the third trimester of pregnancy.

Recurrent episodes occur in about 50% of patients. HSV-1 is less likely to cause recurrent disease than HSV-2. Recurrences are shorter, lasting 5–10 days, less severe, and are usually unilateral. Prodromal symptoms preceding the outbreak by 1–2 days consist of neuralgic-type pain in the buttocks, ankles or groin, or hyperaesthesia at the site

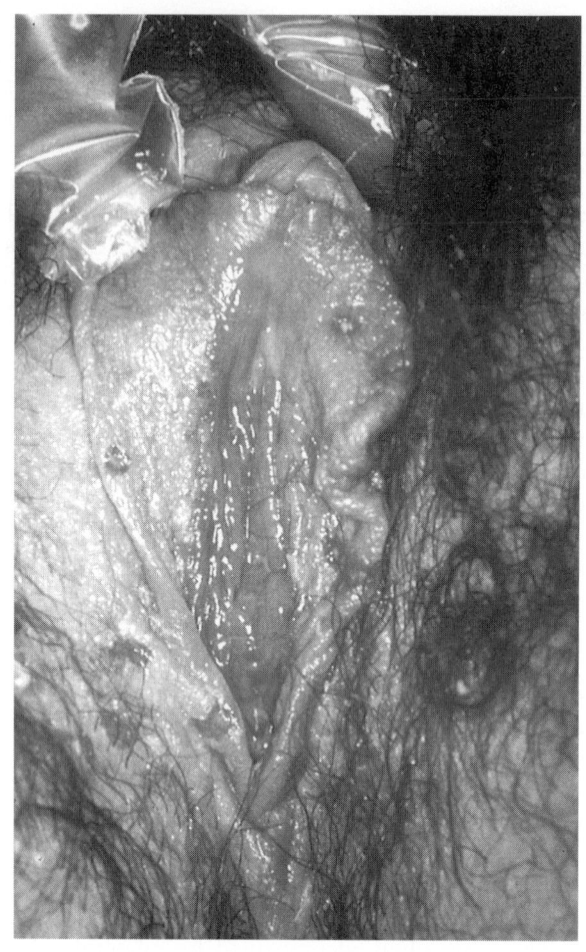

Fig. 56.13 Primary genital herpes: multiple painful ulcers are present on the labia minora.

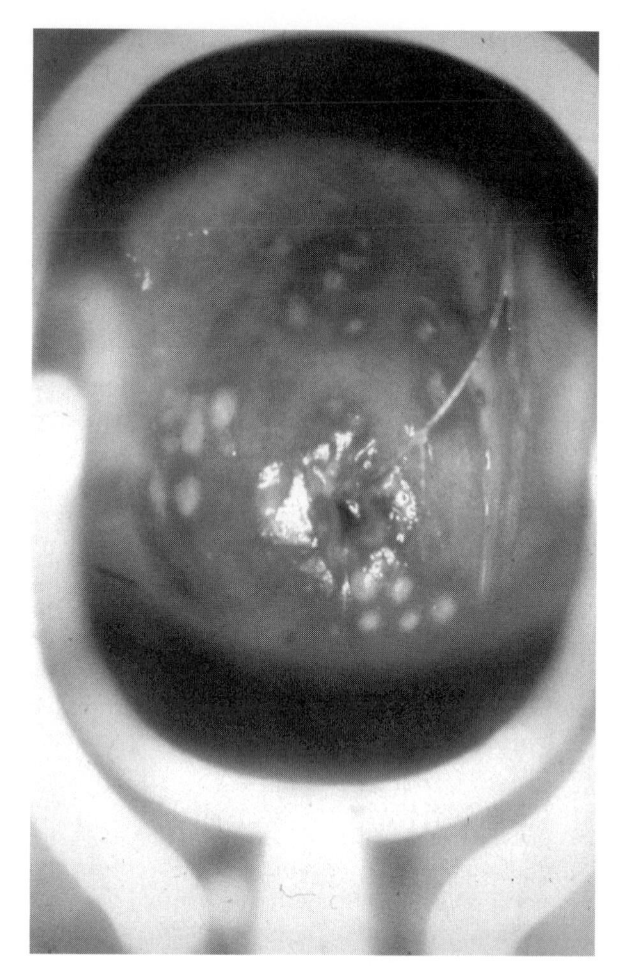

Fig. 56.14 Primary genital herpes: ulcers on the cervix.

of the lesion. Constitutional symptoms are less frequent. Psychological symptoms are often marked in those with frequent recurrences, and may be accompanied by emotional and relationship difficulties. Recurrences may be precipitated by stress, dietary factors, menstruation, exposure to sunlight or sunbeds, and local trauma associated with intercourse.

Diagnosis

The diagnosis should be confirmed by isolation of the virus in tissue culture or by detection of virus antigen in immunofluorescent or ELISA assays. Recently assays have been developed which detect type-specific antibodies to HSV-2 glycoprotein G; these have proved useful in epidemiological studies. Screening tests for other STDs are essential, but may have to be delayed in first episodes because of severe discomfort preventing adequate examination.

Treatment

The general management should be as for other STDs. Patients need counselling as well as both symptomatic and specific therapy. Bed rest, and systemic and local analgesia are important. Antibiotics to control secondary bacterial infection may be required in first episodes, although frequent saline bathing is not only soothing but also controls infection in most cases. Passing urine in the bath reduces pain and lessens the risk of retention.

Specific therapy is with acyclovir, a potent antiviral drug administered either intravenously or, preferably, orally in first episodes, within 6 days of the appearance of lesions. Episodic treatment with acyclovir is also useful in recurrent disease, although the effect is less marked. The drug should be started within 1 day of onset. In patients with very frequent attacks long-term oral acyclovir, 800 mg daily, suppresses the disease. The need for such therapy should be re-evaluated after 6–12 months. New antiviral prodrugs, famciclovir and valaciclovir, with improved pharmacodynamic properties allowing the advantage of less frequent dosing, appear as effective.

Neonatal herpes

Neonatal herpes is a well recognized complication of

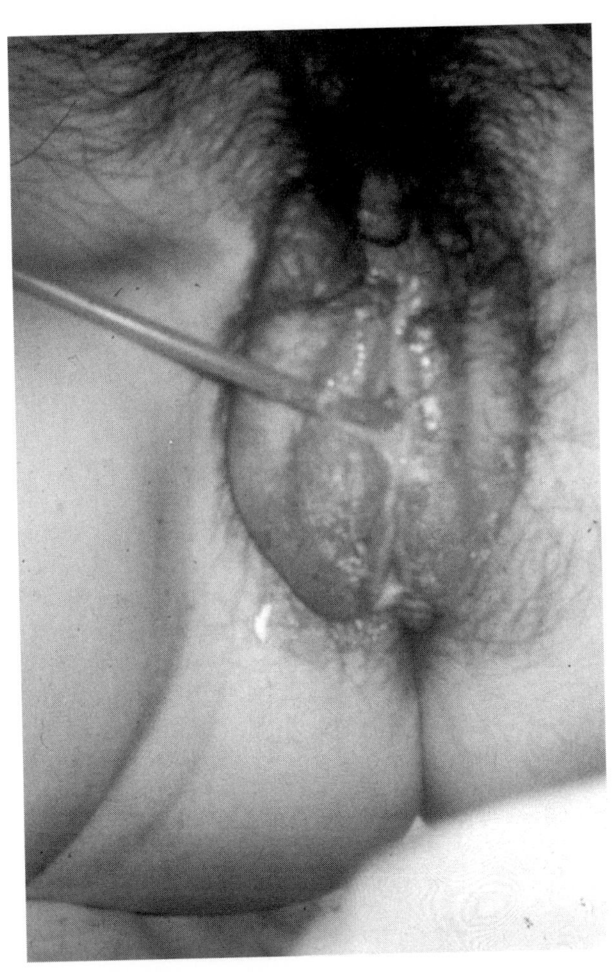

Fig. 56.15 Primary genital herpes: urinary retention and vulval oedema.

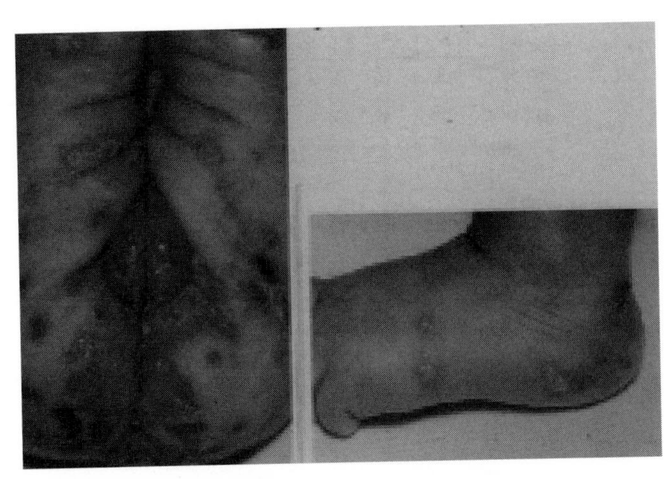

Fig. 56.16 Disseminated neonatal herpes: the lesions on the napkin area are haemorrhagic and ulcerated but vesicles are present on the foot.

maternal genital herpes at the time of labour. The majority of cases of neonatal HSV infection arise from primary, often undetected, maternal infection (Fig. 56.16); the risk of transmission from a recurrent attack or from asymptomatic shedding is much lower (1–4%). Transmission is more likely if the neonate has suffered skin trauma from scalp electrodes or instrumental delivery. The recommendations for the management of herpes in pregnancy have recently been re-evaluated, although much controversy remains.

The most useful current strategy is careful examination of the vulva and cervix for herpes lesions in all women in labour. In cases of primary genital herpes a caesarean section should be performed. Where there is a history of genital herpes most would recommend a caesarean section if the woman has a clinically apparent recurrence or prodromal symptoms at delivery. Others feel that with recurrent lesions the risk of transmission is so low that vaginal delivery is safe. If this approach is taken, the neonate should be monitored closely and viral cultures taken; if HSV is isolated acyclovir should be started. Another approach being evaluated is the use of acyclovir in late pregnancy to suppress recurrences and asymptomatic shedding. Acyclovir appears to be safe and may be effective, although it is not yet licensed for this purpose.

The new type-specific antibody assays have shown the seroprevalence of HSV-2 to be around 30%; this adds weight to the evidence that the risk of transmission from non-primary maternal HSV infection is very low. The possibility of identifying high-risk women who are seronegative for HSV-2 but whose partners are seropositive, holds much promise for the future. Several subunit vaccines have been developed and are currently being evaluated for the prophylaxis of HSV infection. The possibility of a therapeutic vaccine is also being investigated.

Molluscum contagiosum

This is caused by a large pox virus. In young adults it occurs on the genitalia as a sexually transmitted infection, although it can occur in children on the face, neck, upper limbs and trunk, spread by non-sexual close contact. Lesions on the genitals are found particularly on the pubis, thigh and labia majora. They are easily mistaken for genital warts, but close inspection of the small papular lesions shows a characteristic central umbilication. Expressed material shows a myriad of inclusion bodies.

Treatment consists of disrupting the papule, expressing the core and applying phenol with a sharpened orangestick to the residual lesion. Cryotherapy is equally successful.

Viral hepatitis

Several viruses can cause hepatitis, including cytomegalovirus and Epstein–Barr virus. The major viral causes are the hepatitis viruses A, B, C, D and E. Great advances in the characterization, diagnosis and management of the hepatitis viruses have been made in recent years. The major characteristics of these viruses are given in

Table 56.5 Characteristics of the known hepatitis viruses

Hepatitis virus	Transmission	Clinical features	Chronic infection
A	Faecal–oral Oroanal in homosexual men	Silent in 90% Fulminant hepatitis very rare	No
B	Parenteral Sexual Vertical Horizontal in endemic areas	Silent in 90% Children more often asymptomatic Fulminant hepatitis in 1%	10% in adults 90% in perinatal infection Can lead to: Chronic active hepatitis Cirrhosis Hepatocellular carcinoma
C	Parenteral Sexual transmission uncommon	Silent in 95% Fulminant hepatitis very rare	60% Chronic hepatitis Cirrhosis Hepatocellular carcinoma
D	Parenteral Sexual Only in those infected with HBV	Coinfection or superinfection with hepatitis B Fulminant hepatitis 20%	60% Effects as for HBV
E	Faecal–oral Oroanal possible	? limited to Africa/Asia Fulminant hepatitis common in pregnant women (10%)	No

Table 56.6 Serological diagnosis of viral hepatitis

Hepatitis virus	Markers of acute infection	Markers of past infection	Markers of chronic infection
A	IgM anti-HAV	IgG anti-HAV	
B	HBV DNA HBsAg HBeAg IgM anti-HBc	IgG anti-HBc anti-HBe anti-HBs infectivity)	HBV DNA HBsAg HBeAg (indicates high infectivity) anti-HBe (indicates low infectivity)
C	anti-HVC	PCR HCV RNA	anti-HCV PCR HCV RNA
D	IgM anti-HDV	IgG anti-HDV	
E	IgM anti-HEV	IgG anti-HEV	

Table 56.5. The parenterally transmitted viruses B, C and D may also be sexually transmitted. This is more common in homosexual men, but heterosexual transmission is also possible.

Diagnosis

Table 56.6 shows the major tests available for the diagnosis of hepatitis infections, and their significance. Epstein–Barr virus and cytomegalovirus infections can be diagnosed by tests for specific serum immunoglobulin M antibodies.

Treatment

Acute viral hepatitis is usually self-limiting and management is largely supportive, with a low-fat high-carbohydrate diet, bed rest and exclusion of alcohol until liver function tests return to normal. Patients who are carriers should be counselled about the risks of transmission and their condition should be monitored. In chronic hepatitis due to HBV and HCV, systemic interferon has been successful in promoting seroconversion in some cases. However, relapse after cessation of therapy is not uncommon, particularly in chronic HCV infection.

Prevention

Until recently the prevention of hepatitis A has depended on high standards of public health and hygiene, together with passive immunization of those at high risk using normal pooled immunoglobulin. A vaccine was developed in 1992; active immunization is advised for those who spend long periods in areas with a high prevalence of hepatitis A. In the UK, haemophiliacs, sewage workers and other groups who may be at risk may be immunized.

Hepatitis B is an occupational hazard for medical and nursing staff. Simple hygienic precautions and safe routine practice in the handling of blood and body fluids will reduce the risk of transmission from infected patients. Passive immunization is possible with hepatitis B immunoglobulin. Active immunization against hepatitis B is now readily available with genetically engineered vaccine or with purified antigen derived from carriers. It should be offered to health care personnel, non-immune individuals whose lifestyle places them at risk of such infection, and the newborn offspring of infected mothers. Recent government guidelines require that surgeons who undertake exposure-prone procedures should provide evidence of immunity to HBV. The interpretation and implementation of these guidelines has varied and the fate of those who fail to respond to the vaccine requires clarification.

Hepatitis C is best prevented by promoting safer drug use practices and by screening all donated blood.

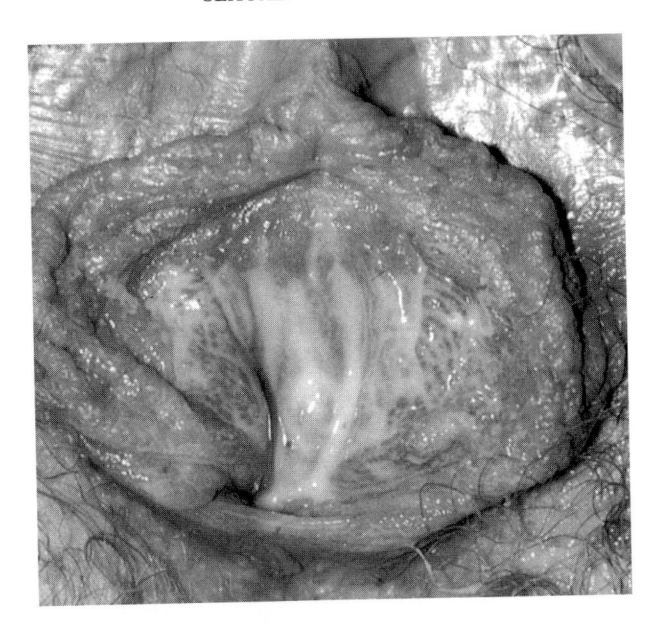

Fig. 56.17 Bacterial vaginosis.

VAGINAL INFECTIONS

Bacterial vaginosis

Bacterial vaginosis, previously known as anaerobic vaginosis and *Gardnerella* vaginitis, is one of the commonest causes of abnormal vaginal discharge. It is a complex condition in which a polymicrobial vaginal flora replaces the normal predominant lactobacilli. The bacteria involved include *Gardnerella vaginalis*, *Bacteroides* species, *Peptostreptococcus* species, *Mycoplasma hominis* and *Mobiluncus* species. Their metabolism produces biologically active metabolites, including volatile amines which cause the characteristic smell of the condition.

Although bacterial vaginosis is more common in sexually active women, it is also found in virgins and lesbians. There is no good evidence that it is an STD. It is more common in users of the IUCD and other non-barrier methods of contraception. Symptoms often develop following menstruation or sexual intercourse, and it is possible that hormonal changes and semen, among other factors, may trigger off the alteration in the vaginal flora.

Clinical features

The cardinal symptom of bacterial vaginosis is a smell, usually described as fishy. This is associated with a thin grey or white homogenous adherent vaginal discharge, which is sometimes frothy (Fig. 56.17). It is seldom associated with mucosal inflammation or with irritation. Many women with bacterial vaginosis are asymptomatic.

Complications

Apart from the psychological distress and disruption to sexual activity suffered by some women with bacterial vaginosis there are few proven complications. There is increasing evidence that bacterial vaginosis is associated with serious pelvic infections in women following surgical procedures, and with preterm labour, prematurity, chorioamnionitis and puerperal fever. However a causal effect has not been proven. Studies of the treatment of bacterial vaginosis in pregnant women are currently being undertaken to assess the impact on pregnancy outcome.

Diagnosis

The clinical diagnosis of bacterial vaginosis can usually be confirmed by simple tests on the vaginal discharge. Typically the pH is greater than 4.5. A drop of 10% potassium hydroxide added to a drop of secretion on a glass slide releases the fishy odour of volatile amines. Microscopy of a wet film shows active motility of *Mobiluncus* spp., and masses of small bacteria coating epithelial cells ('clue cells'). On a Gram stain preparation clue cells can also be identified; the bacteria are Gram-variable. Lactobacilli and pus cells are usually absent. Culture can be misleading as *G. vaginalis* can be found in 40% of women without evidence of the disease. Newer methods of diagnosis, such as gas–liquid chromatography and the detection of proline aminopeptidase in vaginal secretions, are mainly used for research purposes at present.

Management

Metronidazole is the drug of choice. A single 2 g dose is effective, although some prefer to repeat this dosage after 24–48 hours. A longer, 7-day, course of 400 mg twice daily is often given in recurrent cases and may be combined with a course of tetracyclines to eradicate other vaginal pathogens. Metronidazole may cause nausea. Alcohol may precipitate a disulfiram reaction and should be avoided during a course of metronidazole. Metronidazole is best avoided in the first trimester of pregnancy.

Clindamycin orally or vaginally appears to be as effective as metronidazole in the treatment of bacterial vaginosis. It also appears to be safe during pregnancy, although it is not yet licensed for this purpose in the UK.

Treatment of the male partner has not reduced the recurrence of bacterial vaginosis in women. However, the temporary use of condoms may be helpful to avoid semen in the vagina, which undoubtedly precipitates recurrences in many women.

Trichomoniasis

This is caused by infection with the protozoon *Trichomonas vaginalis*, which is actively motile by virtue of its four unipolar flagellae. The condition is usually sexually transmitted and may lie in a dormant state for months or years. Vertical transmission also occurs, and although non-sexual transmission is theoretically possible, owing to the organism's survival in moist secretions, mineral baths and toilets for several hours, it is likely to be an exceptional means of acquisition. Trichomoniasis is frequently associated with other STDs.

Unlike the other causes of vaginitis, the incidence of trichomoniasis has fallen in the past decade. *T. vaginalis* is more common in young sexually active girls, in women in their 40s and in users of non-hormonal, non-barrier methods of contraception.

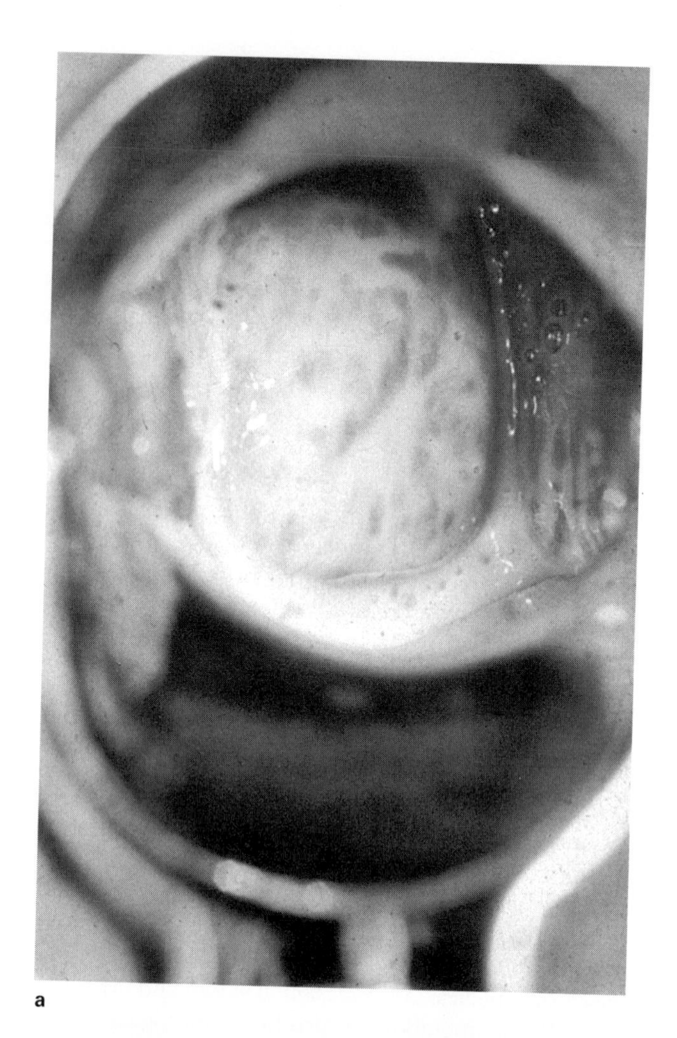

a

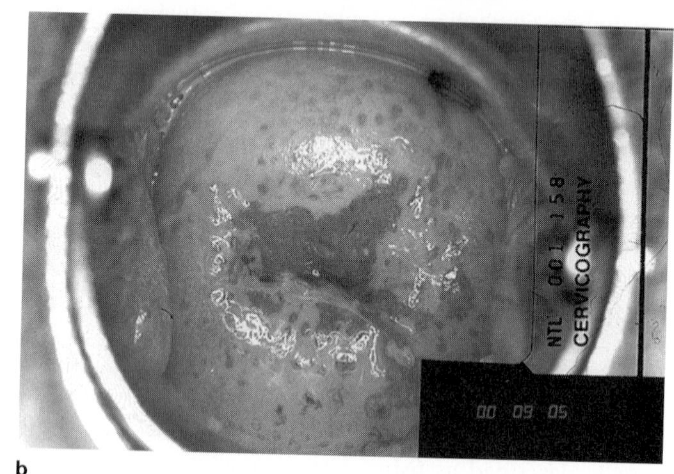

b

Fig. 56.18 Trichomoniasis: **(a)** grey, watery discharge and **(b)** 'strawberry cervix' with petechial haemorrhage.

Clinical features

The condition is typified by a foul-smelling mucopurulent vaginal discharge with accompanying symptoms of dysuria and vulval soreness. Examination will often reveal a severe vulvovaginitis, with perivulval intertrigo and petechial haemorrhage on the vaginal wall and ectocervix (Fig. 56.18).

Diagnosis

The diagnosis is most easily proved by the microscopic identification of the causative protozoon in a wet film. It can also readily be seen in cervical smears. Swabs sent in a transport medium, such as Feinberg–Whittington, can also be cultured. Clinical diagnosis is unreliable in milder cases as the discharge can be mistaken for bacterial vaginosis, especially in IUCD users.

Treatment

Metronidazole is the drug of choice using regimens similar to those in bacterial vaginosis. Other nitroimidazole drugs, such as tinidazole, are also successful in single- or multiple-dose therapy. True metronidazole resistance in *T. vaginalis* is extremely rare. Failures are more often related to utilization and degradation of the drug by other vaginal bacteria, or by failure to absorb the drug after oral administration. Combination broad-spectrum antibiotic–metronidazole regimens will usually eradicate the organism. Occasionally it proves necessary to give intravenous metronidazole on 5 consecutive days. During the first trimester of pregnancy, when metronidazole should be avoided, high-dose imidazole pessaries such as clotrimazole 500 mg nocte for a week may be effective in controlling symptoms.

Male partners usually have asymptomatic urethral infection with *T. vaginalis* but some develop urethritis or balanitis. Detailed investigations will reveal the organism in at least one-third of all sexual partners, hence the desirability of routinely treating the partner with metronidazole. A single 2 g dose is preferred, as this minimizes the period of alcohol abstinence recommended.

Candidiasis

Vulvovaginal candidiasis occurs worldwide. About 75% of women will experience an episode at some time, usually in relation to pregnancy or following antibiotic therapy. About 1 in 10 of these will suffer recurrent attacks, when the physical symptoms are often accompanied by profound psychological upset and sexual dysfunction. Although sexual acquisition probably plays only a small role in the aetiology of vulvovaginal candidiasis, the infection can be passed to male partners, who may act as asymptomatic reservoirs of reinfection or may develop symptomatic balanitis. The commonest causative yeast is *Candida albicans*. Other *Candida* spp. and *Torulopsis glabrata* account for less than 10% of cases, but may be more resistant to treatment. About 20% of women attending GUM clinics harbour vaginal yeasts. In most of these it represents asymptomatic carriage.

Predisposing causes

C. albicans is an opportunistic pathogen which requires an underlying deficit in host local or systemic immunity in order to invade the vagina and cause disease. Local immunity is compromised by the disturbance of commensal bacterial flora induced by broad-spectrum antibiotics; by other genital infections causing inflammation or ulceration of epithelial surfaces; by local trauma induced by intercourse or skin sensitizers; and by genital dermatoses.

Vulvovaginal candidiasis is a well recognized complication of the reduced cellular immunity in late pregnancy, and in all pathological states associated with immunosuppression. It is also more common in endocrine disorders such as diabetes mellitus and thyroid, parathyroid and adrenal disease. Although iron deficiency and other anaemias predispose to chronic mucocutaneous candidiasis, their association with vulvovaginal candidiasis is unproven.

The role of the male in reinfection has probably been overemphasized: in less than one-quarter of cases is the consort the major source of reinfection. Other more common sources are the gastrointestinal tract and the deeper layers of the vagina itself, which are penetrated by yeasts but which are relatively impervious to topical vaginal treatments.

Clinical features

The cardinal symptom is an intense vulval itch, worse with warmth and at night. This may be associated with external dysuria and dyspareunia. Excessive vaginal discharge is not a consistent feature. When present it is classically thick 'cottage cheese' in type, but in some women can be thin and mucopurulent.

The physical signs vary widely – some women with disabling symptoms have little to see other than mild vulval erythema and a few introital fissures. In the most acute cases there is a pronounced vulvovaginitis, with peripheral vulval satellite lesions, vulval oedema and vaginitis with adherent mycotic plaques on the vaginal wall and ectocervix (Figs 56.19 and 56.20).

Diagnosis

Clinical features should not be relied upon. The diagnosis should be confirmed and other pathogens excluded by thorough microbiological investigation. Microscopy of the vaginal discharge shows fungal elements in either 10% potassium hydroxide or Gram stain. A high vaginal swab cultured for *Candida* will give a positive result in carriers, as well as from women with symptomatic vulvovaginal candidiasis.

Treatment

Underlying causes should be corrected if possible. Drugs of the polyene group, such as nystatin, or of the imidazole

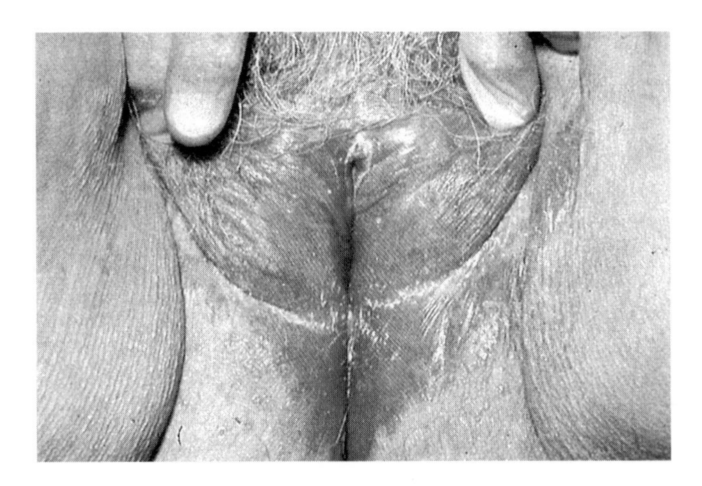

Fig. 56.19 Candida vulvitis. (See opposite.)

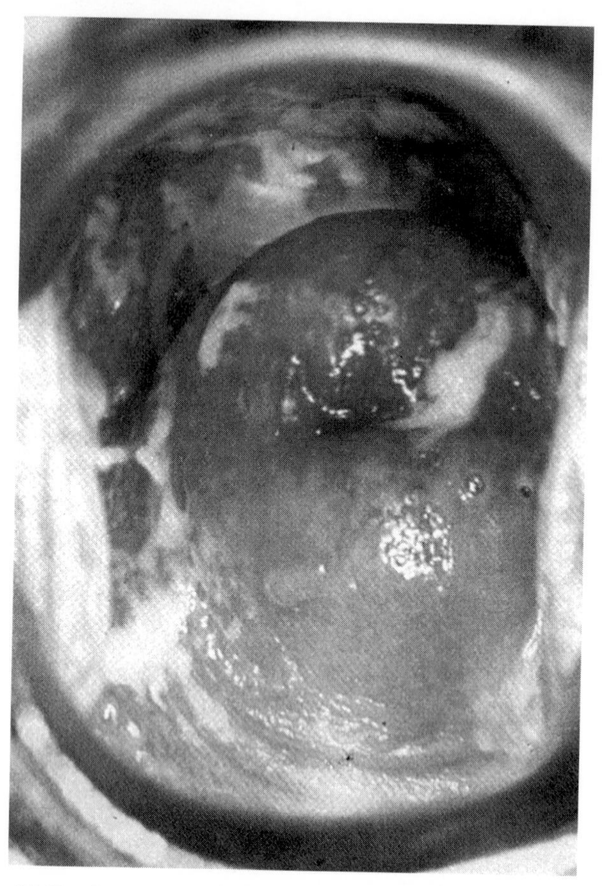

Fig. 56.20 Candida vaginitis: note the thick adherent discharge.

group, such as clotrimazole, miconazole and econazole, are commonly employed as creams and pessaries in topical treatments lasting 1–14 days. Yeast resistance to these drugs is virtually unknown and topical sensitivity is rarely encountered. Acute isolated episodes are usually successfully treated in this way. The systemic antifungal drugs fluconazole and itraconazole are effective in a single oral treatment and appear to be free from serious toxicity. Many patients find these drugs more acceptable than topical treatments, although they are considerably more expensive.

Chronic recurrent candidiasis is often a therapeutic problem, even after the consort has received concurrent penile treatment. Reinfection from underwear can be overcome by steam ironing or by prewash overnight soaks in candidacidal solutions. Eradication of gut and vaginal reservoirs would require systemic antifungal therapy. Good results have been obtained in recurrent vulvovaginal candidiasis by employing an initial 7-day course of fluconazole 50 mg daily, followed by prophylactic treatment with 150 mg single doses at fortnightly or monthly intervals for 3–6 months.

ECTOPARASITIC INFESTATIONS

Both pediculosis pubis and scabies are common infestations in sexually active adults. Their presence should stimulate investigation for accompanying STD.

Pediculosis pubis

The pubic louse, *Phthirus pubis*, has greatly enlarged middle and hind legs with claws adapted to match the diameter of pubic and axillary hair. The louse has also been recovered from the beard area, eyelashes and eyebrows. Adult lice are sedentary, move slowly and survive up to 24 hours when removed from their host. The adult female lays up to four eggs daily, cemented to hairs, and these hatch within 5–10 days. Sexual transmission is usual, although infestations acquired from shared beds and clothing are recorded.

Clinical features

Allergic sensitization to louse bites results in itching, which develops within a week in some individuals whereas others remain asymptomatic for weeks or months. Characteristic blue spots occur at bite sites. Adult lice situated at the base of hairs are often mistaken for freckles or crusts. Nits on hair shafts are more obvious.

Treatment

Topical pediculocide preparations should kill both adults and their eggs. After application, the drug should remain in contact with eggs for at least 1 hour. There are several proprietary preparations which, as lotions, creams or shampoos, usually have as their active constituents either γ-benzene hexachloride or malathion. Vaseline applied to the eyelashes and eyebrows will smother lice by obstructing their breathing apparatus.

Scabies

Scabies is caused by the itch mite *Sarcoptes scabiei*. Adult females measure 400 μm in length, move rapidly, and burrow into the horny layer of the skin where they lay up to three eggs daily. These develop, via larval stages, into adult mites within 10 days.

Epidemiology

Scabies affects all age groups. Non-sexual transmission occurs in families and particularly affects children. Sexual transmission should be suspected in young adults, especially when genital lesions occur.

Clinical features

Although individuals may remain asymptomatic for months, the usual development of intense itching, which is worse at night, occurs 1–8 weeks after infestation. A rash develops symmetrically on the trunk and limbs. Lesions on the head and neck rarely occur. Thread-like linear burrows, crossing skin creases, most commonly affect the fingers, wrists, axillae and nipples. Characteristic excoriated papules occur on the genitals.

Complications include secondary bacterial infection of excoriated lesions. In the mentally retarded, steroid-treated or immunologically compromised individual, massive infestations resulting in a generalized psoriasiform dermatosis may occur. The diagnosis is readily confirmed by identification of the mite on microscopy of material removed from burrows.

Treatment

It is important to treat the patient and all close family and sexual contacts. Topical applications are applied with a paintbrush to all skin areas from the neck down and left for 24 hours. Prior bathing should be avoided as it may increase the risk of systemic toxicity.

γ-benzene hexachloride does not sting and can be used on eczematized skin, but should be avoided in children and pregnant women because of possible neurotoxicity. Malathion, in aqueous or alcoholic solution, has an unpleasant smell and stings on application to broken skin. Monosulfiram, 25% solution in methylated spirit, is diluted in 2–3 parts of water and applied on 3 successive nights. Alcohol should be avoided during treatment because of the risk of 'Antabuse-like' reactions.

Secondary bacterial infection will require appropriate antibiotics. Post-treatment pruritus will usually respond to topical hydrocortisone and reassurance.

KEY POINTS

1. STDs are not necessarily related to social class, to educational attainment or to standards of personal hygiene.
2. A patient with one STD is likely to have another; screening for other infections is essential.
3. STDs are common in women undergoing termination of pregnancy, and are associated with an increased risk of sepsis.
4. The incidence of bacterial STDs in developed countries is declining, whereas viral STDs are increasing.
5. Antenatal screening for syphilis remains cost effective.
6. The commonest sexually transmitted pathogen in developed countries is *Chlamydia trachomatis*.
7. Chlamydial infections are often silent and may remain so for months, and possibly years. Long-standing infection is a frequent cause of tubal damage and infertility.
8. Genital warts are the commonest viral STD; subclinical HPV infection is even more common.
9. The majority of cases of neonatal HSV infection arise from maternal first-episode genital herpes. Classic lesions may be absent.
10. All pregnant women should be examined at delivery for evidence of herpes lesions. If present, delivery should be by caesarean section.
11. The commonest vaginal infections are associated with bacterial vaginosis, *Candida albicans* ('thrush') and *Trichomonas vaginalis*.
12. STDs increase transmission of HIV; STD control is an essential element of an AIDS control programme.

FURTHER READING

Adler M W 1995 ABC of sexually transmitted diseases, 2nd edn. British Medical Journal, London

Arya O P, Osoba A O, Bennett F J 1988 Tropical venereology, 2nd edn. Churchill Livingstone, Edinburgh

Center for Disease Control 1989 Sexually transmitted diseases treatment guidelines. Morbidity and Mortality Weekly Report 38 (suppl)

Holmes K K, Mardh P A, Sparling P F, Weisner P J 1989 Sexually transmitted diseases, 2nd edn. McGraw Hill, New York

Kinghorn G R, Spencer R C (eds) 1993 Sexually transmitted diseases. Medicine International 21: 73–148

Morse S A, Moreland A A, Thompson S E 1989 Atlas of Sexually Transmitted Diseases. Gower, Aldershot

Robertson D H H, McMillan A, Young H 1989 Clinical practice in sexually transmitted disease. Churchill Livingstone, Edinburgh

Sweet R L (ed) 1993 Bacterial vaginosis. American Journal of Obstetrics and Gynecology (suppl) 169: 441–482

Thin R H 1988 Management of genital herpes simplex infections. American Journal of Medicine 85: 3–6

White T S, Coda F A, Ingram D L, Pearson A 1983 Sexually transmitted diseases in sexually abused children. Paediatrics 72: 16–20

Wisdom A 1989 A colour atlas of sexually transmitted diseases. Wolfe, London

Zurhausen H 1987 Papillomaviruses in human cancer. Cancer 15: 1692–1696

57

HIV

F. Johnstone

INTRODUCTION

There are no major specific gynaecological problems associated with HIV, but this disease does impinge heavily on gynaecological practice. With progressing immunoincompetence, vaginal candidiasis, HPV infection and cervical intraepithelial neoplasia are more common and more difficult to treat. HIV does also introduce quite complex considerations in the routine management of menstrual problems, contraception and infertility. In addition, HIV has had an important effect in changing attitudes to infection control during surgery.

BACKGROUND

The aetiological agent of AIDS, HIV, contains two copies of a single-stranded RNA genome and it is only with conversion of the genetic material into DNA that the viral genes can be transcribed and translated into proteins in the usual way. This is accomplished by a viral DNA polymerase with a ribonuclease (together called reverse transcriptase), and it is this reversal of the normal flow of genetic information that classifies HIV as a retrovirus. Once in the form of double-stranded DNA, the viral genetic information is spliced into the DNA of the host cell. It then serves as a template for viral gene transcription leading to the production of new virus. Infection of that cell and its progeny is permanent.

Target cells have the CD4 receptor, a T-cell surface glycoprotein which characterizes the T helper subset of lymphocytes. These cells interact with antigen-presenting cells, which display antigen on their own cell membrane together with class II major histocompatibility complex glycoproteins. Helper T cells then initiate an immune response against other cells bearing the antigen, and thus occupy a pivotal position in overall cell-mediated immune response. However, although the CD4 lymphocyte is the main target, a proportion of peripheral monocytes (which mature to become macrophages), follicular dendritic cells and Langerhans' cells express CD4 and can be infected by HIV. Microglial cells can also be infected and may produce very small amounts of CD4. These other cells do not seem to be destroyed by infection in the way that CD4 lymphocytes are, and may act as a reservoir of virus.

Early infection with HIV is characterized by a very high viral load. After antibodies are formed the viral load is greatly reduced. Typically there is a long quiescent asymptomatic phase, but even in this phase most individuals show a steady loss of CD4 lymphocytes (about 60/mm^3/year), and there are signs of 'activation' in response to HIV. It has become clear that during this period the virus is not latent but is chronically produced at a low level, and that this phase is characterized by interaction between HIV and the immune system. During this time there appears to be enormous diversity of viral species, and antigenic variation may be used by HIV to escape neutralization. With time the immune system gradually collapses, and this allows a higher viral load and also selection of more virulent 'fast' variants, that form high-replicating syncytium-inducing isolates. The CD4 lymphocyte population is then critically reduced, and major clinical disease supervenes.

For most infected women this is a fatal disease, characterised by a long phase without major symptoms, and an average time of about 12 years between infection and death. However, a small proportion of women appear to remain fairly well without major immune compromise for long periods of time, and there are hopes that with advances in treatment, longer survival for most women can be achieved. A number of markers have been shown to be independent predictors of disease progression. The most important is the CD4 lymphocyte count, but p24 antigenaemia reflects viral load indirectly, and β_2 microglobulin reflects activation of the immune system.

Although HIV has now spread throughout the world there is still great variation in prevalence, with more than 10% of women of reproductive age infected in parts of Africa, and very low levels in Egypt and other Arab countries in the Middle East. Because of this variation, HIV is the leading cause of death in young women in Africa and in large urban areas in the USA, but has still to make a substantial impact in many countries.

TRANSMISSION

HIV is predominantly a sexually transmitted disease. Women appear more biologically vulnerable than men, perhaps because as the receptive partner women have a larger mucosal surface exposed during sexual intercourse, and because semen contains a higher concentration of HIV than vaginal fluid.

Discussion of the risks of transmission is often appropriate when a woman does not have a stable sexual relationship or when a couple are discordant for infection. Transmission is more likely when viral levels are high, either closely following infection or late in the course of disease. The presence of other sexually transmitted disease, especially one causing ulceration, is an important risk factor.

Male condom use is highly, though not entirely, protective. In one cohort study of couples where one partner was initially seronegative and the other seropositive, there was no seroconversion among the 124 couples who used condoms consistently (de Vincenzi et al 1994). On theoretical grounds, the Femidom should be protective. Local antiviral preparations may also be protective, but there are as yet no data confirming this. Nevertheless, because of its potential importance, this is a subject of intense research interest (Elias & Heise 1994).

TESTING FOR HIV

The decision to take an HIV antibody test must be an individual decision. HIV testing must not be undertaken without acquiring the patient's fully informed consent. Pre-test counselling should inform the woman of what the test entails and enable her to explore whether this is the right time for her to have information about her HIV status. A positive HIV result confers the (irreversible) knowledge that one is infected with an incurable, progressive life-threatening condition. Since the stigma surrounding HIV and AIDS can lead to rejection and discrimination, this is information that some women would rather not know, especially if they have no symptoms. However, despite the disadvantages, increasingly there are clear advantages to the individual in diagnosing HIV infection. These mainly concern informed decision-making about pregnancy and protection of sexual partners, but increasingly, it is hoped that early treatment will be helpful. The interventions which may protect against vertical transmission (see below) have dramatically increased the perceptions of advantage of knowledge of serostatus as far as pregnancy is concerned.

The principles of HIV testing have been well described (Holman 1992, Sher 1993). High-risk groups for selective HIV testing are shown in Table 57.1 and the issues covered in pretest counselling in Table 57.2.

TREATMENT OF GYNAECOLOGICAL SYMPTOMATOLOGY

Before discussing specific problems we should consider the framework defining treatment. Women infected with

Table 57.1 High-risk groups for selective HIV testing in pregnant women. Not all these groups may readily be determined by direct questioning

- Sexual partners of men who have had sex with other men at any time since 1977
- Drug users or sexual partners of drug users who have injected themselves with drugs at any time since 1977
- Women who have had sex at any time since 1977 with people living in African countries except those on the Mediterranean, or who have sexual partners who have done so
- Sexual partners of haemophiliacs
- Women who are prostitutes

Table 57.2 Issues covered in pretest counselling (From Holman 1992)

Information
Explanation of HIV infection and its relationship to AIDS
Modes of transmission
Sexual and drug-related risk reduction behaviours
The purpose of HIV antibody testing
The meaning of HIV antibody test results
The importance of knowing one's HIV antibody status, particularly with regard to treatment, pregnancy and perinatal transmission
Documentation and reporting of test results

Assessment of patient
Who are the supportive people in her life?
If HIV positive, who could she confide in, who would be supportive and keep her confidence?
How has she generally reacted to stressful situations?
How does she think she might deal with a positive test result?

HIV may have a lot to cope with in terms of social disruption, relationship problems, family fragmentation and the knowledge that they have a fatal disease; then, as the disease progresses, they have chronic ill health punctuated by serious acute episodes of illness. Additional discomforts from gynaecological symptoms may superimpose an intolerable burden. For this reason, particular efforts should be made to resolve symptoms simply and with as little extra investigation or inconvenience as possible. By and large, treatments are unaffected by HIV status, although there are a few caveats to this which are discussed below. As with many issues in the management of HIV, good communication with accurate information is essential in quality care. This should include written material and there are excellent booklets dealing with gynaecological problems and with pregnancy (Mercey et al 1993). As well as standard medical treatments, the woman may want to consider the range of complementary approaches which have been suggested. Although any evidence of effectiveness from controlled trials is usually lacking, individual women undoubtedly benefit from some of these therapies and it is important that they should at least be aware of these options. There is a helpful and comprehensive booklet describing complementary and alternative therapies in the management of HIV disease (NAM 1994).

REPRODUCTIVE TRACT FUNCTION

Menstrual pattern

There are several theoretical reasons why an upset in menstrual pattern might be anticipated in HIV disease. In particular, advancing disease and weight loss might be accompanied by anovulatory bleeding or amenorrhoea; pelvic sepsis could become more symptomatic as immune function declines; and there are possibly differences in endometrial lymphoid cell populations which are not classical endometritis (Johnstone et al 1994b).

Nevertheless, although surprisingly few data have been published, there is no secure evidence that menstrual upset does commonly result directly from HIV infection. Menstrual symptoms were not commonly reported in one large descriptive study (Carpenter et al 1991) and the only published controlled study, of 55 HIV infected women, did not demonstrate any effect of HIV status (Shah et al 1994). The clinical impression persists that there is a high prevalence of menstrual problems, in particular amenorrhoea, with advancing disease, but this impression may largely be due to confounding by drug use, or to more attentive health care.

Little information is available on endocrine function in females with HIV. In men, no striking differences have been found when the men are well, but hypogonadotrophic hypogonadism has been reported as a common feature in those who have AIDS. It has been suggested that this may relate specifically to weight loss rather than to HIV infection itself.

Menometrorrhagia and dysmenorrhoea can often be successfully managed with hormone treatment. Theoretical suggestions that the effect of hormone treatment on the immune system could increase the rate of progression of disease are not supported by evidence from natural history studies, though this is an under-researched area (Howe et al 1994). The risk of exacerbating hepatitis C infection, which is very common in women who became infected through injection drug use, needs to be considered on an individual basis. Hormone replacement in amenorrhoeic women can often improve quality of life and sexual function.

Fertility

Fertility does not seem to be affected by HIV infection. Despite expectations that women with HIV would avoid pregnancy, this has not been local experience. The only large study to address this, in African women, showed only small differences in fertility rates between HIV-infected and non-infected women, which were easily ascribable to intention or relationship breakdown (Ryder et al 1991).

GENITAL INFECTION

Vaginitis

Recurrent vaginal candidiasis is reported to be the most common initial clinical manifestation of HIV infection (Carpenter et al 1991) and has been reported to be a problem at relatively well maintained CD4 counts. Thus Iman et al (1990) suggested a hierarchy of risk of candidal infection, with recurrent vaginal candidiasis becoming more common with early systemic immunosuppression, oral candidiasis becoming common at moderate immunosuppression, and oesophageal candidiasis (an AIDS-defining diagnosis) typically occurring with severe forms of immunosuppression. Not only are HIV-infected women more prone to recurrence, but yeasts other than *Candida albicans* (e.g. *Torulopsis glabrata*) are isolated more frequently, and there is a shorter time before recurrence (Spinollo et al 1994).

Response to treatment is usually good, but relapses frequently require retreatment or maintenance therapy in a majority of patients. This requires a combination of topical and oral antifungal agents, e.g. a short course of an oral imidazole (ketoconazole, fluconazole) followed by clotrimazole 500 mg intravaginally weekly or monthly. There is an ongoing clinical trial (ACTG981) to determine the efficacy of fungal prophylaxis in HIV infection.

Women may also like to try a range of complementary or alternative treatments.

Other vaginal infections, such as bacterial vaginosis,

have not been examined in detail but do not appear to be a major problem.

Pelvic sepsis

Pelvic sepsis is probably more common, or at least more symptomatic, as HIV disease progresses. However, there are no controlled studies demonstrating this, and there are inevitably problems of bias in follow-up studies. HIV-infected women have been shown to present with more severe disease and more symptoms and signs than control women, but to have the expected resolution with antibiotics (Hoegsburg et al 1990, Korn et al 1993). Other studies have pointed to the lower white blood cell count in HIV-infected women, and a greater need for surgical intervention. In general terms early or pre-emptive treatment with antibiotics is indicated in women with HIV disease, and standard treatment is appropriate.

Genital warts

Condyloma acuminata due to HPV (human papilloma virus), usually types 6–11, are common in HIV-infected women and may be more extensive and aggressive than is typical in non-immunocompromised patients. The usual sources of bias and the absence of controlled studies have to be acknowledged. Treatment is along standard lines, with recurrence being common.

NEOPLASMS

There is a risk that as there is a breakdown of the immune system, so there will be an increased risk of tumours, as cells are released from intensive immune surveillance. This is well recognized for non-Hodgkin's lymphomas, which occur in more than 5% of AIDS cases. Gynaecological oncology may become more of a concern as treatments for advanced disease improve. This may mean much longer survival in an immunocompromised state.

Cancer of the cervix

An excess risk of CIN (cervical intraepithelial neoplasia) has been demonstrated in several controlled studies (Schafer et al 1991, Adachi et al 1993, Johnstone et al 1994a). This has been shown on a population basis (Johnstone et al 1994a) and is believed to relate to immune compromise (Adachi et al 1993, Smith et al 1993, Johnstone et al 1994a). However, the exact relationship between HIV and CIN has not been fully explained. There are reports that HPV expression is increased and some reports that recurrence of CIN after treatment is much more common.

There have been concerns about the usefulness of cervical cytology in HIV-infected women, and for this reason some workers have recommended routine colposcopy for follow-up (Maiman et al 1991). However, most studies have validated the use of cervical smears, and La Guardia (1993) advocates 6-monthly review with visual inspection of the lower genital tract and cervical cytology as primary screening. Each centre will have to define a protocol for follow-up in the light of patient numbers, resources and acceptability. This will involve more intensive screening than usual for non-infected women, perhaps initially with cervical smears but with colposcopy performed very readily for any abnormality. Where resources allow, and particularly where CD4 count is less than 300/mm^3, colposcopic assessment should be carried out.

There are case reports of rapidly progressive invasive cervical cancer that did not respond to appropriate therapy. However, so far there are no convincing population data showing an increase in invasive carcinoma of the cervix. Perhaps this may simply be a question of time (or that pre-cancers are being picked up by attentive health care).

Other genital neoplasms

Vulval and anal intraepithelial neoplasia have also been reported more commonly in HIV-infected women (Palevsky 1994). However, there are no reports showing an increase in endometrial or ovarian lesions.

ADVICE ABOUT PREGNANCY

Issues surrounding pregnancy frequently arise in gynaecological practice, in the context of advice about contraception, induced abortion or infertility. It is very important that information is accurate and up to date, as significant new data accrue rapidly.

Pregnancy does not appear to have any major effect on the rate of progression of HIV disease. Nor does HIV in relatively well women have any major effect on pregnancy outcome, although there may be small increases in the rate of spontaneous abortion and small decreases in birthweight. Intuitively, it seems likely that when women are ill and severely immunocompromised there must be some effect on pregnancy, on both fetal growth and chorioamnionitis, leading to preterm labour. There are some data in support of this.

The main concern of mothers is the risk of the baby becoming HIV infected. Of infected babies, about one-third present early with symptoms and progress rapidly, but the remainder have a more chronic infection more similar in scale to the adult. In developed countries most studies have shown a transmission rate of 15–25%. The largest study, the European Collaborative Study (1992), showed a transmission rate of 14.7%. This figure is affected by viral load (higher rates of transmission with early or late infection, or with markers such as low CD4 count).

There is current excitement about the ACTG076 randomized placebo-controlled trial of AZT (Connor et al 1994). Interim analysis on 365 pregnancies revealed a transmission rate of 8.3% in the AZT arm of the study and 25.3% among those receiving placebo. Both mothers and infants tolerated the AZT treatment well, with no significant short-term side effects other than reversible mild anaemia in some infants.

With accumulating circumstantial evidence that a considerable proportion of infection may occur around the time of delivery, attention has focused on labour ward management. Caesarean section may be protective. The analysis published from the European Collaborative Study (1994) does not report a randomized trial but great efforts were made to assess confounding factors associated with transmission risk, and the odds of infection were all around 0.5 in those pregnancies where caesarean section was performed. However, not all studies have found this effect, and a meta-analysis of 11 studies suggests a lesser effect with an odds ratio around 0.80 (Dunn et al, 1994). Routine elective caesarean sections can not be recommended for all HIV-positive women on present information.

The estimated extra 14% risk of transmission, or odds ratio of ×2.3, due to breastfeeding means that breastfeeding is contraindicated where a safe alternative exists (Dunn et al 1992).

Many difficult issues remain about different interventions, including the possibility that effects might be different in women with more advanced disease; that there might be synergy or antagonism between interventions; that future trials may be greatly constrained by existing beliefs; and that management plans for individuals, depending on multiple effective interventions, all with some risk, will be problematic. Nevertheless, there is considerable optimism that with a combination of interventions, perinatal transmission will be substantially reduced.

PREGNANCY CONTROL

Contraception

This area has caused confusion among patients because of the double message of prevention of infection and transmission (condoms) and prevention of pregnancy (often another contraceptive method).

There have been concerns expressed about oral contraceptive pill use because this may be associated with increased viral load in the cervical mucus, hence increasing the risk of onward transmission, and because the pill does have effects on the immune system and hence could increase HIV disease progression (Howe et al 1994). At present these are theoretical concerns unsubstantiated by good clinical evidence, and combined pill use appears a reasonable option for most HIV-infected women.

The intrauterine contraceptive device has a higher risk of endometrial infection and pelvic sepsis, and on theoretical grounds is probably not ideal for HIV-infected women.

Sterilization

Sterilization should be undertaken under the same guidelines as apply to other women. However, care needs to be taken around the time of diagnosis. Some women elect for sterilization at this time when they have not had sufficient opportunity to adjust to the diagnosis, and they may subsequently regret the procedure. HIV itself is not an indication for sterilization and it is important that women make a careful, unhurried decision about their future childbearing. The prevalence of regret following sterilization in our population has been high.

Termination of pregnancy

HIV-infected women should be aware of the possibility of termination of pregnancy where this is legally available. Good communication of all the different issues is important. This includes the understanding that, because of illness or death, the woman may not be able to look after the child until adolescence.

Nevertheless, HIV itself is not usually seen as a reason to terminate a wanted pregnancy (Selwyn et al 1989, Johnstone et al 1990). The complex, interconnected and at best still poorly understood factors in determining the decision to continue or terminate pregnancy made by HIV-infected women are very well explored by Selwyn and Antoniello (1993). This can be a very difficult decision for a woman to take, and once it has been finally reached, whatever it is, she needs empathetic support.

INFERTILITY

This is a contentious but important area because this is a frequent reason for consultation. One consensus view is that on both ethical and legal grounds infertility treatment is contraindicated where a woman is HIV infected (Smith et al 1991). These authors explained their reasons for stopping clomiphene treatment on discovering a woman's seropositive status, and against her wishes. However, theirs is not a unanimous view. Indeed, many HIV screening programmes have the implicit understanding that medical treatment will not be withheld dependent on serostatus, and withdrawal of care is itself ethically problematic. Some gynaecologists (including the author) would argue that discussion and investigation are often essential aspects of care, and that women should not be automatically denied access to treatment because of serostatus.

Infertility may present in a number of different situations. Both partners may be HIV infected, or only one of them. Each situation requires a different approach. As with infertility in other circumstances, continuing childlessness can be extremely distressing, and in HIV infection there may be additional pressing concerns.

Fundamental to all three situations described is the need for thorough discussion about the disease and the meaning of this for the family relationships. Infected individuals have a shortened life expectancy and a number of markers may help to give some idea of this (clinical status, CD4 count, p24 antigenaemia, etc.). In many cases an infected partner will not, owing to progressive illness or death, be able to look after a child up to primary or secondary school age. The risks of infection to the child also need to be clarified. The basic risk of 14% from the ECS needs to be qualified by clinical stage and markers of viral load. However, as discussed above, there is encouraging information that some transmission may be preventable. The issues here are complex and need very well informed and up-to-date information.

In the imaginary case where both partners are infected, both are clinically well, both have a clear understanding of the issues, there are no other contraindications and both are keen to attempt a pregnancy, then the decision about investigation and possible treatment needs to be carefully weighed. There must be awareness of the one published consensus view that treatment should not be given for ethical and legal reasons (Smith et al 1991). Perhaps one way forward is for discussion and early non-invasive investigation to take place, so that there is a good basis for knowing what treatment may be indicated. If specific treatment is required, and the clinician thinks this may be justifiable, then perhaps the decision should be shared with colleagues or even a small committee including local ethicists.

There are particular issues where only one partner is infected. Here, there is the advantage that at least one partner should be alive as the child grows older, but there is also the additional risk of that partner becoming infected. Where the woman is infected this leaves the entirely safe option of artificial insemination by the husband using a syringe. Where only the man is infected, there have been attempts to process semen by gradient centrifugation followed by a swim-up procedure. Semprini et al (1992) reported on 29 women where 17 pregnancies were achieved with no seroconversion. However, as pointed out in subsequent correspondence, the 95% confidence intervals included an infection rate of 6.25 transmissions per 100 inseminations. In addition, Dussaix et al (1993) showed under experimental conditions that HIV could incorporate into the acrosomal head of the spermatozoa and still be capable of infecting CD4 lymphocytes. This is a very important area, but with major uncertainties remaining.

PREPARATION FOR GYNAECOLOGICAL SURGERY

Most HIV-infected women will tolerate surgery well, even though their CD4 count is very low. Chest infection and wound infection are more common, but with prophylactic antibiotics and intensive physiotherapy will not usually present serious problems. Therefore, if surgery is clearly indicated, HIV status should not affect the decision to operate. Nevertheless, there are extra morbidity risks, and where there is doubt about the need for surgery HIV infection should prompt consideration of alternative management.

NOSOCOMIAL TRANSMISSION

Occupational transmission to health care workers

Most occupational transmission has occurred following needlestick or other sharps injury, but there have been a very few documented seroconversions after contamination of broken skin or mucous membranes.

Up to October 1992, seroconversion following a specific exposure incident had been reported in 51 cases, with a further 91 instances of presumed occupational source (Cockroft 1993). Most of the patients had CDC Stage 4 HIV disease. Most of the documented exposures were needlestick injuries and most of those involved a hollow needle containing infected blood. No seroconversion after an injury from a suture needle or other solid needle used in the operating theatre had been reported. Although this will inevitably be a considerable underestimate of the total number of health care workers infected by occupational risk, nevertheless the number is small in relation to the huge number of contacts between health care workers and HIV-infected individuals.

The risk of acquiring HIV from a single accidental exposure to infected blood has been estimated at 0.38% (95% CI 0.18–0.70%). The risk for non-parenteral exposure is thought to be much less, but no figure has been established.

Even at these low levels of risk the estimated lifetime risks to surgeons can be substantial, depending on local prevalence of HIV, the number of operations being performed and needlestick injury rate. Parenteral exposure occurs in 1–7% of surgical procedures. Glove perforation is commonplace, with a rate of 30–50% in gynaecological surgery. However, calculation of lifetime risk is dependent on estimates of seroconversion from solid surgical needle trauma, which may not be realistic. So far, studies of health care workers have not indicated any major excess risk of HIV infection.

Infection control procedures

Although the risk of patient-to-patient transmission may

Table 57.3 Precautions recommended for health care staff (From Joint Working Party 1992)

Invasive procedures in all patients
Have vaccination against hepatitis B
Cover all cuts and abrasions with waterproof dressings
Do not pass sharps hand to hand
Do not use hand needles
Do not guide needles with fingers
Do not resheath needles
Dispose of all sharps safely into approved containers
Put disposables and waste into yellow clinical waste bags for incineration
Additional precautions when caring for known HIV and hepatitis B virus-positive and high-risk patients
Consider non-operative management
Remove unnecessary equipment from theatre
Observe highest level of theatre discipline
Have only experienced surgeons and healthcare workers in theatre
Use: double gloves, high efficiency masks, eye protection, boots, impervious gowns, closed wound drainage
Use: disposable anaesthetic circuitry or appropriate method of decontamination
Disinfect theatre floor with hypochlorite (refer to local policies)

seem remote with appropriate infection control procedures, vigilance is constantly required. Infected women should be reminded about care with blood and the disposal of bloodstained material; showers are preferred to baths. Basic precautions have been well reviewed (RCOG 1990, Joint Working Party 1992). Current opinion favours a high level of universal precautions in gynaecological surgery, but with risk assessment and additional precautions for high-risk patients and procedures. Recommendations are shown in Table 57.3. The debate about whether particular precautions should be universal or selective will continue, although it seems clear that some intermediate position will be adopted by most health care workers. What is often not stressed is that the infected woman should not be subjected to any unnecessary and discriminatory infection control procedures which could isolate her or draw attention to her before other patients or relatives.

There are several changes in surgical practice which will help minimize operator risk of trauma. Blunt-tipped needles are an important advance because they are much less likely to puncture skin, but they do usually pass through the tissues involved in gynaecological surgery without difficulty. A needle guard as part of the needle holder is easy to use and likely to be helpful (Smith, personal communication). Increasing use of staples, double-gloving, avoiding passing sharps from hand to hand, totally avoiding resheathing, and better instrument design, will all help minimize risks. Increased awareness is important because HIV is not the only concern. Hepatitis C is a common infection, an important source of morbidity, and is much more readily transmitted than HIV. Other viral infections transmissible through blood can be expected.

Management of accidental exposures

Immediately after a percutaneous or mucous membrane exposure to potentially HIV-infected blood, thorough washing with warm running water and soap and clinical evaluation of the injury should be performed. Any bleeding should be encouraged.

There have been suggestions, based initially on animal experiments, that AZT may reduce the risk of transmission. This remains unproven: infections certainly have occurred despite AZT prophylaxis, further animal experiments have produced conflicting results, and at present the unproven possibility that AZT might prevent transmission thus has to be weighed against the unproven possibility that AZT could have long-term mutagenic or other effects. There are no compelling data to support or discourage the use of AZT in this situation. This thought should be borne in mind and considered electively by health care workers because, if there is a significant exposure, and AZT is to be taken, it should be taken within an hour of the accident in a dosage of 200 mg every 4 hours for 6 weeks.

Such injuries should be reported to the occupational health service, to allow discussion and assessment of recent up-to-date evidence and also to ensure that the individual has a baseline blood sample for storage and follow-up samples at 3 and 12 months. These could be tested for HIV if requested by the health care worker.

The significance of concern about HIV transmission, even though the risks of becoming infected following solid needle-stick injury at surgery are believed to be extremely low, should not be underestimated. This can be a psychologically stressful time, with the health worker making a decision about AZT, enduring months of uncertainty, and during that time taking great care to prevent sexual transmission.

HIV-infected health care workers

There is only one recorded case of probable transmission from practitioner to patient, where a Florida dentist with AIDS seems to have infected five patients. The overall risk of such transfer is thought to be extremely low, but this belief is based on relatively small, incomplete patient follow-up (Bird et al 1991). Gynaecology is also a high-risk specialty, being overrepresented among outbreaks of hepatitis B infection transmitted from health care workers to patients. Despite the lack of evidence of risk, and in view of the seriousness, the Department of Health and the Medical Defence Union are clear that HIV-positive health workers should not take part in invasive procedures. In addition, the General Medical Council recommends that staff who think they have been at risk should be confidentially tested. There have also been calls (resisted by the profession) for mandatory testing of surgeons, as occurs already for hepatitis B. The risks and issues presented by these two viral infections are, of course, different.

KEY POINTS

1. HIV is the leading cause of death in young women in Africa and large urban areas in the USA, but has still to make a substantial impact insome countries.
2. Worldwide, HIV is predominantly a heterosexually transmitted disease, with transmission more likely when viral levels are high, and in the presence of other sexually transmitted disease. Male condom use is highly, though not entirely, protective.
3. Testing for HIV should be accessible to women in gynaecology clinics, where wanted, and after appropriate counselling.
4. Recurrent vaginal candidiasis is the most common initial manifestation of HIV infection, and after treatment there is a shorter time before recurrence.
5. Genital warts are common in HIV-infected women, and may be more extensive and aggressive than is typical in non-immunocompromised patients.
6. There is an excess rise of CIN in HIV-infected women. It is believed that this relates to immune compromise and that recurrence after treatment is more common. There are isolated reports of rapidly progressive invasive cervical carcinoma, but so far no convincing data showing population increases in invasive disease.
7. VIN and AIN are more common and may become of more concern as treatments for advanced HIV disease improve and there is longer survival in an immunocompromised state.
8. Pregnancy does not have a major effect on progression of HIV disease, and nor does HIV have a major effect on pregnancy.
9. In developed countries 14–25% of babies acquire HIV from their mothers, and this probably relates to maternal viral load.
10. There is evidence that transmission can be reduced by maternal and neonatal treatment with AZT, by avoiding breastfeeding, and probably (although this is not yet clear) by elective caesarean section.
11. Investigation and possible treatment of infertility where the woman is HIV infected is contentious. Some consider this to be contraindicated on legal and ethical grounds.
12. Where a couple are discordant for infection, there is no risk of horizontal transmission where artificial insemination by husband with syringe is used. Where the man is infected, preliminary results using processed semen by gradient centrifugate followed by a swim-up procedure are encouraging, but the safety of this has not been established.
13. Infection control procedures must be rigorous. There are several new developments in surgery which should reduce risk of percutaneous exposure for surgeons.
14. Most documented seroconversions in health care staff have followed needlestick injuries with a hollow needle containing infected blood from a patient with CDC Stage 4 disease. The risk from needlestick injury is estimated at 0.38%.

ADDENDUM

This chapter was completed and submitted in December 1994. It therefore reflects the literature base at that time.

Since then there have been very important breakthroughs in understanding the virology and immunopathogenesis of HIV. Combination anti-viral therapy, titrated against viral load measurements, seem to hold great promise. Some of the new issues relating to pregnancy have been reviewed recently (Johnstone 1996).

Recommendations about chemoprophylaxis after occupational exposure have also been made for the US (MMWR 1996; 45: 468–472). In a retrospective case controlled study, zidovudine prophylaxis was associated with a 79% reduction in the risk of seroconversion after percutaneous exposure to HIV-infected blood (MMWR 1995; 44: 929–933). Because of concern about zidovudine-resistant strains, the recommendation (although not based on secure data) is for health care workers to be offered zidovudine (ZDV) 200 mg tid, lamivudine (3TC) 150 mg bd and, where there is very high risk (e.g. deep injury with large diameter hollow bore needle previously in patient's vein or artery, and a source patient with acute retroviral illness or end stage AIDS) to add indinavir (IDV) 800 mg tid. The recommended regime is for 4 weeks, starting within 1–2 hours of exposure. Because of (1) this short time to consider, (2) the uncertainties of the available data and (3) the complicated risk/benefit considerations, it is important for health care workers to read the above publications and organise their thoughts about chemoprophylaxis before any such needle stick incident. It goes without saying that precautions to prevent exposure remain the priority.

REFERENCES

Adachi A, Fleming I, Burk R D, Ho C Y F, Klein R S 1993 Women with human immunodeficiency virus infection and abnormal Papanicolaou smears: a prospective study of colposcopy and clinical outcome. Obstetrics and Gynecology 81: 372–377

Bird A G, Gore S M, Leigh-Brown A J et al 1991 Escape from collective denial: HIV transmission during surgery. British Medical Journal 303: 351–352

Carpenter C C J, Mayer K H, Stein M D, Leibman B D, Fisher A, Fiore T C 1991 Human immunodeficiency virus infection in North American women: experience with 200 cases and a review of the literature. Medicine 70: 307–325

Cockcroft A 1993 Nosocomial infection and infection control procedures. In: Johnson M A and Johnstone F D (Eds), HIV Infection in Women. Churchill Livingstone, Edinburgh, pp 275–286

Connor E M, Sperling R S, Gelber R et al 1994 Reduction of maternal–infant transmission of human immunodeficiency virus type 1 with zidovudine treatment. New England Journal of Medicine 331: 1173–1180

de Vincenzi I, for the European Study Group on Heterosexual Transmission of HIV 1994 A longitudinal study of human immunodeficiency virus transmission by heterosexual partners. New England Journal of Medicine 331: 341–346

Dunn D T, Newell M L, Aden A E, Peckham C S 1992 Risk of human immunodeficiency virus type 1 transmission through breast feeding. Lancet 340: 585–588

Dunn D T, Newell M L, Mayaux M J et al 1994 Mode of delivery and vertical transmission of HIV-1: a review of prospective studies. Journal of AIDS 7(10): 1064–1066

Dussaix E, Guetard D, Dauguet C et al 1993 Spermatozoa as potential carriers of HIV. Research in Virology 144: 487–495

Elias C J, Heise L L 1994 Challenges for the development of female-controlled vaginal microbicides. AIDS 8: 1–9

European Collaborative Study 1992 Risk factors for mother-to-child transmission of HIV-1. Lancet 339: 1007–1012

European Collaborative Study 1994 Caesarian section and risk of vertical transmission of HIV-1 infection. Lancet 343: 1464–1467

Hoegsburg B, Abulafia O, Sedlis A et al 1990 Sexually transmitted diseases and human immunodeficiency virus infection among women with pelvic inflammatory disease. American Journal of Obstetrics and Gynecology 163: 1135–1139

Holman S 1992 HIV counselling for women of reproductive age. Baillière's Clinical Obstetrics and Gynaecology 6: 53–68

Howe J E, Minkoff H L, Duerr A C 1994 Contraceptives and HIV. AIDS 8: 861–871

Iman N, Carpenter C C J, Mayer K et al 1990 Hierarchical pattern of mucosal Candida infections in HIV-seropositive women. American Journal of Medicine 89: 142–146

Johnstone F D, Brettle R P et al 1990 Women's knowledge of their HIV antibody state: its effect on their decision whether to continue the pregnancy. British Medical Journal 300: 23–24

Johnstone F D, McGoogan E, Smart G E, Brettle R P, Prescott R J 1994a A population-based, controlled study of the relation between HIV infection and cervical neoplasia. British Journal of Obstetrics and Gynaecology 101: 986–991

Johnstone F D, Williams A R W, Bird A G, Bjornsson S 1994b Immunohistochemical characterisation of endometrial lymphoid cell populations in women infected with HIV. Obstetrics and Gynecology 83: 586–593

Johnstone F D 1996 HIV and pregnancy. British Journal of Obstetrics and Gynaecology (in press)

Joint Working Party of the Hospital Infection Society and the Surgical Infection Study Group 1992 Risks to surgeons and patients from HIV and hepatitis: guidelines on precautions and management of exposure to blood or body fluids. British Medical Journal 305: 1337–1343

Korn A P, Landers D V, Green J R, Sweet R L 1993 Pelvic inflammatory disease in human immunodeficiency virus-infected women. Obstetrics and Gynecology 82: 765–768

La Guardia K D 1993 Other sexually transmitted disease: cervical intraepithelial neoplasia. In: Johnson M A, Johnstone F D (eds) HIV infection in women. Churchill Livingstone, Edinburgh, pp 247–261

Maiman M, Tarricone N, Viera J et al 1991 Colposcopic evaluation of human immunodeficiency virus-seropositive women. Obstetrics and Gynecology 78: 84–88

Mercey D, Bewley S, Brocklehurst P 1993 A guide to symptoms and treatments for women living with HIV and AIDS: a guide to HIV infection and childbearing. AVERT, Horsham (obtainable from AVERT, 11 Denne Parade, Horsham, West Sussex RH12 1JD)

NAM 1994 Directory of complementary and alternative therapies in HIV/AIDS. London (obtainable from NAM, 52 Gurling Centre, 49 Effra Road, London SW2 1BZ)

Palevsky J M 1994 Anal human papillomavirus infection and anal cancer in HIV-positive individuals: an emergency problem. AIDS 8: 283–295

Positively Women/Terence Higgins Trust December 1994 Positive women. A guide to symptoms and treatments for women living with HIV and AIDS (obtainable from the Terence Higgins Trust, 52–54 Grays Inn Road, London WC1X 8JU)

Royal College of Obstetricians and Gynaecologists 1990 HIV infection in maternity care and gynaecology. Royal College of Obstetricians and Gynaecologists, London

Ryder R W, Batter V L, Nsuami M et al 1991 Fertility rates in 238 HIV-1 seropositive women in Zaire followed for 3 years post partum. AIDS 5: 1521–1527

Schafer A, Friedmann W, Meikle M, Schwartlander B, Koch M A 1991 The increased frequency of cervical dysplasia–neoplasia in women infected with the human immunodeficiency virus is related to the degree of immunosuppression. American Journal of Obstetrics and Gynecology 164: 593–599

Selwyn P A, Antoniello P 1993 Reproductive decision-making among women with HIV infection. In: Johnstone F D, Johnson M (eds) HIV and women. Churchill Livingstone, Edinburgh

Selwyn P A, Carter R J, Schoenbaum E E, Robertson V J, Klein R S, Rogers M F 1989 Knowledge of HIV antibody status and decisions to continue or terminate pregnancy among intravenous drug users. JAMA 261: 3567–3571

Semprini A E, Leui-Setti P, Bozzo M et al 1992 Insemination of HIV-negative women with processed semen of HIV-positive partners. Lancet 340: 1317–1319

Shah P N, Smith J R, Wells C et al 1994 Menstrual symptoms in women infected by the human immunodeficiency virus. Obstetrics and Gynecology 83: 397–400

Sher L 1993 Counselling around HIV testing in women of reproductive age. In: Johnson M A, Johnstone F D (eds) HIV and women. Churchill Livingstone, Edinburgh

Smith J R, Kitchen V S, Botcherby M et al 1993 Is HIV infection associated with an increase in the prevalence of cervical neoplasia? British Journal of Obstetrics and Gynaecology 100: 316–318

Smith J R, Forster G E, Kitchen V S et al 1991 Infertility management in HIV seropositive couples: a dilemma. British Medical Journal 302: 1447–1450

Spinollo A, Michelone G, Cavanna C, Colonna L, Cadyzzi E, Bucika S 1994 Clinical and microbiological characterisation of symptomatic vulvovaginal candidiasis in HIV-seropositive women. Genitourinary Medicine 70: 268–272

SECTION 6

Legal and general

58

Medicolegal aspects

E. M. Symonds

Indemnity cover for doctors in the UK has been provided by the medical defence organizations for more than 100 years. Since 1990 the broad mass of litigation within the health service has been covered by the local Health Authorities and Trusts. These organizations are not insurance companies and originally arose, as stated in the original memorandum of the Medical Defence Union, out of the need:

1. To support and protect the character and interests of medical practitioners practising in the UK.
2. To promote honourable practice and to suppress or prosecute unauthorized practitioners.
3. To advise and defend or assist in defending members of the Union in cases where proceedings involving questions of professional principle or otherwise are brought against them.

Clifford Hawkins (1985), in his history of the medical defence organizations, refers to the original trigger for the formation of these societies as the case of Dr David Bradley, who in 1884 was found guilty of attempted criminal assault against a woman patient who alleged that Bradley had raped her. A letter from Lawson Tait to the *British Medical Journal* drew attention to the unsatisfactory nature of this judgment. The case was re-examined and the Home Secretary eventually granted a free pardon. It was the lack of proper expert evidence that had resulted in the initial conviction. It was apparent that some proper organization was necessary to defend the interests of doctors and dentists in resisting this type of claim.

THE MEDICAL DEFENCE ORGANIZATIONS

The Medical Defence Union

This was the first of the defence organizations, founded in 1887 with Lawson Tait as the first President. He was a man of great presence and a distinguished surgeon and gynaecologist. In 1893 he resigned as President because of his difficult personality and because of internal difficulties, and the Medical Defence Union moved its office from Birmingham to London.

The Medical Protection Society

The new constitution of the Medical Defence Union introduced by Lawson Tait led to internal dissent on the Council of the MDU, as it proposed to concentrate too much power in too few hands running the organization. Dr Hugh Woods led a dissenting group and, in conjunction with a group of dissatisfied members, he formed the London and Counties Medical Protection Society Ltd (1892). The title was subsequently changed after the Second World War to the Medical Protection Society.

The Medical and Dental Defence Union of Scotland

The Medical and Dental Defence Union of Scotland was formed in 1902 specifically to serve graduates from Scottish schools and doctors working in Scottish hospitals.

Despite the establishment of three different organizations, the essential purpose of the societies has remained constant to the original functions described by the constitution of the Medical Defence Union.

THE MEDICAL DEFENCE ORGANIZATIONS AND INSURANCE COMPANIES

In 1974, the Insurance Companies Act defined a system of requirements and powers for the Secretary of State to regulate the affairs of insurance companies. In many countries doctors are covered by insurance companies, and whereas the medical defence organizations are mutual, non-profit-making defence associations which provide effectively unlimited cover for any person in membership at the time of a specific event, whenever the claim is initiated, insurance companies can load premiums, refuse membership because of multiple claims, settle claims out of court if there is a pecuniary advantage, and require additional insurance to cover retired members and their estates.

This was far removed from the generous cover and support given by the defence organizations. Scrutiny of events over the last 8 years shows that the medical defence organizations are indeed being forced into pathways that are rapidly becoming indistinguishable from the activities of ordinary insurance companies.

THE MEDICOLEGAL FRAMEWORK IN THE UK

Under English law, professional negligence and liability are covered under the laws of civil tort. Until recently, actions against a doctor for negligence could also be based on breach of contract, but the judiciary have in recent years largely removed this option. Thus, in English law all legal issues for the recovery of damages in medical practice fall within the law of negligence. What exactly constitutes negligence is difficult to define. The most widely accepted definition, and the one most commonly applied in the courts, arises from the direction given by Mr Justice McNair in 1957 in the case of *Bolam v. Friern Hospital Management Committee*, and this reads as follows:

> In the ordinary case which does not involve any special skill, negligence in law means this: some failure to do some act which a reasonable man in the circumstances would do, or doing some act which a reasonable man in the circumstances would not do: and if that failure or doing of that act results in injury, then there is a cause of action.
>
> How do you test whether this act or failure is negligent?
>
> In an ordinary case it is generally said that you judge that by the action of the man in the street. He is the ordinary man. In one case it has been said that you judge it by the conduct of the man on the top of a Clapham omnibus. He is the ordinary man. But where you get a situation which involves the use of some special skill or competence, then the test whether there has been negligence or not is not the test of the man on the top of a Clapham omnibus, because he has not got this special skill. The test is the standard of the ordinary skilled man exercising and professing to have that special skill.
>
> A man need not possess the highest expert skill to be at risk of being found negligent. It is well established law that it is sufficient if he exercises the ordinary skill of an ordinary competent man exercising that particular art.

As Butcher (1990) has pointed out, this judgment failed to take account of the status of the doctor involved. The matter was eventually addressed by the Court of Appeal in the case of *Wilsher v. Essex Health Authority*, when it was decided that:

> it must be recognised that different facts make different demands. If it is borne in mind that the structure of hospital medicine envisages that the lower ranks will be occupied by those of whom it would be wrong to expect too much, the risk of abuse by litigious patients can be mitigated.

Nevertheless, the level of skill to be expected of a doctor in training as a specialist is still a grey area, and the desire for courts to compensate plaintiffs has led to unrealistic expectations of clinical skills.

There are also serious difficulties in deciding where complications of particular procedures are acceptable and where the complications are considered to arise from unsatisfactory skills.

The procedure of a claim

Anyone may commence proceedings against any other person and there is no real way by which this process can be screened. The initial claim made by the plaintiff leads to the issuing of a writ of summons from the court, and this must contain a summary of the nature of the claim. It does not have to be precise. The action is usually initiated at the solicitor's request for the production of case notes as an indication of threatened legal action.

The service of a claim has to be personal, but in the past the service has generally been accepted by the doctor's defence organization. It is not clear who will accept service in the future, as this has not been stated by the Department of Health, but one assumes it will be accepted by the health authorities' and Trust hospitals' solicitors. After the service of a statement of claim, the defendant has to serve a defence. Under the Scottish system considerable detail must be supplied and both sides are then entitled to ask for further and better particulars of the statement of claim.

Before the case comes to court, there is a process of discovery of documents which have not already been revealed, the exchange of expert report, and sometimes a meeting of experts to define the areas of agreement and disagreement. The action is then set down for trial and a date is fixed.

Legal aid

The availability of legal aid is determined by the disposable income of the applicant. The opinion of one expert adviser is then sought, as well as counsel's opinion on the likelihood of the claim being successful. If this opinion is favourable, then the certificate is extended to summons for directness, and if the advisers still advise that the claim should succeed then the certificate is extended to trial.

The statute of limitations

In the case of obstetricians, the course of legislation in this field has been entirely adverse.

Claims alleging brain damage can be commenced up to 21 years after birth, and longer if there is mental incapacity.

This effectively makes defence of any case impossible because the case notes will often not be available or will be indecipherable, and the medical and midwifery staff involved will almost certainly have no recollection of the nature of the events involved in the management of the case.

Actions for negligence causing injury have to be commenced within 3 years of the event, but this period can be extended if it can be shown that there was no knowledge within the 3-year period that the injury was significant, or if the plaintiff is under the age of 18 years.

MEDICAL LITIGATION IN THE USA

The system of litigation in the USA is adversarial and cases are heard in front of a judge and jury. In the UK, cases are heard in front of a judge but no jury, and since 1988 this also applies in Eire.

The decision made by both judge and jury is, therefore, highly dependent on the presentation of the case and the experts on either side. It has to be said that this principle also applies in the UK, although not to the same degree.

Contingency fees are a feature of the American system: this means that the lawyers take up to 40% of the award if the case is won by the plaintiff, but do not charge if the case is lost.

Although it is generally believed that this process entirely favours the plaintiff, this is probably not true. Unless the courts are strongly biased against the medical profession, there is a real risk that the lawyers may lose heavily if a frivolous claim is taken to court. Experienced lawyers, therefore, tend to avoid situations where they are unlikely to have a successful case. Moves towards a similar process in the UK have so far largely been resisted, but it is uncertain whether in the British courts such changes would favour the plaintiff or the defendant.

The cost of settlements in the USA has been substantially enhanced by the fact that these matters are determined by the juries, and that there appears to be no limit to the sums awarded for pain, suffering and loss of amenity. This has so far been restricted in the UK because the awards are determined by judges within proscribed agreements. Many of the American states now have a cap on damages in order to limit professional liability. In two states, West Virginia and Florida, a system of no-fault compensation has been introduced for claims concerning birth-related injuries, as a result of the virtual breakdown of the obstetric services.

It seems likely that at some stage the whole structure of civil tort and professional indemnity will have to be changed towards a genuine insurance system, with costs being met by a consortium of insurers involving the state legislature, doctors and hospital insurers.

The cost of litigation simply diverts revenue away from patients suffering disabilities related to their illnesses, and greatly increases the cost of overall medical care.

NO-FAULT COMPENSATION

New Zealand

The first system of no-fault compensation was introduced in New Zealand in 1974 (Blain 1983). It has much broader connotations than medical malpractice and was specifically designed to avoid the inefficiencies of the common law system which, in subjects which always carry an element of uncertainty on causality, carries some of the features of a lottery. Does the woman who bears a child with cerebral palsy need any less support if the condition is congenital than if the child's injury is apparently birth-related? In the case of *Whitehouse v. Jordan*, Lord Justice Lawton stated in 1981: 'The victim of medical mishaps of the present kind should be cared for by the community, not by the hazards of litigation'.

The New Zealand system has taken account of these problems and has now been functioning for 16 years. The scheme is administered by the Accident Compensation Corporation Scheme and part of the funds are provided from general taxation and part from employers' contributions and a levy on the self-employed.

Payments are based on loss of earnings, reasonable medical expenses and other out-of-pocket expenses. There is no contribution for pain and suffering. If the Commission rejects the claim the plaintiff may bring action in court for negligence, but if compensation is accepted the right to go to court is lost.

The Swedish patient insurance scheme

Sweden introduced a patient insurance scheme in 1975 (Oldertz 1984). Decisions are made on objective facts and on the nature of the injury and the disabilities resulting from it. The circumstances leading to the injury are considered to be of little importance, although disciplinary actions can be invoked by other mechanisms where this is considered to be appropriate. Decisions are made by a consortium of Swedish insurers, and if the patient wishes to appeal against the level of compensation he or she can apply to a consulting claims panel.

The main concern with patient insurance systems is the relatively low level of compensation and the cost to the community generally. However, overall, with the removal of legal costs, there seems little doubt that this is a much more efficient method of compensation and ensures that medical practice and new developments are not distorted by the legal process.

TYPES OF GYNAECOLOGICAL CASES IN LITIGATION

General surgical problems

Litigation arises from the general problems that beset all surgical procedures. There is no defence to leaving swabs, packs or instruments in the abdominal cavity or the vagina, and these matters almost invariably attract an out-of-court settlement. Fortunately, gynaecological procedures are rarely subject to the problem of performing the wrong operation. However, occasionally a patient is sterilized when her name is put on the operating list for diagnostic laparoscopy one ahead of or one behind a patient put on the operating list for sterilization.

These are all matters that can be avoided by good practice, and the responsibility lies with the theatre staff and the surgeon to ensure that swab and instrument counts are correct at the end of the operation and that the lists are correct, with the patient receiving the correct operation. One common source of litigation results from the retention of swabs after repair of an episiotomy. In this situation swab counts are often forgotten, and the obstetrician usually relies on directly checking the vaginal cavity at the end of the procedure.

Complications of sterilization

Failed sterilization

Most claims in relation to sterilization relate to failure of the procedure. Until the 1980s it was uncommon to advise patients of the risk of failure of sterilization. Indeed, even today the only reasons for telling the patient of this possibility are medicolegal and to make the patient aware of the possibility of failure, so that early termination of pregnancy can be sought should this happen. In the Particulars of Negligence, it is often alleged that had the patient been informed of the risk of failure she would not have been sterilized, or would have persuaded her partner to have a vasectomy, or would have continued to use contraception. In practice, since gynaecologists began to advise patients of the risk of failure, there is no evidence that women in any way change their intention to be sterilized.

In the case of *Gold v. Haringey Health Authority* (1987) these issues were thoroughly rehearsed and it was agreed after resort to the Court of Appeal that a significant body of gynaecologists did not warn of the risk of failure in 1979 (Brahams 1987). In his original judgment, Mr Justice Schiemann held that there was a duty to counsel the patient about alternative methods of family planning, including vasectomy. As a result of these cases, it is generally agreed that a statement should be included in the consent form to the effect that 'there is a possibility that I may not become or remain sterile'. In fact, it is difficult to sustain an argument that signing a form that acknowledges that the failure to render a patient sterile in the first instance has any value in protecting the surgeon from accusations of negligence.

Claims have also been made in relation to the failure to warn the patient of the risk of ectopic pregnancy.

The other source of claims rests with the accusation that the procedure was faulty. It is now generally recognized and acknowledged by the courts that all tubal occlusive techniques may fail because of recanalization of the tube, but this rarely occurs less than 1 year after the procedure has been performed. Early failure usually indicates that the technique was faulty. In the case of clip sterilization, this means that either one or both clips were applied to the wrong structure, or that the clip fell off or extruded the tube.

Different forms of sterilization tend to have different failure rates, but provided the technique is generally acceptable to practising consultants, its use can be defended. In the case of *Gold v. Haringey Health Authority*, it was alleged that placement of clips across the proximal part of the ampulla instead of the isthmus was negligent, even though there was evidence that the clip completely enclosed the tube. This allegation was not successful. It is particularly helpful to the courts if the tubes are photographed in cases of failed sterilization if a second procedure is undertaken.

Implantation before sterilization

In some cases actions have been brought for failure of sterilizations performed in the second half of the menstrual cycle, where implantation has already occurred even though the period has not been missed. Such allegations can usually be defended provided that the period is not actually overdue. In this case, modern pregnancy tests can detect the presence of human chorionic gonadotrophin within 7 days of the last menstrual period, and if serum human chorionic gonadotrophin measurements are available this may indicate a pregnancy before the last period is missed. An alternative scenario is to perform a diagnostic curettage in all patients sterilized in the second half of the menstrual cycle, but this theoretically raises the risk of performing an illegal termination of pregnancy.

Hazards of laparoscopy

The risks of laparoscopy are well established and have been known since the Royal College of Obstetricians and Gynaecologists report on laparoscopy in 1978 (Chamberlain & Carron-Brown 1978). In general terms, problems such as bowel perforation, damage to vessels and difficulties with insufflation can be defended provided that the surgeon is known to have adequate experience or to be properly supervised if inexperienced. Claims commonly arise from the failure to recognize damage to the gut, with consequent delayed recognition of the development of peritonitis. The use of unipolar diathermy within the peritoneal cavity also leads to delayed perforation of the bowel and claims of negligence. With the extensive use of clips or other occlusive devices instead of diathermy, these claims are now becoming very rare.

Minimally invasive surgery and transcervical endometrial resection

Since the introduction of Crown Indemnity there have been no national UK statistics on claims for minimally invasive surgery, yet it is apparent that numerous serious complications have arisen as a result of inadequate training in these new procedures. From 1990 to 1994, the Medical Defence Union has been notified of 87 claims concerning laparoscopic procedures, 12 of which are being related to laparoscopically assisted surgery (C. James, Medical Defence Union, personal communication). The remaining cases related to laparoscopic sterilization procedures and, clearly, these still represent the bulk of laparoscopic procedures. Of the 12 cases resulting from laparoscopic surgery, one related to an allegation of non-consent, one to an incorrect diagnosis, one was a result of haemorrhage during laparoscopic hysterectomy, three related to fistula formation after laparoscopic hysterectomy, and there was one case of pelvic and vaginal abscesses following laparoscopic hysterectomy. The other cases were related to various haemorrhagic complications.

Over the same period there were 10 claims relating to endometrial resection. There was a 1:7 ratio in claims compared to other forms of hysterectomy. This seems to indicate a higher than expected number of claims for endometrial resection, although there are no actual figures available for the total number of these procedures performed in the population covered by the Medical Defence Union over this period of time. Of the 10 endometrial resections, nine cases related to uterine perforations, three of which also involved bowel damage. Two of the patients died, one from septicaemia and one from a coagulopathy associated with the glycine infusion.

These reports give no indication of the overall complication rate following these procedures, but they do emphasize the potential hazards associated with minimally invasive surgery.

Green and Keddie (1995) reviewed the number of claims reported to the Medical Defence Union concerning laparoscopic cholecystectomy and reported an increasing number of claims associated with bile duct injuries. They emphasized the need for structured training programmes and the need to proceed with caution in adopting new procedures. The issues raised in this report are entirely relevant to the problems arising from minimally invasive surgery in gynaecology.

Termination of pregnancy

In view of the number of terminations that are performed, it is not surprising that the defence organizations have received a large number of claims involving termination of pregnancy. Claims may arise from interpretation of the 1967 Abortion Act or from complications in performing the abortion. In fact, the vast majority of claims are related to the abortion procedure. These difficulties were reviewed by Symonds (1985) in the Royal College of Obstetricians and Gynaecologists' working party on litigation.

'Failed termination'

Continuation of a pregnancy after attempted termination is a common source of litigation. The problem usually arises in early terminations, where the gestation sac is missed by the suction curette, but sometimes occurs with later pregnancies. It is usually possible to recognize products of conception in the suction curette or in the suction flask, but sometimes these can be obscured by blood and decidual material. A common defence offered in these cases is that the uterus was bicornuate, and that a fetus was removed from one horn but left intact on the other side. This defence is unlikely to succeed unless there is proven evidence that the woman does have a double uterus. It is often alleged by solicitors for plaintiffs that the products of conception should have been submitted for histological confirmation, but this is not standard procedure in the UK and most laboratories would not welcome such a policy.

The only way that the consequences of mishaps of this type can be avoided is to ensure that all women have a 6-week follow-up visit to the consultant clinic or to the general practitioner, so that there will be a chance to recognize an ongoing pregnancy.

Incomplete evacuations

Incomplete evacuations are common and sometimes lead to claims, particularly where they cause severe secondary complications from haemorrhage or infection. However, provided the proper steps are taken to complete the evacuation of the uterus, these claims can generally be resisted as the retention of placental tissue or fetal parts is not evidence of negligent management.

Damage to viscera

Perforation of the uterus often occurs during evacuation, either during the performance of a therapeutic termination or following a spontaneous abortion. Injuries may affect the cervix or the body of the uterus. Excessive dilatation of the cervix may result in damage and may be difficult to defend, but the commonest injuries result from perforation of the uterine fundus by the dilators or polyp forceps, or by the curette. It is possible to defend claims based on these accidents provided that the problem is recognized and that the appropriate action is taken.

However, extensive damage to the uterus and bowel as a result of these procedures may be difficult to defend if it is considered that the surgeon's performance was substandard.

Oral contraception

Claims related to oral contraception are not particularly common, and this is perhaps surprising in view of their widespread usage. However, patients should be advised of the diminished efficacy of the pill if they are taking anticonvulsants, some antibiotics and tranquillizers and anti-inflammatory compounds. Furthermore, with the modern low-dose pills missing a pill may result in ovulation and pregnancy.

Good advice can identify these problems and ensure that the doctor is not blamed if failure occurs. It is, perhaps, a reflection on the fact that information about the pill has been widely disseminated that there is a relatively low rate of claims in this field.

Intrauterine devices

Contraception with intrauterine devices enjoyed a time of popularity which is now in decline. Product liability is slowly removing intrauterine devices from the market, despite the fact that for those women whom they suit they are a particularly useful form of contraception. Claims commonly arise from perforation of the uterus, either at the time of insertion or at a later date. If the loop strings cannot be seen in the vagina then it is essential to ascertain the whereabouts of the device and to make a decision about its removal. Some claims have arisen concerning long-term problems with pelvic infections and subfertility.

It is important that care is taken to keep the patient properly informed of potential complications. Correct procedure in inserting a device is also important if a defence is to be sustained against allegations arising from uterine perforation.

Complications arising from hysterectomy

Damage to adjacent viscera

The proximity of bladder and bowel to the uterus means that damage to the bladder, ureters and bowel is a recognized hazard of either vaginal or abdominal hysterectomy.

Urinary fistulae are commonly the basis for medicolegal claims. Despite the fact that vesicovaginal and ureterovaginal fistulae are a recognized complication, can it be assumed that they can always be defended? If one ureter is damaged during a difficult hysterectomy where there is extensive pelvic disease, then it should be possible to defend this action as being the sort of complication that any competent gynaecological surgeon can have and almost invariably has met in a professional lifetime. However, if both ureters are ligated during the performance of a routine hysterectomy, it is unlikely that any expert would want to defend such a case in court. The same considerations apply to damage of the bladder or bowel.

Procedures undertaken for urinary incontinence may also result in bladder damage. This may be an acceptable complication, depending on the nature of the disease and the skill of the surgeon.

Cervical cytology and carcinoma of the cervix

Various claims have arisen in recent years where abnormal cervical smears have been filed without any decision or action being taken until an invasive carcinoma has developed, or where the interpretation of the smear has itself been faulty.

The latter event is relatively uncommon, whereas the failure to act on abnormal cytology occurs relatively frequently, usually as a result of reports being filed in case notes without receiving proper attention. It is therefore essential that a good chain of command is established to make certain that all abnormal smear tests are drawn to the attention of the general practitioner or gynaecologist, so that appropriate action can be taken.

These items form the common basis of claims in gynaecology. There are many other less common sources of litigation which have not been listed.

VALUATION OF A CLAIM – THE QUANTUM

Trials are commonly held to decide on both liability and quantum, but sometimes these events may be split. In forming a judgment about quantum, the judge may take account of the following factors:

1. Pain, suffering and loss of amenity: these factors are difficult to quantify and in the USA this has resulted in unrealistic damages being set by juries. However, damages in British courts tend to be agreed at reasonably fixed levels.

2. Medical and nursing care costs, including those incurred by the relatives in looking after the plaintiff.
3. Future costs of accommodation.
4. Loss of earnings because of incapacity.

The cost of settlements for long-term disabilities is therefore very high, depending on the extent of the disability and life expectancy. This particularly applies to birth-related injuries.

CROWN INDEMNITY

The 1980s witnessed a massive escalation in malpractice litigation. This is reflected in the subscriptions paid and the income of the Medical Defence Union over the last decade (Fig. 58.1). By 1989 it was becoming apparent that the costs could not be contained within the salary structure of full-time consultants and staff in training. This problem was brought to crisis point by the proposal to introduce differential rates for high-risk specialties. Effectively, this meant that doctors working in high-risk disciplines such as obstetrics, orthopaedics, anaesthesia and neurosurgery would be unable to pay the subscription rates, and that these disciplines would become untenable within a relatively short time span. The government therefore introduced Crown Indemnity. Liability for patients treated within the National Health Service will be met by the Department of Health.

Examination of the costs for settlement, and for legal services and disbursements, shows the problem that health authorities have assumed by taking over these responsibilities (Fig. 58.2). This takes no account of the time and effort that will need to be made for defendants and expert witnesses under the civil tort system in the future. In other words, Crown Indemnity provides a short-term solution for the malpractice crisis, but it will eventually distort patient services and medical recruitment in specific high-risk disciplines. In obstetrics, it must be remembered that the processes of litigation apply to anyone attending upon the labour of any mother.

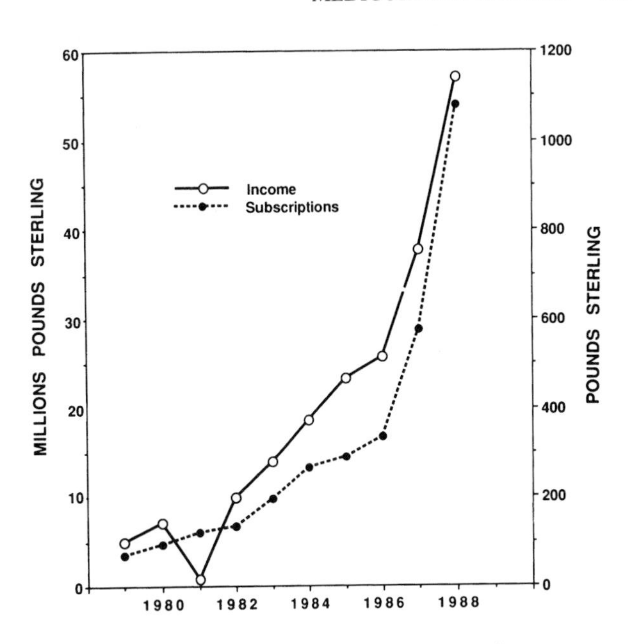

Fig. 58.1 The cost of members' subscriptions and subscription income 1979–1988, derived from Medical Defence Union annual reports.

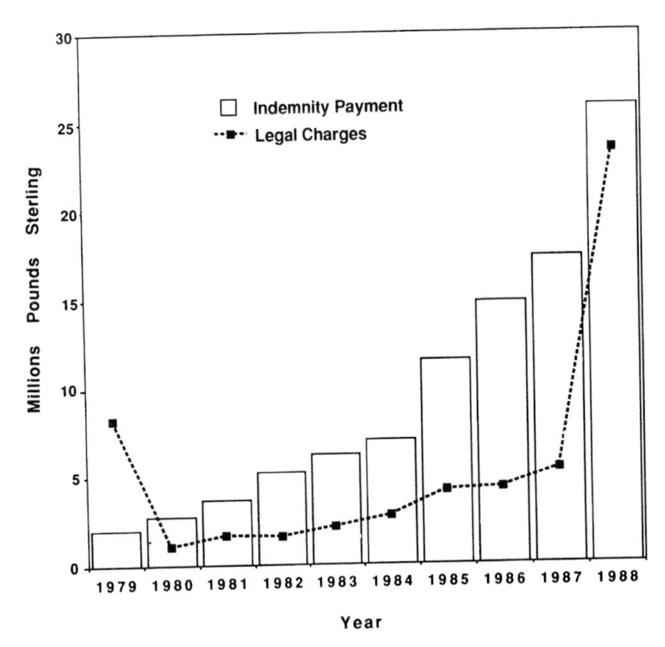

Fig. 58.2 Indemnity payments and legal charges and disbursements 1979–1988, derived from Medical Defence Union annual reports.

RISK MANAGEMENT

The continuing escalation of claims in litigation for medical accidents makes some type of medical risk management essential. Senior and Symonds (1995) have described a prototype proactive risk management system which has been implemented at the Queen's Medical Centre in Nottingham. The group, which is chaired by a lawyer, includes the clinical director of obstetrics and gynaecology, a senior registrar, a representative of the midwifery and gynaecological nursing staff, a consultant paediatrician, a consultant anaesthetist, the hospital litigationofficer and a risk management coordinator. The group meets on a monthly basis to discuss case management based on a list of complications likely to carry a high risk of litigation. The cases are initially notified to a management coordinator, who records details of the incident, where possible within 48 hours. The coordinator also traces the medical records and ensures that they are dated and signed correctly. Medical and nursing staff are never asked to appear before the group and, where some action is indicated, this is initiated by the clinical director. An assessment is made as to liability and quantum where relevant, and assurance is obtained that the patient and relatives are given a full explanation of the problem. This system is proving to be valuable both in identifying unsatisfactory practice and in supporting staff and patients in dealing with complications of operative procedures.

It is time-consuming and requires financial investment, but these factors need to be weighed against the money saved in dealing with potentially litigious problems and by avoiding the development of similar future complications.

KEY POINTS

1. Negligence is judged by the standard of the ordinary skilled doctor exercising that special skill, and should take into account the level of training of the doctor.
2. For brain damage at birth, the statute of limitations extends up to 21 years after delivery. Other actions for negligence have to be commenced within 3 years of the event causing injury.
3. Surgical litigation can be minimized by good theatre practice.
4. It is the obstetrician's responsibility to check the vagina after repair of episiotomy, to ensure that no swabs are left behind.
5. It is important to counsel every patient undergoing sterilization about the risks of failure and ectopic pregnancy.
6. A follow-up visit after termination of pregnancy will enable an ongoing pregnancy to be detected.
7. It is important to inform the patient about likely complications, risks and success rates of any procedure.
8. With an abnormal cervical smear it is prudent to ensure that the general practitioner is also informed of the results.

REFERENCES

Blain A P 1983 Accident compensation in New Zealand, 2nd edn. Butterworth, Wellington, New Zealand

Bolam v. Friern Hospital Management Committee. All England Law Report 1957, pp 118, 121

Brahams D 1987 Pregnancy following sterilisation: two cases fail. Lancet i: 638

Butcher C 1990 In: Chamberlain G, Orr C (eds) How to avoid problems in obstetrics and gynaecology. Members of the Joint Medicolegal Committee of the Royal College of Obstetricians and Gynaecologists and the Medical Defence Organisations. Royal College of Obstetricians and Gynaecologists, London

Chamberlain G, Carron-Brown J 1978 In: Gynaecological laparoscopy. Royal College of Obstetricians and Gynaecologists, London

Chamberlain G, Orr C 1990 How to avoid medico-legal problems in obstetrics and gynaecology. Royal College of Obstetricians and Gynaecologists, London

Green S, Keddie N 1995 Bile duct injury in patients undergoing laparoscopic cholecystectomy: a review. Journal of the Medical Defence Union II(1): 10

Hawkins C 1985 Mishap or malpractice. Blackwell Scientific Publications, Oxford, pp 1–2

Lawton Lord Justice In *Whitehouse v. Jordan.* All England Law Reports 1 1981: 267

Oldertz C 1984 The Swedish patient insurance system – 8 years of experience. Medico-legal Journal 52: 43–59

Senior O E, Symonds E M Medical risk management, a prototype. Current Obstetrics and Gynaecology 5(2): (In press)

Symonds E M 1985 Medico-legal aspects of therapeutic abortion. In: Chamberlain G W P, Orr C J B, Sharp F (eds) Litigation and obstetrics and gynaecology, Proceedings of the 14th study group of the RCOG. Royal College of Obstetricians and Gynaecologists, London, pp 123–129

Wilsher v. Essex Health Authority. Weekly Law Reports 1987, p 466

59

The gynaecologist as defendant and expert witness

Roger V. Clements Margaret Puxon

THE LEGAL FRAMEWORK

Criminal and civil liability

Gynaecologists, like any other citizens, may find themselves in legal conflict with the law, either criminal or civil, but gynaecologists run particular risks in both these areas. In the criminal field they are at risk under the abortion legislation; although prosecutions are rare since the liberalization of the law by the Abortion Act 1967 there are still traps for the unwary, as when a patient is found to be pregnant during a laparotomy and the pregnancy is terminated without the necessary documentary support.

The recent cases where doctors have been prosecuted for manslaughter underline a particular risk to those who undertake surgery beyond their skill, and the legislation against female circumcision puts the doctor in a strange position when he comes to effect a perineal repair on a patient who has suffered such a mutilation.

In the area of civil law doctors may become embroiled with their patients when anything goes wrong with the professional relationship.

Two main types of action may arise: breach of contract and negligence, which is a breach of duty. Less common are actions against doctors for assault and battery: any invasion of a patient's body without consent, or even a threat of such an act, is an assault at common law; where there is actual invasion, it is also battery. In any such case there will also be negligence, but whereas assault and battery are criminal offences as well as civil torts, negligence is purely civil. There may be technical advantages in bringing a case in assault rather than negligence; such cases are almost entirely limited to operations carried out without the patient's consent, for example, where the surgeon removes the uterus or ovaries from a woman without her consent.

Breach of contract

Whenever a practitioner agrees to advise or treat a patient, it is an implied term of that agreement that he will 'bring a fair, reasonable and competent degree of skill' to the care of that patient:

> An attorney does not undertake that at all events you shall gain your case, neither does a surgeon undertake that he will perform a cure; nor does he undertake to use the highest possible degree of skill (Tindal 1838).

But if the surgeon fails to comply with the standards of

that profession he will be in breach of the contract and liable for the return of any fees that may have been paid and damages for any resultant loss or suffering to the patient. The surgeon will also be liable to compensate the patient for any such loss (such as loss of earnings) or expenses incurred, including the cost of further treatment.

Negligence

In practice, most actions against doctors are brought in negligence, which is a tort – a wrongful act at common law, for which the law provides a remedy. The test of fault, however, is the same whether the alleged breach is of the contract or of the duty all professional people have to their clients.

It is not always appreciated that the doctor is in the same position before the law as any other professional person who offers skills, whether they be lawyer, accountant, surveyor or architect. The level of skill required is that which other members of that particular profession regarded as fair and reasonable at the time of the alleged act of negligence. Thus the standard imposed is that of one's peers, not of the public, nor of the judge, although it will be the judge's decision, after hearing all the evidence, to decide what was in fact the accepted standard of care at the time.

This has been the position for at least 30 years, and it was finally given the accolade of the House of Lords in the case of *Whitehouse v. Jordan* (1980), when Lord Edmond-Davies said this:

> Doctors and surgeons fall into no special category and . . . I would have it accepted that the true doctrine was enunciated by *McNair J in Bolam v. Friern Hospital Management Committee* (1957) in the following words: . . . where you get a situation which involves the use of some special skill or competence, then the test as to whether there has been negligence or not is not the test of the man on the top of a Clapham omnibus (a well known figure in law) because he has not got this special skill. The test is the standard of the ordinary skilled man exercising and professing to have that special skill.
>
> If a surgeon fails to measure up to that standard in *any* respect ('clinical judgement' or otherwise), he has been negligent and should be so adjudged.

Such, then, is the test for *all* professional people and, short of legislation, that ruling of the House of Lords will remain the touchstone of medical liability at every level, from the most eminent down to the newly qualified. It must be emphasized that in deciding whether a doctor has been negligent, the law is not concerned with general ethics but only with the interest of the patient within the bounds already defined.

That does not necessarily mean that the same standards will apply to the consultant gynaecologist as to the junior house officer, but if a service is offered then the practitioner who carries out that service will be judged by the standards expected by the profession for that particular service; if there is no one adequately trained to do the job properly, it will not be a defence for the provider unit or even the doctor concerned if something goes wrong because of the doctor's inexperience. The provision of adequate skilled staff is a problem for Parliament rather than for the law (*Wilsher v. Essex Area Health Authority* (1987)): if no one properly trained is available, the operation should not be carried out.

Burden of proof and causation

To succeed with an action, the plaintiff must prove on the balance of probabilities that the defendant was negligent. The defendant does not have to prove that he was *not* negligent.

Even if negligence is proved, there can be no finding of liability against the doctor unless the plaintiff can also prove, again on the balance of probabilities, that the injuries and loss complained of were directly caused by that particular negligence. The plaintiff in a medical negligent claim thus has a difficult task. It is right that this should be so, but it is also right that when there is negligence, the patient should be properly compensated.

Expert witness

In deciding whether the defendant has been negligent the judge will have to hear expert evidence called by both the plaintiff and the defendant. If the experts on both sides differ in their views of what was the proper course of action for the defendant to take in the particular circumstances, as frequently happens when a case comes to court, this will usually indicate that there is a competent body of medical opinion holding the contrary view to that put forward by the plaintiff in her allegation that the defendant fell below the appropriate standards. It may be that the experts on the two sides will come together during the process of questioning and cross-examination during the trial; if not, the judge can accept or reject the medical evidence on one side or the other, assessing the credibility of the witnesses. But the judge must not choose between the two views put forward simply because he prefers the opinion of one expert to the other (see the House of Lords' ruling in *Maynard v. West Midlands Regional Health Authority* 1985).

Would it not be better if the experts on both sides could come together without a time-consuming and expensive hearing in court, thrash out their differences and resolve the issues as to whether the management of the case could or could not be supported by a reasonable body of the profession, and whether the resulting injuries were in fact caused by the failure of the surgeon? Under Rules of Court provision is made for experts to meet before the hearing.

This should happen, but it is uncommon for such meetings to take place: if they do and it appears to both sides that there is a substantial support for the treatment given by the defendant, the plaintiff will almost certainly be advised not to pursue her claim, or perhaps to settle for a modest sum where there is an element of doubt as to her chances of discharging the burden of proof.

It is certainly very important, both from the public's point of view and that of the medical profession, that experts of high calibre should be readily available to give their independent disinterested opinions on these cases. Good opinions, given at an early stage, will often avert litigation or produce a reasonable settlement without a court hearing.

Consent

An increasingly important risk area for all doctors is the question of consent. No-one may lay hands on another against their will without running the risk of criminal prosecution for assault and, if injury results, a civil action for damages for trespass or negligence. In the case of a doctor, consent to any physical interference will readily be implied: a woman must be assumed to consent to a normal physical examination if she consults a gynaecologist, in the absence of clear evidence of her refusal or restriction of such examination. The problems arise when the gynaecologist's intervention results in unfortunate side effects or permanent interference with function, whether or not any part of the body is removed. For example, if the gynaecologist agrees with the patient to perform a hysterectomy and removes the ovaries without her specific consent, that will be a trespass and an act of negligence. The only available defence will be that it was necessary for the life of the patient to proceed at once to remove the ovaries because of some perceived pathology in them.

What is meant by consent? The term 'informed consent' is often used, but there is no such concept in English law. The consent must be *real*: that is to say, the patient must have been given sufficient information for her to understand the nature of the operation, its likely effects, and any complications which may arise and which the surgeon in the exercise of his duty to the patient considers she should be made aware of; only then can she reach a proper decision. But the surgeon need not warn the patient of remote risks, any more than an anaesthetist need warn the patient that a certain small number of those anaesthetized will suffer cardiac arrest or never recover consciousness. Only where there is a recognized risk, rather than a rare complication, is the surgeon under an obligation to warn the patient of that risk. He is not under a duty to warn the patient of the possible results of hypothetical negligent surgery.

The duty to inform the patient before she consents to any physical intrusion is judged by the same criteria as apply to all other aspects of treatment. Lord Diplock, in the House of Lords in 1985, said:

> The doctor's relationship with his patient which gives rise to the normal duty of care to exercise his skill and judgement to improve the patient's health . . . is . . . a single comprehensive duty covering all the ways in which a doctor is called upon to exercise his skill and judgement . . . including warning of something going wrong however skilfully the treatment advised is carried out (*Sidaway v. Board of Governors of Bethlem Royal Hospital* 1985).

In advising an operation, therefore, the doctor must do so in the way in which a competent gynaecologist exercising reasonable skill and care in similar circumstances would have done. In doing this he will take into account the personality of the patient and the importance of the operation to her future wellbeing. It may be good practice not to warn a very nervous patient of any possible complications if she requires immediate surgery for, say, a malignant condition. The doctor must decide how much to say to her taking into account his assessment of her personality, the questions she asks and his view of how much she understands. If the patient asks a direct question, she must be given a truthful answer.

To take the example of hysterectomy: although the surgeon will tell the patient that it is proposed to remove her uterus and perhaps her ovaries, and describe what that will mean for her future wellbeing (sterility, premature menopause), she will not be warned of the possibility of damage to the ureter, vesicovaginal fistula, fatal haemorrhage or anaesthetic death. Where the surgeon feels that there is information which should be imparted to the patient, but her condition and the urgency of the matter make it advisable and in her interest not to go into much detail, it is wise to tell her partner or a close relative of any possible complication. In such circumstances, and where the patient is unable to give consent because she is unconscious or under the influence of drugs, it is essential to keep the family informed, but they must never be given the impression that they are consenting to the treatment. The important thing is not to mislead the patient in any way without some very cogent reason, and then only after careful consideration and discussion with colleagues and perhaps relatives. Where the surgeon feels in a dilemma, in the end he must resolve it alone, but should always make a contemporaneous note recording the reasons for his decision. This will be strong support for his evidence in rebutting any later charge of assault or negligence.

The consent form

The signing of a consent form is some evidence that the patient has been given an opportunity to decide whether or not to undergo the operation after full information, but it is not as important as the evidence of the surgeon as to what he said to the patient and whether or not she understood. The 'catch-all' clause giving the surgeon permission to do anything necessary does not give roving authority to remove whatever he fancies may be for the good of the patient. The surgeon cannot, for example, construe a consent to termination of pregnancy as a licence to sterilize the patient. Explanation of the law on consent is provided in a DHS publication, A Guide to Consent for Examination or Treatment: NHS Management Executive 1990, which includes model consent forms.

The surgeon needs no consent for any emergency procedure. But as one of the aims of good medical practice is to avoid misunderstandings later, it is wise to discuss any emergency with relatives if this is practicable, as part of the general policy of open communication which is so important in the avoidance of litigation.

Consent by third parties

Only the individual concerned can, strictly, give consent for any interference with her body. It is the practice to obtain the consent of a parent for operation on a minor (i.e. under 18), but since the Family Law of Form Act of 1969 a minor who has attained the age of 16 years can given effective consent to any surgical, medical or dental treatment without parental consent. If such consent is refused for an operation on a girl under 16 years, and that operation is regarded as essential for the wellbeing of the girl, the only recourse is for her to be made a ward of court and the court's consent obtained. Sometimes a local authority would take this step, or a parent or medical practitioner may do so. Where the minor is a ward of court, even if she is over 16, the court's consent must be obtained to any intervention. This is something of an anomaly.

A minor under the age of 16 may, in appropriate cases, be competent to consent to treatment. In *Gillick v. West Norfolk and Wisbech Area Health Authority and Another* (1986) the House of Lords held, by a majority of three to two, that a girl under 16 did not lack authority to consent to advice and treatment merely by reason of her age. Such treatment – and the decision applies to *all* types of treatment – could lawfully be given by a doctor without a parent's consent, provided that the patient was old enough to have sufficient understanding and intelligence to enable him or her to understand fully what was being proposed. Thus 'parental right yields to the child's right to make his own decisions' (Lord Scarman) when he achieves understanding; but while his consent to treatment will then override his parent's wishes, the minor's *refusal* of treatment will not override the parental consent or the consent given by the court in the case of a ward (*re W. (a minor)* 1992). This distinction between 'positive' and 'negative' consent is bewildering but well established in law.

In the UK (although not in some states of America) the courts cannot order a surgeon to operate. Nor can a court override a valid refusal of consent given by a competent adult. But there have been cases where the courts have intervened to save the life of a patient where the refusal was *not* valid because the patient was incapable of making a proper judgement by reason of illness or medication or, in one case, because of another's influence. Yet in a case which caused considerable stir a court did override a mother's refusal to have a caesarean section, in order to save the lives of both a mother and child (*re S. (adult: refusal of treatment)* 1992) but it is very doubtful whether this case would be followed, since the decision was made in a situation of great urgency with no time for proper argument. In a case of great authority (*re F. (in utero)* 1988) the Court of Appeal stated that it would be for Parliament, not the courts, to decide whether a mother's refusal of treatment which would save her unborn child should be interfered with by the courts. In any event, no obstetrician should override a mother's refusal of consent, however necessary the treatment for her and the fetus, without a declaration from the courts that it would be lawful for him to do so. Otherwise he would lay himself open to a prosecution for assault, as well as a claim for damages for negligence.

Consent for the mentally handicapped

A further problem as to consent arises in those cases where an adult is incapable of giving consent by reason of mental disability. In the case of *F. v. West Berkshire Health Authority* (1985) the House of Lords ruled that no court has jurisdiction to give or withhold consent to such an operation in such an adult (unlike the position with a minor) but that a court can make a declaration that the proposed operation is lawful 'in the circumstances in the best interests of the woman'. They went on to say that although such a declaration is not necessary to establish the lawfulness of the operation, 'in practice the court's jurisdiction should be invoked whenever such an operation is to be performed'. In view of this ruling, any gynaecologist who believes such a patient requires sterilization, having come to that decision applying the standards laid down in the Bolam test (*Bolam v. Friern HMC* 1957), should ensure that an application is made to the court for approval of the lawfulness of the operation. Lord Brandon said:

> The applicant should normally be those responsible for the care of the patient or those intending to carry out the proposed operation or other treatment if it is declared to be lawful – i.e. the health authority or the surgeon (*F. v. West Berkshire Health Authority* 1985).

But their lordships stressed that the doctor would have a common-law duty to operate in such circumstances if it was in the best interests of the patient. If, therefore, for some reason no application to the court were made, it would seem that a surgeon could not be held guilty of trespass or negligence, if he went on to operate, always keeping within the Bolam principle.

Husband's consent

The consent of a husband is never required for surgery on his wife, not even for sterilization. Nor can he prevent her from having an abortion within the law. But if the woman is unable to give real consent because of her condition it is a wise precaution to discuss the case fully with the husband, always provided that she waives the duty of confidentiality. However, if he does not give his consent the surgeon must decide independently whether or not to operate, and it will be the surgeon's duty to do so if he believes it necessary.

Abortion

The gynaecologist who undertakes to terminate a pregnancy or to sterilize a patient will be liable in damages if the child is nevertheless born alive, or if the woman becomes pregnant as a result of negligence. But there is no right of action in English law for permitting a 'wrongful life'.

In a case in 1982 (*McKay v. Essex Health Authority* 1982) the Court of Appeal decided that a gynaecologist who failed to diagnose rubella in the mother, and thus failed to terminate her pregnancy as she would have wished if she had been told of the risks, was not liable to the child for the handicaps he suffered.

A negligent failed abortion can give rise to a claim for damages. In 1979 an unmarried woman was awarded damages for pain and suffering, loss of earnings and reduced chance of marriage because she went to term after an attempted aspiration abortion in the 7th week (*Sciuriaga v. Powell* 1979). She did not claim the expense of bringing up the child, as she had an affiliation order. The judge held that the gynaecologist had been negligent and rejected the defence that she should have mitigated her damages by having a mid-term abortion when it was discovered that she was still pregnant, saying that it was reasonable for her to refuse termination after she had felt fetal movements. The defence that has been raised in such cases, that it is contrary to public policy to allow a mother to claim damages for the birth of a child who is a source of joy and satisfaction to her, has been rejected by the courts.

The Abortion Act 1967 was modified by the Human Fertilization and Embryology Act 1990, which clarified, for the first time, the upper limit for 'social' abortion at 24 weeks. The Act, however, permits abortion at any gestation where there is a serious threat to the life or health of the mother, or where there is a 'substantial risk' of a 'seriously' handicapped child. These qualifying phrases have never been defined and it is not yet clear how the courts will interpret them. The major dilemma for the clinician who decides to terminate a pregnancy for fetal handicap after the stage of viability is to prevent the live birth of a handicapped fetus which would add prematurity to the baby's problems. The Act does not of course change the status of the child once born: a handicapped fetus born under such circumstances has precisely the same rights in law as any other newborn child; it is only the unborn child who has no rights (except under the Congenital Disabilities (Civil Liability) Act 1976, and then only if it survives for 48 hours).

Sterilization

Failed sterilization claims have become frequent and most of them settle before coming to court. Lack of advice as to the risk of failure of the operation has caused particular problems. The question as to whether the standard of information before consent is obtained for the operation should be different when it has been performed on contraceptive rather than therapeutic grounds was considered in a case brought in 1987 by a woman who became pregnant after a sterilization (properly performed), alleging that she had not been warned of the risks of failure (*Gold v. Haringey Health Authority* 1987). She claimed that if she had been so warned and had been properly advised as to the alternatives, she and her husband would have elected for him to have a vasectomy. The Court of Appeal held that the standard of care required of a doctor was the same whatever the context in which the advice was given, and although the experts agreed that at the date of the hearing (1987) they personally would have advised as to the risks of failure, at the date of the operation (1979) there was a responsible body of doctors who would not have done so. The plaintiff therefore failed. If the failure to give such advice had occurred more recently it would probably have succeeded – depending entirely on the medical evidence.

Since 1980 the courts have, in general, taken the view that there was an obligation to warn about the possibility of failure. The main problem for the plaintiff, however, is causation: that is to say, what difference would it have made to her decision had she known? In practice most women would not be able to say that they would have declined the operation, given the information about failure; but in the absence of such a warning a woman might justifiably claim that she did not understand the significance of amenorrhoea and therefore did not seek abortion in time.

The costs of medical litigation

Although all practitioners are covered either by insurance through their medical defence organizations or by NHS indemnity, it is not only the legal costs of fighting a case that have to be considered. The harassment, the waste of time and the emotional strain of threatened and actual litigation are things that every professional person would wish to avoid, and it bears particularly hard upon the surgeon. The doctor–patient relationship is a precious one, but the price that is paid for it includes the risk of conflict arising. The best way to avoid litigation is to ensure that no medical accidents occur, but this is a counsel of perfection. The next best thing is to ensure that the patient understands before any operation what is entailed, and, if something goes wrong, that she is properly treated and given all the information necessary for her to understand what has gone wrong and what is being done to put it right.

Many claims for medical negligence arise because the patient has been kept in the dark; lack of knowledge and understanding breed suspicion, and even when there has been no error on the part of the doctor, the patient and her friends and relations can come to believe that there is something wrong because information has been kept away from her. Good communication between doctor and patient in this case, as in many others, will avoid trouble. Defensive medicine is not the answer: cooperation with the patient throughout, when this is practicable, combined with the courage to take decisions in the interests of the patient, will always be respected by the courts, and hopefully the claim will not get as far as that.

The Central Fund

In the spring of 1994 the Department of Health published the consultant document *Clinical Negligence: Proposed Creation of a Central Fund in England.* In November 1994 the Department appointed the Medical Protection Society, in collaboration with the insurers Willis Coroon, to design and implement a scheme for the pooling of clinical negligence costs; there are plans to set up a special health authority for its control and administration. The Fund came into operation in April 1995 but at present there is no clear indication as to how the fund will affect the control of malpractice litigation. Much will depend on how many provider units volunteer to take part in the Fund and the extent to which the special health authority influences decisions about settlements at unit level. There have been disturbing suggestions that the administrators of the Fund might seek to prevent local units moving rapidly to early settlement in cases which might, at least in theory, be defended, even though their defence might be more expensive than settlement.

THE GYNAECOLOGIST AS DEFENDANT

A doctor's first duty is always to the patient: duty to his peers comes second. After a medical accident the doctor is naturally concerned about his own responsibility, criticism by peers, the possibility of litigation, fear of appearing in court, and ultimately a finding of negligence. However, the clinician's first concern should be for the consequences of the accident for the patient. One's duty is to establish what went wrong, find out why, explain to the patient, seek to rectify the damage and see that she is properly advised about her legal rights. Only after these duties have been discharged should peer loyalty arise.

The practitioner's duty of care does not cease, and indeed may increase, when a suspicion of an accident arises. The doctor should appreciate the injured patient's difficulty in understanding her legal position and in pursuing any claim she may have.

Any professional person has a duty to inform the client when injury may be the result of negligence, so that he or she may take independent advice. More than 10 years ago the Master of the Rolls (Donaldson 1985), in an address to the Medico-Legal Society, raised the issue, to which he has recently returned in the foreword to a new textbook (Donaldson 1994).

> Both branches of the legal profession have a salutary rule of professional ethics requiring them to advise their client to consult another practitioner if they consider that they may have been in breach of their duty of care and that this breach has led to loss or damage on the part of their client. They are not required to admit to negligence – they may after all be mistaken. However, they must give the client the materials upon which to be advised by another lawyer and this duty will normally be fulfilled simply by handing over the papers.
>
> The position in relation to the medical profession is, or should be, in many respects the same. The duty of care does not involve the doctor in making a definitive judgement upon his own professional conduct and communicating that judgement to the patient. Save in a clear case, he may be less likely than the lawyer to be the person best able to decide. But, in contrast to the position of the lawyer, he has a very special duty of disclosure. He must never conceal from the patient or the patient's advisers precisely what he did and when and why he did it. Such concealment is all too easy in a medical context. The patient, even if conscious, is often in no position to know precisely what treatment he has received. It is to the discharge of this duty, as much as to the protection of the doctor, that the requirement for full and accurate note-taking and, in appropriate cases, for making those notes available to the patient's professional advisers is directed.

Avoidance of litigation

Many doctors feel that the courts set unreasonable standards for them and that this forces them into diagnostic and therapeutic measures which are for the protection of the doctor and not for the good of the patient. However, the standards set by the courts are those of the experts called to give independent evidence; there is no danger that the doctor will be found negligent if the care given is to a standard acceptable to that doctor's peers.

The maintenance of a reasonable standard of care will ultimately avoid a finding of negligence.

A proper standard of notekeeping will make it easier for an independent assessor to understand the care given. To that end, meticulous contemporary notekeeping, including a full history, the advice given in relation to surgery, a precise account of surgical technique or other treatment, and full details of postoperative management is essential. The discharge letter (or summary) in particular requires meticulous care and accuracy, remembering that at some later stage it may be subjected to a critical, even adversarial, examination.

However, in the last resort, although the maintenance of a reasonable standard of care and meticulous notekeeping will defeat litigation, good communication will obviate it. In respect of the standard of care, good communication will often prevent the injured patient from becoming a litigant. Only a tiny percentage of medical negligence ends in litigation: the vast majority is forgiven by the patient. The patient must be kept informed at all times. Part of the duty of care is to ensure that the patient understands as far as possible the options available for treatment. It is sometimes necessary to canvass with the patient the possibility of poor outcome, particularly if the procedure is elective. When things go wrong, a full and frank disclosure to the patient is not only desirable but prudent. A full explanation of the circumstances of an accident is not the same as an admission of liability. However, when liability is undeniable, it is clearly right, and indeed in their own interest, that the provider unit (or in a private case the medical defence organization) should admit liability and settle the case as soon as possible. Where there is no other satisfactory explanation (e.g. a retained swab) admission of fault is appropriate.

In matters relating to consent it is essential that the explanatory material given to the patient is fully reported in her notes and that the patient's questions are properly answered. The limited value of the consent form is dealt with on pages 867–868.

RISK MANAGEMENT

Until 1989 the defence of all medical malpractice concerning doctors was in the hands of the medical defence organizations who, separately from their hospitals, defended doctors. NHS Indemnity, explained in HC (89) 34, was introduced on 1 January 1990, making every health authority responsible for indemnifying all doctors for negligent actions arising out of their NHS practice. With the introduction of Trusts in April 1991, the responsibility was further devolved. Each NHS Trust is responsible for indemnifying successful plaintiffs for any action arising after the creation of that Trust. Liability must at present be met from the Trust's revenue, up to a maximum of 0.5% of annual income. For any sum above that ceiling, arrangements exist for the Trust to borrow from the Treasury and to repay it over a 10-year period. For that Trust this inevitably means an increase in prices and a competitive disadvantage.

Thus, successful medical negligence actions have a serious impact on Trust finances. In practice, the first intimation of an action from medical negligence comes from the 'letter before action'. Since the plaintiff has 3 years from the date of knowledge in which to bring the action for medical negligence, the Trust may experience considerable difficulty in defending the action if, at the first intimation of the likely action, the junior doctors and nurses concerned have left its employment. There will then only be the (often inadequate) medical records upon which to rely. It is against this background that the impetus for clinical risk management has arisen. Many adverse outcomes are clearly identifiable *at the time*, and if the incident is adequately investigated the Trust will not be at a disadvantage if subsequently called to account for its actions. The principles of risk management, i.e. identification, analysis, control and funding, can be applied in the clinical situation.

Adverse outcome reporting is the keystone to any system of risk management. It is necessary to identify in each directorate those incidents most likely to result in litigation. Every department should create its own list of trigger events; in gynaecology these would probably include:

- Unexpected return to the operating theatre.
- Perforation of the uterus during curettage/evacuation.
- Postoperative fistula.
- Surgery exceeding consent.
- Readmission to hospital after early pregnancy intervention.

Once an adverse outcome has been identified its immediate analysis brings two advantages: an opportunity to correct poor practice, and a full and early assessment of all the facts to assess vulnerability.

Following assessment, the response to the injured patient can be swift and appropriate. A good risk management system does not operate to the detriment of the patient for, whereas a defensible case may be better defended, those in which there is clear evidence of liability may be rapidly settled.

A full explanation of clinical risk management can be found in the standard texts (Hirst & Clements 1995, Vincent 1995).

Complaints and litigation

Whereas complaints relate to the 'how does it feel?' aspect of quality (client quality), litigation is much more likely to arise out of a serious adverse outcome (professional quality). In fact, there is little crossover between the two and only 10% of 'letters before action' have previously been notified as complaints.

Letter before action

When a patient seeks to initiate litigation the first intimation is usually a letter from the plaintiff's legal adviser warning the defendant of the intention to pursue a claim. The letter should set out sufficient facts of the event, together with an indication of the likely allegations to be pursued. The purpose of the letter is to seek preaction disclosure of the medical records.

Such a letter requires a prompt response if unnecessary delays and accompanying legal charges are to be avoided. The doctor should not correspond with the patient's solicitors, except to acknowledge the letter: a defensible action may be prejudiced as a result of inappropriate correspondence. Within the health service the doctor should immediately pass on the letter to the appropriate manager, who will consult with the Trust's legal advisers. In private practice the doctor should pass on the letter to his defence organization. Most such letters nowadays state that the plaintiff's solicitors will not agree to restriction of disclosure of notes to a medical adviser, but require disclosure to themselves and their client. The plaintiff's solicitors can obtain a court order for full disclosure if this is refused, provided certain conditions are fulfilled (*Lask v. Gloucester Health Authority* 1985). There is no legal basis for restriction of disclosure: it is essential that the lawyers see the records in order to be able to advise on liability.

Documents to be disclosed

Correspondence and other communications between the solicitors and the client are privileged from production to the plaintiff, even though no litigation was contemplated or pending at the time they were written, provided that they are of confidential nature and the solicitor was acting in a professional capacity, giving legal advice or obtaining it on behalf of the client (e.g. from counsel).

The general principle is that communications between a solicitor and a third party, whether directly or through an agent, which are written after litigation is contemplated or commenced for the purpose of giving or obtaining advice or evidence in regard to that litigation, are privileged. This privilege includes documents which are obtained by a solicitor with a review to enabling him to prosecute or defend an action, or to give advice with reference to existing or contemplated litigation.

However, risk management reports, like reports of accidents and similar documents, are made before litigation is commenced and are not usually protected. This is because the reports have a dual purpose, that of producing as clear an account of the incident as possible so that the facts may be ascertained and any necessary action taken, as well as that of providing a basis on which solicitors may be instructed as necessary and proceedings defended (or settled) if they are instituted. In general, such documents are not privileged.

Meeting legal advisers

It is essential at an early stage in the proceedings that the defendant doctor should give a full explanation of his part in the case, the reasons for acting as he did and an assessment of his own and others' responsibilities. The doctor should have some say in the choice of expert and should try to ensure that the expert chosen to help the defence has appropriate recent experience in circumstances similar to those of the defendant. If he works in a busy district general hospital, it may be little help to have a retired academic to give expert evidence.

It is essential that the defendant doctor should understand the expert evidence which is to be given on his behalf. He should read the expert's report and make sure he agrees with it, or comment accordingly. The defendant should read all of the authorities on which the expert seeks to rely.

When the case is to be defended, the doctor must ensure that he attends a conference with counsel at which the experts are also present, so that it is certain that due weight is given to the doctor's own experience and that it corresponds with the experts' view.

Appearing in court

Before appearing in court the defendant doctor will have the opportunity to read the expert evidence from the plaintiff. This will indicate where the main thrust of cross-examination will lie. The doctor should become familiar with the authorities upon which the plaintiff's experts rely, and make sure that his own experts fully understand the case. Although a witness of fact, the defendant doctor is inevitably an expert in his own field; nevertheless, he should be encouraged to concentrate upon facts.

In giving evidence the defendant doctor must be modest, succinct and intelligible.

THE GYNAECOLOGIST AS EXPERT WITNESS

Definition

The salient feature of an expert witness is that he is unconnected with the case in question and can give an independent opinion of the standards of care provided by the defendant. He must have specialized knowledge and experience in the particular field relevant to the facts under investigation: in a gynaecological case, for example, although the principal expert will himself be a gynaecologist in the same field of practice, other additional experts may be appropriate, such as a general practitioner, or perhaps a scientist working within a much narrower area, such as immunology or genetics. Thus several experts may be called in any one case to deal with different aspects of management.

It is desirable that the expert should have current practical contact with his specialty, although often an eminent practitioner who has retired may have the additional assets of time and opportunity to apply a lifetime's experience to an area in which he is familiar. The expert should not be tempted to stray outside his own particular field of expertise.

The role of the expert

When the expert is first asked for an opinion he should approach the analysis of the case in an objective fashion, forming an opinion without fear or favour. He must give a clear indication of an assessment of the standards of care, but once that opinion has been formed he cannot be disinterested, although he should at all times remain balanced. In an adversarial system the expert who gives evidence on behalf of either plaintiff or defendant becomes part of the team assembled to conduct the litigation, and will have a responsibility to assemble evidence and advise the lawyers on the best way of presenting it. He will be expected not only to justify his own opinion, but also to deal with contrary arguments advanced by the other side.

When giving evidence in court the expert will be subjected to cross-examination in which his views will be challenged and contrary views advanced; he must be able to marshall the evidence in such a way that the independent opinions advanced can be justified. The expert should be able to support these views from textbooks, the literature and acceptable statistics.

The medical report

It is an essential prerequisite for a plaintiff's expert to interview the plaintiff while in possession of all the medical records, so as to compare her version of events with the written record. Similarly, it is unrealistic to expect a defence expert to fulfil his role without the opportunity of discussing management with the doctors concerned.

The first and largest part of the report is a careful analysis of all the hospital records. If the notes are incomplete, the expert must advise the solicitors to inquire for the missing documents, and should not take no for an answer. The expert should then reconstruct the events in his report in a way which an intelligent educated layman will understand. Although it is not essential to include all the details of the events of the case in the report, it is often helpful to the court to do so in a detailed and explicit form.

In the second part, the expert should go on to explain the technical matters involved. For instance, where a urinary fistula has developed as a result of gynaecological surgery, it is essential to explain in the report how such injuries may be caused, the anatomical arrangements (if necessary with diagrams) and their possible sequelae for the plaintiff. Such explanatory material may well be separated from the main narrative, into appendices.

The third part of the report should relate to the case in point to this technical explanation. It should give a critical appraisal of the standards of care. Finally, the expert should give an unequivocal assessment of standards of care and, if he believes these to be defective, should list the areas in which care fell short of the reasonable standard to be expected. In this discussion the expert should avoid the use of the term 'negligence', since this is a question of law and may be misunderstood by doctors; in any event, it is for the court to decide after hearing evidence as to what is acceptable to the profession and hence whether the care has been negligent.

In forming this opinion the expert will refer to standard textbooks, for they define what is an acceptable standard. It is sometimes useful to refer to learned scientific papers, but they often reflect matters that are still under debate and on which there may well be more than one opinion. Such articles can be particularly useful to rebut the view that a particular practice is not acceptable, or conversely to establish that there is a responsible body of medical opinion of a contrary view. It is important that such reference should antedate the accident.

Disclosure of reports

The initial report is prepared for the use of counsel in drafting or rebutting the statement of claim. It will often need to deal with contrary arguments and discuss controversial areas. After the pleadings are closed there will at some stage before the trial be an exchange of experts' reports in accordance with the recent changes in the Rules of Courts (Order 38, Rule 37). In all personal injury cases the court may order disclosure of experts' written reports to the other party or parties:

> When in any cause or matter an application is made in respect of oral expert evidence, then, unless the Court considers that there are special reasons for not doing so, it shall direct that the substance of the evidence be disclosed in the form of a written report or reports to such other parties and within such period as the Court may specify.

There may already have been voluntary exchange or exchange within the provisions for automatic disclosure under Order 25, Rule 8, but in any event parties are now bound to disclose their evidence in medical negligence cases well before the trial, and may not rely on any evidence that has not been disclosed to the other side.

The initial report may not be suitable for disclosure, and

both expert and counsel should be aware that it is not intended for such a purpose. Should the matter reach the courts, a separate report, often shorter and perhaps modified in the light of disclosure of further facts or documents, would be appropriate for exchange. Counsel may wish to draft this final report independently, but the doctor must ensure that it represents his own views.

The court also has the power to order a 'without prejudice' meeting between the experts (Order 38, Rule 38):

> In any cause or matter the Court may, if it thinks fit, direct that there be a meeting 'without prejudice' of such experts within such periods before or after the disclosure of their reports as the Court may specify, for the purpose of identifying those parts of their evidence which are in issue. Where such a meeting takes place the experts may prepare a joint statement indicating those parts of their evidence on which they are, and those on which they are not, in agreement.

The effect of these changes in the rules should be to resolve many cases before trial, or at best narrow the issue. Unfortunately, in gynaecological cases the 'without prejudice' meeting is seldom employed.

Conference

The earlier the expert is involved in a meeting with solicitors and counsel, the better. If possible this should take place before any report is written: this will ensure that the expert's mind is directed to the legal issues, what has to be proved, and where the other side will direct its attack. This will mean that counsel has a report on which to draft the pleadings with confidence, and there should then be no need to amend them later. Time spent in conference is thus well worth the time and expense, as it saves both in the long run. Neither the plaintiff nor the defence can mount their cases properly without early and full consultation between the lawyers, the expert (or experts – there may be more than one) and the client, either patient or doctor.

The pleadings

The pleadings are the formal statements of each party's case. Their importance is that they set out the case on each side, define the allegations and limit the area of dispute, for no evidence can be given that does not relate to allegations in the pleadings. The plaintiff's statement of claim sets out the main events relating to the complaint, then lists the 'particulars of negligence' alleged and gives an account of the damages suffered. The defendant doctor and any other defendant (often the health authority or provider unit) will then prepare their defence.

The next stage in pleading will probably be a request for 'further and better particulars' of the statement of claim or the defence. Those particulars will almost certainly need to be drafted with the expert's help; in any event they should not be served without his approval, as the advocates will be bound by these particulars in the conduct of the case.

Evidence in court

To the uninitiated the giving of expert evidence is often a daunting experience, but there are some simple rules which help. It should be remembered that most judges today, especially in the High Court, have a basic scientific knowledge which enables them to understand even the most difficult medical problem; the judge will probably have read the medical reports and done the necessary 'homework'; above all, he will have empathy with the expert and some common professional understanding.

On a more practical level, the expert must understand that the judge will take down in longhand all the germane points of the evidence, often word for word. It must therefore be given to the judge in a way that he can comprehend and note. The expert should face the judge when giving evidence, and do it in a modest though firm manner and at a speed commensurate with the judge's requirement to take notes.

In cross-examination the expert's views will be attacked with varying degrees of effectiveness. Sometimes it will be necessary to concede a point in cross-examination. To do so gracefully will enhance the expert's authority and credibility. The expert should take time to answer questions if necessary. He should bear in mind the 'bottom line' beyond which he is not prepared to retreat. If the expert's opinion has been stated clearly in the report and he has thought out the implications fully, there should be no difficulty in withstanding cross-examination.

It is important that the expert should hear the evidence given by the expert on the other side, and he should be readily available to counsel during cross-examination; without expert advice, counsel may be unable to cross-examine effectively.

Responsibilities of the expert witness

In *National Justice Compania Naviera SA v. Prudential Assurance Co. Ltd.* (*Ikarian Reefer*) [1993] (*The Times*, 5 March), Cresswell recently summarized the responsibilities of the expert witness in the civil courts. Although the judgement concerns marine insurance, the principles are no less applicable to medical negligence litigation:

> Responsibility of the expert witness
>
> 1. Expert evidence presented to the Court should be, and should be seen to be, the independent product of the expert uninfluenced as to form or content by the exigencies of litigation.
> 2. Independent assistance should be provided to the Court by

way of objective unbiased opinion regarding matters within the expertise of the expert witness. An expert witness in the High Court should never assume the role of advocate.
3. Facts or assumptions upon which the opinion was based should be stated together with material facts which could detract from the concluded opinion.
4. An expert witness should make it clear when a question or issue fell outside his expertise.
5. If the opinion was not properly researched because it was considered that insufficient data was available then that had to be stated with an indication that the opinion was provisional. If the witness could not assert that the report contained the truth, the whole truth and nothing but the truth then the qualification should be stated on the report.
6. If, after exchange of reports, an expert witness changed his mind on a material matter then the change of view should be communicated to the other side through legal representatives without delay and, when appropriate, to the Court.
7. Documents referred to in the expert evidence had to be provided to the other side at the same time as the exchange of reports.

FUTURE TRENDS

Rising expectations, increase in public awareness of scientific and specifically of medical progress, avid interest in the more lurid aspects of professional conduct of all kinds – greatly encouraged by the media – have all increased medical litigation. The profession's own tendency to raise expectations of new techniques fuels the process. Escalating damages in all accident claims, not only those for medical mishap, are inevitable as the costs and potential of caring increase. These are widely publicized, naturally making patients more aware of the significance of many unfortunate sequelae of treatment.

The development of risk management programmes has the potential both to improve quality of care (thus reducing medical accidents) and to improve the handling of litigation so as to reduce costs. Nevertheless, it would be unrealistic to deny that claims will continue to increase in both number and value. In this chapter we have tried to show how these can best be dealt with, to abort those based on ignorance or misunderstanding, and to handle the serious ones in such a way as to minimize the injury to both the plaintiff and the defendant.

In gynaecology there are several areas which threaten to become fertile fields for the disaffected patient; there are also some hopeful signs of change, some of which are controversial but should be examined with a view to progress.

Procedural reform

One of the greatest defects of negligence litigation at present is delay. As a judge said despairingly in a recent case where the plaintiff sought to amend pleadings at the trial, 7 years after issue of the writ and 9 years since the operation: 'I never seem to try a case that is less than 9 years old!' This is scandalous: memories fade, documents are lost, registrars are in the Antipodes; worse than these practical defects, the years may have caused deprivation of rightful damages much needed by the plaintiff, and will almost certainly have built up resentment and even bitterness on both sides.

The new Rules of Courts (p. 873–874), if properly used, could narrow issues and avoid delays which result from neither side understanding what the case is about; as Lord Justice Mustill (1987) said in the Court of Appeal:

> The parties realised, soon after the case began, that they had misunderstood what the case was about. As was stated before us, it was fought 'in the dark'. It lasted four weeks instead of the allotted five days, which not only imposed great pressure of time on all concerned, but meant that the scheduling of the expert witness was put quite out of joint . . . Nearly 150 pages of medical literature were put in, without prior exchange, or any opportunity for proper scrutiny.
>
> All this could have been avoided if there had been adequate clarification of these issues before the trial . . . I believe that practitioners do their clients and the interests of justice no service by continuing to pursue this policy of concealment . . . To me it seems wrong that in this area of the law, more than in any other, this kind of forensic blind-man's buff should continue to be the norm.

This should not happen, again, but unhappily delays can occur for many different reasons (Leigh & Leigh 1994); some of these lie in the control of doctors and their legal advisers, but probably more are the responsibility of plaintiff's lawyers. All the surgeon can do, whether as defendant or expert, is to cooperate fully and promptly with the lawyers, and if appropriate bring such pressure to bear as is possible to hasten matters.

Any action taken to expedite will have the full support of the judges, who will in future be increasingly vigilant to ensure that both sides not only get justice, but get it quickly.

No-fault compensation

Hopes have been fixed by many on the possibility of 'no-fault compensation'. The experiences of those countries who have adopted some such system have not been encouraging, mainly because it has been found impossible to avoid the investigation of causation, and the results of financing such a scheme have been catastrophic (Vennell 1994). It is highly unlikely that it will ever be introduced in the UK. Another method of funding medical negligence claims has however been introduced; lawyers are now able to take on cases, in certain circumstances, on a 'no win, no fee' basis. The uptake in medical negligence has been small because of the difficulty of obtaining insurance to cover defendant costs, in the event that they are awarded against the unsuccessful plaintiff.

New areas of risk in gynaecology

A few cases are now beginning to come before the courts brought by women who complain that their surgery was unnecessary. Several have been widely publicized, including hysterectomy where consent was obtained only for endometrial resection, and of oophorectomy specifically against a patient's wishes, clearly expressed on the consent form. As women become more conscious of their rights to control their own bodies, such cases are likely to increase unless gynaecologists respect their patients' wishes to be treated as responsible adults and to be involved in decisions about their 'disposable' reproductive assets.

The major new area of concern over the past 2 or 3 years has been minimal-access surgery. Whereas for the general surgeon the newer techniques of laparoscopic cholecystectomy and bowel surgery have been the subject of dramatic press reports, for the gynaecologist the procedure of endometrial laser ablation, transcervical endometrial resection and laser laparoscopy have been equally notorious in the public mind. The background to this spate of accidents is complex. A generation of established gynaecologists has been slow to appreciate the importance of thorough basic training in the new techniques; the hand–eye coordination required to achieve safe practice in minimal-access surgery is entirely different from that learned by a generation of surgeons trained in the 1960s and 1970s; 20 years' practice of open abdominal surgery is no assurance of competence with newer techniques, any more than possession of a driving licence and 20 years' practice on the roads fits a driver to fly an aeroplane. The public clamour for the new techniques because the profession, through the media, teaches them to expect them. Purchasing health authorities press for them to be introduced because of the accompanying reduction in the length of stay and a perceived saving in costs. Pressure on all sides leads to short-cuts in training, and hence a series of disasters. Only when a new generation of surgeons brought up with the new techniques comes to maturity will sanity be restored.

Those who break barriers will always attract criticism, and this easily crystallizes into litigation. The whole area of artificial conception is a potential minefield: at present no specific law exists (save for a minimal piece of reactive legislation in a feeble attempt to control surrogacy) (Surrogacy Arrangements Act 1985), but this does not mean that practitioners are immune from the civil law.

Communication is the watchword, as always, but in these new fields, where surgery is neither life-saving nor truly necessary, and often fails, communication becomes vital to a happy outcome on all sides.

Assisted reproduction

From October 1991 most forms of assisted reproduction were brought under the control of the Human Fertilization and Embryology Authority (HFEA). This was set up by the Human Fertilization and Embryology Act 1990, which defined the legal limits and conditions which were in future to govern all medical services for the purpose of 'assisting women to carry children' ('treatment services') and the storage of and research upon gametes and embryos.

The Act does *not* control surrogacy, save to spell out that surrogacy contracts are unenforceable. It does amend the Abortion Act and the Infant Life (Preservation) Act to legalize termination of pregnancy up to term under certain circumstances (see p. 869).

Under the Act no creation, storage or implantation of embryos, or research thereon, is legal unless licensed by the HFEA, which has the power to grant, vary or revoke licences (subject to appeal to the High Court or the Court of Session), to inspect the premises and activities of licensees, and to advise them. The HFEA must also publish a Code of Practice for the guidance of licensees, setting out the manner in which treatment services should be carried out. It is important to distinguish between the edicts of the Act and those of the Code of Practice: the former are mandatory, the latter persuasive; a breach of the former is a criminal offence, which will result in the loss of the licence and possible prosecution, whereas a breach of the Code is *not* a criminal offence, although it may result in the loss or suspension of the licence.

Licences for treatment services – which include in-vitro fertilization, other embyro implantations, artificial insemination and egg donation – are granted to the 'responsible person' in charge of the unit (both being specified in the licence) and continue in force until suspended or revoked. Licences for research are granted for each specific project, and the Authority requires that the protocol should be approved by the appropriate ethics committee. Thus any unit conducting research requires an ethics committee, whereas a unit providing treatment services only is not required by the Code to have one, although most will wish to do so for their own protection and for guidance through a complicated Act and the Code of Conduct, which will undoubtedly be revised frequently.

Any gynaecologist undertaking treatment services as defined in the Act will be well advised to familiarize himself, directly or through his ethics committee, with the provisions of the Act and the current Code. Since undertaking such treatment without a licence, or in breach of its terms, is liable on conviction to a fine or a term of imprisonment for up to 2 years, the rules governing these licences are of vital interest to all practitioners carrying out any sort of assisted reproduction.

The removal of ova for research, or for egg donation,

and oophorectomy to facilitate hormone replacement therapy will require meticulous adherence to professional standards in the giving of advice. In all these cases, and others involving any element of experiment, full discussion with colleagues as well as the patient and detailed note-keeping, together with reasoned correspondence with the general practitioner and perhaps other workers in the same field, will minimize the risks of litigation or even complaint.

KEY POINTS

1. The surgeon does not necessarily undertake to perform a cure but must employ a standard of care appropriate to the time. He will be judged as the ordinary skilled man exercising and professing to have that special skill.
2. For consent for surgery to be real, the patient must be given sufficient information for her to understand the operation, its likely effects and recognized complications.
3. A minor can be made a ward of court if parents refuse permission for surgery. A child under the age of 16 having sufficient understanding may, under appropriate circumstances, consent to treatment.
4. For a mentally handicapped person, a court can declare an operation lawful if it comes to the conclusion that the operation is in the best interests of the patient.
5. In emergency circumstances no consent for surgery is required.
6. A failed termination or sterilization can be the basis for a claim for negligence, especially when advice about risk of failure has not been given.
7. The doctor's first duty is to his patient, and only afterwards to his peers.
8. Litigation is greatly reduced by maintaining a reasonable standard of care and the keeping of meticulous notes; it may be avoided completely by good communication.
9. Risk management is about the avoidance of litigation: it improves quality and reduces costs, but does not disadvantage the plaintiff with a just cause.

REFERENCES

Bolam v. Friern Hospital Management Committee 1957 2 All England Law Reports pp 118, 121
Donaldson M R 1985 The Court of Appeal. Medico-Legal Journal 53: 148–163
Donaldson, Lord 1994 Foreword. In: Clements R V Safe practice in obstetrics and gynaecology: a medico-legal handbook. Churchill Livingstone, Edinburgh
F. v. West Berkshire Health Authority 1985 (Mental Health Act Commission intervening) 2 All England Law Reports 2: 545
Gillick v. West Norfolk and Wisbech Area Health Authority and Another 1986 Appeal Cases 112
Gold v. Haringey Health Authority 1987 2 All England Law Reports p 888
Hirst D, Clements R V 1995 Clinical directors' handbook. Churchill Livingstone, Edinburgh
Lask v. Gloucester Health Authority 1985 The Times 13 December
Leigh S, Leigh M A M S 1994 Medical negligence from the point of view of plaintiff and defendant in safe practice in obstetrics and gynaecology. Churchill Livingstone, Edinburgh
Maynard v. West Midlands Regional Health Authority 1985 1 All England Law Reports p 635
McKay v. Essex Health Authority 1982 2 All England Law Reports p 771
Mustill L J 1987 Medical Protection Society Annual Report p 461
Re F. (in utero) 1988 2 All England Law Reports p 193
Re S. (Adult: Refusal of Treatment) 1992 4 All England Law Reports p 671
Re W. (A minor) 1992 All England Law Reports p 614
Sciuriaga v. Powell 1979 Solicitors Journal 406; considered in Emeh v. Kensington and Chelsea and Westminster AHA 1984 3 All England Law Reports p 1044
Sidaway v. Bethlem Royal Hospital Governors 1985 1 All England Law Reports p 643
Tindal, Chief Justice. In: Lanphier v. Phipos 1838 Carrington and Paynes Reports, pp 475, 479
Vennell M A M 1994 The Commonwealth perspective: New Zealand in safe practice in obstetrics and gynaecology. Churchill Livingstone, Edinburgh
Vincent C 1995 Clinical risk management. BMJ Publications, London
Whitehouse v. Jordan 1980 1 All England Law Reports p 650
Wilsher v. Essex Area Health Authority 1987 2 Weekly Law Reports p 466

60

Forensic gynaecology

R. E. Roberts MBE *F. Lewington* OBE

RAPE

Nature of assault

Sexual assaults on older girls and adult women may involve rape (vaginal penetration), buggery (anal penetration), oral assault (involving both masturbation and ejaculation) and attempts at these assaults, as well as a range of other indecent and degrading acts on various parts of the body. All may be accompanied by threats or actual physical injury. However, it is extremely rare for such victims to be severely wounded, although some may bear defence wounds on the hands, or knife-tip wounds, particularly on the neck. It is not unusual for victims to have no injuries whatsoever through fear or intimidation. Women may be subjected to a variety of indecent and physical assaults and may be made to perform indecent acts themselves. It is important to remember that the outcome is known when the person presents to the hospital or doctor, but at the time of the attack extreme fear of death or serious mutilation may well have precluded rational behaviour.

The true frequency of these assaults will never be known, since many women will not even seek help from a friend or relative or consult their general practitioner. The data for the charts in Figures 60.1–60.4 are taken from actual referrals to St Mary's Centre, Manchester, a special hospital-based centre which offers a comprehensive service basis to adults who have been sexually assaulted. The Centre provides examination facilities for persons reporting to the police and for self-referrals, some of whom may later wish the police to be informed. Crisis and longer-term counselling, and medical care including a sexually transmitted disease clinic and the advice of a consultant gynaecologist, are provided. Over 3000 women have attended the Centre since it opened in 1986.

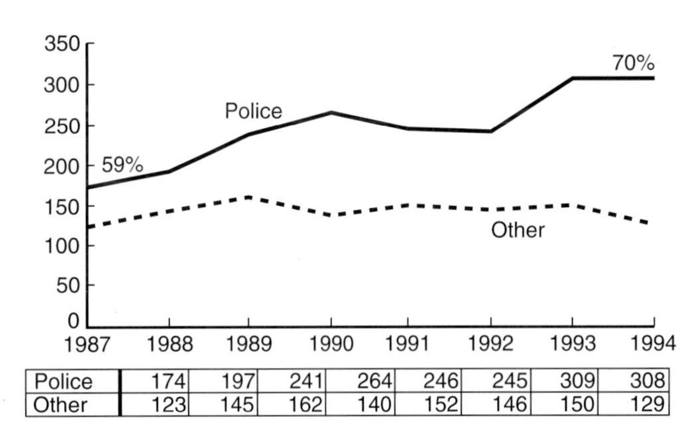

	1987	1988	1989	1990	1991	1992	1993	1994
Police	174	197	241	264	246	245	309	308
Other	123	145	162	140	152	146	150	129

Fig. 60.1 Sources of referral to St Mary's Centre, Manchester. Cases reported to Greater Manchester police are investigated at the Centre. The same service is offered to those reporting directly to the Centre and those who are referred by other agencies, such as doctors or social workers.

Immediate assessment

Management

Women who are injured are likely to report to the police or to a casualty department shortly after the assault. Many women are shocked and unsure as to what they should do. After a few days they may tell their family doctor, or go to a family planning, well woman or sexually transmitted disease clinic. Patients seeking help from the medical profession should be asked if they wish the police to be informed; if so this should be done without delay.

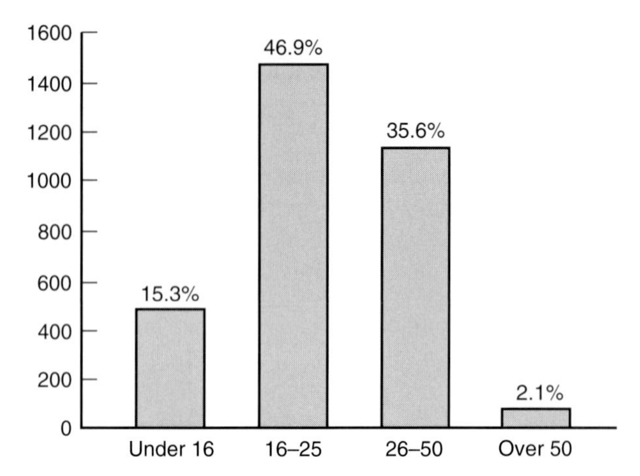

Fig. 60.2 The ages of patients examined at St Mary's Centre, Manchester.

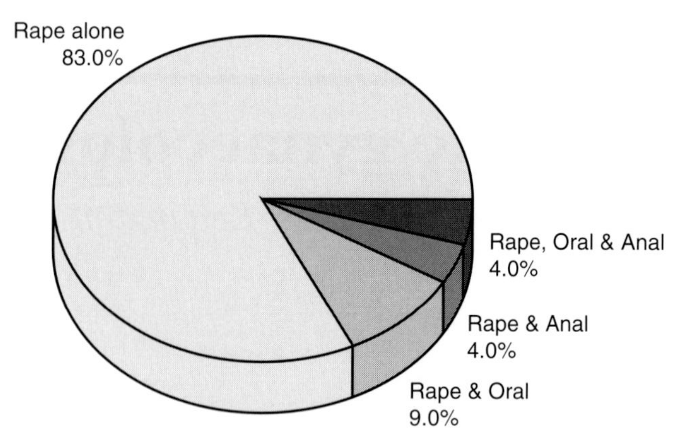

Fig. 60.4 The frequency of rape and other offences among patients examined at St Mary's Centre, Manchester.

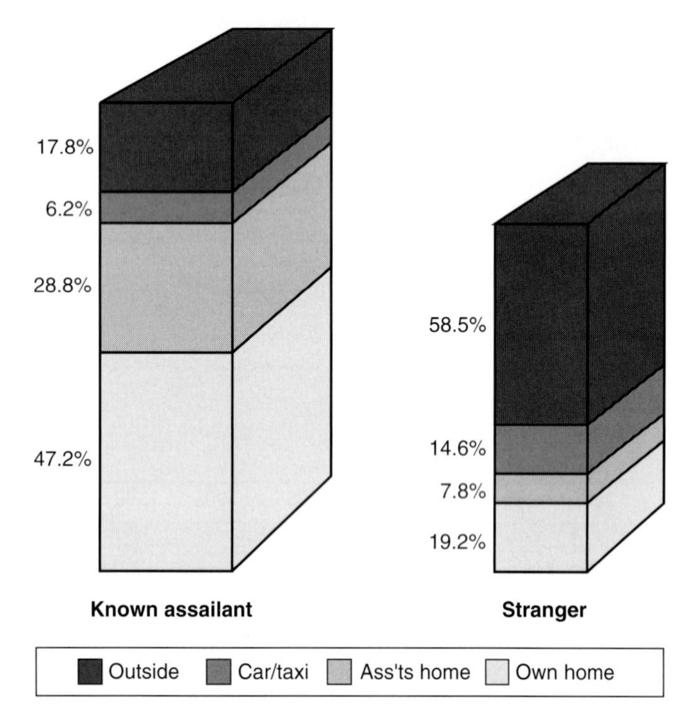

Fig. 60.3 The location of assaults on patients examined at St Mary's Centre, Manchester.

Reporting to the police

Police forces should have a team of trained forensic physicians (of both sexes) to carry out the forensic medical examination. The woman should have the choice of gender of the examiner. She will usually be examined in a special examination suite or in the doctor's surgery. Alternatively, the forensic physician will attend the hospital and take all forensic specimens in the casualty department, ward or theatre as appropriate.

While awaiting the arrival of the forensic physician the hospital staff should avoid removing clothing or cleaning away evidence, but must remember that the patient may be injured and need medical care.

In many parts of the world there will be no forensic examiner and untrained staff will have to carry out the investigation. A brief outline of the procedures to be followed is given here, but staff should have reference to more detailed information (McLay 1990).

The forensic medical examination

The reasons for the medical examination should be explained and consent obtained for it. Therapeutic intentions must be clearly distinguished from forensic ones, both in the mind of the examining doctor and in the understanding of the patient.

If the assault has been reported to the police it is important that the woman understands the role of the doctor. Confidentiality is implied in most medical situations. If the doctor is carrying out the examination at the request of the police, the complainant must be told at the outset that the medical findings will be reported to them and written consent must be obtained for this. It is also important to be aware that disclosure of all information gathered at the initial examination could be ordered by a court.

Partial and delayed reporting to police

If the woman wants to be examined but has not decided whether to report, confidentiality must be respected even if the doctor becomes aware that a serious offence has been committed. Often a woman will allow limited information such as time, place and nature of the attack to be reported, but will not at this stage feel able to be interviewed by a police officer. Such wishes must be respected. In these cases a full and careful examination should be made so that evidence is preserved should the offence be reported later.

When the woman has regained some control of her life after sympathetic and skilled care at the crisis point, she may well decide of her own free will to report to the police, but she should not be pressurized to do so.

Later presentations

It is worth carrying out a full forensic examination, including the gathering of specimens, if up to a week has elapsed after the assault, but the chances of obtaining forensic evidence are much diminished after 48 hours. There may be evidence of previous injuries, such as bruises, scars or bite marks.

A woman presenting to a gynaecologist with vague symptoms may have been the subject of rape or previous abuse in childhood. Sometimes she may wish to report the matter to the police even after many years. Many women are repeatedly assaulted by their partners. They often feel that serious harm has been done and seek medical investigation.

Notes on the medical examination

The doctor should record carefully everything that has been observed and remember that rape is not a medical diagnosis. Careful recording of observations is what is required, and not a value judgement based on incomplete knowledge of the facts.

It is most important that notes are clear, legible, full and contemporaneous. They are the doctor's evidence and the basis on which a statement will be written if required. The notes remain the doctor's personal property but may be called for in court for inspection by the judge and counsel, and may be shown to the jury. Specific questions may be asked regarding particular entries.

The following details should be recorded:

1. Day, date, time (start and finish) and place of the examination and persons present.
2. Who requested the examination.
3. Written consent to the examination, permission for photographs of relevant injuries to be taken and for findings to be reported to the police.
4. History of the attack:
   (a) Physical assault.
   (b) Removal of or damage to clothing.
   (c) Sexual assault.
   (d) Drugs/alcohol involved.
   (e) Actions afterwards (washing, bathing, urination, defecation, drinks, medication).
   (f) Previous sexual intercourse (if within 2 weeks).
   (g) Alcohol or drugs taken immediately prior to the assault.
5. General history:
   (a) Previous health.
   (b) Operations.
   (c) Medications.
   (d) Gynaecological history.
   (e) Obstetric history.
6. State of clothing:
   (a) Torn or damaged.
   (b) Obvious materials adhering (e.g. dust, soil).
   (c) Obvious stains (position, colour, wet, dry).
7. Ask how she feels – record what she says.
8. Examine the whole body and inside the mouth. Measure and chart the injuries. Measure to fixed body points. Photograph if possible.

The medical examination should be of the whole body. It is important to remember that a woman who has been sexually assaulted may not be injured physically. In a sexually active woman there is unlikely to be any sign of trauma in the vulval area unless excessive force was used or objects inserted. Studies have shown that genital injuries are found in 20–30% of rape complainants (Solola et al 1983) and our experience at St Mary's is similar, slight splits and grazes of the fourchette and bruising of the labia being the most common.

The various important possible signs of injury to the head, the front of the body, the vulva and anus are indicated in Figures 60.5–60.7.

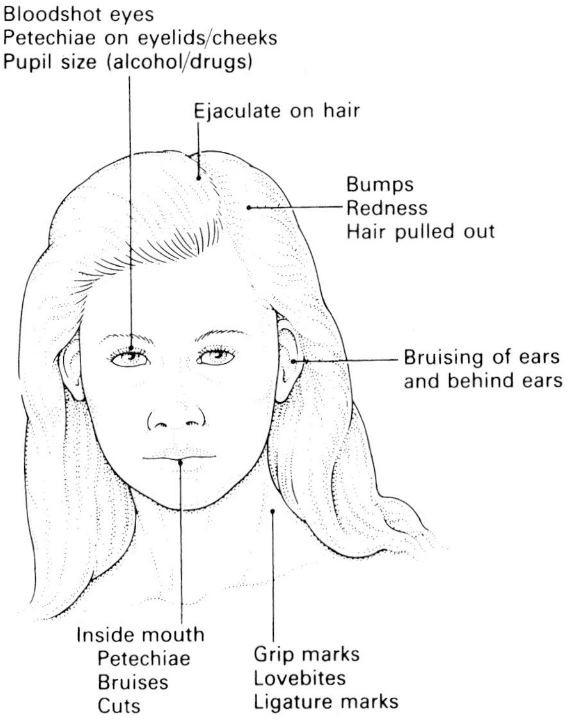

Fig. 60.5 The signs of injury to the head which may be found following sexual assaults.

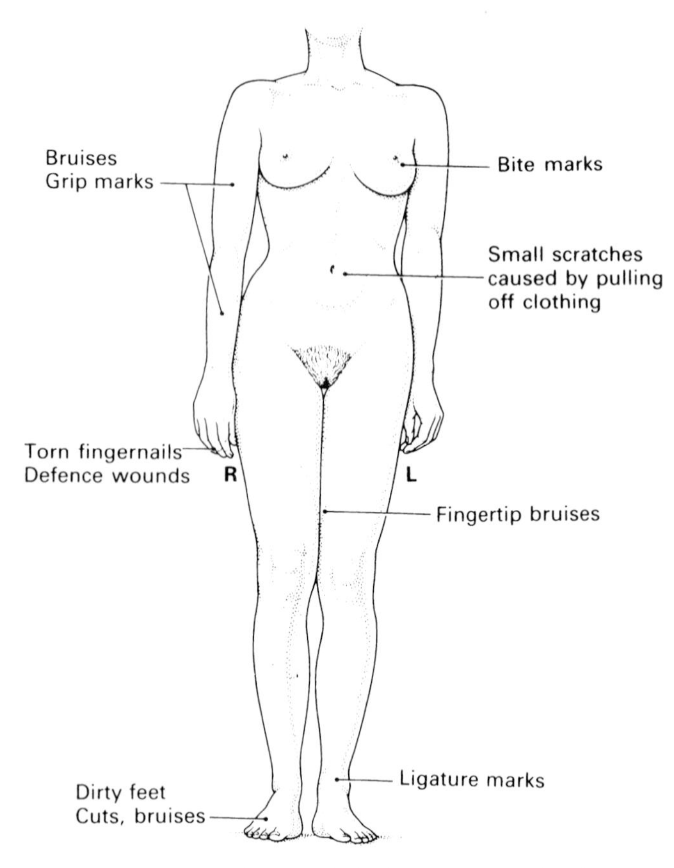

Fig. 60.6 The signs of injury to the body which may be found following sexual assaults.

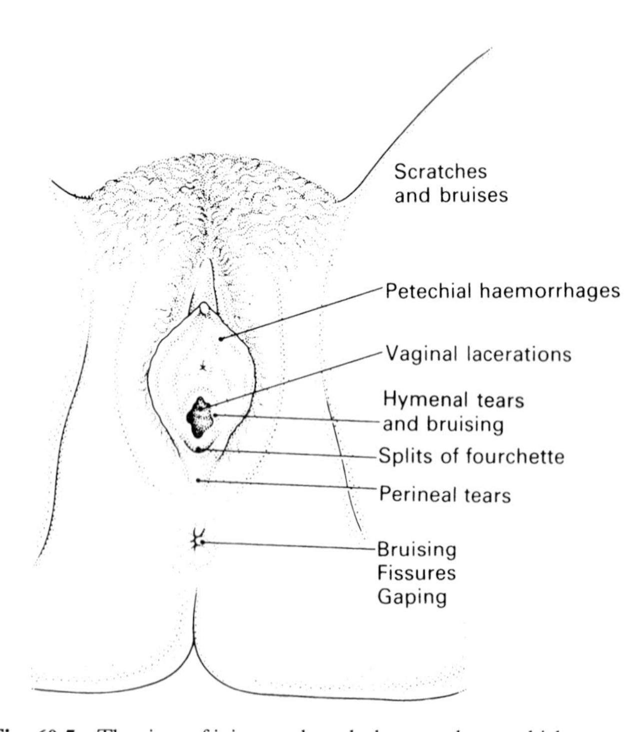

Fig. 60.7 The signs of injury to the vulval area and anus which may be found following sexual assaults.

Forensic samples

The doctor must record exactly how samples were obtained, their labelling, sample number and sealing, and to whom they were handed. Also the times when vaginal swabs, preserved blood and urine samples were taken should be recorded.

The forensic samples fall into two categories: evidential samples and control samples (hair, blood and saliva) for comparison purposes. The usefulness of evidential samples will depend not only on the nature of the indecent acts but also on the time since the assault and the woman's actions subsequently.

Time limits for the survival and detection of spermatozoa and seminal fluid from the vagina, anus and mouth and on unwashed clothing and bedding are given in Table 60.1.

Taking the specimens

Clothing. Complainants should stand on a sheet of paper when undressing so that any debris which falls can be collected. The paper should be folded and retained as a sample. Place each item of clothing in a separate paper bag as it is removed. Secure obvious tufts of fibres in place with clear adhesive tape.

Skin swabs. Skin should be swabbed with a slightly moistened swab (water not saline): use an ampoule of sterile water.

1. For blood, if and where seen.
2. For semen, from areas where assailant ejaculated or wiped his penis.
3. For saliva, from areas licked, bitten or spat upon.

A control swab should be taken from an unstained area of skin.

Mouth swab and saliva sample. Swabs from inside the mouth and around the teeth and gums should be taken if oral assault is alleged within the past 24 hours. A liquid saliva sample (10 ml) should also be taken.

Fingernail samples. Cuttings should be taken if blood, fibres or other debris are seen.

External vaginal and anal swabs. These should be taken from around the introitus and anal margin. The vulval and anal areas should then be washed and dried.

Low vaginal swab. This should be taken by separating the labia.

Vaginal examination. A warmed, moistened (but not lubricated) small disposable speculum should be inserted and the walls inspected for injury. Take one or more high vaginal swabs from above the speculum. If a pool of fluid is present, use a pipette to obtain a larger sample. Take an endocervical swab.

Internal anal swab. If buggery is alleged, take internal anal swabs using a small disposable proctoscope. It is

Table 60.1 Time limits for the detection of spermatozoa and seminal fluid

	Spermatozoa	Reference	Seminal fluid	Reference
Vagina	6 days	Davies and Wilson (1974)	12–18 h	Davies and Wilson (1974)
Anus	65 hours	Willott and Allard (1982)	3 h	MPFSI* unpublished
Mouth	21 h	Davies (1986)	–	
Clothing/bedding	Until washed	–	Until washed	–

*Metropolitan Police Forensic Science Laboratory, London

usually not possible to insert a proctoscope without a lubricant. Take swabs from above the proctoscope to ensure that they are not contaminated. Vaginal swabs must be taken in all suspected buggery cases to establish whether semen found on anal swabs could have drained from the vagina.

Hair samples. Comb the pubic hairs for debris and loose hairs which could have come from the assailant. Cut about 10 pubic hairs close to the skin as a control sample. Similarly, take head hair combings and at least 10 pulled hairs from different parts of the head.

Blood samples. Two blood samples are required, one with preservative (sodium fluoride) and anticoagulant (potassium oxalate) for alcohol assay and one with ethylenediaminetetraacetic acid for grouping and DNA profiling.

Urine samples. If drugs are thought to have been involved in the assault, a urine sample should be taken.

Dirt and debris. Swab any areas of dirt or debris.

Control. An unused control swab should be included with the specimens and a sample of any lubricant used.

Labelling and sealing specimens

Label each specimen with the following:

1. Name of the patient.
2. Date taken.
3. Person taking sample.
4. Type of sample.
5. Sample number.

The accepted way to number samples incorporates the doctor's initials followed by the number of the specimen, e.g. ABC/1 saliva sample; ABC/2 mouth swab.

It is most important to be able to confirm in court that specimens were transferred intact between the doctor and the forensic scientist. Police forces issue individual sealing instructions, all of which are basically as follows. After labelling, the container or bag is fastened with clear adhesive tape. Freezer tape should be used for blood, urine and saliva bottles, swabs and any other items to be refrigerated or frozen. The tape must be wound completely around the neck of bottles and swab caps. When sealing bags the top should be turned over at least 2.5 cm, turned overagain and fastened with a strip of adhesive tape sufficiently long for the free ends to be fastened to the reverse of the bag. Many police forces are introducing specially manufactured tamperproof bags which incorporate a court label in the self-adhesive flap of the bag.

If a woman police officer is present during the examination she will often label and seal specimens as they are taken by the doctor.

Storage of items

Forensic specimens can be stored for months or years in a freezer and used as evidence later if properly packaged and identified.

The following can be frozen:

1. Swabs.
2. Saliva samples.
3. Preserved blood for solvent analysis.

The following should be refrigerated:

1. Preserved blood for drugs/alcohol assay.
2. Blood for grouping and DNA profiling (short term; for long-term storage freeze the specimen).
3. Urine samples.
4. Fingernail cuttings.

The following should be kept at room temperature:

1. Clothing.
2. Hair samples.

Sexually transmitted diseases

After the forensic specimens have been taken swabs should be taken for sexually transmitted diseases, not because one would expect to find evidence of disease which had been transmitted in a recent rape, but for the medical care of the woman. A high vaginal swab for *Trichomonas,* endocervical swabs for gonococci and *Chlamydia,* and urethral, anal and oral swabs can easily be taken and placed in the appropriate transport media.

Follow-up is essential and a thorough sexually transmitted disease screening should be carried out about 7 days later. The question of human immunodeficiency virus infection should be thoroughly considered and discussed at that stage.

Women are increasingly expressing worries about HIV and if they raise the matter it should be discussed at the initial examination, but it is probably better for the doctor not to bring up the subject while the patient is in a state of shock, when she might seriously misinterpret what the doctor has said and worry unnecessarily about whether she has been infected. It is appropriate to advise that the likelihood of infection from a rape is very small (Lacey 1990).

Pregnancy

The question of pregnancy must be discussed and appropriate measures taken. Oral postcoital contraception should be offered if within 72 hours of the attack, or the insertion of a coil should be considered if less than 5 days has elapsed.

Reassurance

Finally, some time should be spent discussing the medical findings and problems.

In ideal circumstances a trained rape counsellor will take over the support of the complainant and trained sympathetic police officers will continue the investigation.

Long-term psychological counselling

To be subjected to sexual assault can be one of life's most traumatic experiences. It forces women to question themselves and their world because it destroys their sense of trust and their sense of control over their lives. The guilt and shame at having been raped are already apparent when women are seen shortly after the offence.

Women often feel guilty about not having struggled or resisted, and it is all too easy for family, friends and professionals such as doctors and police officers to give the impression that not enough was done to avoid being raped.

The degree of psychological trauma is not proportional to the physical injuries sustained, and may even be greater in those who are given the impression that they should have done more to prevent the assault than in those who have injuries.

It is important to reassure the woman that the responsibility lies with the offender, whatever the circumstances.

In the few weeks following the attack severe emotional reactions are common and may necessitate medical help. Many women seek some form of help during the early weeks but may not be able to talk about the real problem. In a hospital clinic they may tell a sympathetic nurse what has really happened, but be unable to tell the doctor. Patients in trouble will offer the doctor a physical complaint such as vague pelvic pain, when the real trouble is too painful to discuss.

Rape trauma

Rape trauma was described by Burgess and Holstrom (1974). It is a post-traumatic stress disorder. The essential feature is the development of characteristic symptoms following a psychologically distressing event outside the range of normal experience, which at the time was accompanied by feelings of intense fear, terror and helplessness.

Symptoms include:

1. Re-experiencing the traumatic event.
2. Avoidance of stimuli associated with the event.
3. Numbing of general responsiveness.
4. Increased arousal.

A prevailing myth about women who have been raped is that they are hysterical and tearful. Many are in a state of shock and disbelief, but may appear to be acting normally, even unconcernedly, and may describe what has occurred in an almost matter-of-fact way. A woman who is used to dealing with strangers, for example a business executive, may present her story in a detached way as though she were dealing with customers.

Women who initially present in a state of shock and appear to be in control will often break down a few days later and become very distressed.

The detailed medical examination does not usually cause distress when conducted immediately after an assault, but if it is carried out a few days later the intimate part of the examination may be very upsetting, and the sensation of the genitalia being touched for the first time since the assault may produce a flashback of the feelings experienced at the time.

Emotional reactions commonly include shame, guilt and self-blame. Some women become very angry and wish for revenge. Perceived lack of concern as well as insensitive remarks will cause disproportionate upset in the traumatized woman. Thoughts continually return to the circumstances of the rape, and the event is relived many times.

Sleep pattern disturbances are common. Difficulty in getting to sleep, waking in the night and nightmares may occur. Eating disorders may also be experienced, but are less common.

Physical symptoms specific to the areas which have been injured may be present, but psychosomatic symptoms related to these may occur later.

Complaints of vaginal soreness, discharge and menstrual irregularities will commonly lead to the woman seeking help.

The long-term effect

Women may appear to have recovered from the attack and be functioning well, only to be set back by situations of stress.

The woman who has been raped will never be quite the same again. She may recover, become a 'survivor' and even be stronger and more able to cope with adversity afterwards, or may be permanently psychologically scarred or disabled by the experience.

A number of factors will influence the outcome:

1. Previous personality, including previous experience of child abuse or rape.
2. The family circumstances and people available for support. Unsupported single women living alone in a large city will find coping much more difficult than those with a supportive family and friends.
3. The way the problem is handled by police officers, medical practitioners, hospital staff and the courts.
4. Those who receive psychological help such as counselling, ideally from trained rape counsellors but also from lay counsellors such as those in victim support schemes or from ministers of religion, are generally thought to recover better than those who do not receive such help. Nurses in gynaecology clinics and casualty departments can be of great help.

Physical symptoms may present years after the rape. Sexual dysfunction is common; fears and phobias may develop. Women become afraid of going out, sleeping alone or going in lifts, and may be unable to stay in their own home if that is where the rape occurred. Many women will move to a different town after the rape.

The partners and family of the woman who has been raped also suffer considerable stress. Parents and husbands may, after initially being supportive, start to blame the woman and, when the rape trauma symptoms persist, become impatient with the continuing disruption of their lives.

Counselling

Where a rape is reported immediately, crisis intervention is indicated. Comfort and support, with a caring attitude being shown, are more important at this stage than specific counselling skills. It is important not to appear to be judgemental or critical.

Those who have been raped in the past may develop psychiatric conditions such as depression, suicidal behaviour, drinking or drug abuse, and will need appropriate professional help for these problems.

The woman who has not reported the rape to anyone may present with severe psychological problems and with complex physical and gynaecological disorders.

We do not know how many people have been raped in the past and have not sought help, and yet have coped and lived effective and reasonably happy lives. Certainly many sexual offences are unreported.

False complaints of rape

Any complaint of rape is a cry for help and the woman making the complaint is in great trouble.

It is almost impossible for a doctor to be able to tell whether a person is lying or not unless the story is so fanciful as to be incapable of being true, or the details of the alleged rape repeatedly change.

The doctor must be careful not to jump to the conclusion that because the circumstances described are outside his or her experience they must be imagined.

Many complaints of rape are based on fact, but the details have been altered, perhaps to offer what is perceived as being a more acceptable story. Sometimes self-inflicted injuries, such as superficial injuries to the face, breasts and arms, will be added by someone who feels dirty and abused, or who feels that she will not be believed unless she is injured.

Sometimes a stranger may be alleged to have committed the rape when the offender is known but the woman does not want him to go to prison.

A common presentation is for the woman to complain of rape when the real reason for feeling degraded is that buggery or oral sex has occurred.

Many women, even sexually experienced ones, find it impossible to talk about these offences and only during the medical examination, when signs of trauma to the anus are found, may the truth emerge.

Some young women may falsely say that they have been raped because their parents are angry at their late arrival home and may already have rung the police. Sympathetic support and understanding from a specially trained police officer and doctor will usually evaluate these cases relatively easily and speedily, and advice and the prescription of emergency contraception will help to resolve the situation. Many genuine allegations of rape are withdrawn or not proceeded with. This is sometimes because there is insufficient evidence on which to proceed to trial, but in many cases it appears that the complainant is unable to cope with the added stress of giving evidence in court many months later, and prefers to retract the allegation.

CHILD SEXUAL ABUSE

Professionals have become increasingly aware of child sexual abuse in recent years. It is not known whether the incidence is rising, but more cases are being reported. Children are now much more likely to be believed when they tell someone about abuse. Spontaneous statements by children are likely to be true and must be treated very seriously indeed.

Child sexual abuse is any use of children for the sexual gratification of others. Most abusers are male, some of them teenagers and a few of them children, who have usually been abused themselves.

It includes:

1. Exposure, e.g. pornographic photography, exposing children to indecent acts by others in real life or on video.
2. Contact, e.g. indecent fondling of the child, masturbation of adult by child, intercrural intercourse.
3. Penetration, oral, vaginal and anal.
4. Penetration with force.

Full sexual intercourse is unusual before the age of 8 or 9, although buggery may occur in younger children. The commonest offences are those of contact, such as indecent fondling progressing to penile contact without penetration. It is unusual for there to be general physical injuries because the child can be abused by a process of seduction and/or intimidation without the need to use force.

Presentation

The matter may present in a number of ways:

1. A direct or indirect statement from the child.
2. Accidental revelation, e.g. when the child is overheard discussing abusive acts.
3. Perceived abuse, where teachers, social workers or others interpret the child's behaviour as indicating abuse.
4. Physical symptoms, e.g. vulval or anal soreness or discharge.
5. Other maltreatment, where the child is physically abused or fails to thrive.
6. Allegations by others, especially in custody disputes.

Where there is a clear statement by the child, the investigation is relatively straightforward. In the other categories the very greatest caution must be exercised, and a careful multidisciplinary assessment is essential before a conclusion can be reached. Often it will be impossible to be certain and this must be accepted. The assessment and diagnosis will never be 100% correct and errors will be made, in both overdiagnosis and underdiagnosis.

Great emphasis has recently been laid on the amount of undiscovered abuse, but the damaging effect on children and their families of overdiagnosis has not always been appreciated.

Most child sexual abuse takes place within the family or is perpetrated by persons – usually men – who are known to the child. Stranger abuse and rape are much less common.

Where a child has recently been raped the forensic investigation will be carried out as for the adult woman. In some cases an examination under anaesthetic will be necessary. The careful gathering of forensic evidence and the recording of injuries are vital.

It may be helpful for joint examinations to be carried out by a forensic examiner and a paediatrician or gynaecologist. This is particularly important where neither doctor has a wealth of experience in child abuse investigations.

Most child sexual abuse does not present as an emergency. It has usually been going on for some time and is escalating in its intrusiveness.

It is important to assure the child that no blame attaches to her, either for allowing or taking part in the abuse, or for not reporting at the outset. It is very difficult for a child, for example in a family where a new stepfather pays her special attention and gives treats, to complain if, when bathing her or putting her to bed, he touches her genitals 'accidentally'. Only when it becomes well outside the range of normal behaviour (and this can be difficult for a child to know) will she tell someone. The child may retract the story when she discovers how seriously the matter is viewed and realizes what the consequences of her disclosure may be. The child and her family must be treated with care and consideration, whatever has happened. Remember that if an allegation of child sexual abuse is made the consequences for the family may be catastrophic, and the mother may see her whole world collapsing about her. Factors which may indicate child sexual abuse are:

1. Change in behaviour, e.g. clinging, irritability, quietness.
2. Regression, e.g. wetting and soiling.
3. Sleep disturbance and nightmares.
4. Poor school performance.
5. Sexualized behaviour.
6. Running away from home.
7. Self-mutilation and parasuicide.
8. Appetite disorders.
9. Drug abuse.
10. Promiscuity.

It is important to remember that there are many other causes of such problems. Medical problems which may indicate child sexual abuse:

1. Recurrent vulval soreness or discharge.
2. Urinary symptoms without infection.
3. Vague complaints, such as abdominal pain.
4. Infections, e.g. gonorrhoea, *Trichomonas*, *Chlamydia*, condylomata acuminata.
5. Signs of injury to genitalia or anus.
6. Pregnancy.

A teenage girl may present with vague gynaecological problems or may ask to go on the pill. Sexual abuse should be suspected if the girl seems evasive or unhappy and is not able to talk about her problem or say who her sexual partner is. Some complaints of rape are masked presentations of child sexual abuse. Injuries to the genitalia may be claimed to be accidental when they are due to abuse.

Medical examination

The medical examination is only one part of the investigation of child sexual abuse. In all cases a careful multidisciplinary approach is essential, with information from a number of professionals being pooled. The findings can only be evaluated in the context of a full assessment, including careful inquiry about family habits and social patterns. It is rarely possible to make a diagnosis on the medical findings alone. Only the presence of semen or pregnancy can prove with certainty that abuse has occurred. If paternity is the issue, e.g. in a suspected incestuous relationship, the police may well ask for release of the fetus for DNA profiling studies if there is a termination.

The child may be referred for medical examination because she has said that abuse has occurred, or because there is medical concern.

It is important that any medical examination does not constitute an abuse of the child. If no penetration has occurred the child may perceive the medical examination as being worse than the alleged abuse. In many cases a careful and thorough inspection, without any touching, may be all that is indicated.

The use of a colposcope enables a detailed but non-intrusive examination to be carried out, and the taking of standard photographs incorporating date recording and a scale should obviate the need for repeated examinations of children. Peer review and second opinions can be obtained and provide more reliable evidence for the courts than has been available hitherto. Where there is no forensic urgency the examination should be arranged for a convenient time within the next few days, but the anxieties of the parents and child and the need for the police to have as much information as possible before they interview the alleged perpetrator indicate that it should be carried out as expeditiously as possible.

The examination should be conducted in quiet, private surroundings and not behind curtains in a busy casualty department.

The child should be treated with consideration and respect. She should be told what is to happen and invited to help. A full general examination should be carried out, both to let the child settle down and to find any general injuries or abnormalities. Height and weight, the state of nutrition and general paediatric information should be recorded.

The behaviour of the child should be noted and the apparent relationship with the parent observed and recorded.

The preschool child is usually most easily examined on the mother's knee, though some will happily lie on the examination couch. A better view of the hymen can often be obtained with the child in the knee–chest position with its bottom in the air. Children often prefer to be examined in this way, as they find it less embarrassing. Older children may wish to be examined without the parent present, but the parent or carer must stay nearby.

Medical findings which may indicate abuse

In many children who have been sexually abused there will be no medical findings. The absence of signs of recent or healed injuries does not negate the allegation or suspicion. Possible findings in the vulval and anal areas are shown in Figure 60.8 (Bays & Chadwick, 1993).

General injuries

There may be signs of previous non-accidental injury or neglect. Bruises, particularly grip marks on the lower face, the arms or legs or over the pelvis, may be seen. Inside the mouth the frenulum may be torn, bruising may be seen inside the cheeks where the face has been gripped, or there may be patchy petechial haemorrhages on the roof of the mouth caused by forceful insertion of the penis. Love bites caused by sucking and tongue pressure are unusual in children, but true bite marks may be found occasionally.

The vulval area

Rubbing and fondling of the genitalia may cause patchy or general redness, and occasionally the skin over the clitoris may be reddened and swollen.

Pushing the penis against the genital area may cause stretching and slight tearing of the hymen. Small splits of

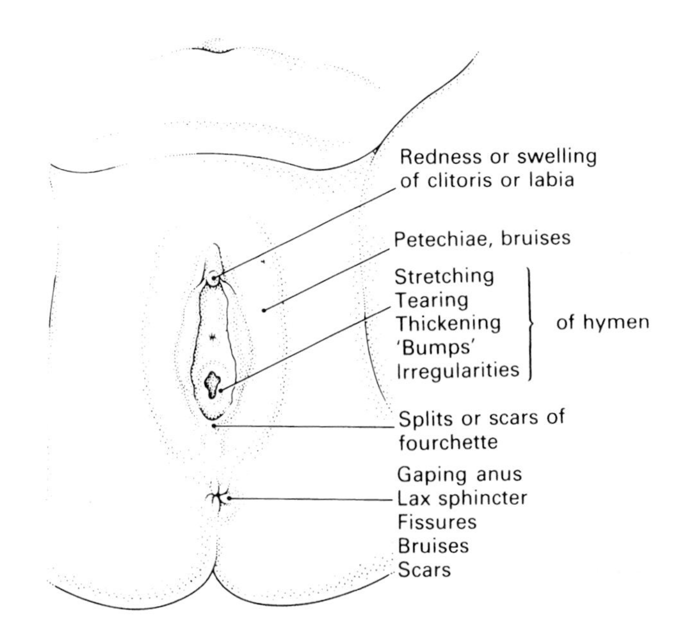

Fig. 60.8 The signs of injury to the vulval area and anus which may be found following child sexual abuse.

the fourchette may be seen, or may heal leaving fine scars, but scarring is not invariable. Friability of the fourchette may occur with non-specific vulvitis as well as with abuse.

The introitus may become stretched and widened by repeated rubbing without there being any tears in the hymen. Care must be taken to distinguish a prominent vestibule from the hymenal opening.

Labial adhesion may sometimes be caused by rubbing which has been sufficient to produce superficial trauma, causing the edges to stick together as they heal, but adhesions are common, associated with low oestrogen status, and are usually innocent.

The area surrounding the urethra may show bruising or petechial haemorrhages when pressure has been exerted there, but it is unusual to find tears of the hymen in the anterior part because the urethra supports and buttresses it. Errors have occurred in mistaking a normal crescentic hymen for tears.

Hymen

As the child relaxes the hymenal orifice will often open up. Its apparent size will vary with the position of the child, the degree of relaxation and the techniques used.

Diameters are usually larger when the child is examined in the knee–chest position. In this position apparent tears, folds and irregularities often smooth out and disappear as the hymen falls forward.

Particular attention should be paid to the posterior half of the hymen, where tears are commonly found and where the width of hymenal tissue present may be reduced by trauma such as rubbing.

If there is still doubt as to whether any tears are present then consideration should be given to using a small glass probe, which can be gently inserted behind the hymen to display its edge.

Slight bumps and notches in the hymen, especially in the anterior part, are now considered to be of less significance than previously, having been observed commonly in children not thought to have been abused (Kerns 1992). There is also less emphasis on the value of measurements of the hymenal orifice, as it becomes apparent that not only does it vary greatly from minute to minute in the same child, but also that there is a considerable degree of overlap between abused and non-abused girls. Great caution should be exercised before ascribing slight variations to abuse.

In young children no attempt should be made to insert a finger into the vagina, but in older girls who are alleging full penetration a finger should be gently placed against the introitus and very gently introduced into the vagina if there is room. Using one finger a good estimate can be obtained of the size of the hymenal orifice, whether the hymenal ring is completely disrupted and whether the vagina has the characteristic roomy smoothed feel which occurs with repeated sexual intercourse. It may be that all that can be said, however, is that either there is or is not room for an object the size of an erect penis to have been inserted. It is often impossible for a doctor to say whether sexual intercourse has or has not occurred (Underhill & Dewhurst 1978).

The anus

The anus should be inspected and the presence of fissures, bruises or scars noted.

Anal dilatation is not usually present unless the examination is carried out within days of the offence, but may occur in unabused children, particularly when there is stool in the rectum. It has proved to be unreliable and misleading as a sign of buggery.

In most cases where buggery has occurred, there will be no medical findings (Heger et al 1992).

Differential diagnosis

Many children are referred to paediatricians and gynaecologists because of vulval soreness or discharge. Some of them have been sexually abused but many have not. During the examination the child can be asked what made her sore and will sometimes make a spontaneous disclosure of abuse. If this occurs the questions, as well as the answers, should be recorded. Care must be taken to avoid leading questions which suggest the answer, and the doctor should not interview the child in depth.

Accidental injuries caused by falling astride bicycle crossbars and other hard objects are common. Usually there is bruising of the outer vulval area, and sometimes splits are seen between the labia minora and majora. The hymen is not damaged in this type of accident but occasionally may be torn if there is a shearing force, such as that caused by being run over by a car wheel, or if there is a fall on to a sharp object. The findings should be entirely consistent with the history given. The ordinary principles of medicine should apply to this subject as to any other, and investigations should be completed before a diagnosis is made. Table 60.2 shows the various conditions which may lead to a mistaken diagnosis of sexual abuse.

Reassurance

After the examination, with the child dressed, the doctor should spend some time talking to both the child and the carers about the examination and findings. Children who have been sexually abused feel guilty and blame themselves for what has happened, and it is important for the doctor, as well as for other investigators, to reassure the child that it is not her fault.

Children often feel that they have been seriously physically damaged and will not be able to grow up normally

Table 60.2 Vulval conditions which have been mistaken for sexual abuse (Bays & Jenny, 1990)

Congenital variations of normal
Cribriform hymen
Crescentic hymen (tears described at 10 o'clock and 2 o'clock)
Midline raphe in fourchette
Traumatic
Straddle injury – usually anterior unilateral
Splits injury
Infective
Non-specific vulvitis
Moniliasis
Streptococcal cellulitis
Dermatological
Seborrhoeic dermatitis
Psoriasis
Lichen sclerosus et atrophicus
Warts
Other
Urethral caruncle
Urethral prolapse

and have babies. A few minutes spent reassuring the child that whatever has occurred, nothing which has happened in the past need affect her future health.

Counselling

At present, services for sexually abused children are patchy and variable. Local authority and voluntary sector social workers are becoming more aware of the problem and training is improving. Long-term counselling for families, including the perpetrator, and for the child may be needed. In some areas treatment programmes under the jurisdiction of the court may be available, such as those of Giaretto et al (1978) in California. Incest survivor groups can often be helpful, provided that their members have come to terms with their own problems.

In many places there will be little, if any, satisfactory long-term help and the damaging effect of child sexual abuse, with its consequences of poor self-image and a failure of the abused person to reach her potential in life, will be apparent for many years and will leave scars not only on the victim, but on her family and friends.

How the problem is handled in the first 48 hours after the matter comes to light, and in particular the therapeutic effect of skilled and sympathetic medical intervention, can do a great deal to minimize these effects and to ensure that the child does not become a permanent loser in life.

INVESTIGATIONS

Laboratory examinations and interpretation of results

The laboratory examination (Keating 1988a, b) is based on Locard's exchange principle 'that every contact leaves a trace' (Locard 1928). The evidential trace materials are of two types: loose debris and stains.

The examination seeks to investigate possible links between the suspect, the victim, the scene of the assault (e.g. child's bed) and items used in the assault (e.g. a bottle neck or broom handle which may have been forced into the vagina or anus).

The materials examined will include those gathered by police investigators in addition to samples taken by doctors examining both victims and suspects.

The amount of evidence detected will depend on the nature of the assault, the time interval since it happened, and subsequent handling of evidential materials, e.g. seminal stains on underwear may have been removed by washing.

The scientific examination may also concern the analysis of preserved blood and urine samples for alcohol, drugs and solvents.

In sexual assaults the most useful materials evidentially are:

1. Semen, blood, saliva, vaginal fluid, lubricants, faeces and urine detected as stains on swabs, clothing, bedding, carpets, etc.
2. Textile fibres, hairs and vegetation detected as loose debris in body samples and on clothing and bedding.
3. Drugs, alcohol and solvents detected in blood and urine samples.

The examination will involve locating the materials, e.g. invisible semen and saliva stains, their identification and comparison with known control samples to establish their origin, e.g. comparison of a DNA profile from a seminal stain with that obtained from a blood sample from a possible suspect, or pubic hairs removed from a child's mouth with those in a pubic hair sample from the suspected perpetrator.

The trace materials are not usually in a good condition. Stains are often small and mixtures frequently occur. A bloodstained vaginal swab could be examined for semen or an external anal swab for lubricants and semen.

The presence of semen provides the most conclusive evidence of sexual intercourse (but not assault) and the laboratory examination will concentrate on the detection and grouping of any seminal stains on swabs, clothing, bedding, etc. Stains may be identified by the presence of spermatozoa or biochemical constituents of the seminal fluid (including acid phosphatase, choline and prostaglandins). Spermatozoa usually persist for much longer (up to 6 days in the vagina) than the chemical constituents (Davies & Wilson 1974), but may be absent (e.g. naturally or after a vasectomy). The longest time-interval for the detection of spermatozoa on anal and rectal swabs is 46 and 65 hours, respectively (Willott & Allard 1982) and from the mouth 21 hours (Davies 1986). It is possible to detect spermatozoa and seminal fluid in stains on unwashed clothing and bedding for many months after the assault.

In an allegation of buggery, anal swabs from a victim should be examined in conjunction with vaginal swabs.

The finding of semen on anal swabs is indicative of buggery only when there is no semen on the vaginal swabs.

Many stains contain relatively large quantities of vaginal material and few spermatozoa. Treatment of stains with a proteinase (to digest epithelial cells) greatly improves the chances of detecting the relatively few spermatozoa present (Chapman et al 1989).

Assay of acid phosphatase activity using *p*-nitrophenyl phosphate as substrate is used to provide more certainty of the presence of seminal fluid on vaginal swabs in the absence of spermatozoa, and for estimation of the time-interval between intercourse and the taking of the swabs in cases where the time of assault is doubtful (Allard & Davies 1978, Davies 1978).

In order to interpret laboratory findings scientists will need to know the exact time when the doctor took the vaginal swabs and preserved blood and urine samples. The laboratory will also require information from the medical examination of the complainant regarding:

1. Previous sexual intercourse (if within 2 weeks of the assault).
2. Contraception on that occasion.
3. Source of any bleeding.
4. Infectious diseases.
5. Current medication.

The advent of DNA profiling and its adaptation for criminal investigations (Gill et al 1985) has made it possible to link seminal stains to a suspect with a high degree of probability.

DNA profiling, also known as genetic fingerprinting or DNA fingerprinting, was originally described by Professor Sir Alec Jeffreys at Leicester University (Jeffreys et al 1985). He discovered that there are hypervariable regions in the DNA structure where the base sequence differs markedly between individuals. Within these hypervariable regions there are short sequences of DNA which are repeated many times, the number of repeats being exactly characteristic of the individual.

These sequences can be visualized by the laboratory process using a radioactive or chemiluminescent DNA probe to reveal a multiple-band pattern on an X-ray film – the DNA profile (Gill et al 1985). In this way, comparison of DNA profiles from the seminal stains can be compared with those of blood samples from suspects. DNA profiling is particularly successful for the elimination of suspects from police enquiries.

DNA profiling is routinely used for seminal stains with a sufficient concentration of spermatozoa. In addition this technique can be used to identify the source of other body fluid stains, such as blood, vaginal fluid, saliva and nasal mucus, provided that they contain sufficient cellular material.

The introduction of DNA profiling initially used multi-locus probes (MLP), but it was found that in the forensic situation many of the samples yielded insufficient DNA for analysis. A new generation of probes, known as single-locus probes (SLP) was then developed and routinely used in forensic examinations. These probes examine the DNA at a single locus and produce a profile of only two bands in any individual. These probes proved particularly useful for the examination of stains containing a mixture of body fluids from more than one person, e.g. a mixture of semen and vaginal fluid on a sheet, or a vaginal swab stained with semen from two or more assailants. Two or more probes can be used sequentially on a single stain to produce, for example, a six-band pattern using three probes.

DNA profiling using both single-locus and multilocus probes is particularly useful in situations of disputed paternity. Successful results can be obtained from fetal material, e.g. after termination in a pregnant teenage girl. In such situations the fetal material is stored frozen until laboratory testing.

DNA profiling using MLP or SLP techniques is not suitable for individualizing seminal stains where there are few or no spermatozoa. The introduction of polymerase chain reaction (PCR) techniques, which enable the small quantity of DNA extracted to replicate until there is sufficient for DNA analysis, has considerably enhanced the range of stains which can be used for DNA analysis. The PCR techniques used most widely for forensic purposes are referred to as STR (short tandem repeat) profiles. The potential also exists using PCR/STR profiling techniques to characterize stains of seminal fluid in which there are no spermatozoa. DNA extracted from epithelial cells present in the seminal fluid can be treated in an exactly similar manner to DNA extracted from a small number of spermatozoa.

The introduction of PCR techniques has reduced the time required to produce a profile to around 1 week. The introduction of further primers for STR typing will greatly enhance the discriminating power of the PCR/STR profiles. This technique has recently been introduced as a routine forensic tool and will provide the basis for a national DNA database to be started in 1995.

Future trends

1. To accumulate further statistics regarding profile frequencies.
2. To accumulate a significant number of entries on a national database of DNA/STR profiles from persons convicted of recordable offences.

COURT PROCEEDINGS

Preparation of the patient for court

It has been said that a woman is raped three times: first by her assailant, secondly by the medical examination and thirdly in the court.

Doctors and police officers are increasingly aware of the problems of raped women and are likely to offer a more understanding and sympathetic approach than has sometimes been the case in the past. The ordeal of giving evidence in court, however, is still considerable, although improved arrangements are now often made to allow witnesses to sit in a private waiting area and to be kept informed at all times of what is happening. A police officer or rape counsellor may take the woman to see the court before the hearing and familiarize her with the procedure.

The period of waiting for the court hearing, which may be many months, can be very stressful, and when the episode has to be relived in the court and the woman's account is perhaps vigorously cross-examined, all the symptoms experienced at the time of the offence may return.

The woman often feels that she is on trial as well as the defendant, and that if he is found not guilty this implies that she is guilty. It is helpful to explain that a criminal trial requires a burden of proof beyond that where there is only the word of one person against another, so that the judge may advise the jury that it is unsafe to convict in such circumstances. This does not mean that she has not been believed.

It is most important for her to be strongly assured that if she tells the truth she has nothing to fear. She can retain her self-respect whether the whole truth comes out in court or not, and whether the defendant is found guilty or not.

When a court case is concluded, whether successfully or not, the woman may suffer an acute episode of stress and, even if under the care of a counsellor, may take an overdose of drugs or need more help.

If the man is convicted she may feel guilt that she has caused him to go to prison. If he is acquitted she may feel that reporting the crime was a waste of time; she may also be afraid of retaliation or revenge from the defendant, or his family or friends.

In the case of child witnesses special arrangements are now made to reduce the stress, but the court proceedings are commonly felt to be the most traumatic event experienced following the disclosure.

Children may now give evidence by live video link or be screened from the alleged perpetrator, and in some countries, including the United Kingdom, prerecorded video evidence is accepted.

At present the legal system appears to safeguard the rights of the defendant but pays insufficient regard to the needs and rights of the aggrieved person. Redressing the balance without removing the inalienable right of the citizen in common law jurisdiction to be regarded innocent until proved guilty is fraught with difficulty.

Presentation of the doctor's evidence (see Ch. 59)

Doctors are often afraid of court and may try to avoid being involved in matters which may require them to give evidence. The subjects of rape and child sexual abuse are distasteful and upsetting, but the people who suffer such violations deserve skilled and professional help. The doctor should not 'pass by on the other side' but should use the skills of medicine and surgery to help.

It is important to remain objective and impartial while offering care and help. It is not possible to remain unaffected by what is seen and heard, but it is important not to become emotionally involved and appear to be biased in favour of the complainant when giving evidence.

The doctor should not try to be a detective or social worker but should approach these problems as any other medical problem, using medical skill and training.

Documentation and reports

Full, clear and legible notes should be made at the time of the examination. The facts that it is important to record in rape examinations have already been listed above. In cases of child abuse the following are essential:

1. The position in which the child was examined.
2. What instruments were used.
3. What the child said during the examination. Record the questions, which should be non-leading, i.e. not suggesting the answer, as well as the answers.

A differential diagnosis should be considered and, if possible, a diagnosis reached. It is important to remember, however, that neither rape nor child sexual abuse is a medical diagnosis, but an opinion should be offered as to whether the findings observed are consistent with the history given, or whether there is another more likely explanation. It is helpful to state whether the findings support the allegation or are neutral as to whether the offence occurred.

The doctor may be called as a professional witness to describe what was found at the time of the examination. Usually, having described the findings, the doctor will be asked to give an opinion as to what may have caused the findings; he then becomes an expert witness.

After the examination-in-chief, which in a criminal trial is usually conducted by counsel for the prosecution, the doctor will be cross-examined by the opposing side. Counsel for the defence is allowed to ask leading questions and can suggest answers to the witness. The doctor should be careful to agree only with that part of the answer which is accurate and not to be led into making statements with which he or she is unhappy.

It is important in giving evidence to keep one's answers simple and as brief as possible. The longer one speaks, the more likely one is to make an error which will be picked up by the opposing counsel.

Before giving evidence in court it is important to read carefully through the notes and refresh one's memory about the case. If there are any points where medical expertise is required, then the appropriate textbooks or journals should be consulted.

Medical evidence is increasingly being challenged in court and medical experts may be retained to advise the defence. It is important to find out a few days before the hearing whether such an expert is involved, and if so to have access to any reports with time to study them carefully before giving evidence.

Always remember that the doctor's task is to assist the court from the basis of his or her special knowledge. If the doctor makes a careful, thorough and unbiased examination at the time, provides thorough and comprehensive notes, refreshes the case thoroughly before giving evidence and, as Bernard Knight (1987) said: 'dresses up, stands up, speaks up and shuts up', there will be nothing to fear.

Truth or the nearest reasonable approach to it that is possible from what is observed is the sole aim. The doctor who properly says he does not know or feels inadequately qualified to advise acquires more respect than one who 'ventures an opinion' (Simpson 1986).

KEY POINTS

1. The frequency of assault on women is unknown.
2. The chances of forensic evidence remaining available are diminished after 48 hours.
3. Careful recording of observations and labelling of samples and specimens are mandatory.
4. It is important to treat the physical and psychological effects of trauma.
5. Most child abuse takes place within the family or by someone known to the child, and usually does not present as an emegency but rather as a chronic situation which has become-worse.
6. In most cases where anal abuse has occurred there will be no medical findings.
7. DNA profiling (genetic fingerprinting) provides great accuracy in detecting source of body fluids, e.g. semen, vaginal fluid, saliva and blood.
8. Single-locus DNA probes are particularly useful when there is disputed paternity.
9. Many women and children will not admit to an assault because of shame and a fear of not being believed.

REFERENCES AND FURTHER READING

Allard J, Davies A 1978 Further information on the use of *p*-nitrophenyl phosphate on vaginal swabs examined in cases of sexual assault. Medicine, Science and the Law 19: 170–172

Bays J, Chadwick D 1993 Medical diagnosis of the sexually abused child. Child Abuse and Neglect 17: 110

Bays J, Jenny C 1990 Genital and anal conditions confused with child sexual abuse trauma. American Journal of Diseases of Children 144: 1319–1322

Burgess A W, Holstrom L L 1974 Rape trauma syndrome. American Journal of Psychiatry 131: 980–986

Chapman R L, Brown N M, Keating S M 1989 The isolation of spermatozoa from sexual assault swabs using proteinase K. Journal of the Forensic Science Society 29: 207–212

Davies A 1978 A preliminary investigation using *p*-nitrophenyl phosphate on vaginal swabs examined in cases of sexual assault. Medicine, Science and the Law 18: 174–178

Davies A 1986 The sexual abuse of children: cases submitted to a police laboratory and the scientific evidence. Medicine, Science and the Law 26: 103–106

Davies A, Wilson E 1974 The persistence of seminal constituents in the human vagina. Forenslc Science 3: 45–55

Giaretto H, Giaretto A, Sgroi S M 1978 In: Sexual assault of children and adolescents. Lexington Books, Lexington, Massachusetts, pp 231–240

Gill P, Jeffreys A J, Werrett D J 1985 Forensic applications of DNA fingerprints. Nature 318: 577–579

Heger A, Emans S J 1992 Evaluation of the sexually abused child. Oxford University Press, Oxford

Jeffreys A J, Wilson V, Thein S L 1985 Individual-specific fingerprints of human DNA. Nature 314: 67–73

Jones D P H 1992 Interviewing the sexually abused child, 2nd edn. Royal College of Psychiatrists, Gaskell, London

Keating S M 1988a The laboratory approach to sexual assault cases. Part I. Sources of information and acts of intercourse. Journal of the Forensic Science Society 28: 35–47

Keating S M 1988b The laboratory approach to sexual assault cases. Part II. Demonstration of the possible offender. Journal of the Forensic Science Society 28: 99–110

Kerns D L et al 1992 Concave hymenal variations in suspected child abuse victims. Pediatrics 90: 265–272

Knight B 1987 Legal aspects of medical practice, 4th edn. Churchill Livingstone, Edinburgh

Lacey H B 1990 Sexually transmitted disease and rape: the experience of a sexual assault centre. International Journal of STD and AIDS 1: 405–409

Locard E 1928 Dust and its analysis. Police Journal 1: 177–192

McLay W D S (ed) 1990 Clinical forensic medicine. Association of Police Surgeons

Mant A K (ed) 1984 Taylor's principles and practice of medical jurisprudence, 13th edn. Churchill Livingstone, Edinburgh

Meadow R (ed) 1993 ABC of child abuse. 2nd edn. British Medical Journal, London

Pierce A M, Robson W J 1993 Genital injury in girls – accidental or not? Paediatric Surgery International 8: 239–243

Simpson K 1986 Textbook of forensic medicine, 9th edn. Edward Arnold, London

Solola A, Scott C, Severs H, Howell J 1983 Rape: Management in an institutional setting. Obstetrics and Gynaecology 61(3): 373–377

Underhill R, Dewhurst C J 1978 The doctor cannot always tell. Medical examination of the 'intact' hymen. Lancet 1: 375

Willott G M, Allard J E 1982 Spermatozoa – their persistence after sexual intercourse. Forensic Science International 19: 135–154

61

Medical ethics

John Friend

ETHICAL CONCEPTS

Hippocrates, like his father and grandfather, was an itinerant healer practising his craft from 'surgeries' while travelling from city to city. His nurses and assistants were bound by an agreement or oath which acted as a code of practice. The oldest available version is from the 10th century AD and resides in the Vatican library (Reiss 1994).

The classic Hippocratic Oath has been displaced over the years by more modern versions, such as the Declaration of Geneva from which evolved the International Code of Medical Ethics. Although the large majority of medical schools in the United States use some form of medical oath it is relatively uncommon on this side of the Atlantic.

The Hippocratic Oath includes the statement: 'I will follow that system of regimen which, according to my ability and judgement, I consider for the benefit of my patients, and abstain from whatever is deleterious and mischievous'. This and other sentiments within the Oath underpin the ethical concepts governing medical practice (BMA 1993).

Ethics is concerned with the problems of action as they exist. The conduct of that action is determined by acceptance of certain principles. Whatever the individual philosophy, politics, religion or other beliefs, there is widespread acceptance of the four main principles: respect for autonomy, beneficence, non-maleficence and justice. Each principle is binding unless in conflict with another moral principle. In this case a choice has to be made (Gillon 1994).

Individual autonomy

Competent people are entitled to make their own decisions on the basis of deliberation as to how they lead their lives, particularly with respect to their bodies and fundamental commitments such as health, family, sexuality and work. This freedom for self-determination is only limited if others are harmed, forced or coerced, or if social stability is undermined. Where any individual or group of individuals is unable to manage the consequences of autonomous decision making, e.g. the very young, disabled or mentally handicapped, then society has a responsibility to protect the vulnerable.

Beneficence and non-maleficence

We have an obligation to practise medicine to the overall benefit of the patient. In professing benefit we need to have the appropriate education and training in order to be in a position to provide beneficial advice and management. We must explain the advantages and disadvantages, and weigh them up so that the result is net benefit and not harm. The information for giving weight to various probabilities comes from effective medical research.

Justice

This can be summarized as the moral obligation to act on

a basis of fairness between competing claims. The persistent question of prioritizing effective medical care within a limited budget is entirely a debate on the fair distribution of scarce resources.

Justice includes a respect for patients' rights. There should, for example, be no reason for personal disapproval of a patient's attitude or lifestyle in deciding the appropriate management. We must try to exclude decisions that have no moral status or justification.

It is not always possible to arrive at a decision between doctor and patient in isolation, as they can impinge on other people. Organizations such as hospital trusts and purchasing health authorities may issue protocols, and indeed society makes its own constraints in the form of statute law. Although our own ethical view might not be entirely coincident with a particular aspect of the law, we are obliged to practise medicine within the law. Indeed, the fact that laws in this country are enacted through a democratic political system which fundamentally respects autonomy and is based on common moral principles, should make that law morally acceptable.

Although the above four principles have been called the 'prima facie' principles (Gillon 1994) there are many subtle strands that flow from them. For example, every member of society is entitled to equal concern and respect, and each life is equally valuable. In the same context, all forms of human life and human tissues should be treated with appropriate respect and sensitivity. Before birth the embryo and fetus do not have 'person' status within the law, and yet they have individual person potential and should be accorded the respect of this status.

In making a judgement in any situation the doctor will rely heavily on not only his medical training but also his developed traits of common sense, a sense of caring, conscience and pragmatism.

Today's young doctors not only have to make ethical decisions in relation to the doctor–patient relationship, but they are also involved in management and organizational decisions. There are many aspects of the organization which are constantly changing and about which each doctor has to come to a conclusion. For example, in the constant search for more efficient and at the same time improved training programmes, the continuity of care for individual patients is being lost. The shorter hours for junior grades and the constant rotation through different training programmes is seen as the right way forward to produce the next generation of expert doctors. As the senior doctors find more time taken up with audit, contract negotiation, business meetings, training supervision, etc., and as cost efficiency requires more assembly-line medical practice, we must guard against confusion and lack of care for the individual patient. We have to decide whether this type of revolution nurtures the best form of medicine and attitudes of care among health workers (Weatherall 1994).

Informed consent

This is a process whereby the knowledgeable professional shares information with the interested patient through effective communication. Its purpose is to make sure that patients are informed; it is not to protect doctors. It is an ethical requirement for medical treatment and participation in medical research.

The information must be factual, adequate for the circumstances and understood, so that the patient can make a reasoned decision.

The consent must be free, which implies the possibility of choosing one of several options or indeed the refusal of all proposed courses of action. It also implies a lack of coercion and deception. Ethically it is based on the respect of the patient as a person, and in particular it respects the patient's moral right to bodily integrity and to self-determination. It makes possible the active involvement of the patient by sharing information, decisions and therefore responsibility for action, and this has clear therapeutic benefits.

Clearly there are limits to any patient's individual right to self-determination on account of the wider needs of others and society in general.

For the practising obstetrician and gynaecologist the process of informed consent sometimes lays down obligations that are not always easy to fulfil. There are areas of our practice where research and audit have provided overwhelming evidence in favour of a certain course of action, e.g. surgical treatment for early-stage ovarian cancer, termination of the pregnancy as a means of preventing further eclampsia, and it is not difficult to communicate this information effectively. There are, however, many aspects of our specialty where the evidence is not so clear-cut, e.g. the various strategies for treating menorrhagia, the statistical nightmare for prenatal diagnosis of chromosome abnormalities where the non-definitive tests are non-invasive and the definitive tests have risks for the integrity of the pregnancy. It remains a duty of the doctor not only to provide the available information but to communicate it in such a way that the patient can make a choice on the basis of fact and not fancy.

Informed consent also has a big part to play in the counselling of patients prior to operation. There is an obligation to provide adequate information not only about the intended procedure, but also about complications and further procedures if these are a significant possibility. Lord Scarman, in the Sidaway case (1985), indicated that the amount of information given is not what the medical profession thinks is appropriate but what the individual patient requires, and failing that, it is what the prudent patient would want to know. For example, counselling before surgery for an apparently benign ovarian cyst must include the possible alternative strategies if it is found at operation that there is evidence of local or more widespread malignancy. Clearly, unexpected problems with a very low chance of occurrence would not be covered.

Respect for choice

The justification for the paternalism previously so prominent in practice was that the ethical principle governing medical care was almost entirely focused on the benefit for the patient as seen through the eyes of the physician.

Within the framework of free consent, however, is the respect for persons and therefore respect for the right to choose, although we recognize that there are limits to the patient's right to choose. For example, a patient with a notifiable infectious disease can be forcibly isolated in hospital against her wishes on account of the public interest.

In the evolution of maternity care there has been increasing participation by the pregnant woman in management decisions, and this has been officially encouraged by government (DoH 1993).

The process is almost universally successful, but very occasionally conflict can arise between the pregnant woman and her health care workers. In 1992, in the only legal case of its kind in this country, the evidence suggested that the life of both the mother and the fetus was in grave danger unless a caesarean section was performed. Following an urgent submission to the President of the Family Division a declaration was made that a caesarean section and any necessary consequential treatment which the hospital and its staff proposed to perform on the patient could be lawfully performed, despite the patient's refusal to give her consent, being vital in the interests of the patient and her unborn child.

Following this judgement there was vigorous discussion in the legal journals regarding the validity of the decision, and both the American College of Obstetricians and Gynecologists and the Royal College of Obstetricians and Gynaecologists have now issued guidelines on medico–maternal–fetal conflict (ACOG 1987, RCOG 1994).

ETHICS COMMITTEES

Although ethical decisions in medicine are taken every day at many different levels, there has been an increasing recognition that medical decisions should be ethically based and, as science advances, particularly in the area of reproductive medicine, new dilemmas are constantly being presented. This has spawned many ethics committees with varying functions and based at local, regional and national level.

Local research ethics committees have been set up throughout the country to regulate and monitor any research activity involving patients. Although these began on a voluntary basis they are now a requirement for each health authority. Guidelines from the Department of Health (Norrie 1993) have slowly led to more uniformity in the assessment of research projects. The role of the committees is to protect the public, and although they do not currently have the force of law, indemnity is likely to be dependent on approval by the committee, so that it is difficult to envisage research being performed without such approval.

It has been traditional in the United Kingdom to set up 'ad hoc' committees to consider specific issues of public concern, and legislation or national guidelines often result from their conclusions. For example, the Warnock Committee was set up in 1982 to consider recent and potential developments in human fertilization and embryology, and the Human Fertilization and Embryology Act was subsequently passed in 1990.

Unlike some European countries such as France, the United Kingdom does not have a government-sponsored national ethics committee.

In 1990 the Nuffield Foundation formed a National Bioethics Committee with a highly distinguished membership. Its terms of reference are:

1. To identify ethical questions raised by advances in medical science in order to respond to and anticipate public concern.
2. To promote public understanding and discussion of relevant questions and to formulate new guidelines where necessary.
3. To publish appropriate reports of its work.

This body has produced several important documents for discussion and the results have become national policy, e.g. the place for gene therapy.

Many medical bodies have their own ethics committees which address problems in their own areas of interest, e.g. the Royal Colleges, the BMA and the pharmaceutical industry. Within obstetrics and gynaecology the International Federation of Gynaecology and Obstetrics (FIGO) has a standing committee for the study of the ethical aspects of human reproduction, and this group discusses mutual problems and issues consensus statements with recommendations on specific ethical issues (FIGO 1994).

The Royal College of Obstetricians and Gynaecologists Ethics Committee was promulgated in 1982 with a remit to consider the ethical aspects and legal implication of matters of concern affecting the practice of obstetrics and gynaecology, so that the Council of the College could provide guidelines.

THERAPEUTIC ABORTION

Consideration of pregnancy termination occurs when conception was accidental or unintentional. For example, there may have been a contraceptive failure. About 150 000 unwanted pregnancies each day, or about 53 million a year, are terminated worldwide (Vanlook & von Hertzen 1993).

There are those who object to abortion under any circumstances, for religious or other reasons. They are of course quite entitled to hold and apply this view to themselves, or indeed to canvas their views more widely: in a democratic country any minority group may promote their cause within the law, but cannot expect their view to form the basis of legislation.

Those who consider that abortion is always wrong believe in the sanctity of all human life, starting from the time of conception. They tend to argue that full moral status is achieved at that time and abortion therefore denies the fetus its rights and constitutes a form of murder. They would have similar views regarding contraceptives that interfered with implantation of the early embryo, e.g. intrauterine devices. They believe that the value of human life following fertilization is so great that any danger from the pregnancy and delivery would remain insignificant. From this position there is no reason for considering abortion for even severe fetal abnormality. Indeed, many feel that abortion on these grounds encourages prejudice against handicapped persons and raises questions over what is and what is not normal.

A second view would permit therapeutic abortion in circumstances where the mother was likely to die if the pregnancy continued. Examples in line with this position include a woman with Eisenmenger's syndrome who has a high chance of dying in pregnancy, or where necessary treatment of a maternal cancer requires the sacrifice or premature delivery of a fetus. This view holds that the moral status or rights of the embryo and fetus are not sufficient to overwhelm those of the mother.

Some people believe that the embryo starts off with very limited rights or status but that these develop during pregnancy, reaching full personhood at the time of birth. In this context abortion which might be acceptable in early pregnancy could be unacceptable towards term. The current law follows this argument to some degree.

The liberal view on abortion does not recognize that the embryo or fetus has rights compared with the woman's rights to decide control over her own body. Under these circumstances a woman still wishing termination of pregnancy following appropriate counselling into the risks associated with the procedure would be offered an abortion. Utilitarians might argue that the abortion decision must depend on the optimal outcome for the happiness and normality of the family. Under this heading they would include termination for a fetal abnormality. Difficulties arise in the measurement and acceptance of the degree of abnormality and the subsequent potential quality of life. Suffice it to say that the solution to an unwanted pregnancy will always be less than perfect, and these difficult decisions are never made without a great deal of emotional stress.

The law

In Britain the fundamental legal position is as defined in the Offences against the Persons Act of 1861, which makes it a felony to terminate a pregnancy unlawfully. In the 1938 case of Rex vs. Bourne the judge ruled that abortion need not be unlawful if it is performed in good faith to preserve the mother's life. The provisions of the Abortion Act 1967, which governs England, Wales and Scotland, spell out the circumstances where an abortion may be carried out without breaking the law. Any doctor can register a conscientious objection to performing an abortion, but he or she is under an obligation to provide necessary treatment if the woman's life is at risk.

The House of Lords discussion of the Janaway case (Janaway 1988) made it clear that the conscientious objection in law only applies to the actual participation in the abortion procedure itself, and that the obligation to counsel, make any necessary arrangements, provide a secondary referral, etc., remained.

The grounds for termination of pregnancy are, 'if two registered medical practitioners are of the opinion, formed in good faith':

1. That the continuance of the pregnancy would involve risk to the life of the pregnant woman, or of injury to the physical or mental health of the pregnant woman or any existing children of her family greater than if the pregnancy were terminated.
2. That there is a substantial risk that if the child were born it would suffer such physical or mental abnormalities as to be seriously handicapped.

Account may also be taken of the pregnant woman's actual or reasonably foreseeable environment.

The Human Fertilization and Embryology Act 1990 provides a statutory limit of 24 weeks for inducing abortion, except in cases where the abortion is performed to save the mother's life, prevent grave permanent injury to her physical or mental health, or where there is a substantial risk of serious fetal handicap. In these circumstances the 24-week limit does not apply.

STERILIZATION

In many countries sterilization is an acceptable form of family planning, provided the individual is adequately counselled into the effects of the procedure and the risks of the surgery. No coercion must be applied to the individual concerned. Some people object to sterilization, either for all or just social indications, on religious or other grounds.

In the United Kingdom consent is required only by the individual being sterilized, though it is wise practice to ensure through that individual that the spouse is agreeable to the intended procedure, as that partner has a right of procreation within marriage.

The patient's agreement to the procedure is valid only if adequate information has been provided and understood, and this must include the reversibility of such a procedure. Consent must be voluntary.

There are no great ethical problems thus far. The main difficulty arises where individuals are not capable of understanding the implications of sterilization. It remains important to respect the autonomy of individuals who have degrees of mental handicap and learning disabilities. If, in the doctor's opinion, the adult patient is unable to understand the full implications of the procedure, then that patient is unable to give consent.

There is no provision in the Mental Health Act 1983 or elsewhere for an appropriate person, such as a nearest relative, to consent to such treatment on behalf of an adult under these conditions.

The case of *Re F.* (1990) concerned the sterilization of an adult with arrested mental development. The House of Lords ruled that the common law allows a doctor to give medical or surgical treatment, e.g. hysterectomy for menorrhagia, to an adult patient who is incapable of consenting only when it is in the patient's own 'best interests'. Thus the action must intend to prevent any deterioration or ensure improvement in the patient's physical or mental health.

This decision allows doctors to treat patients who are incapable of giving consent without recourse to the courts in most circumstances, and indeed doctors may have a common law duty to provide necessary treatment for adults who cannot consent. Sterilization for therapeutic reasons is included in this category.

At times there is a difficulty in defining therapeutic and non-therapeutic indications, and many people remain concerned that individuals with disabilities are being sterilized wrongly without judicial review.

Where the intervention proposed is sterilization for non-therapeutic purposes it is recommended that an application is made to the court. These proceedings are designed to establish that the operation is lawful and is in the patient's interests, rather than those of the applicants, relatives or carers, or at the public's convenience. The Official Solicitor has detailed a recommended procedure (BMA 1992).

Sterilization of a minor to prevent pregnancy falls within a special category. The Official Solicitor advises that the sterilization of a minor, whether they are capable of consenting or not, will require the prior sanction of the court whatever the parents', or indeed the minor's, wishes. This advice embodies good practice but is not law. If such treatment is proposed for a minor an application should be made to the court within the wardship jurisdiction for leave to carry it out (BMA 1992).

CONTRACEPTION AND YOUNG PEOPLE

In 1992 the Secretary of State for Health published a document entitled *The Health of the Nation*, which included objectives and targets (DHSS 1992). One of the key aims was to reduce the incidence of sexually transmitted disease and teenage pregnancies. The specific target in relation to the latter was to reduce the rate of conception among the under 16s by at least 50% by the year 2000 (from 9.5 per 1000 girls aged 13–15 in 1989 to no more than 4.8). The strategy to achieve this target must include the dissemination of information regarding sex education and contraception by various groups of teachers and health care workers, and much greater accessibility to both the information and the contraception.

Contraception includes pre- and postcoital methods, such as oestrogens and/or progestogens, given in different ways, as well as intrauterine devices. These and other drugs are now available and can be used in ways that prevent the establishment of a pregnancy following fertilization. Some doctors and patients may feel uneasy about the use of methods which in their view cause abortion. Others will argue that conception is a process which includes fertilization and implantation, and the prevention of implantation is not therefore abortion. This view is supported by the British Council of Churches, which has stated that 'a woman cannot abort until the fertilized egg has nidated and thus become attached to her body' (British Council of Churches 1962).

There may be both ethical and legal problems in providing contraception to the under-16 age group. Minors who seek contraception are usually sexually active or intending to start a sexual relationship. Most young people today know about contraception but may well not understand the full implications of the treatment. It is obviously important that health care workers should provide full and appropriate counselling in such cases where the patient understands the treatment being provided, informed consent is obtained and autonomy is respected. In counselling an underage girl it is always advisable to persuade her to involve one of her parents or a guardian at an early stage in the consultation. With full understanding by the minor and agreement of all the parties involved there is little ethical difficulty in providing contraception in these circumstances.

If the patient refuses parental involvement then the BMA recommends that the patient's autonomy should be respected and confidentiality should be maintained unless there are very exceptional circumstances for disclosing information without consent, e.g. in cases where there is sexual exploitation or abuse (Gillick 1985).

In such very exceptional circumstances the doctor's duty may lie in protection of the patient, which might best be achieved through a breach of confidentiality. It is possible that with supportive counselling the patient may agree to disclosure.

CONSENT TO CONTRACEPTION AND ABORTION

In 1982 Mrs Gillick wanted the health authority to instruct doctors not to give contraceptive or abortion advice or treatment to any of her daughters without parental consent, and in contradiction to DHSS advice. Subsequently in 1985 the House of Lords ruled that patients under 16 can legally consent to therapeutic treatment without reference to their parents or guardian. In deciding whether to prescribe contraception the following recommendations should be taken into account (Gillick 1985):

1. Whether the patient understands the advice and implications.
2. The doctor should encourage parental involvement and explore the reasons for not involving the parents.
3. The doctor should take into account whether sexual intercourse is likely to take place without contraception.
4. The doctor should assess whether the patient's physical or mental health is likely to suffer if she does not receive contraception.
5. The doctor must consider whether the patient's best interests require the provision of contraception without parental consent.

These guidelines still leave difficulties for the doctor trying to do the right thing, and not least in trying to decide whether the patient has the ability to understand and has complete comprehension of the relevant features (Dyer 1992).

HUMAN IMMUNODEFICIENCY VIRUS

Sexual transmission has been the greatest reason for the spread of AIDS. Latex condoms, and possibly the female condom, are currently the only method of contraception considered adequate to prevent HIV transmission (Olaitan & Johnson 1994). Unfortunately, this is not the most acceptable and effective method of preventing unwanted pregnancies. The doctor therefore has a difficulty in providing satisfactory contraceptive advice. Not many couples will wish to use two methods in order to optimize pregnancy prevention and minimize HIV transmission.

Women are now becoming infected with HIV faster than men in the western world. Anonymous unlinked testing in antenatal patients in the London area shows an increase in prevalence from 1 in 500 in 1990 to 1 in 300 in 1993 (Nicoll et al 1994).

HIV may have a role in modifying gynaecological disease processes, e.g. genital tract infections, or even a direct aetiological effect, e.g. the production of genital tract dysplasia and tumours.

There are particular problems in relation to the prevention of HIV-positive doctors infecting their patients and HIV-positive patients infecting their medical attendants.

Doctors' duty towards their patients

All doctors should extend the same high standard of medical care to patients whether they are HIV positive or negative. Referral to centres with appropriate facilities should take place as for any medical condition, but it is not ethical to withhold investigation or treatment merely because of some perceived personal risk to the doctor or disapproval of an individual's lifestyle.

Although the risk to the general public from an HIV-positive doctor is very small, any doctor who thinks he might be HIV positive should seek counselling and diagnostic testing and, if positive, appropriate medical supervision.

Doctors who are HIV positive should seek advice on the extent of their medical practice, e.g. from a consultant in occupational health or the UK Advisory Panel of the Expert Advisory Group on AIDS (GMC 1993).

Consent and confidentiality

One ethical problem is in relation to the informed consent of a patient prior to testing blood or other samples for the virus. The fear of hearing that an HIV test is positive is based on the lack of effective treatment and the fatal prognosis, together with the stigmatization of homosexuality, drug abuse or promiscuity. Infected patients are also liable to insurance and other financial penalties.

There remains a conflict between the confidential nature of a positive test and the public good of using that knowledge to protect others who might be at risk. For example, if the patient refuses to allow the information to be transmitted to their general practitioner, the investigating doctor has to balance his obligation to maintain confidentiality against the obligations towards other health care workers whose health may be put unnecessarily at risk.

Occasionally a doctor may be faced with a patient who refuses to disclose their HIV status to a sexual partner or other person who could be at risk. The BMA advises as follows (BMA 1993):

> If the patient understands the implications of behaviour which endangers others but refuses to modify it or to share information with sexual partners so depriving them of making an informed choice, there is a strong case for the doctor breaching confidentiality after warning the patient of his intention. Doctors must first seek to persuade the patient to either discontinue all behaviour which puts others at risk, to disclose the information voluntarily or to consent to the doctor so doing. The doctor may be considered to have a duty in very exceptional circumstances to disclose the information to a particular individual or to a responsible authority capable of restraining the patient's behaviour.

Obviously, before any such disclosure the doctor would have to consider the degree of risk to any other persons and be prepared to take responsibility for the results of the decision.

Although some people will argue that blood is often taken from patients and submitted for a number of tests without explicit consent, testing for HIV is significantly different and requires the explicit consent of the individual. Once tested, there are consequences for the individual whatever the result, as the very act of being tested has had influence with some insurance and mortgage companies.

It is important, therefore, prior to removal of blood or other tissues for investigation of HIV, that the patient is fully counselled as to the possible consequences, and then consent obtained. Only in exceptional circumstances, where a test is required to secure the safety of persons other than the patient, or where it is not possible for the prior consent of the patient to be obtained, can testing without explicit consent be justified.

INFERTILITY

Although there is no evidence that pregnancy accelerates the course of HIV infection there is a risk of transmission to the offspring of the order of 15% (European Collaborative Study 1992). At present there is no way of predicting which children will be affected, but advanced maternal disease, delivery before 34 weeks and breastfeeding all make it more likely.

The dilemma facing a doctor who has been consulted by a couple with infertility, where one or both are HIV positive, includes possible transmission to the offspring with all its consequences, and the possible early death of one or both parents.

After full and sympathetic counselling the doctor, who is in the business of trying to help create a new human being, has to decide whether investigation or treatment should be offered. The couple may also eventually require ovulation induction, donor insemination, in-vitro fertilization and other assisted conception techniques, and there may then be further ethical dilemmas over priorities of resource allocation.

In assisted conception techniques where donor gametes, either sperm or ova, are used, then HIV testing of the donors is always necessary to prevent transmission of the virus.

ASSISTED REPRODUCTION

Most gynaecologists, and indeed the majority of the general public, now accept that infertility is not dissimilar to other areas of medical misfortune where doctors legitimately try and relieve the suffering caused by the condition.

The initial investigation and treatment involves the gynaecologist and the infertile couple alone, and at this stage the process is the same as for other medical conditions. A proportion of couples will, however, require the help of in-vitro fertilization and/or the help of a third party for donation of egg, sperm or embryo, or the use of a host uterus for surrogacy.

There are those who object to in-vitro fertilization on religious grounds, believing that a human being is created at the time of conception and that the unitive or procreative aspects of intercourse should not be separated, and who would not seek this type of treatment for themselves. Others fear that tampering with eggs and sperm in a laboratory will lead to abhorrent types of research and experimentation, and object to it on those grounds.

HUMAN FERTILIZATION AND EMBRYOLOGY AUTHORITY (HFEA)

It was following the birth of Louise Brown, a pregnancy established by IVF in July 1978, and on account of the public concerns in the whole area of assisted conception, that the UK Government in 1982 set up a committee under the chairmanship of Dame Mary Warnock 'to consider recent potential developments in medicine and science related to human fertilization and embryology; to consider what policies and safeguards should be applied, including consideration of the social, ethical and legal implications of these developments; and to make recommendations' (DHSS 1984). Their report, published in 1984, recommended the establishment of a statutory licensing authority to regulate research and infertility services where fertilization takes place in vitro and where donor gametes are used for treatment. It was after further public debate and the passage of the Human Fertilization and Embryology Act 1990 that the HFEA was established to control and regulate this area of reproductive medicine, taking over from the Interim Licensing Authority in the summer of 1991. Under the Act certain activities can only be carried out once a licence has been granted. These include:

1. The creation of an embryo in vitro.
2. The storage of gametes and embryos.
3. Embryo replacement within a woman.
4. Mixing sperm with the egg of a hamster or other animal for the sole purpose of testing the sperm for fertility or normality.
5. The creation and use of embryos for research only until the formation of the primitive streak, i.e. within 14 days from the mixing of gametes and excluding any storage time, and only for specific acceptable purposes.

It is a criminal offence for any person to place a live embryo other than a human embryo, or any live gametes other than human gametes, in a woman.

The Act sets out the statutory framework within which centres must operate and the Authority expects licensed centres to operate within their Code of Practice.

In framing the Code of Practice the Authority have been guided by the Act and by:

- The respect which is due to human life at all stages in its development.
- The right of people who are or may be infertile to the proper consideration of their request for treatment.
- A concern for the welfare of children, which cannot always be adequately protected by concern for the interests of the adults involved.
- A recognition of the benefits, both to individuals and to society, which can flow from the responsible pursuit of medical and scientific knowledge.

Licences can be issued by the Authority for treatment, storage and research. Although centres providing treatment and undertaking research do not have to apply for a separate storage licence, each research project requires a separate licence.

All licences are subject to certain conditions, which may be specific to the centre. Review inspection visits occur on an annual basis and the licence committee has the power to revoke the licence under certain circumstances, such as if the person responsible fails to comply with the directions of the Authority. To persist with the activity would then contravene the law.

The rapid advances in the understanding and treatment possibilities in the field of reproductive medicine have inevitably thrown up an enormous number of difficult ethical dilemmas.

Each one of us, at least if intimately involved in this area of work, will have to make up our own minds as to where we stand on any particular issue. Besides this individual stance it is incumbent upon the community to come to a conclusion for the sake of pragmatism and progress to define an acceptable path through these thorny issues. It was for this purpose that the HFE Act reached the statute book and the Authority was promulgated, and its success can be measured by the majority support it enjoys both from the general public and the medical profession, especially those closely involved in assisted conception techniques.

There have been and will continue to be new and challenging questions which need to be answered by individuals and society, but this Act has been a giant step forward in arranging and controlling these affairs amicably. It is impossible that all the ethical dilemmas can be addressed in this chapter, as so many questions arise:

- What is the moral status of the gametes and early conceptus?
- What is the best way of disposing of spare embryos?
- Should embryos be available for research, and if so under what conditions?
- Should embryos be created for research?
- Should frozen embryos be available for treatment or research after the death of one or both parents?
- How many embryos should be implanted per treatment cycle?
- Is superovulation, with its potential hazards, justified rather than using natural ovulation for IVF?
- Is selective reduction of embryos in a multiple pregnancy ethical and legal?
- From what sources is it justified to use donor oocytes?
- How closely should donor gametes be matched to the commissioning parent?
- Should there be an age limit for the recipient of donor oocytes or sperm?
- Is it ever right to use one woman's uterus to produce another woman's baby?
- Does every couple have a moral right to procreate, and what priority should they have for public funding?

In some of these recent dilemmas the Human Fertilization and Embryology Authority has catalysed responsible public debate and then incorporated the results of the widespread debate into their direction for licensed centres. For example, at this time it is not considered ethical to carry out sex selection for social reasons by means of IVF. Likewise, oocyte donation is not permitted from fetuses, even if it were currently possible.

We will now consider some of the more important areas of assisted conception in greater detail.

Donor insemination

This treatment is suitable where the male partner has no sperm DNA capable of fertilizing an oocyte. Although in the natural world this process has always been available, it was frowned on as a form of treatment until the 1970s. A Church of England report in 1948 was highly critical of the practice of AID (artificial insemination by donor), recommending that it should be made a criminal offence, and in 1960 the Feversham Committee (HMSO 1960) set up by the Government considered that AIH (artificial insemination by husband) was acceptable but that AID was opposed by most of the medical profession and society at large – 'an undesirable practice strongly to be discouraged'. In 1973 a BMA Committee under the Chairmanship of Sir John Peel (BMA 1973) recommended that AID should be available under the NHS at accredited centres for appropriate couples.

It has now become an accepted practice available for the 1 in 25 couples where there is a particular male factor problem. As the donor samples need to be frozen the conception rate for this treatment does not approach that of a naturally fertile couple, being around 10% per cycle overall and up to 16–18% per cycle for the best centres. Although there are many arguments that can be advanced both for and against maintaining the anonymity of the donors of gametes (Council for Science and Society 1984) the reasons for such anonymity currently prevail and such a policy is enshrined in the 1990 HFE Act. At present it is difficult to obtain a sufficient number of donors under the present protocols, and there is evidence that many of these donors would be unwilling to offer gamete donation if they were not guaranteed anonymity.

Counselling and the supply of correct information must play a large role for such infertile couples. Many couples do not wish to advertise the cause of their infertility, and confidentiality must be maintained as strictly as requested by the couple. The HFEA also have detailed regulations in this area. Couples will wish to discuss whether any child born following this technique should remain in ignorance of their biological father or not. There is a growing openness in this form of assisted conception and awareness of the advantages of informing children about their genetic origin. Sympathetic organizations are available to help parents in their approach to this problem (e.g. DI Network). In a small proportion of cases AID is performed to avoid the inheritance of an abnormal genetic trait, and it is naturally advisable that any future child should understand that they could not be a carrier of the abnormal family gene.

There is some evidence that AID couples are, if anything, better at parenting than the average (Golombok et al 1993) and the concern of potential fathers that they will not 'bond' with a child to which they have had no genetic input is invalid provided that the child is much wanted.

In law now (HFE Act 1990) the male partner has the same responsibilities and obligations as a natural father, although hereditary titles and some estates cannot be passed on to a male heir.

If the male partner has oligospermia it has been suggested that his sample should be mixed with the donor sperm, but this seems practically and ethically unsound. If there is a chance of natural conception then natural intercourse may achieve that, and I have also known conception to take place during an AID cycle when the woman had also had a relationship with a third party.

Single women without a male partner who may or may not be in a lesbian relationship sometimes feel it is their wish and 'right' to have a child, and will seek medical help from AID centres. Treatment for such individuals is not outlawed, but one of the conditions for issuing a treatment licence by the HFEA is that 'a woman shall not be provided with treatment services unless account has been taken of the welfare of any child who may be born as a result of the treatment (including the need of that child for a father), and of any other child who may be affected by the birth'.

The Ethics Committee of the Royal Collage of Obstetricians and Gynaecologists considered the question of assisted conception and the single woman (RCOG 1991) and strongly reiterated their support for the traditional family unit. They concluded that the potential risks to the child outweighed the perceived benefit, and discouraged such a procedure. Similar difficult decisions have to be made where requests are made for artificial insemination using the husband's sperm (e.g. in cases where semen is collected and stored prior to cancer treatment) following his death.

Ovum and embryo donation

Ovum donation is, mutatis mutandis, an exact biological parallel to sperm donation and the same ethical arguments and dilemmas apply (Abdalla 1994). Ovum donation is different, however, in the case of access to the gametes. The demand for donor oocytes far outstrips the current means of supply, which includes the use of spare oocytes from IVF programmes and volunteers offering oocytes following superovulation at the time of sterilization, hysterectomy, etc. There are risks attendant on the induction of ovulation and egg collection. In time it may be possible to mature eggs in vitro from biopsies of the ovaries, and hence reduce the problem of supply.

Following public consultation the use of donated ovarian tissue in embryo research and assisted conception in January 1994, the HFEA concluded that it was acceptable for fetal ovarian tissue and ovarian tissues from cadavers to be used for licensed research, but not for treatment

Ovum donation, and indeed embryo donation, also differs from AID in that it is likely to be associated with in-vitro fertilization and embryo replacement. It is therefore more demanding and stressful for both patients and doctors.

Few people would have ethical difficulty in accepting ovum donation and IVF for a woman who had had spontaneous premature menopause, but difficulties arise when women seek such assistance after the menopause, in their fifth and sixth decades.

The risks of pregnancy when there is also a possibility of more than one fetus, together with the welfare of any offspring born to a mother at an older than average reproductive age, have been debated. There is little current restriction on paternal age, and established couples can often provide a more stable and secure home for any offspring. At present there are no specific regulations in place concerning this problem, which is likely to remain numerically very small.

In-vitro fertilization

Since the birth of Louise Brown in 1978 the technique of in-vitro fertilization is now widely used and accepted to help infertile couples to overcome many conception faults which cannot be overcome in other ways, e.g. blocked fallopian tubes, resistant ovulation induction, abnormal sperm function and unexplained infertility. In the best circumstance conception rates can reach 25% per cycle, which is equivalent to natural conception rates in normally fertile couples, but the average fertility rates are nearer 10–15% per cycle.

The process involves drug therapy for the woman to induce superovulation, perhaps together with downregulation of her abnormal gonadotrophin output. These drugs have risks of hyperstimulation and multiple pregnancy under certain circumstances, in spite of careful monitoring, and in this country one death has been recorded from hyperstimulation.

Techniques of oocyte collection have become less invasive, and success rates to the point of fertilization and embryo replacement are now good. The largest area of failure remains implantation of the embryo.

The latest techniques for male factor problems, such as intracytoplasmic sperm injection (ICSI), hold out tremendous hope for men who previously had little hope of procreation. There are those who do not agree with the idea of perpetuating the genetic make-up of men who are known to be grossly subnormal in relation to sperm quality.

The development of IVF is constantly throwing up new problems. A few are mentioned below.

1. *Detection of abnormalities.* At the early stage of formation it is possible to perform an embryo biopsy without detriment to the developing potential human being. This technique has already been used in sex-linked disorders to ensure the replacement of an embryo without the defect, and no doubt will be used in the future for many such genetic abnormalities. Most people accept this concept of ensuring the omission of substantial abnormality, although others will argue that it undermines respect for those in society either born or acquiring a disability. There will be a much fiercer debate when it is possible to exclude genetic groupings which some might not consider 'abnormal' at all. Exactly the same arguments apply to gene therapy.

Somatic cell gene therapy which attempts to correct defective genes, in particular tissues in the postnatal person, is not carried forward into the subsequent generation and is a permitted technique.

Any modification of the very early embryo where the cells are pluripotential would effectively modify the reproductive cells and constitute germline therapy. In view of the possible risks associated with this, such as genetic damage during the modification process, it is currently prohibited in the UK, but it may yet have an acceptable place in the future.

2. *Gender selection.* As we have seen, it is quite possible to select the gender of an embryo before placement in the uterus, and this is acceptable to avoid a sex-linked disorder. Claims have been made for successful sperm sorting pre-fertilization, and a gender selection clinic was established in London in 1993. This does not require a licence in order to operate, as it deals with the male partner's fresh sperm samples and no storage function is involved.

Although there is little argument against the use of gender selection for medical reasons, there has been a continuing debate as to whether it should be available for purely social reasons. The arguments (BMA 1993) range over the rights of individuals, the effect of an alteration in the sex ratio on the members of society, and a dangerous step on the slippery slope to 'designer babies'.

In a society where numerous measures are designed to prevent the false devaluation of one or other sex, the Ethics Committee of the RCOG urged a strong presumption against the practice of sex selection for social reasons (RCOG 1993).

The HFEA has currently banned gender selection for social reasons in licensed centres.

3. *Embryo research.* The Human Fertilization and Embryology Act 1990 permits research on the embryo up to 14 days after fertilization, at the time when the primitive streak appears. This is perhaps a compromise position which is acceptable to the majority. It is far too liberal for those who believe that human life starts at fertilization, and that any embryo should therefore be given the chance of development within the womb and that it would be wrong to submit such an early embryo for research. Others would say that sperms and eggs are alive and fertilization is only a process along the path towards a new human person, who arrives at birth. Again, among the many shades of opinion a reasonable view states that the degree of moral status and therefore protection advances slowly towards term, and the degree of invasive research must take this into account. It is on these lines that the current law has been framed.

Embryos used for research may have been created as part of an IVF procedure but are now surplus to requirements. They can then either be donated to others, allowed to perish or used for research. Alternatively, they can be created with the specific intention of research. Some may accept the former position but reject the idea of creating embryos specially for research.

In the UK there is no legislation restricting the creation of embryos for research, provided that the HFEA regulations are upheld. The view prevails that if it is acceptable to use embryos for research, then it is acceptable to produce them for research.

Licences for embryo research are only granted by the HFEA where the aim of the research fits one of the following endeavours:

- Promoting advances in the treatment of infertility.
- Increasing knowledge about the causes of congenital disease.
- Increasing knowledge about the causes of miscarriage.
- Developing more effective techniques of contraception.
- Developing methods for detecting the presence of gene or chromosome abnormalities in embryos before implantation.

- Endeavouring to increase knowledge about the creation and development of embryos, enabling such knowledge to be applied.

SURROGACY

This is an arrangement whereby a woman agrees to carry and give birth to a child on the understanding that the child will be given up after birth to the care of others. The child might or might not be genetically related to the carrying mother. It provides a possible solution for women who have no satisfactory uterus, or for whom a pregnancy and delivery would be too dangerous. With the development of in-vitro techniques fertilization can take place either in vitro or in vivo, depending on the required source of gametes.

Such arrangements have raised concerns over the exploitation of women and their bodies, particularly if sums of money are involved. On the other hand, some women believe that 'lending' their womb for the creation of a family for an infertile couple is the greatest gift they could confer. The Surrogacy Arrangements Act 1985 essentially outlawed commercial surrogacy in the UK (Norrie 1993).

Any act designed to establish a surrogacy arrangement is a criminal offence if that arrangement is made on a commercial basis. Advertising in connection with surrogacy is also a criminal offence. The Act covers third parties only, and is designed to prevent such parties acting for profit. Doctors or others can act as assisting third parties, provided there is no commercial interest. Private arrangements between the commissioning couple and the surrogate mother do not constitute an offence, even if money passes.

The Act also points out that in law the child of the surrogate mother remains her child and her husband's or, if she was unmarried, the genetic father's. Unless the child is adopted by the commissioning couple they have no legal relationship with the child, or rights in law.

A quicker form of adoption was made available under the Human Fertilization and Embryology Act 1990. A court order can be obtained soon after birth declaring that the child is to be treated for all purposes of law as if he or she were the child of the commissioning couple. Certain conditions have to be satisfied:

1. The order must be applied for jointly by a married couple.
2. The child must have been gestated in the womb of a surrogate who has been artificially impregnated.
3. Either the husband and/or the wife must be genetically related to the child as parent.
4. The application must be made within 6 months of birth, and the child must have its home with the applicants.
5. All parties must have given full and unconditional consent.
6. No money, other than reasonable expenses, must have been given or received.

All agree that the welfare of the potential child should be paramount. Doctors can take part in the surrogacy arrangements if they believe they are ethically sound and they are sure that all parties are fully aware of the different risks of such an arrangement, which includes the risks of pregnancy and the possible changing feelings towards the future child during pregnancy and following delivery. Counselling should include discussion of potential pregnancy complications and fetal abnormality, and the relationship between the surrogate mother and the commissioning parents. The former often wish the relationship to be long term, whereas the latter usually wish to sever all connections soon after birth.

An ethical report from the BMA gives helpful conclusions and recommendations in this very difficult area (BMA 1990).

REFERENCES

Abdalla H I 1994 Ethical aspects of oocyte donation. British Journal of Obstetrics and Gynaecology 101: 567–570

ACOG Committee 1987 Patient choice: Maternal fetal conflict No 55

British Council of Churches 1962 Human Reproduction

British Medical Association 1990 Surrogacy: Ethical considerations. BMA, London

British Medical Association 1992 Rights and responsibilities of doctors. BMA, London

British Medical Association 1993 Medical ethics today. BMJ Publishing, London

British Medical Journal Supplement 1973, 1 British Medical Association annual report of the Council: Appendix V: Report of the panel on human artificial insemination (chairman: Sir John Peel). Vol. II 3–5

Council for Science and Society 1984 Human procreation: ethical aspects of the new techniques: report of a working party. Oxford University Press, Oxford

DHSS 1984 Report of the committee of inquiry into human fertilisation and embryology

DHSS 1992 The health of the nation: a strategy for health in England. HMSO, London

Department of Health 1993 Changing childbirth. Report of the Expert Maternity Group. HMSO, London

Dyer C (ed) 1992 Doctors, patients and the law. Ch. 3: Consent to treatment and the capable person. Blackwell Scientific Publications, Oxford.

European Collaborative Study 1992 Risk factors for mother to child transmission of HIV. Lancet 339: 1007–1012

FIGO Committee for the Study of Ethical Aspects of Human Reproduction 1994 Recommendations on ethical issues in obstetrics and gynaecology

General Medical Council 1993 Statement on HIV infection and AIDS: the ethical consideration. GMC, London

Gillick 1985 House of Lords Hearing: 3 All ER at 413

Gillon R 1994 Medical ethics. Four principles plus attention to scope. British Medical Journal 309: 148–188
Golombok S, Cook R, Bish A, Murray C 1993 Quality of parenting in families created by the new reproductive technologies. Journal of Psychosomatic Obstetrics and Gynecology 14 (Suppl): 17–22
HMSO 1960 Home Office with Scottish Home Department: departmental committee on human artificial insemination report (chairman, The Earl of Feversham). Cmnd 1105
Janaway v Salford H A 1988 3 All ER 1079 HL
Nicoll A, McGarrigle C, Heptanstall J et al 1994 Prevalence of HIV infections in pregnant women in London and elsewhere in England. British Medical Journal 309: 376–377
Norrie K McK 1993 The law and ethics of surrogacy. Current Obstetrics and Gynaecology 3: 116–117
Olaitan A, Johnson M A 1994 Gynaecological problems in women infected with HIV. Current Obstetrics and Gynaecology 4: 189–192
RCOG 1991 Assisted conception and the single woman: Ethics Committee report
RCOG 1993 Sex selection: Ethics Committee Report. RCOG Press
RCOG guidelines April 1994 Ethics: 'A consideration of the law and ethics in relation to court authorised obstetric intervention'
Reiss H 1994 Hippocratic Oath. British Medical Journal 309: 952
Sidaway v Board of Governors of the Bethlem Royal Hospital and the Maudsley Hospital 1985 AC 871, 1 All ER 643
Vanlook P F A, Von Hertzen H 1993 Current Obstetrics and Gynaecology 3: 2–10
Weatherall D J 1994 The inhumanity of medicine. British Medical Journal 309: 24–31

62

Lower intestinal tract disease

M. M. Henry

Functional disorders of the anorectum are frequently the consequence of the same aetiopathological mechanisms as those giving rise to a disturbance of function within the genitourinary tract, and therefore a brief account can be justified in a text largely concerned with gynaecological disease. Patients frequently have symptoms referrable to both systems, suggesting that a combined approach to management should be offered whenever possible. In practice, as a consequence of ever-increasing degrees of specialization, this is rarely achieved.

PELVIC FLOOR AND ANORECTAL CONTINENCE (Table 62.1)

It is generally believed by proctologists that the pelvic floor plays a key role in the maintenance of anorectal continence in the normal state. If a pressure probe is inserted into the rectum and withdrawn caudally through the anal canal at centimetre intervals a stepwise increase in pressure is recorded over an area approximately corresponding to the internal anal sphincter (IAS) (Fig. 62.1). Resting anal pressure has been shown to be largely a functional IAS contraction with a small contribution made by the external anal sphincter (EAS) (Bennett & Duthie 1964). If the subject is requested to contract the EAS maximally, the intra-anal pressure increases by a factor of 100%. The role of the IAS and EAS in anorectal control continues to be disputed. Surgical division of the IAS rarely gives rise to any significant functional deficit. Internal sphincter loss in most patients usually leads to only a minor degree of incontinence, mostly restricted to loss of control to flatus and to liquid stool. On the other hand, some patients who

Table 62.1 Factors responsible for normal anorectal continence

Anal sphincters	Internal sphincter Innervated hypogastric and sacral parasympathetic nerves External sphincter Innervated pudendal nerves
Pelvic floor	Anorectal angle (flap-valve) Innervated from above by direct branches of the sacral plexus
Sensory factors	Receptors inthe pelvic floor Rectosphincteric inhibitory reflex (sampling)
Miscellaneous factors	Valves of Houston Anal cushions Vectors acting in the cephalad direction

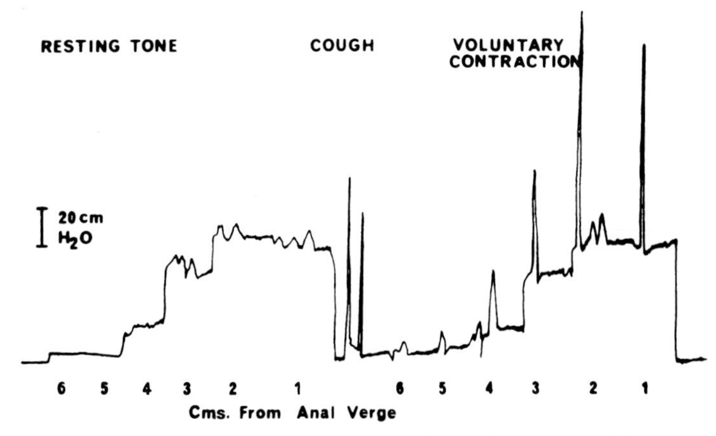

Fig. 62.1 A normal anal pressure profile. In the first section of the tracing the pressure probe has been inserted into the rectum and is withdrawn at centimetre intervals with the patient in the resting state and lying in the left lateral position. The internal sphincter is responsible for a zone of high pressure (maximum 60 cm water) over the distal 4 cm. The pressure profile is repeated but on this occasion the patient is requested to contract the external anal sphincter. Intra-anal pressures are thereby increased during contraction by at least a factor of two times.

develop severe faecal incontinence may on physiological testing be found to have idiopathic IAS deficiency as the primary abnormality, with relative sparing of the EAS and pelvic floor muscles. Similarly, the true function of the EAS as a separate entity remains uncertain, since in most patients division of the muscle ring does not give rise to significant anorectal incontinence other than urgency and soiling in the presence of diarrhoea. However, some patients with neuropathic damage of the EAS (see below), where the pelvic floor is relatively spared, may experience severe functional disturbance.

The puborectalis, because of its intimate relationship to the lower rectum and upper anal canal, is the most relevant of the levator muscles. In company with the remainder of the muscles which comprise the pelvic floor and the EAS, this muscle displays the unusual property (for skeletal muscle) of continuous resting electrical tone. This function is maintained without conscious effort and during sleep (Floyd & Walls 1953), and has been demonstrated to be the consequence of a spinal reflex (Parks et al 1962). Hence disruption of any limb of this reflex (e.g. in tabes dorsalis) will result in complete cessation of resting tone and anorectal incontinence.

Contraction of the puborectalis muscle in turn generates an angle between the lower rectum and upper anal canal – the anorectal angle (Fig. 62.2). There is again dispute concerning the true importance of this anatomical entity. Parks (1975) believed that the angle is a prime importance for the maintenance of normal control because it permits a flap-valve mechanism to operate. He believed that intra-abdominal pressure was conducted via the anterior rectal wall such that any increase (e.g. from coughing or sneezing) caused it to close over the top of the anal canal and effectively excluded the anus from the intrarectal contents. However, Bartolo (1986) failed to demonstrate by radiographic techniques any increase in the angle in a group of normal controls in whom intra-abdominal pressure was increased by performing the Valsalva manoeuvre. There is no question, however, that during a cough impulse there is a considerable recordable reflex increase in the pelvic floor muscle electrical activity (presumably to cause an increase in anorectal angulation), and on sigmoidoscopy the anterior rectal wall can be clearly seen moving downwards as it is forced on to the upper part of the anal canal.

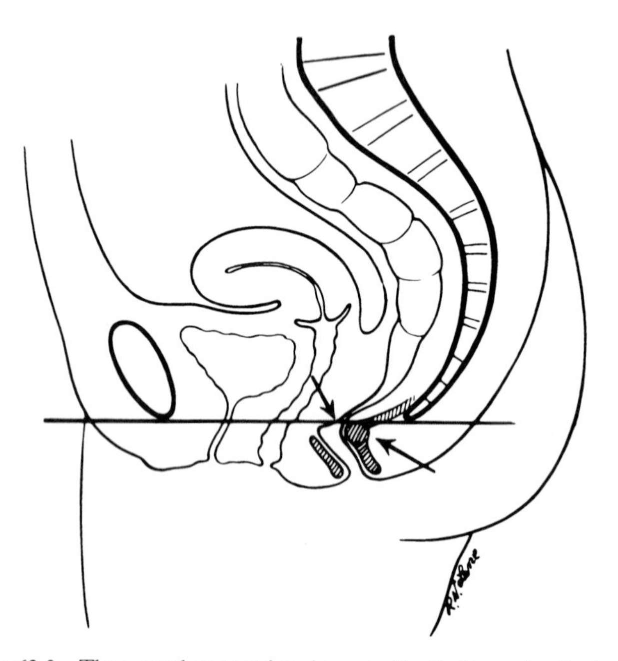

Fig. 62.2 The normal anorectal angle created by the forward pull of the puborectalis muscle (lower arrow). Abdominal pressure is conducted onto the anterior rectal wall (upper arow) helping to prevent leakage of rectal contents when intra-abdominal pressure is raised (e.g by coughing, lifting, etc).

The sensation of a full rectum, alerting the individual to the possibility of an impending need to defecate, is also an important element of normal continence. Sensory receptors have never been clearly identified within the wall or mucosa of the rectum itself, and sensation seems to be preserved in patients undergoing rectal excision and coloanal anastomosis (Lane & Parks 1977). These lines of evidence suggest that the requisite receptors probably reside within the pelvic floor muscles, which cradle and lie in intimate contact with the rectum. Evidence in favour is the demonstration of stretch receptors (Winkler 1958) and muscle spindles (Walls 1959) in these muscles.

An important contributing factor to sensation facilitating a locally mediated visceral reflex is referred to as the rectosphincteric inhibitory reflex. The reflex, first described by Gowers (1877) refers to inhibition of the internal anal sphincter as a consequence of rectal distension, e.g. by flatus or by faeces. The reflex can be shown to be independent of extrinsic neural sources and is abolished by rectal myotomy (Lubowski et al 1987), confirming that the reflexes are mediated via the intramural neural pathways. Under normal conditions the reflex acts to permit a small amount of rectal contents to enter the proximal anal canal in response to IAS relaxation. At the dentate line the contents make contact with the profuse sensory receptors which are concentrated at this level, and therefore permit discrimination between faeces and flatus. If faeces are perceived to be present there is vigorous contraction of the EAS and the anal contents are propelled back to the rectum until the time is propitious for defecation to proceed. Sampling occurs at a regular and frequent basis during the daytime in all normal individuals.

There are certainly other factors that may play a part, and these have yet to be elucidated. For example, the role of haemorrhoids in providing cushions of tissue has never been properly explained, but minor degrees of incontinence are common after haemorrhoidectomy and this cannot be explained on the basis of damage to either of the sphincters.

DEFECATION

When the patient is ready to defecate complex physiological mechanisms are instituted which, like those responsible for continence, are incompletely understood. There is no dispute that, under normal and ideal circumstances, defecation is preceded by a reflex inhibition of electrical activity within the pelvic floor and EAS. This in turn facilitates defecation by causing increased obliquity of the anorectal angle. The passage of the faecal bolus is further assisted by reflex relaxation of the IAS in response to rectal distension. The actual vector forces responsible for evacuation probably arise from increased intra-abdominal pressure, rather than from peristaltic activity within the rectum itself. At the completion of the defecatory effort there is a rapid burst of electrical activity within the EAS and pelvic floor to restore the anorectal angle. At the same time, tone is regained within the IAS. Central mechanisms in the nervous control of defecation are ill understood. Urge incontinence is a feature of inflammatory conditions of the rectum and of spinal and cerebral disorders alike. Recent evidence suggests that there is a fast-conducting direct pyramidal pathway to the sacral anterior horn cells supplying the pelvic floor and EAS; this suggests that the cortex plays an important role in the normal control of these muscles.

INVESTIGATION OF PELVIC FLOOR DISORDERS

Over recent years there has been a marked development in techniques designed to provide an objective assessment of pelvic floor function. This has been a direct consequence of an accelerating interest in the treatment of these conditions.

Manometry

This is the most endurable method, since it is simple, cheap and a relatively non-invasive means of assessing IAS and EAS function. Pressures can be recorded simply by using either water-filled balloons or a water-perfusion system. The latter is vulnerable because the intrusion of faecal contents may introduce artefact. More accurate measurement of complex systems are available, e.g. using transducers and radiotransmitters. However, these are generally only required in units where research commitments are predominant. Recording systems should then be connected via a suitable transducer to a device capable of producing a clear and preferably permanent tracing.

Manometry is currently the only practical method for assessing IAS function, and also the only means of testing the integrity of the rectosphincteric inhibitory reflex. Assessment of the EAS manometrically is less satisfactory, as it requires the patient's subjective ability to comprehend and cooperate during maximal voluntary contraction.

Electromyography

A more accurate approach to the assessment of EAS and pelvic floor function is gained by conventional, and more especially by single-fibre, electromyography (EMG). The former uses either surface electrodes or relatively broad-diameter needle electrodes, both of which record from a wide surface area, and is largely useful in identifying skeletal muscle. The identification of muscle and its anatomical position may be particularly relevant after muscle has been divided (e.g. following a third-degree perineal tear) providing the surgeon with precise anatomical detail of the position of the retracted EAS prior to its repair. In children, EMG exploration may be helpful in identifying the pelvic floor in rectal atresia prior to pullthrough surgery.

To determine whether the skeletal muscle under investigation has undergone denervation (see below) the more sophisticated technique of single-fibre EMG must be used. With concentric needle electrodes individual muscle fibre action potentials cannot be recognized reliably within the motor unit action potential. Single muscle fibre action potentials can be recorded extracellularly by using an electrode whose recording service consists of a central wire, which opens at the midshaft of the electrode in a small circular leading-off surface 25 mm in diameter (Fig. 62.3). In normal muscle, recordings of motor units are made in which one or two single muscle fibre action potentials are obtained within the uptake area of the electrode. In muscle which has been denervated and subsequently reinnervated, the number of components will be increased. An average of the positive components is taken from 20 different sites in the muscle and the figure is referred to as the

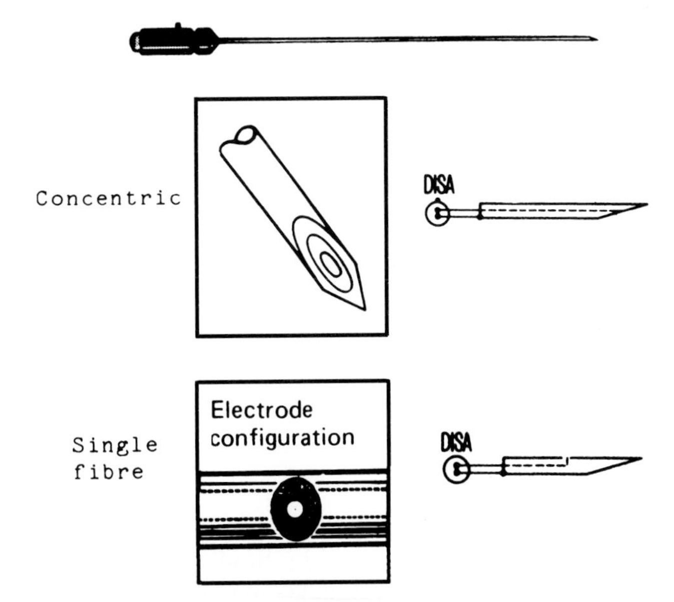

Fig. 62.3 Electrodes employed for electromyography. Upper electrode is of conventional concentric type with its recording surface at the tip. The lower electrode is of single-fibre type with its recording surface situated on the surface of its shank near the tip.

fibre density for that muscle. The normal values obtained in the external anal sphincter are 1.3 in men, 1.5 in women (Jameson et al 1994a).

Nerve stimulation studies

Having established that denervation has occurred within the pelvic floor muscles it may be relevant to determine whether the anatomical site of the neurological damage is central (cauda equina) or peripheral (pudendal nerves).

The central component can be studied by means of transcutaneous lumbar spinal stimulation (Merton et al 1982). A single impulse of 800–1500 V decaying with a time constant of 50 ms is delivered through an electrode placed on the spinous process of L1 and repeated at L4. The evoked contraction associated with the pelvic floor response can be detected either by surface or by needle electrode. Pathology affecting the cauda equina will give rise to a more pronounced delay at L1 than at L4. If the neuronal damage results from peripheral disease, the delay at L1 and L4 will be increased to a similar degree (Snooks et al 1985a).

The peripheral component (i.e. the pudendal nerves) is tested by means of a disposable glove stimulating electrode, which comprises a glove consisting of two stimulating electrodes at the tip and two recording electrodes at the base. The glove is inserted into the rectum and, with the patient in the left lateral position, the tip is brought into contact with the pudendal nerve at the level of the ischial spine. The nerve is then stimulated electrically with a square-wave stimulus of 0.1 ms duration and 50 V amplitude, and the evoked response in the EAS is detected electrically by the surface recording electrodes situated at the base of the glove. The procedure is then repeated for the opposite side and the latency of the EAS muscle responses is measured on the paper printout of the EMG apparatus, from the onset of the stimulus to the onset of the response. The normal value of the pudendal response is 1.9 ms. Recording electrodes can also be mounted on to a Foley catheter and the urinary sphincter contraction response to direct stimulation of the pudendal nerve can be recorded. This is particularly relevant in the investigation of patients with stress incontinence of urine. In a recent study by Vernava et al (1993) it was found that the pudendal nerve terminal latency was much more accurate in determining evidence of denervation than the application of manometric techniques.

Sacral reflexes

Using the technique described by Bradley (1972), reflex anal contraction following stimulation of the bladder neck can be recorded, and these reflexes are found to be increased in neuropathic disorders affecting the pelvic floor as well as in cauda equina disease. The bulbocavernosus reflex, whereby the latent interval between stimulation of the bulbocavernosus muscle, the clitoris and the evoked response within the anal sphincter, has been investigated by Vernava et al (1986), and has been shown to be helpful in detecting motor neuron lesions.

Evoked potentials

Stimulation of the pudendal nerve, from either the anal sphincter or the bladder, can lead to potentials which, by computer averaging, can be distinguished by electrodes placed over the cerebral cortex. Recording of such evoked potentials could be delayed in the presence of spinal disorders, and this is therefore a method for detecting possible spinal disease. However, there is considerable variation in the latencies considered by different groups (Loening-Baucke & Reid 1990). In a study carried out at St Mark's Hospital of 13 patients and 16 healthy controls, reproducible evoked potentials could be recorded after anorectal stimulation only in a minority of subjects, and when recordable they showed a marked inter- and intrasubject variation (Speakman et al 1990).

Anal endosonography

Although information relating to the structure and function of the anal sphincters may be obtained from tests of anorectal physiology, the development of anal endosonography has enabled direct imaging of the sphincters to take place (Law & Bartram 1989). Anal endosonography has been particularly valuable in studying the effects of parturition on the pelvic floor (Sultan et al 1993).

Evacuation proctography

The dynamics of the pelvic floor can be studied digitally by employing cineradiographic techniques using video films on which have been superimposed simultaneous EMG and anal pressure recordings (Womack et al 1985). These techniques may be of specific value in the investigation of a constipated patient to identify the subgroup with pelvic floor spasticity. However, the main drawback of this technique is that it involves considerable radiation to the pelvis, and this may be hazardous as many patients with pelvic floor disease are young and of childbearing age.

PATHOPHYSIOLOGY OF FUNCTIONAL ANORECTAL DISEASE

Porter (1962), employing conventional EMG techniques, made the observation that many patients with rectal prolapse and faecal incontinence could be shown to have abnormal electrical activity of the pelvic floor. The explanation for these changes was clarified by histochemical studies of pelvic floor muscle biopsies in which features consistent with denervation were demonstrated by Parks et al (1977). That these muscles have been denervated in patients with rectal prolapse and anal incontinence was later confirmed by electrophysiological studies (Neil & Swash 1980). Application of nerve stimulation studies showed that the site of neuronal damage was peripheral, i.e. pudendal, in most patients (Snooks et al 1985a). Denervation has since also been demonstrated to have been an important feature in patients with constipation (Snooks et al 1985b), solitary rectal ulcer syndrome (Snooks et al 1985c), urinary incontinence (Snooks & Swash 1984) and the descending perineum syndrome (Henry et al 1982).

The source of the denervation is almost certainly multifactorial and is still a subject for speculation. There seems to be no doubt that many patients develop pelvic floor failure as a consequence of traumatic childbirth (Snooks et al 1984). The innervation of the pelvic floor may be damaged by vaginal delivery, but it appears to be less damaged by caesarean section. Damage is most prominent in multiparae, and correlates most strongly with a prolonged second stage of labour and with forceps delivery. Pudendal nerve injury may also be the consequence of a peripheral neuropathy occurring in diabetes mellitus (Rogers et al 1988), or in direct injury from surgery or road traffic accident. Lower motor neuron lesions may result from disease affecting the cauda equina, but these are generally considered to be rare.

DISORDERS OF THE PELVIC FLOOR

Faecal incontinence

The consequences for the individual affected by anorectal incontinence are often serious, since such patients may perceive themselves to be in a state of social and professional isolation. At St Mark's Hospital, London, of those patients who presented for treatment the disorder appears to be most common in middle age and is eight times more common in women than in men.

Minor faecal incontinence is defined as the inadvertent passage of flatus or soiling in the presence of diarrhoea. This state is usually associated with poor internal anal sphincter function, which in turn is often the consequence of previous anal surgery (anal stretch, haemorrhoidectomy), or may accompany minor anal rectal disorders such as condylomata or second-degree haemorrhoids. Sometimes the condition may occur spontaneously, and this is associated with pharmacological disorders of the internal anal sphincter (Speakman et al 1993). Partial denervation of the pelvic floor and EAS may similarly give rise to lesser degrees of incontinence in which the deficit is only present when challenged by the presence of liquid stool.

These patients are not usually greatly restricted by this handicap, and their management is largely conservative. Anorectal pathology should be looked for on clinical examination and treated accordingly. Where impaction occurs normal function can frequently be readily restored by the use of aperients and rectal washouts. If the IAS alone is deficient, surgery is unlikely to benefit the patient and management usually consists of a combination of codeine phosphate (to constipate) and an irritant suppository to induce complete rectal evacuation.

Major faecal incontinence is defined as the inadvertent passage of formed stool on at least a twice-weekly basis. As discussed above, the majority of patients will be of middle age with a history of obstetric trauma which precedes the onset of incontinence by a period varying from several days to several decades. Sultan et al (1993) found in a study of 202 consecutive women that 35% of primiparous women developed an anal sphincter defect demonstrated by ultrasonography during vaginal delivery. The defect persisted in all women when they were studied 6 months later. Of the 48 multiparous women in the study 40% had a sphincter defect demonstrated before delivery, and this increased to 44% following delivery. None of the 23 women who underwent caesarean section developed a sphincter defect following delivery. In a later study Sultan et al (1994) showed that vaginal delivery resulted in significant prolongation of the pudendal nerve latency bilaterally in primiparous women. In multiparous women (n = 32) six admitted to anal incontinence dating back to previous deliveries, and similarly the pudendal nerve latencies were significantly increased bilaterally following vaginal delivery. There was greater damage recorded on the left side rather than on the right, and the pudendal nerve latency was not altered in those women who were delivered by elective caesarean section. When the obstetric variables were analysed in detail it was found that both a heavy fetus and a long stage of labour strongly correlated with the significant prolongation of pudendal latency. After the sixth decade the muscle denervates as a normal physiological response to ageing, and this contributes further to the loss of anal function and helps to explain why some patients fail to develop problems until later life. Previous trauma responsible for division of the anal sphincter ring (e.g. fracture of the bony pelvis, third-degree perineal tear, anal fistula surgery or sexual assault) may be relevant, and if there is a history of incontinence associated with a history of perineal pain and/or disseminated neurological symptoms, a neurological cause should be considered.

Examination of patients with anorectal incontinence is customarily conducted with the patient in the left lateral position, having first examined the abdomen. On inspection, soiling of the perianal skin with faecal matter may be apparent and when the patient is requested to strain there may be perineal descent associated with genital and/or rectal prolapse. The anal canal itself may gape (if there is

IAS deficiency), and on digital examination of the anus both resting tone (IAS and squeeze tone EAS) may be deficient. The anal reflex will be absent to clinical testing and there may be diminished sensation in the perianal skin.

Before embarking on treatment these patients should be investigated by anorectal physiology tests and, if a neurological or sensory cause is suspected, lumbar myelography should be included. All patients with rectal symptoms should undergo sigmoidoscopy and, where relevant, a barium enema to exclude malignancy. If there are urological symptoms urodynamics, including videocystourethrography, should be considered.

Treatment

By virtue of the degree of their disability these patients require energetic, and often surgical, treatment. Where there is complete rectal prolapse rectopexy is indicated. The majority of patients with prolapse regain near-normal anorectal continence if the prolapse is successfully controlled. In a small subgroup who remain incontinent, pelvic floor surgery can be considered as a secondary procedure.

Anal sphincter repair

Anal sphincter repair can be responsible for near-total recovery of function in 80% of patients, provided that there is no coincidental denervation of the muscle (Lauerberg et al 1988). Engel and colleagues (1994), however, found no evidence to suggest that a prolonged preoperative pudendal latency was necessarily related to a poor outcome for anal sphincter repair in a series of 55 patients from St Mark's Hospital, London. In this series improvement in function was more closely related to the success in obtaining an anatomically intact external anal sphincter ring as judged by anal ultrasound examination.

Before surgery patients should be investigated physiologically to determine whether there is denervation, and also by anal ultrasound to locate the anatomical positions of the retracted ends of the EAS. The operation is usually performed with the patient in the lithotomy position, and some surgeons prefer to carry out a defunctioning colostomy to permit the repair to heal in a relatively uncontaminated environment. The fibrous scar filling the space between the retracted muscle is excised and the mucosa approximated with an absorbable suture. The muscle is then repaired by an overlapping technique using non-absorbable suture material (Fig. 62.4). The wound is left open to heal by secondary intention.

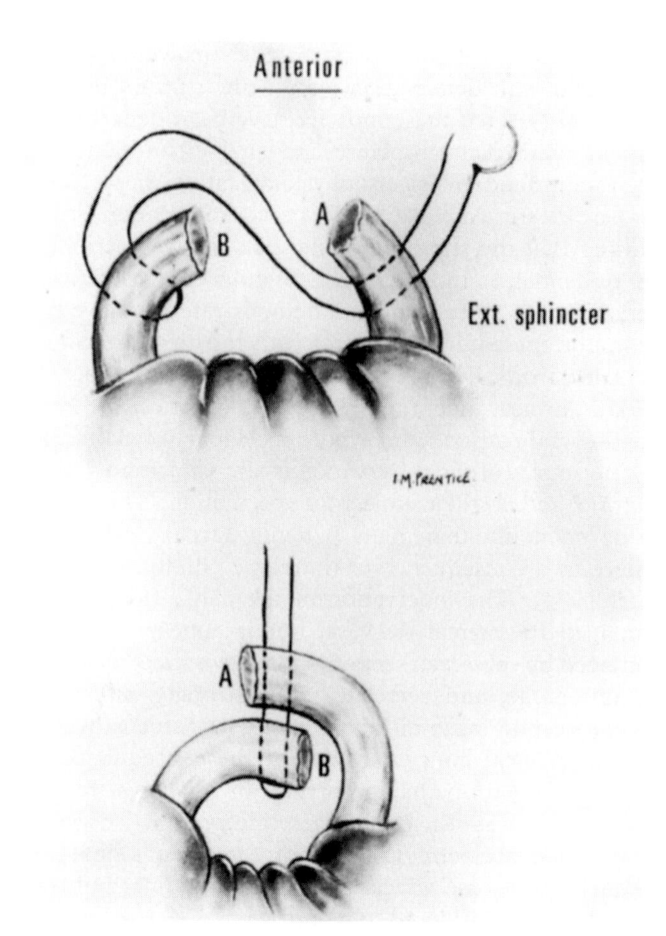

Fig. 62.4 External anal sphincter repair. The muscle ends are overlapped and sutured with a non-absorbable material.

Post anal repair

In the presence of established denervation of the pelvic floor, the preferred procedure in the UK is the operation devised by the late Sir Alan Parks (1975). The procedure can restore continence in about 80% of patients initially, but falls to about 60% after 3 years (Jameson et al 1994b). Parks originally believed that the anorectal angle could be restored, but there is little evidence to support this. It seems more likely that improved function is the consequence of increasing the length of the anal canal and of improving the mechanical advantage of the muscle fibres (Womack et al 1988).

A V-shaped incision is created just behind the anus and the space between the IAS and EAS dissected until Waldeyer's fascia is reached. The fascia has to be divided to obtain access to the pelvis. The levator muscles and EAS are then plicated sequentially using non-absorbable suture material. The skin is partially closed, leaving a portion of the wound to heal by secondary intention (Henry & Porter 1988).

Neuromuscular stimulated gracilis transplant

In the USA attempts have been made to treat anal incontinence by transposing the tendon of the gracilis muscle around the anal canal to create a neosphincter (Pickrell et al 1954). The operation has severe limitations because the gracilis muscle does not possess tonic activity. Williams et al (1990) have attempted to solve this problem by implanting an electrical stimulator into the gracilis muscle, whose tendon is then transplanted around the anus. A constant stimulation is provided to the muscle so that the gracilis is converted into a slow twitch muscle capable of continuous contraction without fatigue. This operation is technically complex and the stimulator expensive. It is too early to comment on the results of this technique, which is still in its experimental phase.

Rectal prolapse

Although this condition is observed at any age, it is most common at the extremes of life. In children the disorder may be associated with mucoviscidosis; if not, it is usually a transient phenomenon requiring minimal treatment. There is no doubt that in adults the majority are associated with pelvic floor denervation (Neill et al 1981). The weak pelvic floor favours prolapse of the anterior rectal wall, which in turn initiates a rectorectal intussusception. In some patients the aetiology remains obscure, although malnutrition and chronic constipation seem to be contributing factors.

The prolapse may develop only during defecation, or alternatively may be permanently down, requiring frequent manual replacement. Sometimes patients are unaware of the prolapse and present with faecal incontinence, occurring as a consequence of pelvic floor denervation and the IAS damage caused by the trauma of the prolapsing four layers of oedematous bowel wall. Rarely, the prolapsing segment may undergo strangulation and subsequent rupture.

Treatment

Most patients require surgical treatment, since persistent prolapse causes cumulative damage to the anal sphincters and the condition itself causes great distress. The preferred procedure in the UK is rectopexy, an operation whereby the rectum is tethered to the sacrum by an inert implant (e.g. Mersilene). The operation can be performed traditionally by an open procedure or, more recently, by laparoscopic methods. For those patients at high anaesthetic risk the procedure described by Delorme (1900) can be attempted. This is a perineal operation in which the redundant mucosa is excised and the underlying muscle plicated.

Descending perineum syndrome, perineal pain syndrome and solitary rectal ulcer syndrome

These uncommon conditions are discussed under a single heading because they are closely allied to each other and may be different manifestations of the same entity. The plane of the perineum normally lies above that of the bony outlet of the pelvis, both in the resting state and during straining. In patients with the descending perineum syndrome, however, the perineum balloons down well below the bony pelvis, particularly during straining (Henry et al 1982). The pelvic muscles are usually denervated and it is far from clear whether this is a primary or secondary event. In other words, it is possible that the pudendal nerves are stretched by elongation caused by the pelvic floor descent. Many patients with this syndrome develop anal incontinence. In the early stages there is prolapse of the anterior rectal wall mucosa into the anal canal. This has the effect of obstructing the passage of the faecal bolus during defecation, and forces the patient to strain excessively to achieve voiding. At the completion of the defecatory effort the redundant mucosa may remain in the anal canal, where it is perceived as retained faecal matter. The patient continues to strain fruitlessly in an effort to void what is in essence part of their own rectal wall.

Because the pudendal nerve is a mixed motor/sensory nerve perineal descent may cause a constant perineal aching pain, which is provoked by prolonged standing and relieved by lying flat.

Perineal descent is also associated with a condition in which there is a shallow, usually solitary, discrete ulcer in the midrectum: solitary rectal ulcer syndrome. The ulcer is usually sited anteriorly or anterolaterally at a level 4–10 cm from the anal verge. These patients similarly strain excessively at defecation, and it is believed that the ulcer is traumatic in origin. The ulcer may be painful and give rise to substantial rectal bleeding.

Treatment

The treatment of these disorders is fequently unsatisfactory. In the early stages the anterior rectal mucosal prolapse may be treated by injection or by surgical excision, combined with advice on improvement in bowel function and, in particular, to avoid straining. Where solitary rectal ulcer syndrome develops in combination with radiological evidence of internal prolapse, rectopexy may prove beneficial (Halligan et al 1995).

Irritable bowel syndrome

The diagnosis of irritable bowel syndrome (IBS) is only made after other pathology has been excluded. The condition represents a spectrum of symptoms, any combination of which can present. There is no objective test by which the condition may be diagnosed and there is no recognizable underlying aetiopathology. There appears to be strong evidence to support the concept that there is a disorder of intestinal motility, but whether this is primary or secondary remains unresolved (Rogers et al 1989). Episodes of pain correlate closely with periods of elevated intraluminal pressure in the colon and small bowel.

Table 62.2 Symptoms associated with irritable bowel syndrome

Symptoms
Severe colicky abdominal pain
Abdominal distension
Constipation
Diarrhoea
Mucus per rectum
Anxiety/depression
Relationship to stress

The range of symptoms associated with IBS is listed in Table 62.2. The site of the abdominal pain can vary from patient to patient and within individual patients. There is usually a clear relationship between symptoms and periods of stress/anxiety. Alteration in bowel habit is almost always present; usually there are periods of constipation alternating with periods of diarrhoea.

Treatment

Treatment should always be medical, since surgery plays no role except as part of the investigative process (i.e. laparoscopy). Some relief may be obtained by a combination of increased dietary fibre and the use of antispasmodics in combination with an antidepressant. Probably the most important role of the clinician is a supportive one.

Constipation

A patient is defined as suffering from constipation if she complains of either infrequent defecation (less than two bowel actions per week) or difficult defecation (straining and difficulty in evacuating the rectum). Under normal conditions the first priority must be the exclusion of an obstructing lesion, such as carcinoma, hence sigmoidoscopy and barium enema should be regarded as mandatory in most patients. A classification of the important causes is given in Table 62.3.

Where no obvious cause can be identified the standard approach is to investigate colonic transit and pelvic floor function in an attempt to distinguish between patients with slow-transit constipation and those with pelvic floor dysfunction (anismus). It is not always possible to differentiate between the two conditions, since some patients will be found to have a combination of both.

Slow-transit constipation

This can be defined by the simple radiological technique described by Hinton and colleagues (1969). A capsule containing 20 radio-opaque solid markers is ingested and on the fifth day a plain abdominal X-ray is performed. Under normal circumstances 80% of the markers should have been voided; if more than 20% remain, the patient can be assumed to have delayed colonic transit.

Table 62.3 Classification of constipation in adults

No structural abnormality of anus, rectum or colon and no associated physical disorder
Faulty diet
Pregnancy
Old age
Idiopathic slow-transit constipation
Irritable bowel syndrome
Structural disease of anus, rectum or colon
Anal pain/stenosis
Colonic stricture
Aganglionosis
Megarectum/megacolon
Secondary to abnormality outside colon
Endocrine/metabolic
Hypothyroidism
Hypercalcaemia
Porphyria
Neurological
Sacral outflow/spinal cord disorders
Cerebral disorders
Systemic sclerosis and other connective tissue disorders
Psychological
Drug side-effect

From Lennard Jones (1985).

This condition is prevalent in women at the time of the menarche and can be associated with severe degrees of constipation, with bowel function proving refractory to laxatives. The colon is of normal diameter, in distinction to primary megacolon, the latter being a functional disorder which occurs in men and women in equal numbers.

Pelvic floor dysfunction

Recently it has been clearly established that some patients have normal transit but are quite unable to empty a full rectum. This occurs in some patients because of increased electrical activity within the pelvic floor musculature during attempted defecation. The aetiology of this paradoxical contraction in the pelvic floor cannot be explained. In some patients this may be a behavioural abnormality which is the consequence of an abnormal pattern of defecation instituted from early childhood. In others the disorder is due to spasticity of the muscle secondary to upper motor neuron lesions; this is frequently observed in patients with multiple sclerosis, for example (Gill et al 1994).

Patients with denervation of the pelvic floor may similarly experience difficulty with defecation, which is aggravated by the presence of a rectocoele. Patients with this disorder frequently need to insert a digit either into the anal canal or into the vagina to assist emptying of a full rectum. The diagnosis of pelvic floor dysfunction is usually made by evacuation proctography (Mahieu et al 1984). A barium paste is introduced into the rectum and cineradiography is performed while the patient attempts defecation. The films are studied for paradoxical puborectalis contraction and intrarectal intussusception. In the latter case obstructed defecation is the consequence of a prolapsing rectum, which may not necessarily be overt and hence cannot be diagnosed by any method other than by defecography.

Treatment of constipation

Under normal circumstances dietary adjustments and/or simple laxatives are adequate means of restoring normal bowel function where there is no underlying obstructive cause. In the severe forms of slow-transit constipation surgery may be indicated. It is now generally accepted that partial resection (e.g. sigmoid colectomy) leads to an early recurrence of symptoms. The treatment of choice is total colectomy and ileorectal anastomosis. This operation restores bowel function at the expense of causing diarrhoea. The abdominal pain these patients describe preoperatively often persists postoperatively, suggesting that the disorder is part of a generalized motility disorder affecting the whole length of the gut.

Patients with pelvic floor dysfunction pose a particular problem in management. Wherever possible, conservative measures to induce liquid stool (by laxatives) and to encourage rectal emptying by the use of irritant suppositories (e.g. glycerine) should be employed. Surgical excision of anterior prolapsing mucosa and repair of rectocoele has been reported as successfully controlling symptoms in up to 50% of patients (Janssen & Van Dijke 1994). Biofeedback techniques to encourage the patient to relax the pelvic floor during attempted defecation are time-consuming but have proved helpful in some cases (Turnbull & Ritvo 1992).

REFERENCES

Bartolo D C C 1986 Flap-valve theory of anorectal continence. British Journal of Surgery 73: 1012–1014

Bennett R C, Duthie H L 1964 The functional importance of the internal sphincter. British Journal of Surgery 51: 355–357

Bradley W E 1972 Urethral electromyelography. Journal of Urology 119: 563–564

Delorme R 1900 Sur le traitement des prolapses du rectum totaux pour l'excision de la muquese rectable au rectocolique. Bulletin des Membres de la Société Chirurgical de Paris 26: 498–499

Engel A F, Kamm M A, Sultan A H, Bartram C I, Nicholls R J 1994 Anterior anal sphincter repair in patients with obstetric trauma. British Journal of Surgery 81: 1231–1234

Floyd W F, Walls E W 1953 Electromyography of the sphincter ani externus in man. Journal of Physiology 122: 599–609

Gill K P, Chia Y W, Henry M M, Shorvon P J 1994 Defecography in multiple sclerosis patients with severe constipation. Radiology 191: 553–556

Gowers W R 1877 The automatic action of the sphincter ani. Proceedings of the Royal Society of London 26: 498–499

Halligan S, Nicholls R J, Bartram C I 1995 Proctographic changes after rectopexy for solitary rectal ulcer syndrome and preoperative predictive factors for a successful outcome. British Journal of Surgery 82: 314–317

Henry M M, Parks A G, Swash M 1982 The pelvic floor muscle in the descending perineum syndrome. British Journal of Surgery 62: 470–472

Henry M M, Porter N H 1988 A colour atlas of faecal incontinence and rectal prolapse. Wolfe Publications, London

Hinton J M, Lennard Jones J E, Young A C 1969 A new method for studying gut transit times using radio-opaque markers. Gut 10: 842–847

Jameson J S, Chia Y W, Kamm M A, Speakman C T M, Chye Y H, Henry M M 1994a Effect of age, sex and parity on anorectal function. British Journal of Surgery 81: 1689–1692

Jameson J S, Speakman C T, Darzi A, Chia Y W, Henry M M 1994b Audit of postanal repair in the treatment of faecal incontinence. Diseases of the Colon and Rectum 37: 369–372

Janssen L W M, Van Dijke C F 1994 Selection criteria for anterior rectal wall repair in symptomatic rectocoele and anterior rectal wall prolapse. Diseases of the Colon and Rectum 37: 1100–1107

Lane R H S, Parks A G 1997 Function of the anal sphincters following colo-anal anastomosis. British Journal of Surgery 64: 596–599

Lauerberg S, Swash M, Henry M M 1988 Delayed external sphincter repair for obstetric tear. British Journal of Surgery 75: 786–788

Law P J, Bartram C I 1989 Anal endosonography – technique and normal anatomy. Gastrointestinal Radiology 14: 349–353

Loening-Baucke V, Read N W 1990 Cortical evoked potentials recorded after electrical endorectal stimulation in human volunteers. Gastroenterology 98: A371

Lubowski D Z, Nicholls R J, Swash M, Jordan M J 1987 Neural control of internal anal sphincter function. British Journal of Surgery 74: 668–670

Mahieu P, Pringot J, Bodart P 1984 Defecography: 1. Description of a new procedure and results in normal patients. Gastrointestinal Radiology 9: 253–261

Merton P A, Hill D K, Morton H B, Marsden C D 1982 Scope of a technique for electrical stimulation of human brain, spinal cord and muscle. Lancet ii: 597–600

Neill M E, Swash M 1980 Increased motor unit fibre density in the external sphincter in anorectal incontinence: a single fibre EMG study. Journal of Neurology, Neurosurgery and Psychiatry 43: 343–347

Neill M E, Parks A G, Swash M 1981 Physiological studies of the anal sphincter musculature in faecal incontinence and rectal prolapse. British Journal of Surgery 68: 531–536

Parks A G 1975 Anorectal incontinence. Proceedings of the Royal Society of Medicine 68: 681–690

Parks A G, Porter N H, Melzack J 1962 Experimental study of the reflex mechanism controlling the muscles of the pelvic floor. Diseases of the Colon and Rectum 5: 407–414

Parks A G, Swash M, Urich H 1977 Sphincter denervation in anorectal incontinence and rectal prolapse. Gut 18: 656–665

Pickrell K, Masters F, Georgiade N, Horton C 1954 Rectal sphincter reconstruction using gracilis muscle transplant. Plastic and Reconstructive Surgery 13: 46–55

Porter N H 1962 Physiological study of the pelvic floor in rectal prolapse. Annals of the Royal College of Surgeons of England 31: 379–404

Rogers J, Levy D M, Henry M M, Misiewicz J J 1988 Pelvic floor neuropathy: a comparative study of diabetes mellitus and idiopathic faecal incontinence. Gut 29: 756–761

Rogers J, Henry M M, Misiewicz J J 1989 Increased segmental activity and intraluminal pressures in the sigmoid colon of patients with irritable bowel syndrome. Gut 30: 634–641

Snooks S J, Swash M 1984 Abnormalities of the innervation of the urethral striated sphincter muscle in incontinence. British Journal of Urology 56: 401–405

Snooks S J, Swash M, Henry M M, Setchell M E 1984 Injury to innervation of pelvic floor sphincter musculature in childbirth. Lancet ii: 546–550

Snooks S J, Swash M, Henry M M 1985a Abnormalities in central and peripheral nerve conduction in patients with anorectal incontinence. Journal of the Royal Society of Medicine 78: 294–300

Snooks S J, Barnes P R H, Swash M, Henry M M 1985b Damage to the innervation of the pelvic floor musculature in chronic constipation. Gastroenterology 89: 977–981
Snooks S J, Nicholls R J, Henry M M, Swash M 1985c Electrophysiological and manometric assessment of the pelvic floor in solitary rectal ulcer syndrome. British Journal of Surgery 72: 131–133
Speakman C T M, Kamm M A, Swash M 1990 Cerebral evoked potentials – are they of value in anorectal disease? Gut 31: A1173
Speakman C T M, Hoyle C H V, Kamm M A, Henry M M, Nicholls R J, Burnstock G 1993 Neuropeptides in the internal anal sphincter in neurogenic faecal incontinence. International Journal of Colorectal Disease 8: 201–205
Sultan A H, Kamm M A, Hudson C N, Thomas J M, Bartram C I 1993 Anal sphincter disruption during vaginal delivery. New England Journal of Medicine 329: 1905–1911
Sultan A H, Kamm M A, Hudson C N 1994 Pudendal nerve damage during labour: prospective study before and after childbirth. British Journal of Obstetrics and Gynaecology 101: 22–28
Turnbull G K, Ritvo P G 1992 Anal sphincter biofeedback relaxation treatment for women with intractable constipation symptoms. Diseases of the Colon and Rectum 35: 530–536
Varma J S, Smith A N, McInnes A 1986 Electrophysiological observations on the human pudendo-anal reflex. Journal of Neurology, Neurosurgery and Psychiatry 227: 135–144
Vernava A M, Longo W E, Daniel R N 1993 Pudendal neuropathy and the importance of EMG evaluation of fecal incontinence. Diseases of the Colon and Rectum 36: 23–27
Walls E W 1959 Recent observations of the anatomy of the anal canal. Proceedings of the Royal Society of Medicine 52 (suppl): 85–87
Williams N S, Hallan R I, Koeze T H, Watkins E S 1990 Construction of a neoanal sphincter by transposition of the gracilis muscle and prolonged neuromuscular stimulation for the treatment of faecal incontinence. Annals of the Royal College of Surgeons of England 72: 108–113
Winkler G 1958 Remarques sur la morphologie et l'innervation du muscle releveur de l'anus. Archives d'Anatomie et Histologie et Embryologie, Strasbourg 41: 77–95
Womack N R, Williams N S, Holmfield J H M, Morrison J F B, Simpkins K C 1985 New method for the dynamic assessment of anorectal function in constipation. British Journal of Surgery 72: 994–997
Womack N R, Morrison J F B, Williams N S 1988 Prospective study of the effects of postanal repair in neurogenic faecal incontinence. British Journal of Surgery 75: 48–52

63

Gynaecology in the elderly

Stuart L. Stanton

Senescence begins and middle age ends, the day your descendants outnumber your friends. *Ogden Nash*

Like all organisms humans are ageing individuals, growing older fastest when youngest. It is only since the beginning of this century that life expectancy has exceeded 50 years in developed countries. The death rate in the elderly has fallen over the last 30 years from 89.1 per 1000 to 67.2 per 1000 for women, and life expectancy for an 80-year-old has risen since 1900 by 7.6 years, probably owing to detection and treatment of disease earlier in life rather than by any direct impact on the health of the elderly.

In animals it is unusual to find a menopause. Whereas most animals show a decline in reproductive capability, there is usually some functioning reproductive tissue at death. Woman is exceptional in having a menopause, perhaps evolving this to limit the effects of harmful environmental factors on future generations.

The link between growth and reproduction is interesting: in the plant world they continue simultaneously. In animals and humans, perhaps because of the competition for resources, growth is completed before reproduction takes place, although few other species have their young born so defenceless and none need potential support for so long. No other organism recognizes its grandparents as family!

The elderly ageing female, although sometimes given pride of place in a matriarchal society, has long been a second-class medical citizen – too old for treatment and accused of disabilities that are a natural consequence of ageing and undeserving of treatment. Terms such as 'senile' vaginitis and 'senile' dementia ought to have been abandoned long ago.

We take the age of 65 years as the starting point for the definition of elderly – the official age of retirement for both sexes, and when pensions are collected and, in some countries, transport is free. The frail elderly may be defined as being above 75 years. The changes found in old age in the female represent those acquired during life and aggravated by withdrawal of oestrogen at the time of menopause.

VULVA

The vulva, like other oestrogen-dependent tissues, atrophies and a mild vulval dystrophy, producing discomfort and irritation, is common. The labia are more readily irritated and more prone to neoplastic change than normal skin. Sexually transmitted diseases, common in the younger age group, may occur, e.g. genital warts and herpes. Non-sexually transmitted herpes (herpes zoster) occurs more frequently. Labial adhesion is not an uncommon abnormality but rarely causes a problem, unless there is vaginal bleeding or incontinence due to uncertain cause. Under a general anaesthetic the labia may be peeled apart and local oestrogen applied to prevent readherence.

Pruritus vulvae is an embarrassing symptom commonly encountered in the elderly.

The important causes include infection, lichen sclerosis, eczema and vulval dystrophy, and underlying systemic skin diseases.

VAGINA

The walls of the vagina become thinner after the menopause owing to the withdrawal of oestrogen, although up to 40% of women will still have oestrogenized vaginal smears for some years. There is a decline in intracellular glycogen production, leading to a decrease in lactobacillae and lactic acid and an increase in the vaginal pH from acid to alkali. These changes lead to an increase in colonization by pathogenic bacteria, accounting for the common occurrence of vaginal infection.

In addition, the decreased oestrogen leads to loss of vaginal tissue elasticity and shrinkage of the vagina, producing dyspareunia and bleeding.

CERVIX AND UTERUS

The squamocolumnar junction of the cervix often recedes into the endocervical canal. This makes it more difficult to obtain an accurate representative cervical smear, so it is important to use a spatula with a narrow enough end to sample the cells from within the lower portion of the endocervical canal.

There is a change in the relative proportion of the cervix to uterus after the menopause: the cervix lengthens by almost 50% and the uterine body becomes smaller, some of this caused by a decrease in cell cytoplasm, again owing to oestrogen withdrawal. The myometrium decreases in bulk and the endometrium becomes thinner. The glands become inactive, mitosis ceases and sometimes cystic dilatation occurs. Unopposed oestrogen (endogenous and exogenous) may lead to endometrial hyperplasia, which may be premalignant.

OVARY

After the menopause the few remaining primordial follicles do not respond to gonadotrophin and oestrogen secretion falls, being only maintained by the stroma. The decline in ovarian function takes place over some 10 years or so. Macroscopically the ovary becomes smaller and more wrinkled with the continuing involution of the cortex, with some relative increase in medullary size.

PELVIC FLOOR

The pelvic floor gradually weakens owing to the combined effects of oestrogen withdrawal and age. The levator ani undergoes increased denervation (Smith et al 1989) and connective tissue, having some dependence on oestrogen, also weakens. This explains the deterioration in pelvic fascia and the increasing likelihood of genital prolapse as age increases. The interdependence of prolapse and age changes have been shown by Smith et al (1989). Lewis (1968) showed that prolapse accounted for 60% of surgery in elderly patients.

URETHRA AND BLADDER

Both the urethra and trigone of the bladder are sensitive to oestrogen and there is deterioration in structure and function as a woman ages.

The urethral lumen becomes more slit-shaped and the folds become coarser. The mucosal lining changes from transitional in the proximal two-thirds to non-keratinizing squamous epithelium.

In the young woman the submucosa contains very rich venous plexuses. In the postmenopausal period the veins become wider and penetrate between the smooth muscle bundles of the longitudinal smooth muscle coat. There are many arteriovenous anastomoses, which decline postmenopausally.

The quantity of elastin increases. The circular muscle coat of the urethra increases in thickness, whereas the whole of the posterior wall of the urethra shows a decline in the amount of striated muscle. With increasing age the diameters of the muscle fibres show a greater variation, whereas the density of the muscle coat greatly decreases (Huisman 1979). All of this makes urethral closure less competent. Urodynamic studies show that the bladder becomes slower, with a reduction in detrusor contraction power during voiding. There is a greater tendency for the detrusor contraction to fade shortly after initiation of voiding, with voiding frequently occurring by means of poorly sustained contractions. The elderly have lower bladder capacities and fullness is experienced at a higher proportion of bladder capacity. This suggests that older people are less sensitive to bladder filling and less inclined to sensory urgency (Malone-Lee 1992). These features account for a greater prevalence of urinary incontinence in the elderly, which varies from 5 to 15% in the community to between 20 and 30% in hospitalized patients, and more than 50% in nursing homes (DuBeau & Resnick 1991).

The pathophysiological changes lead to a higher prevalence of detrusor instability (between 75 and 85%) than in the younger population. Withdrawal of oestrogen may lead to a high prevalence of urinary tract infection in the elderly (20% at 70 years or more; Dantas et al 1981), which is aggravated by voiding difficulty and may lead to symptoms of stress and voiding difficulty. Monga and Stanton (1996) reviewed 280 elderly women with incontinence and found a prevalence of 39% due to urethral sphincter incompetence, 29% due to detrusor instability and 6% with voiding difficulty. The remainder had a mix of urethral sphincter incompetence and detrusor instability.

Any discussion on the bladder and pelvic floor in the elderly should note the important differences between the geriatric and the younger patient. First, the disease presentation in the elderly may be altered by constricted physiological reserves. Secondly, incontinence is more likely to be secondary to different diseases and to have multiple causes. Thirdly, treatment goals and expectations differ widely, and individualized management structures must be evolved (DuBeau & Resnick 1991).

The investigation of urinary symptoms is controversial. Algorithms may be a simple non-invasive and cost-effective approach, yielding a diagnostic accuracy of 83% and a therapeutic accuracy of 95% (Hilton & Stanton 1981), but they lack the precision of urodynamic studies. The latter are invasive, often uncomfortable, costly, and may not yield a great deal more. It is sensible to use an algorithmic approach initially and use urodynamics when simple conservative measures fail and surgery appears likely.

TREATMENT

Caring for the elderly may be compromised by a high default rate to follow-up. Monga and Stanton (1996) reviewed 280 patients who were followed up for 5 years and found that 34 (12%) defaulted before treatment and 92 (32%) defaulted after treatment. Other difficulties included the high prevalence of medical conditions needing treatment. Vaz and Seymour (1989) found that only 20% of general surgical patients over 65 years of age were free of preoperative medical problems, and 30% had three or more problems, the latter group having three times the postoperative morbidity of the former. In patients undergoing colonic surgery, it was preoperative disease rather than age which was the main determinant of immediate postoperative outcome. In a small matched series of 289 patients undergoing colposuspension for incontinence, with 50 women over 65 years, the outcome in terms of length of stay, success rate, postoperative pyrexia and wound infection rates was similar to the remaining patients under 65 years (Baker & Drutz 1992). However, this changes with increasing age: Pollock and Evans (1987) audited major abdominal surgery outcomes in patients over 80 and found increased morbidity and mortality, which were further increased in those patients admitted as emergencies.

Because of slow drug metabolism in the elderly and the tendency of some drugs to have cardiotoxic side effects, it is wiser to use small doses (e.g. 2.5 mg of oxybutynin hydrochloride daily for detrusor instability) and combine this with bladder retraining. The dose can gradually be increased and titrated against side effects and improvement.

SURGERY

Normally, elderly patients tolerate vaginal operations better than abdominal operations. However, care should be taken to avoid short-lived expediency by recommending an inferior and painfree operation with a short-lived success, rather than a more extensive and painful suprapubic operation with a greater chance of cure. The demands of the patient's lifestyle and quality of life must be taken into account. The proportion of elective and emergency gynaecological surgery may vary according to age. In a district general hospital, for example, 6.5% of gynaecological patients over 65 were admitted for elective surgery, whereas 2.4% were admitted for emergency gynaecological surgery (Holmes 1995, personal communication).

The case mix of admissions varies: Lewis (1968) found that 19% had malignancy and 68% had prolapse or incontinence. Isaacs and Baquero (1987) found that 62% had malignancy and 22% were being treated for prolapse and incontinence. Old age should not debar surgery. The elderly will have more age-associated pathology and a higher postoperative morbidity and mortality, and therefore need a more individualized approach to preoperative assessment and postoperative management. The former should include a discussion with the patient and her carers about expectations, risk benefits and expected progress. Risk prediction is important but difficult. A past or present medical problem may increase postoperative morbidity and mortality threefold. Emergency surgery is associated with a three- to fourfold increase in mortality. In addition, some surgical complications present atypically in the elderly, so confusing and delaying the diagnosis. The APACHE III system, with a database of 17 440 adults, has predictions to guide therapy but must be used in conjunction with clinical judgement. The CEPOD Audit (Buck et al 1987) found that 79% of perioperative mortality occurred in patients over 65 years of age. Intercurrent disease was thought to contribute to death in between 44 and 52% of cases. It is important to note that morbidity may be prolonged beyond the stay in hospital, and Jaluvka (1980) found that 80% of deaths had occurred by the 15th day.

The majority of mortality and morbidity may be attributed to respiratory, cardiovascular or neurological disease. About 28% of elderly patients have symptoms of preoperative respiratory disease. The risk factors for postoperative morbidity include preoperative chest disease, a high abdominal wound and smoking. The peak incidence for respiratory complications is between the second and fourth postoperative days. Recent studies with a pulse oximeter have shown that a high proportion of elderly patients have postoperative hypoxaemia, and that this may be responsible for arrhythmias leading to sudden death which in the past has been attributed to occult cardiac disease. Hypothermia can be a significant problem for the elderly. Heat loss through an open peritoneal cavity, inadequate warmth within a cool theatre, and cold intravenous fluid may unexpectedly lower core temperature. Uncontrolled hypothermia can lead to hypotension and cardiac arrhythmia. Frequent temperature recording and the use of foil insulation around the patient are important.

Preoperative cardiovascular disease has been found in 50% of elderly patients. About 1–3% are likely to have a myocardial infarct and 5–10% will have cardiovascular failure postoperatively. The risk factors include age over 70 years, a myocardial infarct within 3–6 months and symptoms of cardiac failure.

About 1% of postoperative patients over 65 develop a cerebrovascular accident. About 10% will have postoperative delirium: of these a third will be due to respiratory infection and other causes will include sedatives and cardiac failure. The high incidence of all these complications in the elderly is an argument for placing postopera-

Table 63.1 Cure rates for urethral sphincter incompetence in the elderly

		n	Cure (%)
Gillon & Stanton (1984)	Colposuspension	35	89 (O)
Peattie & Stanton (1988)	Stamey	44	39 (O)
Griffiths Jones & Abrams (1990)	Stamey	21	65 (S)
Kato et al (1990)	Stamey	33	88 (S)
Nitti et al (1993)	Raz	92	88 (S)
Stanton et al (1995)	Raz	39	46 (O)

O, objective; S, subjective

tive elderly patients on a medical rather than a surgical ward, where the insidious postoperative onset of respiratory, cerebrovascular and neurological failure is likely to be better detected.

The preoperative assessment was discussed in Chapter 7 by Van Besouw and Tidy. The additional investigations recommended for the elderly include serum urea and electrolytes, ECG, chest X-ray and a random blood sugar test.

Vaginal prolapse surgery, such as vaginal hysterectomy and anterior and posterior repair, are usually safer and non-traumatic operations and are reasonable alternatives to a ring pessary if the latter is inadequate. If there is coexisting urethral sphincter incompetence, either a Raz endoscopic procedure combined with an anterior colporrhaphy can be performed or, alternatively, if the patient is fit and has adequate vaginal capacity and mobility, a colposuspension may be used. Cure rates for sphincter incompetence in the elderly are shown in Table 63.1.

SEXUALITY

There is no upper age limit for the expression of sexuality, which may vary from generation to generation. In a probability sample survey of couples in the community over 60 years of age, 56% of married and 5% of unmarried women and 74% of married and 31% of unmarried men were still sexually active (Diokno et al 1990). Sexual activity is an important part of marital stability which in turn may play a role in stabilizing society, in which the older person as grandparent has an important role. The Kinsey Reports (1948, 1953) are the largest detailed study of human sexual behaviour but have small samples of those over 65. Whereas the prevalence of intercourse falls to less than three times a week by the age of 60, the quality and degree of sexual satisfaction rises after the age of 50. When activity does cease for a couple, it is usually a decision of the male owing to involuntary erectile failure.

The physical changes in the female may correspond to the withdrawal of oestrogen and progesterone at the menopause (unless hormone replacement therapy is given), although testosterone secretion is maintained through ovarian and adrenal androgen production. In the elderly the distinction between the excitatory and plateau phases is less well marked.

In the excitatory phase the swelling and parting of the labia majora is rare after the age of 50. Lubrication is delayed and less prolific, but nipple erection occurs and is well maintained.

In the plateau phase skin flushing is less common and the clitoris shows less glans swelling than in the younger woman. The orgasm contractions are slighter and there may be no accompanying rectal contractions. The resolution phase proceeds rapidly.

The elderly woman still remains more flexible than her male partner, and able to enjoy orgasm long after the time that her partner can penetrate; however, the loss of sexual activity is more easily accepted than in the male. Intimate physical contact still remains an important feature of their partnership.

SUMMARY

Women of all ages have a right to expect health care treatment. It is wrong to imply that disorders of the elderly are, per se, due to age and are therefore not treatable. Many of the conditions in this chapter may be managed by appropriate hormone replacement therapy. Surgery should not be withheld when the patient is fit.

KEY POINTS

1. Oestrogen deprivation adversely affects pelvic floor and urethral sphincter function and may promote urinary infection.
2. The elderly have a high default rate and need care with follow-up.
3. Surgery in the elderly has higher morbidity and mortality than in the young.
4. There is no upper age limit for expression of sexuality.

REFERENCES

Baker K, Drutz H 1992 Age as a risk factor in major genitourinary surgery. Canadian Journal of Surgery 35: 188–191

Buck N, Devlin H, Lunn J 1987 Report of a confidential enquiry into perioperative deaths (CEPOD); London. Nuffield Provinces Hospital Trust, London

Dantas A, Kasviki-Charvati P, Papanawiotou P, Marketos S 1981

Bacteriuria and survival in old age. New England Journal of Medicine 304: 939–943
Diokno A, Brown M, Herzog R 1990 Sexual function in the elderly. Archives of Internal Medicine 150: 197–200
DuBeau C, Resnick N 1991 Evaluation of the causes and severity of geriatric incontinence. Urologic Clinics of North America 18: 243–256
Gillon G, Stanton S L 1984 Long term follow-up for surgery for urinary incontinence in elderly women. British Journal of Urology 56: 478–481
Griffiths Jones M, Abrams P 1990 The Stamey endoscopic bladder neck suspension in the elderly. British Journal of Urology 65: 170–172
Hilton P, Stanton S L 1981 Algorithmic methods for assessing urinary incontinence in elderly women. British Medical Journal 282: 940–942
Huisman A 1979 Morphology of the female urethra. MD Thesis, University of Groningen
Isaacs J H, Baquero I O 1987 Good reasons for surgery in older patients. Contemporary Obstetrics and Gynecology 29: 153–168
Jaluvka V 1980 Surgical geriatric gynaecology. A contribution to geriatric gynaecology with particular consideration of post-operative mortality. Gynecology and Obstetrics 7: 171–173
Kato K, Kondo A, Saito M, Otani T 1990 Stamey's procedure for stress urinary incontinence: surgical results between the elderly and adults. Neurourology and Urodynamics 9: 399–400
Kinsey A, Pomeroy W, Martin C 1948 Sexual behaviour in the human male. Saunders, Philadelphia
Kinsey A, Pomeroy W, Martin C, Gebhard P 1953 Sexual behaviour in the human female. Saunders, Philadelphia
Lewis A 1968 Major gynaecological surgery in the elderly. Journal of the International Federation for Gynecology and Obstetrics 6: 244–258
Malone-Lee J 1992 Urinary incontinence. Reviews in Clinical Gerontology 2: 123–139
Monga A, Madjar S, Stanton S L 1996. A comparative study of urinary incontinence in women below and above 65 years. (Submitted)
Nitti V, Bregg K, Sussman E, Raz S 1993 The Raz bladder neck suspension in patients 65 years and older. Journal of Urology 149: 802–807
Peattie A, Stanton S L 1988 The Stamey operation for correction of genuine stress incontinence in the elderly. Neurourology and Urodynamics 7: 287–288
Pollock A, Evans M 1987 Major abdominal operations on patients aged 80 or over: an audit. British Medical Journal 295: 1522
Smith A, Hosker G, Warrell D 1989 The role of partial denervation of the pelvic floor and the aetiology of genito-urinary prolapse and stress incontinence of urine: a neurophysiological study. British Journal of Obstetrics and Gynaecology 99: 24–28
Stanton S L, Reynolds S, Creighton S 1995 The modified Pereyra (Raz) procedure for genuine stress incontinence – a useful option in the elderly or frail patient? International Urogynecology Journal 6: 222–225
Vaz F, Seymour D 1989 A prospective study of elderly general surgical patients in Cardiff. Methodology and preoperative problems. Age and Ageing 18: 309–315

64

Effective care in gynaecology

G. Jarvis

INTRODUCTION

When Chalmers et al (1989) published their textbook *Effective Care in Pregnancy and Childbirth,* the editor of the *British Journal of Obstetrics and Gynaecology* described it in an editorial as 'probably the most important book in obstetrics to appear this century' (Paintin 1990). This was the first textbook in any specialty of medicine which consisted entirely of structured reviews of selected topics, but perhaps even more importantly, it contained a detailed account of the methodology that could be adopted in the preparation of such a structured review.

Why a structured review rather than a detailed review? One reason is that a structured review makes a strenuous attempt to minimize bias, especially selection bias. In a review the author analyses the available scientific information and selects from that information the publications that illustrate the concepts and details under discussion. In a structured review there is no selection – the author must present all of the information which is available in an easily assimilable fashion, but must also describe the methodology by which that information was obtained and analysed.

The first part of this chapter will make a critical assessment of the technique of structured review; the second part will select structured reviews from within gynaecology to illustrate how such a process may make the management of our patients more effective.

Systematic reviews are not confined to obstetrics and gynaecology. They have been widely used, for instance, in neonatology (the prevention of neonatal respiratory distress syndrome using surfactant; Enhorning et al 1985), cardiology (fibrinolytic therapy in the prevention of mortality in acute myocardial infarction; Yusuf et al 1985) and orthopaedic surgery (the prevention of venous thromboembolism; Imperiale & Speroff 1994). The Cochrane Database of Systematic Reviews is arguably the most comprehensive collection of such reviews currently available (Cochrane Library 1996).

PREPARATION AND MAINTENANCE OF A STRUCTURED REVIEW

A structured review means exactly what it says. Whatever the exact style chosen by the author in the presentation of the structured review, the following eight principles must be an integral part of the exercise:

1. State objective.
2. State eligibility criteria.
3. Identify all potentially eligible studies.
4. Assemble complete set of potentially eligible studies.
5. Apply eligibility criteria.
6. Analyse data.
7. Prepare report.
8. Maintain the review.

Each of these will now be discussed in turn.

State objective

There must be a very clear statement of the objective of the exercise: a general title, as used in a review, is unsatisfactory for this purpose. This clear statement of the objective, both in the text and in the title, not only acts as a control on clarity of thought in the author and the reader, but it also allows the structured review to be identified from a search of the literature at a later date. Thus, for example, the publication by Yusuf et al (1985) referred to above is entitled 'Intravenous and intracoronary fibrinolytic therapy in acute myocardial infarction – overview of results on mortality, reinfarction and side-effects from 33 randomised control trials'. In gynaecology, Hughes et al (1992) entitled their structured review 'The routine use of gonadotrophin-releasing hormone agonists prior to in vitro fertilisation and gamete intrafallopian transfer – a meta-analysis of randomised controlled trials'.

Apply eligibility criteria

All clinical trials carry eligibility criteria and those from one trial may not be the same as those from another on the same subject. This allows for some degree of heterogeneity and may leave the concept of a structured review open to the criticism that it is comparing apples with oranges.

Although heterogeneity may be tested mathematically (and this is discussed in the section of the analysis of data) the reasons why each and every identified study should be included or excluded from the final analysis must be made clear to the reader, who may or may not agree with the criteria supplied.

There are several examples from the gynaecological literature which illustrate the importance of stating such eligibility criteria.

Fantl et al (1994) identified 166 scientific articles which assessed oestrogen therapy in the management of urinary incontinence in postmenopausal women. Some 143 of these did not meet the entry criteria, even though the entry criteria as stated by Fantl and his colleagues were relatively simple. They chose to include only articles which appeared in a peer-reviewed journal; subjects with a confirmed diagnosis of urinary incontinence based on either clinical or urodynamic evaluation, a named oestrogen, together with its dosage and whether used in the presence or absence of a progestin; it had to be stated whether the findings were subjective (symptoms or signs) or objective (pad test or urodynamic assessment); and comparison had to be included with either a control group in controlled trials or an estimated change in uncontrolled trials. Another example of the importance of eligibility criteria comes from the scientific assessment of the literature on infertility. Vandekerckhove et al (1993) identified 501 randomized trials in male and female infertility treatment, yet pregnancy was only assessed as an outcome in 291 (58%).

Identify all potentially eligible studies

The identification of all potentially eligible studies is the most difficult, time-consuming yet important part of the preparation of a structured review.

In an ideal world this ought really to be the simplest. The reviewer should expect to go to the nearest computer terminal linked to a database of scientific publications, key in perhaps three accepted MeSH terms, and return a little later to pick up the printout of all potentially eligible studies. However, the reviewer who adopts this technique will produce a most incomplete study for several reasons.

Publication bias

Unpublished studies may not have appeared in peer-review journals, not because their methodology was inferior, but because their results were negative. The published literature may therefore overestimate the strength of effectiveness of any given treatment compared to non-intervention (Easterbrook et al 1991, Dickersin et al 1994). The existence of such studies can only be assessed at present by such techniques as searching abstracts of international scientific meetings, or by knowing work which currently exists but has not been published in a journal. This is clearly an unsatisfactory and biasing situation, and perhaps will only be overcome by the establishment of a trial register wherein every clinical trial commenced is registered with a central body which can then be accessed by other workers.

Problems of electronic searches

All the information currently available in peer-reviewed journals may not always be identified by an electronic search. This is partly because those organizations that cull the literature in order to produce a database of scientific publications may do so in an incomplete manner, and partly because the search strategy by the reviewer is suboptimal.

The risks that electronic databases give incomplete information may be minimized by simple improvements. A reviewer cannot expect to retrieve a randomized clinical trial if the author of the publication or the editor of the journal does not classify the study as such. Such a statement may be obvious, but nevertheless important. It is only in the last 4 years that the *British Journal of Obstetrics and Gynaecology*, for instance, has carried a specific index item of randomized controlled trials, yet this journal is well ahead of the field, with many mainline journals not carrying such an index title. There needs to be improved training and quality control by those who cull the literature, such as the National Library of Congress which is aware of the problem and taking great steps to minimize it. Searches can improve retrieval of trials electronically by adopting a structured strategy, which includes taking advice from those who are used to electronic searches in such aspects as the choice of MeSH headings and free text terms. Even in units which pride themselves on an ability to produce an optimal search strategy, electronic searching is still incomplete. One of our Research Fellows searched for trials in gynaecological oncology within the *British Journal of Obstetrics and Gynaecology* and the *American Journal of Obstetrics and Gynecology*. This electronic search was then checked by a hand search. If the total number of publications available by combined electronic and hand searching was 100%, the electronic search revealed only 69% of available publications within the British journal, whereas the hand search revealed 94%. Similarly, the electronic search revealed 61% of those publications within the American journal, whereas the hand search revealed 83%. It is therefore clear that a search strategy must include both electronic and hand searching.

Hand searching

Hand searching is neither glamorous nor rapid. It is a long and tedious process and is not 100% complete because of observer fatigue. Moreover, it is not practical to hand search all potential journals for appropriate scientific publications. In the British Library there are approximately 18 000 biomedical journals. It is therefore appropriate to limit hand searching to those journals the reviewer knows will have a satisfactory yield of appropriate publications, and to augment this with a hand search of journals regularly represented within the electronic search. Without such a strategy, the law of diminishing returns will apply (Cooke 1996).

Restriction to randomized controlled trials

Some structured reviews are confined only to randomized controlled clinical trials, whereas other reviews allow a wider brief and include case control studies or even open studies. The randomized controlled trial is the 'gold standard' of medical treatment evaluation, and where a search has provided sufficient controlled trials to allow a conclusion to be reached, even if that conclusion is that the available information is incomplete and additional studies are required, it is appropriate to analyse only these controlled trials and to state this in the methodology.

Unfortunately, if this idea was applied to gynaecology huge sections of knowledge would not be represented. There are sufficient randomized controlled trials in certain areas, for example infertility and chemotherapy for ovarian cancer, for this stance to be taken with scientific credibility, but there are other areas of gynaecology where to exclude all but randomized controlled trials would mean that large sections of available information would be ignored. Perhaps the best example of this relates to the assessment of increased risk of breast cancer in women receiving hormone replacement therapy. There are currently some 37 such case controlled studies known to this author, and no randomized trial. It is also most improbable that a randomized trial to assess the risk of breast cancer in women receiving hormone replacement therapy will ever take place. It is therefore appropriate that such studies are analysed as the basis of a structured review, and this must be made clear in the methodology. There are other areas of gynaecology where small numbers of randomized trials exist, but do not allow firm conclusions to be based purely on their own evidence. In such a situation it is appropriate to analyse the data from randomized controlled trials and from open studies, making it clear in the methodology that this is the situation. For instance, in a recent review of the objective incidence of continence following different surgical treatments for genuine stress incontinence, some 213 studies were identified but only seven involved randomized trials. To have analysed only the studies with randomized trials would have meant that the results would have been identified in only 556 out of 20 481 patients (Jarvis 1994). A more recent structured review has identified a further 5 randomized trials of surgery for this condition (Downs and Black 1996).

It is therefore better that the deficiencies of the available literature are identified in a structured review, for this may act as a stimulus in further research.

Assemble complete set of potentially eligible studies

This requires no further amplification.

Apply eligibility criteria

It is in this section that the clarity of thought in devising the objective or objectives becomes important. There is little relevance, for instance, in analysing those trials of the treatment of infertility which do not take pregnancy as an outcome, where this objective is being studied. Such trials may be worthy of analysis by a different outcome, for instance complication rates, but should not be included in the pregnancy outcome assessments.

A further example of the importance of such clarity of eligibility criteria was illustrated in a recent review of the efficacy of progesterone support for pregnancy in women with recurrent miscarriage (Daya 1989). This reviewer identified 34 potentially eligible studies, yet analysed only three that met the criteria. Some studies had to be excluded because they reported on patients with threatened miscarriage without a previous history of recurrent miscarriage; some had to be excluded because there were incomplete data available on the previous miscarriages which made meaningful comparison impossible; and other studies had to be excluded after points of clarification were made following direct contact with the authors of the published studies. This illustrates an important point in the preparation of a structured overview. There will be times when the studies identified do not give the information necessary to decide whether or not they fulfil the eligibility criteria. The reviewer should have no hesitation in making contact with the first-named author of the study and seeking detailed clarification.

Analysis of data

Data may be analysed in a number of ways, and one commonly used technique in contemporary practice is meta-analysis.

Inevitably, different trials will vary in the magnitude and sometimes even in the direction of the observed treatment compared with the controlled group, especially if the trials are small. Small trials may demonstrate an apparent difference between measured outcome and expected outcome where none exists, or may fail to demonstrate such a difference where a difference does exist. The technique of meta-analysis involves the combining of results of studies in order to produce a single estimate of outcome, the difference between observed and expected outcome being analysed using such techniques as confidence intervals, relative risk or odds ratios (Altman & Elbourne 1988, Morris & Gardner 1988, Simes 1990, Hughes 1992).

When such a meta-analysis takes place the size of the population under study increases and the 95% confidence intervals become narrower. The result of this assessment is that whereas individual trials may fail to demonstrate a statistical significance between observed and expected outcome because they are not sufficiently powerful, the meta-analysis may suggest such a difference in that the 95% confidence intervals no longer straddle unity. An example of this is the meta-analysis referred to above by Daya, on the efficacy of progesterone support for pregnancy in women with recurrent miscarriages. The three trials that satisfied the eligibility criteria all had 95% confidence intervals which straddled unity, whereas the overall estimate from meta-analysis suggested a statistically significant improvement in outcome with treatment in this situation.

There is also the technique of cumulative meta-analysis, in which the results of each trial in order of publication date are cumulatively analysed with all previous trials, rather than as a single baseline. The advantage of such a technique is that it becomes possible to indicate the date by which a statistically significant improvement in outcome was demonstrable, even though individual trials rarely had the power to produce such a narrow confidence interval. Although confirmatory studies are then required before the benefit is finally accepted, the technique illustrates the point at which further published studies added little to the information other than further narrowing of the confidence intervals. This technique has been used to assess the application of intravenous streptokinase as a thrombolytic therapy for acute myocardial infarction (Lau et al 1992). These authors identified 33 trials evaluating this therapy between 1959 and 1988. By 1973, an accumulated 2432 patients had been involved in trials which, when analysed together, first demonstrated a statistically significant outcome favouring treatment. The remaining 26 trials, involving over 34 000 patients, merely served to narrow the 95% confidence intervals while presumably approximately 17 000 of these patients were denied streptokinase intervention.

Meta-analysis, however, is not a technique without its problems or its critics. The single most important potential criticism is that trials with different entry criteria, and therefore potentially different patient populations, may be combined and thereby produce a result which may not be clinically applicable. This is termed clinical heterogeneity, and the size of this heterogeneity can be assessed either empirically by the reviewer comparing entry criteria and excluding those trials where clear non-compatibility is present, or mathematically and statistically using known formulae (Eysenck 1994, Thompson 1994). If statistical heterogeneity cannot be demonstrated, it does not mean that clinical heterogeneity is not present, but if statistical heterogeneity can be demonstrated then it is probably inappropriate for the meta-analysis to have been carried out in the first place. This is really a criticism of the reviewer rather than a criticism of the technique.

Prepare report

The report should detail the points made in this description of the production of a systematic review. It is particularly important for eligibility criteria to be stated, those studies excluded to be identified, and a full reference list given. This may cause a potential conflict between the reviewer and the editor of the journal, since a publication bearing perhaps 200–300 references may mean that the reference section is actually larger than the paper itself, and editorial boards may need to be convinced of the importance of the reference section in its entirety.

It is also appropriate that the reviewer should discuss the implications for clinical practice based on the findings and the implications, if any, for future research.

Maintain the review

When a structured review is published it is merely a snapshot of the available information at the time when the review was assembled. It is important that the reviewer keeps the analysis complete and up to date, especially in reviews which have failed to demonstrate a benefit from a given method of treatment. With further studies it may be that the confidence intervals shorten and a benefit then becomes apparent. When this happens it should be communicated to the journal which published the original study. It is also possible that original meta-analyses which suggested a benefit of a given treatment may ultimately fail to confirm that benefit with increasing information, although this is less likely especially in the presence of either a relatively powerful effect or of relatively close confidence intervals.

FURTHER EXAMPLES IN GYNAECOLOGY

Examples of the results from structured overviews and their clinical implications have already been given above. However, there are a relatively small but increasing number of structured reviews available in the gynaecological literature and these have significant implications for gynaecological practice. Examples of some of these will now be given. Since this is not a structured review of structured reviews in gynaecology, the author has selected overviews within gynaecology to illustrate areas of clinical importance. Constraints on space must obviously allow this review to be incomplete.

Infertility

There are more randomized control trials assessing procedures within assisted conception than in other areas of infertility or reproductive medicine. Such studies have been reviewed by Vandekerckhove et al (1993). Perhaps three recent structured overviews should be detailed.

Gonadotrophin-releasing hormone agonists and ovulation induction

Hughes et al (1992) analysed 10 trials comparing clinical pregnancy rates per treatment cycle following the use of gonadotrophin-releasing hormone (GnRH) agonists associated with different techniques of ovulation induction protocols, with techniques that did not involve the use of such agonists. This analysis suggested that the routine use of GnRH agonists may increase the incidence of clinical pregnancy by between 80 and 127%, although the authors state that these results should be accepted with some degree of caution since the quality of randomization in the studies concerned was not as high as it might have been. Several of the trials included did not use satisfactory randomization (telephone randomization, sealed envelopes, random number sequences), but either used quasi randomization (allocation by alternating day, patient, hospital record number) or failed to describe a technique of randomization at all. It is appropriate that if quasi randomization is used or the technique of randomization is not described, trials should be excluded from the analysis.

Luteal phase support

Soliman et al (1994) used meta-analysis to assess the role of luteal phase support in infertility treatment based on randomized trials. This assessment suggested a reduced spontaneous abortion rate when progesterone or hCG were used for luteal phase support in IVF cycles, but not with other infertility treatments.

Hysterosalpingography

Sometimes meta-analysis demonstrates a surprising result which then requires the establishment of a hypothesis, which will itself then need to be tested. Watson et al (1994) described a significant increase in pregnancy rates following hysterosalpingography performed using an oil-soluble contrast medium compared to pregnancy rates following use of a water-soluble contrast medium. This apparent benefit was greatest for patients with unexplained infertility. The authors concluded that oil-soluble media may be better able to 'flush out' mucous plugs within the fallopian tubes than can water-based media, and this would account for the results in unexplained infertility. Such a meta-analysis has therefore produced a hypothesis which itself can now be scientifically tested.

Recurrent spontaneous miscarriage

Progesterone and recurrent miscarriage

The structured review by Daya (1989) on the efficacy of progesterone support for pregnancy in women with recurrent miscarriage has already been described.

Immunotherapy

Fraser et al (1993) reviewed the value of immunization with either leukocyte immunotherapy or trophoblast membrane infusion in the treatment of recurrent spontaneous miscarriage. Whereas earlier studies had suggested a benefit, subsequent randomized trials, including a meta-analysis which included the original data, have failed to demonstrate a benefit (the 95% confidence intervals for the odds ratio of benefit ranging from 0.44 to 3.8). With such wide confidence intervals it is not possible to draw the conclusion of benefit.

Visual display units

There has been much media speculation on the potential association between the use of a visual display terminal (VDU) and the outcome of pregnancy. Parazzini et al (1993) identified seven studies which analysed the relationship between VDU use and the risk of spontaneous miscarriage. The confidence intervals of the odds ratios for spontaneous abortion in women exposed to VDUs during pregnancy range between 0.9 and 1.2, with identical confidence intervals for the risk of congenital malformations. Women can therefore be reassured that there is no evidence for increased risk following exposure to VDUs.

Infections

Prophylactic antibiotics and hysterectomy

It is probably no longer justifiable to omit prophylactic antibiotic therapy in women undergoing total abdominal hysterectomy for benign disease. Mittendorf et al (1993) identified 25 randomized controlled trials of antibiotic prophylaxis which satisfied rigorous protocols. Overall, 21% of patients who did not receive antibiotic prophylaxis had a serious infection after abdominal hysterectomy, compared to 9.0% who did receive antibiotics. The 95% confidence intervals for the odds ratio did not straddle unity. It may now be difficult, both clinically and medicolegally, to omit prophylactic antibiotics unless there is a specific reason for doing so.

Treatment of pelvic inflammatory disease

A common clinical situation is the recurrence of acute pelvic inflammatory disease when the causative microorganism has not been identified. Walker et al (1993) identified 34 treatment studies, of which 21 met the criteria for evaluation. This study identified several treatment regimens, all of which used a combination of more than one antimicrobial agent, which would carry a clinical cure rate of between 75 and 94% in acute pelvic inflammatory disease.

Urinary infections

Single-dose antibiotic treatment for urinary tract infection is an attractive alternative to the conventional 5–14-day course, and is associated with increased patient acceptability, decreased cost and decreased side effects. Leibovici and Wysenbeek (1991) identified 25 randomized controlled trials which compared single-dose antibiotics with a more conventional therapy and concluded that single-dose antibiotic therapy was inadequate when compared with multidose regimens. There is now a need for increased numbers of trials which compare a 3–5-day regimen with a 7–10-day regimen.

Urinary incontinence

Surgical techniques for stress incontinence

The need for an increased number of randomized trials that compare different techniques of surgical treatment for genuine stress incontinence has already been stated. Although it is highly probable that suprapubic techniques will carry an increased continence rate balanced by an increased incidence of side effects, there are only two randomized studies that compare these techniques, and the appropriate arms of those trials involve less than 300 patients. The need for one large trial is clear.

Role of HRT

The use of oestrogen in the management of urinary incontinence in postmenopausal women has been assessed (Fantl et al 1994). These authors were able to demonstrate convincing evidence that the use of oestrogen subjectively improves urinary incontinence in postmenopausal women, together with objective evidence for a significant effect on the maximum urethral closure pressure but no significant overall effect on the quantity of urine lost by incontinent postmenopausal women. It is therefore unlikely that oestrogen alone represents an acceptable form of treatment for such patients.

Nocturnal enuresis

There has been increased interest in the use of synthetic vasopressin (desmopressin or DDAVP) in the treatment of nocturnal enuresis. Most of the good-quality scientific evidence available relates to paediatric studies, and Moffatt et al (1993) analysed the data from 18 randomized controlled trials involving different treatment modalities. They were able to demonstrate that DDAVP significantly reduced the number of wet nights in children receiving this preparation, but that the treatment was not as effective as conditioning alarms as a primary therapy.

Prevention of postoperative venous thromboembolism

Much of the evidence for the potential benefits in the prevention of thromboembolic disease following gynaecological surgery has to be extrapolated from abdominal surgery in general or orthopaedic surgery, rather than gynaecological surgery in particular. Wells et al (1994) analysed 11 studies which assessed the use of graduated compression stockings in the prevention of postoperative venous thromboembolism in patients undergoing abdominal, gynaecological, urological or neurosurgical procedures. The 95% confidence intervals for the odds ratio of reduced risk of thromboembolism were 0.23–0.42 when compared with controls. This would suggest a risk reduction of between 53 and 73% for patients wearing such stockings, and it may now be difficult to justify why patients should not receive such prophylaxis.

The use of heparin, both unfractionated and low molecular weight, in the prevention of perioperative thrombosis has been assessed by Leizorovicz et al (1992) from an assessment of 52 randomized controlled trials (29 in general surgery and 23 in orthopaedic surgery). They were able to demonstrate that both types of heparin were associated with a significant reduction in thromboembolic complication, and that low molecular weight heparin appeared to have a greater benefit than did unfractionated heparin in prevention, without any significant increase in the incidence of major haemorrhage.

Hormone replacement therapy and breast cancer

The large number of case controlled studies in this area has already been discussed. There have now been five meta-analyses identified by this author in the assessment of the risk of breast cancer in women receiving long-term hormone replacement therapy. From these the following conclusions may be drawn. Overall, there is either a neutral risk for carcinoma of the breast in women receiving hormone replacement therapy, or at most a small increased relative risk in the order of 1.06. There is no increased risk for carcinoma of the breast yet demonstrated in women receiving hormone replacement therapy who have a past history of benign breast disease, but there is a small statistically relevant increased relative risk of carcinoma in the breast in women receiving hormone replacement therapy who have a family history of carcinoma of the breast. Although there is a trend towards an increased relative risk with an increased oestrogen dosage and duration of effect, the range of this relative risk is so wide that no firm conclusion can be drawn. At the current state of knowledge, patients should be reassured that there is no convincing evidence for an increased risk of carcinoma in the breast in women receiving long-term hormone replacement therapy, but they should also be counselled that this conclusion may need to be altered with the accumulation of further information. What is yet to be assessed is whether women who have used long-term oral contraception, especially when below the age of 25, then have a further increase in the risk of carcinoma of the breast should they subsequently use hormone replacement therapy.

Gynaecological oncology

Treatment of early cervical carcinoma

It is unlikely now that the relative benefits and risks of radical surgery and radical radiotherapy will ever be compared in women with early carcinoma of the cervix, especially before the menopause. In one of the earliest meta-analyses reported, Brady (1979) conducted a survey of US institutions with regard to their treatment for Stage Ib disease. He showed that of the 93 institutions favouring primary surgery, 6815 patients treated surgically had an 81% 5-year survival rate, whereas 6446 patients were treated with radiotherapy with a 70% 5-year disease-free survival. Of 26 institutions favouring radiotherapy, 3430 patients treated with radiotherapy had a 75% 5-year disease-free survival. It is likely that the choice of treatment modality in Stage Ib carcinoma of the cervix will be based upon a comparison of side effects rather than treatment efficacy.

Chemotherapy regimens in ovarian cancer

There have been several meta-analyses which have compared randomized trials of different chemotherapy regimens in the presence of ovarian cancer. Levin and Hryniuk (1987) analysed 33 such trials and concluded that multiple-agent regimens were associated with a distinct survival advantage over single alkylating agent regimens, and that multiagent regimens containing cisplatinum had particular advantage. Peto and Easton (1989) concluded that non-platinum combinations were probably not significantly superior to non-platinum single-agent regimens, whereas cisplatinum regimens were significantly superior to non-cisplatinum regimens. They also concluded that cisplatinum in multiagent regimens was statistically superior to cisplatinum alone. Such conclusions have been reinforced by the largest meta-analysis available, the Advanced Ovarian Cancer Triallist Group (1991).

Menorrhagia

There are relatively few randomized controlled trials, involving small numbers of patients, in the medical management of menorrhagia due to so-called dysfunctional uterine bleeding. Those trials which do exist suggest that tranexamic acid reduces mean menstrual blood loss by 45% whilst norethisterone reduces the loss by 20% (Preston et al 1995), yet clinicians consistently prescribe the less effective agent more commonly (Coulter et al 1995, Farquar & Kimble 1996).

CONCLUSION

The only purpose in producing a systematic review is to improve clinical practice, either directly by the results of that review or indirectly by identifying areas for research. Clinical guidelines based on systematic reviews will only be as good as the information identified and analysed within that review. However, if the structured review is appropriately performed and the research upon which it is based appropriately reported, good-quality consensus clinical guidelines can result (Feder 1994). Such guidelines do not inhibit clinical freedom, although they may well identify areas of suboptimal clinical practice. They allow the busy clinician to have a full assessment of the available clinical information without the need to rely on incomplete and random identification of information in the local medical library (Laupacis et al 1988). There is no doubt that good-quality randomized clinical trials and structured reviews will have beneficial effects upon clinical practice (Lamas et al 1992; Sackett & Rosenberg 1995).

REFERENCES

Advanced Ovarian Cancer Triallist Group 1991 Chemotherapy in advanced ovarian cancer – overview of randomised clinical trials. British Medical Journal 303: 884–893

Altman D J, Elbourne D 1988 Combining results from several clinical trials. British Journal of Obstetrics and Gynaecology 95: 1–2

Brady L W 1979 Surgery or radiotherapy for carcinoma of the cervix. International Journal of Radiation, Oncology, Biology and Physics 51: 877–879

Chalmers I, Enkin M W, Keirse M J N C 1989 Effective care in pregnancy and childbirth. Oxford University Press, Oxford

Cochrane Library 1996. The Cochrane Database of Systematic Reviews. British Medical Journal Publishing Group, London.

Cooke I E 1996 Finding the evidence. Baillière's Clinical Obstetrics and Gynaecology 10, 551–67

Coulter A, Kelland J, Peto R et al 1995 Treating menorrhagia in primary care; an overview of drug trials and a survey prescribing practice. International Journal of Health Technology Assessment 11, 456–71

Crowley P 1996 Using an overview. Baillière's Clinical Obstetrics and Gynaecology 10, 585–97

Daya S 1989 Efficacy of progesterone support for pregnancy in women with recurrent miscarriage. A meta-analysis of controlled trials. British Journal of Obstetrics and Gynaecology 96: 275–280

Dickersin K et al 1994 Identifying relevant studies for systematic reviews. British Medical Journal 309: 1286–1291

Downs S, Black N 1996 Systematic review of the literature on the effectiveness of the surgery for genuine stress incontinence. London School of Hygiene and Tropical Medicine 47–50

Easterbrook P J, Berlin J A, Jopalan R et al 1991 Publication by clinic research. Lancet 337: 867–872

Enhorning G, Sherman A, Possmayer F et al 1985 Prevention of neonatal respiratory distress syndrome by tracheal instillation of surfactant. Pediatrics 76: 145–153

Eysenck H J 1994 Meta-analysis and its problems. British Medical Journal 309: 789–792

Fantl J A, Cardozo L, McClish D et al 1994 Oestrogen therapy and the management of urinary incontinence in postmenopausal women and meta-analysis. Obstetrics and Gynecology 83: 12–18

Farquhar C, Kimble R 1996 How do New Zealand gynaecologists treat menorrhagia? Australian and New Zealand Journal of Obstetrics and Gynaecology 36, 1–4

Feder G 1994 Clinical guidelines in 1994. British Medical Journal 309: 1457–1458

Fraser E J, Grimes D A, Schulz K F 1993 Immunisation as therapy for recurrent spontaneous abortion – review and meta-analysis. Obstetrics and Gynecology 82: 854–859

Hughes E G 1992 Meta-analysis and the critical appraisal of infertility literature. Fertility and Sterility 57: 275–277

Hughes E G, Fedorkow D M, Daya S et al 1992 The use of gonadotrophin releasing hormone agonists prior to in vitro fertilisation and gamete intrafallopian transfer – meta-analysis of randomised control trials. Fertility and Sterility 58: 888–896

Imperiale T F, Speroff T 1994 A meta-analysis of methods to prevent venus thromboembolism following total hip replacement. Journal of the American Medical Association 271: 1780–1785

Jarvis G J 1994 Surgery for genuine stress incontinence. British Journal of Obstetrics and Gynaecology 101: 371–374

Lamas G A, Pfeffer M A, Hamm P et al 1992 Do results of randomised clinical trials of cardiovascular drugs influence medical practice? New England Journal of Medicine 327: 241–247

Lau G, Antman E N, Jimenez-Silva J et al 1992 Cumulative meta-analysis of therapeutic trials for myocardial infarction. New England Journal of Medicine 327: 248–254

Laupacis A, Sackett D, Roberts R S 1988 An assessment of clinical useful measures of the consequences of treatment. New England Journal of Medicine 318: 1728–1733

Leibovici L, Wysenbeek A J 1991 Single dose antibiotic treatment for urinary tract infection in women – a meta-analysis of randomised trials. Quarterly Journal of Medicine 285: 43–57

Leizorovicz A, Haugh M C, Chapuis F R et al 1992 Low molecular weight heparin in prevention of perioperative thrombosis. British Medical Journal 305: 913–920

Levin L, Hryniuk W M 1987 Dose intensity analysis of chemotherapy regimes in ovarian carcinoma. Journal of Clinical Oncology 57: 56–67

Mittendorf R, Aronson M P, Berry R E et al 1993 Avoiding serious infections associated with abdominal hysterectomy – meta-analysis of antibiotic prophylaxis. American Journal of Obstetrics and Gynecology 169: 1119–1124

Moffatt M E K, Harlos S, Karshen A J et al 1993 Desmopressin acetate and nocturnal enuresis. Pediatrics 92: 420–425

Morris J A, Gardner M J 1988 Calculating confidence intervals for relative risks (odds ratios) and standardised ratios and rates. British Medical Journal 296: 1313–1316

Paintin D B 1990 Effective care in pregnancy and childbirth. (Editorial) British Journal of Obstetrics and Gynaecology 97: 967–969

Parazzini F, Luchini L, La Vechia C et al 1993 Video display terminal use during pregnancy and reproductive outcome – a meta-analysis. Journal of Epidemiology and Community Health 47: 265–268

Peto R, Easton D 1989 Cancer treatment trials. Cancer Surveys 8: 511–533

Sackett D L, Rosenberg W M C 1995 The need for evidenced based medicine. Journal of the Royal Society of Medicine 88, 620–4

Preston J T, Cameron I T, Adams E J et al. Comparative study of tranexamic acid and norethisterone in the treatment of ovulatory menorrhagia. British Journal of Obstetrics and Gynaecology 102, 401–6

Simes J 1990 Meta-analysis – its importance in cost effectiveness studies. Medical Journal of Australia 153: S13–S16

Soliman S, Daya S, Collins J et al 1994 The role of luteal phase support in infertility treatment – a meta-analysis of randomised trials. Fertility and Sterility 61: 1068–1076

Stoll B A, Parbhoo S 1988 Treatment of menopausal symptoms in breast cancer patients. Lancet 1: 1278–1279

Thompson S G 1994 Why sources of heterogeneity in meta-analysis should be investigated. British Medical Journal 309: 1351–1355

Vandekerckhove P, O'Donovan P A, Lilford R J et al 1993 Infertility treatment – from cookery to science. The epidemiology of randomised controlled trials. British Journal of Obstetrics and Gynaecology 100: 1005–1036

Walker C K, Cahn J G, Washington A E et al 1993 Pelvic inflammatory disease – meta-analysis of anti-microbial regimen efficiency. Journal of Infectious Diseases 168: 969–978

Watson A, Vandekerckhove P, Lilford R et al 1994 Meta-analysis of the therapeutic role of oil-soluble contrast media at hysterosalpingography. Fertility and Sterility 61: 470–477

Wells P S, Lensing A W A, Hirsh J 1994 Graduated compression stockings in the prevention of postoperative venous thromboembolism. Archives of Internal Medicine 154: 67–72

Yusuf S, Collins R, Peto R et al 1985 Intravenous and intracoronary fibrinolytic therapy in acute myocardial infarction – an overview of results on mortality, reinfarction and side-effects from 33 randomised controlled trials. European Heart Journal 65: 56–85

Index

Abbreviations: CIN: cervical intraepithelial neoplasia; GnRH: gonadotrophin releasing hormone; HIV: human immunodeficiency virus; HPV: human papilloma viruses; HRT: hormone replacement therapy; IUCD: intrauterine contraceptive device; IVF: *in vitro* fertilization; PID: pelvic inflammatory disease; PMS: premenstrual syndrome; STD: sexually transmitted disease; VAIN: vaginal intraepithelial neoplasia; VIN: vulval intraepithelial neoplasia.